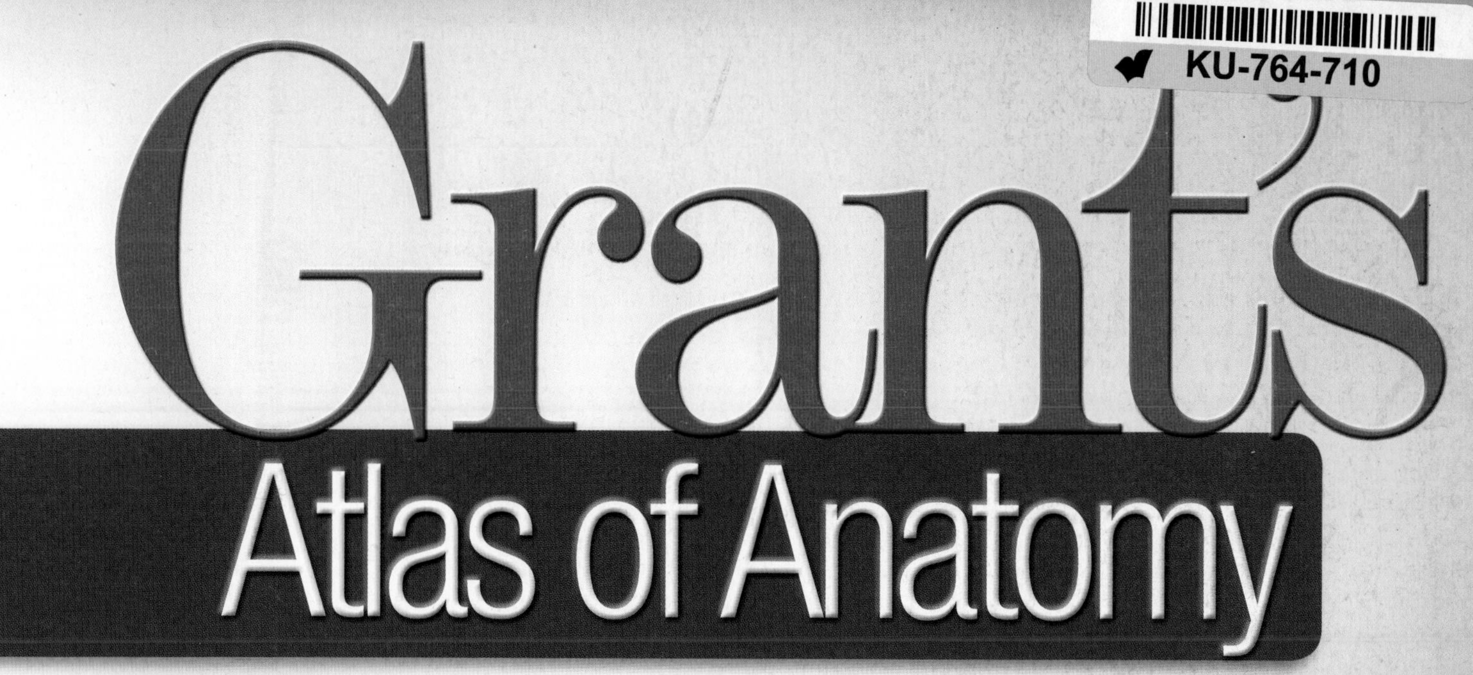
Grant's
Atlas of Anatomy

THIRTEENTH EDITION

Anne M.R. Agur, B.Sc. (OT), M.Sc., Ph.D

Professor, Division of Anatomy, Department of Surgery, Faculty of Medicine
Department of Physical Therapy, Department of Occupational Therapy
Division of Biomedical Communications, Institute of Medical Science
Graduate Department of Rehabilitation Science, Graduate Department of Dentistry
University of Toronto
Toronto, Ontario, Canada

Arthur F. Dalley II, Ph.D.

Professor, Department of Cell & Developmental Biology
Adjunct Professor, Department of Orthopaedics and Rehabilitation
Vanderbilt University School of Medicine
Adjunct Professor of Anatomy
Belmont University School of Physical Therapy
Nashville, Tennessee

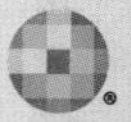
Wolters Kluwer | Lippincott Williams & Wilkins
Health

Philadelphia • Baltimore • New York • London
Buenos Aires • Hong Kong • Sydney • Tokyo

Acquisitions Editor: Crystal Taylor
Product Manager: Julie Montalbano
Marketing Manager: Joy Fisher Williams
Designer: Holly McLaughlin
Compositor: SPi Global

Thirteenth Edition

By J.C.B. Grant:
First Edition, 1943 Second Edition, 1947 Third Edition, 1951
Fourth Edition, 1956 Fifth Edition, 1962 Sixth Edition, 1972

By J.E. Anderson:
Seventh Edition, 1978 Eighth Edition, 1983

By A.M.R. Agur:
Ninth Edition, 1991 Tenth Edition, 1999
Eleventh Edition, 2005

By A.M.R. Agur and A.F. Dalley:
Twelfth Edition, 2009

351 West Camden Street
Baltimore, MD 21201

Two Commerce Square
2001 Market Street
Philadelphia, PA 19103

Printed in China

ISBN: 978-1-4511-1031-9

To purchase additional copies of this book, call our customer service department at **(800) 638-3030** or fax orders to **(301) 223-2320**. International customers should call **(301) 223-2300**.

Visit Lippincott Williams & Wilkins on the Internet: http://www.lww.com. Lippincott Williams & Wilkins customer service representatives are available from 8:30 am to 6:00 pm, EST.

9 8 7 6 5 4 3 2 1

CCS0112

To my husband Enno and my children Erik and Kristina
for their support and encouragement
(A.M.R.A.)

To Muriel
My bride, best friend, counselor, and mother of our sons;
To my family
Tristan, Lana, Elijah, Finley, Sawyer,
Denver, and Skyler
With great appreciation for their support, humor, and patience
(A.F.D.)

And with sincere appreciation for the anatomical donors
Without whom our studies would not be possible

DR. JOHN CHARLES BOILEAU GRANT • 1886–1973

by Dr. Carlton G. Smith, M.D., Ph.D. (1905–2003)
Professor Emeritus, Division of Anatomy, Department of Surgery
Faculty of Medicine, University of Toronto, Toronto, Ontario, Canada

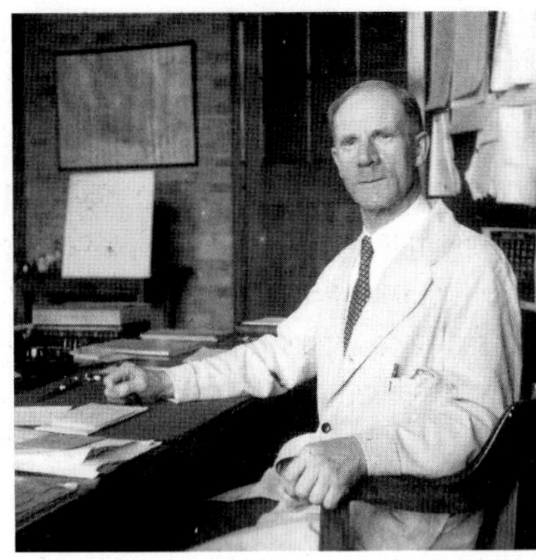

Dr. J.C. Boileau Grant in his office, McMurrich Building, University of Toronto, 1946. Through his textbooks, Dr. Grant made an indelible impression on the teaching of anatomy throughout the world. *(Courtesy of Dr. C. G. Smith.)*

The life of Dr. J.C. Boileau Grant has been likened to the course of the seventh cranial nerve as it passes out of the skull: complicated, but purposeful.[1] He was born in the parish of Lasswade in Edinburgh, Scotland, on February 6, 1886. Dr. Grant studied medicine at the University of Edinburgh from 1903 to 1908. Here, his skill as a dissector in the laboratory of the renowned anatomist, Dr. Daniel John Cunningham (1850–1909), earned him a number of awards.

Following graduation, Dr. Grant was appointed the resident house officer at the Infirmary in Whitehaven, Cumberland. From 1909 to 1911, Dr. Grant demonstrated anatomy in the University of Edinburgh, followed by two years at the University of Durham, at Newcastle-on-Tyne in England, in the laboratory of Professor Robert Howden, editor of *Gray's Anatomy.*

With the outbreak of World War I in 1914, Dr. Grant joined the Royal Army Medical Corps and served with distinction. He was mentioned in dispatches in September 1916, received the Military Cross in September 1917 for "conspicuous gallantry and devotion to duty during attack," and received a bar to the Military Cross in August 1918.[1]

In October 1919, released from the Royal Army, he accepted the position of Professor of Anatomy at the University of Manitoba in Winnipeg, Canada. With the frontline medical practitioner in mind, he endeavored to "bring up a generation of surgeons who knew exactly what they were doing once an operation had begun."[1] Devoted to research and learning, Dr. Grant took interest in other projects, such as performing anthropometric studies of Indian tribes in northern Manitoba during the 1920s. In Winnipeg, Dr. Grant met Catriona Christie, whom he married in 1922.

Dr. Grant was known for his reliance on logic, analysis, and deduction as opposed to rote memory. While at the University of Manitoba, Dr. Grant began writing *A Method of Anatomy, Descriptive and Deductive,* which was published in 1937.[2]

In 1930, Dr. Grant accepted the position of Chair of Anatomy at the University of Toronto. He stressed the value of a "clean" dissection, with the structures well defined. This required the delicate touch of a sharp scalpel, and students soon learned that a dull tool was anathema. Instructive dissections were made available in the Anatomy Museum, a means of student review on which Dr. Grant placed a high priority. Illustrations of these actual dissections are included in *Grant's Atlas of Anatomy.*

The first edition of the *Atlas*, published in 1943, was the first anatomical atlas to be published in North America.[3] *Grant's Dissector* preceded the *Atlas* in 1940.[4]

Dr. Grant remained at the University of Toronto until his retirement in 1956. At that time, he became Curator of the Anatomy Museum in the University. He also served as Visiting Professor of Anatomy at the University of California at Los Angeles, where he taught for 10 years.

Dr. Grant died in 1973 of cancer. Through his teaching method, still presented in the Grant's textbooks, Dr. Grant's life interest—human anatomy—lives on. In their eulogy, colleagues and friends Ross MacKenzie and J. S. Thompson said, "Dr. Grant's knowledge of anatomical fact was encyclopedic, and he enjoyed nothing better than sharing his knowledge with others, whether they were junior students or senior staff. While somewhat strict as a teacher, his quiet wit and boundless humanity never failed to impress. He was, in the very finest sense, a scholar and a gentleman."[1]

This edition of *Grant's Atlas* has, like its predecessors, required intense research, market input, and creativity. It is not enough to rely on a solid reputation; with each new edition, we have adapted and changed many aspects of the *Atlas* while maintaining the commitment to pedagogical excellence and anatomical realism that has enriched its long history. Medical and health sciences education, and the role of anatomy instruction and application within it, continually evolve to reflect new teaching approaches and educational models. The health care system itself is changing, and the skills and knowledge that future health care practitioners must master are changing along with it. Finally, technologic advances in publishing, particularly in online resources and electronic media, have transformed the way students access content and the methods by which educators teach content. All of these developments have shaped the vision and directed the execution of this thirteenth edition of *Grant's Atlas*, as evidenced by the following key features.

Classic "Grant's" images updated for today's students. A unique feature of *Grant's Atlas* is that, rather than providing an idealized view of human anatomy, the classic illustrations represent actual dissections that the student can directly compare with specimens in the lab. Because the original models used for these illustrations were real cadavers, the accuracy of these illustrations is unparalleled, offering students the best introduction to anatomy possible. Over the years and in this edition, we have made many changes to the illustrations to match the shifting expectations of students, adding more vibrant colors and updating the style. All figures were carefully analyzed to ensure that label placement remained effective and that the illustration's relevance was still clear.

Schematic illustrations. Full-color schematic illustrations and orientation figures supplement the dissection figures to clarify anatomical concepts, show the relationships of structures, and give an overview of the body region being studied. The illustrations conform to Dr. Grant's admonition to "keep it simple": extraneous labels were deleted, and some labels were added to identify key structures and make the illustrations as useful as possible to students.

Legends with easy-to-find clinical applications. Admittedly, artwork is the focus of any atlas; however, the *Grant's* legends have long been considered a unique and valuable feature of the *Atlas*. The observations and comments that accompany the illustrations draw attention to salient points and significant structures that might otherwise escape notice. Their purpose is to interpret the illustrations without providing exhaustive description. Readability, clarity, and practicality were emphasized in the editing of this edition. Clinical comments, which deliver practical "pearls" that link anatomic features with their significance in health care practice, appear in blue text within the figure legends. New clinical comments have been added in this edition, providing even more relevance for students searching for medical application of anatomical concepts.

Enhanced diagnostic imaging and surface anatomy. Because medical imaging has taken on increased importance in the diagnosis and treatment of injuries and illnesses, diagnostic images are used liberally throughout the chapters, and a special imaging section appears at the end of each chapter. Over 100 clinically relevant magnetic resonance images (MRIs), computed tomography (CT) scans, ultrasound scans, and corresponding orientation drawings are included in this edition. Labeled surface anatomy photographs with ethnic diversity continue to be an important feature in this new edition.

Updated and improved tables. Tables help students organize complex information in an easy-to-use format ideal for review and study. In addition to muscles, tables featuring nerves, arteries, and other relevant structures are included. The table format in this edition received a substantial update; a consistent color code is used to clearly demarcate columns. Tables are strategically placed on the same page as the illustrations that demonstrate the structures listed in the tables.

Logical organization and layout. The organization and layout of the *Atlas* have always been determined with ease-of-use as the goal. Although the basic organization by body region was maintained in this edition, the order of plates within every chapter was scrutinized to ensure that it is logical and pedagogically effective. Sections within each chapter further organize the region into discrete subregions; these subregions appear as headings on the pages. Readers need only glance at these headings to orient themselves to the region and subregion that the figures on the page belong to. A chapter table of contents comprises the first page of each chapter.

Helpful learning and teaching tools. The thirteenth edition of *Grant's Atlas* offers a wide range of online resources for both the student and the instructor on Lippincott Williams & Wilkins' thePoint site: http://thePoint.lww.com/GrantsAtlas13e. Students have access to an online e-book, an interactive atlas containing all of the atlas images, an interactive question bank, and selected video clips from the best-selling *Acland's Video Atlas of Human Anatomy* collection. For instructors, online ancillaries include an interactive atlas with slideshow and image-export functions as well as an image bank.

We hope that you enjoy using this thirteenth edition of *Grant's Atlas* and that it becomes a trusted partner in your educational experience. We believe that this new edition safeguards the *Atlas's* historical strengths while enhancing its usefulness to today's students.

Anne M.R. Agur
Arthur F. Dalley II

ACKNOWLEDGMENTS

Starting with the first edition of this *Atlas* published in 1943, many people have given generously of their talents and expertise and we acknowledge their participation with heartfelt gratitude. Most of the original carbon-dust halftones on which this book is based were created by Dorothy Foster Chubb, a pupil of Max Brödel and one of Canada's first professionally trained medical illustrators. She was later joined by Nancy Joy, who is Professor Emeritus in the Division of Biomedical Communications, University of Toronto. Mrs. Chubb was mainly responsible for the artwork of the first two editions and the sixth edition; Miss Joy, for those in between. In subsequent editions, additional line and halftone illustrations by Elizabeth Blackstock, Elia Hopper Ross, and Marguerite Drummond were added. In recent editions, the artwork of Valerie Oxorn and the surface anatomy photography of Anne Rayner of Vanderbilt University Medical Center's Medical Art Group have augmented the modern look and feel of the atlas.

Much credit is also due to Charles E. Storton for his role in the preparation of the majority of the original dissections and preliminary photographic work. We also wish to acknowledge the work of Dr. James Anderson, a pupil of Dr. Grant, under whose stewardship the seventh and eighth editions were published.

The following individuals also provided invaluable contributions to previous editions of the atlas and are gratefully acknowledged: C.A. Armstrong, P.G. Ashmore, D. Baker, D.A. Barr, J.V. Basmajian, S. Bensley, D. Bilbey, J. Bottos, W. Boyd, J. Callagan, H.A. Cates, S.A. Crooks, M. Dickie, C. Duckwall, R. Duckwall, J.W.A. Duckworth, F.B. Fallis, J.B. Francis, J.S. Fraser, P. George, R.K. George, M.G. Gray, B.L. Guyatt, C.W. Hill, W.J. Horsey, B.S. Jaden, M.J. Lee, G.F. Lewis, I.B. MacDonald, D.L. MacIntosh, R.G. MacKenzie, S. Mader, K.O. McCuaig, D. Mazierski, W.R. Mitchell, K. Nancekivell, A.J.A. Noronha, S. O'Sullivan, W. Pallie, W.M. Paul, D. Rini, C. Sandone, C.H. Sawyer, A.I. Scott, J.S. Simpkins, J.S. Simpson, C.G. Smith, I.M. Thompson, J.S. Thompson, N.A. Watters, R.W. Wilson, B. Vallecoccia, and K. Yu.

THIRTEENTH EDITION

We are indebted to our colleagues and former professors for their encouragement—especially Dr. Keith L. Moore for his expert advice and Drs. Daniel O. Graney, Lawrence Ross, Ryan Splittgerber, Lily Cabellon, and Douglas J. Gould for their invaluable input.

We extend our gratitude to our medical illustrator Valerie Oxorn, whose artistic skills and anatomical insights made substantial contributions to this edition. We would also like to acknowledge Jennifer Clements, Art Director at Lippincott Williams & Wilkins, who managed the art program for this edition.

Special thanks go to everyone at **Lippincott Williams & Wilkins**—especially Crystal Taylor, Acquisitions Editor, and Julie Montalbano, Product Manager. All of your efforts and expertise are much appreciated.

We would like to thank the hundreds of instructors and students who have over the years communicated via the publisher and directly with the editor their suggestions for how this *Atlas* might be improved. Finally, we would like to acknowledge the reviewers who reviewed previous editions of the *Atlas* as well as the following reviewers who reviewed the twelfth edition and provided expert advice on the development of this edition in particular:

FACULTY REVIEWERS

Belinda Beck, Griffith University, Queesnsland, Australia
Juliette Cooper, University of Manitoba, Winnipeg, Manitoba, Canada
Donald Fletcher, East Carolina State University, Greenville, North Carolina
Georgina Fyfe, Curtin University, Perth, Australia
Doug Gould, The Ohio State University, Columbus, Ohio
Rod Green, Latrobe University, Victoria, Australia
Jan Smit, Queen's University Belfast, United Kingdom
Mark Stringer, University of Otago, New Zealand
Marjan Vandersteen, Universiteit Hasselt, Diepenbeek, Belgium
Bruce Wainman, McMaster University, Hamilton, Ontario, Canada
Robert Whitaker, University of Cambridge, United Kingdom

STUDENT REVIEWERS

Merrian Brooks
Tameka Byrd
Daniel Choi
Terry Dean
Stephen Goldberg
Peter Hakim
Andrew Jensen
Daniel Kou
Malini Kumar
Janelle Lum
Leah Phillabaum

We hope that readers and reviewers will find many of their suggestions incorporated into the twelfth edition and will continue to provide their valuable input.

Anne M.R. Agur
Arthur F. Dalley II

CONTENTS

Dr. John Charles Boileau Grant vi
Preface vii
Acknowledgments viii
List of Tables xi
Table and Figure Credits xiii

1 Thorax 1

Pectoral Region 2
Breast 4
Bony Thorax and Joints 12
Thoracic Wall 19
Thoracic Contents 27
Pleural Cavities 30
Mediastinum 31
Lungs and Pleura 32
Bronchi and Bronchopulmonary Segments 38
Innervation and Lymphatic Drainage of Lungs 44
External Heart 46
Coronary Vessels 56
Conduction System of Heart 60
Internal Heart and Valves 61
Superior Mediastinum and Great Vessels 68
Diaphragm 75
Posterior Thorax 76
Overview of Autonomic Innervation 86
Overview of Lymphatic Drainage of Thorax 88
Sectional Anatomy and Imaging 90

2 Abdomen 97

Overview 98
Anterolateral Abdominal Wall 100
Inguinal Region 110
Testis 120
Peritoneum and Peritoneal Cavity 122
Digestive System 132
Stomach 133
Pancreas, Duodenum, and Spleen 136
Intestines 140
Liver and Gallbladder 150
Biliary Ducts 160
Portal Venous System 164
Posterior Abdominal Viscera 166
Kidneys 169
Posterolateral Abdominal Wall 173
Diaphragm 178
Abdominal Aorta and Inferior Vena Cava 179
Autonomic Innervation 180
Lymphatic Drainage 186
Sectional Anatomy and Imaging 190

3 Pelvis and Perineum 197

Pelvic Girdle 198
Ligaments of Pelvic Girdle 205
Floor and Walls of Pelvis 206
Sacral and Coccygeal Plexuses 210
Peritoneal Reflections in Pelvis 212
Rectum and Anal Canal 214
Organs of Male Pelvis 220
Vessels of Male Pelvis 228
Lymphatic Drainage of Male Pelvis and Perineum 232
Innervation of Male Pelvic Organs 234
Organs of Female Pelvis 236
Vessels of Female Pelvis 242
Lymphatic Drainage of Female Pelvis and Perineum 248
Innervation of Female Pelvic Organs 250
Subperitoneal Region of Pelvis 254
Surface Anatomy of Perineum 256
Overview of Male and Female Perineum 258
Male Perineum 265
Female Perineum 273
Imaging and Sectional Anatomy of Pelvis and Perineum 280

4 Back 289

Overview of Vertebral Column 290
Cervical Spine 298
Craniovertebral Joints 302
Thoracic Spine 304
Lumbar Spine 306
Ligaments and Intervertebral Discs 308
Bones, Joints, and Ligaments of Pelvic Girdle 313
Anomalies of Vertebrae 320
Muscles of Back 322
Suboccipital Region 332
Spinal Cord and Meninges 336
Vertebral Venous Plexuses 344
Components of Spinal Nerves 345
Dermatomes and Myotomes 348
Autonomic Nerves 350
Imaging of Vertebral Column 354

5 Lower Limb 357

Systemic Overview of Lower Limb: Bones 358
Systemic Overview of Lower Limb: Nerves 362
Systemic Overview of Lower Limb: Blood Vessels 370

Systemic Overview of Lower Limb: Lymphatics 374
Systemic Overview of Lower Limb: Musculofascial Compartments 376
Retro-Inguinal Passage and Femoral Triangle 378
Anterior and Medial Compartments of Thigh 382
Lateral Thigh 389
Bones and Muscle Attachments of Thigh 390
Gluteal Region and Posterior Compartment of Thigh 392
Hip Joint 402
Knee Region 410
Knee Joint 416
Anterior and Lateral Compartments of Leg, Dorsum of Foot 430
Posterior Compartment of Leg 440
Tibiofibular Joints 450
Sole of Foot 451
Ankle, Subtalar, and Foot Joints 456
Arches of Foot 474
Bony Anomalies 475
Imaging and Sectional Anatomy 476

6 Upper Limb 481

Systemic Overview of Upper Limb: Bones 482
Systemic Overview of Upper Limb: Nerves 488
Systemic Overview of Upper Limb: Arteries 494
Systemic Overview of Upper Limb: Veins and Lymphatics 496
Systemic Overview of Upper Limb: Musculofascial Compartments 500
Pectoral Region 502
Axilla, Axillary Vessels, and Brachial Plexus 509
Scapular Region and Superficial Back 520
Arm and Rotator Cuff 524
Joints of Shoulder Region 538
Elbow Region 546
Elbow Joint 552
Anterior Aspect of Forearm 558
Anterior Aspect of Wrist and Palm of Hand 562
Posterior Aspect of Forearm 582
Posterior Aspect of Wrist and Dorsum of Hand 586
Lateral Aspect of Wrist and Hand 592
Medial Aspect of Wrist and Hand 595
Bones and Joints of Wrist and Hand 596
Function of Hand: Grips and Pinches 604
Imaging and Sectional Anatomy 605

7 Head 611

Cranium 612
Face and Scalp 632
Meninges and Meningeal Spaces 641
Cranial Base and Cranial Nerves 646
Blood Supply of Brain 652
Orbit and Eyeball 656
Parotid Region 668
Temporal Region and Infratemporal Fossa 670
Temporomandibular Joint 678
Tongue 682
Palate 688
Teeth 691
Nose, Paranasal Sinuses, and Pterygopalatine Fossa 696
Ear 709
Lymphatic Drainage of Head 722
Autonomic Innervation of Head 723
Imaging of Head 724
Neuroanatomy: Overview and Ventricular System 728
Telencephalon (Cerebrum) and Diencephalon 731
Brainstem and Cerebellum 740
Imaging of Brain 746

8 Neck 751

Subcutaneous Structures and Cervical Fascia 752
Skeleton of Neck 756
Regions of Neck 758
Lateral Region (Posterior Triangle) of Neck 760
Anterior Region (Anterior Triangle) of Neck 764
Neurovascular Structures of Neck 768
Visceral Compartment of Neck 774
Root and Prevertebral Region of Neck 778
Submandibular Region and Floor of Mouth 784
Posterior Cervical Region 789
Pharynx 792
Isthmus of Fauces 798
Larynx 804
Sectional Anatomy and Imaging of Neck 812

9 Cranial Nerves 817

Overview of Cranial Nerves 818
Cranial Nerve Nuclei 822
Cranial Nerve I: Olfactory 824
Cranial Nerve II: Optic 825
Cranial Nerves III, IV, and VI: Oculomotor, Trochlear, and Abducent 827
Cranial Nerve V: Trigeminal 830
Cranial Nerve VII: Facial 837
Cranial Nerve VIII: Vestibulocochlear 838
Cranial Nerve IX: Glossopharyngeal 840
Cranial Nerve X: Vagus 843
Cranial Nerve XI: Spinal Accessory 844
Cranial Nerve XII: Hypoglossal 845
Summary of Autonomic Ganglia of Head 846
Summary of Cranial Nerve Lesions 847
Sectional Imaging of Cranial Nerves 848

REFERENCES 851

INDEX 853

LIST OF TABLES

1 THORAX

1.1 Muscles of Thoracic Wall 23
1.2 Muscles of Respiration 26
1.3 Surface Markings of Parietal Pleura (Blue) and Surface Markings of Lungs Covered with Visceral Pleura (Pink) 33

2 ABDOMEN

2.1 Principal Muscles of Anterolateral Abdominal Wall 108
2.2 Boundaries of Inguinal Canal 112
2.3 Characteristics of Inguinal Hernias 119
2.4 Terms Used to Describe Parts of Peritoneum 124
2.5 Parts and Relationships of Duodenum 137
2.6 Schema of Terminology for Subdivisions of the Liver 155
2.7 Principal Muscles of Posterior Abdominal Wall 176
2.8 Autonomic Innervation of Abdominal Viscera (Splanchnic Nerves) 183

3 PELVIS AND PERINEUM

3.1 Differences Between Male and Female Pelves 202
3.2 Muscles of Pelvic Walls and Floor 207
3.3 Nerves of Sacral and Coccygeal Plexuses 211
3.4 Arteries of Male Pelvis 229
3.5 Lymphatic Drainage of Male Pelvis and Perineum 233
3.6 Effect of Sympathetic and Parasympathetic Stimulation on Urinary Tract, Genital System, and Rectum 234
3.7 Arteries of Female Pelvis 247
3.8 Lymphatic Drainage of Structures of Female Pelvis and Perineum 249
3.9 Muscles of Perineum 260

4 BACK

4.1 Typical Cervical Vertebrae (C3–C7) 298
4.2 Thoracic Vertebrae 304
4.3 Lumbar Vertebrae 306
4.4 Intrinsic Back Muscles 331
4.5 Muscles of Atlanto-Occipital and Atlanto-Axial Joints 334

5 LOWER LIMB

5.1 Motor Nerves of Lower Limb 363
5.2 Cutaneous Nerves of Lower Limb 365
5.3 Nerve Lesions 366
5.4 Nerve Root (Anterior Ramus) Lesions 367
5.5 Muscles of Anterior Thigh 385
5.6 Muscles of Medial Thigh 386
5.7 Muscles of Gluteal Region 394
5.8 Muscles of Posterior Thigh (Hamstring) 395
5.9 Nerves of Gluteal Region 400
5.10 Arteries of Gluteal Region and Posterior Thigh 401
5.11 Bursae Around Knee 423
5.12 Muscles of Anterior Compartment of Leg 431
5.13 Common, Superficial, and Deep Fibular (Peroneal) Nerves 432
5.14 Arterial Supply to Dorsum of Foot 435
5.15 Muscles of Lateral Compartment of Leg 437
5.16 Muscles of Posterior Compartment of Leg 440
5.17 Arterial Supply of Leg and Foot 449
5.18 Muscles in Sole of Foot—First Layer 452
5.19 Muscles in Sole of Foot—Second Layer 453
5.20 Muscles in Sole of Foot—Third Layer 454
5.21 Muscles in Sole of Foot—Fourth Layer 455
5.22 Joints of Foot 467

6 UPPER LIMB

6.1 Cutaneous Nerves of Upper Limb 491
6.2 Clinical Manifestations of Nerve Root Compression: Upper Limb (UL) 492
6.3 Dermatomes of Upper Limb 493
6.4 Anterior Axio-Appendicular Muscles 507
6.5 Arteries of Proximal Upper Limb (Shoulder Region and Arm) 512
6.6 Brachial Plexus 515
6.7 Superficial Back (Posterior Axio-Appendicular) and Deltoid Muscles 521
6.8 Movements of Scapula 523
6.9 Scapulohumeral Muscles 525
6.10 Arm Muscles 528
6.11 Arteries of Forearm 558
6.12 Muscles of Anterior Aspect of Forearm 561
6.13 Muscles of Hand 573
6.14 Arteries of Hand 581
6.15 Muscles of Posterior Surface of Forearm 583
6.16 Lesions of Nerves of Upper Limb 603

7 HEAD

7.1 Foramina and other Apertures of Cranial Fossae, and Contents 620
7.2 Main Muscles of Facial Expression 635
7.3 Nerves of Face and Scalp 637
7.4 Arteries of Superficial Face and Scalp 638
7.5 Veins of Face 639
7.6 Openings by Which Cranial Nerves Exit Cranial Cavity 647
7.7 Arterial Supply to Brain 653
7.8 Actions of Muscles of Orbit Starting from Primary Position 662
7.9 Muscles of Orbit 663
7.10 Arteries of Orbit 665
7.11 Muscles of Mastication (Acting on Temporomandibular Joint) 678
7.12 Movements of Temporomandibular Joint 679
7.13 Muscles of Tongue 683
7.14 Muscles of Soft Palate 690
7.15 Primary and Secondary Dentition 695

8 NECK

8.1 Platysma 752
8.2 Cervical Regions and Contents 758
8.3 Sternocleidomastoid and Trapezius 759
8.4 Suprahyoid and Infrahyoid Muscles 767
8.5 Arteries of Neck 770
8.6 Prevertebral and Scalene Muscles 780
8.7 Lateral Vertebral Muscles 783
8.8 Muscles of Posterior Cervical Region 789
8.9 Muscles of Pharynx 794
8.10 Muscles of Larynx 808

9 CRANIAL NERVES

9.1 Summary of Cranial Nerves 821
9.2 Olfactory Nerve (CN I) 824
9.3 Optic Nerve (CN II) 825

LIST OF TABLES

9.4 Oculomotor (CN III), Trochlear (CN IV), and Abducent (CN VI) Nerves 828
9.5 Trigeminal Nerve (CN V) 830
9.6 Branches of Ophthalmic Nerve (CN V_1) 831
9.7 Branches of Maxillary Nerve (CN V_2) 832
9.8 Branches of Mandibular Nerve (CN V_3) 834
9.9 Facial Nerve (CN VII), Including Motor Root and Intermediate Nerve 836
9.10 Vestibulocochlear Nerve (CN VIII) 838
9.11 Glossopharyngeal Nerve (CN IX) 840
9.12 Vagus Nerve (CN X) 843
9.13 Spinal Accessory Nerve (CN XI) 844
9.14 Hypoglossal Nerve (CN XII) 845
9.15 Autonomic Ganglia of Head 846
9.16 Summary of Cranial Nerve Lesions 847

TABLE AND FIGURE CREDITS

CHAPTER 1

1.26 Courtesy of Dr. E.L. Lansdown, University of Toronto, Canada
1.36A Courtesy of Dr. D.E. Sanders, University of Toronto, Canada
1.36C Courtesy of Dr. E.L. Lansdown, University of Toronto, Canada
1.36 Courtesy of I. Verschuur, Joint Department of Medical Imaging, UHN/Mount Sinai Hospital, Toronto, Canada
1.43B,E Courtesy of I. Verschuur, Joint Department of Medical Imaging, UHN/Mount Sinai Hospital, Toronto, Canada
1.43C and 1.52 Moore KL, Dalley AF, Clinically Oriented Anatomy, 5th ed, 2006:170 (Fig. 155). A is based on Torrent-Guasp F, Buckberg GD, Clemente C et al. The Structure and Function of the Helical Heart and Its Buttress Wrapping. I. The normal macroscopic structure of the heart. Sem. Thor. Cardiovasc Surgery. 13 (4): 301–319, 2001.
1.46D Dean D, Herbener TE. Cross-Sectional Human Anatomy, 2000:25 (Plate 2.9).
1.49C Courtesy of I. Verschuur, Joint Department of Medical Imaging: UHN/Mount Sinai Hospital, Toronto, Canada
1.50B,D Courtesy of I. Morrow, University of Manitoba, Canada
1.51B Courtesy of Dr. J. Heslin, Toronto, Canada
1.52C Feigenbaum H, Armstrong WF, Ryan T. Feigenbaum's Echocardiography. 5th ed, 2005:116.
1.57 Courtesy of I. Verschuur, Joint Department of Medical Imaging, UHN/Mount Sinai Hospital, Toronto, Canada
1.64B Courtesy of Dr. E.L. Lansdown, University of Toronto, Canada
1.79A-F MRIs courtesy of Dr. M.A. Haider, University of Toronto, Canada
1.80A-C MRIs courtesy of Dr. M.A. Haider, University of Toronto, Canada
1.81AB MRIs courtesy of Dr. M.A. Haider, University of Toronto, Canada

CHAPTER 2

2.7B Lockhart, RD, Hamilton, GF., Fyfe FW. Anatomy of the Human Body, Philadelphia, Lippincott, 1959.
2.9 Clay JH, Pounds DM. Basic Clinical Massage Therapy: Integrating Anatomy and Treatment. 2nd ed, 2008:275. (Fig. 7.2)
2.26B MRI courtesy of Dr. M.A. Haider, University of Toronto, Canada
2.32C Dudek RW, Louis TM, *High-Yield Gross Anatomy,* 4th edition, 2010:106. (Fig. 11.2)
2.34A Dudek RW, Louis TM, *High-Yield Gross Anatomy,* 4th edition, 2010:103. (Fig. 11.1)
2.34B Courtesy of Dr. J. Heslin, Toronto, Canada
2.34C,D Courtesy of Dr. E.L. Lansdown, University of Toronto, Canada
2.36 Courtesy of Dr. J. Heslin, Toronto, Canada
2.42A Courtesy of Dr. C.S. Ho, University of Toronto, Canada
2.42B Courtesy of Dr. E.L. Lansdown, University of Toronto, Canada
2.45A Courtesy of Dr. E.L. Lansdown, University of Toronto, Canada
2.45B Courtesy of Dr. J. Heslin, Toronto, Canada
2.47 Courtesy of Dr. K. Sniderman, University of Toronto, Canada
2.53B Courtesy of A. M. Arenson, University of Toronto, Canada
2.59D Courtesy of Dr. G.B. Haber, University of Toronto, Canada
2.61AB Courtesy of Dr. J. Heslin, Toronto, Canada
2.63AB Courtesy of Dr. G.B. Haber, University of Toronto, Canada
2.66B Radiograph courtesy of G.B.Haber, University of Toronto, Canada; photo courtesy of Mission Hospital Regional Center, Mission Viejo, California
2.73B Courtesy of M. Asch, University of Toronto, Canada
2.72B Courtesy of E.L. Lansdown, University of Toronto, Canada
2.68B (right) Courtesy of M. Asch, University of Toronto, Canada
2.91A-C Courtesy of Dr. M.A. Haider, University of Toronto, Canada
2.91D The Visible Human Project; National Library of Medicine; Visible Man Image number 1625.
2.91E,G Dean D, Herbener TE. Cross Sectional Human Anatomy**,** 2000:45,53 (Plates 3.9, 3.13)
2.92A-D Courtesy of Dr. M.A. Haider, University of Toronto, Canada
2.93A-D Courtesy of Dr. M.A. Haider, University of Toronto, Canada

CHAPTER 3

3.7 Snell, R. Clinical Anatomy by Regions, 9th edition, 2011. (Figs. 7.39 and 7.41)
3.13C Dudek RW, Louis TM, *High-Yield Gross Anatomy,* 4th edition, 2010:189. (Fig. 18.4)
3.24 (left) from Dauber W, Pocket Atlas of Human Anatomy Rev 5e, NY, Thieme 2007, p. 195
3.26C,D Bickley LS, Bates' Guide to Physical Examination and History Taking, 10th edition, p. 563.
3.33B,C Bickley LS, Bates' Guide to Physical Examination and History Taking, 10th edition, p. 540, 541
3.33D Courtesy of RE Bristow, Johns Hopkins School of Medicine, Baltimore, MD
3.68A-D Courtesy of Dr. M.A. Haider, University of Toronto, Canada
3.68E Courtesy of The Visible Human Project; National Library of Medicine; Visible Man Image number 1940
3.69 Uflacker R. Atlas of Vascular Anatomy: An Angiographic Approach, 1997:611.
3.70A-C Courtesy of Dr. M.A. Haider, University of Toronto, Canada
3.71 MRIs courtesy of Dr. M.A. Haider, University of Toronto, Canada
3.72A-G MRIs courtesy of Dr. M.A. Haider, University of Toronto, Canada; sectioned specimens from The Visible Human Project; National Library of Medicine; Visible Woman Image numbers 1870 and 1895
3.73AB Courtesy of Dr. M.A. Haider, University of Toronto, Canada.
3.74A-D Ultrasounds courtesy of A.M. Arenson, University of Toronto, Canada
3.75D Reprinted with permission from Stuart GCE, Reid DF. Diagnostic studies. In Copeland LJ (ed.): Textbook of Gynecology. Philadelphia, WB Saunders, 1993.

CHAPTER 4

4.1B Courtesy of D. Salonen, University of Toronto, Canada
4.7B,D,F and 4.8E Courtesy of Drs. E. Becker and P. Bobechko, University of Toronto, Canada
4.8C,D Courtesy of E. Becker, University of Toronto, Canada
4.11A,B Courtesy of J. Heslin, Unitersity of Toronto, Canada
4.11C,D Courtesy of D. Armstrong, University of Toronto, Canada
4.12C Courtesy of D. Salonen, University of Toronto, Canada
4.15B and 4.16B Courtesy of E. Becker, University of Toronto, Canada
4.40C Clay JH, Pounds DM. Basic Clinical Massage Therapy: Integrating Anatomy and Treatment. 2003:92 (Fig. 3.40)
4.49B Courtesy of D. Salonen, University of Toronto, Canada
4.56AB Courtesy of The Visible Human Project; National Library of Medicine; Visible Man 1168.
4.56C Courtesy of D. Armstrong, University of Toronto, Canada
4.57A,B Courtesy of The Visible Human Project; National Library of Medicine; Visible Man 1715.
4.58A,B Courtesy of The Visible Human Project; National Library of Medicine; Visible Man 1805.
4.59A-D Courtesy of D. Salonen, University of Toronto, Canada

CHAPTER 5

5.3B,D Courtesy of P. Babyn, University of Toronto, Canada
5.8A-D A and B are based on Foerster, O.: The Dermatomes in Man. Brain 56(1):1-39, 1933.C and D are based on Keefan JJ, Garrett FD. The segmental distribution of the cutaneous nerves in the limbs of man. Anat Rec 1948;102:409
5.12B Rassner: Dermatologie. Lehrbuch und Atlas © Urban & Schwarzenberg Verlag München. (Appeared in Moore KL, Dalley AF. Clincally Oriented Anatomy. 4th Ed., 1999:527.)
5.14B Courtesy of Dr. E.L. Lansdown, University of Toronto, Canada
5.22A-D Modified from Clay JH, Pounds DM. Basic Clinical Massage Therapy: Integrating Anatomy and Treatment. 2002:301 (Plate 9.2).
5.22E,H Modified from Clay JH, Pounds DM. Basic Clinical Massage Therapy: Integrating Anatomy and Treatment. 2002:280,312 (Figs. 8.10, 9.10)
5.34A Courtesy of E. Becker, University of Toronto, Canada
5.39C Daffner RH. Clinical Radiology: The Essentials. Baltimore: Williams & Wilkins, 1993:491 (Fig. 11.99)
5.40B Courtesy of Dr. D. Salonen, University of Toronto, Canada
5.51 (inset) Courtesy of Dr. Robert Peroutka, Cockeysville, MD
5.56A,B Courtesy of Dr. P. Bobechko, University of Toronto, Canada
5.56C Courtesy of Dr. D. Salonen, University of Toronto, Canada
5.57B,C Courtesy of Dr. D. Salonen, University of Toronto, Canada
5.58 Courtesy of Dr. P. Bobechko, University of Toronto, Canada
5.59B,C Courtesy of Dr. D. Salonen, University of Toronto, Canada

5.65C,D Clay JH, Pounds DM. Basic Clinical Massage Therapy: Integrating Anatomy and Treatment. 2002:352,354 (Figs. 10.16 & 10.18)
5.73A Courtesy of Dr. D. K. Sniderman, University of Toronto, Canada
5.81B and 5.86A Courtesy of Dr. E. Becker, University of Toronto, Canada
5.86B Courtesy of Dr. P. Bobechko, University of Toronto, Canada
5.87B Courtesy of E. Becker, University of Toronto, Canada
5.89B Courtesy of Dr. W. Kucharczyk, University of Toronto, Canada
5.90B Courtesy of Dr. W. Kucharczyk, University of Toronto, Canada
5.98C Courtesy of Dr. P. Bobechko, University of Toronto, Canada
5.100C Courtesy of The Visible Human Project; National Library of Medicine; Visible Man 2105.
5.100D-F MRIs courtesy of Dr. D. Salonen, University of Toronto, Canada
5.102C Courtesy of The Visible Human Project; National Library of Medicine; Visible Man 2551.
5.102D-F MRIs courtesy of Dr. D. Salonen, University of Toronto, Canada
Table 5.3 (unnumbered figures) Dudek RW, Louis TM, *High-Yield Gross Anatomy,* 4th edition, 2010:228. (Table 21-1)

CHAPTER 6
6.7A,B Based on Foerster, O.: The Dermatomes in Man. Brain 56(1):1-39,1933. (Appeared in Moore KL, Dalley AF. Clinically Oriented Anatomy. 4th ed, 1999:682,683.)
6.7C,D Based on Keegan JJ, Garrett FD. The segmental distribution of the cutaneous nerves in the limbs of man. Anat Rec 1948;102:409
6.10 Tank W, Gest TR: KWW Atlas of Anatomy. Baltimore: Lippincott Williams & Wilkins, 2008. Pl. 2-53, p. 82.
6.21L Courtesy of D. Armstrong, University of Toronto, Canada
6.24C Courtesy of D. Armstrong, University of Toronto, Canada
6.29B Rowland LP, Merritt's Textbook of Neurology, 9th ed. Baltimore, Williams & Wilkins, 1995
6.31ABD Clay JH, Pounds DM. Basic Clinical Massage Therapy: Integrating Anatomy and Treatment. 2002:113,136,132 (Plates 4.4, 4.31, 4.24)
6.33B,D Clay JH, Pounds DM. Basic Clinical Massage Therapy: Integrating Anatomy and Treatment. 2002:144,138 (Figs. 4.44, 4.33)
6.48A Courtesy of E. Becker, University of Toronto, Canada
6.48C,E Courtesy of D. Salonen, University of Toronto, Canada
6.48D Courtesy of R. Leekam, University of Toronto and West End Diagnostic Imaging, Canada
6.53C Courtesy of E. Becker, University of Toronto, Canada
6.54 Radiographs courtesy of J. Heslin, Toronto, Canada;
6.55B Courtesy of D. Salonen, University of Toronto, Canada
6.56B Courtesy of E. Becker, University of Toronto, Canada
6.63A, 6.64A, 6.65A, 6.66A Clay JH, Pounds DM. Basic Clinical Massage Therapy: Integrating Anatomy and Treatment. 2002:170 (Plate 5.3)
6.72A-D Clay JH, Pounds DM. Basic Clinical Massage Therapy: Integrating Anatomy and Treatment. 2002:174 (Plate 5.55)
6.83 Clay JH, Pounds DM. Basic Clinical Massage Therapy: Integrating Anatomy and Treatment. 2002:127 (Plate 5.5)
6.89F Courtesy of E. Becker, University of Toronto, Canada
6.92A,B Courtesy of E. Becker, University of Toronto, Canada
6.93B Courtesy of D. Armstrong, University of Toronto, Canada
6.99 A-C Courtesy of D. Salonen, University of Toronto, Canada
6.100C-E Courtesy of D. Salonen, University of Toronto, Canada
6.101A-C Courtesy of D. Salonen, University of Toronto, Canada
6.102 B Courtesy of R. Leekam, University of Toronto and West End Diagnostic Imaging, Canada
6.35A,B Clay JH, Pounds DM. Basic Clinical Massage Therapy: Integrating Anatomy and Treatment. 2002:170,171,173,179 (Plates 5.3, 5.4, 5.6, and Fig. 5.1)

CHAPTER 7
7.1B,E,F Courtesy of Dr. D. Armstrong, University of Toronto, Canada
7.7A,B Courtesy of Dr. E. Becker, University of Toronto, Canada
7.29A-C Courtesy of Dr. D. Armstrong, University of Toronto, Canada
7.35A,B Courtesy of I. Verschuur, Joint Department of Medical Imaging, UHN/Mount Sinai Hospital, Toronto, Canada
7.38D Courtesy of Dr. W. Kucharczyk, University of Toronto, Canada
7.39B Melloni,R. Melloni's Illustrated Review of Human Anatomy by Structures-Arteries, Bones, Muscles, Nerves, Veins, 1988, p. 198
7.42A-D Modified from Girard, Louis, Anatomy of the Huma Eye. II. The Extra-ocular Muscles. Teaching Films, Inc. Houston, TX
7.45C Melloni,R. Melloni's Illustrated Review of Human Anatomy by Structures-Arteries, Bones, Muscles, Nerves, Veins, 1988, p. 189.
7.46A Courtesy of J.R. Buncic, University of Toronto, Canada
7.56 CTs and MRIs from Langland OE, Langlais RP, Preece JW. Principles of Dental Imaging, 2002:278 (Figs. 11.32A, B; 11.33A, B).
7.65A Langland OE, Langlais RP, Preece JW. Principles of Dental Imaging, 2002:334 (Fig. 14.1).
7.65B Courtesy of M.J. Phatoah, University of Toronto, Canada.
7.66E Courtesy of Dr. B. Libgott, Division of Anatomy/Department of Surgery, University of Toronto, Ontario, Canada
7.67B,C Woelfel JB, Scheid RC. Dental Anatomy: Its Relevance to Dentistry. 6th ed, 2002:86,46 (Figs. 3.5 & 3.6).
7.76B Courtesy of D. Armstrong, University of Toronto, Canada
7.76C Courtesy of E. Becker, University of Toronto, Canada
7.77C Courtesy of E. Becker, University of Toronto, Canada
7.78B Modified from Paff, GH Anatomy of the Head & Neck. Philadelphia: WB Sanders Co., 1973. figs 238–240, p. 142–143.
7.84D Courtesy of Welch Allyn, Inc. Skaneateles Falls, NY. (Appeared in Moore KL, Dalley AF. Clinically Oriented Anatomy. 4th ed, 1999:966 (Fig. 8.2)
7.94B-D Courtesy of W. Kucharczyk, University of Toronto, Canada
7.95B Courtesy of Dr. W. Kucharczyk, University of Toronto, Canada
7.96A-C All photos courtesy of The Visible Human Project; National Library of Medicine; Visible Man 1107 and 1168.
7.99–7.102, 7.104, 7.105B,C and 7.106 Colorized from photographs provided courtesy of Dr. C.G. Smith, which appears in Smith CG. Serial Dissections of the Human Brain. Baltimore: Urban & Schwarzenber, Inc. and Toronto: Gage Publishing Ltd., 1981 (© Carlton G. Smith)
7.103A-F MRIs courtesy of Dr. D. Armstrong, University of Toronto, Canada
7.107A-E MRIs courtesy of Dr. D. Armstrong, University of Toronto, Canada
7.108A-F MRIs courtesy of Dr. D. Armstrong, University of Toronto, Canada
7.109A-C MRIs courtesy of Dr. D. Armstrong, University of Toronto, Canada
7.53 Illustrations from Clay JH, Pounds DM. Basic Clinical Massage Therapy: Integrating Anatomy and Treatment. 2002:76,74,79 (Figs.3.17, 3.15, 3.19).
7.64 (bottom left illustration) Clay JH, Pounds DM. Basic Clinical Massage Therapy: Integrating Anatomy and Treatment, 2002:80 (Fig. 3.22).

CHAPTER 8
8.5B Courtesy of J. Heslin, University of Toronto, Canada
8.7 Modified from Clay JH, Pounds DM. Basic Clinical Massage Therapy: Integrating Anatomy and Treatment. 2003:90,91 (Figs. 3.36, 3.48)
8.12A Modified from Clay JH, Pounds DM. Basic Clinical Massage Therapy: Integrating Anatomy and Treatment. 2003:88 (Fig. 3.34)
8.15B Courtesy of Dr. D. Armstrong, University of Toronto, Canada
8.24B Modified from Clay JH, Pounds DM. Basic Clinical Massage Therapy: Integrating Anatomy and Treatment. 2003:92 (Fig. 3.40)
8.25A Clay JH, Pounds DM. Basic Clinical Massage Therapy: Integrating Anatomy and Treatment. 2003:101,128 (Figs. 3.53, 4.17)
8.25B Clay JH, Pounds DM. Basic Clinical Massage Therapy: Integrating Anatomy and Treatment. 2nd ed, 2008:103. (Fig. 3.40)
8.25C Clay JH, Pounds DM. Basic Clinical Massage Therapy: Integrating Anatomy and Treatment. 2nd ed, 2008:140. (Fig. 4.17)
8.25D Clay JH, Pounds DM. Basic Clinical Massage Therapy: Integrating Anatomy and Treatment. 2nd ed, 2008:67. (Fig. 3.6)
8.28 Clay JH, Pounds DM. Basic Clinical Massage Therapy: Integrating Anatomy and Treatment. 2003:96,100,104 (Figs. 3.48, 3.52, 3.56)
8.34A Abrahams P. The Atlas of the Human Body. San Diego, CA: Thunder Bay Press, 2002, p. 86.
8.34B From Liebgott B. The Anatomical Basis of Dentistry. Philadelphia, PA: Mosby, 1982.
8.41A Rohen JW, Yokochi C, Lutjen-DrecollE, Romrell LJ. Color Atlas of Anatomy: A Photographic Study of the Human Body. 5th ed, 2002.
8.41C Courtesy of Dr. D. Salonen, University of Toronto, Canada.
8.44A-C Courtesy of Dr. D. Salonen, University of Toronto, Canada;
8.46B Courtesy of Dr. E. Becker, University of Toronto, Canada
8.47 Siemens Medical Solutions USA, Inc.

CHAPTER 9
9.23A-F Courtesy of Dr. W. Kucharczyk, University of Toronto, Canada
9.24A-C Photos courtesy of Dr. W. Kucharczyk, University of Toronto, Canada

Thorax

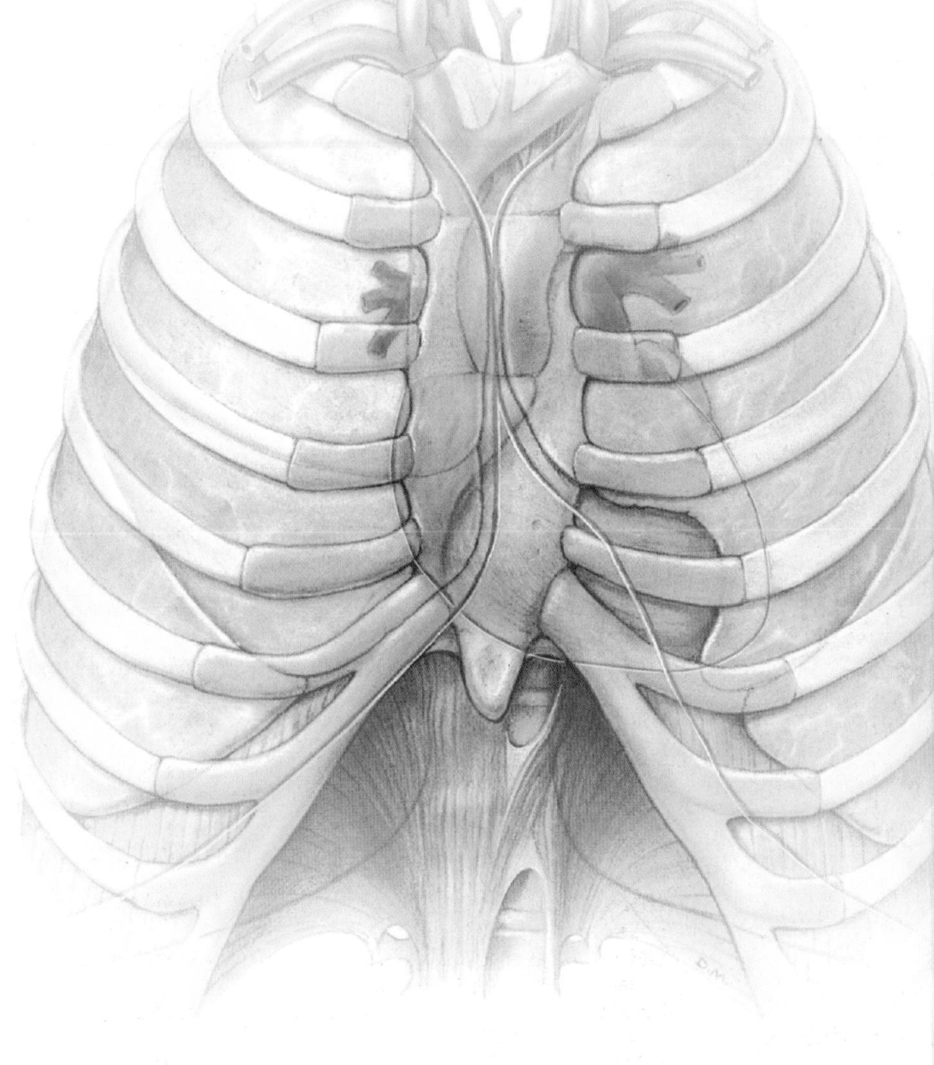

Pectoral Region	2
Breast	4
Bony Thorax and Joints	12
Thoracic Wall	19
Thoracic Contents	27
Pleural Cavities	30
Mediastinum	31
Lungs and Pleura	32
Bronchi and Bronchopulmonary Segments	38
Innervation and Lymphatic Drainage of Lungs	44
External Heart	46
Coronary Vessels	56
Conduction System of Heart	60
Internal Heart and Valves	61
Superior Mediastinum and Great Vessels	68
Diaphragm	75
Posterior Thorax	76
Overview of Autonomic Innervation	86
Overview of Lymphatic Drainage of Thorax	88
Sectional Anatomy and Imaging	90

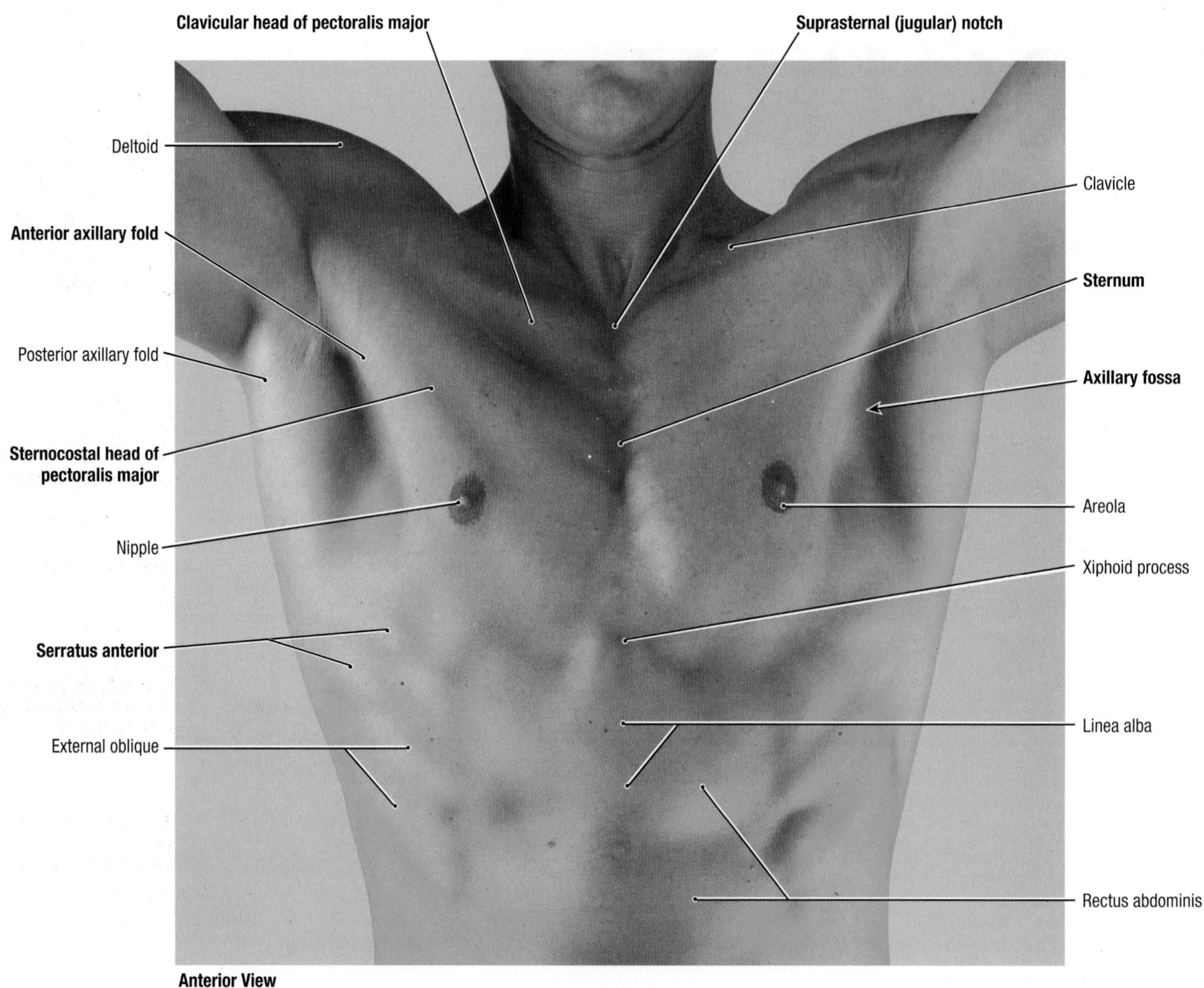
Clavicular head of pectoralis major
Suprasternal (jugular) notch
Deltoid
Clavicle
Anterior axillary fold
Sternum
Posterior axillary fold
Axillary fossa
Sternocostal head of pectoralis major
Areola
Nipple
Xiphoid process
Serratus anterior
Linea alba
External oblique
Rectus abdominis
Anterior View

1.1 SURFACE ANATOMY OF MALE PECTORAL REGION

- The subject is adducting the shoulders against resistance to demonstrate the pectoralis major muscle.
- The sternum (breastbone) lies subcutaneously in the anterior median line and is palpable throughout its length.
- The suprasternal notch can be palpated between the prominent medial ends of the clavicle.
- The pectoralis major muscle has two parts, the sternocostal and clavicular heads.
- The inferior border of the sternocostal head of the pectoralis major muscle forms the anterior axillary fold. The axillary fossa ("armpit") is a surface feature overlying a fat-filled space, the axilla, posterior to the anterior fold.
- The male nipple overlies the fourth intercostal space.

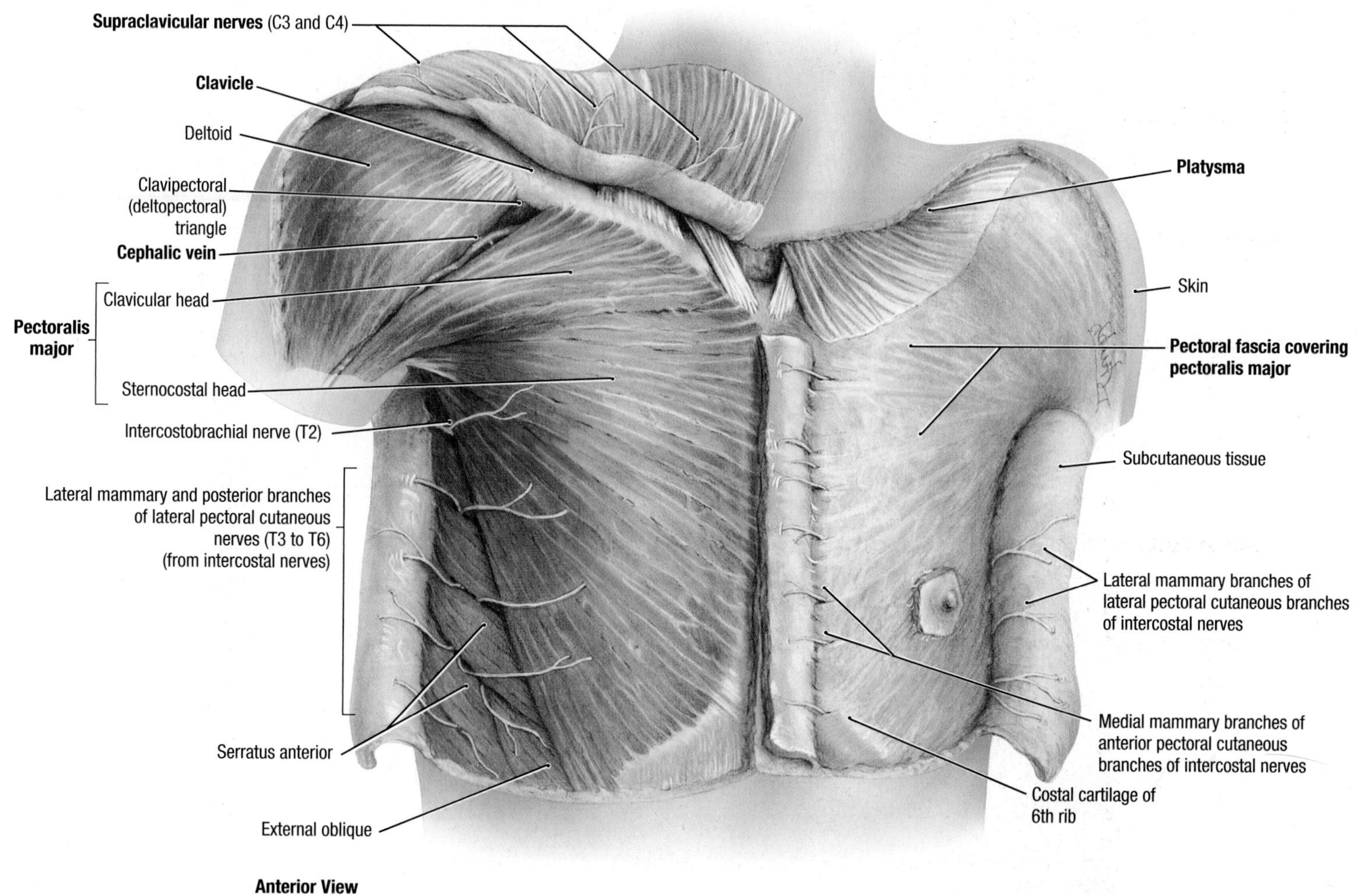
Supraclavicular nerves (C3 and C4)
Clavicle
Deltoid
Clavipectoral (deltopectoral) triangle
Cephalic vein
Pectoralis major
Clavicular head
Sternocostal head
Intercostobrachial nerve (T2)
Lateral mammary and posterior branches of lateral pectoral cutaneous nerves (T3 to T6) (from intercostal nerves)
Serratus anterior
External oblique
Anterior View
Platysma
Skin
Pectoral fascia covering pectoralis major
Subcutaneous tissue
Lateral mammary branches of lateral pectoral cutaneous branches of intercostal nerves
Medial mammary branches of anterior pectoral cutaneous branches of intercostal nerves
Costal cartilage of 6th rib

1.2 SUPERFICIAL DISSECTION, MALE PECTORAL REGION

- The platysma muscle, which descends to the 2nd or 3rd rib, is cut short on both sides of the specimen; together with the supraclavicular nerves, it is reflected superiorly on the right side.
- The pectoral fascia covers the pectoralis major.
- The clavicle lies deep to the subcutaneous tissue and the platysma muscle.
- The cephalic vein passes deeply in the clavipectoral (deltopectoral) triangle to join the axillary vein.
- Supraclavicular (C3 and C4) and upper thoracic nerves (T2 to T6) supply cutaneous innervation to the pectoral region.
- The clavipectoral (deltopectoral) triangle, bounded by the clavicle superiorly, the deltoid muscle laterally, and the clavicular head of the pectoralis major muscle medially, underlies a surface depression called the infraclavicular fossa.

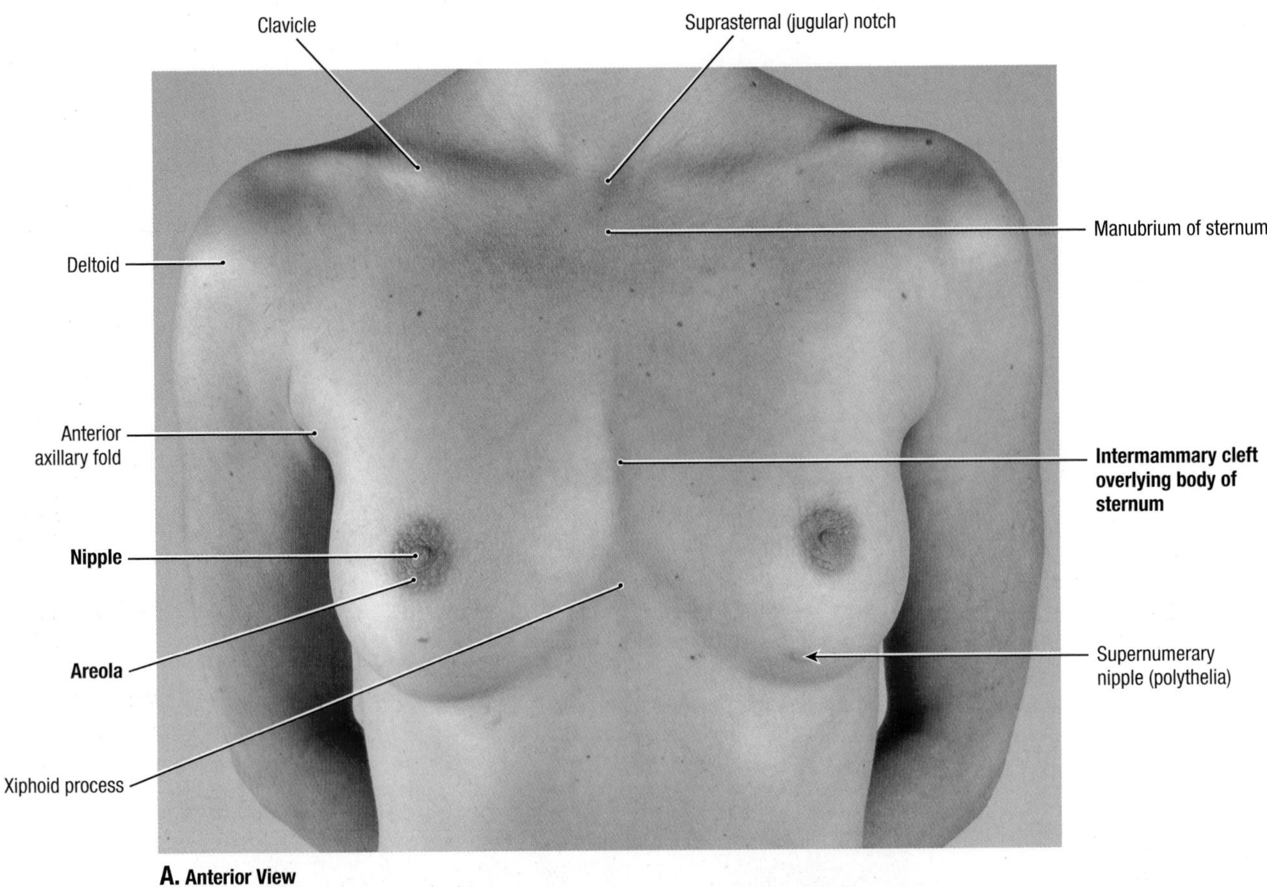
Clavicle
Suprasternal (jugular) notch
Manubrium of sternum
Deltoid
Anterior axillary fold
Intermammary cleft overlying body of sternum
Nipple
Areola
Supernumerary nipple (polythelia)
Xiphoid process

A. Anterior View

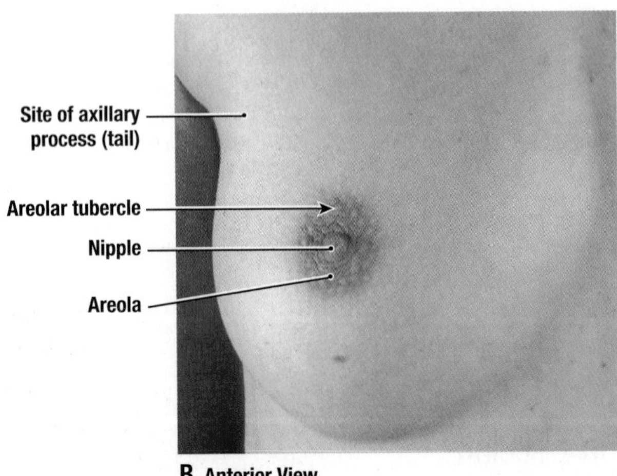
Site of axillary process (tail)
Areolar tubercle
Nipple
Areola

B. Anterior View

1.3 SURFACE ANATOMY OF FEMALE PECTORAL REGION

A. Overview. **B.** Breast. The roughly circular base of the female breast extends transversely from the lateral border of the sternum to the midaxillary line and vertically from the 2nd to 6th ribs. A small part of the breast may extend along the inferolateral edge of the pectoralis major muscle toward the axillary fossa, forming an axillary process or tail (of Spence).

Polymastia (supernumerary breasts) or **polythelia** (accessory nipples) may occur superior or inferior to the normal pair, occasionally developing in the axillary fossa or anterior abdominal wall. Supernumerary breasts usually consist of only a rudimentary nipple and areola, which may be mistaken for a mole (nevus) until they change pigmentation with the normal nipples during pregnancy.

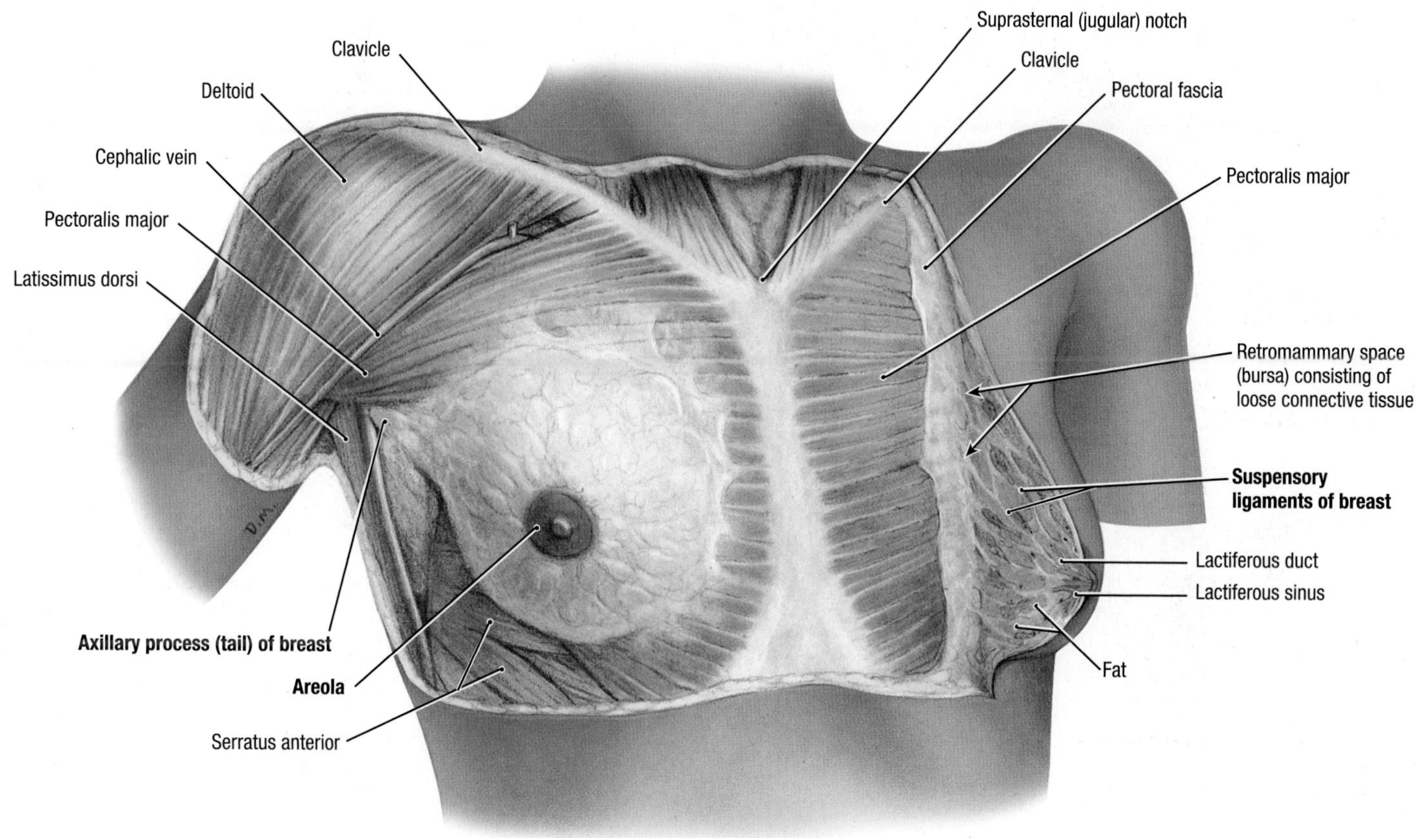
Clavicle
Deltoid
Cephalic vein
Pectoralis major
Latissimus dorsi
Axillary process (tail) of breast
Areola
Serratus anterior
Suprasternal (jugular) notch
Clavicle
Pectoral fascia
Pectoralis major
Retromammary space (bursa) consisting of loose connective tissue
Suspensory ligaments of breast
Lactiferous duct
Lactiferous sinus
Fat

A. **Anterior View**

1.4 SUPERFICIAL DISSECTION, FEMALE PECTORAL REGION

A. Dissection.

- On the specimen's right side, the skin is removed; on the left side, the breast is sagittally sectioned.
- Two thirds of the breast rests on the pectoral fascia covering the pectoralis major; the other third rests on the fascia covering the serratus anterior muscle.
- The region of loose connective tissue between the pectoral fascia and the deep surface of the breast, the retromammary space (bursa), permits the breast to move on the deep fascia.

Cancer can spread by contiguity (invasion of adjacent tissue). When **breast cancer** cells invade the retromammary space, attach to or invade the pectoral fascia overlying the pectoralis major, or metastasize to the interpectoral nodes (Fig. 1.7), the breast elevates when the muscle contracts. This movement is a clinical sign of advanced cancer of the breast.

B. Breast Quadrants. For the anatomical location and description of tumors and cysts, the surface of the breast is divided into four quadrants. For example: "A hard irregular mass was felt in the superior medial quadrant of the breast at the 2 o'clock position, approximately 2.5 cm from the margin of the areola."

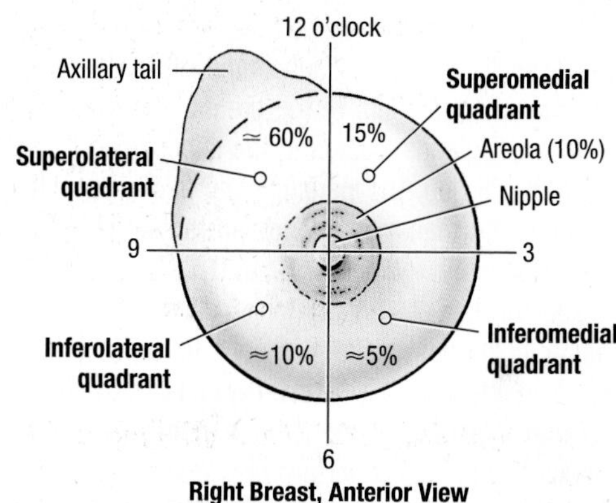
12 o'clock
Axillary tail
Superomedial quadrant
≈ 60%
15%
Areola (10%)
Superolateral quadrant
Nipple
9
3
Inferolateral quadrant
≈10%
≈5%
Inferomedial quadrant
6
Right Breast, Anterior View

B. **Quadrants of Breast: Percentage of Malignant Tumors**

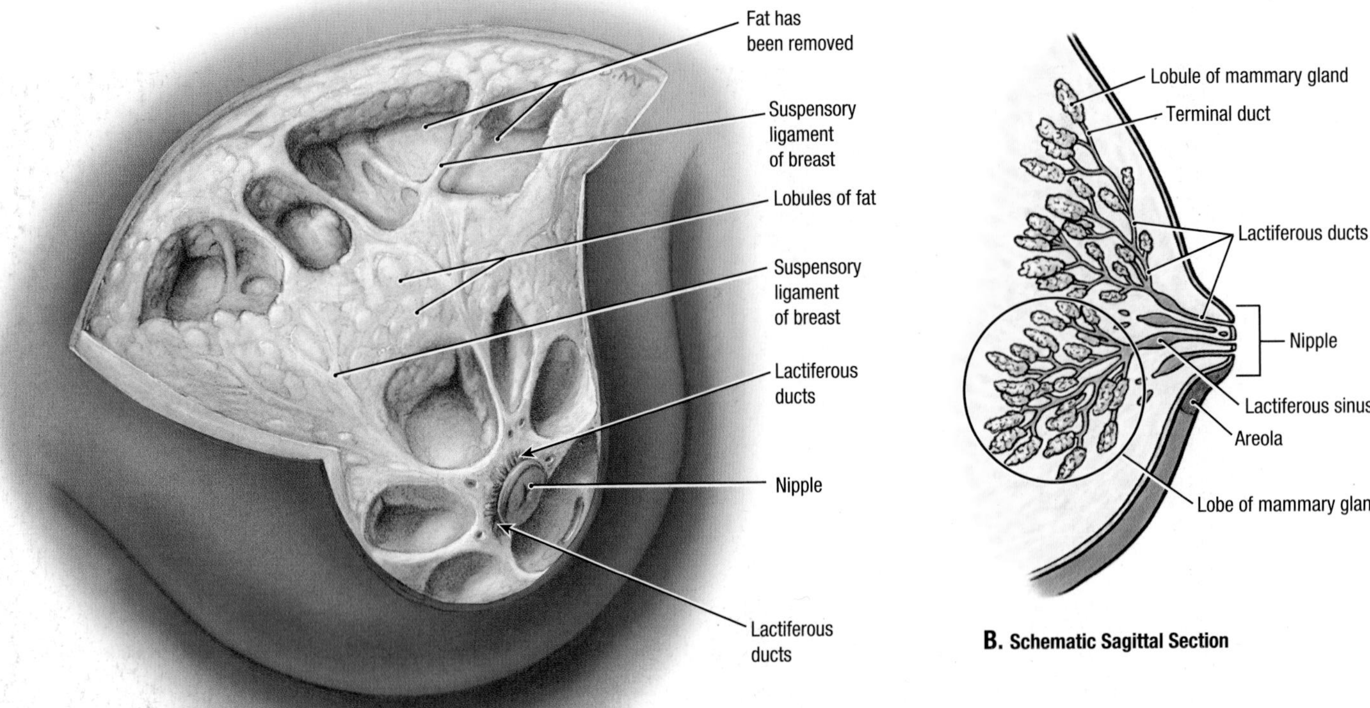
Fat has been removed
Suspensory ligament of breast
Lobules of fat
Suspensory ligament of breast
Lactiferous ducts
Nipple
Lactiferous ducts
Lobule of mammary gland
Terminal duct
Lactiferous ducts
Nipple
Lactiferous sinus
Areola
Lobe of mammary gland

A. Anterior View

B. Schematic Sagittal Section

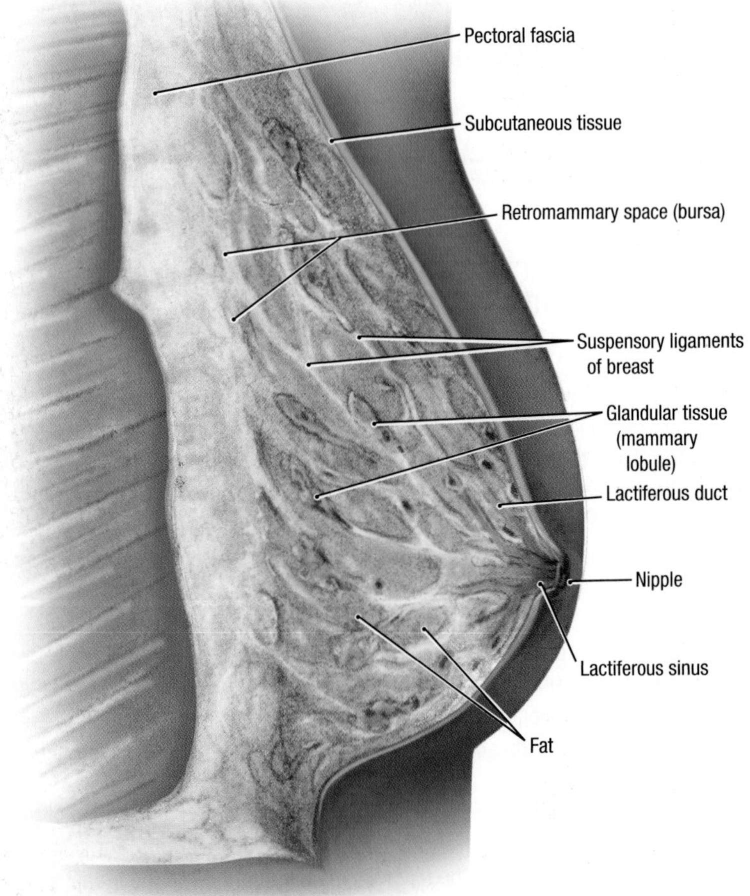
Pectoral fascia
Subcutaneous tissue
Retromammary space (bursa)
Suspensory ligaments of breast
Glandular tissue (mammary lobule)
Lactiferous duct
Nipple
Lactiferous sinus
Fat

C. Sagittal Section of Breast

1.5 FEMALE MAMMARY GLAND

A. Dissection. Areas of subcutaneous fat were removed to show the suspensory ligaments of the breast. The mammary glands are modified sweat glands located in the subcutaneous tissue. They consist of glandular tissue, the parenchyma, and supporting fibrous tissue, the stroma. The mammary glands are attached to the dermis of the skin by suspensory ligaments. **B. and C.** Sagittal sections. The glandular tissue consists of 15 to 20 lobes, each composed of lobules. Each lobe has a lactiferous duct that widens to form the lactiferous sinus before opening on the nipple. **Interference with the lymphatic drainage by cancer** may cause lymphedema (edema, excess fluid in the subcutaneous tissue), which in turn may result in deviation of the nipple and a leathery, thickened appearance of the breast skin. Prominent (puffy) skin between dimpled pores may develop, which gives the skin an orange-peel appearance (*peau d'orange* sign). Larger dimples may form if pulled by cancerous invasion of the suspensory ligaments of the breast.

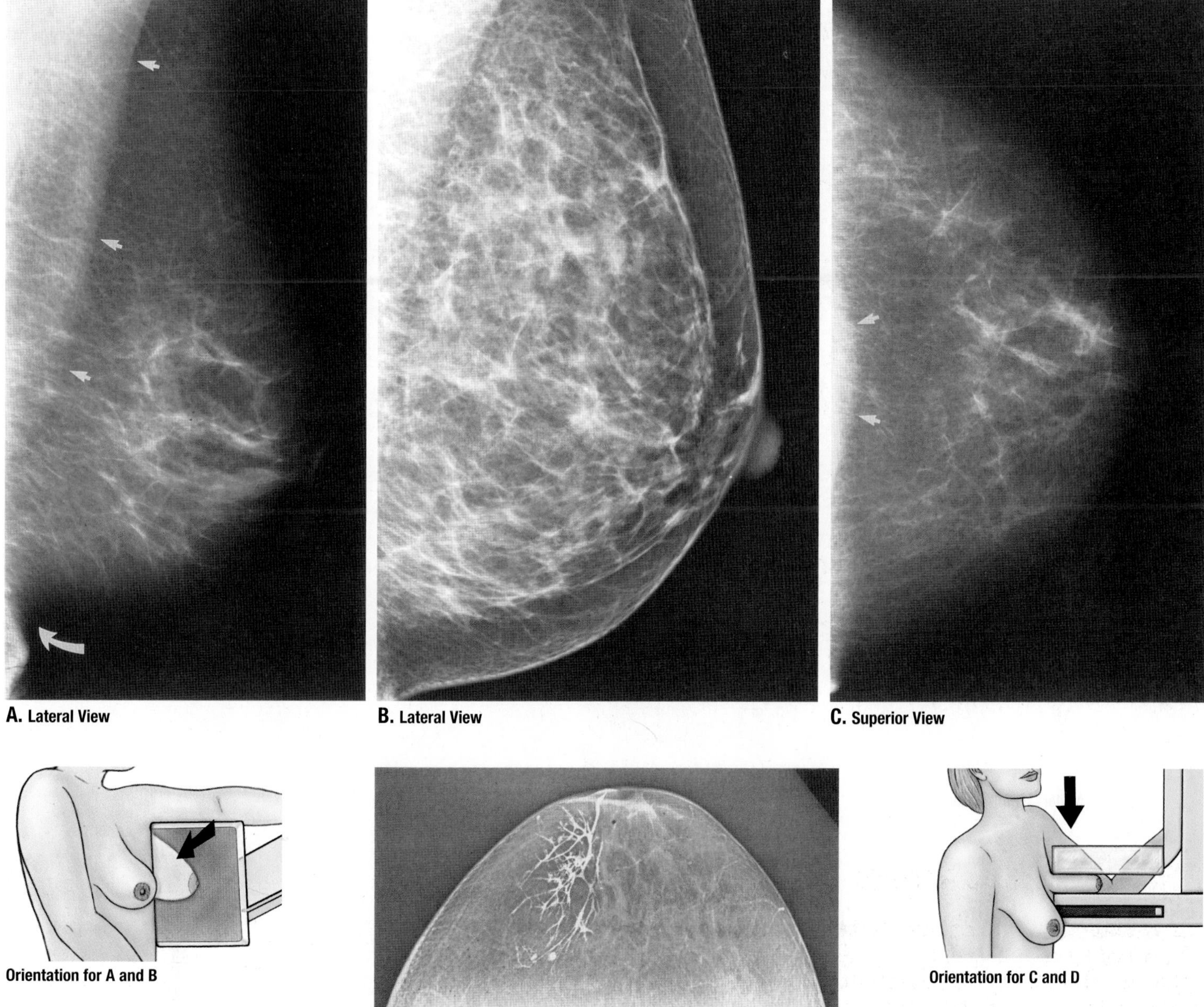
A. Lateral View
B. Lateral View
C. Superior View
Orientation for A and B
Orientation for C and D
D. Superior View

1.6 IMAGING OF BREAST

A. Mediolateral oblique (MLO) mammogram of left breast. The pectoralis major muscle is indicated with *white arrowheads* and the inframammary fold with a *curved white arrow.* The nipple is seen in profile. Observe the connective tissue network of the breast. The stroma is radiopaque and changes with age and during lactation. **B.** Digital mammogram. **C.** Craniocaudal (CC) mammogram of left breast. Pectoralis major (*white arrows*). **D.** Glactogram. Contrast has been injected into a lactiferous duct, outlining the branching pattern of its tributaries.

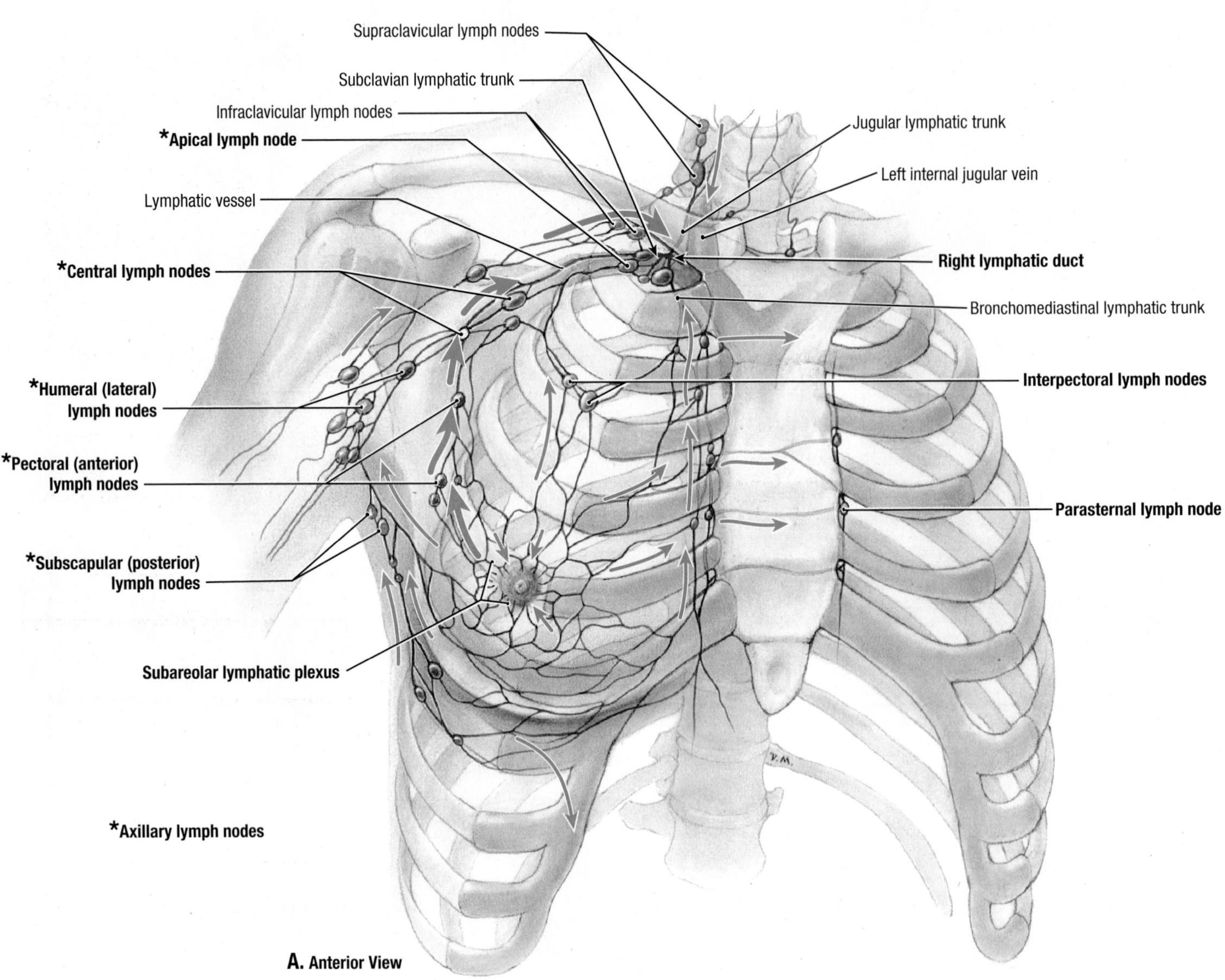
Supraclavicular lymph nodes
Subclavian lymphatic trunk
Infraclavicular lymph nodes
*Apical lymph node
Lymphatic vessel
*Central lymph nodes
*Humeral (lateral) lymph nodes
*Pectoral (anterior) lymph nodes
*Subscapular (posterior) lymph nodes
Subareolar lymphatic plexus
*Axillary lymph nodes
Jugular lymphatic trunk
Left internal jugular vein
Right lymphatic duct
Bronchomediastinal lymphatic trunk
Interpectoral lymph nodes
Parasternal lymph node

A. Anterior View

1.7 LYMPHATIC DRAINAGE OF BREAST

A. Overview. Lymph drained from the upper limb and breast passes through nodes arranged irregularly in groups of axillary lymph nodes: (1) pectoral, along the inferior border of the pectoralis minor muscle; (2) subscapular, along the subscapular artery and veins; (3) humeral, along the distal part of the axillary vein; (4) central, at the base of the axilla, embedded in axillary fat; and (5) apical, along the axillary vein between the clavicle and the pectoralis minor muscle. Most of the breast drains via the pectoral, central, and apical axillary nodes to the subclavian lymph trunk, which joins the venous system at the junction of the subclavian and internal jugular veins. The medial part of the breast drains to the parasternal nodes, which are located along the internal thoracic vessels.

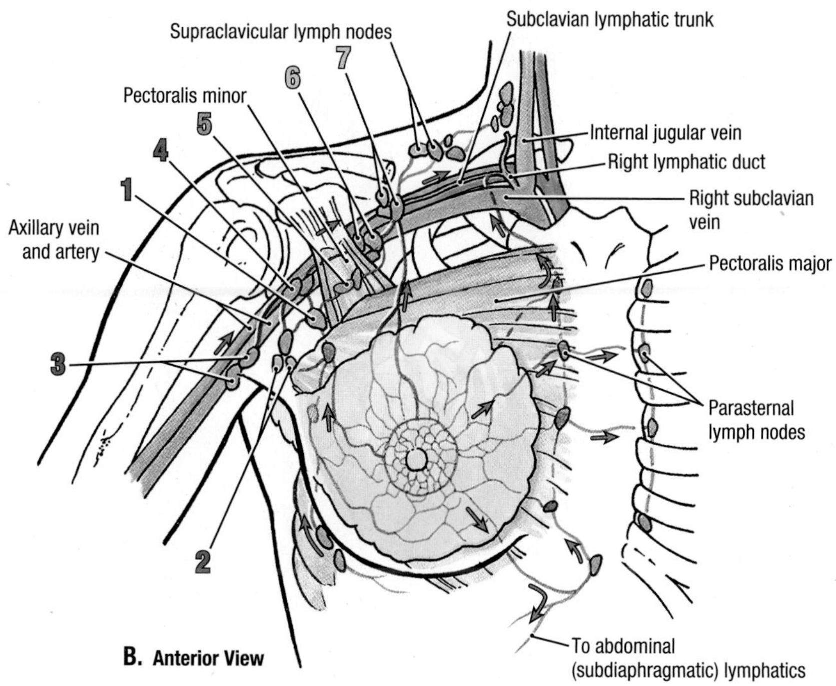
Supraclavicular lymph nodes
Subclavian lymphatic trunk
7
6
Pectoralis minor
5
4
1
Axillary vein
and artery
Internal jugular vein
Right lymphatic duct
Right subclavian
vein
Pectoralis major
3
Parasternal
lymph nodes
2
To abdominal
(subdiaphragmatic) lymphatics

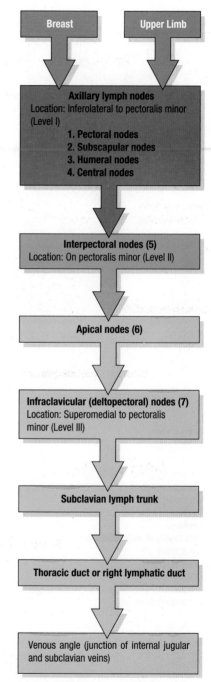

B. Anterior View

Breast → **Upper Limb** →

Axillary lymph nodes
Location: Inferolateral to pectoralis minor (Level I)

1. **Pectoral nodes**
2. **Subscapular nodes**
3. **Humeral nodes**
4. **Central nodes**

↓

Interpectoral nodes (5)
Location: On pectoralis minor (Level II)

↓

Apical nodes (6)

↓

Infraclavicular (deltopectoral) nodes (7)
Location: Superomedial to pectoralis minor (Level III)

↓

Subclavian lymph trunk

↓

Thoracic duct or right lymphatic duct

↓

Venous angle (junction of internal jugular and subclavian veins)

C. Flow of lymph from the breast and upper limb to the venous angle.

1.7 LYMPHATIC DRAINAGE OF BREAST *(CONTINUED)*

B. Pattern of lymphatic drainage. **Breast cancer** typically spreads by means of lymphatic vessels (lymphogenic metastasis), which carry cancer cells from the breast to the lymph nodes, chiefly those in the axilla. The cells lodge in the nodes, producing nests of tumor cells (metastases). Abundant communications among lymphatic pathways and among axillary, cervical, and parasternal nodes may also cause metastases from the breast to develop in the supraclavicular lymph nodes, the opposite breast, or the abdomen. The prognosis of breast cancer has been correlated with the level of metastasis (I, II, or III) and to the number of involved axillary lymph nodes. **C.** Flow of lymph from the breast and upper limb to the venous angle.

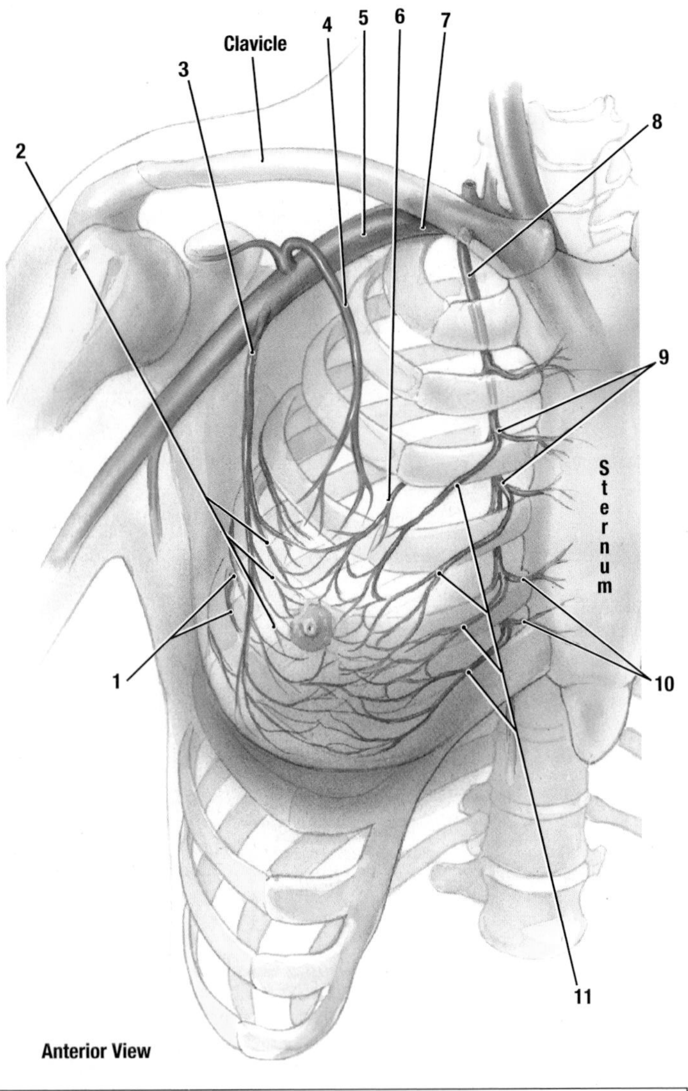
Clavicle
1
2
3
4
5
6
7
8
9
10
11
Sternum
Anterior View

Arteries:

1. Lateral mammary branches of lateral cutaneous branches of posterior intercostal arteries
2. Lateral mammary branches of lateral thoracic artery
3. Lateral thoracic artery
4. Pectoral branch of thoraco-acromial artery
5. Axillary artery
6. Mammary branch of anterior intercostal artery
7. Subclavian artery
8. Internal thoracic artery
9. Perforating branches
10. Sternal branches
11. Medial mammary branches

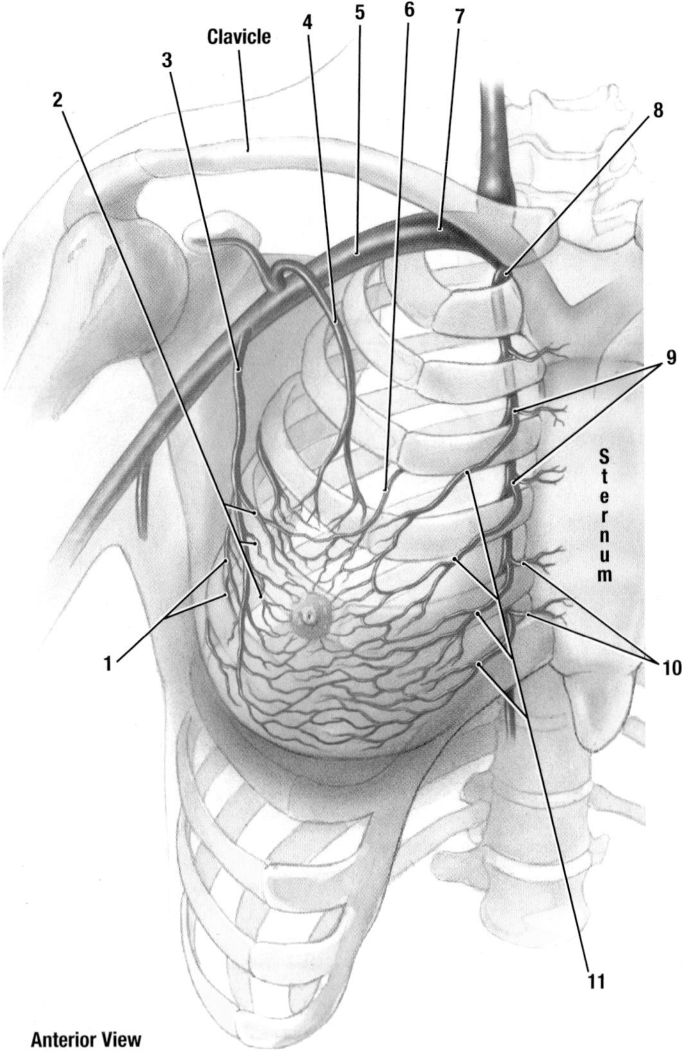
Clavicle
1
2
3
4
5
6
7
8
9
10
11
Sternum
Anterior View

Veins:

1. Lateral mammary branches of lateral cutaneous branches of posterior intercostal veins
2. Lateral mammary branches of lateral thoracic vein
3. Lateral thoracic vein
4. Pectoral branch of thoraco-acromial vein
5. Axillary vein
6. Mammary branch of anterior intercostal vein
7. Subclavian vein
8. Internal thoracic vein
9. Perforating branches
10. Sternal branches
11. Medial mammary veins

1.8 ARTERIAL SUPPLY AND VENOUS DRAINAGE OF BREAST

Arteries enter and veins drain the breast from its superomedial and superolateral aspects; vessels also penetrate the deep surface of the breast. The vessels branch profusely and anastomose with each other.

Breast incisions are placed in the inferior breast quadrants when possible because these quadrants are less vascular than the superior ones.

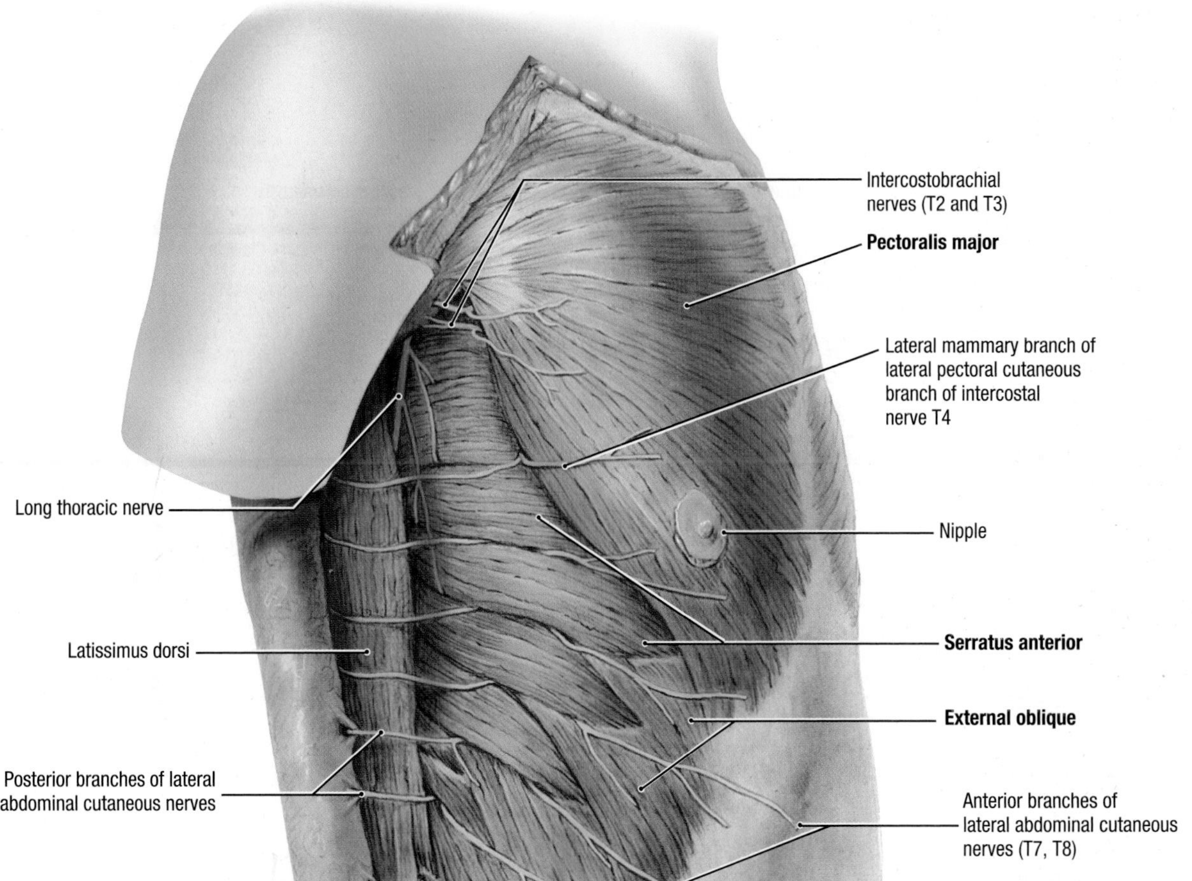
Intercostobrachial nerves (T2 and T3)
Pectoralis major
Lateral mammary branch of lateral pectoral cutaneous branch of intercostal nerve T4
Long thoracic nerve
Nipple
Latissimus dorsi
Serratus anterior
External oblique
Posterior branches of lateral abdominal cutaneous nerves
Anterior branches of lateral abdominal cutaneous nerves (T7, T8)

A. **Anterolateral View (Male)**

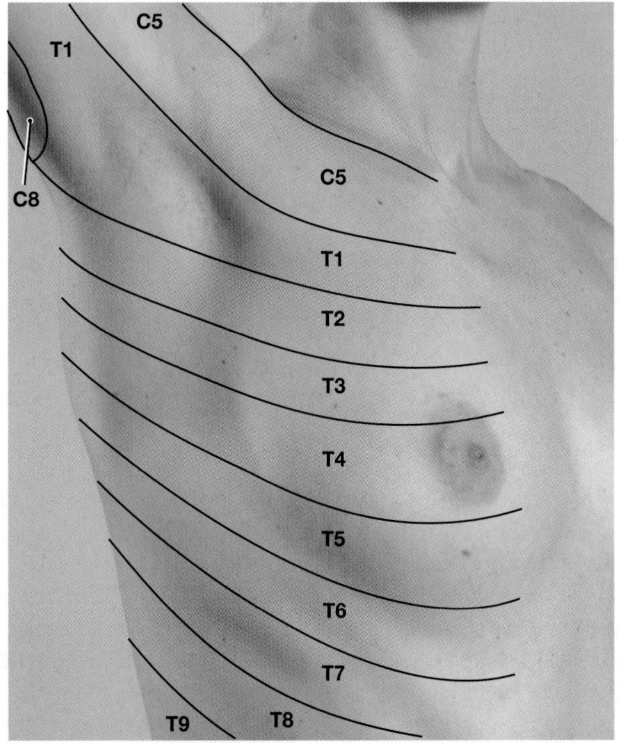
C5
T1
C8
C5
T1
T2
T3
T4
T5
T6
T7
T9
T8

B. **Anterolateral View (Female)**

1.9 MUSCLES AND NERVES OF BED OF BREAST

A. Muscles comprising bed and cutaneous nerves. **B.** Dermatomes.

Local anesthesia of an intercostal space (intercostal nerve block) is produced by injecting a local anesthetic agent around the intercostal nerves between the paravertebral line and the area of required anesthesia. Because any particular area of skin usually receives innervation from two adjacent nerves, considerable overlapping of contiguous dermatomes occurs. Therefore, complete loss of sensation usually does not occur unless two or more intercostal nerves are anesthetized.

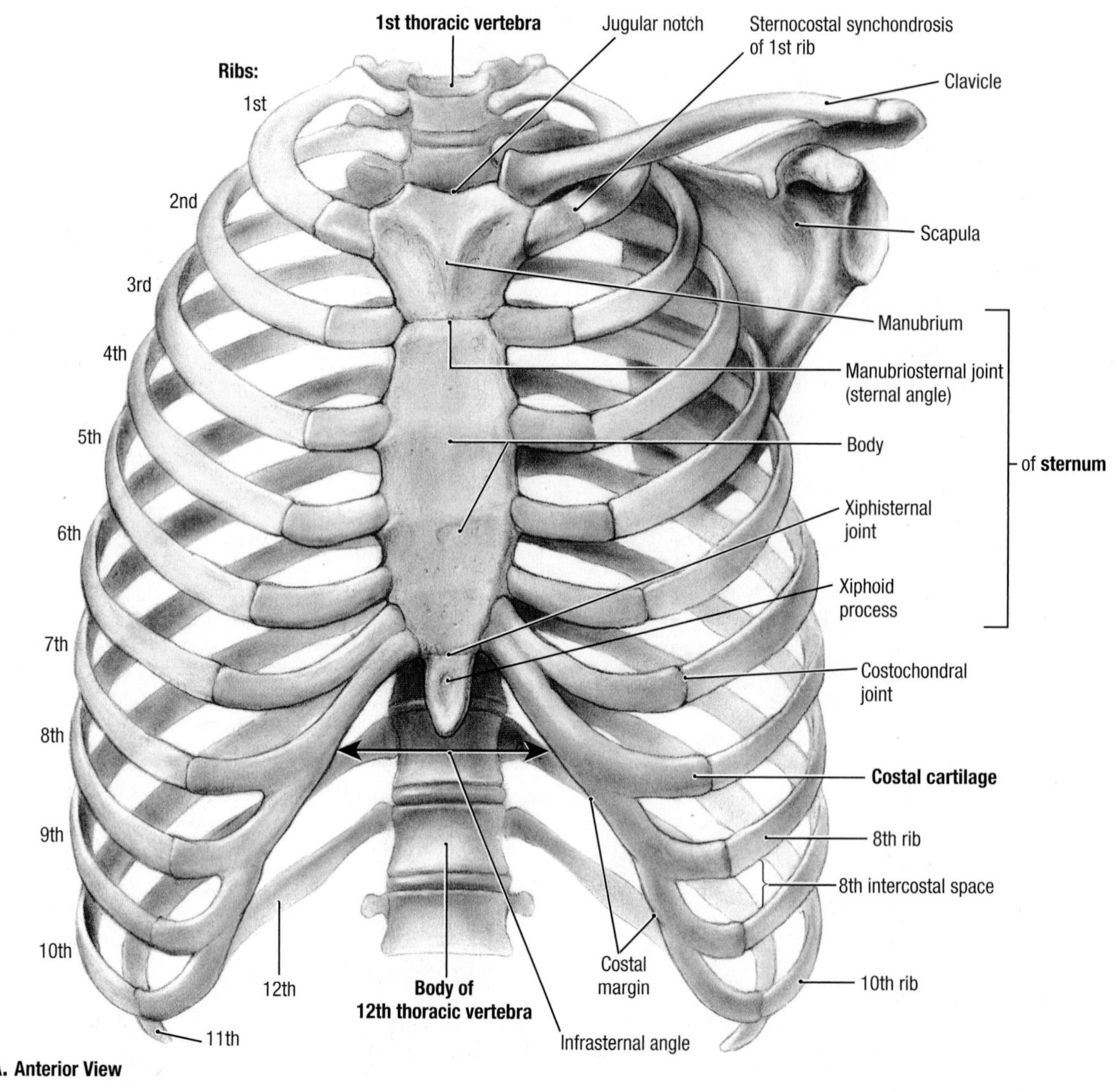
1st thoracic vertebra
Jugular notch
Sternocostal synchondrosis of 1st rib
Clavicle
Ribs:
1st
2nd
3rd
4th
5th
6th
7th
8th
9th
10th
11th
12th
Scapula
Manubrium
Manubriosternal joint (sternal angle)
Body
of sternum
Xiphisternal joint
Xiphoid process
Costochondral joint
Costal cartilage
8th rib
8th intercostal space
10th rib
Costal margin
Body of 12th thoracic vertebra
Infrasternal angle

A. Anterior View

1.10 BONY THORAX

- The thoracic cage consists of 12 thoracic vertebrae, 12 pairs of ribs and costal cartilages, and the sternum.
- Anteriorly, the superior seven costal cartilages articulate with the sternum; the 8th, 9th, and 10th cartilages articulate with the cartilage above forming the costal margin; the 11th and 12th are "floating" ribs, that is, their cartilages do not articulate anteriorly.
- The clavicle lies over the 1st rib, making it difficult to palpate. The 2nd rib is easily palpable because its costal cartilage articulates with the sternum at the sternal angle, located at the junction of the manubrium and body of the sternum.
- The 3rd to 10th ribs can be palpated in sequence inferolaterally from the 2nd rib; the fused costal cartilages of the 7th to 10th ribs form the costal arch (margin), and the tips of the 11th and 12th ribs can be palpated posterolaterally.
- A **rib dislocation** is the displacement of a costal cartilage from the sternum; a **rib separation** refers to dislocation of the costochondral joint.

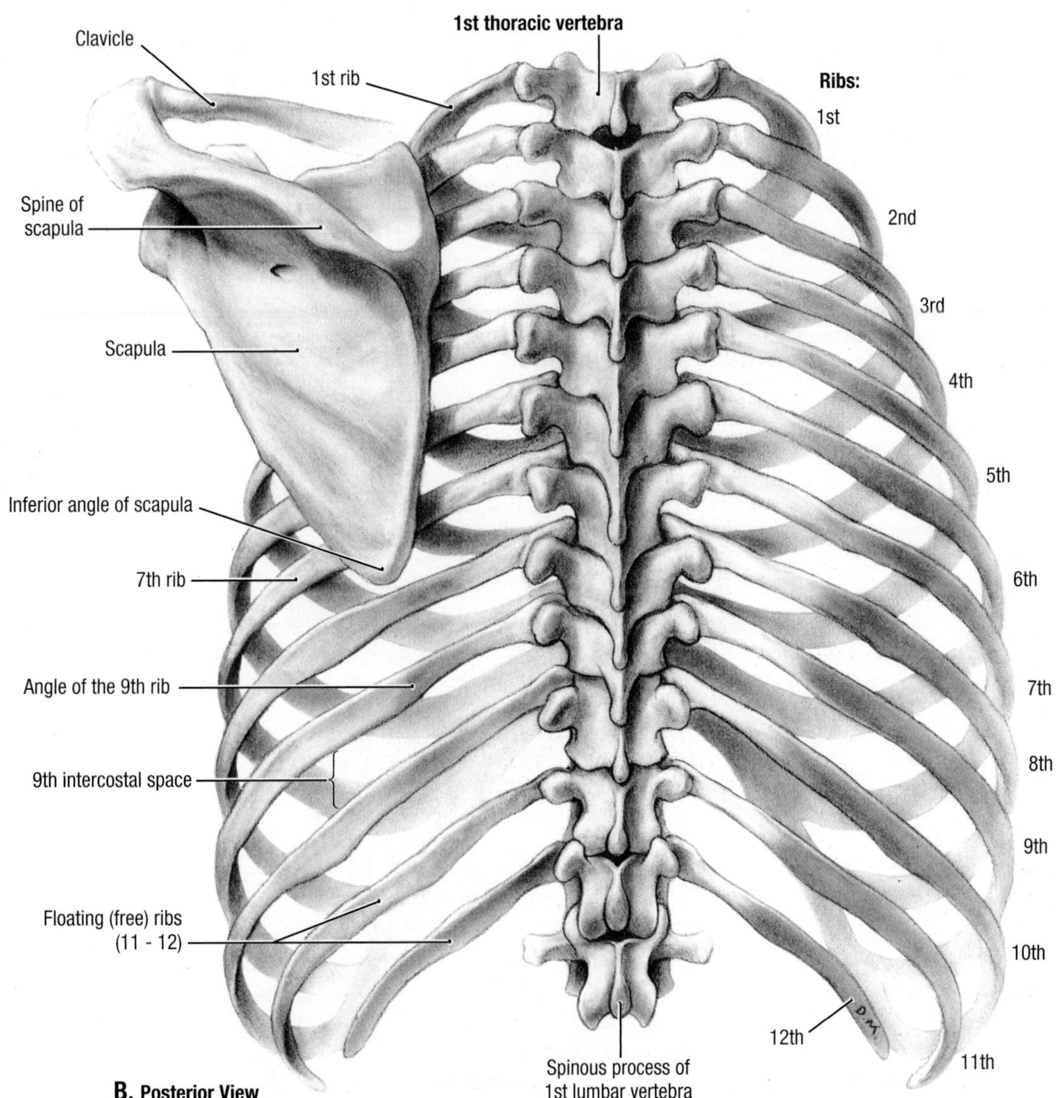
Clavicle
1st thoracic vertebra
1st rib
Ribs:
1st
Spine of scapula
2nd
3rd
Scapula
4th
5th
Inferior angle of scapula
6th
7th rib
Angle of the 9th rib
7th
9th intercostal space
8th
9th
Floating (free) ribs (11 - 12)
10th
12th
D.M.
11th
Spinous process of 1st lumbar vertebra

B. Posterior View

1.10 BONY THORAX (*CONTINUED*)

- The superior thoracic aperture (thoracic inlet) is the doorway between the thoracic cavity and the neck region; it is bounded by the 1st thoracic vertebra, the 1st ribs and their cartilages, and the manubrium of the sternum.
- Each rib articulates posteriorly with the vertebral column.
- Posteriorly, all ribs angle inferiorly; anteriorly, the 3rd to 10th costal cartilages angle superiorly.
- The scapula is suspended from the clavicle and extends across the 2nd to 7th ribs posteriorly.
- When clinicians refer to the superior thoracic aperture as the thoracic "outlet," they are emphasizing the important nerves and arteries that pass through this aperture into the lower neck and upper limb. Hence, various types of **thoracic outlet syndromes** exist, such as the costoclavicular syndrome—pallor and coldness of the **skin of the upper limb** and diminished radial pulse—resulting from compression of the subclavian artery between the clavicle and the 1st rib.

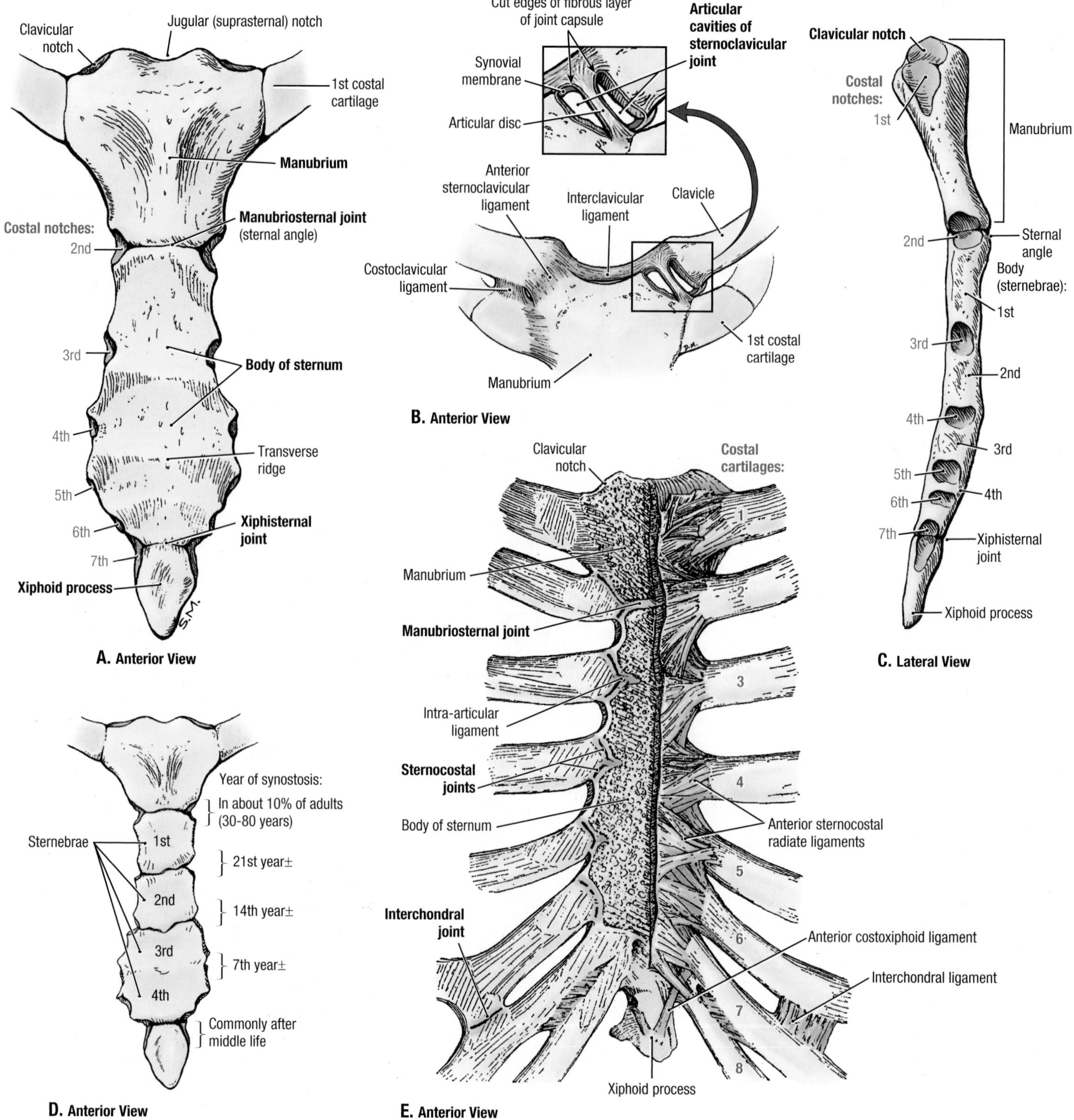
Clavicular notch
Jugular (suprasternal) notch
1st costal cartilage
Manubrium
Costal notches:
2nd
Manubriosternal joint (sternal angle)
3rd
Body of sternum
4th
Transverse ridge
5th
6th
Xiphisternal joint
7th
Xiphoid process
A. Anterior View
Cut edges of fibrous layer of joint capsule
Articular cavities of sternoclavicular joint
Synovial membrane
Articular disc
Anterior sternoclavicular ligament
Interclavicular ligament
Clavicle
Costoclavicular ligament
1st costal cartilage
Manubrium
B. Anterior View
Clavicular notch
Costal notches:
1st
Manubrium
2nd
Sternal angle
Body (sternebrae):
1st
3rd
2nd
4th
3rd
5th
4th
6th
7th
Xiphisternal joint
Xiphoid process
C. Lateral View
Year of synostosis:
In about 10% of adults (30-80 years)
Sternebrae
1st
21st year±
2nd
14th year±
3rd
7th year±
4th
Commonly after middle life
D. Anterior View
Clavicular notch
Costal cartilages:
1
Manubrium
2
Manubriosternal joint
3
Intra-articular ligament
Sternocostal joints
4
Body of sternum
Anterior sternocostal radiate ligaments
5
Interchondral joint
6
Anterior costoxiphoid ligament
Interchondral ligament
7
8
Xiphoid process
E. Anterior View

1.11 STERNUM AND ASSOCIATED JOINTS

A. Parts of sternum. **B.** Sternoclavicular joint. **C.** Features of the lateral aspect of the sternum. **D.** Ages of ossification of sternum. **E**. Sternocostal, manubriosternal, and interchondral joints. On the right side of the specimen, the cortex of the sternum and the external surface of the costal cartilages have been shaved away.

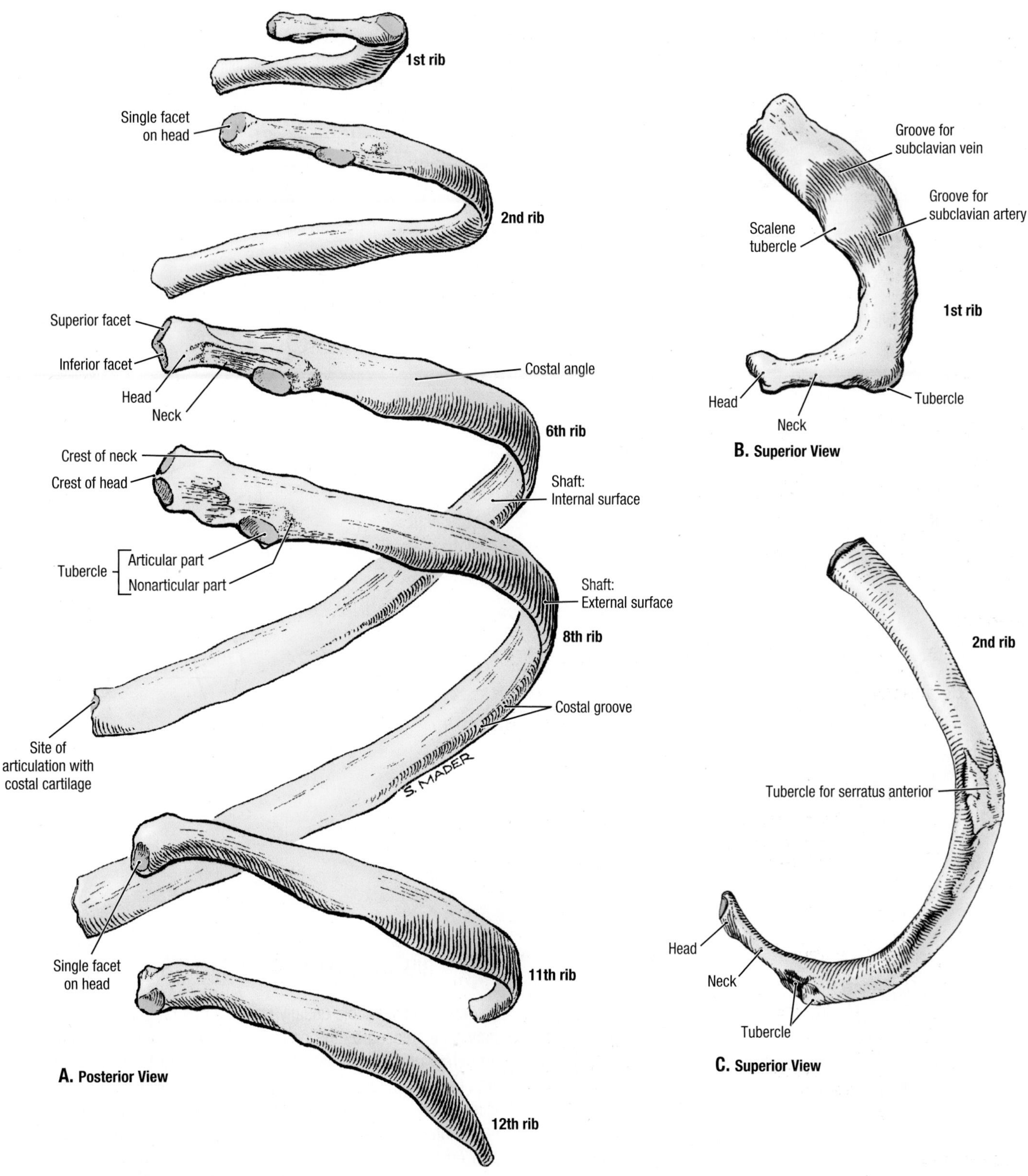
1st rib
Single facet on head
2nd rib
Superior facet
Inferior facet
Head
Neck
Costal angle
6th rib
Crest of neck
Crest of head
Shaft: Internal surface
Tubercle
Articular part
Nonarticular part
Shaft: External surface
8th rib
Costal groove
Site of articulation with costal cartilage
S. MADER
Single facet on head
11th rib
12th rib
A. Posterior View
Groove for subclavian vein
Groove for subclavian artery
Scalene tubercle
1st rib
Head
Neck
Tubercle
B. Superior View
2nd rib
Tubercle for serratus anterior
Head
Neck
Tubercle
C. Superior View

1.12 RIBS

A. "Typical" (6th and 8th) and "atypical" (1st and 2nd and 11th and 12th) ribs. **B.** First rib. **C.** Second rib.

Rib fractures. The weakest part of a rib is immediately anterior to its angle. The middle ribs are most commonly fractured.

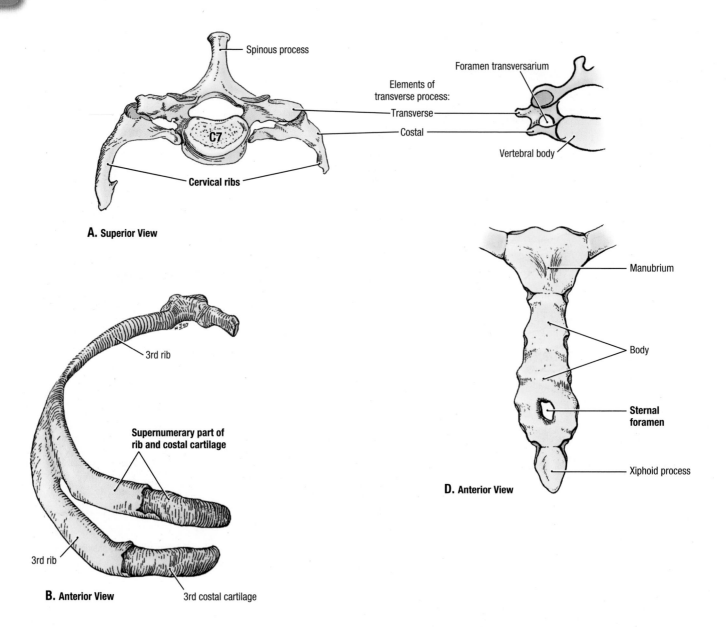

Spinous process
Foramen transversarium
Elements of transverse process:
Transverse
Costal
Vertebral body
C7
Cervical ribs

A. **Superior View**

Manubrium
Body
Sternal foramen
Xiphoid process

D. **Anterior View**

3rd rib
Supernumerary part of rib and costal cartilage
3rd rib
3rd costal cartilage

B. **Anterior View**

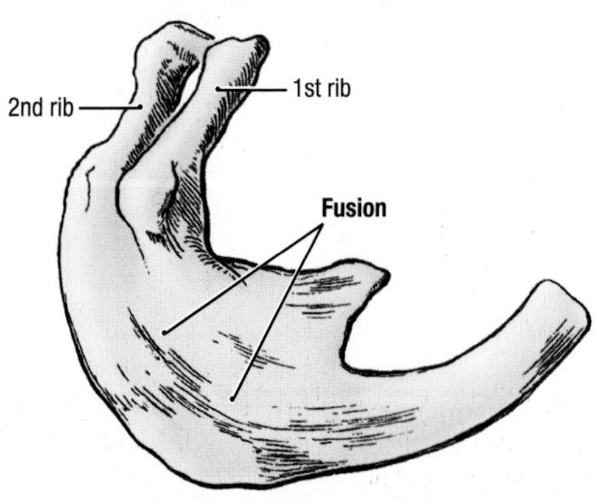
2nd rib
1st rib
Fusion

C. **Superior View**

1.13 RIB AND STERNUM ANOMALIES

A. Cervical ribs. People usually have 12 ribs on each side, but the number may be increased by the presence of cervical and/or lumbar ribs (supernumerary ribs) or decreased by a failure of the 12th pair to form. **Cervical ribs** (present in up to 1% of people) articulate with the C7 vertebra and are clinically significant because they may compress spinal nerves C8 and T1 or the inferior trunk of the brachial plexus supplying the upper limb. Tingling and numbness may occur along the medial border of the forearm. They may also compress the subclavian artery, resulting in **ischemic muscle pain** (caused by poor blood supply) in the upper limb. **Lumbar ribs** are less common than cervical ribs, but have clinical significance in that they may confuse the identity of vertebral levels in diagnostic images. **B.** Bifid rib. The superior component of this 3rd rib is supernumerary and articulated with the lateral aspect of the 1st sternebra. The inferior component articulated at the junction of the 1st and 2nd sternebrae. **C.** Bicipital rib. In this specimen, there has been partial fusion of the first two thoracic ribs. **D.** Sternal foramen.

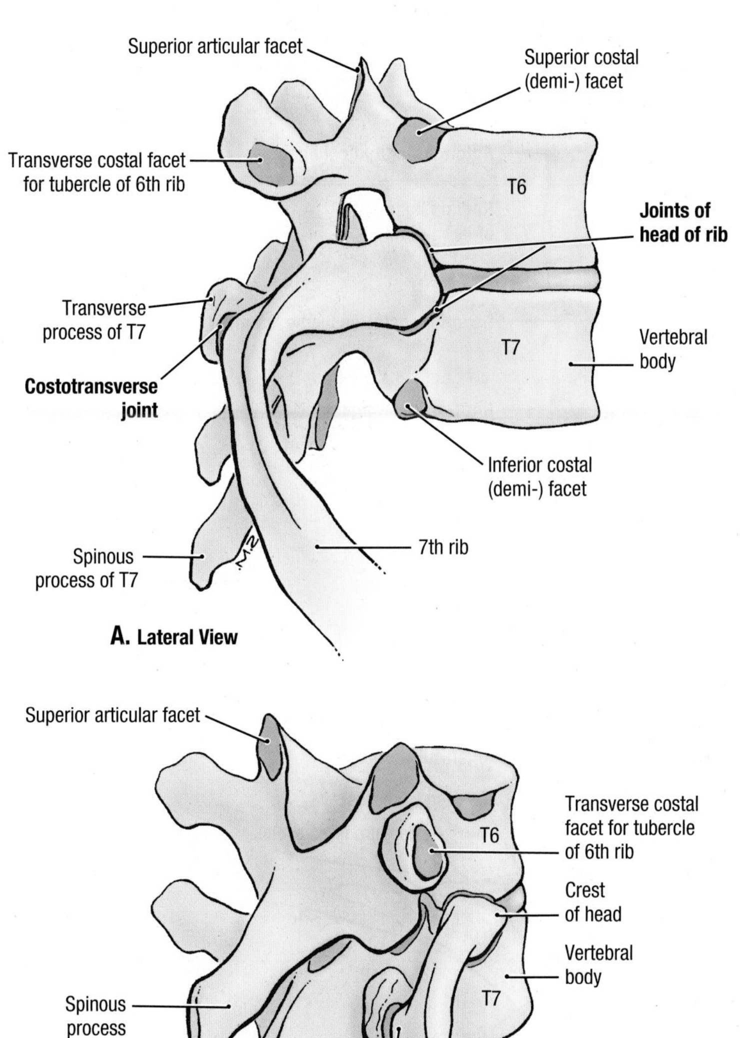
Superior articular facet
Superior costal (demi-) facet
Transverse costal facet for tubercle of 6th rib
T6
Joints of head of rib
Transverse process of T7
T7
Vertebral body
Costotransverse joint
Inferior costal (demi-) facet
Spinous process of T7
7th rib
Superior articular facet
Transverse costal facet for tubercle of 6th rib
T6
Crest of head
Vertebral body
Spinous process of T6
T7
7th rib
Tubercle of 7th rib

A. Lateral View

B. Posterolateral View

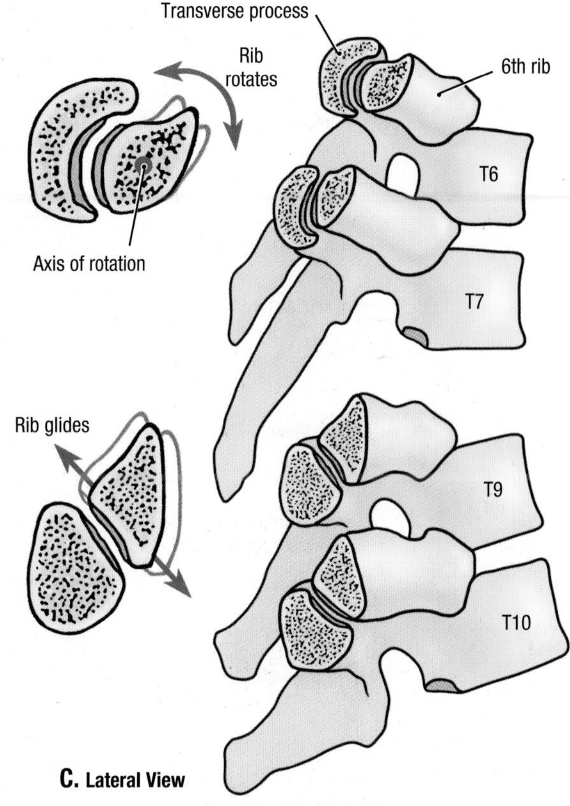
Transverse process
Rib rotates
6th rib
T6
Axis of rotation
T7
Rib glides
T9
T10

C. Lateral View

1.14 COSTOVERTEBRAL ARTICULATIONS

A. and B. Articulating structures.

- There are two articular facets on the head of the rib: a larger, inferior costal facet for articulation with the vertebral body of its own number, and a smaller, superior costal facet for articulation with the vertebral body of the vertebra superior to the rib.
- The crest of the head of the rib separates the superior and inferior costal facets.
- The smooth articular part of the tubercle of the rib, the transverse costal facet, articulates with the transverse process of the same numbered vertebra at the costotransverse joint.

C. Movements at the costotransverse joints. At the 1st to 7th costotransverse joints, the ribs rotate, increasing the anteroposterior diameter of the thorax; at the 8th, 9th, and 10th, they glide, increasing the transverse diameter of the upper abdomen.

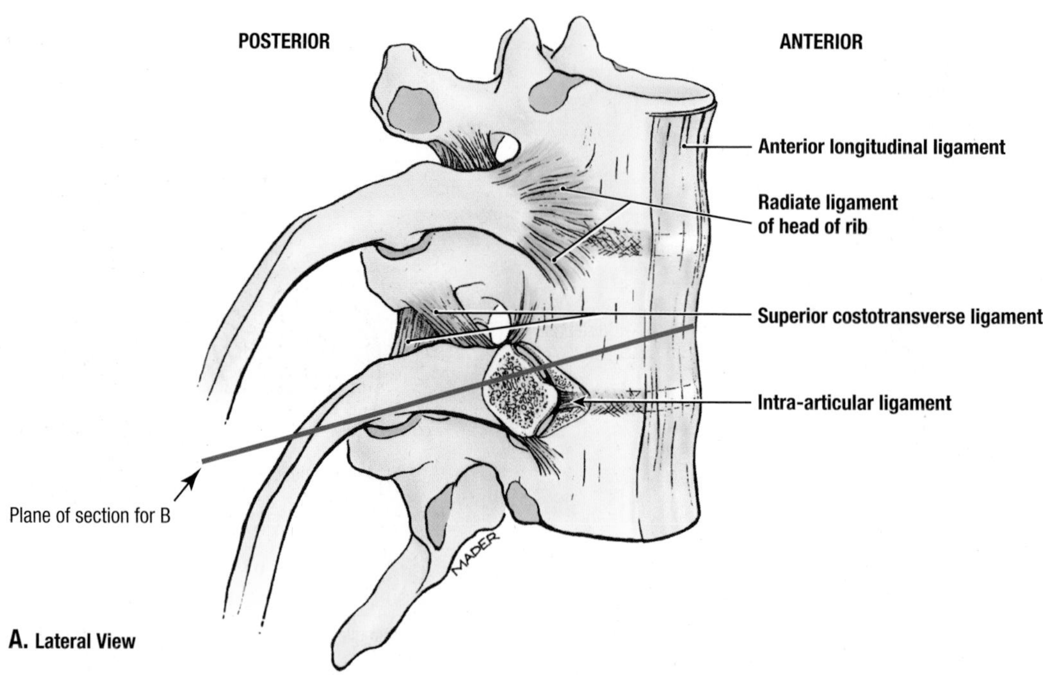
POSTERIOR
ANTERIOR
Anterior longitudinal ligament
Radiate ligament of head of rib
Superior costotransverse ligament
Intra-articular ligament
Plane of section for B
MADER
A. Lateral View

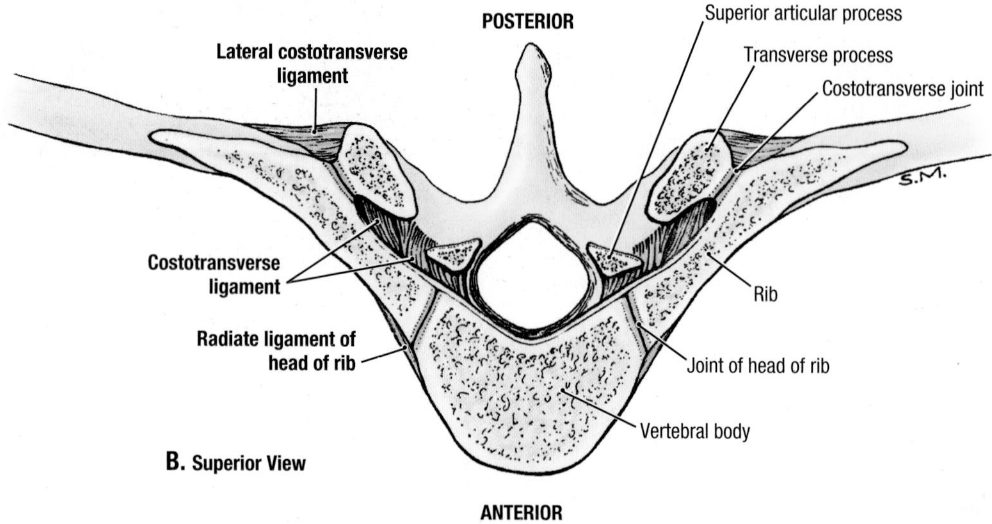
POSTERIOR
Superior articular process
Lateral costotransverse ligament
Transverse process
Costotransverse joint
S.M.
Costotransverse ligament
Rib
Radiate ligament of head of rib
Joint of head of rib
Vertebral body
B. Superior View
ANTERIOR

1.15 LIGAMENTS OF COSTOVERTEBRAL ARTICULATIONS

A. External and internal ligaments.

- The radiate ligament joins the head of the rib to two vertebral bodies and the interposed intervertebral disc.
- The superior costotransverse ligament joins the crest of the neck of the rib to the transverse process above.
- The intra-articular ligament joins the crest of the head of the rib to the intervertebral disc.

B. Transverse section.

- The vertebral body, transverse processes, superior articulating processes, and posterior elements of the articulating ribs have been transversely sectioned to visualize the joint surfaces and ligaments.
- The costotransverse ligament joins the posterior aspect of the neck of the rib to the adjacent transverse process.
- The lateral costotransverse ligament joins the nonarticulating part of the tubercle of the rib to the tip (apex) of the transverse process.

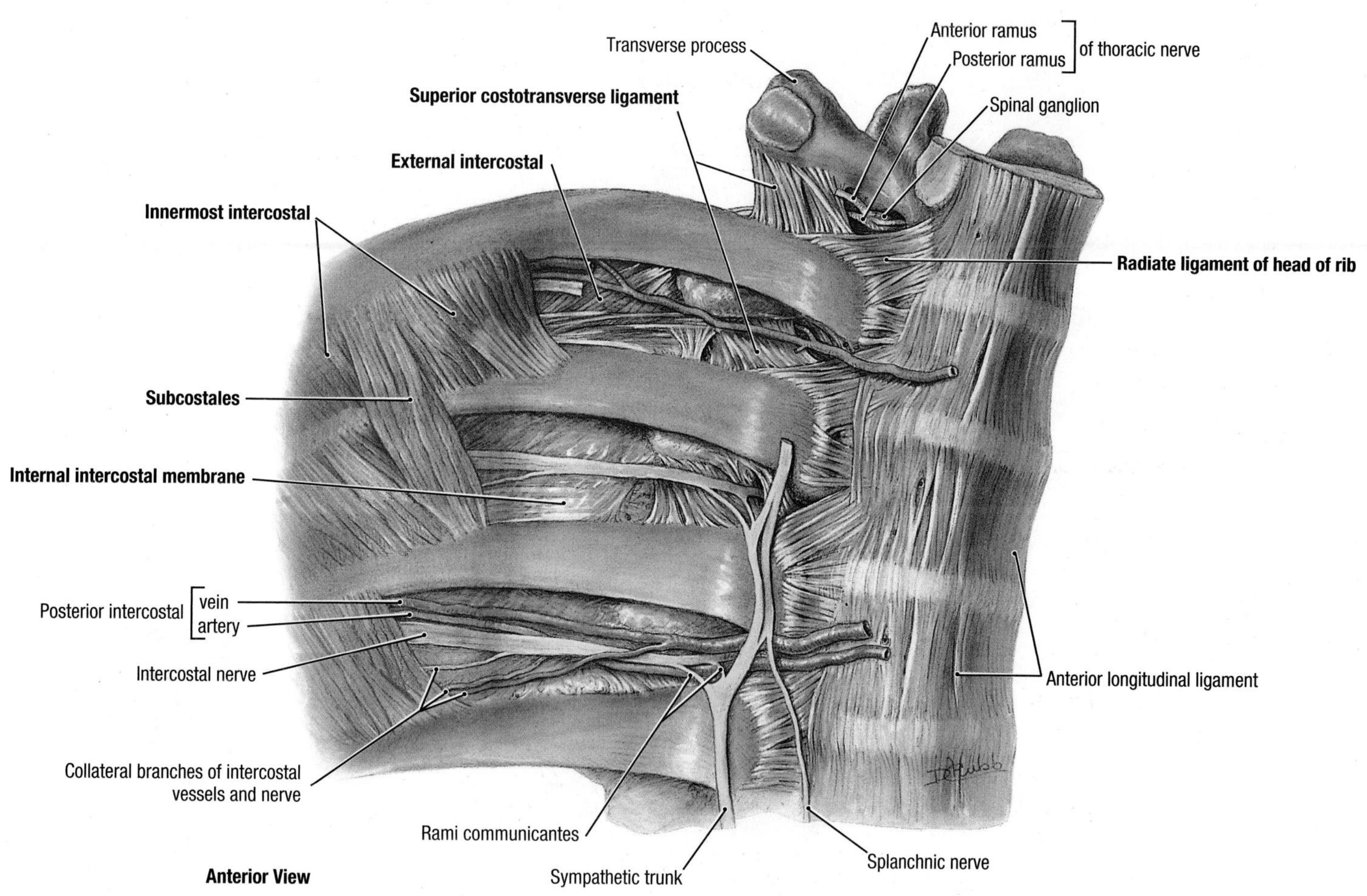
Transverse process
Anterior ramus
Posterior ramus
of thoracic nerve
Superior costotransverse ligament
Spinal ganglion
External intercostal
Innermost intercostal
Radiate ligament of head of rib
Subcostales
Internal intercostal membrane
Posterior intercostal
vein
artery
Intercostal nerve
Anterior longitudinal ligament
Collateral branches of intercostal vessels and nerve
Rami communicantes
Splanchnic nerve
Anterior View
Sympathetic trunk

1.16 VERTEBRAL ENDS OF INTERNAL ASPECT OF INTERCOSTAL SPACES

- Portions of the innermost intercostal muscle that bridge two intercostal spaces are called subcostales muscles.
- The internal intercostal membrane, in the middle space, is continuous medially with the superior costotransverse ligament.
- Note the order of the structures in the most inferior space: posterior intercostal vein and artery, and intercostal nerve; note also their collateral branches.
- The anterior ramus crosses anterior to the superior costotransverse ligament; the posterior ramus is posterior to it.
- The intercostal nerves attach to the sympathetic trunk by rami communicantes; the splanchnic nerve is a visceral branch of the trunk.

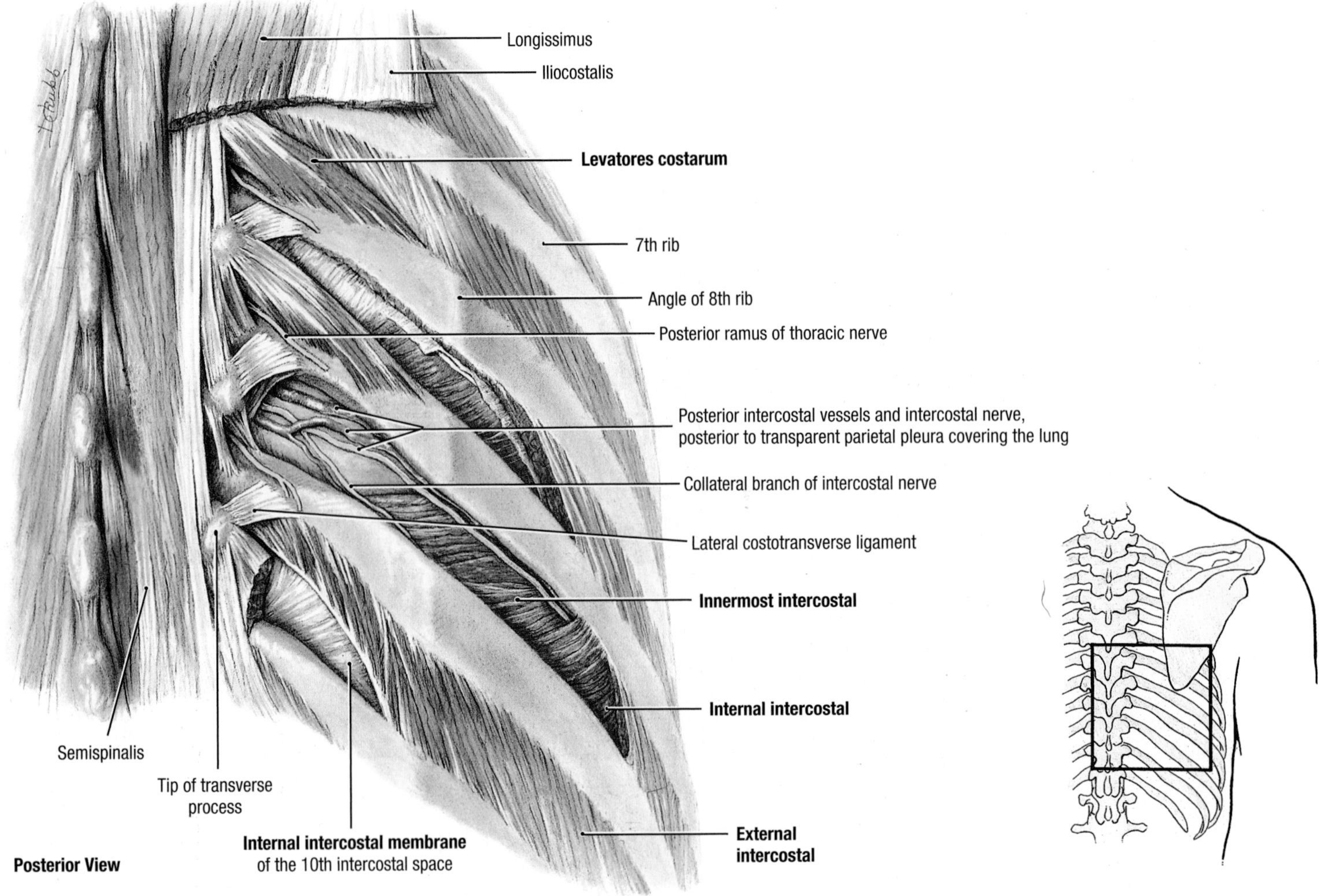

Longissimus
Iliocostalis
Levatores costarum
7th rib
Angle of 8th rib
Posterior ramus of thoracic nerve
Posterior intercostal vessels and intercostal nerve, posterior to transparent parietal pleura covering the lung
Collateral branch of intercostal nerve
Lateral costotransverse ligament
Innermost intercostal
Internal intercostal
Semispinalis
Tip of transverse process
Internal intercostal membrane of the 10th intercostal space
External intercostal
Posterior View

1.17 VERTEBRAL ENDS OF EXTERNAL ASPECT OF INFERIOR INTERCOSTAL SPACES

- The iliocostalis and longissimus muscles have been removed, exposing the levatores costarum muscle. Of the five intercostal spaces shown, the superior two (6th and 7th) are intact. In the 8th and 10th spaces, varying portions of the external intercostal muscle have been removed to reveal the underlying internal intercostal membrane, which is continuous with the internal intercostal muscle. In the 9th space, the levatores costarum muscle has been removed to show the posterior intercostal vessels and intercostal nerve.
- The intercostal vessels and nerve disappear laterally between the internal and innermost intercostal muscles.
- The intercostal nerve is the most inferior of the neurovascular trio (posterior intercostal vein and artery and intercostal nerve) and the least sheltered in the intercostal groove; a collateral branch arises near the angle of the rib.
- **Thoracocentesis.** Sometimes it is necessary to insert a hypodermic needle through an intercostal space into the pleural cavity (see Fig. 1.27) to obtain a sample of pleural fluid or to remove blood or pus. To avoid damage to the intercostal nerve and vessels, the needle is inserted superior to the rib, high enough to avoid the collateral branches.

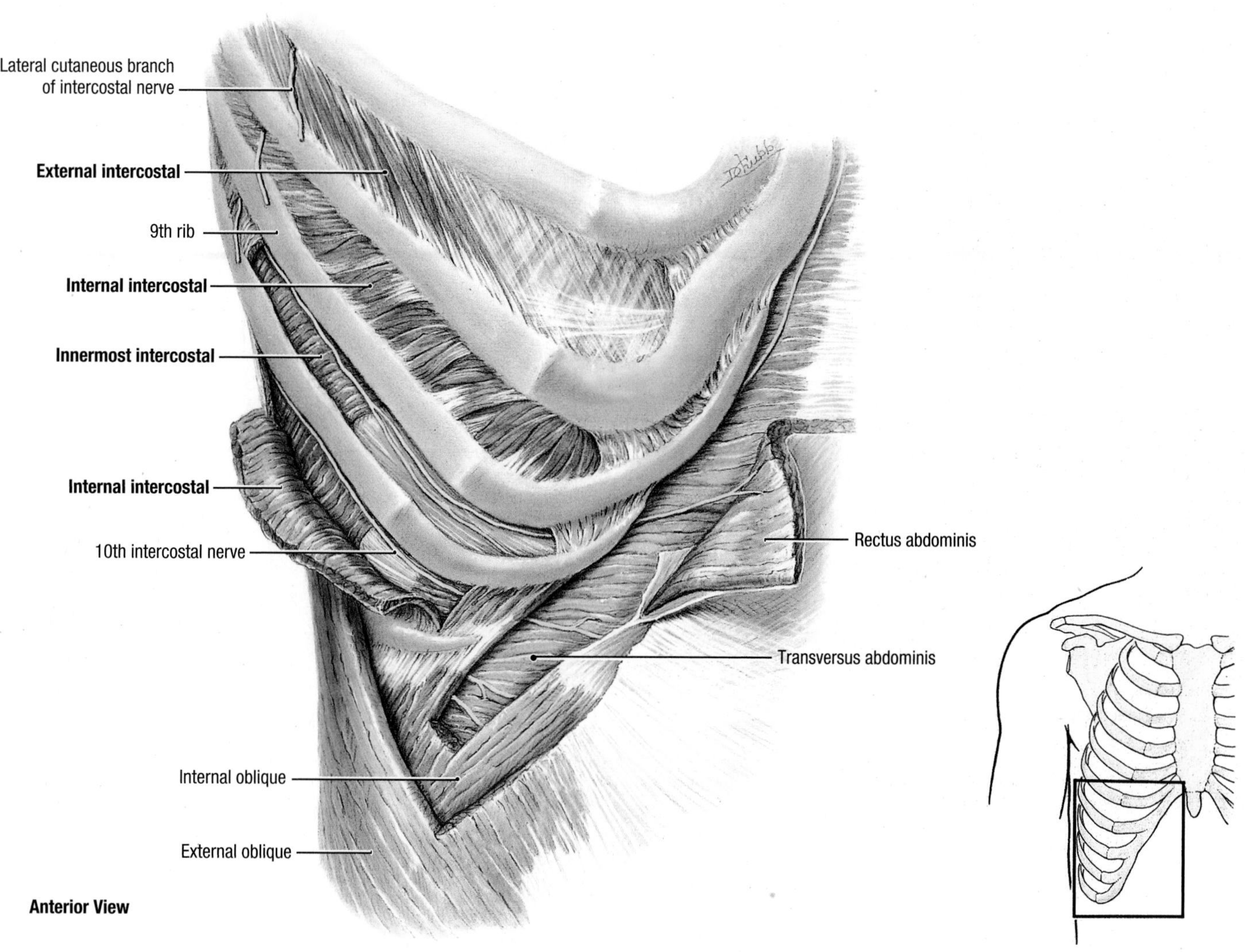
Lateral cutaneous branch of intercostal nerve
External intercostal
9th rib
Internal intercostal
Innermost intercostal
Internal intercostal
10th intercostal nerve
Rectus abdominis
Transversus abdominis
Internal oblique
External oblique
Anterior View

1.18 ANTERIOR ENDS OF INFERIOR INTERCOSTAL SPACES

- The fibers of the external intercostal and external oblique muscles run inferomedially.
- The internal intercostal and internal oblique muscles are in continuity at the ends of the 9th, 10th, and 11th intercostal spaces.
- The intercostal nerves lie deep to the internal intercostal muscle but superficial to the innermost intercostal muscle; anteriorly, these nerves lie superficial to the transversus thoracis or transversus abdominis muscles.
- Intercostal nerves run parallel to the ribs and costal cartilages; on reaching the abdominal wall, nerves T7 and T8 continue superiorly, T9 continues nearly horizontally, and T10 continues inferomedially toward the umbilicus. These nerves provide cutaneous innervation in overlapping segmental bands.

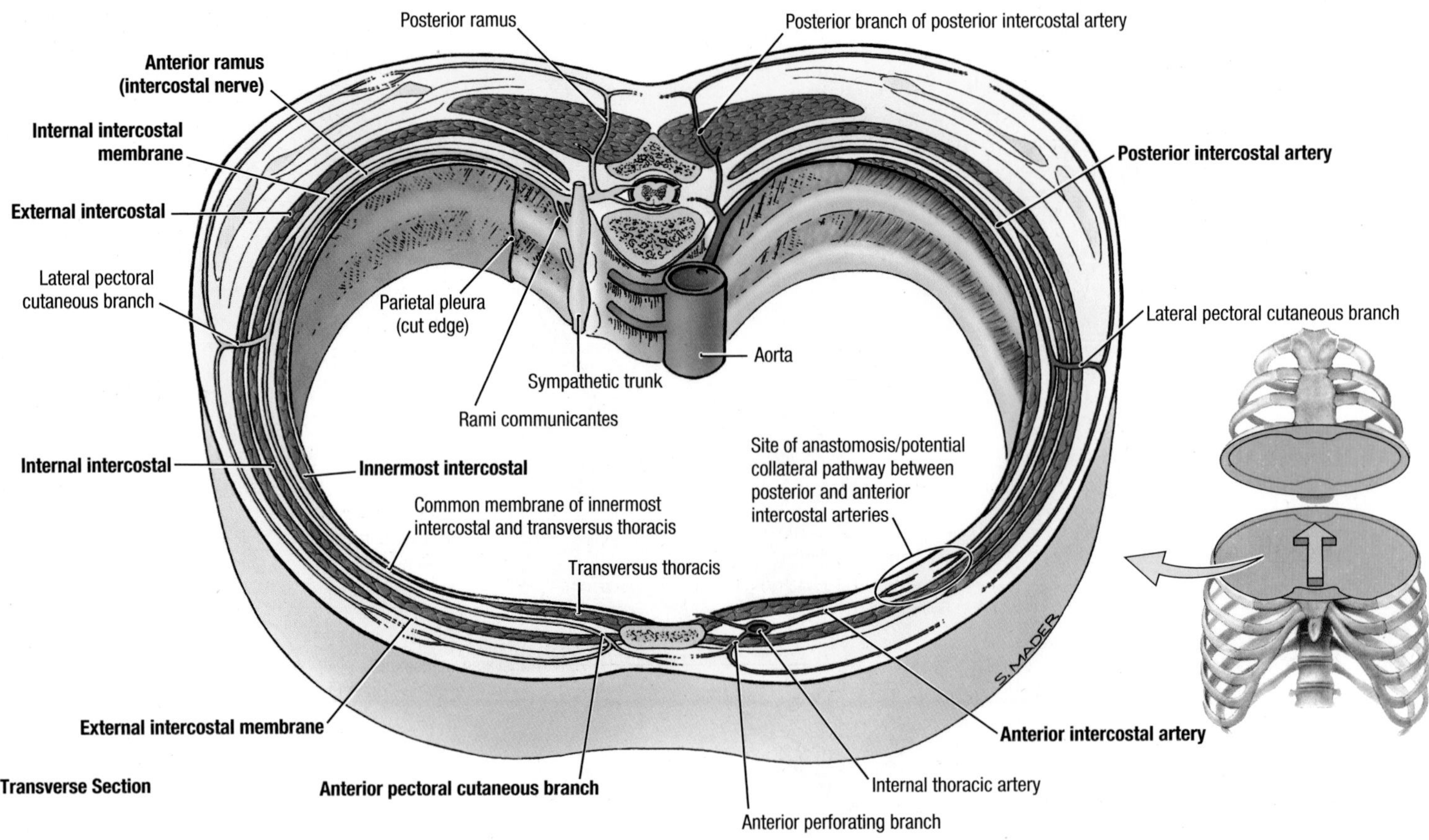
Posterior ramus
Posterior branch of posterior intercostal artery
Anterior ramus (intercostal nerve)
Internal intercostal membrane
Posterior intercostal artery
External intercostal
Lateral pectoral cutaneous branch
Parietal pleura (cut edge)
Lateral pectoral cutaneous branch
Aorta
Sympathetic trunk
Rami communicantes
Site of anastomosis/potential collateral pathway between posterior and anterior intercostal arteries
Internal intercostal
Innermost intercostal
Common membrane of innermost intercostal and transversus thoracis
Transversus thoracis
S. MADER
External intercostal membrane
Anterior intercostal artery
Transverse Section
Anterior pectoral cutaneous branch
Internal thoracic artery
Anterior perforating branch

1.19 CONTENTS OF INTERCOSTAL SPACE, TRANSVERSE SECTION

- The diagram is simplified by showing nerves on the right and arteries on the left.
- The three musculomembranous layers are the external intercostal muscle and membrane, internal intercostal muscle and membrane, and the innermost intercostal muscle, transversus thoracis muscle, and the membrane connecting them.
- The intercostal nerves are the anterior rami of spinal nerves T1 to T11; the anterior ramus of T12 is the subcostal nerve.
- Posterior intercostal arteries are branches of the aorta (the superior two spaces are supplied from the superior intercostal branch of the costocervical trunk); the anterior intercostal arteries are branches of the internal thoracic artery or its branch, the musculophrenic artery.
- The posterior rami innervate the deep back muscles and skin adjacent to the vertebral column.

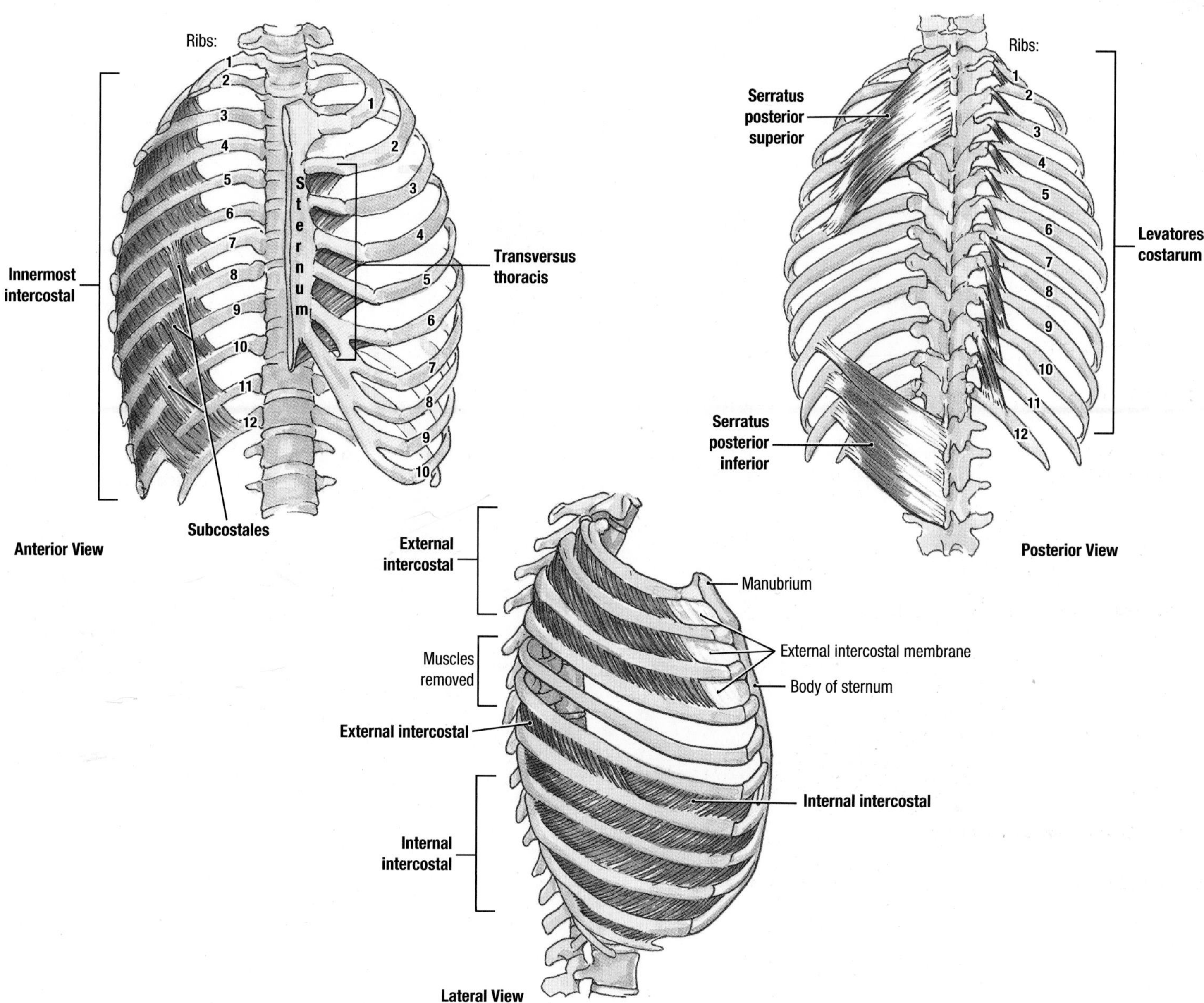
Ribs:
1
2
3
4
5
6
7
8
9
10
11
12
Innermost intercostal
Sternum
Transversus thoracis
Subcostales
Anterior View
Serratus posterior superior
Serratus posterior inferior
Levatores costarum
Posterior View
External intercostal
Muscles removed
External intercostal
Internal intercostal
Manubrium
External intercostal membrane
Body of sternum
Internal intercostal
Lateral View

1.20 MUSCLES OF THORACIC WALL

TABLE 1.1 MUSCLES OF THORACIC WALL

Muscle	Superior Attachment	Inferior Attachment	Innervation	Action[a]
External intercostal	Inferior border of ribs	Superior border of rib below	Intercostal nerve	Elevate ribs
Internal intercostal				Depress ribs
Innermost intercostal				Probably elevate ribs
Transversus thoracis	Posterior surface of lower sternum	Internal surface of costal cartilages 2–6		Depress ribs
Subcostales	Internal surface of lower ribs near their angles	Superior borders of 2nd or 3rd ribs below		
Levatores costarum	Transverse processes of C7–T11	Subjacent ribs between tubercle and angle	Posterior rami of C8–T11 nerves	Elevate ribs
Serratus posterior superior	Nuchal ligament, spinous processes of C7–T3	Superior borders of 2nd–4th ribs	Second to fifth intercostal nerves	Depress ribs
Serratus posterior inferior	Spinous processes of T11–L2	Inferior borders of 8th–12th ribs near their angles	Anterior rami of T9–T12 nerves	

[a]The tonus of all intercostal muscles keep intercostal spaces rigid, thereby preventing them from bulging out during expiration and from being drawn in during inspiration. Role of individual intercostal muscles and accessory muscles of respiration in moving the ribs is difficult to interpret despite many electromyographic studies. The role of the respiratory muscles depends on which accessory muscles are contracting at the same time.

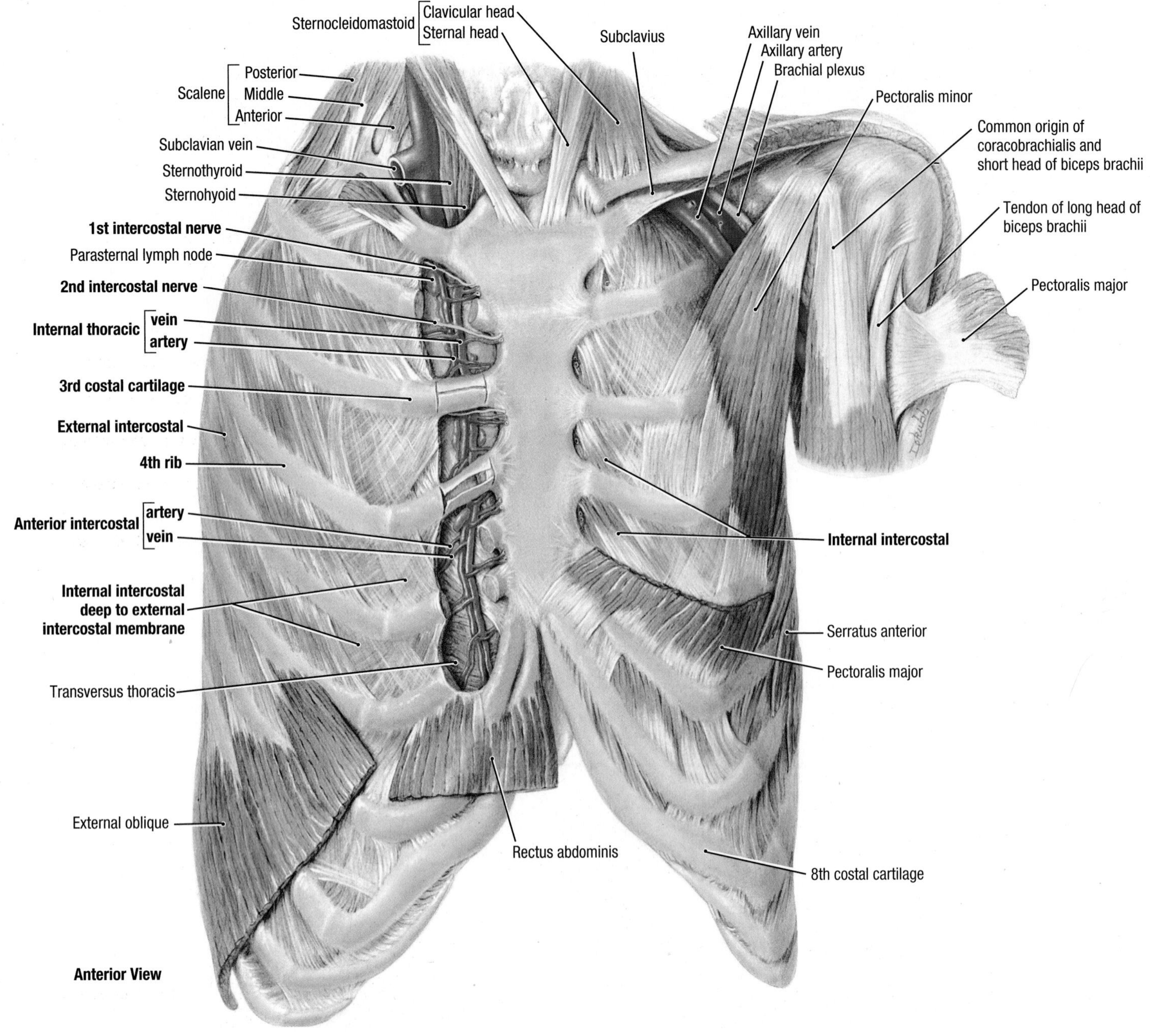
Sternocleidomastoid
Clavicular head
Sternal head
Subclavius
Axillary vein
Axillary artery
Brachial plexus
Pectoralis minor
Common origin of coracobrachialis and short head of biceps brachii
Tendon of long head of biceps brachii
Pectoralis major
Scalene
Posterior
Middle
Anterior
Subclavian vein
Sternothyroid
Sternohyoid
1st intercostal nerve
Parasternal lymph node
2nd intercostal nerve
Internal thoracic
vein
artery
3rd costal cartilage
External intercostal
4th rib
Anterior intercostal
artery
vein
Internal intercostal
Internal intercostal deep to external intercostal membrane
Serratus anterior
Pectoralis major
Transversus thoracis
External oblique
Rectus abdominis
8th costal cartilage
Anterior View

1.21 EXTERNAL ASPECT OF THORACIC WALL

- H-shaped cuts were made through the perichondrium of the 3rd and 4th costal cartilages to shell out segments of cartilage. During surgery, retaining perichondrium promotes regrowth of removed cartilages.
- The internal thoracic (internal mammary) vessels run inferiorly deep to the costal cartilages and just lateral to the edge of the sternum, providing anterior intercostal branches.
- The parasternal lymph nodes (*green*) receive lymphatic vessels from the anterior parts of intercostal spaces, the costal pleura and diaphragm, and the medial part of the breast.
- The subclavian vessels are "sandwiched" between the 1st rib and clavicle and are "padded" by the subclavius.
- **Surgical access to thorax**. To gain access to the thoracic cavity for surgical procedures, the sternum is divided in the median plane (median sternotomy) and retracted (spread apart). After surgery, the halves of the sternum are held together with wire structures.

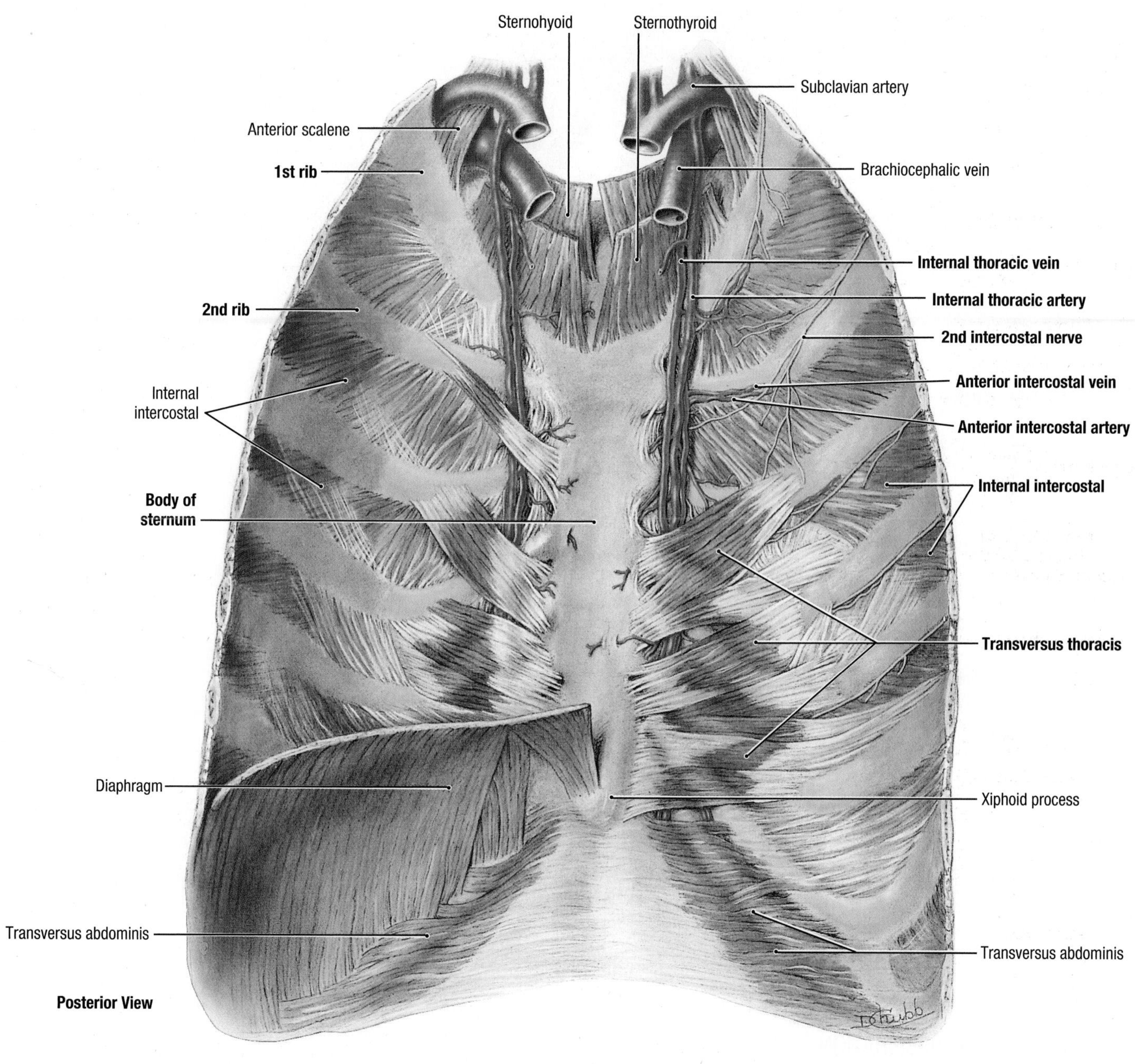
Sternohyoid
Sternothyroid
Subclavian artery
Anterior scalene
1st rib
Brachiocephalic vein
Internal thoracic vein
Internal thoracic artery
2nd rib
2nd intercostal nerve
Anterior intercostal vein
Internal intercostal
Anterior intercostal artery
Internal intercostal
Body of sternum
Transversus thoracis
Diaphragm
Xiphoid process
Transversus abdominis
Transversus abdominis
Posterior View

1.22 INTERNAL ASPECT OF THE ANTERIOR THORACIC WALL

- The inferior portions of the internal thoracic vessels are covered posteriorly by the transversus thoracis muscle; the superior portions are in contact with the parietal pleura (removed).
- The transversus thoracis muscle (superior to diaphragm) is continuous with the transversus abdominis muscle (inferior to diaphragm); these form the innermost layer of the three flat muscles of the thoracoabdominal wall.
- The internal thoracic (internal mammary) artery arises from the subclavian artery and is accompanied by two venae comitantes up to the 2nd costal cartilage in this specimen and, superior to this, by the single internal thoracic vein, which drains into the brachiocephalic vein.

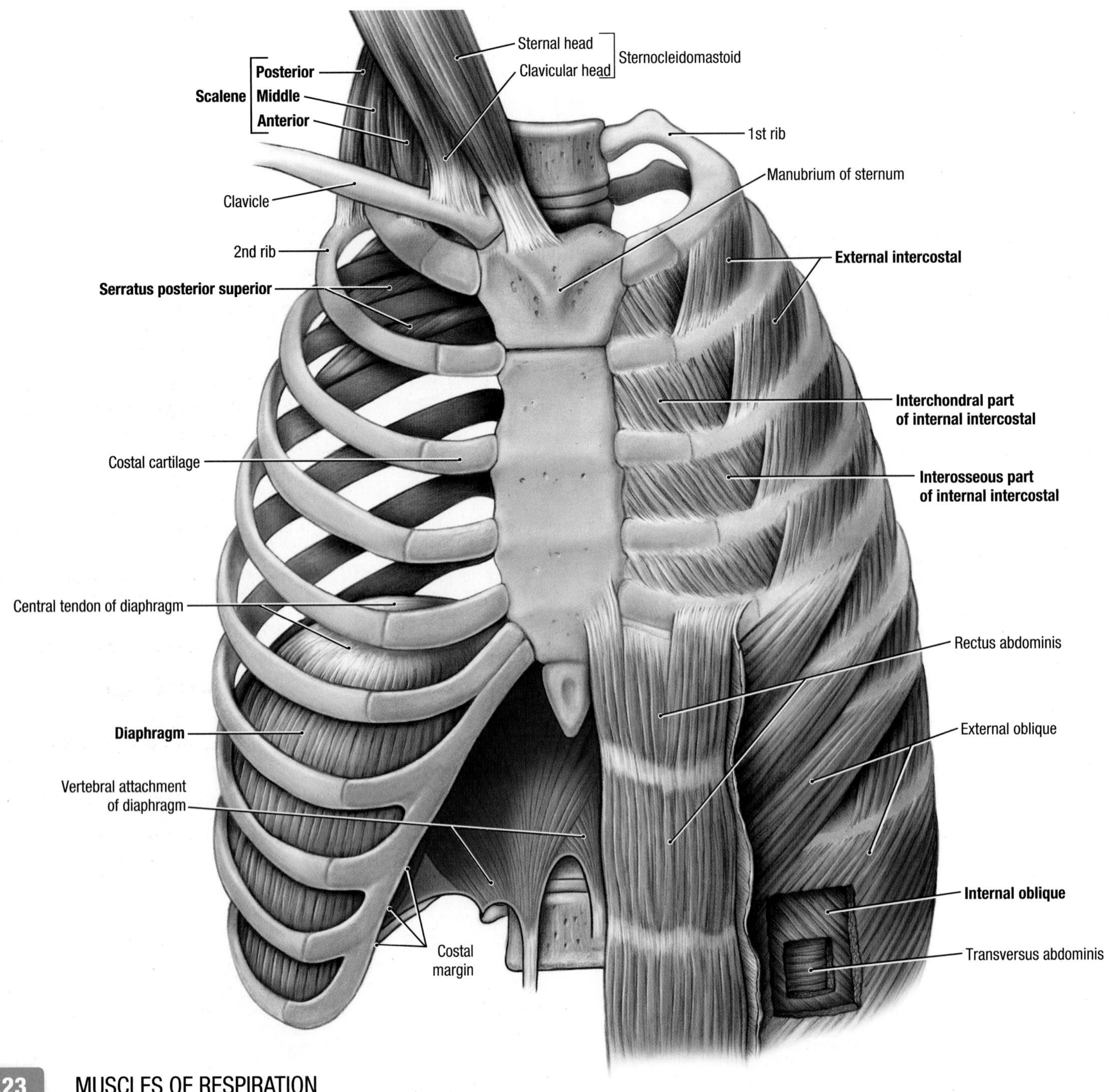

Sternal head
Clavicular head
Sternocleidomastoid
Scalene
Posterior
Middle
Anterior
1st rib
Manubrium of sternum
Clavicle
2nd rib
External intercostal
Serratus posterior superior
Interchondral part of internal intercostal
Costal cartilage
Interosseous part of internal intercostal
Central tendon of diaphragm
Rectus abdominis
Diaphragm
External oblique
Vertebral attachment of diaphragm
Internal oblique
Costal margin
Transversus abdominis

1.23 MUSCLES OF RESPIRATION

TABLE 1.2 MUSCLES OF RESPIRATION

Inspiration			Expiration
Normal (Quiet)	Major	Diaphragm (Active Contraction)	Passive (Elastic) Recoil of Lungs and Thoracic Cage
	Minor	*Tonic contraction* of external intercostals and interchondral portion of internal intercostals to resist negative pressure	*Tonic contraction* of muscles of anterolateral abdominal walls (rectus abdominis, external and internal obliques, transversus abdominis) to antagonize diaphragm by maintaining intra-abdominal pressure
Active (Forced)		In addition to the above, *active contraction* of sternocleidomastoid, descending (superior) trapezius, pectoralis minor, and scalenes, to elevate and fix upper rib cage	In addition to the above, *active contraction* of muscles of anterolateral abdominal wall (antagonizing diaphragm by increasing intra-abdominal pressure and by pulling inferiorly and fixing inferior costal margin): rectus abdominis, external and internal obliques, and transversus abdominis
		External intercostals, interchondral portion of internal intercostals, subcostales, levatores costarum, and serratus posterior superior[a] to elevate ribs	Internal intercostal (interosseous part) and serratus posterior inferior[a] to depress ribs

[a]Recent studies indicate that the serratus posterior superior and inferior muscles may serve primarily as organs of proprioception rather than motion.

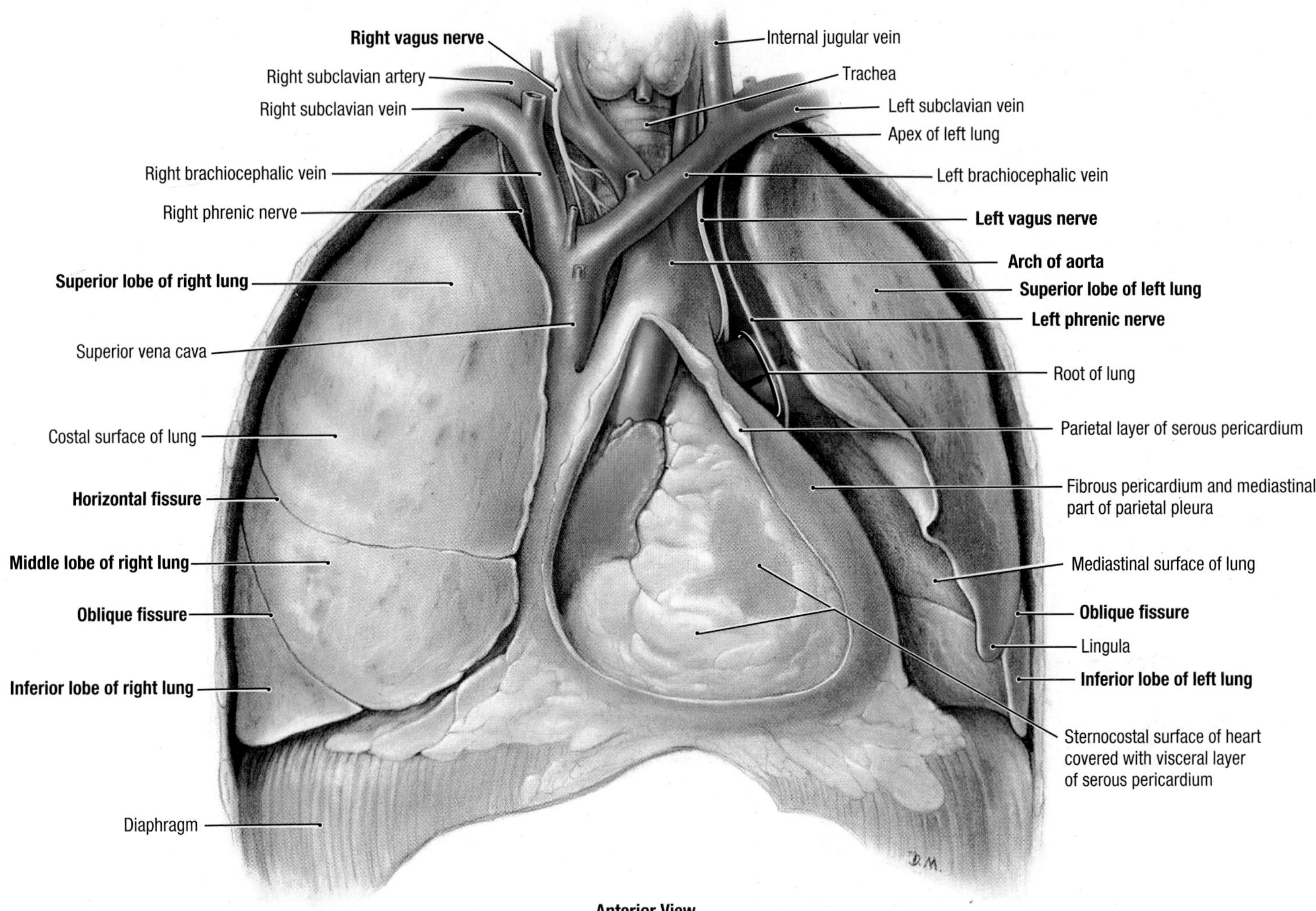
Right vagus nerve
Right subclavian artery
Right subclavian vein
Right brachiocephalic vein
Right phrenic nerve
Superior lobe of right lung
Superior vena cava
Costal surface of lung
Horizontal fissure
Middle lobe of right lung
Oblique fissure
Inferior lobe of right lung
Diaphragm
Internal jugular vein
Trachea
Left subclavian vein
Apex of left lung
Left brachiocephalic vein
Left vagus nerve
Arch of aorta
Superior lobe of left lung
Left phrenic nerve
Root of lung
Parietal layer of serous pericardium
Fibrous pericardium and mediastinal part of parietal pleura
Mediastinal surface of lung
Oblique fissure
Lingula
Inferior lobe of left lung
Sternocostal surface of heart covered with visceral layer of serous pericardium
D.M.

Anterior View

1.24 THORACIC CONTENTS IN SITU

- The fibrous pericardium, lined by the parietal layer of serous pericardium, is removed anteriorly to expose the heart and great vessels.
- The right lung has three lobes; the superior lobe is separated from the middle lobe by the horizontal fissure, and the middle lobe is separated from the inferior lobe by the oblique fissure. The left lung has two lobes, superior and inferior, separated by the oblique fissure.
- The anterior border of the left lung is reflected laterally to visualize the phrenic nerve passing anterior to the root of the lung and the vagus nerve lying anterior to the arch of the aorta and then passing posterior to the root of the lung.
- As the right vagus nerve passes anterior to the right subclavian artery, it gives rise to the recurrent branch and then divides to contribute fibers to the esophageal, cardiac, and pulmonary plexuses.

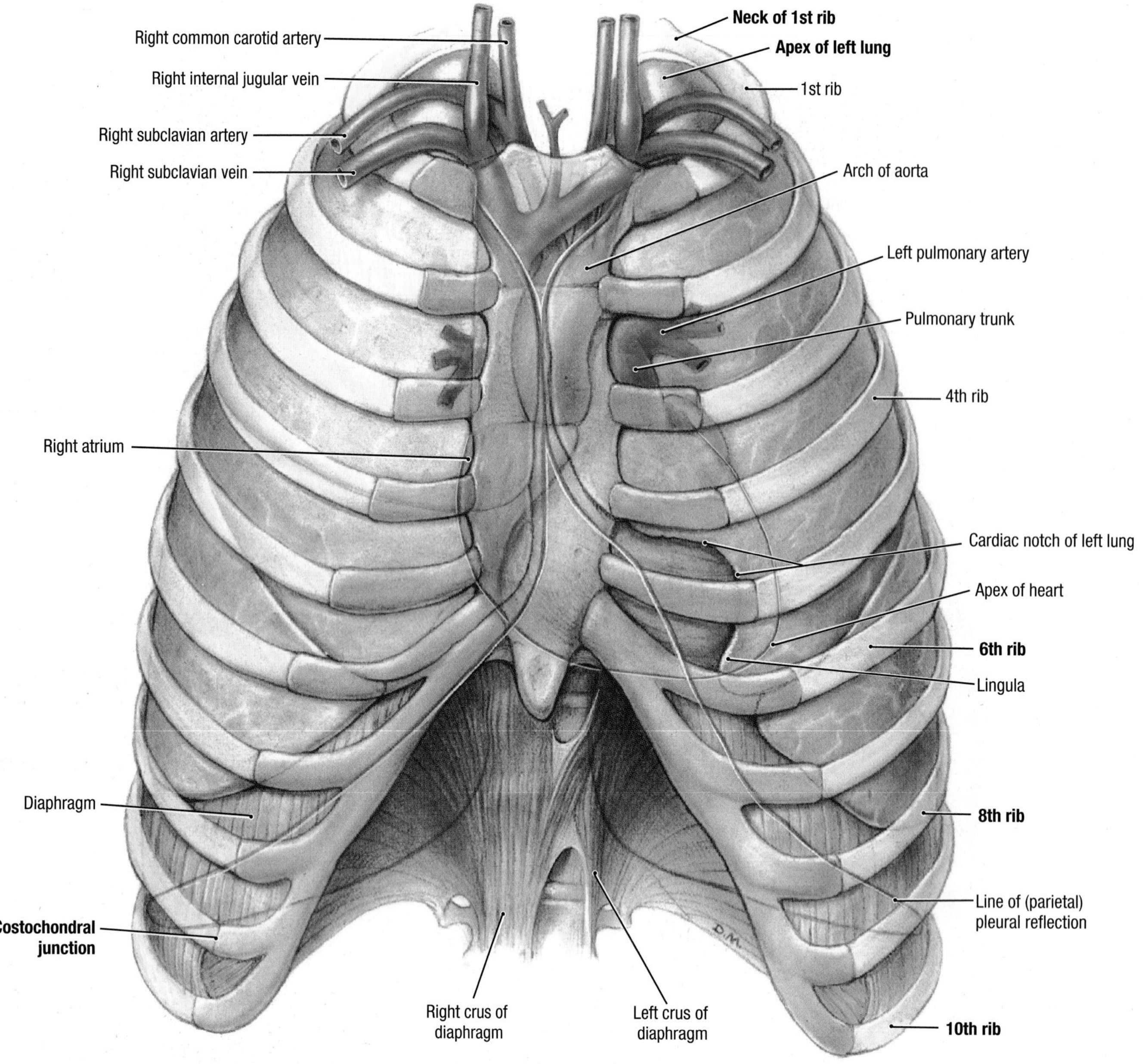

Right common carotid artery
Right internal jugular vein
Right subclavian artery
Right subclavian vein
Right atrium
Diaphragm
Costochondral junction
Right crus of diaphragm
Left crus of diaphragm
Neck of 1st rib
Apex of left lung
1st rib
Arch of aorta
Left pulmonary artery
Pulmonary trunk
4th rib
Cardiac notch of left lung
Apex of heart
6th rib
Lingula
8th rib
Line of (parietal) pleural reflection
10th rib
D.M.

1.25 TOPOGRAPHY OF THE LUNGS AND MEDIASTINUM

- The mediastinum is located between the pleural cavities and is occupied by the heart and the tissues anterior, posterior, and superior to the heart.
- The apex of the lungs is at the level of the neck of the 1st rib, and the inferior border of the lungs is at the 6th rib in the left midclavicular line and the 8th rib at the lateral aspect of the bony thorax at the midaxillary line.
- The cardiac notch of the left lung and the corresponding deviation of the parietal pleura are away from the median plane toward the left side.
- The inferior reflection of parietal pleura is at the 8th costochondral junction in the midclavicular line, at the 10th rib in the midaxillary line.
- The apex of the heart is in the 5th intercostal space at the left midclavicular line.
- The right atrium forms the right border of the heart and extends just beyond the lateral margin of the sternum.
- The branches of the great vessels pass through the superior thoracic aperture.

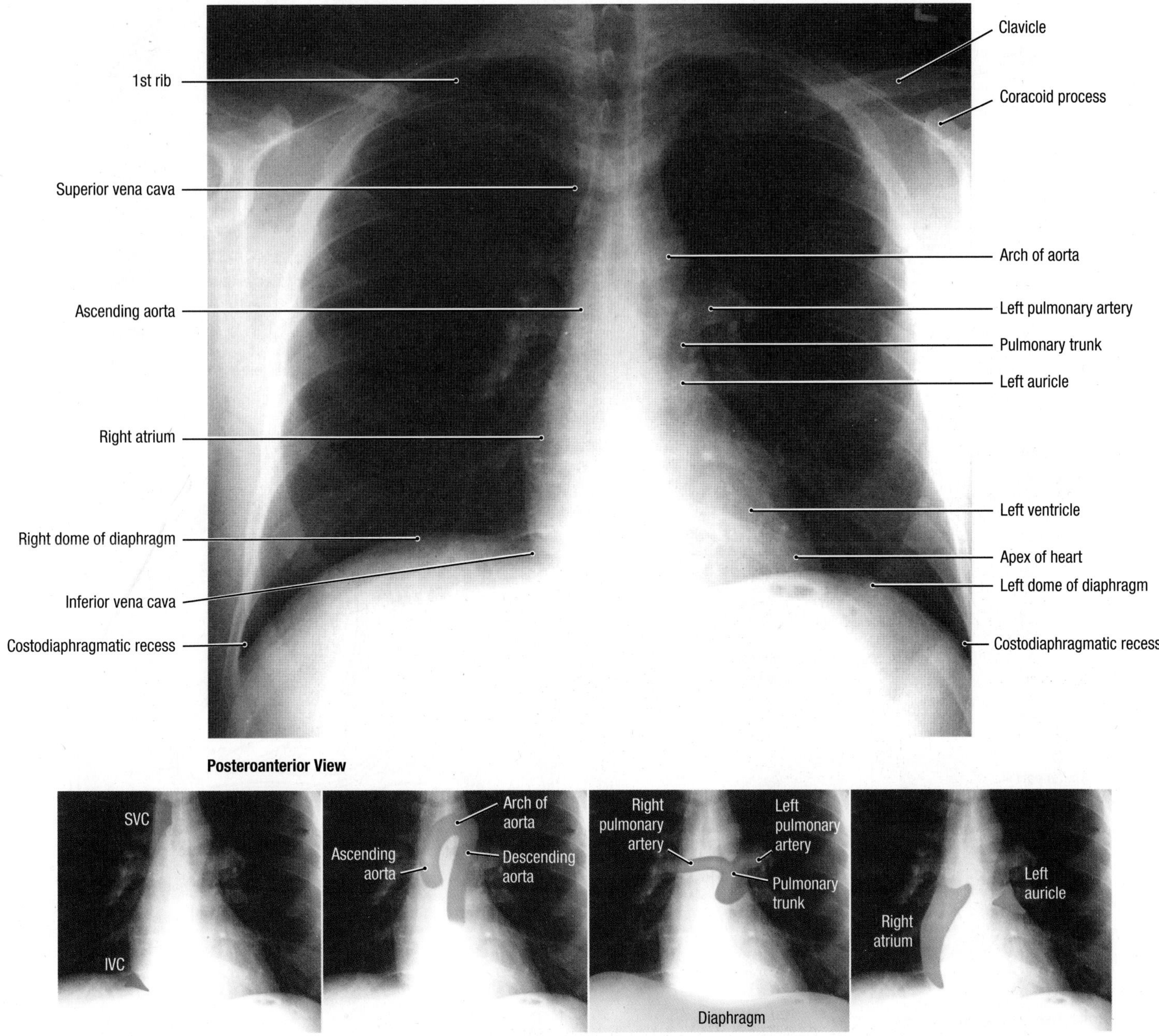
1st rib
Superior vena cava
Ascending aorta
Right atrium
Right dome of diaphragm
Inferior vena cava
Costodiaphragmatic recess
Clavicle
Coracoid process
Arch of aorta
Left pulmonary artery
Pulmonary trunk
Left auricle
Left ventricle
Apex of heart
Left dome of diaphragm
Costodiaphragmatic recess
Posteroanterior View
SVC
IVC
Arch of aorta
Ascending aorta
Descending aorta
Right pulmonary artery
Left pulmonary artery
Pulmonary trunk
Diaphragm
Left auricle
Right atrium

1.26 RADIOGRAPH OF CHEST

- The right dome of the diaphragm is higher than the left dome due primarily to the large underlying liver.
- The convex right mediastinal border of the heart is formed by the right atrium; above this, the superior vena cava and ascending aorta produce less convex borders.
- The left border of the mediastinal silhouette is formed by the arch of the aorta, pulmonary trunk, left auricle (normally not prominent), and left ventricle.
- Follow the 1st rib to where it curves laterally and then medially to cross inferior to the clavicle.
- Any structure in the mediastinum may contribute to **pathological widening of the mediastinal silhouette**, e.g., after trauma that produces hemorrhage into the mediastinum, malignant lymphoma (cancer of lymphatic tissue) that produces massive enlargement of mediastinal lymph nodes, or enlargement (hypertrophy) of the heart occurring with congestive heart failure.

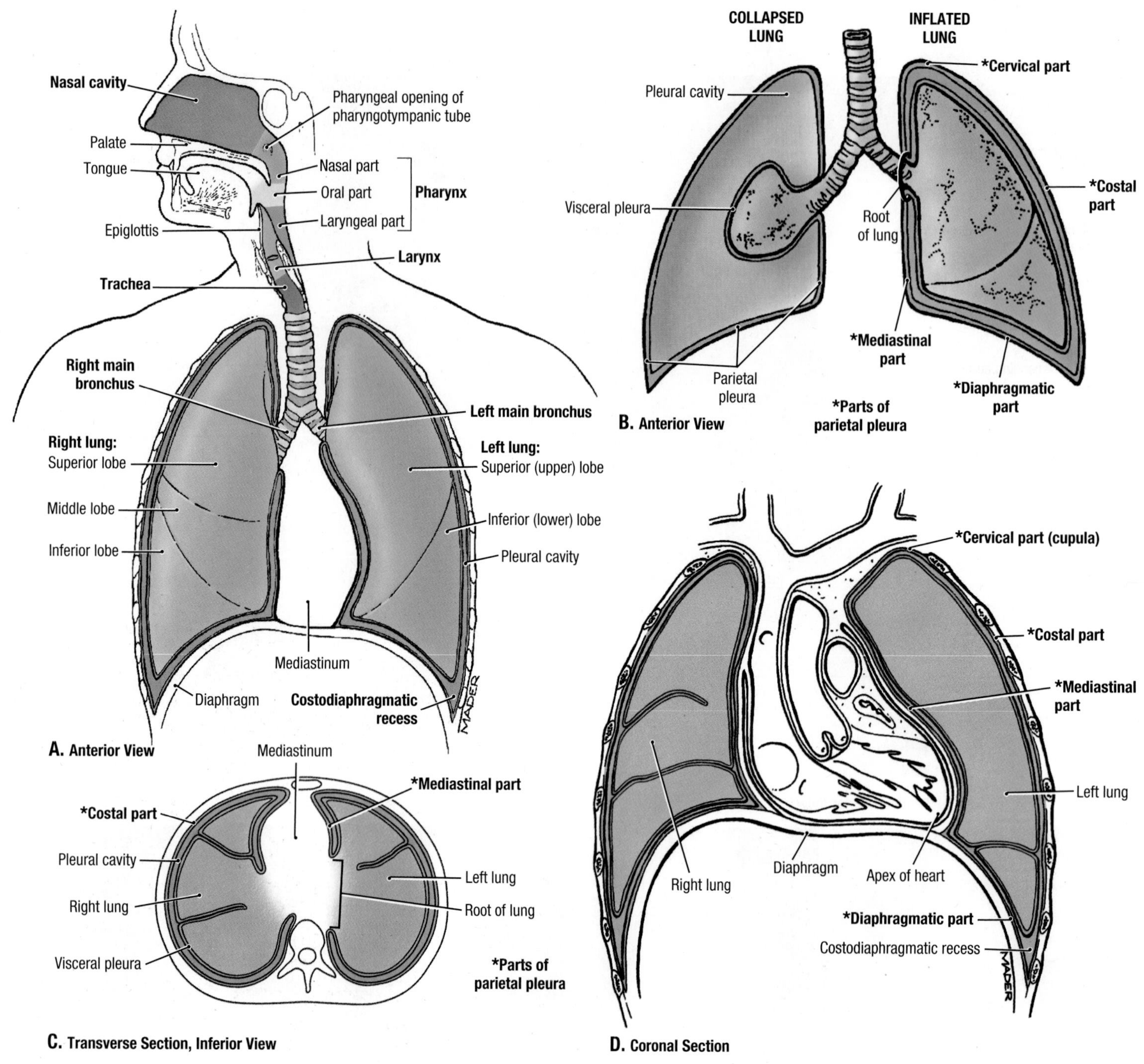
Nasal cavity
Palate
Tongue
Pharyngeal opening of pharyngotympanic tube
Nasal part
Oral part
Laryngeal part
Pharynx
Epiglottis
Larynx
Trachea
Right main bronchus
Left main bronchus
Right lung:
Superior lobe
Middle lobe
Inferior lobe
Left lung:
Superior (upper) lobe
Inferior (lower) lobe
Pleural cavity
Mediastinum
Diaphragm
Costodiaphragmatic recess
MADER
A. Anterior View
COLLAPSED LUNG
INFLATED LUNG
*Cervical part
Pleural cavity
Visceral pleura
Root of lung
*Costal part
*Mediastinal part
Parietal pleura
*Diaphragmatic part
B. Anterior View
*Parts of parietal pleura
Mediastinum
*Mediastinal part
*Costal part
Pleural cavity
Right lung
Left lung
Root of lung
Visceral pleura
*Parts of parietal pleura
C. Transverse Section, Inferior View
*Cervical part (cupula)
*Costal part
*Mediastinal part
Left lung
Right lung
Diaphragm
Apex of heart
*Diaphragmatic part
Costodiaphragmatic recess
MADER
D. Coronal Section

1.27 RESPIRATORY SYSTEM

A. Overview. **B.** Pleural cavity and pleura. **C.** Transverse section. **D**. Coronal section through heart and lungs.

- The lungs invaginate a continuous membranous pleural sac; the visceral (pulmonary) pleura covers the lungs, and the parietal pleura lines the thoracic cavity; the visceral and parietal pleurae are continuous around the root of the lung.
- The parietal pleura can be divided regionally into the costal, diaphragmatic, mediastinal, and cervical parts; note the costodiaphragmatic recess.
- The pleural cavity is a potential space between the visceral and parietal pleurae that contains a thin layer of fluid. If a sufficient amount of air enters the pleural cavity, the surface tension adhering visceral to parietal pleura (lung to thoracic wall) is broken, and the lung collapses (**atelectasis**) because of its inherent elasticity (elastic recoil). When a lung collapses, the pleural cavity—normally a potential space—becomes a real space (**B**) and may contain air (**pneumothorax**), blood (**hemothorax**), etc.

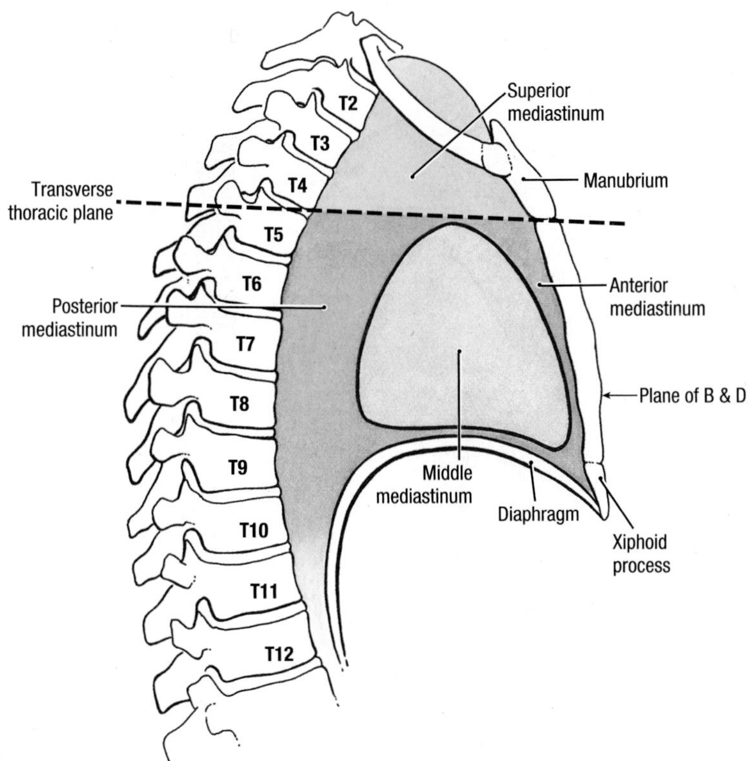
T2
T3
T4
T5
T6
T7
T8
T9
T10
T11
T12
Superior mediastinum
Manubrium
Transverse thoracic plane
Anterior mediastinum
Posterior mediastinum
Plane of B & D
Middle mediastinum
Diaphragm
Xiphoid process

A. Median Section, Left Lateral View

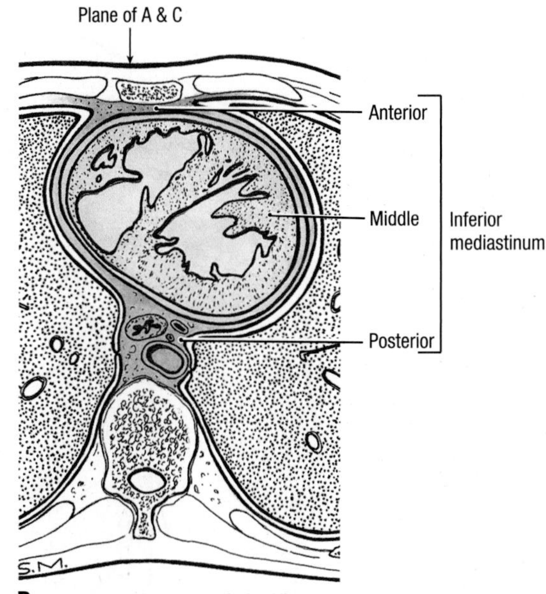
Plane of A & C
Anterior
Middle
Inferior mediastinum
Posterior
S.M.

B. Transverse Section, Inferior View

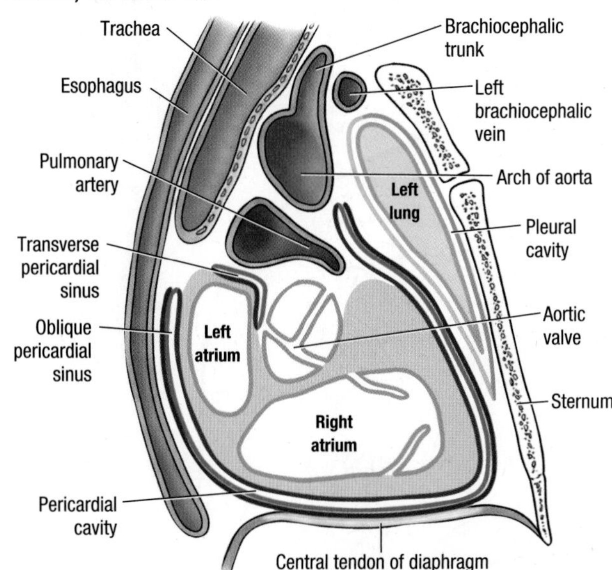
Trachea
Esophagus
Brachiocephalic trunk
Left brachiocephalic vein
Arch of aorta
Pulmonary artery
Left lung
Pleural cavity
Transverse pericardial sinus
Aortic valve
Oblique pericardial sinus
Left atrium
Sternum
Right atrium
Pericardial cavity
Central tendon of diaphragm

C. Median Section, Right Lateral View

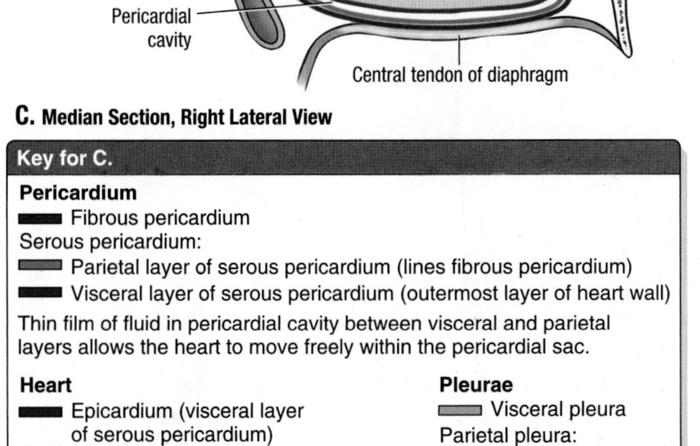

Key for C.

Pericardium

Fibrous pericardium

Serous pericardium:

Parietal layer of serous pericardium (lines fibrous pericardium)

Visceral layer of serous pericardium (outermost layer of heart wall)

Thin film of fluid in pericardial cavity between visceral and parietal layers allows the heart to move freely within the pericardial sac.

Heart

Epicardium (visceral layer of serous pericardium)

Myocardium

Endocardium

Pleurae

Visceral pleura

Parietal pleura:

Mediastinal

Costal

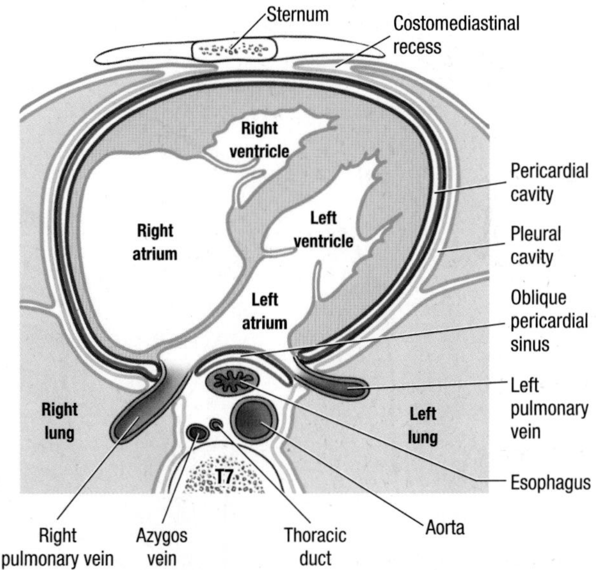
Sternum
Costomediastinal recess
Right ventricle
Pericardial cavity
Left ventricle
Right atrium
Pleural cavity
Left atrium
Oblique pericardial sinus
Left pulmonary vein
Right lung
Left lung
T7
Esophagus
Right pulmonary vein
Azygos vein
Thoracic duct
Aorta

D. Transverse Section, Inferior View

1.28 MEDIASTINUM AND PERICARDIUM

A. and B. Subdivisions of mediastinum. **C. and D.** Layers of pericardium and heart.

Cardiac tamponade (heart compression) is a potentially lethal condition because heart volume is increasingly compromised by the fluid outside the heart but inside the pericardial cavity. The heart is increasingly compressed and circulation fails. Blood in the pericardial cavity, **hemopericardium**, produces cardiac tamponade.

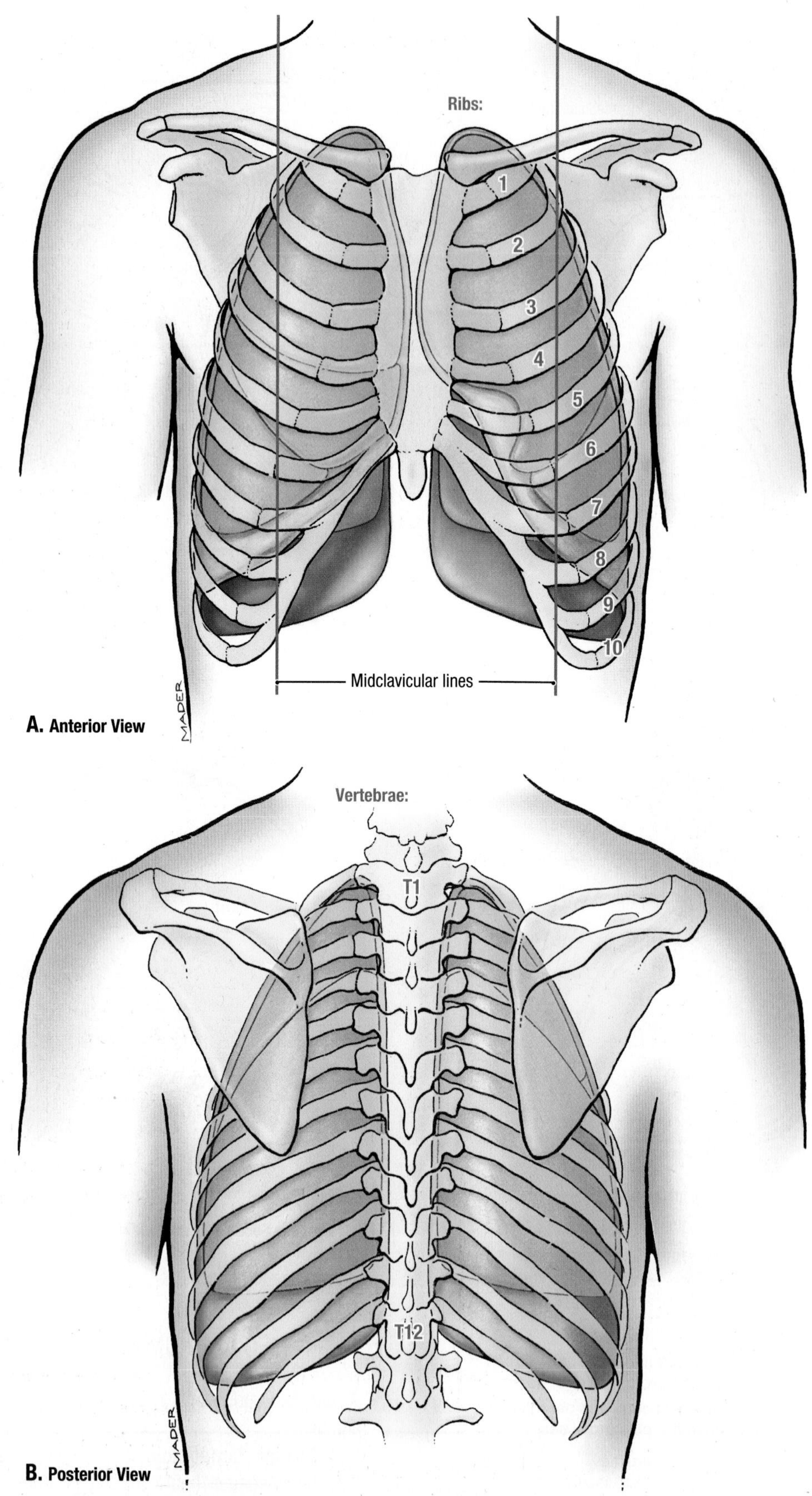
Ribs:
1
2
3
4
5
6
7
8
9
10
Midclavicular lines
MADER
A. Anterior View
Vertebrae:
T1
T12
MADER
B. Posterior View

1.29 EXTENT OF PARIETAL PLEURA AND LUNGS

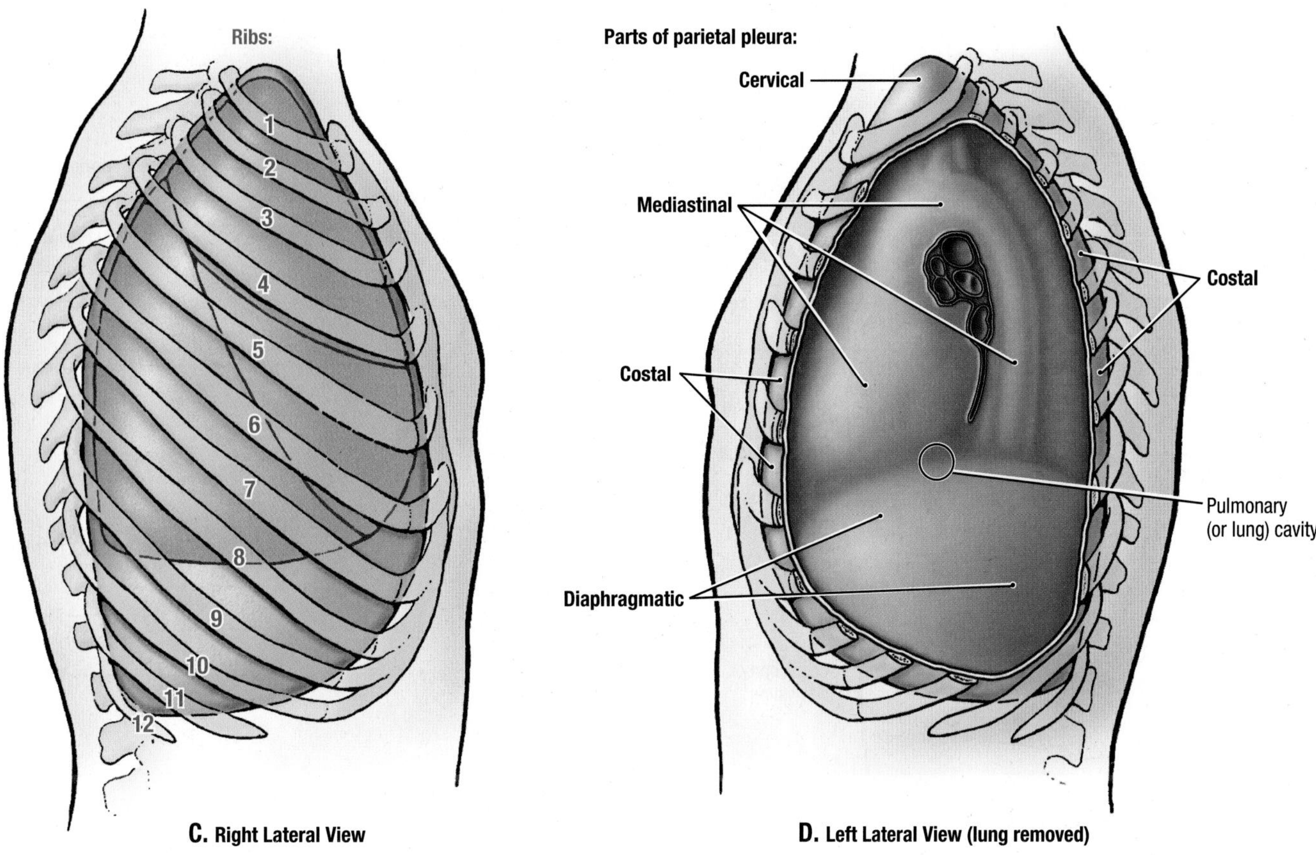
Ribs:
1
2
3
4
5
6
7
8
9
10
11
12
Parts of parietal pleura:
Cervical
Mediastinal
Costal
Costal
Pulmonary
(or lung) cavity
Diaphragmatic

C. Right Lateral View

D. Left Lateral View (lung removed)

1.29 EXTENT OF PARIETAL PLEURA AND LUNGS (*CONTINUED*)

TABLE 1.3 SURFACE MARKINGS OF PARIETAL PLEURA (BLUE)

Level	Left Pleura	Right Pleura
Apex	About 4 cm superior to middle of clavicle	About 4 cm superior to middle of clavicle
4th costal cartilage	Midline (anteriorly)	Midline (anteriorly)
6th costal cartilage	Lateral margin of sternum	Midline (anteriorly)
8th costal cartilage	Midclavicular line	Midclavicular line
10th rib	Midaxillary line	Midaxillary line
11th rib	Line of inferior angle of scapula	Line of inferior angle of scapula
12th rib	Lateral border of erector spinae to T12 spinous process (slightly lower level than right pleura)	Lateral border of erector spinae to T12 spinous process

SURFACE MARKINGS OF LUNGS COVERED WITH VISCERAL PLEURA (PINK)

Level	Left Lung	Right Lung
Apex	About 4 cm superior to middle of clavicle	About 4 cm superior to middle of clavicle
2nd costal cartilage	Midline (anteriorly)	Midline (anteriorly)
4th costal cartilage	Lateral margin of sternum	Lateral margin of sternum
6th costal cartilage	Follows 4th costal cartilage, turns inferiorly to 6th costal cartilage in the midclavicular line (cardiac notch)	Midclavicular line
8th rib	Midaxillary line	Midaxillary line
10th rib	Line of inferior angle of scapula to T10 spinous process	Line of inferior angle of scapula to T10 spinous process

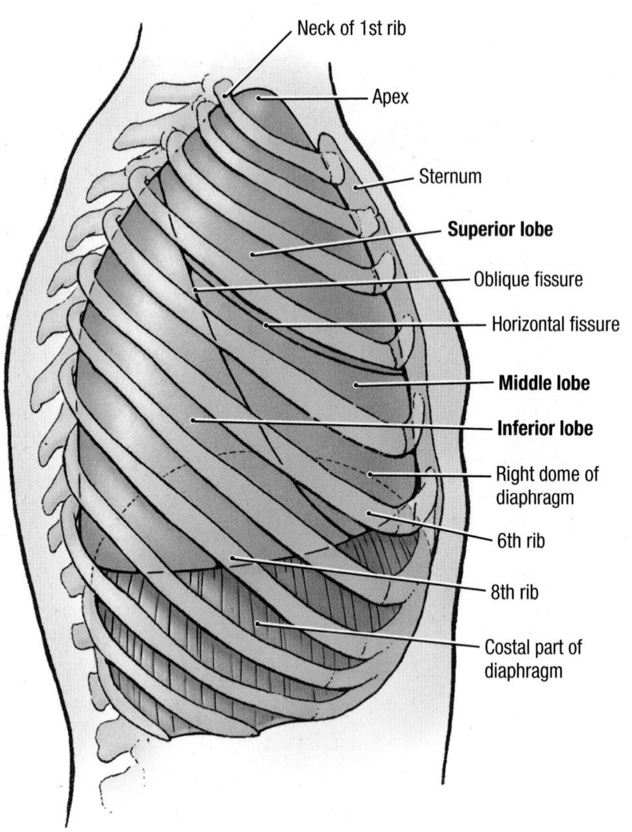
Neck of 1st rib
Apex
Sternum
Superior lobe
Oblique fissure
Horizontal fissure
Middle lobe
Inferior lobe
Right dome of diaphragm
6th rib
8th rib
Costal part of diaphragm

A. **Lateral View**

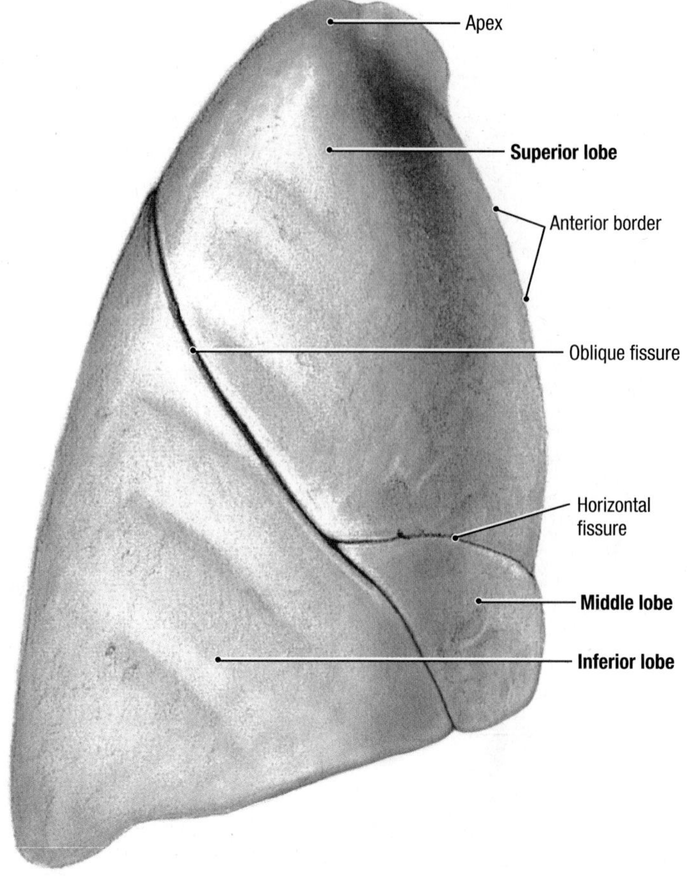
Apex
Superior lobe
Anterior border
Oblique fissure
Horizontal fissure
Middle lobe
Inferior lobe

B. **Lateral View**

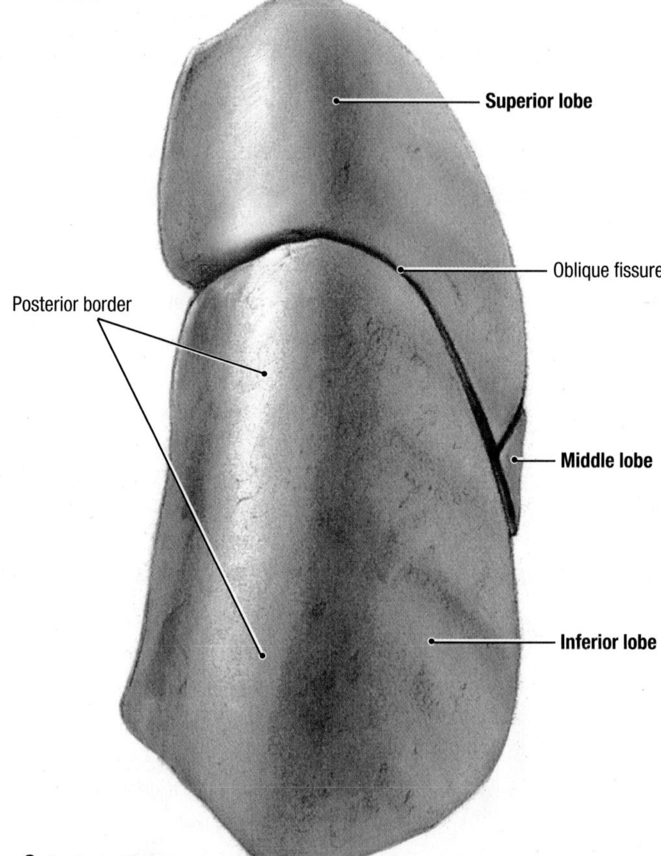
Superior lobe
Oblique fissure
Posterior border
Middle lobe
Inferior lobe

C. **Posterior View**

1.30 RIGHT LUNG

- The oblique and horizontal fissures divide the right lung into three lobes: superior, middle and inferior.
- The right lung is larger and heavier than the left, but is shorter and wider because the right dome of the diaphragm is higher and the heart bulges more to the left.
- Cadaveric lungs may be shrunken, firm and discolored, whereas healthy lungs in living people are normally soft, light and spongy.
- Each lung has an apex and base, three surfaces (costal, mediastinal and diaphragmatic) and three borders (anterior, inferior and posterior).

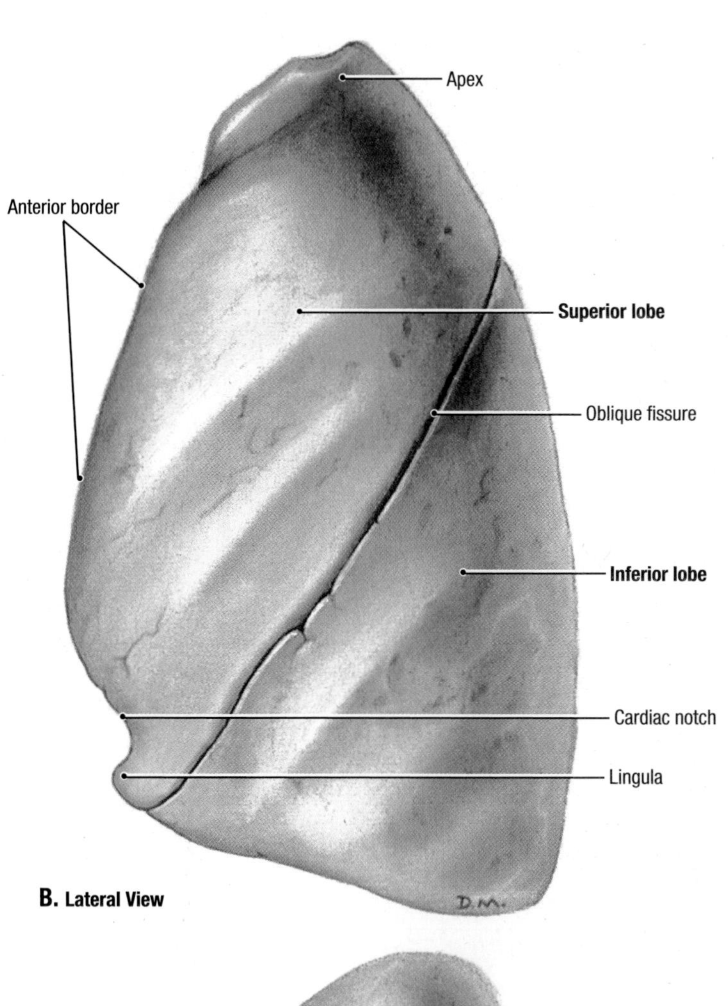
Apex
Anterior border
Superior lobe
Oblique fissure
Inferior lobe
Cardiac notch
Lingula

B. Lateral View

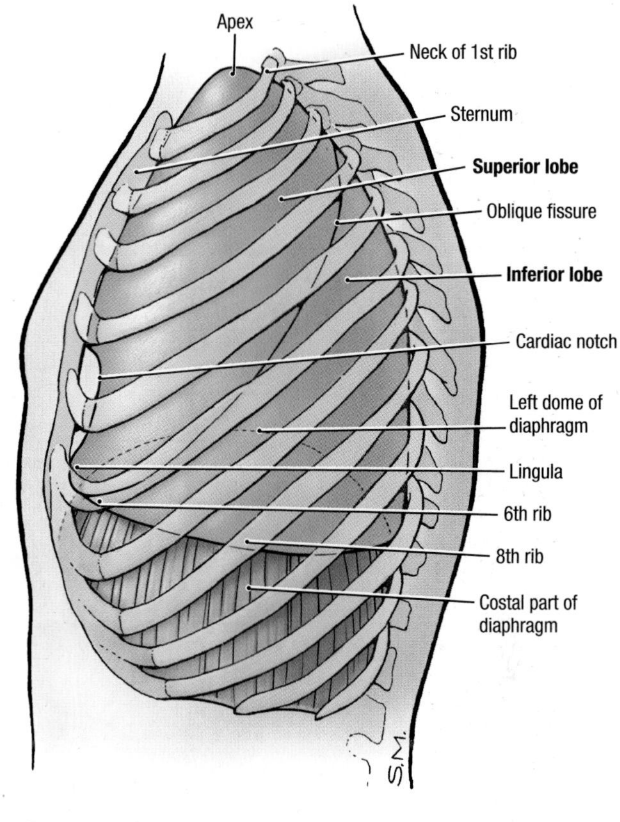
Apex
Neck of 1st rib
Sternum
Superior lobe
Oblique fissure
Inferior lobe
Cardiac notch
Left dome of diaphragm
Lingula
6th rib
8th rib
Costal part of diaphragm

A. Lateral View

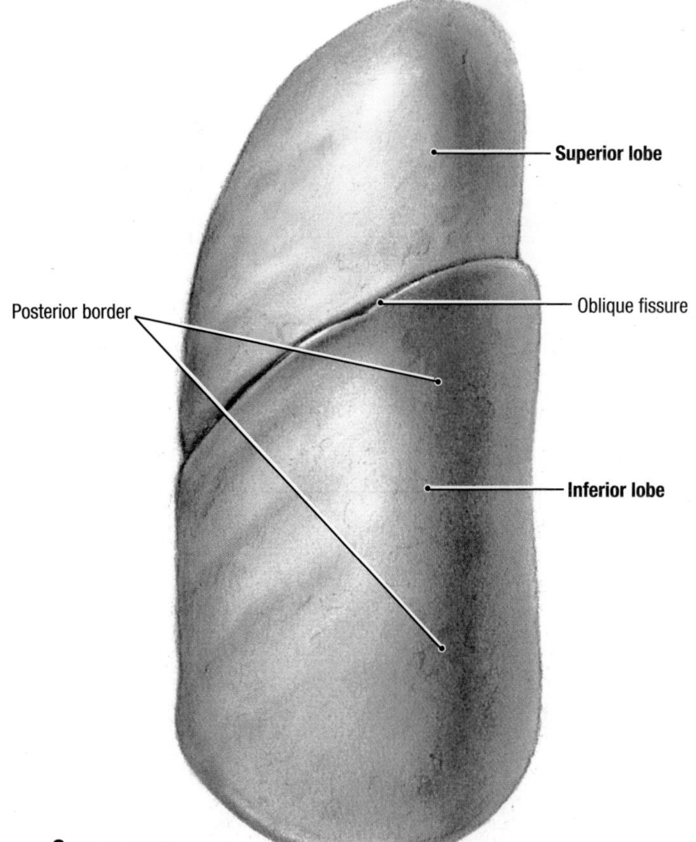
Superior lobe
Oblique fissure
Posterior border
Inferior lobe

C. Posterior View

1.31 LEFT LUNG

- The left lung has two lobes, superior and inferior, separated by the oblique fissure.
- The anterior border has a deep cardiac notch that indents the antero-inferior aspect of the superior lobe.
- The lingula, a tonguelike process of the superior lobe, extends below the cardiac notch and slides in and out of the costomediastinal recess during inspiration and expiration.
- The lungs of an embalmed cadaver usually retain impressions of structures that lie adjacent to them, such as the ribs and heart.

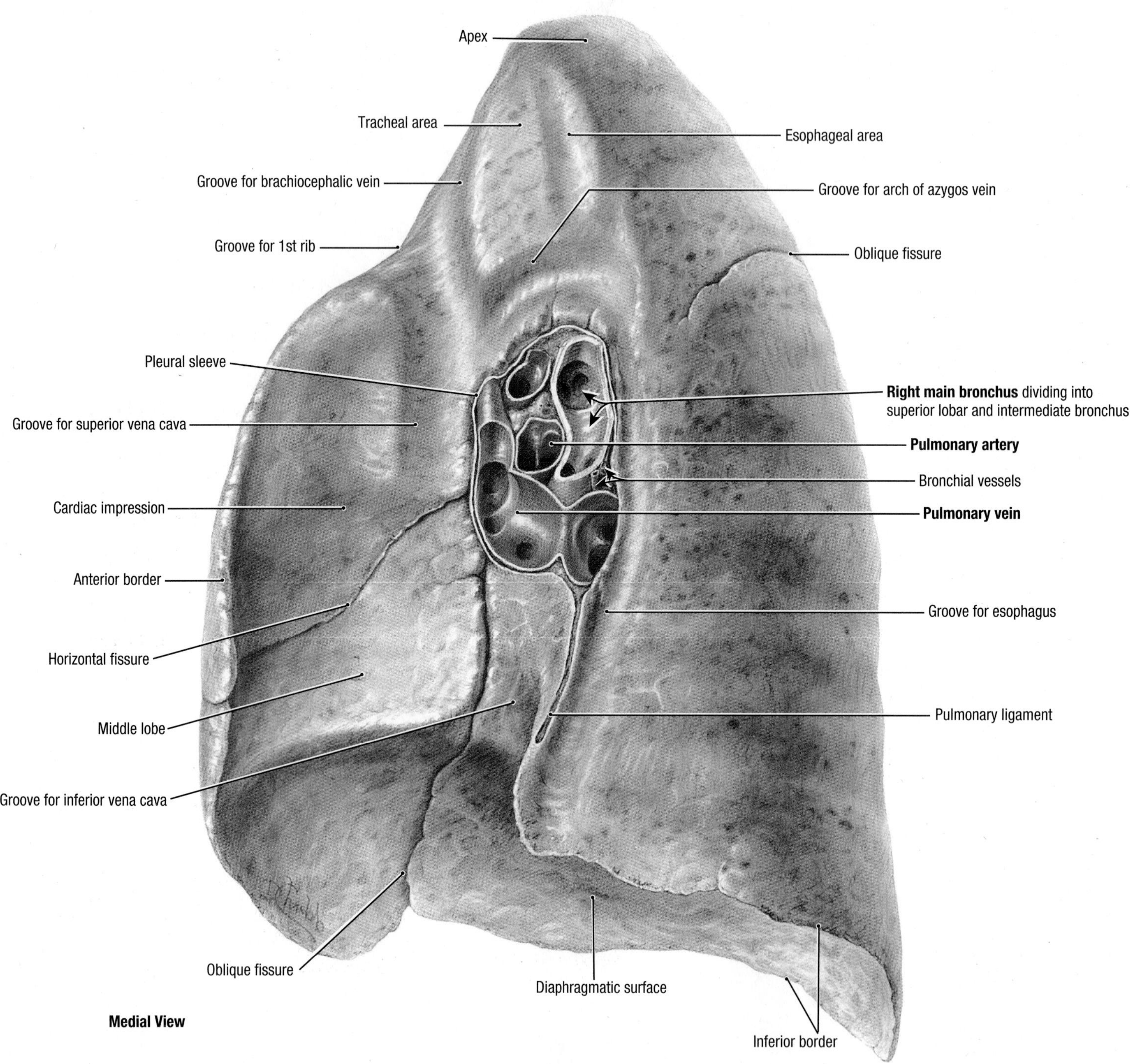

Apex
Tracheal area
Esophageal area
Groove for brachiocephalic vein
Groove for arch of azygos vein
Groove for 1st rib
Oblique fissure
Pleural sleeve
Right main bronchus dividing into superior lobar and intermediate bronchus
Groove for superior vena cava
Pulmonary artery
Bronchial vessels
Cardiac impression
Pulmonary vein
Anterior border
Groove for esophagus
Horizontal fissure
Middle lobe
Pulmonary ligament
Groove for inferior vena cava
Oblique fissure
Diaphragmatic surface
Medial View
Inferior border

1.32 MEDIASTINAL (MEDIAL) SURFACE AND HILUM OF RIGHT LUNG

The embalmed lung shows impressions of the structures with which it comes into contact, clearly demarcated as surface features; the base is contoured by the domes of the diaphragm; the costal surface bears the impressions of the ribs; distended vessels leave their mark, but nerves do not. The oblique fissure is incomplete here.

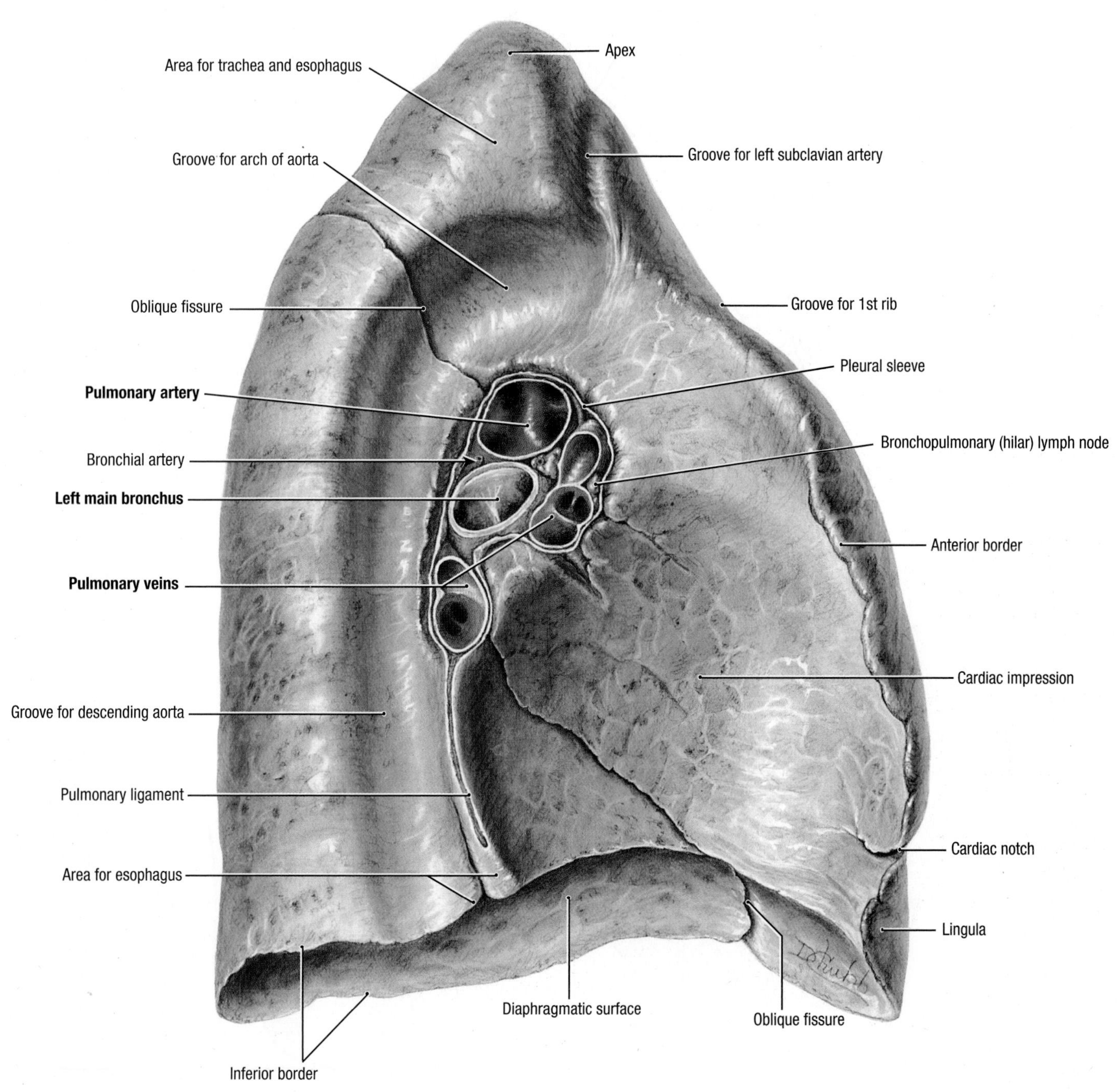
Apex
Area for trachea and esophagus
Groove for arch of aorta
Groove for left subclavian artery
Oblique fissure
Groove for 1st rib
Pleural sleeve
Pulmonary artery
Bronchial artery
Bronchopulmonary (hilar) lymph node
Left main bronchus
Anterior border
Pulmonary veins
Cardiac impression
Groove for descending aorta
Pulmonary ligament
Cardiac notch
Area for esophagus
Lingula
Diaphragmatic surface
Oblique fissure
Inferior border

Medial View

1.33 MEDIASTINAL (MEDIAL) SURFACE AND HILUM OF LEFT LUNG

Note the site of contact with esophagus, between the descending aorta and the inferior end of the pulmonary ligament. In the right and left roots, the artery is superior, the bronchus is posterior, one vein is anterior, and the other is inferior; in the right root, the bronchus to the superior lobe (also called the *eparterial bronchus*) is the most superior structure.

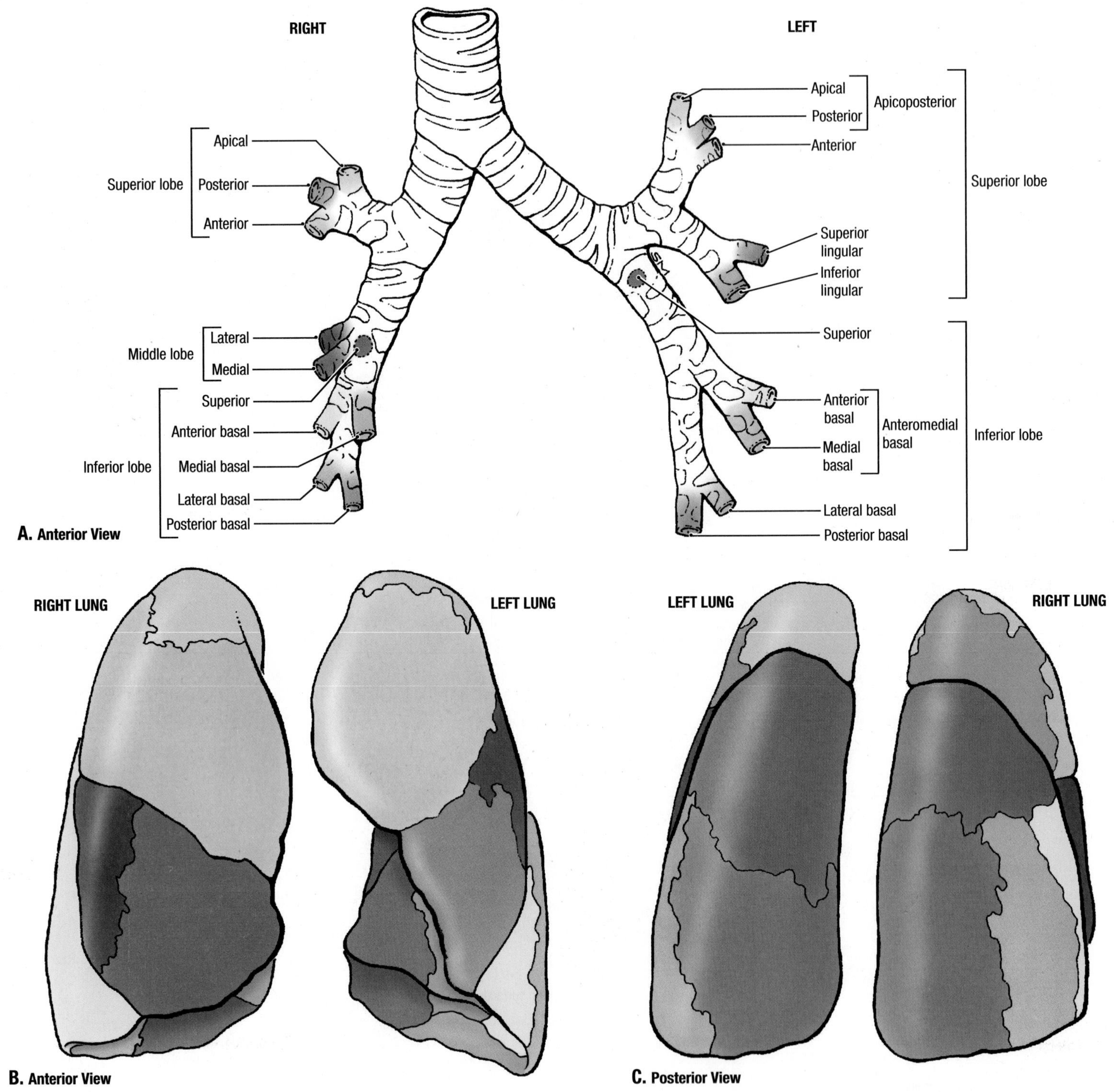

RIGHT
LEFT
Superior lobe
Apical
Posterior
Anterior
Middle lobe
Lateral
Medial
Inferior lobe
Superior
Anterior basal
Medial basal
Lateral basal
Posterior basal
Apical
Posterior
Apicoposterior
Anterior
Superior lobe
Superior lingular
Inferior lingular
Superior
Anterior basal
Medial basal
Anteromedial basal
Inferior lobe
Lateral basal
Posterior basal
A. Anterior View
RIGHT LUNG
LEFT LUNG
LEFT LUNG
RIGHT LUNG
B. Anterior View
C. Posterior View

1.34 SEGMENTAL BRONCHI AND BRONCHOPULMONARY SEGMENTS

A. There are 10 tertiary or segmental bronchi on the right, and 8 on the left. Note that on the left, the apical and posterior bronchi arise from a single stem, as do the anterior basal and medial basal. **B.–F.** A bronchopulmonary segment consists of a tertiary bronchus, pulmonary vein and artery, and the portion of lung they serve. These structures are surgically separable to allow segmental resection of the lung. To prepare these specimens, the tertiary bronchi of fresh lungs were isolated within the hilum and injected with latex of various colors. Minor variations in the branching of the bronchi result in variations in the surface patterns.

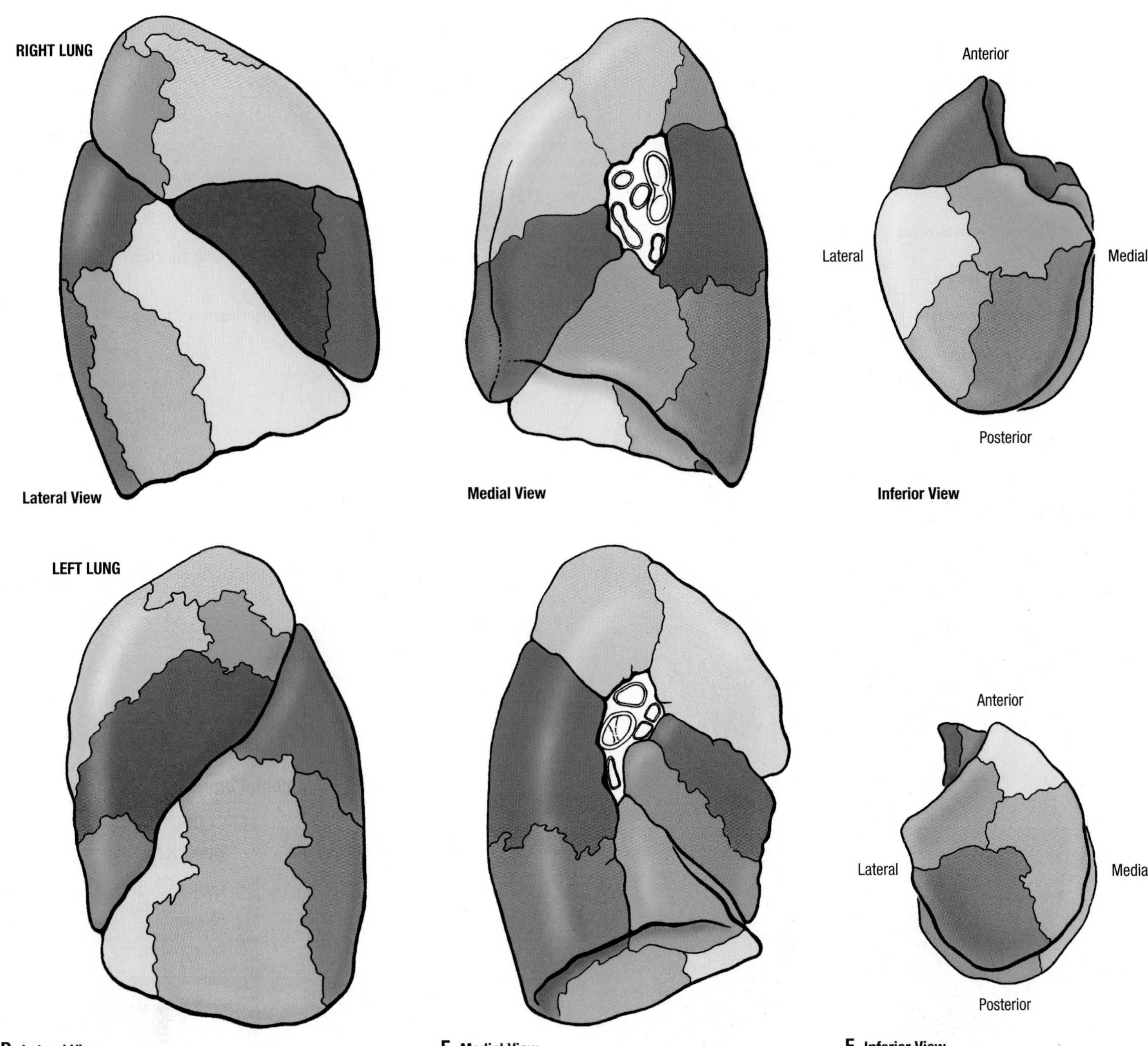
RIGHT LUNG
Lateral View
Medial View
Anterior
Lateral
Medial
Posterior
Inferior View
LEFT LUNG
Anterior
Lateral
Medial
Posterior

D. Lateral View

E. Medial View

F. Inferior View

1.34 SEGMENTAL BRONCHI AND BRONCHOPULMONARY SEGMENTS (*CONTINUED*)

Knowledge of the anatomy of the bronchopulmonary segments is essential for precise interpretations of diagnostic images of the lungs and for surgical resection (removal) of diseased segments. During the treatment of lung cancer, the surgeon may remove a whole lung (**pneumonectomy**), a lobe (**lobectomy**), or one or more bronchopulmonary segments (**segmentectomy**). Knowledge and understanding of the bronchopulmonary segments and their relationship to the bronchial tree are also essential for planning drainage and clearance techniques used in physical therapy for enhancing drainage from specific areas (e.g., in patients with pneumonia or cystic fibrosis).

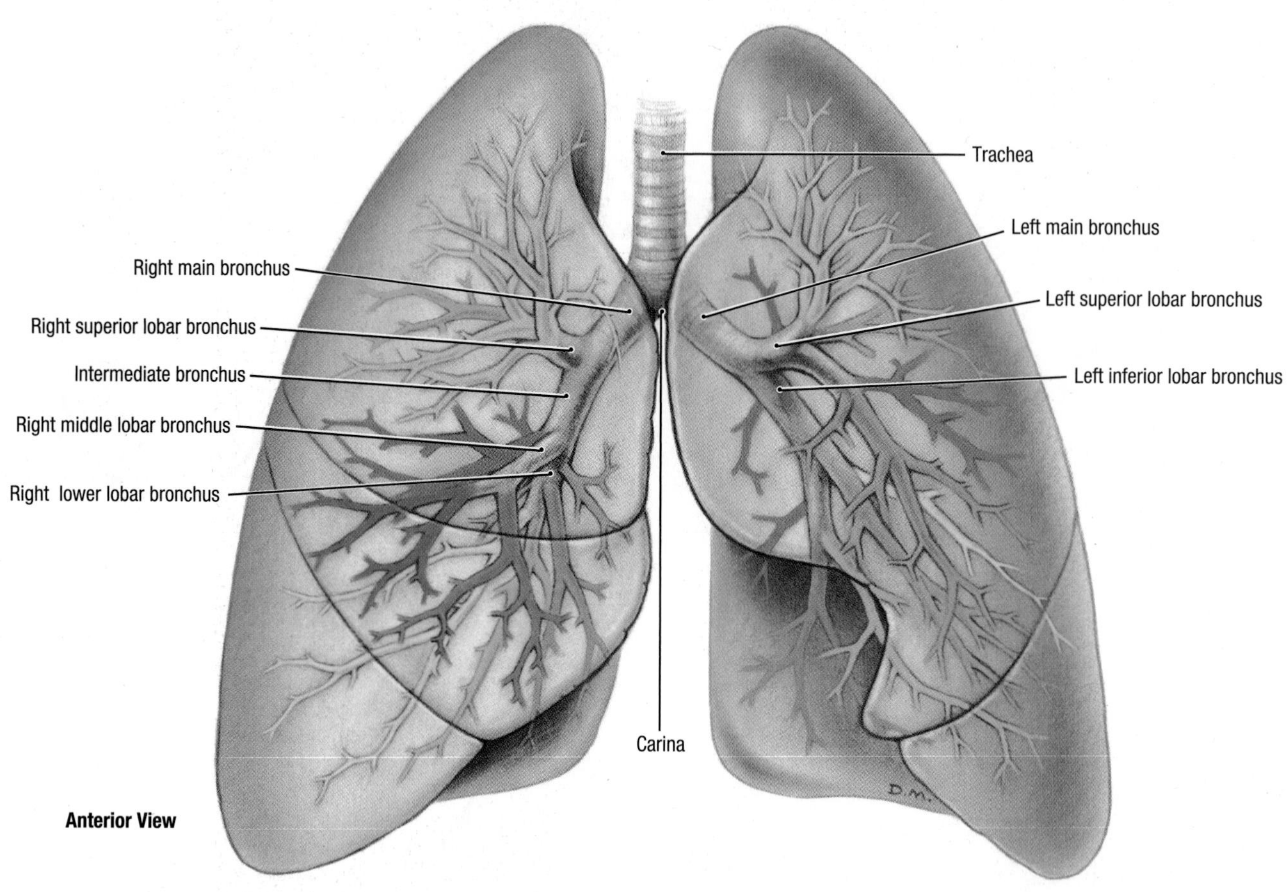
Trachea
Left main bronchus
Left superior lobar bronchus
Left inferior lobar bronchus
Right main bronchus
Right superior lobar bronchus
Intermediate bronchus
Right middle lobar bronchus
Right lower lobar bronchus
Carina
Anterior View
D.M.

Segmental bronchi:

RIGHT LUNG	LEFT LUNG
Superior Lobe	**Superior Lobe**
Apical	Apical (Apicoposterior)
Posterior	Posterior (Apicoposterior)
Anterior	Anterior
	Superior lingular
	Inferior lingular
Middle Lobe	
Lateral	
Medial	
Inferior Lobe	**Inferior Lobe**
Superior	Superior
Anterior basal	Anterior basal (Anteromedial basal)
Medial basal	Medial basal (Anteromedial basal)
Lateral basal	Lateral basal
Posterior basal	Posterior basal

1.35 TRACHEA AND BRONCHI IN SITU

- The segmental (tertiary) bronchi are color coded.
- The trachea bifurcates into right and left main (primary) bronchi; the right main bronchus is shorter, wider, and more vertical than the left. Therefore, it is more likely that **aspirated foreign bodies** will enter and lodge in the right main bronchus or one of its descending branches.
- The right main bronchus gives off the right superior lobe bronchus (eparterial bronchus) before entering the hilum (hilus) of the lung; after entering the hilum, the continuing intermediate bronchus divides into the right middle and inferior lobar bronchi.
- The left main bronchus divides at the hilum into the left superior and left inferior lobar bronchi; the lobar bronchi further divide into segmental (tertiary) bronchi.

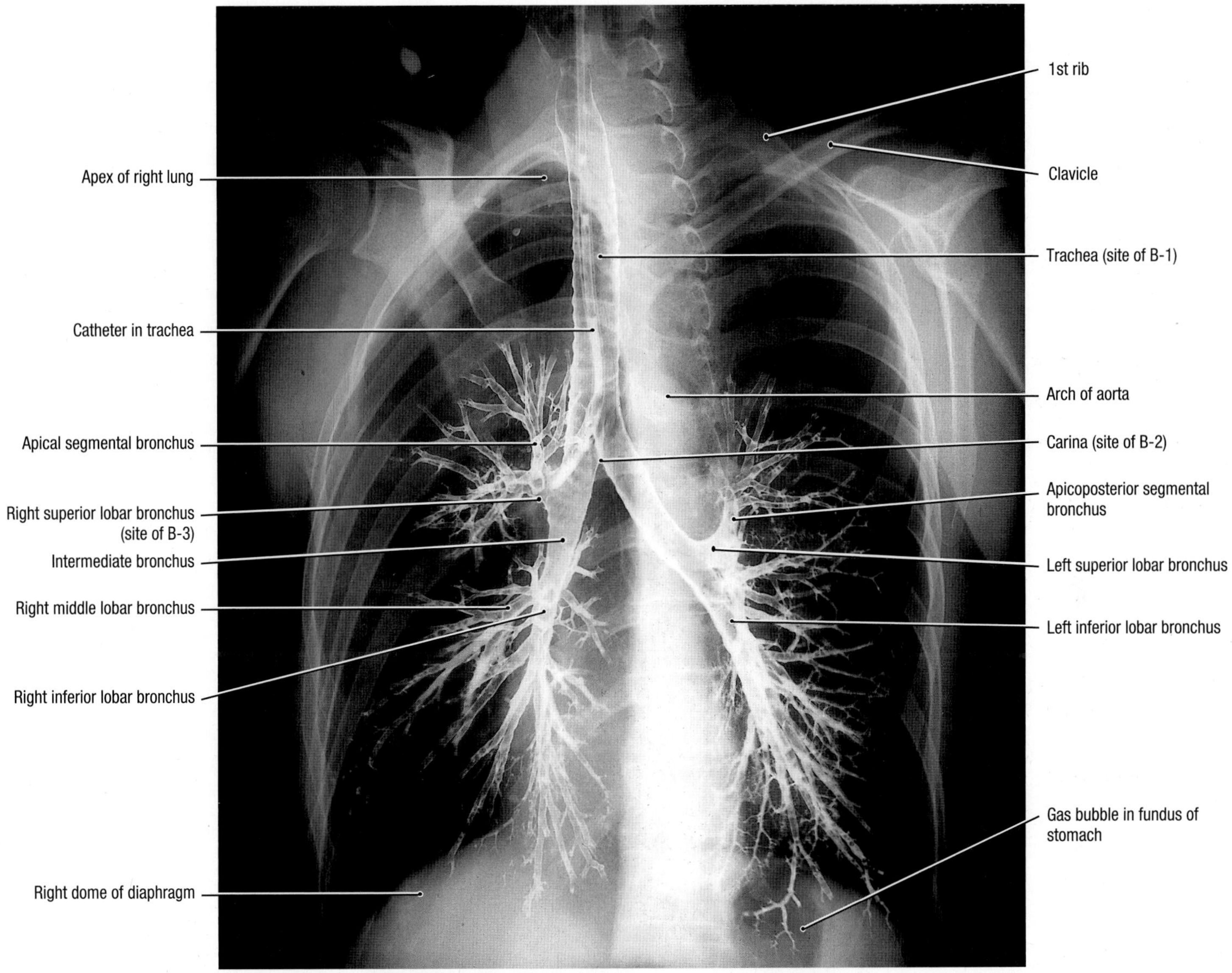

1st rib
Apex of right lung
Clavicle
Trachea (site of B-1)
Catheter in trachea
Arch of aorta
Apical segmental bronchus
Carina (site of B-2)
Apicoposterior segmental bronchus
Right superior lobar bronchus (site of B-3)
Intermediate bronchus
Left superior lobar bronchus
Right middle lobar bronchus
Left inferior lobar bronchus
Right inferior lobar bronchus
Gas bubble in fundus of stomach
Right dome of diaphragm

A. **Slightly Oblique Anteroposterior View**

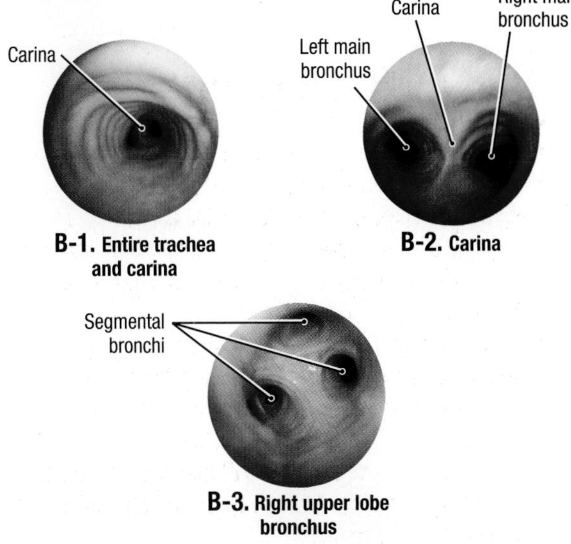
Carina
Left main bronchus
Carina
Right main bronchus
Segmental bronchi

B-1. **Entire trachea and carina**

B-2. **Carina**

B-3. **Right upper lobe bronchus**

B. **Bronchoscopic Views**

1.36 BRONCHOGRAMS

A. Bronchogram of tracheobronchial tree. **B.** Bronchoscopy.

When examining the bronchi with a *bronchoscope*—an endoscope for inspecting the interior of the tracheobronchial tree for diagnostic purposes—one can observe a ridge, the *carina*, between the orifices of the main bronchi. If the tracheobronchial lymph nodes in the angle between the main bronchi are enlarged because cancer cells have metastasized from a bronchogenic carcinoma, for example, the carina is distorted, widened posteriorly, and immobile.

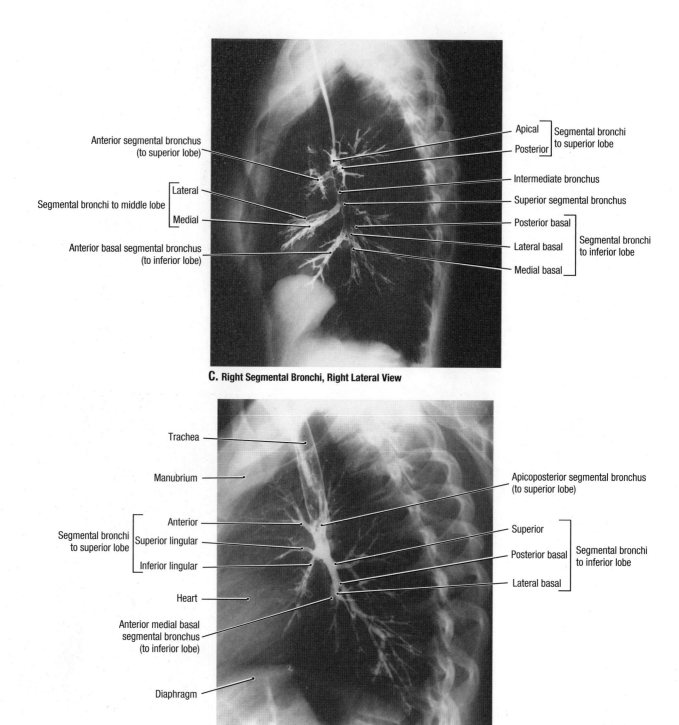

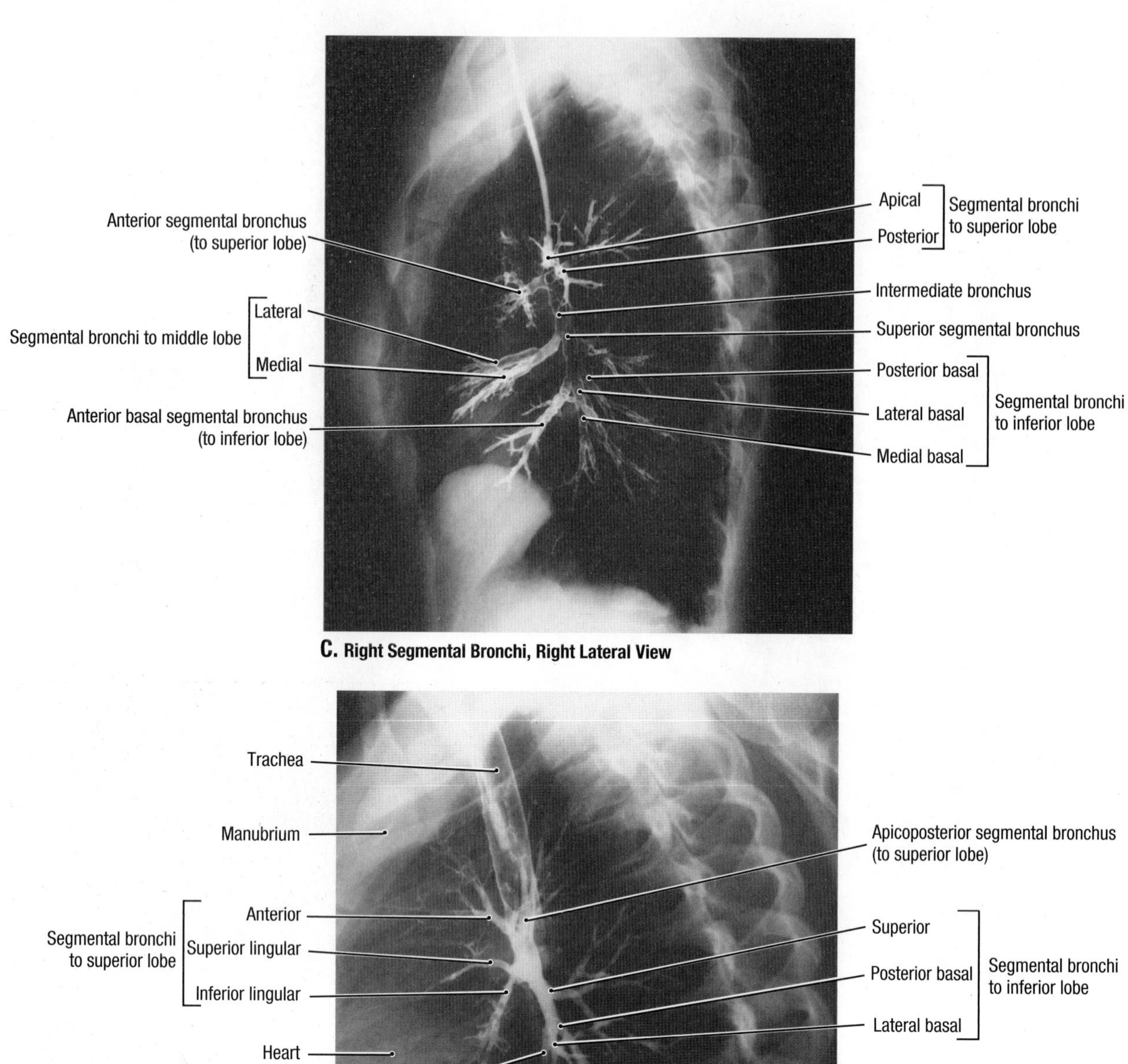
Anterior segmental bronchus (to superior lobe)
Segmental bronchi to middle lobe
Lateral
Medial
Anterior basal segmental bronchus (to inferior lobe)
Apical
Posterior
Segmental bronchi to superior lobe
Intermediate bronchus
Superior segmental bronchus
Posterior basal
Lateral basal
Medial basal
Segmental bronchi to inferior lobe

C. **Right Segmental Bronchi, Right Lateral View**

Trachea
Manubrium
Segmental bronchi to superior lobe
Anterior
Superior lingular
Inferior lingular
Heart
Anterior medial basal segmental bronchus (to inferior lobe)
Diaphragm
Apicoposterior segmental bronchus (to superior lobe)
Superior
Posterior basal
Lateral basal
Segmental bronchi to inferior lobe

D. **Left Segmental Bronchi, Left Lateral View**

1.36 BRONCHOGRAMS (*CONTINUED*)

C. Right lateral bronchogram, showing segmental bronchi. **D.** Left lateral bronchogram, showing segmental bronchi.

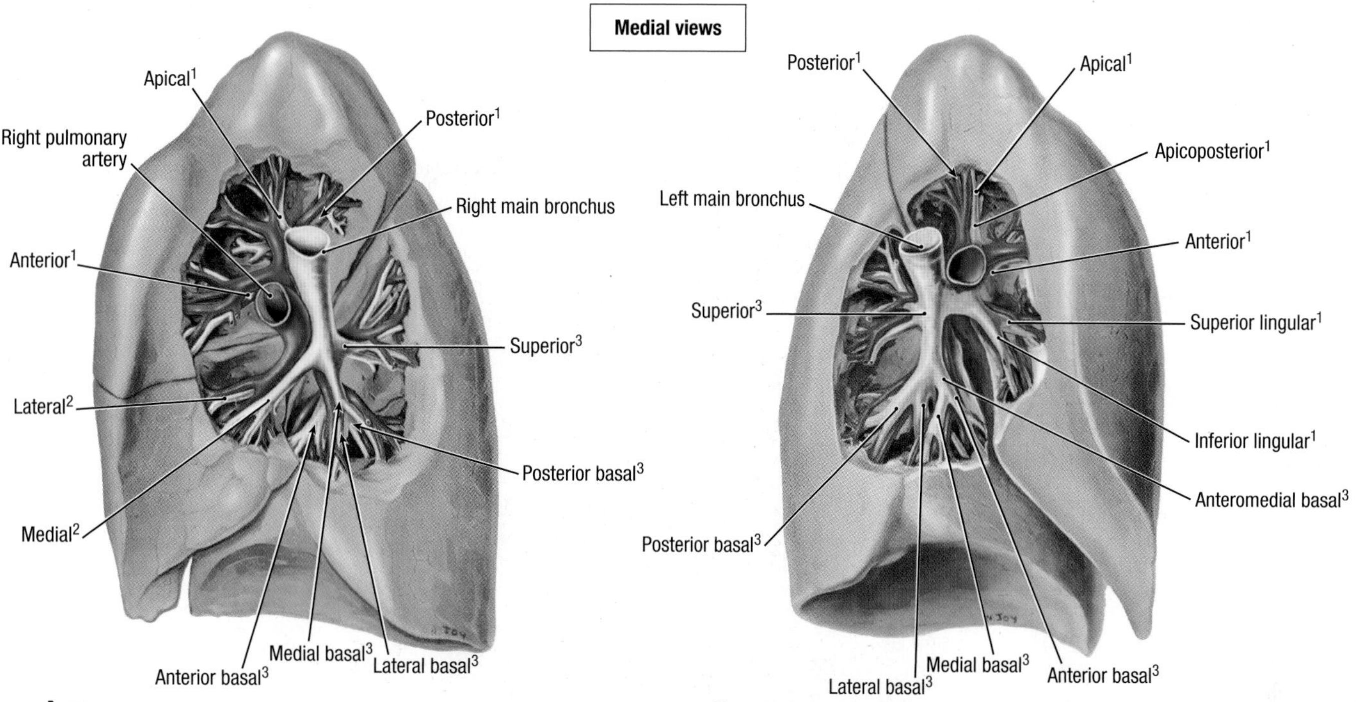
Medial views
Apical[1]
Right pulmonary artery
Posterior[1]
Right main bronchus
Anterior[1]
Superior[3]
Lateral[2]
Posterior basal[3]
Medial[2]
Medial basal[3]
Lateral basal[3]
Anterior basal[3]
A. Right Lung
Posterior[1]
Apical[1]
Apicoposterior[1]
Left main bronchus
Anterior[1]
Superior[3]
Superior lingular[1]
Inferior lingular[1]
Anteromedial basal[3]
Posterior basal[3]
Medial basal[3]
Anterior basal[3]
Lateral basal[3]
B. Left Lung

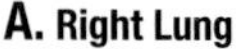

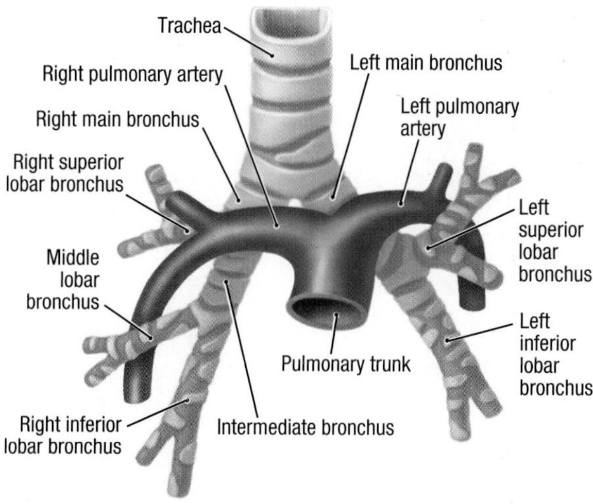
Trachea
Right pulmonary artery
Left main bronchus
Right main bronchus
Left pulmonary artery
Right superior lobar bronchus
Left superior lobar bronchus
Middle lobar bronchus
Left inferior lobar bronchus
Pulmonary trunk
Right inferior lobar bronchus
Intermediate bronchus

C. Anterior View

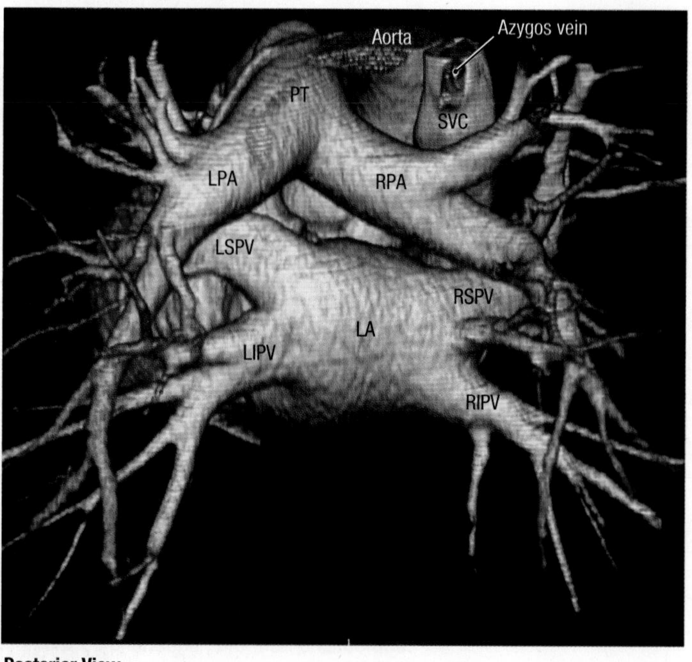
Aorta
Azygos vein
PT
SVC
LPA
RPA
LSPV
RSPV
LA
LIPV
RIPV

Posterior View

1.37 RELATIONSHIP OF BRONCHI AND PULMONARY ARTERIES

A. Right lung. **B.** Left lung. **C.** Pulmonary arteries and main bronchii. Superscripts indicate segmental bronchi to the [1]superior lobe, [2]middle lobe, and [3]inferior lobe. The pulmonary arteries of fresh lungs were filled with latex, the bronchi were inflated with air. The tissues surrounding the bronchi and vessels were removed.

Obstruction of a pulmonary artery by a blood clot (**pulmonary embolism**) results in partial or complete obstruction of blood flow to the lung.

1.38 3D VOLUME RECONSTRUCTION (3DVR) OF PULMONARY ARTERIES AND VEINS AND LEFT ATRIUM

The pulmonary trunk (*PT*) divides into a longer right pulmonary artery (*RPA*) and shorter left pulmonary artery (*LPA*); the left superior (*LSPV*) and inferior (*LIPV*) and the right superior (*RSPV*) and inferior (*RIPV*) pulmonary veins drain into the left atrium (*LA*). Superior vena cava (*SVC*).

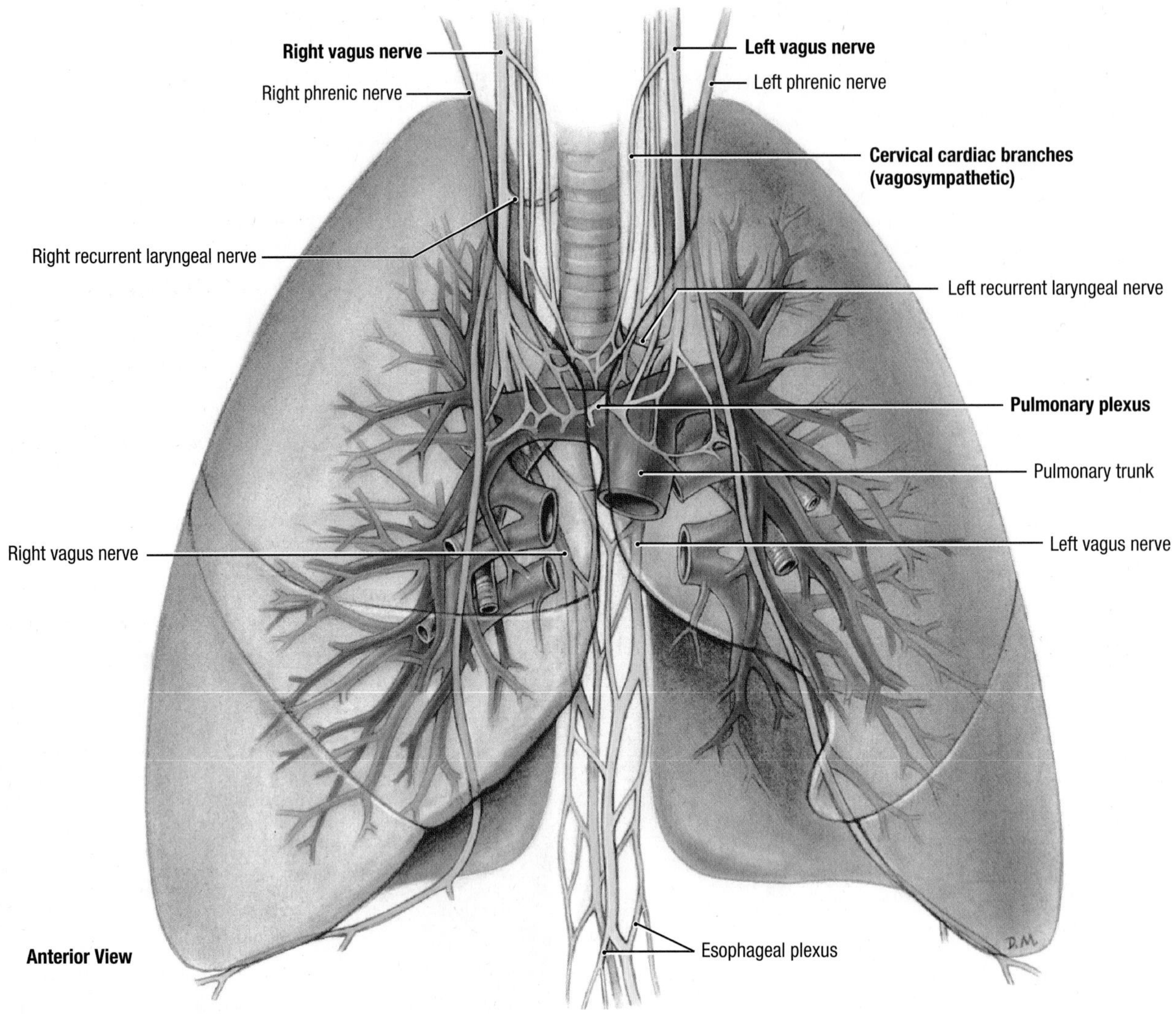
Right vagus nerve
Right phrenic nerve
Left vagus nerve
Left phrenic nerve
Cervical cardiac branches (vagosympathetic)
Right recurrent laryngeal nerve
Left recurrent laryngeal nerve
Pulmonary plexus
Pulmonary trunk
Right vagus nerve
Left vagus nerve
Esophageal plexus
Anterior View
D.M.

1.39 INNERVATION OF LUNGS

- The pulmonary plexuses, located anterior and posterior to the roots of the lungs, receive sympathetic contributions from the right and left sympathetic trunks (2nd to 5th thoracic ganglia, not shown) and parasympathetic contributions from the right and left vagus nerves; cell bodies of postsynaptic parasympathetic neurons are in the pulmonary plexuses and along the branches of the pulmonary tree.
- The right and left vagus nerves continue inferiorly from the posterior pulmonary plexus to contribute fibers to the esophageal plexus.
- The phrenic nerves pass anterior to the root of the lung on their way to the diaphragm.
- **Pleurisy/pleuritis.** The visceral pleura is insensitive to pain. The autonomic nerves reach the visceral pleura in company with the bronchial vessels. The visceral pleura receives no nerves of general sensation.
- The parietal pleura is sensitive to pain because it is richly supplied by branches of the somatic intercostal and phrenic nerves. Irritation of the parietal pleura produces local pain and referred pain to the areas sharing innervation by the same segments of the spinal cord.

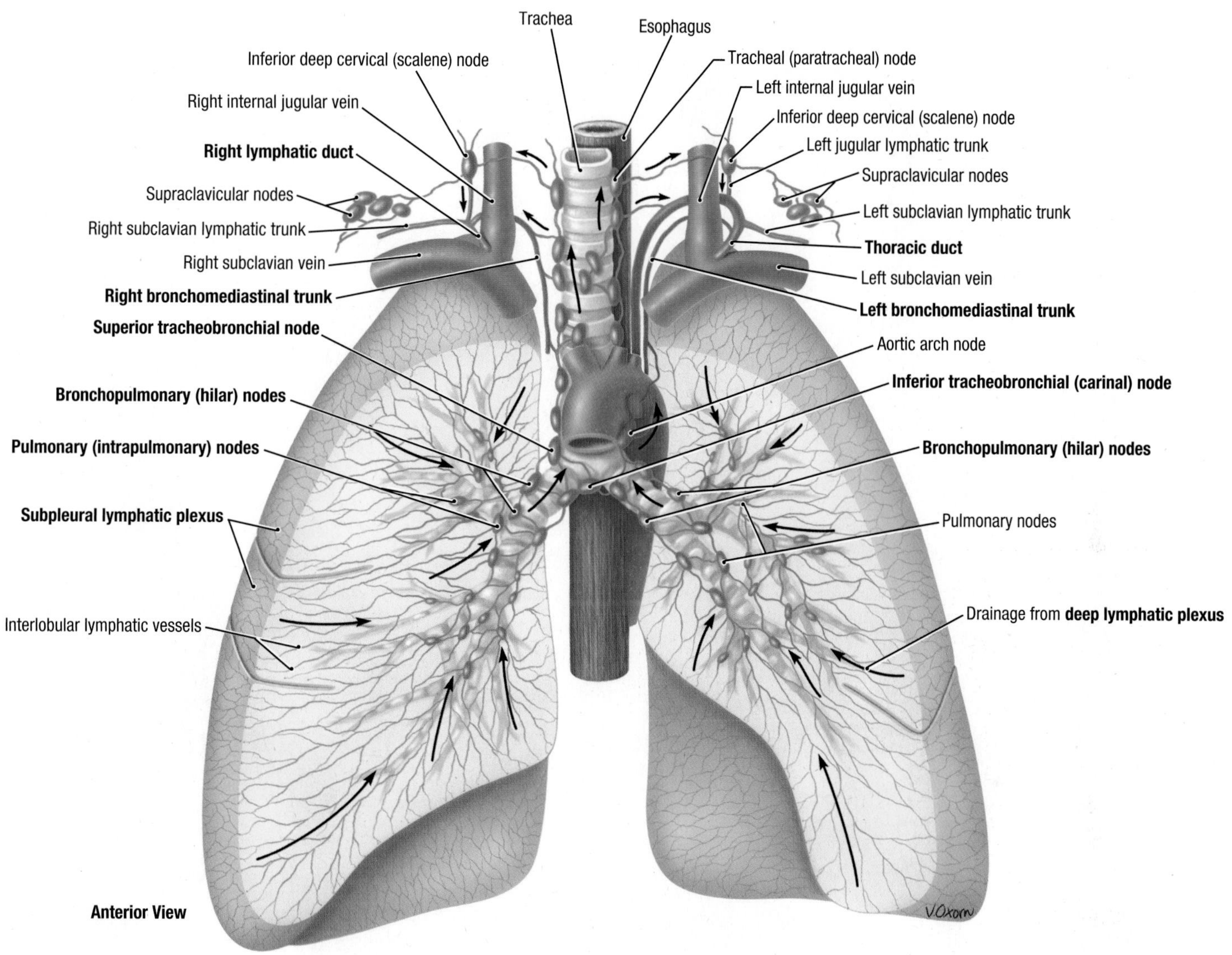
Trachea
Esophagus
Inferior deep cervical (scalene) node
Tracheal (paratracheal) node
Right internal jugular vein
Left internal jugular vein
Inferior deep cervical (scalene) node
Right lymphatic duct
Left jugular lymphatic trunk
Supraclavicular nodes
Supraclavicular nodes
Right subclavian lymphatic trunk
Left subclavian lymphatic trunk
Thoracic duct
Right subclavian vein
Left subclavian vein
Right bronchomediastinal trunk
Left bronchomediastinal trunk
Superior tracheobronchial node
Aortic arch node
Inferior tracheobronchial (carinal) node
Bronchopulmonary (hilar) nodes
Bronchopulmonary (hilar) nodes
Pulmonary (intrapulmonary) nodes
Subpleural lymphatic plexus
Pulmonary nodes
Interlobular lymphatic vessels
Drainage from deep lymphatic plexus
Anterior View
V.Oxorn

1.40 LYMPHATIC DRAINAGE OF LUNGS

- Lymphatic vessels originate in the subpleural (superficial) and deep lymphatic plexuses.
- The subpleural lymphatic plexus is superficial, lying deep to the visceral pleura, and drains lymph from the surface of the lung to the bronchopulmonary (hilar) nodes.
- The deep lymphatic plexus is in the lung and follows the bronchi and pulmonary vessels to the pulmonary, and then bronchopulmonary, nodes located at the root of the lung.
- All lymph from the lungs enters the inferior (carinal) and superior tracheobronchial nodes and then continues to the right and left bronchomediastinal trunks to drain into the venous system via the right lymphatic and thoracic ducts; lymph from the left inferior lobe passes largely to the right side.
- Lymph from the parietal pleura drains into lymph nodes of the thoracic wall (Fig. 1.71).

Lung cancer (carcinoma) metastasizes early to the bronchopulmonary lymph nodes and subsequently to the other thoracic lymph nodes. Common sites of **hematogenous metastases** (spreading through the blood) of cancer cells from a bronchogenic carcinoma are the brain, bones, lungs, and suprarenal glands. Often the lymph nodes superior to the clavicle—the supraclavicular lymph nodes—are enlarged when lung (bronchogenic) carcinoma develops owing to metastasis of cancer cells from the tumor. Consequently, the supraclavicular nodes were once referred to as sentinel lymph nodes. More recently, the term sentinel lymph node has been applied to a node or nodes that first receive lymph drainage from a cancer-containing area, regardless of location, following injection of blue dye containing radioactive tracer (technetium-99).

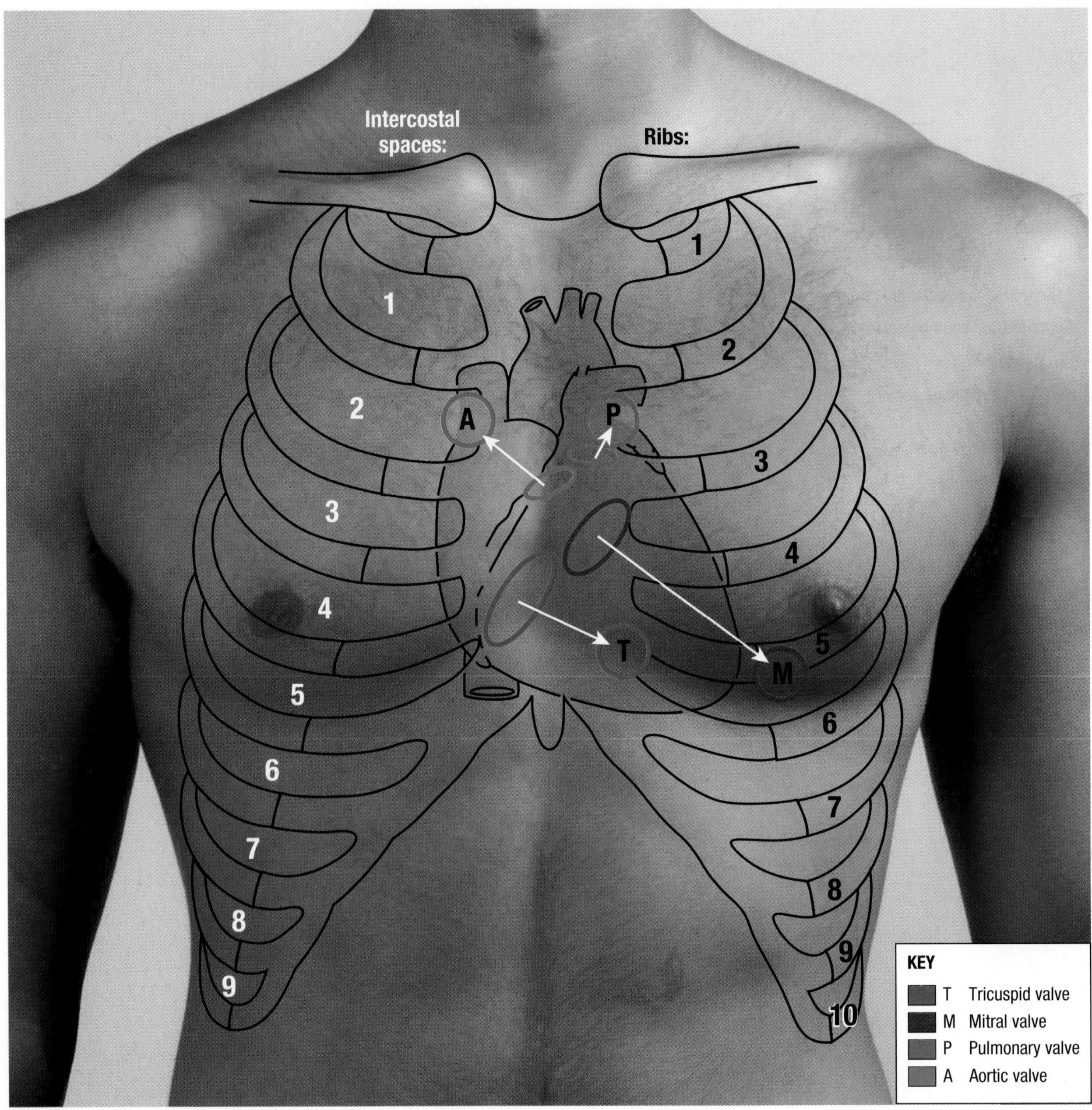
Intercostal spaces:
Ribs:
1
2
3
4
5
6
7
8
9
10
A
P
T
M
KEY
T Tricuspid valve
M Mitral valve
P Pulmonary valve
A Aortic valve

Anterior View

1.41 SURFACE MARKINGS OF THE HEART, HEART VALVES, AND THEIR AUSCULTATION AREAS

- The location of each heart valve in situ is indicated by a colored oval and the area of auscultation of the valve is indicated as a circle of the same color containing the first letter of the valve name.
- The auscultation areas are sites where the sounds of each of the heart's valves can be heard most distinctly through a stethoscope (*cardiac auscultation*).
- The aortic (*A*) and pulmonary (*P*) auscultation areas are in the 2nd intercostal space to the right and left of the sternal border; the tricuspid area (*T*) is near the left sternal border in the 5th or 6th intercostal space; the mitral valve (*M*) is heard best near the apex of the heart in the 5th intercostal space in the midclavicular line.

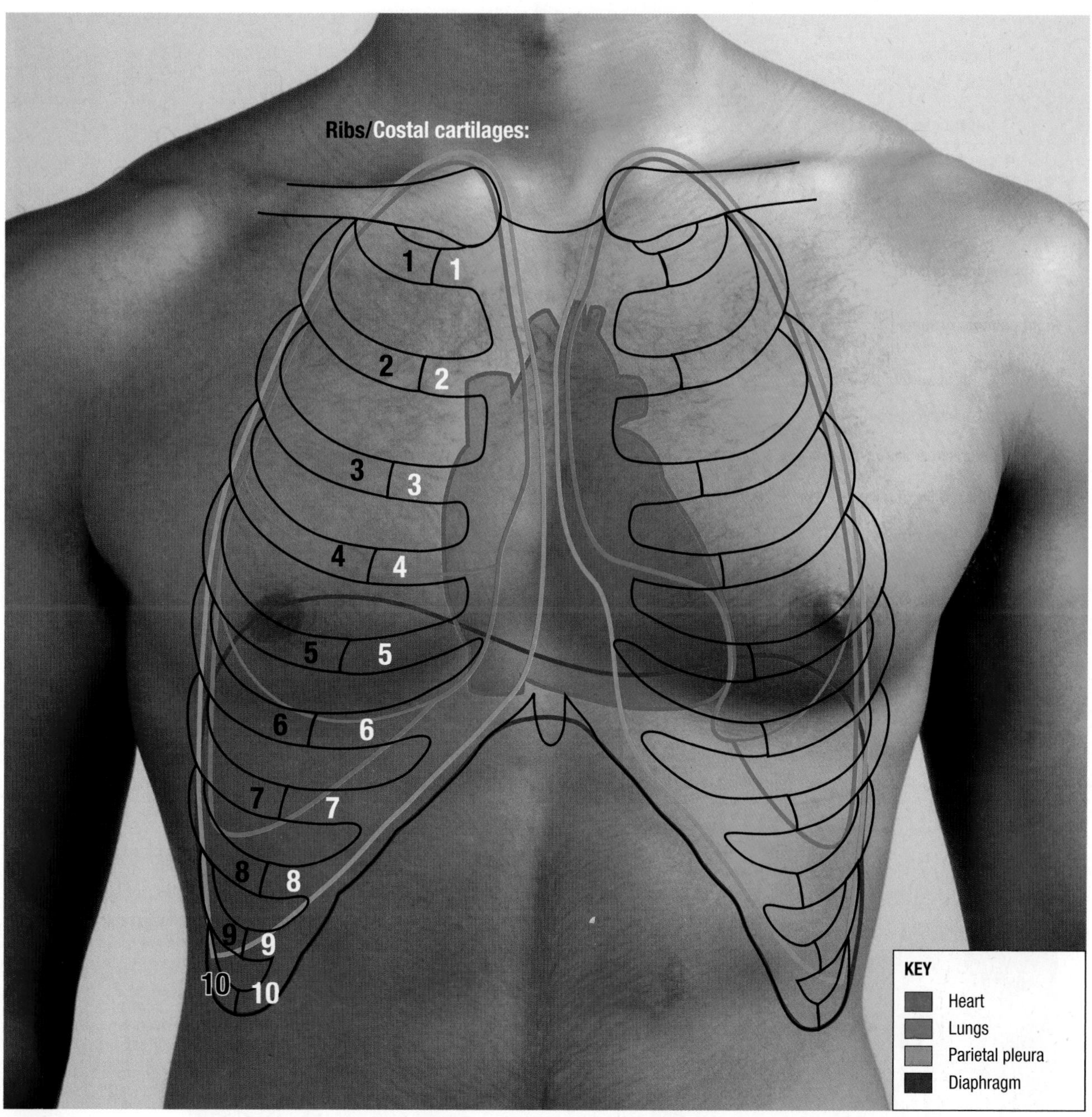
Ribs/Costal cartilages:
1 1
2 2
3 3
4 4
5 5
6 6
7 7
8 8
9 9
10 10
KEY
Heart
Lungs
Parietal pleura
Diaphragm

Anterior View

1.42 SURFACE MARKINGS OF THE HEART, LUNGS, AND DIAPHRAGM

- The superior border of the heart is represented by a slightly oblique line joining the 3rd costal cartilages; the convex right side of the heart projects lateral to the sternum and inferiorly, lying at the 6th or 7th costochondral junction; the inferior border of the heart is lying superior to the central tendon of the diaphragm and sloping slightly inferiorly to the apex at the 5th interspace at the midclavicular line.
- The right dome of the diaphragm is higher than the left because of the large size of the liver inferior to the dome; during expiration the right dome reaches as high as the 5th rib and the left dome ascends to the 5th intercostal space.
- The left pleural cavity is smaller than the right because of the projection of the heart to the left side.

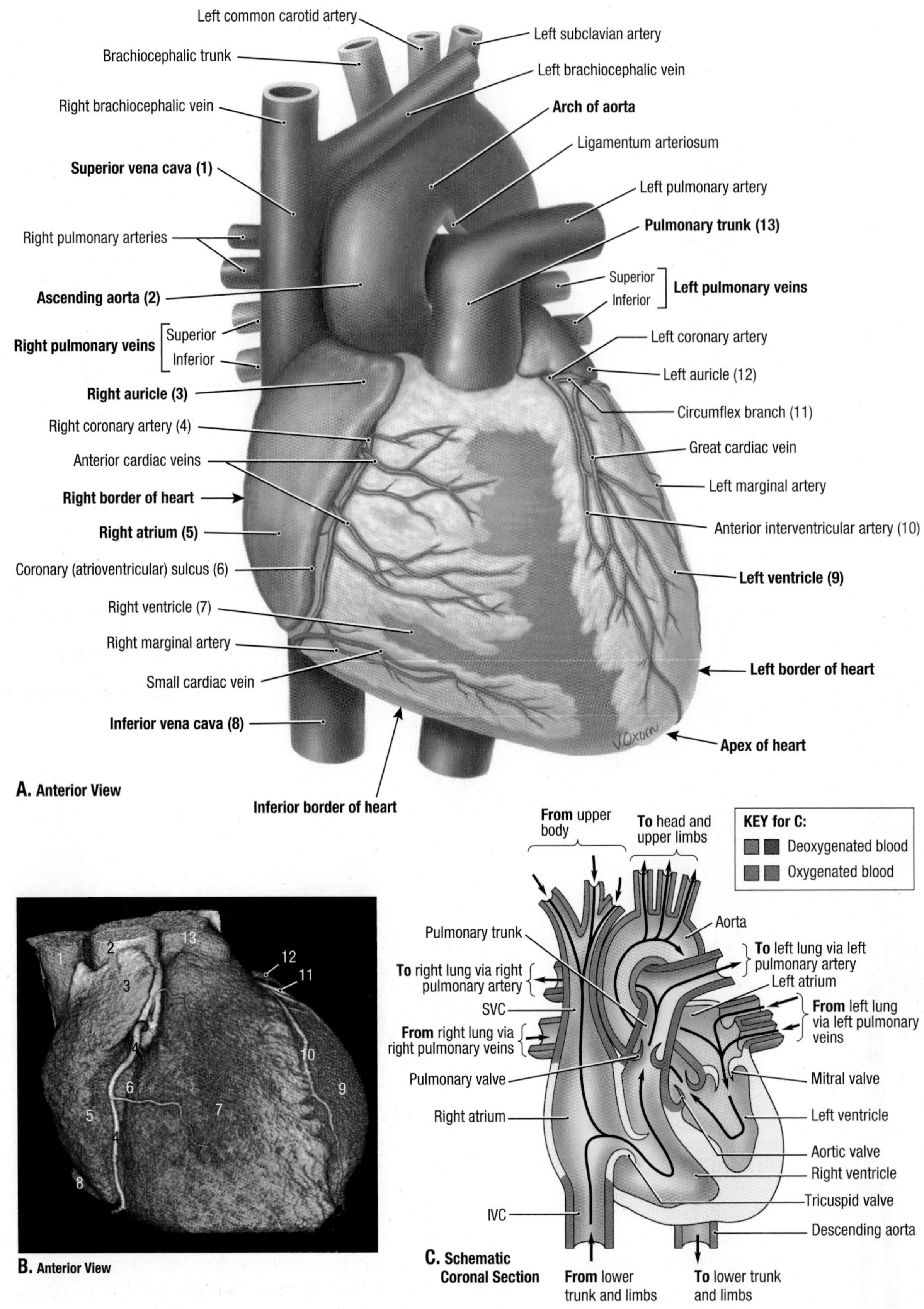
Left common carotid artery
Brachiocephalic trunk
Right brachiocephalic vein
Superior vena cava (1)
Right pulmonary arteries
Ascending aorta (2)
Right pulmonary veins
Superior
Inferior
Right auricle (3)
Right coronary artery (4)
Anterior cardiac veins
Right border of heart
Right atrium (5)
Coronary (atrioventricular) sulcus (6)
Right ventricle (7)
Right marginal artery
Small cardiac vein
Inferior vena cava (8)
Inferior border of heart
Left subclavian artery
Left brachiocephalic vein
Arch of aorta
Ligamentum arteriosum
Left pulmonary artery
Pulmonary trunk (13)
Superior
Inferior
Left pulmonary veins
Left coronary artery
Left auricle (12)
Circumflex branch (11)
Great cardiac vein
Left marginal artery
Anterior interventricular artery (10)
Left ventricle (9)
Left border of heart
Apex of heart
V.Oxorn
From upper body
To head and upper limbs
KEY for C:
Deoxygenated blood
Oxygenated blood
Pulmonary trunk
To right lung via right pulmonary artery
SVC
From right lung via right pulmonary veins
Pulmonary valve
Right atrium
IVC
Aorta
To left lung via left pulmonary artery
Left atrium
From left lung via left pulmonary veins
Mitral valve
Left ventricle
Aortic valve
Right ventricle
Tricuspid valve
Descending aorta
From lower trunk and limbs
To lower trunk and limbs
1
2
13
12
11
3
4
10
6
9
5
7
4
8

A. Anterior View

B. Anterior View

C. Schematic Coronal Section

1.43 HEART AND GREAT VESSELS

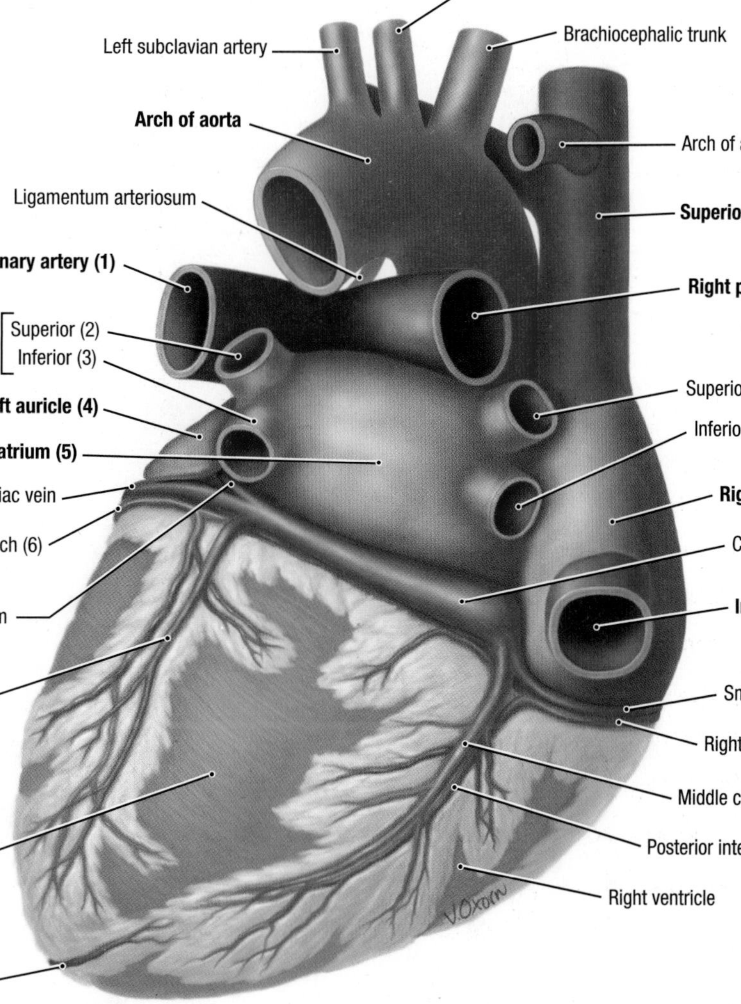

Left common carotid artery
Left subclavian artery
Brachiocephalic trunk
Arch of aorta
Arch of azygos vein
Ligamentum arteriosum
Superior vena cava
Left pulmonary artery (1)
Right pulmonary artery (15)
Left pulmonary veins Superior (2) Inferior (3)
Superior (14) Inferior (13) **Right pulmonary veins**
Left auricle (4)
Left atrium (5)
Great cardiac vein
Right atrium (12)
Circumflex branch (6)
Coronary sinus (11)
Oblique vein of left atrium
Inferior vena cava
Left posterior ventricular vein
Small cardiac vein
Right coronary artery (10)
Middle cardiac vein (9)
Left ventricle (7)
Posterior interventricular artery (8)
Right ventricle
Anterior interventricular artery

D. Posteroinferior View

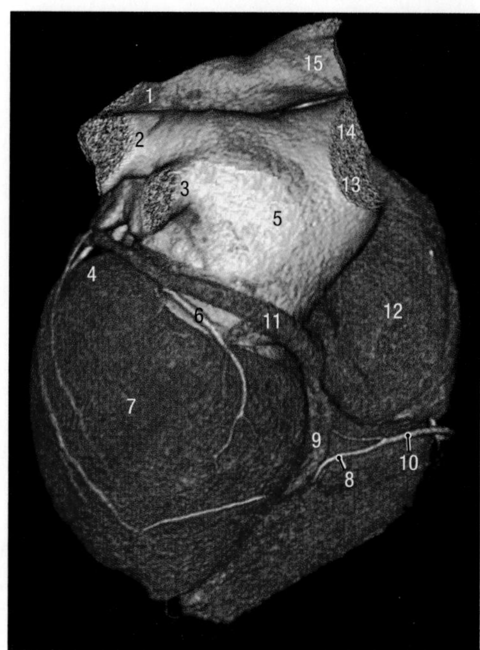
15
1
14
2
3
13
5
4
12
6
11
7
9
8
10

E. Posteroinferior View

1.43 HEART AND GREAT VESSELS (*CONTINUED*)

A. Anatomical specimen

- The right border of the heart, formed by the right atrium, is slightly convex and almost in line with the superior vena cava.
- The inferior border is formed primarily by the right ventricle and part of the left ventricle.
- The left border is formed primarily by the left ventricle and part of the left auricle.

B. 3D volume reconstruction from MRI of heart and coronary vessels (living patient). Numbers refer to structures in **A.**

C. Circulation of blood through the heart

D. Anatomical specimen, posterior view.

- Most of the left atrium and left ventricle are visible in this posteroinferior view.
- The right and left pulmonary veins open into the left atrium.
- The arch of the aorta extends superiorly, posteriorly and to the left, in a nearly sagittal planes.

E. 3D volume reconstruction from MRI of heart and coronary vessels. Numbers refer to structures in **D.**

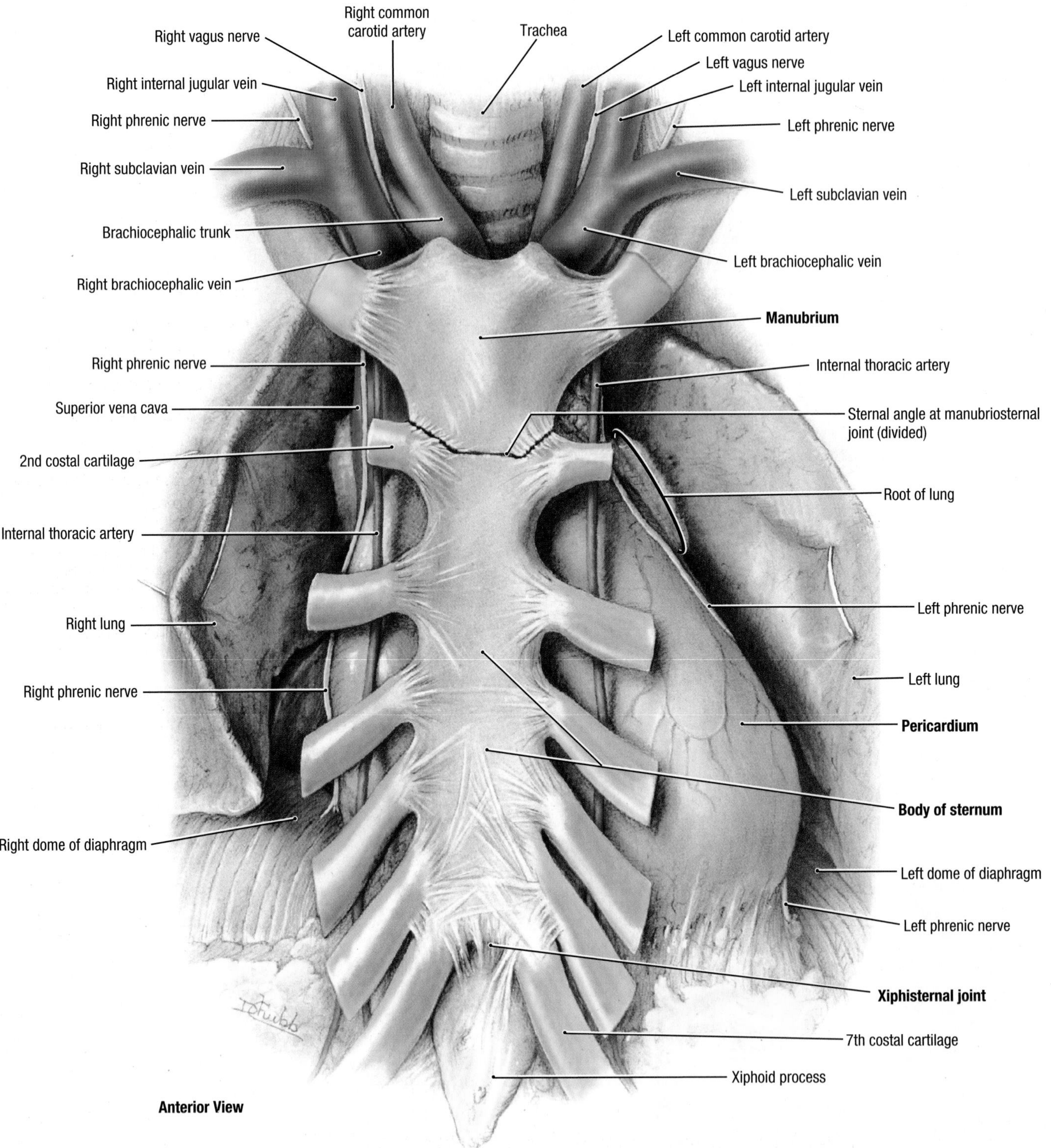
Right vagus nerve
Right common carotid artery
Trachea
Left common carotid artery
Left vagus nerve
Left internal jugular vein
Right internal jugular vein
Right phrenic nerve
Left phrenic nerve
Right subclavian vein
Left subclavian vein
Brachiocephalic trunk
Left brachiocephalic vein
Right brachiocephalic vein
Manubrium
Right phrenic nerve
Internal thoracic artery
Superior vena cava
Sternal angle at manubriosternal joint (divided)
2nd costal cartilage
Root of lung
Internal thoracic artery
Left phrenic nerve
Right lung
Left lung
Right phrenic nerve
Pericardium
Body of sternum
Right dome of diaphragm
Left dome of diaphragm
Left phrenic nerve
Xiphisternal joint
7th costal cartilage
Xiphoid process

Anterior View

1.44 PERICARDIUM IN RELATION TO STERNUM

- The pericardium lies posterior to the body of the sternum, extending from just superior to the sternal angle to the level of the xiphisternal joint; approximately two thirds lies to the left of the median plane.
- The heart lies between the sternum and the anterior mediastinum anteriorly and the vertebral column and the posterior mediastinum posteriorly. In **cardiac compression**, the sternum is depressed 4 to 5 cm, forcing blood out of the heart and into the great vessels.
- Internal thoracic arteries arise from the subclavian arteries and descend posterior to the costal cartilages, running lateral to the sternum and anterior to the pleura.

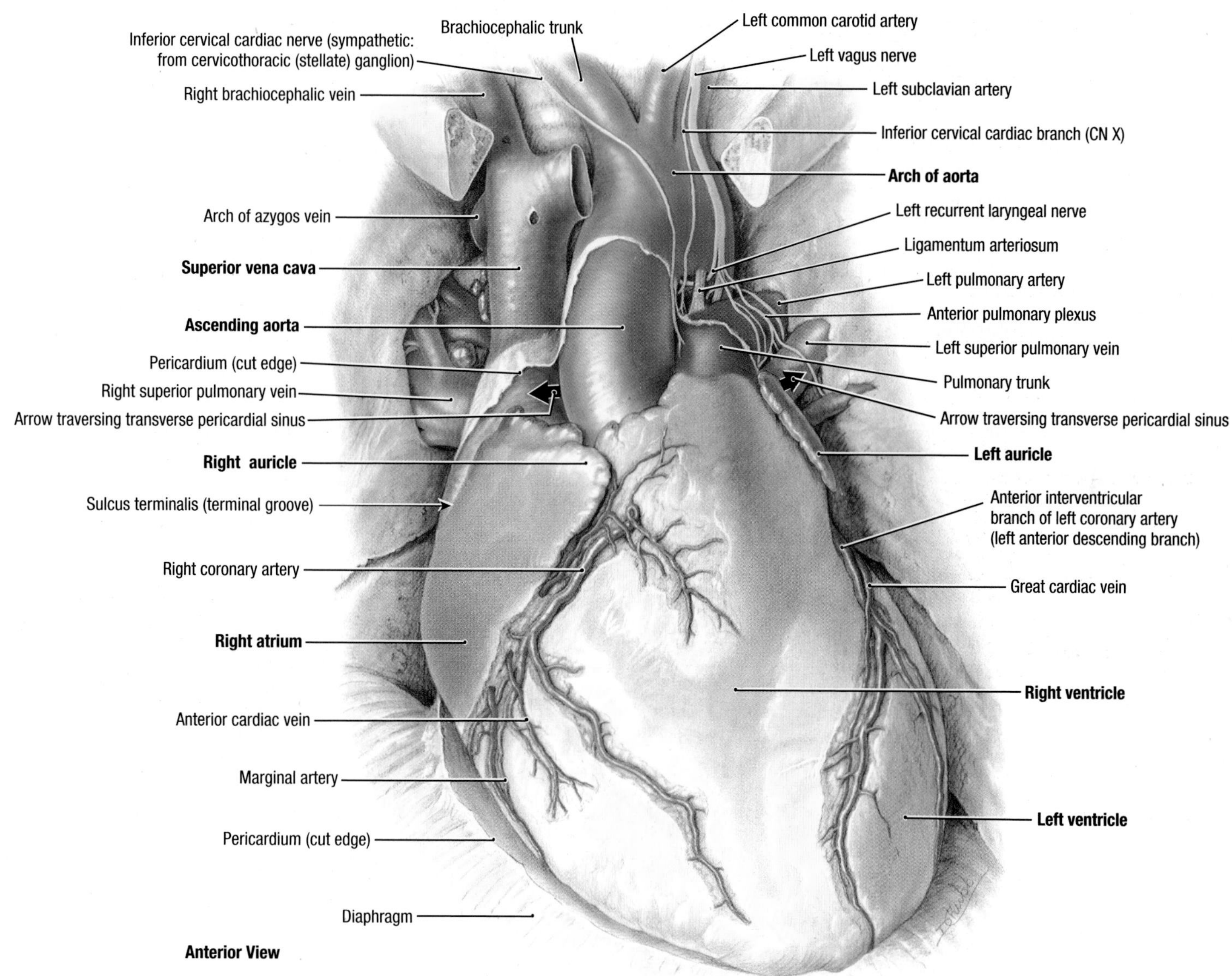
Inferior cervical cardiac nerve (sympathetic: from cervicothoracic (stellate) ganglion)
Brachiocephalic trunk
Left common carotid artery
Left vagus nerve
Left subclavian artery
Right brachiocephalic vein
Inferior cervical cardiac branch (CN X)
Arch of aorta
Arch of azygos vein
Left recurrent laryngeal nerve
Ligamentum arteriosum
Superior vena cava
Left pulmonary artery
Anterior pulmonary plexus
Ascending aorta
Left superior pulmonary vein
Pericardium (cut edge)
Pulmonary trunk
Right superior pulmonary vein
Arrow traversing transverse pericardial sinus
Arrow traversing transverse pericardial sinus
Left auricle
Right auricle
Sulcus terminalis (terminal groove)
Anterior interventricular branch of left coronary artery (left anterior descending branch)
Right coronary artery
Great cardiac vein
Right atrium
Right ventricle
Anterior cardiac vein
Marginal artery
Left ventricle
Pericardium (cut edge)
Diaphragm
Anterior View

1.45 STERNOCOSTAL (ANTERIOR) SURFACE OF HEART AND GREAT VESSELS IN SITU

- The right ventricle forms most of the sternocostal surface.
- The entire right auricle and much of the right atrium are visible anteriorly, but only a small portion of the left auricle is visible; the auricles, like a closing claw, grasp the origins of the pulmonary trunk and ascending aorta from a posterior approach.
- The ligamentum arteriosum passes from the origin of the left pulmonary artery to the arch of the aorta.
- The right coronary artery courses in the anterior atrioventricular groove, and the anterior interventricular branch of the left coronary artery (anterior descending branch) courses in or parallel to the anterior interventricular groove (see Fig. 1.43B).
- The left vagus nerve passes lateral to the arch of the aorta and then posterior to the root of the lung; the left recurrent laryngeal nerve passes inferior to the arch of the aorta posterior to the ligamentum arteriosum.
- The great cardiac vein ascends beside the anterior interventricular branch of the left coronary artery to drain into the coronary sinus posteriorly.

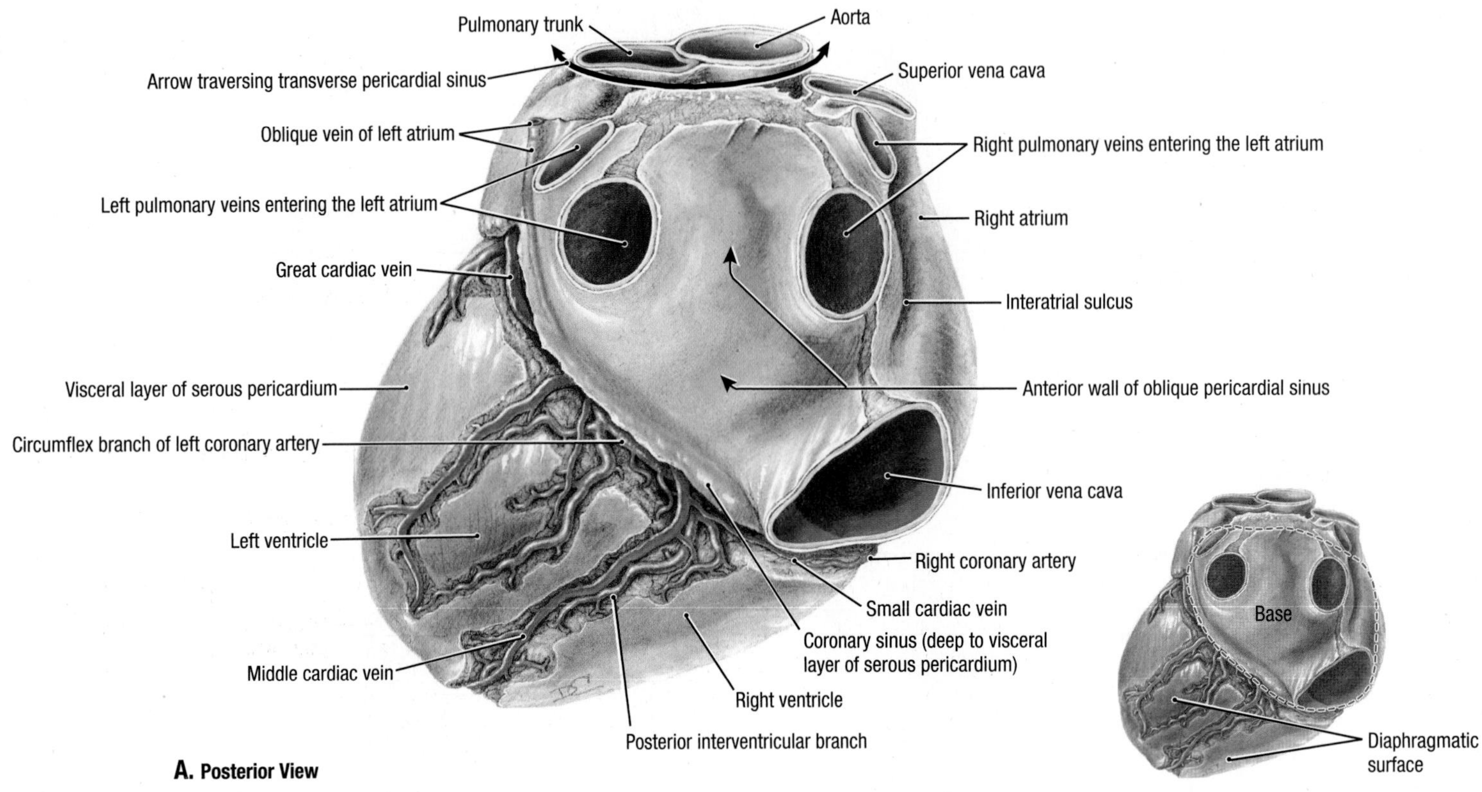
Pulmonary trunk
Aorta
Arrow traversing transverse pericardial sinus
Superior vena cava
Oblique vein of left atrium
Right pulmonary veins entering the left atrium
Left pulmonary veins entering the left atrium
Right atrium
Great cardiac vein
Interatrial sulcus
Visceral layer of serous pericardium
Anterior wall of oblique pericardial sinus
Circumflex branch of left coronary artery
Inferior vena cava
Left ventricle
Right coronary artery
Small cardiac vein
Coronary sinus (deep to visceral layer of serous pericardium)
Middle cardiac vein
Right ventricle
Posterior interventricular branch
Base
Diaphragmatic surface

A. Posterior View

1.46 HEART AND PERICARDIUM

- This heart **(A)** was removed from the interior of the pericardial sac **(B).**
- The entire base, or posterior surface, and part of the diaphragmatic or inferior surface of the heart are in view.
- The superior vena cava and larger inferior vena cava join the superior and inferior aspects of the right atrium.
- The left atrium forms the greater part of the base (posterior surface) of the heart.
- The left coronary artery in this specimen is dominant, since it supplies the posterior interventricular branch.
- Most branches of cardiac veins cross branches of the coronary arteries superficially.
- The visceral layer of serous pericardium (epicardium) covers the surface of the heart and reflects onto the great vessels; from around the great vessels, the serous pericardium reflects to line the internal aspect of the fibrous pericardium as the parietal layer of serous pericardium. The fibrous pericardium and the parietal layer of serous pericardium form the pericardial sac that encases the heart.
- Note the cut edges of the reflections of serous pericardia around the arterial vessels (the pulmonary trunk and aorta) and venous vessels (the superior and inferior venae cavae and the pulmonary veins).
- **Surgical isolation of cardiac outflow.** The transverse pericardial sinus is especially important to cardiac surgeons. After the pericardial sac has been opened anteriorly, a finger can be passed through the transverse pericardial sinus posterior to the aorta and pulmonary trunk. By passing a surgical clamp or placing a ligature around these vessels, inserting the tubes of a coronary bypass machine, and then tightening the ligature, surgeons can stop or divert the circulation of blood in these large arteries while performing cardiac surgery.

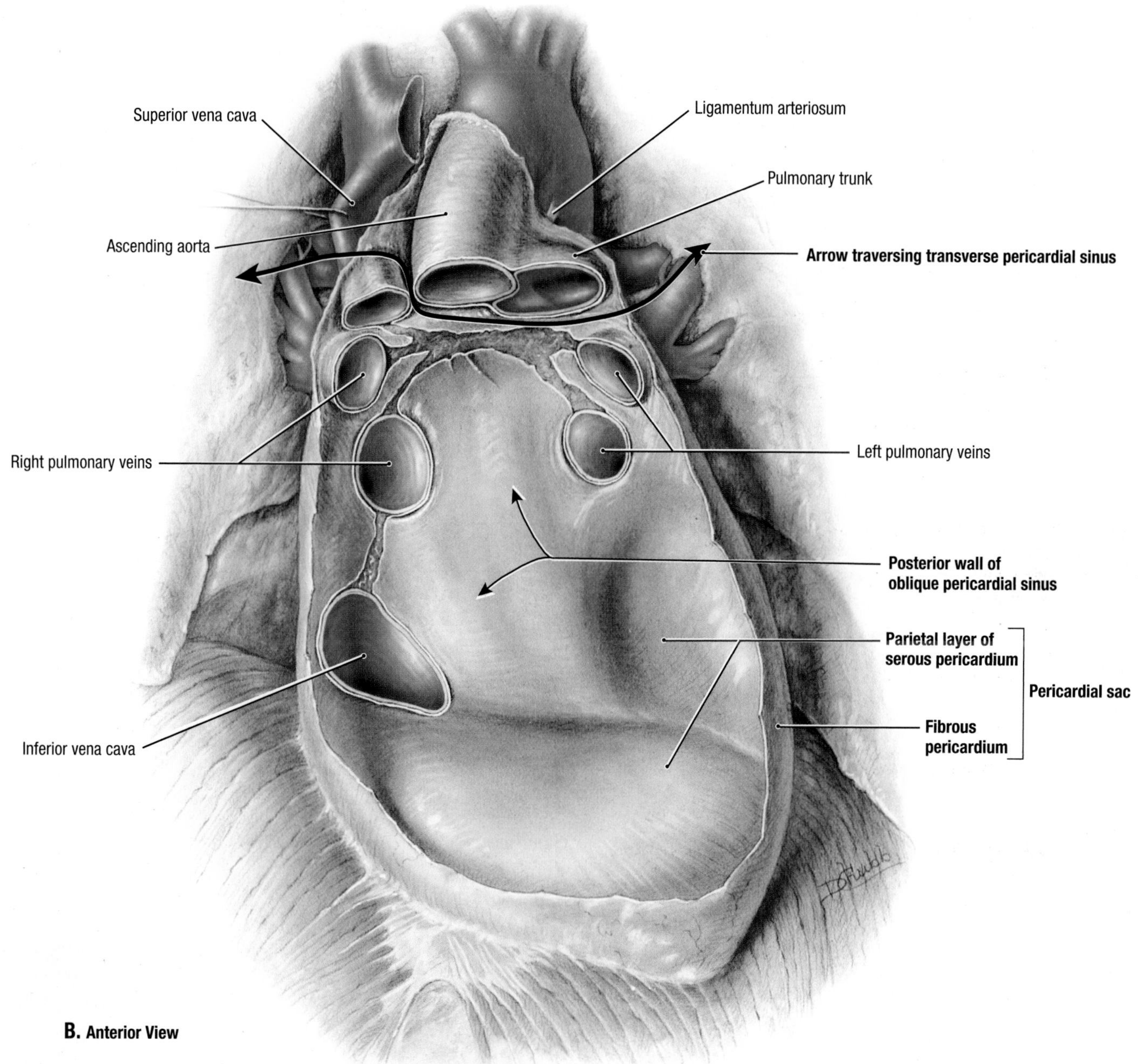
Superior vena cava
Ligamentum arteriosum
Pulmonary trunk
Ascending aorta
Arrow traversing transverse pericardial sinus
Right pulmonary veins
Left pulmonary veins
Posterior wall of oblique pericardial sinus
Parietal layer of serous pericardium
Pericardial sac
Fibrous pericardium
Inferior vena cava

B. **Anterior View**

1.46 HEART AND PERICARDIUM (*CONTINUED*)

- Interior of pericardial sac. Eight vessels were severed to excise the heart: superior and inferior venae cavae, four pulmonary veins, and two pulmonary arteries.
- The oblique sinus is bounded anteriorly by the visceral layer of serous pericardium covering the left atrium **(A)**, posteriorly by the parietal layer of serous pericardium lining the fibrous pericardium, and superiorly and laterally by the reflection of serous pericardium around the four pulmonary veins and the superior and inferior venae cavae **(B)**.
- The transverse sinus is bounded anteriorly by the serous pericardium covering the posterior aspect of the pulmonary trunk and aorta, and posteriorly by the visceral pericardium reflecting from the atria **(A)** inferiorly and the superior vena cava superiorly on the right.
- Blood in the pericardial cavity, **hemopericardium**, produces *cardiac tamponade*. Hemopericardium may result from perforation of a weakened area of the heart muscle owing to a previous **myocardial infarction (MI)** or heart attack, from bleeding into the pericardial cavity after cardiac operations, or from stab wounds. Heart volume is increasingly compromised and circulation fails.

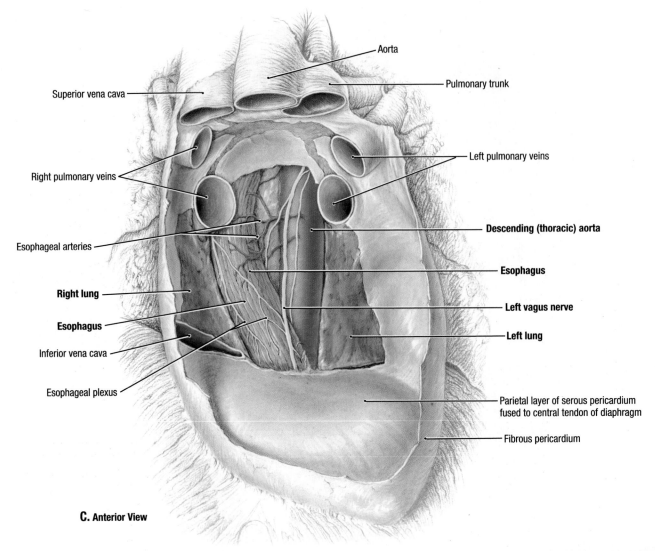

Aorta
Superior vena cava
Pulmonary trunk
Right pulmonary veins
Left pulmonary veins
Esophageal arteries
Descending (thoracic) aorta
Esophagus
Right lung
Left vagus nerve
Esophagus
Left lung
Inferior vena cava
Esophageal plexus
Parietal layer of serous pericardium fused to central tendon of diaphragm
Fibrous pericardium

C. **Anterior View**

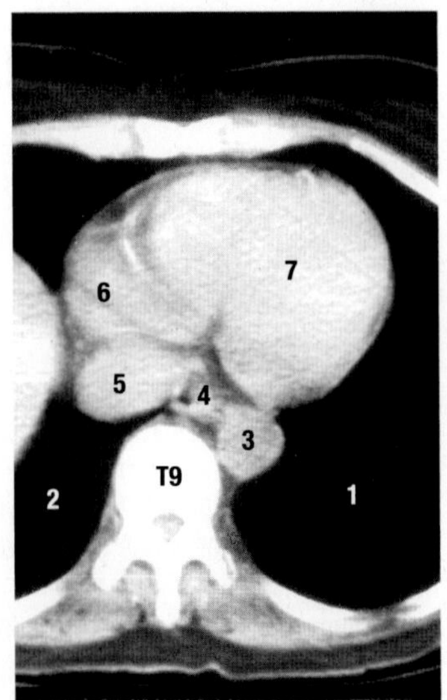

7
6
5
4
3
T9
2
1

D. **Axial CT Scan, Inferior View**

1.46 HEART AND PERICARDIUM (*CONTINUED*)

C. Posterior relationships; dissection. The fibrous and parietal layers of serous pericardium have been removed from posterior and lateral to the oblique sinus. The esophagus in this specimen is deflected to the right; it usually lies in contact with the aorta, forming primary posterior relationships of the heart. **D**. Posterior relationships of heart. Axial computed tomographic (CT) scan at level of T9 vertebra. *1*, left lung; *2*, right lung; *3*, descending aorta; *4*, esophagus; *5*, inferior vena cava; *6*, right atrium; *7*, left ventricle.

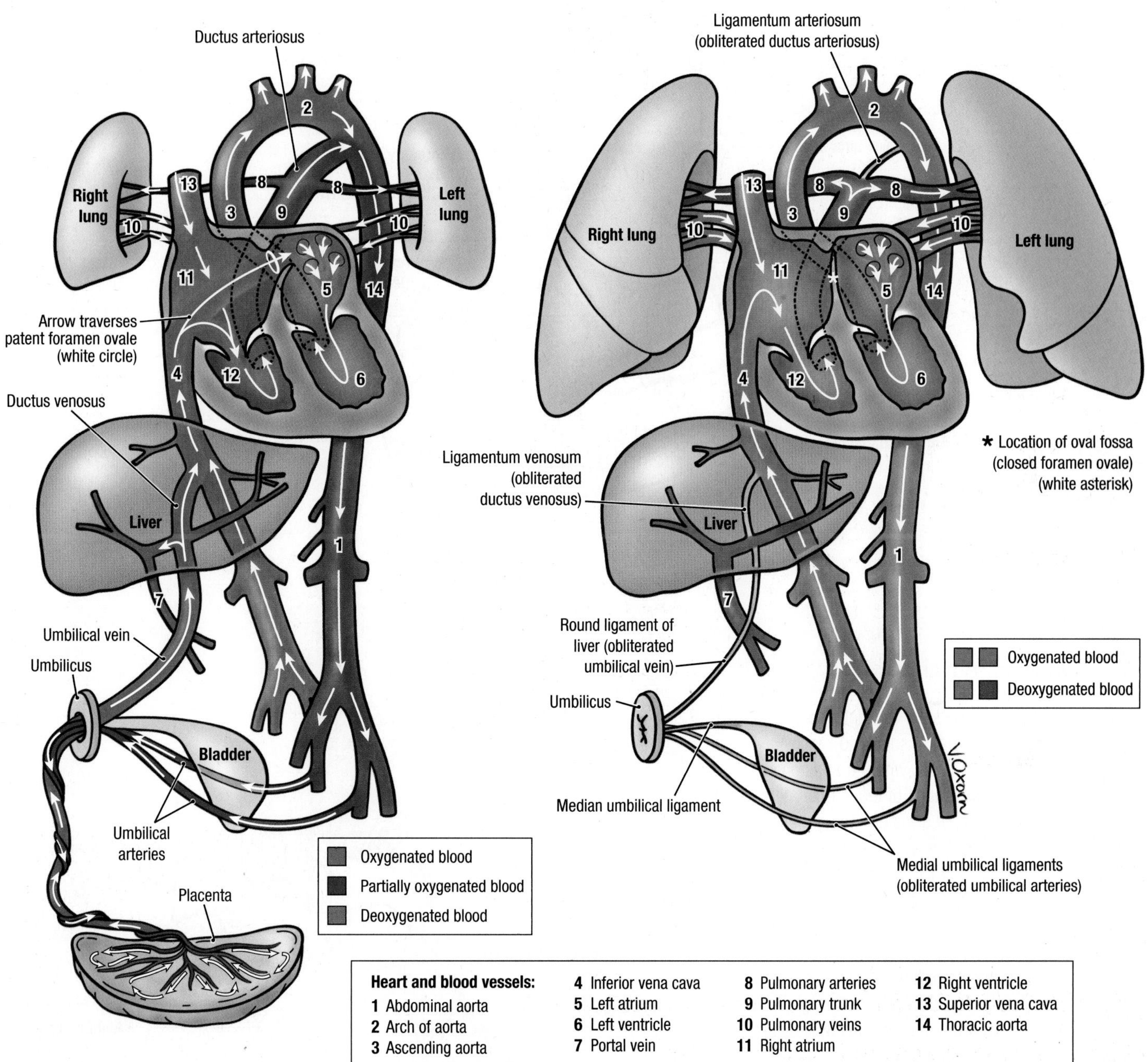
Ductus arteriosus
Right lung
Left lung
Arrow traverses patent foramen ovale (white circle)
Ductus venosus
Liver
Umbilical vein
Umbilicus
Bladder
Umbilical arteries
Placenta
Oxygenated blood
Partially oxygenated blood
Deoxygenated blood
Ligamentum arteriosum (obliterated ductus arteriosus)
Right lung
Left lung
Ligamentum venosum (obliterated ductus venosus)
Liver
* Location of oval fossa (closed foramen ovale) (white asterisk)
Round ligament of liver (obliterated umbilical vein)
Umbilicus
Oxygenated blood
Deoxygenated blood
Bladder
Median umbilical ligament
Medial umbilical ligaments (obliterated umbilical arteries)
V.Oxorn
Heart and blood vessels:
1 Abdominal aorta
2 Arch of aorta
3 Ascending aorta
4 Inferior vena cava
5 Left atrium
6 Left ventricle
7 Portal vein
8 Pulmonary arteries
9 Pulmonary trunk
10 Pulmonary veins
11 Right atrium
12 Right ventricle
13 Superior vena cava
14 Thoracic aorta

1.47 PRE- AND POSTNATAL CIRCULATION

At birth two major changes take place: (1) pulmonary respiration starts and (2) after the umbilical cord is ligated, the umbilical arteries (except the most proximal part), umbilical vein, and ductus venosus are occluded and become ligaments.

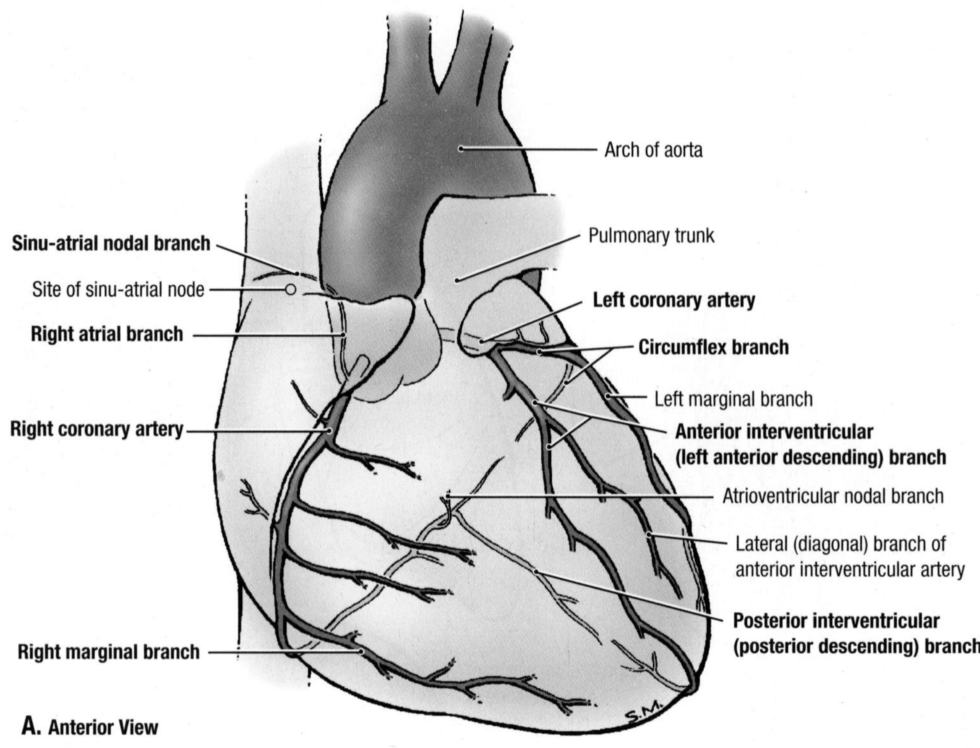
Arch of aorta
Pulmonary trunk
Sinu-atrial nodal branch
Site of sinu-atrial node
Left coronary artery
Right atrial branch
Circumflex branch
Left marginal branch
Right coronary artery
Anterior interventricular (left anterior descending) branch
Atrioventricular nodal branch
Lateral (diagonal) branch of anterior interventricular artery
Posterior interventricular (posterior descending) branch
Right marginal branch
S.M.

A. Anterior View

1.48 CORONARY ARTERIES

- In the most common pattern, the right coronary artery travels in the coronary sulcus to reach the posterior surface of the heart, where it anastomoses with the circumflex branch of the left coronary artery. Early in its course, it gives off the right atrial branch, which supplies the sinu-atrial (SA) node via its sinu-atrial nodal branch. Major branches are a marginal branch supplying much of the anterior wall of the right ventricle, an atrioventricular (AV) nodal branch given off near the posterior border of the interventricular septum, and a posterior interventricular branch in the interventricular groove that anastomoses with the anterior interventricular branch of the left coronary artery.
- The left coronary artery divides into a circumflex branch that passes posteriorly to anastomose with the right coronary artery on the posterior aspect of the heart and an anterior descending branch in the interventricular groove; the origin of the SA nodal branch is variable and may be a branch of the left coronary artery.
- The interventricular septum receives its blood supply from septal branches of the two interventricular (descending) branches: typically the anterior two thirds from the left coronary, and the posterior one third from the right (see Fig. 1.51A).

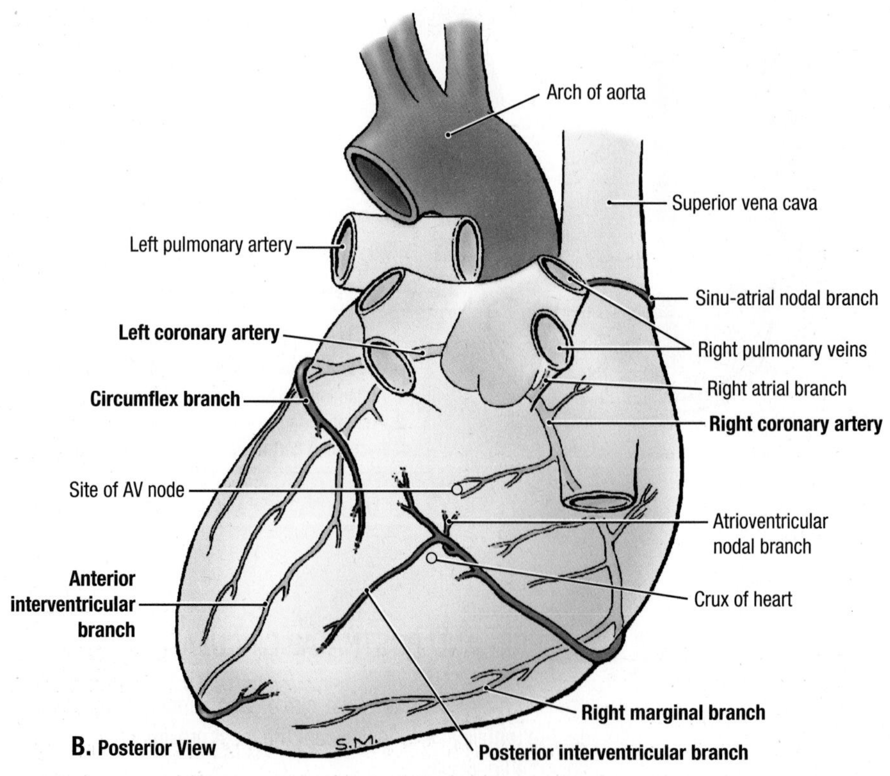
Arch of aorta
Superior vena cava
Left pulmonary artery
Sinu-atrial nodal branch
Left coronary artery
Right pulmonary veins
Right atrial branch
Circumflex branch
Right coronary artery
Site of AV node
Atrioventricular nodal branch
Anterior interventricular branch
Crux of heart
Right marginal branch
Posterior interventricular branch
S.M.

B. Posterior View

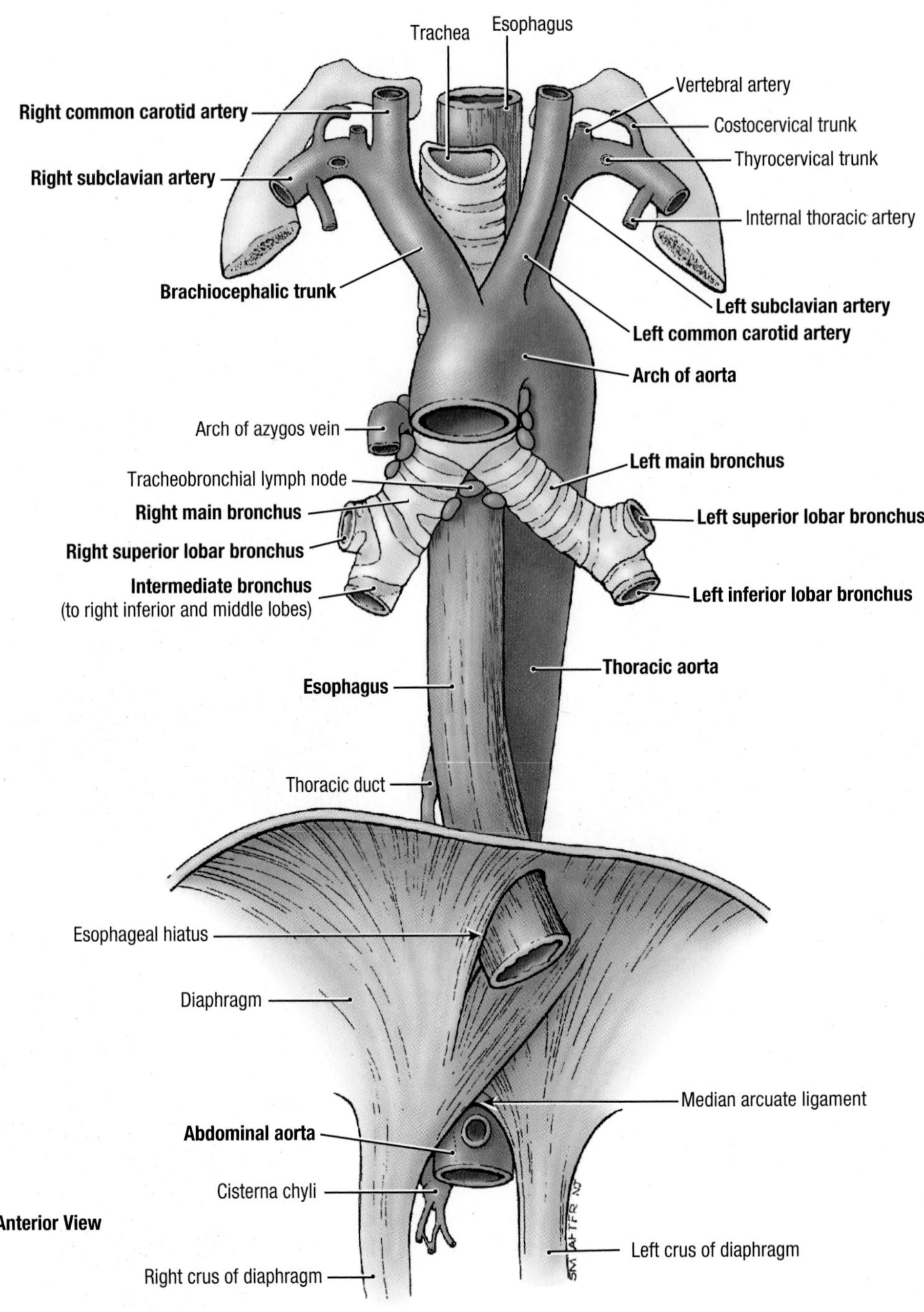
Trachea
Esophagus
Right common carotid artery
Right subclavian artery
Vertebral artery
Costocervical trunk
Thyrocervical trunk
Internal thoracic artery
Brachiocephalic trunk
Left subclavian artery
Left common carotid artery
Arch of aorta
Arch of azygos vein
Tracheobronchial lymph node
Left main bronchus
Right main bronchus
Left superior lobar bronchus
Right superior lobar bronchus
Intermediate bronchus
(to right inferior and middle lobes)
Left inferior lobar bronchus
Thoracic aorta
Esophagus
Thoracic duct
Esophageal hiatus
Diaphragm
Median arcuate ligament
Abdominal aorta
Cisterna chyli
Anterior View
Left crus of diaphragm
Right crus of diaphragm

1.68 ESOPHAGUS, TRACHEA, AND AORTA

- The anterior relations of the thoracic part of the esophagus from superior to inferior are the trachea (from origin at cricoid cartilage to bifurcation), right and left bronchi, inferior tracheobronchial lymph nodes, pericardium (not shown) and, finally, the diaphragm.
- The arch of the aorta passes posterior to the left of these four structures as it arches over the left main bronchus; the arch of the azygos vein passes anterior to their right as it arches over the right main bronchus.
- The impressions produced in the esophagus by adjacent structures (aorta, left main bronchus, and esophageal hiatus) are of clinical interest because of the slower passage of substances at these sites. The impressions indicate where swallowed foreign objects are most likely to lodge and where a stricture may develop after the accidental drinking of a caustic liquid such as lye.

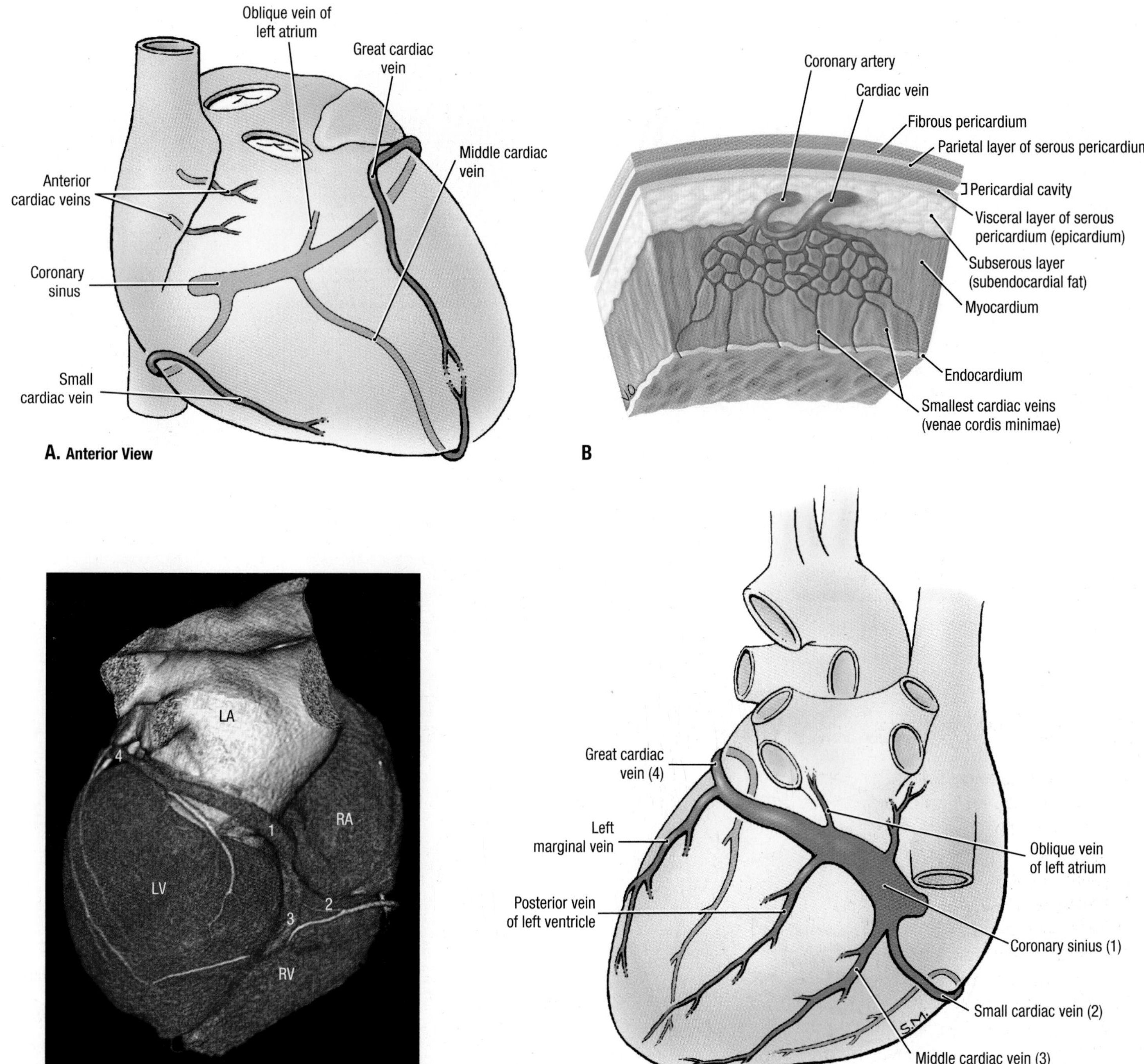
Oblique vein of left atrium
Great cardiac vein
Middle cardiac vein
Anterior cardiac veins
Coronary sinus
Small cardiac vein
Coronary artery
Cardiac vein
Fibrous pericardium
Parietal layer of serous pericardium
Pericardial cavity
Visceral layer of serous pericardium (epicardium)
Subserous layer (subendocardial fat)
Myocardium
Endocardium
Smallest cardiac veins (venae cordis minimae)
LA
RA
LV
RV
1
2
3
4
Great cardiac vein (4)
Left marginal vein
Posterior vein of left ventricle
Oblique vein of left atrium
Coronary sinius (1)
Small cardiac vein (2)
Middle cardiac vein (3)

A. **Anterior View**

B

C. **Posteroinferior View**

D. **Posteroinferior View**

1.49 CARDIAC VEINS

A. Anterior aspect. **B.** Smallest cardiac veins. **C.** 3D volume reconstruction. Numbers refer to veins in **D.** *LA*, left atrium; *RA*, right atrium; *LV*, left ventricle; *RV*, right ventricle. **D.** Posteroinferior aspect.

The coronary sinus is the major venous drainage vessel of the heart; it is located posteriorly in the atrioventricular (coronary) groove and drains into the right atrium. The great, middle, and small cardiac veins; the oblique vein of the left atrium; and the posterior vein of the left ventricle are the principal vessels draining into the coronary sinus. The anterior cardiac veins drain directly into the right atrium. The smallest cardiac veins (venae cordis minimae) drain the myocardium directly into the atria and ventricles **(B).** The cardiac veins accompany the coronary arteries and their branches.

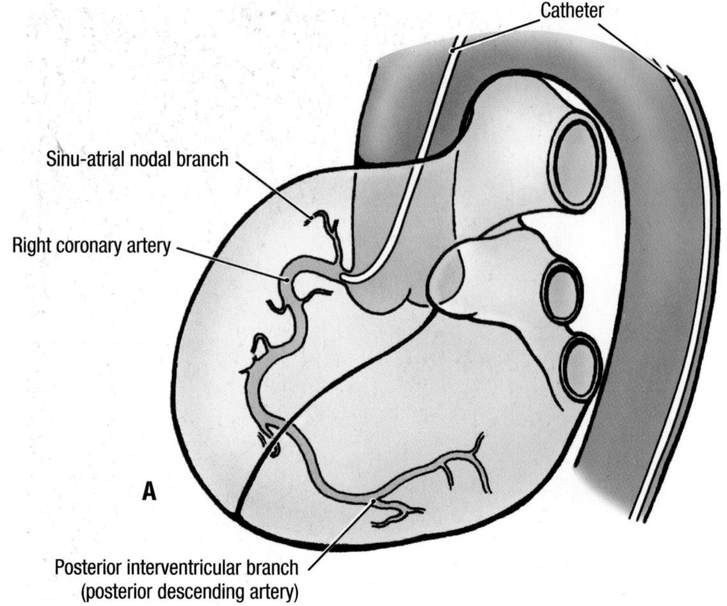
Catheter
Sinu-atrial nodal branch
Right coronary artery
A
Posterior interventricular branch
(posterior descending artery)

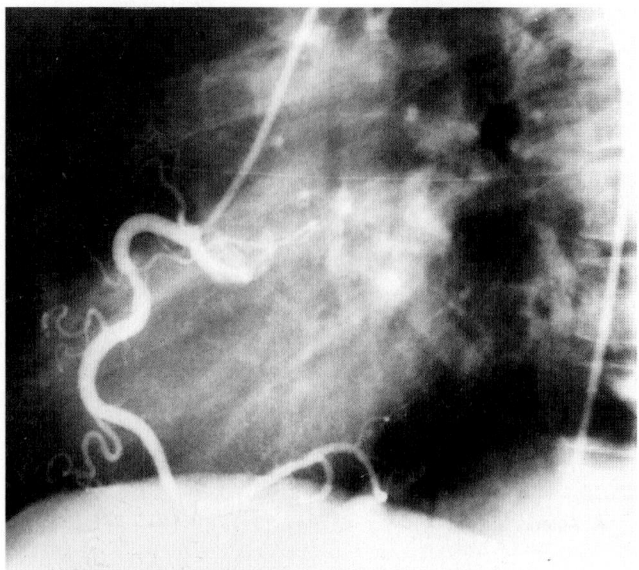

B. **Left Anterior Oblique View**

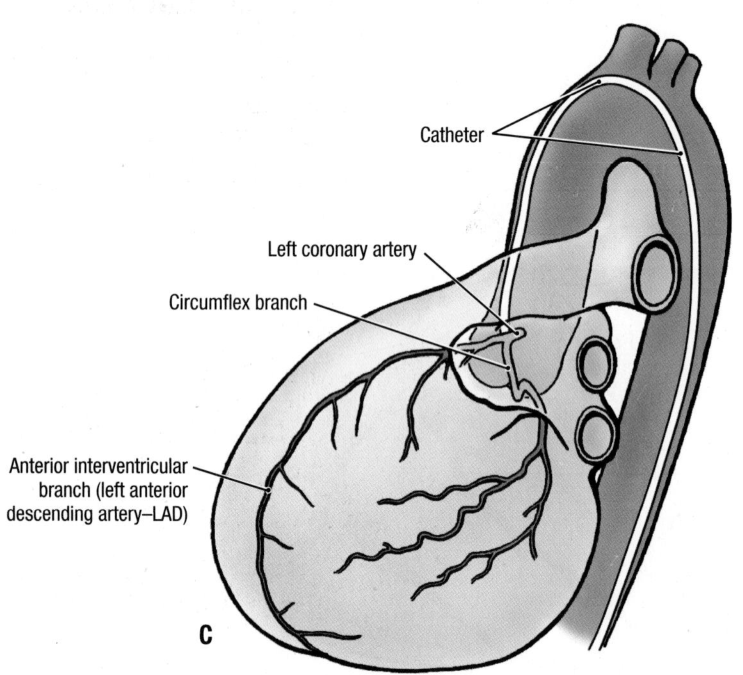
Catheter
Left coronary artery
Circumflex branch
Anterior interventricular
branch (left anterior
descending artery–LAD)
C

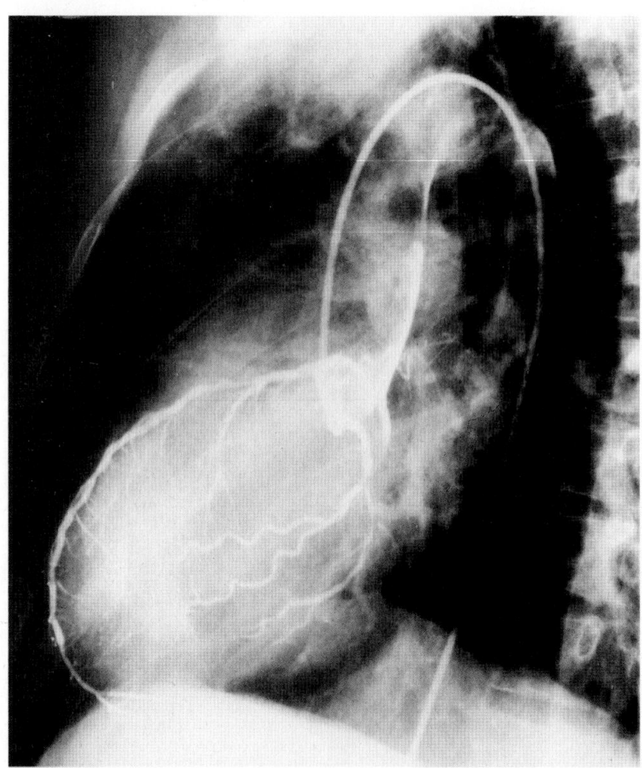

D. **Left Anterior Oblique View**

1.50 CORONARY ARTERIOGRAMS WITH ORIENTATION DRAWINGS

Right (**A** and **B**) and left (**C** and **D**) coronary arteriograms.

Coronary artery disease (CAD), one of the leading causes of death, results in a reduced blood supply to the vital myocardial tissue. The three most common sites of coronary artery occlusion and the approximate percentage of occlusions involving each artery are the (1) anterior interventricular (clinically referred to as LAD) branch of the left coronary artery (LCA) (40% to 50%); (2) right coronary artery (RCA), (30% to 40%); (3) circumflex branch of the LCA (15% to 20%).

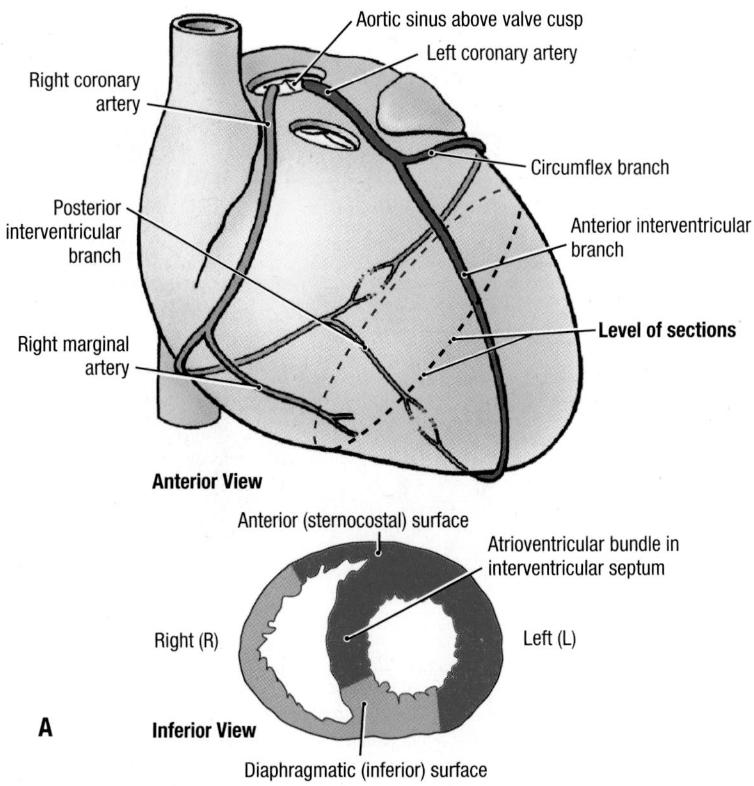
Aortic sinus above valve cusp
Left coronary artery
Right coronary artery
Circumflex branch
Posterior interventricular branch
Anterior interventricular branch
Level of sections
Right marginal artery
Anterior View
Anterior (sternocostal) surface
Atrioventricular bundle in interventricular septum
Right (R)
Left (L)
A
Inferior View
Diaphragmatic (inferior) surface

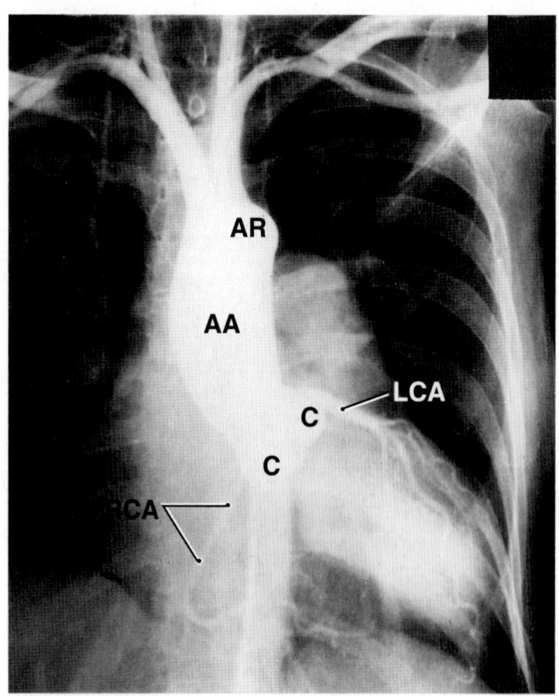
AR
AA
LCA
C
C
RCA

B. Coronary Angiogram, Anteroposterior View

KEY for B:			
AA	Ascending aorta	LCA	Left coronary artery
AR	Arch of aorta	RCA	Right coronary artery
C	Cusp of aortic valve		

A. and B. Most common pattern (67%). Right coronary artery is dominant, giving rise to the posterior interventricular branch.

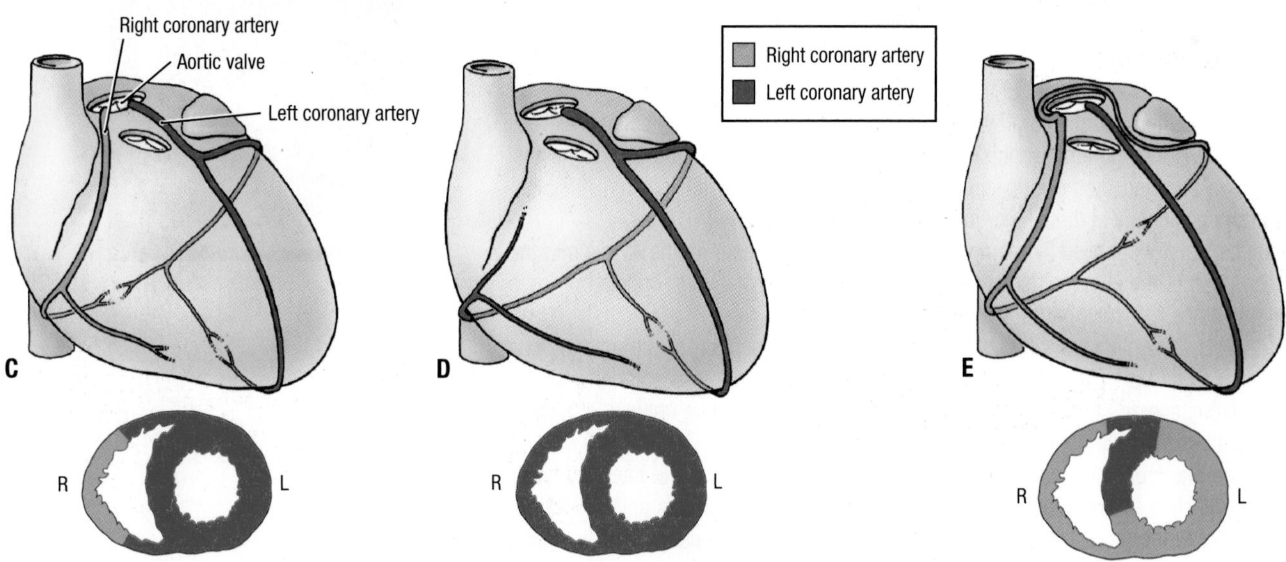
Right coronary artery
Aortic valve
Left coronary artery
Right coronary artery
Left coronary artery
C
D
E
R
L
R
L
R
L

C. and D. Left coronary artery gives rise to the posterior interventricular branch (15%).

E. Circumflex branch emerging from right coronary sinus.

1.51 CORONARY CIRCULATION

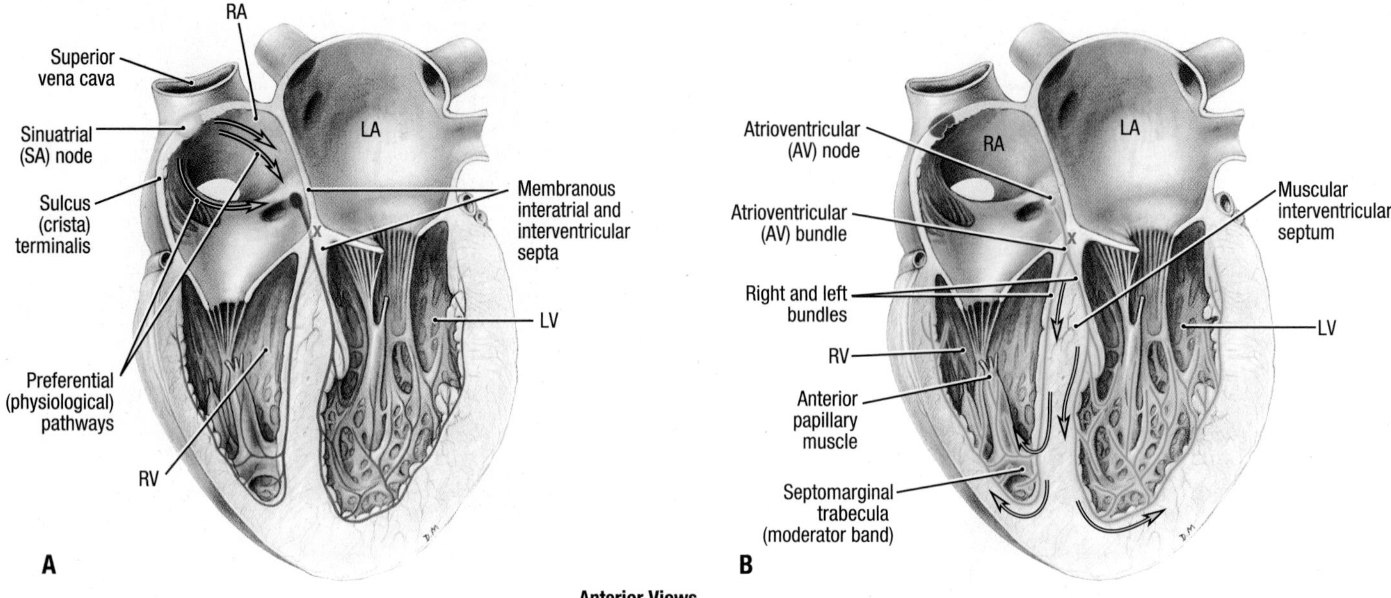
RA
Superior vena cava
Sinuatrial (SA) node
Sulcus (crista) terminalis
Preferential (physiological) pathways
RV
LA
Membranous interatrial and interventricular septa
LV
A
Atrioventricular (AV) node
Atrioventricular (AV) bundle
Right and left bundles
RV
Anterior papillary muscle
Septomarginal trabecula (moderator band)
RA
LA
Muscular interventricular septum
LV
B

Anterior Views

RV Right ventricle	LV Left ventricle
x Crux of heart	
RA Right atrium	LA Left atrium

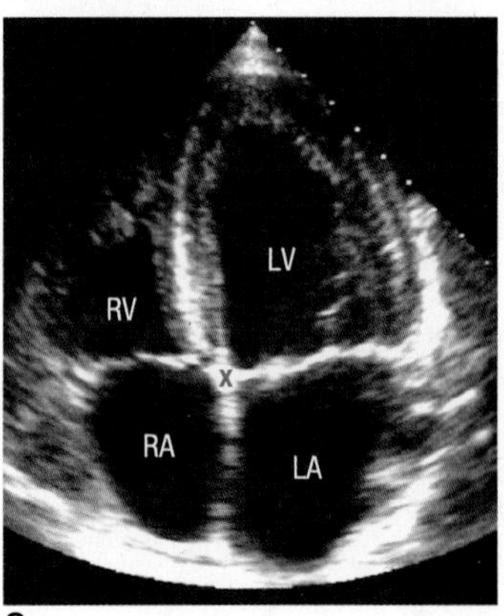
LV
RV
RA
LA
x

C

1.52 CONDUCTION SYSTEM OF HEART, CORONAL SECTION

A. Impulses (*arrows*) initiated at the sinu-atrial node. **B.** Atrioventricular (AV) node, AV bundle, and bundle branches. **C.** Echocardiogram, apical four-chamber view.

- The sinu-atrial (SA) node in the wall of the right atrium near the superior end of the sulcus terminalis (internally crista terminalis) extends over the opening of the superior vena cava. The SA node is the "pacemaker" of the heart because it initiates muscle contraction and determines the heart rate. It is supplied by the sinuatrial nodal artery, usually a branch of the right atrial branch of the right coronary artery, but it may arise from the left coronary artery.
- Contraction spreads through the atrial wall (myogenic induction) until it reaches the atrioventricular (AV) node in the interatrial septum superomedial to the opening of the coronary sinus. The AV node is supplied by the atrioventricular nodal artery, usually arising from the right coronary artery posteriorly at the inferior margin of the interatrial septum.
- The AV bundle, usually supplied by the right coronary artery, passes from the AV node in the membranous part of the interventricular septum, dividing into right and left bundle branches on either side of the muscular part of the interventricular septum.
- The right bundle branch travels inferiorly in the interventricular septum to the anterior wall of the ventricle, with part passing via the septomarginal trabecula to the anterior papillary muscle; excitation spreads throughout the right ventricular wall through a network of subendocardial branches from the right bundle (Purkinje fibers).
- The left bundle branch lies beneath the endocardium on the left side of the interventricular septum and branches to enter the anterior and posterior papillary muscles and the wall of the left ventricle; further branching into a plexus of subendocardial branches (Purkinje fibers) allows the impulses to be conveyed throughout the left ventricular wall. The bundle branches are mostly supplied by the left coronary artery except the posterior limb of the left bundle branch, which is supplied by both coronary arteries.
- **Damage to the cardiac conduction system** (often by compromised blood supply as in coronary artery disease) leads to disturbances of muscle contraction. Damage to the AV node results in "heart block" because the atrial excitation wave does not reach the ventricles, which begin to contract independently at their own slower rate. Damage to one of the bundle branches results in "bundle branch block," in which excitation goes down the unaffected branch to cause systole of that ventricle; the impulse then spreads to the other ventricle, producing later asynchronous contraction.

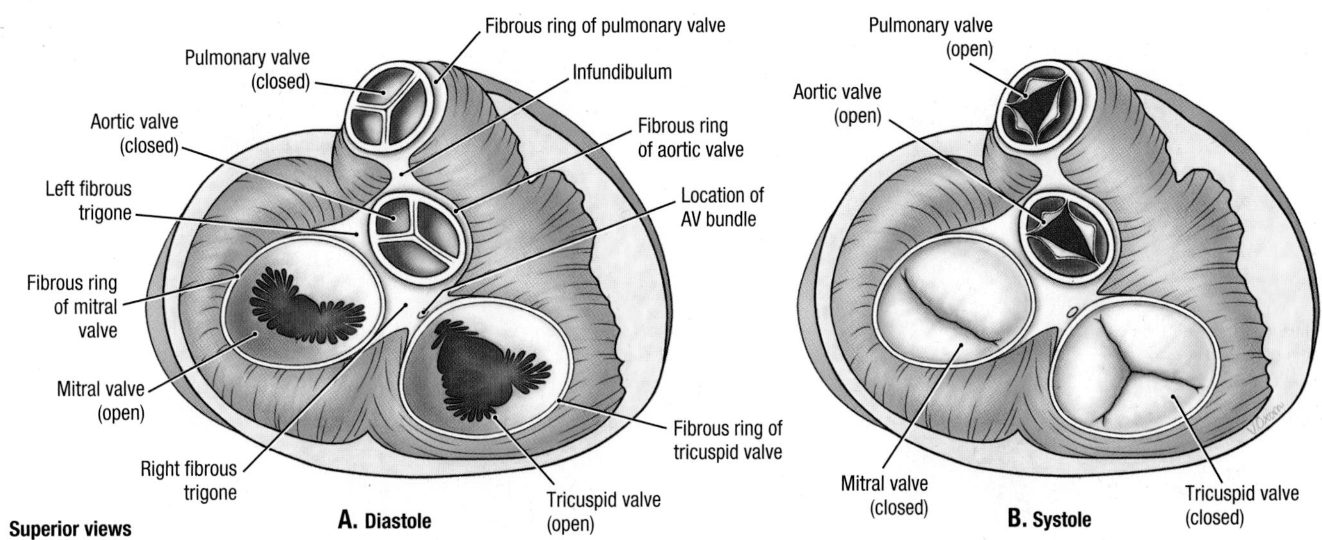
Fibrous ring of pulmonary valve
Pulmonary valve (closed)
Infundibulum
Aortic valve (closed)
Fibrous ring of aortic valve
Left fibrous trigone
Location of AV bundle
Fibrous ring of mitral valve
Mitral valve (open)
Fibrous ring of tricuspid valve
Right fibrous trigone
Tricuspid valve (open)
Superior views
A. Diastole
Pulmonary valve (open)
Aortic valve (open)
Mitral valve (closed)
B. Systole
Tricuspid valve (closed)

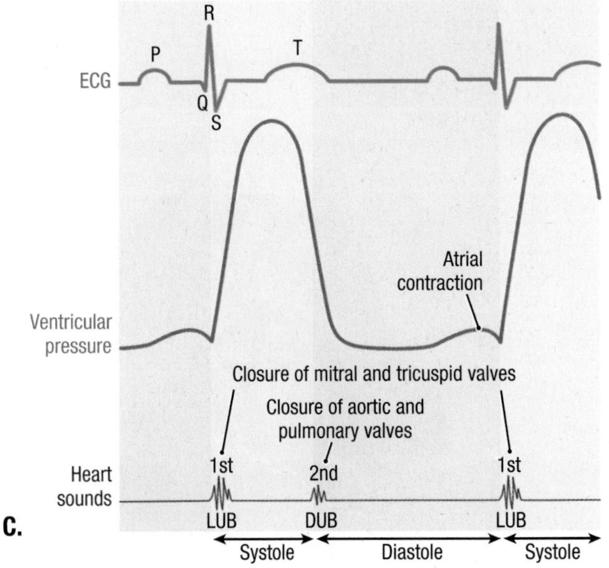
R
P
T
ECG
Q
S
Atrial contraction
Ventricular pressure
Closure of mitral and tricuspid valves
Closure of aortic and pulmonary valves
Heart sounds
1st
2nd
1st
LUB
DUB
LUB
Systole
Diastole
Systole
C.

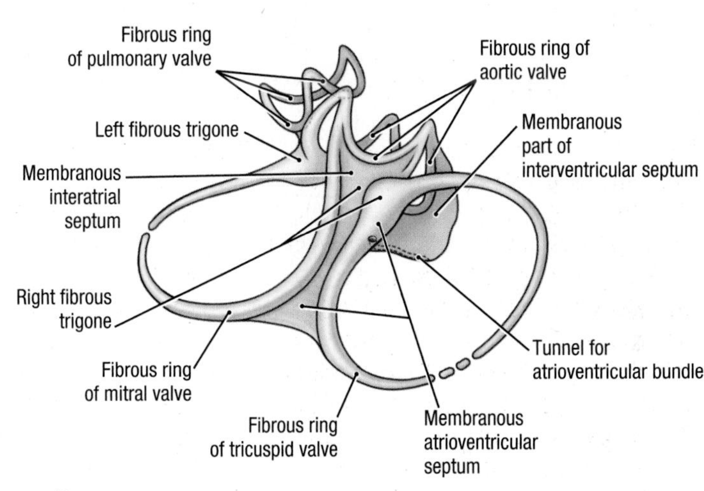
Fibrous ring of pulmonary valve
Fibrous ring of aortic valve
Left fibrous trigone
Membranous part of interventricular septum
Membranous interatrial septum
Right fibrous trigone
Tunnel for atrioventricular bundle
Fibrous ring of mitral valve
Fibrous ring of tricuspid valve
Membranous atrioventricular septum
D. Posteroinferior view

1.53 CARDIAC CYCLE AND CARDIAC SKELETON

A. Ventricular diastole. **B.** Ventricular systole. **C.** Correlation of ventricular pressure, electrocardiogram (ECG), and heart sounds. The cardiac cycle describes the complete movement of the heart or heartbeat and includes the period from the beginning of one heartbeat to the beginning of the next one. The cycle consists of diastole (ventricular relaxation and filling) and systole (ventricular contraction and emptying). The right heart is the pump for the pulmonary circuit; the left heart is the pump for the systemic circuit. (see Fig. 1.43C). **D.** Cardiac skeleton. The fibrous framework of dense collagen forms four fibrous rings, which provide attachment for the leaflets and cusps of the valves, and two fibrous trigones that connect the rings, and the membranous parts of the interatrial and interventricular septa. The fibrous skeleton keeps the orifices of the valves patent and separates the myenterically conducted impulses of the atria.

Disorders involving the valves of the heart disturb the pumping efficiency of the heart. **Valvular heart disease** produces either stenosis (narrowing) or insufficiency. **Valvular stenosis** is the failure of a valve to open fully, slowing blood flow from a chamber. **Valvular insufficiency**, or regurgitation, is the failure of the valve to close completely, usually owing to nodule formation on (or scarring and contraction of) the cusps so that the edges do not meet or align. This allows a variable amount of blood (depending on the severity) to flow back into the chamber it was just ejected from. Both stenosis and insufficiency result in an increased workload for the heart. Because valvular diseases are mechanical problems, damaged or defective cardiac valves are often replaced surgically in a procedure called **valvuloplasty**.

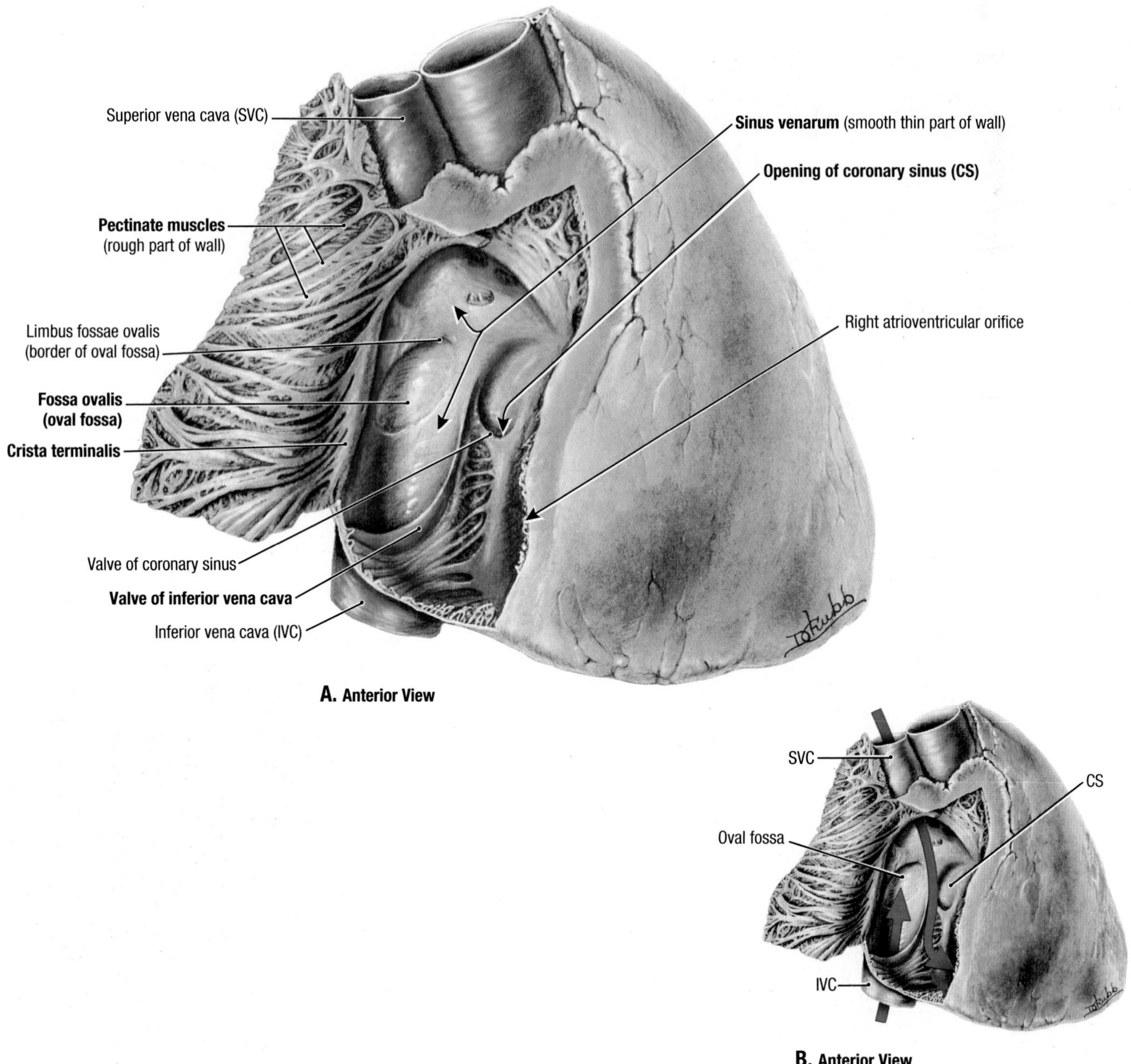
Superior vena cava (SVC)
Sinus venarum (smooth thin part of wall)
Opening of coronary sinus (CS)
Pectinate muscles (rough part of wall)
Right atrioventricular orifice
Limbus fossae ovalis (border of oval fossa)
Fossa ovalis (oval fossa)
Crista terminalis
Valve of coronary sinus
Valve of inferior vena cava
Inferior vena cava (IVC)
SVC
CS
Oval fossa
IVC

A. Anterior View

B. Anterior View

1.54 RIGHT ATRIUM

A. Interior of right atrium. The anterior wall of the right atrium is reflected. **B.** Blood flow into atrium from the superior and inferior vena cavae.

- The smooth part of the atrial wall is formed by the absorption of the right horn of the sinus venosus, and the rough part is formed from the primitive atrium.
- Crista terminalis, the valve of the inferior vena cava, and the valve of the coronary sinus separate the smooth part from the rough part.
- The pectinate muscle passes anteriorly from the crista terminalis; the crista underlies the sulcus terminalis (not shown), a groove visible externally on the posterolateral surface of the right atrium between the superior and inferior venae cavae.
- The superior and inferior venae cavae and the coronary sinus open onto the smooth part of the right atrium; the anterior cardiac veins and venae cordis minimae (not visible) also open into the atrium.
- The floor of the fossa is the remnant of the fetal septum primum; the crescent-shaped ridge (limbus fossae ovalis) partially surrounding the fossa is the remnant of the septum secundum.
- In **B,** the inflow from the superior vena cava is directed toward the tricuspid orifice, whereas blood from the inferior vena cava is directed toward the fossa ovalis.
- Congenital anomalies of the interatrial septum, most often incomplete closure of the oval foramen (patent foramen ovale), are **atrial septal defects (ASDs)**. A probe-size patency is present in the superior part of the oval fossa in 15% to 25% of adults (Moore and Persaud, 2008). These small openings, by themselves, cause no hemodynamic abnormalities. Large ASDs allow oxygenated blood from the lungs to be shunted from the left atrium through the ASD into the right atrium, causing enlargement of the right atrium and ventricle and dilation of the pulmonary trunk.

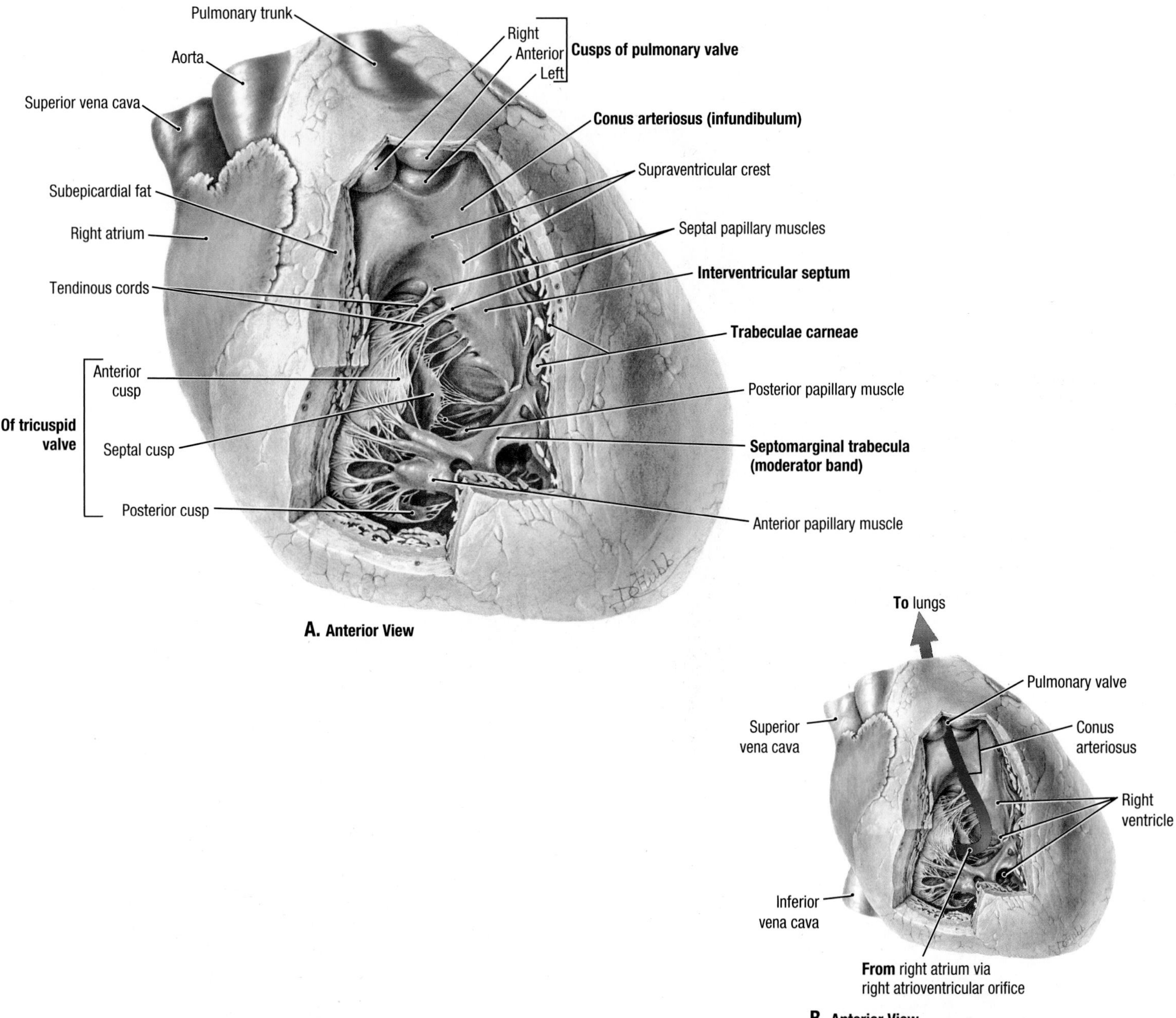
Pulmonary trunk
Aorta
Superior vena cava
Right
Anterior
Left
Cusps of pulmonary valve
Conus arteriosus (infundibulum)
Supraventricular crest
Subepicardial fat
Right atrium
Septal papillary muscles
Interventricular septum
Tendinous cords
Trabeculae carneae
Anterior cusp
Posterior papillary muscle
Of tricuspid valve
Septal cusp
Septomarginal trabecula (moderator band)
Posterior cusp
Anterior papillary muscle
To lungs
Pulmonary valve
Superior vena cava
Conus arteriosus
Right ventricle
Inferior vena cava
From right atrium via right atrioventricular orifice

A. Anterior View

B. Anterior View

1.55 RIGHT VENTRICLE

A. Interior of right ventricle. **B.** Blood flow through right heart.

- The entrance to this chamber, the right atrioventricular or tricuspid orifice, is situated posteriorly; the exit, the orifice of the pulmonary trunk, is superior.
- The outflow portion of the chamber inferior to the pulmonary orifice (conus arteriosus or infundibulum) has a smooth, funnel-shaped wall; the remainder of the ventricle is rough with fleshy trabeculae.
- There are three types of trabeculae: mere ridges, bridges attached only at each end, and fingerlike projections called papillary muscles. The anterior papillary muscle rises from the anterior wall, the posterior (papillary muscle) from the posterior wall, and a series of small septal papillae from the septal wall.
- The septomarginal trabecula, here thick, extends from the septum to the base of the anterior papillary muscle.
- The membranous part of the interventricular septum develops separately from the muscular part and has a complex embryological origin (Moore and Persaud, 2008). Consequently, this part is the common site of *ventricular septal defects* (VSDs), although defects also occur in the muscular part. VSDs rank first on all lists of cardiac defects. The size of the defect varies from 1 to 25 mm. A VSD causes a left-to-right shunt of blood through the defect. A large shunt increases pulmonary blood flow, which causes severe pulmonary disease (*pulmonary hypertension*, or increased blood pressure) and may cause *cardiac failure*.

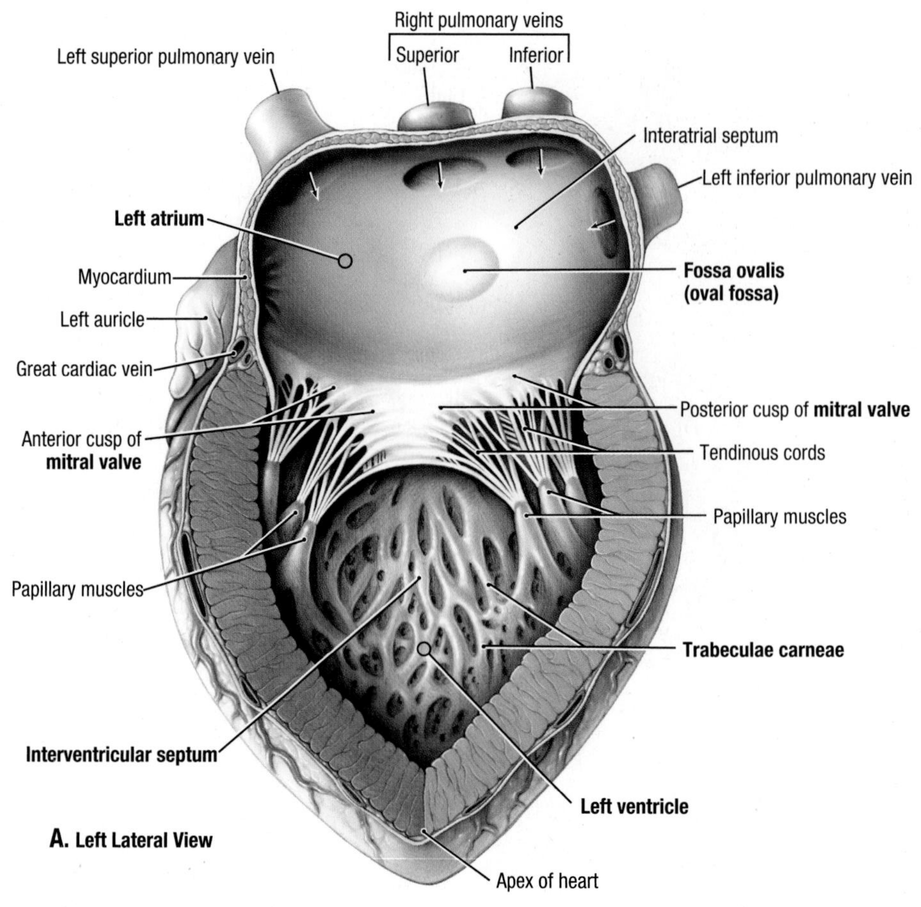
Right pulmonary veins
Superior
Inferior
Left superior pulmonary vein
Interatrial septum
Left inferior pulmonary vein
Left atrium
Myocardium
Left auricle
Great cardiac vein
Fossa ovalis (oval fossa)
Posterior cusp of mitral valve
Anterior cusp of mitral valve
Tendinous cords
Papillary muscles
Papillary muscles
Trabeculae carneae
Interventricular septum
Left ventricle
Apex of heart

A. Left Lateral View

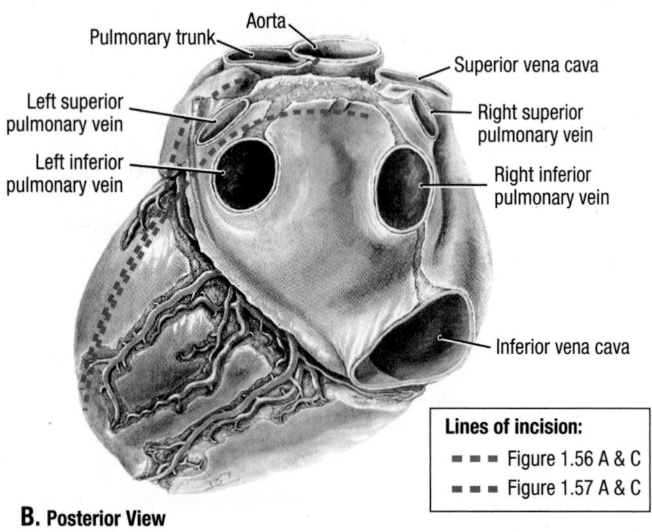
Aorta
Pulmonary trunk
Superior vena cava
Left superior pulmonary vein
Right superior pulmonary vein
Left inferior pulmonary vein
Right inferior pulmonary vein
Inferior vena cava
Lines of incision:
Figure 1.56 A & C
Figure 1.57 A & C

B. Posterior View

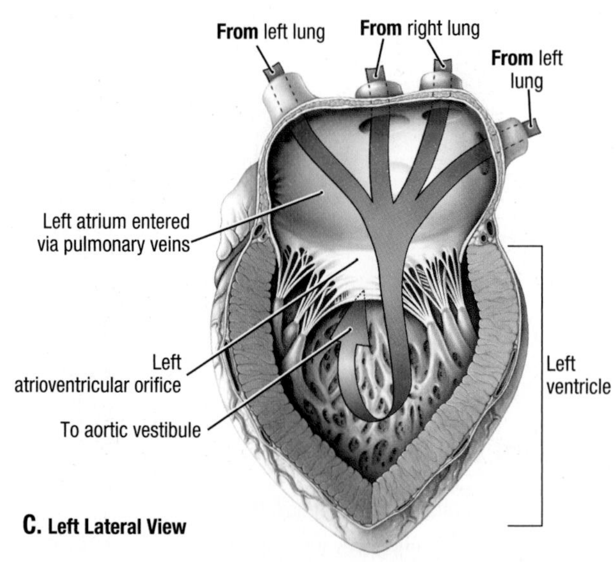
From left lung
From right lung
From left lung
Left atrium entered via pulmonary veins
Left atrioventricular orifice
To aortic vestibule
Left ventricle

C. Left Lateral View

1.56 LEFT ATRIUM AND LEFT VENTRICLE

A. Interior of left heart. **B.** Blood flow through the left heart.

- A diagonal cut was made from the base of the heart to the apex, passing between the superior and inferior pulmonary veins and through the posterior cusp of the mitral valve, followed by retraction (spreading) of the left heart wall on each side of the incision.
- The entrances (pulmonary veins) to the left atrium are posterior, and the exit (left atrioventricular or mitral orifice) is anterior.
- The left side of the fossa ovalis is also seen on the left side of the interatrial septum, although the left side is not usually as distinct as the right side is within the right atrium.
- Except for that of the auricle, the atrial wall is smooth.

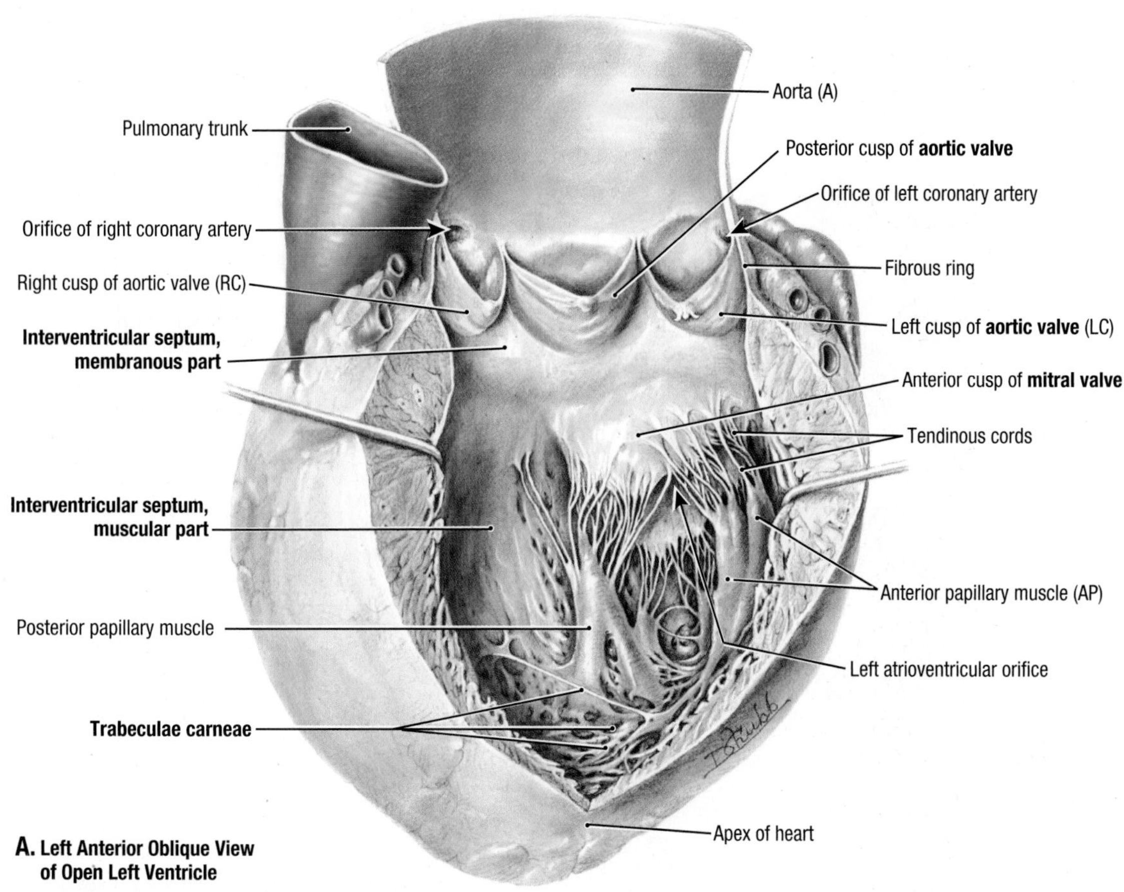
Aorta (A)
Pulmonary trunk
Posterior cusp of **aortic valve**
Orifice of left coronary artery
Orifice of right coronary artery
Fibrous ring
Right cusp of aortic valve (RC)
Left cusp of **aortic valve** (LC)
Interventricular septum, membranous part
Anterior cusp of **mitral valve**
Tendinous cords
Interventricular septum, muscular part
Anterior papillary muscle (AP)
Posterior papillary muscle
Left atrioventricular orifice
Trabeculae carneae
Apex of heart

A. **Left Anterior Oblique View of Open Left Ventricle**

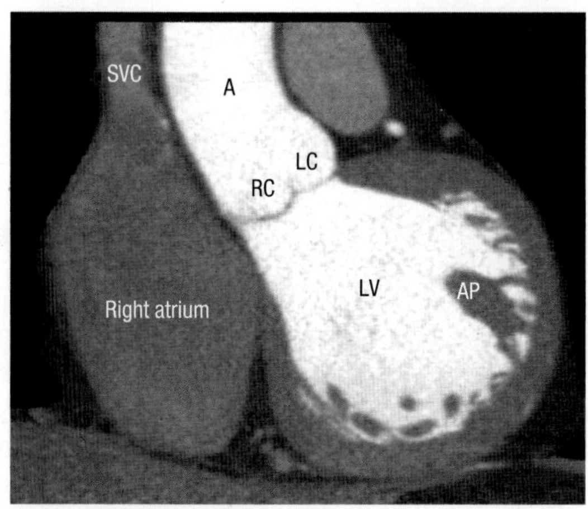
SVC
A
LC
RC
Right atrium
LV
AP

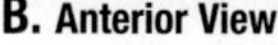

B. **Anterior View**

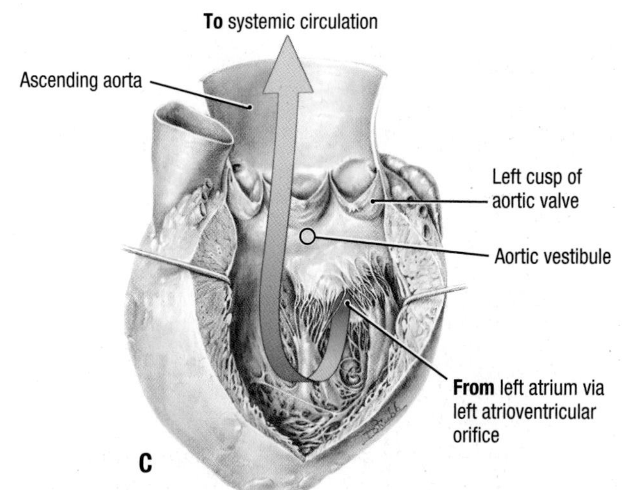
To systemic circulation
Ascending aorta
Left cusp of aortic valve
Aortic vestibule
From left atrium via left atrioventricular orifice

C

1.57 LEFT VENTRICLE

A. Interior of left ventricle. **B.** Coronal CT angiogram. Letters refer to structures in **A. C.** Blood flow through the left ventricle.

- A cut was made from the apex along the left margin of the heart, passing posterior to the pulmonary trunk, to open the aortic vestibule and ascending aorta.
- The chamber has a conical shape.
- The entrance (left atrioventricular, bicuspid, or mitral orifice) is situated posteriorly, and the exit (aortic orifice) is superior.
- The left ventricular wall is thin and muscular near the apex, thick and muscular superiorly, and thin and fibrous (nonelastic) at the aortic orifice.
- Two large papillary muscles, the anterior from the anterior wall and the posterior from the posterior wall, control the adjacent halves of two cusps of the mitral valve with tendinous cords (chordae tendineae).
- The anterior cusp of the mitral valve lies between the inlet (mitral orifice) and the outlet (aortic orifice).

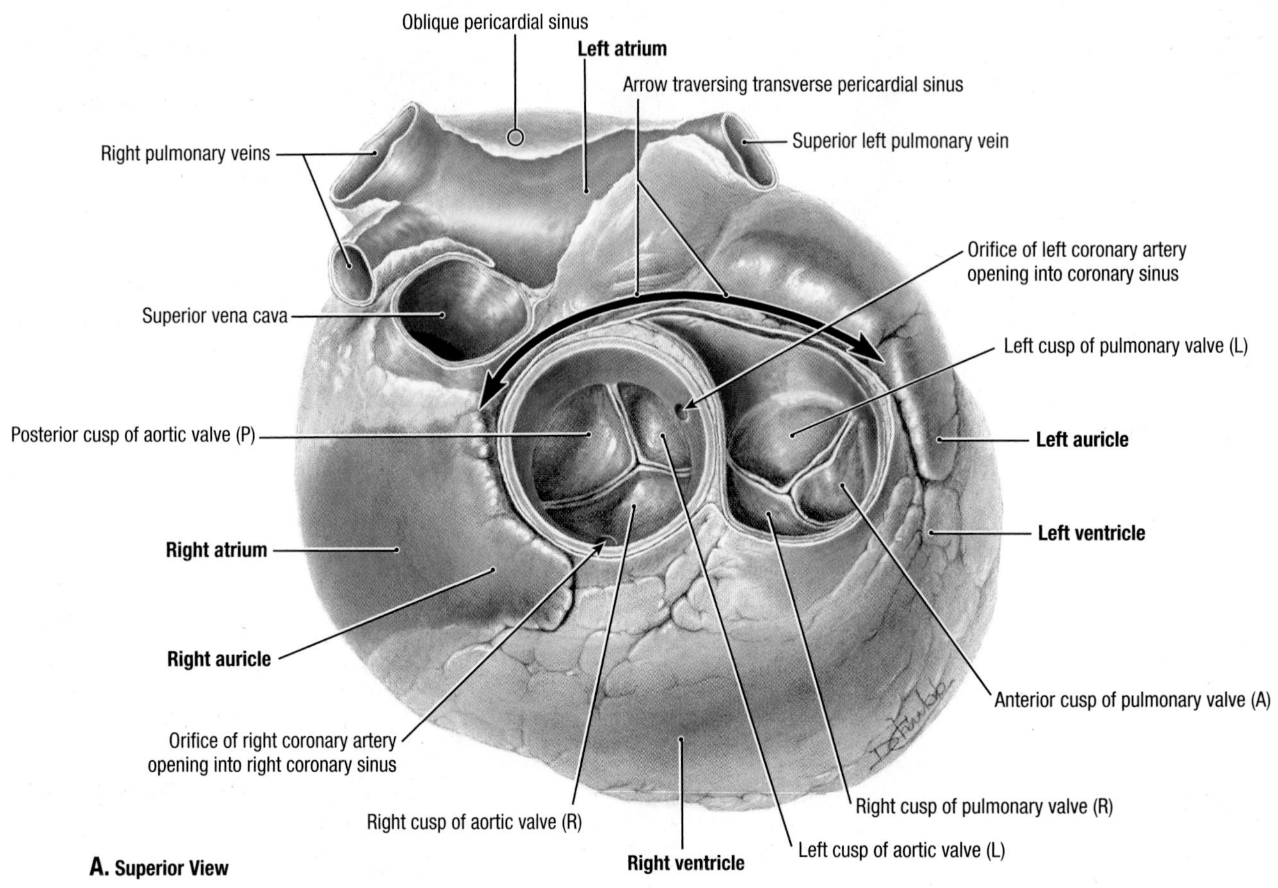
Oblique pericardial sinus
Left atrium
Arrow traversing transverse pericardial sinus
Right pulmonary veins
Superior left pulmonary vein
Orifice of left coronary artery opening into coronary sinus
Superior vena cava
Left cusp of pulmonary valve (L)
Posterior cusp of aortic valve (P)
Left auricle
Left ventricle
Right atrium
Right auricle
Anterior cusp of pulmonary valve (A)
Orifice of right coronary artery opening into right coronary sinus
Right cusp of pulmonary valve (R)
Right cusp of aortic valve (R)
Left cusp of aortic valve (L)
Right ventricle

A. Superior View

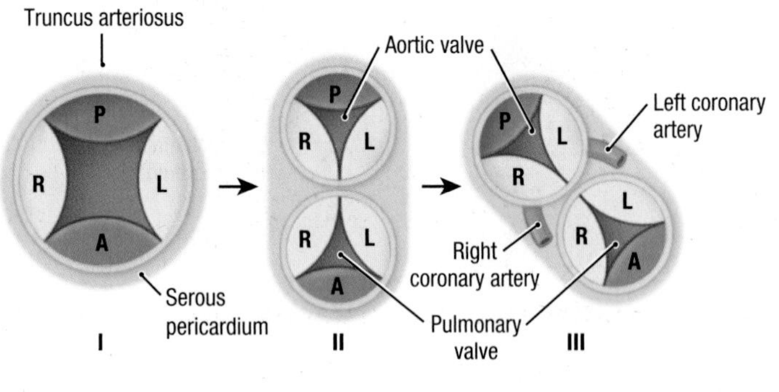
Truncus arteriosus
P
R
L
A
Serous pericardium
I
Aortic valve
P
R
L
R
L
A
II
Left coronary artery
Right coronary artery
Pulmonary valve
P
L
R
L
R
A
III
Semilunar valves:
R Right
A Anterior
L Left
P Posterior

B

1.58 VALVES OF HEART

A. Excised heart.

- The ventricles are positioned anteriorly and to the left, the atria posteriorly and to the right.
- The roots of the aorta and pulmonary artery, which conduct blood from the ventricles, are placed anterior to the atria and their incoming blood vessels (the superior and inferior vena cava and pulmonary veins).
- The aorta and pulmonary artery are enclosed within a common tube of serous pericardium and partly embraced by the auricles of the atria.
- The transverse pericardial sinus curves posterior to the enclosed stems of the aorta and pulmonary trunk and anterior to the superior vena cava and upper limits of the atria.
- The three cusps of the aortic and pulmonary valves. Immediately superior to each semilunar cusp, the walls of the origins of the pulmonary trunk and aorta are slightly dilated, forming a sinus. The aortic sinuses and sinuses of the pulmonary trunk (pulmonary sinuses) are the spaces at the origin of the pulmonary trunk and ascending aorta between the dilated wall of the vessel and each cusp of the semilunar valves.

B. Developmental basis for naming of pulmonary and aortic valve cusps.

- The names of these cusps have a developmental origin (**B**) the truncus arteriosus with four cusps **(I)** splits to form two valves, each with three cusps **(II)**. The heart undergoes partial rotation to the left on its axis, resulting in the arrangement of cusps shown in **(III)** and in Figure 1.58B.

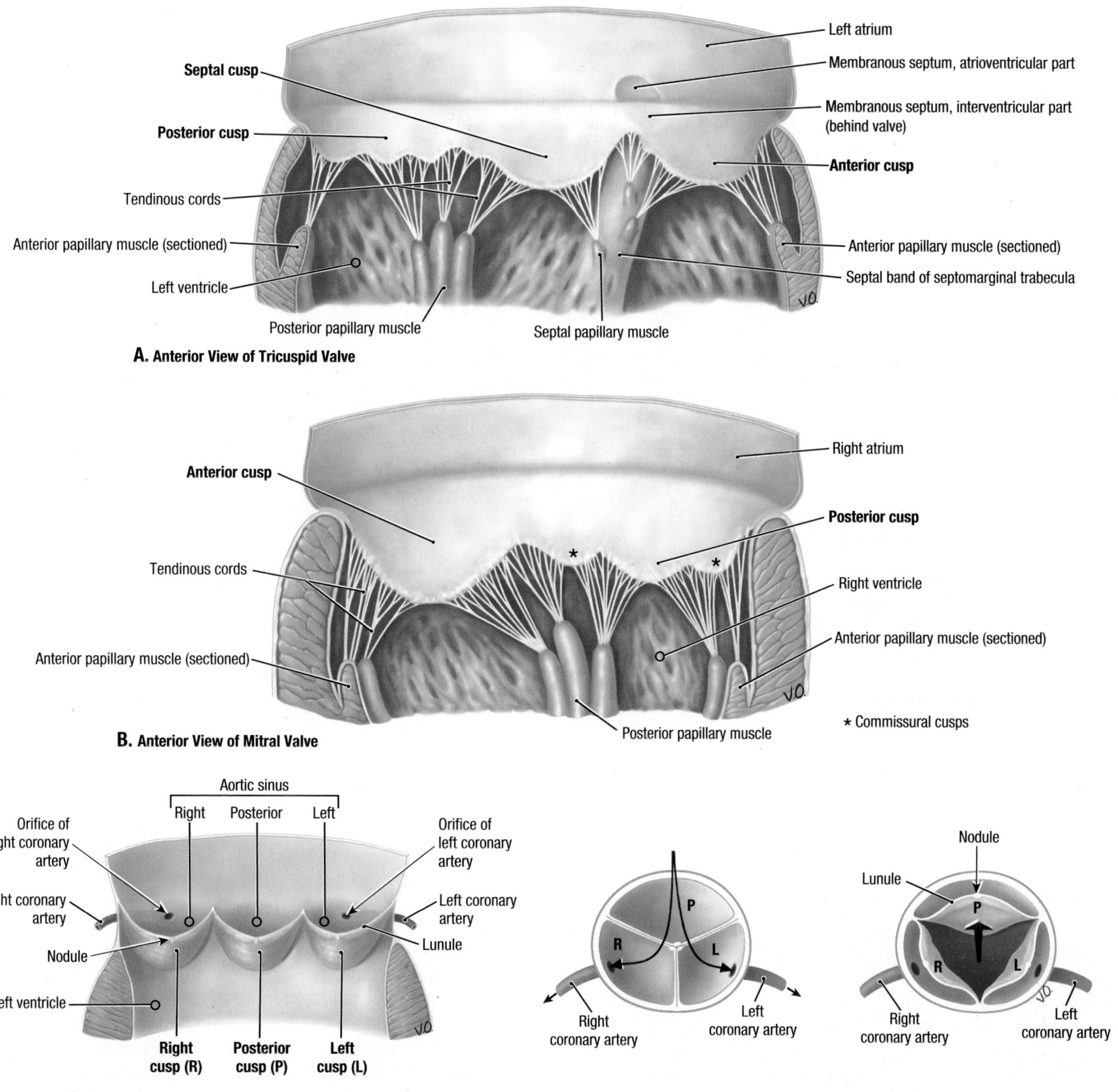
Left atrium
Septal cusp
Membranous septum, atrioventricular part
Membranous septum, interventricular part (behind valve)
Posterior cusp
Anterior cusp
Tendinous cords
Anterior papillary muscle (sectioned)
Anterior papillary muscle (sectioned)
Left ventricle
Septal band of septomarginal trabecula
Posterior papillary muscle
Septal papillary muscle
Right atrium
Anterior cusp
Posterior cusp
Tendinous cords
Right ventricle
Anterior papillary muscle (sectioned)
Anterior papillary muscle (sectioned)
Posterior papillary muscle
* Commissural cusps
Aortic sinus
Right
Posterior
Left
Orifice of right coronary artery
Orifice of left coronary artery
Right coronary artery
Left coronary artery
Nodule
Lunule
Left ventricle
Right cusp (R)
Posterior cusp (P)
Left cusp (L)
P
R
L
Right coronary artery
Left coronary artery
Nodule
Lunule
P
R
L
Right coronary artery
Left coronary artery

A. Anterior View of Tricuspid Valve

B. Anterior View of Mitral Valve

C. Left Posterior Oblique View of Aortic Valve

D. Superior Views of Aortic Valve (Arrows indicate direction of blood flow)

1.59 VALVES OF THE HEART

A. and B. Atrioventricular valves. **C. and D.** Semilunar valves.

Tendinous cords pass from the tips of the papillary muscles to the free margins and ventricular surfaces of the cusps of the tricuspid **(A)** and mitral **(B)** valves. Each papillary muscle or muscle group controls the adjacent sides of two cusps, resisting valve prolapse during systole. In **(C),** as in Figure 1.57A, the anulus of the aortic valve has been incised between the right and left cusps and spread open. Each cusp of the semilunar valves bears a nodule in the midpoint of its free edge, flanked by thin connective tissue areas (lunules). When the ventricles relax to fill (diastole), backflow of blood from aortic recoil or pulmonary resistance fills the sinus (space between cusp and dilated part of the aortic or pulmonary wall), causing the nodules and lunules to meet centrally, closing the valve **(D, *left*).** Filling of the coronary arteries occurs during diastole (when ventricular walls are relaxed) as backflow "inflates" the cusps to close the valve.

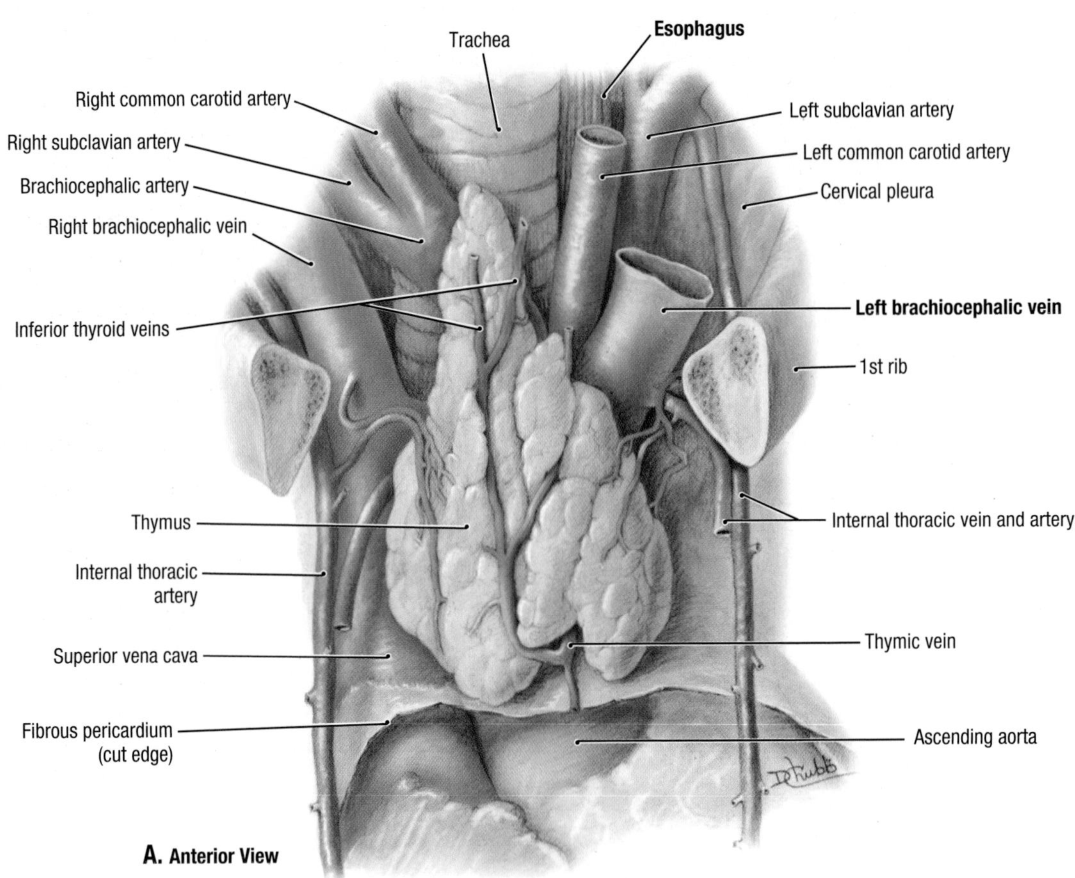
Trachea
Esophagus
Right common carotid artery
Right subclavian artery
Brachiocephalic artery
Right brachiocephalic vein
Inferior thyroid veins
Left subclavian artery
Left common carotid artery
Cervical pleura
Left brachiocephalic vein
1st rib
Thymus
Internal thoracic artery
Internal thoracic vein and artery
Superior vena cava
Thymic vein
Fibrous pericardium (cut edge)
Ascending aorta

A. Anterior View

1.60 SUPERIOR MEDIASTINUM I AND II: SUPERFICIAL DISSECTIONS

A. Thymus in situ. The sternum and ribs have been excised and the pleurae removed. It is unusual in an adult to see such a discrete thymus, which is large during puberty but subsequently regresses and is for the most part replaced by fat and fibrous tissue. **B.** Thymus removed. **C.** Relationship of nerves and vessels. The right vagus nerve (CN X) crosses anterior to the right subclavian artery and gives off the right recurrent laryngeal nerve, which passes medially to reach the trachea and esophagus. The left recurrent laryngeal nerve passes inferior and then posterior to the arch of the aorta and ascends between the trachea and esophagus to the larynx.

The distal part of the ascending aorta receives a strong thrust of blood when the left ventricle contracts. Because its wall is not reinforced by fibrous pericardium (the fibrous pericardium blends with the aortic adventitia at the beginning of the arch), an aneurysm may develop. An **aortic aneurysm** is evident on chest film (radiograph of the thorax) or a magnetic resonance angiogram as an enlarged area of the ascending aorta silhouette. Individuals with an aneurysm usually complain of chest pain that radiates to the back. The aneurysm may exert pressure on the trachea, esophagus, and recurrent laryngeal nerve, causing difficulty in breathing and swallowing.

The recurrent laryngeal nerves supply all the intrinsic muscles of the larynx, except the cricothyroid. Consequently, any investigative procedure or disease process in the superior mediastinum may involve these nerves and affect the voice. Because the left recurrent laryngeal nerve hooks around the arch of the aorta and ascends between the trachea and the esophagus, it may be involved when there is a bronchial or esophageal carcinoma, enlargement of mediastinal lymph nodes, or an aneurysm of the arch of the aorta.

The thymus is a prominent feature during infancy and childhood. In some infants, the thymus may compress the trachea. The thymus plays an important role in the development and maintenance of the immune system. As puberty is reached, the thymus begins to diminish in relative size. By adulthood, it is replaced by adipose tissue.

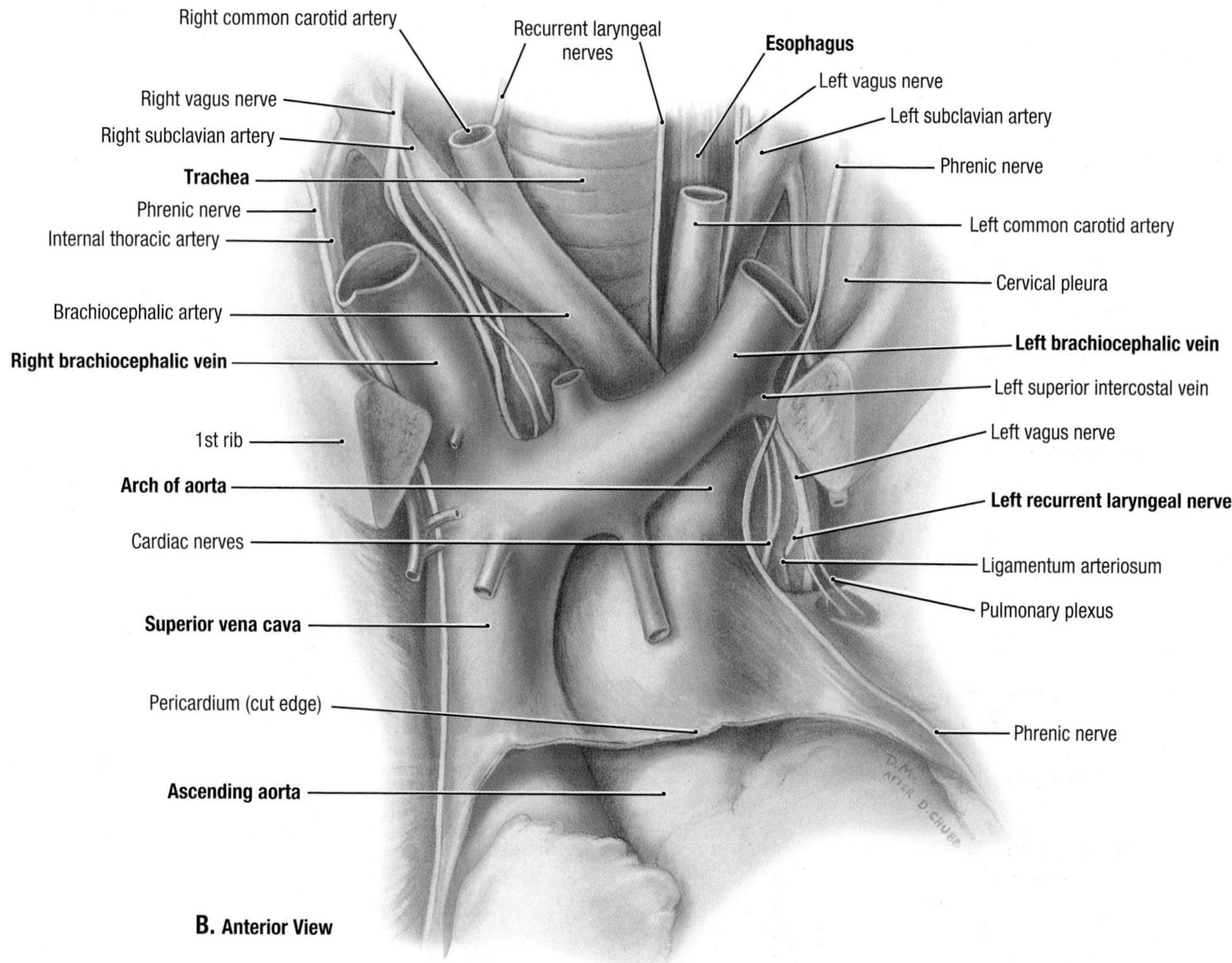
Right common carotid artery
Recurrent laryngeal nerves
Esophagus
Left vagus nerve
Right vagus nerve
Left subclavian artery
Right subclavian artery
Trachea
Phrenic nerve
Phrenic nerve
Internal thoracic artery
Left common carotid artery
Cervical pleura
Brachiocephalic artery
Left brachiocephalic vein
Right brachiocephalic vein
Left superior intercostal vein
1st rib
Left vagus nerve
Arch of aorta
Left recurrent laryngeal nerve
Cardiac nerves
Ligamentum arteriosum
Pulmonary plexus
Superior vena cava
Pericardium (cut edge)
Phrenic nerve
Ascending aorta

B. **Anterior View**

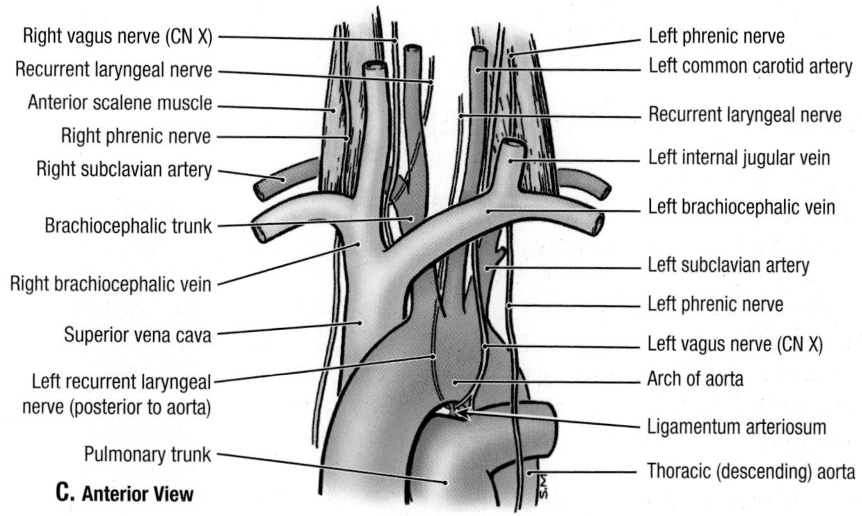
Right vagus nerve (CN X)
Left phrenic nerve
Recurrent laryngeal nerve
Left common carotid artery
Anterior scalene muscle
Recurrent laryngeal nerve
Right phrenic nerve
Left internal jugular vein
Right subclavian artery
Brachiocephalic trunk
Left brachiocephalic vein
Left subclavian artery
Right brachiocephalic vein
Left phrenic nerve
Superior vena cava
Left vagus nerve (CN X)
Left recurrent laryngeal nerve (posterior to aorta)
Arch of aorta
Ligamentum arteriosum
Pulmonary trunk
Thoracic (descending) aorta

C. **Anterior View**

1.60 SUPERIOR MEDIASTINUM I AND II (*CONTINUED*)

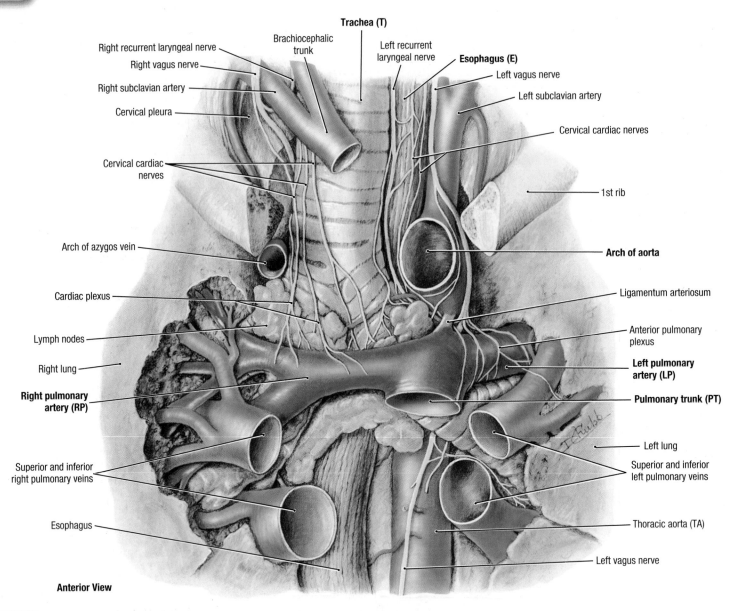

Trachea (T)
Brachiocephalic trunk
Right recurrent laryngeal nerve
Right vagus nerve
Right subclavian artery
Cervical pleura
Left recurrent laryngeal nerve
Esophagus (E)
Left vagus nerve
Left subclavian artery
Cervical cardiac nerves
Cervical cardiac nerves
1st rib
Arch of azygos vein
Arch of aorta
Cardiac plexus
Ligamentum arteriosum
Lymph nodes
Anterior pulmonary plexus
Right lung
Left pulmonary artery (LP)
Right pulmonary artery (RP)
Pulmonary trunk (PT)
Left lung
Superior and inferior right pulmonary veins
Superior and inferior left pulmonary veins
Esophagus
Thoracic aorta (TA)
Left vagus nerve
Anterior View

1.61 SUPERIOR MEDIASTINUM III: CARDIAC PLEXUS AND PULMONARY ARTERIES

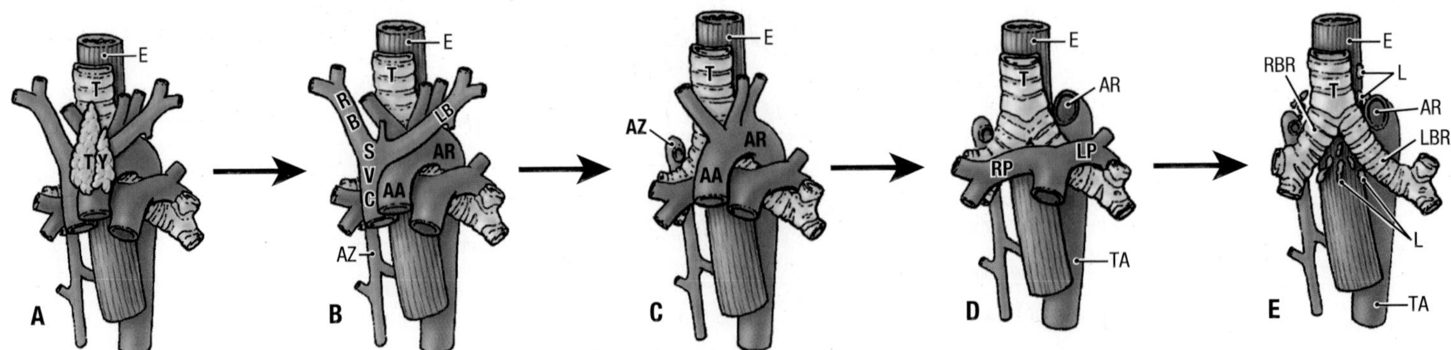
E
T
TY
A
RB
LB
S
V
C
AA
AR
AZ
B
AZ
T
AA
AR
C
E
T
AR
RP
LP
TA
D
RBR
L
AR
LBR
L
TA
E

1.62 RELATIONS OF GREAT VESSELS AND TRACHEA

Observe, from superficial to deep: **(A)** Thymus (*TY*); **(B)** the right (*RB*) and left (*LB*) brachiocephalic veins form the superior vena cava (*SVC*) and receive the arch of the azygos vein (*AZ*) posteriorly; **(C)** the ascending aorta (*AA*) and arch of the aorta (*AR*) arch over the right pulmonary artery and left main bronchus; **(D)** the right and left pulmonary arteries (*RP* and *LP*); and **(E)** the tracheobronchial lymph nodes (*L*) at the tracheal bifurcation (*T*).

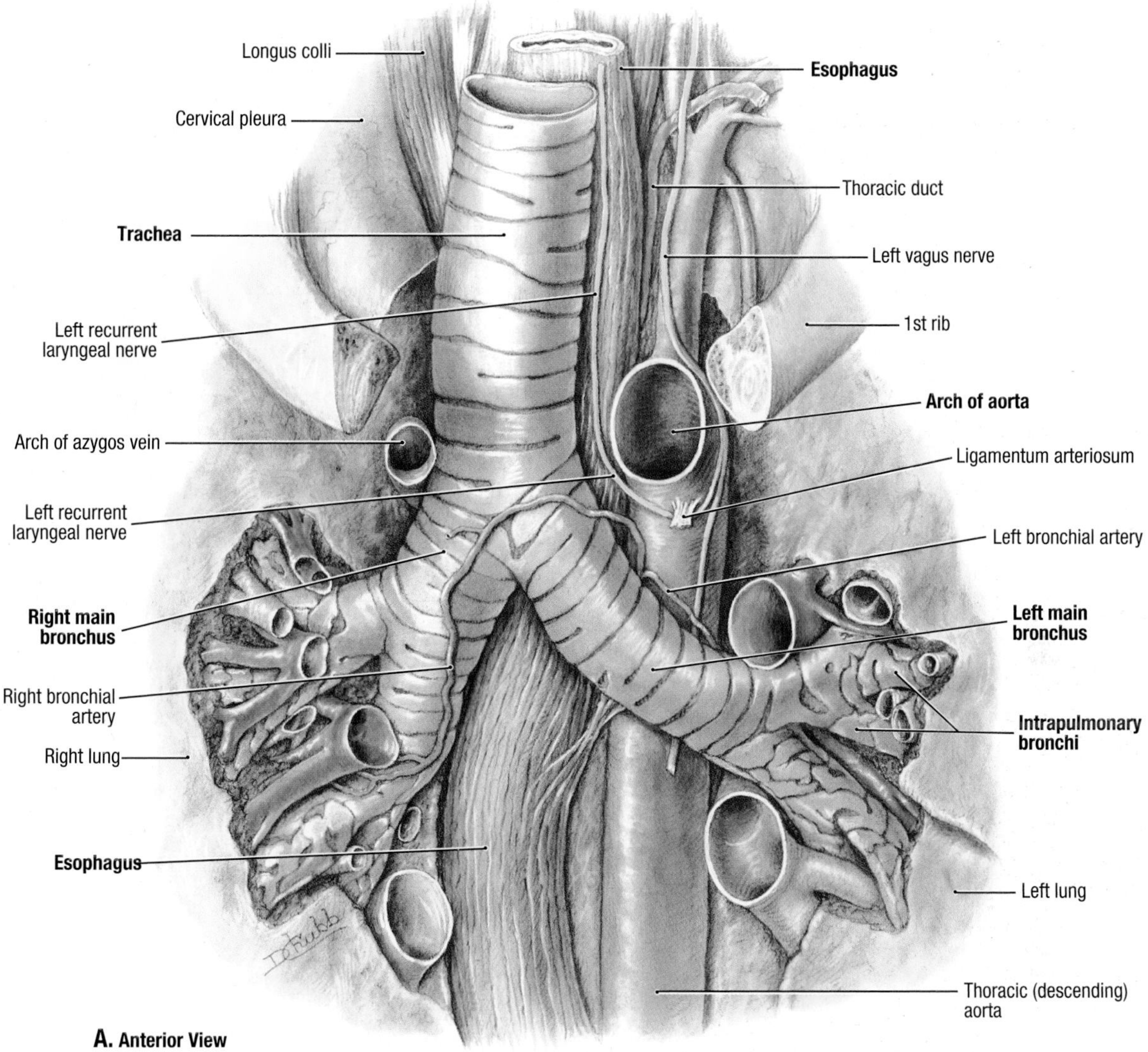

Longus colli
Esophagus
Cervical pleura
Thoracic duct
Trachea
Left vagus nerve
Left recurrent laryngeal nerve
1st rib
Arch of aorta
Arch of azygos vein
Ligamentum arteriosum
Left recurrent laryngeal nerve
Left bronchial artery
Right main bronchus
Left main bronchus
Right bronchial artery
Intrapulmonary bronchi
Right lung
Esophagus
Left lung
Thoracic (descending) aorta

A. Anterior View

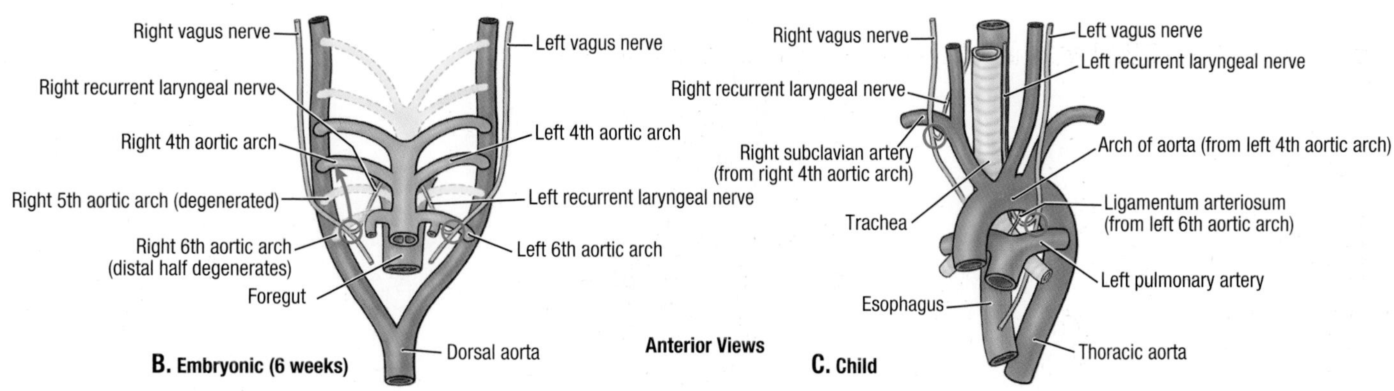
Right vagus nerve
Left vagus nerve
Right recurrent laryngeal nerve
Right 4th aortic arch
Left 4th aortic arch
Right 5th aortic arch (degenerated)
Left recurrent laryngeal nerve
Right 6th aortic arch (distal half degenerates)
Left 6th aortic arch
Foregut
Dorsal aorta
Right vagus nerve
Left vagus nerve
Left recurrent laryngeal nerve
Right recurrent laryngeal nerve
Right subclavian artery (from right 4th aortic arch)
Arch of aorta (from left 4th aortic arch)
Trachea
Ligamentum arteriosum (from left 6th aortic arch)
Left pulmonary artery
Esophagus
Thoracic aorta

B. Embryonic (6 weeks) **Anterior Views** **C. Child**

1.63 SUPERIOR MEDIASTINUM IV: TRACHEAL BIFURCATION AND BRONCHI

A. Dissection. **B.** Asymmetrical course of right and left recurrent laryngeal nerves. Arch VI disappears on the right, leaving the right recurrent laryngeal nerve to pass under arch IV, which becomes the right subclavian artery. Arch VI becomes part of the ductus arteriosus on the left side, and arch IV "descends" to become the arch of the aorta; thus the left recurrent laryngeal nerve is pulled into the thorax.

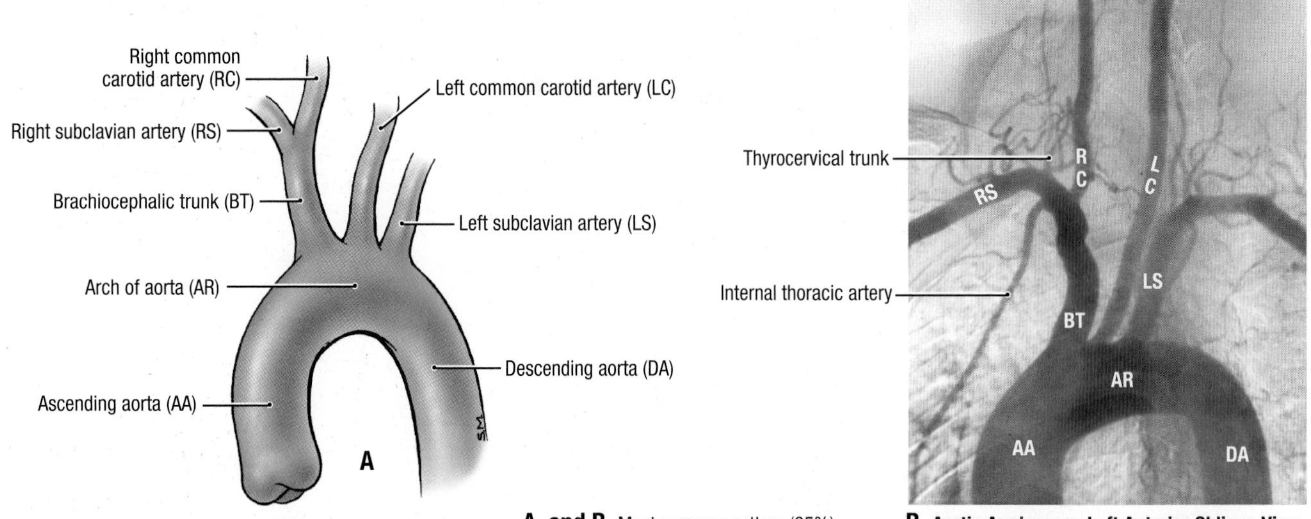
Right common carotid artery (RC)
Left common carotid artery (LC)
Right subclavian artery (RS)
Brachiocephalic trunk (BT)
Left subclavian artery (LS)
Arch of aorta (AR)
Descending aorta (DA)
Ascending aorta (AA)
A
Thyrocervical trunk
Internal thoracic artery
RS
R
C
L
C
LS
BT
AR
AA
DA

A. and B. Most common pattern (65%)

B. Aortic Angiogram, Left Anterior Oblique View

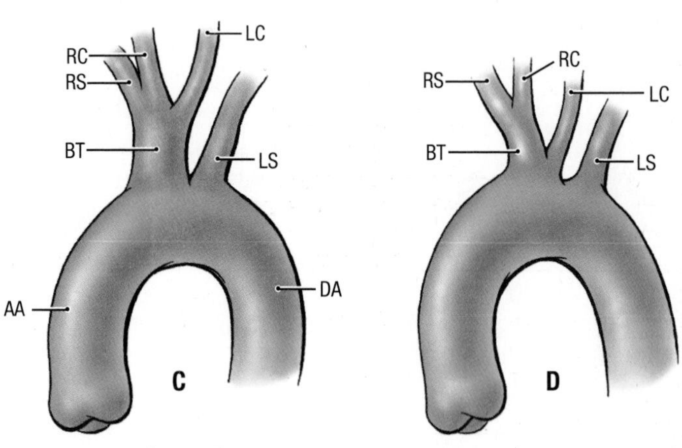
LC
RC
RS
BT
LS
AA
DA
C
RC
RS
LC
BT
LS
D

C. and D. Left common carotid artery originating from the brachiocephalic trunk (27%)

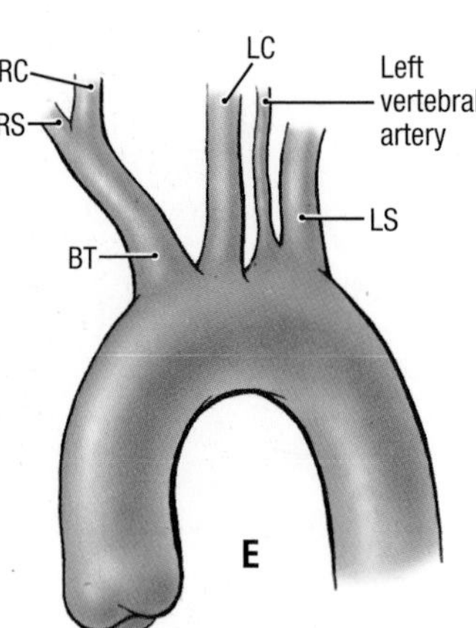
LC
RC
RS
Left vertebral artery
LS
BT
E

E. Four arteries originating independently from the arch of the aorta (2.5%)

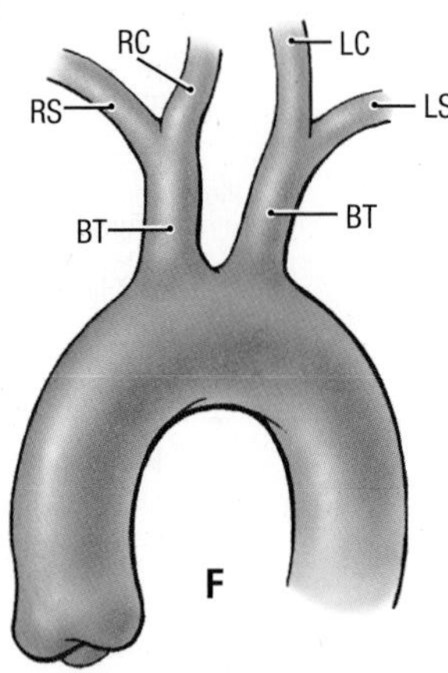
RC
LC
RS
LS
BT
BT
F

F. Right and left brachiocephalic trunks originating from the arch of the aorta (1.2%)

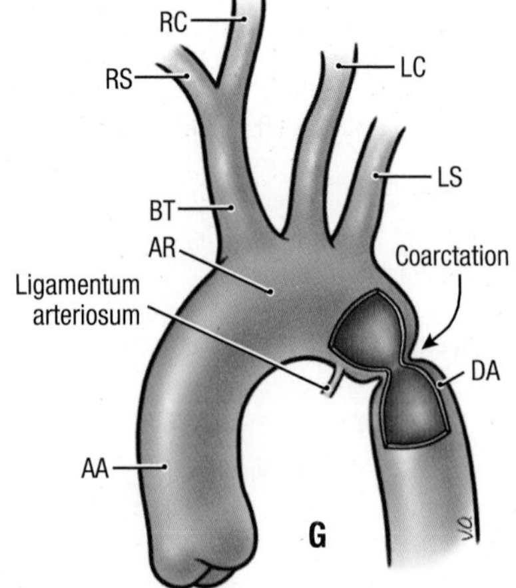
RC
RS
LC
LS
BT
AR
Coarctation
Ligamentum arteriosum
DA
AA
G

KEY

AA	Ascending aorta
AR	Arch of aorta
DA	Descending aorta
BT	Brachiocephalic trunk (artery)
LC	Left common carotid artery
LS	Left subclavian artery
RC	Right common carotid artery
RS	Right subclavian artery

1.64 BRANCHES OF AORTIC ARCH

A. and B. Most common pattern (65%). **C.–F.** Variations. **G.** In **coarctation of the aorta,** the arch or descending aorta has an abnormal narrowing (stenosis) that diminishes the caliber of the aortic lumen, producing an obstruction to blood flow. The most common site is near the ligamentum arteriosum. When the coarctation is inferior to this site (postductal coarctation), a good collateral circulation usually develops between the proximal and distal parts of the aorta through the intercostal and internal thoracic arteries.

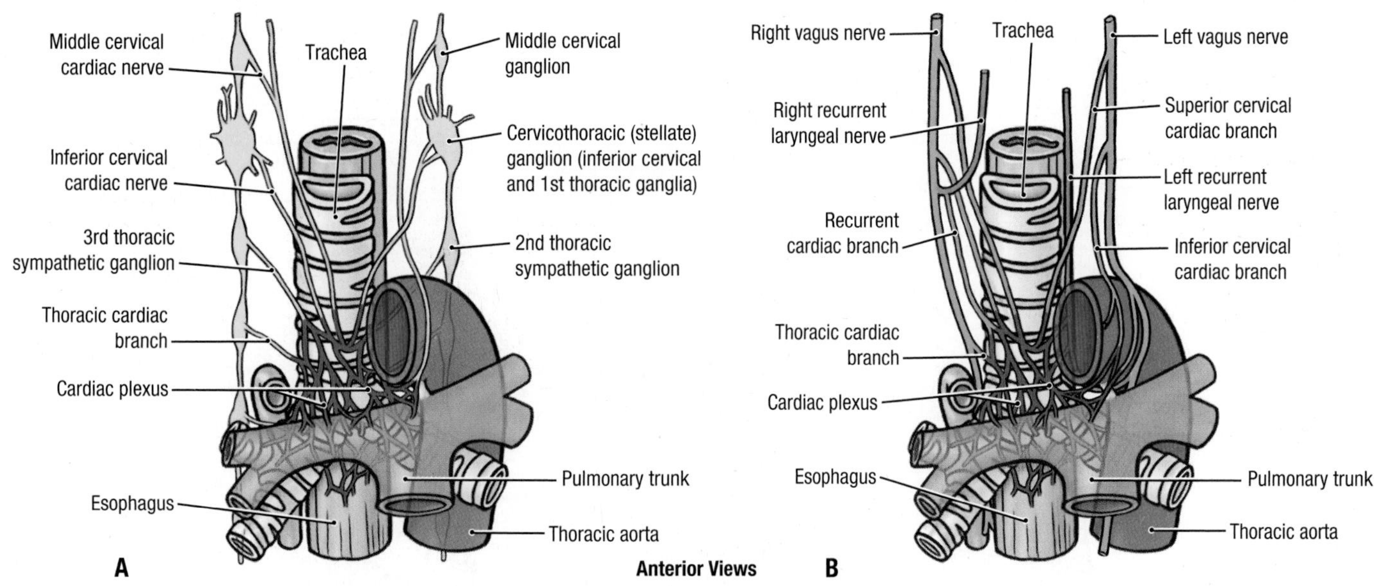
Middle cervical cardiac nerve
Trachea
Middle cervical ganglion
Cervicothoracic (stellate) ganglion (inferior cervical and 1st thoracic ganglia)
Inferior cervical cardiac nerve
3rd thoracic sympathetic ganglion
2nd thoracic sympathetic ganglion
Thoracic cardiac branch
Cardiac plexus
Pulmonary trunk
Esophagus
Thoracic aorta
A
Anterior Views
B
Right vagus nerve
Trachea
Left vagus nerve
Right recurrent laryngeal nerve
Superior cervical cardiac branch
Left recurrent laryngeal nerve
Recurrent cardiac branch
Inferior cervical cardiac branch
Thoracic cardiac branch
Cardiac plexus
Esophagus
Pulmonary trunk
Thoracic aorta

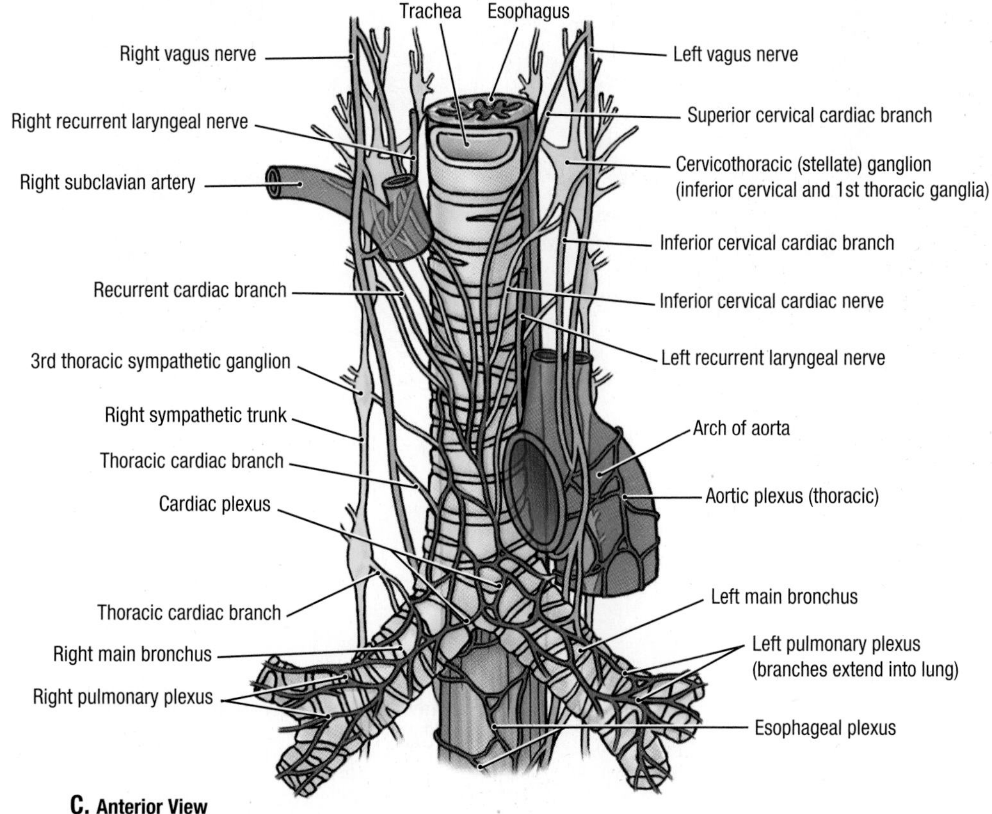
Trachea
Esophagus
Right vagus nerve
Left vagus nerve
Right recurrent laryngeal nerve
Superior cervical cardiac branch
Right subclavian artery
Cervicothoracic (stellate) ganglion (inferior cervical and 1st thoracic ganglia)
Inferior cervical cardiac branch
Recurrent cardiac branch
Inferior cervical cardiac nerve
3rd thoracic sympathetic ganglion
Left recurrent laryngeal nerve
Right sympathetic trunk
Arch of aorta
Thoracic cardiac branch
Cardiac plexus
Aortic plexus (thoracic)
Left main bronchus
Thoracic cardiac branch
Right main bronchus
Left pulmonary plexus (branches extend into lung)
Right pulmonary plexus
Esophageal plexus
C. Anterior View

1.65 CARDIAC AND PULMONARY PLEXUSES

A. Sympathetic contribution. **B.** Parasympathetic contribution. **C.** Overview. *Yellow*, sympathetic; *blue*, parasympathetic; *green*, mixed sympathetic and parasympathetic nerves.

Heart: Sympathetic stimulation increases the heart's rate and the force of its contractions. Parasympathetic stimulation slows the heart rate, reduces the force of contraction, and constricts the coronary arteries, saving energy between periods of increased demand. While the cardiac plexus is shown in relation to the bifurcation of the trachea, note that it lies directly posterior to the superior margin of the heart (see Fig. 1.28C) and in close proximity to the nodal tissue and origins of the coronary arteries.

Lungs: Sympathetic fibers are inhibitory to the bronchial muscle (bronchodilator), motor to pulmonary vessels (vasoconstrictor) and inhibitory to the alveolar glands of the bronchial tree. Parasympathetic fibers from CN X are bronchoconstrictors, secretory to the glands of the bronchial tree (secretomotor).

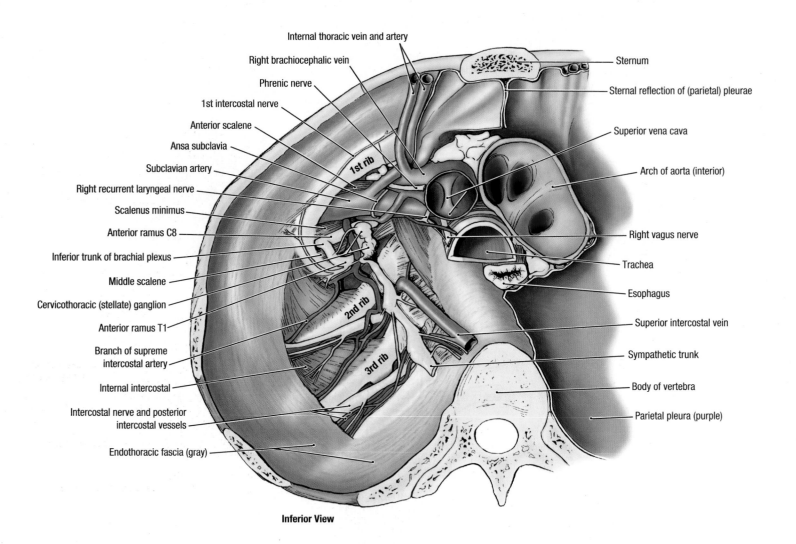

Internal thoracic vein and artery
Right brachiocephalic vein
Phrenic nerve
1st intercostal nerve
Anterior scalene
Ansa subclavia
Subclavian artery
Right recurrent laryngeal nerve
Scalenus minimus
Anterior ramus C8
Inferior trunk of brachial plexus
Middle scalene
Cervicothoracic (stellate) ganglion
Anterior ramus T1
Branch of supreme intercostal artery
Internal intercostal
Intercostal nerve and posterior intercostal vessels
Endothoracic fascia (gray)
1st rib
2nd rib
3rd rib
Sternum
Sternal reflection of (parietal) pleurae
Superior vena cava
Arch of aorta (interior)
Right vagus nerve
Trachea
Esophagus
Superior intercostal vein
Sympathetic trunk
Body of vertebra
Parietal pleura (purple)

Inferior View

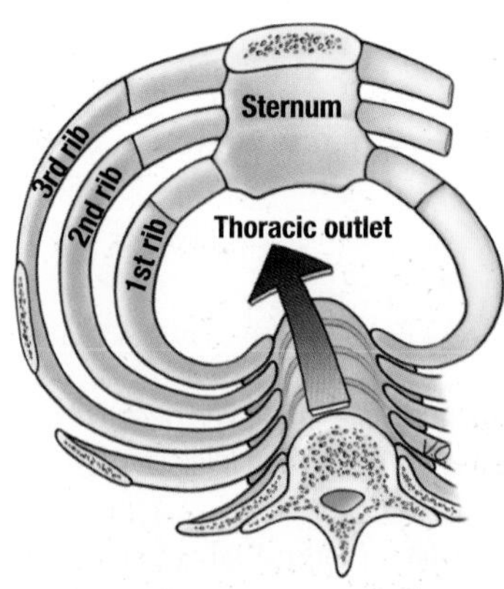
Sternum
3rd rib
2nd rib
1st rib
Thoracic outlet

1.66 SUPERIOR MEDIASTINUM AND ROOF OF PLEURAL CAVITY

- The cervical, costal, and mediastinal parietal pleura (*purple*) and portions of the endothoracic fascia (*gray*) have been removed from the right side of the specimen to demonstrate structures traversing the superior thoracic aperture.
- The first part of the subclavian artery disappears as it crosses the first rib anterior to the anterior scalene muscle.
- The ansa subclavia from the sympathetic trunk and right recurrent laryngeal nerve from the vagus are seen looping inferior to the subclavian artery.
- The anterior rami of C8 and T1 merge to form the inferior trunk of the brachial plexus, which crosses the first rib posterior to the anterior scalene muscle.

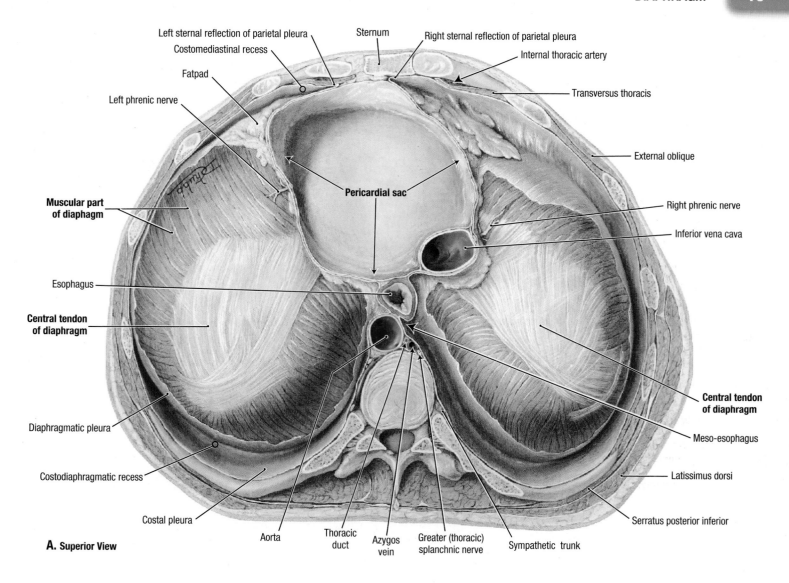

Left sternal reflection of parietal pleura
Sternum
Right sternal reflection of parietal pleura
Costomediastinal recess
Internal thoracic artery
Fatpad
Transversus thoracis
Left phrenic nerve
External oblique
Pericardial sac
Muscular part of diaphagm
Right phrenic nerve
Inferior vena cava
Esophagus
Central tendon of diaphragm
Central tendon of diaphragm
Diaphragmatic pleura
Meso-esophagus
Costodiaphragmatic recess
Latissimus dorsi
Costal pleura
Serratus posterior inferior
Aorta
Thoracic duct
Azygos vein
Greater (thoracic) splanchnic nerve
Sympathetic trunk

A. Superior View

1.67 DIAPHRAGM AND PERICARDIAL SAC

A. The diaphragmatic pleura is mostly removed. The pericardial sac is situated on the anterior half of the diaphragm; one third is to the right of the median plane, and two thirds to the left. Note also that anterior to the pericardium, the sternal reflection of the left pleural sac approaches but fails to meet that of the right sac in the median plane; and on reaching the vertebral column, the costal pleura becomes the mediastinal pleura. Irritation of the parietal pleura produces local pain and referred pain to the areas sharing innervation by the same segments of the spinal cord. Irritation of the costal and peripheral parts of the diaphragmatic pleura results in local pain and referred pain along the intercostal nerves to the thoracic and abdominal walls. Irritation of the mediastinal and central diaphragmatic areas of the parietal pleura results in pain that is referred to the root of the neck and over the shoulder (C3–C5 dermatomes). **B.** Between the inferior part of the esophagus and the aorta, the right and left layers of mediastinal pleura form a dorsal meso-esophagus, especially when the body is in the prone position.

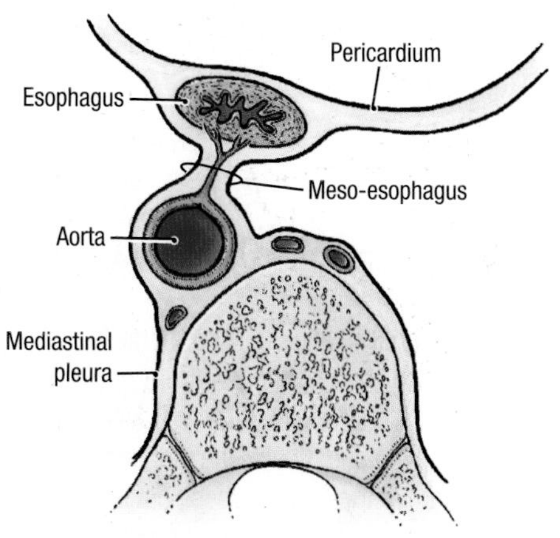
Pericardium
Esophagus
Meso-esophagus
Aorta
Mediastinal pleura

B. Superior View

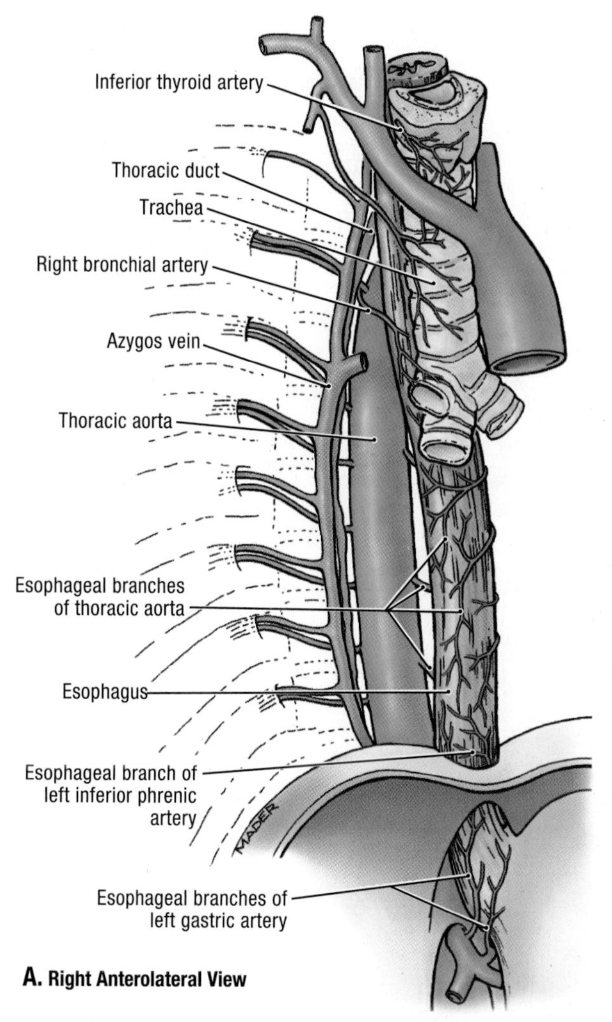
Inferior thyroid artery
Thoracic duct
Trachea
Right bronchial artery
Azygos vein
Thoracic aorta
Esophageal branches of thoracic aorta
Esophagus
Esophageal branch of left inferior phrenic artery
Esophageal branches of left gastric artery
MADER

A. **Right Anterolateral View**

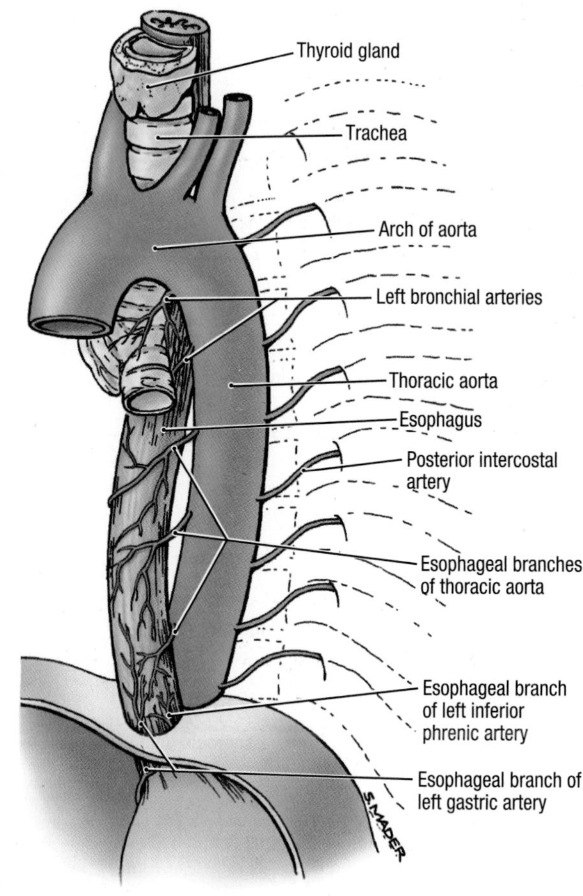
Thyroid gland
Trachea
Arch of aorta
Left bronchial arteries
Thoracic aorta
Esophagus
Posterior intercostal artery
Esophageal branches of thoracic aorta
Esophageal branch of left inferior phrenic artery
Esophageal branch of left gastric artery
S. MADER

B. **Left Anterolateral View**

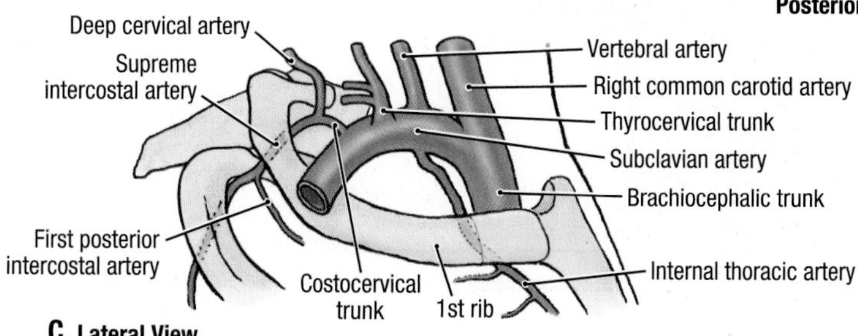
Deep cervical artery
Supreme intercostal artery
First posterior intercostal artery
Costocervical trunk
1st rib
Vertebral artery
Right common carotid artery
Thyrocervical trunk
Subclavian artery
Brachiocephalic trunk
Internal thoracic artery

C. **Lateral View**

Posterior intercostal arteries:
1st
2nd
3rd
4th
5th
6th
7th
8th
9th
10th
11th
Subcostal artery
Deep cervical artery
Costocervical trunk
1st rib
Ligamentum arteriosum
Bronchial arteries
* Coronary arteries
Esophageal branches
Posterior intercostal arteries
Superior phrenic arteries
Subcostal artery
Diaphragm
Celiac trunk

D. **Anterior View**

1.69 ARTERIAL SUPPLY TO TRACHEA AND ESOPHAGUS

A. and B. The continuous anastomotic chain of arteries on the esophagus is formed (1) by branches of the right and left inferior thyroid and right supreme intercostal arteries superiorly, (2) by the unpaired median aortic (bronchial and esophageal) branches, and (3) by branches of the left gastric and left inferior phrenic arteries inferiorly. The right bronchial artery usually arises from the superior left bronchial or 3rd right posterior intercostal artery (here the 5th) or from the aorta directly. The unpaired median aortic branches also supply the trachea and bronchi. **C.** Origin of supreme intercostal artery. **D.** Branches of the thoracic aorta.

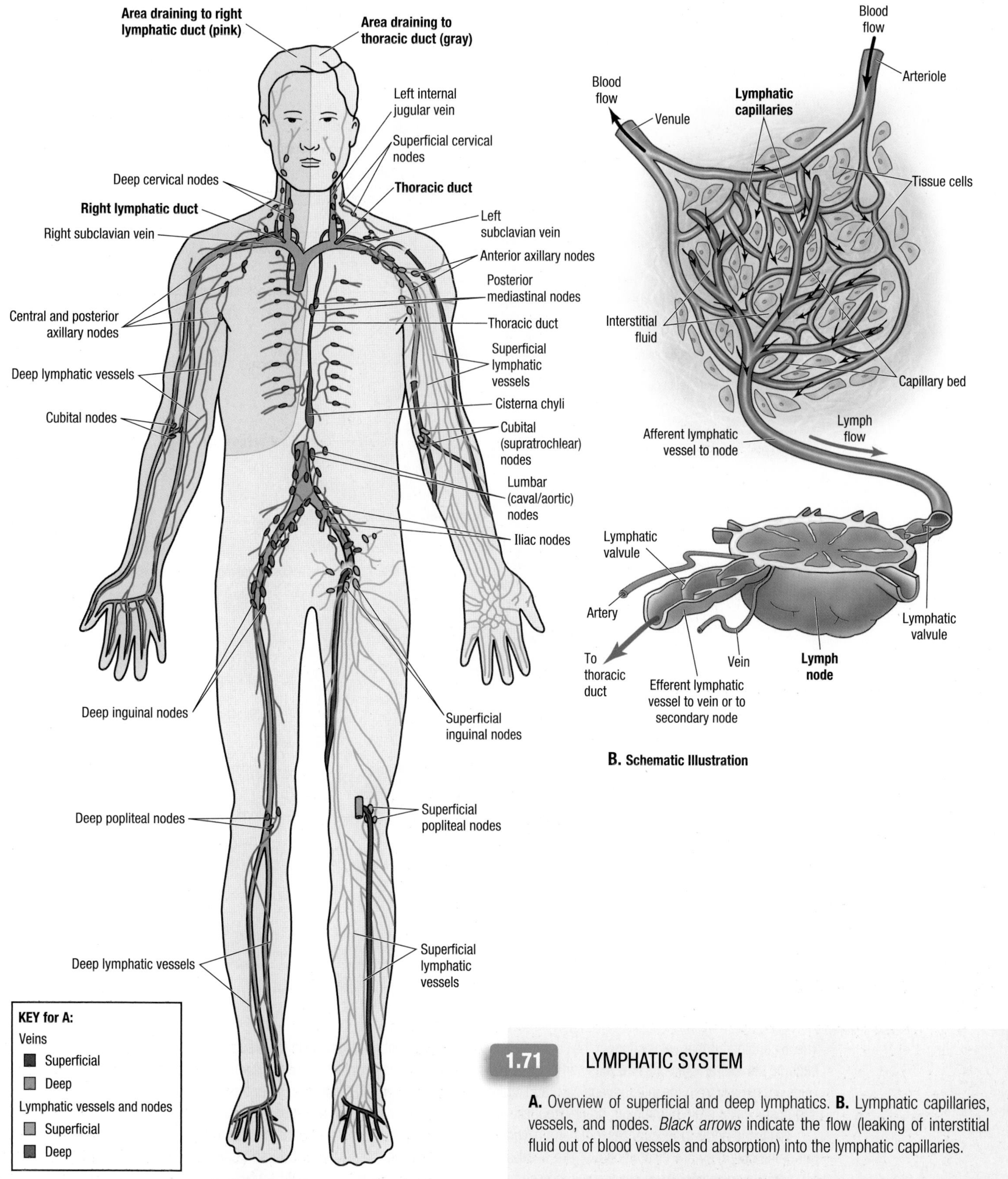
Area draining to right lymphatic duct (pink)
Area draining to thoracic duct (gray)
Left internal jugular vein
Superficial cervical nodes
Deep cervical nodes
Thoracic duct
Right lymphatic duct
Left subclavian vein
Right subclavian vein
Anterior axillary nodes
Posterior mediastinal nodes
Central and posterior axillary nodes
Thoracic duct
Superficial lymphatic vessels
Deep lymphatic vessels
Cisterna chyli
Cubital nodes
Cubital (supratrochlear) nodes
Lumbar (caval/aortic) nodes
Iliac nodes
Deep inguinal nodes
Superficial inguinal nodes
Deep popliteal nodes
Superficial popliteal nodes
Deep lymphatic vessels
Superficial lymphatic vessels
KEY for A:
Veins
Superficial
Deep
Lymphatic vessels and nodes
Superficial
Deep
A. Anterior View
Blood flow
Arteriole
Blood flow
Venule
Lymphatic capillaries
Tissue cells
Interstitial fluid
Capillary bed
Lymph flow
Afferent lymphatic vessel to node
Lymphatic valvule
Artery
Lymphatic valvule
To thoracic duct
Vein
Lymph node
Efferent lymphatic vessel to vein or to secondary node
B. Schematic Illustration

1.71 LYMPHATIC SYSTEM

A. Overview of superficial and deep lymphatics. **B.** Lymphatic capillaries, vessels, and nodes. *Black arrows* indicate the flow (leaking of interstitial fluid out of blood vessels and absorption) into the lymphatic capillaries.

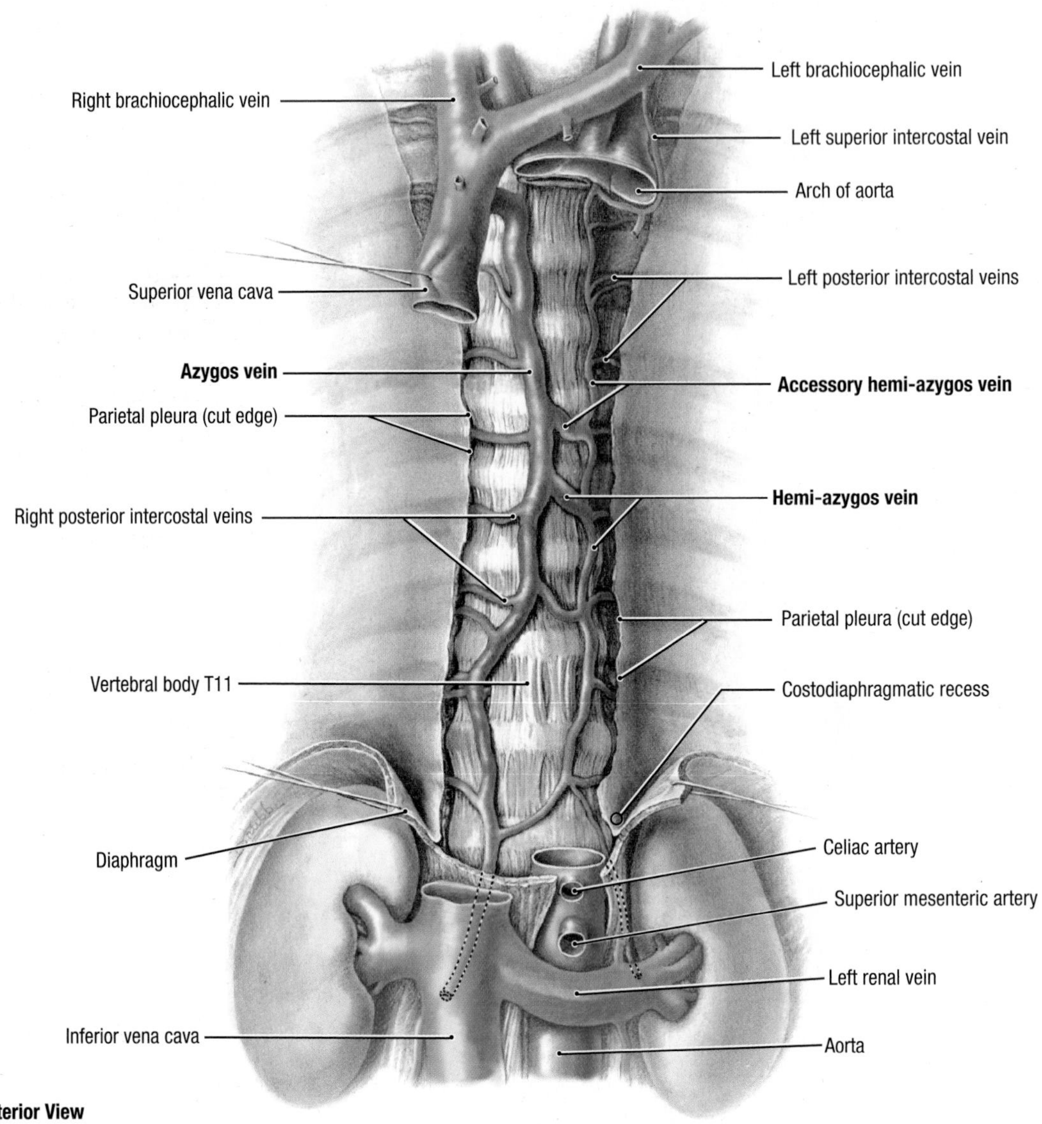

Right brachiocephalic vein
Left brachiocephalic vein
Left superior intercostal vein
Arch of aorta
Superior vena cava
Left posterior intercostal veins
Azygos vein
Accessory hemi-azygos vein
Parietal pleura (cut edge)
Hemi-azygos vein
Right posterior intercostal veins
Parietal pleura (cut edge)
Vertebral body T11
Costodiaphragmatic recess
Diaphragm
Celiac artery
Superior mesenteric artery
Left renal vein
Inferior vena cava
Aorta

A. Anterior View

1.72 AZYGOS SYSTEM OF VEINS

The ascending lumbar veins connect the common iliac veins to the lumbar veins and join the subcostal veins to become the lateral roots of the azygos and hemi-azygos veins; the medial roots of the azygos and hemi-azygos veins are usually from the inferior vena cava and left renal vein, if present. Typically the upper four left posterior intercostal veins drain into the left brachiocephalic vein, directly and via the left superior intercostal veins.

In **A,** the hemi-azygos, accessory hemi-azygos, and left superior intercostals veins are continuous here, but commonly they are discontinuous. The hemi-azygos vein crosses the vertebral column at approximately T9, and the accessory hemi-azygos vein crosses at T8, to enter the azygos vein. In **A,** there are four cross-connecting channels between the azygos and hemi-azygos systems. The azygos vein arches superior to the root of the right lung at T4 to drain into the superior vena cava.

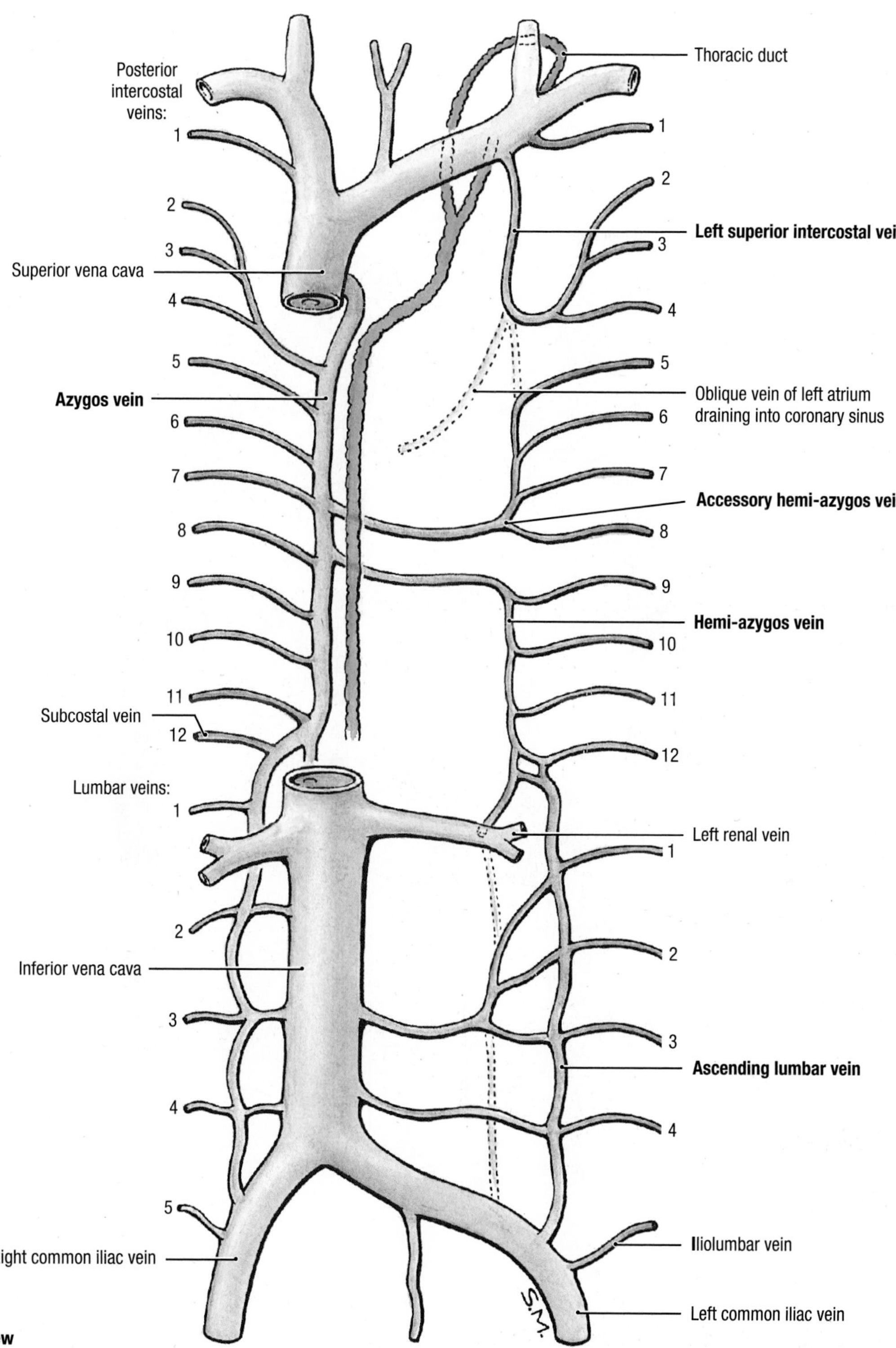
Posterior intercostal veins:
1
2
3
4
5
6
7
8
9
10
11
12
Superior vena cava
Azygos vein
Subcostal vein
Lumbar veins:
1
2
3
4
5
Inferior vena cava
Right common iliac vein
Thoracic duct
1
2
Left superior intercostal vein
3
4
5
Oblique vein of left atrium draining into coronary sinus
6
7
Accessory hemi-azygos vein
8
9
Hemi-azygos vein
10
11
12
Left renal vein
1
2
3
Ascending lumbar vein
4
Iliolumbar vein
Left common iliac vein
S.M.

B. **Anterior View**

1.72 AZYGOS SYSTEM OF VEINS (*CONTINUED*)

The azygos, hemi-azygos, and accessory hemi-azygos veins offer alternate means of venous drainage from the thoracic, abdominal, and back regions when **obstruction of the IVC** occurs. In some people, an accessory azygos vein parallels the main azygos vein on the right side. Other people have no hemi-azygos system of veins. A clinically important variation, although uncommon, is when the azygos system receives all the blood from the IVC, except that from the liver. In these people, the azygos system drains nearly all the blood inferior to the diaphragm, except that from the digestive tract. When **obstruction of the SVC** occurs superior to the entrance of the azygos vein, blood can drain inferiorly into the veins of the abdominal wall and return to the right atrium through the IVC and azygos system of veins.

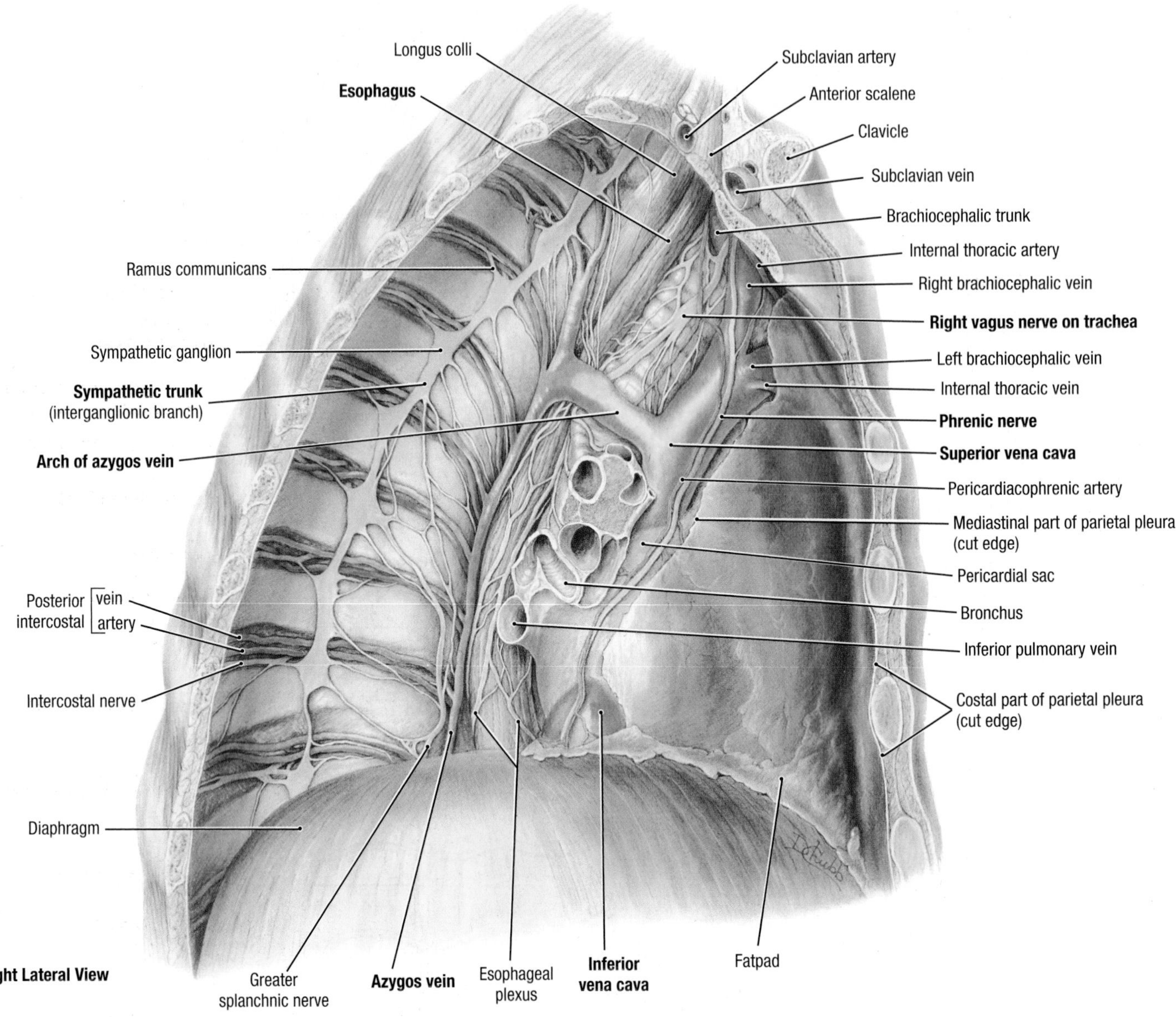
Longus colli
Esophagus
Subclavian artery
Anterior scalene
Clavicle
Subclavian vein
Brachiocephalic trunk
Internal thoracic artery
Right brachiocephalic vein
Right vagus nerve on trachea
Left brachiocephalic vein
Internal thoracic vein
Phrenic nerve
Superior vena cava
Pericardiacophrenic artery
Mediastinal part of parietal pleura (cut edge)
Pericardial sac
Bronchus
Inferior pulmonary vein
Costal part of parietal pleura (cut edge)
Ramus communicans
Sympathetic ganglion
Sympathetic trunk (interganglionic branch)
Arch of azygos vein
Posterior intercostal vein
Posterior intercostal artery
Intercostal nerve
Diaphragm
Greater splanchnic nerve
Azygos vein
Esophageal plexus
Inferior vena cava
Fatpad
Right Lateral View

1.73 MEDIASTINUM, RIGHT SIDE

- The costal and mediastinal pleurae have mostly been removed, exposing the underlying structures. Compare with the mediastinal surface of the right lung in Figure 1.32.
- The right side of the mediastinum is the "blue side," dominated by the arch of the azygos vein and the superior vena cava.
- Both the trachea and the esophagus are visible from the right side.
- The right vagus nerve descends on the medial surface of the trachea, passes medial to the arch of the azygos vein, posterior to the root of the lung, and then enters the esophageal plexus.
- The right phrenic nerve passes anterior to the root of the lung lateral to both venae cavae.

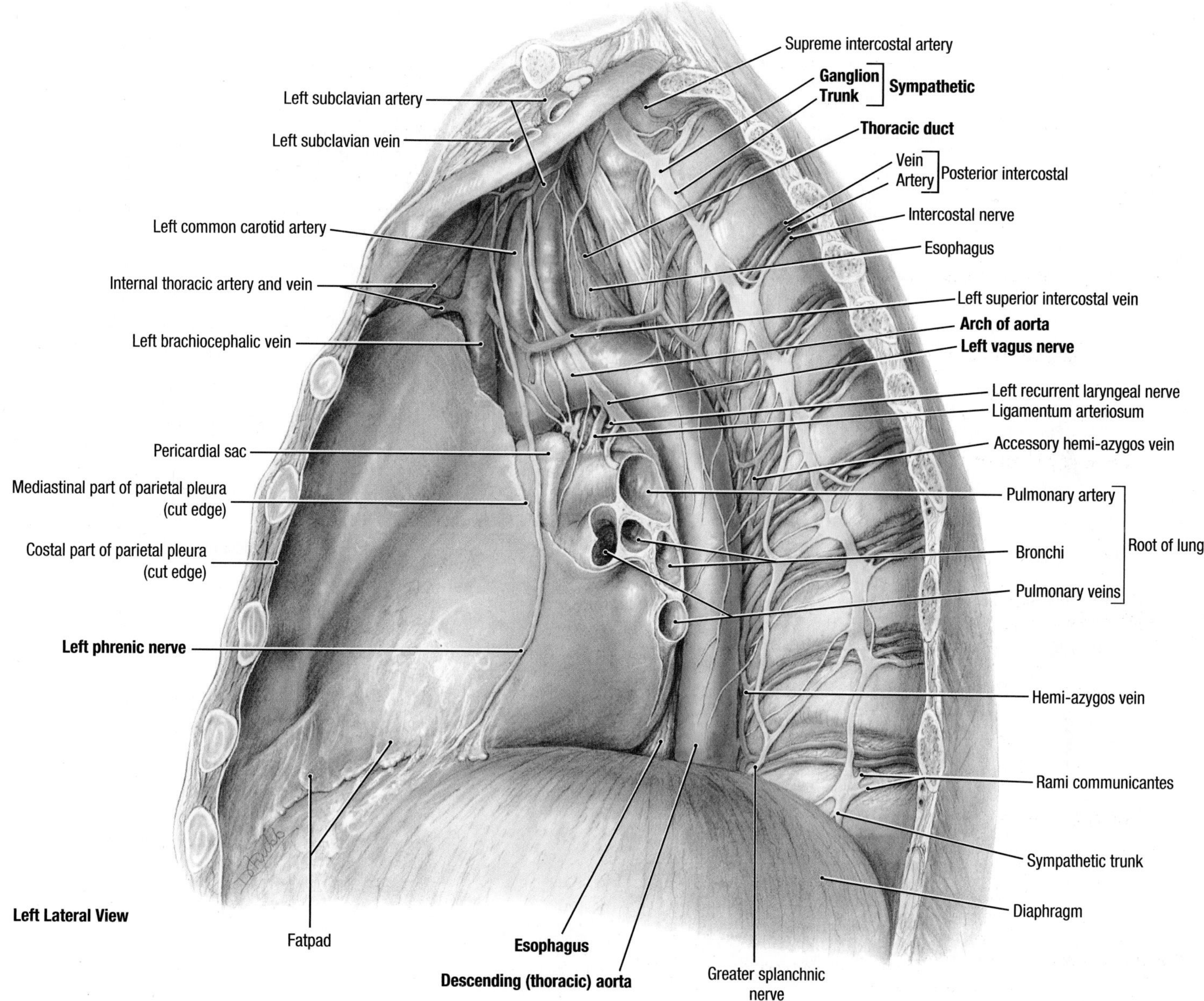
Supreme intercostal artery
Ganglion
Trunk
Sympathetic
Thoracic duct
Vein
Artery
Posterior intercostal
Intercostal nerve
Esophagus
Left superior intercostal vein
Arch of aorta
Left vagus nerve
Left recurrent laryngeal nerve
Ligamentum arteriosum
Accessory hemi-azygos vein
Pulmonary artery
Bronchi
Pulmonary veins
Root of lung
Hemi-azygos vein
Rami communicantes
Sympathetic trunk
Diaphragm
Greater splanchnic nerve
Descending (thoracic) aorta
Esophagus
Fatpad
Left Lateral View
Left phrenic nerve
Costal part of parietal pleura (cut edge)
Mediastinal part of parietal pleura (cut edge)
Pericardial sac
Left brachiocephalic vein
Internal thoracic artery and vein
Left common carotid artery
Left subclavian vein
Left subclavian artery

1.74 MEDIASTINUM, LEFT SIDE

- Compare with the mediastinal surface of the left lung in Figure 1.33.
- The left side of the mediastinum is the "red side," dominated by the arch and descending portion of the aorta, the left common carotid and subclavian arteries; the latter obscure the trachea from view.
- The thoracic duct can be seen on the left side of the esophagus.
- The left vagus nerve passes posterior to the root of the lung, sending its recurrent laryngeal branch around the ligamentum arteriosum inferior and then medial to the aortic arch.
- The phrenic nerve passes anterior to the root of the lung and penetrates the diaphragm more anteriorly than on the right side.

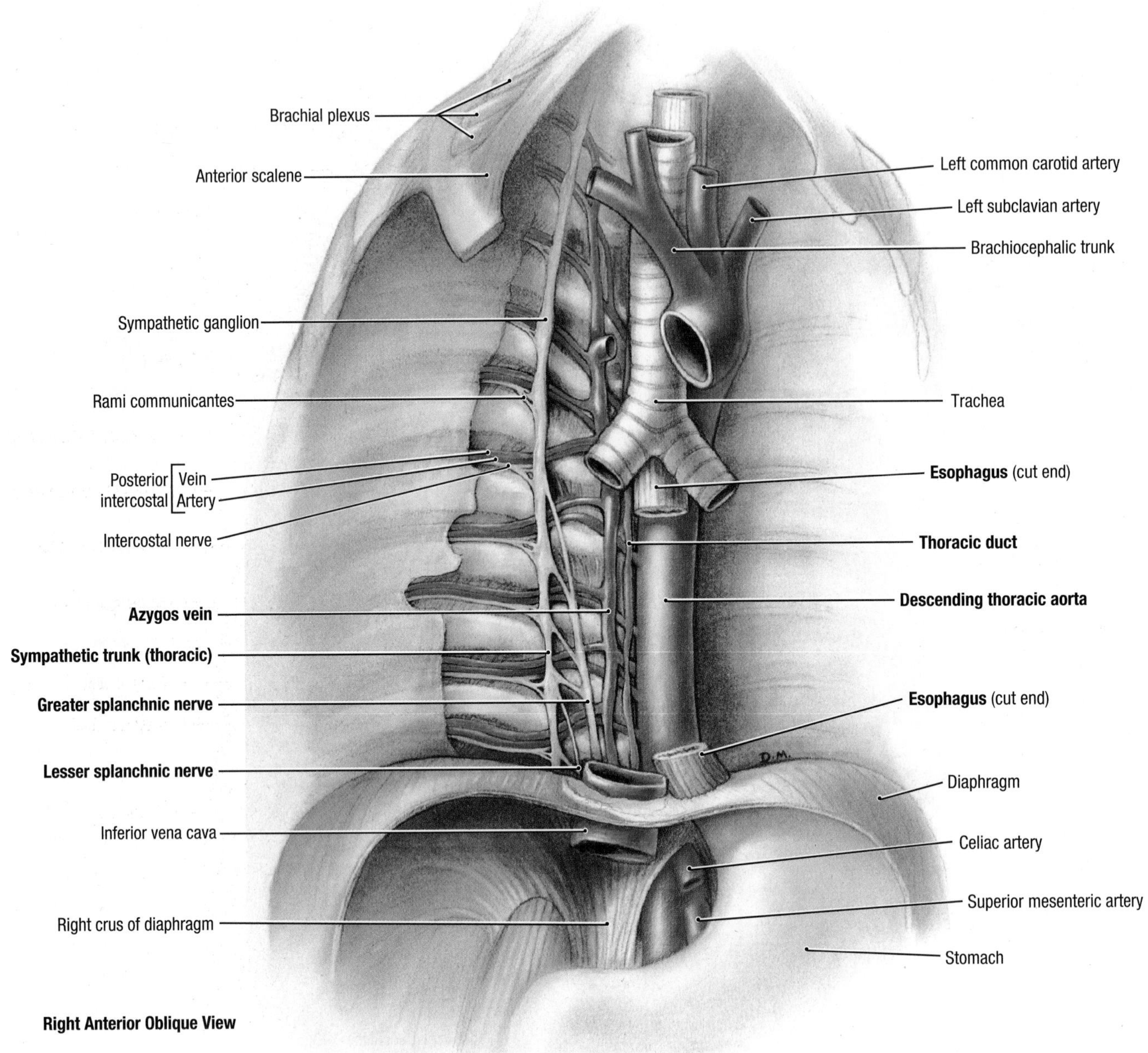
Brachial plexus
Anterior scalene
Sympathetic ganglion
Rami communicantes
Posterior intercostal Vein
Artery
Intercostal nerve
Azygos vein
Sympathetic trunk (thoracic)
Greater splanchnic nerve
Lesser splanchnic nerve
Inferior vena cava
Right crus of diaphragm
Left common carotid artery
Left subclavian artery
Brachiocephalic trunk
Trachea
Esophagus (cut end)
Thoracic duct
Descending thoracic aorta
Esophagus (cut end)
Diaphragm
Celiac artery
Superior mesenteric artery
Stomach
D.M.

Right Anterior Oblique View

1.75 STRUCTURES OF POSTERIOR MEDIASTINUM I

- In this specimen, the parietal pleura is intact on the left side and partially removed on the right side. A portion of the esophagus, between the bifurcation of the trachea and the diaphragm, is also removed.
- The thoracic sympathetic trunk is connected to each intercostal nerve by rami communicantes.
- The greater splanchnic nerve is formed by fibers from the 5th to 10th thoracic sympathetic ganglia, and the lesser splanchnic nerve receives fibers from the 10th and 11th thoracic ganglia. Both nerves contain presynaptic and visceral afferent fibers.
- The azygos vein ascends anterior to the intercostal vessels and to the right of the thoracic duct and aorta and drains into the superior vena cava.

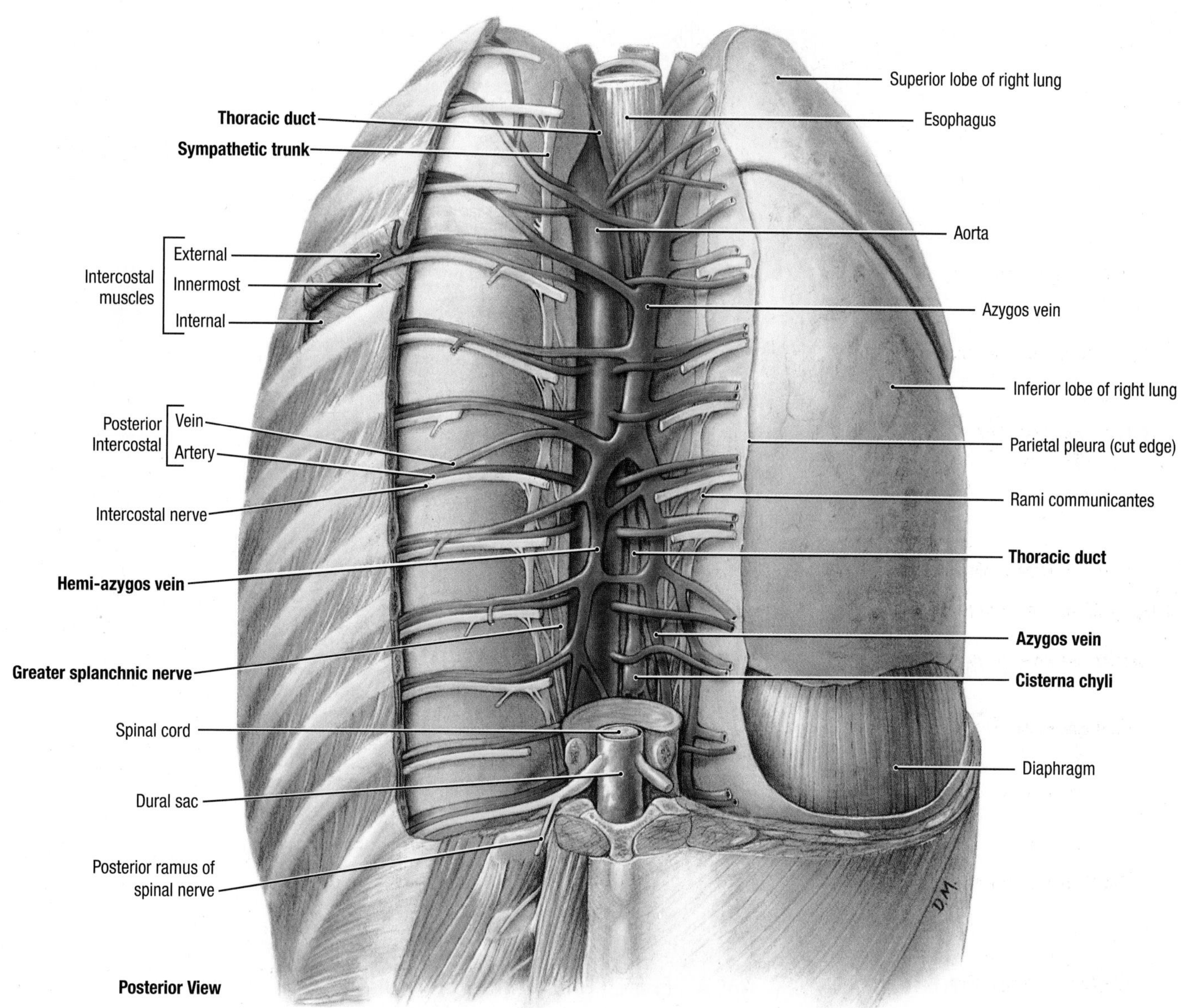
Thoracic duct
Sympathetic trunk
Intercostal muscles
External
Innermost
Internal
Posterior Intercostal
Vein
Artery
Intercostal nerve
Hemi-azygos vein
Greater splanchnic nerve
Spinal cord
Dural sac
Posterior ramus of spinal nerve
Superior lobe of right lung
Esophagus
Aorta
Azygos vein
Inferior lobe of right lung
Parietal pleura (cut edge)
Rami communicantes
Thoracic duct
Azygos vein
Cisterna chyli
Diaphragm
D.M.

Posterior View

1.76 STRUCTURES OF POSTERIOR MEDIASTINUM II

- The thoracic vertebral column and thoracic cage are removed on the right. On the left, the ribs and intercostal musculature are removed posteriorly as far laterally as the angles of the ribs. The parietal pleura is intact on the left side but partially removed on the right to reveal the visceral pleura covering the right lung.
- The azygos vein is on the right side, and the hemi-azygos vein is on the left, crossing the midline (usually at T9, but higher in this specimen) to join the azygos vein. The accessory hemi-azygos vein is absent in this specimen; instead, three most superior posterior intercostal veins drain directly into the azygos vein.

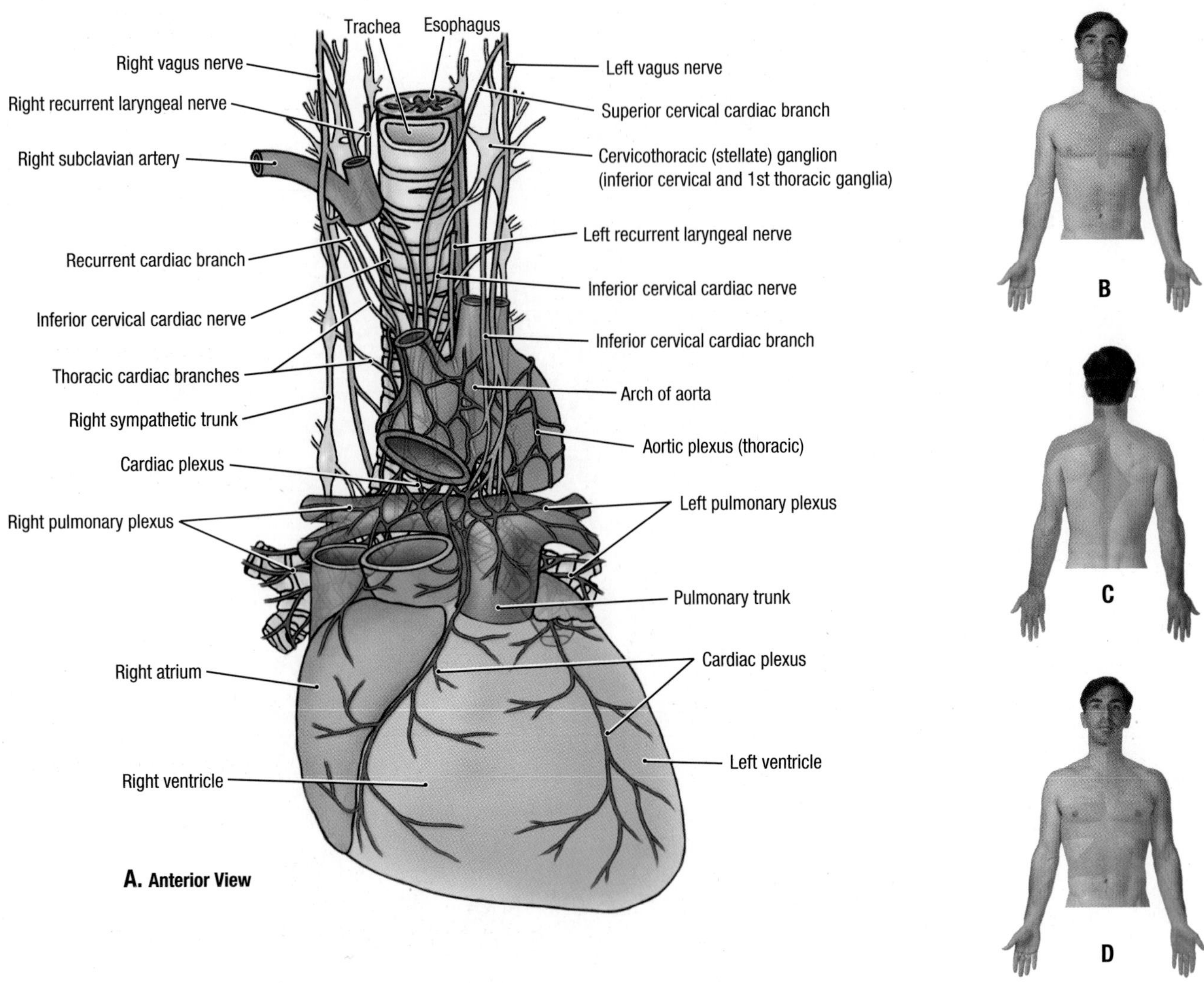
Trachea
Esophagus
Right vagus nerve
Right recurrent laryngeal nerve
Right subclavian artery
Recurrent cardiac branch
Inferior cervical cardiac nerve
Thoracic cardiac branches
Right sympathetic trunk
Cardiac plexus
Right pulmonary plexus
Right atrium
Right ventricle
Left vagus nerve
Superior cervical cardiac branch
Cervicothoracic (stellate) ganglion
(inferior cervical and 1st thoracic ganglia)
Left recurrent laryngeal nerve
Inferior cervical cardiac nerve
Inferior cervical cardiac branch
Arch of aorta
Aortic plexus (thoracic)
Left pulmonary plexus
Pulmonary trunk
Cardiac plexus
Left ventricle
A. Anterior View
B
C
D

1.77 OVERVIEW OF AUTONOMIC AND VISCERAL AFFERENT INNERVATION OF THORAX

A. Innervation of heart. **B.–D.** Areas of cardiac referred pain (*red*). **E.** Innervation of posterior and superior mediastina.

The heart is insensitive to touch, cutting, cold, and heat; however, ischemia and the accumulation of metabolic products stimulate pain endings in the myocardium. The afferent pain fibers run centrally in the middle and inferior cervical branches and especially in the thoracic cardiac branches of the sympathetic trunk. The axons of these primary sensory neurons enter spinal cord segments T1 through T4 or T5, especially on the left side.

Cardiac referred pain is a phenomenon whereby noxious stimuli originating in the heart are perceived by a person as pain arising from a superficial part of the body—the skin on the left upper limb, for example. Visceral referred pain is transmitted by visceral afferent fibers accompanying sympathetic fibers and is typically referred to somatic structures or areas such as a limb having afferent fibers with cell bodies in the same spinal ganglion, and central processes that enter the spinal cord through the same posterior roots (Hardy and Naftel, 2001).

Anginal pain is commonly felt as radiating from the substernal and left pectoral regions to the left shoulder and the medial aspect of the left upper limb (**B**). This part of the limb is supplied by the medial cutaneous nerve of the arm. Often the lateral cutaneous branches of the 2nd and 3rd intercostal nerves (the intercostobrachial nerves) join or overlap in their distribution with the medial cutaneous nerve of the arm. Consequently, cardiac pain is referred to the upper limb because the spinal cord segments of these cutaneous nerves (T1–T3) are also common to the visceral afferent terminations for the coronary arteries. Synaptic contacts may also be made with commissural (connector) neurons, which conduct impulses to neurons on the right side of comparable areas of the spinal cord. This occurrence explains why pain of cardiac origin, although usually referred to the left side, may be referred to the right side, both sides, or the back (**C and D**).

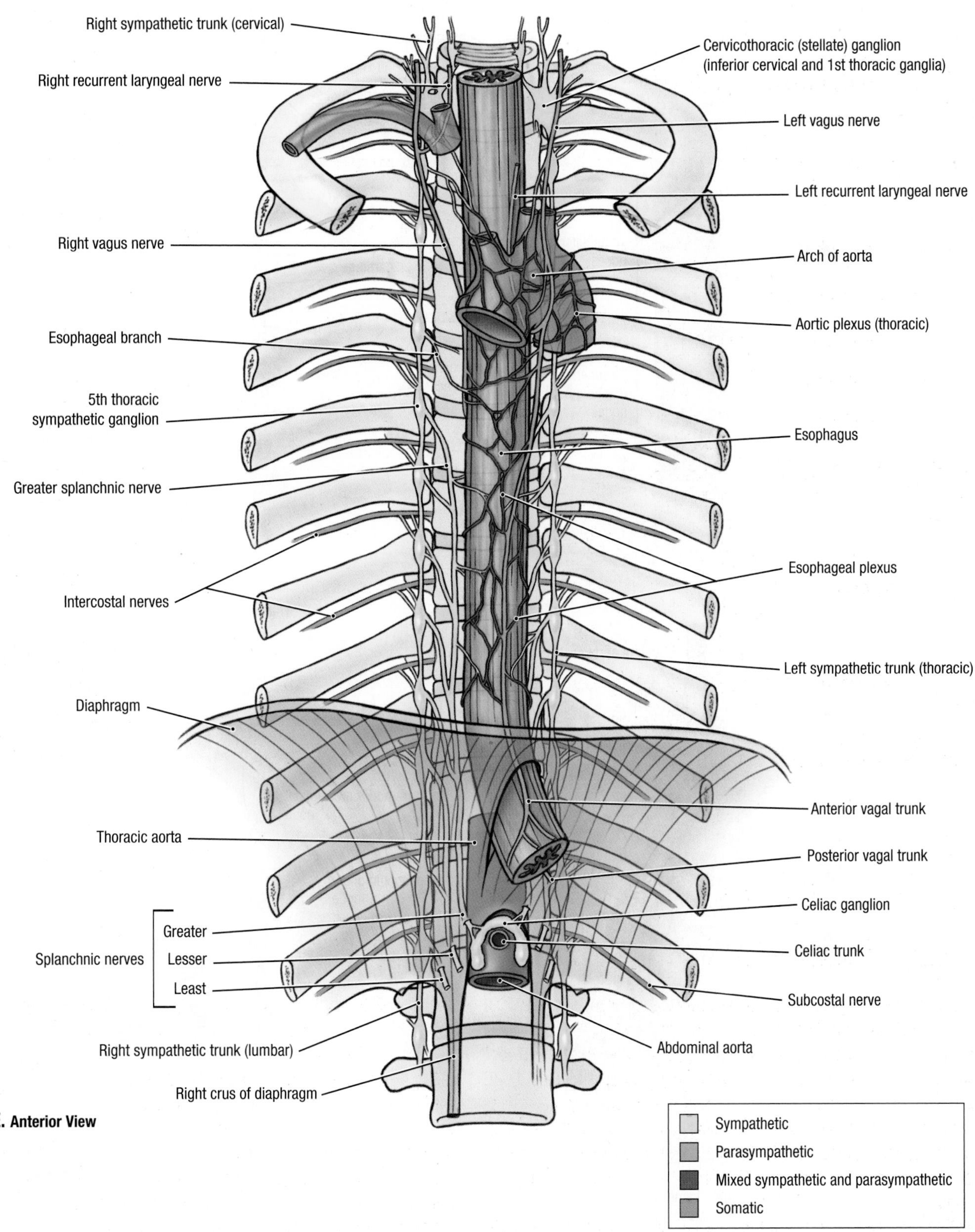
Right sympathetic trunk (cervical)
Right recurrent laryngeal nerve
Cervicothoracic (stellate) ganglion (inferior cervical and 1st thoracic ganglia)
Left vagus nerve
Left recurrent laryngeal nerve
Right vagus nerve
Arch of aorta
Aortic plexus (thoracic)
Esophageal branch
5th thoracic sympathetic ganglion
Esophagus
Greater splanchnic nerve
Esophageal plexus
Intercostal nerves
Left sympathetic trunk (thoracic)
Diaphragm
Anterior vagal trunk
Thoracic aorta
Posterior vagal trunk
Celiac ganglion
Splanchnic nerves
Greater
Lesser
Least
Celiac trunk
Subcostal nerve
Right sympathetic trunk (lumbar)
Abdominal aorta
Right crus of diaphragm
Sympathetic
Parasympathetic
Mixed sympathetic and parasympathetic
Somatic

E. **Anterior View**

1.77 OVERVIEW OF AUTONOMIC INNERVATION OF THE THORAX (*CONTINUED*)

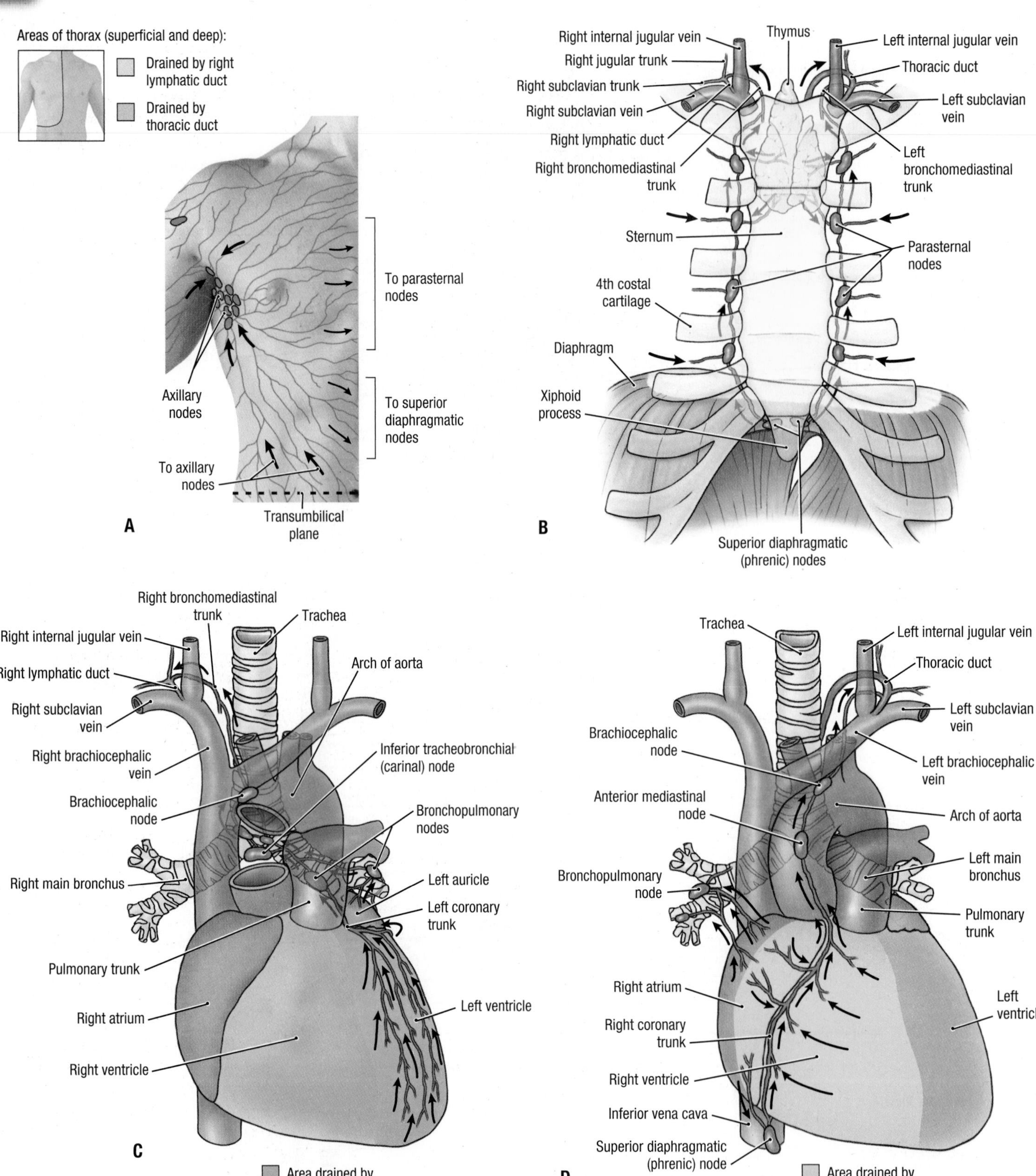
Areas of thorax (superficial and deep):
Drained by right lymphatic duct
Drained by thoracic duct
To parasternal nodes
Axillary nodes
To superior diaphragmatic nodes
To axillary nodes
Transumbilical plane
A
Right internal jugular vein
Thymus
Left internal jugular vein
Right jugular trunk
Thoracic duct
Right subclavian trunk
Left subclavian vein
Right subclavian vein
Right lymphatic duct
Left bronchomediastinal trunk
Right bronchomediastinal trunk
Sternum
Parasternal nodes
4th costal cartilage
Diaphragm
Xiphoid process
B
Superior diaphragmatic (phrenic) nodes
Right bronchomediastinal trunk
Trachea
Right internal jugular vein
Arch of aorta
Right lymphatic duct
Right subclavian vein
Right brachiocephalic vein
Inferior tracheobronchial (carinal) node
Brachiocephalic node
Bronchopulmonary nodes
Right main bronchus
Left auricle
Left coronary trunk
Pulmonary trunk
Left ventricle
Right atrium
Right ventricle
C
Area drained by left coronary trunk
Anterior Views
Trachea
Left internal jugular vein
Thoracic duct
Left subclavian vein
Brachiocephalic node
Left brachiocephalic vein
Anterior mediastinal node
Arch of aorta
Left main bronchus
Bronchopulmonary node
Pulmonary trunk
Right atrium
Left ventricle
Right coronary trunk
Right ventricle
Inferior vena cava
Superior diaphragmatic (phrenic) node
D
Area drained by right coronary trunk

1.78 OVERVIEW OF LYMPHATIC DRAINAGE OF THORAX

A. Superficial lymphatic drainage. **B.** Deep lymphatic drainage of parasternal nodes. **C.** Lymphatic drainage of left side of heart. **D.** Lymphatic drainage of right side of heart.

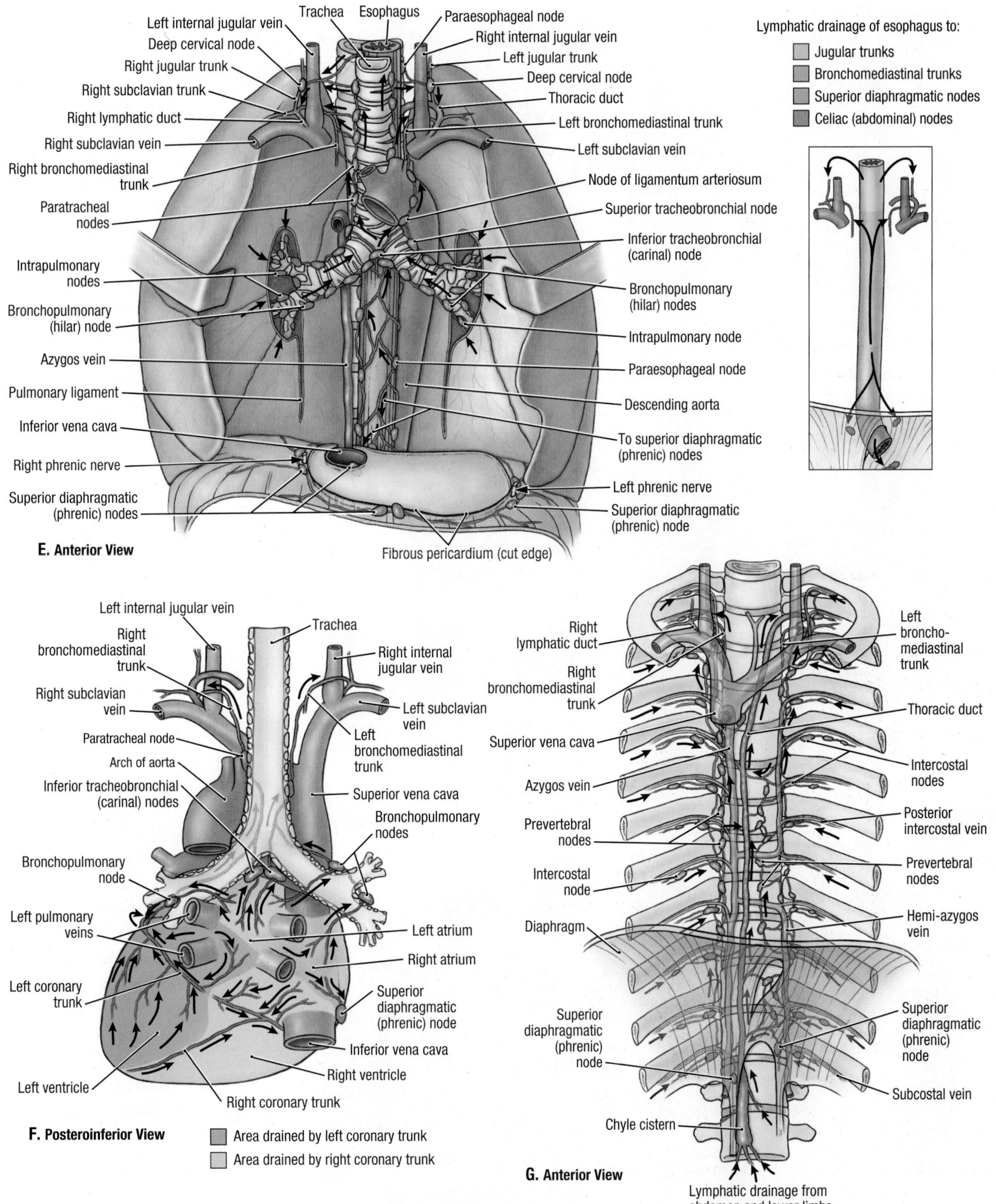
Trachea
Esophagus
Left internal jugular vein
Deep cervical node
Right jugular trunk
Right subclavian trunk
Right lymphatic duct
Right subclavian vein
Right bronchomediastinal trunk
Paratracheal nodes
Intrapulmonary nodes
Bronchopulmonary (hilar) node
Azygos vein
Pulmonary ligament
Inferior vena cava
Right phrenic nerve
Superior diaphragmatic (phrenic) nodes
Paraesophageal node
Right internal jugular vein
Left jugular trunk
Deep cervical node
Thoracic duct
Left bronchomediastinal trunk
Left subclavian vein
Node of ligamentum arteriosum
Superior tracheobronchial node
Inferior tracheobronchial (carinal) node
Bronchopulmonary (hilar) nodes
Intrapulmonary node
Paraesophageal node
Descending aorta
To superior diaphragmatic (phrenic) nodes
Left phrenic nerve
Superior diaphragmatic (phrenic) node
Fibrous pericardium (cut edge)
E. Anterior View
Lymphatic drainage of esophagus to:
Jugular trunks
Bronchomediastinal trunks
Superior diaphragmatic nodes
Celiac (abdominal) nodes
Left internal jugular vein
Right bronchomediastinal trunk
Right subclavian vein
Paratracheal node
Arch of aorta
Inferior tracheobronchial (carinal) nodes
Bronchopulmonary node
Left pulmonary veins
Left coronary trunk
Left ventricle
Trachea
Right internal jugular vein
Left subclavian vein
Left bronchomediastinal trunk
Superior vena cava
Bronchopulmonary nodes
Left atrium
Right atrium
Superior diaphragmatic (phrenic) node
Inferior vena cava
Right ventricle
Right coronary trunk
F. Posteroinferior View
Area drained by left coronary trunk
Area drained by right coronary trunk
Right lymphatic duct
Right bronchomediastinal trunk
Superior vena cava
Azygos vein
Prevertebral nodes
Intercostal node
Diaphragm
Superior diaphragmatic (phrenic) node
Chyle cistern
Left broncho-mediastinal trunk
Thoracic duct
Intercostal nodes
Posterior intercostal vein
Prevertebral nodes
Hemi-azygos vein
Superior diaphragmatic (phrenic) node
Subcostal vein
G. Anterior View
Lymphatic drainage from abdomen and lower limbs

1.78 OVERVIEW OF LYMPHATIC DRAINAGE OF THORAX (*CONTINUED*)

E. Lymphatic drainage of lungs, esophagus, and superior surface of diaphragm. **F.** Lymphatic drainage of posterior and inferior surfaces of heart. **G.** Lymphatic drainage of posterior mediastinum.

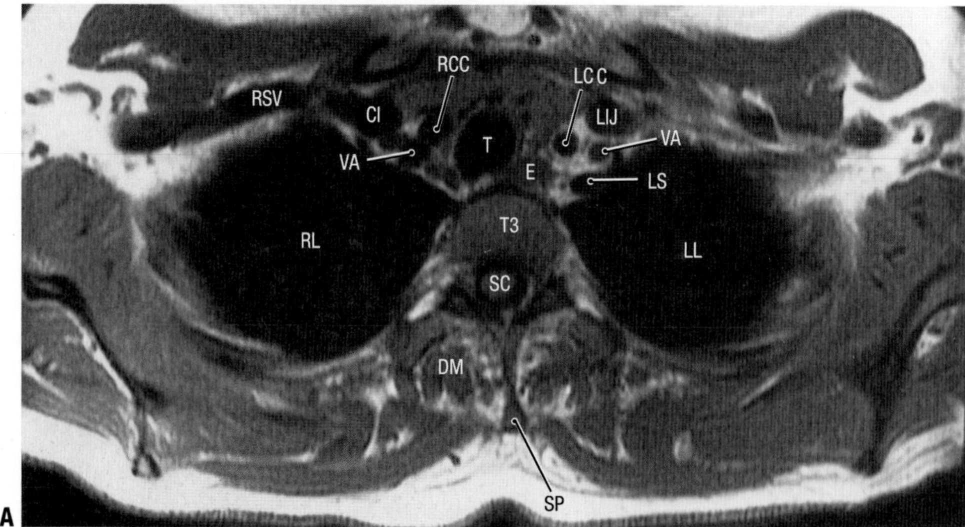

A
RSV
CI
RCC
LCC
LIJ
VA
T
E
VA
LS
RL
T3
LL
SC
DM
SP

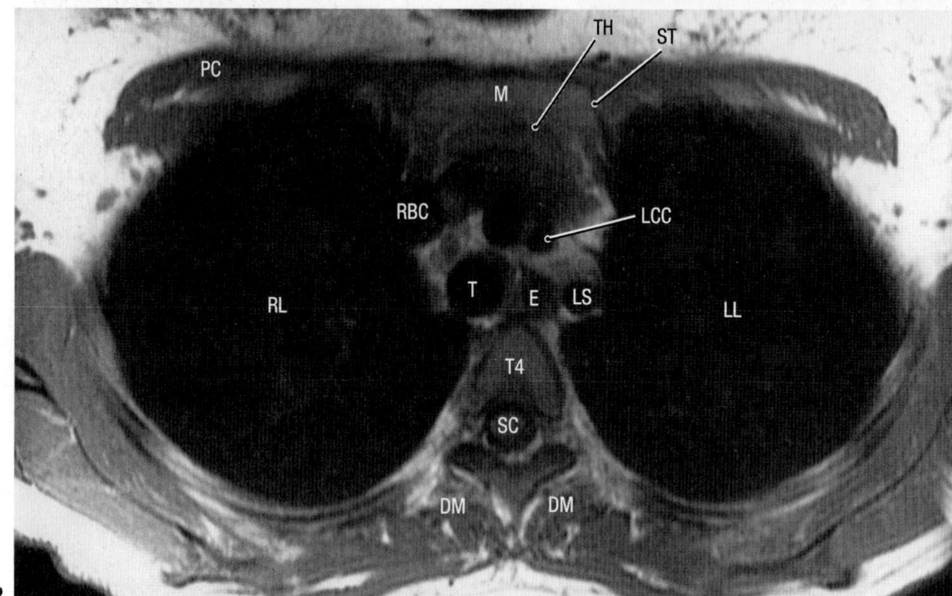

B
PC
TH
ST
M
RBC
LCC
RL
T
E
LS
LL
T4
SC
DM
DM

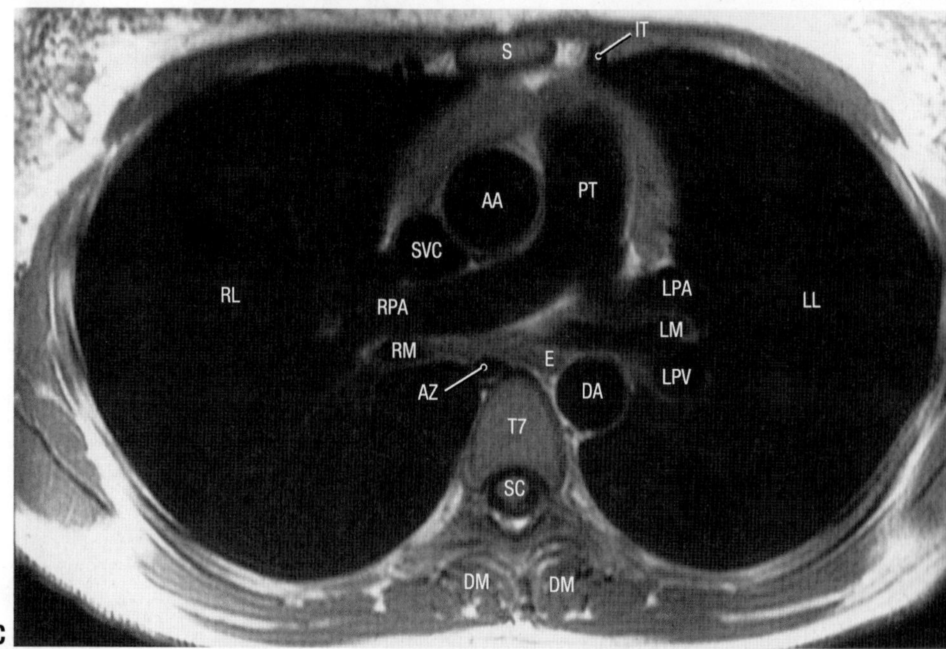

C
S
IT
AA
PT
SVC
RL
RPA
LPA
LL
LM
RM
E
LPV
AZ
DA
T7
SC
DM
DM

AA	Ascending aorta
AI	Anterior interventricular artery
AZ	Azygos vein
CA	Cusp of aortic valve
CI	Confluence of internal jugular vein
DA	Descending aorta
DM	Deep back muscles
E	Esophagus
HR	Head of rib
HZ	Hemi-azygos vein
IT	Internal thoracic vessels
IVS	Interventricular septum
LA	Left atrium
LC	Left coronary artery
LCC	Left common carotid artery
LIJ	Left internal jugular vein
LL	Left lung
LM	Left main bronchus
LPA	Left pulmonary artery
LPV	Left pulmonary vein
LS	Left subclavian artery
LV	Left vertebral artery
M	Manubrium
P	Pericardium
PC	Pectoralis major
PI	Pulmonary infundibulum
PM	Papillary muscle
PT	Pulmonary trunk
RA	Right atrium
RBC	Right brachiocephalic vein
RCC	Right common carotid artery
RL	Right lung
RM	Right middle lobar bronchus
RPA	Right pulmonary artery
RPV	Right pulmonary vein
RSV	Right subclavian vein
RV	Right vertebral artery
S	Sternum
SC	Spinal cord
SP	Spinous process
ST	Sternoclavicular joint
SVC	Superior vena cava
T3-T10	Vertebral body
T	Trachea
TH	Thymus
VA	Vertebral artery

1.79 TRANSVERSE (AXIAL) MRIs OF THORAX (A–F)

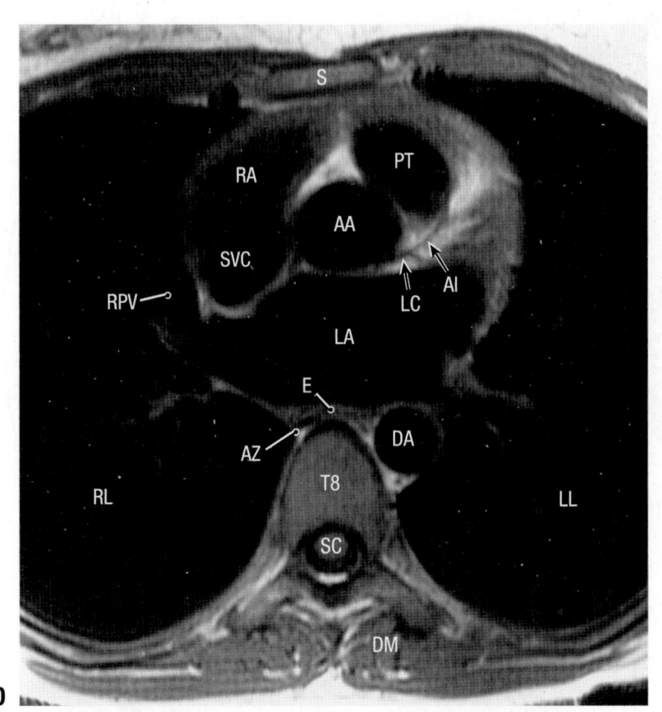
S
RA
PT
AA
SVC
RPV
LC
AI
LA
E
AZ
DA
T8
RL
LL
SC
DM
D

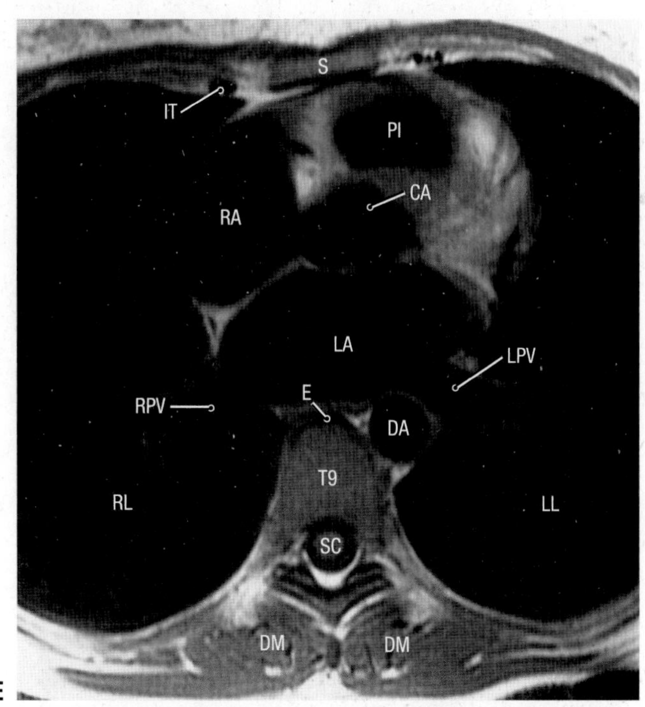
S
IT
PI
CA
RA
LA
LPV
RPV
E
DA
T9
RL
LL
SC
DM
DM
E

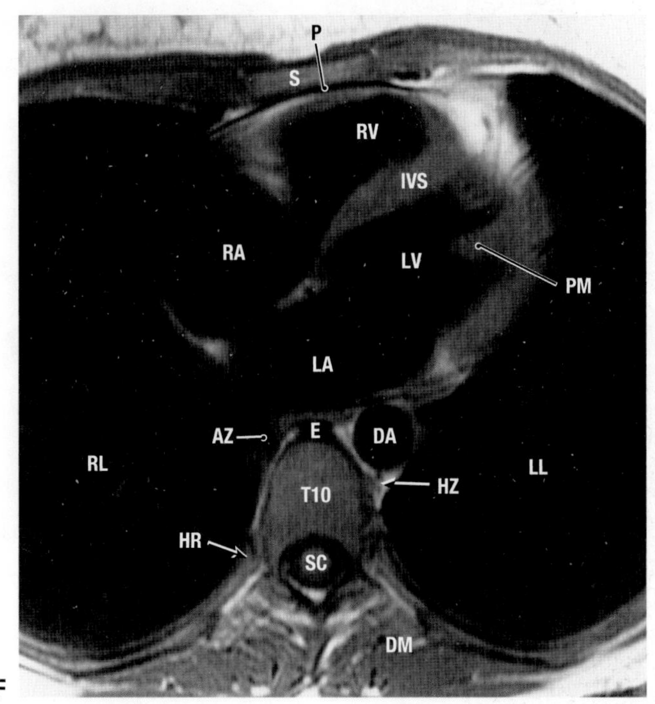
P
S
RV
IVS
RA
LV
PM
LA
AZ
E
DA
RL
LL
HZ
T10
HR
SC
DM
F

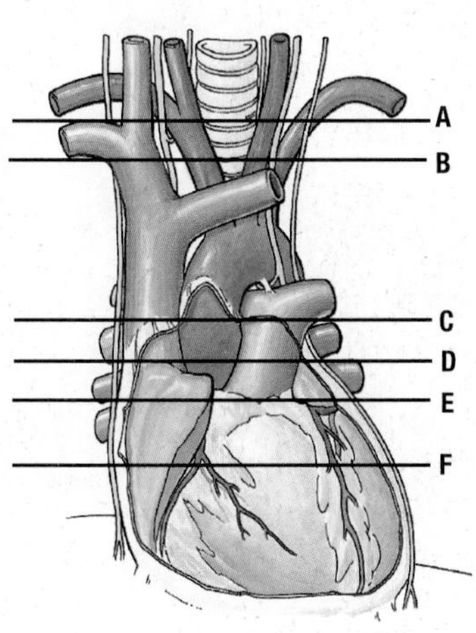
A
B
C
D
E
F

1.79 TRANSVERSE (AXIAL) MRIs OF THORAX (*CONTINUED*)

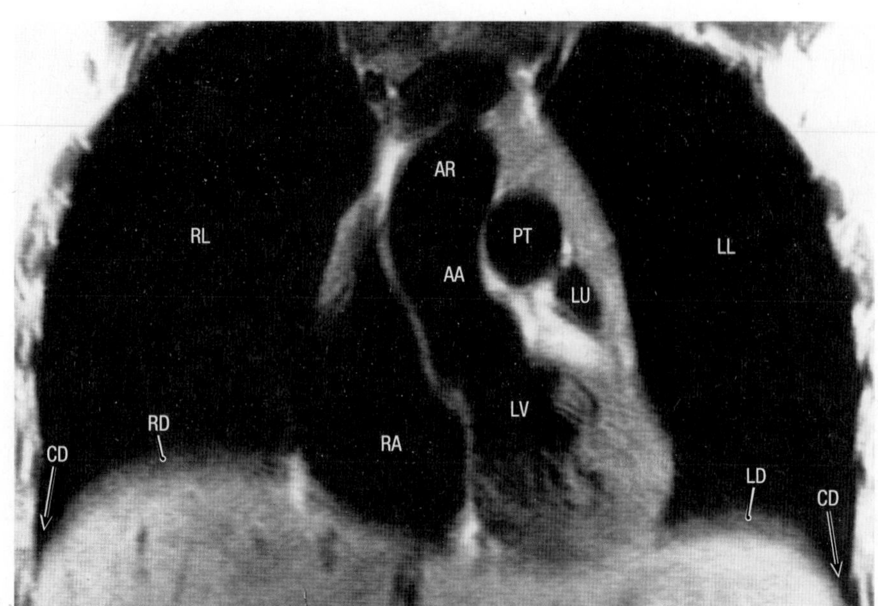
AR
PT
AA
LU
RL
LL
LV
RA
RD
CD
LD
CD
A

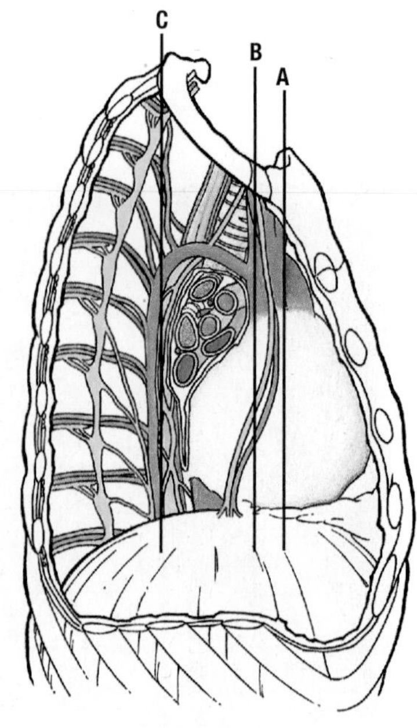
C
B
A

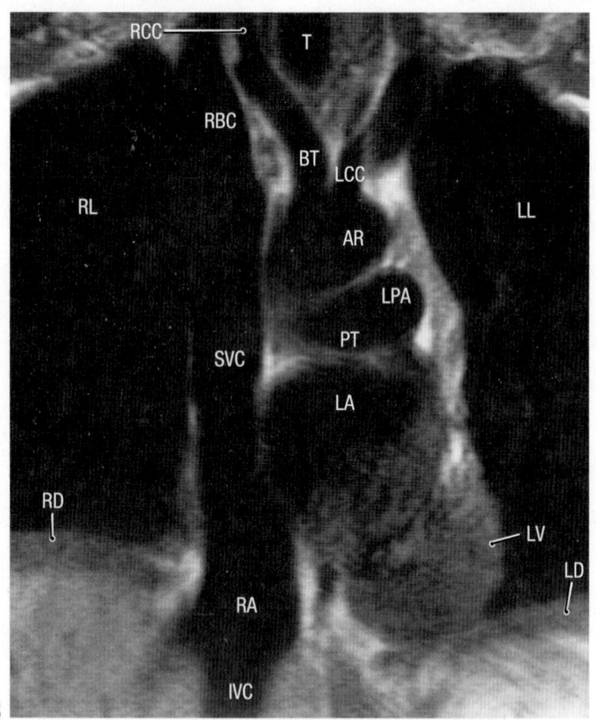
RCC
T
RBC
BT
LCC
RL
LL
AR
LPA
PT
SVC
LA
RD
LV
LD
RA
IVC
B

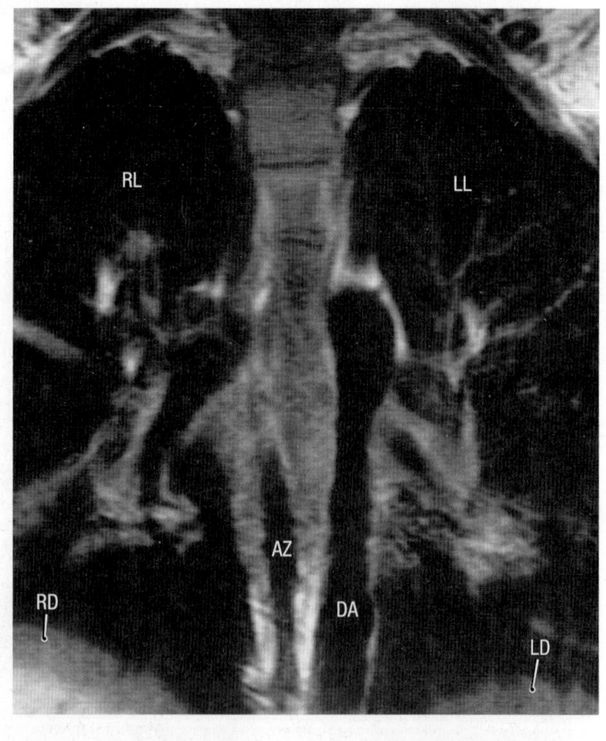
RL
LL
AZ
RD
DA
LD
C

AA	Ascending aorta	IVC	Inferior vena cava	LU	Left auricle	RD	Right dome of diaphragm
AR	Arch of aorta	LA	Left atrium	LV	Left ventricle	RL	Right lung
AZ	Azygos vein	LCC	Left common carotid artery	PT	Pulmonary trunk	RV	Right ventricle
BT	Brachiocephalic trunk	LD	Left dome of diaphragm	RA	Right atrium	SVC	Superior vena cava
CD	Costodiaphragmatic recess	LL	Left lung	RBC	Right brachiocephalic vein	T	Trachea
DA	Descending aorta	LPA	Left pulmonary artery	RCC	Right common carotid artery	V	Vertebral body

1.80 CORONAL MRIs OF THORAX

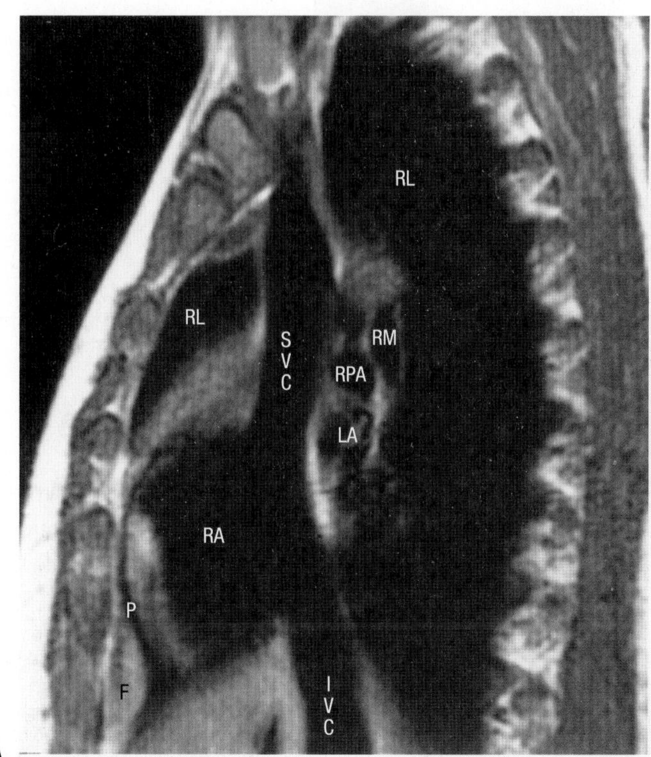
RL
RL
SVC
RM
RPA
LA
RA
P
F
IVC
A

AR	Arch of aorta
AA	Ascending aorta
DA	Descending aorta
F	Fat
IVC	Inferior vena cava
LA	Left atrium
LBC	Left brachiocephalic vein
LCC	Left common carotid artery
LL	Left lung
LM	Left main bronchus
LS	Left subclavian artery
LV	Left ventricle
P	Pericardium
RA	Right atrium
RL	Right lung
RM	Right main bronchus
RPA	Right pulmonary artery
RV	Right ventricle
SVC	Superior vena cava

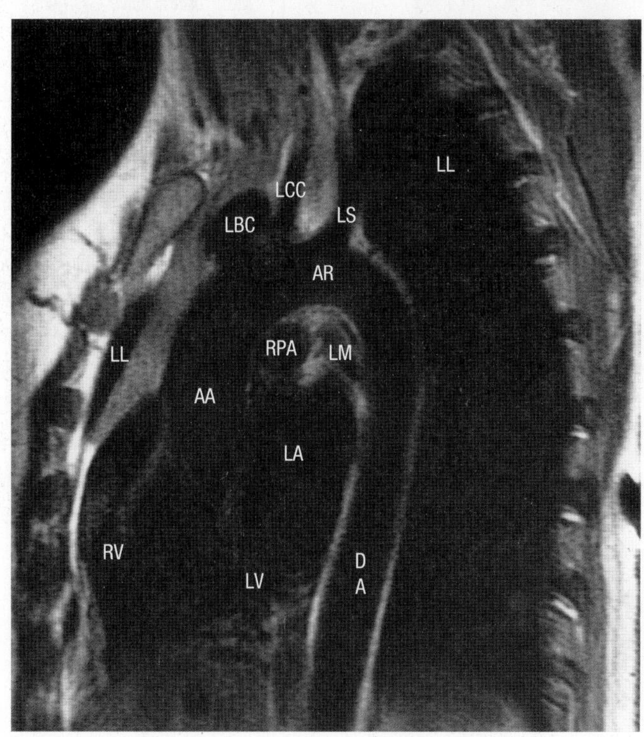
LL
LCC
LBC
LS
AR
RPA
LM
LL
AA
LA
RV
LV
DA
B

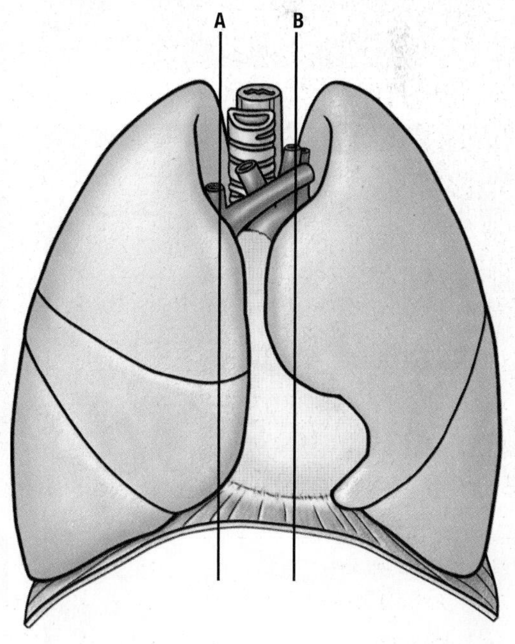
A
B

1.81 SAGITTAL MRIs OF THORAX

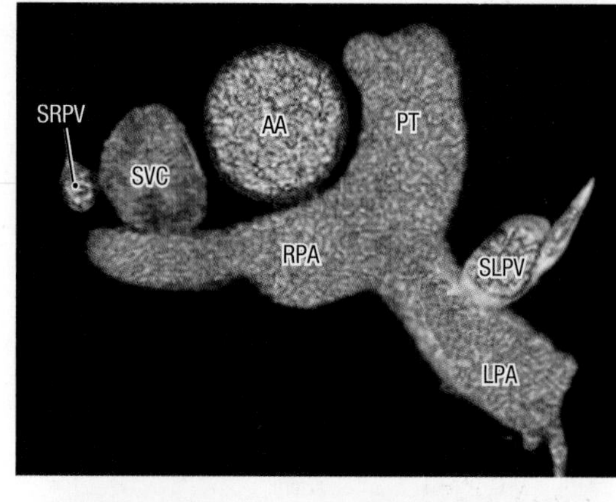
SRPV
SVC
AA
PT
RPA
SLPV
LPA

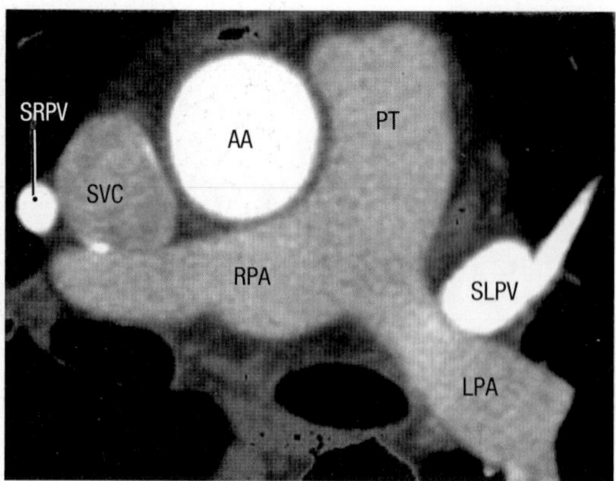
SRPV
SVC
AA
PT
RPA
SLPV
LPA

A

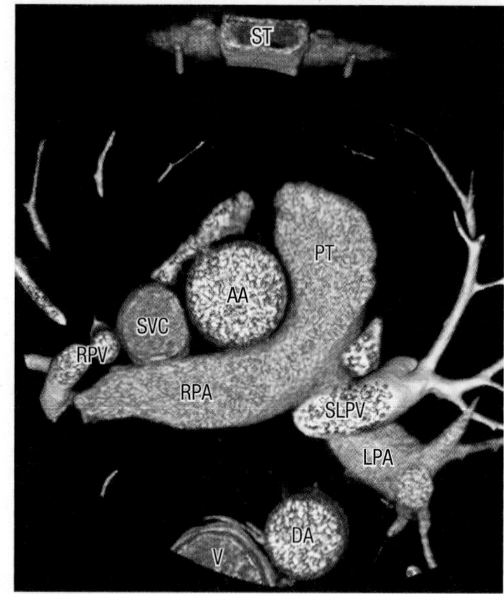
ST
PT
AA
SVC
RPV
RPA
SLPV
LPA
DA
V

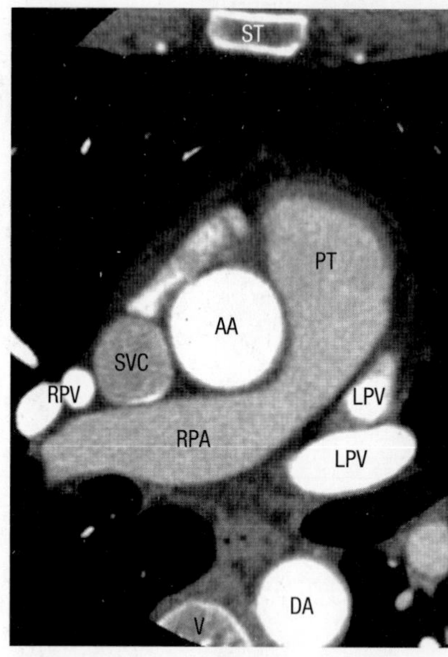
ST
PT
AA
SVC
RPV
RPA
LPV
LPV
DA
V

B

AA	Ascending aorta
AZ	Azygos vein
DA	Descending aorta
E	Esophagus
ILPV	Inferior left pulmonary vein
IRPV	Inferior right pulmonary vein
IS	Interventricular septum
LA	Left atrium
LCA	Left coronary artery
LPA	Left pulmonary artery
LPV	Left pulmonary vein
LV	Left ventricle
MV	Mitral valve
PT	Pulmonary trunk
RA	Right atrium
RCA	Right coronary artery
RPA	Right pulmonary artery
RPV	Right pulmonary vein
RV	Right ventricle
SLPV	Superior left pulmonary vein
SRPV	Superior right pulmonary vein
SVC	Superior vena cava
V	Vertebra
ST	Sternum

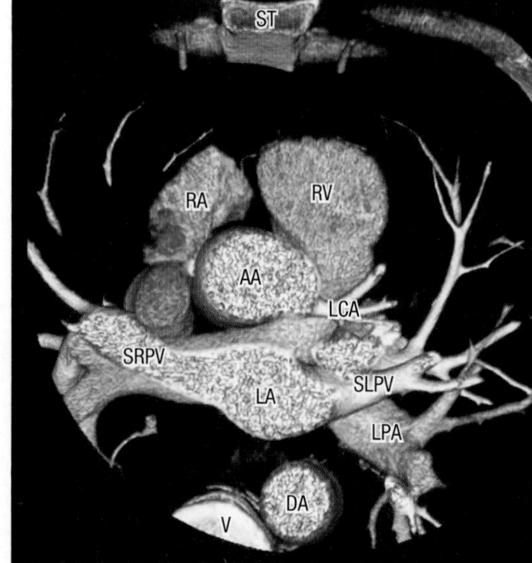
ST
RA
RV
AA
LCA
SRPV
LA
SLPV
LPA
DA
V

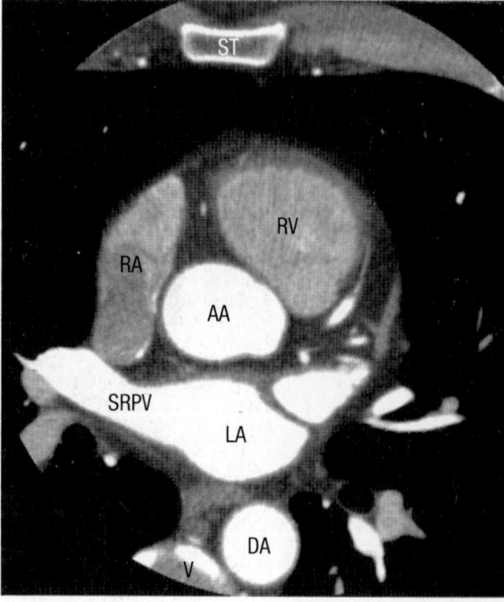
ST
RV
RA
AA
SRPV
LA
DA
V

C

1.82 TRANSVERSE OR HORIZONTAL (AXIAL) 3D VOLUME RECONSTRUCTIONS (ON LEFT SIDE OF PAGE) AND CT ANGIOGRAMS OF THORAX (A–F)

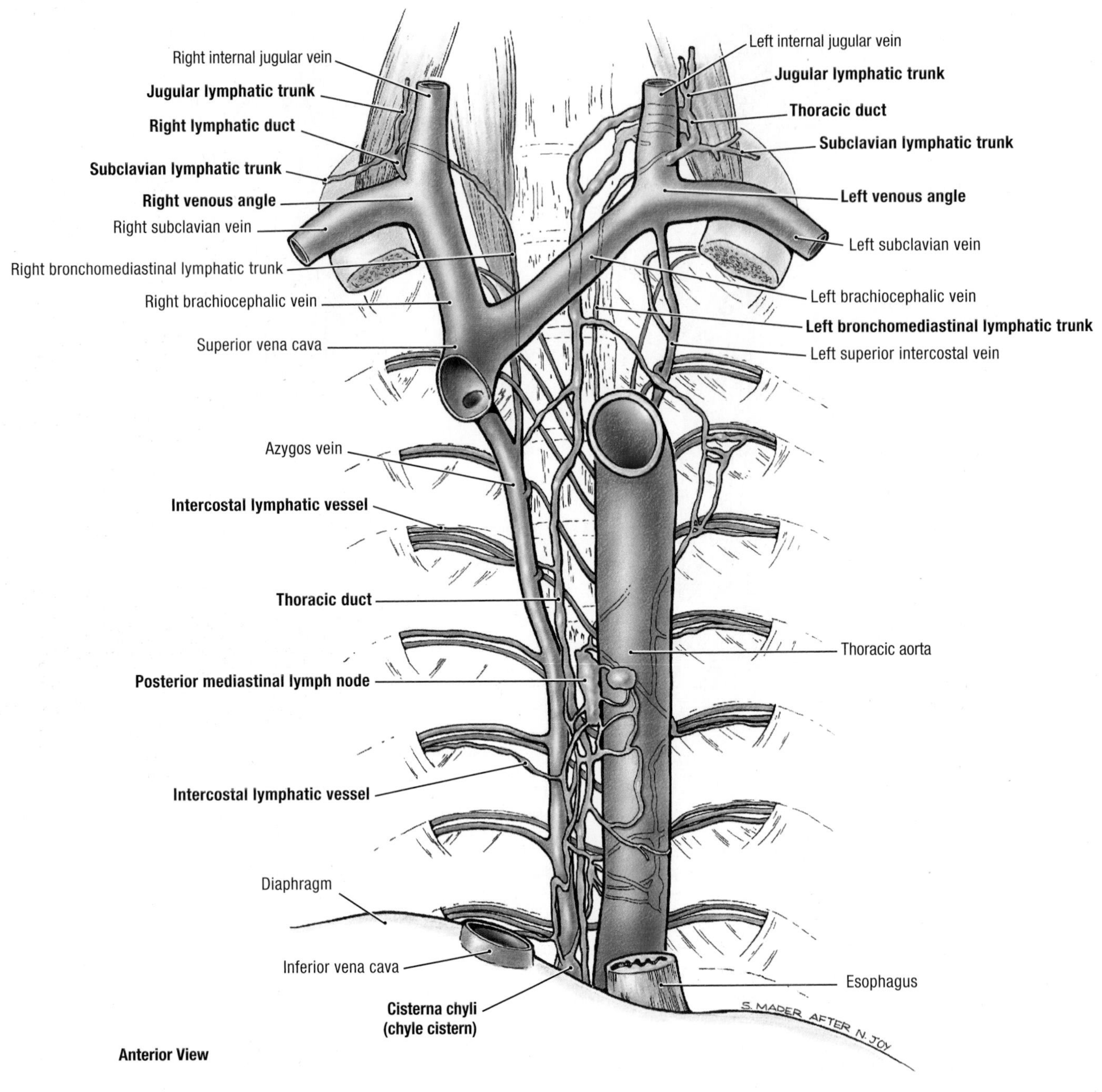
Right internal jugular vein
Jugular lymphatic trunk
Right lymphatic duct
Subclavian lymphatic trunk
Right venous angle
Right subclavian vein
Right bronchomediastinal lymphatic trunk
Right brachiocephalic vein
Superior vena cava
Azygos vein
Intercostal lymphatic vessel
Thoracic duct
Posterior mediastinal lymph node
Intercostal lymphatic vessel
Diaphragm
Inferior vena cava
Cisterna chyli
(chyle cistern)
Left internal jugular vein
Jugular lymphatic trunk
Thoracic duct
Subclavian lymphatic trunk
Left venous angle
Left subclavian vein
Left brachiocephalic vein
Left bronchomediastinal lymphatic trunk
Left superior intercostal vein
Thoracic aorta
Esophagus
S. MADER AFTER N. JOY
Anterior View

1.70 THORACIC DUCT

- The descending aorta is located to the left, and the azygos vein slightly to the right of the midline.
- The thoracic duct (1) originates from the cisterna chyli at the T12 vertebral level, (2) ascends on the vertebral column between the azygos vein and the descending aorta, (3) passes to the left at the junction of the posterior and superior mediastina, and continues its ascent to the neck, where (4) it arches laterally to enter the venous system near or at the angle of union of the left internal jugular and subclavian veins (left venous angle).
- The thoracic duct is commonly plexiform (resembling a network) in the posterior mediastinum.
- The termination of the thoracic duct typically receives the left jugular, subclavian, and bronchomediastinal trunks.
- The right lymph duct is short and formed by the union of the right jugular, subclavian, and bronchomediastinal trunks.
- **Because the thoracic duct is thin walled and may be colorless, it may not be easily identified. Consequently, it is vulnerable to inadvertent injury during investigative and/or surgical procedures in the posterior mediastinum. Laceration of the thoracic duct results in chyle escaping into the thoracic cavity. Chyle may also enter the pleural cavity, producing chylothorax.**

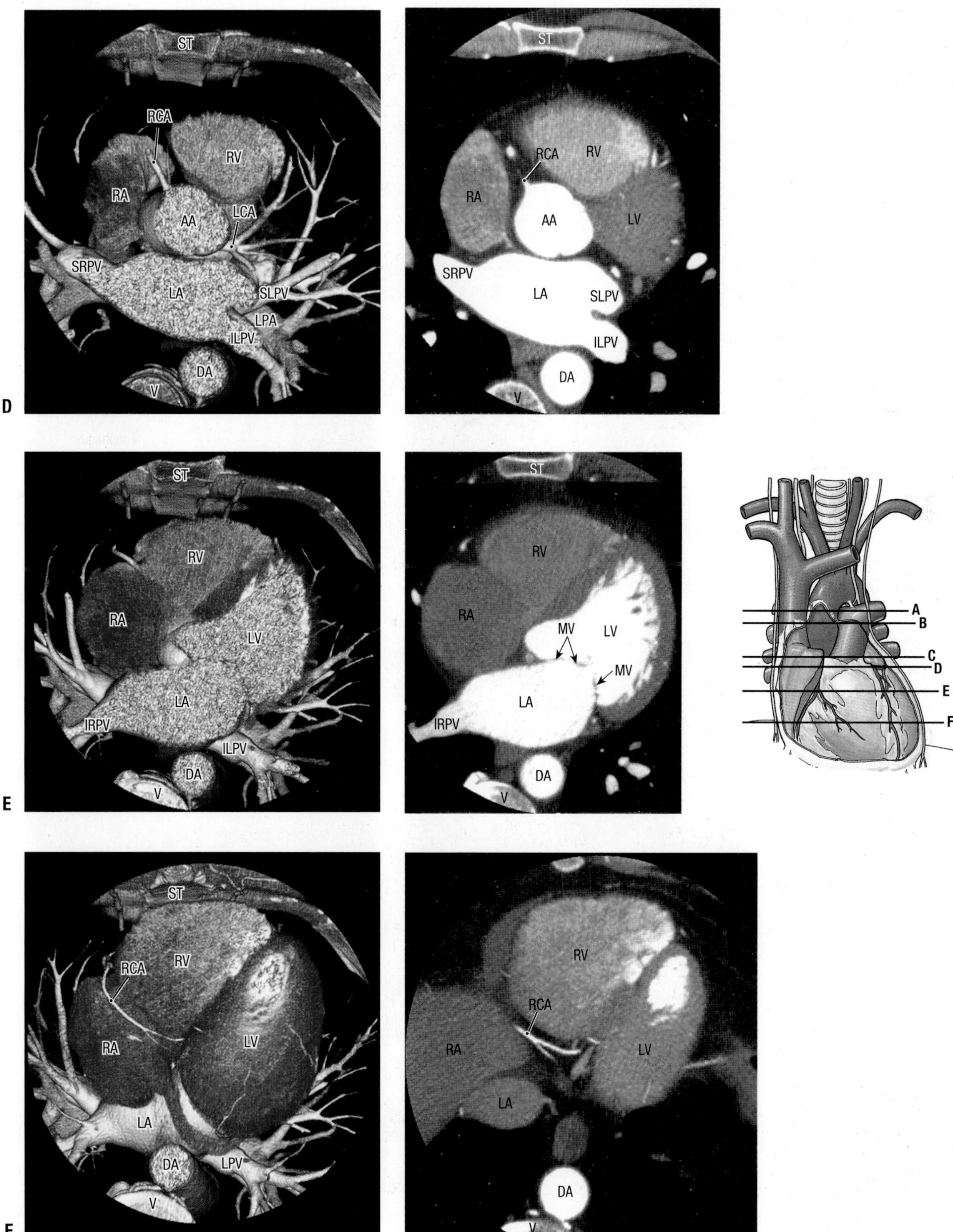
ST
RCA
RV
RA
AA
LCA
LV
SRPV
LA
SLPV
LPA
ILPV
DA
V
D
MV
IRPV
E
LPV
F
A
B
C

1.82 TRANSVERSE OR HORIZONTAL (AXIAL) 3D VOLUME RECONSTRUCTIONS (ON LEFT SIDE OF PAGE) AND CT ANGIOGRAMS OF THORAX (A–F) (*CONTINUED*)

Abdomen

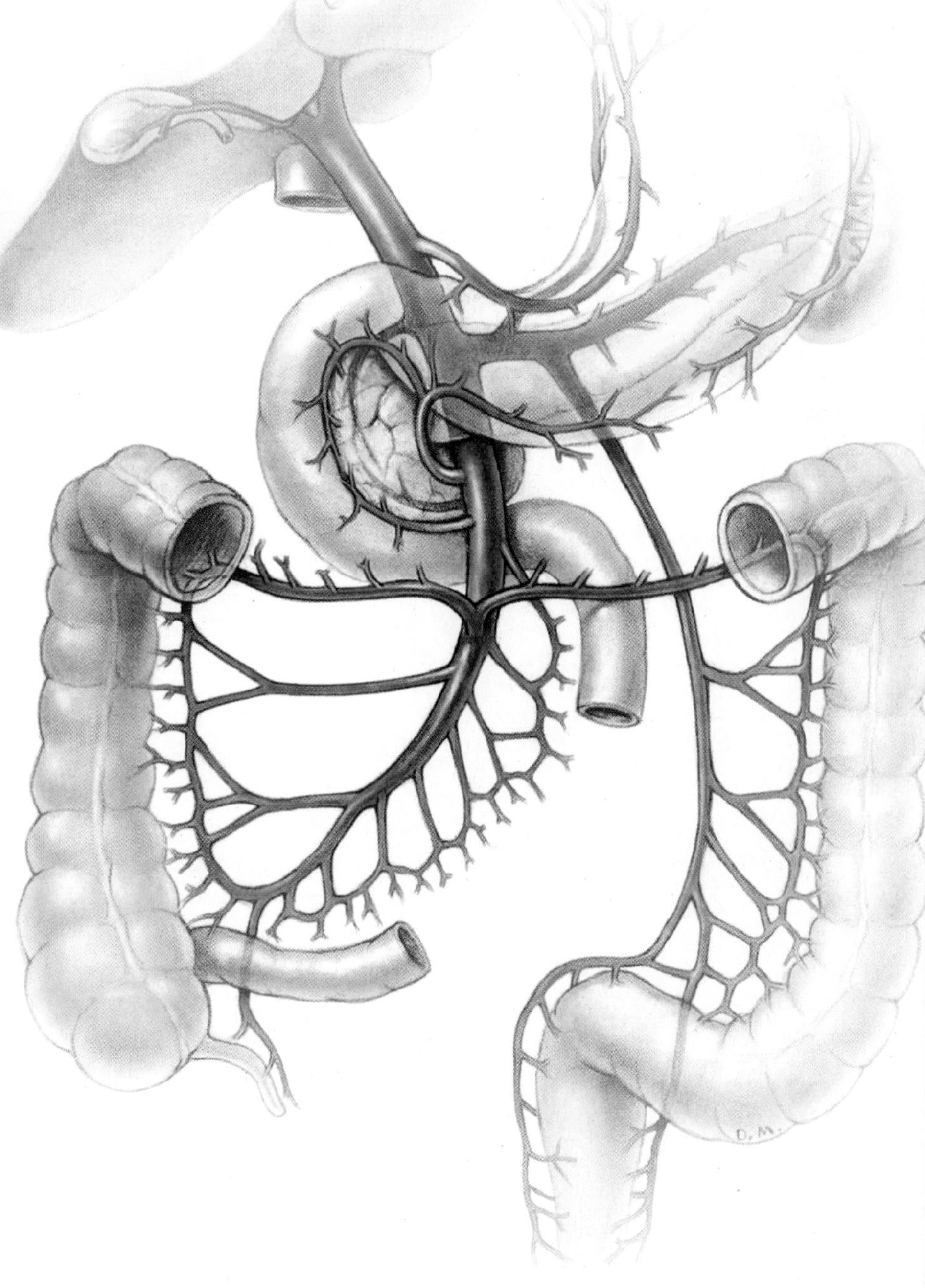
D.M.

Overview	98
Anterolateral Abdominal Wall	100
Inguinal Region	110
Testis	120
Peritoneum and Peritoneal Cavity	122
Digestive System	132
Stomach	133
Pancreas, Duodenum, and Spleen	136
Intestines	140
Liver and Gallbladder	150
Biliary Ducts	160
Portal Venous System	164
Posterior Abdominal Viscera	166
Kidneys	169
Posterolateral Abdominal Wall	173
Diaphragm	178
Abdominal Aorta and Inferior Vena Cava	179
Autonomic Innervation	180
Lymphatic Drainage	186
Sectional Anatomy and Imaging	190

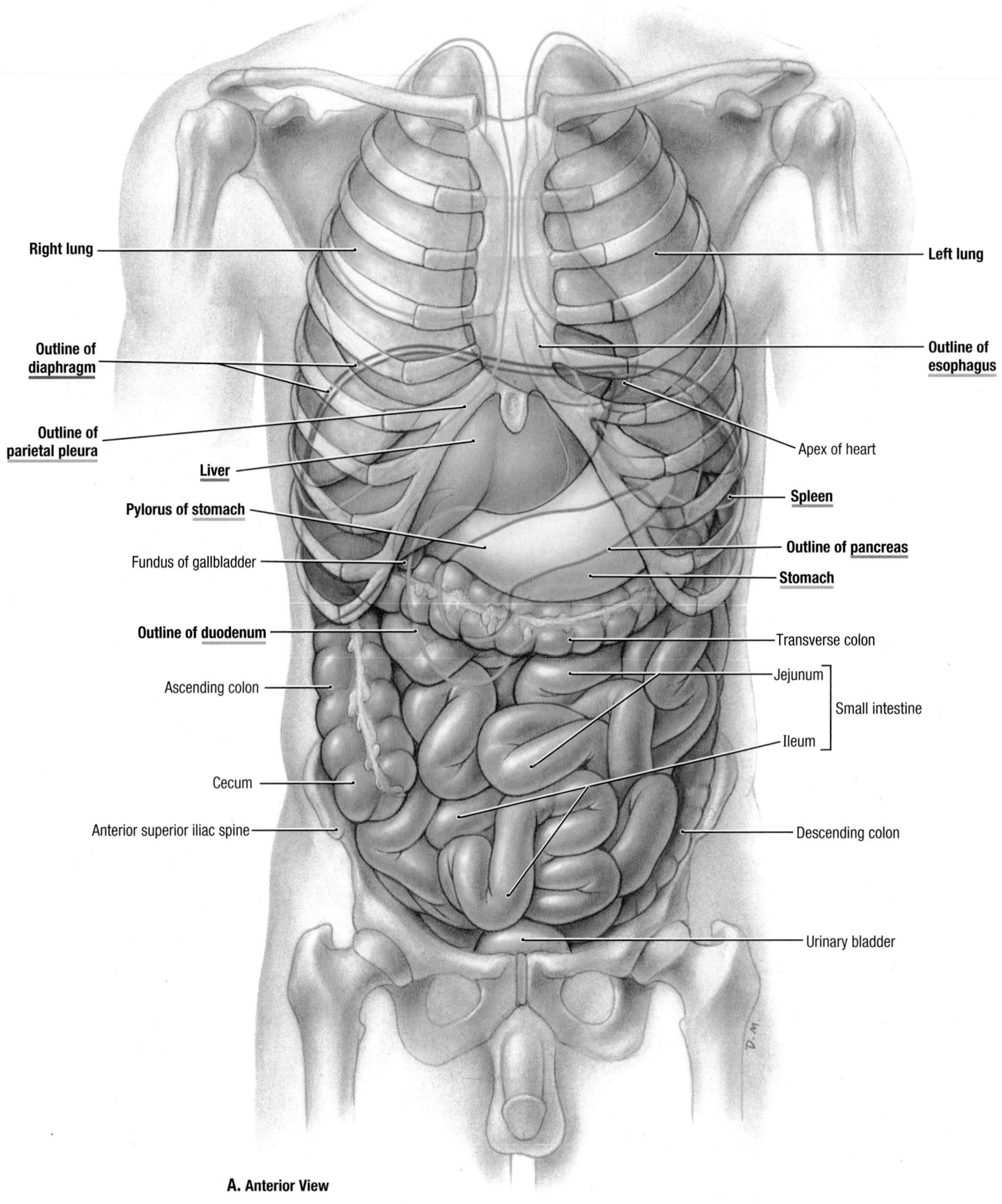
Right lung
Left lung
Outline of diaphragm
Outline of esophagus
Outline of parietal pleura
Apex of heart
Liver
Spleen
Pylorus of stomach
Outline of pancreas
Fundus of gallbladder
Stomach
Outline of duodenum
Transverse colon
Jejunum
Small intestine
Ileum
Ascending colon
Cecum
Anterior superior iliac spine
Descending colon
Urinary bladder
D.M.

A. Anterior View

2.1 ABDOMINAL VISCERA IN SITU

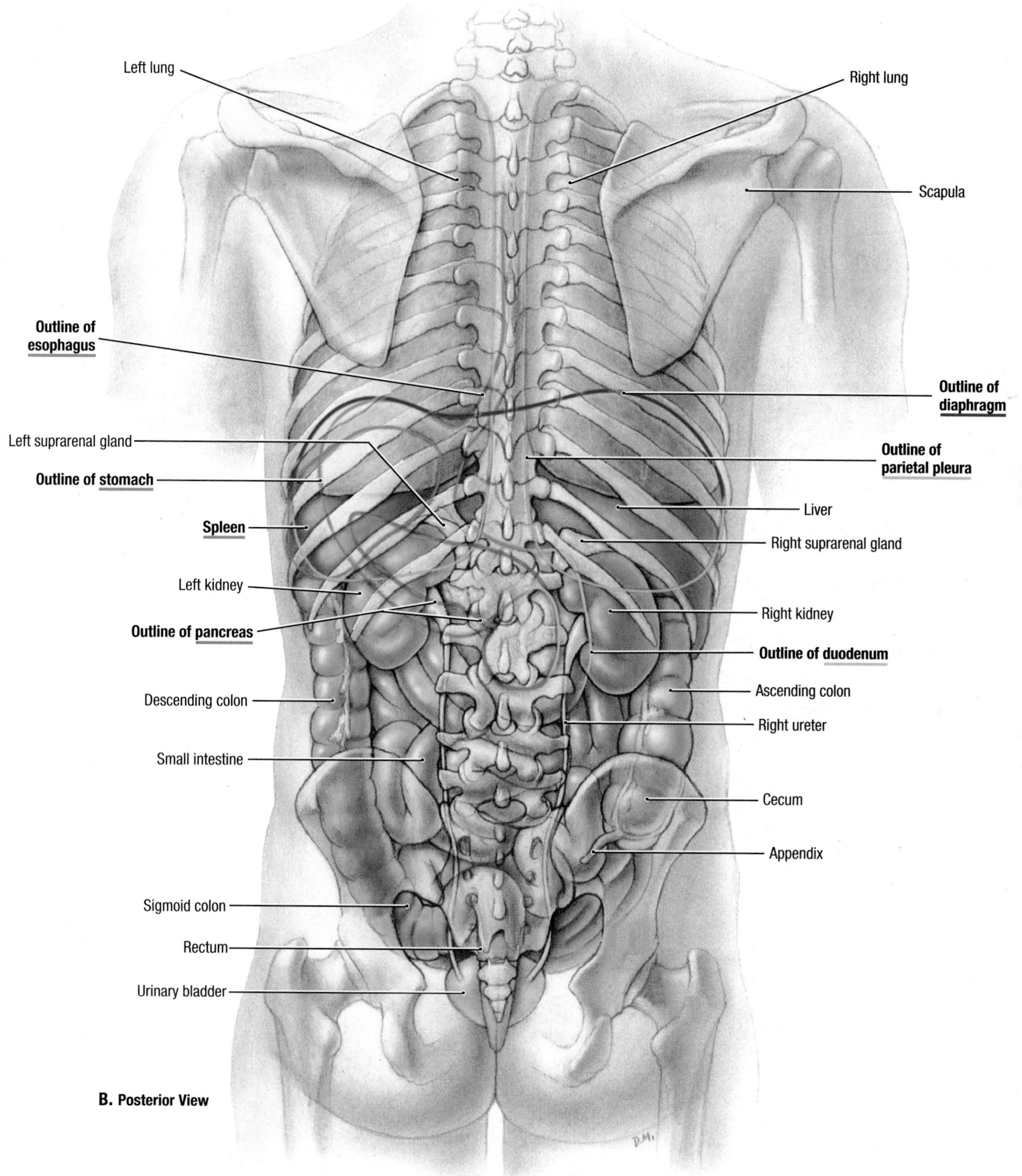
Left lung
Right lung
Scapula
Outline of esophagus
Outline of diaphragm
Left suprarenal gland
Outline of parietal pleura
Outline of stomach
Liver
Spleen
Right suprarenal gland
Left kidney
Right kidney
Outline of pancreas
Outline of duodenum
Descending colon
Ascending colon
Right ureter
Small intestine
Cecum
Appendix
Sigmoid colon
Rectum
Urinary bladder
D.M.

B. Posterior View

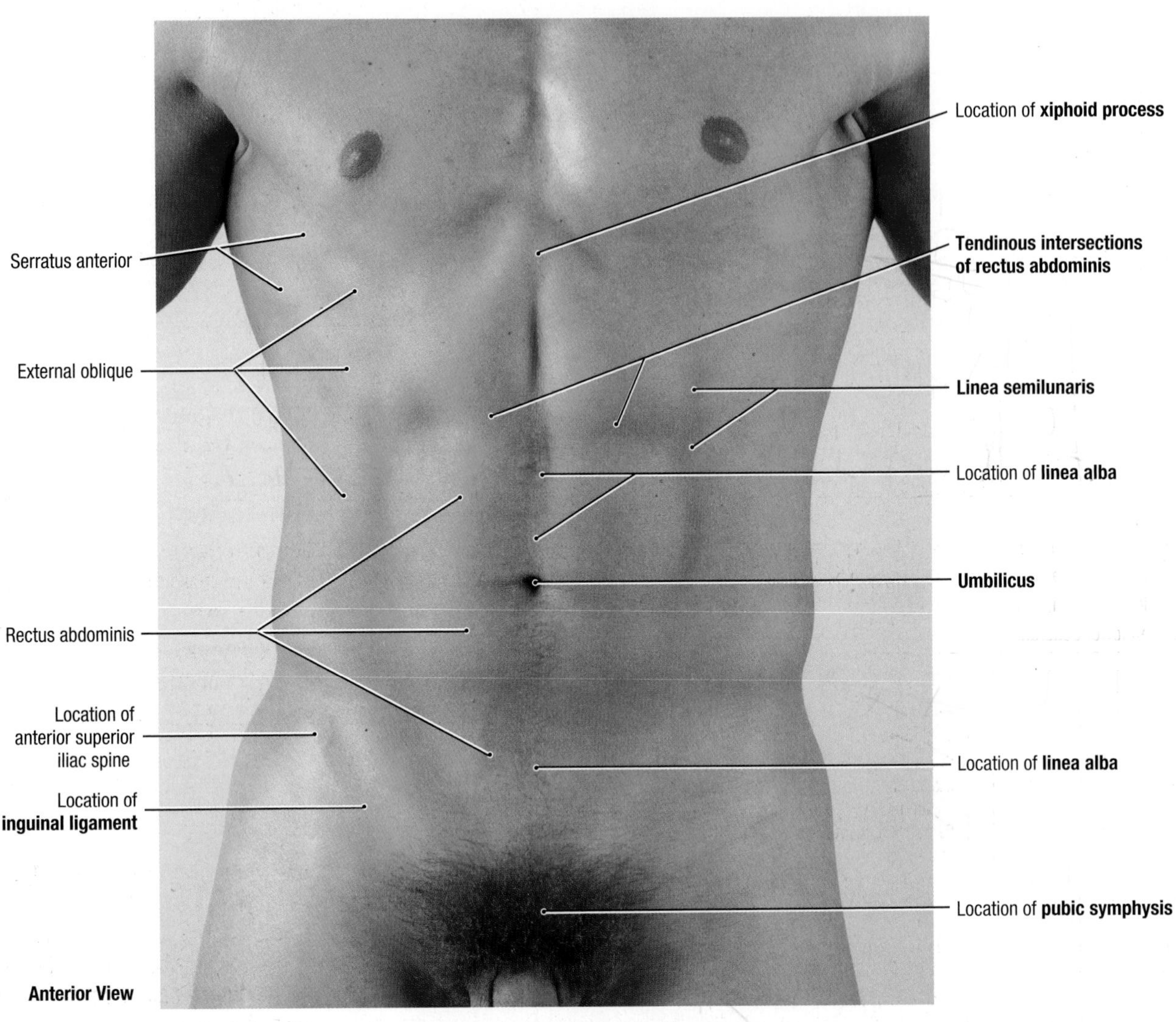
Location of xiphoid process
Serratus anterior
Tendinous intersections of rectus abdominis
External oblique
Linea semilunaris
Location of linea alba
Umbilicus
Rectus abdominis
Location of anterior superior iliac spine
Location of linea alba
Location of inguinal ligament
Location of pubic symphysis
Anterior View

2.2 SURFACE ANATOMY

A. Surface features.

- The umbilicus is where the umbilical cord entered the fetus and indicates the anterior level of the T10 dermatome, typically at the level of the IV disc between the L3 and L4 vertebrae.
- The linea alba is a fibrous band extending from the xiphoid process to the pubic symphysis that is demarcated superficially by a midline vertical skin groove as far inferiorly as the umbilicus.
- Curved skin grooves, the linea semilunaris, demarcate the lateral borders of the rectus abdominis muscle and rectus sheath.
- In lean individuals with good muscle development, three transverse skin grooves overlie the tendinous intersections of the rectus abdominis muscle.
- The site of the inguinal ligament is indicated by a skin crease, the inguinal groove, just inferior and parallel to the ligament, marking the division between the anterolateral abdominal wall and the thigh.

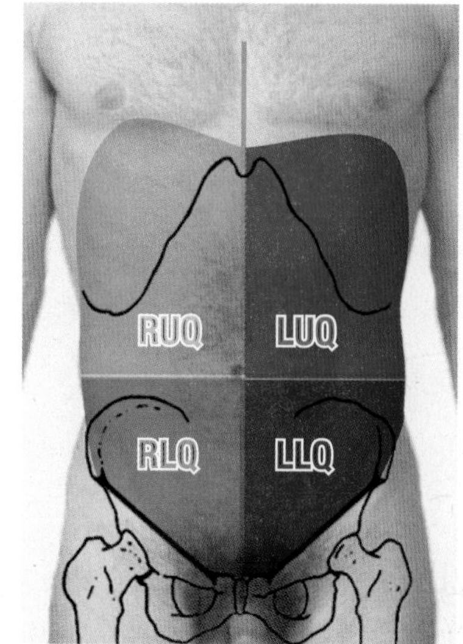
RUQ
LUQ
RLQ
LLQ

Abdominal Quadrants:

RUQ Right upper quadrant
LUQ Left upper quadrant
RLQ Right lower quadrant
LLQ Left lower quadrant

Median plane
Transumbilical plane

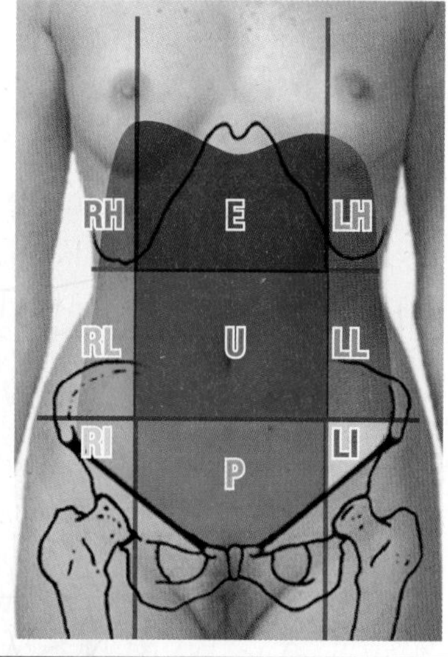
RH
E
LH
RL
U
LL
RI
P
LI

Abdominal Regions:

RH Right hypochondrium
RL Right flank (lateral region)
RI Right inguinal (groin)
LH Left hypochondrium
LL Left flank (lateral region)
LI Left inguinal (groin)

E Epigastric
U Umbilical
P Pubic

Midclavicular plane
Transtubercular plane
Subcostal plane

Right upper quadrant (RUQ)
Liver: right lobe Gallbladder Stomach: pylorus Duodenum: parts 1-3 Pancreas: head Right suprarenal gland Right kidney Right colic (hepatic) flexure Ascending colon: superior part Transverse colon: right half

Left upper quadrant (LUQ)
Liver: left lobe Spleen Stomach Jejunum and proximal ileum Pancreas: body and tail Left kidney Left suprarenal gland Left colic (splenic) flexure Transverse colon: left half Descending colon: superior part

Right lower quadrant (RLQ)
Cecum Appendix Most of ileum Ascending colon: inferior part Right ovary Right uterine tube Right ureter: abdominal part Right spermatic cord: abdominal part Uterus (if enlarged) Urinary bladder (if very full)

Left lower quadrant (LLQ)
Sigmoid colon Descending colon: inferior part Left ovary Left uterine tube Left ureter: abdominal part Left spermatic cord: abdominal part Uterus (if enlarged) Urinary bladder (if very full)

2.3 ABDOMINAL REGIONS AND QUADRANTS

A. Quadrants. **B.** Regions. It is important to know what organs are located in each abdominal region or quadrant so that one knows where to auscultate, percuss, and palpate them and to record the locations of findings during a physical exam.

The six common causes of **abdominal protrusion** begin with the letter F: food, fluid, fat, feces, flatus, and fetus. Eversion of the umbilicus may be a sign of increased intra-abdominal pressure, usually resulting from ascites (abdominal accumulation of serous fluid in the peritoneal cavity), or a large mass (e.g., a tumor, fetus, or enlarged organ such as the liver [hepatomegaly]).

Warm hands are important when palpating the abdominal wall because cold hands make the anterolateral abdominal muscles tense, producing involuntary muscle spasms known as guarding. Intense guarding, boardlike reflexive muscular rigidity that cannot be willfully suppressed, occurs during palpation when an organ (such as the appendix) is inflamed and in itself constitutes a clinically significant sign of **acute abdomen.** The involuntary muscular spasms attempt to protect the viscera from pressure, which is painful when an abdominal infection is present. The common nerve supply of the skin and muscles of the wall explains why these spasms occur.

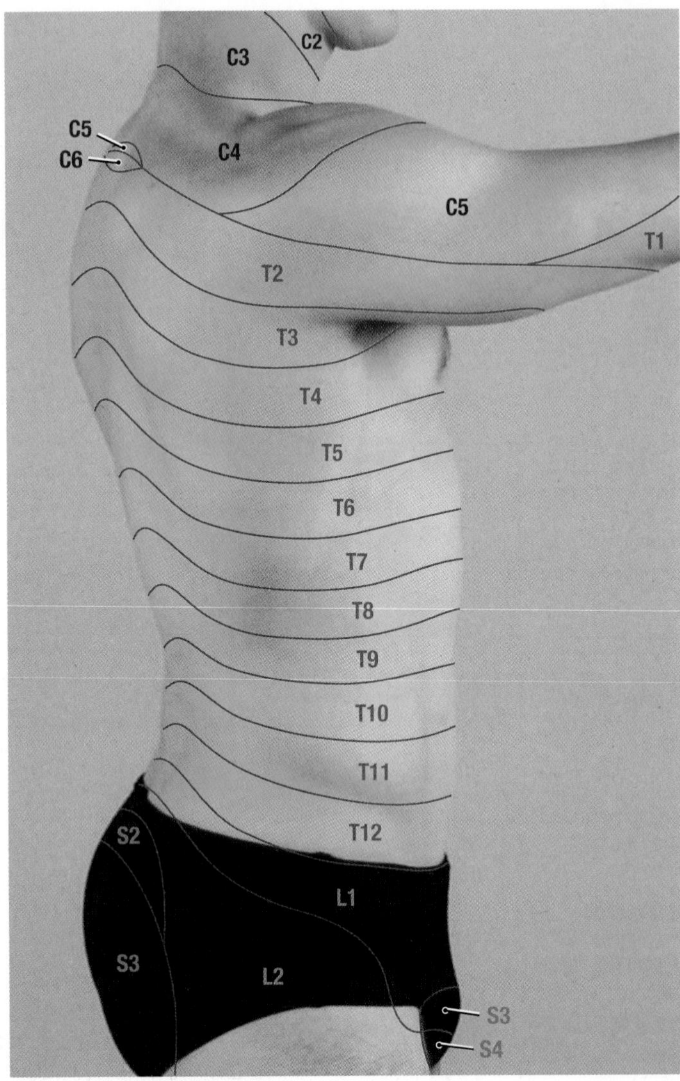
C2
C3
C5
C6
C4
C5
T1
T2
T3
T4
T5
T6
T7
T8
T9
T10
T11
T12
S2
L1
S3
L2
S3
S4

Lateral View

2.4 DERMATOMES

The thoraco-abdominal (T7–T11) nerves run between the external and internal oblique muscles to supply sensory innervation to the overlying skin. The T10 nerve supplies the region of the umbilicus. The subcostal nerve (T12) runs along the inferior border of the 12th rib to supply the skin over the anterior superior iliac spine and hip. The iliohypogastric nerve (L1) innervates the skin over the iliac crest and hypogastric region and the ilio-inguinal nerve (L1) the skin of the medial aspect of the thigh, the scrotum or labium majus, and mons pubis.

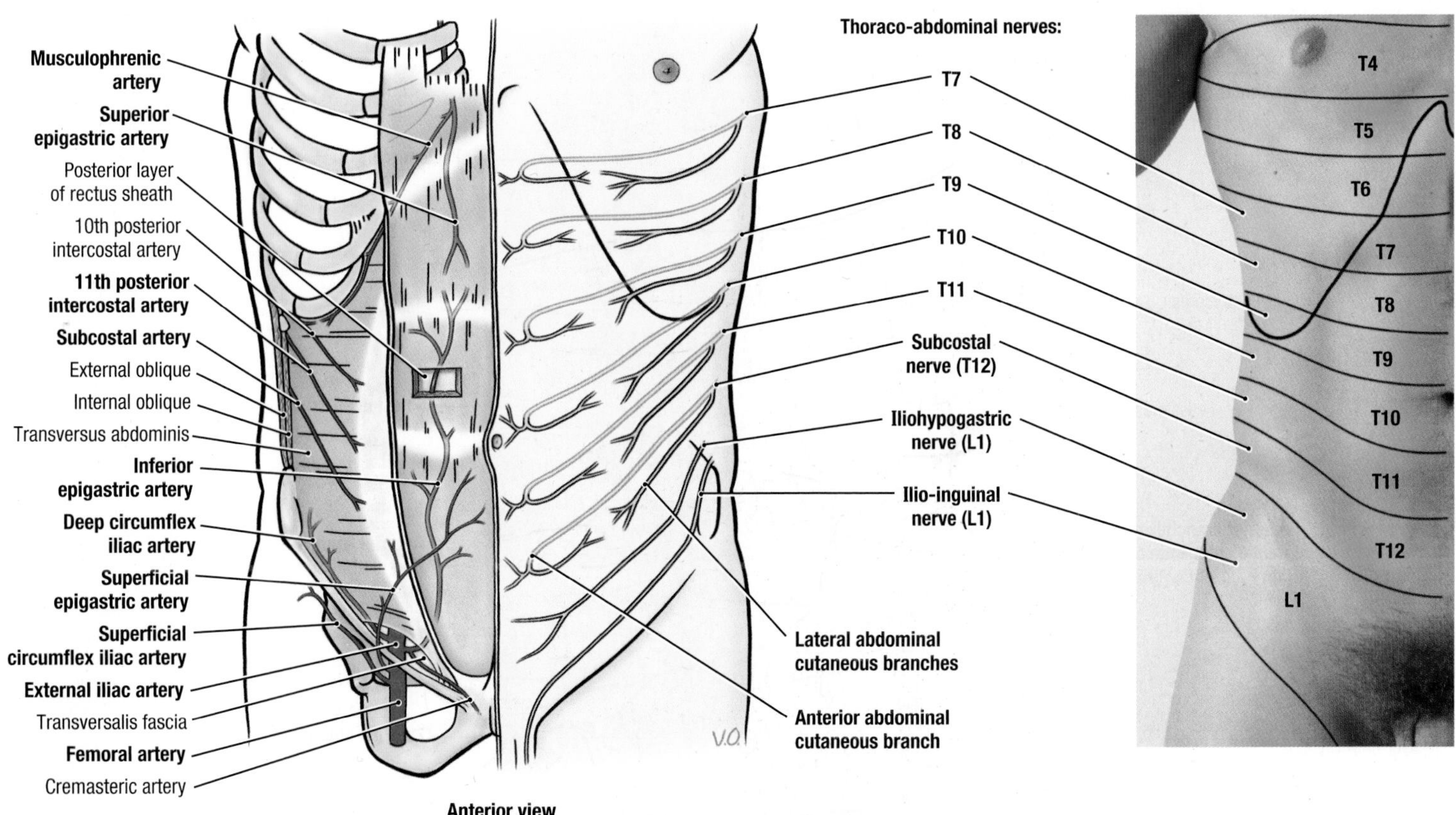
Musculophrenic artery
Superior epigastric artery
Posterior layer of rectus sheath
10th posterior intercostal artery
11th posterior intercostal artery
Subcostal artery
External oblique
Internal oblique
Transversus abdominis
Inferior epigastric artery
Deep circumflex iliac artery
Superficial epigastric artery
Superficial circumflex iliac artery
External iliac artery
Transversalis fascia
Femoral artery
Cremasteric artery
Thoraco-abdominal nerves:
T7
T8
T9
T10
T11
Subcostal nerve (T12)
Iliohypogastric nerve (L1)
Ilio-inguinal nerve (L1)
Lateral abdominal cutaneous branches
Anterior abdominal cutaneous branch
V.O.
T4
T5
T6
T7
T8
T9
T10
T11
T12
L1

Anterior view

2.5 ARTERIES AND NERVES OF ANTEROLATERAL ABDOMINAL WALL

The skin and muscles of the anterolateral abdominal wall are supplied mainly by the:

- Thoraco-abdominal nerves: distal, abdominal parts of the anterior rami of the inferior six thoracic spinal nerves (T7–T11), which have muscular branches and anterior and lateral abdominal cutaneous branches. The anterior abdominal cutaneous branches pierce the rectus sheath a short distance from the median plane, after the rectus abdominis muscle has been supplied. Spinal nerves T7–T9 supply the skin superior to the umbilicus; T10 innervates the skin around the umbilicus.
- Subcostal nerve: large anterior ramus of spinal nerve T12.
- Iliohypogastric and ilio-inguinal nerves: terminal branches of the anterior ramus of spinal nerve L1.
- Spinal nerve T11, plus the cutaneous branches of the subcostal (T12), iliohypogastric, and ilio-inguinal (L1) nerves: supply the skin inferior to the umbilicus.

The blood vessels of the anterolateral abdominal wall are the:

- Superior epigastric vessels and branches of the musculophrenic vessels from the internal thoracic vessels.
- Inferior epigastric and deep circumflex iliac vessels from the external iliac vessels.
- Superficial circumflex iliac and superficial epigastric vessels from the femoral artery and great saphenous vein.
- Posterior intercostal vessels in the 11th intercostal space and anterior branches of subcostal vessels.

Incisional nerve injury. The inferior thoracic spinal nerves (T7–T12) and the iliohypogastric and ilio-inguinal nerves (L1) approach the abdominal musculature separately to provide the multisegmental innervation of the abdominal muscles. Thus they are distributed across the anterolateral abdominal wall, where they run oblique but mostly horizontal courses. They are susceptible to injury in surgical incisions or from trauma at any level of the abdominal wall. Injury to them may result in weakening of the muscles. In the inguinal region, such a weakness may predispose an individual to development of an inguinal hernia.

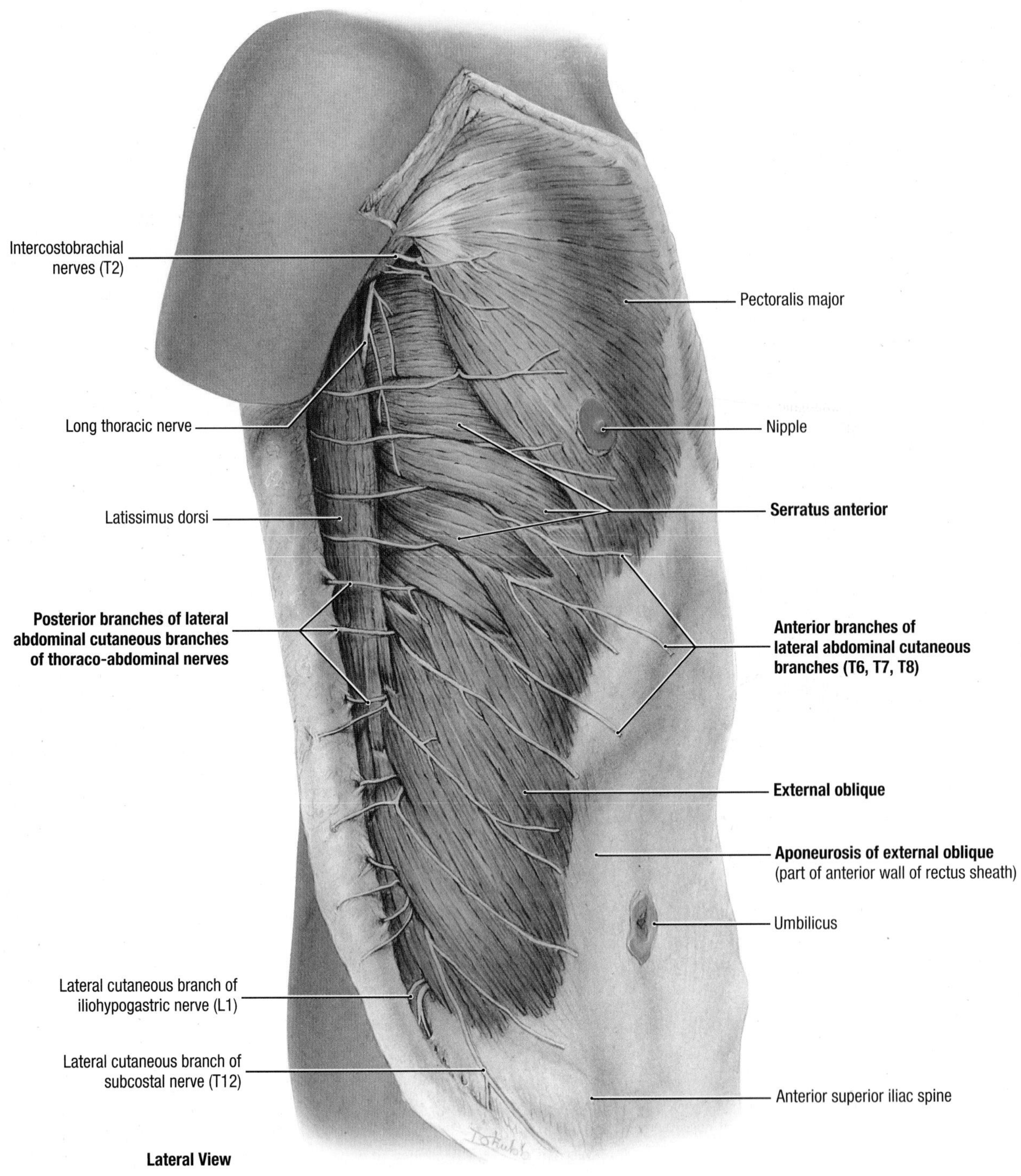
Intercostobrachial nerves (T2)
Pectoralis major
Long thoracic nerve
Nipple
Latissimus dorsi
Serratus anterior
Posterior branches of lateral abdominal cutaneous branches of thoraco-abdominal nerves
Anterior branches of lateral abdominal cutaneous branches (T6, T7, T8)
External oblique
Aponeurosis of external oblique (part of anterior wall of rectus sheath)
Umbilicus
Lateral cutaneous branch of iliohypogastric nerve (L1)
Lateral cutaneous branch of subcostal nerve (T12)
Anterior superior iliac spine
Lateral View

2.6 ANTEROLATERAL ABDOMINAL WALL, SUPERFICIAL DISSECTION

The muscular portion of the external oblique muscle interdigitates with slips of the serratus anterior muscle, and the aponeurotic portion contributes to the anterior wall of the rectus sheath. The anterior and posterior branches of the lateral abdominal cutaneous branches of the thoraco-abdominal nerves course superficially in the subcutaneous tissue.

- **Umbilical hernias** are usually small protrusions of extraperitoneal fat and/or peritoneum and omentum and sometimes bowel. They result from increased intra-abdominal pressure in the presence of weakness or incomplete closure of the anterior abdominal wall after ligation of the umbilical cord at birth, or may be acquired later, most commonly in women and obese people.
- The lines along which the fibers of the abdominal aponeurosis interlace (see Fig. 2.10A,B,D) are also potential sites of herniation. These gaps may be congenital, the result of the stresses of obesity and aging, or the consequence of surgical or traumatic wounds.

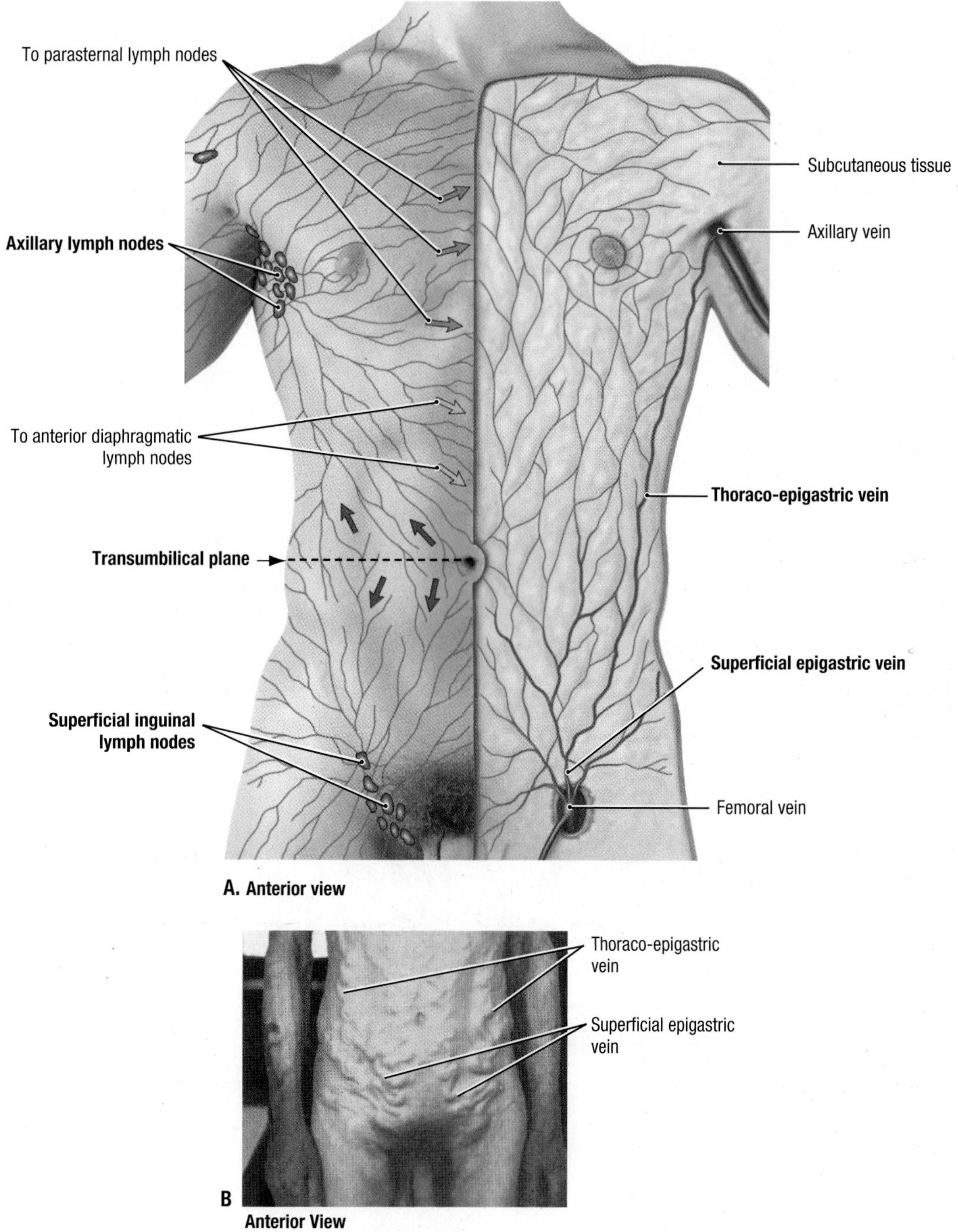
To parasternal lymph nodes
Subcutaneous tissue
Axillary lymph nodes
Axillary vein
To anterior diaphragmatic lymph nodes
Thoraco-epigastric vein
Transumbilical plane
Superficial epigastric vein
Superficial inguinal lymph nodes
Femoral vein
Thoraco-epigastric vein
Superficial epigastric vein

A. Anterior view

B Anterior View

2.7 LYMPHATIC DRAINAGE AND SUBCUTANEOUS (SUPERFICIAL) VENOUS DRAINAGE OF ANTEROLATERAL ABDOMINAL WALL

A. Overview.

- The skin and subcutaneous tissue of the abdominal wall are served by an intricate subcutaneous venous plexus, draining superiorly to the internal thoracic vein medially and the lateral thoracic vein laterally and inferiorly to the superficial and inferior epigastric veins, tributaries of the femoral and external iliac veins, respectively.
- Superficial lymphatic vessels accompany the subcutaneous veins; those superior to the transumbilical plane drain mainly to the axillary lymph nodes; however, a few drain to the parasternal lymph nodes. Superficial lymphatic vessels inferior to the transumbilical plane drain to the superficial inguinal lymph nodes.

B. Enlargement of subcutaneous veins.

- **Liposuction** is a surgical method for removing unwanted subcutaneous fat using a percutaneously placed suction tube and high vacuum pressure. The tubes are inserted subdermally through small skin incisions.
- When flow in the superior or inferior vena cava is obstructed, anastomoses between the tributaries of these systemic veins, such as the thoraco-epigastric vein, may provide **collateral pathways** by which the obstruction may be bypassed, allowing blood to return to the heart. The veins become enlarged and tortuous **(B).**

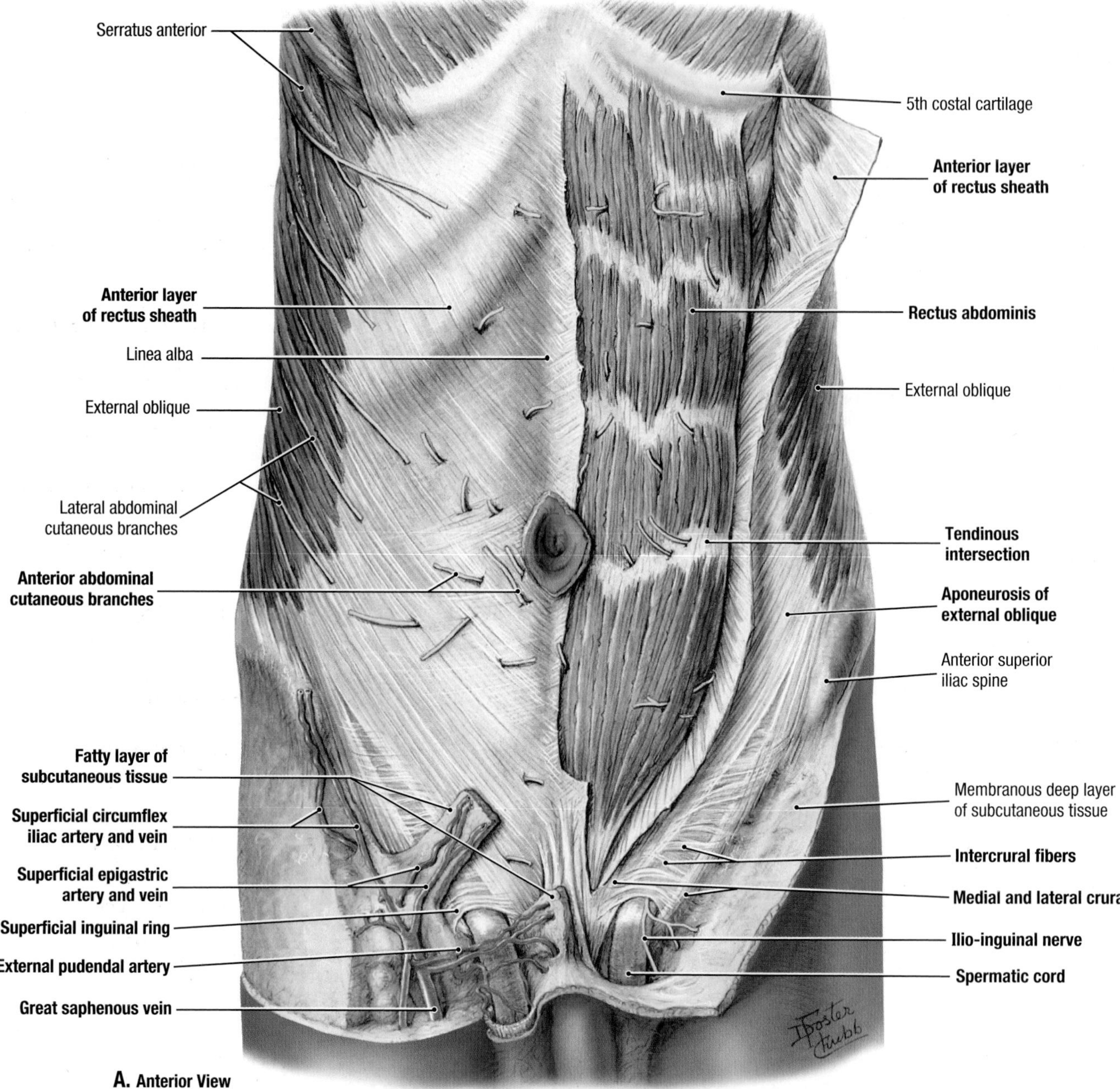
Serratus anterior
5th costal cartilage
Anterior layer of rectus sheath
Anterior layer of rectus sheath
Rectus abdominis
Linea alba
External oblique
External oblique
Lateral abdominal cutaneous branches
Tendinous intersection
Anterior abdominal cutaneous branches
Aponeurosis of external oblique
Anterior superior iliac spine
Fatty layer of subcutaneous tissue
Membranous deep layer of subcutaneous tissue
Superficial circumflex iliac artery and vein
Intercrural fibers
Superficial epigastric artery and vein
Medial and lateral crura
Superficial inguinal ring
Ilio-inguinal nerve
External pudendal artery
Spermatic cord
Great saphenous vein

A. Anterior View

2.8 ANTERIOR ABDOMINAL WALL

A. Superficial dissection demonstrating the relationship of the cutaneous nerves and superficial vessels to the musculoaponeurotic structures. The anterior wall of the left rectus sheath is reflected, revealing the rectus abdominis muscle, segmented by tendinous intersections.

- After the T7 to T12 spinal nerves supply the muscles, their anterior abdominal cutaneous branches emerge from the rectus abdominis muscle and pierce the anterior wall of its sheath.
- The three superficial inguinal branches of the femoral artery (superficial circumflex iliac artery, superficial epigastric artery, and external pudendal artery) and the great saphenous vein lie in the fatty layer of subcutaneous tissue.
- The fibers of the external oblique aponeurosis separate into medial and lateral crura, which, with the intercrural fibers that unite them, form the superficial inguinal ring. The spermatic cord of the male (shown here), or round ligament of the female, exits the inguinal canal through the superficial inguinal ring along with the ilio-inguinal nerve.

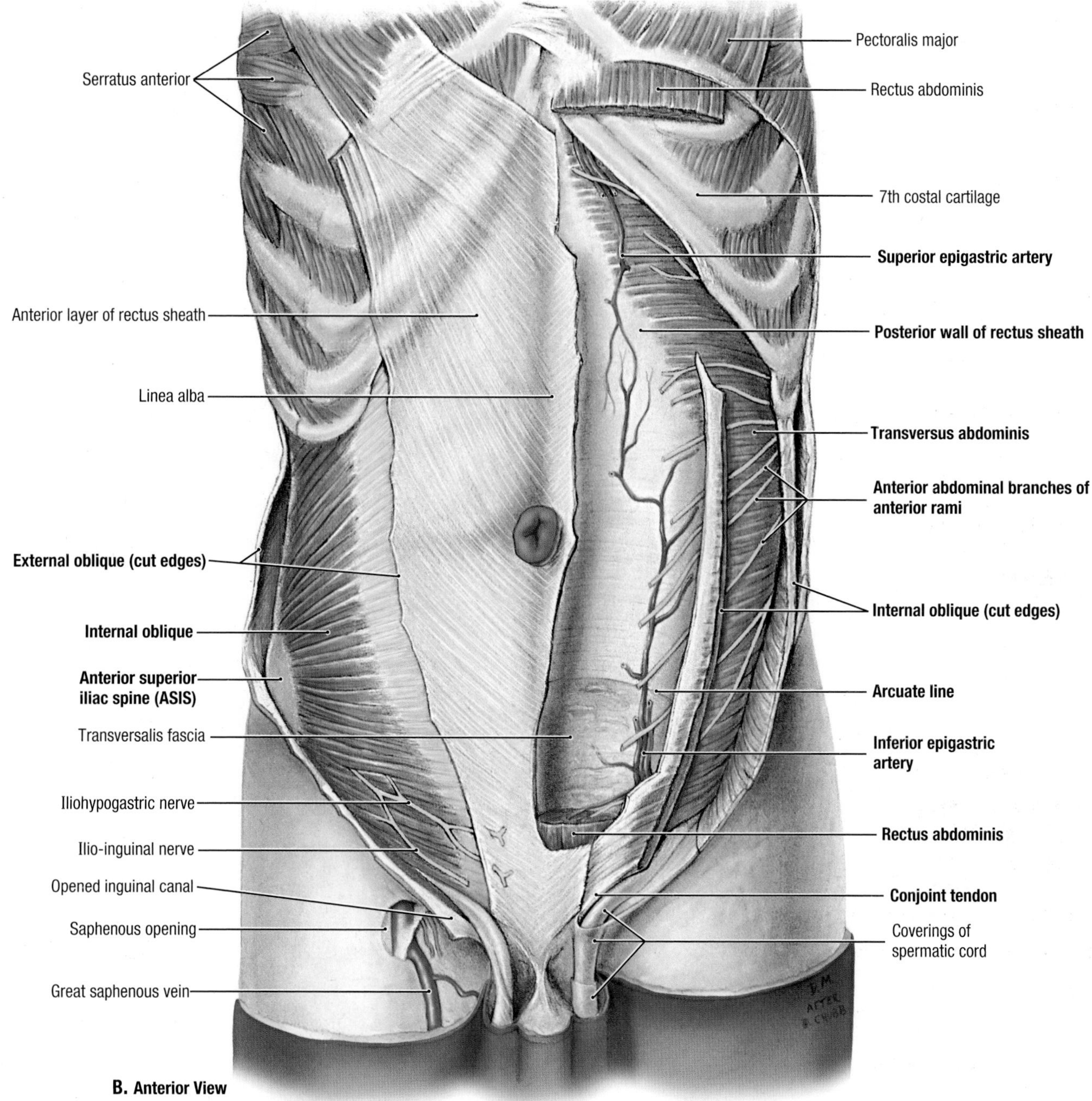
Serratus anterior
Pectoralis major
Rectus abdominis
7th costal cartilage
Superior epigastric artery
Anterior layer of rectus sheath
Posterior wall of rectus sheath
Linea alba
Transversus abdominis
Anterior abdominal branches of anterior rami
External oblique (cut edges)
Internal oblique (cut edges)
Internal oblique
Anterior superior iliac spine (ASIS)
Arcuate line
Transversalis fascia
Inferior epigastric artery
Iliohypogastric nerve
Rectus abdominis
Ilio-inguinal nerve
Opened inguinal canal
Conjoint tendon
Saphenous opening
Coverings of spermatic cord
Great saphenous vein

B. Anterior View

2.8 ANTERIOR ABDOMINAL WALL (*CONTINUED*)

B. Deep dissection. On the right side of the specimen, most of the external oblique muscle is excised. On the left, the internal oblique muscle is divided and the rectus abdominis muscle is excised, revealing the posterior wall of the rectus sheath.

- The fibers of the internal oblique muscle run horizontally at the level of the anterior superior iliac spine (ASIS), obliquely upward superior to the ASIS, and obliquely downward inferior to the ASIS.
- The arcuate line is at the level of the ASIS; inferior to the line, only transversalis fascia lies posterior to the rectus abdominis muscle.
- Initially, the anterior abdominal branches of the anterior rami course between the internal oblique and transversus abdominis muscles.
- The anastomosis between the superior and inferior epigastric arteries indirectly unites the subclavian artery of the upper limb to the external iliac arteries of the lower limb. The anastomosis can become functionally patent in response to **slowly developing occlusion of the aorta.**

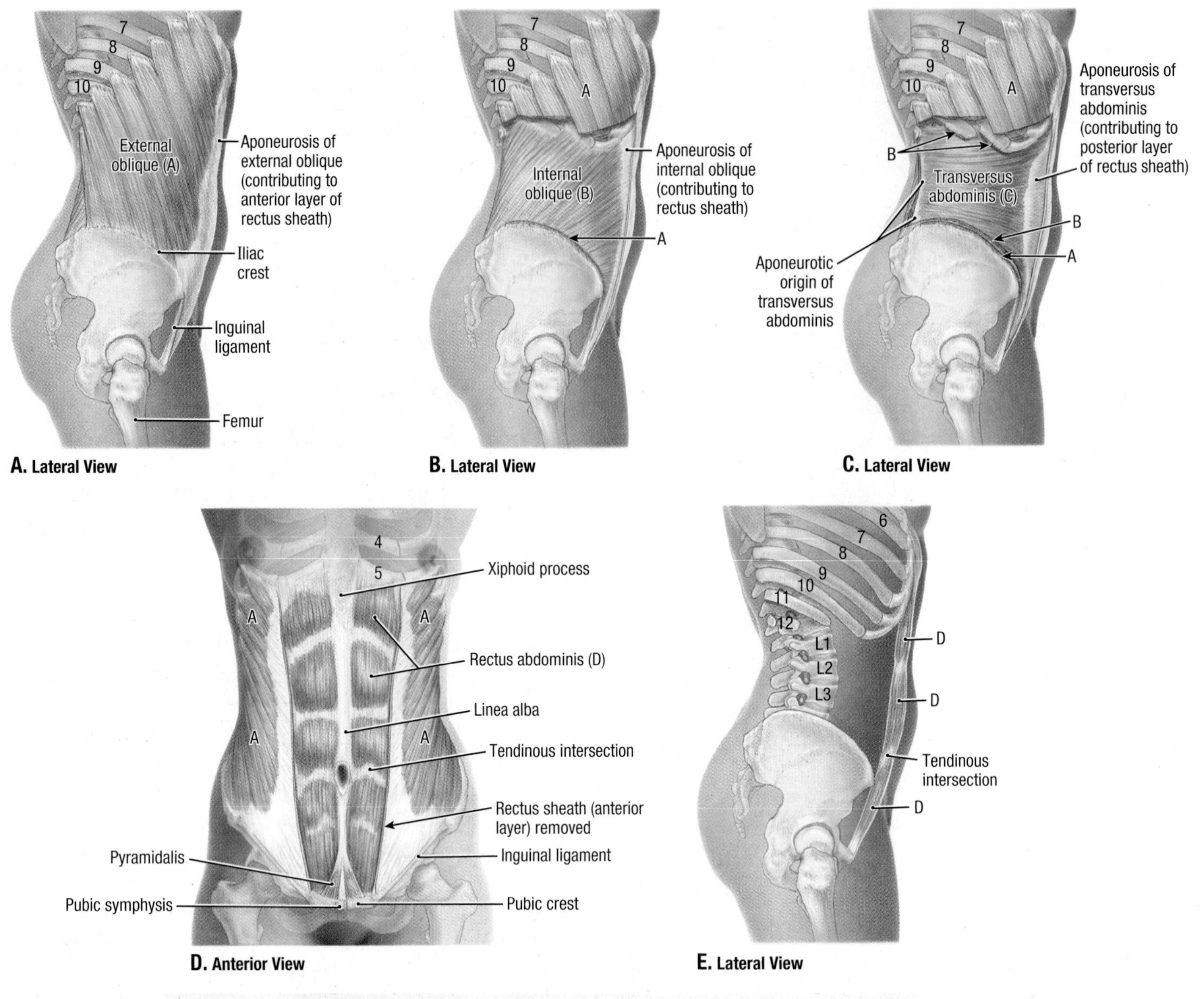
7
8
9
10
External oblique (A)
Aponeurosis of external oblique (contributing to anterior layer of rectus sheath)
Iliac crest
Inguinal ligament
Femur
A. Lateral View
A
Internal oblique (B)
Aponeurosis of internal oblique (contributing to rectus sheath)
B. Lateral View
B
Transversus abdominis (C)
Aponeurosis of transversus abdominis (contributing to posterior layer of rectus sheath)
Aponeurotic origin of transversus abdominis
C. Lateral View
4
5
Xiphoid process
Rectus abdominis (D)
Linea alba
Tendinous intersection
Rectus sheath (anterior layer) removed
Inguinal ligament
Pyramidalis
Pubic symphysis
Pubic crest
D. Anterior View
6
11
12
L1
L2
L3
D
Tendinous intersection
E. Lateral View

2.9 MUSCLES OF ANTEROLATERAL ABDOMINAL WALL

A. External oblique. **B.** Internal oblique. **C.** Transversus abdominis. **D. and E.** Rectus abdominis and pyramidalis.

TABLE 2.1 PRINCIPAL MUSCLES OF ANTEROLATERAL ABDOMINAL WALL

Muscles[a]	Origin	Insertion	Innervation	Action(s)
External oblique **(A)**	External surfaces of 5th–12th ribs	Linea alba, pubic tubercle, and anterior half of iliac crest	Thoraco-abdominal nerves (anterior rami of T7–T11) and subcostal nerve	Compresses and supports abdominal viscera; flexes and rotates trunk
Internal oblique **(B)**	Thoracolumbar fascia, anterior two thirds of iliac crest, and connective tissue deep to inguinal ligament	Inferior borders of 10th–12th ribs, linea alba, and pubis via conjoint tendon	Thoraco-abdominal nerves (anterior rami of T7–T11), subcostal nerve, and first lumbar nerve	
Transversus abdominis **(C)**	Internal surfaces of 7th–12th costal cartilages, thoracolumbar fascia, iliac crest, and connective tissue deep to inguinal ligament (iliopsoas fascia)	Linea alba with aponeurosis of internal oblique, pubic crest, and pectin pubis via conjoint tendon		Compresses and supports abdominal viscera (external oblique ipsilaterally, internal oblique contralaterally)
Rectus abdominis **(D)**	Pubic symphysis and pubic crest	Xiphoid process and 5th–7th costal cartilages	Thoraco-abdominal nerves (T7–T11) and subcostal nerve	Flexes trunk (lumbar vertebrae) and compresses abdominal viscera;[b] stabilizes and controls tilt of pelvis (antilordosis)

[a]Approximately 80% of people have a *pyramidalis muscle,* which is located in the rectus sheath anterior to the most inferior part of the rectus abdominis. It extends from the pubic crest of the hip bone to the linea alba. This small muscle tenses the linea alba.

[b]In so doing, these muscles act as antagonists of the diaphragm to produce expiration.

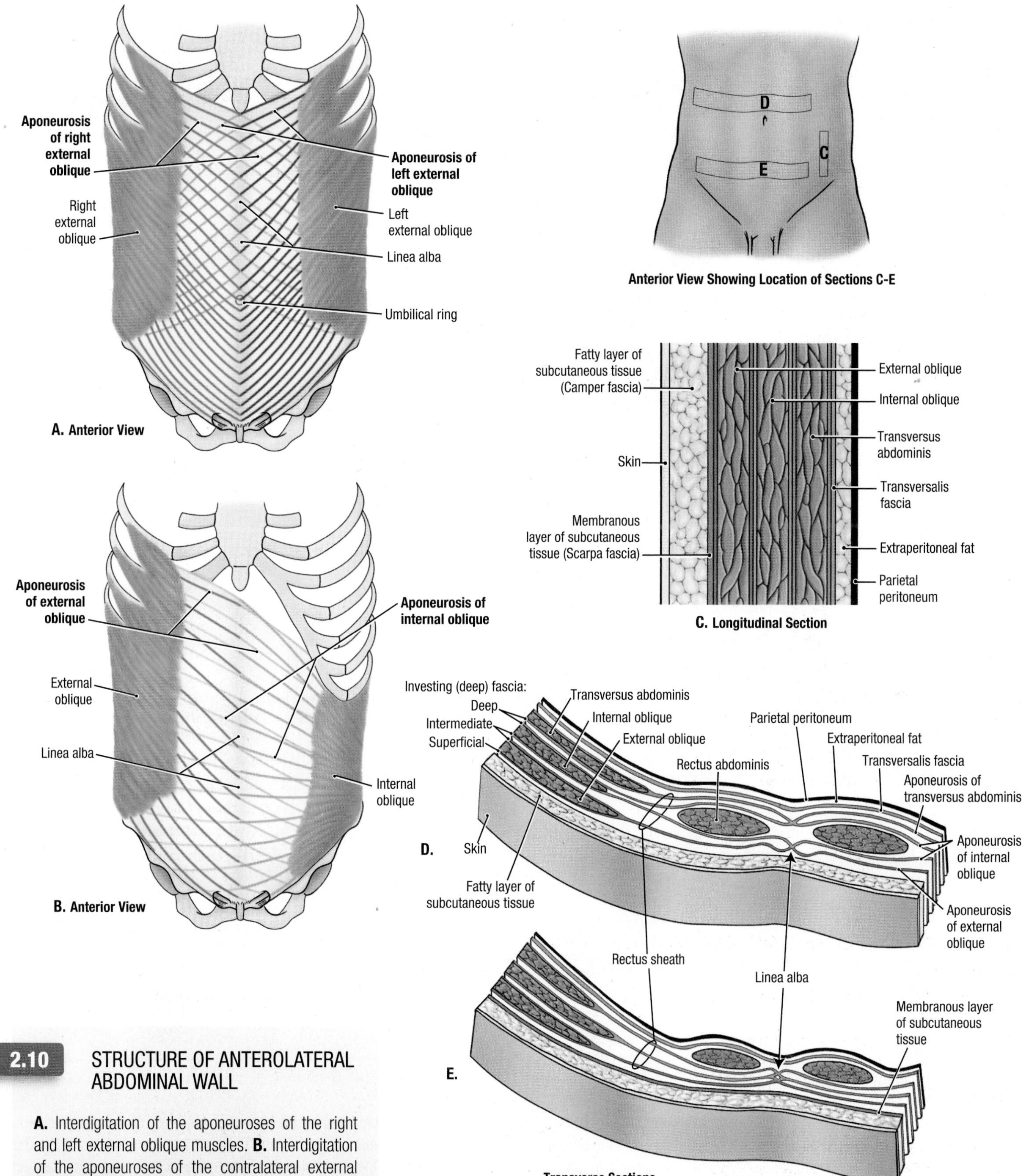
Aponeurosis of right external oblique
Aponeurosis of left external oblique
Right external oblique
Left external oblique
Linea alba
Umbilical ring
A. Anterior View
Aponeurosis of external oblique
Aponeurosis of internal oblique
External oblique
Linea alba
Internal oblique
B. Anterior View
D
E
C
Anterior View Showing Location of Sections C-E
Fatty layer of subcutaneous tissue (Camper fascia)
Skin
Membranous layer of subcutaneous tissue (Scarpa fascia)
External oblique
Internal oblique
Transversus abdominis
Transversalis fascia
Extraperitoneal fat
Parietal peritoneum
C. Longitudinal Section
Investing (deep) fascia:
Deep
Intermediate
Superficial
Transversus abdominis
Internal oblique
External oblique
Rectus abdominis
Parietal peritoneum
Extraperitoneal fat
Transversalis fascia
Aponeurosis of transversus abdominis
Aponeurosis of internal oblique
Aponeurosis of external oblique
D.
Skin
Fatty layer of subcutaneous tissue
Rectus sheath
Linea alba
Membranous layer of subcutaneous tissue
E.
Transverse Sections

2.10 STRUCTURE OF ANTEROLATERAL ABDOMINAL WALL

A. Interdigitation of the aponeuroses of the right and left external oblique muscles. **B.** Interdigitation of the aponeuroses of the contralateral external and internal oblique muscles. **C.–E.** Layers of the abdominal wall and the rectus sheath.

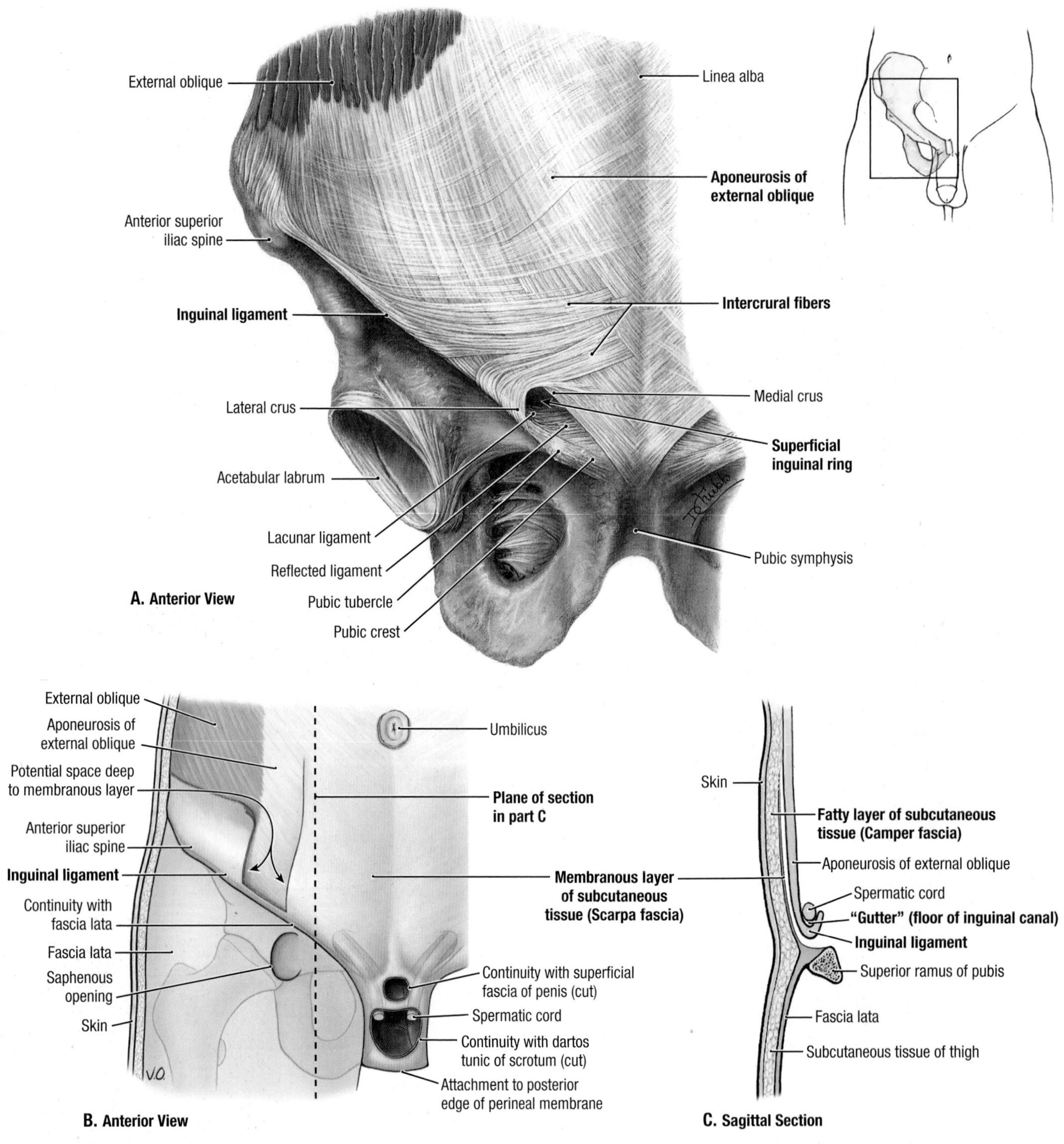
External oblique
Linea alba
Aponeurosis of external oblique
Anterior superior iliac spine
Inguinal ligament
Intercrural fibers
Medial crus
Lateral crus
Superficial inguinal ring
Acetabular labrum
Lacunar ligament
Pubic symphysis
Reflected ligament
A. Anterior View
Pubic tubercle
Pubic crest
External oblique
Aponeurosis of external oblique
Umbilicus
Potential space deep to membranous layer
Plane of section in part C
Skin
Fatty layer of subcutaneous tissue (Camper fascia)
Anterior superior iliac spine
Aponeurosis of external oblique
Inguinal ligament
Membranous layer of subcutaneous tissue (Scarpa fascia)
Continuity with fascia lata
Spermatic cord
"Gutter" (floor of inguinal canal)
Inguinal ligament
Fascia lata
Superior ramus of pubis
Saphenous opening
Continuity with superficial fascia of penis (cut)
Skin
Spermatic cord
Fascia lata
Continuity with dartos tunic of scrotum (cut)
Subcutaneous tissue of thigh
Attachment to posterior edge of perineal membrane
B. Anterior View
C. Sagittal Section

2.11 INGUINAL REGION OF MALE I

A. Formations of the aponeurosis of the external oblique muscle. **B. and C.** Membranous (deep) layer of subcutaneous tissue. Inferior to the umbilicus, the subcutaneous tissue is composed of two layers: a superficial fatty layer and a deep membranous layer. Laterally, the membranous layer fuses with the fascia lata of the thigh about a finger's breadth inferior to the inguinal ligament. Medially, it fuses with the linea alba and pubic symphysis in the midline, and inferiorly, it continues as the membranous layer of the subcutaneous tissue of the perineum and penis and the dartos fascia of the scrotum. The inferior margin of the external oblique aponeurosis is thickened and turned internally forming the inguinal ligament. The superior surface of the in-turning inguinal ligament forms a shallow trough or "gutter" that is the floor of the inguinal canal.

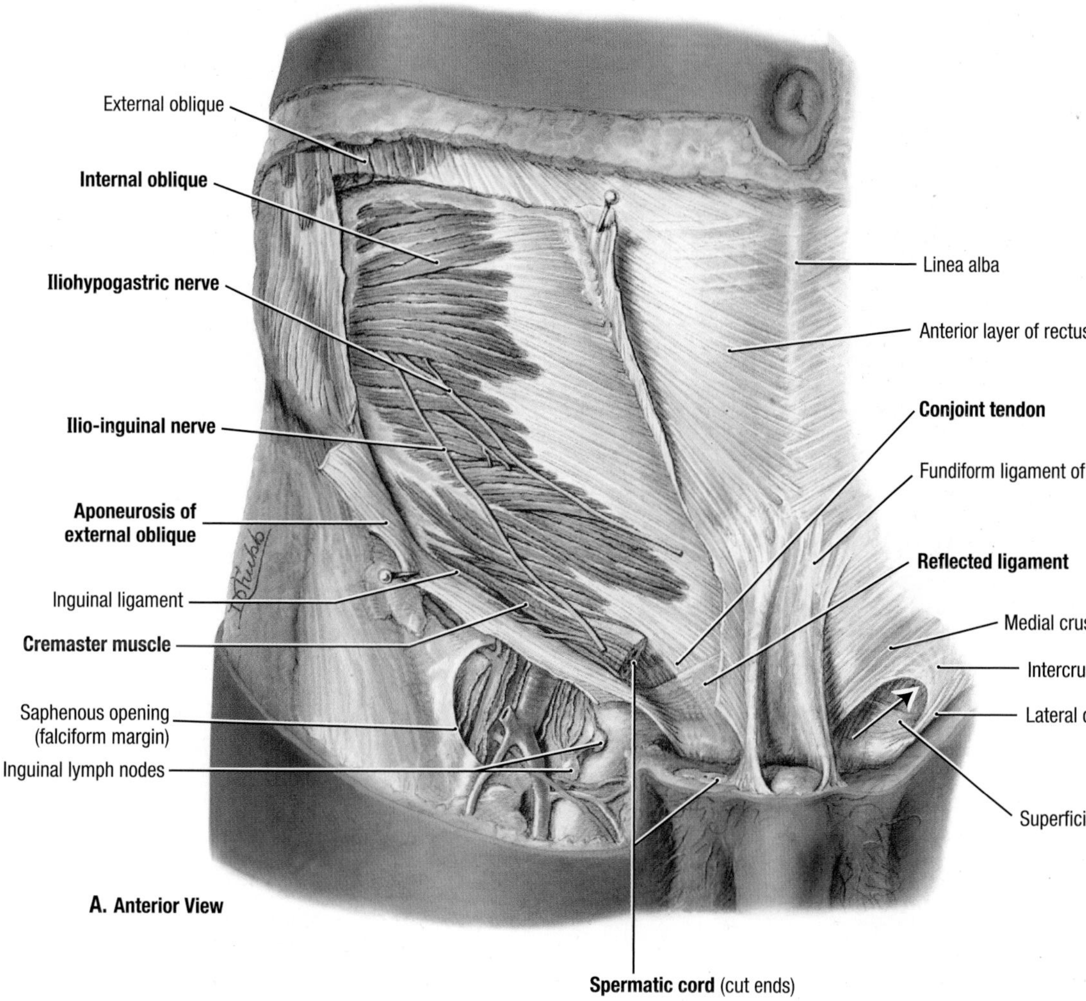

External oblique
Internal oblique
Iliohypogastric nerve
Ilio-inguinal nerve
Aponeurosis of external oblique
Inguinal ligament
Cremaster muscle
Saphenous opening (falciform margin)
Inguinal lymph nodes
Linea alba
Anterior layer of rectus sheath
Conjoint tendon
Fundiform ligament of penis
Reflected ligament
Medial crus
Intercrural fibers
Lateral crus
Of aponeurosis of external oblique
Superficial inguinal ring
Spermatic cord (cut ends)

A. Anterior View

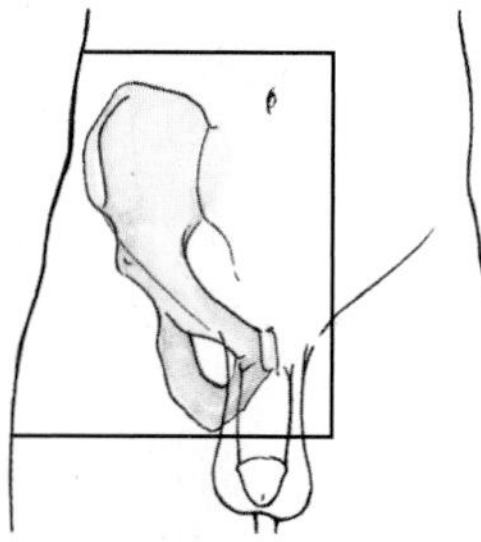

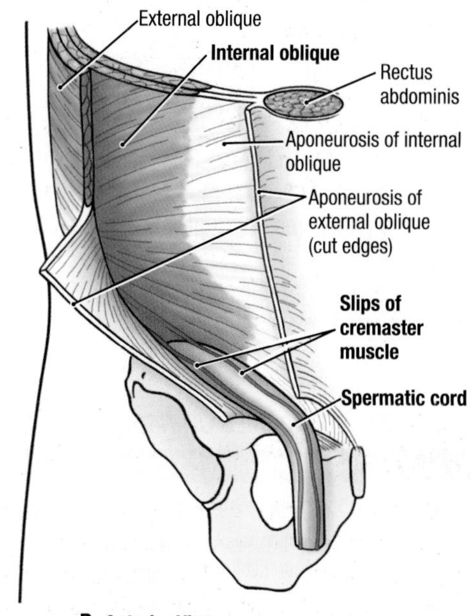
External oblique
Internal oblique
Rectus abdominis
Aponeurosis of internal oblique
Aponeurosis of external oblique (cut edges)
Slips of cremaster muscle
Spermatic cord

B. Anterior View

2.12 INGUINAL REGION OF MALE II

A. Internal oblique and cremaster muscle. Part of the aponeurosis of the external oblique muscle is cut away, and the spermatic cord is cut short. **B.** Schematic illustration.

- The cremaster muscle covers the spermatic cord.
- The reflected ligament is formed by aponeurotic fibers of the external oblique muscle and lies anterior to the conjoint tendon. The conjoint tendon is formed by the fusion of the aponeurosis of the internal oblique and transversus abdominis muscles.
- The cutaneous branches of the iliohypogastric and ilio-inguinal nerves (L1) course between the internal and external oblique muscles and must be avoided when an **appendectomy (gridiron) incision** is made in this region.

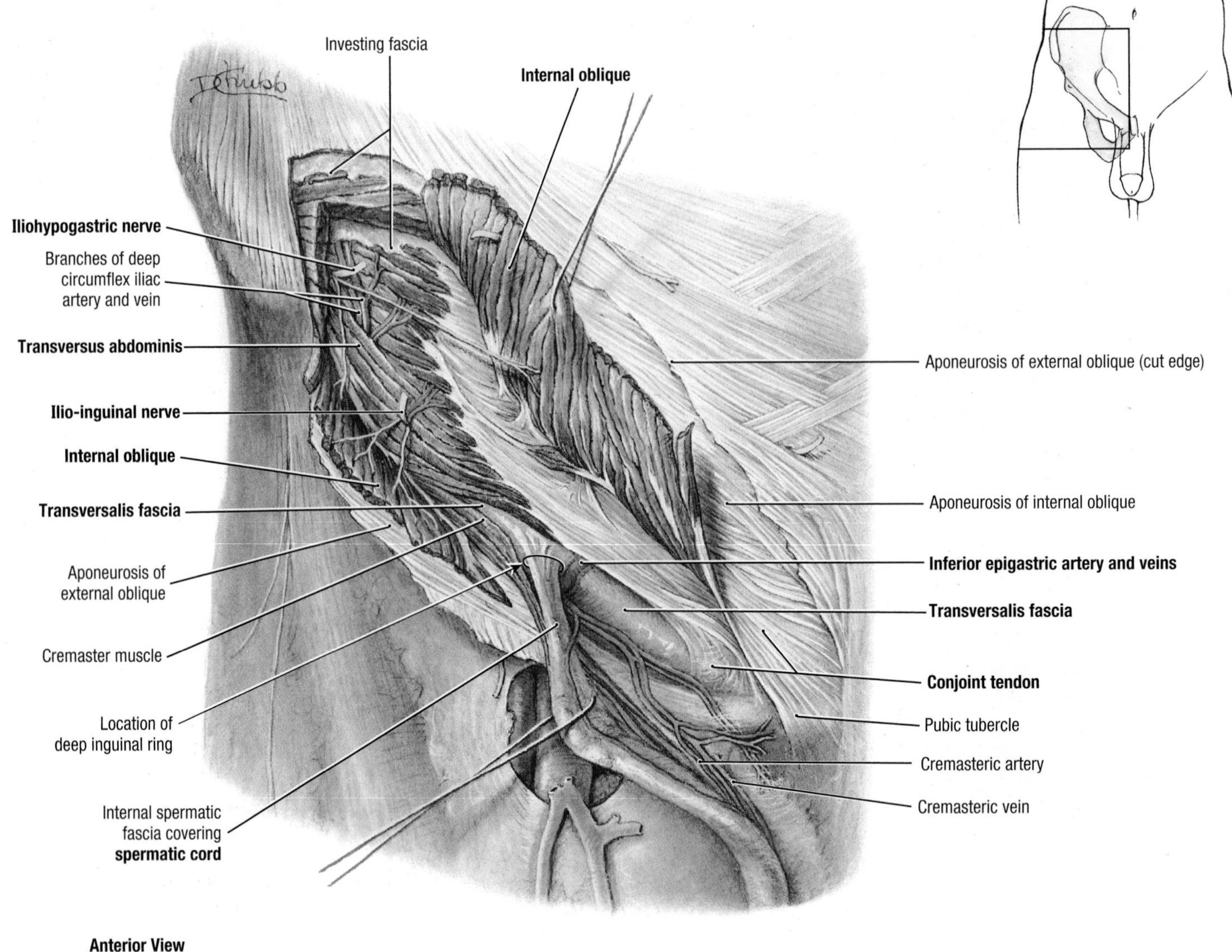

Investing fascia
Internal oblique
Iliohypogastric nerve
Branches of deep circumflex iliac artery and vein
Transversus abdominis
Ilio-inguinal nerve
Internal oblique
Transversalis fascia
Aponeurosis of external oblique
Cremaster muscle
Location of deep inguinal ring
Internal spermatic fascia covering spermatic cord
Aponeurosis of external oblique (cut edge)
Aponeurosis of internal oblique
Inferior epigastric artery and veins
Transversalis fascia
Conjoint tendon
Pubic tubercle
Cremasteric artery
Cremasteric vein

Anterior View

2.13 INGUINAL REGION OF MALE III

The internal oblique muscle is reflected, and the spermatic cord is retracted.

- The internal oblique muscle portion of the conjoint tendon is attached to the pubic crest, and the transversus abdominis portion to the pectineal line.
- The iliohypogastric and ilio-inguinal nerves (L1) supply the internal oblique and transversus abdominis muscles.
- The transversalis fascia is evaginated to form the tubular internal spermatic fascia. The mouth of the tube, called the deep inguinal ring, is situated lateral to the inferior epigastric vessels.

TABLE 2.2 BOUNDARIES OF INGUINAL CANAL

Boundary	Deep Ring/Lateral Third	Middle Third	Lateral Third/Superficial Ring
Posterior wall	Transversalis fascia	Transversalis fascia	Inguinal falx (conjoint tendon) plus reflected inguinal ligament
Anterior wall	Internal oblique plus lateral crus of aponeurosis of external oblique	Aponeurosis of external oblique (lateral crus and intercrural fibers)	Aponeurosis of external oblique (intercrural fibers), with fascia of external oblique continuing onto cord as external spermatic fascia
Roof	Transversalis fascia	Musculoa-poneurotic arches of internal oblique and transversus abdominis	Medial crus of aponeurosis of external oblique
Floor	Iliopubic tract	Inguinal ligament	Lacunar ligament

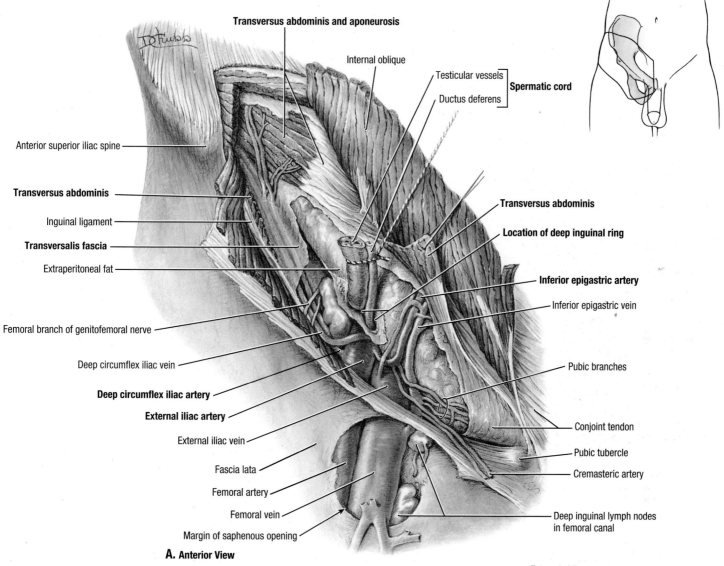

Transversus abdominis and aponeurosis
Internal oblique
Testicular vessels
Ductus deferens
Spermatic cord
Anterior superior iliac spine
Transversus abdominis
Inguinal ligament
Transversalis fascia
Extraperitoneal fat
Transversus abdominis
Location of deep inguinal ring
Inferior epigastric artery
Inferior epigastric vein
Femoral branch of genitofemoral nerve
Deep circumflex iliac vein
Deep circumflex iliac artery
External iliac artery
External iliac vein
Fascia lata
Femoral artery
Femoral vein
Margin of saphenous opening
Pubic branches
Conjoint tendon
Pubic tubercle
Cremasteric artery
Deep inguinal lymph nodes in femoral canal

A. Anterior View

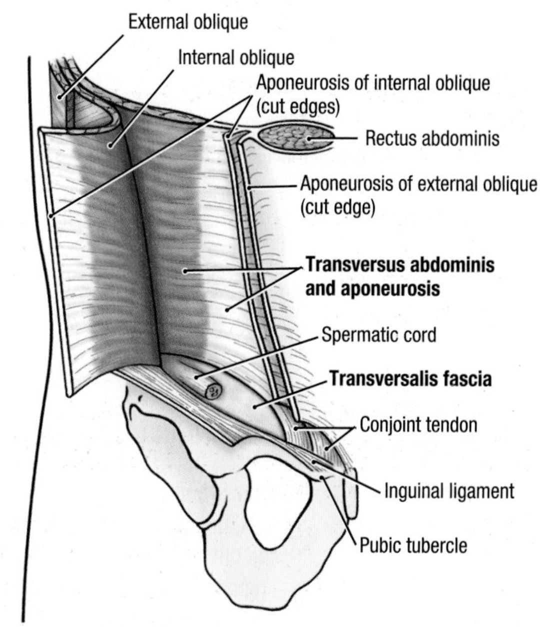
External oblique
Internal oblique
Aponeurosis of internal oblique (cut edges)
Rectus abdominis
Aponeurosis of external oblique (cut edge)
Transversus abdominis and aponeurosis
Spermatic cord
Transversalis fascia
Conjoint tendon
Inguinal ligament
Pubic tubercle

B. Anterior View

2.14 INGUINAL REGION OF MALE IV

A. The inguinal part of the transversus abdominis muscle and transversalis fascia is partially cut away, the spermatic cord is excised, and the ductus deferens is retracted. **B.** Schematic illustration.

- The deep inguinal ring is located superior to the inguinal ligament at the midpoint between the anterior superior iliac spine and pubic tubercle.
- The external iliac artery has two branches, the deep circumflex iliac and inferior epigastric arteries. Note also the cremasteric artery and pubic branch arising from the latter.

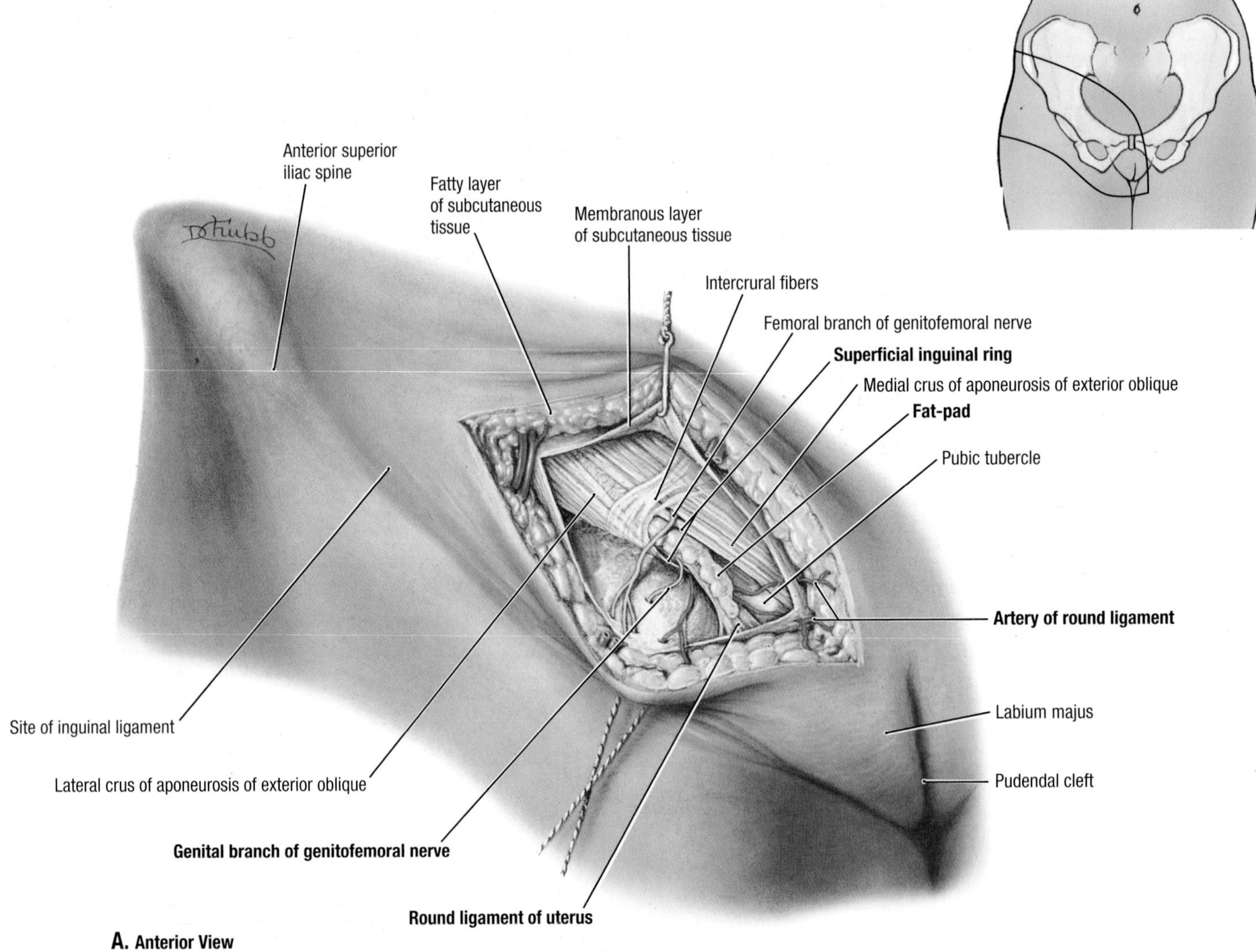

Anterior superior iliac spine
Fatty layer of subcutaneous tissue
Membranous layer of subcutaneous tissue
Intercrural fibers
Femoral branch of genitofemoral nerve
Superficial inguinal ring
Medial crus of aponeurosis of exterior oblique
Fat-pad
Pubic tubercle
Artery of round ligament
Labium majus
Pudendal cleft
Site of inguinal ligament
Lateral crus of aponeurosis of exterior oblique
Genital branch of genitofemoral nerve
Round ligament of uterus

A. Anterior View

2.15 INGUINAL CANAL OF FEMALE

Progressive dissections of the female inguinal canal **(A.–D)**.

- In **A,** the superficial inguinal ring is small. Passing through the superficial inguinal ring are the round ligament of the uterus, a closely applied fat pad, the genital branch of the genitofemoral nerve, and the artery of the round ligament of the uterus. The ilio-inguinal nerve may also pass through the ring.
- The round ligament breaks up into strands as it leaves the inguinal canal and approaches the labium majus **(C).**
- The external iliac artery and vein are exposed deep to the inguinal canal by excising the transversalis fascia **(D).**

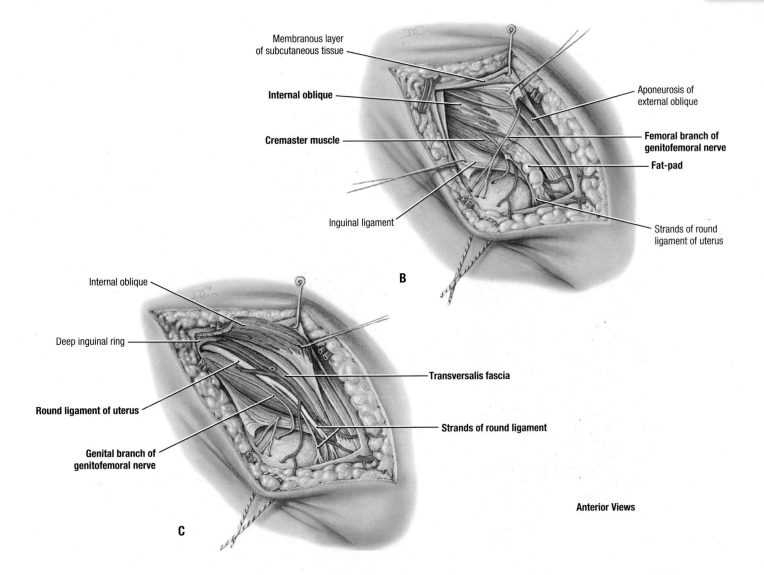

Membranous layer of subcutaneous tissue
Internal oblique
Cremaster muscle
Inguinal ligament
Aponeurosis of external oblique
Femoral branch of genitofemoral nerve
Fat-pad
Strands of round ligament of uterus
B

Internal oblique
Deep inguinal ring
Round ligament of uterus
Genital branch of genitofemoral nerve
Transversalis fascia
Strands of round ligament
C

Anterior Views

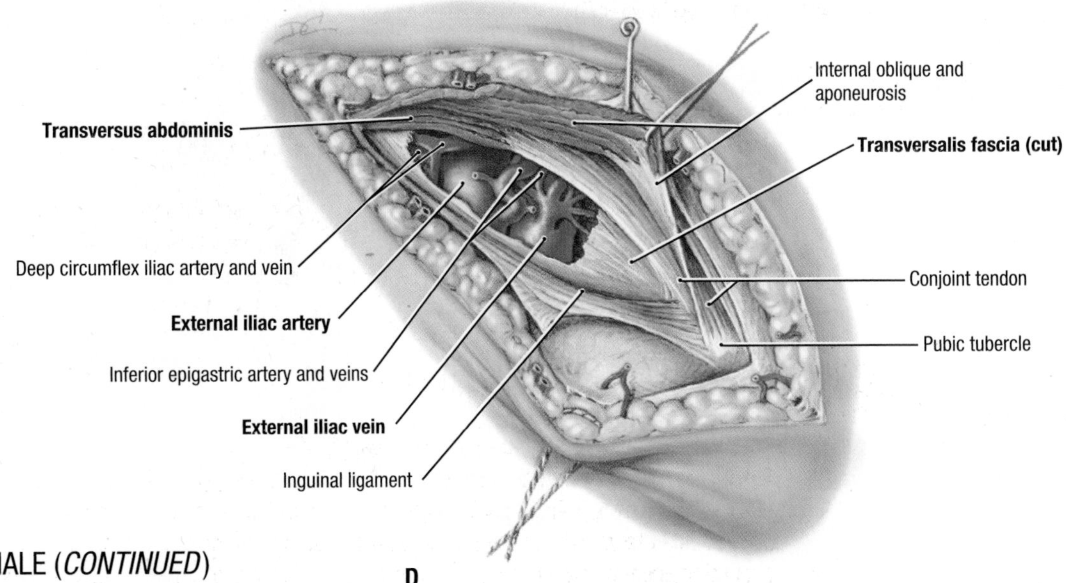
Transversus abdominis
Deep circumflex iliac artery and vein
External iliac artery
Inferior epigastric artery and veins
External iliac vein
Inguinal ligament
Internal oblique and aponeurosis
Transversalis fascia (cut)
Conjoint tendon
Pubic tubercle
D

2.15 INGUINAL CANAL OF FEMALE (*CONTINUED*)

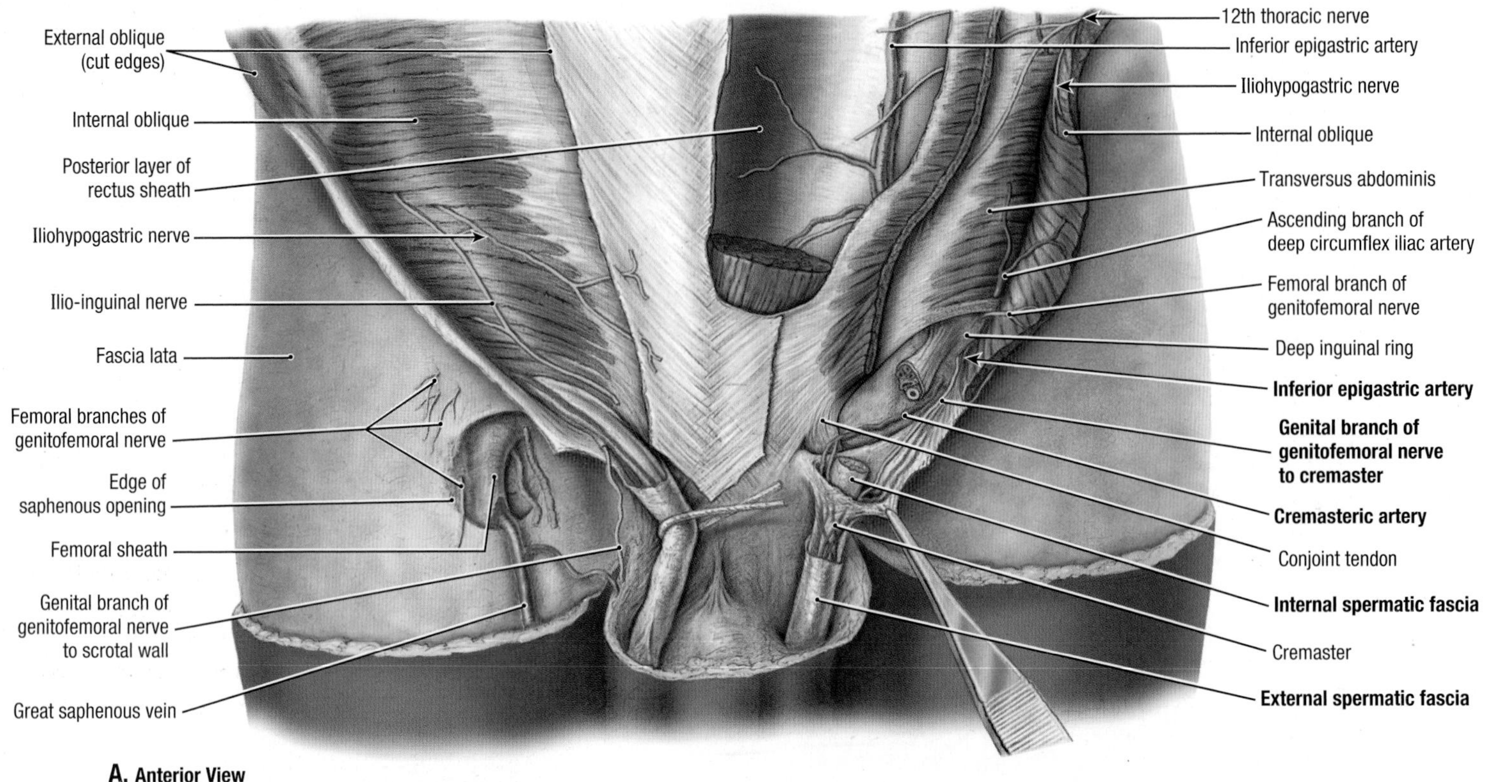

External oblique (cut edges)
Internal oblique
Posterior layer of rectus sheath
Iliohypogastric nerve
Ilio-inguinal nerve
Fascia lata
Femoral branches of genitofemoral nerve
Edge of saphenous opening
Femoral sheath
Genital branch of genitofemoral nerve to scrotal wall
Great saphenous vein
12th thoracic nerve
Inferior epigastric artery
Iliohypogastric nerve
Internal oblique
Transversus abdominis
Ascending branch of deep circumflex iliac artery
Femoral branch of genitofemoral nerve
Deep inguinal ring
Inferior epigastric artery
Genital branch of genitofemoral nerve to cremaster
Cremasteric artery
Conjoint tendon
Internal spermatic fascia
Cremaster
External spermatic fascia

A. **Anterior View**

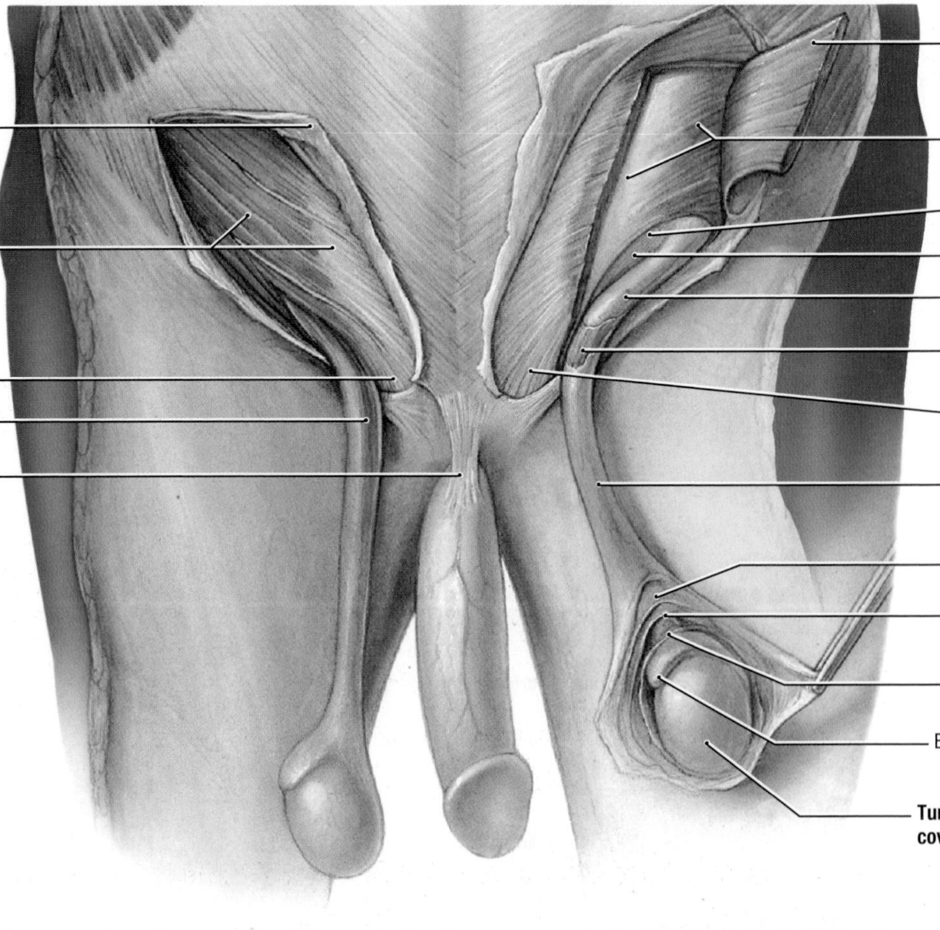

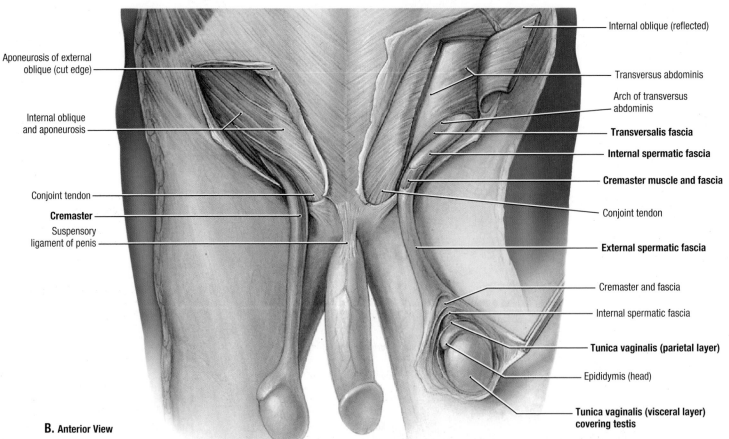

Aponeurosis of external oblique (cut edge)
Internal oblique and aponeurosis
Conjoint tendon
Cremaster
Suspensory ligament of penis
Internal oblique (reflected)
Transversus abdominis
Arch of transversus abdominis
Transversalis fascia
Internal spermatic fascia
Cremaster muscle and fascia
Conjoint tendon
External spermatic fascia
Cremaster and fascia
Internal spermatic fascia
Tunica vaginalis (parietal layer)
Epididymis (head)
Tunica vaginalis (visceral layer) covering testis

B. **Anterior View**

2.16 INGUINAL CANAL, SPERMATIC CORD, AND TESTIS

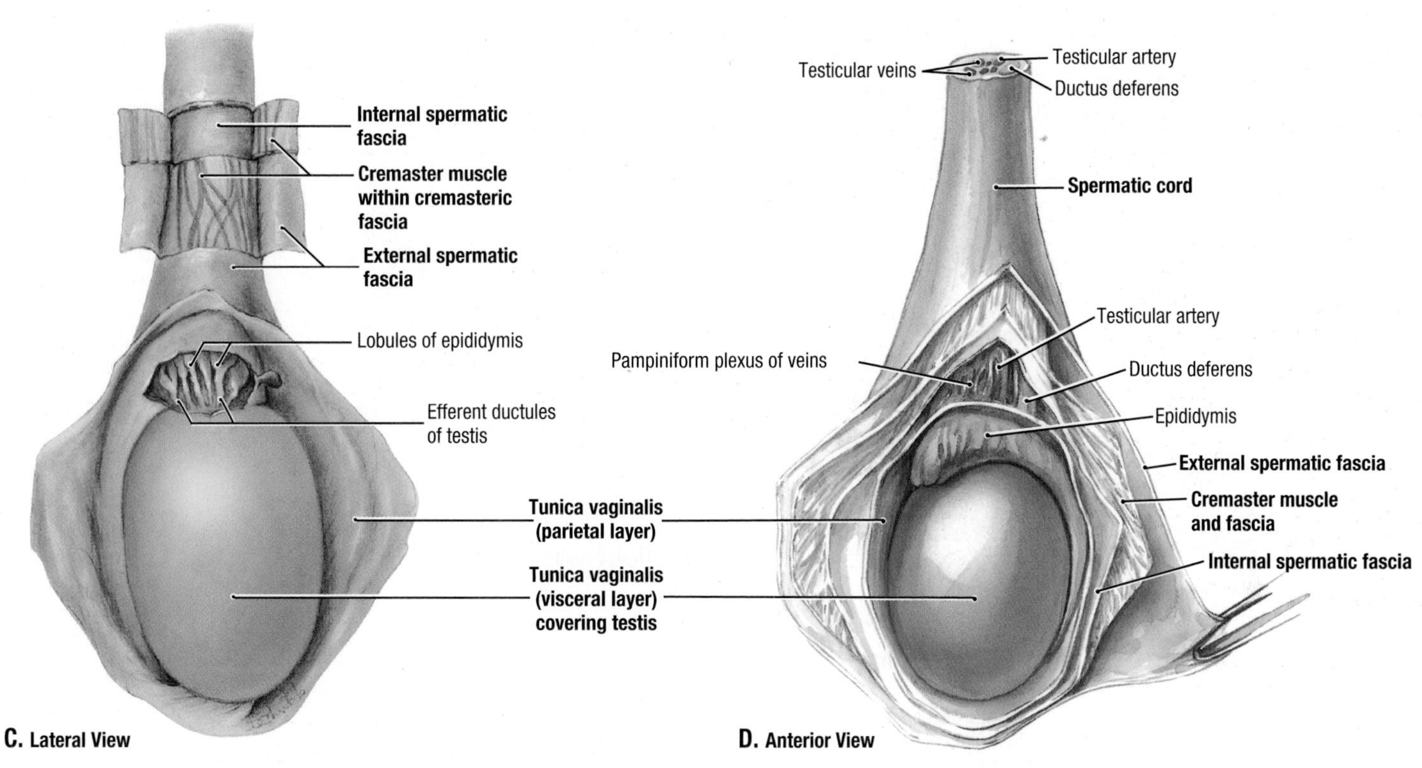
Internal spermatic fascia
Cremaster muscle within cremasteric fascia
External spermatic fascia
Lobules of epididymis
Efferent ductules of testis
Tunica vaginalis (parietal layer)
Tunica vaginalis (visceral layer) covering testis
Testicular veins
Testicular artery
Ductus deferens
Spermatic cord
Testicular artery
Pampiniform plexus of veins
Ductus deferens
Epididymis
External spermatic fascia
Cremaster muscle and fascia
Internal spermatic fascia

C. Lateral View

D. Anterior View

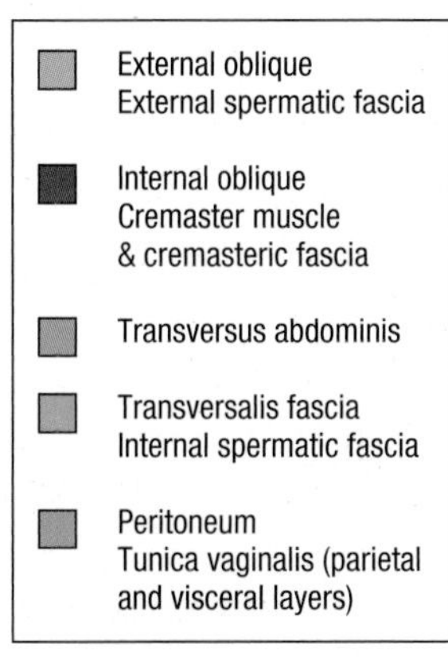
External oblique
External spermatic fascia
Internal oblique
Cremaster muscle
& cremasteric fascia
Transversus abdominis
Transversalis fascia
Internal spermatic fascia
Peritoneum
Tunica vaginalis (parietal and visceral layers)

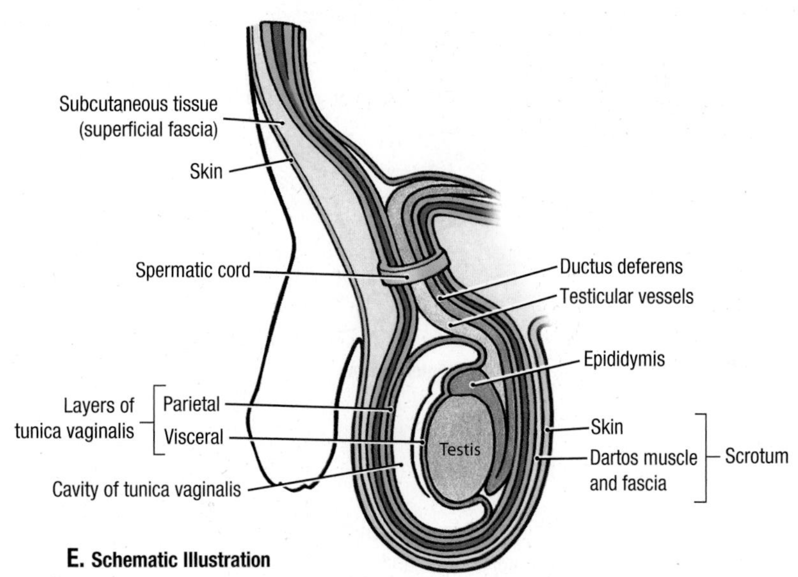
Subcutaneous tissue (superficial fascia)
Skin
Spermatic cord
Ductus deferens
Testicular vessels
Epididymis
Layers of tunica vaginalis
Parietal
Visceral
Testis
Skin
Dartos muscle and fascia
Scrotum
Cavity of tunica vaginalis

E. Schematic Illustration

2.16 INGUINAL CANAL, SPERMATIC CORD, AND TESTIS (*CONTINUED*)

A. Dissection of inguinal canal. **B.** Dissection of inguinal region and coverings of the spermatic cord and testis. **C.–E.** Coverings of spermatic cord and testis.

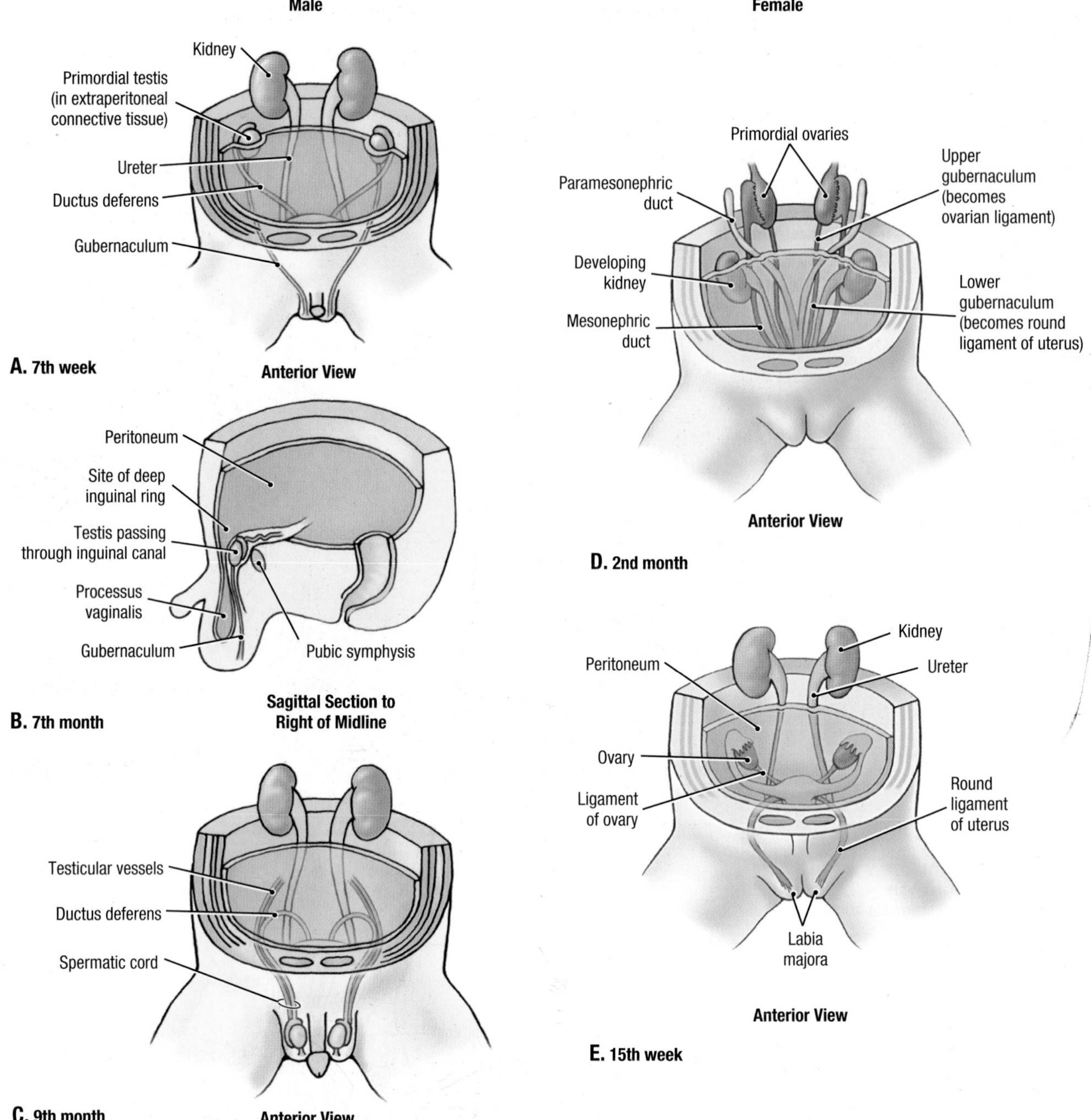

Male
Kidney
Primordial testis (in extraperitoneal connective tissue)
Ureter
Ductus deferens
Gubernaculum
A. 7th week
Anterior View
Peritoneum
Site of deep inguinal ring
Testis passing through inguinal canal
Processus vaginalis
Gubernaculum
Pubic symphysis
B. 7th month
Sagittal Section to Right of Midline
Testicular vessels
Ductus deferens
Spermatic cord
C. 9th month
Anterior View
Female
Primordial ovaries
Paramesonephric duct
Upper gubernaculum (becomes ovarian ligament)
Developing kidney
Mesonephric duct
Lower gubernaculum (becomes round ligament of uterus)
Anterior View
D. 2nd month
Kidney
Peritoneum
Ureter
Ovary
Ligament of ovary
Round ligament of uterus
Labia majora
Anterior View
E. 15th week

2.17 DESCENT OF GONADS

The inguinal canals in females are narrower than those in males, and the canals in infants of both sexes are shorter and much less oblique than in adults. For a complete description of the embryology of the inguinal region, see Moore and Persaud (2008).

The fetal testes descend from the dorsal abdominal wall in the superior lumbar region to the deep inguinal rings during the 9th to 12th fetal weeks. This movement probably results from the growth of the vertebral column and pelvis. The male gubernaculum, attached to the caudal pole of the testis and accompanied by an outpouching of peritoneum, the processus vaginalis, projects into the scrotum. The testis descends posterior to the processus vaginalis. The inferior remnant of the processus vaginalis forms the tunica vaginalis covering the testis. The ductus deferens, testicular vessels, nerves, and lymphatics accompany the testis. The final descent of the testis usually occurs before or shortly after birth.

The fetal ovaries also descend from the dorsal abdominal wall in the superior lumbar region during the 12th week but pass into the lesser pelvis. The female gubernaculum attaches to the caudal pole of the ovary and projects into the labia majora, attaching en route to the uterus; the part passing from the uterus to the ovary forms the ovarian ligament, and the remainder of it becomes the round ligament of the uterus. Because of the attachment of the ovarian ligaments to the uterus, the ovaries do not descend to the inguinal region; however, the round ligament passes through the inguinal canal and attaches to the subcutaneous tissue of the labium majus.

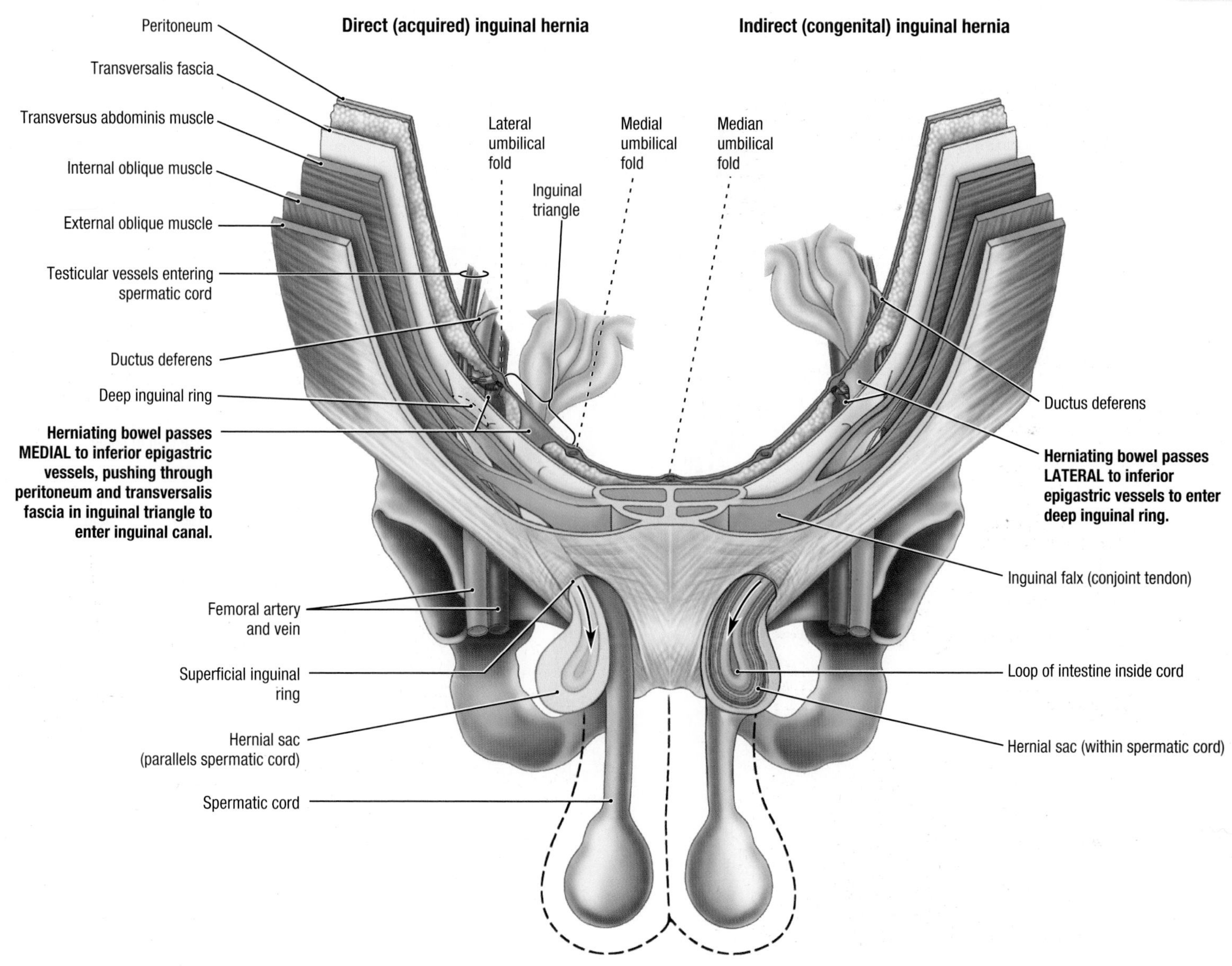
Direct (acquired) inguinal hernia
Indirect (congenital) inguinal hernia
Peritoneum
Transversalis fascia
Transversus abdominis muscle
Internal oblique muscle
External oblique muscle
Testicular vessels entering spermatic cord
Ductus deferens
Deep inguinal ring
Herniating bowel passes MEDIAL to inferior epigastric vessels, pushing through peritoneum and transversalis fascia in inguinal triangle to enter inguinal canal.
Lateral umbilical fold
Inguinal triangle
Medial umbilical fold
Median umbilical fold
Ductus deferens
Herniating bowel passes LATERAL to inferior epigastric vessels to enter deep inguinal ring.
Inguinal falx (conjoint tendon)
Femoral artery and vein
Superficial inguinal ring
Loop of intestine inside cord
Hernial sac (parallels spermatic cord)
Hernial sac (within spermatic cord)
Spermatic cord

2.18 COURSE OF DIRECT AND INDIRECT INGUINAL HERNIAS

An **inguinal hernia** is a protrusion of parietal peritoneum and viscera, such as the small intestine, through the abdominal wall in the inguinal region. There are two major categories of inguinal hernia: indirect and direct. More than two thirds are indirect hernias, most commonly occurring in males.

TABLE 2.3 CHARACTERISTICS OF INGUINAL HERNIAS

Characteristics[a]	Direct (Acquired)	Indirect (Congenital)
Predisposing factors	Weakness of anterior abdominal wall in inguinal triangle (e.g., owing to distended superficial ring, narrow conjoint tendon, or attenuation of aponeurosis in males >40 years of age)	Patency of processus vaginalis (complete or at least of superior part) in younger persons, the great majority of whom are males
Frequency	Less common (one third to one fourth of inguinal hernias)	More common (two third to three fourth of inguinal hernias)
Coverings at exit from abdominal cavity (**A** and **B**)	Peritoneum plus transversalis fascia (lies outside inner one or two fascial coverings of cord)	Peritoneum of persistent processus vaginalis plus all three fascial coverings of cord/round ligament
Course **(C)**	Usually traverses only medial third of inguinal canal, external and parallel to vestige of processus vaginalis	Traverses inguinal canal (entire canal if it is sufficient size) within processus vaginalis
Exit from anterior abdominal wall	Via superficial ring, lateral to cord; rarely enters scrotum	Via superficial ring inside cord, commonly passing into scrotum/labium majus

[a]Letters in parentheses refer to the figure parts.

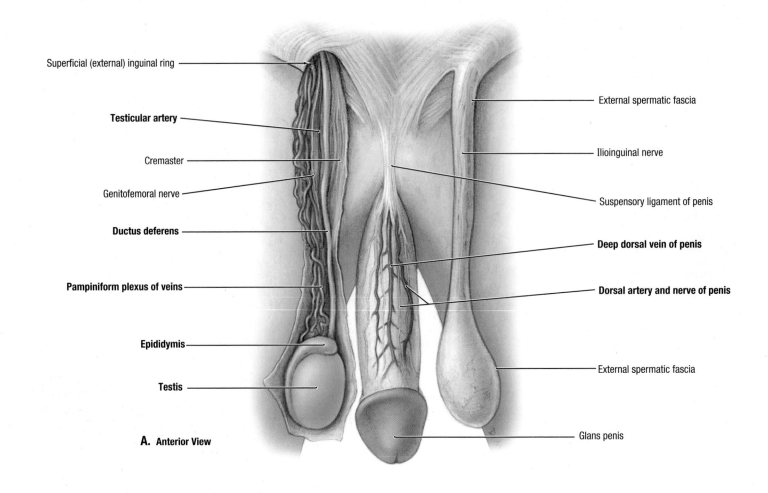

Superficial (external) inguinal ring
Testicular artery
Cremaster
Genitofemoral nerve
Ductus deferens
Pampiniform plexus of veins
Epididymis
Testis
External spermatic fascia
Ilioinguinal nerve
Suspensory ligament of penis
Deep dorsal vein of penis
Dorsal artery and nerve of penis
External spermatic fascia
Glans penis

A. Anterior View

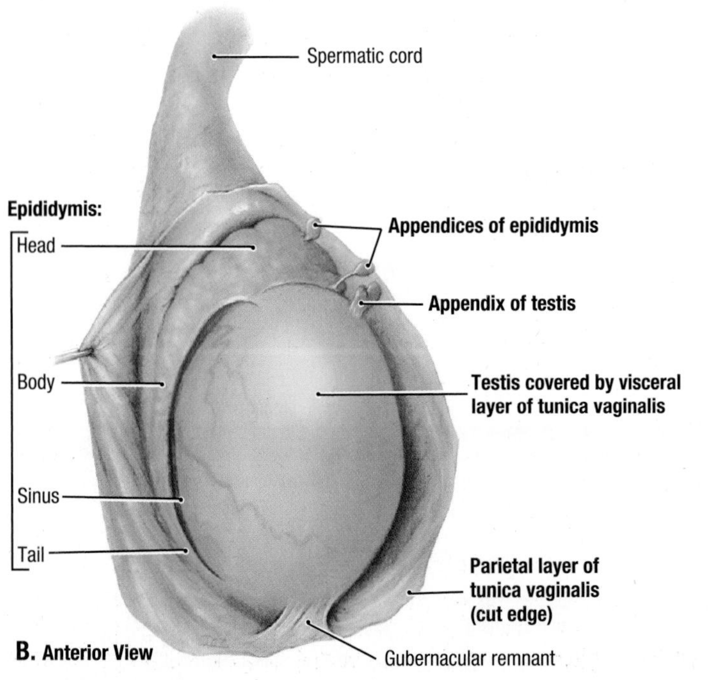
Spermatic cord
Epididymis:
Head
Body
Sinus
Tail
Appendices of epididymis
Appendix of testis
Testis covered by visceral layer of tunica vaginalis
Parietal layer of tunica vaginalis (cut edge)
Gubernacular remnant

B. Anterior View

2.19 SPERMATIC CORD, TESTIS, AND EPIDIDYMIS

A. Dissection of spermatic cord. The subcutaneous tissue (dartos fascia) covering the penis has been removed and the deep fascia rendered transparent to demonstrate the median deep dorsal vein and the bilateral dorsal arteries and nerves of the penis. On the specimen's right, the coverings of the spermatic cord and testis are reflected, and the contents of the cord are separated. The testicular artery has been separated from the pampiniform plexus of veins that surrounds it as it courses parallel to the ductus deferens. Lymphatic vessels and autonomic nerve fibers (not shown) are also present. **B.** The tunica vaginalis has been incised longitudinally to expose its cavity, surrounding the testis anteriorly and laterally, and extending between the testis and epididymis at the sinus of the epididymis. The epididymis is located posterolateral to the left testis, that is, on the right side of the right testis and on the left side of the left testis. The appendices of the testis and epididymis may be observed in some specimens. These structures are small remnants of the embryonic genital (paramesonephric) duct.

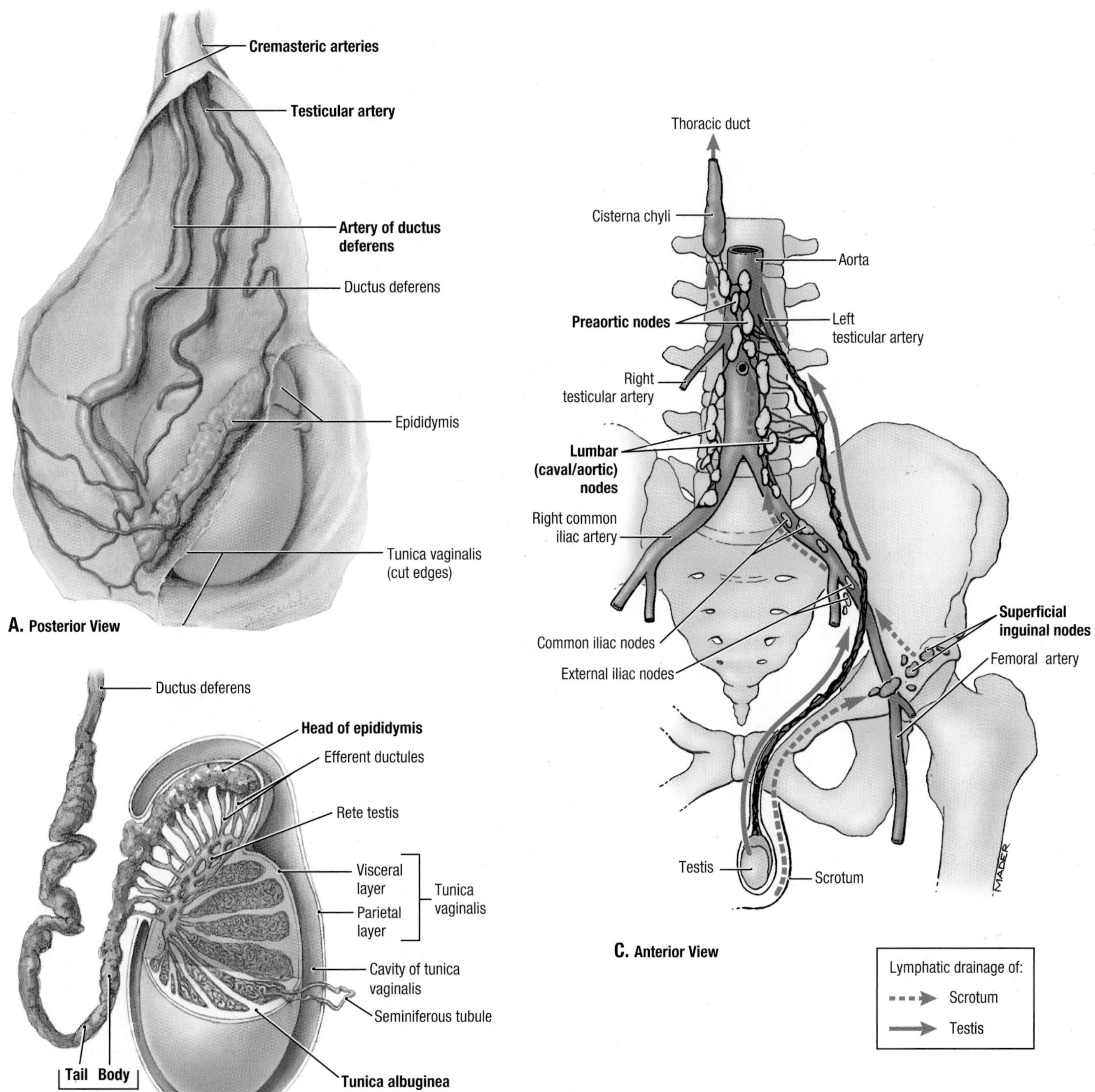
Cremasteric arteries
Testicular artery
Artery of ductus deferens
Ductus deferens
Epididymis
Tunica vaginalis (cut edges)
Ductus deferens
Head of epididymis
Efferent ductules
Rete testis
Visceral layer
Parietal layer
Tunica vaginalis
Cavity of tunica vaginalis
Seminiferous tubule
Tunica albuginea
Tail Body
of epididymis
Thoracic duct
Cisterna chyli
Aorta
Preaortic nodes
Left testicular artery
Right testicular artery
Lumbar (caval/aortic) nodes
Right common iliac artery
Common iliac nodes
External iliac nodes
Superficial inguinal nodes
Femoral artery
Testis
Scrotum
Lymphatic drainage of:
Scrotum
Testis

A. Posterior View

B. Longitinal Section of Tunica Vaginalis; Testis Sectioned in Sagittal and Transverse Planes

C. Anterior View

2.20 BLOOD SUPPLY AND LYMPHATIC DRAINAGE OF TESTIS

A. Blood supply. **B.** Internal structure. **C.** Lymphatic drainage. Because the testes descend from the posterior abdominal wall into the scrotum during fetal development, their lymphatic drainage differs from that of the scrotum, which is an outpouching of the abdominal skin. Consequently, **cancer of the testis** metastasizes initially to the lumbar lymph nodes, and **cancer of the scrotum** metastasizes initially to the superficial inguinal lymph nodes.

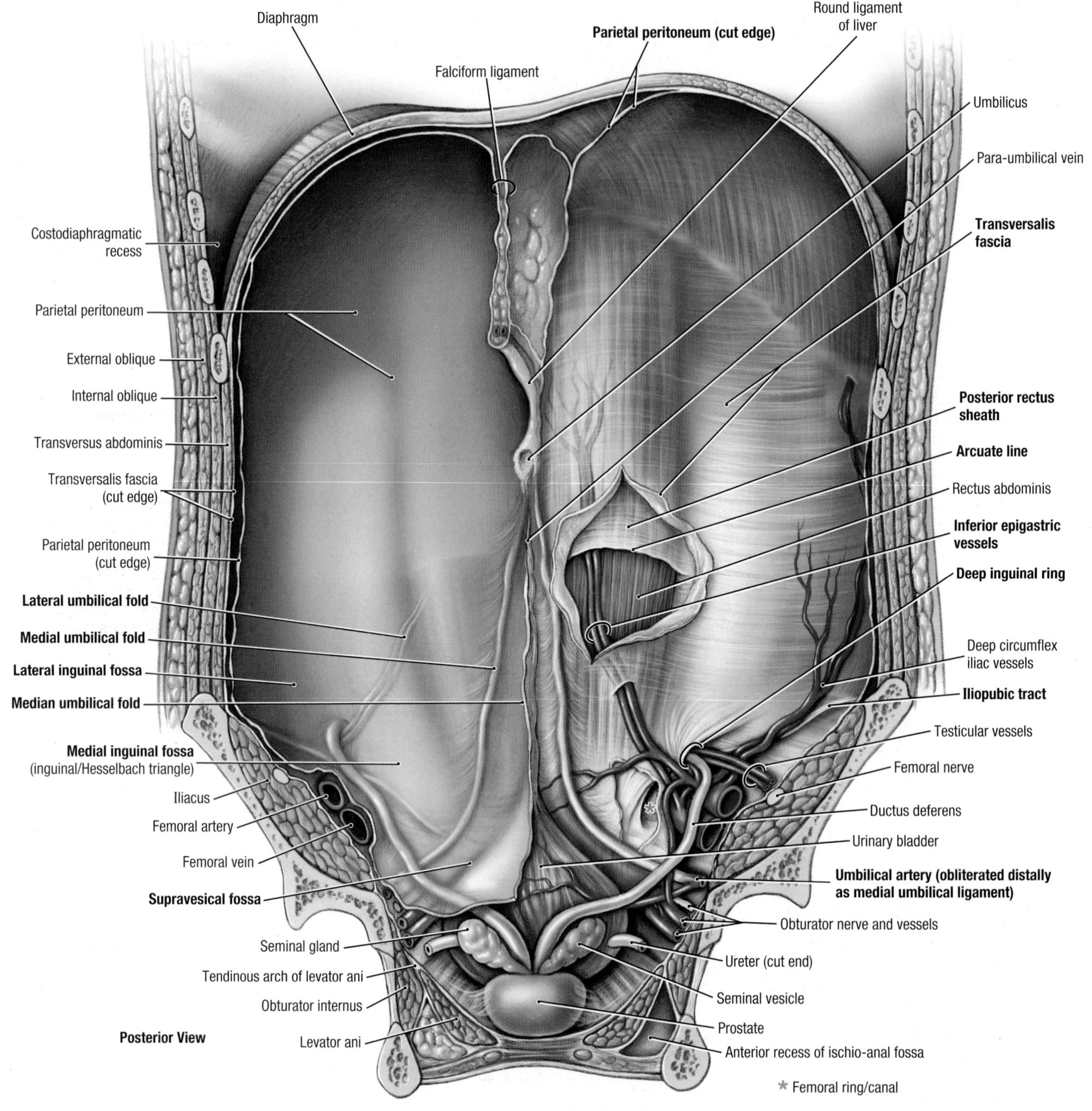
Diaphragm
Parietal peritoneum (cut edge)
Round ligament of liver
Falciform ligament
Umbilicus
Para-umbilical vein
Transversalis fascia
Costodiaphragmatic recess
Parietal peritoneum
External oblique
Internal oblique
Transversus abdominis
Transversalis fascia (cut edge)
Parietal peritoneum (cut edge)
Lateral umbilical fold
Medial umbilical fold
Lateral inguinal fossa
Median umbilical fold
Medial inguinal fossa (inguinal/Hesselbach triangle)
Iliacus
Femoral artery
Femoral vein
Supravesical fossa
Seminal gland
Tendinous arch of levator ani
Obturator internus
Posterior View
Levator ani
Posterior rectus sheath
Arcuate line
Rectus abdominis
Inferior epigastric vessels
Deep inguinal ring
Deep circumflex iliac vessels
Iliopubic tract
Testicular vessels
Femoral nerve
Ductus deferens
Urinary bladder
Umbilical artery (obliterated distally as medial umbilical ligament)
Obturator nerve and vessels
Ureter (cut end)
Seminal vesicle
Prostate
Anterior recess of ischio-anal fossa
* Femoral ring/canal

2.21 POSTERIOR ASPECT OF THE ANTEROLATERAL ABDOMINAL WALL

Umbilical folds (median, medial, and lateral) are reflections of the parietal peritoneum that are raised from the body wall by underlying structures. The median umbilical fold extends from the urinary bladder to the umbilicus and covers the median umbilical ligament (the remnant of the urachus). The two medial umbilical folds cover the medial umbilical ligaments (occluded remnants of the fetal umbilical arteries). Two lateral umbilical folds cover the inferior epigastric vessels. The supravesical fossae are between the median and medial umbilical folds, the medial inguinal fossae (inguinal triangles) are between the medial and lateral umbilical folds, and the lateral inguinal fossae and deep inguinal rings are lateral to the lateral umbilical folds.

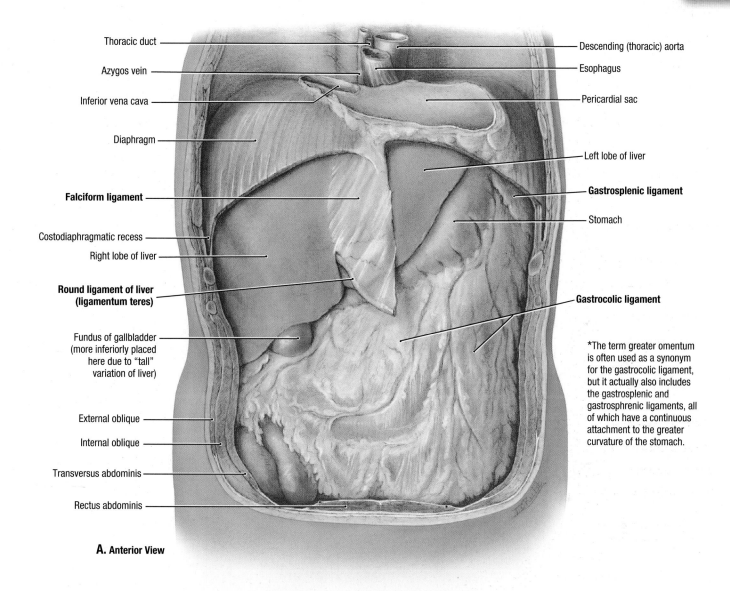

Thoracic duct
Azygos vein
Inferior vena cava
Diaphragm
Falciform ligament
Costodiaphragmatic recess
Right lobe of liver
Round ligament of liver (ligamentum teres)
Fundus of gallbladder (more inferiorly placed here due to "tall" variation of liver)
External oblique
Internal oblique
Transversus abdominis
Rectus abdominis
Descending (thoracic) aorta
Esophagus
Pericardial sac
Left lobe of liver
Gastrosplenic ligament
Stomach
Gastrocolic ligament

A. Anterior View

*The term greater omentum is often used as a synonym for the gastrocolic ligament, but it actually also includes the gastrosplenic and gastrosphrenic ligaments, all of which have a continuous attachment to the greater curvature of the stomach.

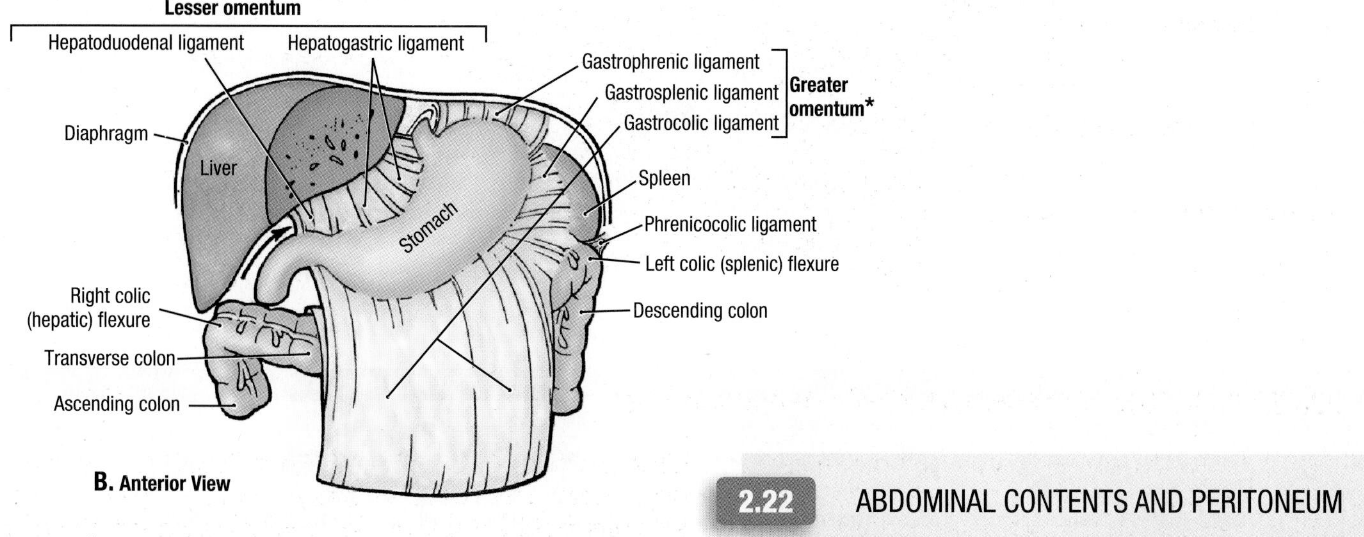
Lesser omentum
Hepatoduodenal ligament
Hepatogastric ligament
Gastrophrenic ligament
Gastrosplenic ligament
Gastrocolic ligament
Greater omentum*
Diaphragm
Liver
Stomach
Spleen
Phrenicocolic ligament
Left colic (splenic) flexure
Descending colon
Right colic (hepatic) flexure
Transverse colon
Ascending colon

B. Anterior View

2.22 ABDOMINAL CONTENTS AND PERITONEUM

A. Dissection. **B.** Components of greater and lesser omentum. *Arrow*, site of omental (epiploic) foramen.

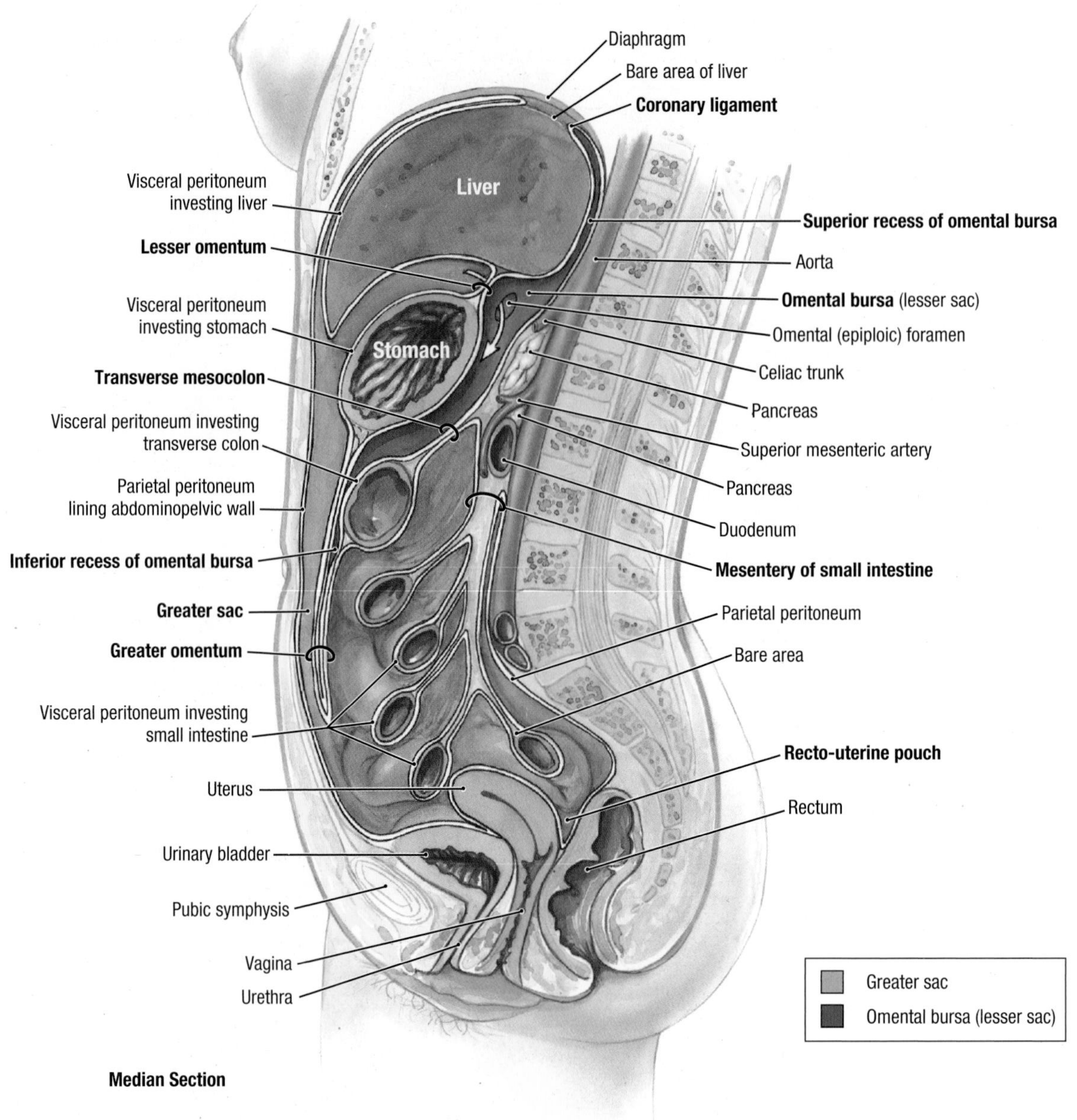
Diaphragm
Bare area of liver
Coronary ligament
Liver
Visceral peritoneum investing liver
Superior recess of omental bursa
Aorta
Lesser omentum
Omental bursa (lesser sac)
Omental (epiploic) foramen
Visceral peritoneum investing stomach
Stomach
Celiac trunk
Pancreas
Transverse mesocolon
Superior mesenteric artery
Visceral peritoneum investing transverse colon
Pancreas
Parietal peritoneum lining abdominopelvic wall
Duodenum
Inferior recess of omental bursa
Mesentery of small intestine
Greater sac
Parietal peritoneum
Greater omentum
Bare area
Visceral peritoneum investing small intestine
Recto-uterine pouch
Uterus
Rectum
Urinary bladder
Pubic symphysis
Vagina
Urethra
Greater sac
Omental bursa (lesser sac)
Median Section

2.23 PERITONEAL FORMATIONS AND BARE AREAS

Various terms are used to describe the parts of the peritoneum that connect organs with other organs or to the abdominal wall and to describe the compartments and recesses that are formed as a consequence. The *arrow* passes through the omental (epiploic) foramen.

TABLE 2.4 TERMS USED TO DESCRIBE PARTS OF PERITONEUM

Term	Definition
Peritoneal ligament	Double layer of peritoneum that connects an organ with another organ or to the abdominal wall.
Mesentery	Double layer of peritoneum that occurs as a result of the invagination of the peritoneum by an organ and constitutes a continuity of the visceral and parietal peritoneum.
Omentum	Double-layered extension of peritoneum passing from the stomach and proximal part of the duodenum to adjacent organs. The greater omentum extends from the greater curvature of the stomach and the proximal duodenum; the lesser omentum from the lesser curvature.
Bare area	Every organ must have an area, the bare area, that is not covered with visceral peritoneum, to allow the entrance and exit of neurovascular structures. Bare areas are formed in relation to the attachments of mesenteries, omenta, and ligaments. Named bare areas, e.g., bare area of liver, are especially extensive in area.

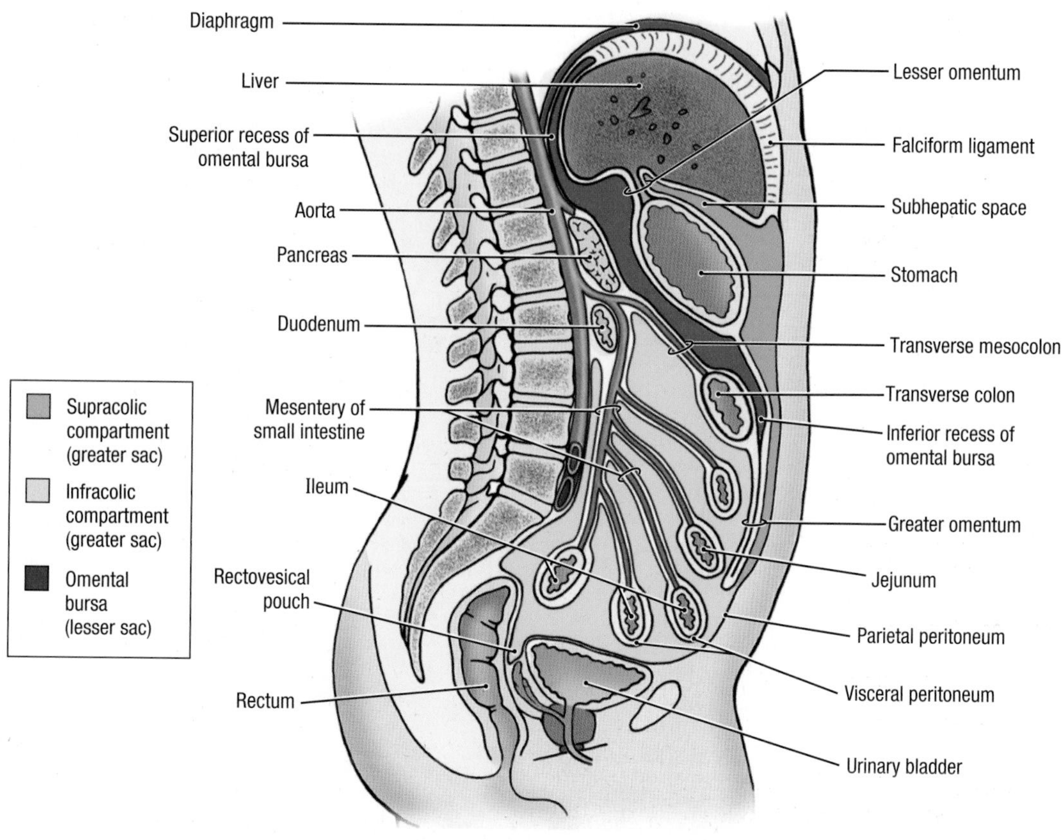
Diaphragm
Liver
Superior recess of omental bursa
Aorta
Pancreas
Duodenum
Mesentery of small intestine
Ileum
Rectovesical pouch
Rectum
Lesser omentum
Falciform ligament
Subhepatic space
Stomach
Transverse mesocolon
Transverse colon
Inferior recess of omental bursa
Greater omentum
Jejunum
Parietal peritoneum
Visceral peritoneum
Urinary bladder
Supracolic compartment (greater sac)
Infracolic compartment (greater sac)
Omental bursa (lesser sac)

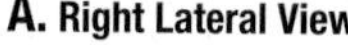

A. Right Lateral View

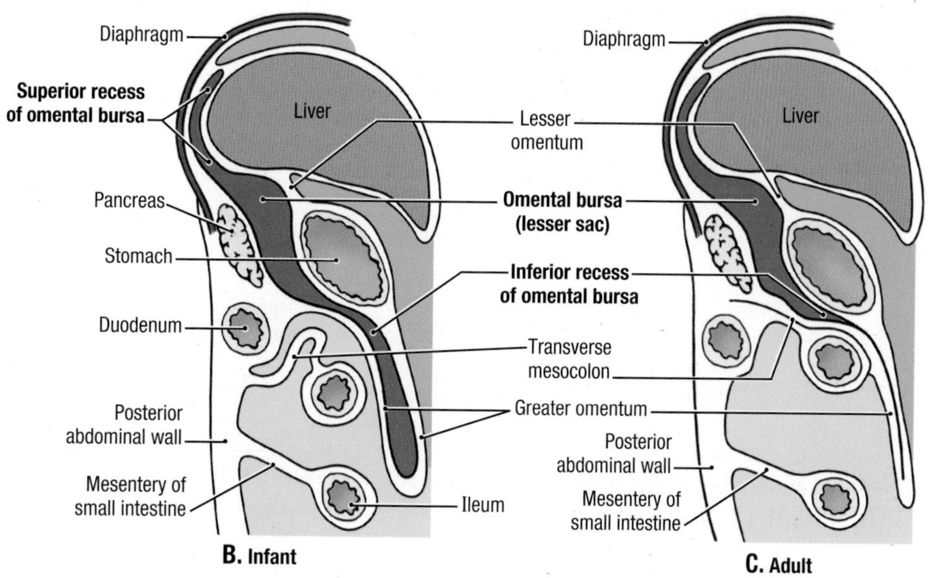
Diaphragm
Superior recess of omental bursa
Liver
Pancreas
Stomach
Duodenum
Posterior abdominal wall
Mesentery of small intestine
Lesser omentum
Omental bursa (lesser sac)
Inferior recess of omental bursa
Transverse mesocolon
Greater omentum
Ileum
Posterior abdominal wall
Mesentery of small intestine

B. Infant

C. Adult

Schematic Sagittal Sections, Lateral View

2.24 SUBDIVISIONS OF PERITONEAL CAVITY

A. Sagittal section. **B.** In an infant, the omental bursa (lesser sac) is an isolated part of the peritoneal cavity, lying dorsal to the stomach and extending superiorly to the liver and diaphragm (superior recess of the omental bursa) and inferiorly between the layers of the greater omentum (inferior recess of the omental bursa). **C.** In an adult, after fusion of the layers of the greater omentum, the inferior recess of the omental bursa now extends inferiorly only as far as the transverse colon. The *red arrows* pass from the greater sac through the omental (epiploic) foramen into the omental bursa.

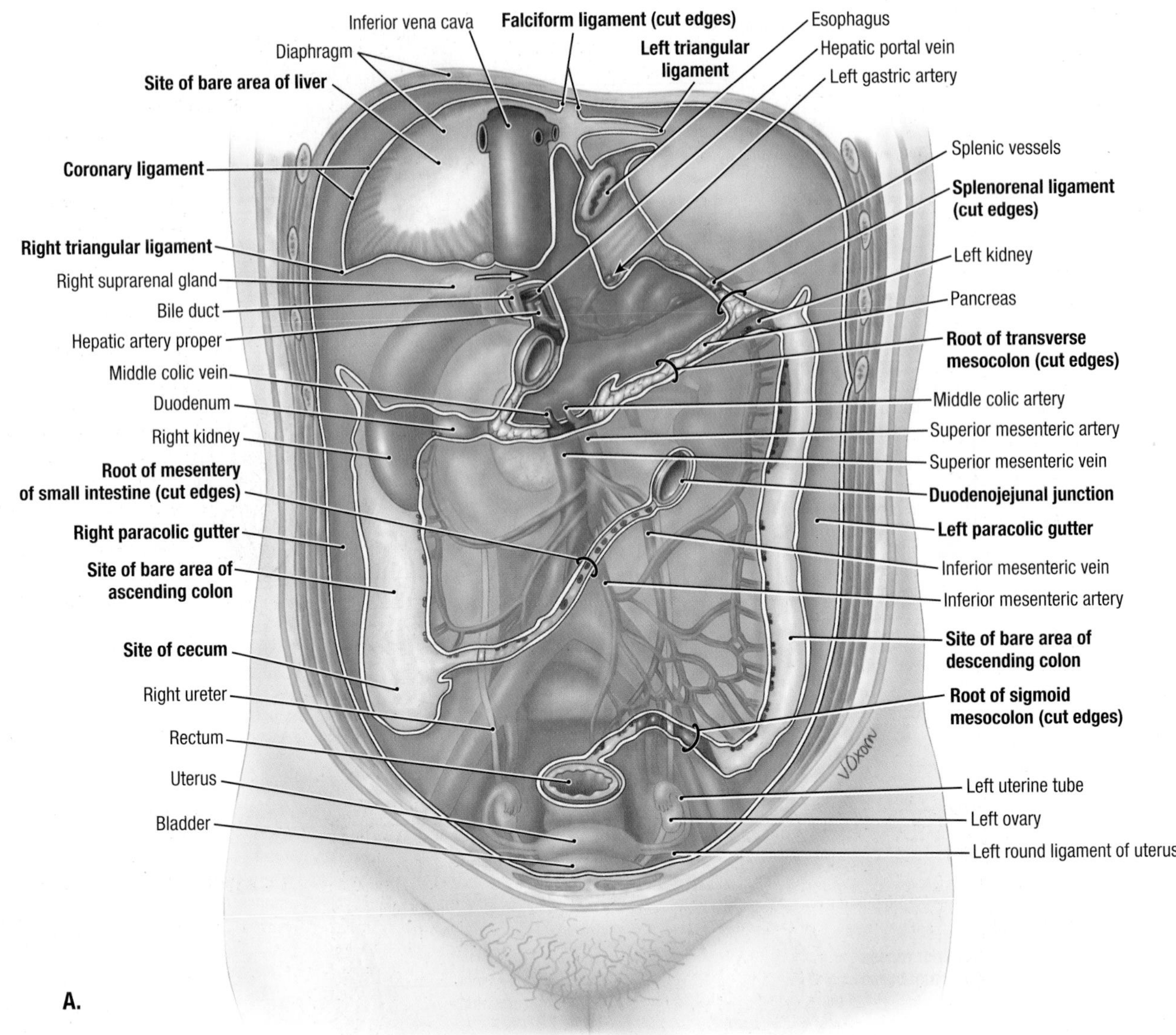
Inferior vena cava
Falciform ligament (cut edges)
Esophagus
Diaphragm
Left triangular ligament
Hepatic portal vein
Site of bare area of liver
Left gastric artery
Coronary ligament
Splenic vessels
Splenorenal ligament (cut edges)
Right triangular ligament
Right suprarenal gland
Left kidney
Bile duct
Pancreas
Hepatic artery proper
Root of transverse mesocolon (cut edges)
Middle colic vein
Middle colic artery
Duodenum
Superior mesenteric artery
Right kidney
Superior mesenteric vein
Root of mesentery of small intestine (cut edges)
Duodenojejunal junction
Right paracolic gutter
Left paracolic gutter
Site of bare area of ascending colon
Inferior mesenteric vein
Inferior mesenteric artery
Site of cecum
Site of bare area of descending colon
Right ureter
Root of sigmoid mesocolon (cut edges)
Rectum
Uterus
Left uterine tube
Left ovary
Bladder
Left round ligament of uterus
A.

Anterior Views

Transverse colon
Supracolic compartment
Transverse mesocolon
Phrenicocolic ligament
Left colic (splenic) flexure
Right colic (hepatic) flexure
Tenia coli
Ascending colon
Root of mesentery of small intestine
Descending colon
Right paracolic gutter
Right infracolic space
Left infracolic space
Left paracolic gutter
Infracolic compartment
B.

2.25 POSTERIOR WALL OF PERITONEAL CAVITY

A. Roots of the peritoneal reflections. The peritoneal reflections from the posterior abdominal wall (mesenteries and reflections surrounding bare areas of liver and secondarily retroperitoneal organs) have been cut at their roots, and the intraperitoneal and secondarily retroperitoneal viscera have been removed. The *white arrow* passes through the omental (epiploic) foramen. **B.** Supracolic and infracolic compartments of the greater sac. The infracolic spaces and paracolic gutters are of clinical importance because they determine the paths (*black arrows*) for the **flow of ascitic fluid with changes in position**, and the spread of intraperitoneal infections.

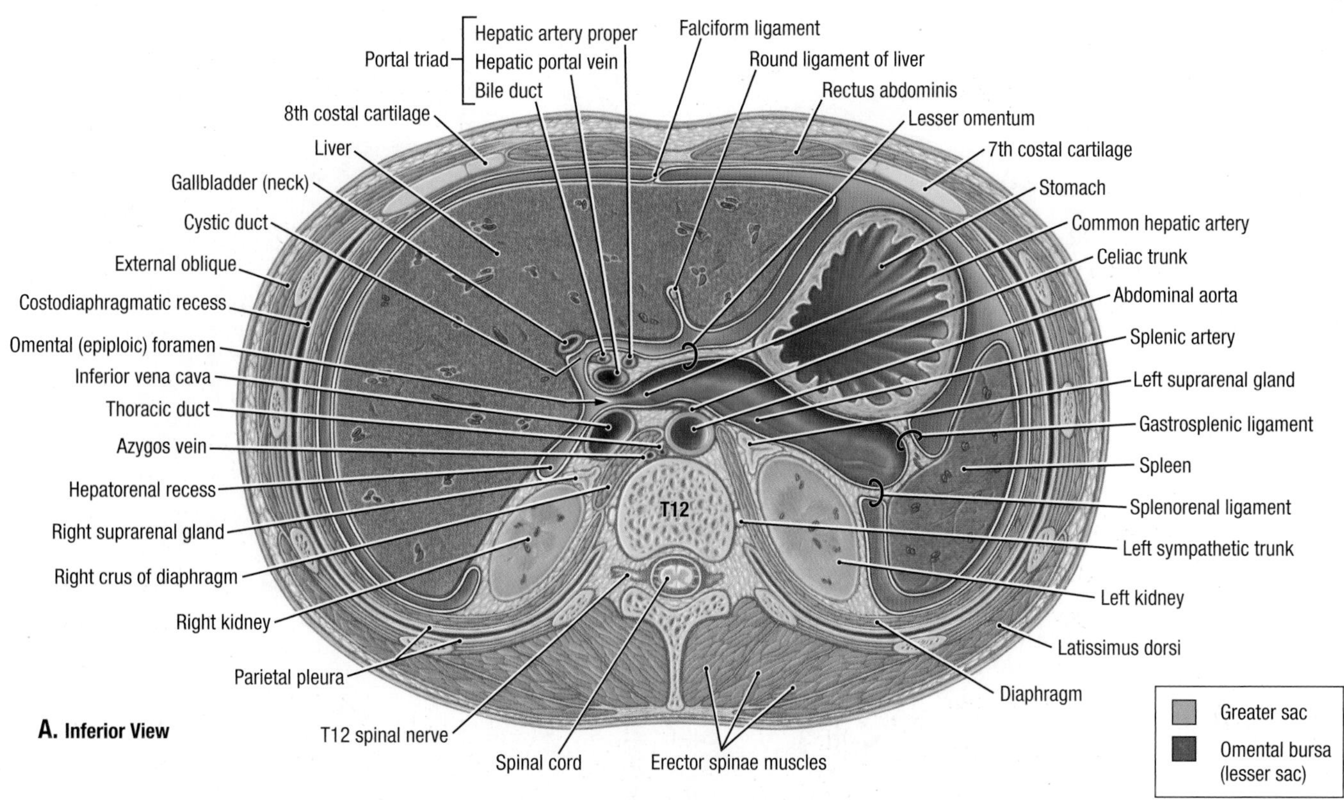
Portal triad
Hepatic artery proper
Hepatic portal vein
Bile duct
Falciform ligament
Round ligament of liver
Rectus abdominis
Lesser omentum
8th costal cartilage
Liver
7th costal cartilage
Gallbladder (neck)
Stomach
Cystic duct
Common hepatic artery
Celiac trunk
External oblique
Abdominal aorta
Costodiaphragmatic recess
Splenic artery
Omental (epiploic) foramen
Left suprarenal gland
Inferior vena cava
Thoracic duct
Gastrosplenic ligament
Azygos vein
Spleen
Hepatorenal recess
Splenorenal ligament
T12
Right suprarenal gland
Left sympathetic trunk
Right crus of diaphragm
Left kidney
Right kidney
Latissimus dorsi
Parietal pleura
Diaphragm
T12 spinal nerve
Spinal cord
Erector spinae muscles
Greater sac
Omental bursa (lesser sac)

A. **Inferior View**

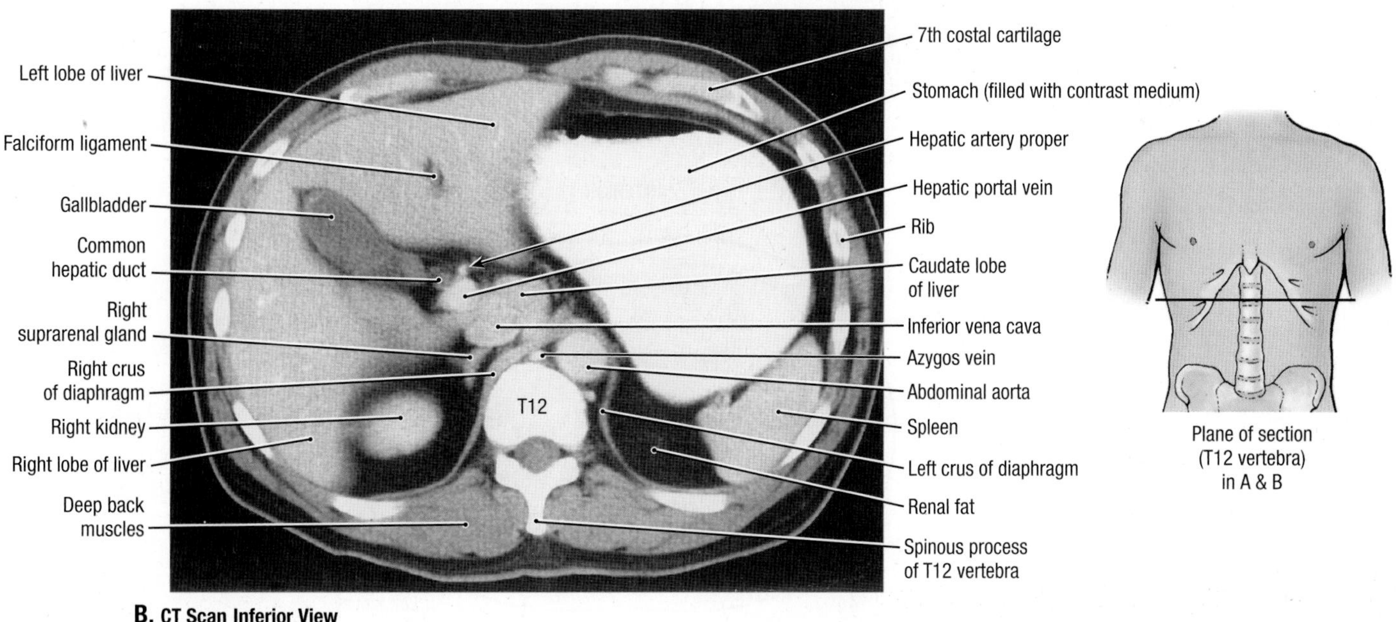
7th costal cartilage
Left lobe of liver
Stomach (filled with contrast medium)
Falciform ligament
Hepatic artery proper
Gallbladder
Hepatic portal vein
Rib
Common hepatic duct
Caudate lobe of liver
Right suprarenal gland
Inferior vena cava
Azygos vein
Right crus of diaphragm
Abdominal aorta
T12
Right kidney
Spleen
Right lobe of liver
Left crus of diaphragm
Renal fat
Deep back muscles
Spinous process of T12 vertebra
Plane of section (T12 vertebra) in A & B

B. **CT Scan Inferior View**

2.26 TRANSVERSE SECTIONS THROUGH GREATER SAC AND OMENTAL BURSA

- When bacterial contamination occurs or when the gut is traumatically penetrated or ruptured as the result of infection and inflammation, gas, fecal matter, and bacteria enter the peritoneal cavity. The result is infection and inflammation of the peritoneum, called **peritonitis**.
- Under certain pathological conditions such as peritonitis, the peritoneal cavity may be distended with abnormal fluid, **ascites**. Widespread metastases (spread) of cancer cells to the abdominal viscera cause exudation (escape) of fluid that is often blood stained. Thus the peritoneal cavity may be distended with several liters of abnormal fluid. Surgical puncture of the peritoneal cavity for the aspiration of drainage of fluid is called **paracentesis**.

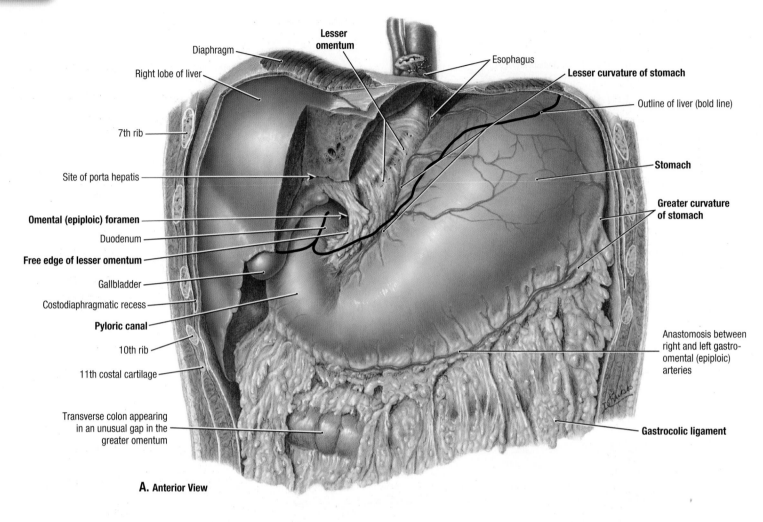

Lesser omentum
Diaphragm
Esophagus
Right lobe of liver
Lesser curvature of stomach
Outline of liver (bold line)
7th rib
Stomach
Site of porta hepatis
Greater curvature of stomach
Omental (epiploic) foramen
Duodenum
Free edge of lesser omentum
Gallbladder
Costodiaphragmatic recess
Pyloric canal
10th rib
Anastomosis between right and left gastro-omental (epiploic) arteries
11th costal cartilage
Transverse colon appearing in an unusual gap in the greater omentum
Gastrocolic ligament

A. Anterior View

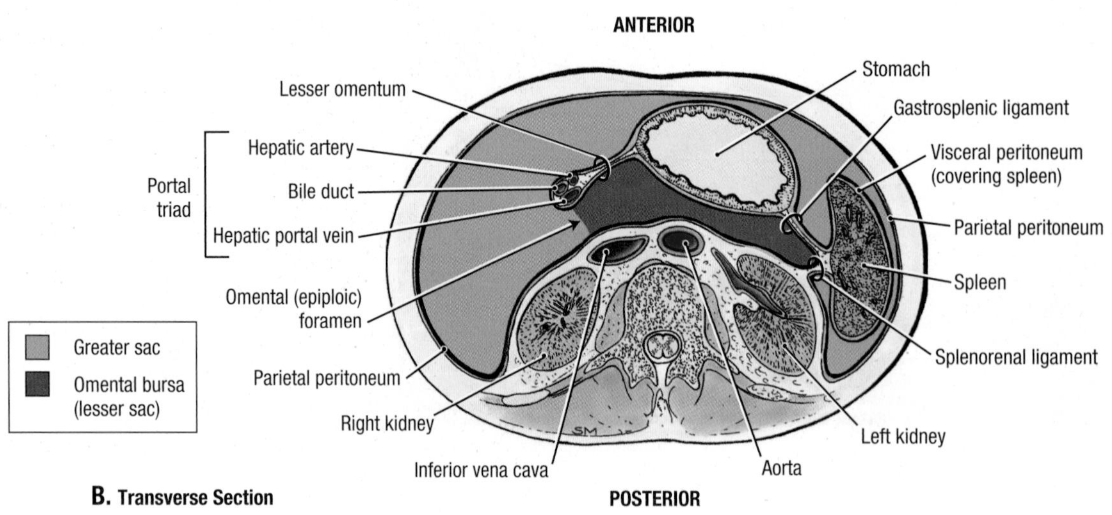
ANTERIOR
Stomach
Lesser omentum
Gastrosplenic ligament
Hepatic artery
Visceral peritoneum (covering spleen)
Portal triad
Bile duct
Parietal peritoneum
Hepatic portal vein
Spleen
Omental (epiploic) foramen
Greater sac
Omental bursa (lesser sac)
Splenorenal ligament
Parietal peritoneum
Right kidney
Left kidney
Inferior vena cava
Aorta
POSTERIOR

B. Transverse Section

2.27 STOMACH AND OMENTA

A. Lesser and greater omenta. The stomach is inflated with air, and the left part of the liver is cut away. The gallbladder, followed superiorly, leads to the free margin of the lesser omentum and serves as a guide to the omental (epiploic) foramen, which lies posterior to that free margin. **B.** Omental bursa (lesser sac), schematic transverse section.

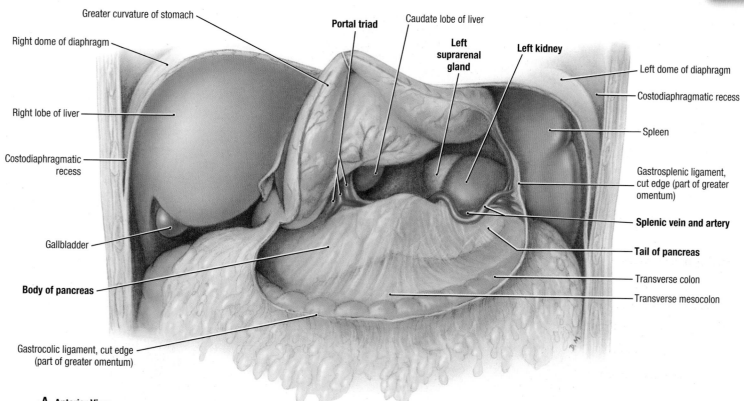

Greater curvature of stomach
Portal triad
Caudate lobe of liver
Right dome of diaphragm
Left suprarenal gland
Left kidney
Left dome of diaphragm
Costodiaphragmatic recess
Right lobe of liver
Spleen
Costodiaphragmatic recess
Gastrosplenic ligament, cut edge (part of greater omentum)
Splenic vein and artery
Gallbladder
Tail of pancreas
Transverse colon
Body of pancreas
Transverse mesocolon
Gastrocolic ligament, cut edge (part of greater omentum)

A. Anterior View

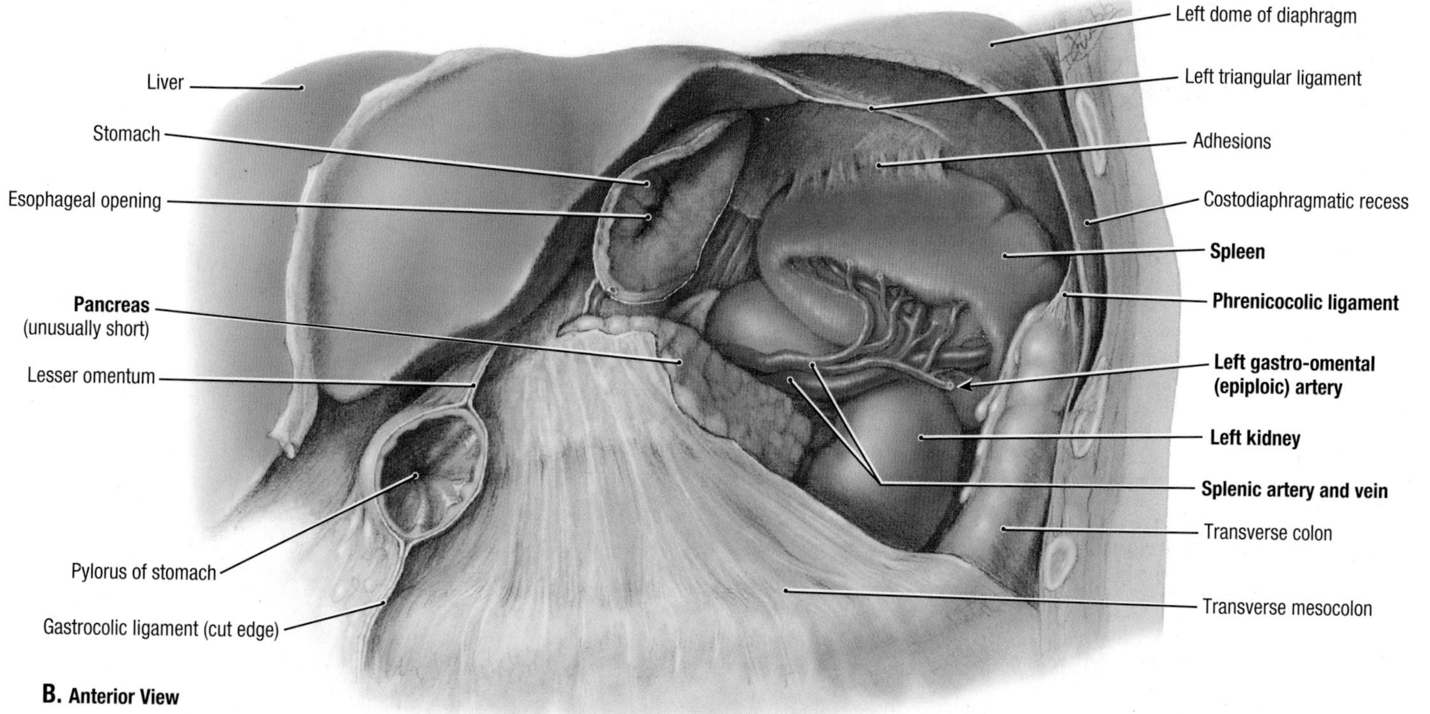
Left dome of diaphragm
Liver
Left triangular ligament
Stomach
Adhesions
Esophageal opening
Costodiaphragmatic recess
Spleen
Pancreas
(unusually short)
Phrenicocolic ligament
Lesser omentum
Left gastro-omental
(epiploic) artery
Left kidney
Splenic artery and vein
Transverse colon
Pylorus of stomach
Transverse mesocolon
Gastrocolic ligament (cut edge)

B. Anterior View

2.28 POSTERIOR RELATIONSHIPS OF OMENTAL BURSA (LESSER SAC)

A. Opened omental bursa. The greater omentum has been cut along the greater curvature of the stomach; the stomach is reflected superiorly. Peritoneum of the stomach bed is partially removed. **B.** Stomach bed. The stomach is excised. Peritoneum covering the stomach bed and inferior part of the kidney and pancreas is largely removed. **Adhesions** binding the spleen to the diaphragm are pathological, but not unusual.

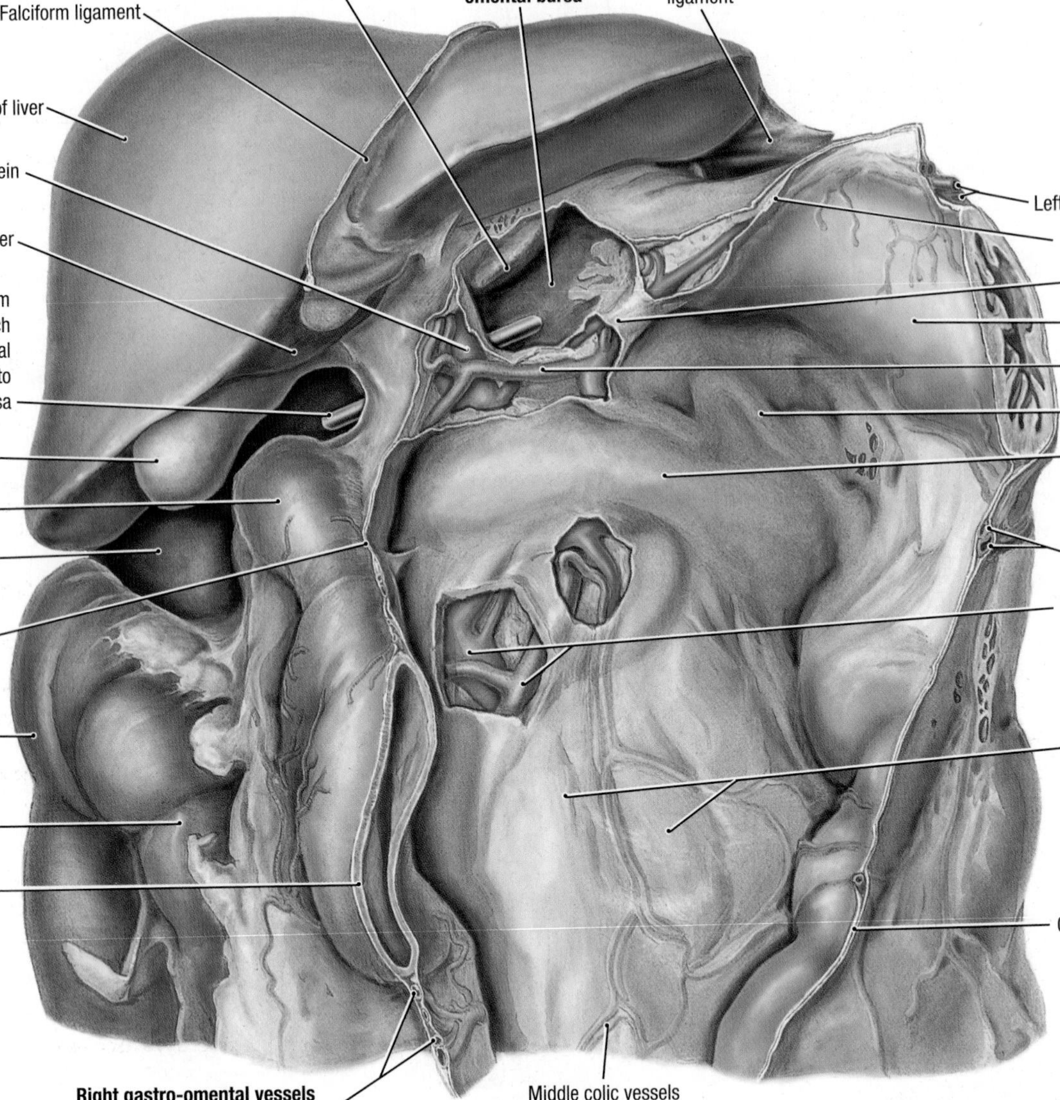

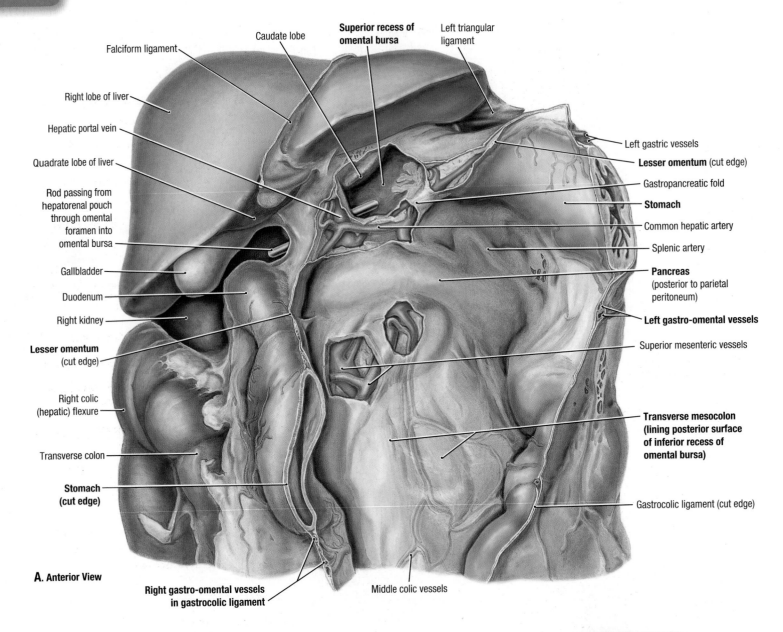

Caudate lobe
Superior recess of omental bursa
Left triangular ligament
Falciform ligament
Right lobe of liver
Hepatic portal vein
Quadrate lobe of liver
Rod passing from hepatorenal pouch through omental foramen into omental bursa
Gallbladder
Duodenum
Right kidney
Lesser omentum (cut edge)
Right colic (hepatic) flexure
Transverse colon
Stomach (cut edge)
Left gastric vessels
Lesser omentum (cut edge)
Gastropancreatic fold
Stomach
Common hepatic artery
Splenic artery
Pancreas (posterior to parietal peritoneum)
Left gastro-omental vessels
Superior mesenteric vessels
Transverse mesocolon (lining posterior surface of inferior recess of omental bursa)
Gastrocolic ligament (cut edge)
Right gastro-omental vessels in gastrocolic ligament
Middle colic vessels

A. Anterior View

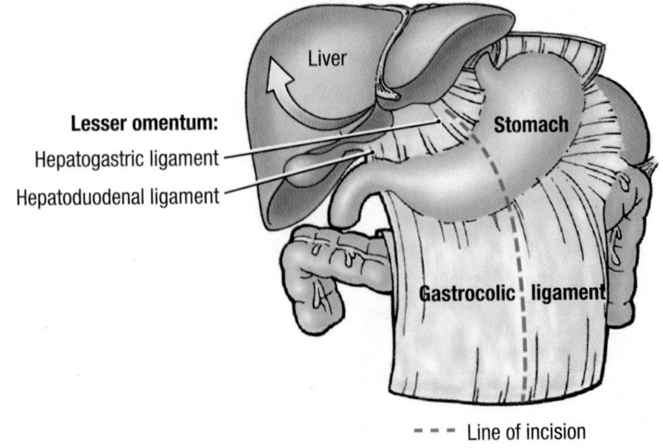
Liver
Stomach
Lesser omentum:
Hepatogastric ligament
Hepatoduodenal ligament
Gastrocolic ligament
Line of incision

B. Anterior View

2.29 OMENTAL BURSA (LESSER SAC), OPENED

A. Dissection. **B.** Line of incision in **A.** The anterior wall of the omental bursa, consisting of the stomach, lesser omentum, anterior layer of the greater omentum, and vessels along the curvatures of the stomach, has been sectioned sagittally. The two halves have been retracted to the left and right: the body of the stomach on the left side, and the pyloric part of the stomach and first part of the duodenum on the right. The right kidney forms the posterior wall of the hepatorenal pouch (part of greater sac), and the pancreas lies horizontally on the posterior wall of the main compartment of the omental bursa (lesser sac). The gastrocolic ligament forms the anterior wall and the lower part of the posterior wall of the inferior recess of the omental bursa. The transverse mesocolon forms the upper part of the posterior wall of the inferior recess of the omental bursa.

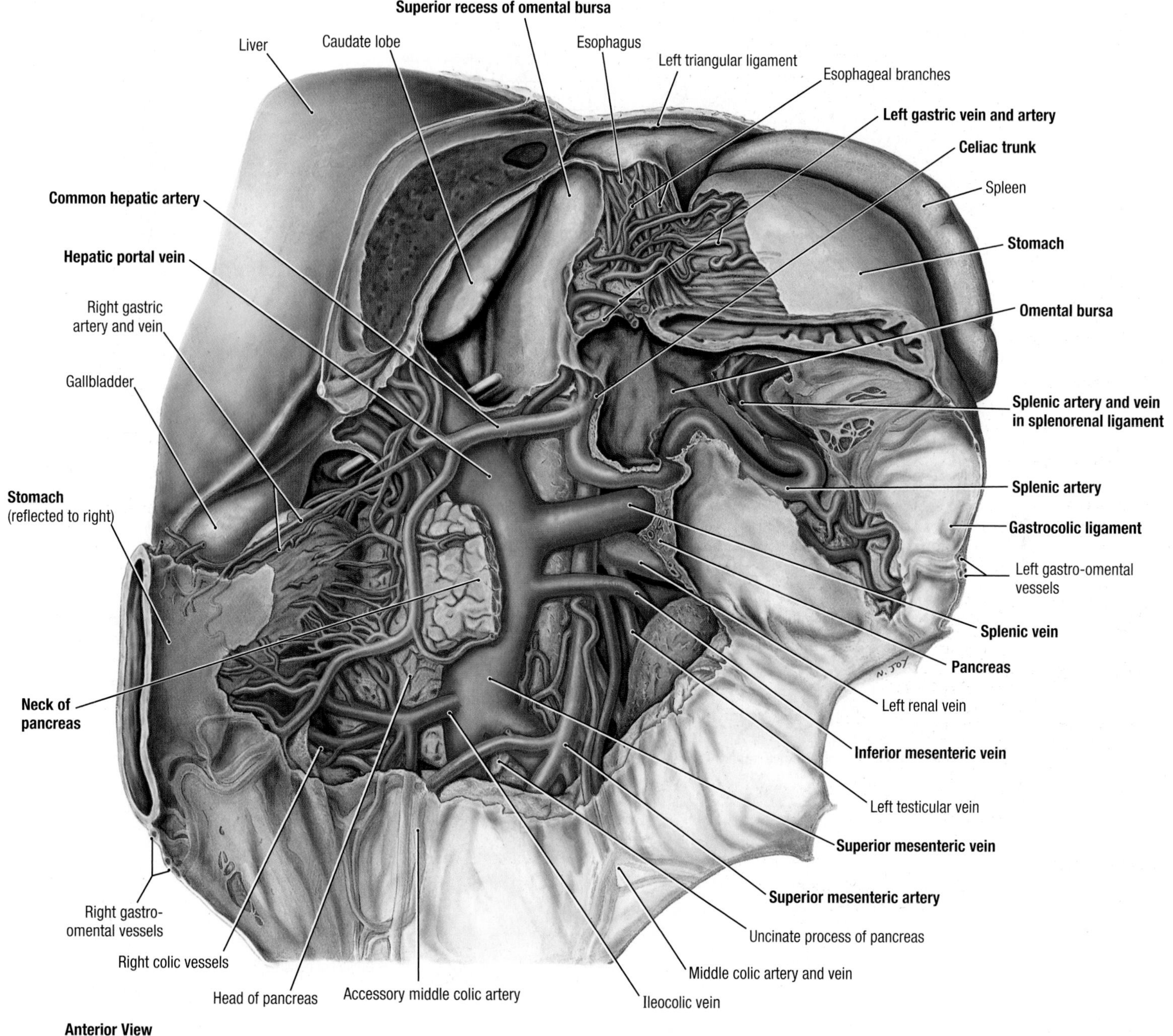
Superior recess of omental bursa
Liver
Caudate lobe
Esophagus
Left triangular ligament
Esophageal branches
Left gastric vein and artery
Celiac trunk
Spleen
Common hepatic artery
Stomach
Hepatic portal vein
Omental bursa
Right gastric artery and vein
Gallbladder
Splenic artery and vein in splenorenal ligament
Splenic artery
Stomach (reflected to right)
Gastrocolic ligament
Left gastro-omental vessels
Splenic vein
Pancreas
Neck of pancreas
Left renal vein
Inferior mesenteric vein
Left testicular vein
Superior mesenteric vein
Superior mesenteric artery
Right gastro-omental vessels
Uncinate process of pancreas
Right colic vessels
Middle colic artery and vein
Head of pancreas
Accessory middle colic artery
Ileocolic vein
Anterior View

2.30 POSTERIOR WALL OF OMENTAL BURSA

The parietal peritoneum of the posterior wall of the omental bursa has been mostly removed, and a section of the pancreas has been excised. The rod passes through the omental foramen.

- The celiac trunk gives rise to the left gastric artery, the splenic artery that runs tortuously to the left, and the common hepatic artery that runs to the right, passing anterior to the hepatic portal vein.
- The hepatic portal vein is formed posterior to the neck of the pancreas by the union of the superior mesenteric and splenic veins, with the inferior mesenteric vein joining at or near the angle of union.
- The left testicular vein usually drains into the left renal vein. Both are systemic veins.
- **Inflammation of the parietal peritoneum** can occur due to an enlarged organ or by the escape of fluid from an organ. The area becomes inflamed and causes pain over the affected region.
- **Rebound tenderness** is a pain that is elicited after pressure over the inflamed area is released.

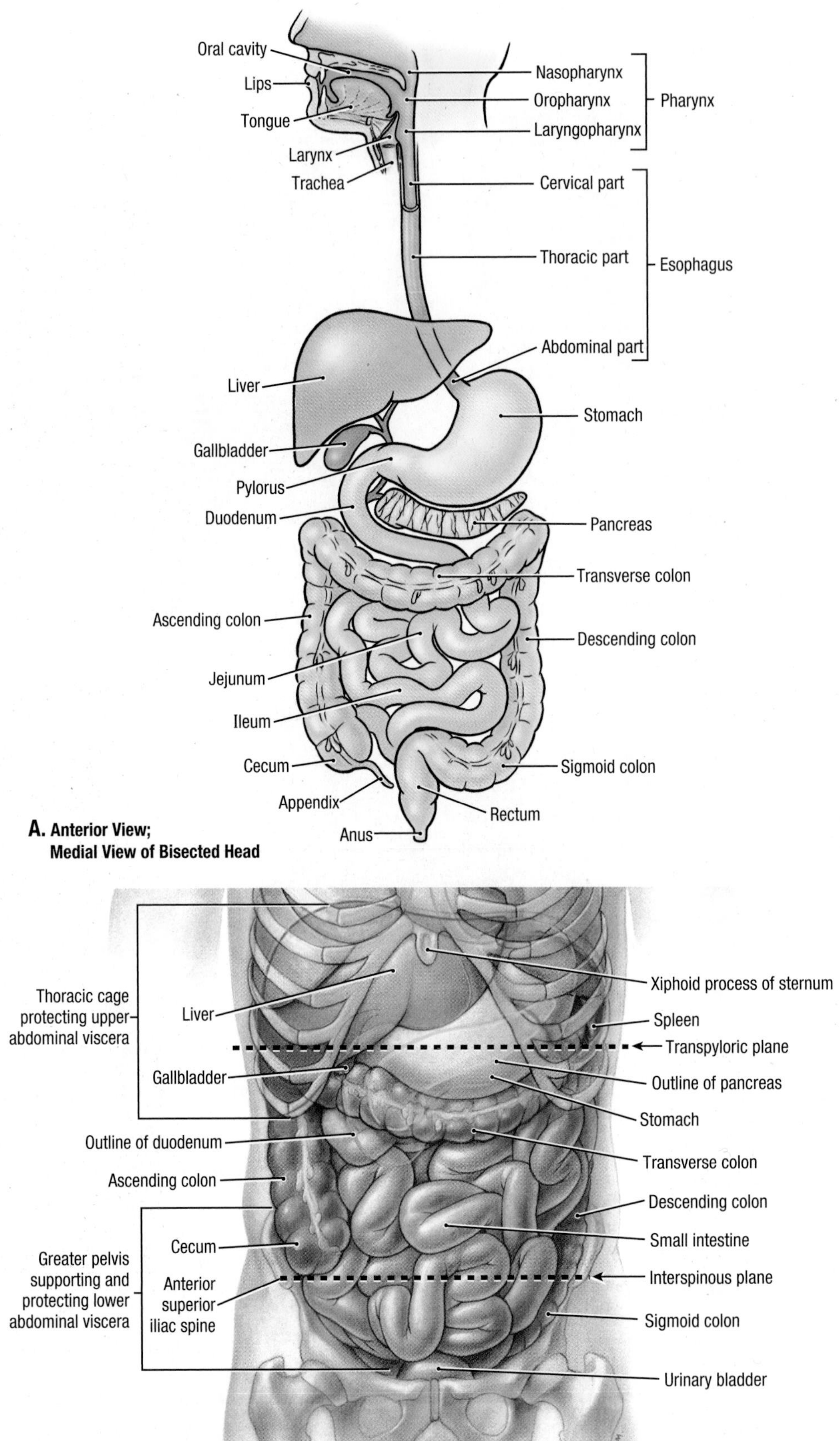
Oral cavity
Lips
Tongue
Larynx
Trachea
Nasopharynx
Oropharynx
Laryngopharynx
Pharynx
Cervical part
Thoracic part
Abdominal part
Esophagus
Liver
Gallbladder
Pylorus
Duodenum
Stomach
Pancreas
Transverse colon
Ascending colon
Descending colon
Jejunum
Ileum
Cecum
Appendix
Sigmoid colon
Rectum
Anus
A. Anterior View;
Medial View of Bisected Head
Thoracic cage protecting upper abdominal viscera
Liver
Gallbladder
Xiphoid process of sternum
Spleen
Transpyloric plane
Outline of pancreas
Stomach
Outline of duodenum
Transverse colon
Ascending colon
Descending colon
Cecum
Small intestine
Greater pelvis supporting and protecting lower abdominal viscera
Anterior superior iliac spine
Interspinous plane
Sigmoid colon
Urinary bladder
B. Anterior View

2.31 DIGESTIVE SYSTEM

A. Schematic illustration. **B.** Abdominal portion. The digestive system extends from the lips to the anus. Associated organs include the liver, gallbladder, and pancreas.

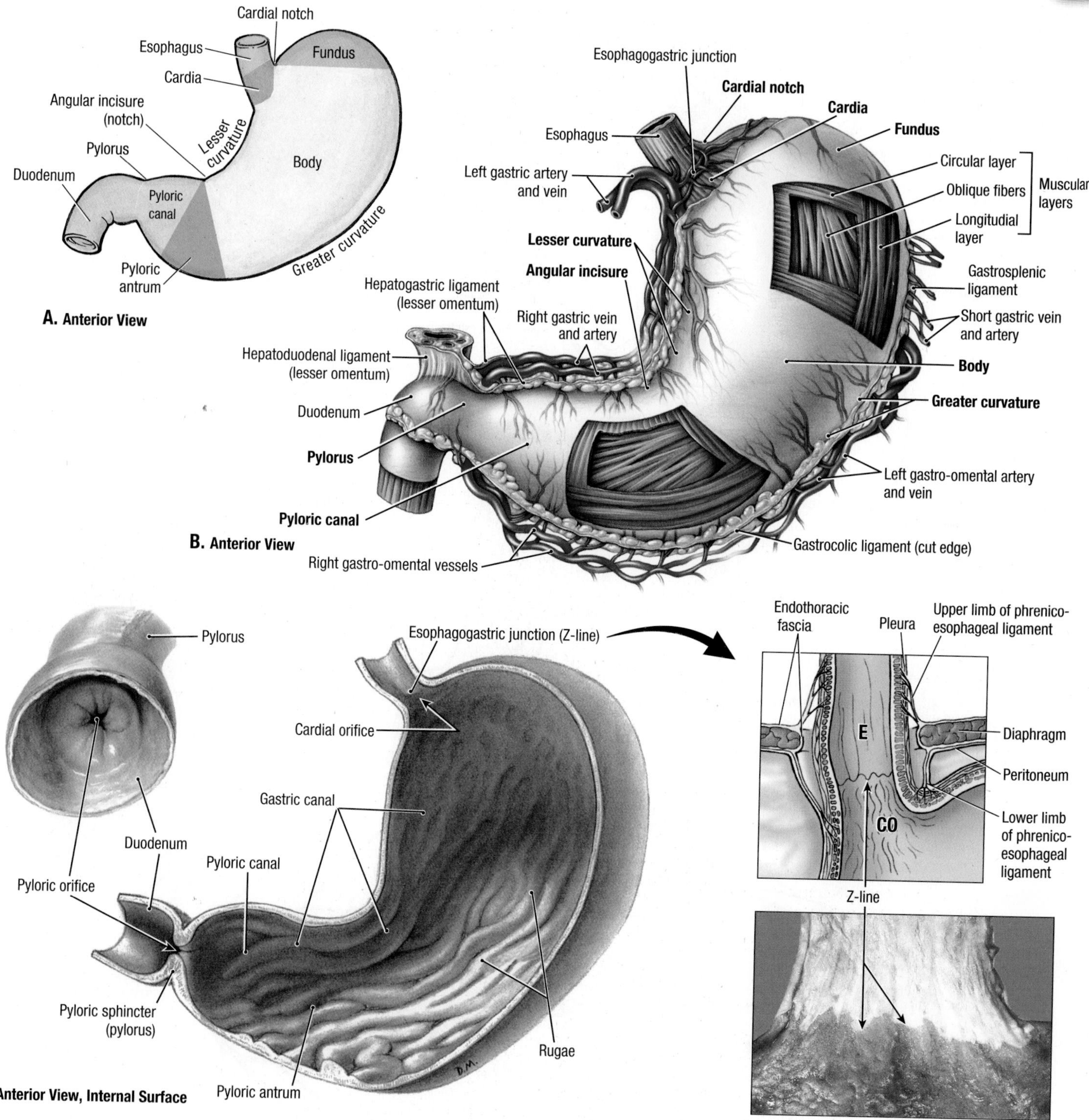
Cardial notch
Esophagus
Fundus
Cardia
Angular incisure (notch)
Lesser curvature
Pylorus
Body
Duodenum
Pyloric canal
Greater curvature
Pyloric antrum
A. Anterior View
Esophagogastric junction
Cardial notch
Cardia
Esophagus
Fundus
Left gastric artery and vein
Circular layer
Oblique fibers
Longitudial layer
Muscular layers
Lesser curvature
Angular incisure
Gastrosplenic ligament
Hepatogastric ligament (lesser omentum)
Right gastric vein and artery
Short gastric vein and artery
Hepatoduodenal ligament (lesser omentum)
Body
Duodenum
Greater curvature
Pylorus
Left gastro-omental artery and vein
Pyloric canal
B. Anterior View
Gastrocolic ligament (cut edge)
Right gastro-omental vessels
Pylorus
Esophagogastric junction (Z-line)
Endothoracic fascia
Pleura
Upper limb of phrenico-esophageal ligament
Cardial orifice
E
Diaphragm
Peritoneum
Gastric canal
CO
Lower limb of phrenico-esophageal ligament
Duodenum
Pyloric canal
Pyloric orifice
Z-line
Pyloric sphincter (pylorus)
Rugae
C. Anterior View, Internal Surface
Pyloric antrum

2.32 STOMACH

A. Parts. **B.** External surface. **C.** Internal surface (mucous membrane), anterior wall removed. Insets: Left side of page—pylorus, viewed from the duodenum. Right side of page—details of the esophagogastric junction. The Z-line is where the stratified squamous epithelium of the esophagus (white portion in photograph) to the simple columnar epithelium of the stomach (dark portion).

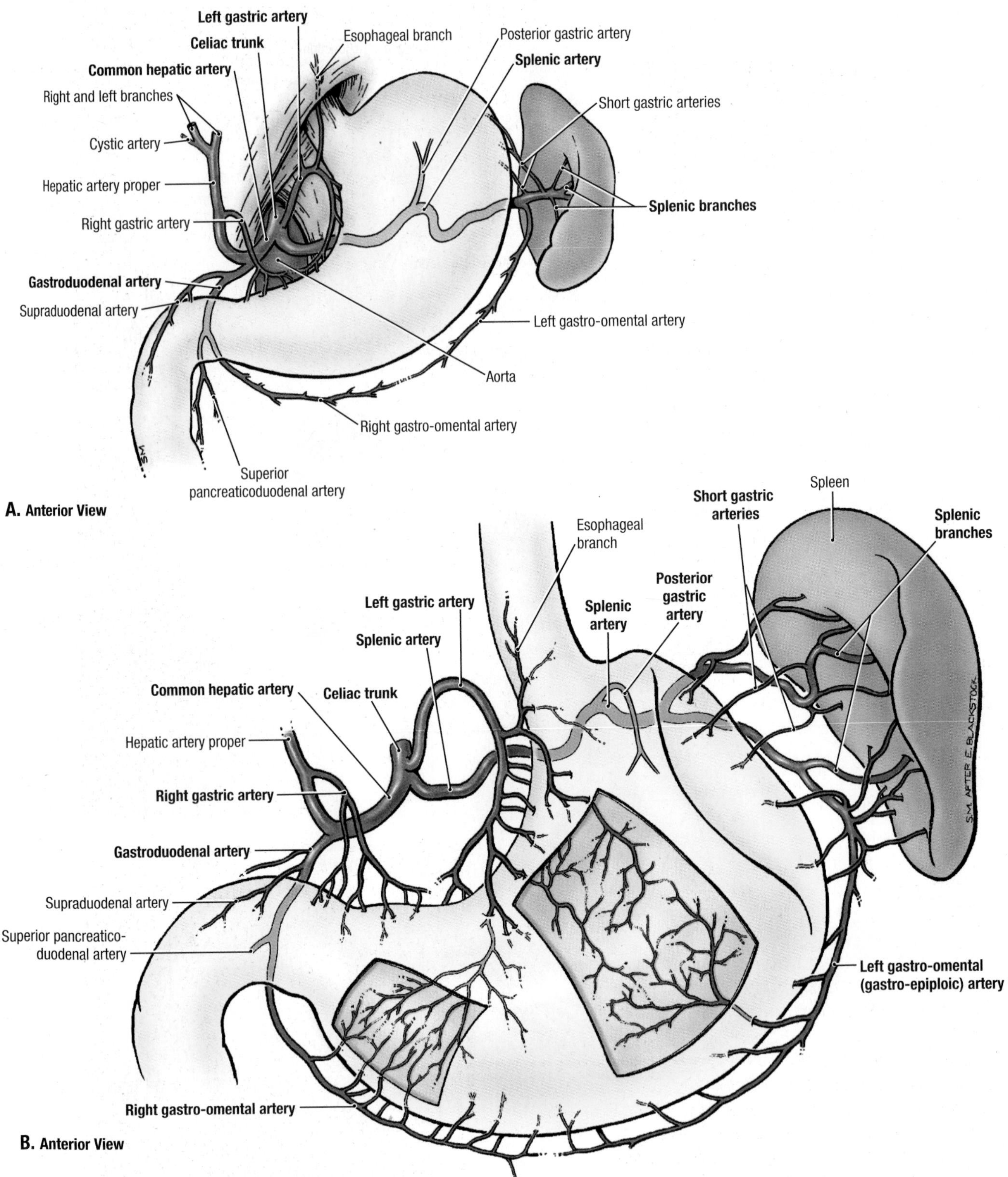

Left gastric artery
Celiac trunk
Common hepatic artery
Right and left branches
Cystic artery
Hepatic artery proper
Right gastric artery
Gastroduodenal artery
Supraduodenal artery
Esophageal branch
Posterior gastric artery
Splenic artery
Short gastric arteries
Splenic branches
Left gastro-omental artery
Aorta
Right gastro-omental artery
Superior pancreaticoduodenal artery
A. Anterior View
Spleen
Short gastric arteries
Splenic branches
Esophageal branch
Posterior gastric artery
Splenic artery
Left gastric artery
Splenic artery
Common hepatic artery
Celiac trunk
Hepatic artery proper
Right gastric artery
Gastroduodenal artery
Supraduodenal artery
Superior pancreatico-duodenal artery
Left gastro-omental (gastro-epiploic) artery
Right gastro-omental artery
B. Anterior View
S.M. AFTER E. BLACKSTOCK

2.33 CELIAC ARTERY

A. Branches of celiac trunk. The celiac trunk is a branch of the abdominal aorta, arising immediately inferior to the aortic hiatus of the diaphragm (T12 vertebral level). The vessel is usually 1 to 2 cm long and divides into the left gastric, common hepatic, and splenic arteries. The celiac trunk supplies the liver, gall bladder, inferior esophagus, stomach, pancreas, spleen, and duodenum. **B.** Arteries of stomach and spleen. The serous and muscular coats are removed from two areas of the stomach, revealing anastomotic networks in the submucous coat.

Five main sites where esophagus is constricted:

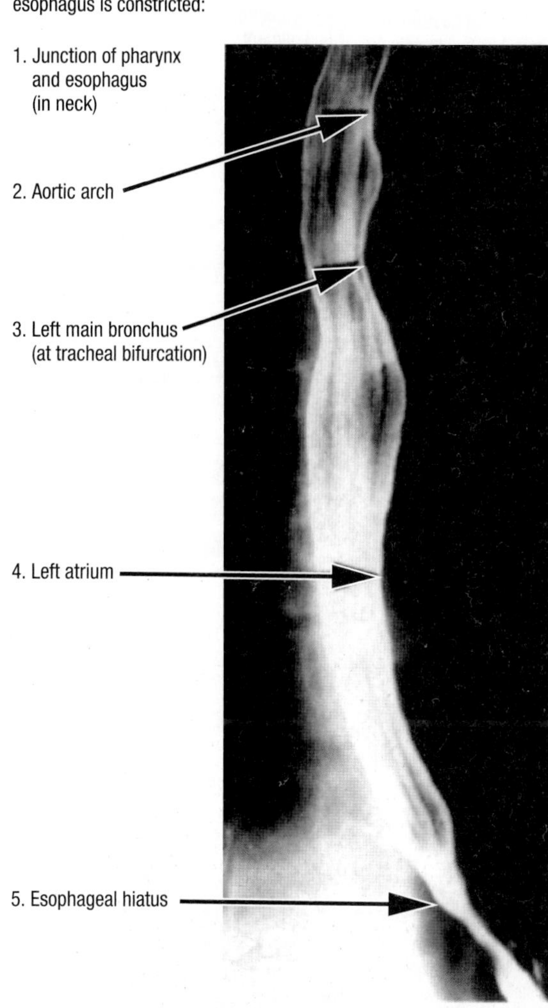
1. Junction of pharynx and esophagus (in neck)
2. Aortic arch
3. Left main bronchus (at tracheal bifurcation)
4. Left atrium
5. Esophageal hiatus

A. Lateral View

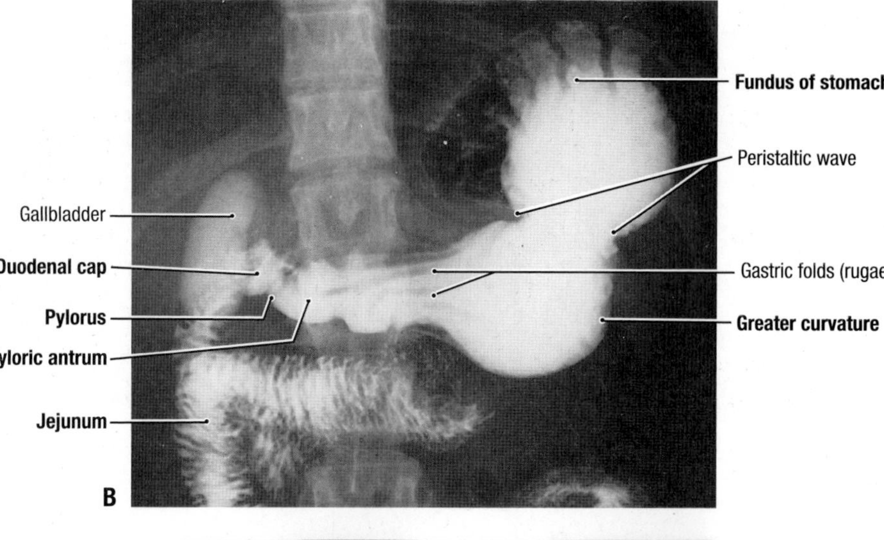
Fundus of stomach
Peristaltic wave
Gallbladder
Duodenal cap
Gastric folds (rugae)
Pylorus
Greater curvature
Pyloric antrum
Jejunum
B

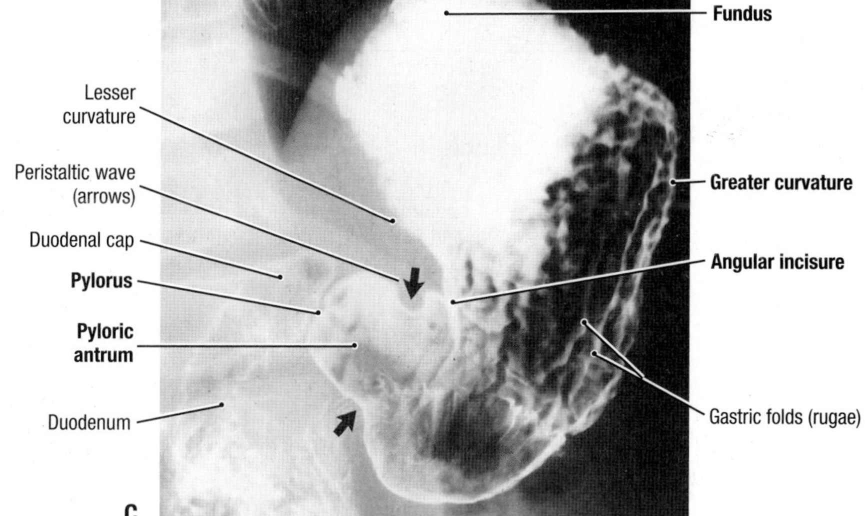
Fundus
Lesser curvature
Greater curvature
Peristaltic wave (arrows)
Duodenal cap
Angular incisure
Pylorus
Pyloric antrum
Gastric folds (rugae)
Duodenum
C

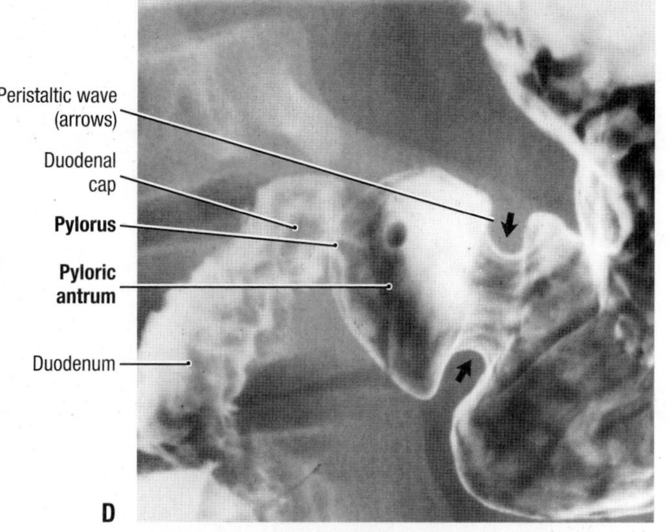
Peristaltic wave (arrows)
Duodenal cap
Pylorus
Pyloric antrum
Duodenum
D

Anterior Views (B–D)

2.34 RADIOGRAPHS OF ESOPHAGUS, STOMACH, DUODENUM (BARIUM SWALLOW)

A. Five sites of normal esophageal constriction. **B.** Stomach, small intestine, and gallbladder. Note additional contrast medium in gallbladder. **C.** Stomach and duodenum. **D.** Pyloric antrum and duodenal cap.

Blockage of esophagus. The impressions produced in the esophagus by adjacent structures are of clinical interest because of the slower passage of substances at these sites. The impressions indicate where swallowed foreign objects are most likely to lodge and where a stricture may develop, for example, after the accidental drinking of a caustic liquid, such as lye.

A **hiatal (hiatus) hernia** is a protrusion of a part of the stomach into the mediastinum through the esophageal hiatus of the diaphragm. The hernias occur most often in people after middle age, possibly because of weakening of the muscular part of the diaphragm and widening of the esophageal hiatus.

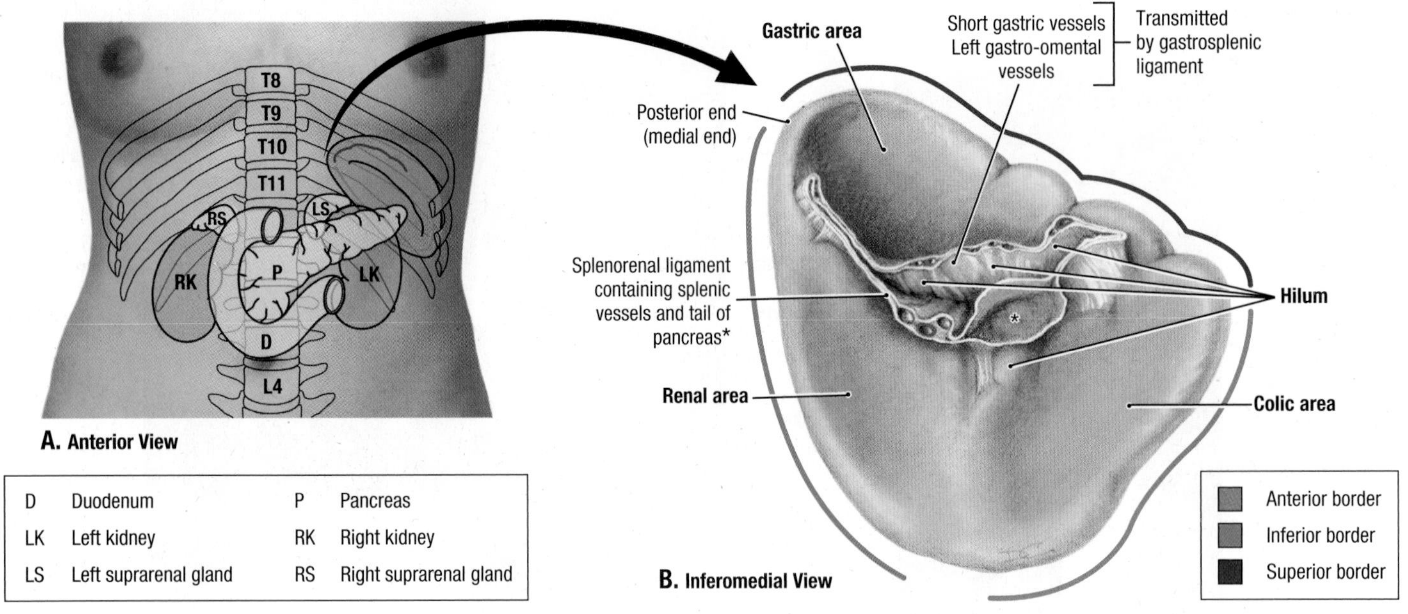

T8
T9
T10
T11
RS
LS
RK
P
LK
D
L4
A. Anterior View
D Duodenum
LK Left kidney
LS Left suprarenal gland
P Pancreas
RK Right kidney
RS Right suprarenal gland
Gastric area
Short gastric vessels
Left gastro-omental vessels
Transmitted by gastrosplenic ligament
Posterior end (medial end)
Splenorenal ligament containing splenic vessels and tail of pancreas*
Hilum
Renal area
Colic area
Anterior border
Inferior border
Superior border
B. Inferomedial View

2.35 SPLEEN

A. The surface anatomy of the spleen. The spleen lies superficially in the left upper abdominal quadrant between the 9th and 11th ribs. **B.** Note the impressions (colic, renal, and gastric areas) made by structures in contact with its visceral surface. The superior border is notched.

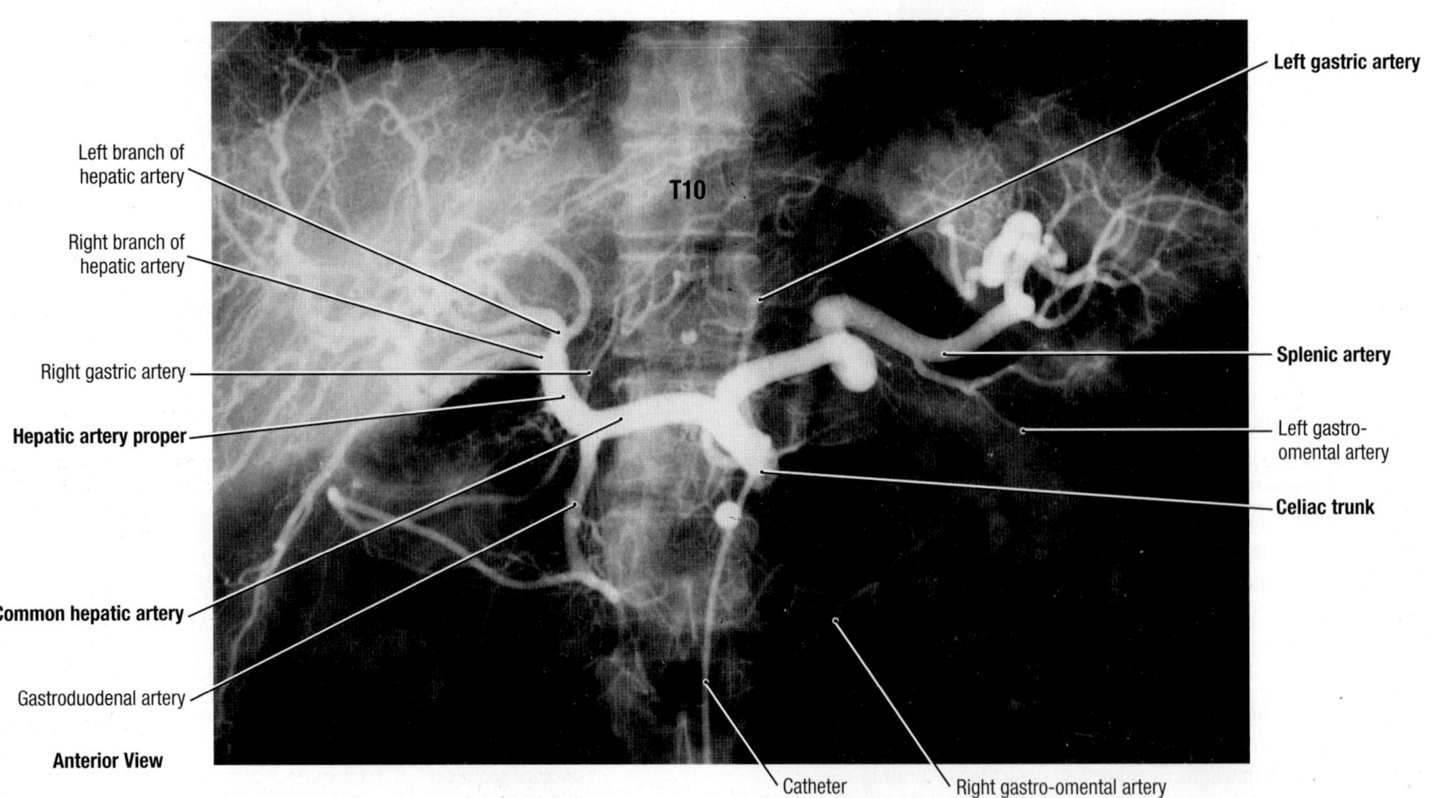

Left gastric artery
Left branch of hepatic artery
T10
Right branch of hepatic artery
Splenic artery
Right gastric artery
Hepatic artery proper
Left gastro-omental artery
Celiac trunk
Common hepatic artery
Gastroduodenal artery
Anterior View
Catheter
Right gastro-omental artery

2.36 CELIAC ARTERIOGRAM

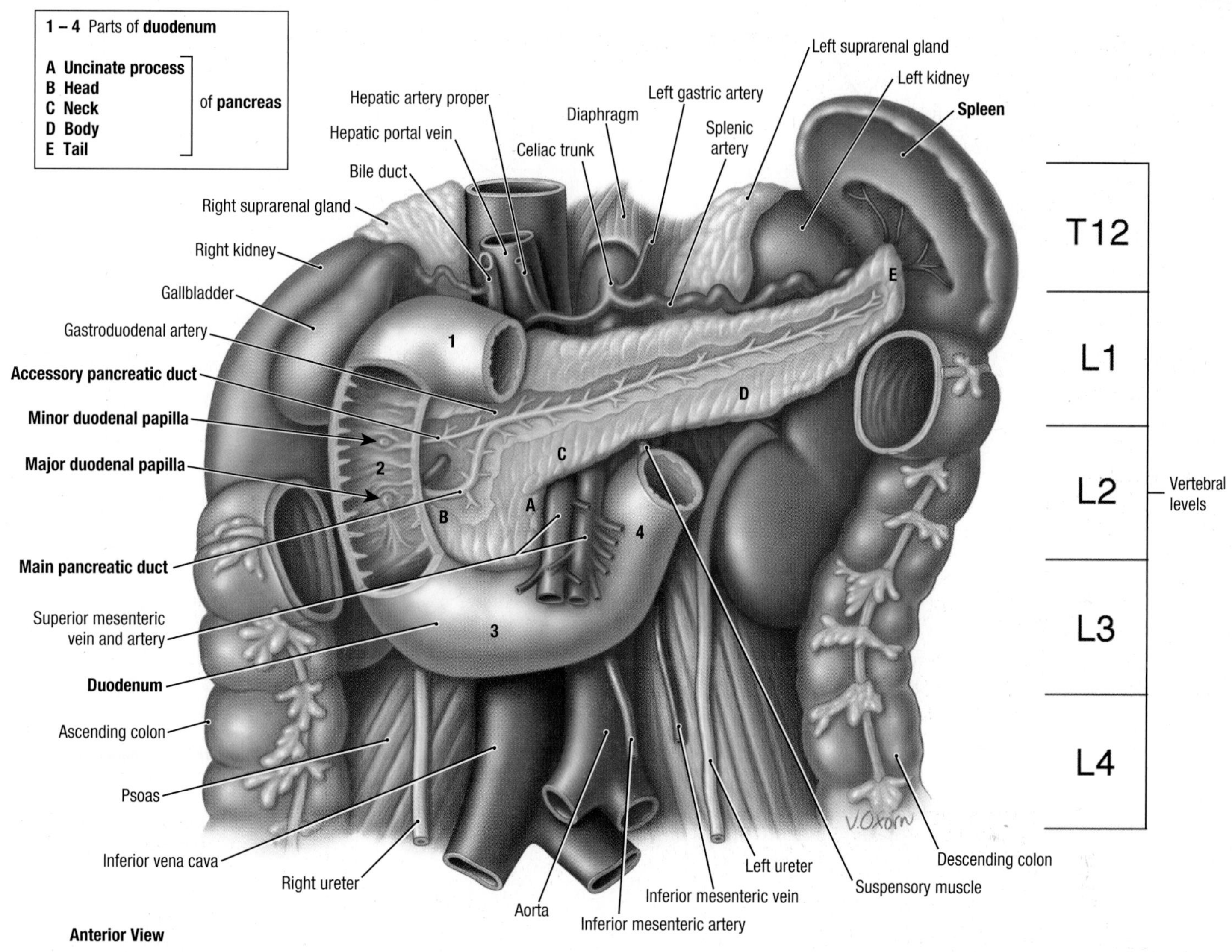
1 – 4 Parts of duodenum
A Uncinate process
B Head
C Neck
D Body
E Tail
of pancreas
Hepatic artery proper
Hepatic portal vein
Bile duct
Right suprarenal gland
Right kidney
Gallbladder
Gastroduodenal artery
Accessory pancreatic duct
Minor duodenal papilla
Major duodenal papilla
Main pancreatic duct
Superior mesenteric vein and artery
Duodenum
Ascending colon
Psoas
Inferior vena cava
Right ureter
Aorta
Inferior mesenteric artery
Inferior mesenteric vein
Left ureter
Suspensory muscle
Descending colon
Diaphragm
Celiac trunk
Left gastric artery
Splenic artery
Left suprarenal gland
Left kidney
Spleen
T12
L1
L2
L3
L4
Vertebral levels
Anterior View

2.37 PARTS AND RELATIONSHIPS OF PANCREAS AND DUODENUM

A. Pancreas and duodenum in situ.

TABLE 2.5 PARTS AND RELATIONSHIPS OF DUODENUM

Part of Duodenum	Anterior	Posterior	Medial	Superior	Inferior	Vertebral Level
Superior (**1**st part)	Peritoneum Gallbladder Quadrate lobe of liver	Bile duct Gastroduodenal artery Hepatic portal vein IVC		Neck of gallbladder	Neck of pancreas	Anterolateral to L1 vertebra
Descending (**2**nd part)	Transverse colon Transverse mesocolon Coils of small intestine	Hilum of right kidney Renal vessels Ureter Psoas major	Head of pancreas Pancreatic duct Bile duct			Right of L2–L3 vertebrae
Inferior (horizontal or **3**rd part)	Superior mesenteric artery Superior mesenteric vein Coils of small intestine	Right psoas major IVC Aorta Right ureter		Head and uncinate process of pancreas Superior mesenteric artery and vein		Anterior to L3 vertebra
Ascending (**4**th part)	Beginning of root of mesentery Coils of jejunum	Left psoas major Left margin of aorta	Superior mesenteric artery and vein	Body of pancreas		Left of L3 vertebra

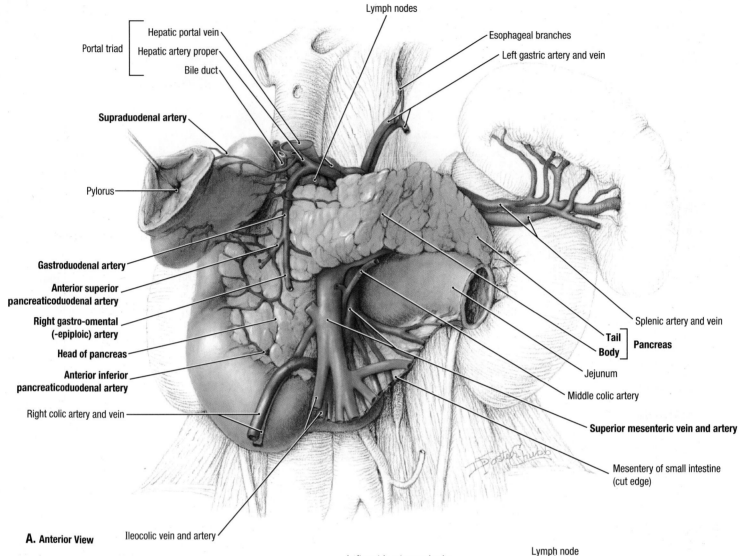

Lymph nodes
Portal triad
Hepatic portal vein
Hepatic artery proper
Bile duct
Esophageal branches
Left gastric artery and vein
Supraduodenal artery
Pylorus
Gastroduodenal artery
Anterior superior pancreaticoduodenal artery
Right gastro-omental (-epiploic) artery
Head of pancreas
Anterior inferior pancreaticoduodenal artery
Right colic artery and vein
Splenic artery and vein
Tail
Body
Pancreas
Jejunum
Middle colic artery
Superior mesenteric vein and artery
Mesentery of small intestine (cut edge)
Ileocolic vein and artery

A. **Anterior View**

2.38 PARTS AND RELATIONSHIPS OF PANCREAS AND DUODENUM (*CONTINUED*)

B. Anterior relationships. The gastroduodenal artery descends anterior to the neck of the pancreas. **C.** Posterior relationships. The splenic artery and vein course on the posterior aspect of the pancreatic tail, which usually extends to the spleen. The pancreas "loops" around the right side of the superior mesenteric vessels so that its neck is anterior, its head is to the right, and its uncinate process is posterior to the vessels. The splenic and superior mesenteric veins unite posterior to the neck to form the hepatic portal vein. The bile duct descends in a fissure (opened up) in the posterior part of the head of the pancreas. Most inflammatory erosions of the duodenal wall, **duodenal (peptic) ulcers**, are in the posterior wall of the superior (1st) part of the duodenum within 3 cm of the pylorus.

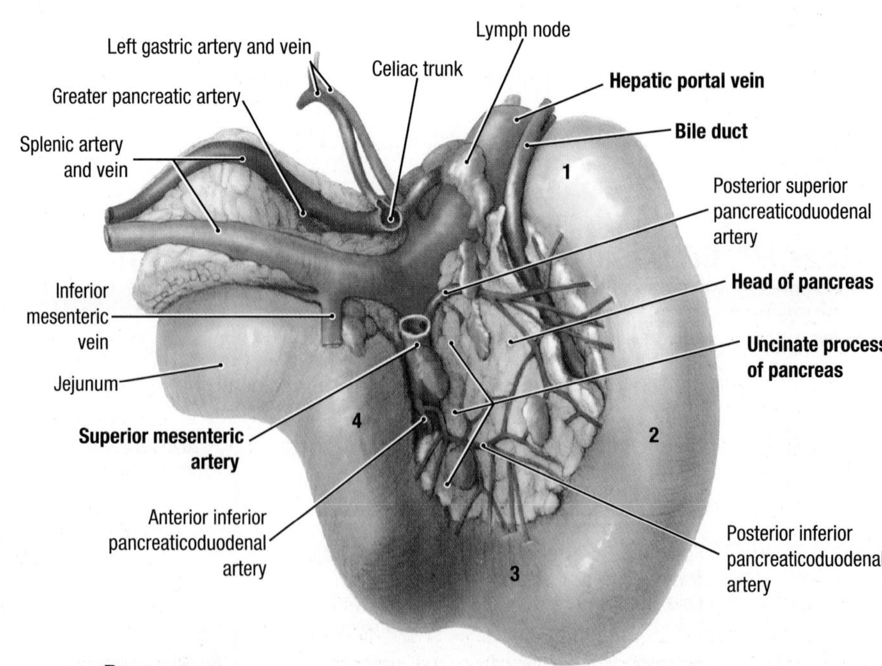
Left gastric artery and vein
Lymph node
Celiac trunk
Greater pancreatic artery
Hepatic portal vein
Bile duct
Splenic artery and vein
1
Posterior superior pancreaticoduodenal artery
Head of pancreas
Inferior mesenteric vein
Uncinate process of pancreas
Jejunum
4
Superior mesenteric artery
2
Anterior inferior pancreaticoduodenal artery
Posterior inferior pancreaticoduodenal artery
3

B. **Posterior View**

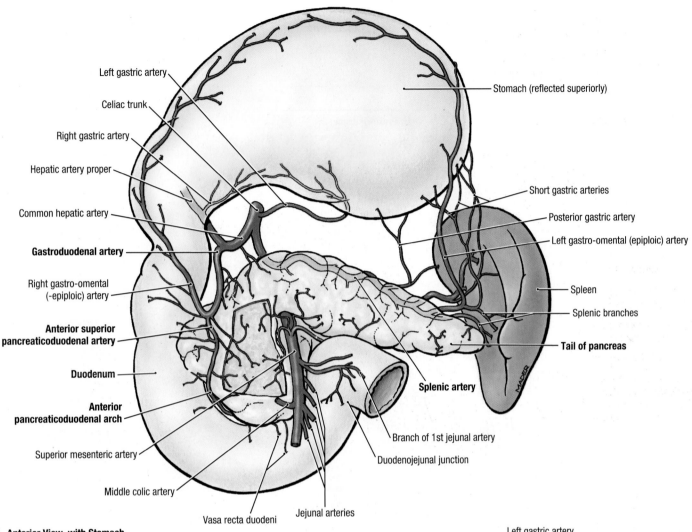

Left gastric artery
Celiac trunk
Right gastric artery
Hepatic artery proper
Common hepatic artery
Gastroduodenal artery
Right gastro-omental (-epiploic) artery
Anterior superior pancreaticoduodenal artery
Duodenum
Anterior pancreaticoduodenal arch
Superior mesenteric artery
Middle colic artery
Vasa recta duodeni
Jejunal arteries
Duodenojejunal junction
Branch of 1st jejunal artery
Splenic artery
Tail of pancreas
Splenic branches
Spleen
Left gastro-omental (epiploic) artery
Posterior gastric artery
Short gastric arteries
Stomach (reflected superiorly)
MADER

A. Anterior View, with Stomach Reflected Superiorly

2.39 BLOOD SUPPLY TO THE PANCREAS, DUODENUM, AND SPLEEN

A. Celiac trunk and superior mesenteric artery. **B.** Pancreatic and pancreaticoduodenal arteries.

- The anterior superior pancreaticoduodenal artery from the gastroduodenal artery and the anterior inferior pancreaticoduodenal artery of the superior mesenteric artery form the anterior pancreaticoduodenal arch anterior to the head of the pancreas. The posterior superior and posterior inferior branches of the same two arteries form the posterior pancreaticoduodenal arch posterior to the pancreas. The anterior and posterior inferior arteries often arise from a common stem.
- Arteries supplying the pancreas are derived from the common hepatic artery, gastroduodenal artery, pancreaticoduodenal arches, splenic artery, and superior mesenteric artery.

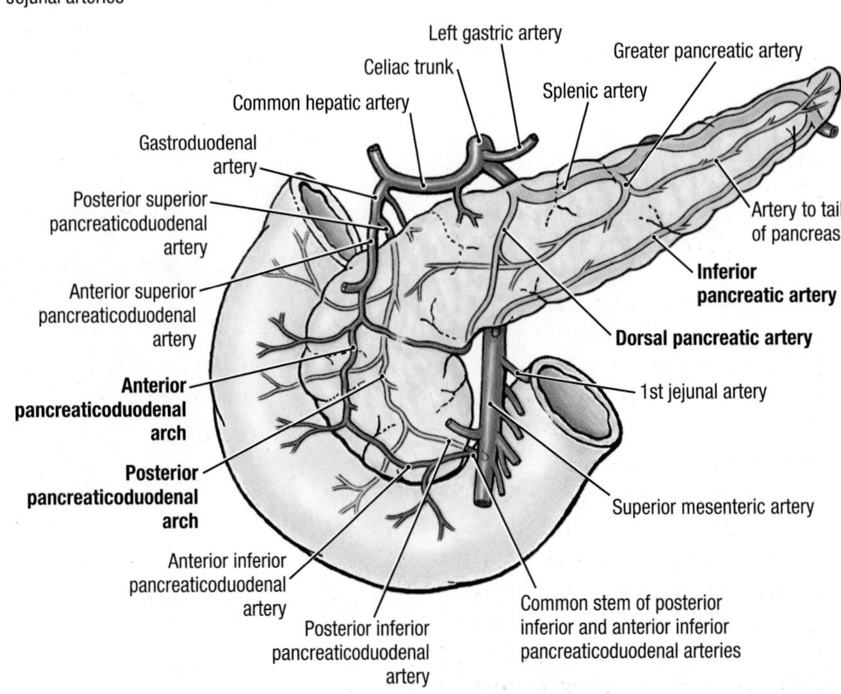
Left gastric artery
Celiac trunk
Greater pancreatic artery
Splenic artery
Common hepatic artery
Gastroduodenal artery
Posterior superior pancreaticoduodenal artery
Anterior superior pancreaticoduodenal artery
Artery to tail of pancreas
Inferior pancreatic artery
Dorsal pancreatic artery
1st jejunal artery
Anterior pancreaticoduodenal arch
Posterior pancreaticoduodenal arch
Superior mesenteric artery
Anterior inferior pancreaticoduodenal artery
Posterior inferior pancreaticoduodenal artery
Common stem of posterior inferior and anterior inferior pancreaticoduodenal arteries

B. Anterior View

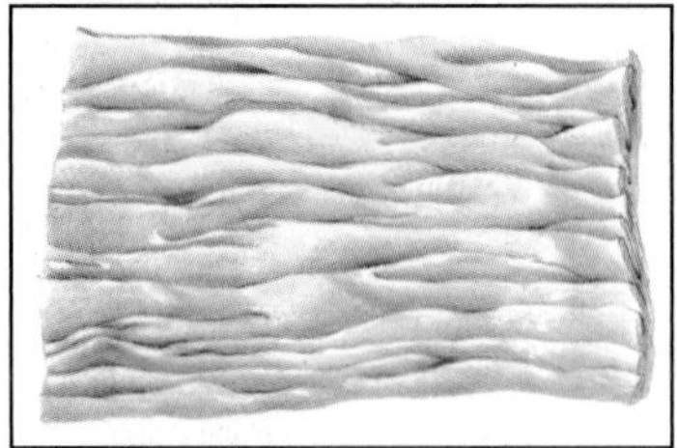

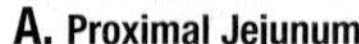

A. Proximal Jejunum

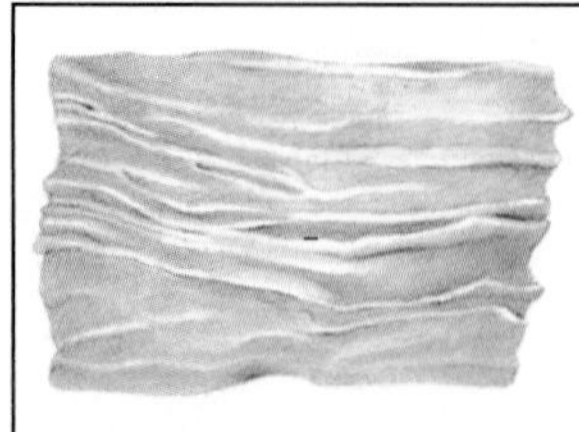

B. Proximal Ileum

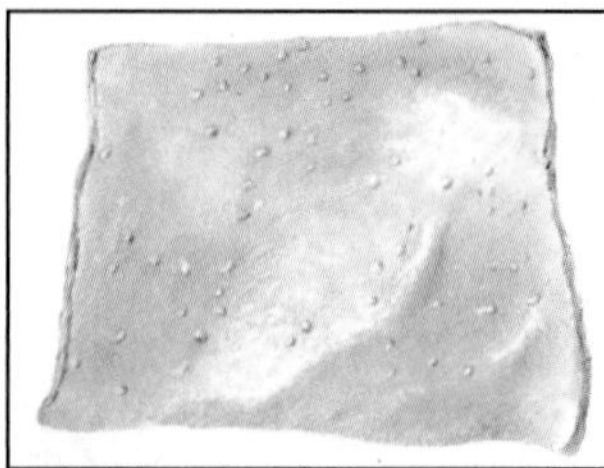

C. Distal Ileum

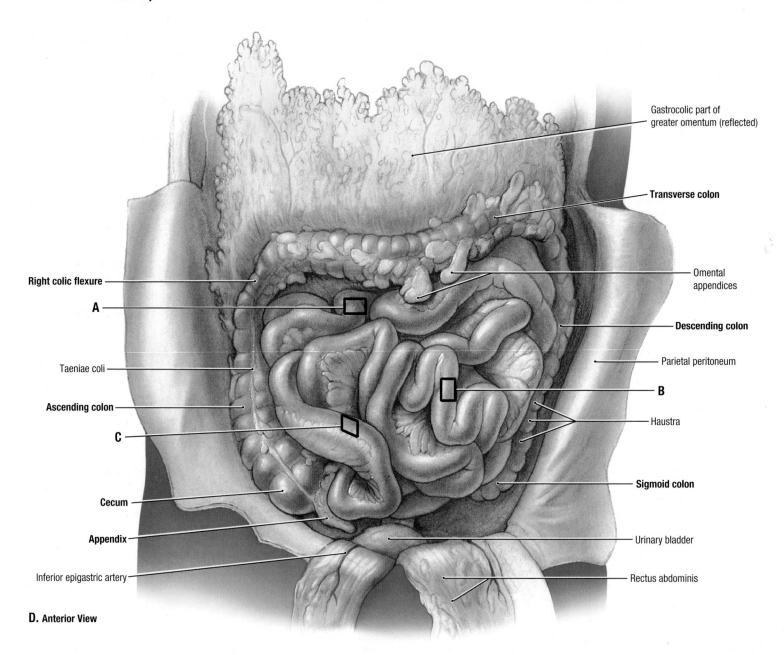

Gastrocolic part of greater omentum (reflected)
Transverse colon
Right colic flexure
Omental appendices
A
Descending colon
Taeniae coli
Parietal peritoneum
B
Ascending colon
Haustra
C
Sigmoid colon
Cecum
Appendix
Urinary bladder
Inferior epigastric artery
Rectus abdominis

D. Anterior View

2.40 INTESTINES IN SITU, INTERIOR OF SMALL INTESTINE

A. Proximal jejunum. The circular folds are tall, closely packed, and commonly branched. **B.** Proximal ileum. The circular folds are low and becoming sparse. The caliber of the gut is reduced, and the wall is thinner. **C.** Distal ileum. Circular folds are absent, and solitary lymph nodules stud the wall.

D. Intestines in situ, greater omentum reflected. The ileum is reflected to expose the appendix. The appendix usually lies posterior to the cecum (retrocecal) or, as in this case, projects over the pelvic brim. The features of the large intestines are the taeniae coli, haustra, and omental appendices.

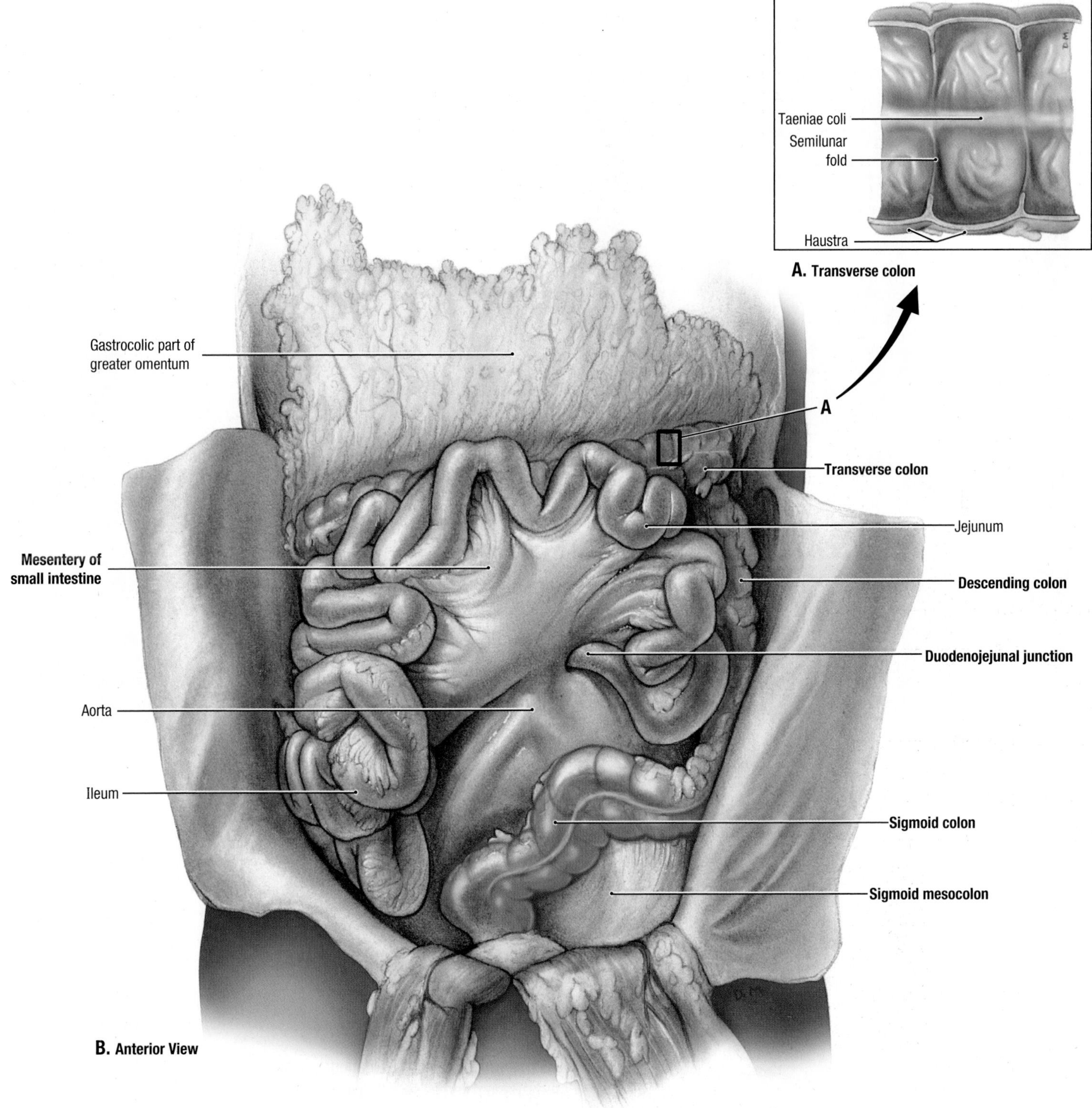
Taeniae coli
Semilunar fold
Haustra
A. Transverse colon
Gastrocolic part of greater omentum
A
Transverse colon
Jejunum
Mesentery of small intestine
Descending colon
Duodenojejunal junction
Aorta
Ileum
Sigmoid colon
Sigmoid mesocolon
B. Anterior View

2.41 SIGMOID MESOCOLON AND MESENTERY OF SMALL INTESTINE, INTERIOR OF TRANSVERSE COLON

A. Transverse colon. The semilunar folds and taeniae coli form prominent features on the smooth-surfaced wall. **B.** Sigmoid mesocolon and mesentery of the small intestine.

- The duodenojejunal junction is situated to the left of the median plane.
- The mesentery of the small intestine fans out extensively from its short root to accommodate the length of jejunum and ileum (~6 m).
- The descending colon is the narrowest part of the large intestine and is retroperitoneal. The sigmoid colon has a mesentery, the sigmoid mesocolon; the sigmoid colon is continuous with the rectum at the point at which the sigmoid mesocolon ends.

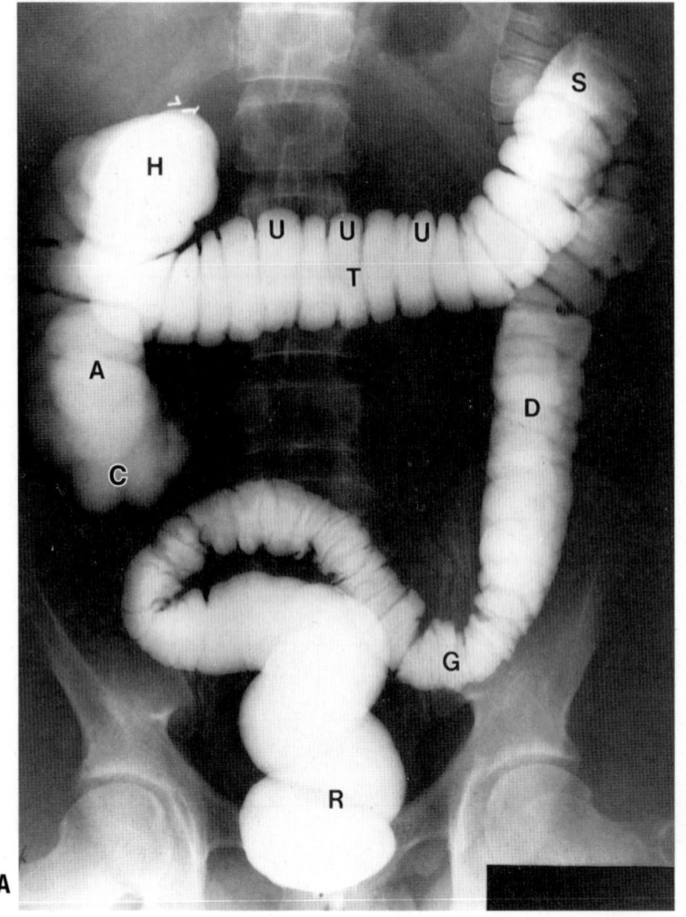
S
H
U
U
U
T
A
D
C
G
R

A

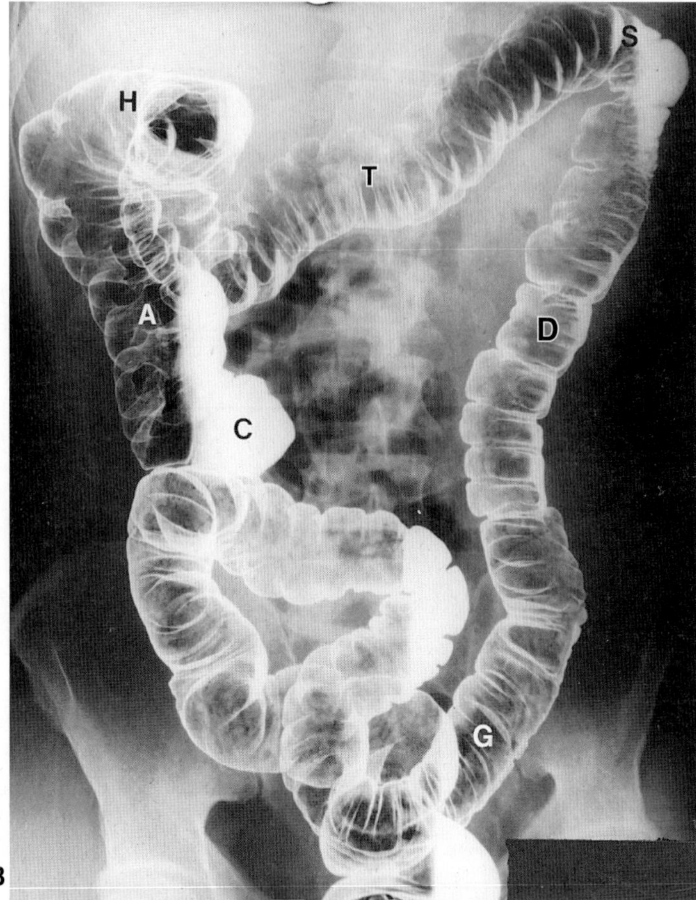
S
H
T
A
D
C
G

B

Postero-anterior Radiographs

A	Ascending colon	G	Sigmoid colon	S	Splenic flexure
C	Cecum	H	Hepatic flexure	T	Transverse colon
D	Descending colon	R	Rectum	U	Haustra

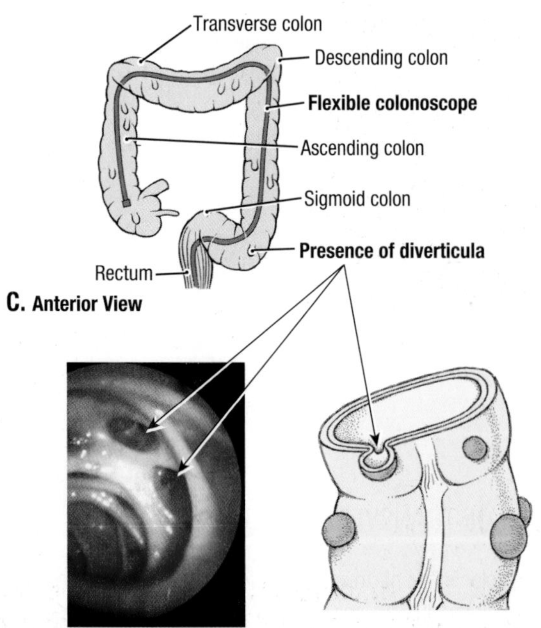
Transverse colon
Descending colon
Flexible colonoscope
Ascending colon
Sigmoid colon
Presence of diverticula
Rectum

C. Anterior View

D. Colonoscopic View

E. Diverticulosis

2.42 BARIUM ENEMA AND COLONOSCOPY OF COLON

A. Single-contrast study. A barium enema has filled the colon. **B. Double-contrast study.** Barium can be seen coating the walls of the colon, which is distended with air, providing a vivid view of the mucosal relief and haustra. C. The interior of the colon can be observed with an elongated endoscope, usually a fiberoptic **flexible colonoscope.** The endoscope is a tube that inserts into the colon through the anus and rectum. **D. Diverticulosis of the colon** can be photographed through a colonoscope. **E. Diverticulosis** is a disorder in which multiple false diverticula (external evaginations or outpocketings of the mucosa of the colon) develop along the intestine. It primarily affects middle-aged and elderly people. Diverticulosis is commonly (60%) found in the sigmoid colon. Diverticula are subject to infection and rupture, leading to **diverticulitis,** and they can distort and erode the nutrient arteries, leading to hemorrhage.

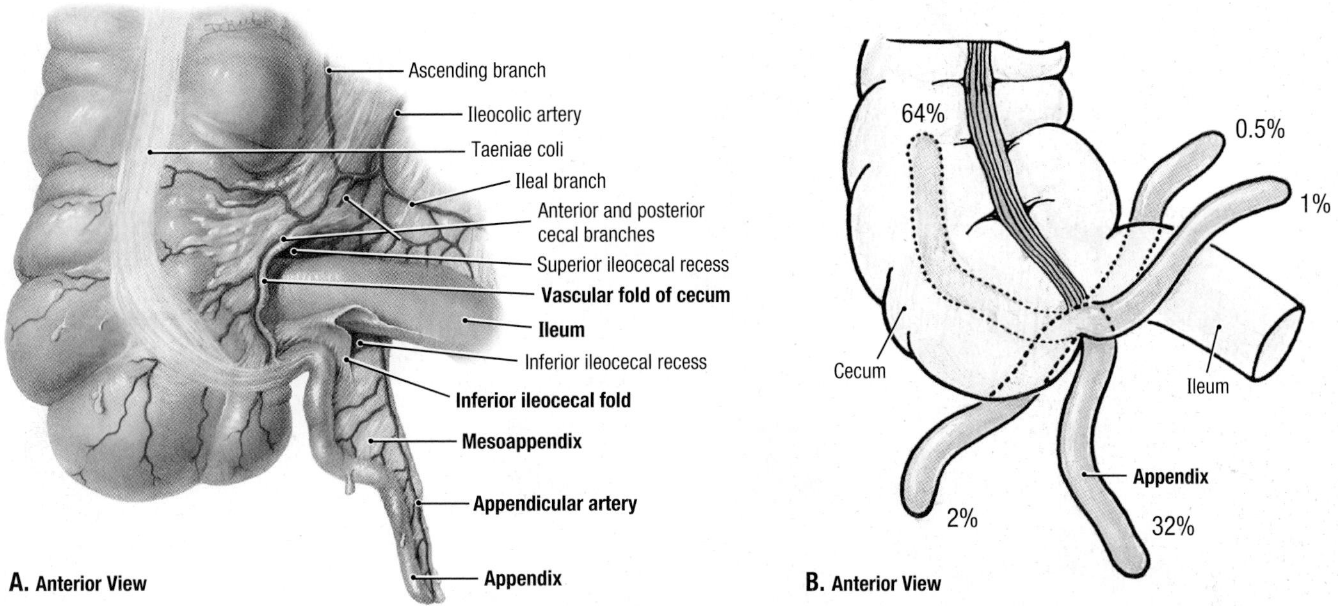
Ascending branch
Ileocolic artery
Taeniae coli
Ileal branch
Anterior and posterior cecal branches
Superior ileocecal recess
Vascular fold of cecum
Ileum
Inferior ileocecal recess
Inferior ileocecal fold
Mesoappendix
Appendicular artery
Appendix
A. Anterior View
64%
0.5%
1%
Cecum
Ileum
Appendix
2%
32%
B. Anterior View

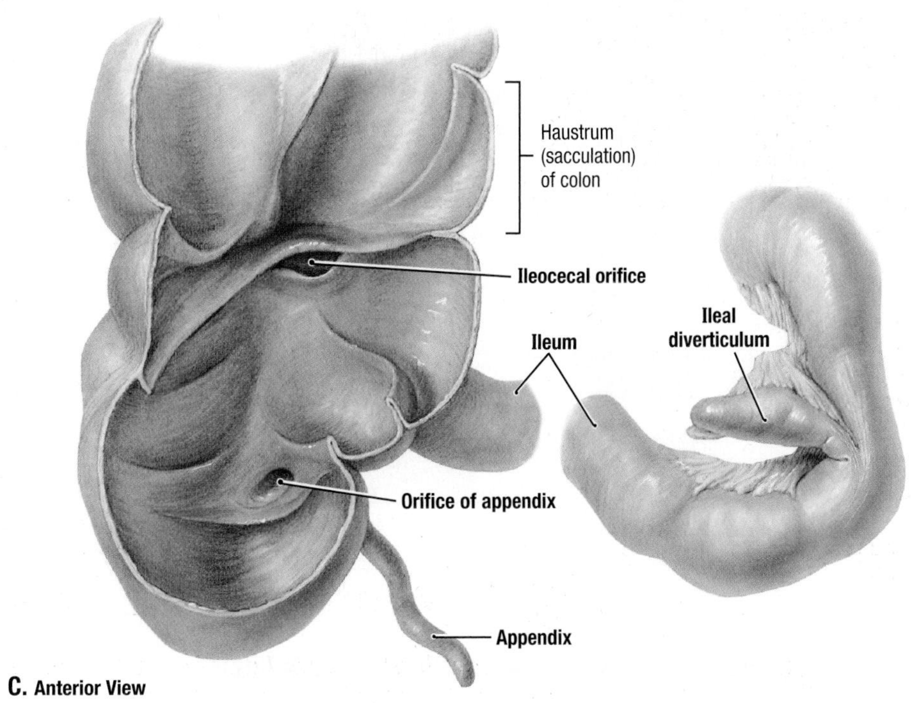
Haustrum (sacculation) of colon
Ileocecal orifice
Ileum
Ileal diverticulum
Orifice of appendix
Appendix
C. Anterior View

2.43 ILEOCECAL REGION AND APPENDIX

A. Blood supply. The appendicular artery is located in the free edge of the mesoappendix. The inferior ileocecal fold is bloodless, whereas the superior ileocecal fold is called the vascular fold of the cecum. **B.** The approximate incidence of various positions of the appendix. **C.** Interior of a dried cecum and ileal diverticulum (of Meckel). This cecum was filled with air until dry, opened, and varnished. **Ileal diverticulum** is a congenital anomaly that occurs in 1% to 2% of persons. It is a pouchlike remnant (3 to 6 cm long) of the proximal part of the yolk stalk, typically within 50 cm of the ileocecal junction. It sometimes becomes inflamed and produces pain that may mimic that produced by appendicitis.

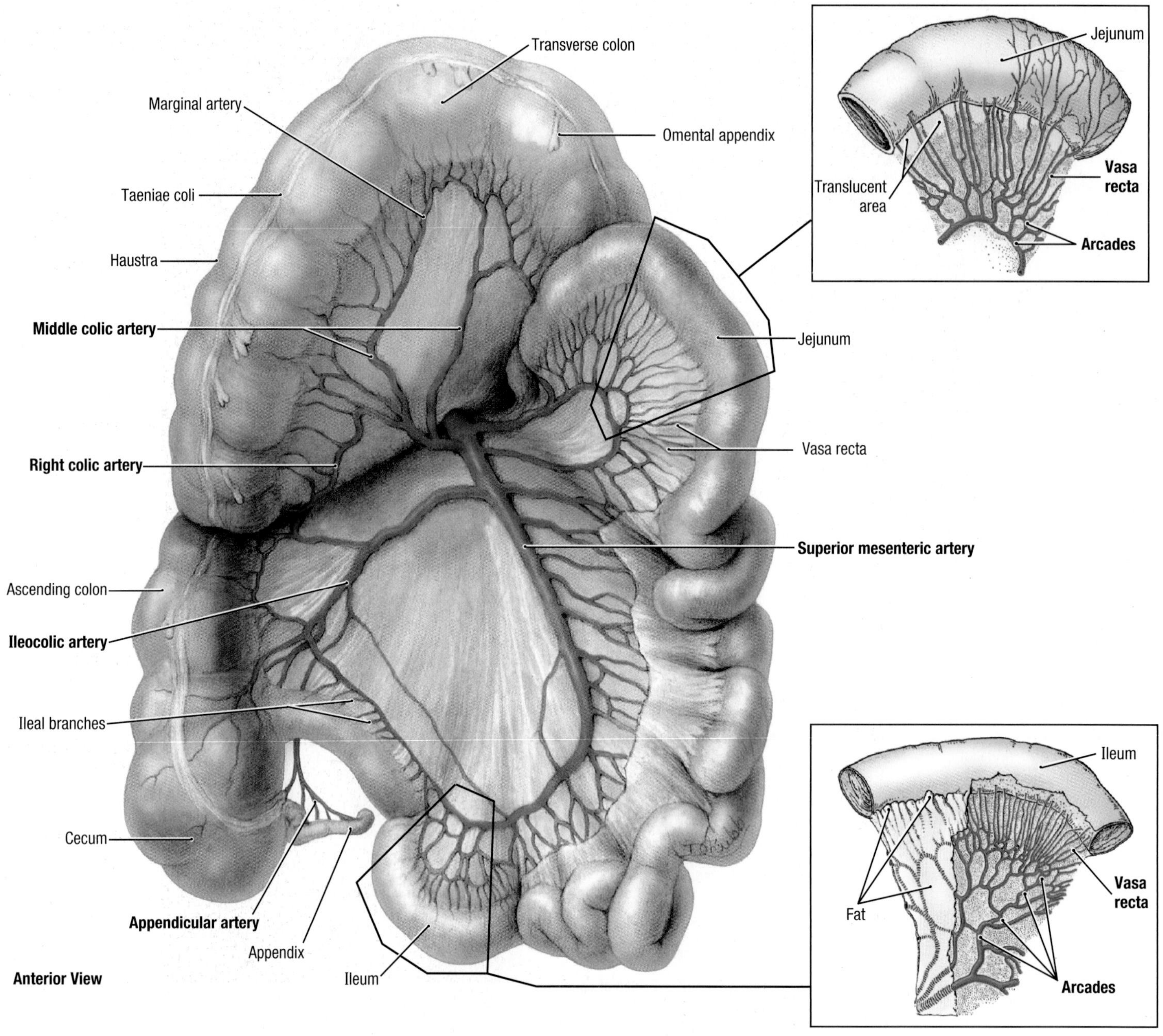

Transverse colon
Marginal artery
Omental appendix
Taeniae coli
Haustra
Middle colic artery
Jejunum
Vasa recta
Right colic artery
Superior mesenteric artery
Ascending colon
Ileocolic artery
Ileal branches
Cecum
Appendicular artery
Appendix
Ileum
Anterior View
Jejunum
Translucent area
Vasa recta
Arcades
Ileum
Fat
Vasa recta
Arcades

2.44 SUPERIOR MESENTERIC ARTERY AND ARTERIAL ARCADES

The peritoneum is partially stripped off.

- The superior mesenteric artery ends by anastomosing with one of its own branches, the ileal branch of the ileocolic artery.
- On the inset drawings of jejunum and ileum compare the diameter, thickness of wall, number of arterial arcades, long or short vasa recta, presence of translucent (fat-free) areas at the mesenteric border, and fat encroaching on the wall of the gut between the jejunum and ileum.
- **Acute inflammation of the appendix** is a common cause of an acute abdomen (severe abdominal pain arising suddenly). The pain of appendicitis usually commences as a vague pain in the periumbilical region because afferent pain fibers enter the spinal cord at the T10 level. Later, severe pain in the right lower quadrant results from irritation of the parietal peritoneum lining the posterior abdominal wall.

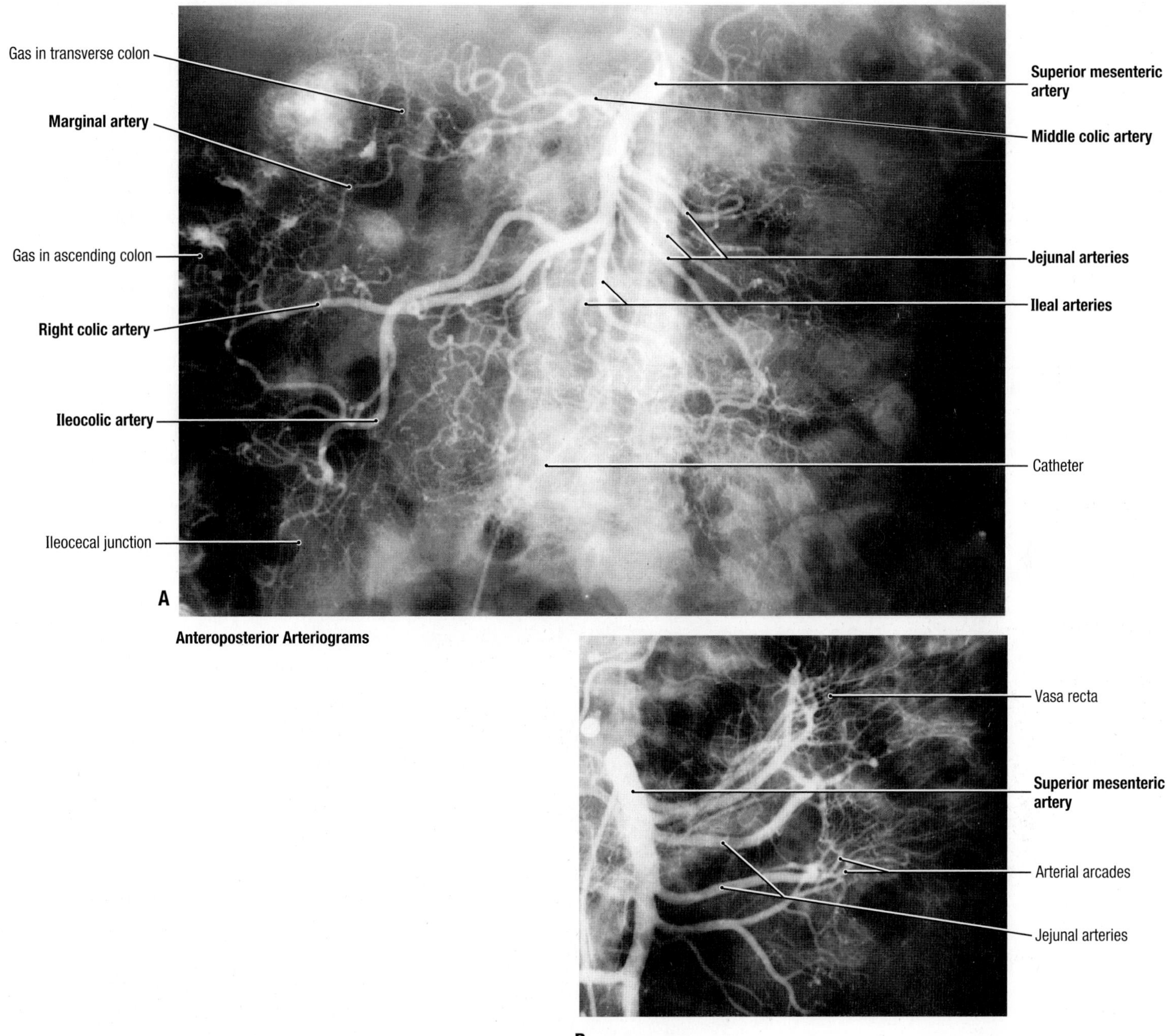
Gas in transverse colon
Marginal artery
Gas in ascending colon
Right colic artery
Ileocolic artery
Ileocecal junction
A
Superior mesenteric artery
Middle colic artery
Jejunal arteries
Ileal arteries
Catheter
Anteroposterior Arteriograms
Vasa recta
Superior mesenteric artery
Arterial arcades
Jejunal arteries
B

2.45 SUPERIOR MESENTERIC ARTERIOGRAMS

A. Branches of superior mesenteric artery. Consult Figure 2.44 to identify the branches. **B.** Enlargement to show the jejunal arteries, arterial arcades, and vasa recta.

- The branches of the superior mesenteric artery include, from its left side, 12 or more jejunal and ileal arteries that anastomose to form arcades from which vasa recta pass to the small intestine and, from its right side, the middle colic, ileocolic, and commonly (but not here) an independent right colic artery that anastomose to form a marginal artery that parallels the mesenteric border at the colon and from which vasa recta pass to the large intestine. **Occlusion of the vasa recta** by emboli results in ischemia of the part of the intestine concerned. If the ischemia is severe, necrosis of the involved segment results and **ileus** (obstruction of the intestine) of the paralytic type occurs. Ileus is accompanied by a severe colicky pain, along with abdominal distension, vomiting, and often fever and dehydration. If the condition is diagnosed early (e.g., using a superior mesenteric arteriogram), the obstructed part of the vessel may be cleared surgically.

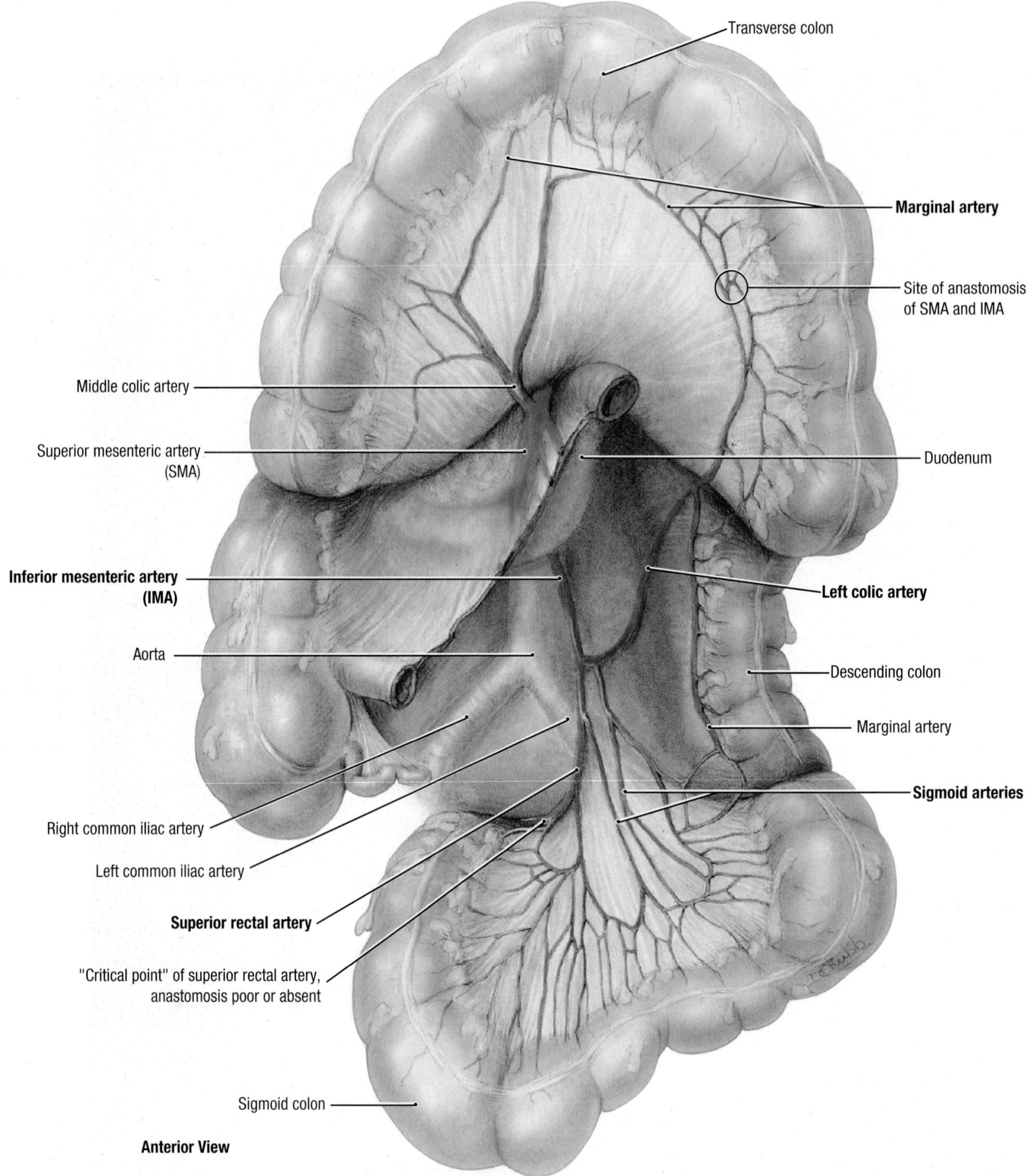

Transverse colon
Marginal artery
Site of anastomosis of SMA and IMA
Middle colic artery
Superior mesenteric artery (SMA)
Duodenum
Inferior mesenteric artery (IMA)
Left colic artery
Aorta
Descending colon
Marginal artery
Sigmoid arteries
Right common iliac artery
Left common iliac artery
Superior rectal artery
"Critical point" of superior rectal artery, anastomosis poor or absent
Sigmoid colon
Anterior View

2.46 INFERIOR MESENTERIC ARTERY

The mesentery of the small intestine has been cut at its root.

- The inferior mesenteric artery arises posterior to the ascending part of the duodenum, about 4 cm superior to the bifurcation of the aorta; on crossing the left common iliac artery, it becomes the superior rectal artery.
- The branches of the inferior mesenteric artery include the left colic artery and several sigmoid arteries; the inferior two sigmoid arteries branch from the superior rectal artery.
- The point at which the last artery to the colon branches from the superior rectal artery is known as the "critical point" of the superior rectal artery; distal to this point, there are poor or no anastomotic connections with the superior rectal artery.

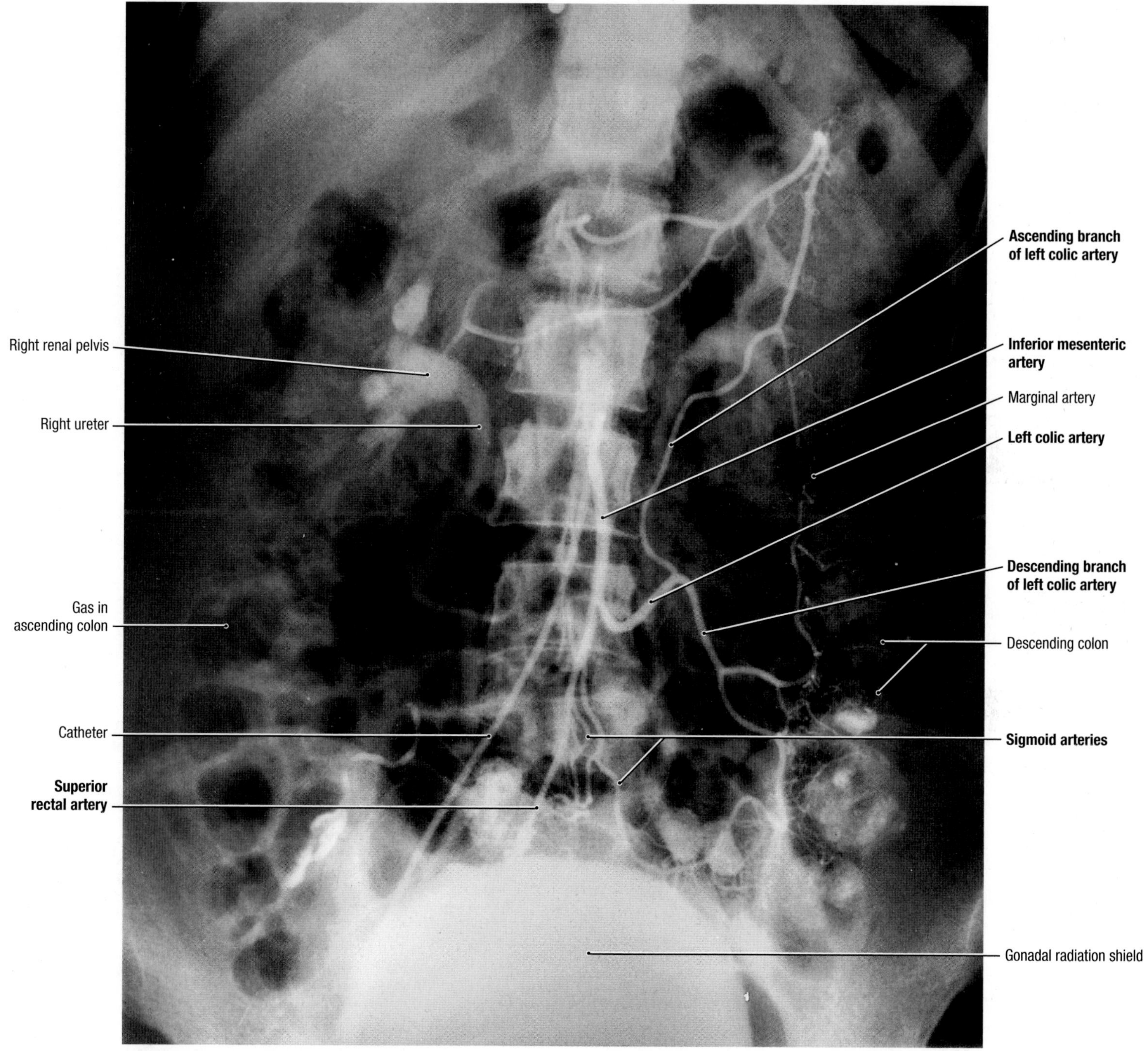
Right renal pelvis
Right ureter
Gas in ascending colon
Catheter
Superior rectal artery
Ascending branch of left colic artery
Inferior mesenteric artery
Marginal artery
Left colic artery
Descending branch of left colic artery
Descending colon
Sigmoid arteries
Gonadal radiation shield

Postero-anterior Arteriogram

2.47 INFERIOR MESENTERIC ARTERIOGRAM

- The left colic artery courses to the left toward the descending colon and splits into ascending and descending branches.
- The sigmoid arteries, two to four in number, supply the sigmoid colon.
- The superior rectal artery, which is the continuation of the inferior mesenteric artery, supplies the rectum; the superior rectal anastomoses are formed by branches of the middle and inferior rectal arteries (from the internal iliac artery).

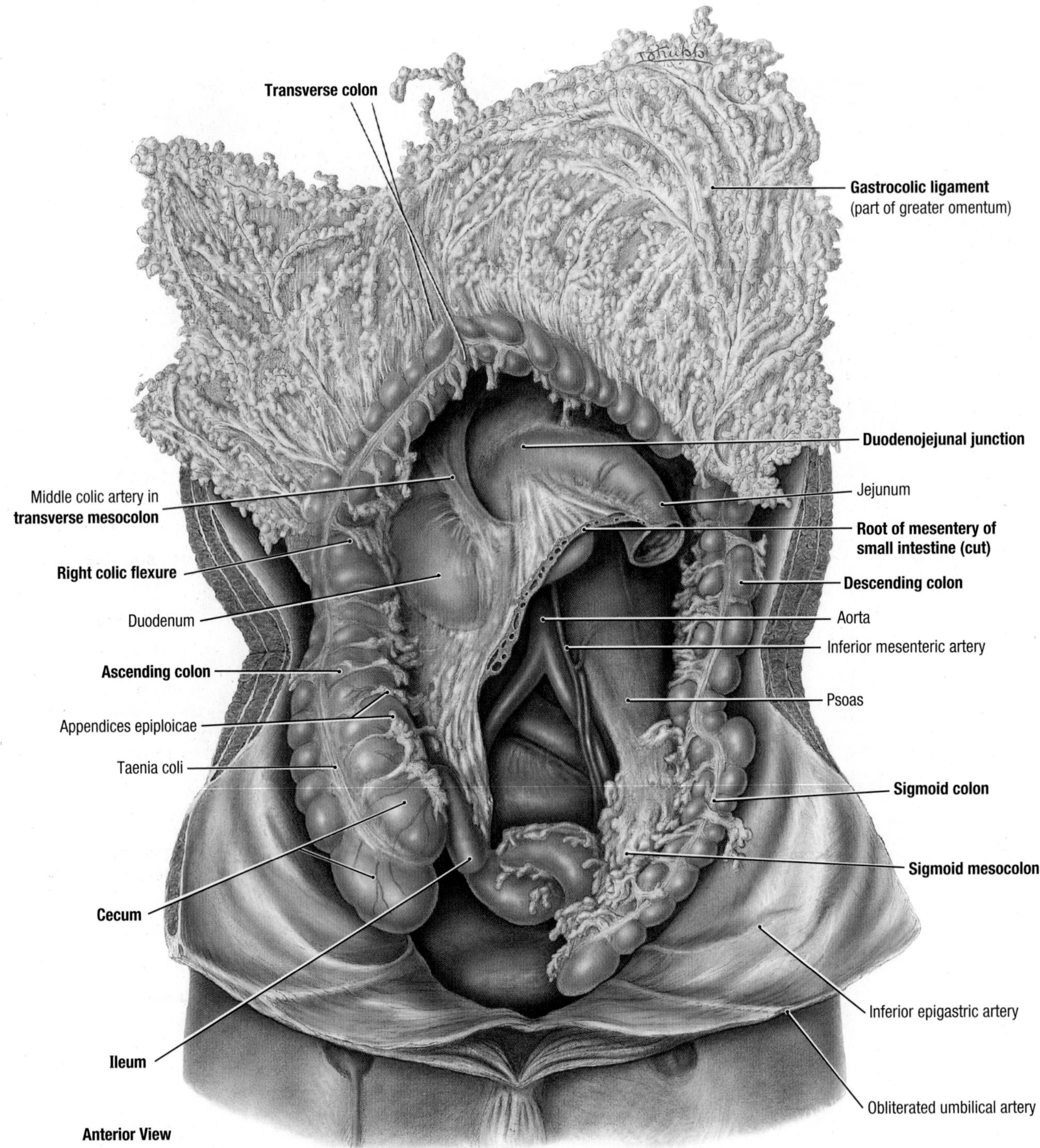
Transverse colon
Gastrocolic ligament
(part of greater omentum)
Duodenojejunal junction
Jejunum
Middle colic artery in
transverse mesocolon
Root of mesentery of
small intestine (cut)
Right colic flexure
Descending colon
Duodenum
Aorta
Inferior mesenteric artery
Ascending colon
Psoas
Appendices epiploicae
Taenia coli
Sigmoid colon
Sigmoid mesocolon
Cecum
Inferior epigastric artery
Ileum
Obliterated umbilical artery
Anterior View

2.48 PERITONEUM OF POSTERIOR ABDOMINAL CAVITY

The gastrocolic ligament is retracted superiorly, along with the transverse colon and transverse mesocolon. The appendix had been surgically removed. This dissection is continued in Figure 2.49.

- The root of the mesentery of the small intestine, approximately 15 to 20 cm in length, extends between the duodenojejunal junction and ileocecal junction.
- The large intestine forms 3½ sides of a square around the jejunum and ileum. On the right are the cecum and ascending colon, superior is the transverse colon, on the left is the descending and sigmoid colon, and inferiorly is the sigmoid colon.
- **Chronic inflammation of the colon (ulcerative colitis, Crohn disease)** is characterized by severe inflammation and ulceration of the colon and rectum. In some patients, a colectomy is performed, during which the terminal ileum and colon as well as the rectum and anal canal are removed. An ileostomy is then constructed to establish an artificial cutaneous opening between the ileum and the skin of the anterolateral abdominal wall.

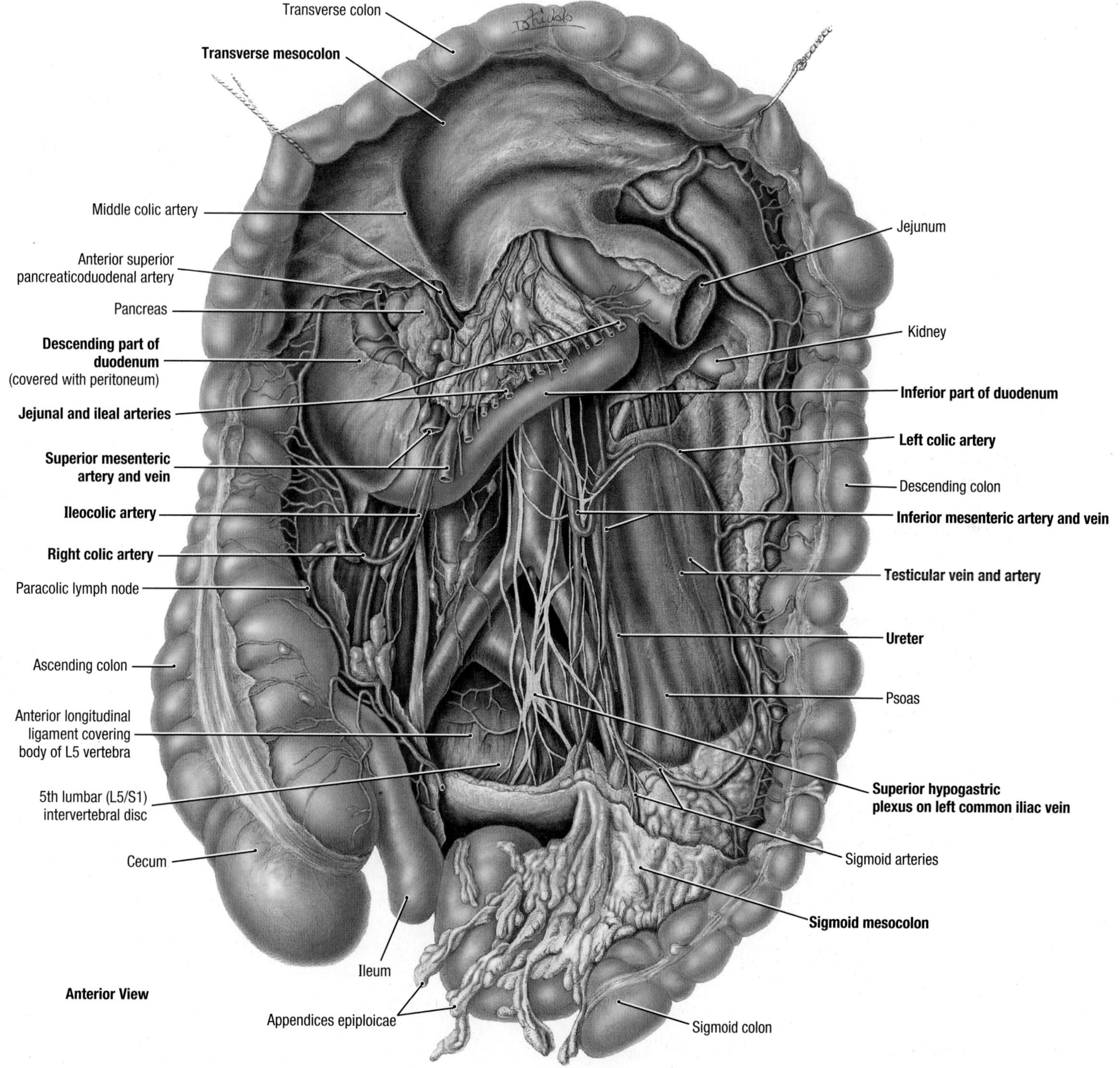
Transverse colon
Transverse mesocolon
Middle colic artery
Anterior superior pancreaticoduodenal artery
Pancreas
Descending part of duodenum (covered with peritoneum)
Jejunal and ileal arteries
Superior mesenteric artery and vein
Ileocolic artery
Right colic artery
Paracolic lymph node
Ascending colon
Anterior longitudinal ligament covering body of L5 vertebra
5th lumbar (L5/S1) intervertebral disc
Cecum
Ileum
Anterior View
Appendices epiploicae
Sigmoid colon
Jejunum
Kidney
Inferior part of duodenum
Left colic artery
Descending colon
Inferior mesenteric artery and vein
Testicular vein and artery
Ureter
Psoas
Superior hypogastric plexus on left common iliac vein
Sigmoid arteries
Sigmoid mesocolon

2.49 POSTERIOR ABDOMINAL CAVITY WITH PERITONEUM REMOVED

The jejunal and ileal branches (cut) pass from the left side of the superior mesenteric artery. The right colic artery here is a branch of the ileocolic artery. This is the same specimen as in Figure 2.48.

- The duodenum is large in diameter before crossing the superior mesenteric vessels and narrow afterward.
- On the right side, there are lymph nodes on the colon, paracolic nodes beside the colon, and nodes along the ileocolic artery, which drain into nodes anterior to the pancreas.
- The intestines and intestinal vessels lie on a resectable plane anterior to that of the testicular vessels; these in turn lie anterior to the plane of the kidney, its vessels, and the ureter.
- The superior hypogastric plexus lie inferior to the bifurcation of the aorta and anterior to the left common iliac vein, the body of the 5th lumbar vertebra, and the 5th intervertebral disc.

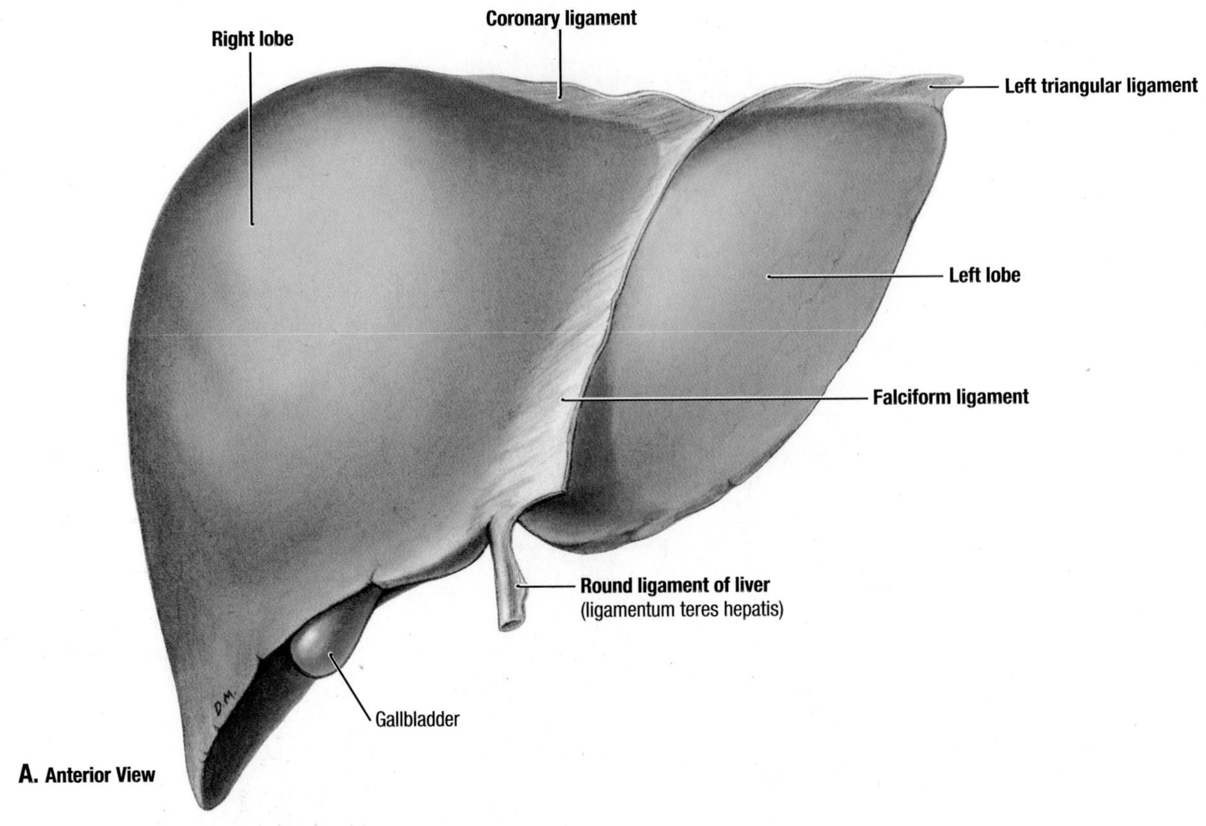

Right lobe
Coronary ligament
Left triangular ligament
Left lobe
Falciform ligament
Round ligament of liver
(ligamentum teres hepatis)
Gallbladder
D.M.

A. Anterior View

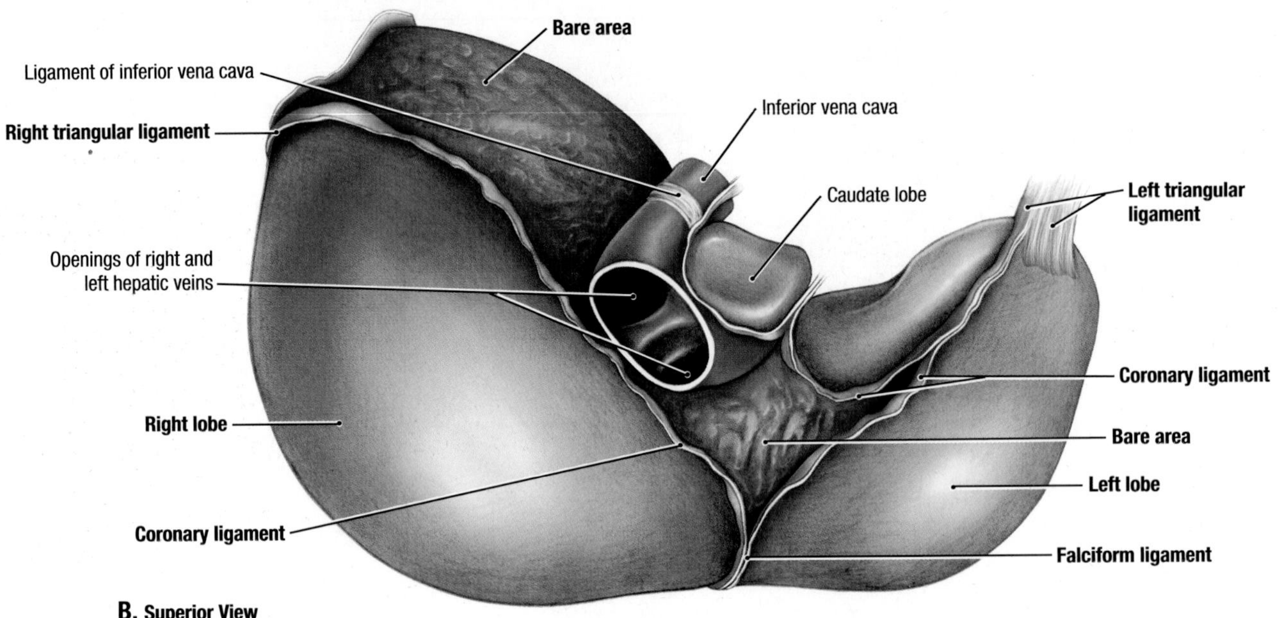

Bare area
Ligament of inferior vena cava
Right triangular ligament
Inferior vena cava
Caudate lobe
Left triangular ligament
Openings of right and left hepatic veins
Coronary ligament
Bare area
Right lobe
Left lobe
Coronary ligament
Falciform ligament

B. Superior View

2.50 DIAPHRAGMATIC (ANTERIOR AND SUPERIOR) SURFACE OF LIVER

A. The falciform ligament has been severed close to its attachment to the diaphragm and anterior abdominal wall and demarcates the right and left lobes of the liver. The round ligament of the liver (ligamentum teres) lies within the free edge of the falciform ligament.

B. The two layers of peritoneum that form the falciform ligament separate over the superior aspect (surrounding the bare area) of the liver to form the superior layer of the coronary ligament and the right and left triangular ligaments.

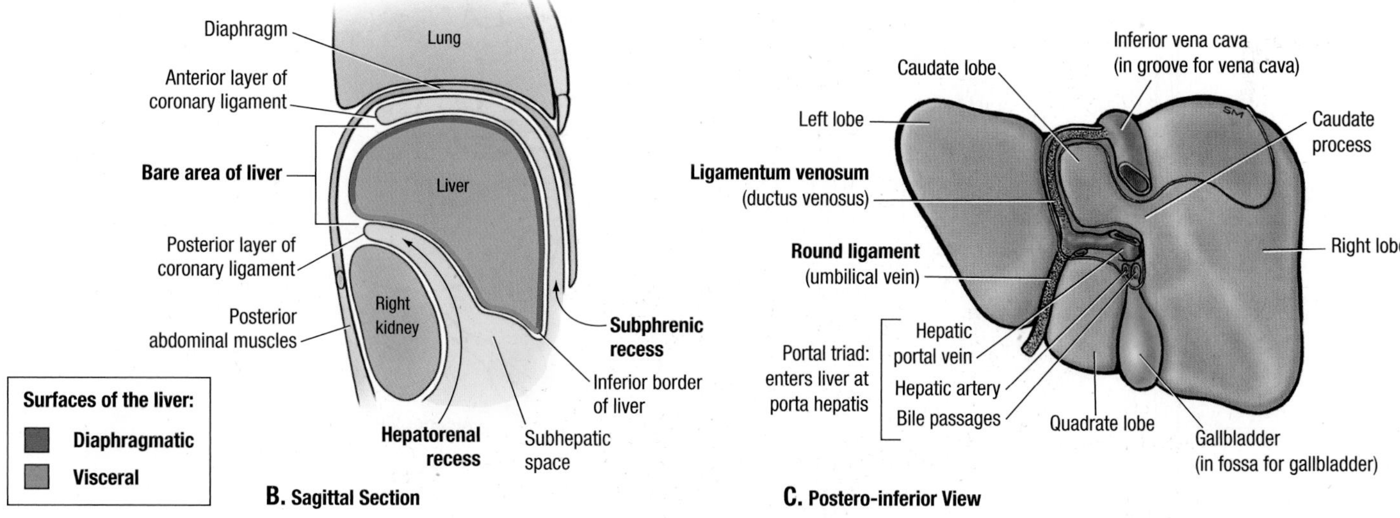
Left triangular ligament
Lesser omentum
Diaphragmatic area
Bare area
Inferior vena cava
Esophageal area
Left lobe
Line separating diaphragmatic and visceral surfaces
Gastric area
Suprarenal area
Caudate lobe
Coronary ligament
Hepatic artery
Renal area
Bile duct
Caudate process
Porta hepatis
Hepatic portal vein
Pyloric area
Right lobe
Quadrate lobe
Duodenal area
Gallbladder
Falciform ligament
Round ligament of liver
A. Postero-inferior View
Colic area
Diaphragm
Lung
Anterior layer of coronary ligament
Bare area of liver
Liver
Posterior layer of coronary ligament
Right kidney
Posterior abdominal muscles
Subphrenic recess
Inferior border of liver
Surfaces of the liver:
Diaphragmatic
Visceral
Hepatorenal recess
Subhepatic space
B. Sagittal Section
Caudate lobe
Inferior vena cava (in groove for vena cava)
Left lobe
Caudate process
Ligamentum venosum (ductus venosus)
Round ligament (umbilical vein)
Right lobe
Portal triad: enters liver at porta hepatis
Hepatic portal vein
Hepatic artery
Bile passages
Quadrate lobe
Gallbladder (in fossa for gallbladder)
C. Postero-inferior View

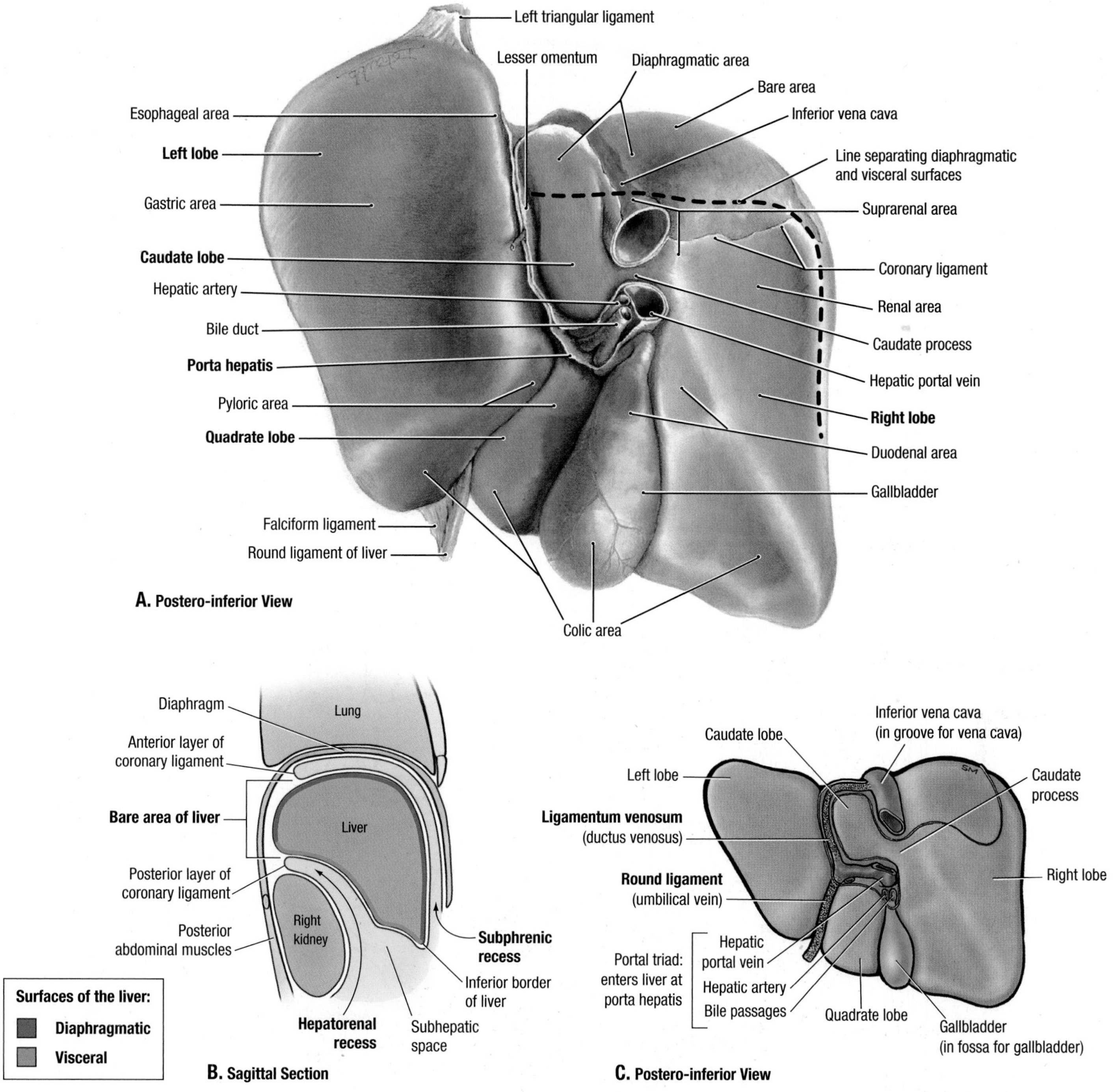

2.51 VISCERAL (POSTERO-INFERIOR) SURFACE OF LIVER

A. Isolated specimen demonstrating lobes, and impressions of adjacent viscera. **B.** Hepatic surfaces and peritoneal recesses. **C.** Round ligament of liver and ligamentum venosum. The round ligament of liver includes the obliterated remains of the umbilical vein that carried well-oxygenated blood from the placenta to the fetus. The ligamentum venosum is the fibrous remnant of the fetal ductus venosus that shunted blood from the umbilical vein to the inferior vena cava, short circuiting the liver. Hepatic tissue may be obtained for diagnostic purposes by **liver biopsy.** The needle puncture is commonly made through the right 10th intercostal space in the midaxillary line. Before the physician takes the biopsy, the person is asked to hold his or her breath in full expiration to reduce the costodiaphragmatic recess and to lessen the possibility of damaging the lung and contaminating the pleural cavity.

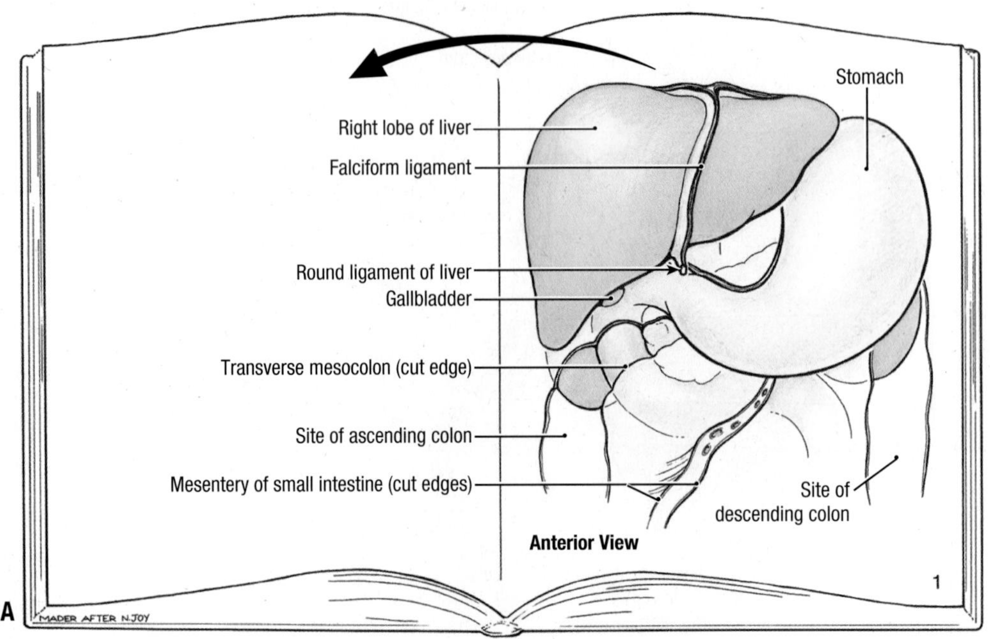
Stomach
Right lobe of liver
Falciform ligament
Round ligament of liver
Gallbladder
Transverse mesocolon (cut edge)
Site of ascending colon
Mesentery of small intestine (cut edges)
Site of descending colon
Anterior View
1
A
MADER AFTER N.JOY

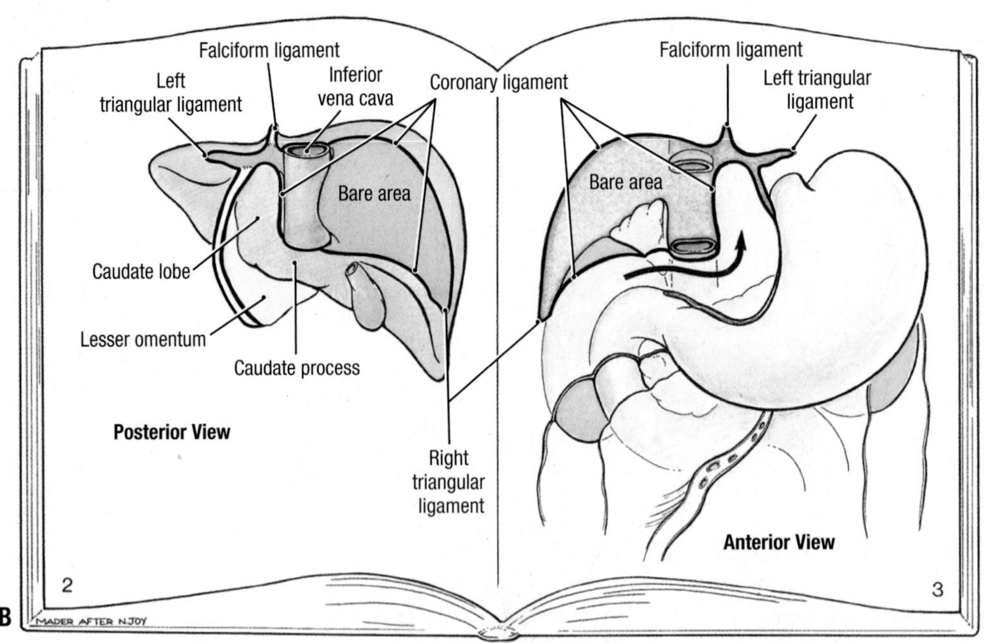
Falciform ligament
Left triangular ligament
Inferior vena cava
Coronary ligament
Falciform ligament
Left triangular ligament
Bare area
Bare area
Caudate lobe
Lesser omentum
Caudate process
Posterior View
Right triangular ligament
Anterior View
2
3
B
MADER AFTER N.JOY

2.52 LIVER AND ITS POSTERIOR RELATIONS, SCHEMATIC ILLUSTRATION

A. Liver in situ. The jejunum, ileum, and the ascending, transverse, and descending colons have been removed. **B.** The liver is drawn schematically on a page in a book, so that as the page is turned (*arrow in A*), the liver is reflected to the right to reveal its posterior surface, and on the facing page, the posterior relations that compose the bed of the liver are viewed. The *arrow in B* traverses the omental (epiploic) foramen to enter the omental bursa and its superior recess (*arrowhead*). The bare area is triangular, hence the coronary ligament that surrounds it is three-sided; its left side, or base, is between the inferior vena cava and caudate lobe, and its apex is at the right triangular ligament, where the superior and inferior layers of the coronary ligament meet.

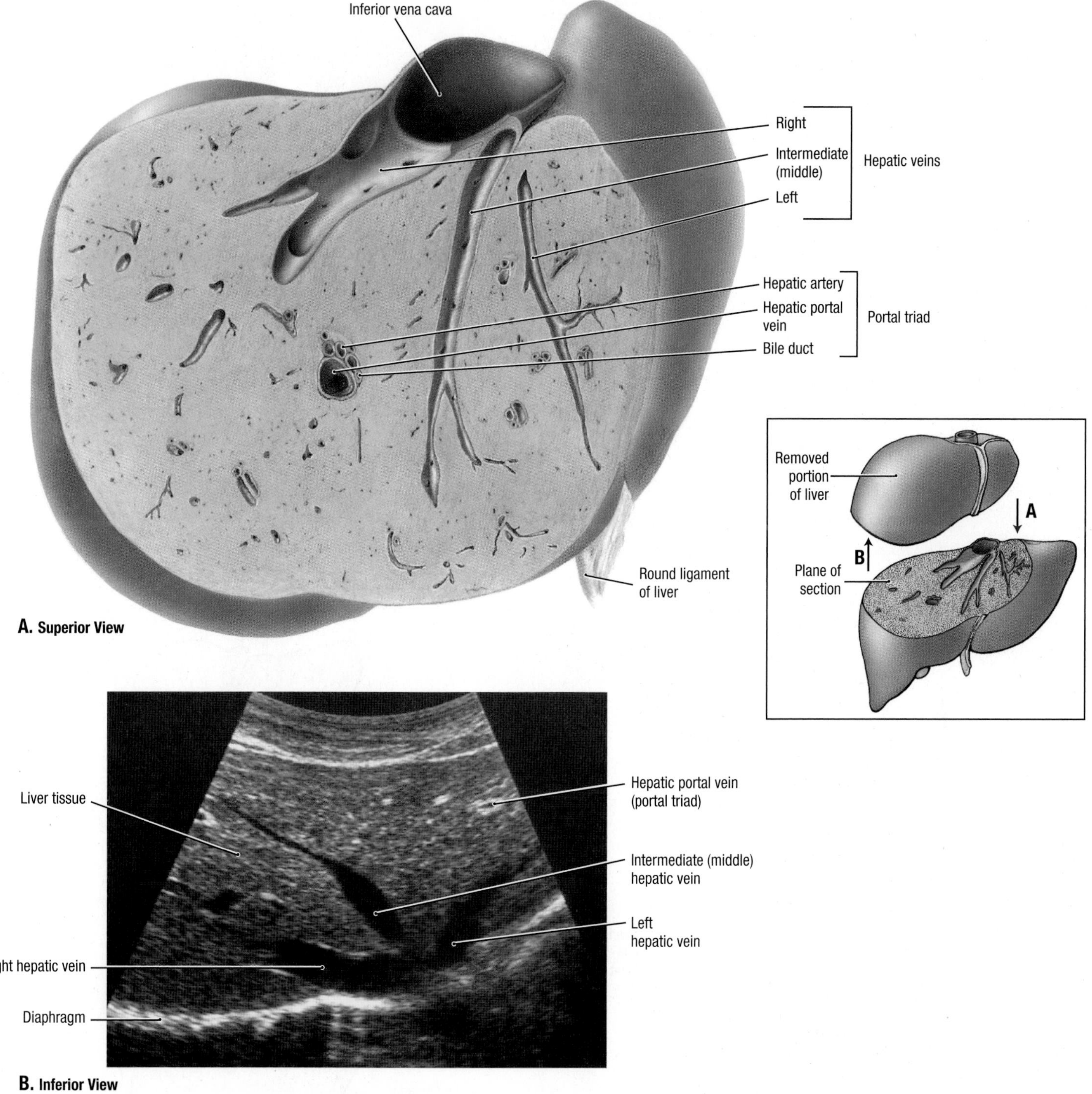
Inferior vena cava
Right
Intermediate (middle)
Left
Hepatic veins
Hepatic artery
Hepatic portal vein
Bile duct
Portal triad
Round ligament of liver
A. Superior View
Removed portion of liver
A
B
Plane of section
Liver tissue
Hepatic portal vein (portal triad)
Intermediate (middle) hepatic vein
Left hepatic vein
Right hepatic vein
Diaphragm
B. Inferior View

2.53 HEPATIC VEINS

A. Approximately horizontal section of liver with the posterior aspect at the top of page. Note the multiple perivascular fibrous capsules sectioned throughout the cut surface, each containing a portal triad (the hepatic portal vein, hepatic artery, bile ductules) plus lymph vessels. Interdigitating with these are branches of the three main hepatic veins (right, intermediate, and left), which, unaccompanied and lacking capsules, converge on the inferior vena cava. **B.** Ultrasound scan. The transducer was placed under the costal margin and directed posteriorly, producing an inverted image corresponding to **A.**

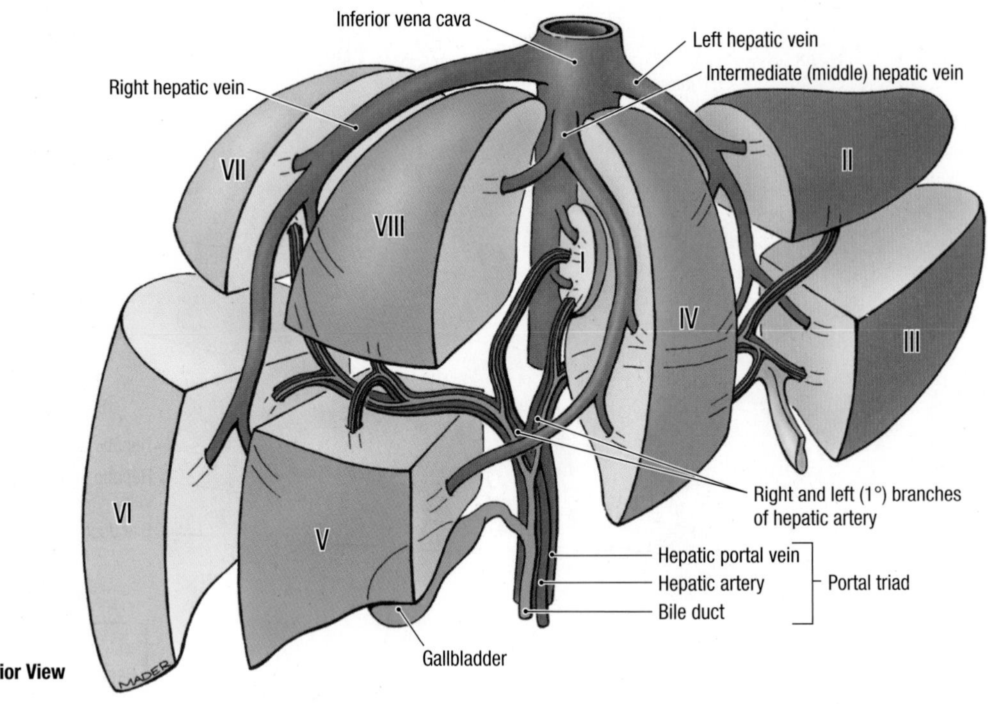

Inferior vena cava
Left hepatic vein
Intermediate (middle) hepatic vein
Right hepatic vein
VII
VIII
I
II
IV
III
VI
V
Right and left (1°) branches of hepatic artery
Hepatic portal vein
Hepatic artery
Bile duct
Portal triad
Gallbladder
MADER

A. Anterior View

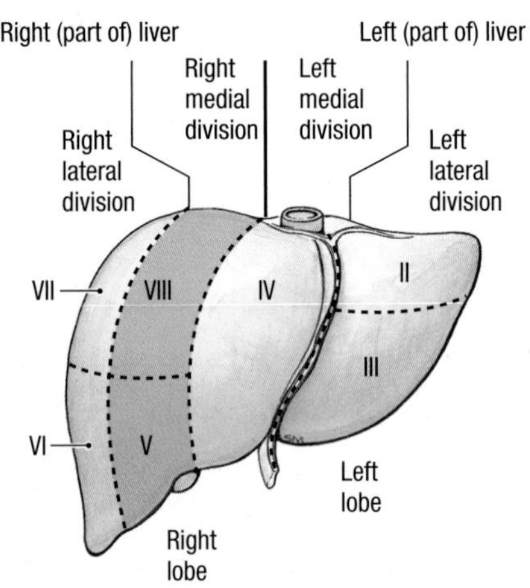

Right (part of) liver
Left (part of) liver
Right medial division
Left medial division
Right lateral division
Left lateral division
VII
VIII
IV
II
III
VI
V
Left lobe
Right lobe

B

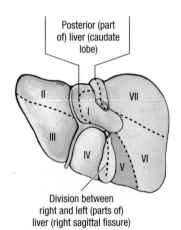

Posterior (part of) liver (caudate lobe)
II
VII
I
III
IV
V
VI
Division between right and left (parts of) liver (right sagittal fissure)

C

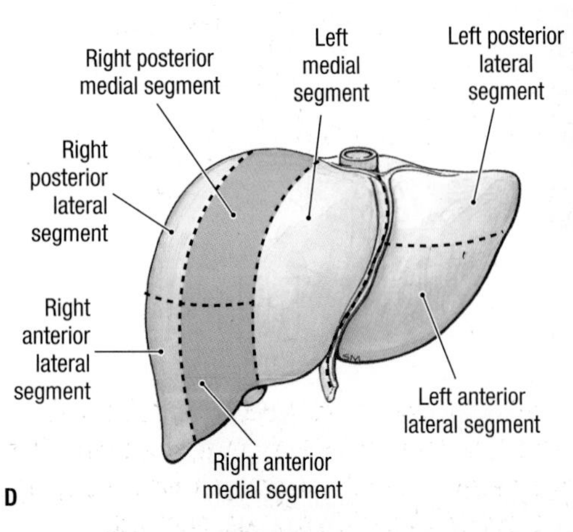

Right posterior medial segment
Left medial segment
Left posterior lateral segment
Right posterior lateral segment
Right anterior lateral segment
Left anterior lateral segment
Right anterior medial segment

D

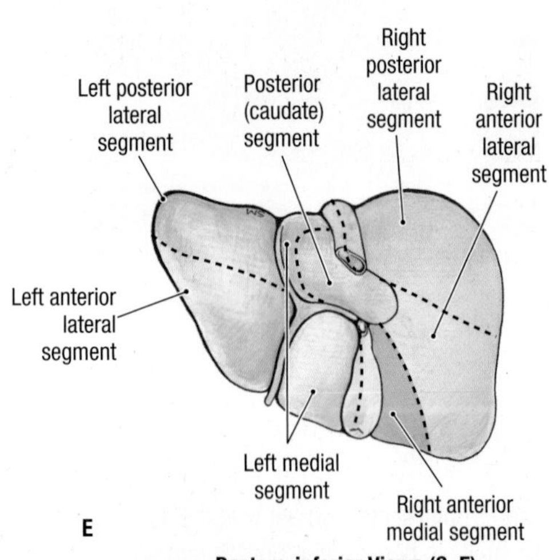

Left posterior lateral segment
Posterior (caudate) segment
Right posterior lateral segment
Right anterior lateral segment
Left anterior lateral segment
Left medial segment
Right anterior medial segment

E

Anterior Views (B, D)

Postero-inferior Views (C, E)

2.54 HEPATIC SEGMENTATION

2.54 HEPATIC SEGMENTATION *(CONTINUED)*

Each segment is supplied by a secondary or tertiary branch of the hepatic artery, bile duct, and portal vein. The hepatic veins interdigitate between the structures of the portal triad and are intersegmental in that they drain adjacent segments. Since the right and left hepatic arteries and ducts and branches of the right and left portal veins do not communicate, it is possible to perform **hepatic lobectomies** (removal of the right or left part of the liver) and **segmentectomies.** Each segment can be identified numerically or by name (Table 2.6).

TABLE 2.6 SCHEMA OF TERMINOLOGY FOR SUBDIVISIONS OF THE LIVER

Anatomical Term	Right Lobe		Left Lobe		Caudate Lobe	
Functional/surgical term[a]	Right (part of) liver [Right portal lobe[b]]		Left (part of) liver [Left portal lobe[c]]		Posterior (part of) liver	
	Right lateral division	Right medial division	Left medial division	Left lateral division	[Right caudate lobe[b]]	[Left caudate lobe[c]]
	Posterior lateral segment **Segment VII** [Posterior superior area]	Posterior medial segment **Segment VIII** [Anterior superior area]	[Medial superior area] Left medial segment **Segment IV**	Lateral segment **Segment II** [Lateral superior area]	Posterior segment **Segment I**	
	Right anterior lateral segment **Segment VI** [Posterior inferior area]	Anterior medial segment **Segment V** [Anterior inferior area]	[Medial inferior area = quadrate lobe]	Left anterior lateral segment **Segment III** [Lateral inferior area]		

[a]The labels in the table and figure above reflect the Terminologia *Anatomica: International Anatomical Terminology.* Previous terminology is in brackets.
[b,c]Under the schema of the previous terminology, the caudate lobe was divided into right and left halves, and [b]the right half of the caudate lobe was considered a subdivision of the right portal lobe; [c]the left half of the caudate lobe was considered a subdivision of the left portal lobe.

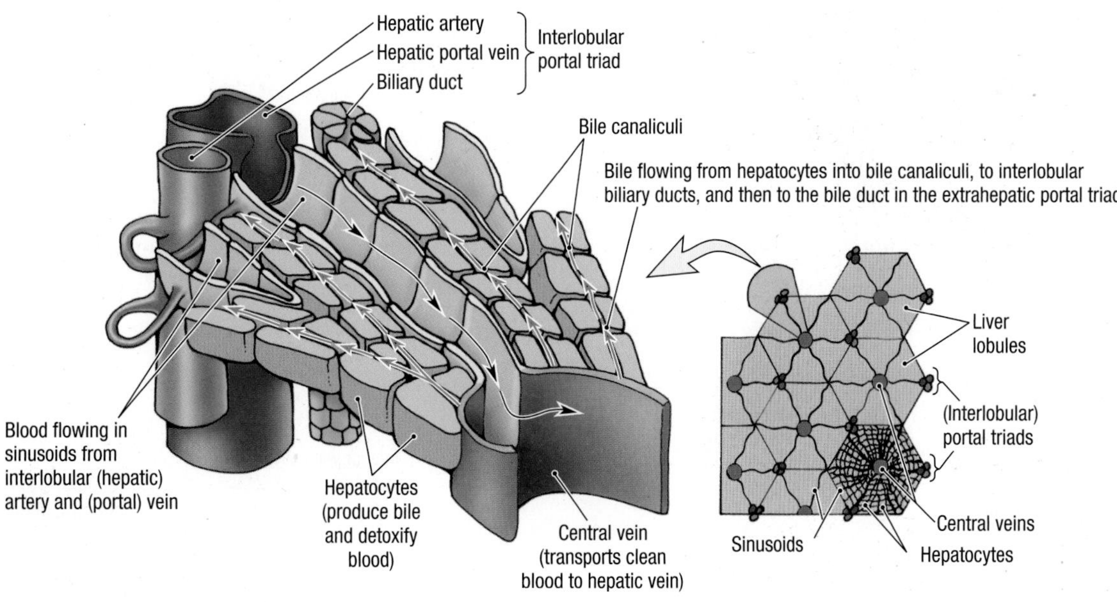
Hepatic artery
Hepatic portal vein
Biliary duct
Interlobular portal triad
Bile canaliculi
Bile flowing from hepatocytes into bile canaliculi, to interlobular biliary ducts, and then to the bile duct in the extrahepatic portal triad
Liver lobules
(Interlobular) portal triads
Central veins
Hepatocytes
Sinusoids
Blood flowing in sinusoids from interlobular (hepatic) artery and (portal) vein
Hepatocytes (produce bile and detoxify blood)
Central vein (transports clean blood to hepatic vein)

2.55 FLOW OF BLOOD AND BILE IN THE LIVER

This small part of a liver lobule shows the components of the interlobular portal triad and the positioning of the sinusoids and bile canaliculi. **Right.** The cut surface of the liver shows the hexagonal pattern of the lobules.

- With the exception of lipids, every substance absorbed by the alimentary tract is received first by the liver, via the hepatic portal vein. In addition to its many metabolic activities, the liver stores glycogen and secretes bile.
- There is progressive destruction of hepatocytes in **cirrhosis of the liver** and replacement of them by fibrous tissue. This tissue surrounds the intrahepatic blood vessels and biliary ducts, making the liver firm and impeding circulation of blood through it.

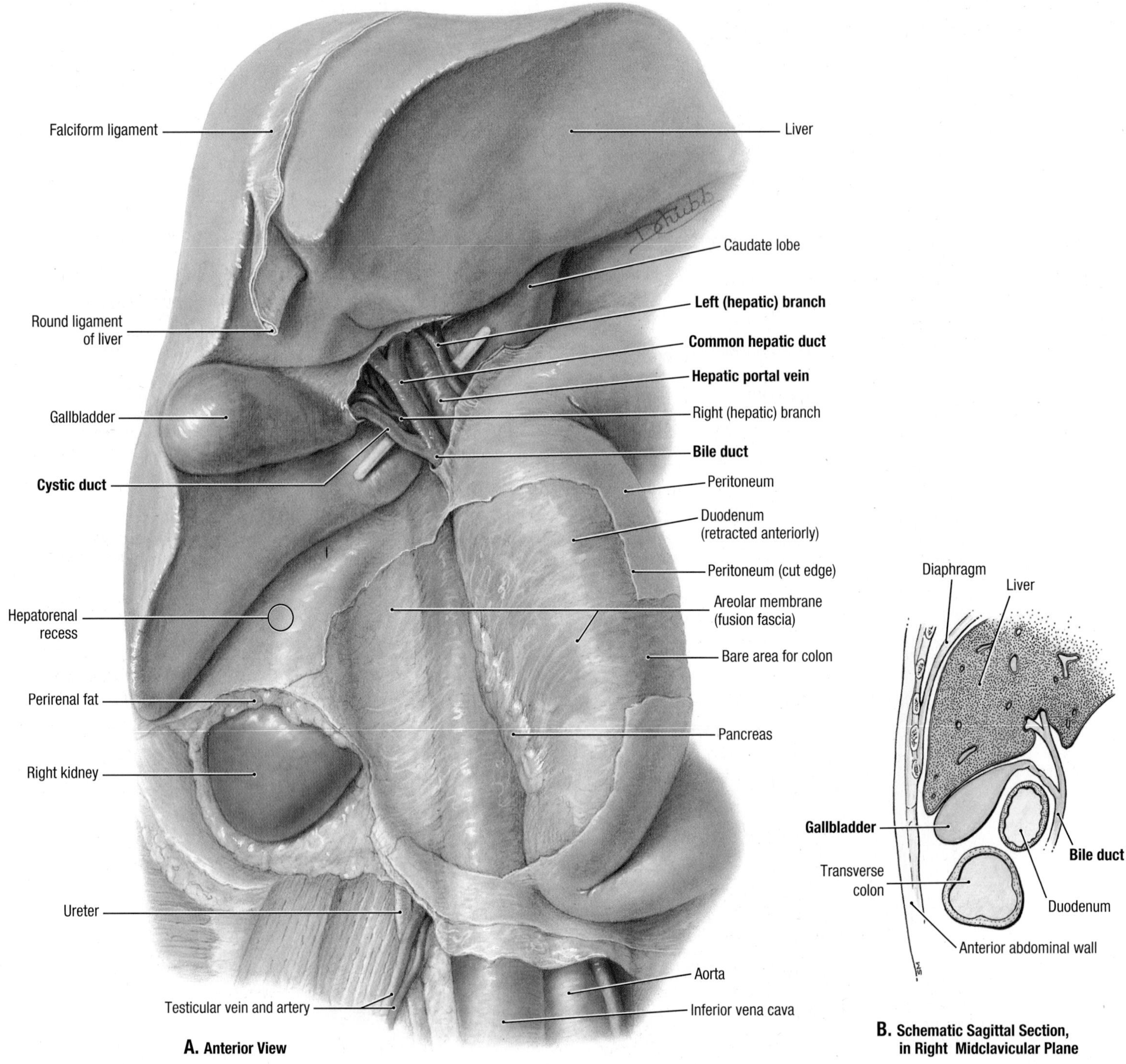
Falciform ligament
Liver
Caudate lobe
Left (hepatic) branch
Round ligament of liver
Common hepatic duct
Hepatic portal vein
Gallbladder
Right (hepatic) branch
Bile duct
Cystic duct
Peritoneum
Duodenum (retracted anteriorly)
Peritoneum (cut edge)
Hepatorenal recess
Areolar membrane (fusion fascia)
Bare area for colon
Perirenal fat
Pancreas
Right kidney
Ureter
Aorta
Testicular vein and artery
Inferior vena cava
Diaphragm
Liver
Gallbladder
Bile duct
Transverse colon
Duodenum
Anterior abdominal wall

A. Anterior View

B. Schematic Sagittal Section, in Right Midclavicular Plane

2.56 EXPOSURE OF THE PORTAL TRIAD

A. The portal triad typically consists of the hepatic portal vein (posteriorly), the hepatic artery proper (ascending from the left), and the bile passages (descending to the right). Here, the hepatic artery proper is replaced by a left hepatic branch, arising directly from the common hepatic artery, and a right hepatic branch, arising from the superior mesenteric artery (a common variation). A rod traverses the omental (epiploic) foramen. The lesser omentum and transverse colon are removed, and the peritoneum is cut along the right border of the duodenum; this part of the duodenum is retracted anteriorly. The space opened up reveals two smooth areolar membranes (fusion fascia) normally applied to each other that are vestiges of the embryonic peritoneum originally covering these surfaces. **B.** Typical relations of gallbladder, cystic duct, and bile duct to the duodenum.

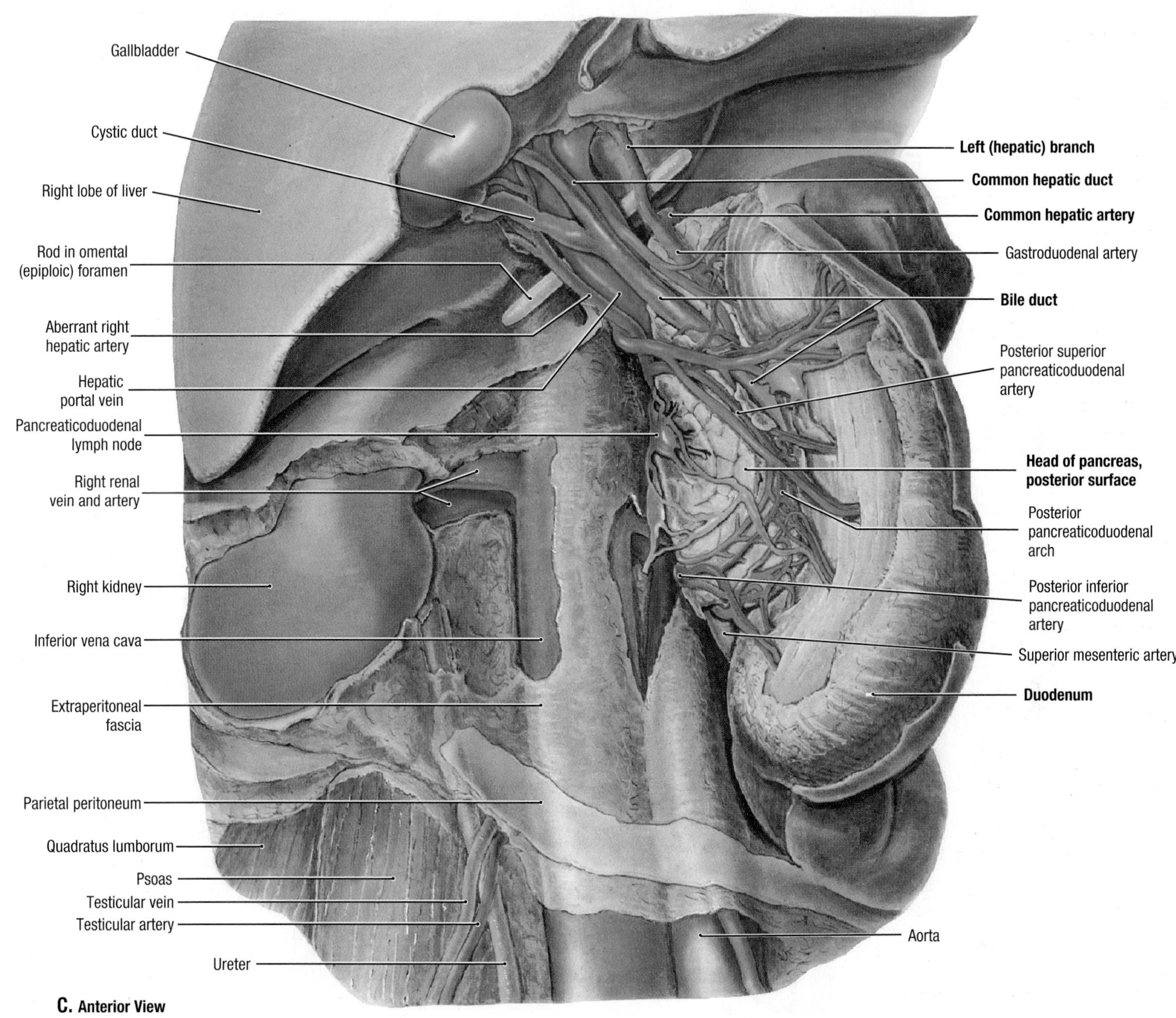
Gallbladder
Cystic duct
Right lobe of liver
Rod in omental (epiploic) foramen
Aberrant right hepatic artery
Hepatic portal vein
Pancreaticoduodenal lymph node
Right renal vein and artery
Right kidney
Inferior vena cava
Extraperitoneal fascia
Parietal peritoneum
Quadratus lumborum
Psoas
Testicular vein
Testicular artery
Ureter
Left (hepatic) branch
Common hepatic duct
Common hepatic artery
Gastroduodenal artery
Bile duct
Posterior superior pancreaticoduodenal artery
Head of pancreas, posterior surface
Posterior pancreaticoduodenal arch
Posterior inferior pancreaticoduodenal artery
Superior mesenteric artery
Duodenum
Aorta

C. Anterior View

2.56 EXPOSURE OF THE PORTAL TRIAD (*CONTINUED*)

C. Continuing the dissection in **A**, the secondarily retroperitoneal viscera (duodenum and head of the pancreas) are retracted anteriorly and to the left. The areolar membrane (fusion fascia) covering the posterior aspect of the pancreas and duodenum is largely removed, and that covering the anterior aspect of the great vessels is partly removed. A common method for **reducing portal hypertension** is to divert blood from the portal venous system to the systemic venous system by creating a communication between the portal vein and the IVC. This **portacaval anastomosis or portosystemic shunt** may be created where these vessels lie close to each other posterior to the liver.

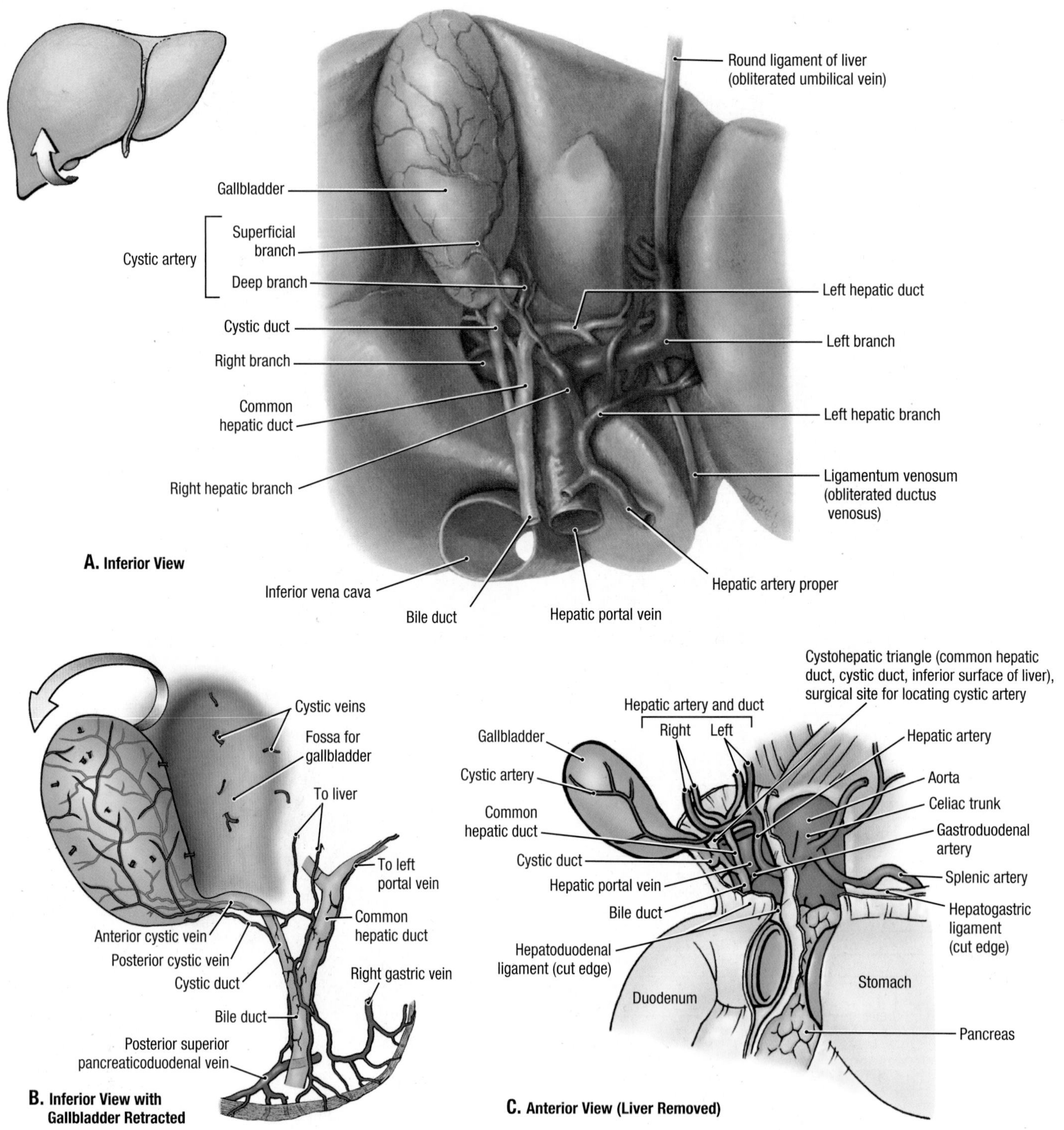
Round ligament of liver (obliterated umbilical vein)
Gallbladder
Cystic artery
Superficial branch
Deep branch
Left hepatic duct
Cystic duct
Left branch
Right branch
Common hepatic duct
Left hepatic branch
Right hepatic branch
Ligamentum venosum (obliterated ductus venosus)
A. Inferior View
Inferior vena cava
Bile duct
Hepatic portal vein
Hepatic artery proper
Cystic veins
Fossa for gallbladder
To liver
To left portal vein
Common hepatic duct
Anterior cystic vein
Posterior cystic vein
Cystic duct
Right gastric vein
Bile duct
Posterior superior pancreaticoduodenal vein
B. Inferior View with Gallbladder Retracted
Cystohepatic triangle (common hepatic duct, cystic duct, inferior surface of liver), surgical site for locating cystic artery
Hepatic artery and duct
Right
Left
Gallbladder
Hepatic artery
Cystic artery
Aorta
Celiac trunk
Common hepatic duct
Gastroduodenal artery
Cystic duct
Splenic artery
Hepatic portal vein
Bile duct
Hepatogastric ligament (cut edge)
Hepatoduodenal ligament (cut edge)
Stomach
Duodenum
Pancreas
C. Anterior View (Liver Removed)

2.57 GALLBLADDER AND STRUCTURES OF PORTA HEPATIS

A. Gallbladder, cystic artery, and extrahepatic bile ducts. The inferior border of the liver is elevated to demonstrate its visceral surface (as in orientation figure). **B.** Venous drainage of the gall bladder and extrahepatic ducts. Most veins are tributaries of the hepatic portal vein, but some drain directly to the liver. **C.** Portal triad within the hepatoduodenal ligament (free edge of lesser omentum). **Gallstones** are concretions, in the gallbladder or extrahepatic biliary ducts. The cystohepatic (hepatobiliary) triangle (Calot), between the common hepatic duct, cystic duct, and liver, is an important endoscopic landmark for locating the cystic artery during **cholecystectomy.**

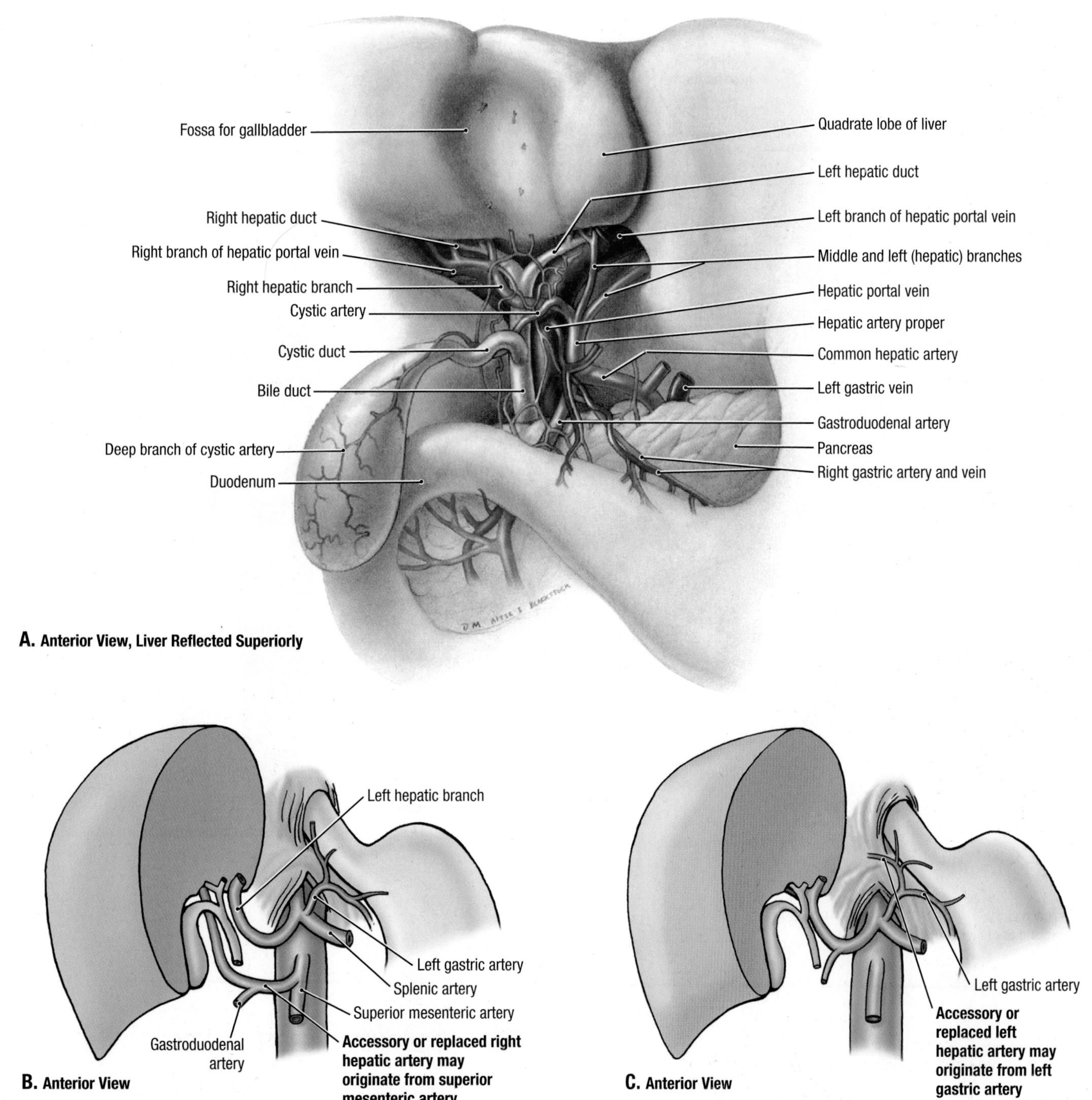
Fossa for gallbladder
Quadrate lobe of liver
Left hepatic duct
Right hepatic duct
Left branch of hepatic portal vein
Right branch of hepatic portal vein
Middle and left (hepatic) branches
Right hepatic branch
Hepatic portal vein
Cystic artery
Hepatic artery proper
Cystic duct
Common hepatic artery
Bile duct
Left gastric vein
Gastroduodenal artery
Deep branch of cystic artery
Pancreas
Duodenum
Right gastric artery and vein
Left hepatic branch
Left gastric artery
Splenic artery
Superior mesenteric artery
Gastroduodenal artery
Accessory or replaced right hepatic artery may originate from superior mesenteric artery
Left gastric artery
Accessory or replaced left hepatic artery may originate from left gastric artery

A. **Anterior View, Liver Reflected Superiorly**

B. **Anterior View**

C. **Anterior View**

2.58 VESSELS IN PORTA HEPATIS

A. Hepatic and cystic vessels. The liver is reflected superiorly. The gallbladder, freed from its bed or fossa, has remained nearly in its anatomical position, pulled slightly to the right. The deep branch of the cystic artery on the deep, or attached, surface of the gallbladder anastomoses with branches of the superficial branch of the cystic artery and sends twigs into the bed of the gallbladder. Veins (not all shown) accompany most arteries. **B.** Aberrant (accessory or replaced) right hepatic artery. **C.** Aberrant left hepatic artery. Awareness of the variations in arteries and bile duct formation is important for surgeons when they ligate the cystic duct during **cholecystectomy** (removal of the gallbladder).

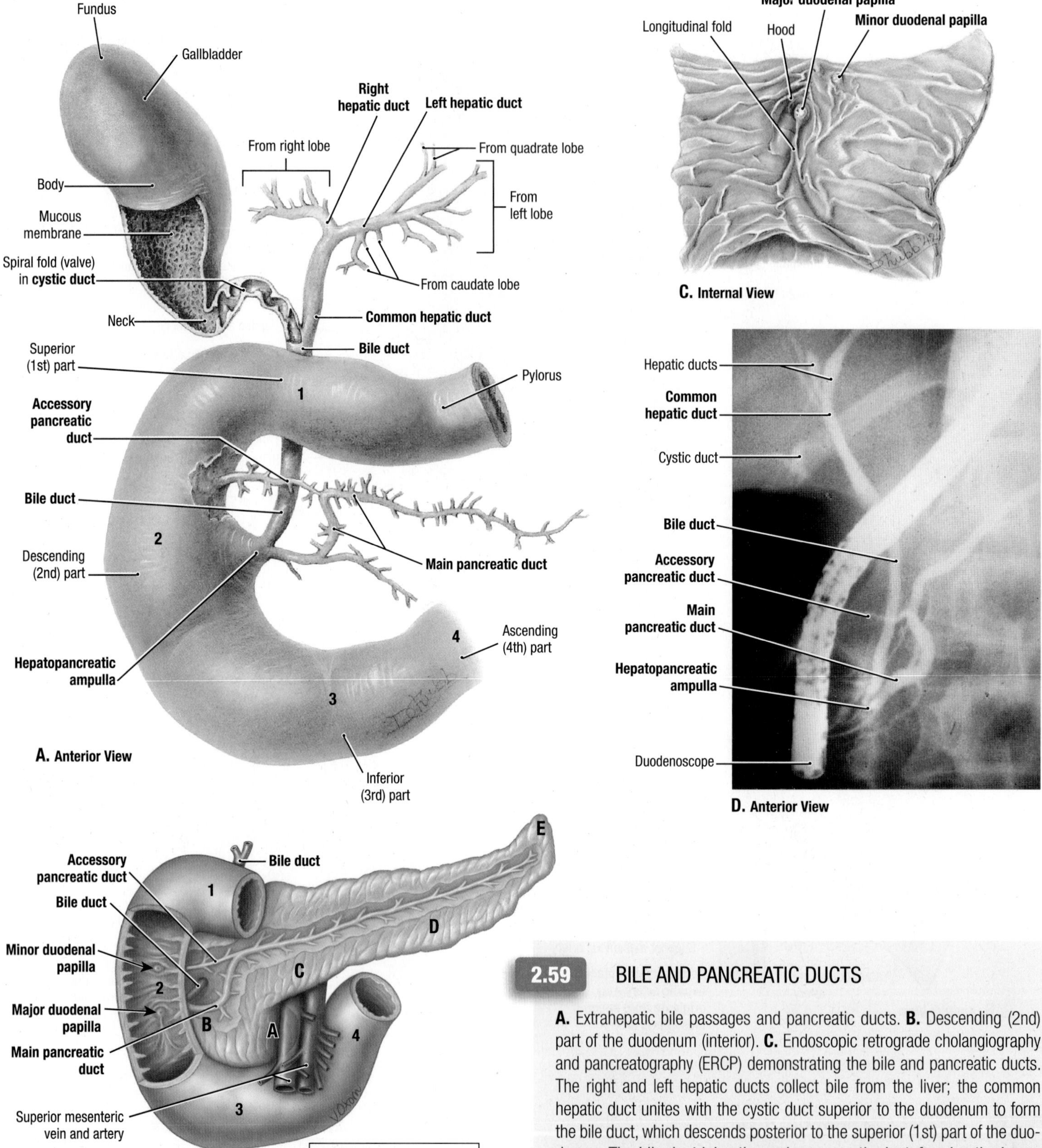

Fundus
Gallbladder
Body
Mucous membrane
Spiral fold (valve) in cystic duct
Neck
Right hepatic duct
Left hepatic duct
From right lobe
From quadrate lobe
From left lobe
From caudate lobe
Common hepatic duct
Bile duct
Superior (1st) part
Pylorus
Accessory pancreatic duct
Bile duct
Descending (2nd) part
Main pancreatic duct
Hepatopancreatic ampulla
Ascending (4th) part
Inferior (3rd) part
1
2
3
4
Major duodenal papilla
Longitudinal fold
Hood
Minor duodenal papilla
Hepatic ducts
Common hepatic duct
Cystic duct
Bile duct
Accessory pancreatic duct
Main pancreatic duct
Hepatopancreatic ampulla
Duodenoscope
Accessory pancreatic duct
Bile duct
Minor duodenal papilla
Major duodenal papilla
Main pancreatic duct
Superior mesenteric vein and artery
A
B
C
D
E
1 – 4 Parts of duodenum
Parts of pancreas:
A Uncinate process (extends posterior to superior mesenteric vein)
B Head
C Neck
D Body
E Tail

A. Anterior View

C. Internal View

D. Anterior View

B. Anterior View

2.59 BILE AND PANCREATIC DUCTS

A. Extrahepatic bile passages and pancreatic ducts. **B.** Descending (2nd) part of the duodenum (interior). **C.** Endoscopic retrograde cholangiography and pancreatography (ERCP) demonstrating the bile and pancreatic ducts. The right and left hepatic ducts collect bile from the liver; the common hepatic duct unites with the cystic duct superior to the duodenum to form the bile duct, which descends posterior to the superior (1st) part of the duodenum. The bile duct joins the main pancreatic duct, forming the hepatopancreatic ampulla, which opens on the major duodenal papilla. This opening is the narrowest part of the biliary passages and is the common site for **impaction of a gallstone.** Gallstones may produce biliary colic (pain in the epigastric region). The accessory pancreatic duct opens on the minor duodenal papilla.

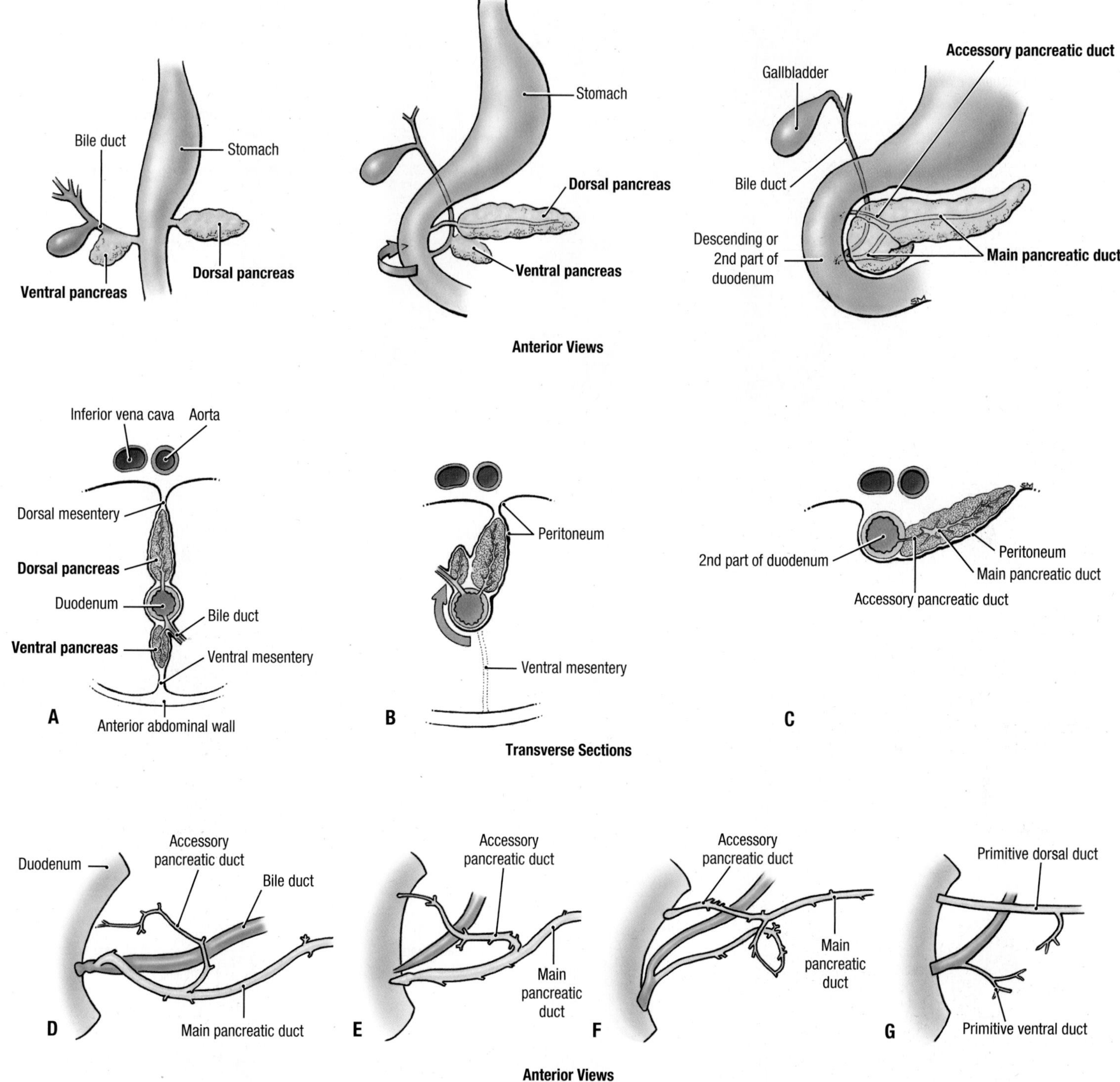
Bile duct
Stomach
Ventral pancreas
Dorsal pancreas
Stomach
Dorsal pancreas
Ventral pancreas
Gallbladder
Accessory pancreatic duct
Bile duct
Descending or 2nd part of duodenum
Main pancreatic duct
Anterior Views
Inferior vena cava
Aorta
Dorsal mesentery
Dorsal pancreas
Duodenum
Bile duct
Ventral pancreas
Ventral mesentery
A
Anterior abdominal wall
Peritoneum
Ventral mesentery
B
2nd part of duodenum
Peritoneum
Main pancreatic duct
Accessory pancreatic duct
C
Transverse Sections
Duodenum
Accessory pancreatic duct
Bile duct
D
Main pancreatic duct
Accessory pancreatic duct
Main pancreatic duct
E
Accessory pancreatic duct
Main pancreatic duct
F
Primitive dorsal duct
G
Primitive ventral duct
Anterior Views

2.60 DEVELOPMENT AND VARIABILITY OF THE PANCREATIC DUCTS

A.–C. Anterior views (*top*) and transverse sections (*bottom*) of the stages in the development of the pancreas. **A.** The small, primitive ventral bud arises in common with the bile duct, and a larger, primitive dorsal bud arises independently from the duodenum. **B.** The 2nd, or descending, part of the duodenum rotates on its long axis, which brings the ventral bud and bile duct posterior to the dorsal bud. **C.** A connecting segment unites the dorsal duct to the ventral duct, whereupon the duodenal end of the dorsal duct atrophies, and the direction of flow within it is reversed. **D.–G.** Common variations of the pancreatic duct. **D.** An accessory duct that has lost its connection with the duodenum. **E.** An accessory duct that is large enough to relieve an obstructed main duct. **F.** An accessory duct that could probably substitute for the main duct. **G.** A persisting primitive dorsal duct unconnected to the primitive ventral duct.

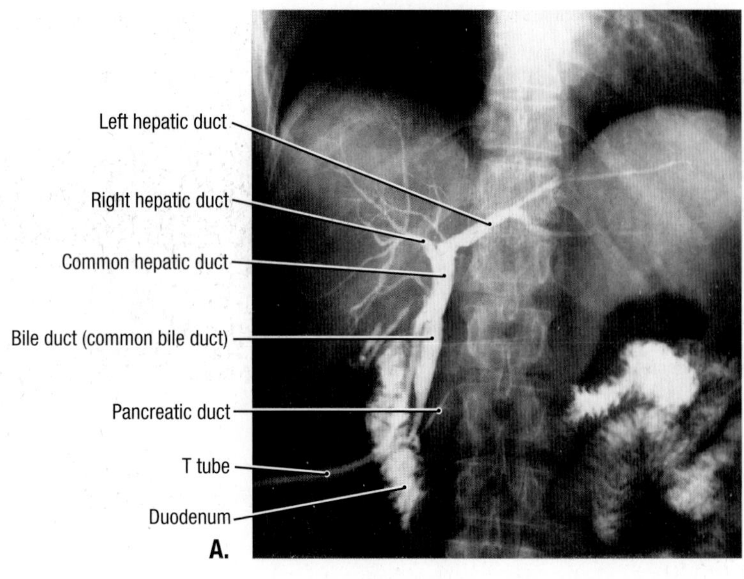
Left hepatic duct
Right hepatic duct
Common hepatic duct
Bile duct (common bile duct)
Pancreatic duct
T tube
Duodenum
A.

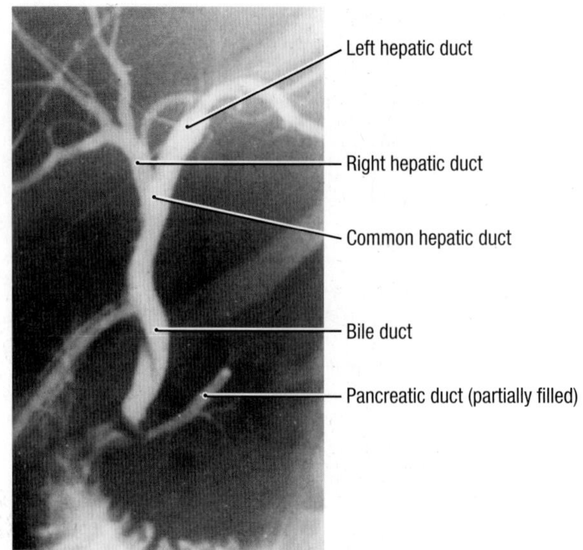
Left hepatic duct
Right hepatic duct
Common hepatic duct
Bile duct
Pancreatic duct (partially filled)
B.

2.61 RADIOGRAPHS OF BILIARY PASSAGES

After a cholecystectomy (removal of the gallbladder), contrast medium was injected with a T tube inserted into the bile passages. The biliary passages are visualized in the superior abdomen in **A** and are more localized in **B.**

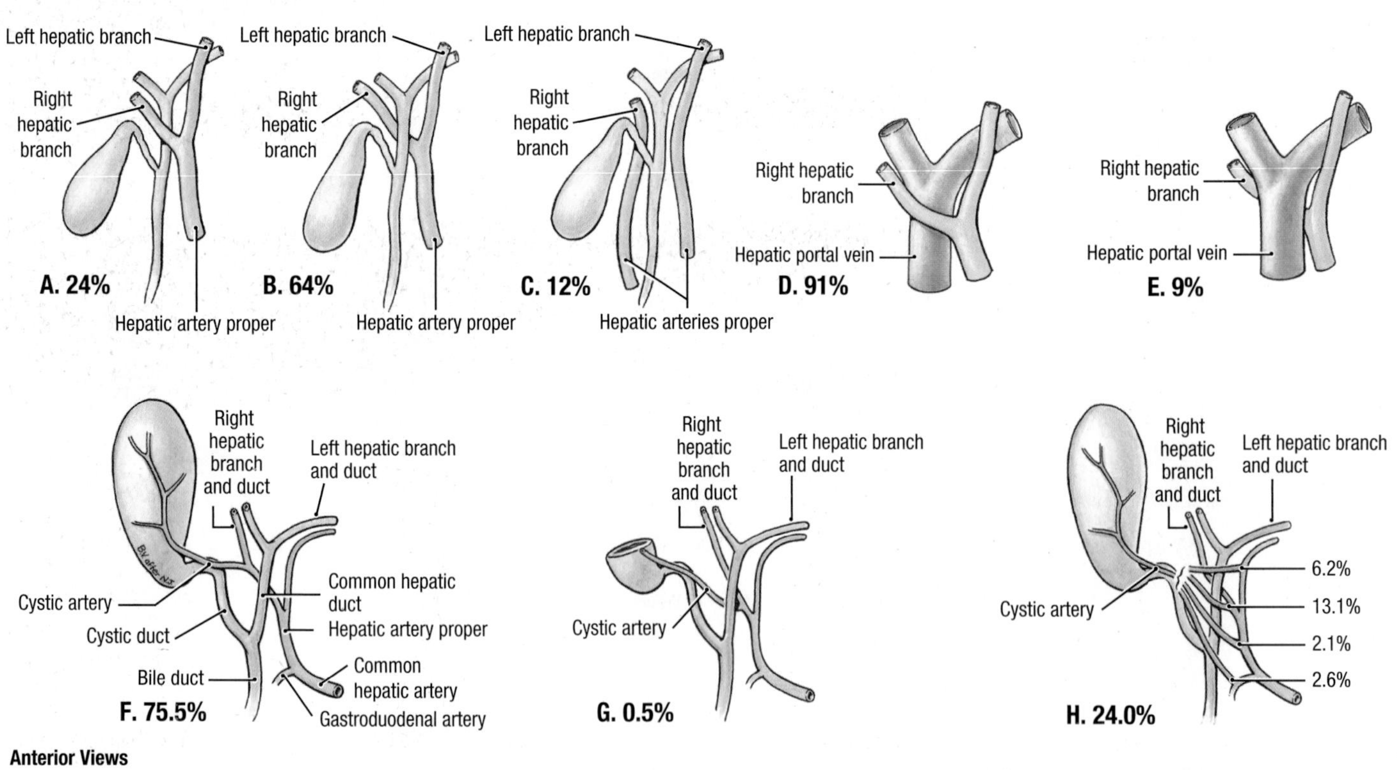
Left hepatic branch
Right hepatic branch
A. 24%
Hepatic artery proper
Left hepatic branch
Right hepatic branch
B. 64%
Hepatic artery proper
Left hepatic branch
Right hepatic branch
C. 12%
Hepatic arteries proper
Right hepatic branch
Hepatic portal vein
D. 91%
Right hepatic branch
Hepatic portal vein
E. 9%
Right hepatic branch and duct
Left hepatic branch and duct
Common hepatic duct
Hepatic artery proper
Cystic artery
Cystic duct
Bile duct
Common hepatic artery
Gastroduodenal artery
F. 75.5%
Right hepatic branch and duct
Left hepatic branch and duct
Cystic artery
G. 0.5%
Right hepatic branch and duct
Left hepatic branch and duct
Cystic artery
6.2%
13.1%
2.1%
2.6%
H. 24.0%
Anterior Views

2.62 VARIATIONS IN HEPATIC AND CYSTIC ARTERIES

In a study of 165 cadavers in Dr. Grant's laboratory, five patterns were observed. **A.** Right hepatic artery crossing anterior to bile passages, 24%. **B.** Right hepatic artery crossing posterior to bile passages, 64%. **C.** Aberrant artery arising from the superior mesenteric artery, 12%. The artery crossed anterior **(D)** to the portal vein in 91% and posterior **(E)** in 9%. The cystic artery usually arises from the right hepatic artery in the angle between the common hepatic duct and cystic duct (see cystohepatic triangle, Fig. 2.57A), without crossing the common hepatic duct **(F. and G)**. However, when it arises on the left of the bile passages, it almost always crosses anterior to the passages **(H)**.

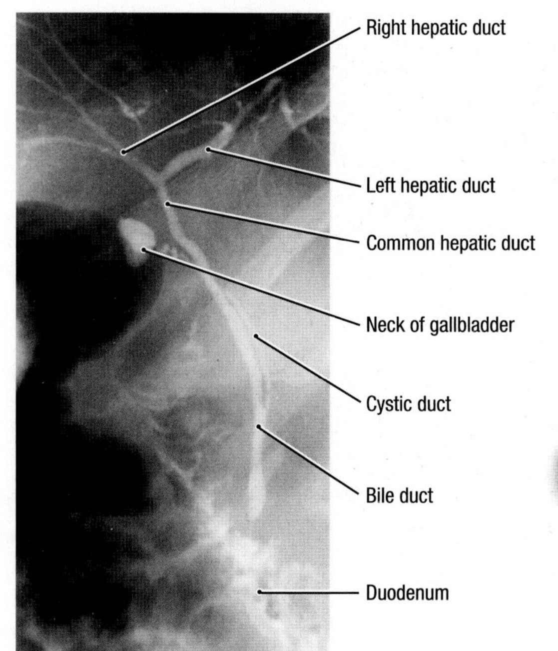
Right hepatic duct
Left hepatic duct
Common hepatic duct
Neck of gallbladder
Cystic duct
Bile duct
Duodenum

A. Anterior View

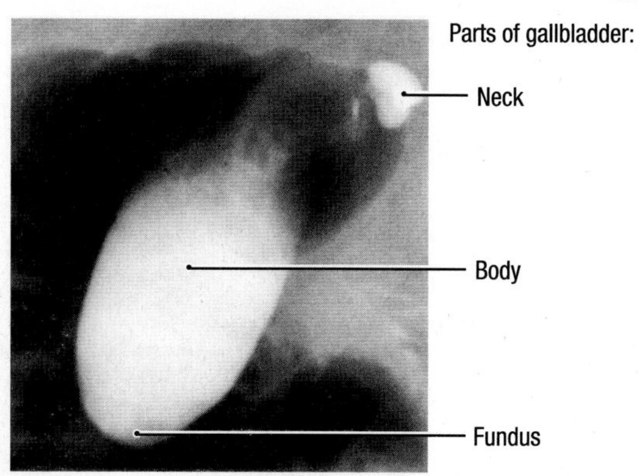
Parts of gallbladder:
Neck
Body
Fundus

B. Anterior View

2.63 ENDOSCOPIC RETROGRADE CHOLANGIOGRAPHY OF GALLBLADDER AND BILIARY PASSAGES

A. Cystic duct. **B.** Parts of gallbladder.

Endoscopic retrograde cholangiography (ERCP) is done by first passing a fiberoptic endoscope through the mouth, esophagus, and stomach. Then the duodenum is entered, and a cannula is inserted into the major duodenal papilla and advanced under fluoroscopic control into the duct of choice (bile duct or pancreatic duct) for injection of radiographic contrast medium.

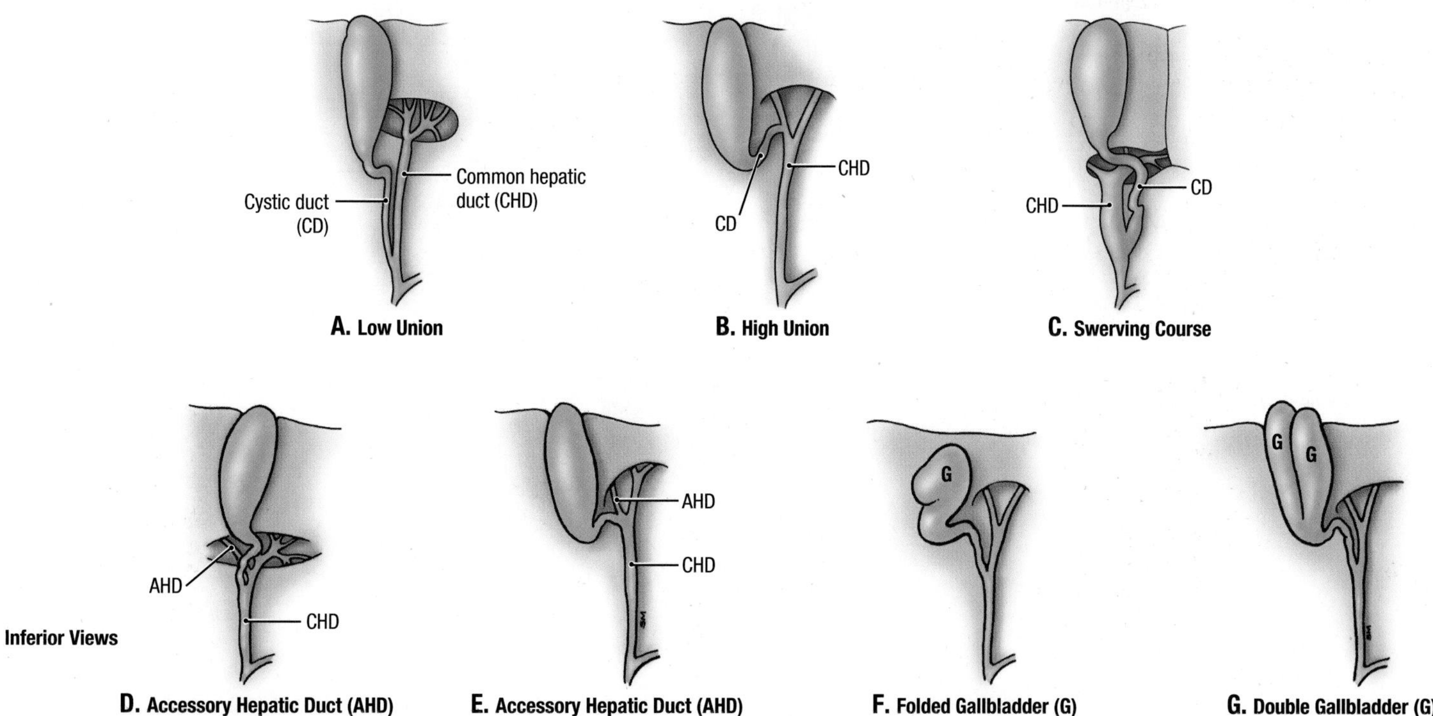
Cystic duct (CD)
Common hepatic duct (CHD)
CHD
CD
CHD
CD
AHD
CHD
AHD
CHD
G
G
G
Inferior Views

A. Low Union **B.** High Union **C.** Swerving Course

D. Accessory Hepatic Duct (AHD) **E.** Accessory Hepatic Duct (AHD) **F.** Folded Gallbladder (G) **G.** Double Gallbladder (G)

2.64 VARIATIONS OF CYSTIC AND HEPATIC DUCTS AND GALLBLADDER

The cystic duct usually lies on the right side of the common hepatic duct, joining it just above the superior (1st) part of the duodenum, but this varies as in **A.–C.** Of 95 gallbladders and bile passages studied in Dr. Grant's laboratory, 7 had accessory ducts. Of these, four joined the common hepatic duct near the cystic duct **(D),** two joined the cystic duct **(E)**, and one was an anastomosing duct connecting the cystic with the common hepatic duct. **F.** Folded gallbladder. **G.** Double gallbladder.

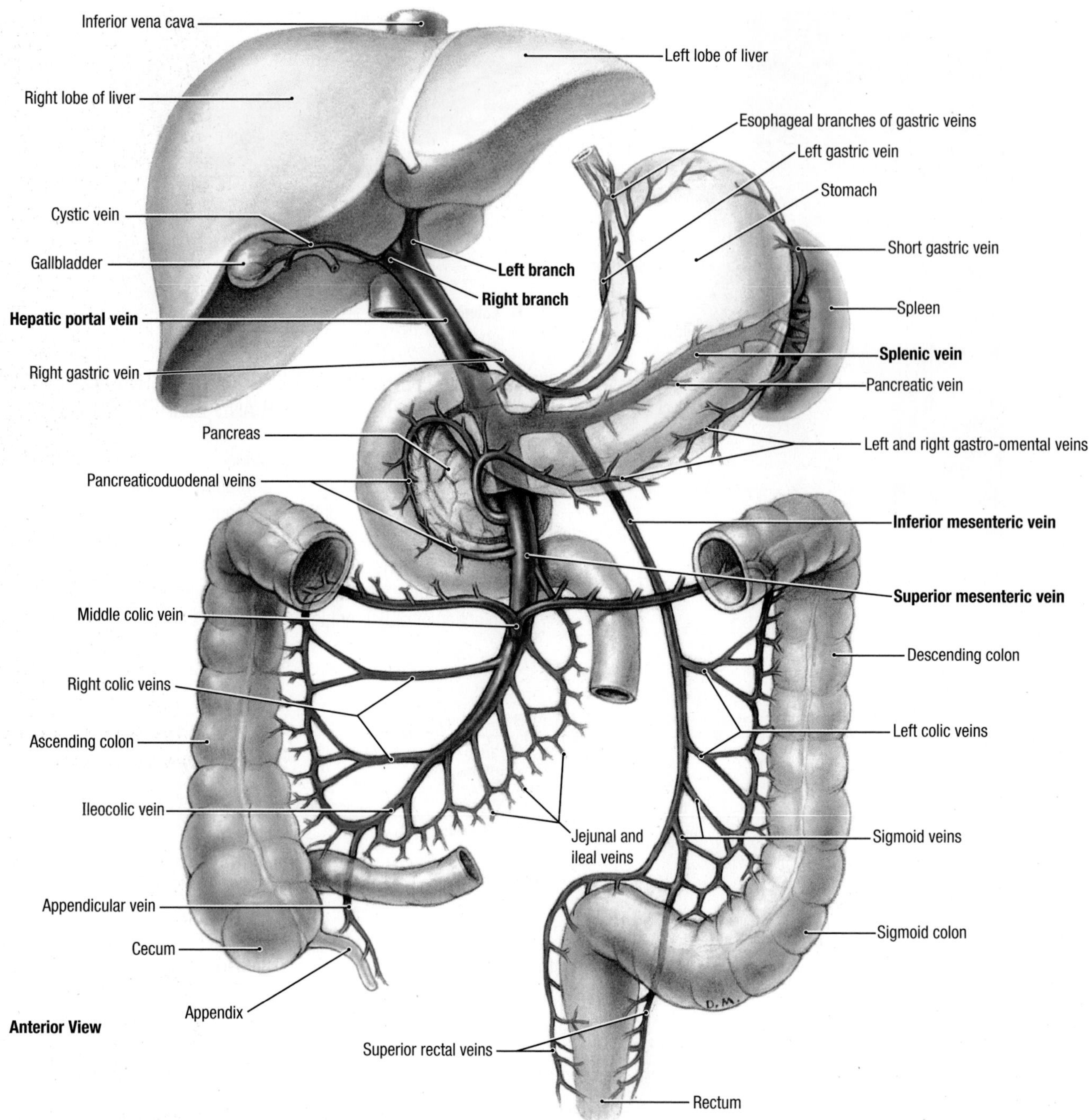
Inferior vena cava
Left lobe of liver
Right lobe of liver
Esophageal branches of gastric veins
Left gastric vein
Stomach
Cystic vein
Short gastric vein
Gallbladder
Left branch
Right branch
Spleen
Hepatic portal vein
Splenic vein
Right gastric vein
Pancreatic vein
Pancreas
Left and right gastro-omental veins
Pancreaticoduodenal veins
Inferior mesenteric vein
Superior mesenteric vein
Middle colic vein
Descending colon
Right colic veins
Ascending colon
Left colic veins
Ileocolic vein
Jejunal and ileal veins
Sigmoid veins
Appendicular vein
Sigmoid colon
Cecum
Appendix
Anterior View
Superior rectal veins
Rectum

2.65 PORTAL VENOUS SYSTEM

- The hepatic portal vein drains venous blood from the gastrointestinal tract, spleen, pancreas, and gallbladder to the sinusoids of the liver; from here, the blood is conveyed to the systemic venous system by the hepatic veins that drain directly to the inferior vena cava.
- The hepatic portal vein forms posterior to the neck of the pancreas by the union of the superior mesenteric and splenic veins, with the inferior mesenteric vein joining at or near the angle of union.
- The splenic vein drains blood from the inferior mesenteric, left gastro-omental (epiploic), short gastric, and pancreatic veins.
- The right gastro-omental, pancreaticoduodenal, jejunal, ileal, right, and middle colic veins drain into the superior mesenteric vein.
- The inferior mesenteric vein commences in the rectal plexus as the superior rectal vein and, after crossing the common iliac vessels, becomes the inferior mesenteric vein; branches include the sigmoid and left colic veins.
- The hepatic portal vein divides into right and left branches at the porta hepatis. The left branch carries mainly, but not exclusively, blood from the inferior mesenteric, gastric, and splenic veins, and the right branch carries blood mainly from the superior mesenteric vein.

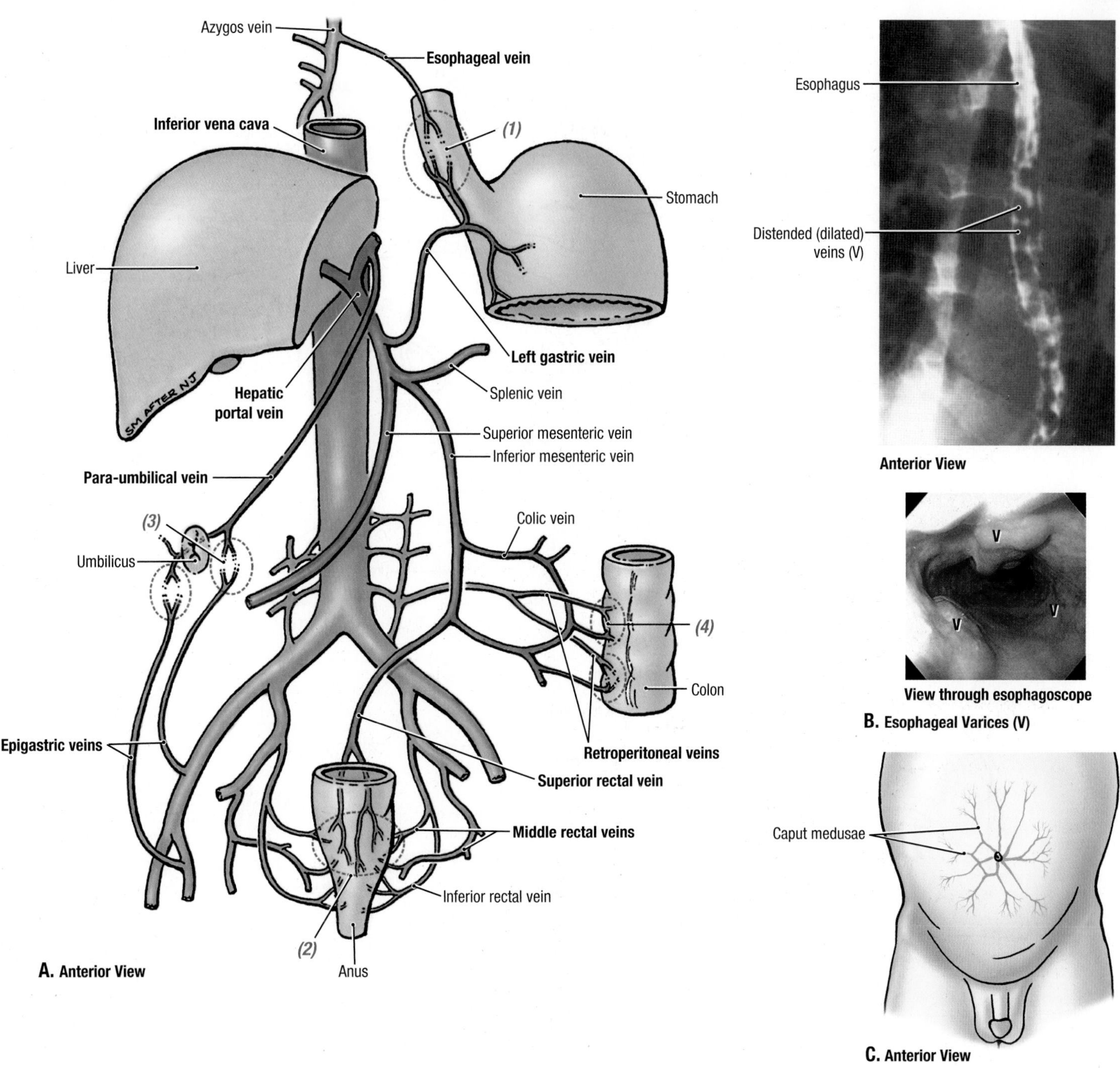
Azygos vein
Esophageal vein
Inferior vena cava
(1)
Stomach
Liver
Left gastric vein
Splenic vein
Hepatic portal vein
SM AFTER NJ
Superior mesenteric vein
Inferior mesenteric vein
Para-umbilical vein
Colic vein
(3)
Umbilicus
(4)
Colon
Epigastric veins
Retroperitoneal veins
Superior rectal vein
Middle rectal veins
Inferior rectal vein
(2)
Anus
Esophagus
Distended (dilated) veins (V)
V
V
V
Caput medusae

A. Anterior View

Anterior View

View through esophagoscope

B. Esophageal Varices (V)

C. Anterior View

2.66 PORTACAVAL SYSTEM

A. Portacaval system. In this diagram, portal tributaries are *dark blue*, and systemic tributaries and communicating veins are *light blue*. In **portal hypertension** (as in hepatic cirrhosis), the portal blood cannot pass freely through the liver, and the portocaval anastomoses become engorged, dilated, or even varicose; as a consequence, these veins may rupture. The sites of the portocaval anastomosis shown are between *(1)* esophageal veins draining into the azygos vein (systemic) and left gastric vein (portal), which when dilated are esophageal varices; *(2)* the inferior and middle rectal veins, draining into the inferior vena cava (systemic) and the superior rectal vein continuing as the inferior mesenteric vein (portal) (hemorrhoids result if the vessels are dilated); *(3)* paraumbilical veins (portal) and small epigastric veins of the anterior abdominal wall (systemic), which when varicose form "caput medusae" (so named because of the resemblance of the radiating veins to the serpents on the head of Medusa, a character in Greek mythology); and *(4)* twigs of colic veins (portal) anastomosing with systemic retroperitoneal veins. **B.** Esophageal varices. **C.** Caput medusae.

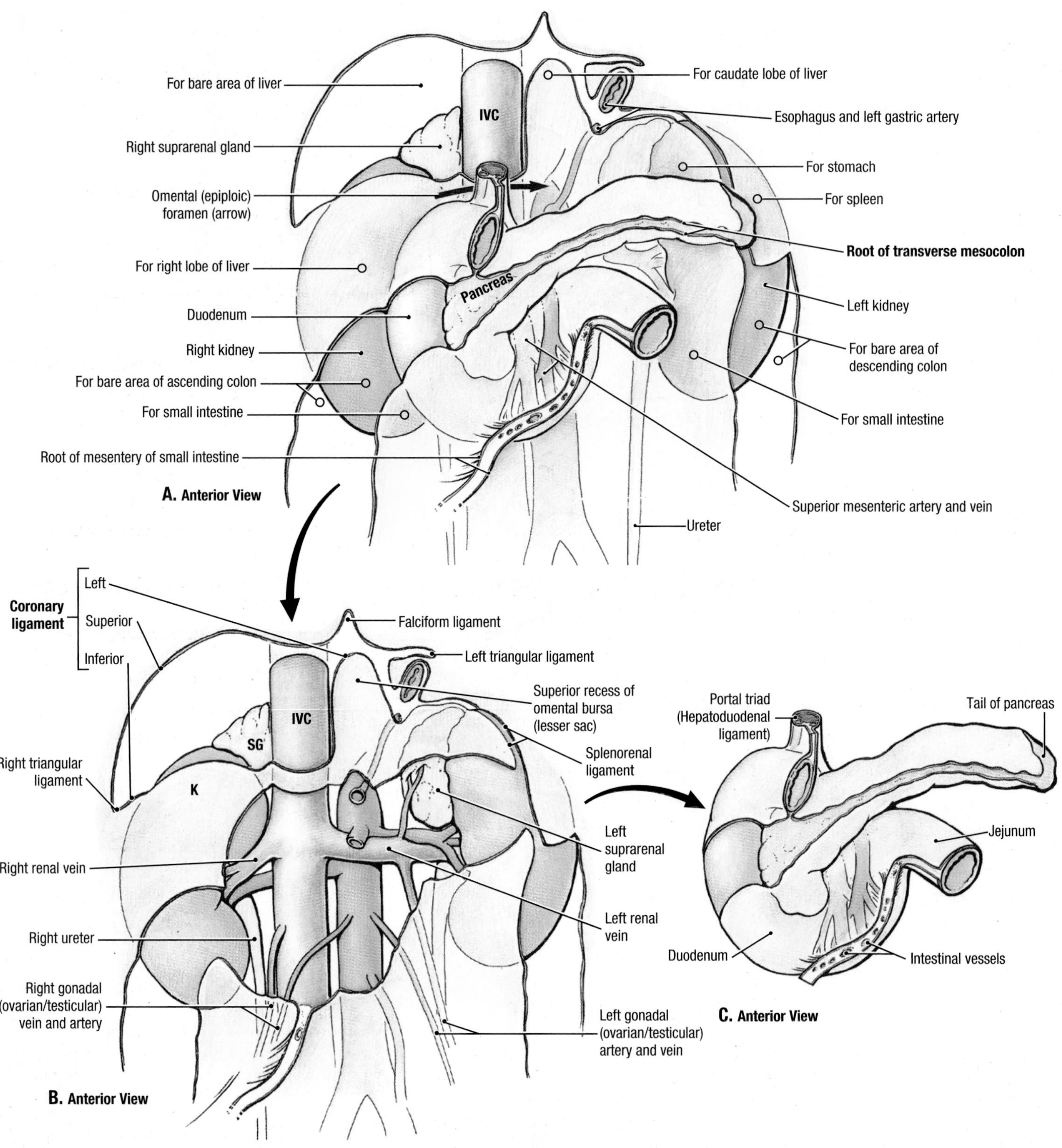
For bare area of liver
Right suprarenal gland
Omental (epiploic) foramen (arrow)
For right lobe of liver
Duodenum
Right kidney
For bare area of ascending colon
For small intestine
Root of mesentery of small intestine
IVC
Pancreas
For caudate lobe of liver
Esophagus and left gastric artery
For stomach
For spleen
Root of transverse mesocolon
Left kidney
For bare area of descending colon
For small intestine
Superior mesenteric artery and vein
Ureter
A. Anterior View
Coronary ligament
Left
Superior
Inferior
Falciform ligament
Left triangular ligament
Superior recess of omental bursa (lesser sac)
Splenorenal ligament
IVC
SG
K
Right triangular ligament
Right renal vein
Right ureter
Right gonadal (ovarian/testicular) vein and artery
Left suprarenal gland
Left renal vein
Left gonadal (ovarian/testicular) artery and vein
B. Anterior View
Portal triad (Hepatoduodenal ligament)
Tail of pancreas
Jejunum
Duodenum
Intestinal vessels
C. Anterior View

2.67 POSTERIOR ABDOMINAL VISCERA AND THEIR ANTERIOR RELATIONS

The peritoneal coverings are yellow. **A.** Duodenum and pancreas in situ. Note the line of attachment of the root of the transverse mesocolon is to the body and tail of the pancreas. The viscera contacting specific regions are indicated by the term "for." The omental (epiploic) foramen is traversed by an arrow. **B.** After removal of duodenum and pancreas. The three parts of the coronary ligament are attached to the diaphragm, except where the inferior vena cava (IVC), suprarenal gland (SG), and kidney (K) intervene. **C.** Pancreas and duodenum removed from **A.**

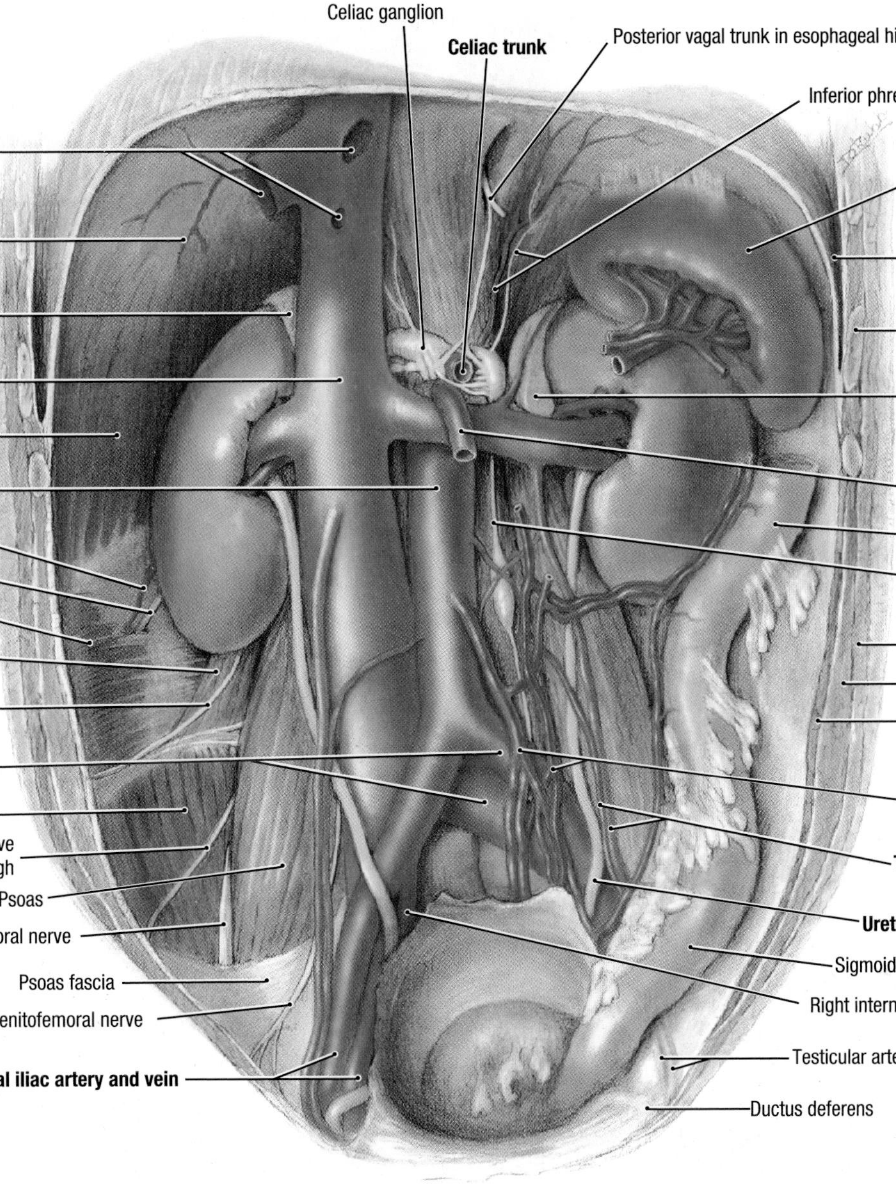

Celiac ganglion
Celiac trunk
Posterior vagal trunk in esophageal hiatus
Inferior phrenic artery and plexus
Hepatic veins
Spleen
Inferior phrenic artery
Costodiaphragmatic recess
Right suprarenal gland
10th rib
Inferior vena cava
Left suprarenal gland
Diaphragm
Abdominal aorta
Superior mesenteric artery
Subcostal artery
Descending colon
Subcostal nerve
Sympathetic trunk
Transversus abdominis
Quadratus lumborum
External oblique
Iliohypogastric and ilio-inguinal nerves
Internal oblique
Transversus abdominis
Left common iliac artery and vein
Inferior mesenteric artery and vein
Iliacus
Lateral cutaneous nerve of thigh
Testicular artery and vein
Psoas
Femoral nerve
Ureter
Sigmoid colon
Psoas fascia
Right internal iliac artery
Genitofemoral nerve
Testicular artery and vein
External iliac artery and vein
Ductus deferens

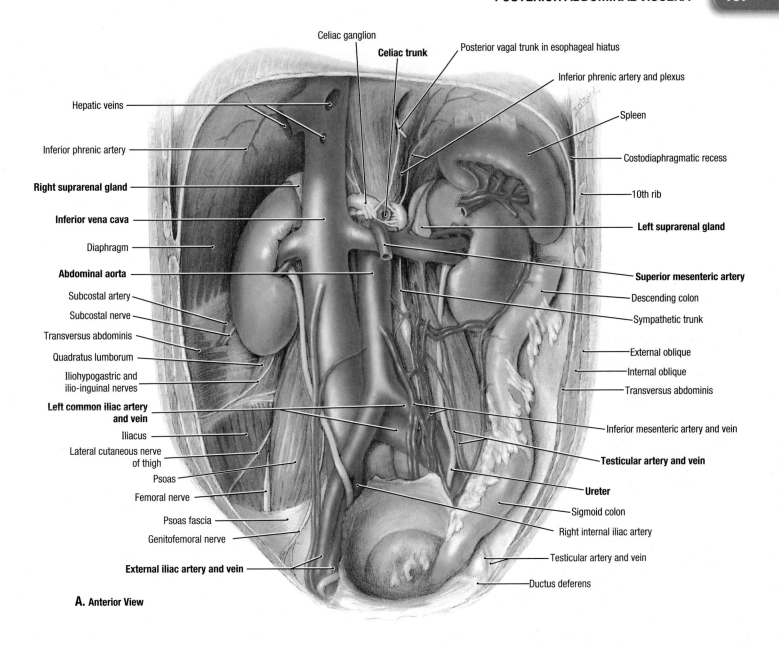

A. Anterior View

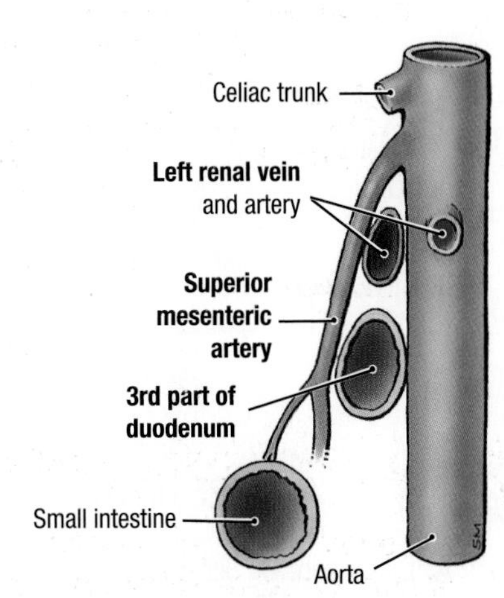
Celiac trunk
Left renal vein
and artery
Superior
mesenteric
artery
3rd part of
duodenum
Small intestine
Aorta

B. Lateral View (from left)

2.68 VISCERA AND VESSELS OF POSTERIOR ABDOMINAL WALL

A. Great vessels, kidneys, and suprarenal glands. **B.** Relationships of left renal vein and inferior (3rd) part of duodenum to aorta and superior mesenteric artery.

- The abdominal aorta is shorter and smaller in caliber than the inferior vena cava.
- The inferior mesenteric artery arises about 4 cm superior to the aortic bifurcation and crosses the left common iliac vessels to become the superior rectal artery.
- The left renal vein drains the left testis, left suprarenal gland, and left kidney; the renal arteries are posterior to the renal veins.
- The ureter crosses the external iliac artery just beyond the common iliac bifurcation.
- The testicular vessels cross anterior to the ureter and join the ductus deferens at the deep inguinal ring.
- In **B**, the left renal vein and duodenum (and uncinate process of pancreas—not shown) pass between the aorta posteriorly and the superior mesenteric artery anteriorly; they may be compressed like nuts in a nutcracker.

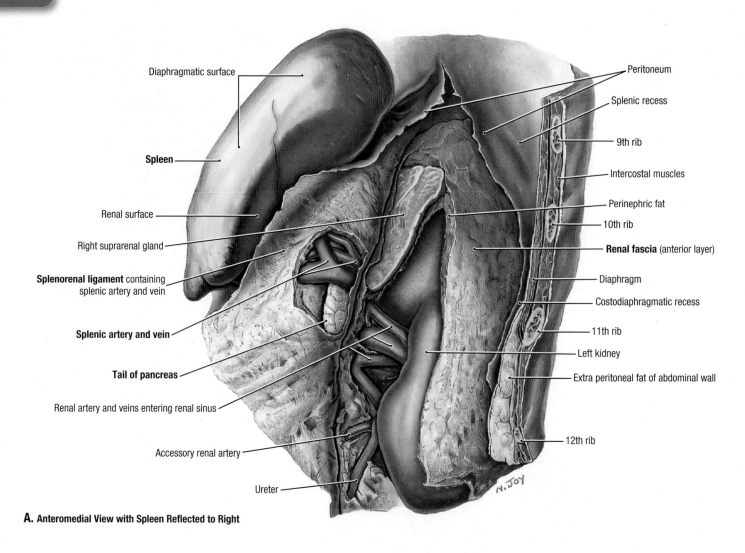

Diaphragmatic surface
Spleen
Renal surface
Right suprarenal gland
Splenorenal ligament containing splenic artery and vein
Splenic artery and vein
Tail of pancreas
Renal artery and veins entering renal sinus
Accessory renal artery
Ureter
Peritoneum
Splenic recess
9th rib
Intercostal muscles
Perinephric fat
10th rib
Renal fascia (anterior layer)
Diaphragm
Costodiaphragmatic recess
11th rib
Left kidney
Extra peritoneal fat of abdominal wall
12th rib
N. Joy

A. Anteromedial View with Spleen Reflected to Right

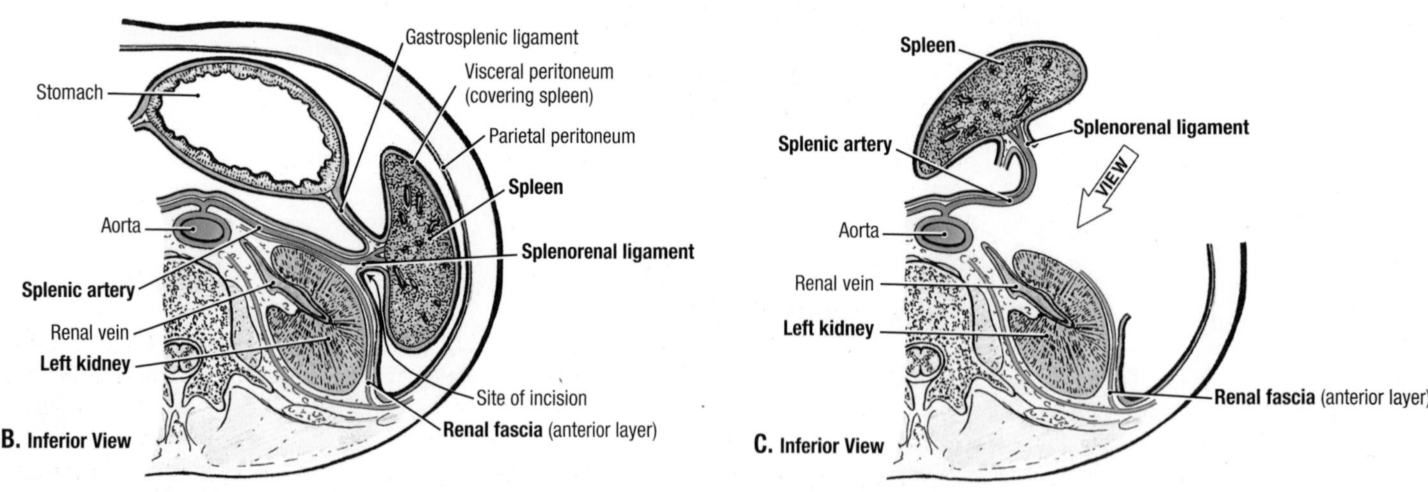
Stomach
Gastrosplenic ligament
Visceral peritoneum (covering spleen)
Parietal peritoneum
Spleen
Aorta
Splenorenal ligament
Splenic artery
Renal vein
Left kidney
Site of incision
Renal fascia (anterior layer)
Spleen
Splenic artery
Splenorenal ligament
VIEW
Aorta
Renal vein
Left kidney
Renal fascia (anterior layer)

B. Inferior View

C. Inferior View

2.69 EXPOSURE OF THE LEFT KIDNEY AND SUPRARENAL GLAND

A. Dissection. **B.** Schematic section with spleen and splenorenal ligament intact. **C.** Procedure used in **A** to expose the kidney. The spleen and splenorenal ligament are reflected anteriorly, with the splenic vessels and tail of the pancreas. Part of the renal fascia of the kidney is removed. Note the proximity of the splenic vein and left renal vein, enabling a **splenorenal shunt** to be established surgically to relieve portal hypertension.

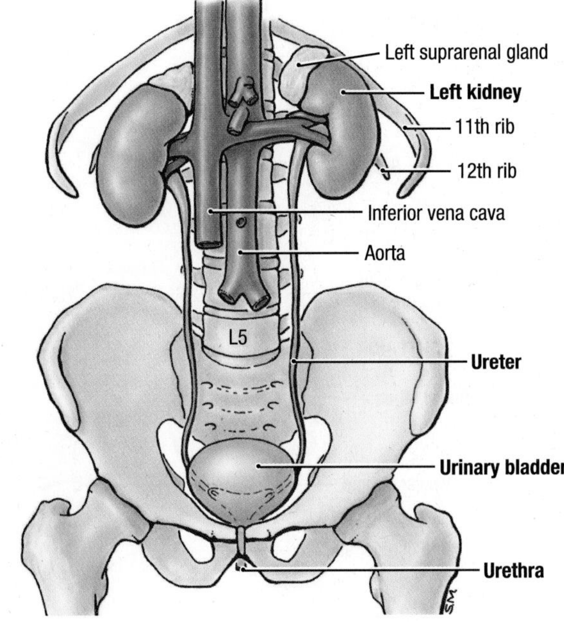
Left suprarenal gland
Left kidney
11th rib
12th rib
Inferior vena cava
Aorta
L5
Ureter
Urinary bladder
Urethra

A. Anterior View

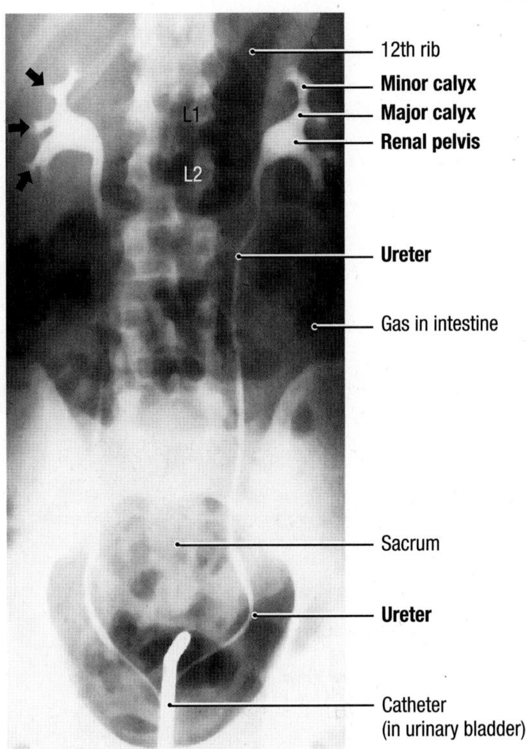
L1
L2
12th rib
Minor calyx
Major calyx
Renal pelvis
Ureter
Gas in intestine
Sacrum
Ureter
Catheter
(in urinary bladder)

B. Anteroposterior Pyelogram

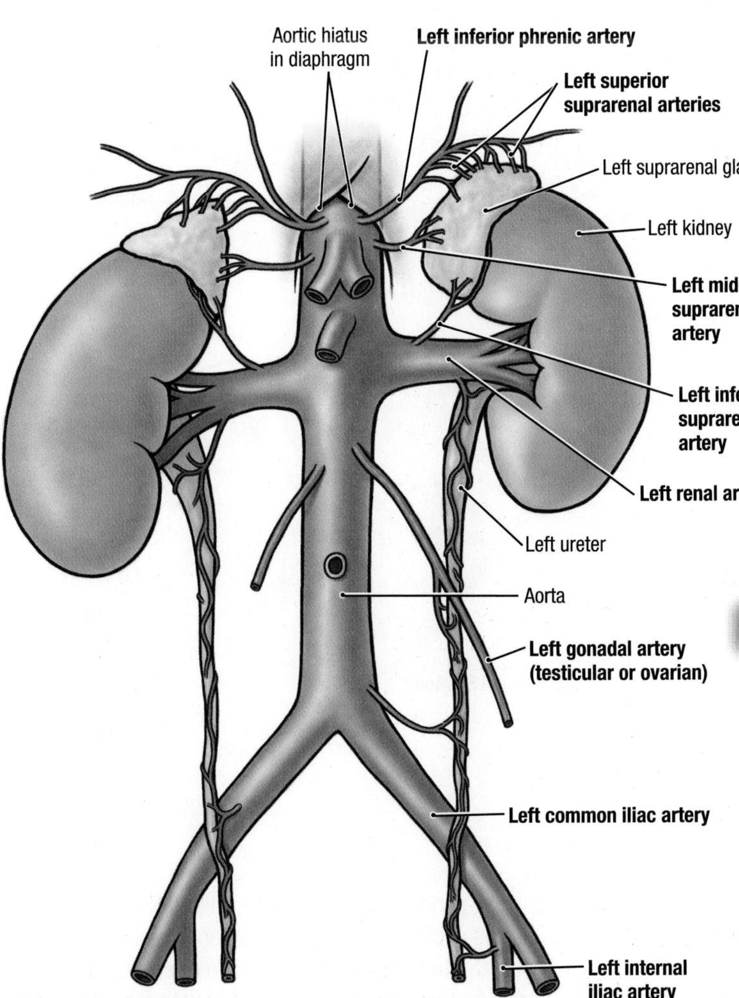
Aortic hiatus
in diaphragm
Left inferior phrenic artery
Left superior
suprarenal arteries
Left suprarenal gland
Left kidney
Left middle
suprarenal
artery
Left inferior
suprarenal
artery
Left renal artery
Left ureter
Aorta
Left gonadal artery
(testicular or ovarian)
Left common iliac artery
Left internal
iliac artery

C. Anterior View

2.70 KIDNEYS AND SUPRARENAL GLANDS

A. Overview of urinary system. **B.** Pyelogram. Radiopaque material occupies the cavities that normally conduct urine. Note the papillae (indicated with *arrows*) bulging into the minor calices, which empty into a major calyx that opens, in turn, into the renal pelvis drained by the ureter. **C.** Arterial supply of the suprarenal glands, kidneys, and ureters.

Renal transplantation is now an established operation for the treatment of selected cases of chronic renal failure. The kidney can be removed from the donor without damaging the suprarenal gland because of the weak septum of renal fascia that separates the kidney from this gland. The site for transplanting a kidney is in the iliac fossa of the greater pelvis. The renal artery and vein are joined to the external iliac artery and vein, respectively, and the ureter is sutured into the urinary bladder.

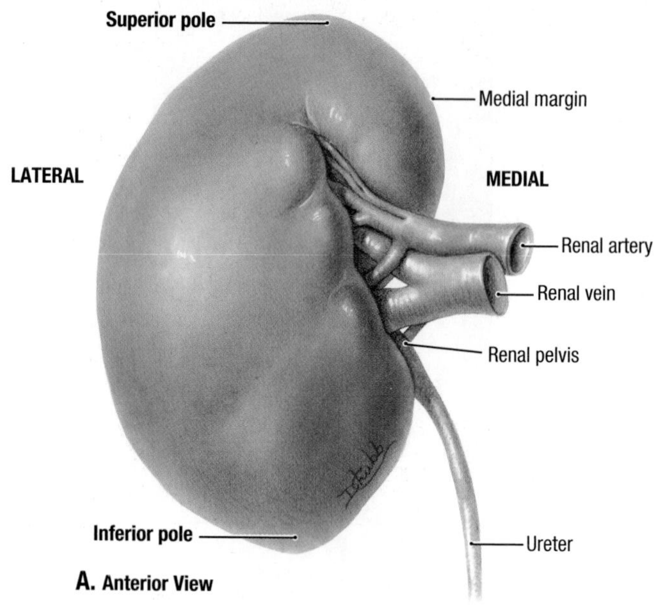
Superior pole
Medial margin
LATERAL
MEDIAL
Renal artery
Renal vein
Renal pelvis
Inferior pole
Ureter

A. Anterior View

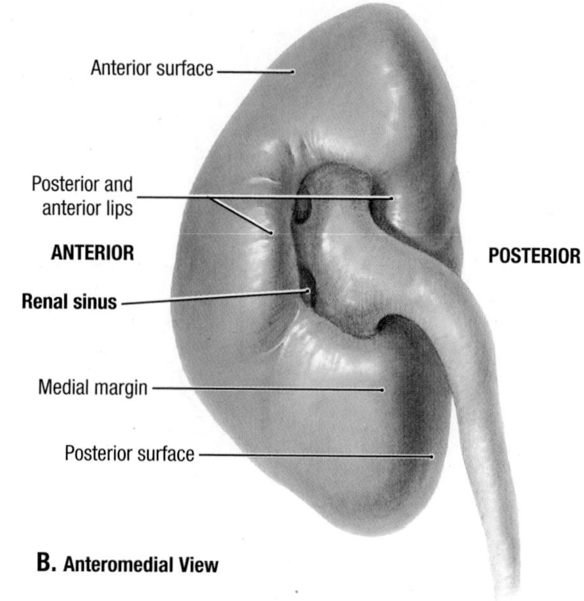
Anterior surface
Posterior and anterior lips
ANTERIOR
POSTERIOR
Renal sinus
Medial margin
Posterior surface

B. Anteromedial View

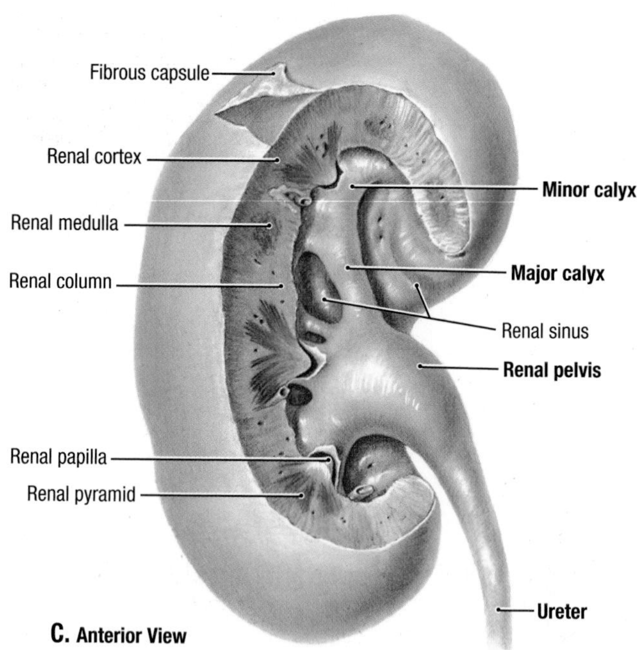
Fibrous capsule
Renal cortex
Minor calyx
Renal medulla
Major calyx
Renal column
Renal sinus
Renal pelvis
Renal papilla
Renal pyramid
Ureter

C. Anterior View

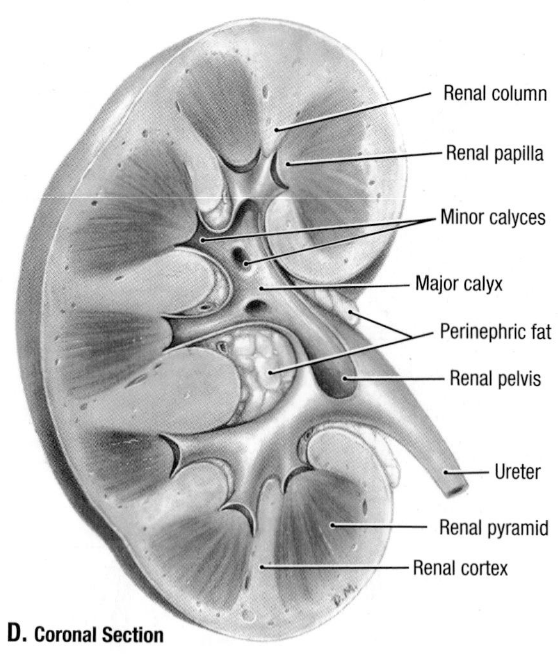
Renal column
Renal papilla
Minor calyces
Major calyx
Perinephric fat
Renal pelvis
Ureter
Renal pyramid
Renal cortex

D. Coronal Section

2.71 STRUCTURE OF KIDNEY

A. External features. The superior pole of the kidney is closer to the median plane than the inferior pole. Approximately 25% of kidneys may have a 2nd, 3rd, and even 4th accessory renal artery branching from the aorta. These multiple vessels enter through the renal sinus or at the superior or inferior pole. **B.** Renal sinus. The renal sinus is a vertical "pocket" opening on the medial side of the kidney. Tucked into the pocket are the renal pelvis and renal vessels in a matrix of perinephric fat. **C.** Renal calices. The anterior wall of the renal sinus has been cut away to expose the renal pelvis and the calices. **D.** Internal features. **Cysts in the kidney**, multiple or solitary, are common and usually benign findings during ultrasound examinations and dissection of cadavers. **Adult polycystic disease** of the kidneys, however, is an important cause of renal failure.

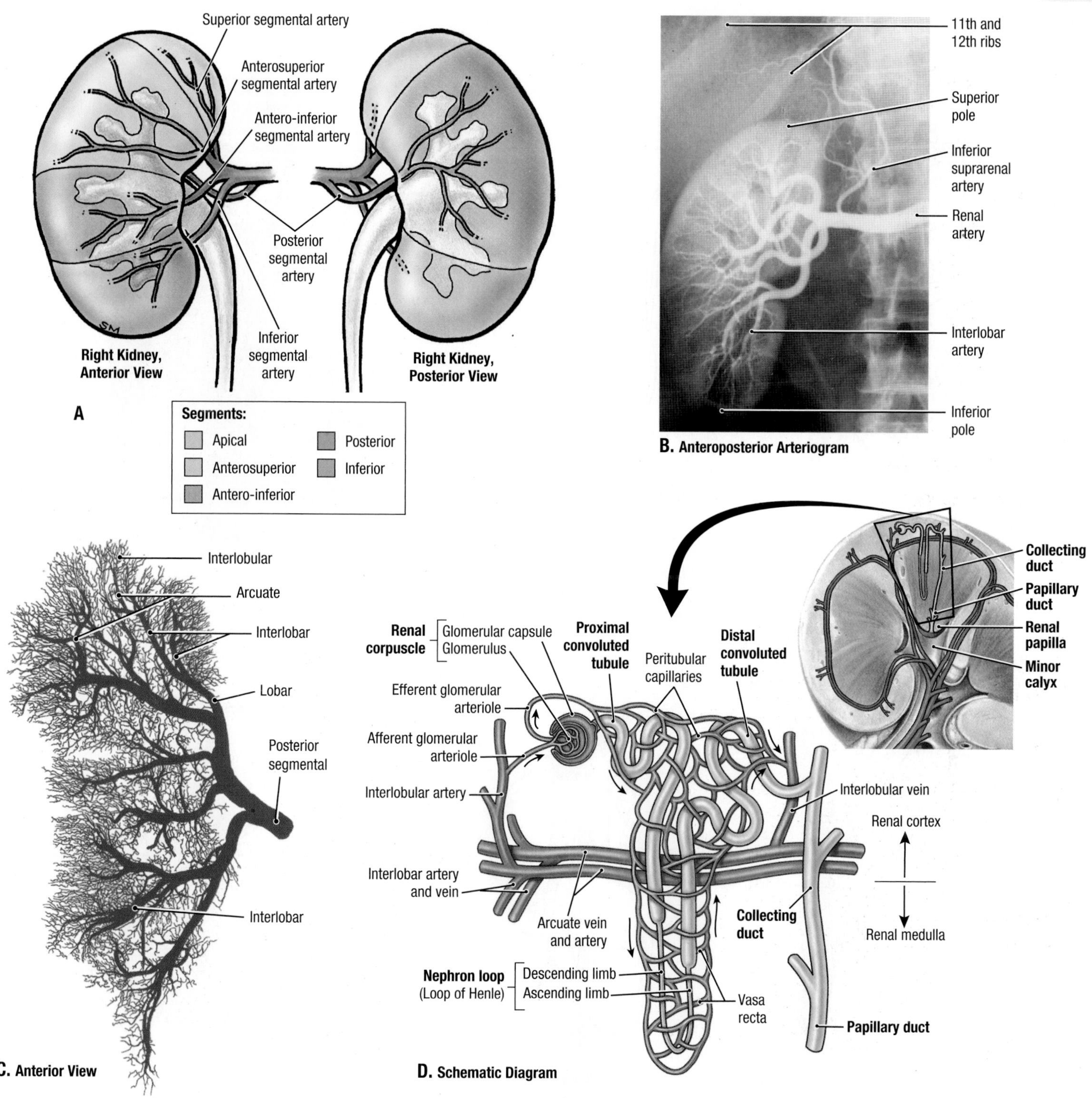
Superior segmental artery
Anterosuperior segmental artery
Antero-inferior segmental artery
Posterior segmental artery
Inferior segmental artery
Right Kidney, Anterior View
Right Kidney, Posterior View
A
Segments:
Apical
Anterosuperior
Antero-inferior
Posterior
Inferior
11th and 12th ribs
Superior pole
Inferior suprarenal artery
Renal artery
Interlobar artery
Inferior pole
B. Anteroposterior Arteriogram
Interlobular
Arcuate
Interlobar
Lobar
Posterior segmental
Interlobar
C. Anterior View
Renal corpuscle
Glomerular capsule
Glomerulus
Proximal convoluted tubule
Peritubular capillaries
Distal convoluted tubule
Efferent glomerular arteriole
Afferent glomerular arteriole
Interlobular artery
Interlobular vein
Renal cortex
Interlobar artery and vein
Arcuate vein and artery
Collecting duct
Renal medulla
Nephron loop (Loop of Henle)
Descending limb
Ascending limb
Vasa recta
Papillary duct
D. Schematic Diagram
Collecting duct
Papillary duct
Renal papilla
Minor calyx

2.72 SEGMENTS OF THE KIDNEYS

A. Segmental arteries. Segmental arteries do not anastomose significantly with other segmental arteries; they are end arteries. The area supplied by each segmented artery is an independent, surgically respectable unit or **renal segment. B.** Renal arteriogram. **C.** Corrosion cast of posterior segmental artery of kidney. **D.** The nephron is the functional unit of the kidney consisting of a renal corpuscle, proximal tubule, nephron loop, and distal tubule. Papillary ducts open onto renal papillae, emptying into minor calices.

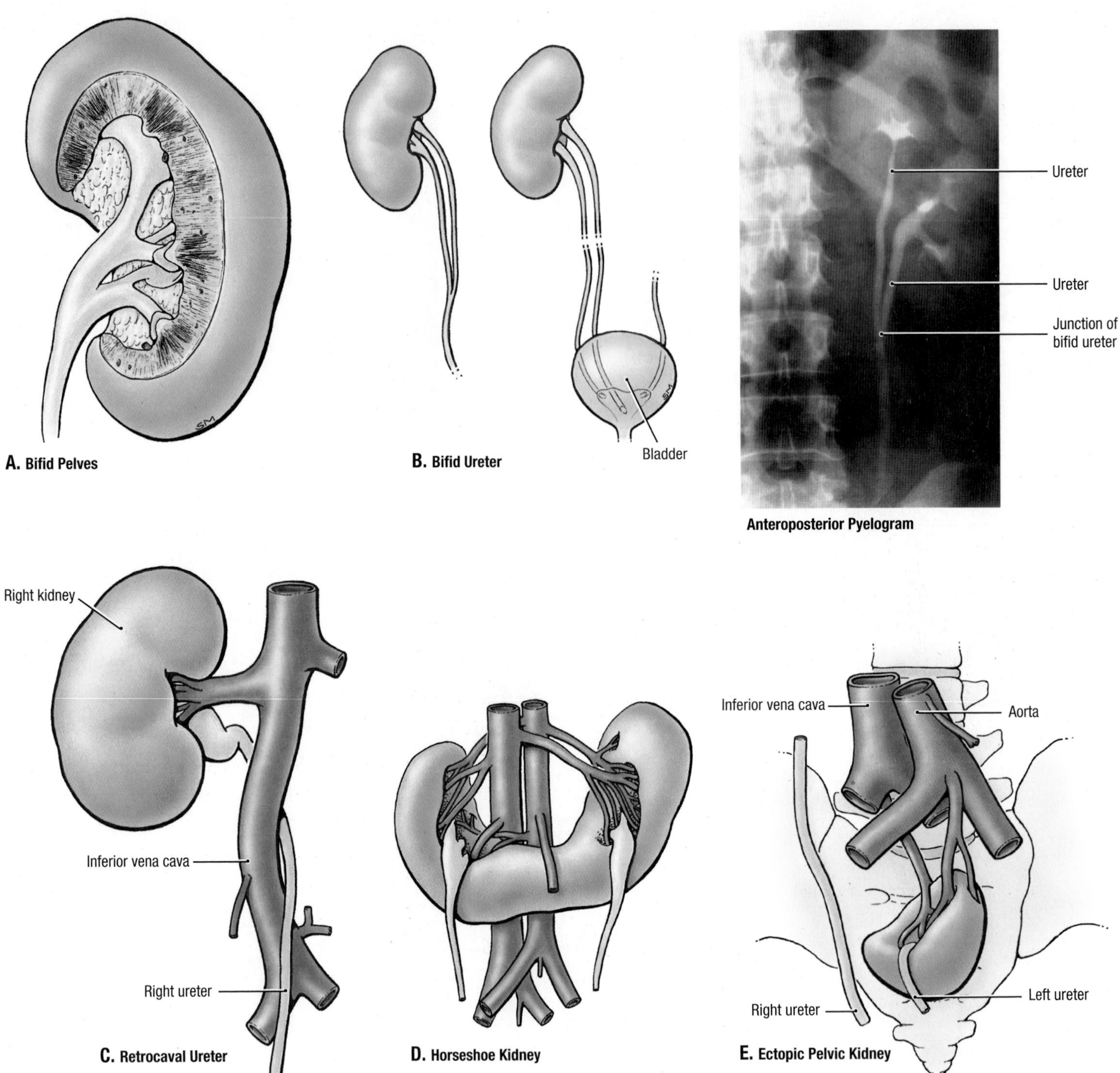
Ureter
Ureter
Junction of
bifid ureter
Bladder
Right kidney
Inferior vena cava
Right ureter
Inferior vena cava
Aorta
Right ureter
Left ureter

A. Bifid Pelves

B. Bifid Ureter

Anteroposterior Pyelogram

C. Retrocaval Ureter

D. Horseshoe Kidney

E. Ectopic Pelvic Kidney

Anterior Views

2.73 ANOMALIES OF KIDNEY AND URETER

A. Bifid pelves. The pelves are almost replaced by two long major calices, which extend outside the sinus. **B. Duplicated, or bifid, ureters**. These can be unilateral or bilateral and complete or incomplete. **C. Retrocaval ureter.** The ureter courses posterior and then anterior to the inferior vena cava. **D. Horseshoe kidney.** The right and left kidneys are fused in the midline. **E. Ectopic pelvic kidney.** Pelvic kidneys have no fatty capsule and can be unilateral or bilateral. During childbirth, they may cause obstruction and suffer injury.

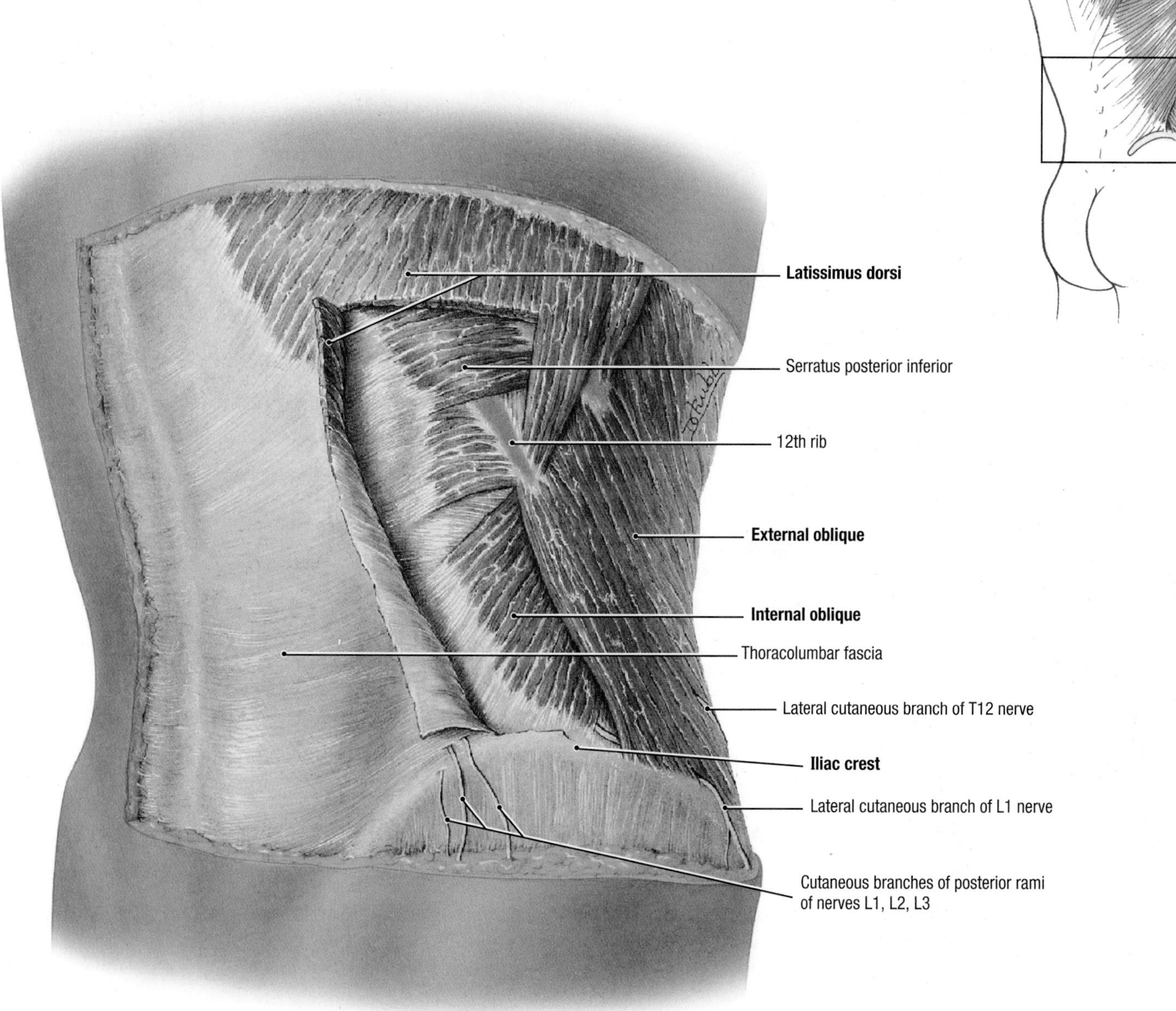
Latissimus dorsi
Serratus posterior inferior
12th rib
External oblique
Internal oblique
Thoracolumbar fascia
Lateral cutaneous branch of T12 nerve
Iliac crest
Lateral cutaneous branch of L1 nerve
Cutaneous branches of posterior rami of nerves L1, L2, L3

Posterolateral View

2.74 POSTEROLATERAL ABDOMINAL WALL: EXPOSURE OF KIDNEY I

The latissimus dorsi is partially reflected.

- The external oblique muscle has an oblique, free posterior border that extends from the tip of the 12th rib to the midpoint of the iliac crest.
- The internal oblique muscle extends posteriorly beyond the border of the external oblique muscle.

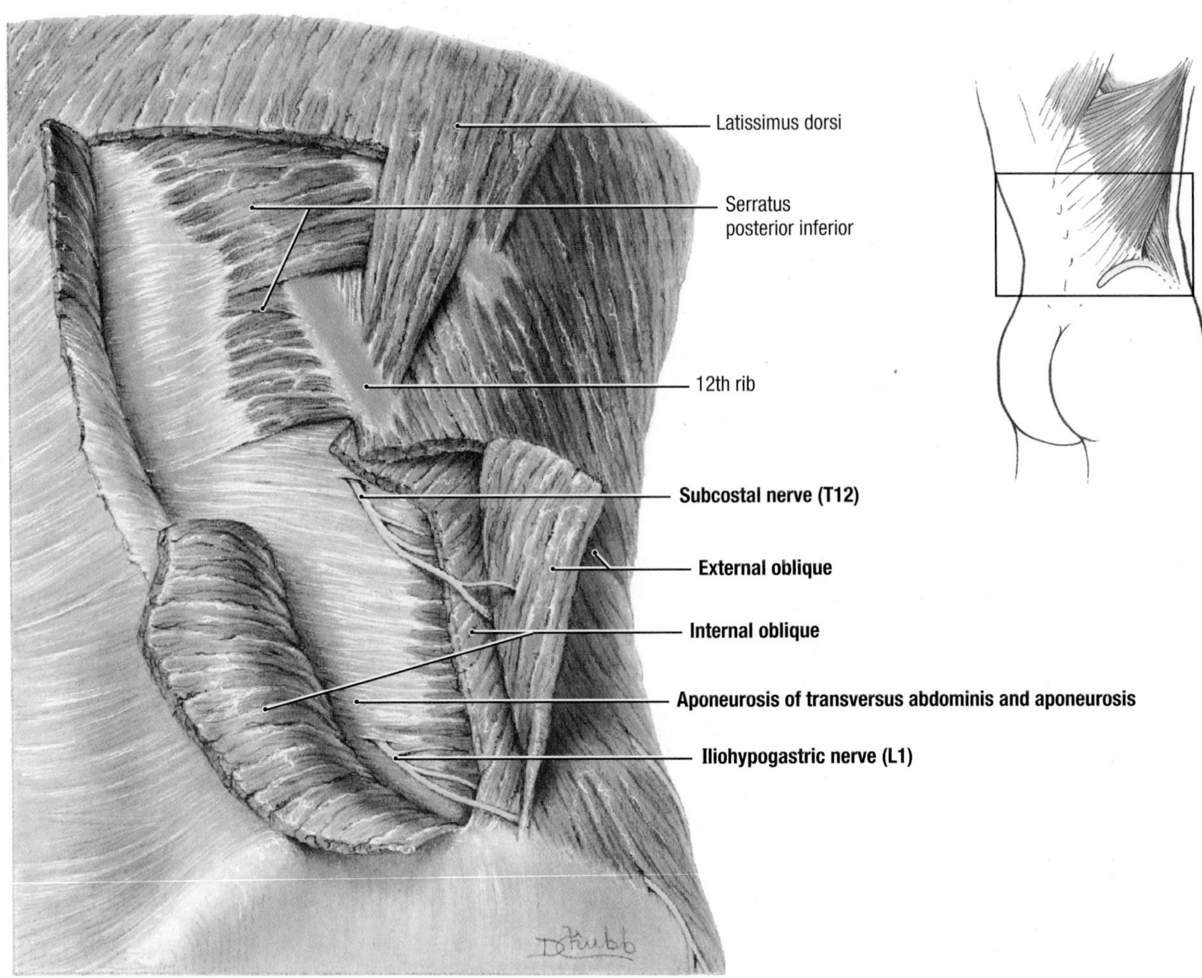
Latissimus dorsi
Serratus posterior inferior
12th rib
Subcostal nerve (T12)
External oblique
Internal oblique
Aponeurosis of transversus abdominis and aponeurosis
Iliohypogastric nerve (L1)
Posterolateral View

2.75 POSTEROLATERAL ABDOMINAL WALL: EXPOSURE OF KIDNEY II

The external oblique muscle is incised and reflected laterally, and the internal oblique muscle is incised and reflected medially; the transversus abdominis muscle and its posterior aponeurosis are exposed where pierced by the subcostal (T12) and iliohypogastric (L1) nerves. These nerves give off motor twigs and lateral cutaneous branches and continue anteriorly between the internal oblique and transversus abdominis muscles.

2.76 POSTEROLATERAL ABDOMINAL WALL: EXPOSURE OF KIDNEY III AND RENAL FASCIA →

A. The posterior aponeurosis of the transversus abdominis muscle is divided between the subcostal and iliohypogastric nerves and lateral to the oblique lateral border of the quadratus lumborum muscle; the retroperitoneal fat surrounding the kidney is exposed. **B.** Renal fascia and retroperitoneal fat, schematic transverse section. The renal fascia is within this fat; the portion of fat internal to the renal fascia is termed perinephric fat (perirenal fat capsule), and the fat immediately external is paranephric fat (pararenal fat body).

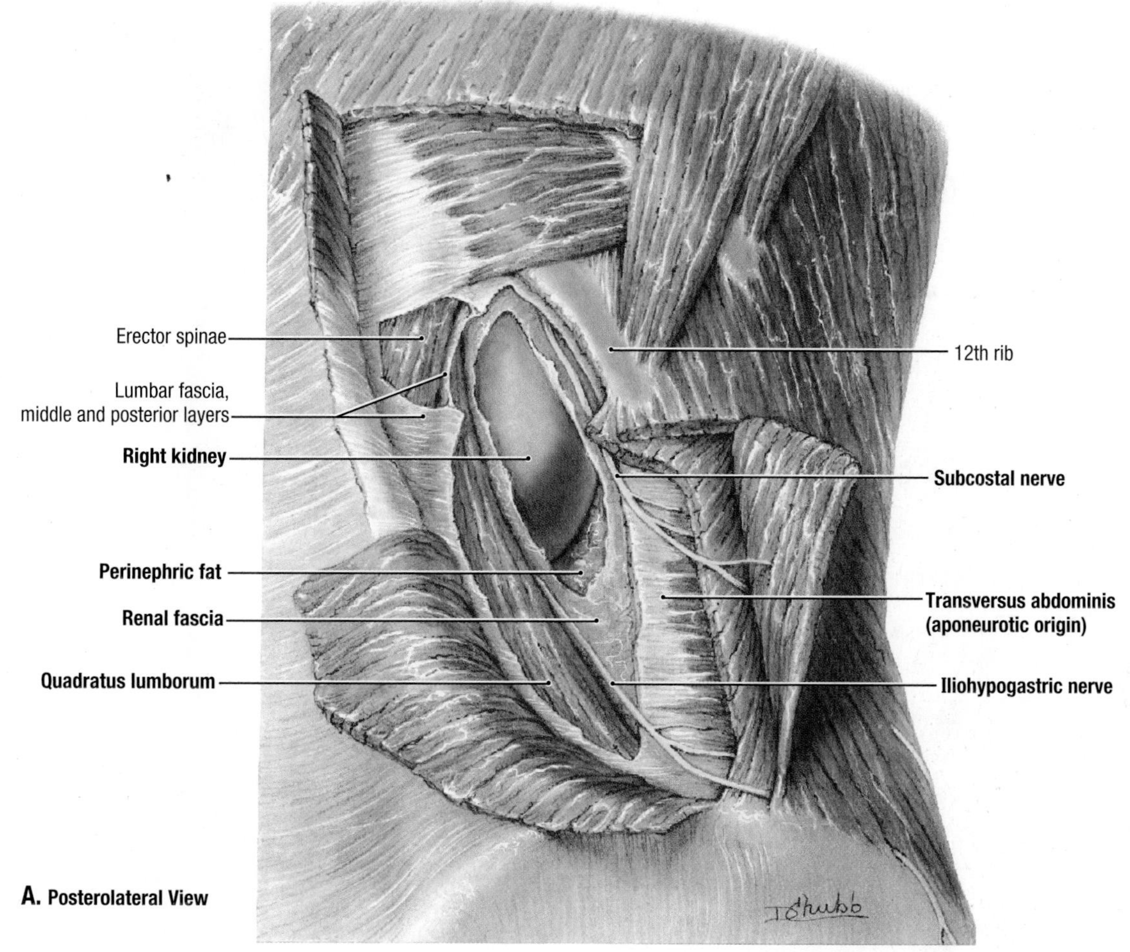
Erector spinae
Lumbar fascia, middle and posterior layers
Right kidney
Perinephric fat
Renal fascia
Quadratus lumborum
12th rib
Subcostal nerve
Transversus abdominis (aponeurotic origin)
Iliohypogastric nerve

A. Posterolateral View

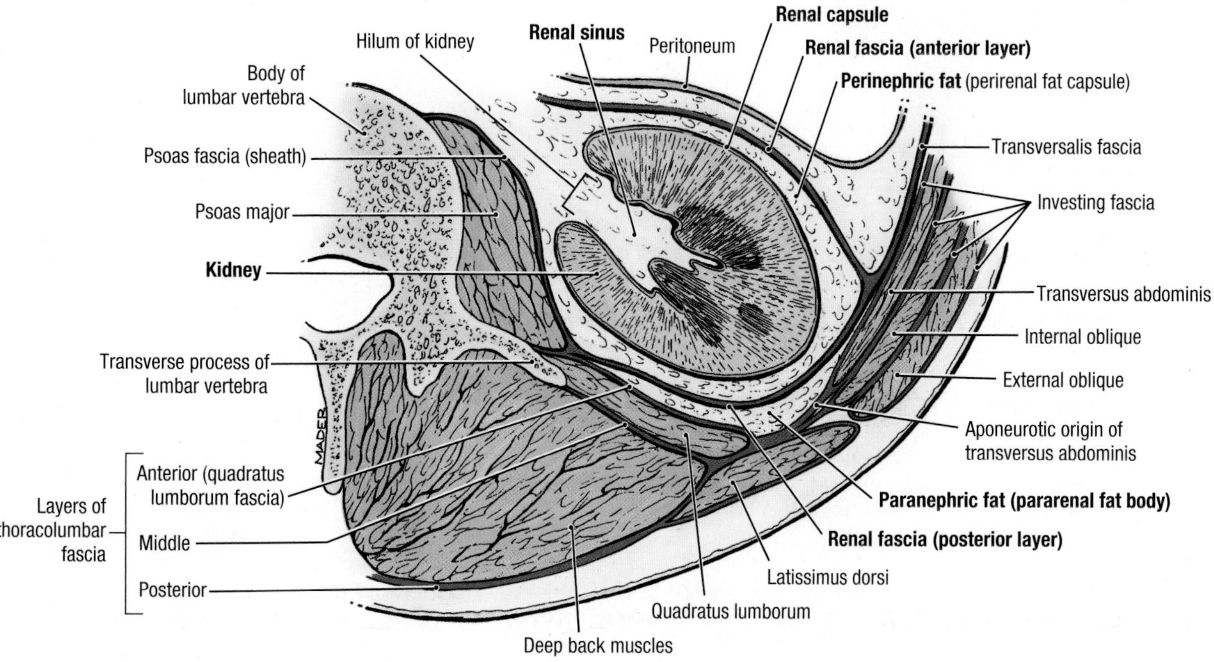
Hilum of kidney
Renal sinus
Peritoneum
Renal capsule
Renal fascia (anterior layer)
Perinephric fat (perirenal fat capsule)
Body of lumbar vertebra
Psoas fascia (sheath)
Psoas major
Kidney
Transverse process of lumbar vertebra
Transversalis fascia
Investing fascia
Transversus abdominis
Internal oblique
External oblique
Aponeurotic origin of transversus abdominis
Paranephric fat (pararenal fat body)
Renal fascia (posterior layer)
Latissimus dorsi
Quadratus lumborum
Deep back muscles
Layers of thoracolumbar fascia
Anterior (quadratus lumborum fascia)
Middle
Posterior
MADER

B. Transverse Section

2.76 POSTEROLATERAL ABDOMINAL WALL: EXPOSURE OF KIDNEY III AND RENAL FASCIA (*CONTINUED*)

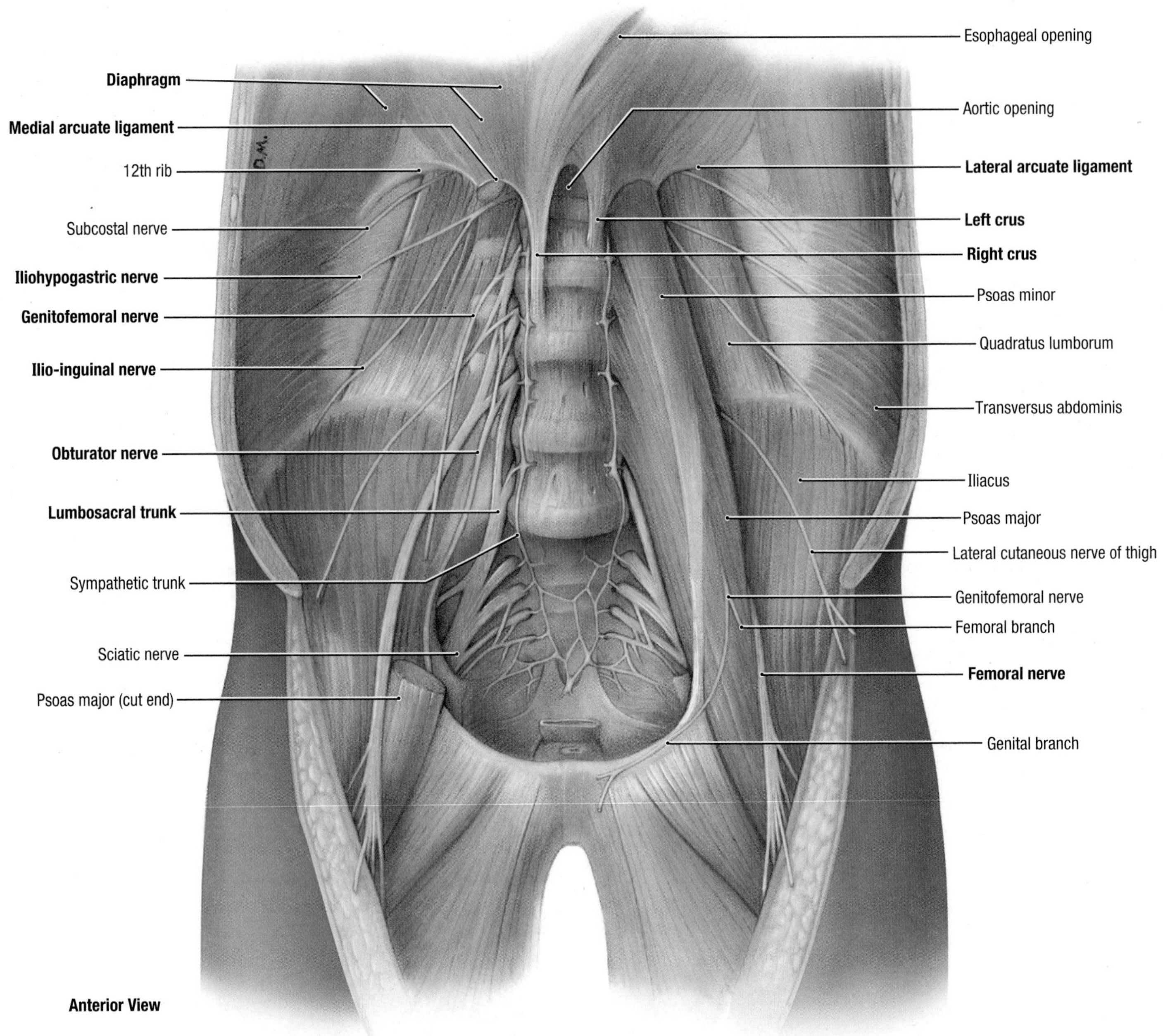

Esophageal opening
Diaphragm
Aortic opening
Medial arcuate ligament
12th rib
Lateral arcuate ligament
Subcostal nerve
Left crus
Right crus
Iliohypogastric nerve
Psoas minor
Genitofemoral nerve
Quadratus lumborum
Ilio-inguinal nerve
Transversus abdominis
Obturator nerve
Iliacus
Lumbosacral trunk
Psoas major
Lateral cutaneous nerve of thigh
Sympathetic trunk
Genitofemoral nerve
Femoral branch
Sciatic nerve
Femoral nerve
Psoas major (cut end)
Genital branch
Anterior View

2.77 LUMBAR PLEXUS AND VERTEBRAL ATTACHMENT OF DIAPHRAGM

TABLE 2.7 PRINCIPAL MUSCLES OF POSTERIOR ABDOMINAL WALL

Muscle	Superior Attachments	Inferior Attachments	Innervation	Actions
Psoas major[a,b]	Transverse processes of lumbar vertebrae; sides of bodies of T12–L5 vertebrae and intervening intervertebral discs	By a strong tendon to lesser trochanter of femur	Anterior rami of lumbar nerves (**L1, L2**, L3)	Acting inferiorly with iliacus, it flexes thigh at hip; acting superiorly, it flexes vertebral column laterally; it is used to balance the trunk; during sitting it acts inferiorly with iliacus to flex trunk
Iliacus[a]	Superior two thirds of iliac fossa, ala of sacrum, and anterior sacro-iliac ligaments	Lesser trochanter of femur and shaft inferior to it, and to psoas major tendon	Femoral nerve (**L2**, L3, L4)	Flexes thigh and stabilizes hip joint; acts with psoas major
Quadratus lumborum	Medial half of inferior border of 12th rib and tips of lumbar transverse processes	Iliolumbar ligament and internal lip of iliac crest	Anterior rami of T12 and L1–L4 nerves	Extends and laterally flexes vertebral column; fixes 12th rib during inspiration

[a]Psoas major and iliacus muscles are often described together as the iliopsoas muscle when flexion of the thigh is discussed.
[b]Psoas minor attaches proximally to the sides of bodies of T12–L1 vertebrae and intervertebral disc and distally to the pectineal line and iliopectineal eminence via the iliopectineal arch; it does not cross the hip joint. It is used to balance the trunk, in conjunction with psoas major. Innervation is from the anterior rami of lumbar nerves (L1, L2).

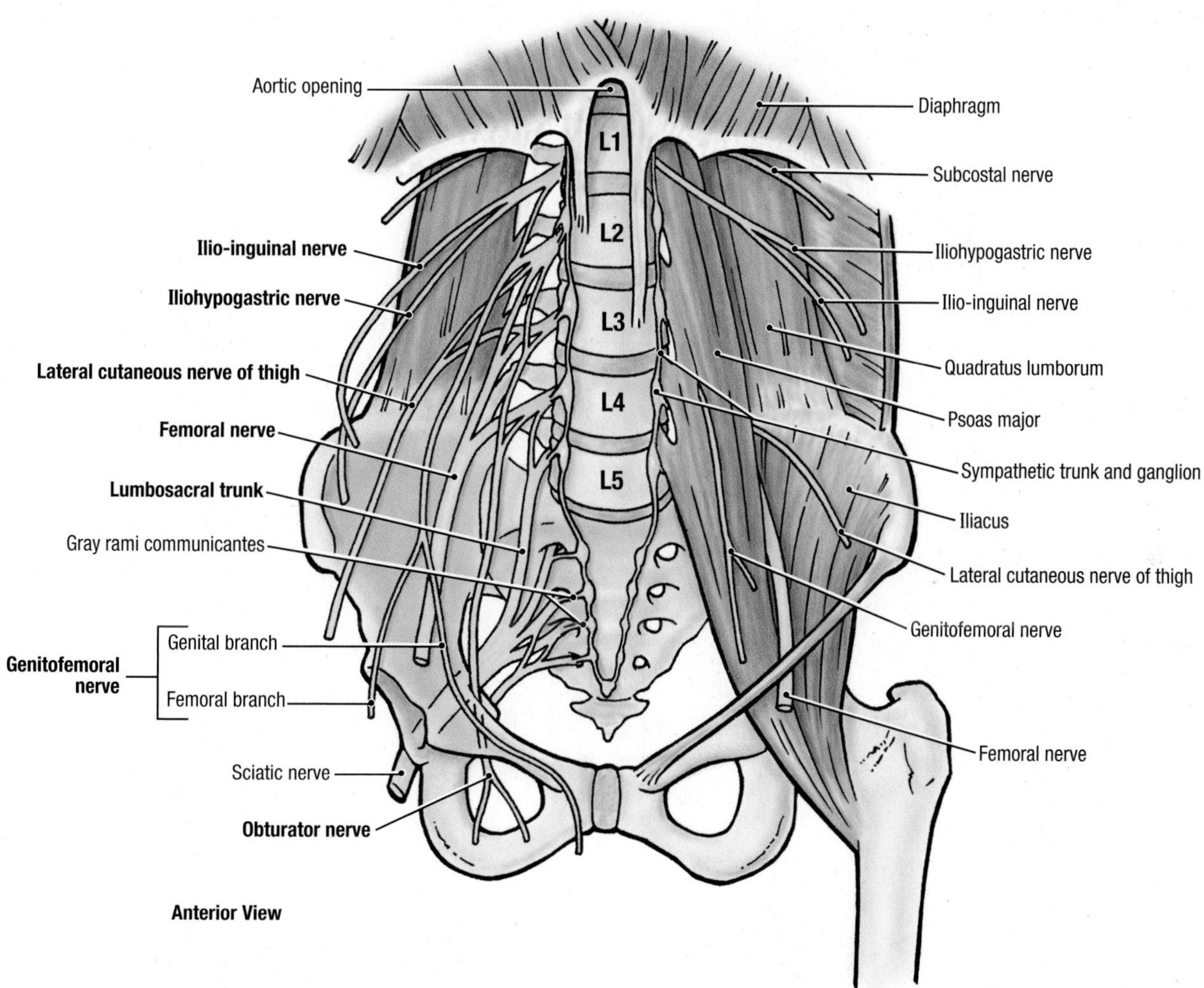
Aortic opening
Diaphragm
Subcostal nerve
L1
L2
L3
L4
L5
Ilio-inguinal nerve
Iliohypogastric nerve
Iliohypogastric nerve
Ilio-inguinal nerve
Lateral cutaneous nerve of thigh
Quadratus lumborum
Psoas major
Femoral nerve
Sympathetic trunk and ganglion
Lumbosacral trunk
Iliacus
Gray rami communicantes
Lateral cutaneous nerve of thigh
Genitofemoral nerve
Genital branch
Genitofemoral nerve
Femoral branch
Femoral nerve
Sciatic nerve
Obturator nerve
Anterior View

2.78 NERVES OF LUMBAR PLEXUS

The lumbar plexus of nerves is in the posterior part of the psoas major, anterior to the lumbar transverse processes. This nerve network is composed of the anterior rami of L1–L4 nerves. All rami receive gray rami communicates from the sympathetic trunks. The following nerves are branches of the lumbar plexus:

- Ilio-inguinal and iliohypogastric nerves (L1) arise from the anterior ramus of L1 and enter the abdomen posterior to the medial arcuate ligaments and pass inferolaterally, anterior to the quadratus lumborum muscle; they pierce the transversus abdominis muscle near the anterior superior iliac spine and pass through the internal and external oblique muscles to supply the skin of the suprapubic and inguinal regions.
- Lateral cutaneous nerve of thigh (L2, L3) runs inferolaterally on the iliacus muscle and enters the thigh posterior to the inguinal ligament, just medial to the anterior superior iliac spine; it supplies the skin on the anterolateral surface of the thigh.
- Femoral nerve (L2–L4) emerges from the lateral border of the psoas and innervates the iliacus muscle and the extensor muscles of the knee.
- Genitofemoral nerve (L1, L2) pierces the anterior surface of the psoas major muscle and runs inferiorly on it deep to the psoas fascia; it divides lateral to the common and external iliac arteries into femoral and genital branches.
- Obturator nerve (L2–L4) emerges from the medial border of the psoas to supply the adductor muscles of the thigh.
- Lumbosacral trunk (L4, L5) passes over the ala (wing) of the sacrum and descends into the pelvis to take part in the formation of the sacral plexus along with the anterior rami of S1–S4 nerves.

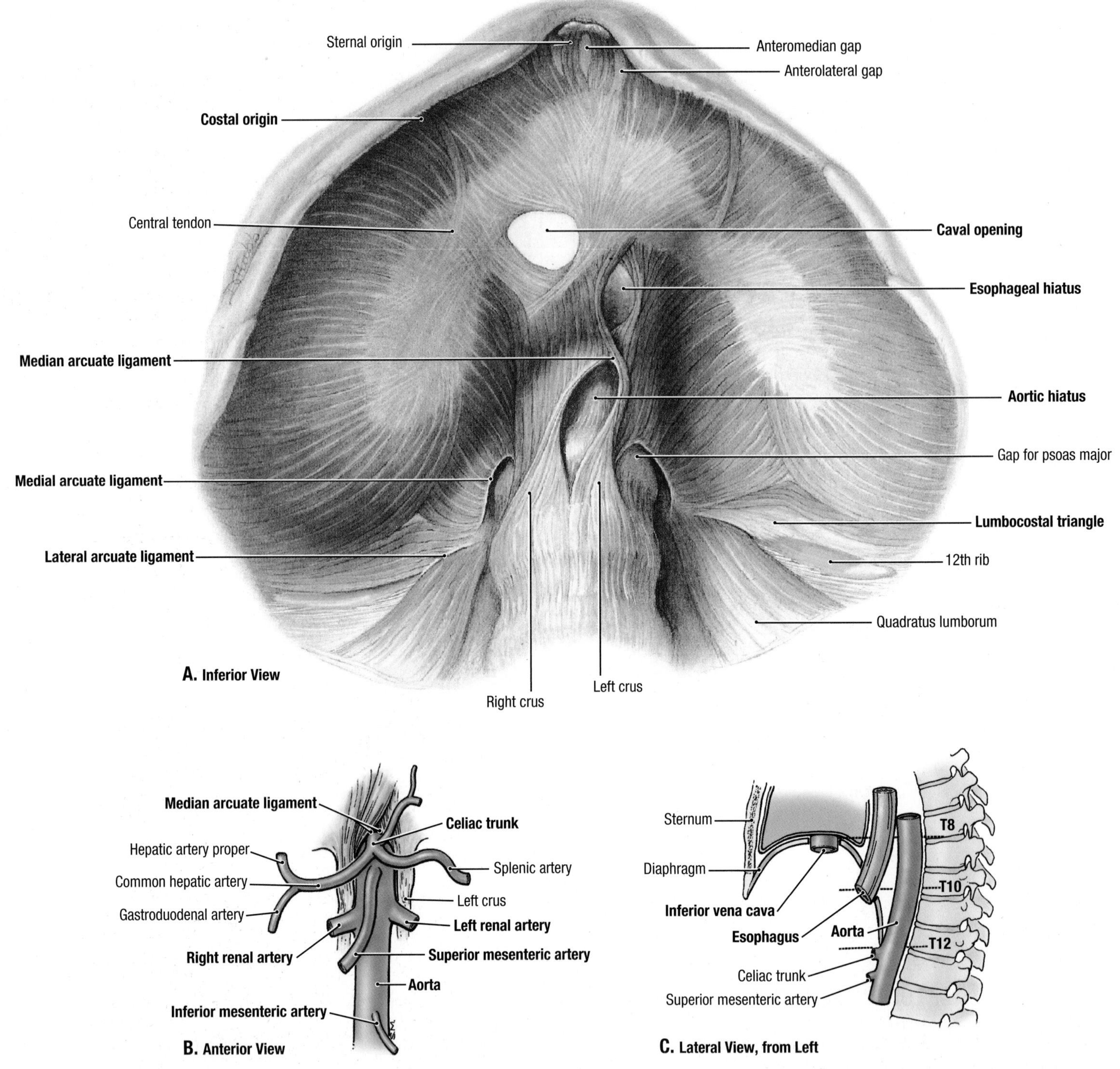
Sternal origin
Anteromedian gap
Anterolateral gap
Costal origin
Central tendon
Caval opening
Esophageal hiatus
Median arcuate ligament
Aortic hiatus
Gap for psoas major
Medial arcuate ligament
Lumbocostal triangle
Lateral arcuate ligament
12th rib
Quadratus lumborum
A. Inferior View
Right crus
Left crus
Median arcuate ligament
Celiac trunk
Hepatic artery proper
Splenic artery
Common hepatic artery
Left crus
Gastroduodenal artery
Left renal artery
Right renal artery
Superior mesenteric artery
Aorta
Inferior mesenteric artery
B. Anterior View
Sternum
T8
Diaphragm
T10
Inferior vena cava
Esophagus
Aorta
T12
Celiac trunk
Superior mesenteric artery
C. Lateral View, from Left

2.79 DIAPHRAGM

A. Dissection. The clover-shaped central tendon is the aponeurotic insertion of the muscle. **Diaphragmatic hernia.** The diaphragm in this specimen fails to arise from the left lateral arcuate ligament, leaving a potential opening, the lumbocostal triangle, through which abdominal contents may be herniated into the thoracic cavity following a sudden increase in intra-thoracic or intra-abdominal pressure. A **hiatal hernia** is a protrusion of part of the stomach into the thorax through the esophageal hiatus.

B. Median arcuate ligament and branches of the aorta. **C.** Openings of the diaphragm. There are three major openings: (1) the caval opening for the inferior vena cava, most anterior, at the T8 vertebral level to the right of the midline; (2) the esophageal hiatus, intermediate, at T10 level and to the left; and (3) the aortic hiatus, which allows the aorta to pass posterior to the vertebral attachment of the diaphragm in the midline at T12.

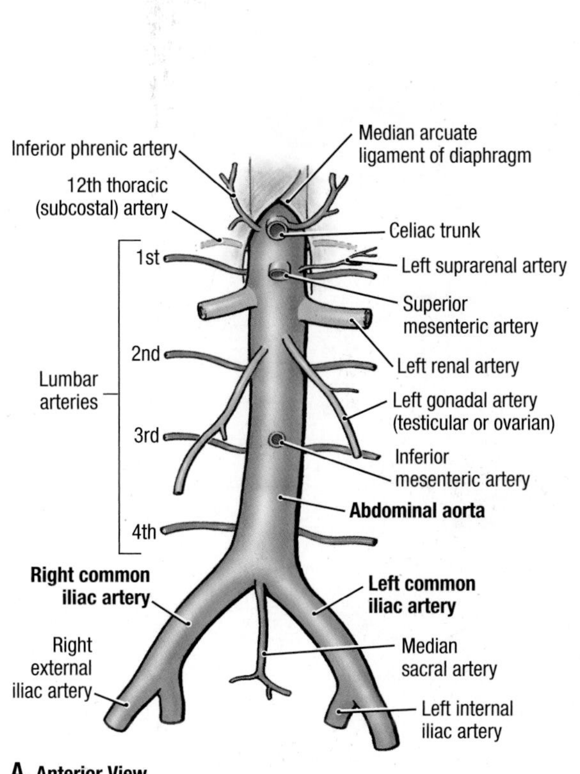
Inferior phrenic artery
Median arcuate ligament of diaphragm
12th thoracic (subcostal) artery
Celiac trunk
1st
Left suprarenal artery
Superior mesenteric artery
2nd
Left renal artery
Lumbar arteries
Left gonadal artery (testicular or ovarian)
3rd
Inferior mesenteric artery
Abdominal aorta
4th
Right common iliac artery
Left common iliac artery
Right external iliac artery
Median sacral artery
Left internal iliac artery

A. Anterior View

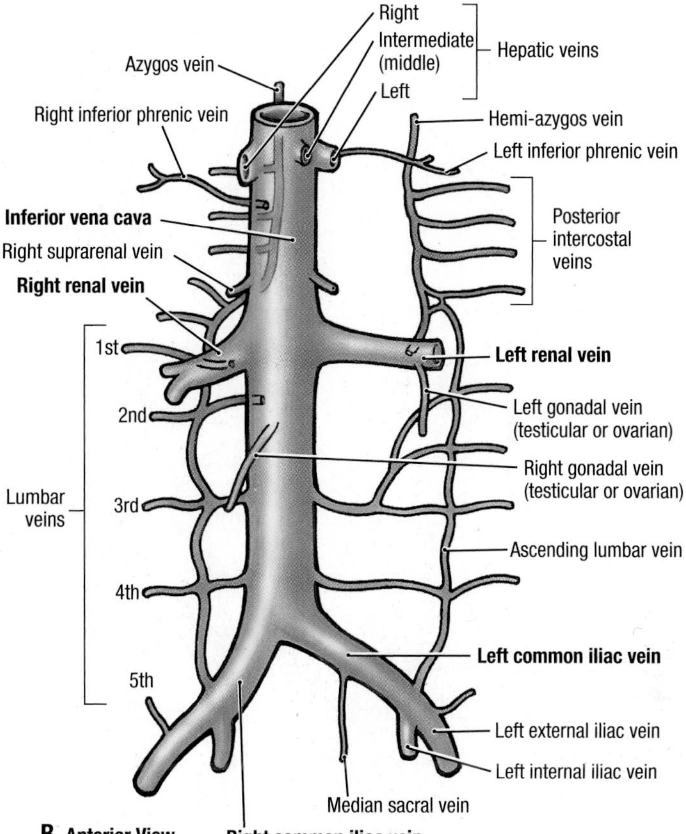
Right
Intermediate (middle)
Left
Hepatic veins
Azygos vein
Right inferior phrenic vein
Hemi-azygos vein
Left inferior phrenic vein
Inferior vena cava
Posterior intercostal veins
Right suprarenal vein
Right renal vein
1st
Left renal vein
2nd
Left gonadal vein (testicular or ovarian)
Right gonadal vein (testicular or ovarian)
Lumbar veins
3rd
Ascending lumbar vein
4th
Left common iliac vein
5th
Left external iliac vein
Left internal iliac vein
Median sacral vein
Right common iliac vein

B. Anterior View

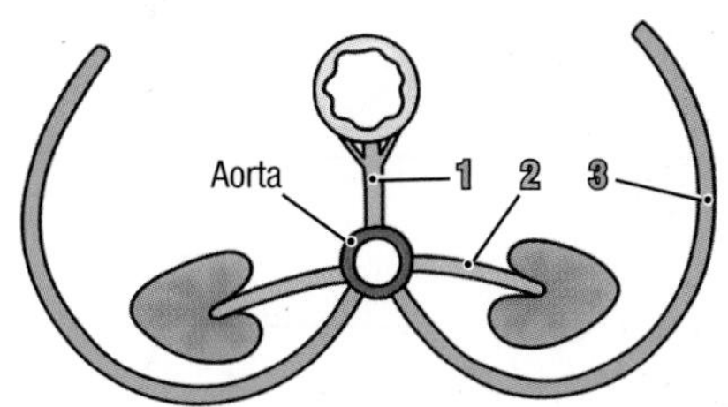
Aorta
1
2
3

Three Vascular Planes

	Origin from Aorta	Class	Distribution	Abdominal Branches (Arteries)	Vertebral Level
1	Anterior midline	Unpaired visceral	Alimentary tract	Celiac	T12
				Superior mesenteric (SMA)	L1
				Inferior mesenteric (IMA)	L3
2	Lateral	Paired visceral	Urogenital and endocrine organs	Suprarenal	L1
				Renal	L1
				Gonadal (testicular or ovarian)	L2
3	Postero-lateral	Paired parietal (segmental)	Diaphragm Body Wall	Subcostal	T12
				Inferior phrenic	T12
				Lumbar	L1–L4

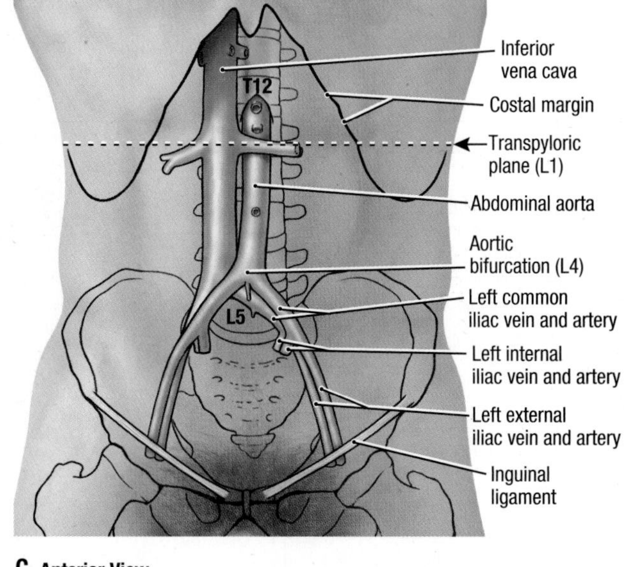
T12
L5
Inferior vena cava
Costal margin
Transpyloric plane (L1)
Abdominal aorta
Aortic bifurcation (L4)
Left common iliac vein and artery
Left internal iliac vein and artery
Left external iliac vein and artery
Inguinal ligament

C. Anterior View

2.80 ABDOMINAL AORTA AND INFERIOR VENA CAVA AND THEIR BRANCHES

A. Branches of abdominal aorta. **B.** Tributaries of the inferior vena cava (IVC). **C.** Surface anatomy.

Rupture of an **aortic aneurysm** (localized enlargement of the abdominal aorta) causes severe pain in the abdomen or back. If unrecognized, a ruptured aneurysm has a mortality of nearly 90% because of heavy blood loss. Surgeons can repair an aneurysm by opening it, inserting a prosthetic graft (such as one made of Dacron), and sewing the wall of the aneurysmal aorta over the graft to protect it. Aneurysms may also be treated by endovascular catheterization procedures.

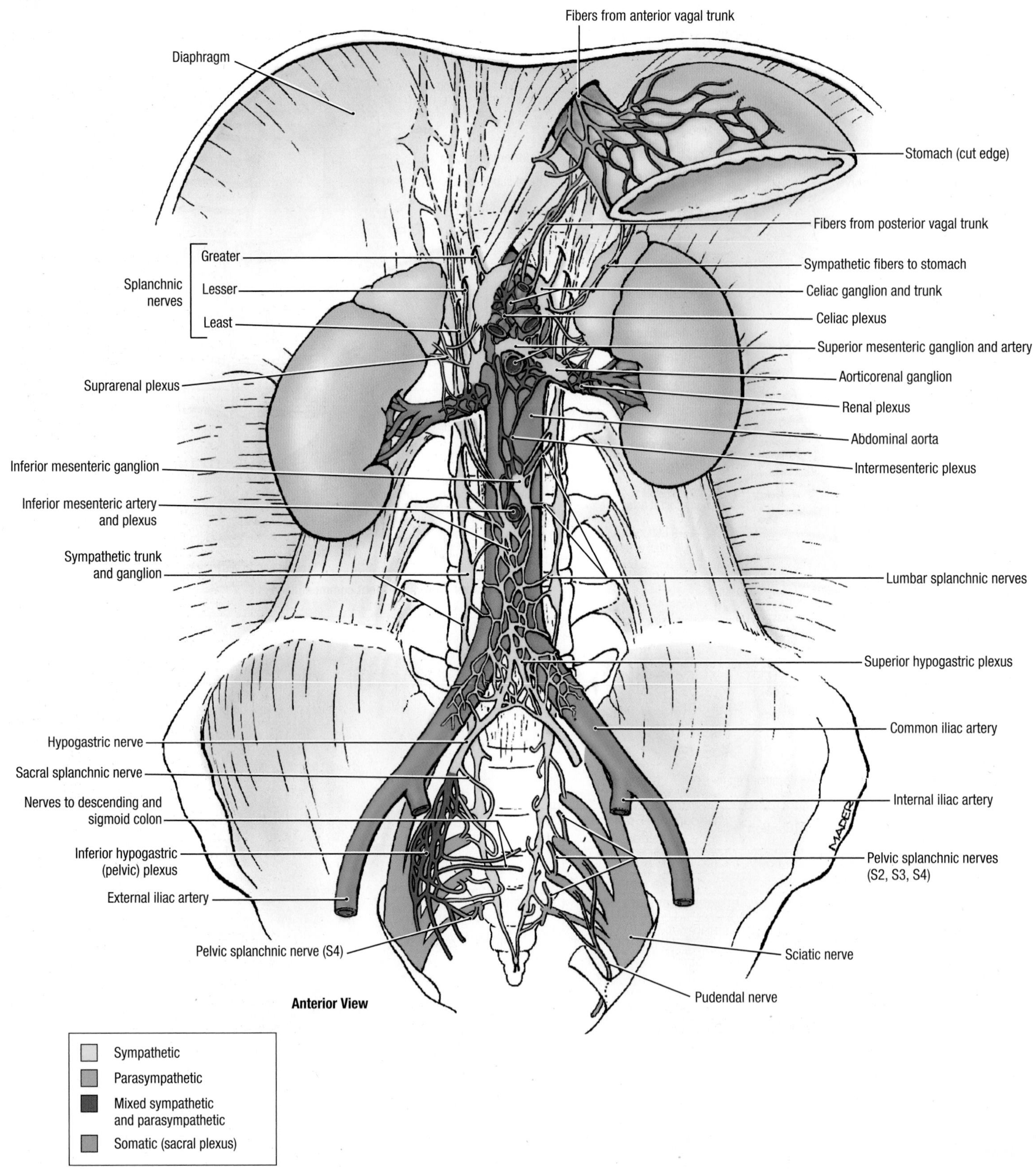
Fibers from anterior vagal trunk
Diaphragm
Stomach (cut edge)
Fibers from posterior vagal trunk
Splanchnic nerves
Greater
Lesser
Least
Sympathetic fibers to stomach
Celiac ganglion and trunk
Celiac plexus
Superior mesenteric ganglion and artery
Aorticorenal ganglion
Suprarenal plexus
Renal plexus
Abdominal aorta
Intermesenteric plexus
Inferior mesenteric ganglion
Inferior mesenteric artery and plexus
Sympathetic trunk and ganglion
Lumbar splanchnic nerves
Superior hypogastric plexus
Common iliac artery
Hypogastric nerve
Sacral splanchnic nerve
Internal iliac artery
Nerves to descending and sigmoid colon
Inferior hypogastric (pelvic) plexus
Pelvic splanchnic nerves (S2, S3, S4)
External iliac artery
Sciatic nerve
Pelvic splanchnic nerve (S4)
Pudendal nerve
MADER
Anterior View
Sympathetic
Parasympathetic
Mixed sympathetic and parasympathetic
Somatic (sacral plexus)

2.81 ABDOMINOPELVIC NERVE PLEXUSES AND GANGLIA

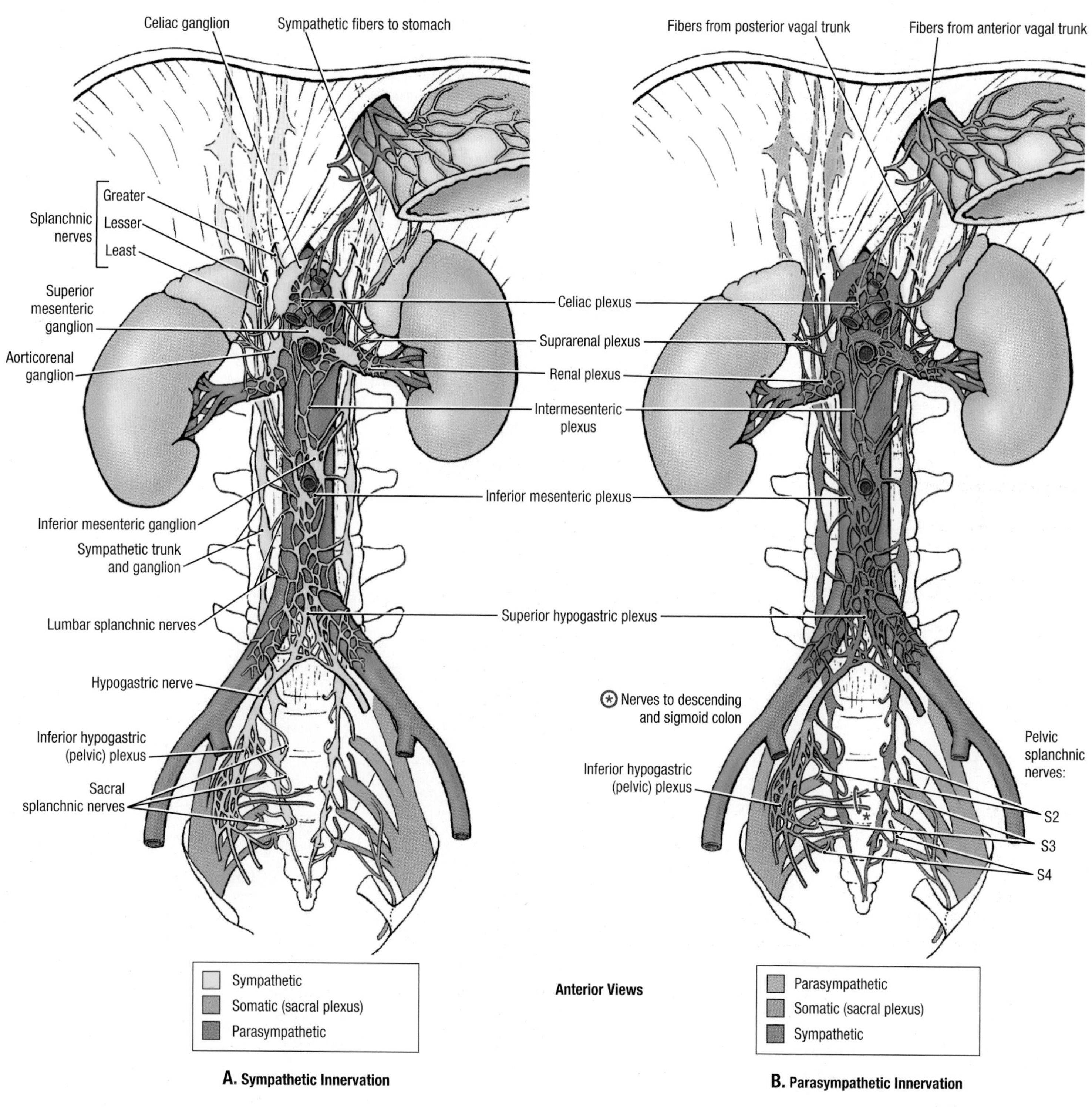
Celiac ganglion
Sympathetic fibers to stomach
Splanchnic nerves
Greater
Lesser
Least
Superior mesenteric ganglion
Aorticorenal ganglion
Inferior mesenteric ganglion
Sympathetic trunk and ganglion
Lumbar splanchnic nerves
Hypogastric nerve
Inferior hypogastric (pelvic) plexus
Sacral splanchnic nerves
Fibers from posterior vagal trunk
Fibers from anterior vagal trunk
Celiac plexus
Suprarenal plexus
Renal plexus
Intermesenteric plexus
Inferior mesenteric plexus
Superior hypogastric plexus
* Nerves to descending and sigmoid colon
Inferior hypogastric (pelvic) plexus
Pelvic splanchnic nerves:
S2
S3
S4
Sympathetic
Somatic (sacral plexus)
Parasympathetic
Anterior Views
Parasympathetic
Somatic (sacral plexus)
Sympathetic
A. Sympathetic Innervation
B. Parasympathetic Innervation

2.82 OVERVIEW OF AUTONOMIC NERVOUS SYSTEM

A. Sympathetic. **B.** Parasympathetic.

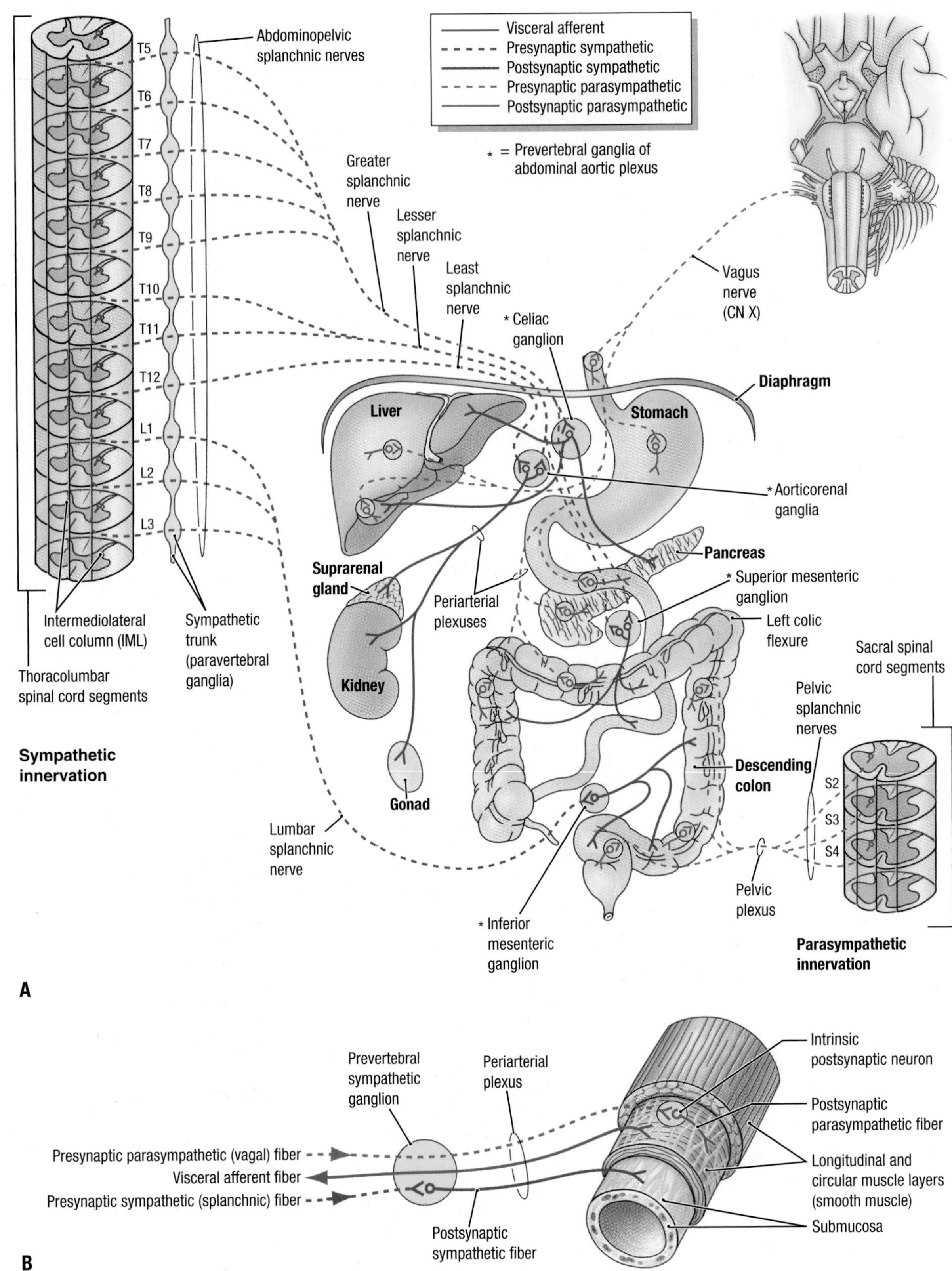

Visceral afferent
Presynaptic sympathetic
Postsynaptic sympathetic
Presynaptic parasympathetic
Postsynaptic parasympathetic
* = Prevertebral ganglia of abdominal aortic plexus
T5
T6
T7
T8
T9
T10
T11
T12
L1
L2
L3
Abdominopelvic splanchnic nerves
Greater splanchnic nerve
Lesser splanchnic nerve
Least splanchnic nerve
* Celiac ganglion
Vagus nerve (CN X)
Diaphragm
Liver
Stomach
* Aorticorenal ganglia
Pancreas
* Superior mesenteric ganglion
Suprarenal gland
Periarterial plexuses
Left colic flexure
Kidney
Gonad
Descending colon
Intermediolateral cell column (IML)
Sympathetic trunk (paravertebral ganglia)
Thoracolumbar spinal cord segments
Sympathetic innervation
Lumbar splanchnic nerve
* Inferior mesenteric ganglion
Pelvic splanchnic nerves
Sacral spinal cord segments
S2
S3
S4
Pelvic plexus
Parasympathetic innervation
A
Prevertebral sympathetic ganglion
Periarterial plexus
Intrinsic postsynaptic neuron
Postsynaptic parasympathetic fiber
Presynaptic parasympathetic (vagal) fiber
Visceral afferent fiber
Presynaptic sympathetic (splanchnic) fiber
Longitudinal and circular muscle layers (smooth muscle)
Submucosa
Postsynaptic sympathetic fiber
B

2.83 ORIGIN AND DISTRIBUTION OF PRESYNAPTIC AND POSTSYNAPTIC SYMPATHETIC AND PARASYMPATHETIC FIBERS, AND GANGLIA INVOLVED IN SUPPLYING ABDOMINAL VISCERA

A. Overview. **B.** Fibers supplying the intrinsic plexuses of abdominal viscera.

TABLE 2.8 AUTONOMIC INNERVATION OF ABDOMINAL VISCERA (SPLANCHNIC NERVES)

Splanchnic Nerves	Autonomic Fiber Type[a]	System	Origin	Destination
A. **Cardiopulmonary** (Cervical and upper thoracic)	Postsynaptic	Sympathetic	Cervical and upper thoracic sympathetic trunk	Thoracic cavity (viscera superior to the level of diaphragm)
B. **Abdominopelvic** 1. Lower thoracic a. Greater b. Lesser c. Least 2. Lumbar 3. Sacral	Presynaptic		Lower thoracic and abdominopelvic sympathetic trunk: 1. Thoracic sympathetic trunk: a. T5–T9 or T10 level b. T10–T11 level c. T12 level 2. Abdominal sympathetic trunk 3. Pelvic (sacral) sympathetic trunk	Abdominopelvic cavity (prevertebral ganglia serving viscera and suprarenal glands inferior to the level of diaphragm) 1. Abdominal prevertebral ganglia: a. Celiac ganglia b. Aorticorenal ganglia c. & 2. Other abdominal prevertebral ganglia (superior and inferior mesenteric and of intermesenteric/hypogastric plexuses) 3. Pelvic prevertebral ganglia
C. **Pelvic**	Presynaptic	Parasympathetic	Anterior rami of S2–S4 spinal nerves	Intrinsic ganglia of descending and sigmoid colon, rectum, and pelvic viscera

[a]Splanchnic nerves also convey visceral afferent fibers, which are not part of the autonomic nervous system.

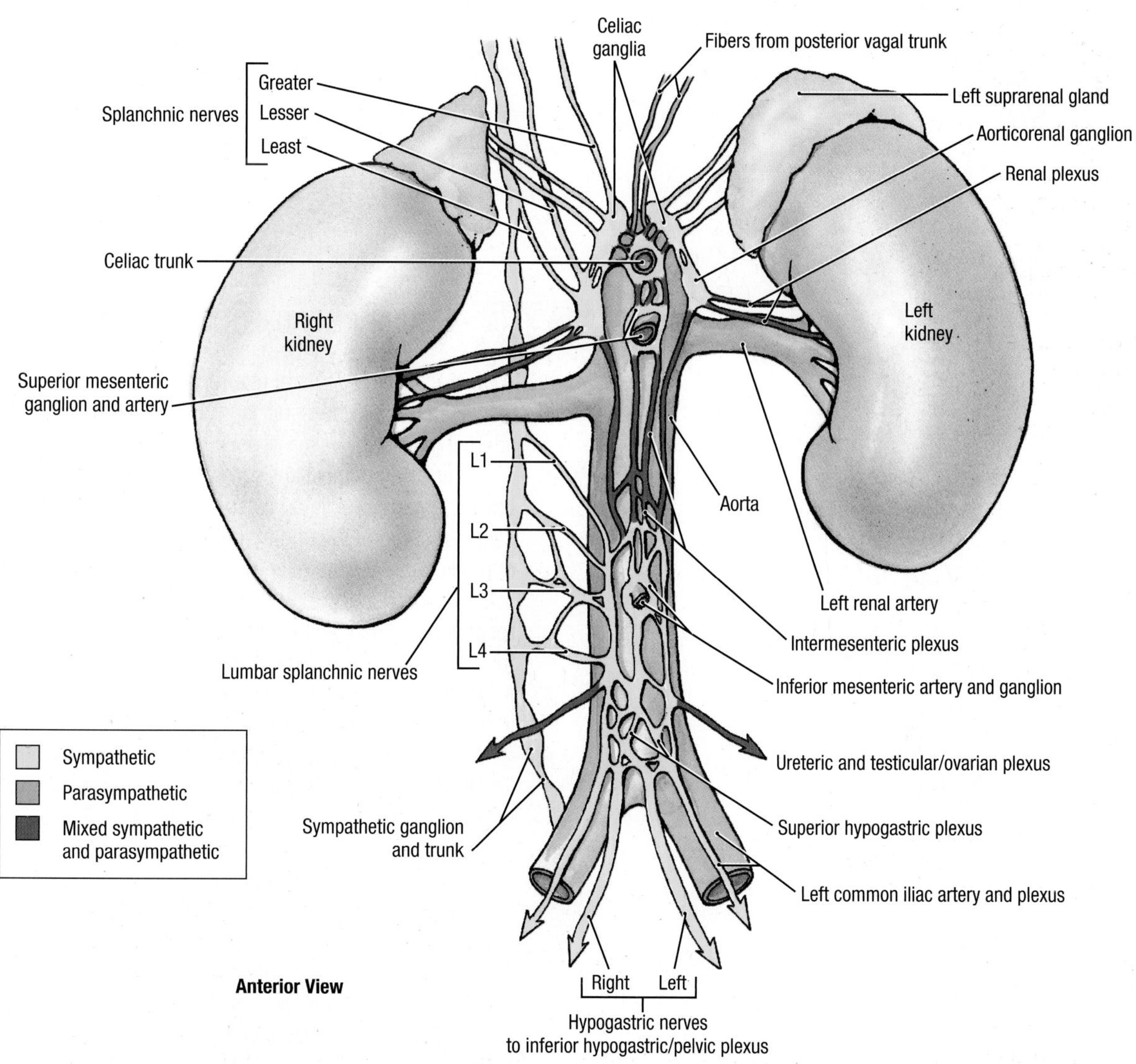
Celiac ganglia
Fibers from posterior vagal trunk
Splanchnic nerves
Greater
Lesser
Least
Left suprarenal gland
Aorticorenal ganglion
Renal plexus
Celiac trunk
Right kidney
Left kidney
Superior mesenteric ganglion and artery
L1
L2
L3
L4
Aorta
Left renal artery
Intermesenteric plexus
Lumbar splanchnic nerves
Inferior mesenteric artery and ganglion
Sympathetic
Parasympathetic
Mixed sympathetic and parasympathetic
Ureteric and testicular/ovarian plexus
Sympathetic ganglion and trunk
Superior hypogastric plexus
Left common iliac artery and plexus
Anterior View
Right
Left
Hypogastric nerves to inferior hypogastric/pelvic plexus

2.84 ABDOMINAL NERVE PLEXUSES AND GANGLIA

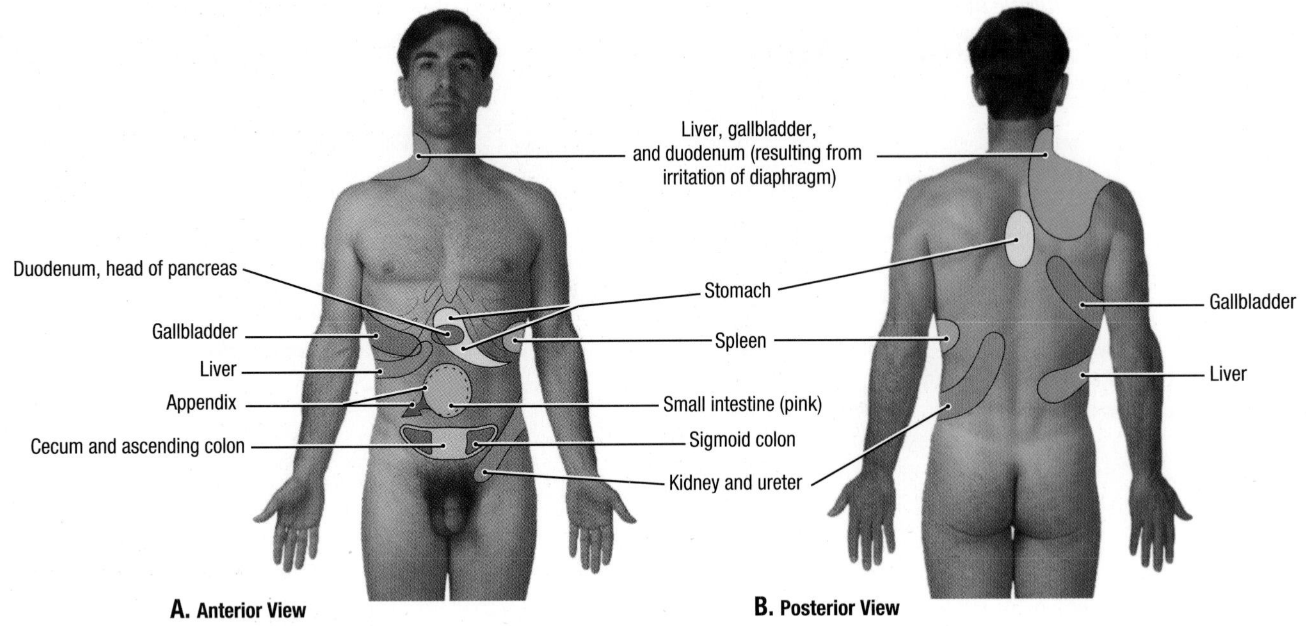
Liver, gallbladder, and duodenum (resulting from irritation of diaphragm)
Duodenum, head of pancreas
Gallbladder
Liver
Appendix
Cecum and ascending colon
Stomach
Spleen
Small intestine (pink)
Sigmoid colon
Kidney and ureter
Gallbladder
Liver

A. Anterior View

B. Posterior View

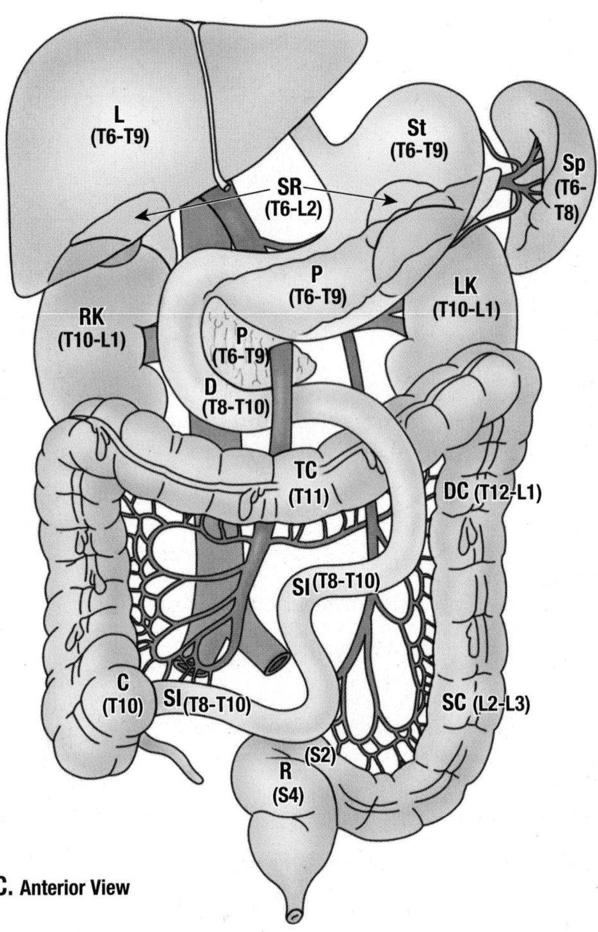
L (T6-T9)
St (T6-T9)
Sp (T6-T8)
SR (T6-L2)
P (T6-T9)
LK (T10-L1)
RK (T10-L1)
P (T6-T9)
D (T8-T10)
TC (T11)
DC (T12-L1)
SI (T8-T10)
C (T10)
SI (T8-T10)
SC (L2-L3)
(S2)
R (S4)

C. Anterior View

C	Cecum	P	Pancreas	Sp	Spleen
D	Duodenum	R	Rectum	SR	Suprarenal gands
DC	Descending colon	RK	Right kidney	St	Stomach
L	Liver	SC	Sigmoid colon	TC	Transverse colon
LK	Left kidney	SI	Small intestine		

2.85 SURFACE PROJECTIONS OF VISCERAL PAIN

A. and B. Sites of visceral referred pain. **C.** Approximate spinal cord segments and spinal sensory ganglia involved in sympathetic and visceral afferent (pain) innervation of abdominal viscera.

Pain is an unpleasant sensation associated with actual or potential tissue damage, mediated by specific nerve fibers to the brain, where its conscious appreciation may be modified. Organic pain arising from an organ such as the stomach varies from dull to severe; however, the pain is poorly localized. It radiates to the dermatome level served by the corresponding sensory ganglion, which receives the visceral afferent fibers from the organ concerned. **Visceral referred pain** from a gastric ulcer, for example, is referred to the epigastric region because the stomach is supplied by pain afferents that reach the T7 and T8 spinal sensory ganglia and spinal cord segments through the greater splanchnic nerve. The brain interprets the pain as though the irritation occurred in the skin of the epigastric region, which is also supplied by the same sensory ganglia and spinal cord segments.

Pain arising from the parietal peritoneum is of the somatic type and is usually severe. The site of its origin can be localized. The anatomical basis for this localization of pain is that the parietal peritoneum is supplied by somatic sensory fibers through thoracic nerves, whereas a viscus such as the appendix is supplied by visceral afferent fibers in the lesser splanchnic nerve. Inflamed parietal peritoneum is extremely sensitive to stretching. When digital pressure is applied to the anterolateral abdominal wall over the site of inflammation, the parietal peritoneum is stretched. When the fingers are suddenly removed, extreme localized pain is usually felt, known as **rebound tenderness.**

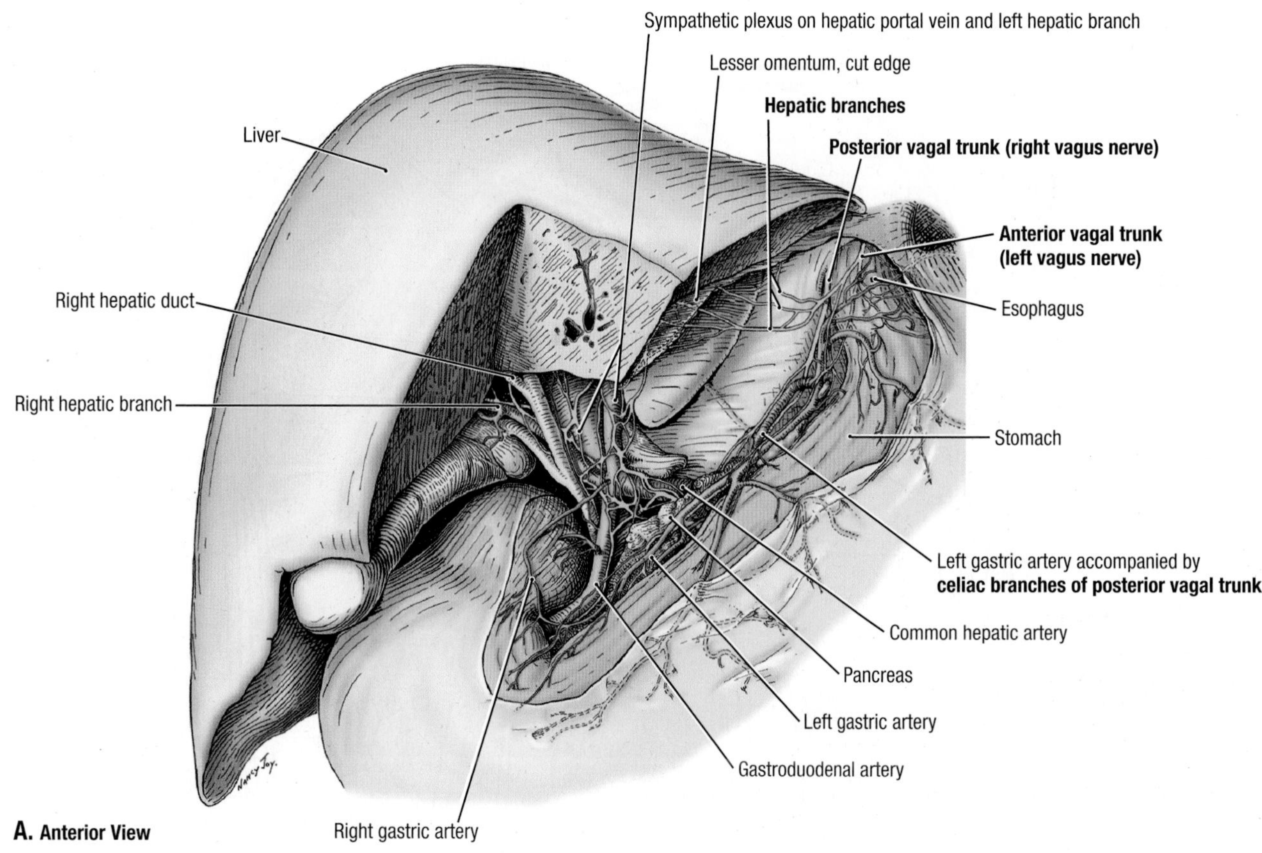
Sympathetic plexus on hepatic portal vein and left hepatic branch
Lesser omentum, cut edge
Hepatic branches
Posterior vagal trunk (right vagus nerve)
Liver
Anterior vagal trunk (left vagus nerve)
Right hepatic duct
Esophagus
Right hepatic branch
Stomach
Left gastric artery accompanied by celiac branches of posterior vagal trunk
Common hepatic artery
Pancreas
Left gastric artery
Gastroduodenal artery
Right gastric artery

A. **Anterior View**

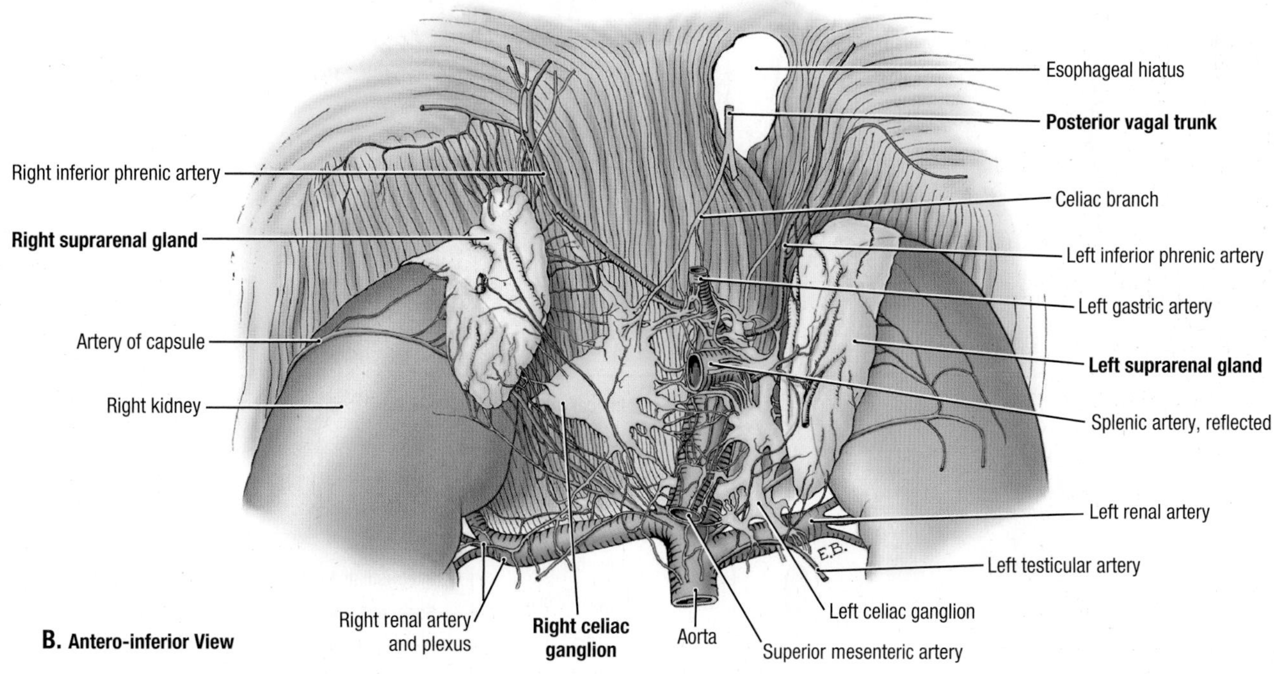
Esophageal hiatus
Posterior vagal trunk
Right inferior phrenic artery
Celiac branch
Right suprarenal gland
Left inferior phrenic artery
Left gastric artery
Artery of capsule
Left suprarenal gland
Right kidney
Splenic artery, reflected
Left renal artery
Left testicular artery
Right renal artery and plexus
Right celiac ganglion
Aorta
Left celiac ganglion
Superior mesenteric artery

B. **Antero-inferior View**

2.86 VAGUS NERVES IN ABDOMEN

A. Anterior and posterior vagal trunks. **B.** Celiac plexus and ganglia and suprarenal glands.

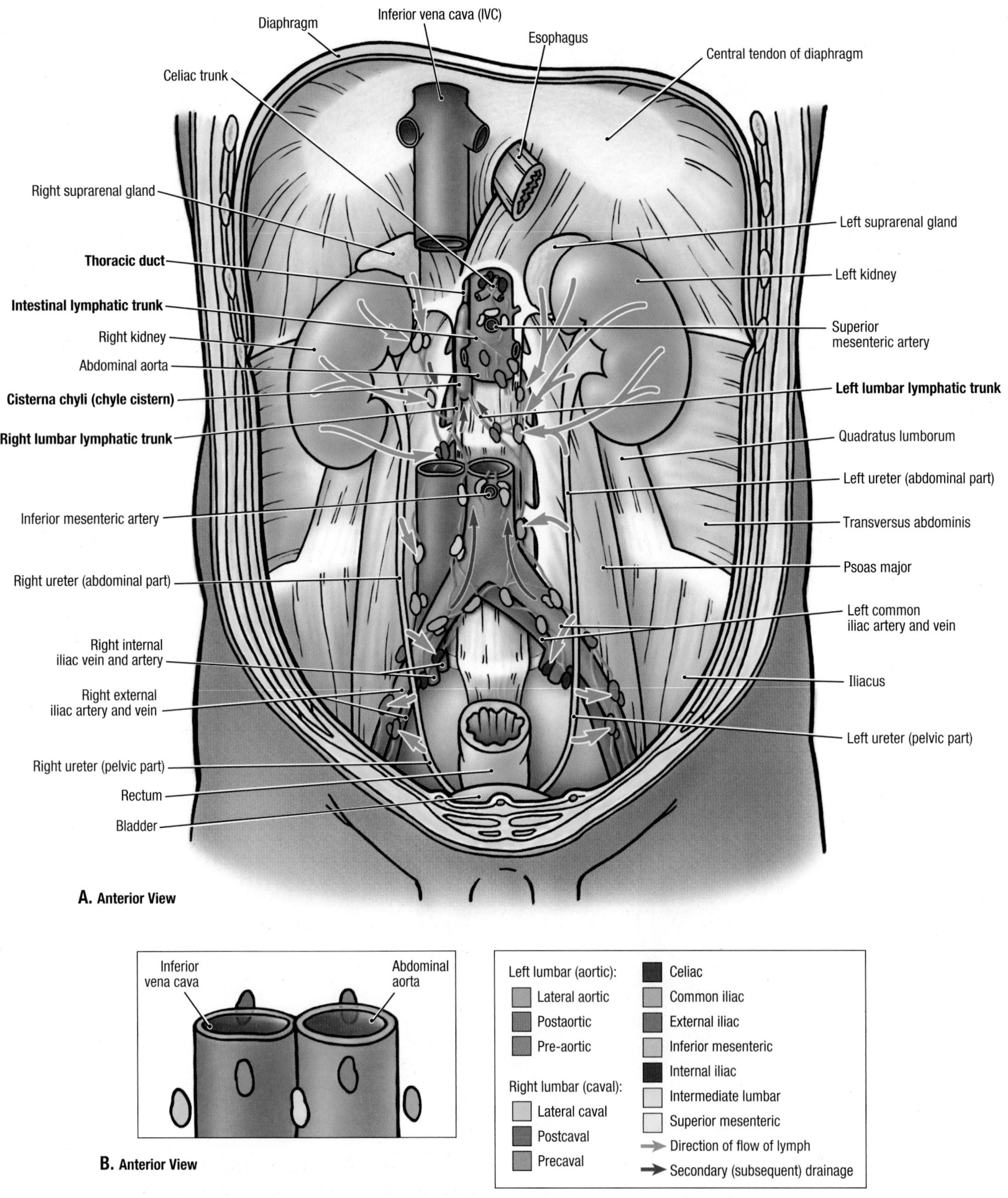

Diaphragm
Inferior vena cava (IVC)
Esophagus
Central tendon of diaphragm
Celiac trunk
Right suprarenal gland
Left suprarenal gland
Thoracic duct
Left kidney
Intestinal lymphatic trunk
Superior mesenteric artery
Right kidney
Abdominal aorta
Cisterna chyli (chyle cistern)
Left lumbar lymphatic trunk
Right lumbar lymphatic trunk
Quadratus lumborum
Left ureter (abdominal part)
Inferior mesenteric artery
Transversus abdominis
Psoas major
Right ureter (abdominal part)
Left common iliac artery and vein
Right internal iliac vein and artery
Iliacus
Right external iliac artery and vein
Left ureter (pelvic part)
Right ureter (pelvic part)
Rectum
Bladder
Inferior vena cava
Abdominal aorta
Left lumbar (aortic):
Lateral aortic
Postaortic
Pre-aortic
Right lumbar (caval):
Lateral caval
Postcaval
Precaval
Celiac
Common iliac
External iliac
Inferior mesenteric
Internal iliac
Intermediate lumbar
Superior mesenteric
Direction of flow of lymph
Secondary (subsequent) drainage

A. Anterior View

B. Anterior View

2.87 LYMPHATIC DRAINAGE OF SUPRARENAL GLANDS, KIDNEYS, AND URETERS

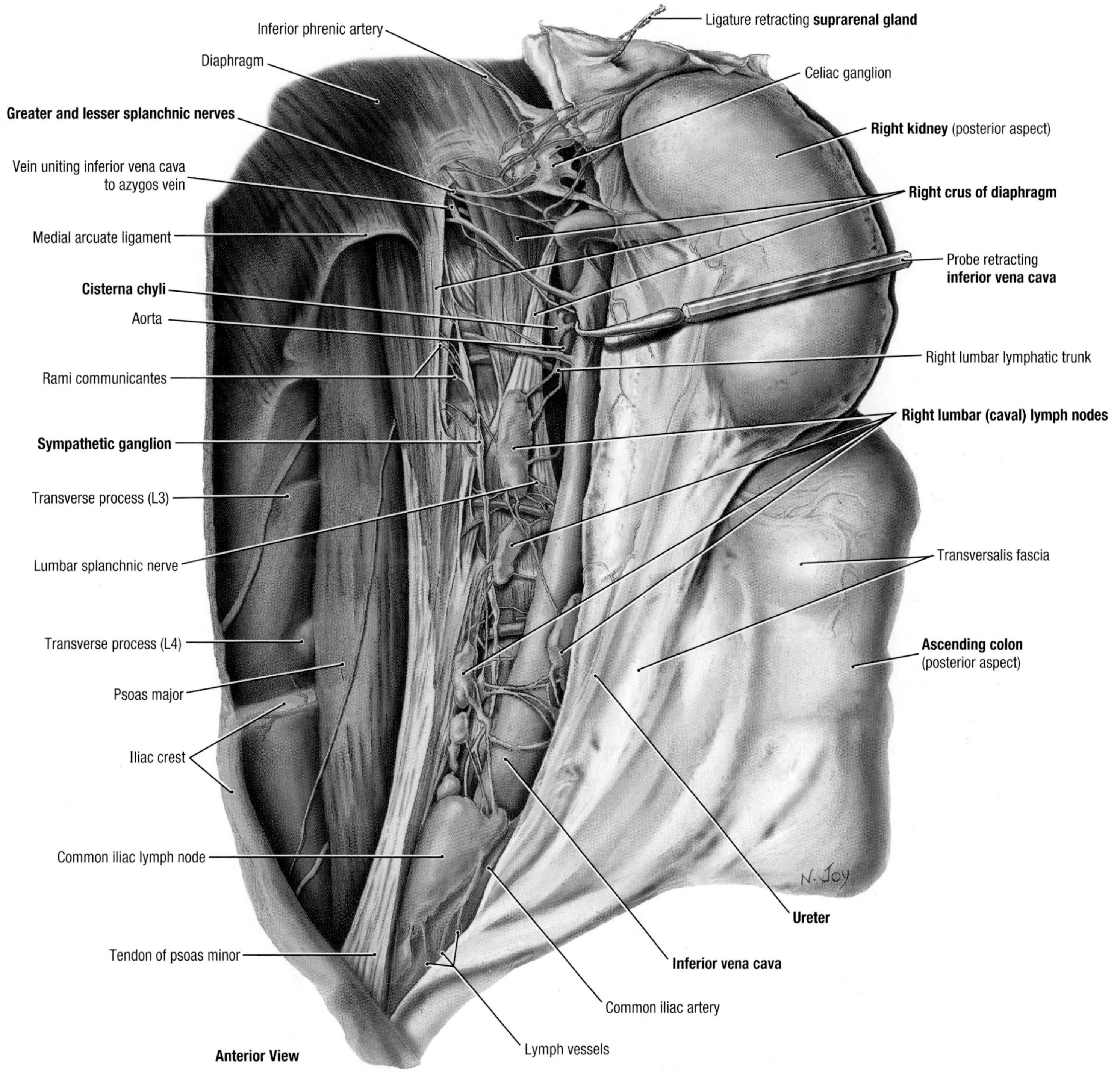
Ligature retracting suprarenal gland
Inferior phrenic artery
Diaphragm
Celiac ganglion
Greater and lesser splanchnic nerves
Right kidney (posterior aspect)
Vein uniting inferior vena cava to azygos vein
Right crus of diaphragm
Medial arcuate ligament
Probe retracting inferior vena cava
Cisterna chyli
Aorta
Right lumbar lymphatic trunk
Rami communicantes
Right lumbar (caval) lymph nodes
Sympathetic ganglion
Transverse process (L3)
Transversalis fascia
Lumbar splanchnic nerve
Transverse process (L4)
Ascending colon (posterior aspect)
Psoas major
Iliac crest
Common iliac lymph node
N. Joy
Ureter
Tendon of psoas minor
Inferior vena cava
Common iliac artery
Anterior View
Lymph vessels

2.88 LUMBAR LYMPH NODES, SYMPATHETIC TRUNK, NERVES, AND GANGLIA

The right suprarenal gland, kidney, ureter, and colon are reflected to the left; the inferior vena cava is pulled medially, and the third and fourth lumbar veins are removed. In this specimen, the greater and lesser splanchnic nerves, the sympathetic trunk, and a communicating vein pass through an unusually wide cleft in the right crus. The splanchnic nerves convey preganglionic fibers arising from the cell bodies in the (thoracolumbar) sympathetic trunk. The greater splanchnic nerve is from thoracic ganglia 5 to 9, and the lesser from thoracic ganglia 10 to 11.

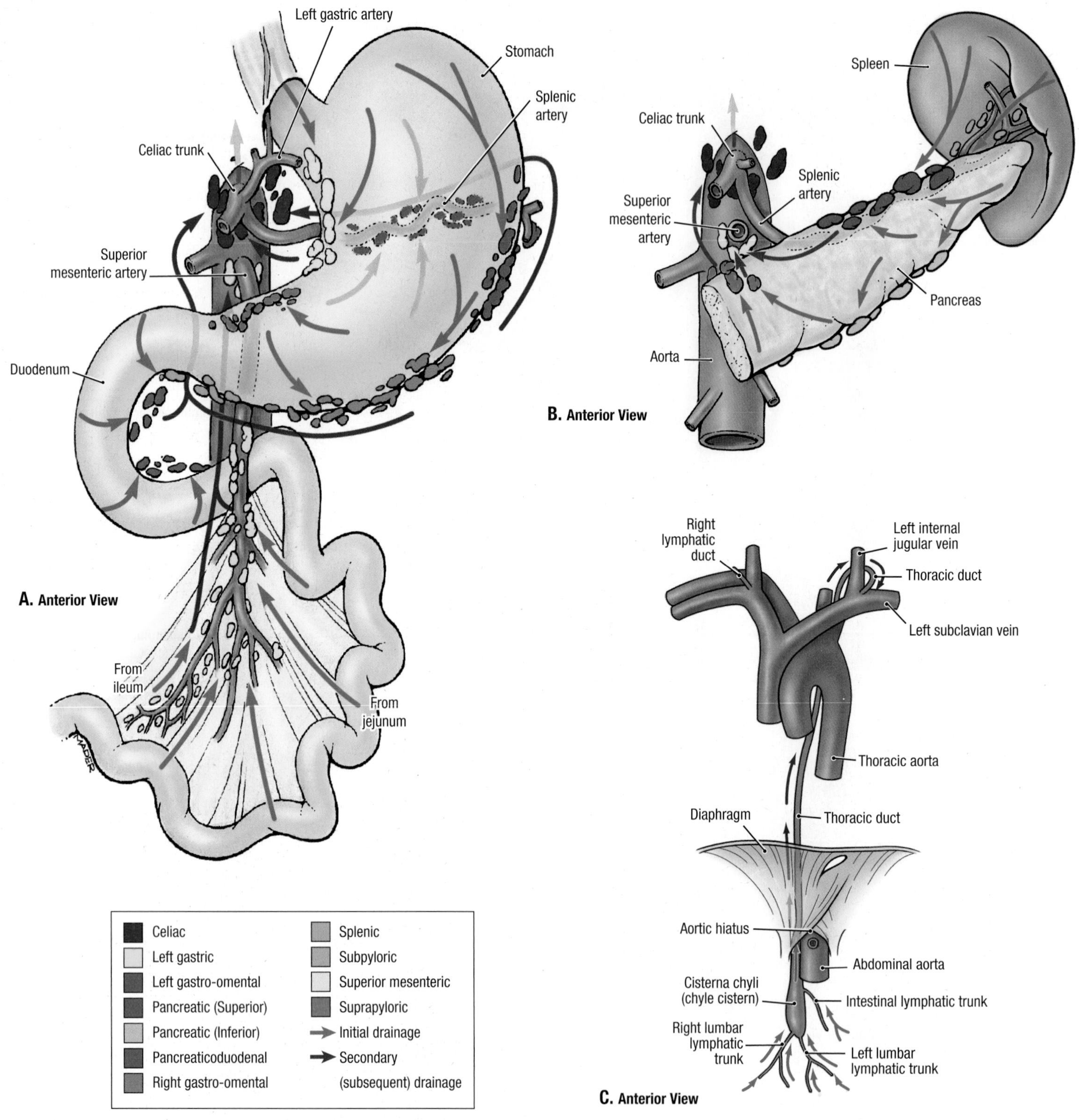

Left gastric artery
Stomach
Splenic artery
Celiac trunk
Superior mesenteric artery
Duodenum
A. Anterior View
From ileum
From jejunum
Spleen
Celiac trunk
Splenic artery
Superior mesenteric artery
Pancreas
Aorta
B. Anterior View
Right lymphatic duct
Left internal jugular vein
Thoracic duct
Left subclavian vein
Thoracic aorta
Diaphragm
Thoracic duct
Aortic hiatus
Abdominal aorta
Cisterna chyli (chyle cistern)
Intestinal lymphatic trunk
Right lumbar lymphatic trunk
Left lumbar lymphatic trunk
C. Anterior View
Celiac
Left gastric
Left gastro-omental
Pancreatic (Superior)
Pancreatic (Inferior)
Pancreaticoduodenal
Right gastro-omental
Splenic
Subpyloric
Superior mesenteric
Suprapyloric
Initial drainage
Secondary (subsequent) drainage

2.89 LYMPHATIC DRAINAGE

A. Stomach and small intestine. **B.** Spleen and pancreas. **C.** Drainage from lumbar and intestinal lymphatic trunks. The *arrows* indicate the direction of lymph flow; each group of lymph nodes is color coded. Lymph from the abdominal nodes drains into the cisterna chyli, origin of the inferior end of the thoracic duct. The thoracic duct receives all lymph that forms inferior to the diaphragm and left upper quadrant (thorax and left upper limb) and empties into the junction of the left subclavian and left internal jugular veins.

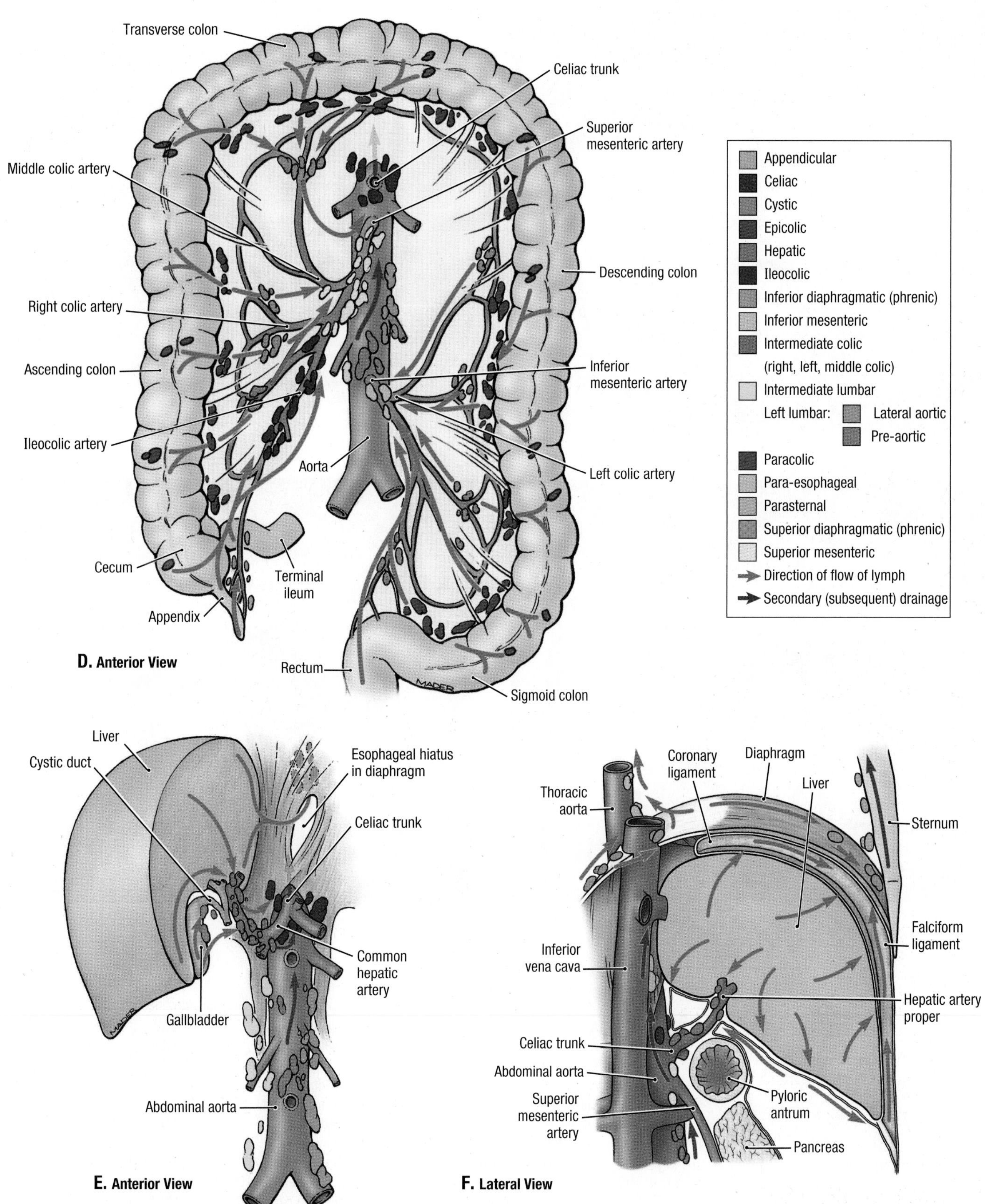
Transverse colon
Celiac trunk
Superior mesenteric artery
Middle colic artery
Descending colon
Right colic artery
Ascending colon
Inferior mesenteric artery
Ileocolic artery
Aorta
Left colic artery
Cecum
Terminal ileum
Appendix
Rectum
Sigmoid colon
D. Anterior View
Appendicular
Celiac
Cystic
Epicolic
Hepatic
Ileocolic
Inferior diaphragmatic (phrenic)
Inferior mesenteric
Intermediate colic
(right, left, middle colic)
Intermediate lumbar
Left lumbar:
Lateral aortic
Pre-aortic
Paracolic
Para-esophageal
Parasternal
Superior diaphragmatic (phrenic)
Superior mesenteric
Direction of flow of lymph
Secondary (subsequent) drainage
Liver
Cystic duct
Esophageal hiatus in diaphragm
Celiac trunk
Common hepatic artery
Gallbladder
Abdominal aorta
E. Anterior View
Coronary ligament
Diaphragm
Liver
Thoracic aorta
Sternum
Falciform ligament
Inferior vena cava
Hepatic artery proper
Celiac trunk
Abdominal aorta
Superior mesenteric artery
Pyloric antrum
Pancreas
F. Lateral View

2.89 LYMPHATIC DRAINAGE (*CONTINUED*)

D. Large intestine. **E.** Liver and gallbladder. **F.** Liver.

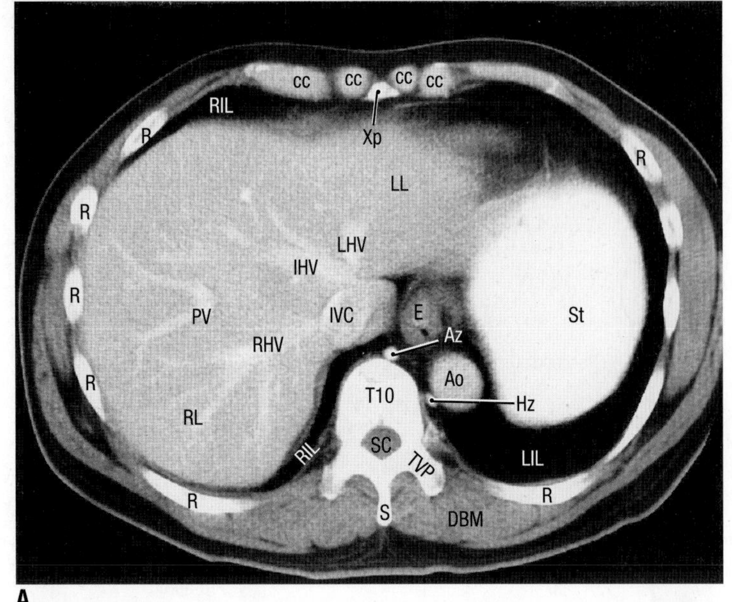
cc
cc
cc
cc
RIL
Xp
R
R
LL
R
LHV
IHV
R
PV
IVC
E
St
Az
RHV
Ao
R
T10
Hz
RL
SC
RIL
TVP
LIL
R
R
S
DBM
A

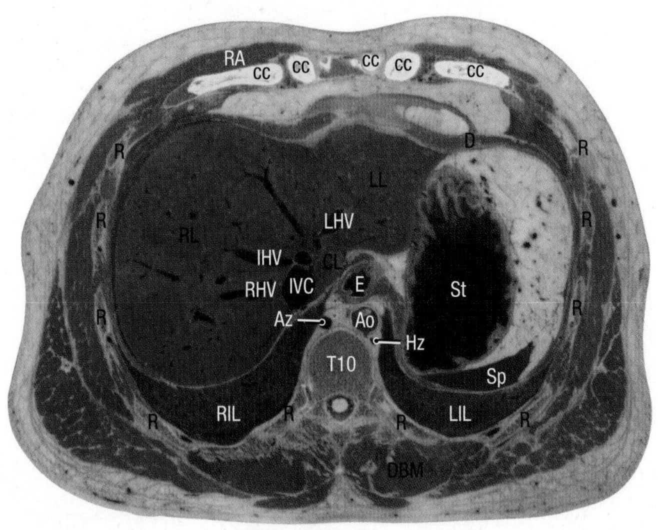
RA
cc
cc
cc
cc
cc
D
R
R
LL
R
RL
LHV
R
IHV
CL
E
St
RHV
IVC
R
Az
Ao
Hz
R
T10
Sp
R
RIL
R
R
LIL
R
DBM
B

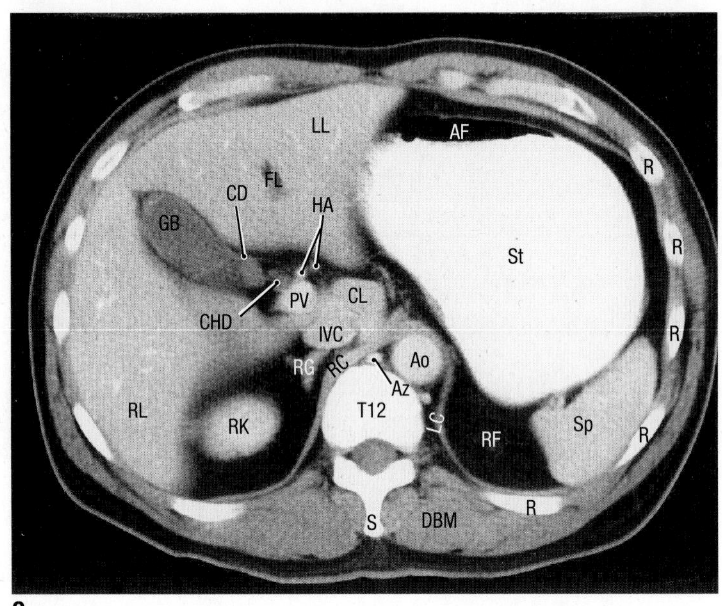
LL
AF
FL
R
CD
HA
GB
St
R
PV
CL
CHD
R
IVC
Ao
RG
RC
Az
RL
RK
T12
LC
RF
Sp
R
S
DBM
R
C

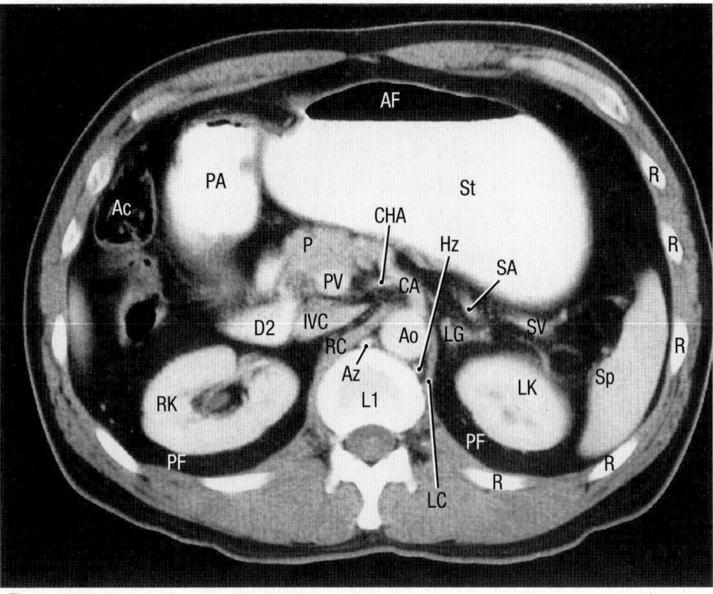
AF
PA
St
R
Ac
CHA
R
P
Hz
SA
PV
CA
D2
IVC
Ao
LG
SV
R
RC
Az
LK
Sp
RK
L1
PF
PF
R
R
LC
D

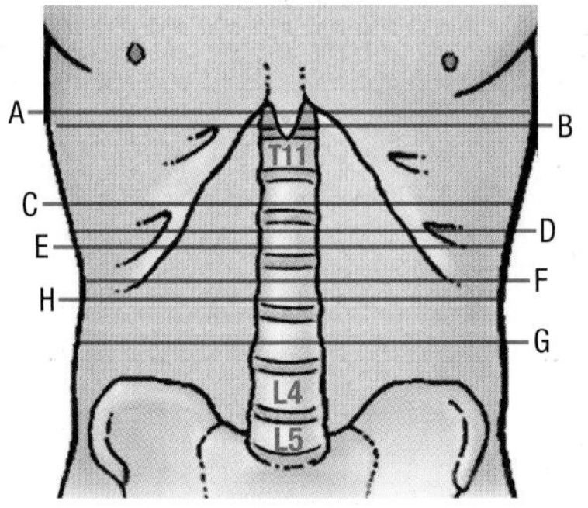
A
B
T11
C
D
E
F
H
G
L4
L5

Ac	Ascending colon	Dc	Descending colon	LHV	Left hepatic vein
AF	Air-fluid level of stomach	D2	Descending part of duodenum	LIL	Left inferior lobe of lung
Ao	Aorta	D3	Inferior part of duodenum	LK	Left kidney
Az	Azygos vein	E	Esophagus	LL	Left lobe of liver
CA	Celiac artery	FL	Falciform ligament	LRV	Left renal vein
cc	Costal cartilage	GB	Gallbladder	LU	Left ureter
CD	Cystic duct	HA	Hepatic artery	IHV	Intermediate hepatic vein
CHA	Common hepatic artery	Hz	Hemi-azygos vein	P	Pancreas
CHD	Common hepatic duct	IMV	Inferior mesenteric vein	PA	Pyloric antrum of stomach
CL	Caudate lobe of liver	IVC	Inferior vena cava	PB	Body of pancreas
D	Diaphragm	LC	Left crus of diaphragm	PC	Portal confluence
DBM	Deep back muscles	LG	Left suprarenal gland		

2.90 TRANSVERSE OR HORIZONTAL (AXIAL) MRIs OF ABDOMEN

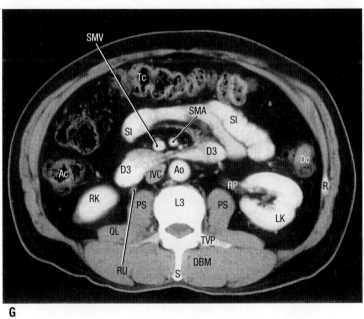

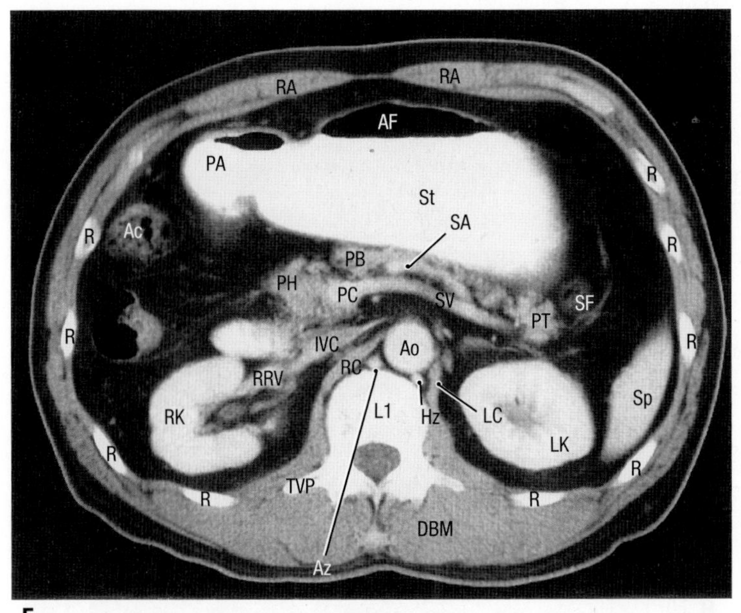
RA
RA
AF
PA
St
SA
R
Ac
PB
PH
PC
SV
SF
PT
IVC
Ao
RRV
RC
L1
Hz
LC
Sp
RK
LK
TVP
DBM
Az

E

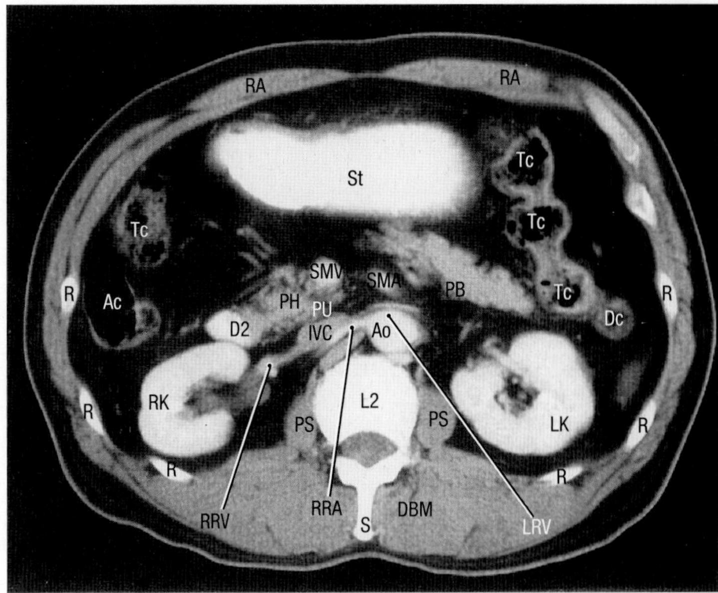
RA
RA
St
Tc
SMV
SMA
PB
PH
PU
Ac
D2
IVC
Ao
Dc
R
RK
L2
PS
LK
RRV
RRA
DBM
S
LRV

F

G

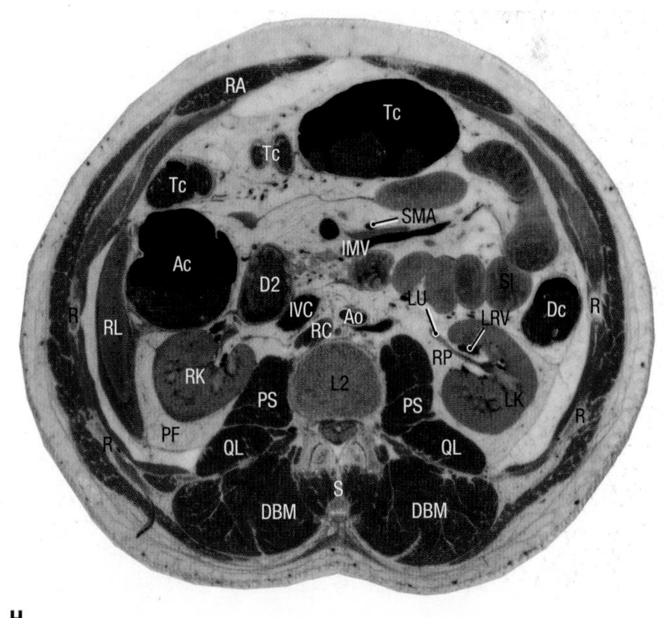
RA
Tc
SMA
IMV
Ac
D2
SI
Dc
R
RL
IVC
RC
Ao
LU
LRV
RP
RK
L2
PS
LK
PF
QL
S
DBM

H

PF	Perinephric fat	RC	Right crus of diaphragm	RRV	Right renal vein	Sp	Spleen
PH	Head of pancreas	RF	Retroperitoneal fat	RU	Right ureter	St	Stomach
PS	Psoas muscle	RG	Right suprarenal gland	S	Spinous process	SV	Splenic vein
PT	Tail of pancreas	RHV	Right hepatic vein	SA	Splenic artery	Tc	Transverse colon
PU	Uncinate process of pancreas	RIL	Right inferior lobe of lung	SC	Spinal cord	TVP	Transverse process
PV	Hepatic portal vein	RK	Right kidney	SF	Splenic flexure	Xp	Xiphoid process
QL	Quadratus lumborum	RL	Right lobe of liver	SI	Small intestine		
R	Rib	RP	Renal pelvis	SMA	Superior mesenteric artery		
RA	Rectus abdominis	RRA	Right renal artery	SMV	Superior mesenteric vein		

2.90 TRANSVERSE OR HORIZONTAL (AXIAL) MRIs OF ABDOMEN (*CONTINUED*)

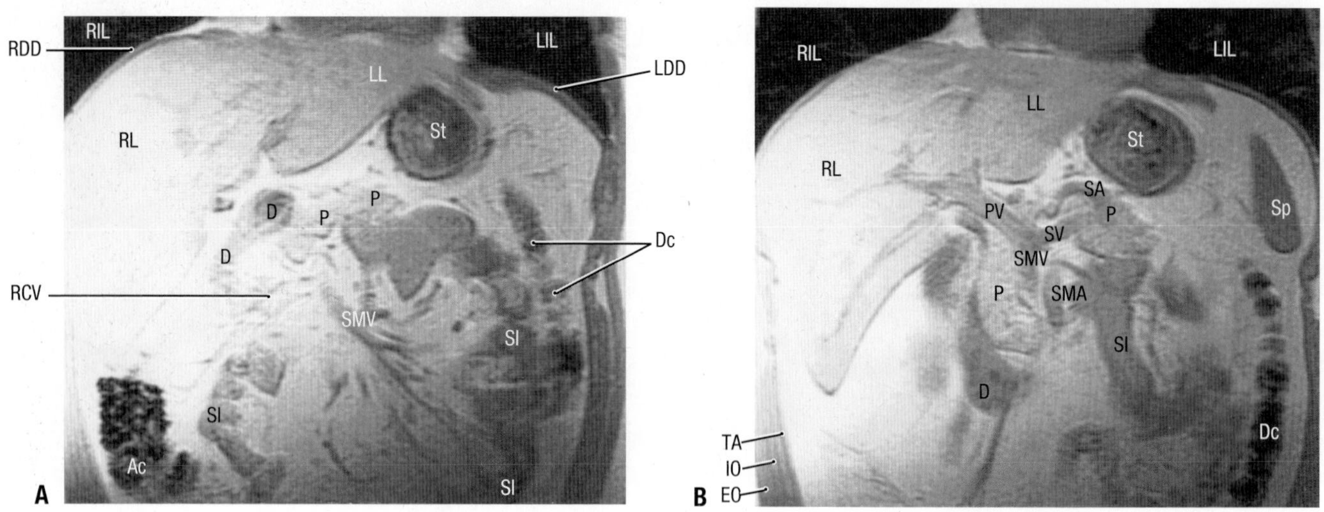
RDD
RIL
LIL
LDD
LL
St
RL
D
P
P
Dc
D
RCV
SMV
SI
SI
Ac
SI
A
RIL
LIL
LL
St
RL
SA
PV
P
Sp
SV
SMV
P
SMA
SI
D
Dc
TA
IO
EO
B

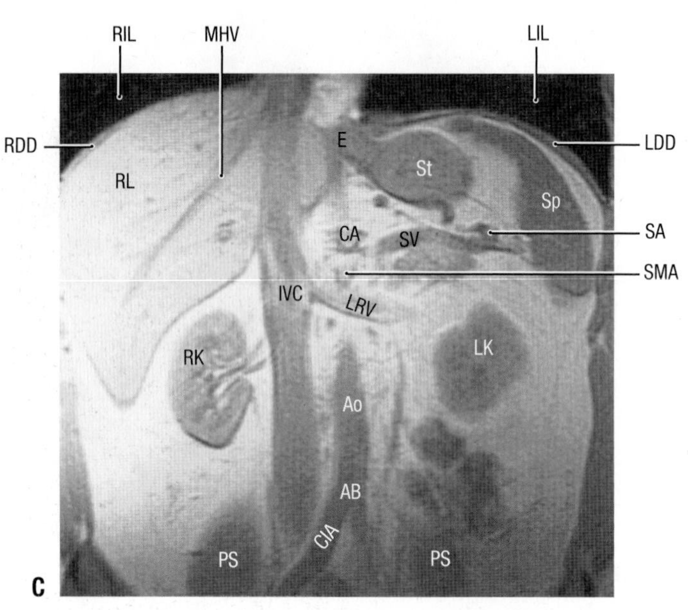
RIL
MHV
LIL
RDD
E
LDD
RL
St
Sp
CA
SV
SA
SMA
IVC
LRV
RK
LK
Ao
AB
CIA
PS
PS
C

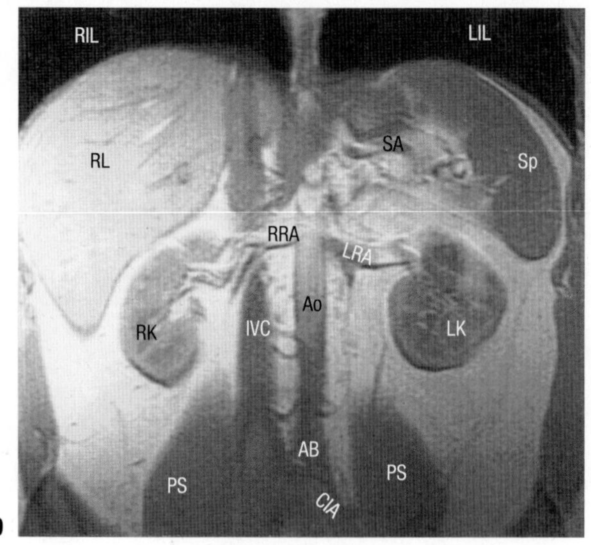
RIL
LIL
RL
SA
Sp
RRA
LRA
Ao
RK
IVC
LK
AB
PS
PS
CIA
D

AB	Aortic bifurcation	IO	Internal oblique	P	Pancreas	SA	Splenic artery
Ac	Ascending colon	IVC	Inferior vena cava	PV	Portal vein	SI	Small intestine
Ao	Aorta	LDD	Left dome of diaphragm	PS	Psoas	SMA	Superior mesenteric artery
CA	Celiac artery	LIL	Left lung (inferior lobe)	RCV	Right colic vein	SMV	Superior mesenteric vein
CIA	Common iliac artery	LK	Left kidney	RDD	Right dome of diaphragm	Sp	Spleen
D	Duodenum	LL	Left lobe of liver	RIL	Right lung (inferior lobe)	St	Stomach
Dc	Descending colon	LRA	Left renal artery	RK	Right kidney	SV	Splenic vein
E	Esophagus	LRV	Left renal vein	RL	Right lobe of liver	TA	Transversus abdominis
EO	External oblique	MHV	Middle hepatic vein	RRA	Right renal artery		

2.91 CORONAL MRIs OF ABDOMEN

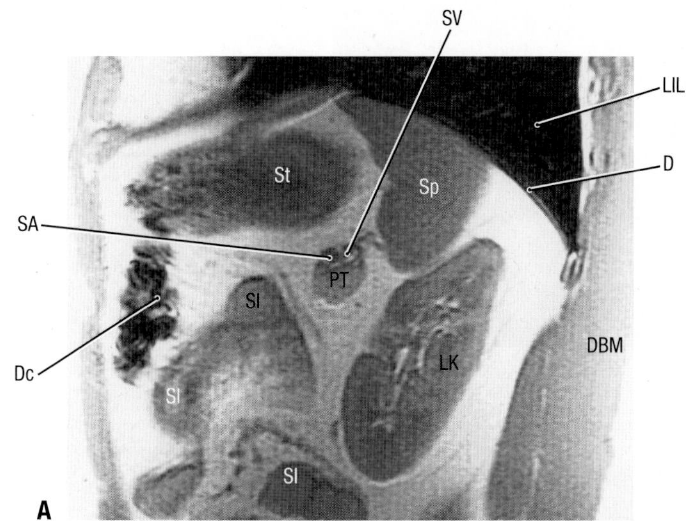
SV
LIL
D
St
Sp
SA
PT
SI
Dc
DBM
LK
SI
SI
A

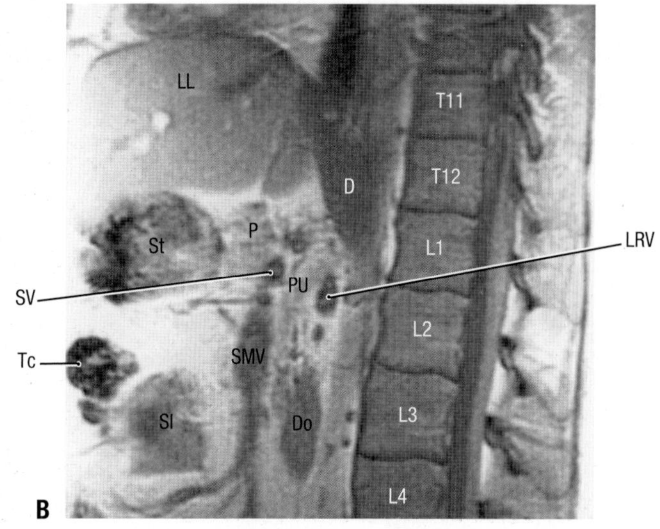
LL
T11
T12
D
St
P
L1
LRV
SV
PU
L2
Tc
SMV
SI
Do
L3
L4
B

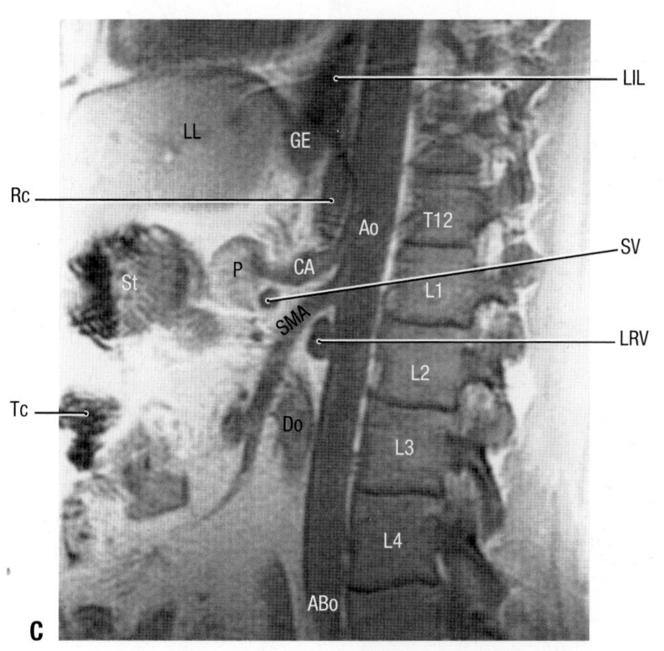
LIL
LL
GE
Rc
Ao
T12
SV
St
P
CA
L1
SMA
LRV
L2
Tc
Do
L3
L4
ABo
C

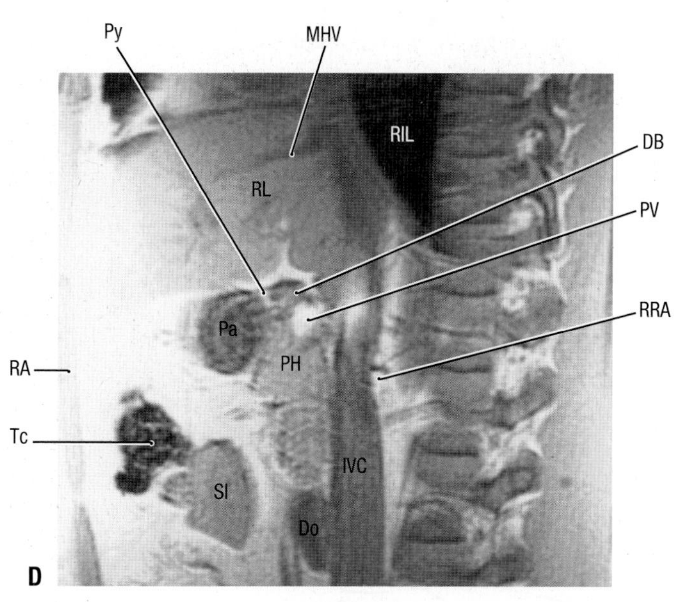
Py
MHV
RIL
DB
RL
PV
RRA
Pa
PH
RA
Tc
IVC
SI
Do
D

Ao	Aorta	IVC	Inferior vena cava	PH	Head of pancreas	RRA	Right renal artery
ABo	Bifurcation of aorta	LIL	Inferior lobe of left lung	PT	Tail of pancreas	SA	Splenic artery
CA	Celiac artery	LK	Left kidney	PV	Portal vein	SI	Small intestine
D	Diaphragm	LL	Left lobe of liver	PU	Uncinate process of pancreas	SMA	Superior mesenteric artery
DB	Bulb of duodenum	LRV	Left renal vein	Py	Pylorus of stomach	SMV	Superior mesenteric vein
Dc	Descending colon	MHV	Middle hepatic vein	RA	Rectus abdominus	Sp	Spleen
Do	Duodenum	P	Pancreas	RC	Right crus	St	Stomach
DBM	Deep back muscles	Pa	Pyloric antrum	RIL	Inferior lobe of right lung	SV	Splenic vein
GE	Gastroesophageal junction	PC	Portal confluence	RL	Right lobe of right liver	Tc	Transverse colon

2.92 SAGITTAL MRIs OF ABDOMEN

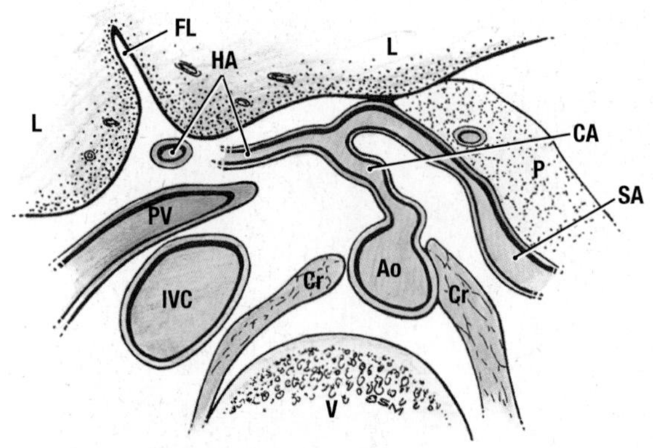
FL
HA
L
L
CA
P
SA
PV
IVC
Cr
Ao
Cr
V

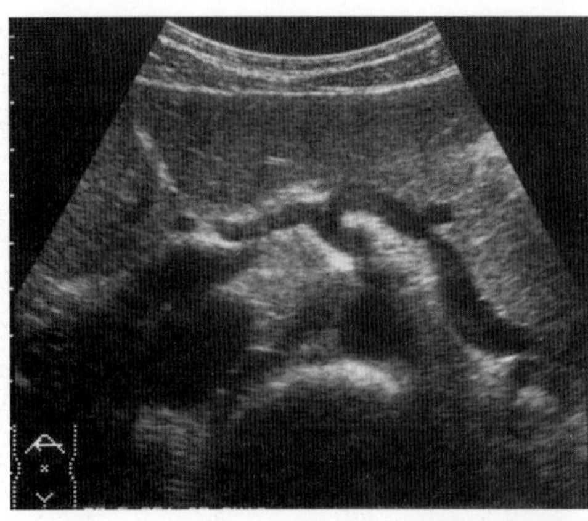

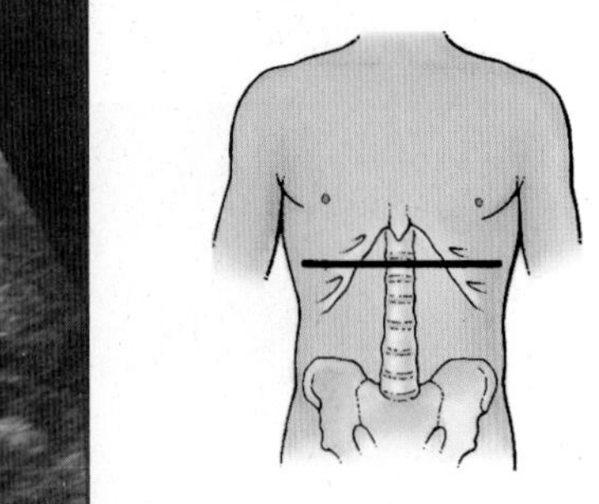

A. Transverse Section, Inferior View

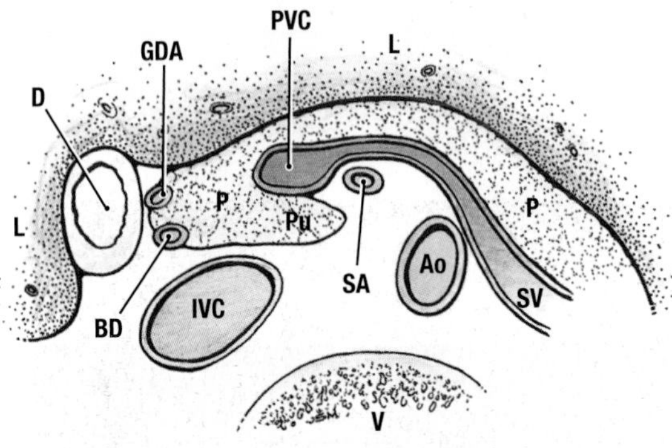
PVC
GDA
L
D
P
Pu
P
L
Ao
SA
SV
IVC
BD
V

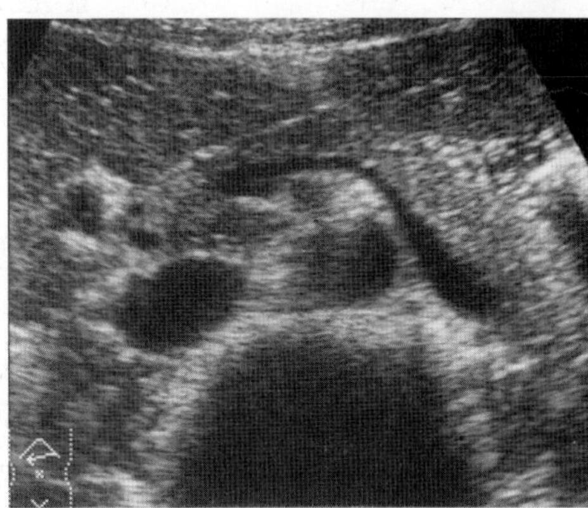

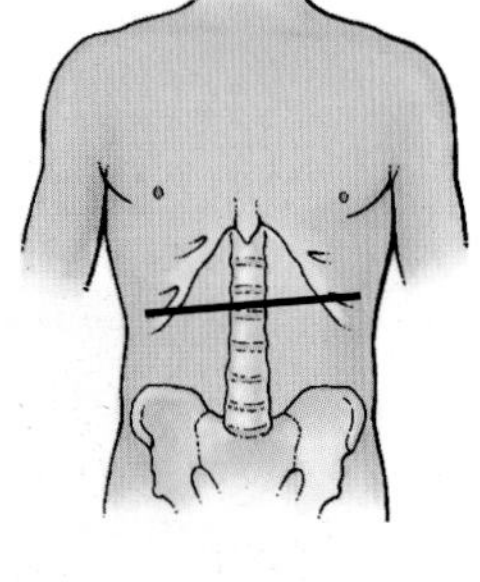

B. Transverse Section, Inferior View

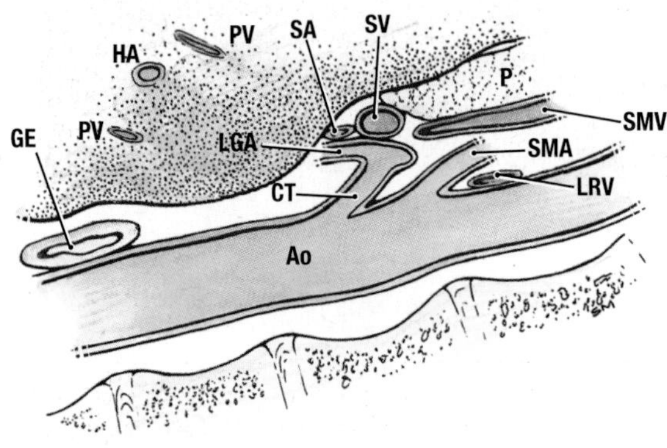
HA
PV
SA
SV
P
SMV
GE
PV
LGA
SMA
CT
LRV
Ao

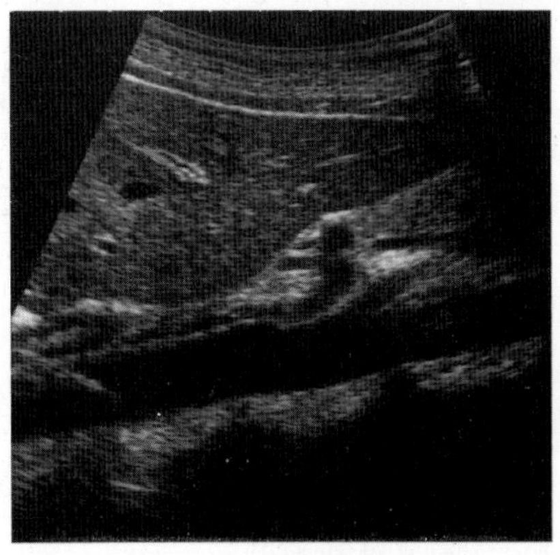

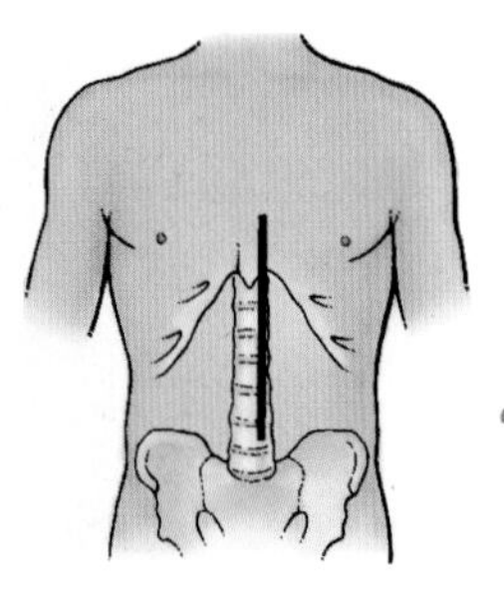

C. Median Section, Right Lateral View

2.93 ULTRASOUND SCANS AND MR ANGIOGRAM OF ABDOMEN

A. Transverse ultrasound scan through celiac trunk. **B.** Transverse ultrasound scan through pancreas. **C. and D.** Sagittal ultrasound scans through the aorta, celiac trunk, and superior mesenteric artery. (**D.** with Doppler.) **E.** MR angiogram of abdominal aorta and branches. **F.** Transverse ultrasound scan at hilum of left kidney with the left renal artery and vein (with Doppler). **G.** Sagittal ultrasound scan of the right kidney.

A major advantage of ultrasonography is its ability to produce real-time images, demonstrating motion of structures and flow within blood vessels. In Doppler ultrasonography (**D** and **F**) the shifts in frequency between emitted ultrasonic waves and their echoes are used to measure the velocities of moving objects. This technique is based on the principle of the Doppler effect. Blood flow through vessels is displayed in color, superimposed on the two-dimensional cross-sectional image (slow flow: *blue*, fast flow: *orange*).

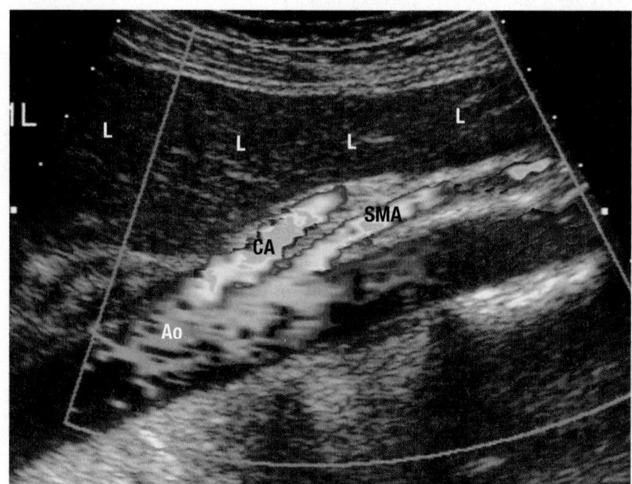
L
L
L
L
L
CA
SMA
Ao

D. **Median Section, Right Lateral View**

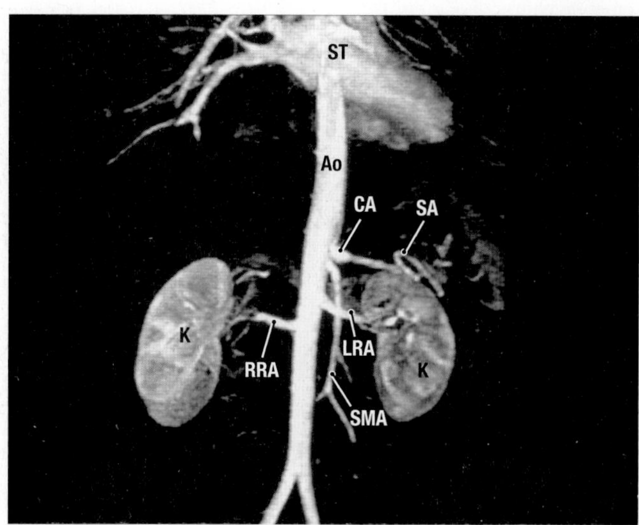
ST
Ao
CA
SA
K
RRA
LRA
K
SMA

E. **Anterior View**

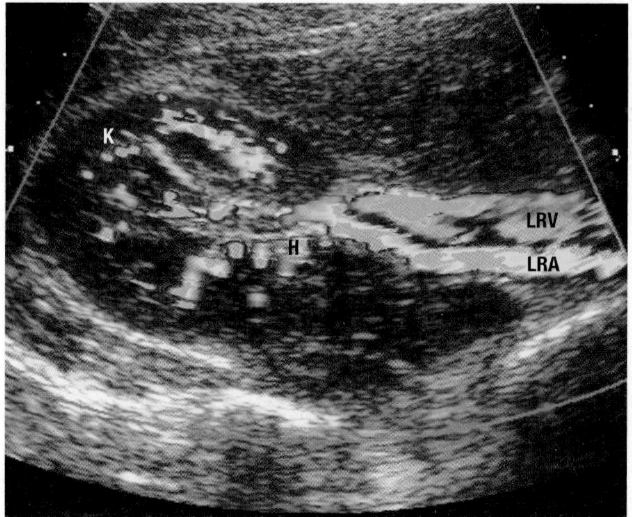
K
H
LRV
LRA

F. **Transverse Section**

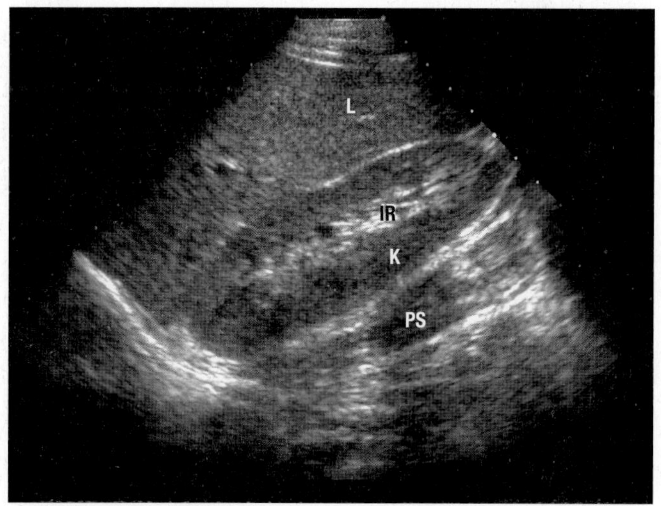
L
IR
K
PS

G. **Sagittal Section, Right Lateral View**

Ao	Aorta	H	Hilum of kidney	LRV	Left renal vein	SMA	Superior mesenteric artery
BD	Bile duct	HA	Hepatic artery	P	Pancreas	SMV	Superior mesenteric vein
CA	Celiac artery	IR	Perirenal fat in renal sinus	PS	Psoas	ST	Stomach
Cr	Crus of diaphragm	IVC	Inferior vena cava	Pu	Uncinate process of pancreas	SV	Splenic vein
D	Duodenum	K	Cortex of kidney	PV	Portal vein	V	Vertebra
FL	Falciform ligament	L	Liver	PVC	Portal venous confluence		
GDA	Gastroduodenal artery	LGA	Left gastric artery	RRA	Right renal artery		
GE	Gastro-esophageal junction	LRA	Left renal artery	SA	Splenic artery		

2.93 ULTRASOUND SCANS AND MR ANGIOGRAM OF ABDOMEN (*CONTINUED*)

CHAPTER 3

Pelvis and Perineum

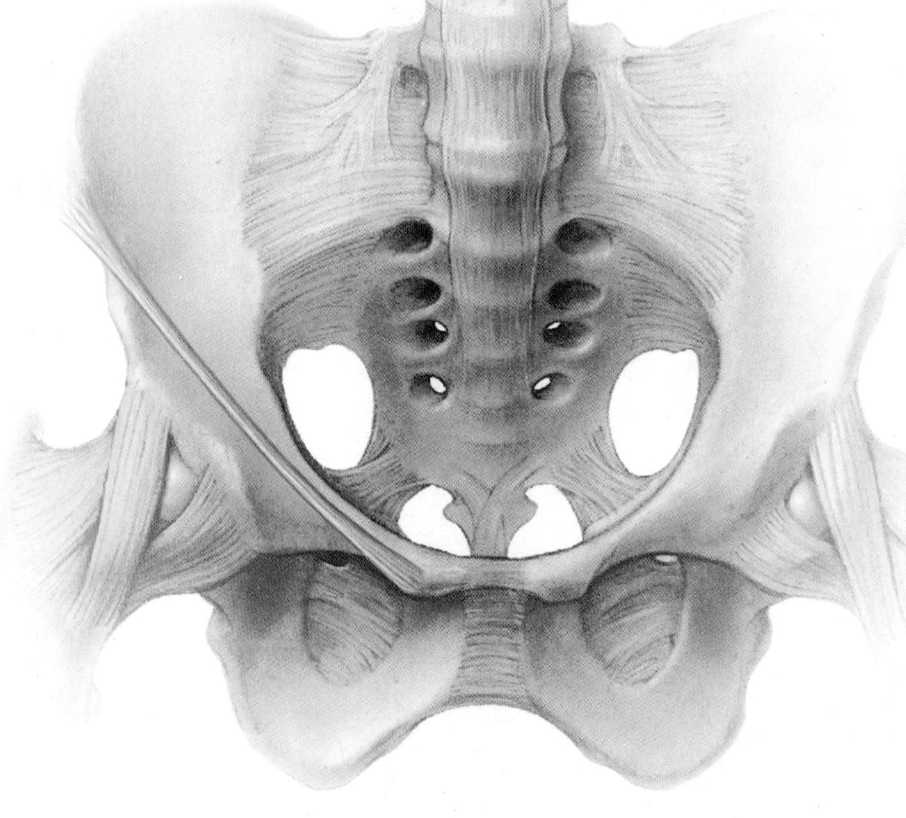

Pelvic Girdle	198
Ligaments of Pelvic Girdle	205
Floor and Walls of Pelvis	206
Sacral and Coccygeal Plexuses	210
Peritoneal Reflections in Pelvis	212
Rectum and Anal Canal	214
Organs of Male Pelvis	220
Vessels of Male Pelvis	228
Lymphatic Drainage of Male Pelvis and Perineum	232
Innervation of Male Pelvic Organs	234
Organs of Female Pelvis	236
Vessels of Female Pelvis	242
Lymphatic Drainage of Female Pelvis and Perineum	248
Innervation of Female Pelvic Organs	250
Subperitoneal Region of Pelvis	254
Surface Anatomy of Perineum	256
Overview of Male and Female Perineum	258
Male Perineum	265
Female Perineum	273
Imaging and Sectional Anatomy of Pelvis and Perineum	280

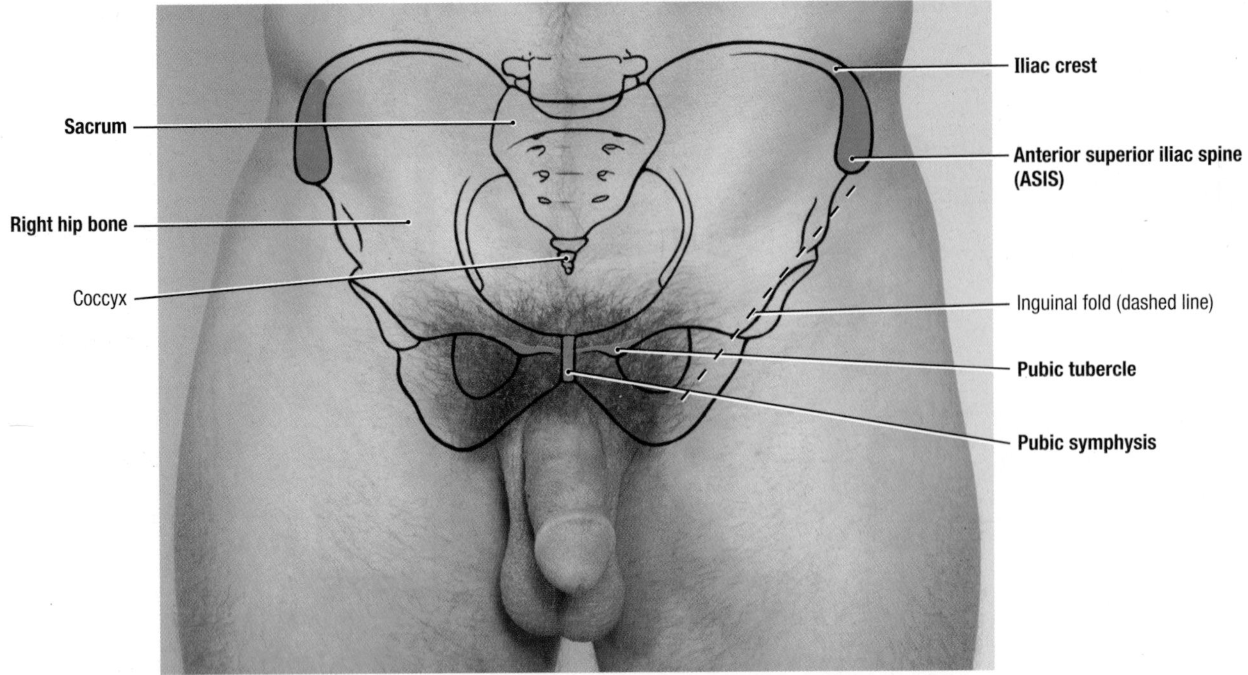
Iliac crest
Sacrum
Anterior superior iliac spine (ASIS)
Right hip bone
Coccyx
Inguinal fold (dashed line)
Pubic tubercle
Pubic symphysis

A. Anterior View

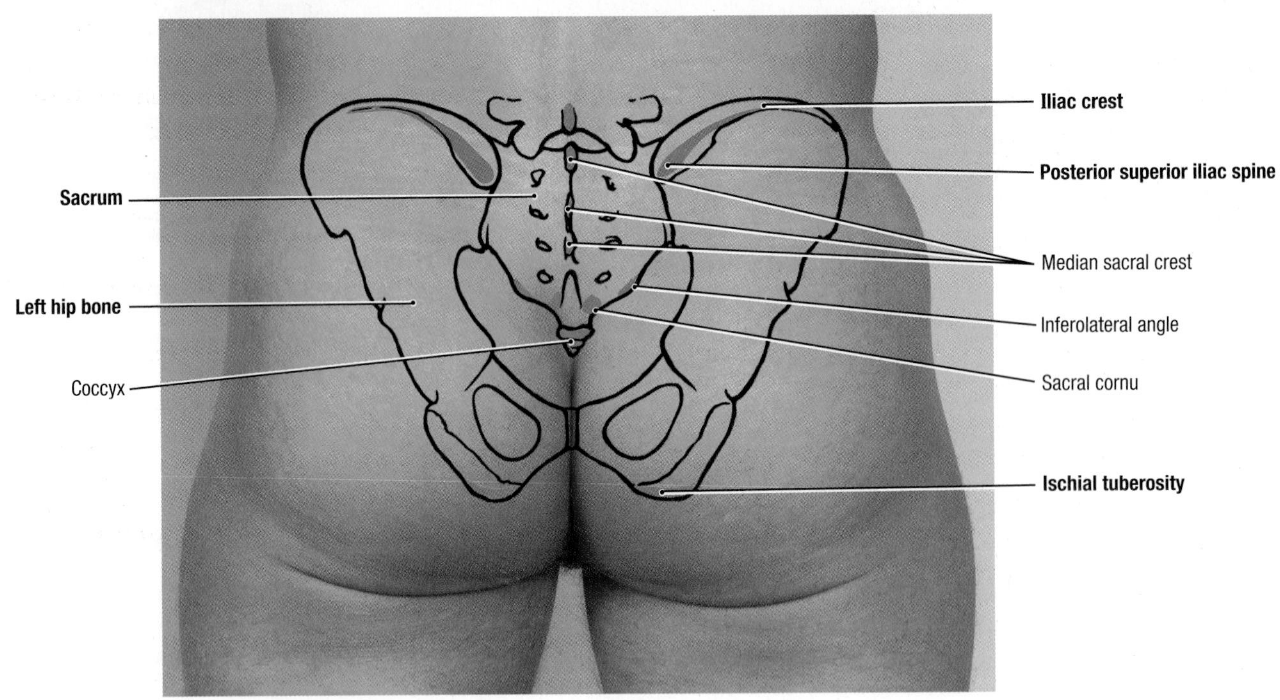
Iliac crest
Posterior superior iliac spine
Sacrum
Median sacral crest
Left hip bone
Inferolateral angle
Coccyx
Sacral cornu
Ischial tuberosity

B. Posterior View

3.1 SURFACE ANATOMY OF MALE PELVIC GIRDLE

The pelvic girdle (bony pelvis) is a basin-shaped ring of three bones (right and left hip bones and sacrum) that connects the vertebral column to the femora. **Palpable features** (*green*) should be symmetrical across the midline. **A.** The anterior third of the iliac crests are subcutaneous and usually easily palpable. The remainder of the crests may also be palpable, depending on the thickness of the overlying subcutaneous tissue (fat). The inguinal ligament spans between the palpable anterior superior iliac spine (ASIS) and pubic tubercle, located superior to the lateral and medial ends of the inguinal fold. **B.** The posterior superior iliac spine (PSIS) is usually palpable and often lies deep to a visible dimple, indicating the S2 vertebral level. The ischial tuberosities may be palpated when the hip joint is flexed.

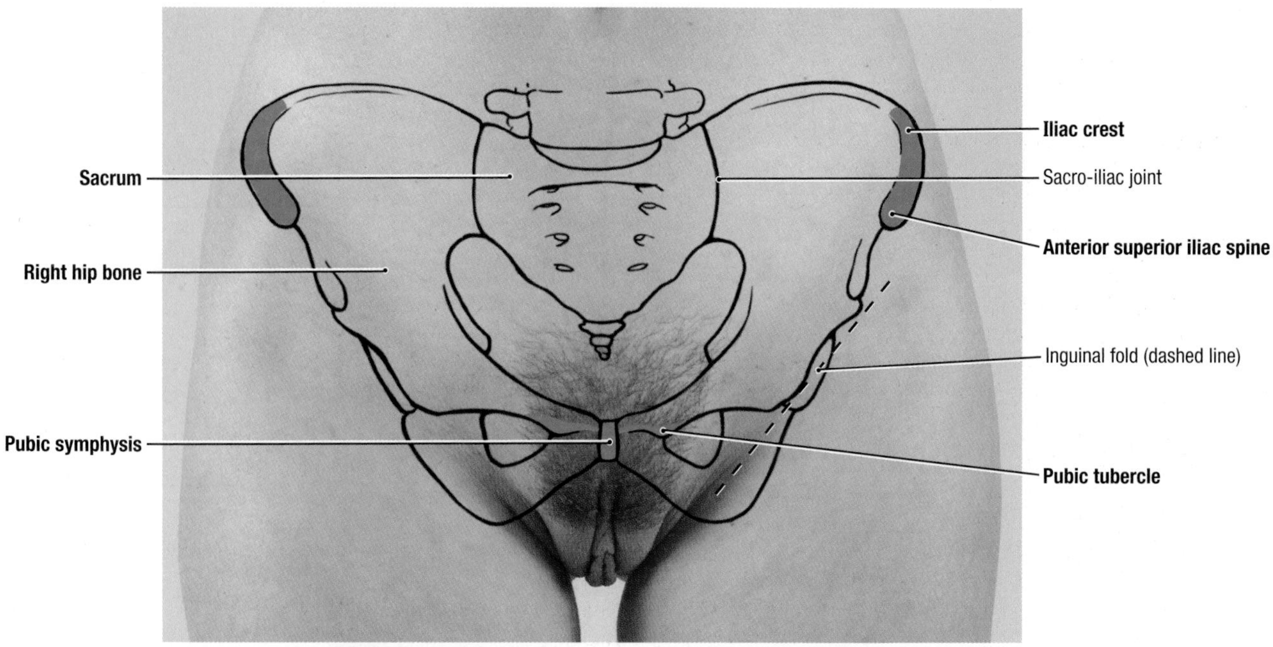
Sacrum
Right hip bone
Pubic symphysis
Iliac crest
Sacro-iliac joint
Anterior superior iliac spine
Inguinal fold (dashed line)
Pubic tubercle

A. Anterior View

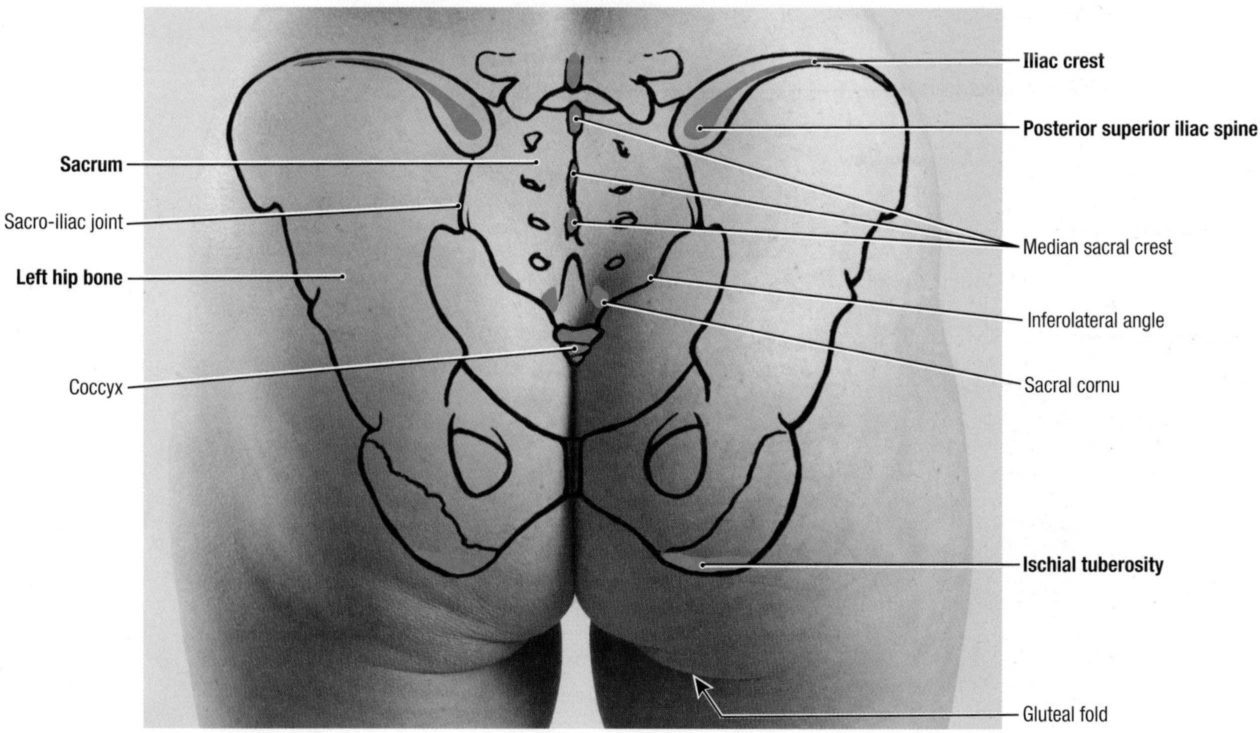
Sacrum
Sacro-iliac joint
Left hip bone
Coccyx
Iliac crest
Posterior superior iliac spine
Median sacral crest
Inferolateral angle
Sacral cornu
Ischial tuberosity
Gluteal fold

B. Posterior View

3.2 SURFACE ANATOMY OF FEMALE PELVIC GIRDLE

The female pelvic girdle is relatively wider and shallower than that of the male, related to its additional roles of bearing the weight of the gravid uterus in late **pregnancy** and allowing passage of the fetus through the pelvic outlet during childbirth **(parturition). A. Palpable features** (*green*): The hip bones are joined anteriorly at the pubic symphysis. The presence of a thick overlying pubic fat pad forming the mons pubis may interfere with palpation of the pubic tubercles and symphysis. **B.** Posteriorly the hip bones are joined to the sacrum at the sacro-iliac joints.

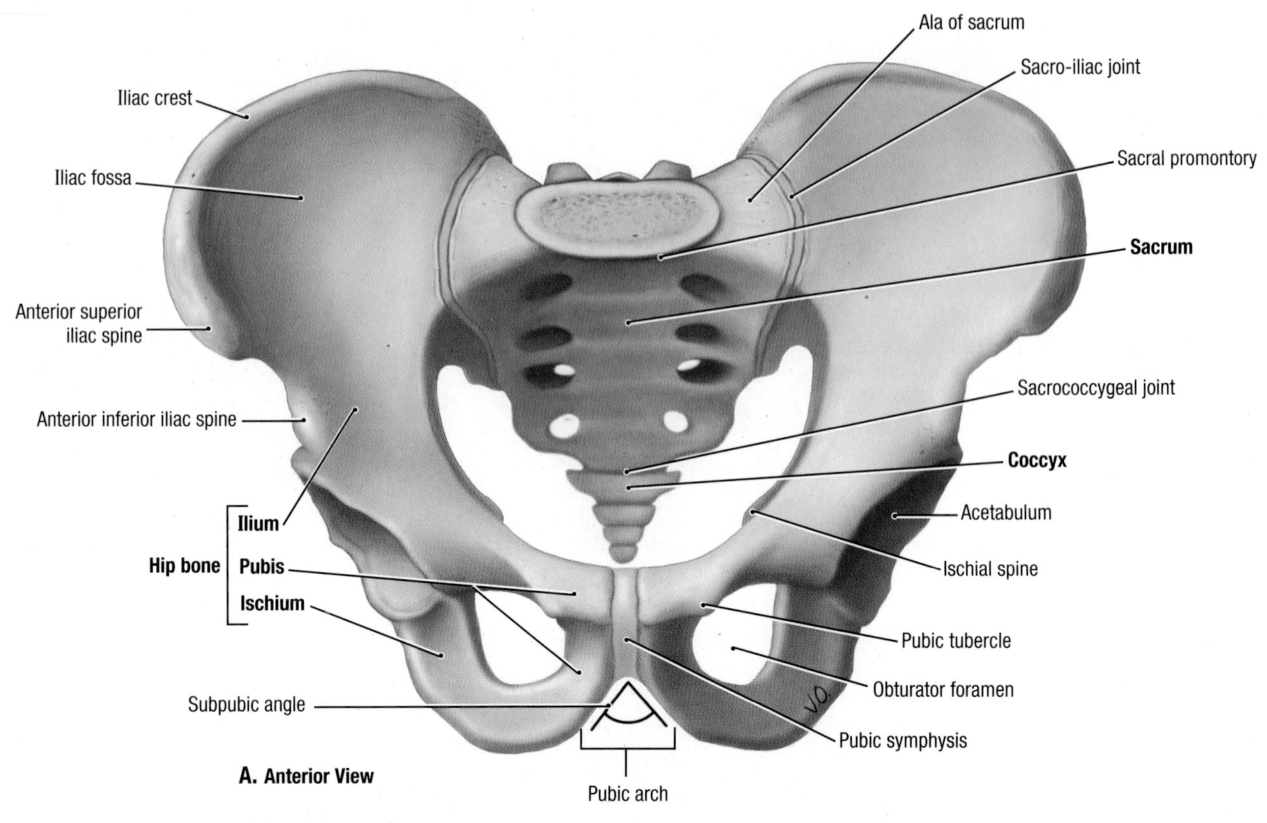
Ala of sacrum
Sacro-iliac joint
Iliac crest
Sacral promontory
Iliac fossa
Sacrum
Anterior superior iliac spine
Sacrococcygeal joint
Anterior inferior iliac spine
Coccyx
Acetabulum
Ilium
Hip bone
Pubis
Ischial spine
Ischium
Pubic tubercle
Obturator foramen
Subpubic angle
Pubic symphysis
Pubic arch

A. Anterior View

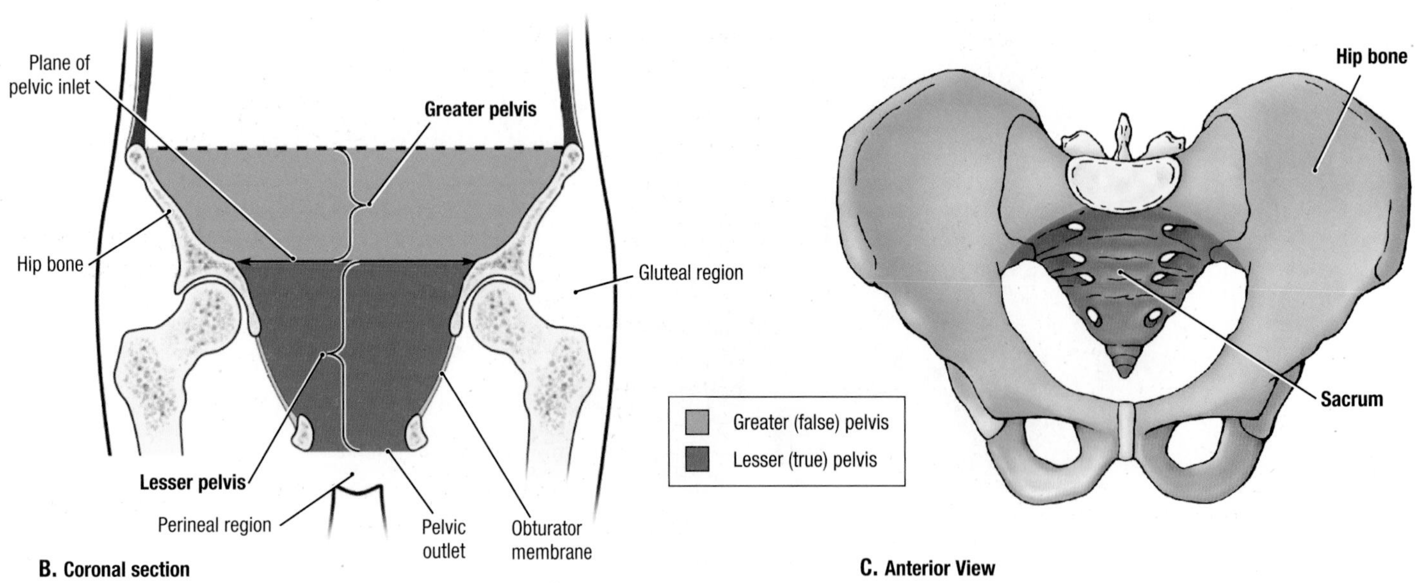
Plane of pelvic inlet
Greater pelvis
Hip bone
Gluteal region
Lesser pelvis
Perineal region
Pelvic outlet
Obturator membrane
Greater (false) pelvis
Lesser (true) pelvis
Hip bone
Sacrum

B. Coronal section

C. Anterior View

3.3 BONES AND DIVISIONS OF PELVIS

A. Bones of pelvis. The three bones composing the pelvis are the pubis, ischium, and ilium. **B. and C.** Lesser and greater pelvis, schematic illustrations. The plane of the pelvic inlet (*double-headed arrow* in *B*) separates the greater pelvis (part of the abdominal cavity) from the lesser pelvis (pelvic cavity).

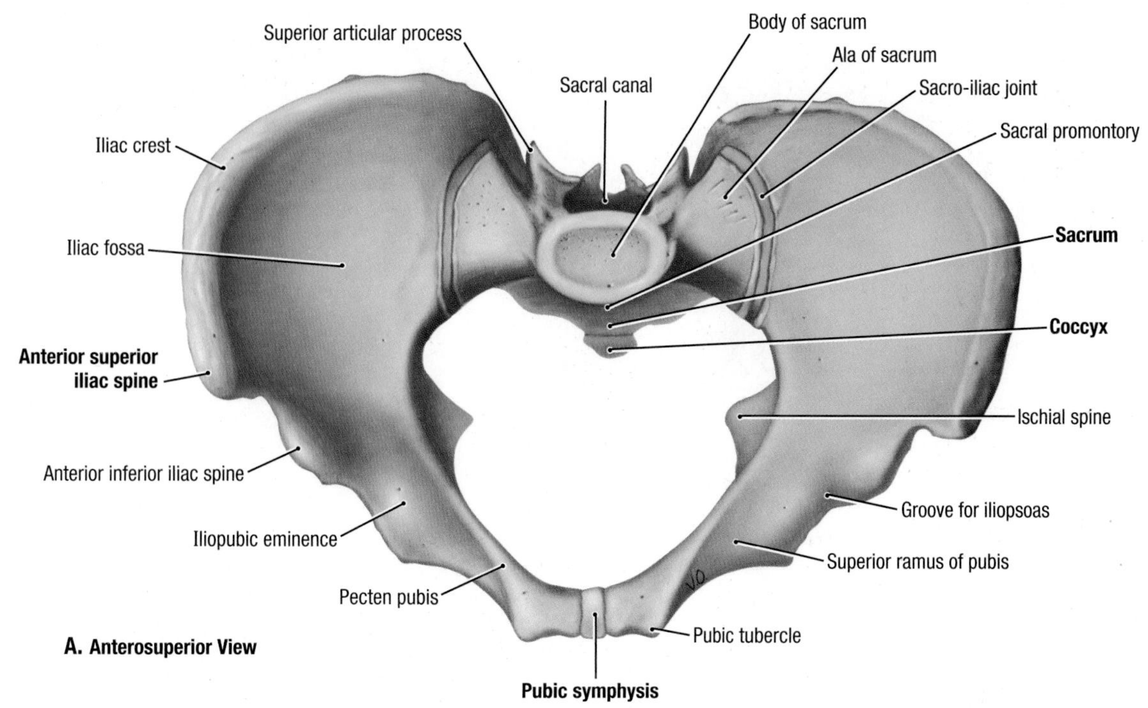
Superior articular process
Body of sacrum
Ala of sacrum
Sacral canal
Sacro-iliac joint
Sacral promontory
Iliac crest
Iliac fossa
Sacrum
Coccyx
Anterior superior iliac spine
Ischial spine
Anterior inferior iliac spine
Groove for iliopsoas
Iliopubic eminence
Superior ramus of pubis
Pecten pubis
Pubic tubercle
Pubic symphysis

A. Anterosuperior View

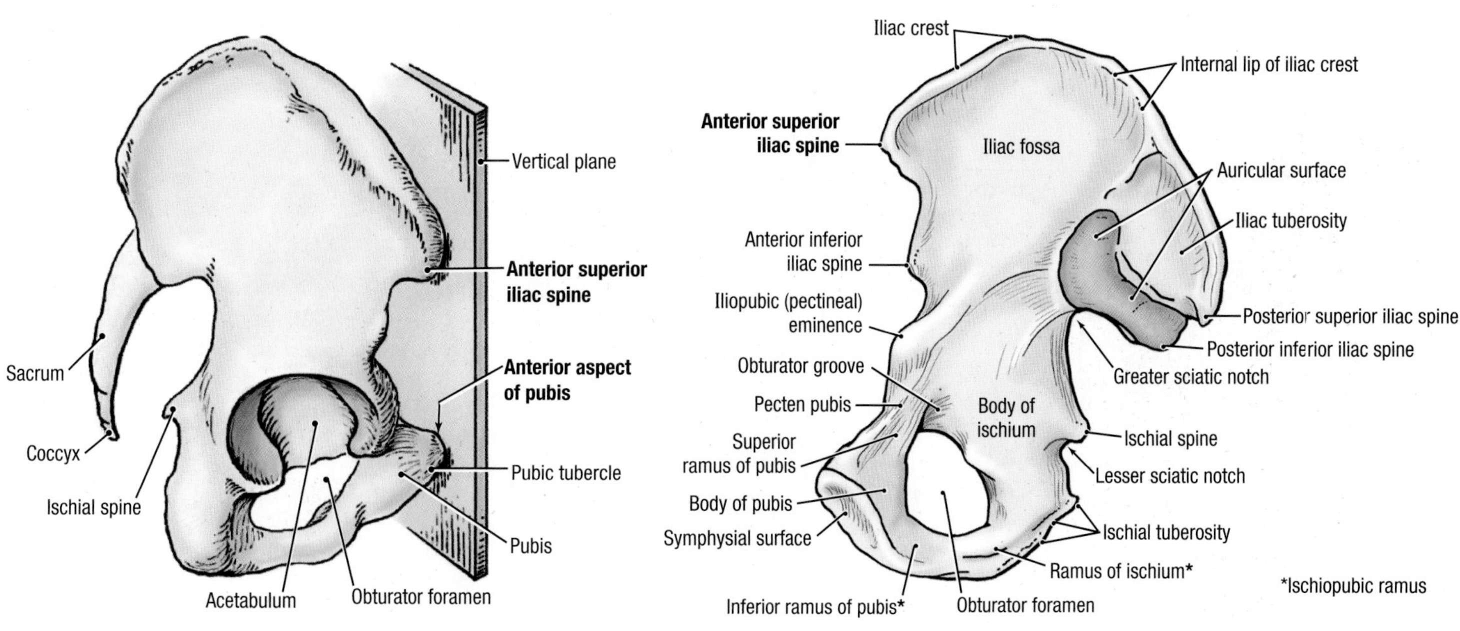
Vertical plane
Anterior superior iliac spine
Anterior aspect of pubis
Sacrum
Coccyx
Pubic tubercle
Ischial spine
Pubis
Acetabulum
Obturator foramen
Iliac crest
Internal lip of iliac crest
Anterior superior iliac spine
Iliac fossa
Auricular surface
Iliac tuberosity
Anterior inferior iliac spine
Iliopubic (pectineal) eminence
Posterior superior iliac spine
Posterior inferior iliac spine
Obturator groove
Greater sciatic notch
Pecten pubis
Body of ischium
Superior ramus of pubis
Ischial spine
Lesser sciatic notch
Body of pubis
Symphysial surface
Ischial tuberosity
Ramus of ischium*
Inferior ramus of pubis*
Obturator foramen
*Ischiopubic ramus

B. Lateral View **C. Medial Aspect**

3.4 PELVIS, ANATOMICAL POSITION

A. Pelvic girdle. **B.** Placement of hip bone in anatomical position. In the anatomical position, (1) the anterior superior iliac spine and the anterior aspect of the pubis lie in the same vertical plane and (2) the sacrum is located superiorly, the coccyx posteriorly, and the pubic symphysis antero-inferiorly. **C.** Features of hip bone.

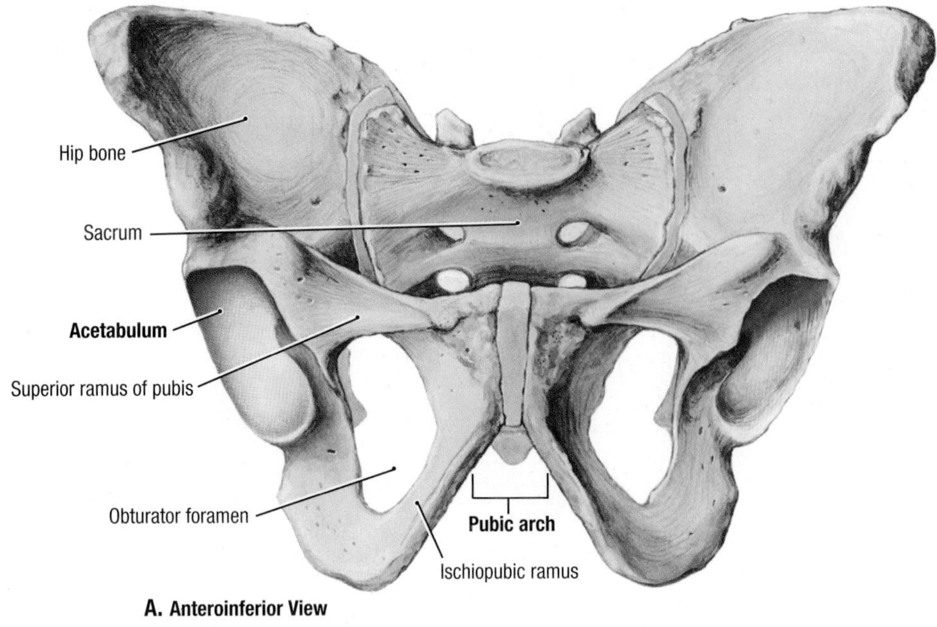
Hip bone
Sacrum
Acetabulum
Superior ramus of pubis
Obturator foramen
Pubic arch
Ischiopubic ramus

A. Anteroinferior View

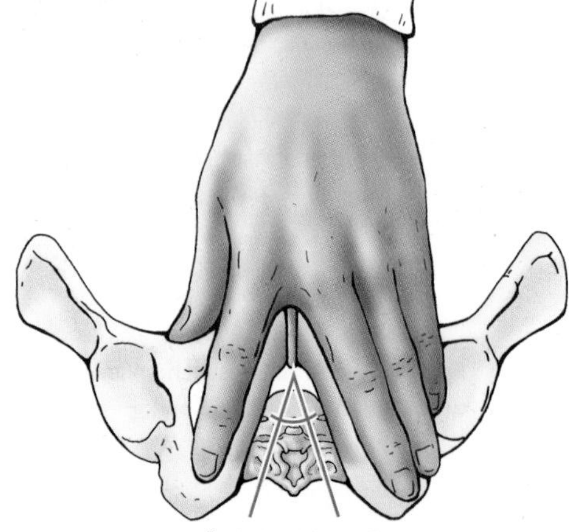

C. Subpubic angle
"V" shaped

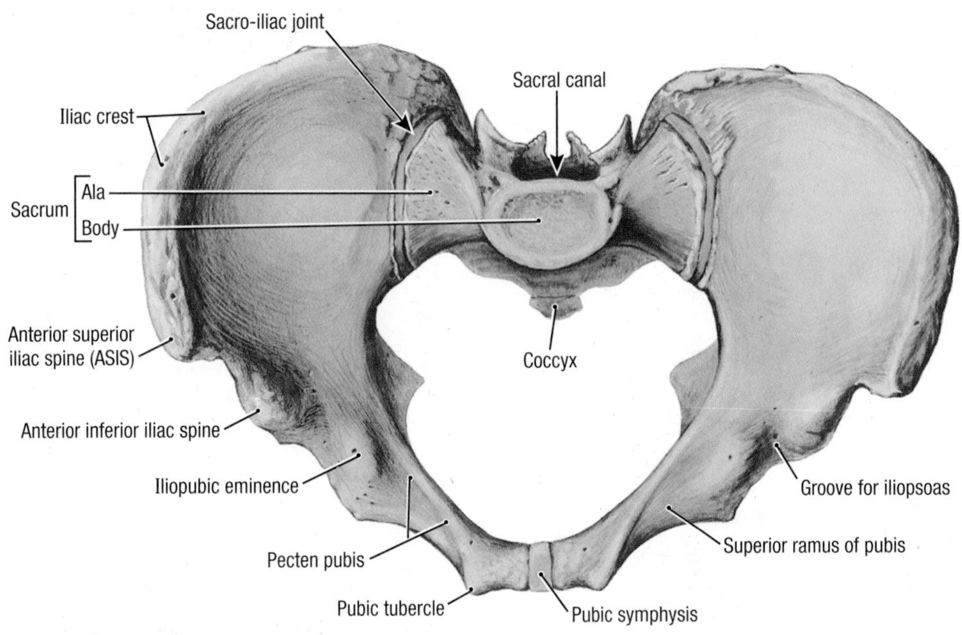
Sacro-iliac joint
Sacral canal
Iliac crest
Sacrum
Ala
Body
Anterior superior iliac spine (ASIS)
Coccyx
Anterior inferior iliac spine
Iliopubic eminence
Groove for iliopsoas
Superior ramus of pubis
Pecten pubis
Pubic tubercle
Pubic symphysis

B. Anterosuperior View

3.5 MALE PELVIC GIRDLE

TABLE 3.1 DIFFERENCES BETWEEN MALE AND FEMALE PELVES

Bony Pelvis	Male	Female
General structure	Thicker and heavier	Thinner and lighter
Greater pelvis (pelvis major)	Deeper	Shallower
Lesser pelvis (pelvis minor)	Narrower and deeper, tapering	Wider and shallower, cylindrical
Pelvic inlet (superior pelvic aperture)	Heart shaped, narrower	More oval or rounded, wider

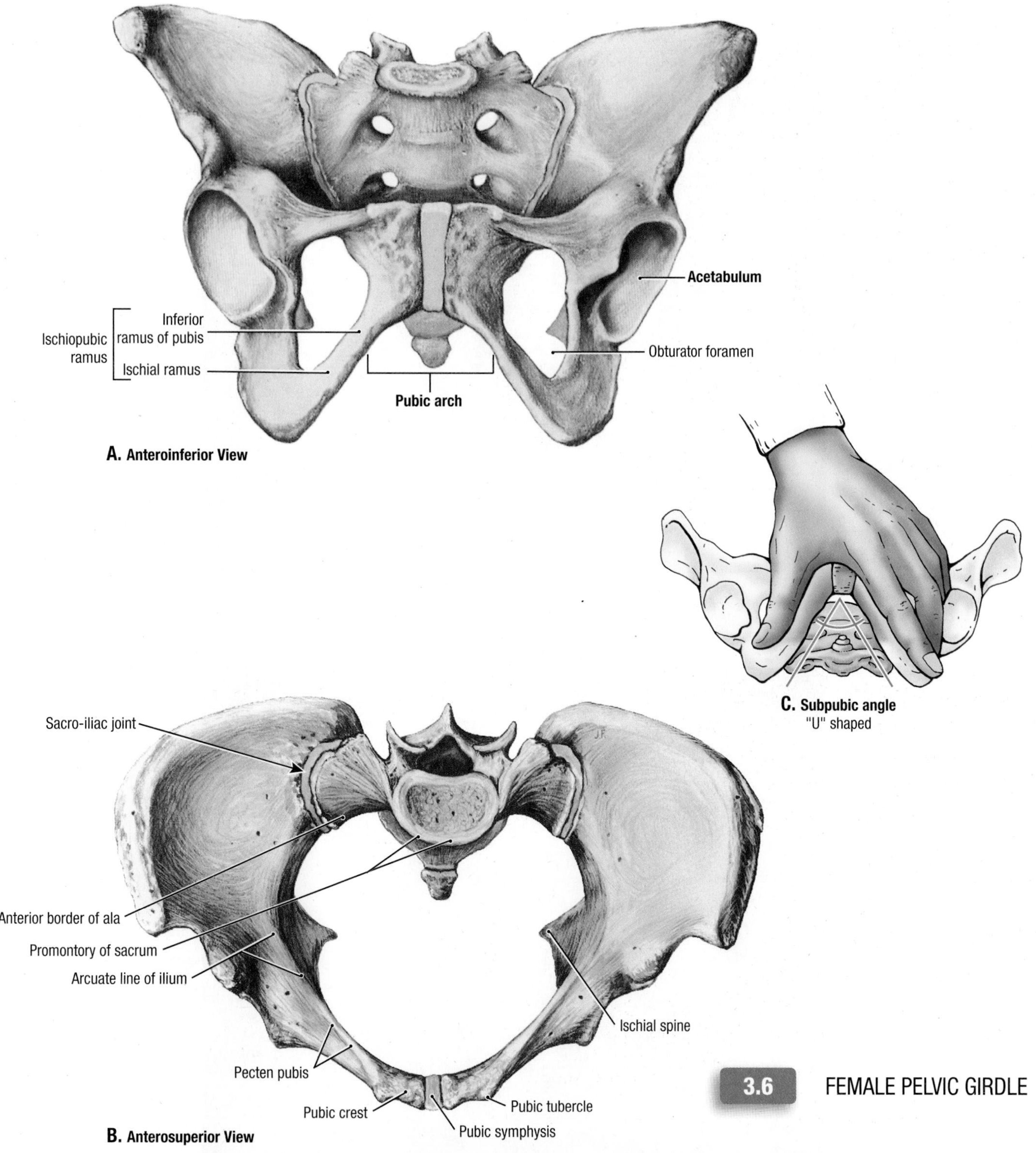
Ischiopubic ramus
Inferior ramus of pubis
Ischial ramus
Pubic arch
Acetabulum
Obturator foramen
Sacro-iliac joint
Anterior border of ala
Promontory of sacrum
Arcuate line of ilium
Ischial spine
Pecten pubis
Pubic crest
Pubic tubercle
Pubic symphysis

A. Anteroinferior View

C. Subpubic angle
"U" shaped

B. Anterosuperior View

3.6 FEMALE PELVIC GIRDLE

TABLE 3.1 DIFFERENCES BETWEEN MALE AND FEMALE PELVES (CONTINUED)

Bony Pelvis	Male	Female
Sacrum/coccyx	More curved	Less curved
Pelvic outlet (inferior pelvic aperture)	Comparatively small	Comparatively large
Pubic arch and subpubic angle	Narrower	Wider
Obturator foramen	Round	Oval
Acetabulum	Large	Small

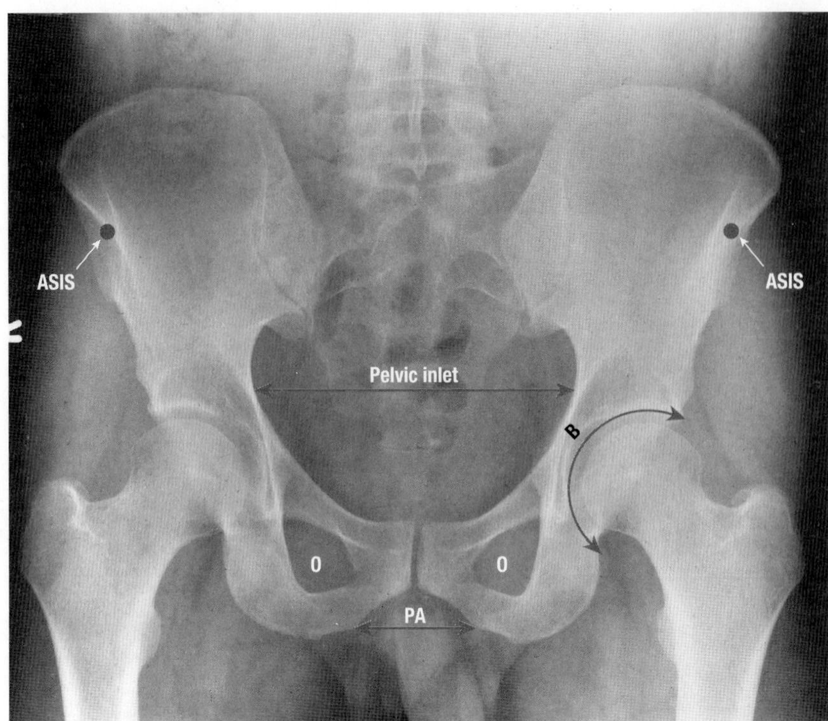
ASIS
ASIS
Pelvic inlet
B
O
O
PA

A. Anteroposterior View, Male Pelvis

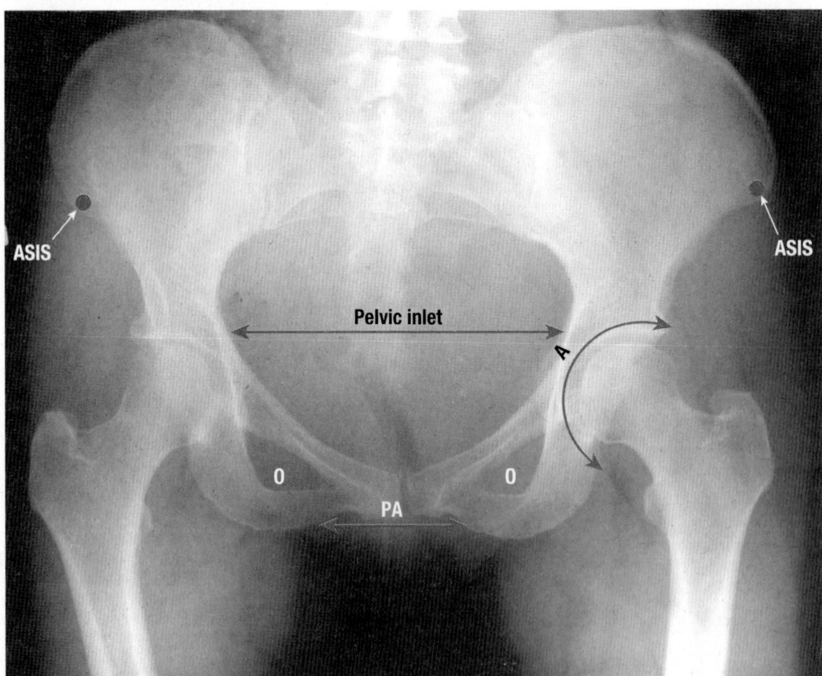
ASIS
ASIS
Pelvic inlet
A
O
O
PA

B. Anteroposterior View, Female Pelvis

3.7 RADIOGRAPHS OF PELVIS

A. Male. **B.** Female. Some of the main differences of male and female pelves are listed in Table 3.1. The radiographs highlight some of these differences. *A,* acetabulum; *ASIS,* anterior superior iliac spine; *O,* obturator foramen; *PA,* pubic arch.

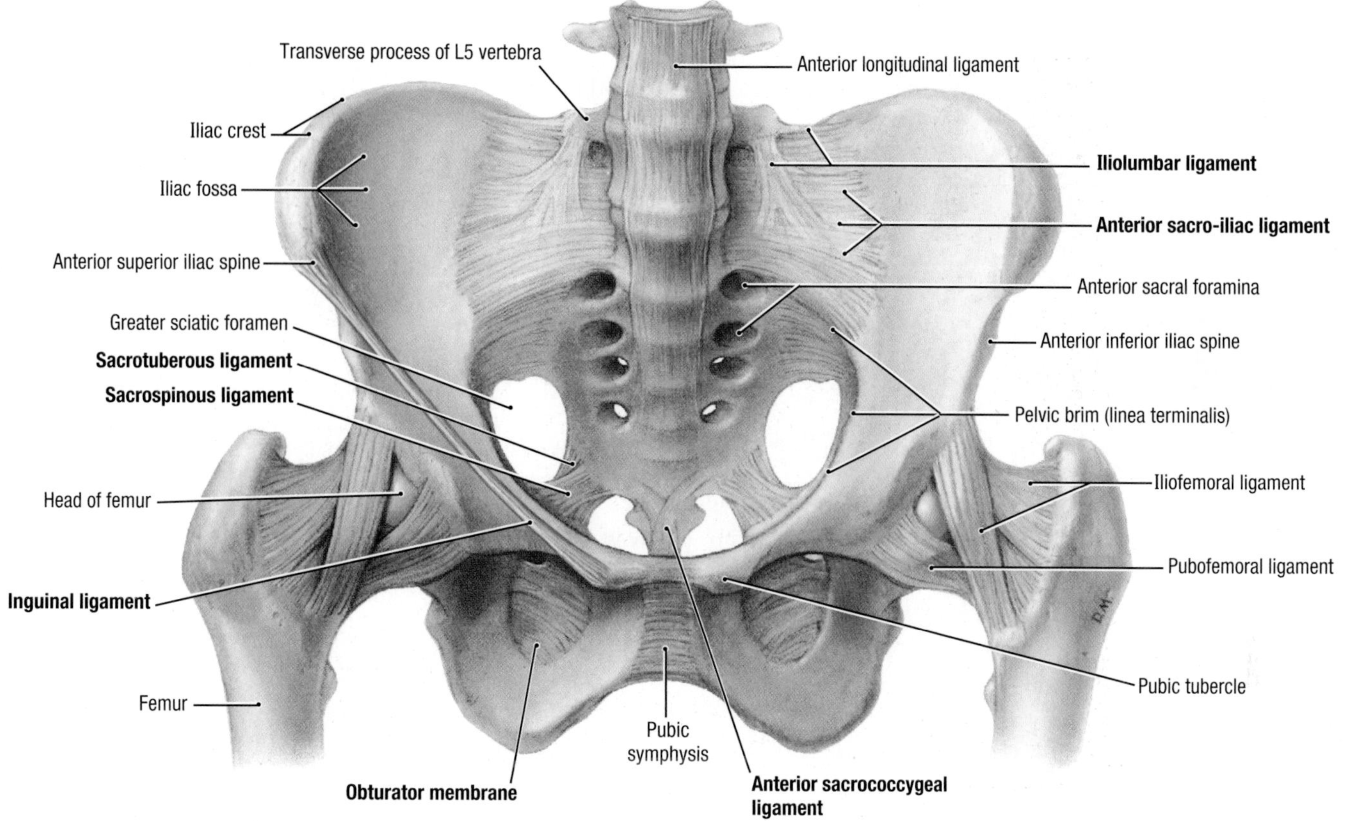
Transverse process of L5 vertebra
Anterior longitudinal ligament
Iliac crest
Iliolumbar ligament
Iliac fossa
Anterior sacro-iliac ligament
Anterior superior iliac spine
Anterior sacral foramina
Greater sciatic foramen
Anterior inferior iliac spine
Sacrotuberous ligament
Sacrospinous ligament
Pelvic brim (linea terminalis)
Iliofemoral ligament
Head of femur
Pubofemoral ligament
Inguinal ligament
Pubic tubercle
Femur
Pubic symphysis
Obturator membrane
Anterior sacrococcygeal ligament

A. Anterior View

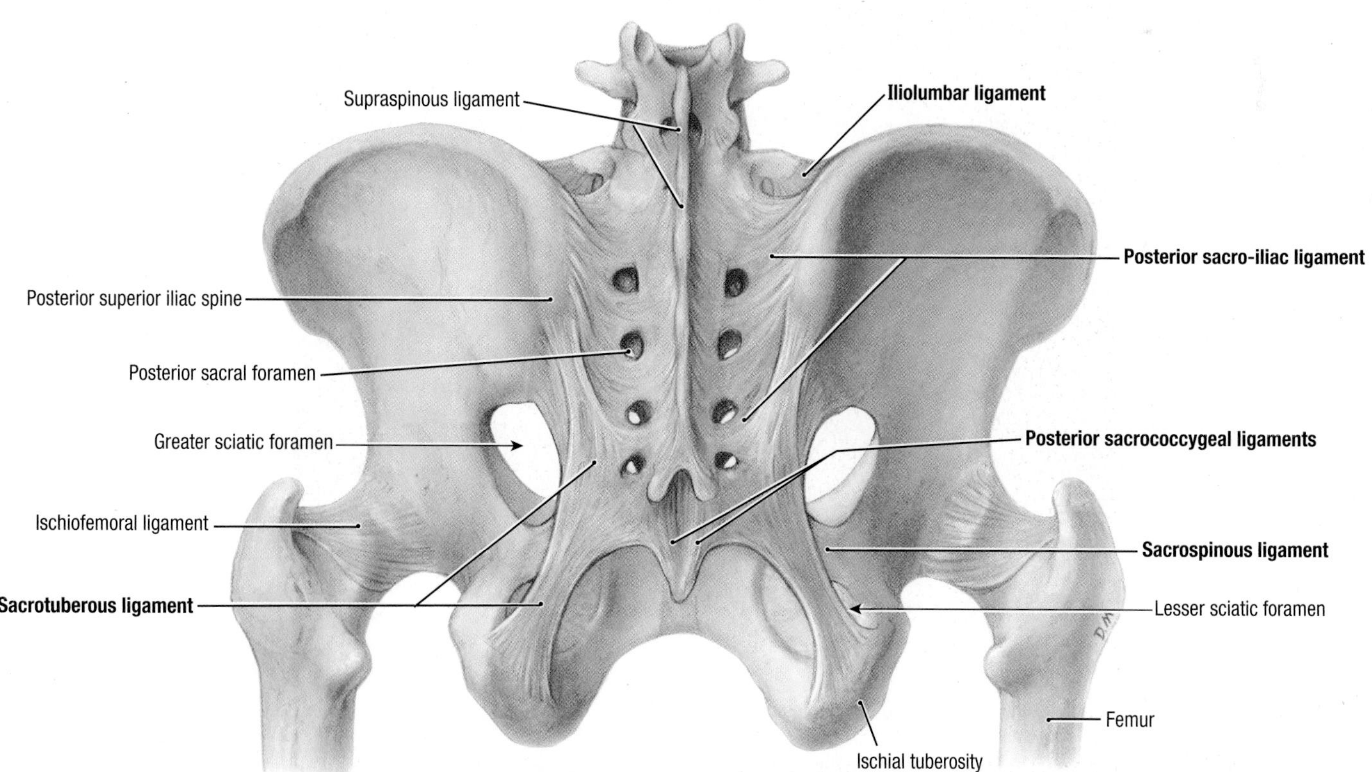
Supraspinous ligament
Iliolumbar ligament
Posterior sacro-iliac ligament
Posterior superior iliac spine
Posterior sacral foramen
Greater sciatic foramen
Posterior sacrococcygeal ligaments
Ischiofemoral ligament
Sacrospinous ligament
Sacrotuberous ligament
Lesser sciatic foramen
Femur
Ischial tuberosity

B. Posterior View

3.8 PELVIS AND PELVIC LIGAMENTS

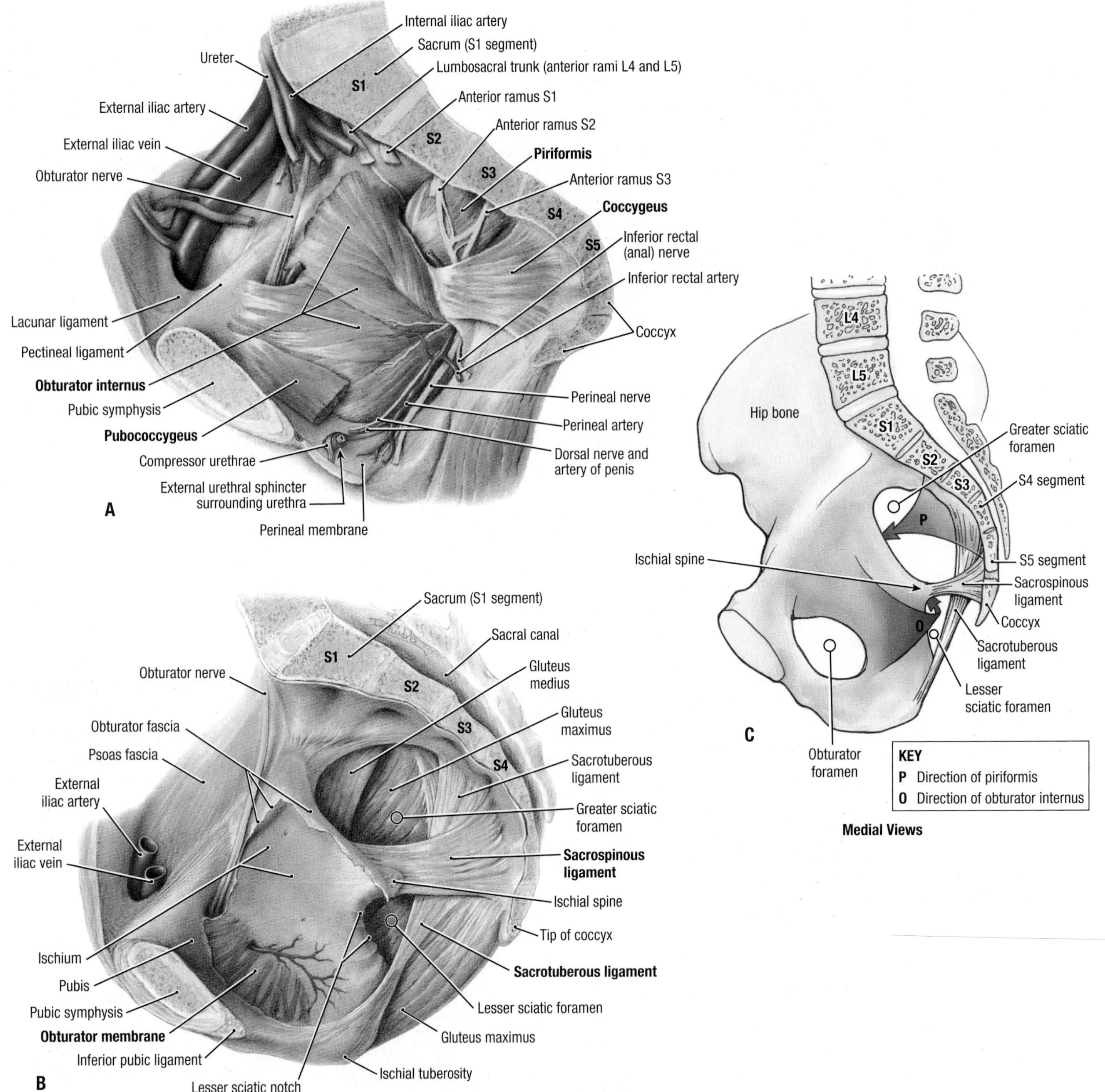
Internal iliac artery
Sacrum (S1 segment)
Ureter
Lumbosacral trunk (anterior rami L4 and L5)
S1
External iliac artery
Anterior ramus S1
External iliac vein
S2
Anterior ramus S2
Piriformis
Obturator nerve
S3
Anterior ramus S3
Coccygeus
S4
S5
Inferior rectal (anal) nerve
Inferior rectal artery
Lacunar ligament
Coccyx
Pectineal ligament
Obturator internus
Perineal nerve
Pubic symphysis
Perineal artery
Pubococcygeus
Dorsal nerve and artery of penis
Compressor urethrae
External urethral sphincter surrounding urethra
A
Perineal membrane
Sacrum (S1 segment)
Sacral canal
S1
Obturator nerve
S2
Gluteus medius
Obturator fascia
S3
Gluteus maximus
Psoas fascia
S4
Sacrotuberous ligament
External iliac artery
Greater sciatic foramen
External iliac vein
Sacrospinous ligament
Ischial spine
Tip of coccyx
Ischium
Sacrotuberous ligament
Pubis
Lesser sciatic foramen
Pubic symphysis
Obturator membrane
Gluteus maximus
Inferior pubic ligament
Ischial tuberosity
B
Lesser sciatic notch
L4
L5
Hip bone
S1
S2
S3
Greater sciatic foramen
S4 segment
P
Ischial spine
S5 segment
Sacrospinous ligament
Coccyx
O
Sacrotuberous ligament
Lesser sciatic foramen
C
Obturator foramen
KEY
P Direction of piriformis
O Direction of obturator internus

Medial Views

3.9 OBTURATOR INTERNUS AND PIRIFORMIS

- On the lateral pelvic wall, the obturator foramen is closed by the obturator membrane; the obturator internus muscle attaches to the obturator membrane and surrounding bone and exits the lesser pelvis through the lesser sciatic foramen; obturator fascia lies on the medial surface of the muscle.
- Piriformis lies on the posterolateral pelvic wall and leaves the lesser pelvis through the greater sciatic foramen.

Muscles of floor of pelvis*:

Pelvic diaphragm (PD) = Levator ani (LA) + Coccygeus (C)
(PD = LA + C)

Levator ani (LA) = Pubococcygeus (PC) + Iliococcygeus (IC)
(LA = PC + IC)

Pubococcygeus (PC♀) = Puborectalis (PR) + Pubovaginalis (PV)
(PC = PR + PV♀)

Pubococcygeus (PC♂) = Puborectalis (PR) + Puboprostaticus (PP)
(PC = PR + PP♂) (Levator prostatae)

*Formulas: Dr. Larry M. Ross.
The University of Texas Medical School at Houston

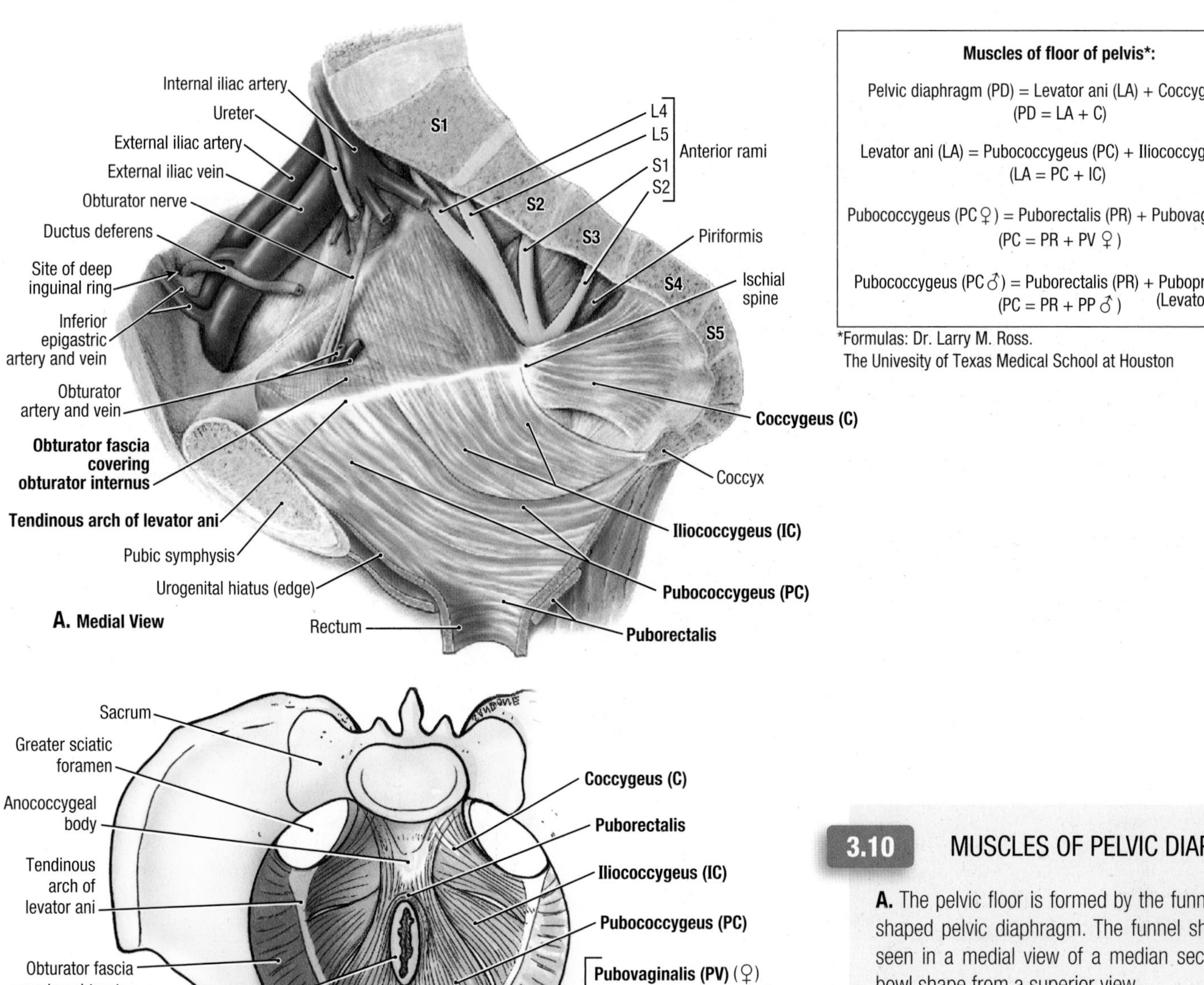
Internal iliac artery
Ureter
External iliac artery
External iliac vein
Obturator nerve
Ductus deferens
Site of deep inguinal ring
Inferior epigastric artery and vein
Obturator artery and vein
Obturator fascia covering obturator internus
Tendinous arch of levator ani
Pubic symphysis
Urogenital hiatus (edge)
Rectum
S1
S2
S3
S4
S5
L4
L5
S1
S2
Anterior rami
Piriformis
Ischial spine
Coccygeus (C)
Coccyx
Iliococcygeus (IC)
Pubococcygeus (PC)
Puborectalis
Sacrum
Greater sciatic foramen
Anococcygeal body
Tendinous arch of levator ani
Obturator fascia covering obturator internus
Rectum
Perineal body
Coccygeus (C)
Puborectalis
Iliococcygeus (IC)
Pubococcygeus (PC)
Pubovaginalis (PV) (♀)
Puboprostaticus (PP) (♂)
Urogenital hiatus
Pubic symphysis

A. Medial View

B. Anterosuperior View

3.10 MUSCLES OF PELVIC DIAPHRAGM

A. The pelvic floor is formed by the funnel- or bowl-shaped pelvic diaphragm. The funnel shape can be seen in a medial view of a median section. **B.** The bowl shape from a superior view.

TABLE 3.2 MUSCLES OF PELVIC WALLS AND FLOOR

Boundary	Muscle	Proximal Attachment	Distal Attachment	Innervation	Main Action
Lateral wall	Obturator internus	Pelvic surfaces of ilium and ischium, obturator membrane	Greater trochanter of femur	Nerve to obturator internus (L5, S1, S2)	Rotates hip joint laterally; assists in holding head of femur in acetabulum
Posterolateral wall	Piriformis	Pelvic surface of S2–S4 segments, superior margin of greater sciatic notch, sacrotuberous ligament		Anterior rami of S1 and S2	Rotates hip joint laterally; abducts hip joint; assists in holding head of femur in acetabulum
Floor	Levator ani (pubococcygeus, puborectalis, and iliococcygeus)	Body of pubis, tendinous arch of obturator fascia, ischial spine	Perineal body, coccyx, anococcygeal ligament, walls of prostate or vagina, rectum, and anal canal	Nerve to levator ani (branches of S4), inferior anal (rectal) nerve, and coccygeal plexus	Forms most of pelvic diaphragm that helps support pelvic viscera and resists increases in intra-abdominal pressure
	Coccygeus (ischiococcygeus)	Ischial spine	Inferior end of sacrum and coccyx	Branches of S4 and S5 spinal nerves	Forms small part of pelvic diaphragm that supports pelvic viscera; flexes sacrococcygeal joints

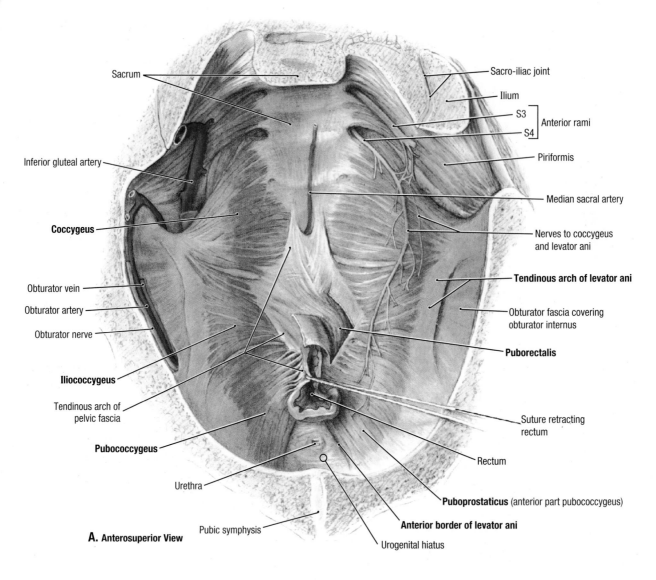

Sacrum
Sacro-iliac joint
Ilium
S3
S4
Anterior rami
Inferior gluteal artery
Piriformis
Median sacral artery
Coccygeus
Nerves to coccygeus and levator ani
Obturator vein
Tendinous arch of levator ani
Obturator artery
Obturator fascia covering obturator internus
Obturator nerve
Puborectalis
Iliococcygeus
Tendinous arch of pelvic fascia
Suture retracting rectum
Pubococcygeus
Rectum
Urethra
Puboprostaticus (anterior part pubococcygeus)
Pubic symphysis
Anterior border of levator ani
Urogenital hiatus

A. Anterosuperior View

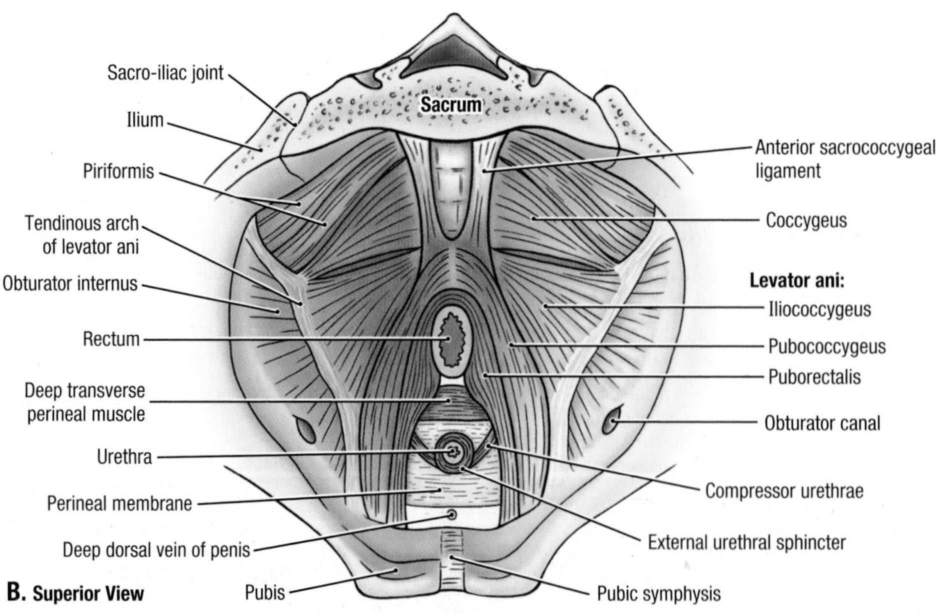
Sacro-iliac joint
Sacrum
Ilium
Anterior sacrococcygeal ligament
Piriformis
Coccygeus
Tendinous arch of levator ani
Levator ani:
Obturator internus
Iliococcygeus
Rectum
Pubococcygeus
Puborectalis
Deep transverse perineal muscle
Obturator canal
Urethra
Compressor urethrae
Perineal membrane
External urethral sphincter
Deep dorsal vein of penis
Pubis
Pubic symphysis

B. Superior View

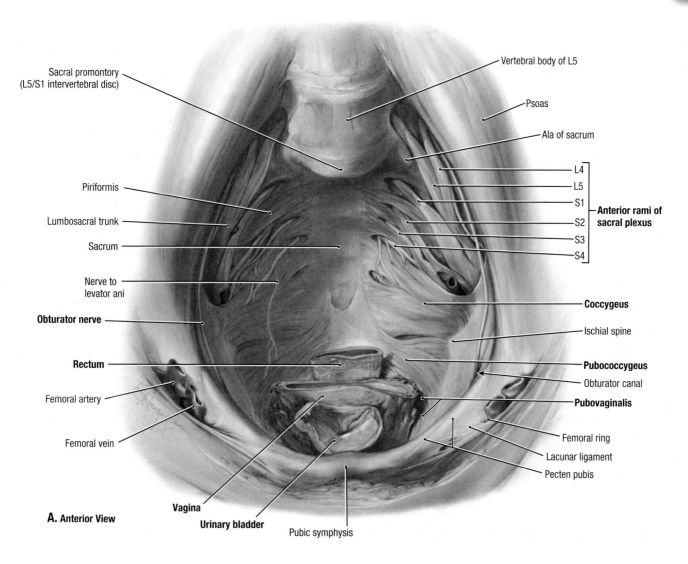

Sacral promontory (L5/S1 intervertebral disc)
Vertebral body of L5
Psoas
Ala of sacrum
Piriformis
Lumbosacral trunk
Sacrum
L4
L5
S1
S2
S3
S4
Anterior rami of sacral plexus
Nerve to levator ani
Obturator nerve
Coccygeus
Ischial spine
Rectum
Pubococcygeus
Obturator canal
Femoral artery
Pubovaginalis
Femoral vein
Femoral ring
Lacunar ligament
Pecten pubis
Vagina
Urinary bladder
Pubic symphysis

A. Anterior View

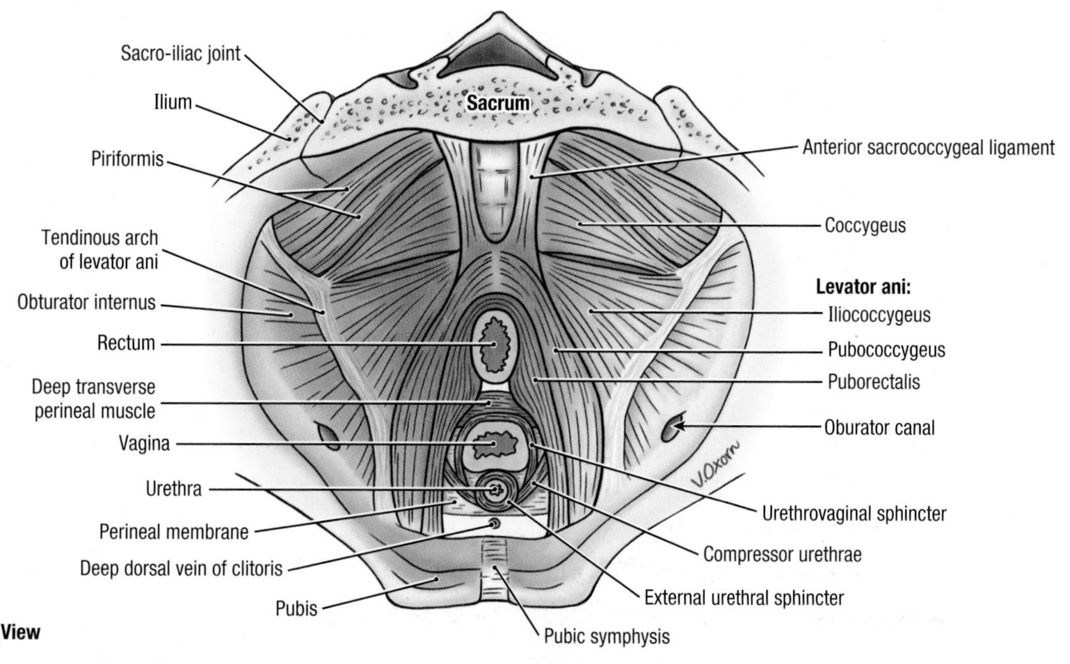
Sacro-iliac joint
Ilium
Sacrum
Piriformis
Anterior sacrococcygeal ligament
Coccygeus
Tendinous arch of levator ani
Levator ani:
Obturator internus
Iliococcygeus
Rectum
Pubococcygeus
Puborectalis
Deep transverse perineal muscle
Oburator canal
Vagina
V.Oxorn
Urethra
Urethrovaginal sphincter
Perineal membrane
Compressor urethrae
Deep dorsal vein of clitoris
External urethral sphincter
Pubis
Pubic symphysis

B. Superior View

3.12 FLOOR AND WALLS OF FEMALE PELVIS

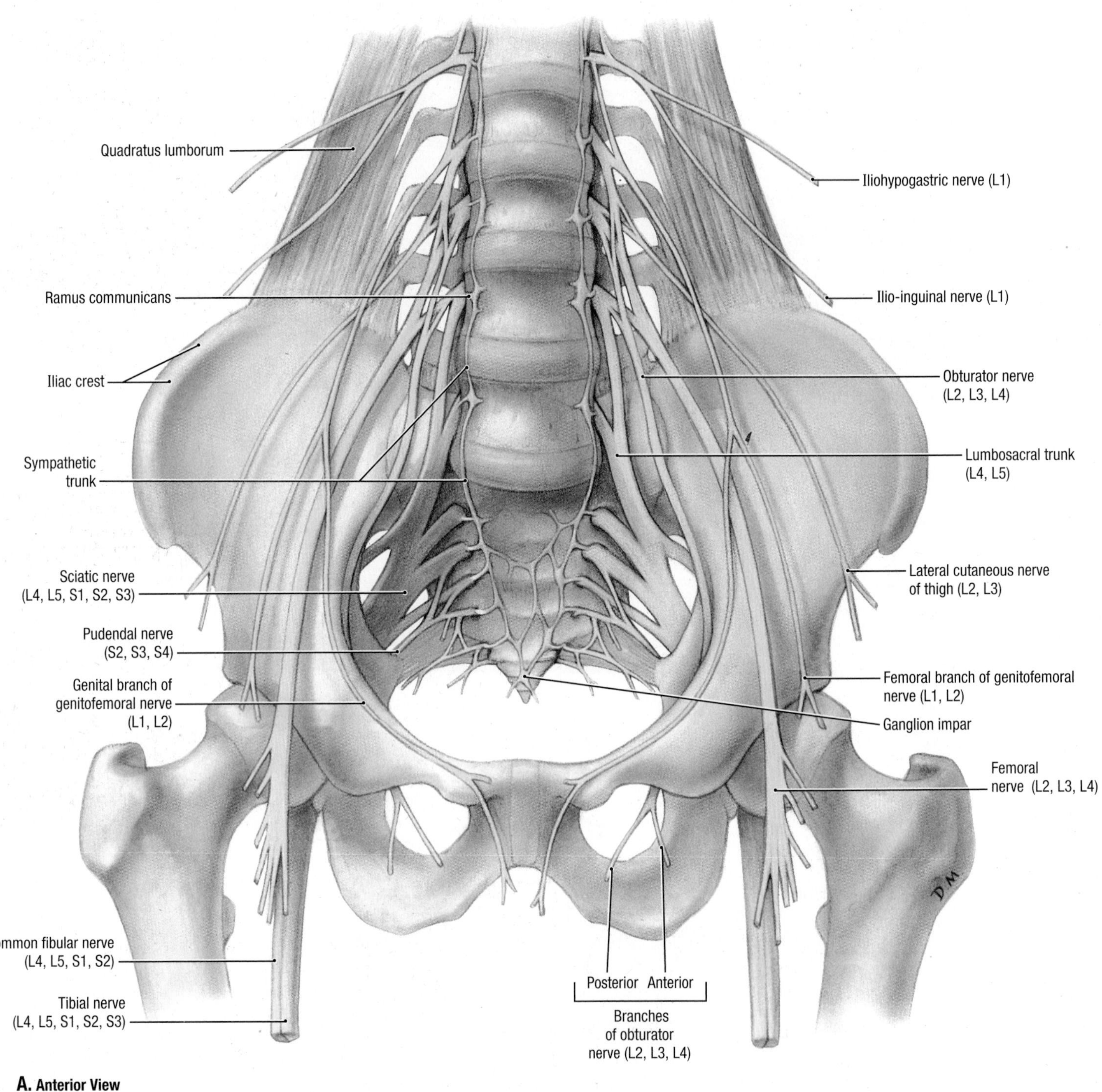
Quadratus lumborum
Iliohypogastric nerve (L1)
Ramus communicans
Ilio-inguinal nerve (L1)
Iliac crest
Obturator nerve
(L2, L3, L4)
Sympathetic
trunk
Lumbosacral trunk
(L4, L5)
Sciatic nerve
(L4, L5, S1, S2, S3)
Lateral cutaneous nerve
of thigh (L2, L3)
Pudendal nerve
(S2, S3, S4)
Genital branch of
genitofemoral nerve
(L1, L2)
Femoral branch of genitofemoral
nerve (L1, L2)
Ganglion impar
Femoral
nerve (L2, L3, L4)
Common fibular nerve
(L4, L5, S1, S2)
Tibial nerve
(L4, L5, S1, S2, S3)
Posterior Anterior
Branches
of obturator
nerve (L2, L3, L4)

A. Anterior View

3.13 SACRAL AND COCCYGEAL NERVE PLEXUSES

A. Dissection

- The sympathetic trunk or its ganglia send rami communicantes to each sacral and coccygeal nerve.
- The anterior ramus from L4 joins that of L5 to form the lumbosacral trunk.

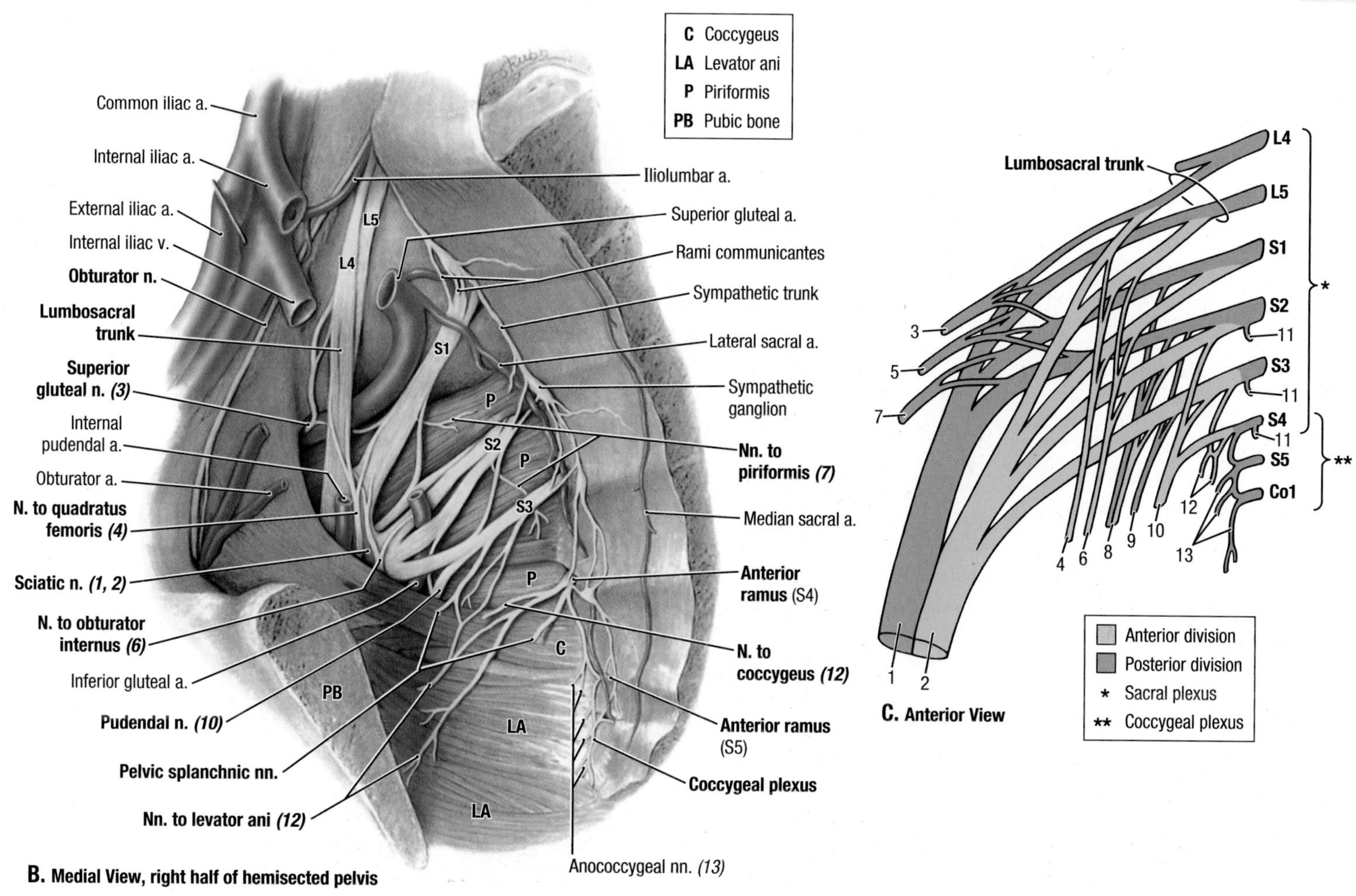
C Coccygeus
LA Levator ani
P Piriformis
PB Pubic bone
Common iliac a.
Internal iliac a.
External iliac a.
Internal iliac v.
Obturator n.
Lumbosacral trunk
Superior gluteal n. (3)
Internal pudendal a.
Obturator a.
N. to quadratus femoris (4)
Sciatic n. (1, 2)
N. to obturator internus (6)
Inferior gluteal a.
Pudendal n. (10)
Pelvic splanchnic nn.
Nn. to levator ani (12)
Iliolumbar a.
Superior gluteal a.
Rami communicantes
Sympathetic trunk
Lateral sacral a.
Sympathetic ganglion
Nn. to piriformis (7)
Median sacral a.
Anterior ramus (S4)
N. to coccygeus (12)
Anterior ramus (S5)
Coccygeal plexus
Anococcygeal nn. (13)
L4
L5
S1
S2
S3
P
C
PB
LA
Lumbosacral trunk
S4
S5
Co1
Anterior division
Posterior division
* Sacral plexus
** Coccygeal plexus

B. Medial View, right half of hemisected pelvis

C. Anterior View

3.13 SACRAL AND COCCYGEAL NERVE PLEXUSES *(CONTINUED)*

B. and C. Schematic illustrations.

TABLE 3.3 NERVES OF SACRAL AND COCCYGEAL PLEXUSES

Nerve	Origin	Distribution
Sciatic:		
1. Common fibular	L4, L5, S1, S2	Articular branches to hip joint and muscular branches to flexors of knee joint in thigh and all muscles in leg and foot
2. Tibial	L4, L5, S1, S2, S3	
3. Superior gluteal	L4, L5, S1	Gluteus medius and gluteus minimus muscles
4. Nerve to quadratus femoris and inferior gemellus	L4, L5, S1	Quadratus femoris and inferior gemellus muscles
5. Inferior gluteal	L5, S1, S2	Gluteus maximus muscle
6. Nerve to obturator internus and superior gemellus	L5, S1, S2	Obturator internus and superior gemellus muscles
7. Nerve to piriformis	S1, S2	Piriformis muscle
8. Posterior cutaneous nerve of thigh	S1, S2, S3	Cutaneous branches to buttock and uppermost medial and posterior surfaces of thigh
9. Perforating cutaneous	S2, S3	Cutaneous branches to medial part of buttock
10. Pudendal	S2, S3, S4	Structures in perineum, sensory to genitalia, muscular branches to perineal muscles, external urethral sphincter, and external anal sphincter
11. Pelvic splanchnic	S2, S3, S4	Pelvic viscera via inferior hypogastric and pelvic plexuses
12. Nerves to levator ani and coccygeus	S3, S4	Levator ani and coccygeus muscles
13. Anococcygeal nerves	S4, S5, Co1	Penetrate coccygeal attachments of sacrospinous/sacrotuberous ligaments to supply overlying skin

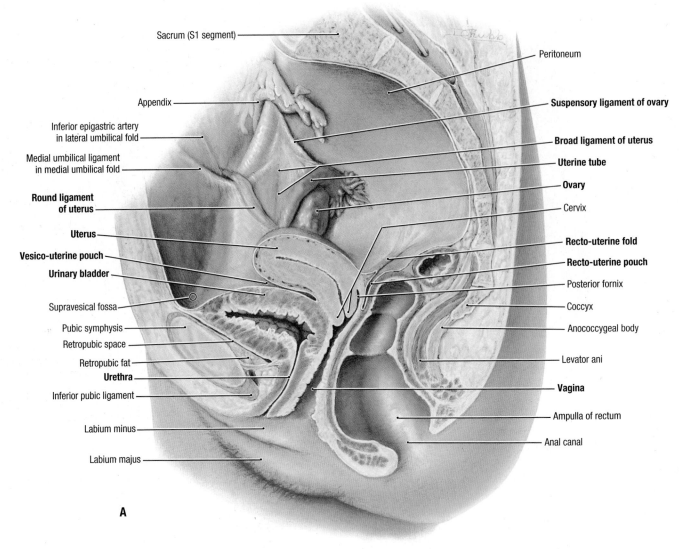

Sacrum (S1 segment)
Appendix
Inferior epigastric artery in lateral umbilical fold
Medial umbilical ligament in medial umbilical fold
Round ligament of uterus
Uterus
Vesico-uterine pouch
Urinary bladder
Supravesical fossa
Pubic symphysis
Retropubic space
Retropubic fat
Urethra
Inferior pubic ligament
Labium minus
Labium majus
Peritoneum
Suspensory ligament of ovary
Broad ligament of uterus
Uterine tube
Ovary
Cervix
Recto-uterine fold
Recto-uterine pouch
Posterior fornix
Coccyx
Anococcygeal body
Levator ani
Vagina
Ampulla of rectum
Anal canal

A

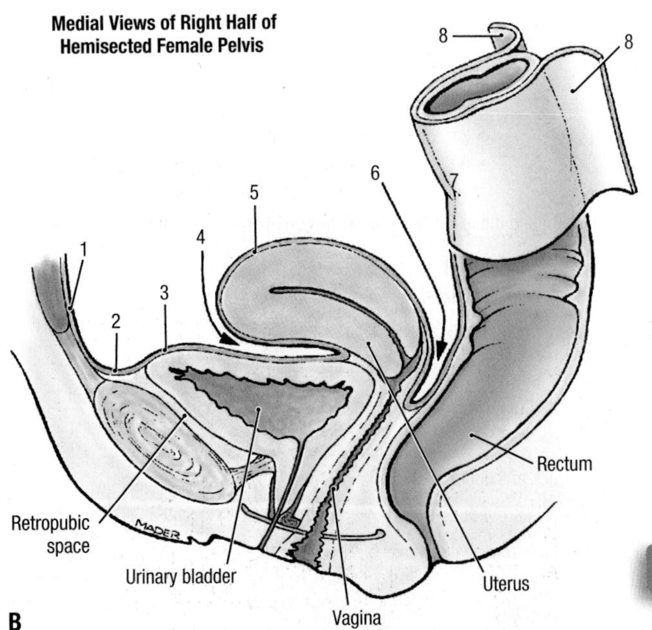
Medial Views of Right Half of Hemisected Female Pelvis
8
8
6
7
5
4
1
3
2
Rectum
Retropubic space
Urinary bladder
Vagina
Uterus
MADER
B

Female:

Peritoneum passes:

- From the anteiror abdominal wall *(1)*
- Superior to the pubic bone *(2)*, forming supravesical fossa
- On the superior surface of the urinary bladder *(3)*
- From the bladder to mid-uterus, forming the vesico-uterine pouch *(4)*
- On the fundus and body of the uterus, and posterior fornix of the vagina *(5)*
- Between the rectum and uterus, forming the recto-uterine pouch *(6)*
- On the anterior and lateral sides of the rectum *(7)*
- Posteriorly to become the sigmoid mesocolon *(8)*

3.14 PERITONEUM COVERING FEMALE PELVIC ORGANS

A. Organs in situ with peritoneal reflections. **B.** Schematic illustration. The level of the supravesical fossa changes with filling and emptying of bladder.

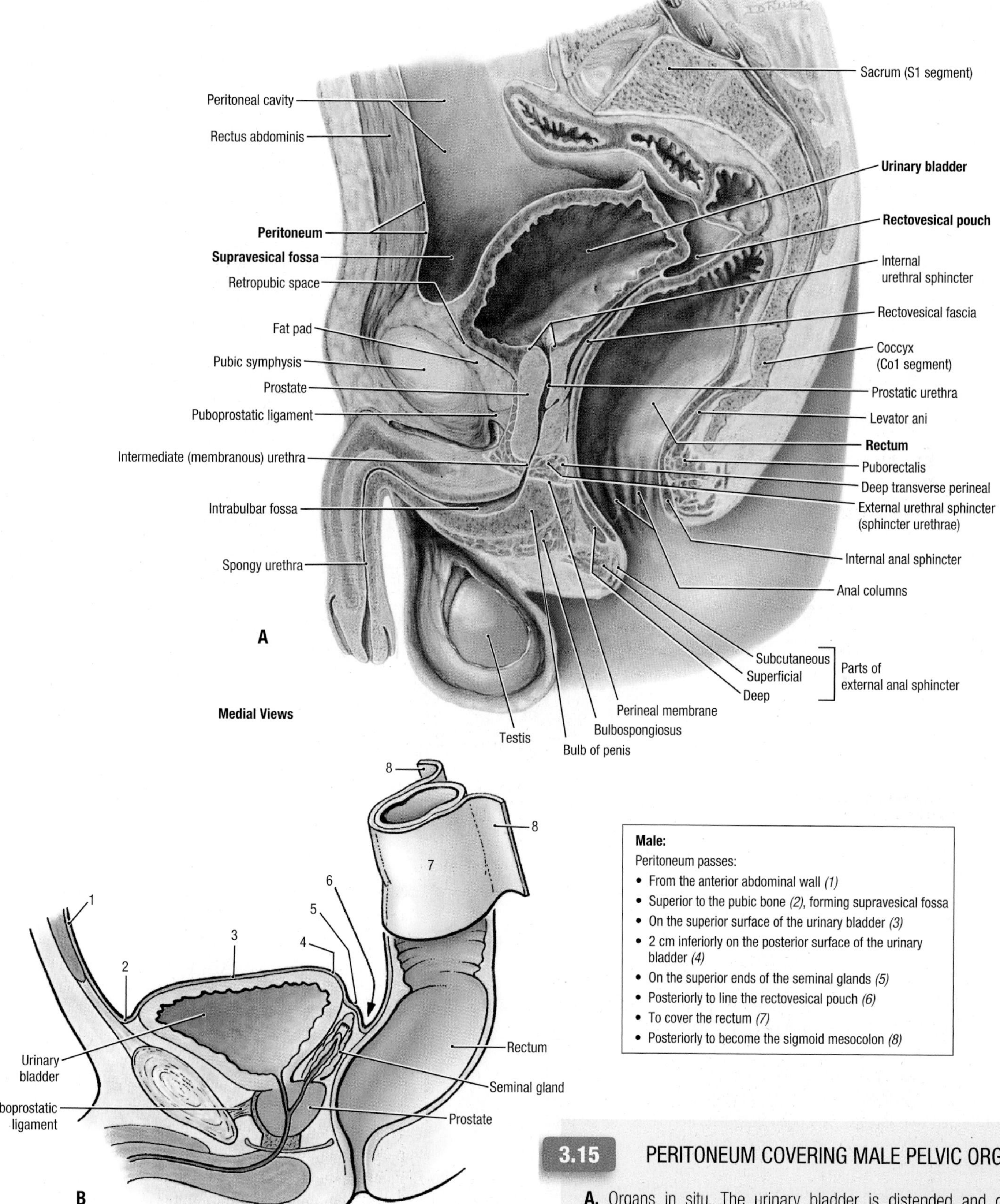
Sacrum (S1 segment)
Peritoneal cavity
Rectus abdominis
Urinary bladder
Rectovesical pouch
Peritoneum
Supravesical fossa
Internal urethral sphincter
Retropubic space
Rectovesical fascia
Fat pad
Coccyx (Co1 segment)
Pubic symphysis
Prostate
Prostatic urethra
Puboprostatic ligament
Levator ani
Rectum
Intermediate (membranous) urethra
Puborectalis
Deep transverse perineal
External urethral sphincter (sphincter urethrae)
Intrabulbar fossa
Spongy urethra
Internal anal sphincter
Anal columns
A
Subcutaneous
Superficial
Deep
Parts of external anal sphincter
Medial Views
Perineal membrane
Bulbospongiosus
Testis
Bulb of penis
8
8
7
6
1
5
3
4
2
Urinary bladder
Rectum
Seminal gland
Puboprostatic ligament
Prostate
B

Male:

Peritoneum passes:

- From the anterior abdominal wall *(1)*
- Superior to the pubic bone *(2)*, forming supravesical fossa
- On the superior surface of the urinary bladder *(3)*
- 2 cm inferiorly on the posterior surface of the urinary bladder *(4)*
- On the superior ends of the seminal glands *(5)*
- Posteriorly to line the rectovesical pouch *(6)*
- To cover the rectum *(7)*
- Posteriorly to become the sigmoid mesocolon *(8)*

3.15 PERITONEUM COVERING MALE PELVIC ORGANS

A. Organs in situ. The urinary bladder is distended and displaced posteriorly in this specimen, not anteriorly as is usual, forming a broad and deep supravesical fossa even when the bladder is full. **B.** Peritoneum covering male pelvic organs. Typically, the location of supravesical fossa changes with filling and emptying of bladder.

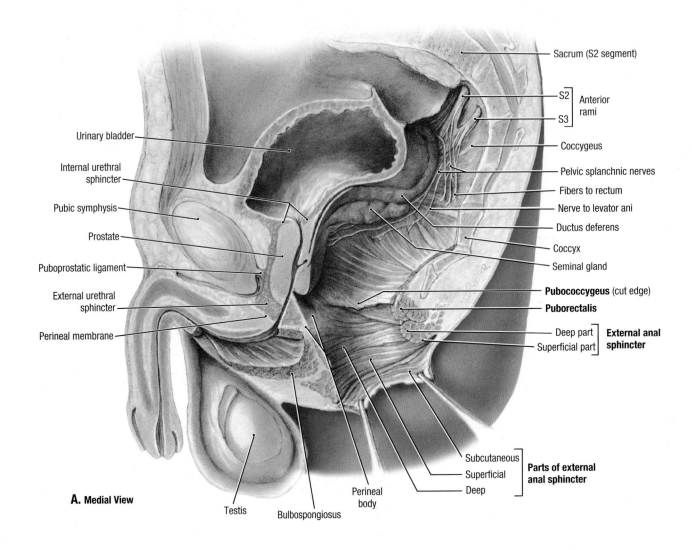

Sacrum (S2 segment)
S2
S3
Anterior rami
Urinary bladder
Coccygeus
Pelvic splanchnic nerves
Internal urethral sphincter
Fibers to rectum
Pubic symphysis
Nerve to levator ani
Ductus deferens
Prostate
Coccyx
Seminal gland
Puboprostatic ligament
Pubococcygeus (cut edge)
External urethral sphincter
Puborectalis
Deep part
Superficial part
External anal sphincter
Perineal membrane
Subcutaneous
Superficial
Deep
Parts of external anal sphincter
Testis
Bulbospongiosus
Perineal body

A. Medial View

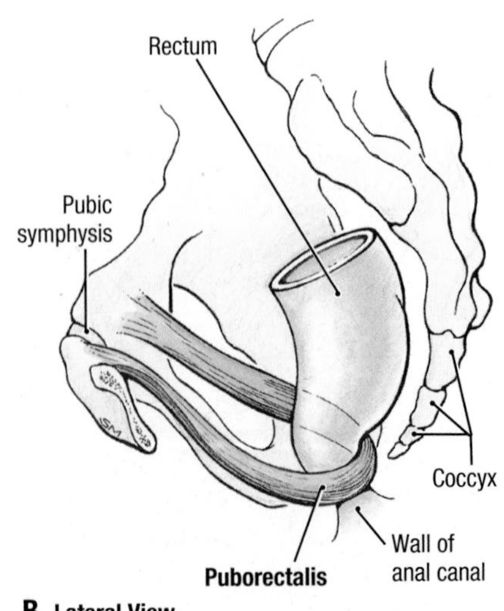
Rectum
Pubic symphysis
Coccyx
Wall of anal canal
Puborectalis

B. Lateral View

3.16 ANAL SPHINCTERS AND ANAL CANAL

A. Levator ani, in right half of hemisected pelvis.

- The subcutaneous fibers of the external anal sphincter and overlying skin are reflected with forceps. The pubococcygeus muscle is cut to reveal the anal canal, to which it is, in part, attached.

B. Puborectalis.

- The innermost part of the pubococcygeus muscle, the puborectalis, forms a U-shaped muscular "sling" around the anorectal junction, which maintains the anorectal (perineal) flexure.

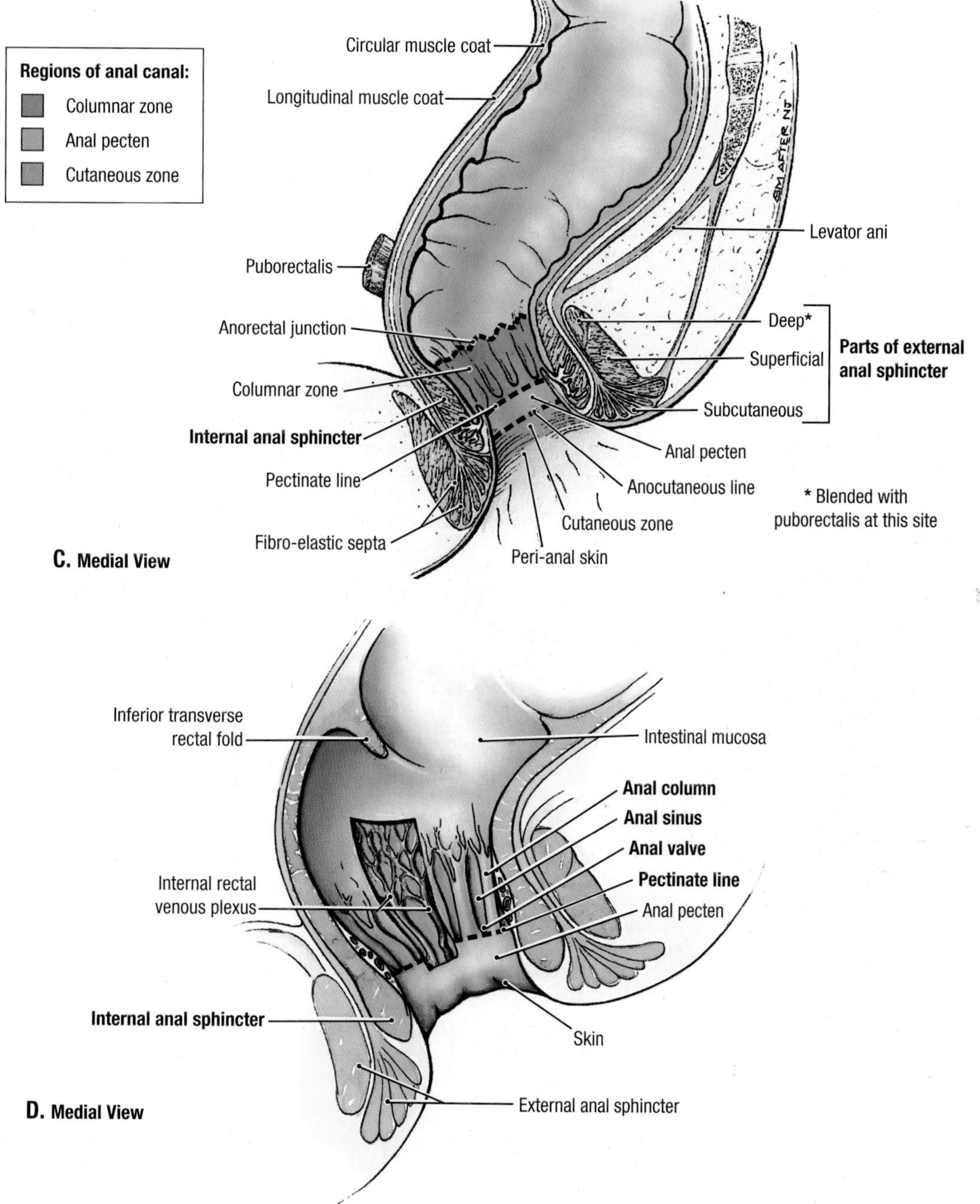
Regions of anal canal:
Columnar zone
Anal pecten
Cutaneous zone
Circular muscle coat
Longitudinal muscle coat
Levator ani
Puborectalis
Anorectal junction
Deep*
Superficial
Subcutaneous
Parts of external anal sphincter
Columnar zone
Internal anal sphincter
Anal pecten
Pectinate line
Anocutaneous line
* Blended with puborectalis at this site
Cutaneous zone
Fibro-elastic septa
Peri-anal skin
C. Medial View
Inferior transverse rectal fold
Intestinal mucosa
Anal column
Anal sinus
Anal valve
Pectinate line
Anal pecten
Internal rectal venous plexus
Skin
Internal anal sphincter
External anal sphincter
D. Medial View

3.16 ANAL SPHINCTERS AND ANAL CANAL *(CONTINUED)*

C. External and internal anal sphincters.

- The internal anal sphincter is a thickening of the inner, circular muscular coat of the anal canal.
- The external anal sphincter has three often indistinct continuous zones: deep, superficial, and subcutaneous; the deep part intermingles with the puborectalis muscle posteriorly.
- The longitudinal muscle layer of the rectum separates the internal and external anal sphincters and terminates in the subcutaneous tissue and skin around the anus.

D. Features of the anal canal.

- The anal columns are 5 to 10 vertical folds of mucosa separated by anal sinuses and valves; they contain portions of the rectal venous plexus.
- The pecten is a smooth area of hairless stratified epithelium that lies between the anal valves superiorly and the inferior border of the internal anal sphincter inferiorly.
- The pectinate line is an irregular line at the base of the anal valves where the intestinal mucosa is continuous with the pecten; this indicates the junction of the superior part of the anal canal (derived from embryonic hindgut) and the inferior part of the anal canal (derived from the anal pit [proctodeum]). Innervation is visceral proximal to the line and somatic distally; lymphatic drainage is to the pararectal nodes proximally and to the superficial inguinal nodes distally.

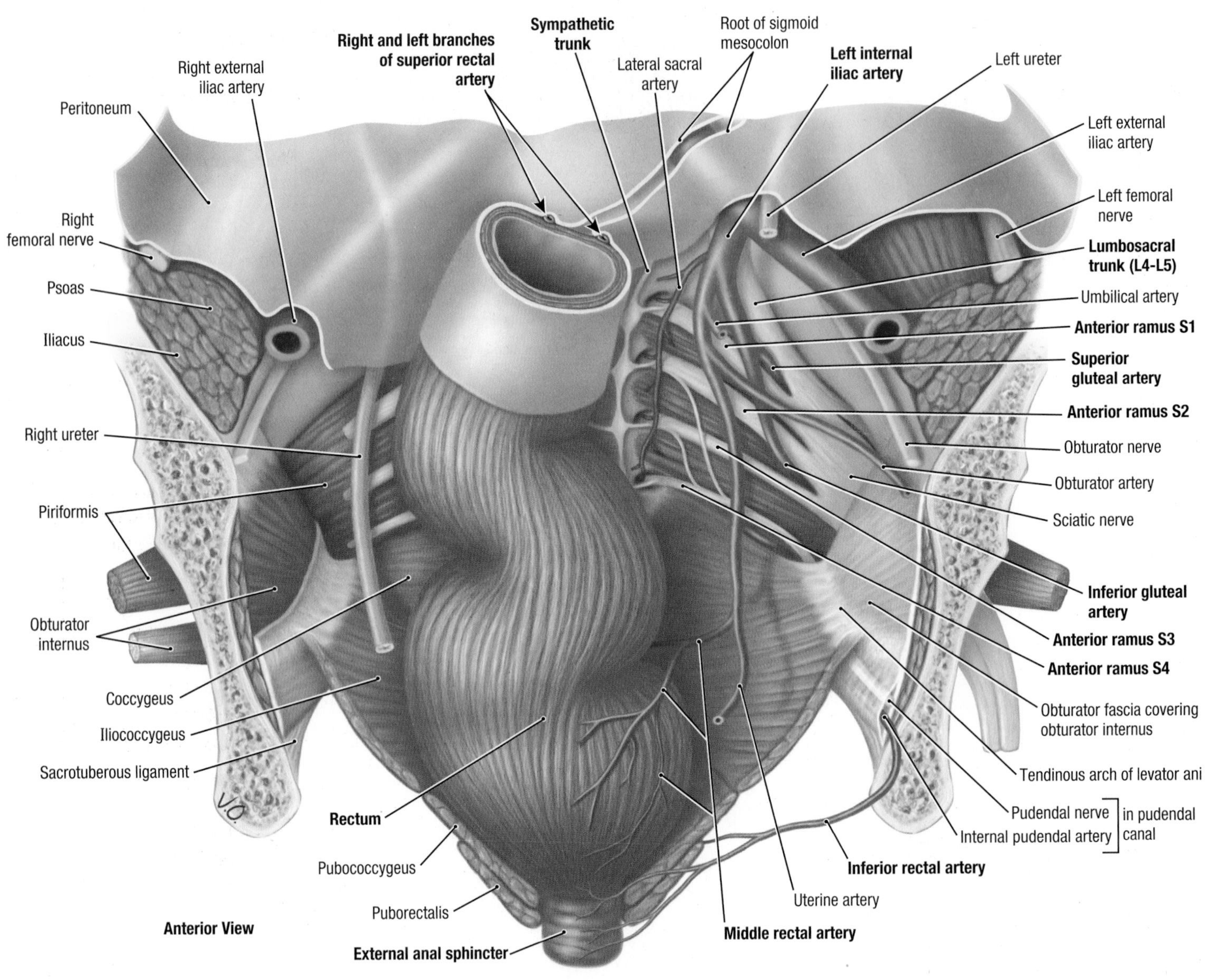
Right and left branches of superior rectal artery
Sympathetic trunk
Root of sigmoid mesocolon
Right external iliac artery
Lateral sacral artery
Left internal iliac artery
Left ureter
Peritoneum
Left external iliac artery
Left femoral nerve
Right femoral nerve
Lumbosacral trunk (L4-L5)
Psoas
Umbilical artery
Anterior ramus S1
Iliacus
Superior gluteal artery
Anterior ramus S2
Right ureter
Obturator nerve
Obturator artery
Piriformis
Sciatic nerve
Inferior gluteal artery
Obturator internus
Anterior ramus S3
Anterior ramus S4
Coccygeus
Obturator fascia covering obturator internus
Iliococcygeus
Sacrotuberous ligament
Tendinous arch of levator ani
Rectum
Pudendal nerve
Internal pudendal artery
in pudendal canal
Pubococcygeus
Inferior rectal artery
Uterine artery
Puborectalis
Anterior View
Middle rectal artery
External anal sphincter
V.O.

3.17 RECTUM, ANAL CANAL, AND NEUROVASCULAR STRUCTURES OF POSTERIOR PELVIS

The pelvis is coronally bisected anterior to the rectum and anal canal. The superior gluteal artery often passes posteriorly between the anterior rami of L5 and S1, and the inferior gluteal artery between S2 and S3.

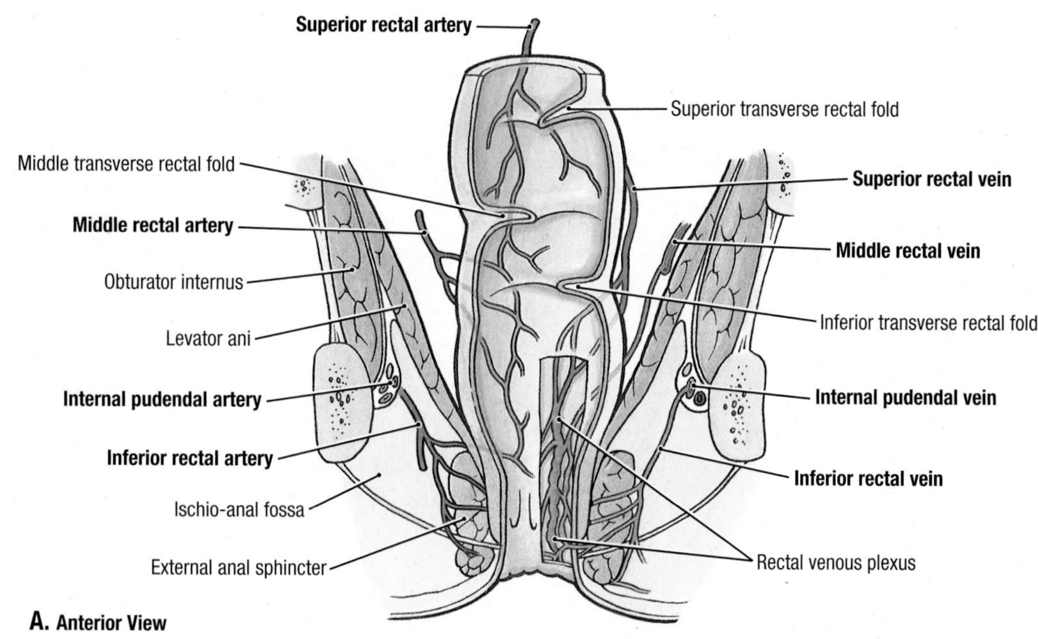
Superior rectal artery
Superior transverse rectal fold
Middle transverse rectal fold
Superior rectal vein
Middle rectal artery
Middle rectal vein
Obturator internus
Inferior transverse rectal fold
Levator ani
Internal pudendal artery
Internal pudendal vein
Inferior rectal artery
Inferior rectal vein
Ischio-anal fossa
External anal sphincter
Rectal venous plexus

A. Anterior View

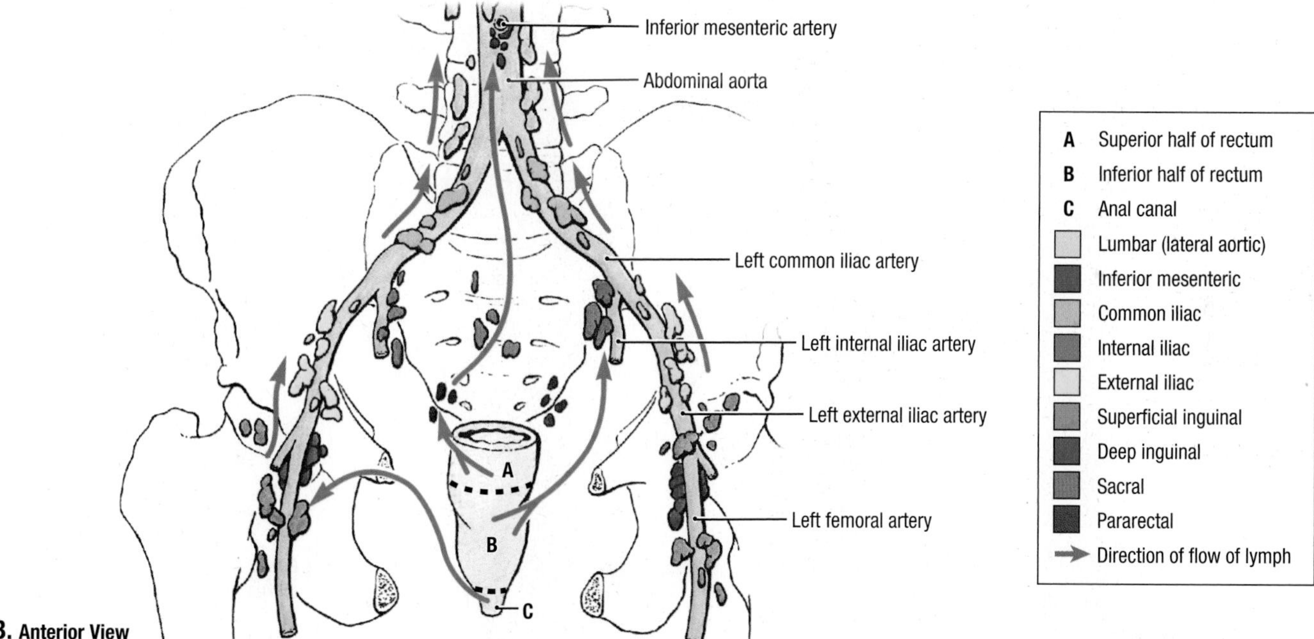
Inferior mesenteric artery
Abdominal aorta
Left common iliac artery
Left internal iliac artery
Left external iliac artery
Left femoral artery
A
B
C
A Superior half of rectum
B Inferior half of rectum
C Anal canal
Lumbar (lateral aortic)
Inferior mesenteric
Common iliac
Internal iliac
External iliac
Superficial inguinal
Deep inguinal
Sacral
Pararectal
Direction of flow of lymph

B. Anterior View

3.18 VASCULATURE OF RECTUM

A. Arterial and venous drainage.

- The continuation of the inferior mesenteric artery, the superior rectal artery, supplies the proximal part of rectum.
- Right and left middle rectal arteries, usually arising from the inferior vesical (male) or uterine (female) arteries, supply the middle and inferior parts of the rectum.
- Inferior rectal arteries, arising from the internal pudendal arteries, supply the anorectal junction and the anal canal.
- The rectal venous plexus surrounds the distal rectum and anal canal and consists of an internal rectal plexus deep to the epithelium of the anal canal and an external rectal plexus external to the muscular coats of the wall of the anal canal.
- The superior rectal vein drains into the portal system, and the middle and inferior veins drain into the systemic system; thus, this is an important area of **portacaval anastomosis** (see information on Hemorrhoids with Fig. 3.30).

B. Lymphatic drainage.

- The superior, middle, and inferior rectal veins drain the rectum and anal canal; there are anastomoses between the plexuses formed by all three veins.

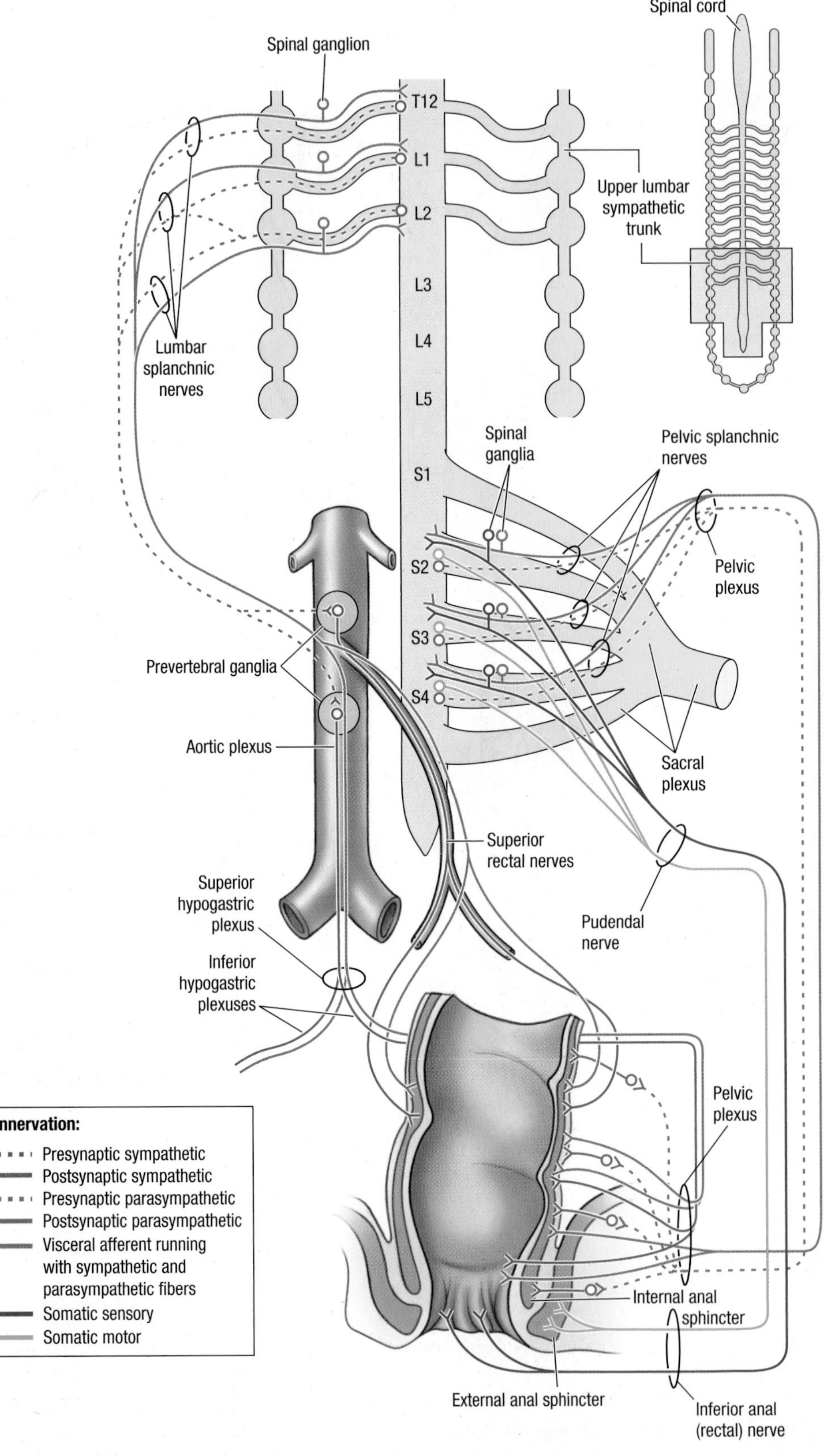
Spinal cord
Spinal ganglion
T12
L1
L2
L3
L4
L5
S1
S2
S3
S4
Upper lumbar sympathetic trunk
Lumbar splanchnic nerves
Spinal ganglia
Pelvic splanchnic nerves
Pelvic plexus
Prevertebral ganglia
Aortic plexus
Sacral plexus
Superior rectal nerves
Superior hypogastric plexus
Pudendal nerve
Inferior hypogastric plexuses
Pelvic plexus
Innervation:
Presynaptic sympathetic
Postsynaptic sympathetic
Presynaptic parasympathetic
Postsynaptic parasympathetic
Visceral afferent running with sympathetic and parasympathetic fibers
Somatic sensory
Somatic motor
Internal anal sphincter
External anal sphincter
Inferior anal (rectal) nerve

3.19 INNERVATION OF RECTUM AND ANAL CANAL

The lumbar and pelvic spinal nerves and hypogastric plexuses have been retracted laterally for clarity.

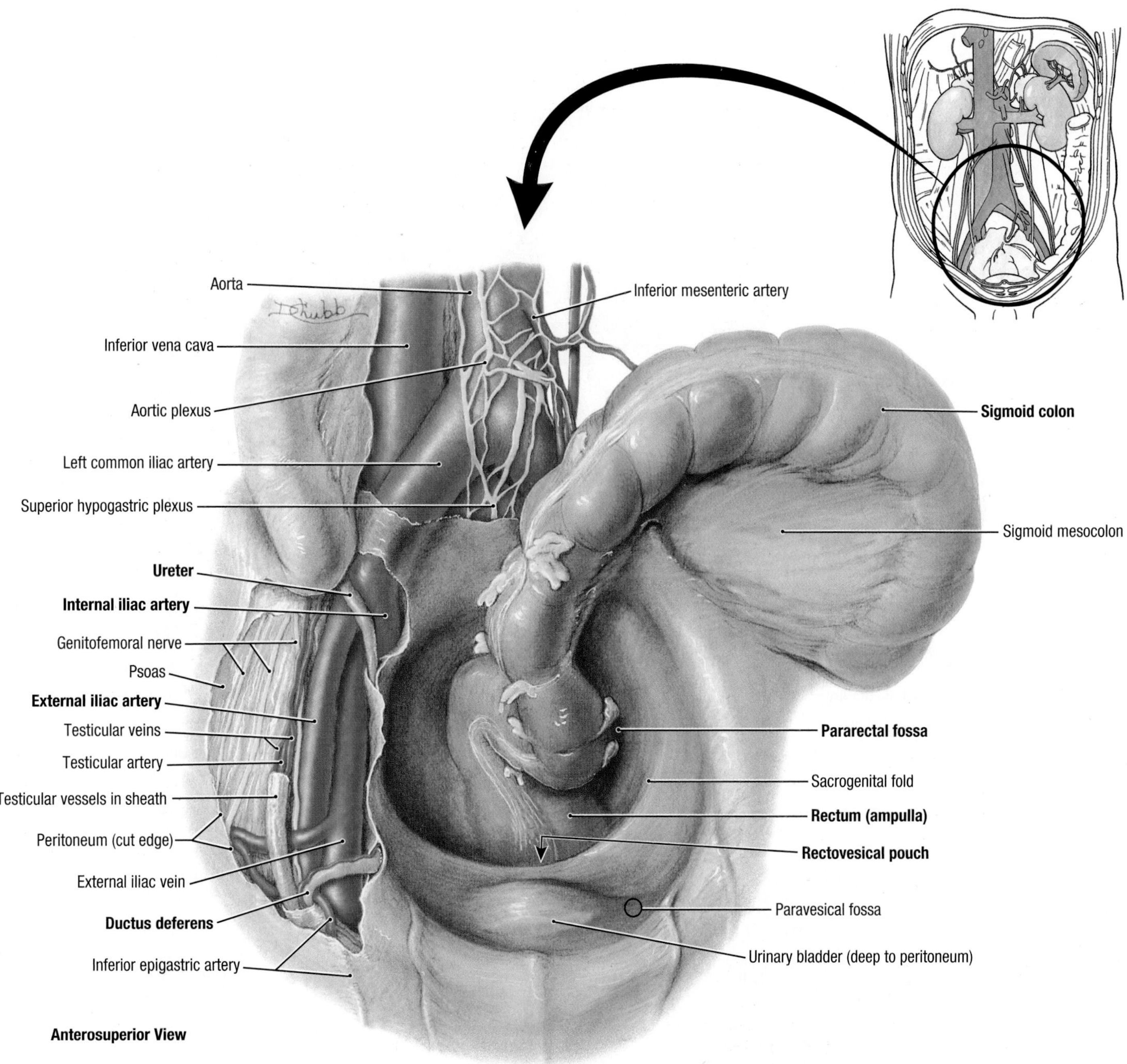
Aorta
Inferior mesenteric artery
Inferior vena cava
Aortic plexus
Sigmoid colon
Left common iliac artery
Superior hypogastric plexus
Sigmoid mesocolon
Ureter
Internal iliac artery
Genitofemoral nerve
Psoas
External iliac artery
Testicular veins
Testicular artery
Testicular vessels in sheath
Peritoneum (cut edge)
External iliac vein
Ductus deferens
Inferior epigastric artery
Pararectal fossa
Sacrogenital fold
Rectum (ampulla)
Rectovesical pouch
Paravesical fossa
Urinary bladder (deep to peritoneum)
Anterosuperior View

3.20 RECTUM IN SITU

- The sigmoid colon begins at the left pelvic brim and becomes the rectum anterior to the third sacral segment in the midline.
- The superior hypogastric plexus lies inferior to the bifurcation of the aorta and anterior to the left common iliac vein.
- The ureter adheres to the external aspect of the peritoneum, crosses the external iliac vessels, and descends anterior to the internal iliac artery. The ductus deferens and its artery also adhere to the peritoneum, cross the external iliac vessels, and then hook around the inferior epigastric artery to join the other components of the spermatic cord.
- The genitofemoral nerve lies on the psoas.

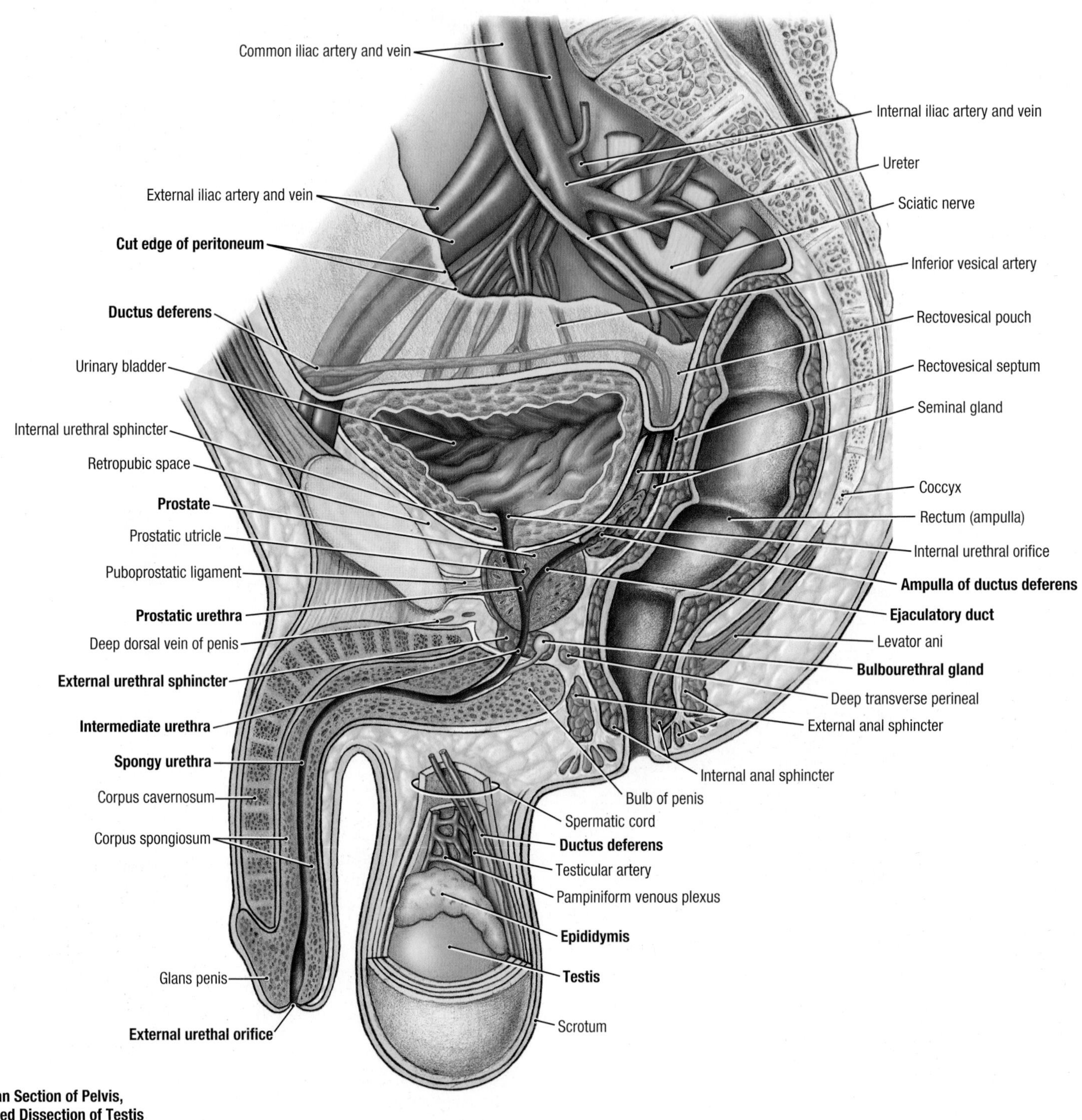
Common iliac artery and vein
Internal iliac artery and vein
Ureter
Sciatic nerve
External iliac artery and vein
Cut edge of peritoneum
Inferior vesical artery
Ductus deferens
Rectovesical pouch
Urinary bladder
Rectovesical septum
Seminal gland
Internal urethral sphincter
Retropubic space
Coccyx
Prostate
Rectum (ampulla)
Prostatic utricle
Internal urethral orifice
Puboprostatic ligament
Ampulla of ductus deferens
Prostatic urethra
Ejaculatory duct
Deep dorsal vein of penis
Levator ani
External urethral sphincter
Bulbourethral gland
Deep transverse perineal
Intermediate urethra
External anal sphincter
Spongy urethra
Internal anal sphincter
Corpus cavernosum
Bulb of penis
Spermatic cord
Corpus spongiosum
Ductus deferens
Testicular artery
Pampiniform venous plexus
Epididymis
Testis
Glans penis
Scrotum
External urethal orifice

Median Section of Pelvis, Stepped Dissection of Testis

3.21 MALE PELVIC ORGANS AND EXTERNAL GENITALIA

- Pelvic viscera are subperitoneal, mostly embedded in a matrix of fatty endopelvic fascia.

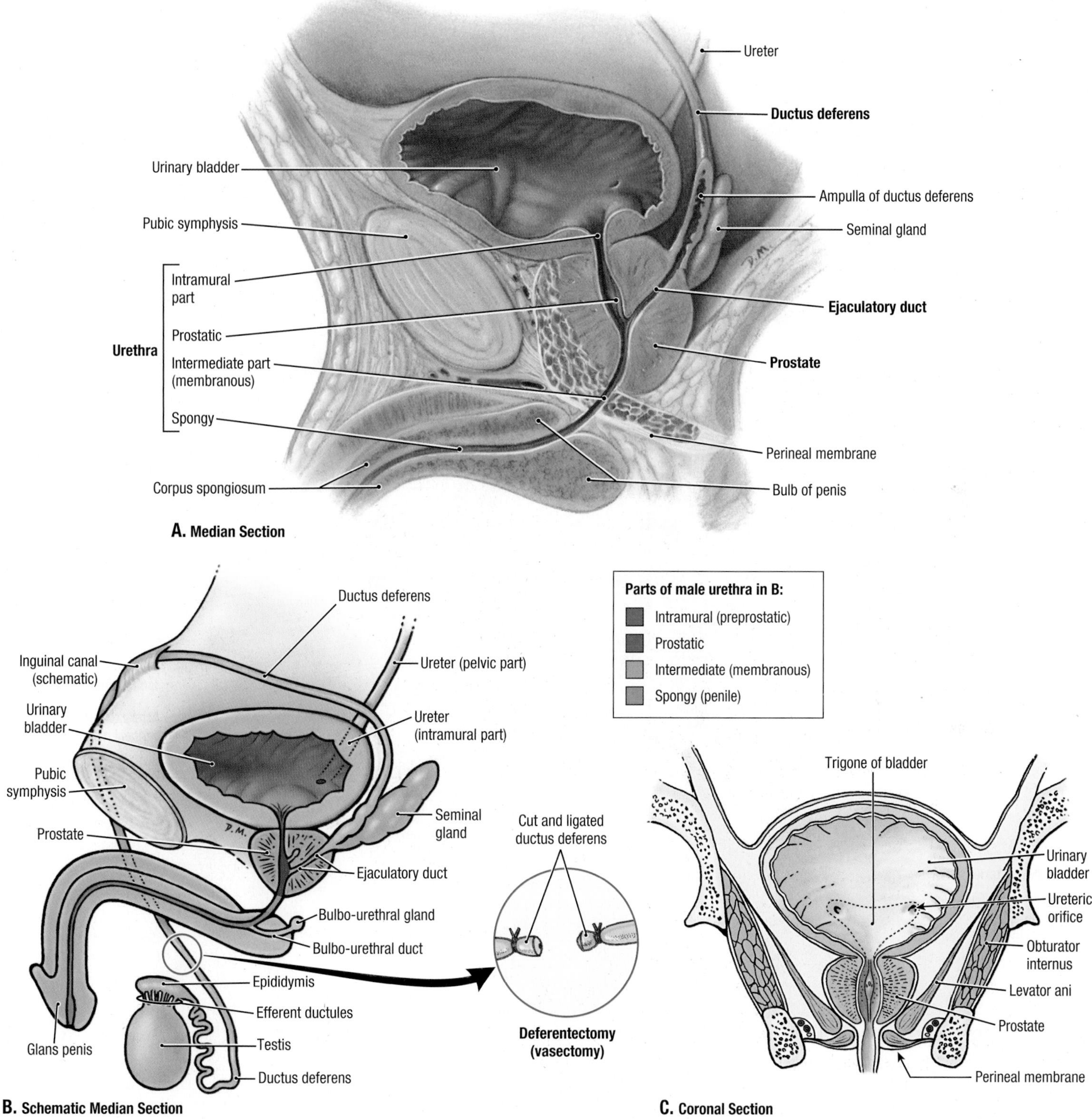
Ureter
Ductus deferens
Urinary bladder
Ampulla of ductus deferens
Pubic symphysis
Seminal gland
Intramural part
Ejaculatory duct
Prostatic
Urethra
Intermediate part (membranous)
Prostate
Spongy
Perineal membrane
Corpus spongiosum
Bulb of penis
A. Median Section
Ductus deferens
Parts of male urethra in B:
Intramural (preprostatic)
Prostatic
Intermediate (membranous)
Spongy (penile)
Inguinal canal (schematic)
Ureter (pelvic part)
Urinary bladder
Ureter (intramural part)
Pubic symphysis
Trigone of bladder
Seminal gland
Cut and ligated ductus deferens
Prostate
Urinary bladder
Ejaculatory duct
Ureteric orifice
Bulbo-urethral gland
Bulbo-urethral duct
Obturator internus
Epididymis
Levator ani
Efferent ductules
Prostate
Testis
Deferentectomy (vasectomy)
Glans penis
Ductus deferens
Perineal membrane
B. Schematic Median Section
C. Coronal Section

3.22 URINARY BLADDER, PROSTATE, AND DUCTUS DEFERENS

A. Dissection. The ejaculatory duct (~2 cm in length) is formed by the union of the ductus deferens and duct of the seminal gland; it passes anteriorly and inferiorly through the substance of the prostate to enter the prostatic urethra on the seminal colliculus. **B.** Overview of urogenital system, schematic illustration. **C.** Coronal section through urinary bladder, prostate, and proximal urethra.

The common method of sterilizing males is a **deferentectomy**, popularly called **vasectomy**. During this procedure, part of the ductus deferens is ligated and/or excised through an incision in the superior part of the scrotum. Hence, the subsequent ejaculated fluid contains no sperms.

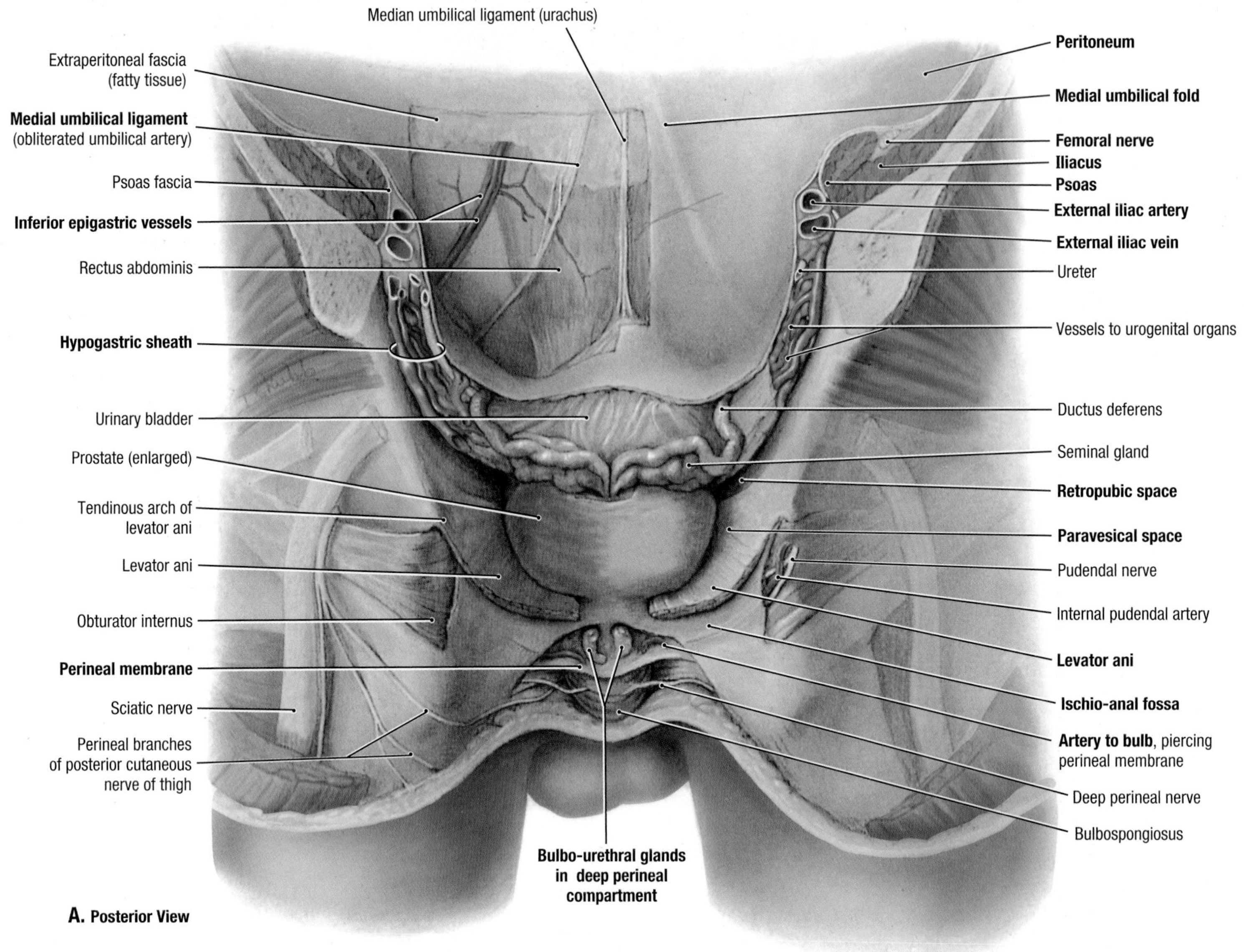
Median umbilical ligament (urachus)
Extraperitoneal fascia (fatty tissue)
Medial umbilical ligament (obliterated umbilical artery)
Psoas fascia
Inferior epigastric vessels
Rectus abdominis
Hypogastric sheath
Urinary bladder
Prostate (enlarged)
Tendinous arch of levator ani
Levator ani
Obturator internus
Perineal membrane
Sciatic nerve
Perineal branches of posterior cutaneous nerve of thigh
Peritoneum
Medial umbilical fold
Femoral nerve
Iliacus
Psoas
External iliac artery
External iliac vein
Ureter
Vessels to urogenital organs
Ductus deferens
Seminal gland
Retropubic space
Paravesical space
Pudendal nerve
Internal pudendal artery
Levator ani
Ischio-anal fossa
Artery to bulb, piercing perineal membrane
Deep perineal nerve
Bulbospongiosus
Bulbo-urethral glands in deep perineal compartment

A. Posterior View

3.23 POSTERIOR APPROACH TO ANTERIOR PELVIC AND PERINEAL STRUCTURES AND SPACES

A. Dissection. The rectovesical septum and all pelvic and perineal structures posterior to it have been removed. **B.** Posterior surface of inferior part of anterior abdominal wall with umbilical folds and ligaments and anterior pelvic viscera. **C.** Schematic coronal section through the anterior pelvis (plane of urinary bladder and prostate) demonstrating pelvic fascia.

- In **A** and **B**, the inferior epigastric artery and accompanying veins enter the rectus sheath, covered posteriorly with peritoneum to form the lateral umbilical fold. The medial umbilical fold is formed by peritoneum overlying the medial umbilical ligament (obliterated umbilical artery), and the median umbilical fold is formed by the median umbilical ligament (urachus).
- In **A**, the femoral nerve lies between the psoas and iliacus muscles, covered on their internal aspects with psoas (membranous parietal) fascia; the external iliac artery and vein lie within the areolar extraperitoneal fascia.
- The pelvic genito-urinary organs are subperitoneal. Near the bladder, the ureter accompanies a "leash" of internal iliac vessels and derivatives within the fibro-areolar hypogastric sheath.
- The levator ani and its fascial coverings separate the retropubic and paravesical spaces of the pelvis from the ischio-anal fossae of the perineum. The fat that occupies these spaces has been removed.
- The bulbo-urethral glands and the initial part of the artery to the bulb lie superior to the perineal membrane in the deep perineal compartment.

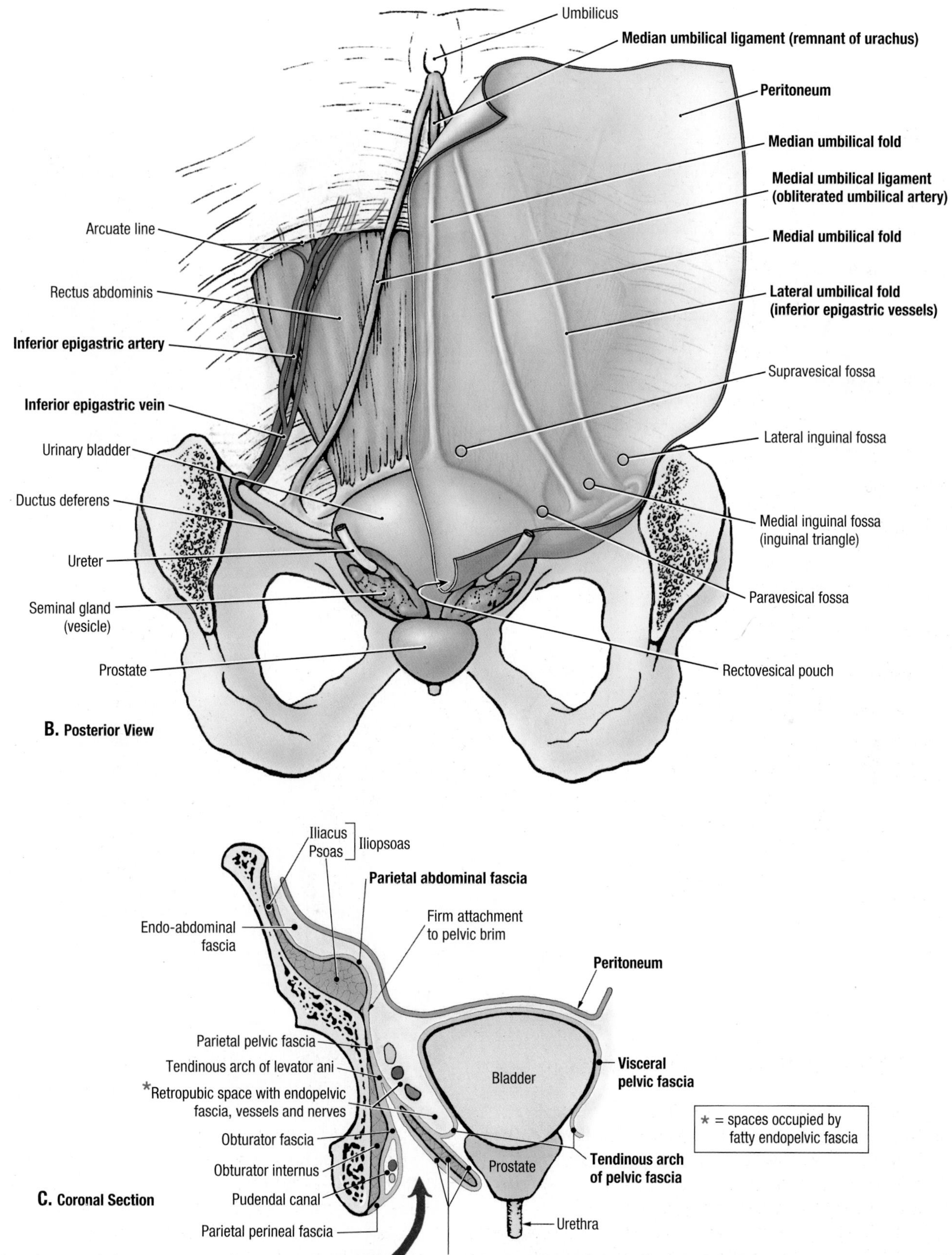
Umbilicus
Median umbilical ligament (remnant of urachus)
Peritoneum
Median umbilical fold
Medial umbilical ligament (obliterated umbilical artery)
Medial umbilical fold
Lateral umbilical fold (inferior epigastric vessels)
Supravesical fossa
Lateral inguinal fossa
Medial inguinal fossa (inguinal triangle)
Paravesical fossa
Rectovesical pouch
Arcuate line
Rectus abdominis
Inferior epigastric artery
Inferior epigastric vein
Urinary bladder
Ductus deferens
Ureter
Seminal gland (vesicle)
Prostate
B. Posterior View
Iliacus
Psoas
Iliopsoas
Parietal abdominal fascia
Endo-abdominal fascia
Firm attachment to pelvic brim
Peritoneum
Parietal pelvic fascia
Tendinous arch of levator ani
*Retropubic space with endopelvic fascia, vessels and nerves
Obturator fascia
Obturator internus
Pudendal canal
Parietal perineal fascia
*Ischio-anal (ischiorectal) fossa
Bladder
Visceral pelvic fascia
* = spaces occupied by fatty endopelvic fascia
Prostate
Tendinous arch of pelvic fascia
Urethra
Levator ani with superior and inferior parietal fascia
C. Coronal Section

3.23 POSTERIOR APPROACH TO ANTERIOR PELVIC AND PERINEAL STRUCTURES AND SPACES *(CONTINUED)*

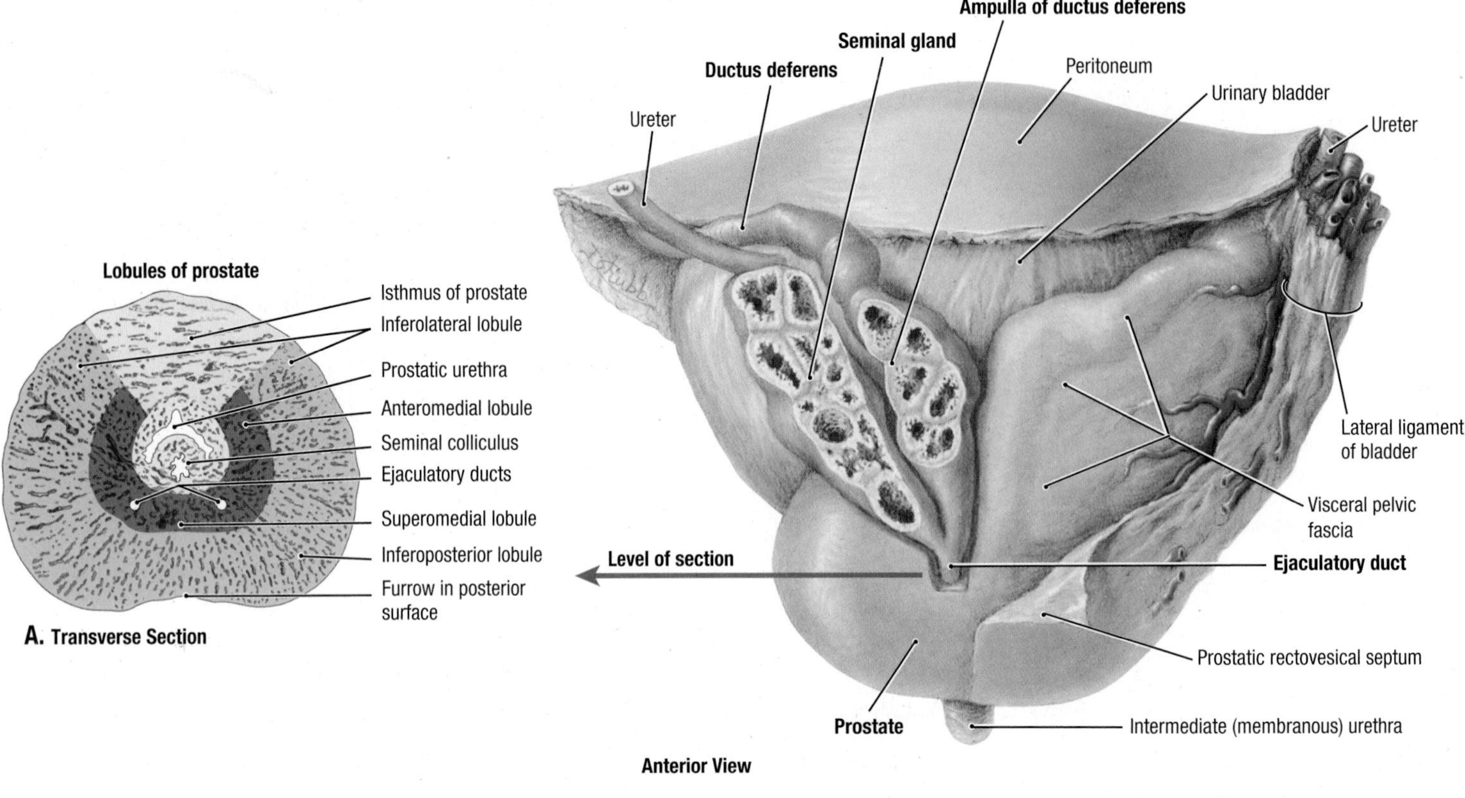

Lobules of prostate
Isthmus of prostate
Inferolateral lobule
Prostatic urethra
Anteromedial lobule
Seminal colliculus
Ejaculatory ducts
Superomedial lobule
Inferoposterior lobule
Furrow in posterior surface
Ampulla of ductus deferens
Seminal gland
Ductus deferens
Peritoneum
Urinary bladder
Ureter
Ureter
Lateral ligament of bladder
Visceral pelvic fascia
Level of section
Ejaculatory duct
Prostatic rectovesical septum
Prostate
Intermediate (membranous) urethra

A. Transverse Section

Anterior View

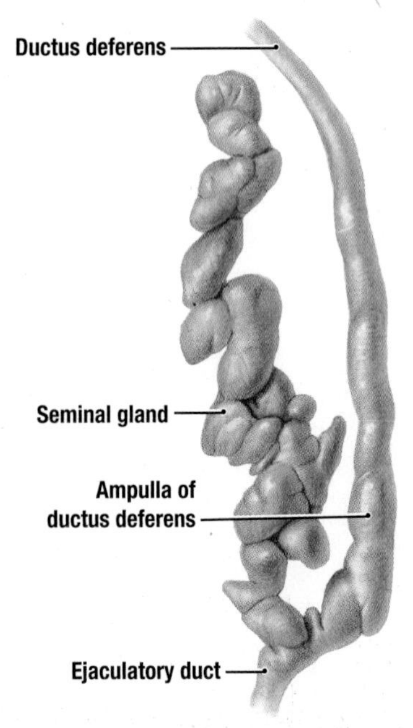

Ductus deferens
Seminal gland
Ampulla of ductus deferens
Ejaculatory duct

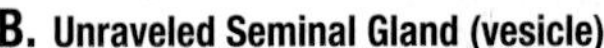
B. Unraveled Seminal Gland (vesicle)

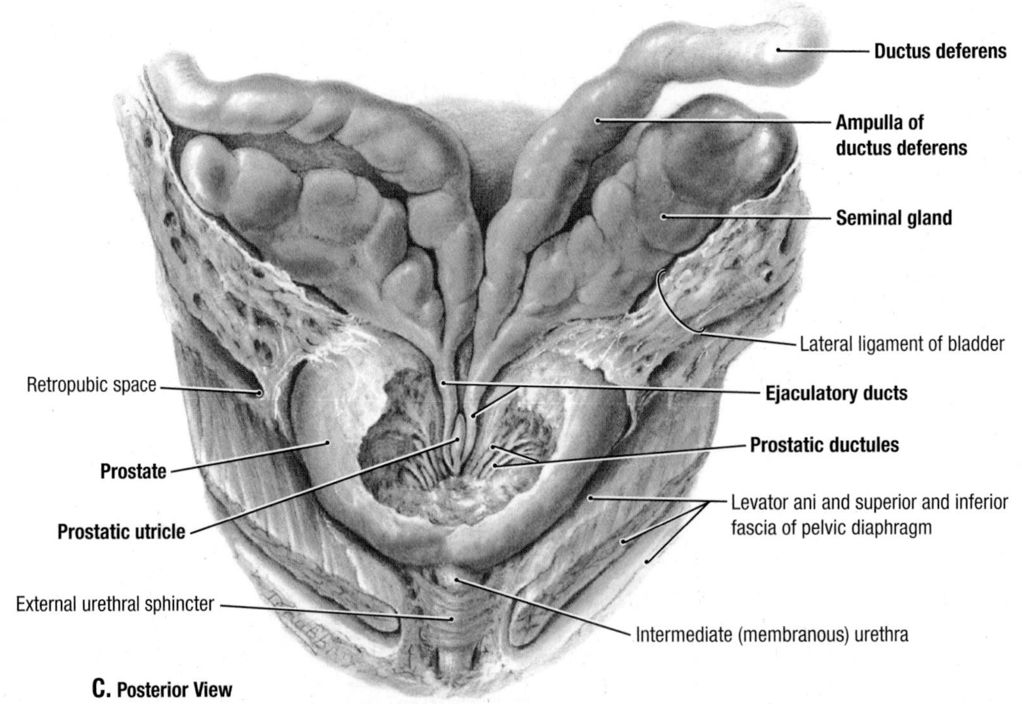

Ductus deferens
Ampulla of ductus deferens
Seminal gland
Lateral ligament of bladder
Retropubic space
Ejaculatory ducts
Prostatic ductules
Prostate
Levator ani and superior and inferior fascia of pelvic diaphragm
Prostatic utricle
External urethral sphincter
Intermediate (membranous) urethra

C. Posterior View

3.24 SEMINAL GLANDS AND PROSTATE

A. Bladder, ductus deferens, seminal glands (vesicles), and lobules of prostate. The left seminal gland and ampulla of the ductus deferens are dissected and opened; part of the prostate is cut away to expose the ejaculatory duct. **B.** Seminal gland unraveled. The gland is a tortuous tube with numerous dilatations. The ampulla of the ductus deferens has similar dilatations. **C.** Prostate, dissected posteriorly. The ejaculatory duct (~2 cm in length) is formed by the union of the ductus deferens and the duct of the seminal gland; it passes anteriorly and inferiorly through the substance of the prostate to enter the prostatic urethra on the seminal colliculus. The prostatic utricle lies between the ends of the two ejaculatory ducts. The prostatic ductules mostly open onto the prostatic sinus.

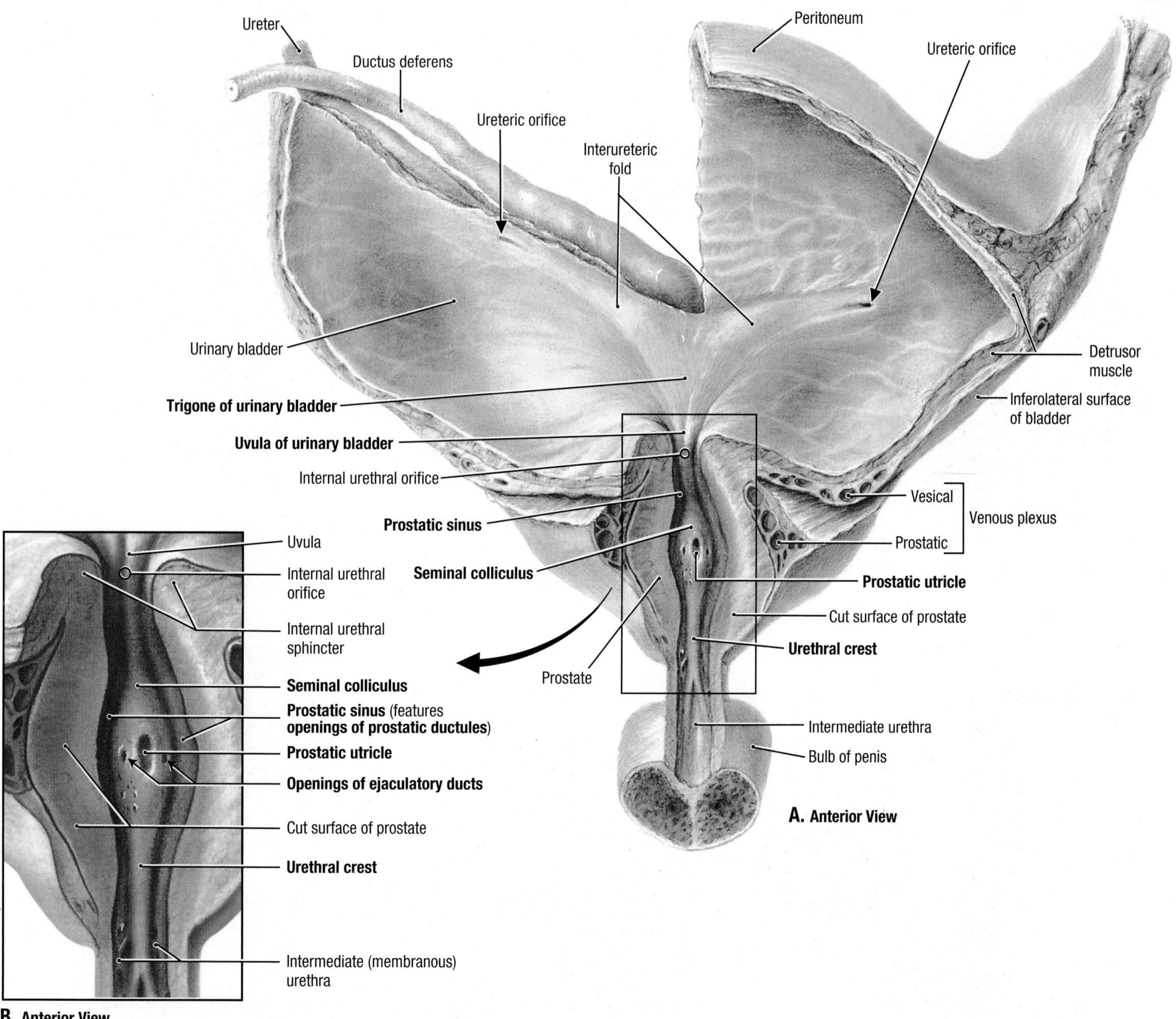
Ureter
Ductus deferens
Ureteric orifice
Interureteric fold
Peritoneum
Ureteric orifice
Urinary bladder
Trigone of urinary bladder
Uvula of urinary bladder
Internal urethral orifice
Prostatic sinus
Seminal colliculus
Detrusor muscle
Inferolateral surface of bladder
Vesical
Venous plexus
Prostatic
Prostatic utricle
Cut surface of prostate
Urethral crest
Prostate
Intermediate urethra
Bulb of penis
A. Anterior View
Uvula
Internal urethral orifice
Internal urethral sphincter
Seminal colliculus
Prostatic sinus (features openings of prostatic ductules)
Prostatic utricle
Openings of ejaculatory ducts
Cut surface of prostate
Urethral crest
Intermediate (membranous) urethra
B. Anterior View

3.25 INTERIOR OF MALE URINARY BLADDER AND PROSTATIC URETHRA

A. Dissection. The anterior walls of the bladder, prostate, and urethra were cut away. **B.** Features of the prostatic urethra.

- The mucous membrane is smooth over the trigone of the urinary bladder (triangular region demarcated by ureteric and internal urethral orifices) but folded elsewhere, especially when the bladder is empty.
- The opening of the vestigial prostatic utricle is in the seminal colliculus on the urethral crest; there is an orifice of an ejaculatory duct on each side of the prostatic utricle. The prostatic fascia encloses a venous plexus.

The prostate is of considerable medical interest because enlargement or **benign hypertrophy of the prostate (BHP)** is common after middle age, affecting virtually every male who lives long enough. An enlarged prostate projects into the urinary bladder and impedes urination by distorting the prostatic urethra. The middle lobule usually enlarges the most and obstructs the internal urethral orifice. The more the person strains, the more the valvelike prostatic mass occludes the urethra.

BHP is a common cause of urethral obstruction, leading to **nocturia** (needing to void during the night), **dysuria** (difficulty and/or pain during urination), and **urgency** (sudden desire to void). BHP also increases the risk of bladder infections (**cystitis**) as well as kidney damage.

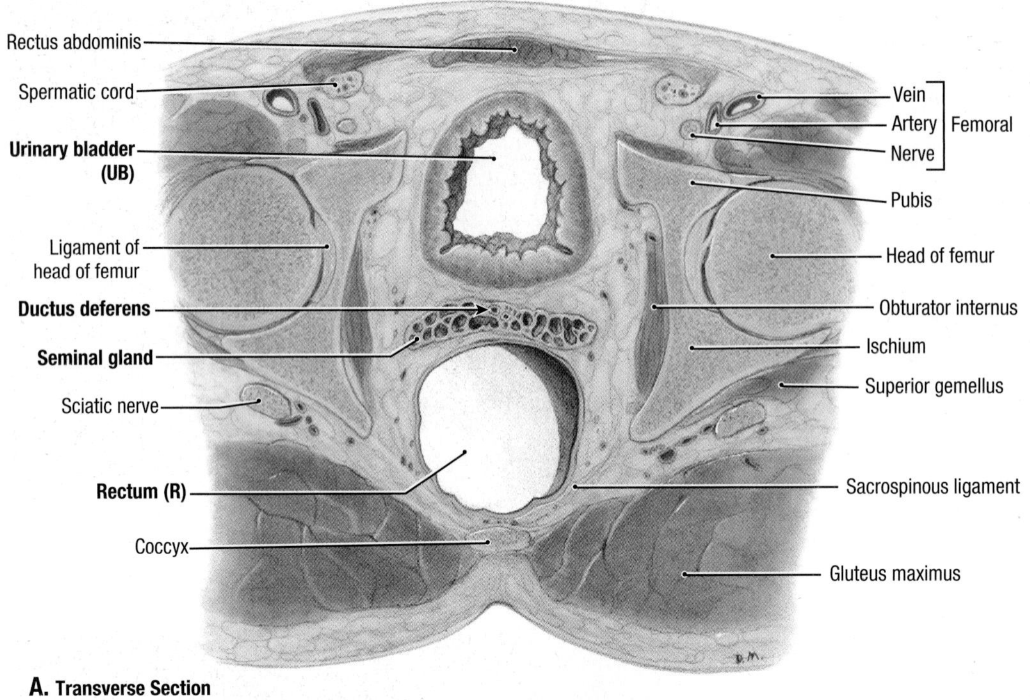
Rectus abdominis
Spermatic cord
Urinary bladder (UB)
Ligament of head of femur
Ductus deferens
Seminal gland
Sciatic nerve
Rectum (R)
Coccyx
Vein
Artery
Nerve
Femoral
Pubis
Head of femur
Obturator internus
Ischium
Superior gemellus
Sacrospinous ligament
Gluteus maximus
D.M.

A. **Transverse Section**

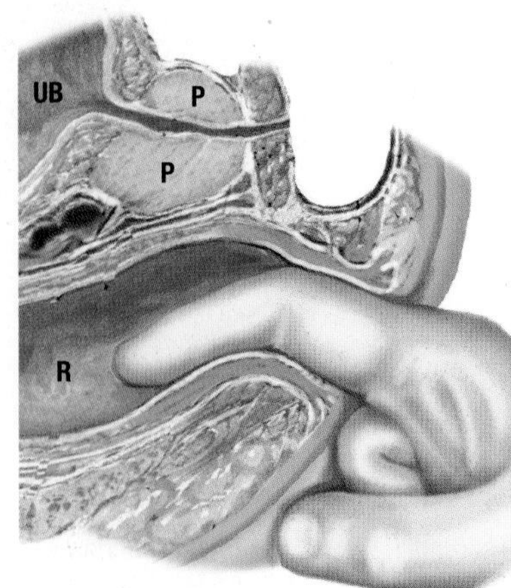
UB
P
P
R

C. **Sagittal Section**

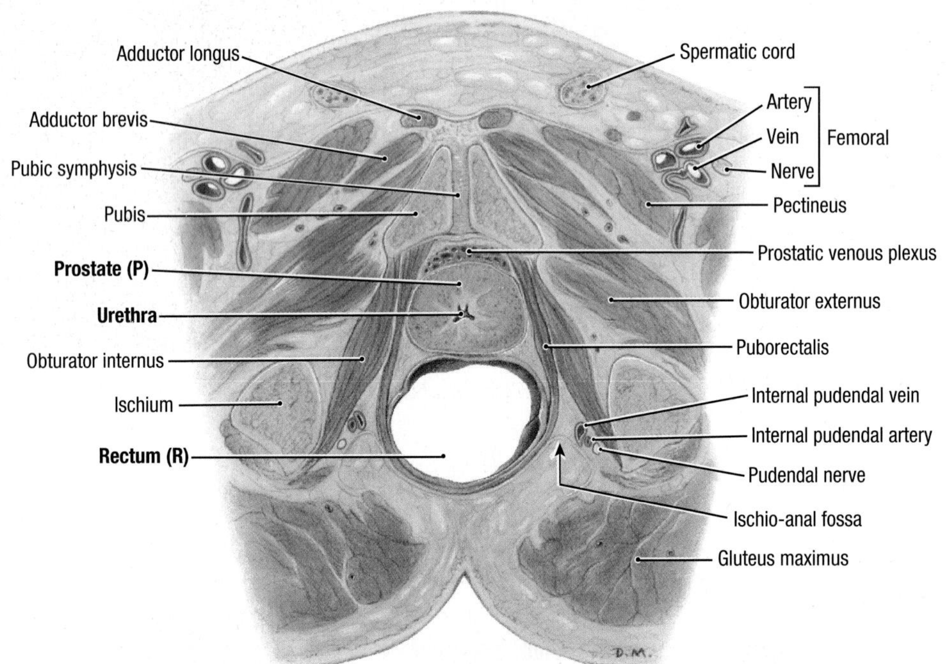
Adductor longus
Adductor brevis
Pubic symphysis
Pubis
Prostate (P)
Urethra
Obturator internus
Ischium
Rectum (R)
Spermatic cord
Artery
Vein
Nerve
Femoral
Pectineus
Prostatic venous plexus
Obturator externus
Puborectalis
Internal pudendal vein
Internal pudendal artery
Pudendal nerve
Ischio-anal fossa
Gluteus maximus
D.M.

B. **Transverse Section**

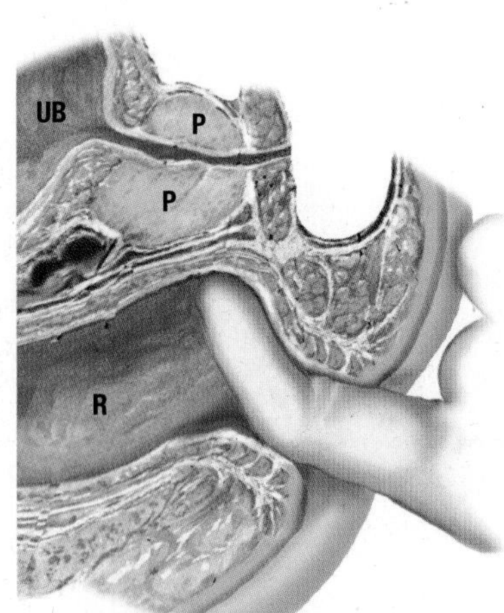
UB
P
P
R

D. **Sagittal Section**

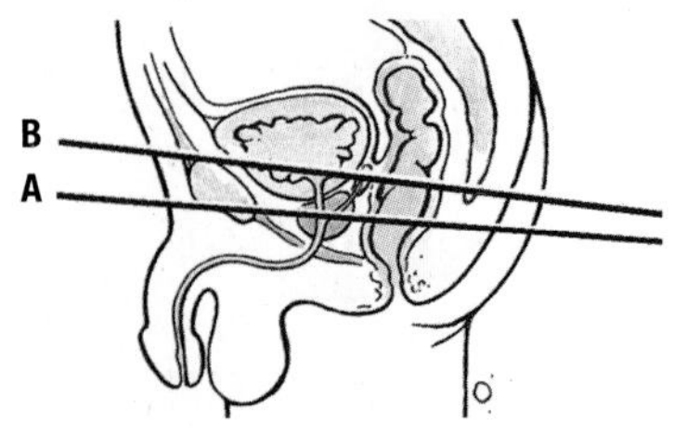
B
A

3.26 MALE PELVIS, TRANSVERSE SECTIONS

A. Section through prostate and puborectalis. **B.** Section through urinary bladder and seminal gland. **C. and D.** The prostate *(P)* is examined for enlargement and tumors (focal masses or asymmetry) by **digital rectal examination**. A full bladder offers resistance, holding the gland in place and making it more readily palpable. The malignant prostate feels hard and often irregular. (*R, rectum).*

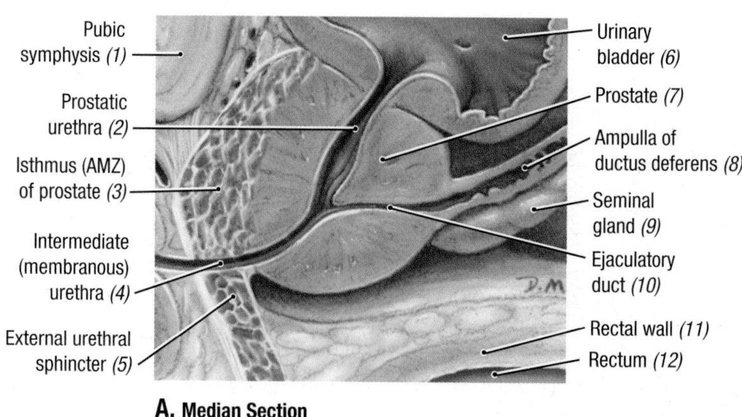
Pubic symphysis (1)
Prostatic urethra (2)
Isthmus (AMZ) of prostate (3)
Intermediate (membranous) urethra (4)
External urethral sphincter (5)
Urinary bladder (6)
Prostate (7)
Ampulla of ductus deferens (8)
Seminal gland (9)
Ejaculatory duct (10)
Rectal wall (11)
Rectum (12)
D.M

A. **Median Section**

Key for US scan:

12 Site of transducer in rectum
13 Concretions surrounding distended and collapsed urethra
14 Calcification in seminal colliculus

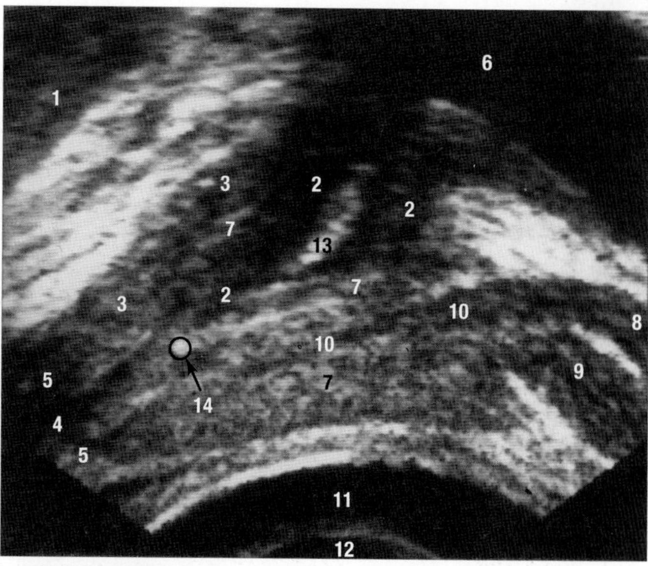
1
6
3
2
2
7
13
3
2
7
10
8
5
10
9
7
14
4
5
11
12

Longitudinal (Median) Scan

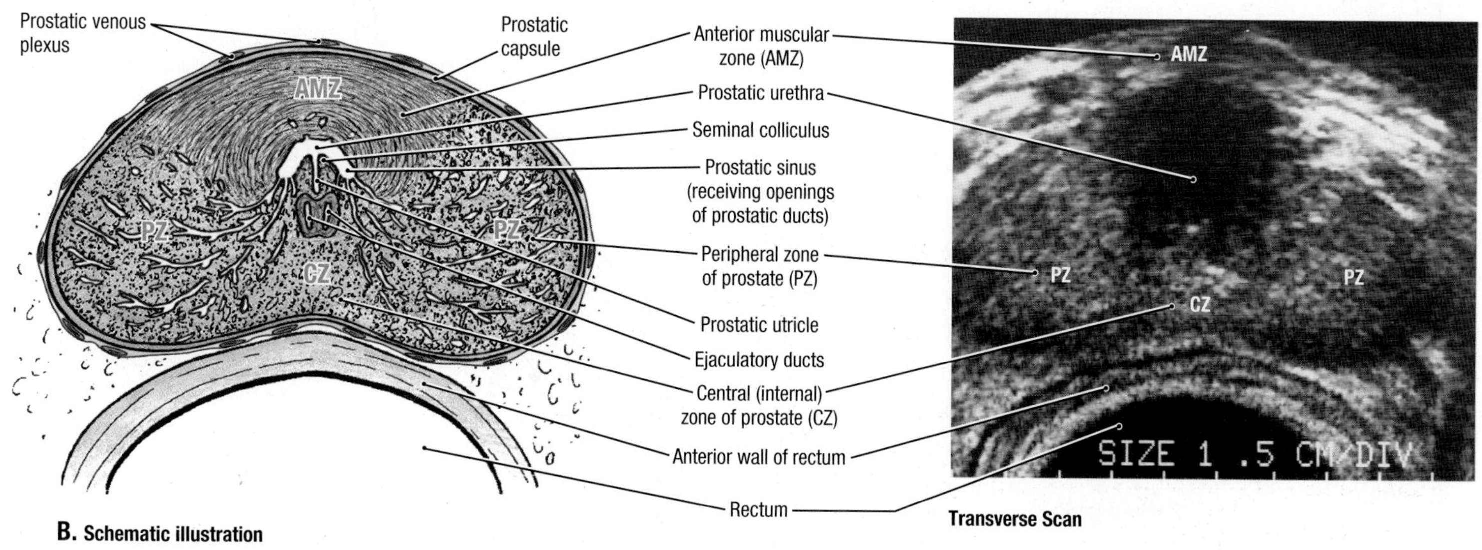
Prostatic venous plexus
Prostatic capsule
AMZ
PZ
PZ
CZ
Anterior muscular zone (AMZ)
Prostatic urethra
Seminal colliculus
Prostatic sinus (receiving openings of prostatic ducts)
Peripheral zone of prostate (PZ)
Prostatic utricle
Ejaculatory ducts
Central (internal) zone of prostate (CZ)
Anterior wall of rectum
Rectum
AMZ
PZ
PZ
CZ
SIZE 1 .5 CM/DIV

B. **Schematic illustration**

Transverse Scan

3.27 TRANSRECTAL ULTRASOUND SCANS OF MALE PELVIS

A. Longitudinal scan. **B.** Transverse scan. The probe was inserted into the rectum to scan the anteriorly located prostate. The ducts of the glands in the peripheral zone open into the prostatic sinuses, whereas the ducts of the glands in the central (internal) zone open into the prostatic sinuses and onto the seminal colliculus.

Because of the close relationship of the prostate to the prostatic urethra, obstructions of the urethra may be relieved endoscopically. The instrument is inserted transurethrally through the external urethral orifice and spongy urethra into the prostatic urethra. All or part of the prostate, or just the hypertrophied part, is removed by **transurethral resection of the prostate (TURP)**. In more serious cases, the entire prostate is removed along with the seminal glands, ejaculatory ducts, and terminal parts of the deferent ducts **(radical prostatectomy)**.

TURP and improved operative techniques (laparoscopic or robotic surgery) attempt to preserve the nerves and blood vessels associated with the capsule of the prostate and adjacent to the seminal vesicles as they pass to and from the penis, increasing the possibility for patients to retain sexual function after surgery, as well as restoring normal urinary control.

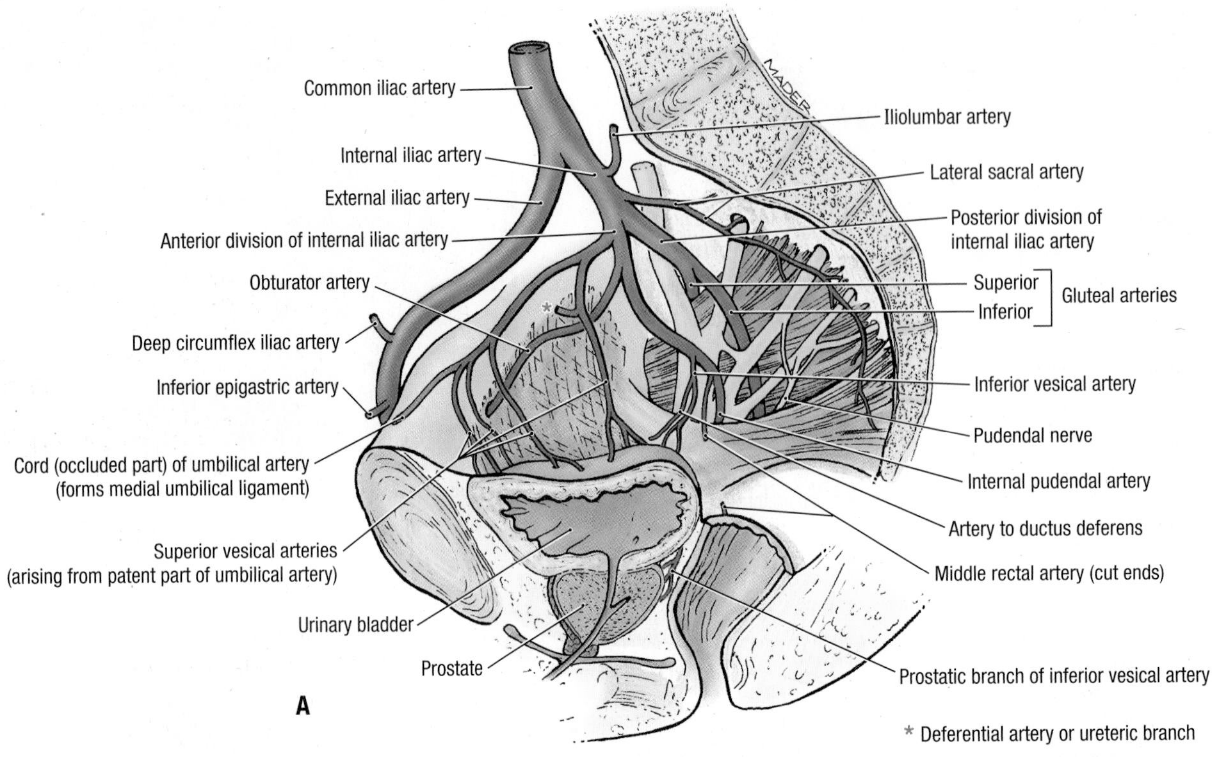

Common iliac artery
Internal iliac artery
External iliac artery
Anterior division of internal iliac artery
Obturator artery
Deep circumflex iliac artery
Inferior epigastric artery
Cord (occluded part) of umbilical artery (forms medial umbilical ligament)
Superior vesical arteries (arising from patent part of umbilical artery)
Urinary bladder
Prostate
A
Iliolumbar artery
Lateral sacral artery
Posterior division of internal iliac artery
Superior
Inferior
Gluteal arteries
Inferior vesical artery
Pudendal nerve
Internal pudendal artery
Artery to ductus deferens
Middle rectal artery (cut ends)
Prostatic branch of inferior vesical artery
* Deferential artery or ureteric branch

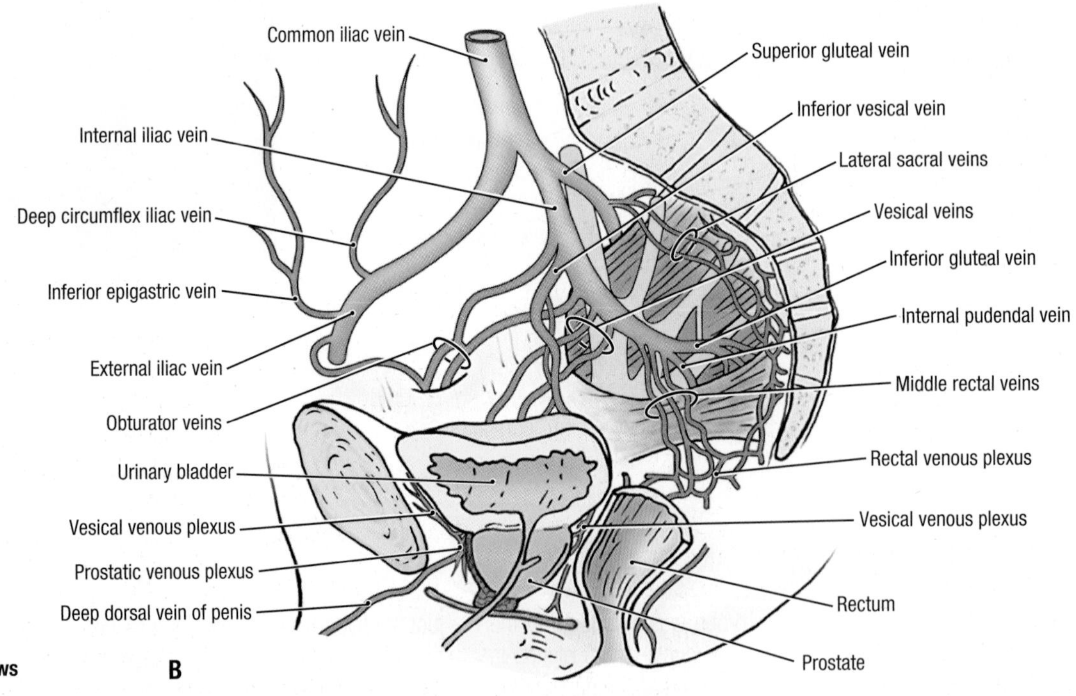

Common iliac vein
Internal iliac vein
Deep circumflex iliac vein
Inferior epigastric vein
External iliac vein
Obturator veins
Urinary bladder
Vesical venous plexus
Prostatic venous plexus
Deep dorsal vein of penis
Superior gluteal vein
Inferior vesical vein
Lateral sacral veins
Vesical veins
Inferior gluteal vein
Internal pudendal vein
Middle rectal veins
Rectal venous plexus
Vesical venous plexus
Rectum
Prostate
Medial Views
B

3.28 ARTERIES AND VEINS OF MALE PELVIS

A. Arteries. **B.** Pelvic veins and venous plexuses.

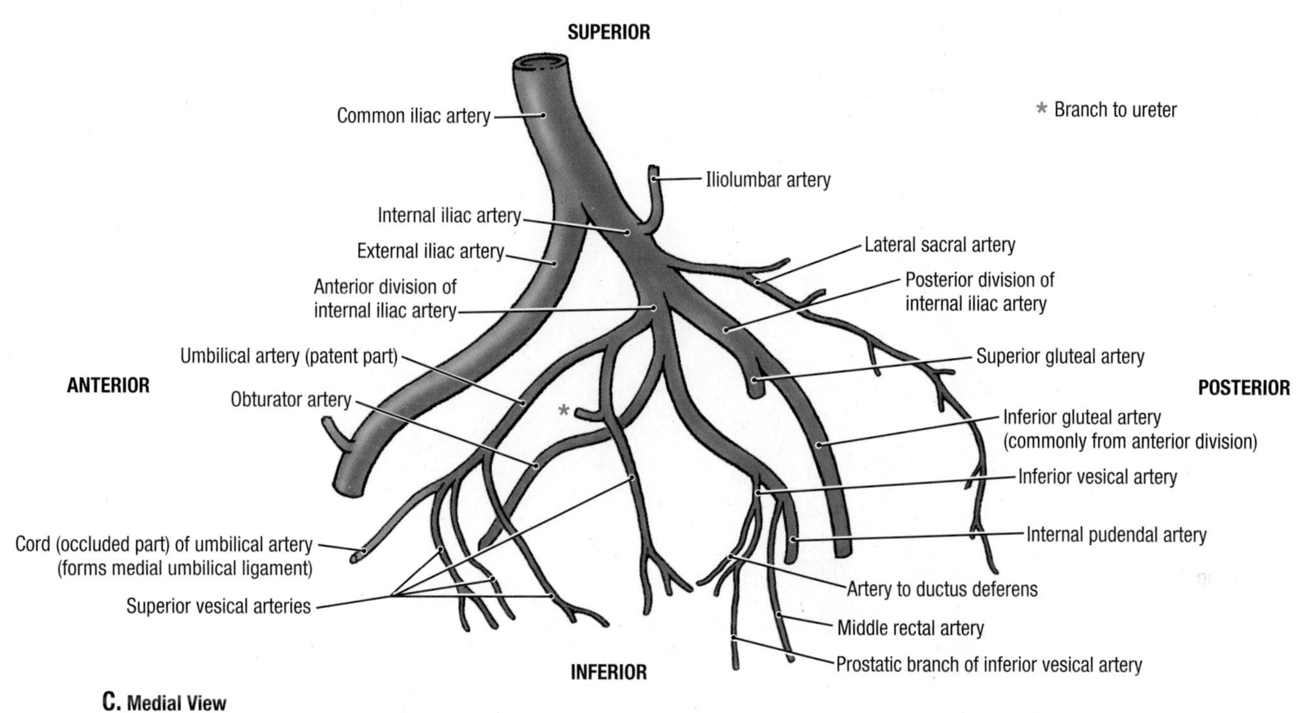
SUPERIOR
Common iliac artery
* Branch to ureter
Iliolumbar artery
Internal iliac artery
External iliac artery
Lateral sacral artery
Anterior division of internal iliac artery
Posterior division of internal iliac artery
Umbilical artery (patent part)
Superior gluteal artery
ANTERIOR
Obturator artery
POSTERIOR
Inferior gluteal artery (commonly from anterior division)
Inferior vesical artery
Internal pudendal artery
Cord (occluded part) of umbilical artery (forms medial umbilical ligament)
Artery to ductus deferens
Superior vesical arteries
Middle rectal artery
Prostatic branch of inferior vesical artery
INFERIOR

C. **Medial View**

3.28 ARTERIES AND VEINS OF MALE PELVIS *(CONTINUED)*

C. Arteries, isolated from **A.**

TABLE 3.4 ARTERIES OF MALE PELVIS

Artery	Origin	Course	Distribution
Internal iliac	Common iliac artery	Passes medially over pelvic brim and descends into pelvic cavity; often forms anterior and posterior divisions	Main blood supply to pelvic organs, gluteal muscles, and perineum
Anterior division of internal iliac artery	Internal iliac artery	Passes laterally along lateral wall of pelvis, dividing into visceral, obturator, and internal pudendal arteries	Pelvic viscera, perineum, and muscles of superior medial thigh
Umbilical	Anterior division of internal iliac artery	Short pelvic course; gives off superior vesical arteries, then obliterates, becoming medial umbilical ligament	Urinary bladder and, in some males, ductus deferens
Superior vesical	Patent part of umbilical artery	Usually multiple; pass to superior aspect of urinary bladder	Superior aspect of urinary bladder and distal ureter
Artery to ductus deferens	Superior or inferior vesical artery	Runs subperitoneally to ductus deferens	Ductus deferens
Obturator	Anterior division of internal iliac artery	Runs antero-inferiorly on lateral pelvic wall	Pelvic muscles, nutrient artery to head of femur and medial compartment of thigh
Inferior vesical		Passes subperitoneally giving rise to prostatic artery and occasionally the artery to the ductus deferens	Inferior aspect of urinary bladder, pelvic ureter, seminal glands, and prostate
Middle rectal		Descends in pelvis to rectum	Seminal glands, prostate, and inferior part of rectum
Internal pudendal		Exits pelvis through greater sciatic foramen and enters perineum via lesser sciatic foramen	Main artery to perineum, including muscles and skin of anal and urogenital triangles; erectile bodies
Posterior division of internal iliac artery	Internal iliac artery	Passes posteriorly and gives rise to parietal branches	Pelvic wall and gluteal region iliac artery
Iliolumbar	Posterior division of internal iliac artery	Ascends anterior to sacro-iliac joint and posterior to common iliac vessels and psoas major	Iliacus, psoas major, quadratus lumborum muscles, and cauda equina in vertebral canal
Lateral sacral (superior and inferior)		Run on anteromedial aspect of piriformis to send branches into pelvic sacral foramina	Piriformis muscle, structures in sacral canal and erector spinae muscles
Testicular (gonadal) [see Fig. 3.28A]	Abdominal aorta	Descends retroperitoneally; traverses inguinal canal and enters scrotum	Abdominal ureter, testis and epididymis

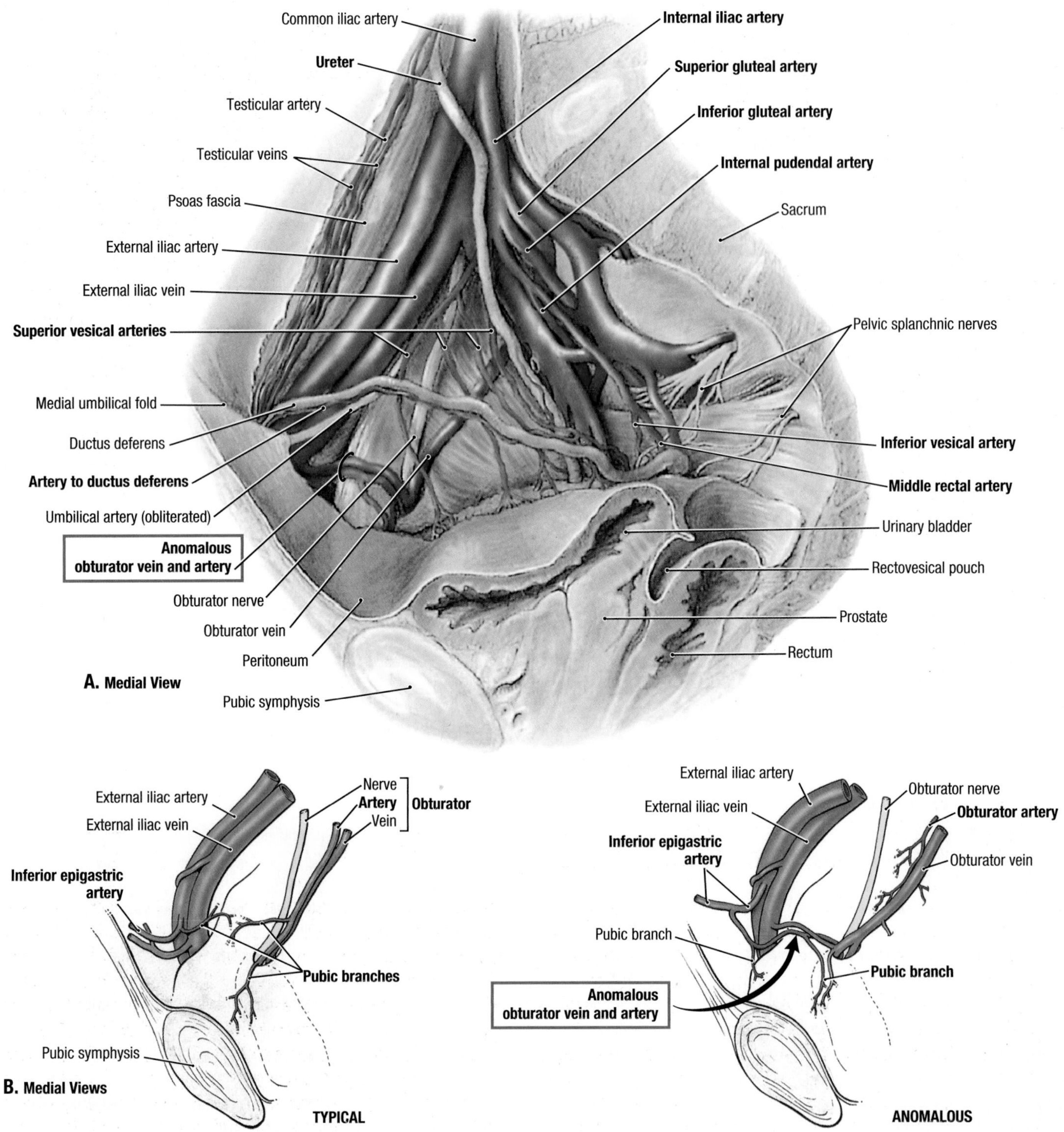
Common iliac artery
Ureter
Testicular artery
Testicular veins
Psoas fascia
External iliac artery
External iliac vein
Superior vesical arteries
Medial umbilical fold
Ductus deferens
Artery to ductus deferens
Umbilical artery (obliterated)
Anomalous obturator vein and artery
Obturator nerve
Obturator vein
Peritoneum
A. Medial View
Pubic symphysis
Internal iliac artery
Superior gluteal artery
Inferior gluteal artery
Internal pudendal artery
Sacrum
Pelvic splanchnic nerves
Inferior vesical artery
Middle rectal artery
Urinary bladder
Rectovesical pouch
Prostate
Rectum
External iliac artery
External iliac vein
Inferior epigastric artery
Nerve
Artery
Vein
Obturator
Pubic branches
Pubic symphysis
B. Medial Views
TYPICAL
External iliac artery
External iliac vein
Inferior epigastric artery
Obturator nerve
Obturator artery
Obturator vein
Pubic branch
Pubic branch
Anomalous obturator vein and artery
ANOMALOUS

3.29 PELVIC VESSELS IN SITU; LATERAL PELVIC WALL

A. Dissection. The ureter crosses the external iliac artery at its origin (common iliac bifurcation), and the ductus deferens crosses the external iliac artery at its termination (deep inguinal ring). The ureter crosses the external iliac artery at its origin (common iliac bifurcation), and the ductus deferens crosses the external iliac artery at its termination (deep inguinal ring). In this speciman, an anomalous (replaced) obturator artery branches from the inferior epigastric artery. **B.** Typical and anomalous obturator arteries.

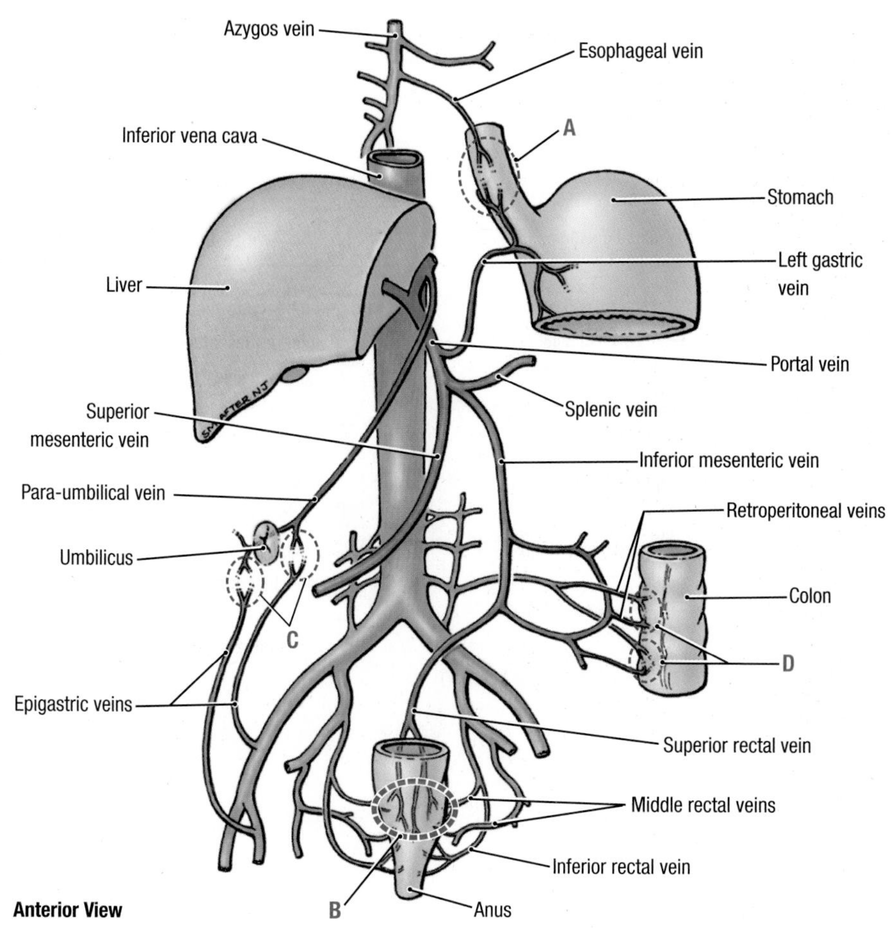
Azygos vein
Esophageal vein
Inferior vena cava
A
Stomach
Liver
Left gastric vein
Portal vein
Superior mesenteric vein
Splenic vein
Inferior mesenteric vein
Para-umbilical vein
Retroperitoneal veins
Umbilicus
Colon
C
D
Epigastric veins
Superior rectal vein
Middle rectal veins
Inferior rectal vein
Anus
B
Anterior View

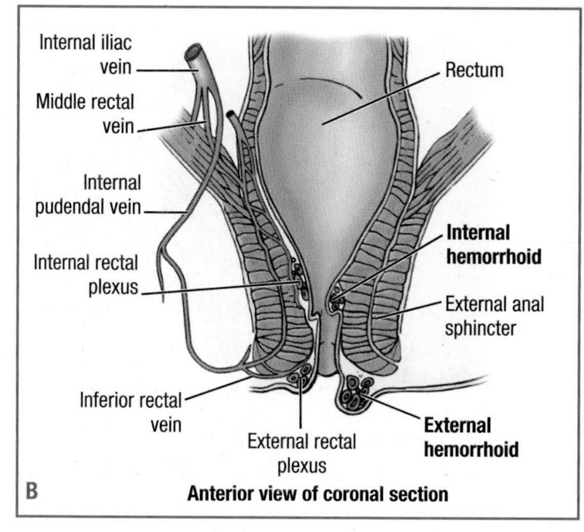
Internal iliac vein
Middle rectal vein
Internal pudendal vein
Internal rectal plexus
Inferior rectal vein
External rectal plexus
Rectum
Internal hemorrhoid
External anal sphincter
External hemorrhoid
B
Anterior view of coronal section

3.30 PORTAL–SYSTEMIC (PORTACAVAL) ANASTOMOSES

A. The portal tributaries are *purple,* and systemic tributaries are *blue. A–D* indicate sites of portal–systemic anastomoses. *A,* between portal and systemic esophageal veins; *B,* between portal and systemic rectal veins; *C,* para-umbilical veins (portal) anastomosing with small epigastric veins of the anterior abdominal wall (systemic); *D,* twigs of colic veins (portal) anastomosing with retroperitoneal veins (systemic).

B. Hemorrhoids. Internal hemorrhoids (piles) are prolapses of rectal mucosa containing the normally dilated veins of the internal rectal venous plexus. Internal hemorrhoids are thought to result from a breakdown of the muscularis mucosae, a smooth muscle layer deep to the mucosa. Internal hemorrhoids that prolapse through the anal canal are often compressed by the contracted sphincters, impeding blood flow. As a result, they tend to strangulate and ulcerate. Because of the presence of abundant arteriovenous anastomoses, bleeding from internal hemorrhoids is characteristically bright red. The current practice is to treat only prolapsed, ulcerated internal hemorrhoids.

External hemorrhoids are thromboses (blood clots) in the veins of the external rectal venous plexus and are covered by skin. Predisposing factors for hemorrhoids include pregnancy, chronic constipation, and any disorder that impedes venous return including increased intra-abdominal pressure. The superior rectal vein drains into the inferior mesenteric vein, whereas the middle and inferior rectal veins drain through the systemic system into the inferior vena cava. Any abnormal increase in pressure in the valveless portal system or veins of the trunk may cause enlargement of the superior rectal veins, resulting in an increase in blood flow or stasis in the internal rectal venous plexus. In **portal hypertension** that occurs in relation to *hepatic cirrhosis,* the portacaval anastomosis (e.g., esophageal) may become varicose and rupture. It is important to note, however, that the veins of the rectal plexuses normally appear varicose (dilated and tortuous), even in newborns, and that internal hemorrhoids occur most commonly in the absence of portal hypertension.

Regarding pain from and the treatment of hemorrhoids, it is important to note that the anal canal superior to the pectinate line is visceral; thus, it is innervated by visceral afferent pain fibers, so that an incision or needle insertion into this region is painless. Internal hemorrhoids are not painful and can be treated without anesthesia. Inferior to the pectinate line, the anal canal is somatic, supplied by the inferior anal (rectal) nerves containing somatic sensory fibers. Therefore, it is sensitive to painful stimuli (e.g., to the prick of a hypodermic needle). External hemorrhoids can be painful, but often resolve in a few days.

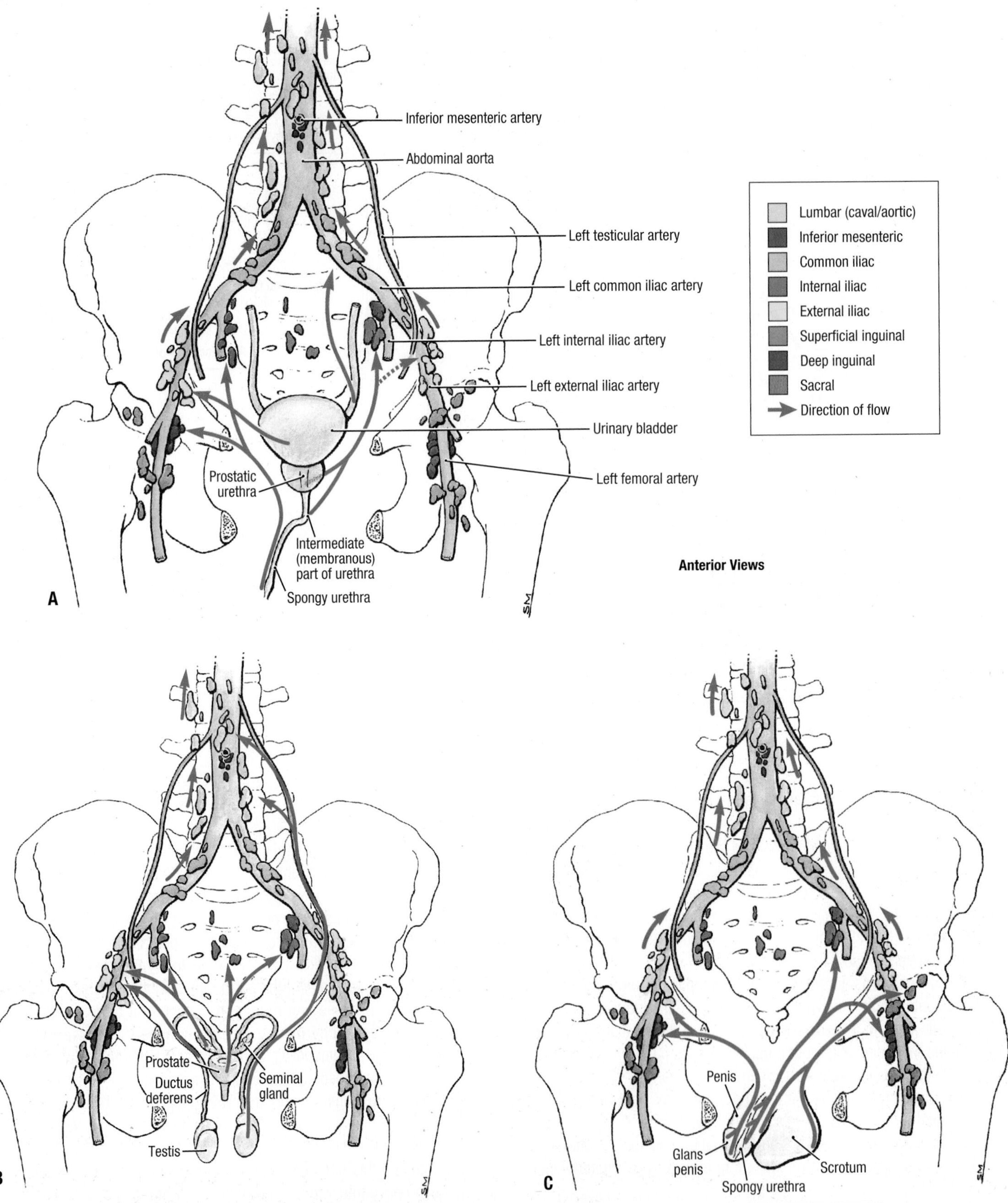

Inferior mesenteric artery
Abdominal aorta
Left testicular artery
Left common iliac artery
Left internal iliac artery
Left external iliac artery
Urinary bladder
Left femoral artery
Prostatic urethra
Intermediate (membranous) part of urethra
Spongy urethra
A
Anterior Views
Lumbar (caval/aortic)
Inferior mesenteric
Common iliac
Internal iliac
External iliac
Superficial inguinal
Deep inguinal
Sacral
Direction of flow
Prostate
Ductus deferens
Seminal gland
Testis
B
Penis
Glans penis
Spongy urethra
Scrotum
C

3.31 LYMPHATIC DRAINAGE OF MALE PELVIS AND PERINEUM

A. Pelvic urinary system. **B.** Internal genital organs. **C.** Penis, spongy urethra, scrotum and testis.

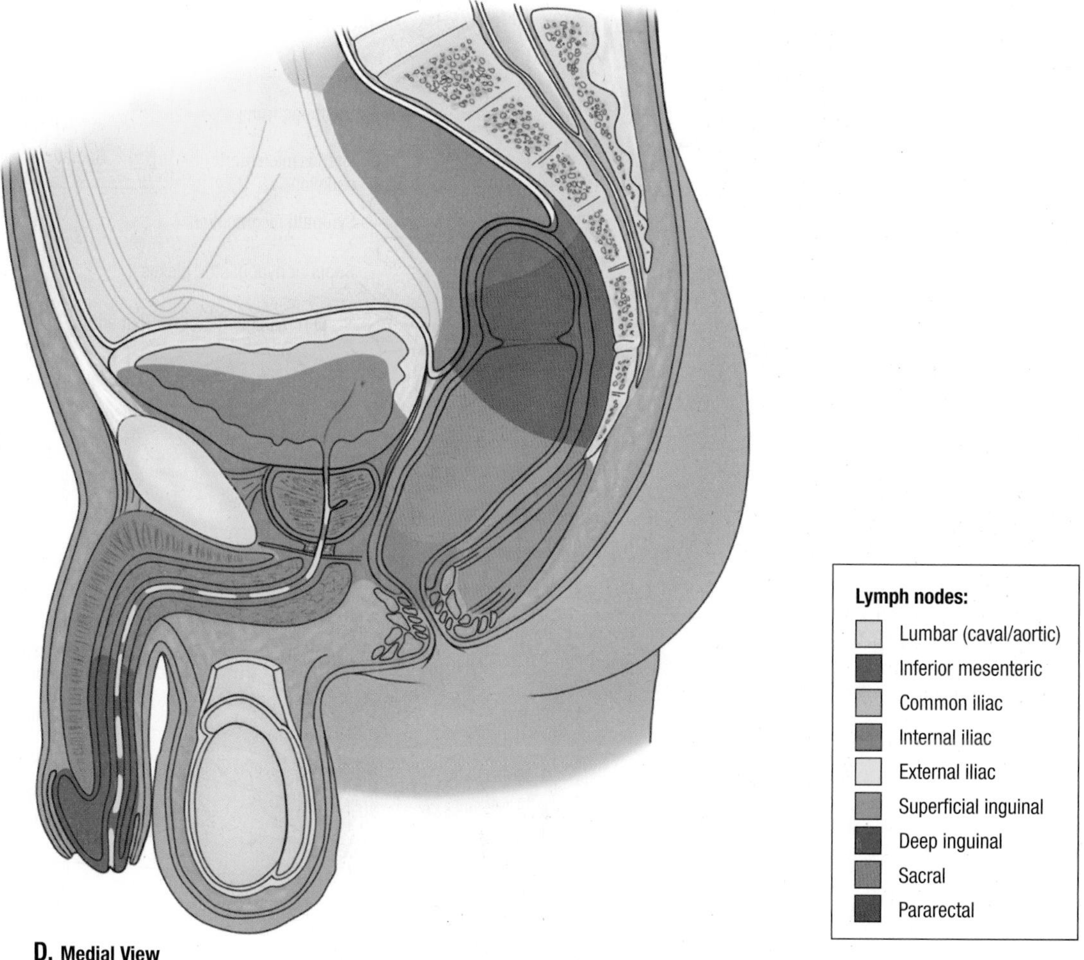
Lymph nodes:
Lumbar (caval/aortic)
Inferior mesenteric
Common iliac
Internal iliac
External iliac
Superficial inguinal
Deep inguinal
Sacral
Pararectal

D. Medial View

3.31 LYMPHATIC DRAINAGE OF MALE PELVIS AND PERINEUM *(CONTINUED)*

D. Zones of pelvis and perineum initially draining into specific groups of lymph nodes.

TABLE 3.5 LYMPHATIC DRAINAGE OF MALE PELVIS AND PERINEUM

Lymph Node Group	Structures Typically Draining to Lymph Node Group
Lumbar	Gonads and associated structures (including testicular vessels), urethra, testis, epididymis, common iliac nodes
Inferior mesenteric nodes	Superiormost rectum, sigmoid colon, descending colon, pararectal nodes
Common iliac nodes	External and internal iliac lymph nodes
Internal iliac nodes	Inferior pelvic structures, deep perineal structures, sacral nodes, prostatic urethra, prostate, base of bladder, inferior part of pelvic ureter, inferior part of seminal glands, cavernous bodies, anal canal (above pectinate line), inferior rectum
External iliac nodes	Anterosuperior pelvic structures, deep inguinal nodes, superior aspect of bladder, superior part of pelvic ureter, upper part of seminal gland, pelvic part of ductus deferens, intermediate and spongy urethra
Superficial inguinal nodes	Lower limb, superficial drainage of inferolateral quadrant of trunk, including anterior abdominal wall inferior to umbilicus, gluteal region, superficial perineal structures, skin of perineum including skin and prepuce of penis, scrotum, perianal skin, anal canal inferior to pectinate line
Deep inguinal nodes	Glans of penis, distal spongy urethra, superficial inguinal nodes
Sacral nodes	Posteroinferior pelvic structures, inferior rectum
Pararectal nodes	Superior rectum

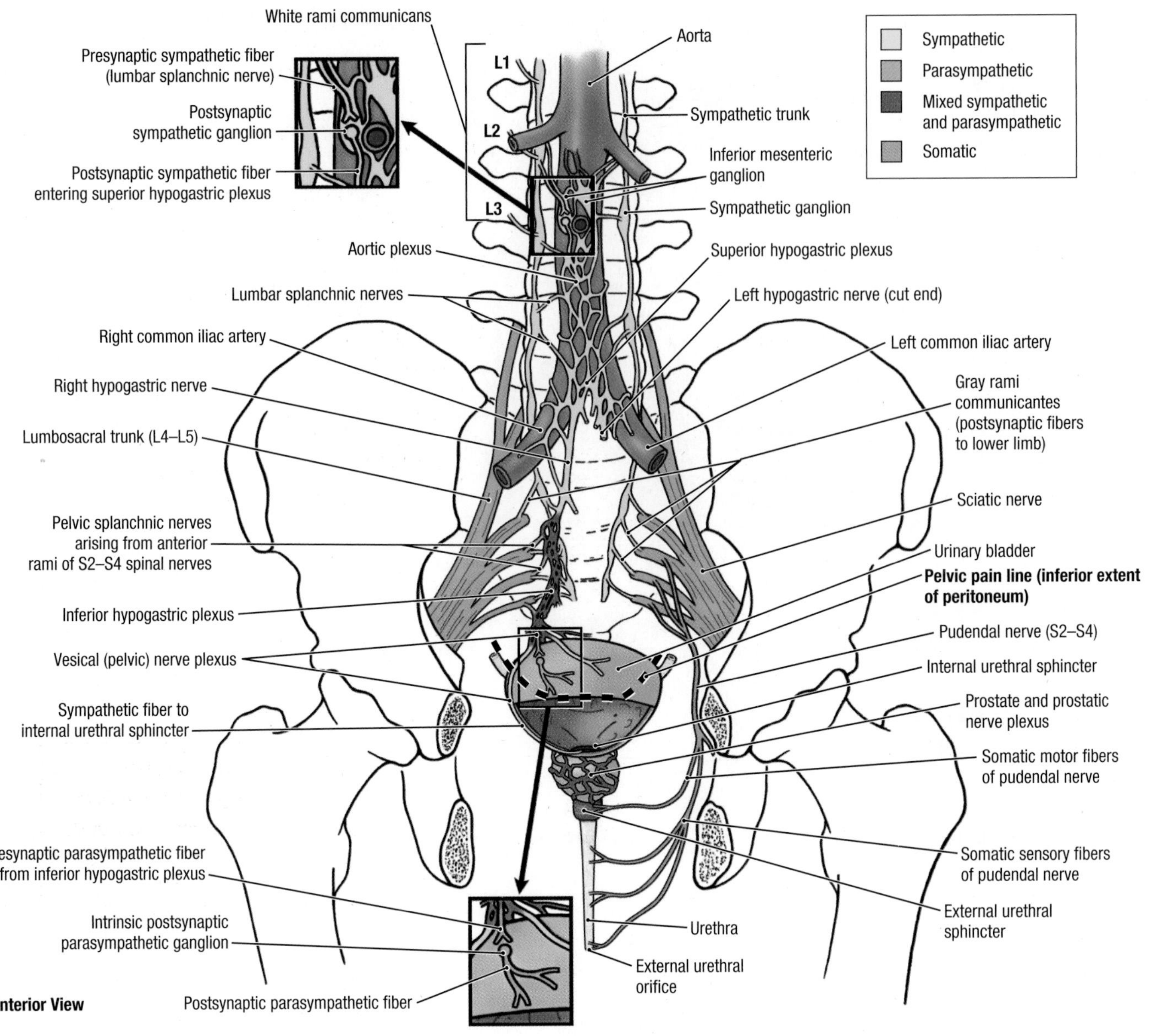

White rami communicans
Aorta
Presynaptic sympathetic fiber (lumbar splanchnic nerve)
Postsynaptic sympathetic ganglion
Postsynaptic sympathetic fiber entering superior hypogastric plexus
L1
L2
L3
Sympathetic trunk
Inferior mesenteric ganglion
Sympathetic ganglion
Sympathetic
Parasympathetic
Mixed sympathetic and parasympathetic
Somatic
Aortic plexus
Superior hypogastric plexus
Lumbar splanchnic nerves
Left hypogastric nerve (cut end)
Right common iliac artery
Left common iliac artery
Right hypogastric nerve
Gray rami communicantes (postsynaptic fibers to lower limb)
Lumbosacral trunk (L4–L5)
Sciatic nerve
Pelvic splanchnic nerves arising from anterior rami of S2–S4 spinal nerves
Urinary bladder
Pelvic pain line (inferior extent of peritoneum)
Inferior hypogastric plexus
Pudendal nerve (S2–S4)
Vesical (pelvic) nerve plexus
Internal urethral sphincter
Sympathetic fiber to internal urethral sphincter
Prostate and prostatic nerve plexus
Somatic motor fibers of pudendal nerve
Somatic sensory fibers of pudendal nerve
Presynaptic parasympathetic fiber from inferior hypogastric plexus
External urethral sphincter
Intrinsic postsynaptic parasympathetic ganglion
Urethra
External urethral orifice
Postsynaptic parasympathetic fiber

A. Anterior View

3.32 INNERVATION OF MALE PELVIS AND PERINEUM

TABLE 3.6 EFFECT OF SYMPATHETIC AND PARASYMPATHETIC STIMULATION ON URINARY TRACT, GENITAL SYSTEM, AND RECTUM

Organ, Tract, or System	Effect of Sympathetic Stimulation	Effect of Parasympathetic Stimulation
Urinary tract	Vasoconstriction of renal vessels slows urine formation; internal sphincter of male bladder contracted to prevent retrograde ejaculation and maintain urinary continence	Inhibits contraction of internal sphincter of bladder in males; contracts detrusor muscle of the bladder wall causing urination
Genital system	Causes ejaculation and vasoconstriction resulting in remission of erection	Produces engorgement (erection) of erectile tissues of the external genitals
Rectum	Maintains tonus of internal anal sphincter; inhibits peristalsis of rectum	Rectal contraction (peristalsis) for defecation; inhibition of contraction of internal anal sphincter

The parasympathetic system is restricted in its distribution to the head, neck, and body cavities (except for erectile tissues of genitalia); otherwise, parasympathetic fibers are never found in the body wall and limbs. Sympathetic fibers, by comparison, are distributed to all vascularized portions of the body.

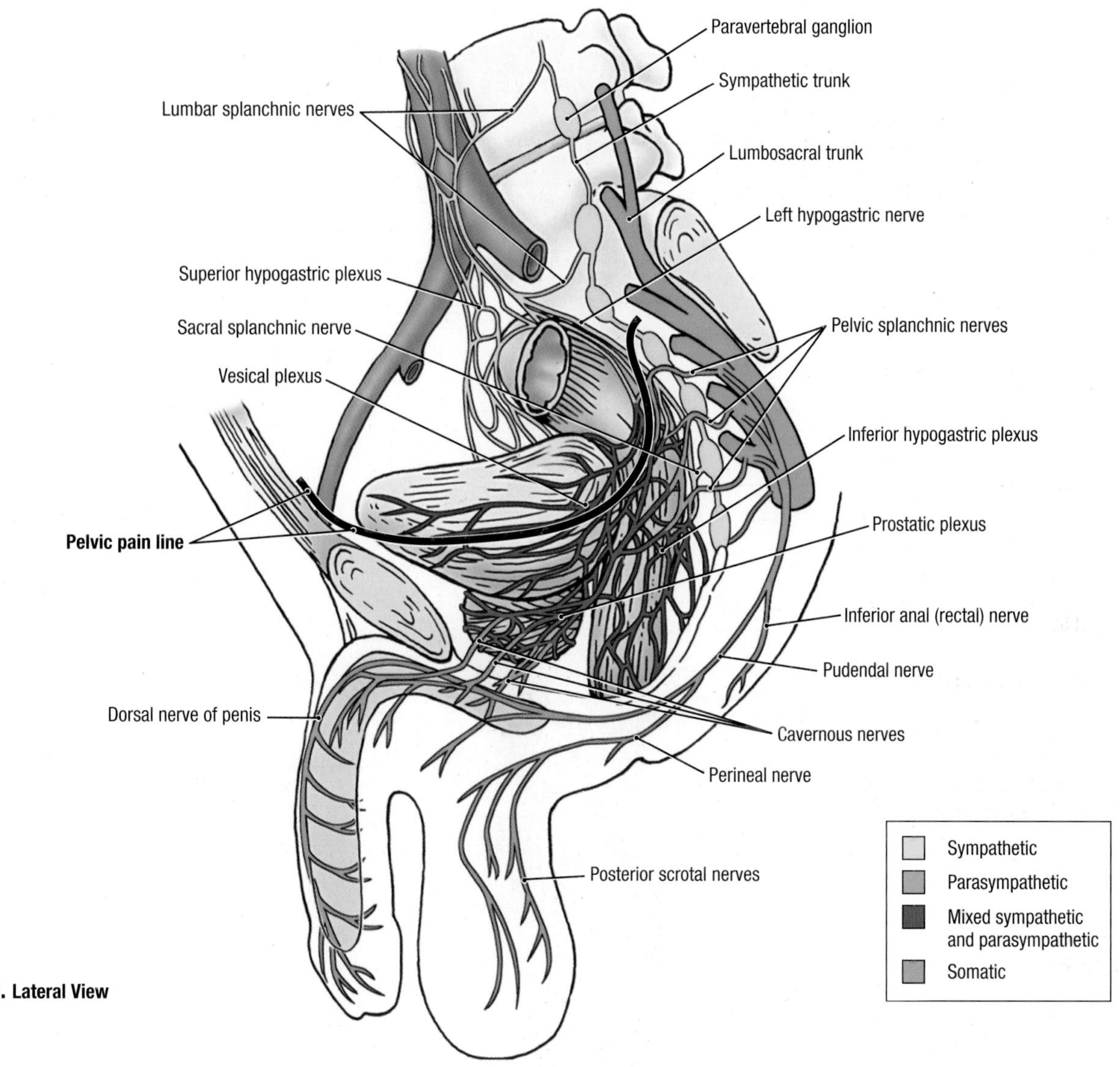
Paravertebral ganglion
Sympathetic trunk
Lumbar splanchnic nerves
Lumbosacral trunk
Left hypogastric nerve
Superior hypogastric plexus
Sacral splanchnic nerve
Pelvic splanchnic nerves
Vesical plexus
Inferior hypogastric plexus
Pelvic pain line
Prostatic plexus
Inferior anal (rectal) nerve
Pudendal nerve
Dorsal nerve of penis
Cavernous nerves
Perineal nerve
Posterior scrotal nerves
Sympathetic
Parasympathetic
Mixed sympathetic and parasympathetic
Somatic

B. Lateral View

3.32 INNERVATION OF MALE PELVIS AND PERINEUM *(CONTINUED)*

A. Overview. **B.** Innervation of prostate and external genitalia.

- The primary function of the sacral sympathetic trunks is to provide postsynaptic fibers to the sacral plexus for sympathetic innervation of the lower limb.
- The peri-arterial plexuses of the ovarian, superior rectal, and internal iliac arteries are minor routes by which sympathetic fibers enter the pelvis. Their primary function is vasomotion of the arteries they accompany.
- The hypogastric plexuses (superior and inferior) are networks of sympathetic and visceral afferent nerve fibers.
- The superior hypogastric plexus carries fibers conveyed to and from the aortic (intermesenteric) plexus by the L3 and L4 splanchnic nerves. The superior hypogastric plexus divides into right and left hypogastric nerves that merge with the parasympathetic pelvic splanchnic nerves to form the inferior hypogastric plexuses.
- The fibers of the inferior hypogastric plexuses continue to the pelvic viscera upon which they form pelvic plexuses, e.g., prostatic nerve plexus.
- The pelvic splanchnic nerves convey presynaptic parasympathetic fibers from the S2–S4 spinal cord segments, which make up the sacral outflow of the parasympathetic system.
- Visceral afferents conveying unconscious reflex sensation follow the course of the parasympathetic fibers retrogradely to the spinal sensory ganglia of S2–S4, as do those transmitting pain sensations from the viscera inferior to the pelvic pain line (structures that do not contact the peritoneum plus the distal sigmoid colon and rectum). Visceral afferent fibers conducting pain from structures superior to the pelvic pain line (structures in contact with the peritoneum, except for the distal sigmoid colon and rectum) follow the sympathetic fibers retrogradely to inferior thoracic and superior lumbar spinal ganglia.

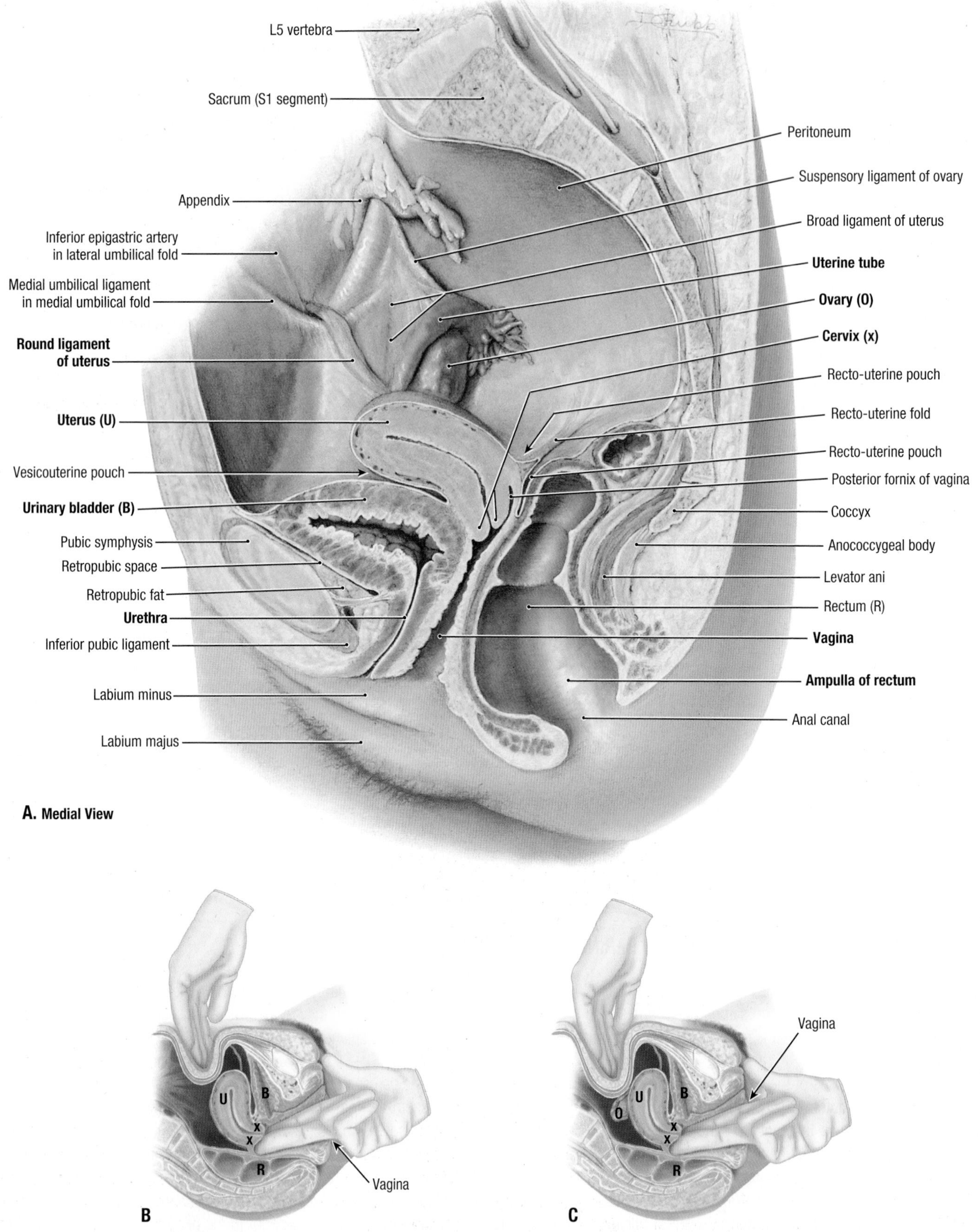

L5 vertebra
Sacrum (S1 segment)
Peritoneum
Suspensory ligament of ovary
Broad ligament of uterus
Uterine tube
Ovary (O)
Cervix (x)
Recto-uterine pouch
Recto-uterine fold
Recto-uterine pouch
Posterior fornix of vagina
Coccyx
Anococcygeal body
Levator ani
Rectum (R)
Vagina
Ampulla of rectum
Anal canal
Appendix
Inferior epigastric artery in lateral umbilical fold
Medial umbilical ligament in medial umbilical fold
Round ligament of uterus
Uterus (U)
Vesicouterine pouch
Urinary bladder (B)
Pubic symphysis
Retropubic space
Retropubic fat
Urethra
Inferior pubic ligament
Labium minus
Labium majus
U
B
x
x
R
Vagina
O
U
B
x
x
R
Vagina

A. **Medial View**

B

C

3.33 FEMALE PELVIC ORGANS IN SITU

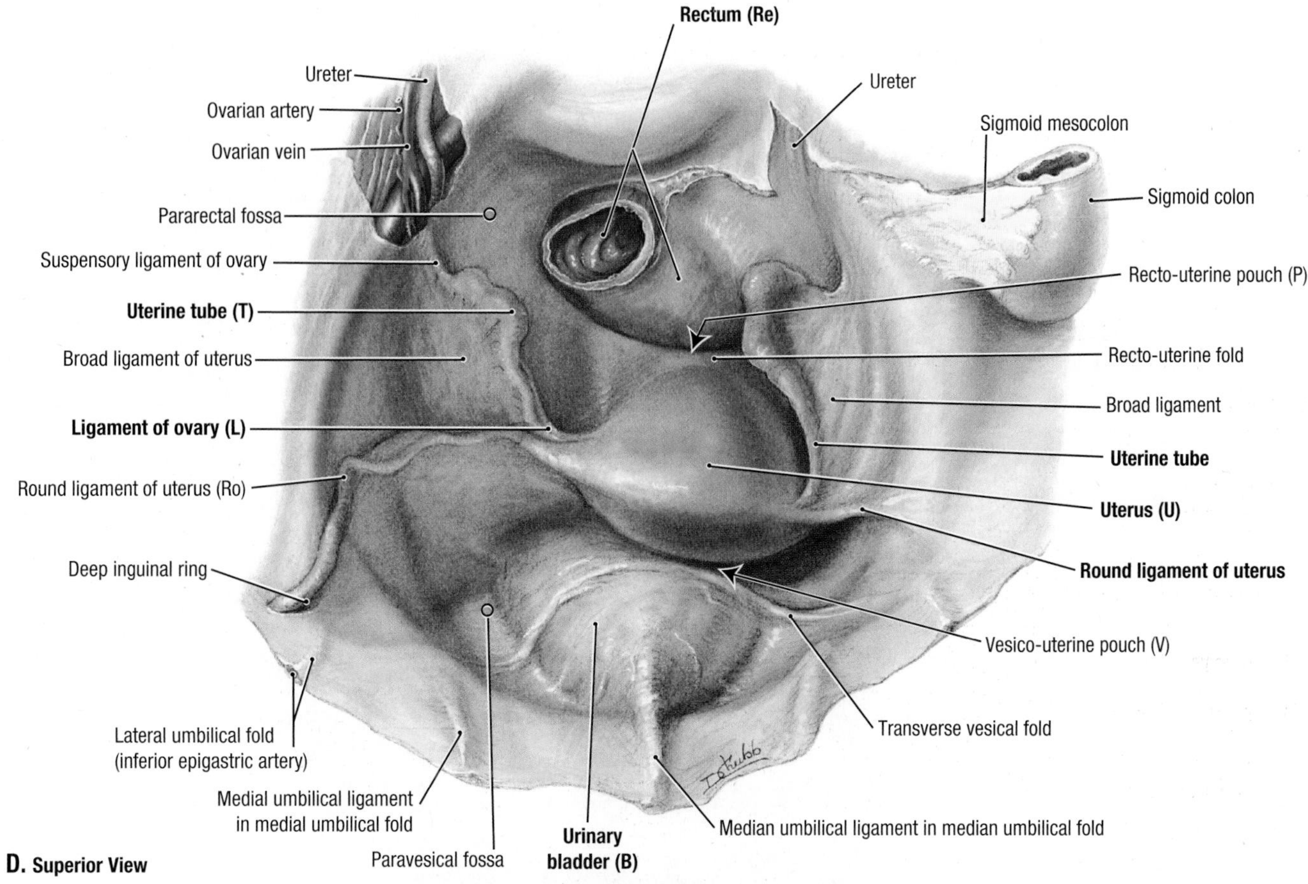
Rectum (Re)
Ureter
Ovarian artery
Ovarian vein
Ureter
Sigmoid mesocolon
Sigmoid colon
Pararectal fossa
Suspensory ligament of ovary
Recto-uterine pouch (P)
Uterine tube (T)
Broad ligament of uterus
Recto-uterine fold
Broad ligament
Ligament of ovary (L)
Uterine tube
Round ligament of uterus (Ro)
Uterus (U)
Deep inguinal ring
Round ligament of uterus
Vesico-uterine pouch (V)
Transverse vesical fold
Lateral umbilical fold
(inferior epigastric artery)
Medial umbilical ligament
in medial umbilical fold
Median umbilical ligament in median umbilical fold
Paravesical fossa
Urinary
bladder (B)

D. Superior View

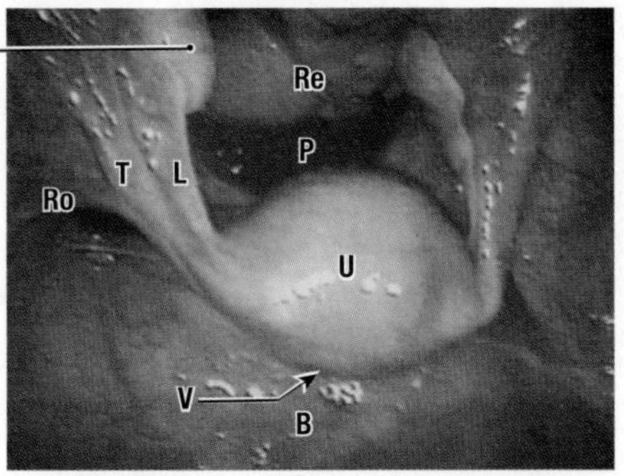
Ovary
(not seen in A
as it lies on the
posterior aspect
of the broad ligament)
Re
P
T
L
Ro
U
V
B

E. Laparoscopic View of Normal Female Pelvis

3.33 FEMALE PELVIC ORGANS IN SITU *(CONTINUED)*

A. Median section. The adult uterus is typically *anteverted* (tipped antereosuperiorly relative to the axis of the vagina) and *anteflexed* (flexed or bent anteriorly relative to the cervix, creating the *angle of flexion*) so that its mass lies over the bladder. The cervix, opening on the anterior wall of the vagina, has a short, round, anterior lip and a long, thin, posterior lip. **B. Bimanual palpation of uterus. C. Bimanual palpation of uterine adnexa** (e.g., ovaries). **D.** True pelvis with peritoneum intact, viewed from above. The uterus is usually asymmetrically placed. The round ligament of the female takes the same subperitoneal course as the ductus deferens of the male.

E. Laparoscopy involves inserting a laparoscope into the peritoneal cavity through a small incision below the umbilicus. Insufflation of inert gas creates a pneumoperitoneum to provide space to visualize the pelvic organs. Additional openings (ports) can be made to introduce other instruments for manipulation or to enable therapeutic procedures (e.g., ligation of the uterine tubes).

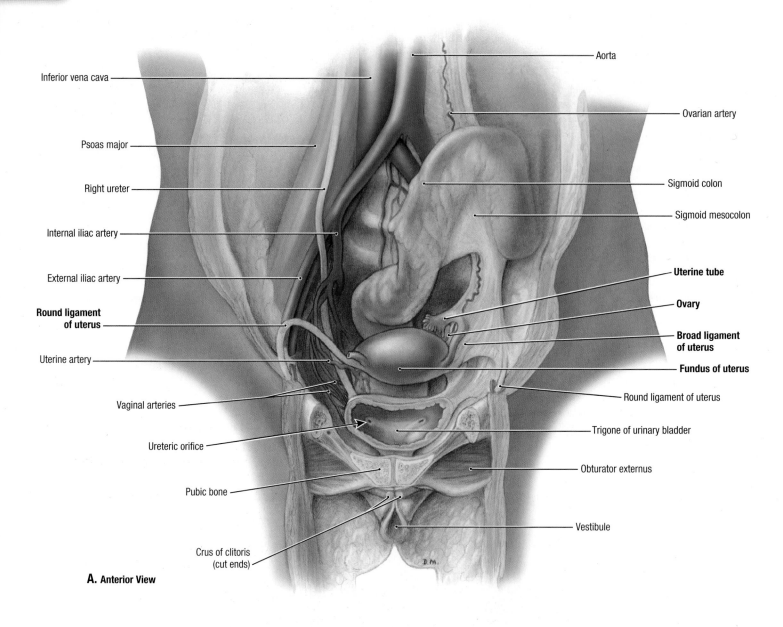

Aorta
Inferior vena cava
Ovarian artery
Psoas major
Sigmoid colon
Right ureter
Sigmoid mesocolon
Internal iliac artery
External iliac artery
Uterine tube
Ovary
Round ligament of uterus
Broad ligament of uterus
Uterine artery
Fundus of uterus
Round ligament of uterus
Vaginal arteries
Trigone of urinary bladder
Ureteric orifice
Obturator externus
Pubic bone
Vestibule
Crus of clitoris (cut ends)

A. Anterior View

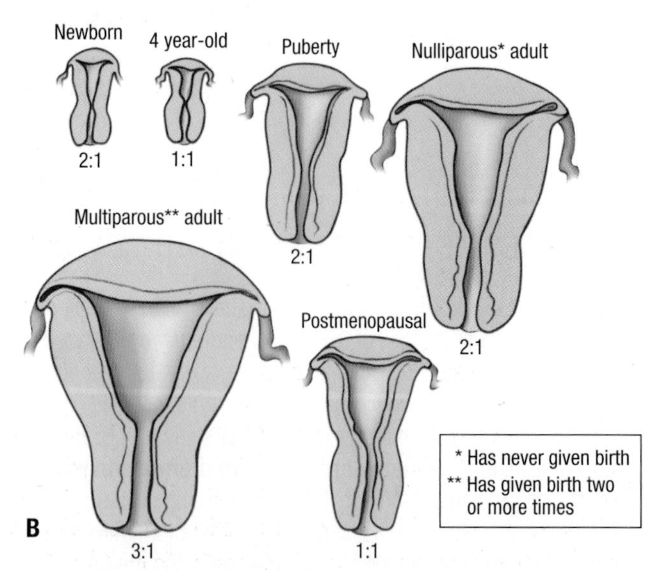

Newborn
2:1
4 year-old
1:1
Puberty
2:1
Nulliparous* adult
2:1
Multiparous** adult
3:1
Postmenopausal
1:1
* Has never given birth
** Has given birth two or more times
B

3.34 FEMALE GENITAL ORGANS

A. Dissection. Part of the pubic bones, the anterior aspect of the bladder, and—on the specimen's right side—the uterine tube, ovary, broad ligament, and peritoneum covering the lateral wall of the pelvis have been removed. **B. Lifetime changes in uterine size and proportion** (body to cervical ratio, e.g., 2:1). All these stages represent normal anatomy for the particular age and reproductive status of the woman.

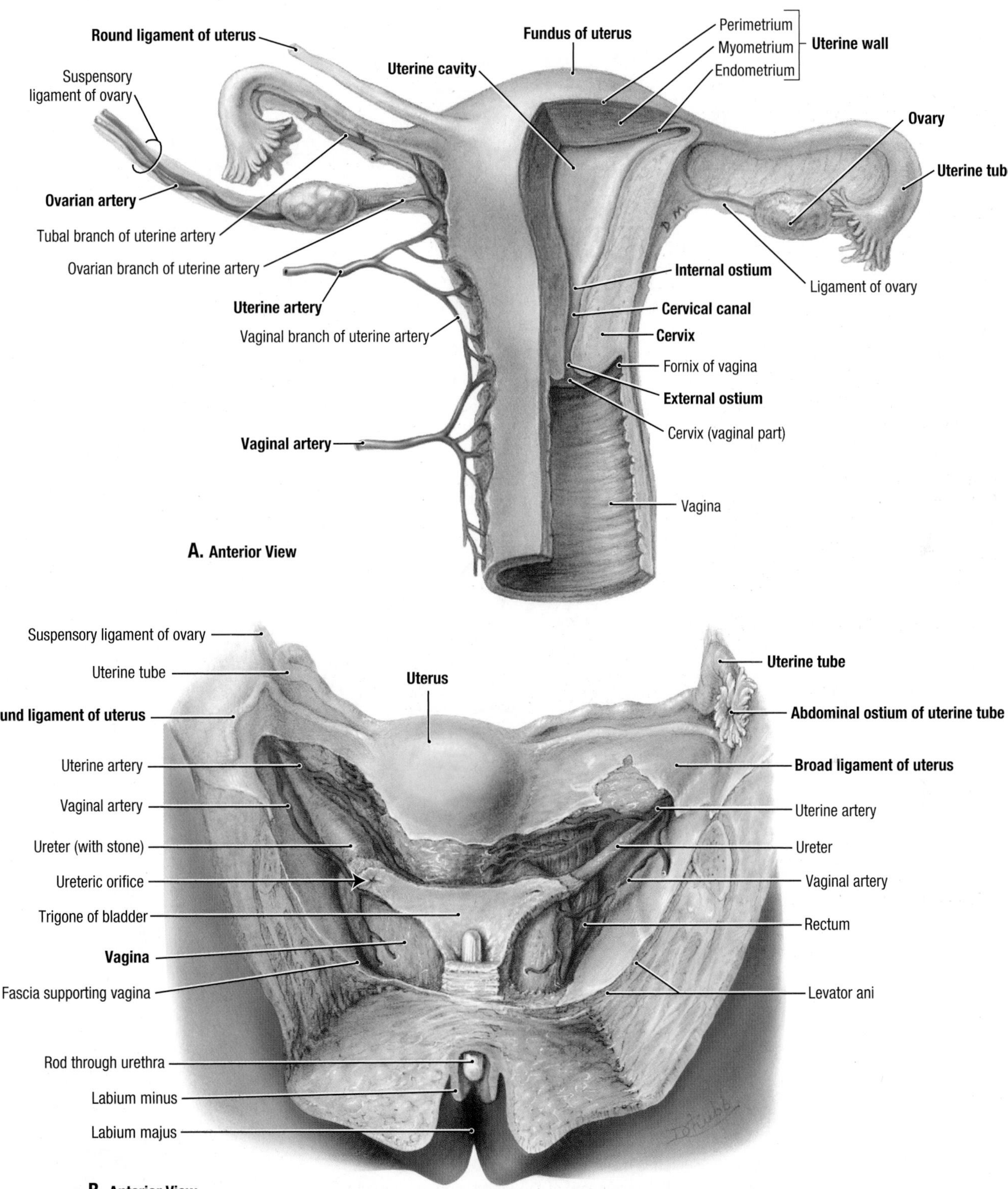
Round ligament of uterus
Suspensory ligament of ovary
Ovarian artery
Tubal branch of uterine artery
Ovarian branch of uterine artery
Uterine artery
Vaginal branch of uterine artery
Vaginal artery
Uterine cavity
Fundus of uterus
Perimetrium
Myometrium
Endometrium
Uterine wall
Ovary
Uterine tube
Ligament of ovary
Internal ostium
Cervical canal
Cervix
Fornix of vagina
External ostium
Cervix (vaginal part)
Vagina
A. Anterior View
Suspensory ligament of ovary
Uterine tube
Round ligament of uterus
Uterine artery
Vaginal artery
Ureter (with stone)
Ureteric orifice
Trigone of bladder
Vagina
Fascia supporting vagina
Rod through urethra
Labium minus
Labium majus
Uterus
Uterine tube
Abdominal ostium of uterine tube
Broad ligament of uterus
Uterine artery
Ureter
Vaginal artery
Rectum
Levator ani
B. Anterior View

3.35 UTERUS AND ITS ADNEXA

A. Blood supply. On the specimen's left side, part of the uterine wall with the round ligament and the vaginal wall have been cut away to expose the cervix, uterine cavity, and thick muscular wall of the uterus, the myometrium. On the specimen's right side, the ovarian artery (from the aorta) and uterine artery (from the internal iliac) supply the ovary, uterine tube, and uterus and anastomose in the broad ligament along the lateral aspect of the uterus. The uterine artery sends a uterine branch to supply the uterine body and fundus and a vaginal branch to supply the cervix and vagina. **B.** Uterus and broad ligament. The pubic bones and bladder, trigone excepted, are removed, as a continued dissection from Figure 3.34.

Uterine tube
Mesosalpinx
Ovarian artery and veins
Ligament of ovary
Suspensory ligament of ovary
Mesovarium
Uterus
Ovary
Round ligament of uterus
Broad ligament
Medial cut in B
Lateral cut in B

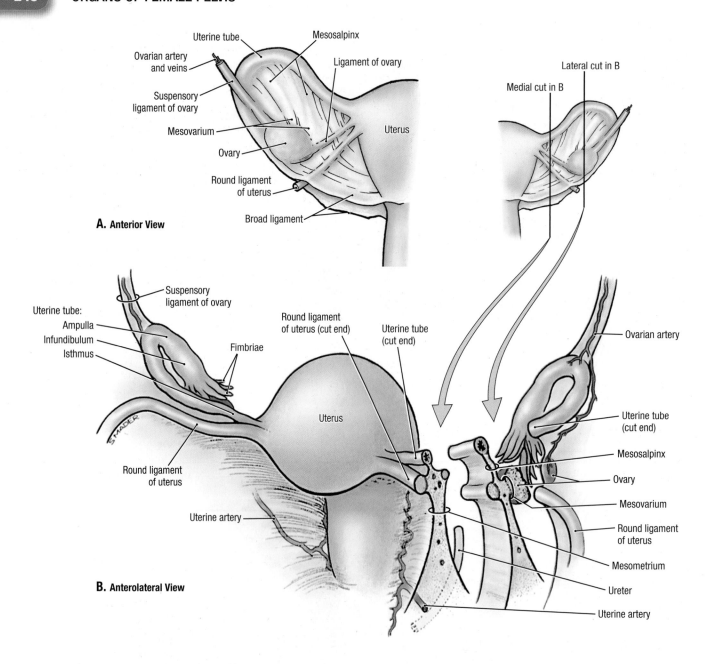

A. Anterior View

Suspensory ligament of ovary
Uterine tube:
Ampulla
Infundibulum
Isthmus
Fimbriae
Round ligament of uterus (cut end)
Uterine tube (cut end)
Uterus
Round ligament of uterus
Uterine artery
Ovarian artery
Uterine tube (cut end)
Mesosalpinx
Ovary
Mesovarium
Round ligament of uterus
Mesometrium
Ureter
Uterine artery

B. Anterolateral View

3.36 UTERUS AND BROAD LIGAMENT

A. and B. Two paramedian sections show "mesenteries" with the prefix meso-. "Salpinx" is the Greek word for trumpet or tube, "metro" for uterus. The mesentery of the uterus and uterine tube is called the broad ligament. The major part of the broad ligament, the *mesometrium*, is attached to the uterus. The ovary is attached to the broad ligament by a mesentery of its own, called the *mesovarium*; to the uterus by the ligament of the ovary; and near the pelvic brim, by the suspensory ligament of the ovary containing the ovarian vessels. The part of the broad ligament superior to the level of the mesovarium is called the *mesosalpinx*. **C. Hysterectomy** (excision of the uterus) is performed through the lower anterior abdominal wall or through the vagina. Because the uterine artery crosses superior to the ureter near the lateral fornix of the vagina, the ureter is in danger of being inadvertently clamped or severed when the uterine artery is tied off during a hysterectomy.

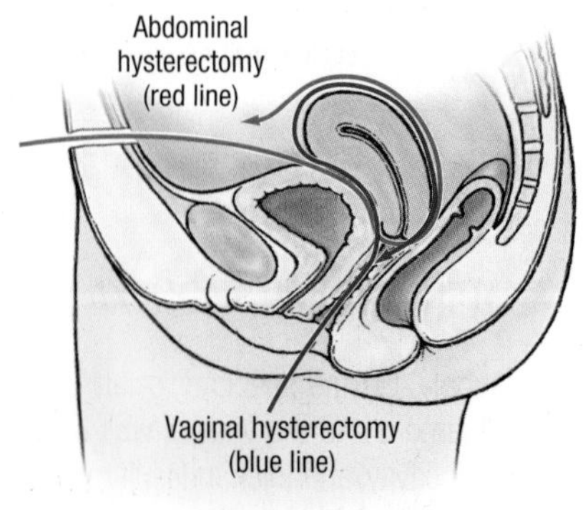
Abdominal hysterectomy (red line)
Vaginal hysterectomy (blue line)

C. Medial View

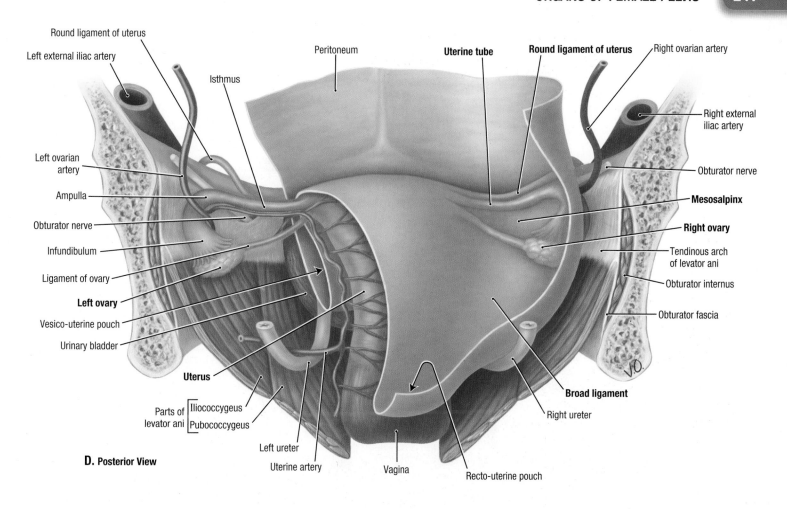

Round ligament of uterus
Left external iliac artery
Peritoneum
Uterine tube
Round ligament of uterus
Right ovarian artery
Isthmus
Right external iliac artery
Left ovarian artery
Obturator nerve
Ampulla
Mesosalpinx
Obturator nerve
Right ovary
Infundibulum
Tendinous arch of levator ani
Ligament of ovary
Obturator internus
Left ovary
Obturator fascia
Vesico-uterine pouch
Urinary bladder
Uterus
Broad ligament
Parts of levator ani
Iliococcygeus
Pubococcygeus
Right ureter
Left ureter
Uterine artery
Vagina
Recto-uterine pouch
V.O.

D. Posterior View

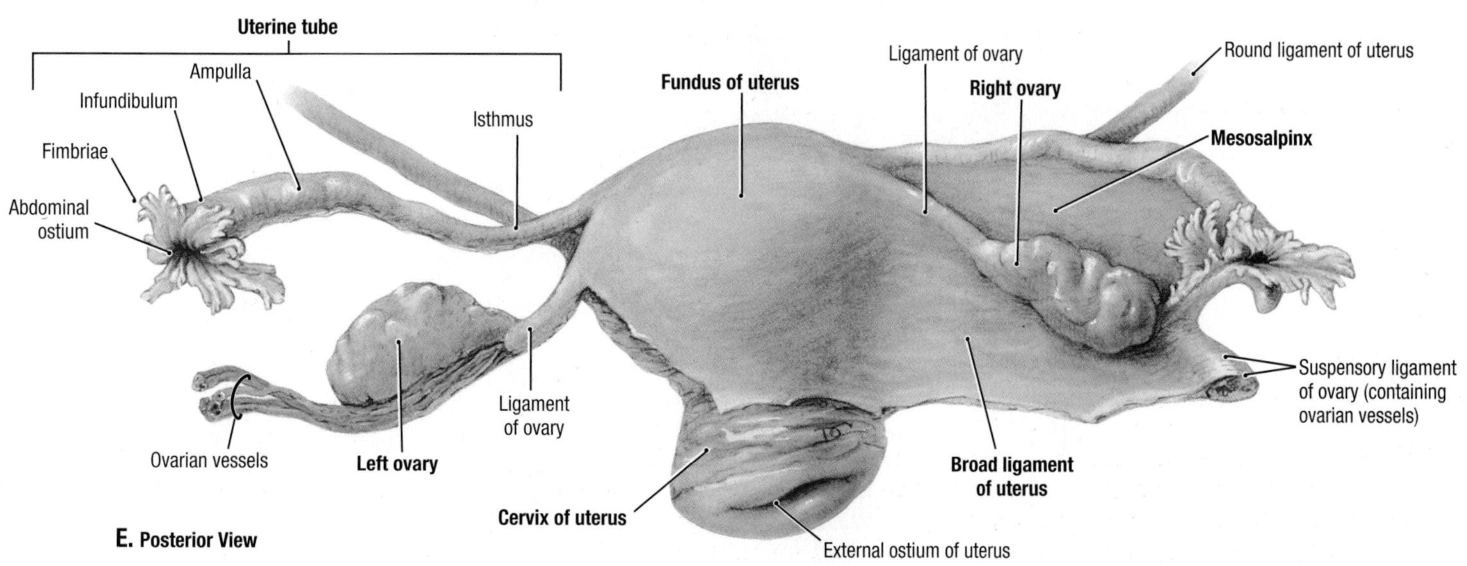
Uterine tube
Ampulla
Infundibulum
Fimbriae
Abdominal ostium
Isthmus
Fundus of uterus
Ligament of ovary
Right ovary
Round ligament of uterus
Mesosalpinx
Suspensory ligament of ovary (containing ovarian vessels)
Ligament of ovary
Ovarian vessels
Left ovary
Broad ligament of uterus
Cervix of uterus
External ostium of uterus

E. Posterior View

3.36 UTERUS AND BROAD LIGAMENT *(CONTINUED)*

D. Uterus in situ. **E.** Uterus and adnexa, removed from cadaver.

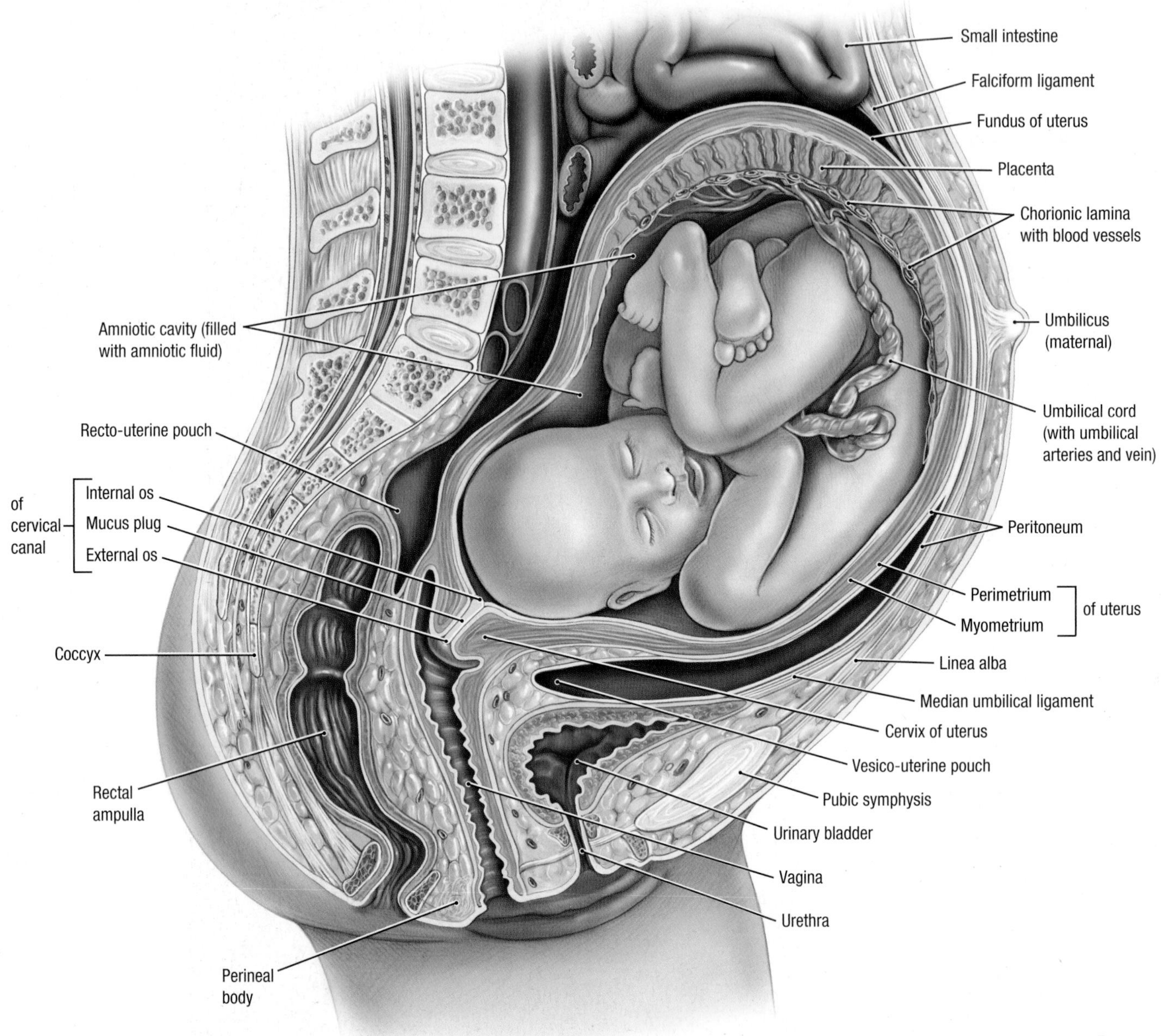
Small intestine
Falciform ligament
Fundus of uterus
Placenta
Chorionic lamina
with blood vessels
Amniotic cavity (filled
with amniotic fluid)
Umbilicus
(maternal)
Umbilical cord
(with umbilical
arteries and vein)
Recto-uterine pouch
of
cervical
canal
Internal os
Mucus plug
External os
Peritoneum
Perimetrium
Myometrium
of uterus
Coccyx
Linea alba
Median umbilical ligament
Cervix of uterus
Vesico-uterine pouch
Pubic symphysis
Rectal
ampulla
Urinary bladder
Vagina
Urethra
Perineal
body
A

3.37 PREGNANT UTERUS

A. Median section; fetus is intact.

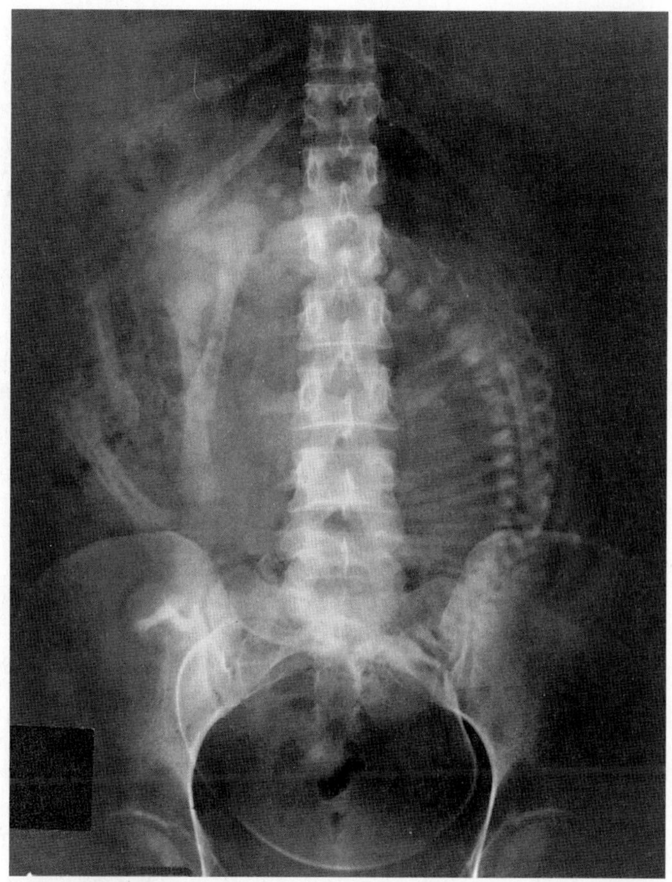

B. **Anteroposterior View**

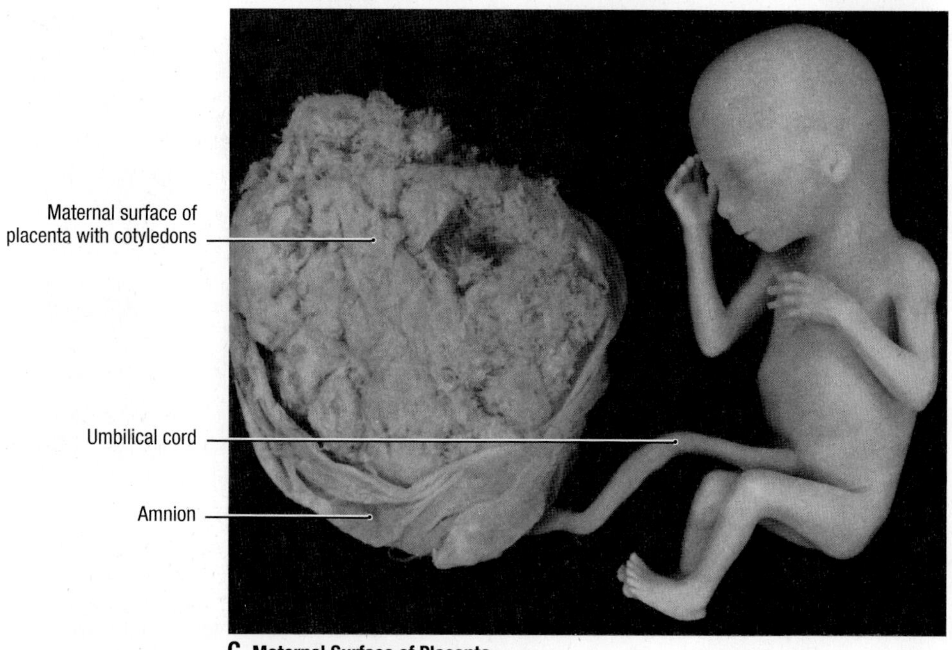
Maternal surface of placenta with cotyledons
Umbilical cord
Amnion

C. **Maternal Surface of Placenta**

3.37 PREGNANT UTERUS *(CONTINUED)*

B. Radiograph of fetus. **C.** Photograph of an 18-week-old fetus connected to the placenta by the umbilical cord.

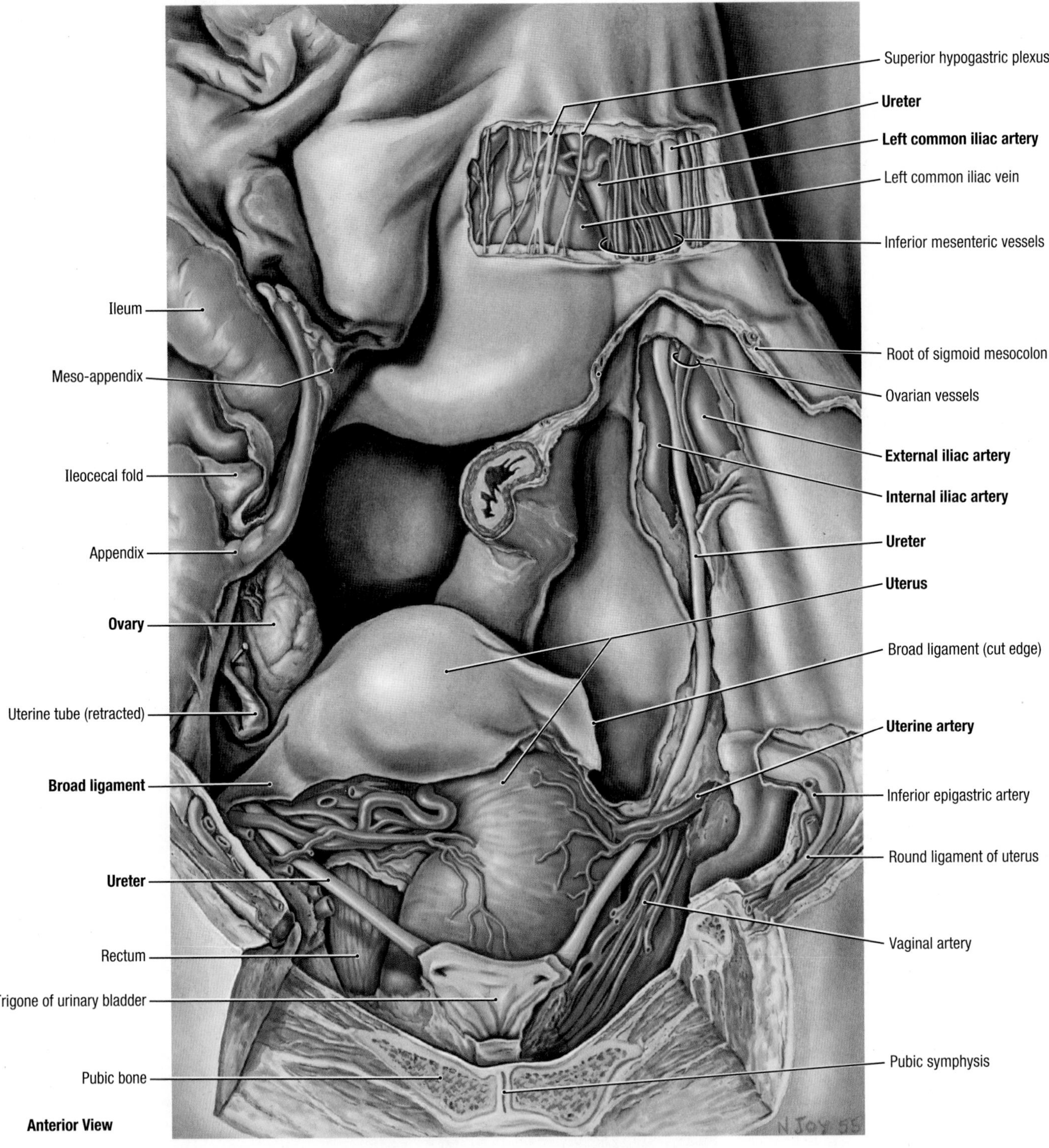
Superior hypogastric plexus
Ureter
Left common iliac artery
Left common iliac vein
Inferior mesenteric vessels
Ileum
Meso-appendix
Root of sigmoid mesocolon
Ovarian vessels
External iliac artery
Ileocecal fold
Internal iliac artery
Appendix
Ureter
Uterus
Ovary
Broad ligament (cut edge)
Uterine tube (retracted)
Uterine artery
Broad ligament
Inferior epigastric artery
Round ligament of uterus
Ureter
Vaginal artery
Rectum
Trigone of urinary bladder
Pubic symphysis
Pubic bone
Anterior View
N. JOY 55

3.38 URETER AND RELATIONSHIP TO UTERINE ARTERY

- Most of the pubic symphysis and most of the bladder (except the trigone) have been removed as in Figure 3.34B.
- The left ureter is crossed by the ovarian vessels and nerves; the apex of the inverted V-shaped root of the sigmoid mesocolon is situated anterior to the left ureter.
- The left ureter crosses the external iliac artery at the bifurcation of the common iliac artery and then descends anterior to the internal iliac artery; its course is subperitoneal from where it enters the pelvis to where it passes deep to the broad ligament and is crossed by the uterine artery. **Injury of the ureter** may occur in this region when the uterine artery is ligated and cut during hysterectomy.

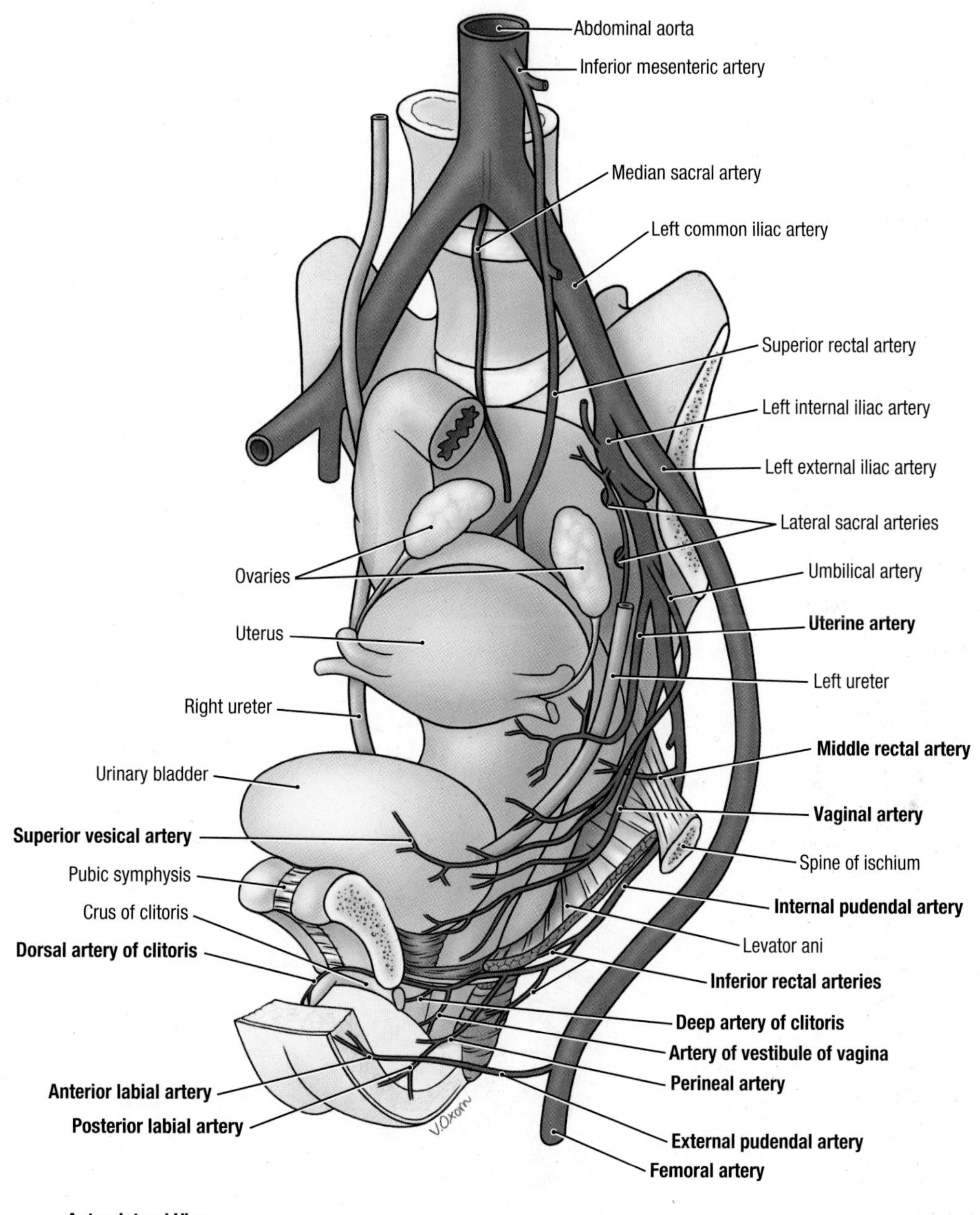
Abdominal aorta
Inferior mesenteric artery
Median sacral artery
Left common iliac artery
Superior rectal artery
Left internal iliac artery
Left external iliac artery
Lateral sacral arteries
Umbilical artery
Uterine artery
Left ureter
Middle rectal artery
Vaginal artery
Spine of ischium
Internal pudendal artery
Levator ani
Inferior rectal arteries
Deep artery of clitoris
Artery of vestibule of vagina
Perineal artery
External pudendal artery
Femoral artery
Ovaries
Uterus
Right ureter
Urinary bladder
Superior vesical artery
Pubic symphysis
Crus of clitoris
Dorsal artery of clitoris
Anterior labial artery
Posterior labial artery
V.Oxorn
Anterolateral View

3.39 ARTERIAL SUPPLY OF FEMALE PELVIS AND PERINEUM

- The blood supply of the uterus is mainly from the *uterine arteries*, with potential collateral supply from the ovarian arteries.
- The arteries supplying the superior part of the vagina derive from the *uterine arteries*; the arteries supplying the middle and inferior parts of the vagina derive from the *vaginal* and *internal pudendal arteries*.
- The superior vesical arteries supply the anterosuperior parts of the bladder; the vaginal arteries supply the postero-inferior parts of the bladder.

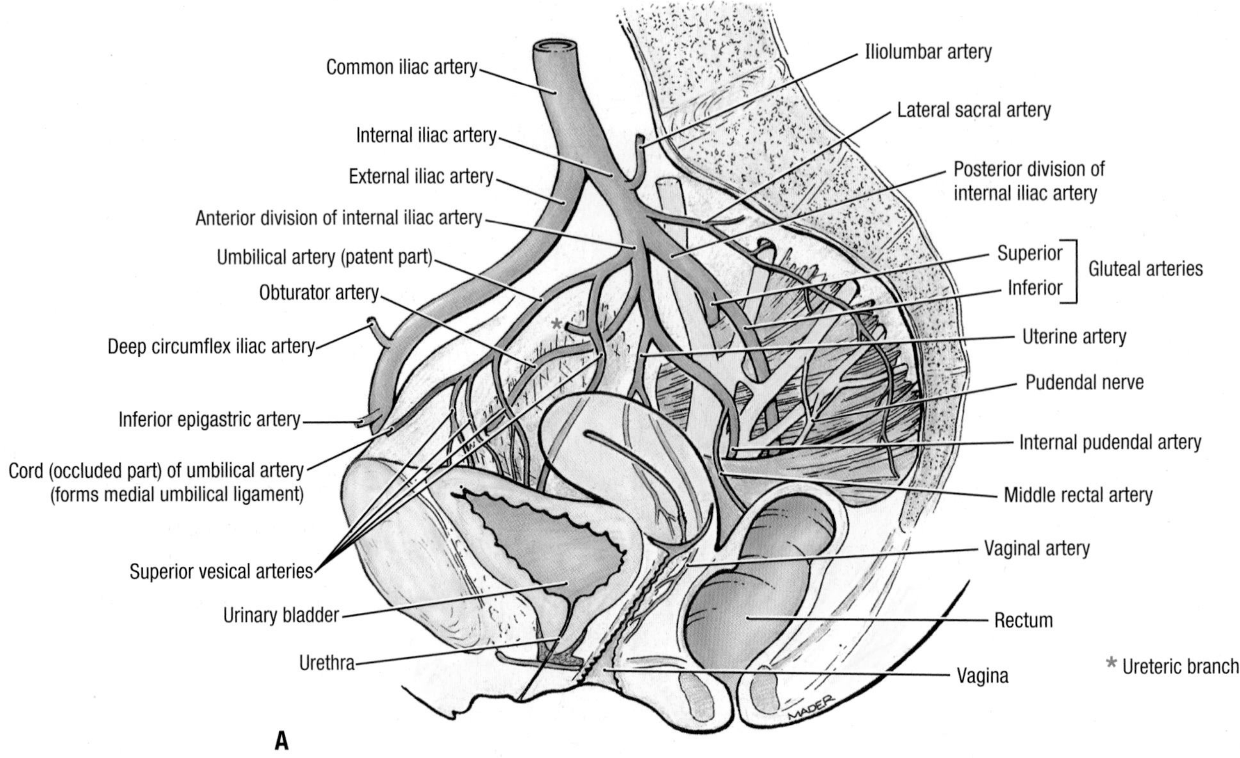
Common iliac artery
Internal iliac artery
External iliac artery
Anterior division of internal iliac artery
Umbilical artery (patent part)
Obturator artery
Deep circumflex iliac artery
Inferior epigastric artery
Cord (occluded part) of umbilical artery
(forms medial umbilical ligament)
Superior vesical arteries
Urinary bladder
Urethra
Iliolumbar artery
Lateral sacral artery
Posterior division of
internal iliac artery
Superior
Inferior
Gluteal arteries
Uterine artery
Pudendal nerve
Internal pudendal artery
Middle rectal artery
Vaginal artery
Rectum
Vagina
* Ureteric branch
A

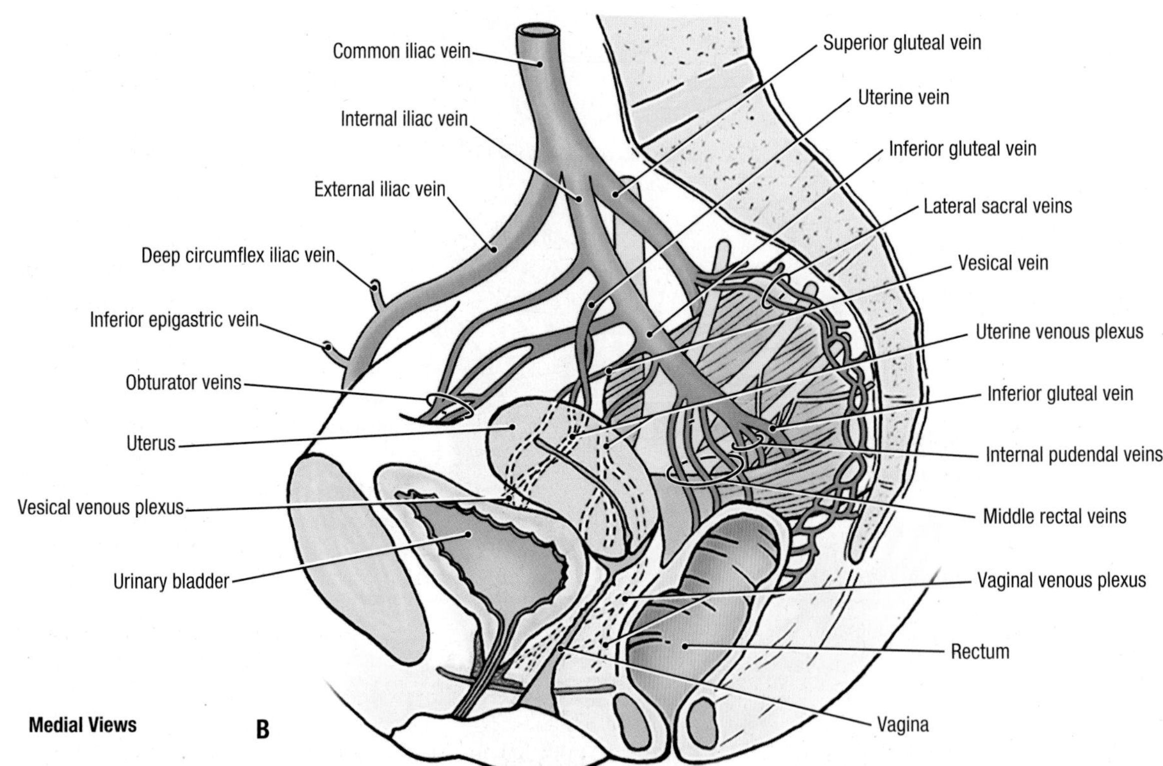
Common iliac vein
Internal iliac vein
External iliac vein
Deep circumflex iliac vein
Inferior epigastric vein
Obturator veins
Uterus
Vesical venous plexus
Urinary bladder
Superior gluteal vein
Uterine vein
Inferior gluteal vein
Lateral sacral veins
Vesical vein
Uterine venous plexus
Inferior gluteal vein
Internal pudendal veins
Middle rectal veins
Vaginal venous plexus
Rectum
Vagina
Medial Views
B

3.40 ARTERIES AND VEINS OF FEMALE PELVIS

A. Arteries in situ. **B.** Pelvic veins and venous plexuses. **C.** Arteries isolated from **A**.

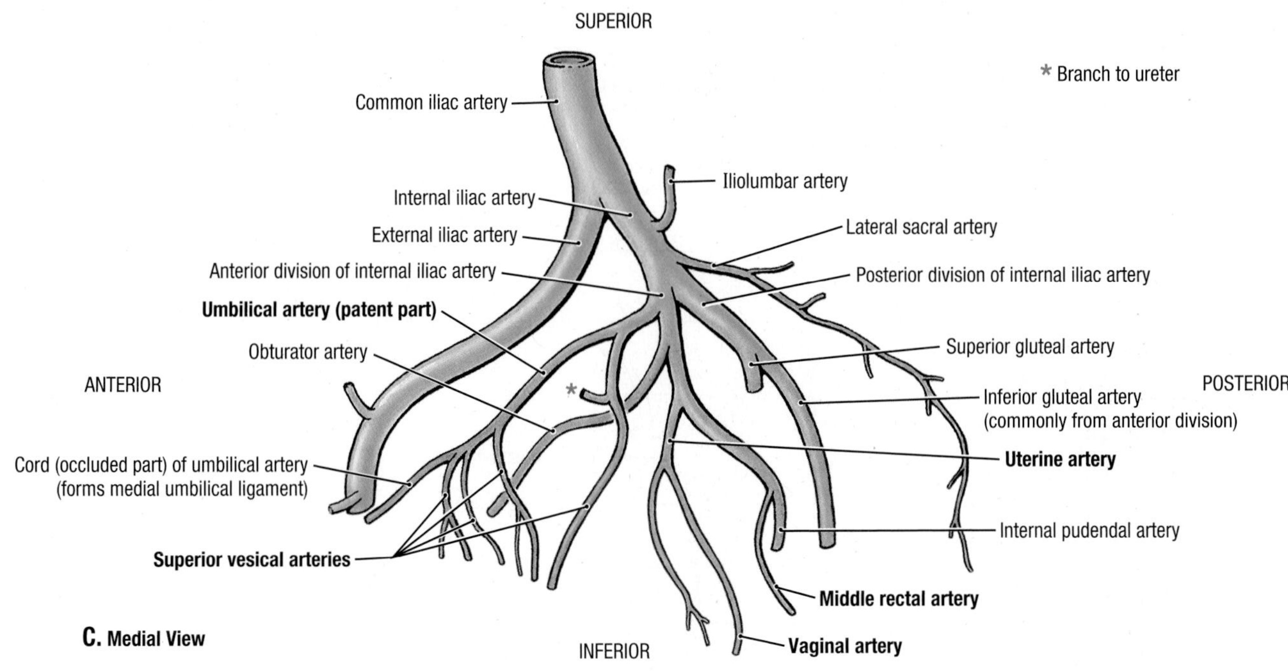
SUPERIOR
* Branch to ureter
Common iliac artery
Iliolumbar artery
Internal iliac artery
External iliac artery
Lateral sacral artery
Anterior division of internal iliac artery
Posterior division of internal iliac artery
Umbilical artery (patent part)
Obturator artery
Superior gluteal artery
ANTERIOR
POSTERIOR
Inferior gluteal artery
(commonly from anterior division)
Cord (occluded part) of umbilical artery
(forms medial umbilical ligament)
Uterine artery
Internal pudendal artery
Superior vesical arteries
Middle rectal artery
INFERIOR
Vaginal artery

C. Medial View

3.40 ARTERIES AND VEINS OF FEMALE PELVIS *(CONTINUED)*

TABLE 3.7 ARTERIES OF FEMALE PELVIS

Artery	Origin	Course	Distribution
Internal iliac	Common iliac artery	Passes over pelvic brim and descends into pelvic cavity	Main blood supply to pelvic organs, gluteal muscles, and perineum
Anterior division of internal iliac artery	Internal iliac artery	Passes anteriorly along lateral wall of pelvis, dividing into visceral, obturator, and internal iliac arteries	Pelvic viscera and muscles of superior medial thigh and perineum
Umbilical	Anterior division of internal iliac artery	Short pelvic course, gives off superior vesical arteries	Superior aspect of urinary bladder
Superior vesical artery	Patent proximal part of umbilical artery	Usually multiple, pass to superior aspect of urinary bladder	Superior aspect of urinary bladder
Obturator	Anterior division of internal iliac artery	Runs antero-inferiorly on lateral pelvic wall	Pelvic muscles, nutrient artery to ilium, head of femur, and muscles of medial compartment of thigh
Uterine		Runs anteromedially in base of broad ligament/superior cardinal ligament; gives rise to vaginal branch, then crosses ureter superiorly to reach lateral aspect of uterine cervix	Uterus, ligaments of uterus, medial parts of uterine tube and ovary, and superior vagina
Vaginal		Divides into vaginal and inferior vesical branches	Vaginal branch: lower vagina, vestibular bulb, and adjacent rectum; inferior vesical branch: fundus of urinary bladder
Middle rectal		Descends in pelvis to inferior part of rectum	Inferior part of rectum
Internal pudendal		Exits pelvis via greater sciatic foramen and enters perineum (ischio-anal fossa) via lesser sciatic foramen	Main artery to perineum including muscles of anal canal and perineum, skin and urogenital triangle and erectile bodies
Posterior division of internal iliac artery	Internal iliac artery	Passes posteriorly and gives rise to parietal branches	Pelvic wall and gluteal region
Iliolumbar	Posterior division of internal iliac artery	Ascends anterior to sacro-iliac joint and posterior to common iliac vessels and psoas major	Iliacus, psoas major, quadratus lumborum muscles, and cauda equina in vertebral canal
Lateral sacral (superior and inferior)		Run on anteromedial aspect of piriformis	Piriformis muscle, structures in sacral canal, and erector spinae muscles
Ovarian	Abdominal aorta	Crosses pelvic brim and descends in suspensory ligament to ovary	Abdominal and/or pelvic ureter, ovary, and ampullary end of uterine tube

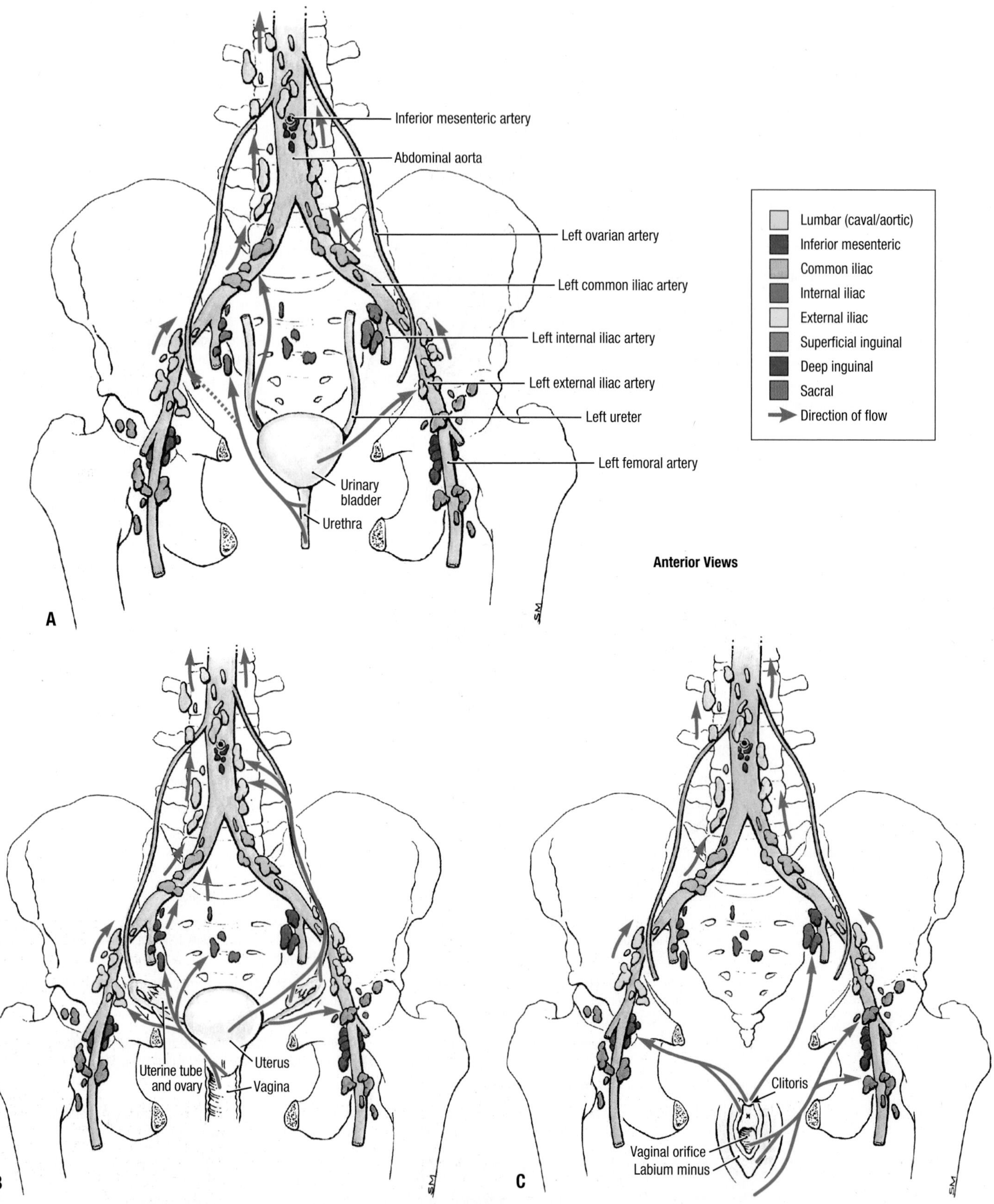
Inferior mesenteric artery
Abdominal aorta
Left ovarian artery
Left common iliac artery
Left internal iliac artery
Left external iliac artery
Left ureter
Left femoral artery
Urinary bladder
Urethra
Lumbar (caval/aortic)
Inferior mesenteric
Common iliac
Internal iliac
External iliac
Superficial inguinal
Deep inguinal
Sacral
Direction of flow
Anterior Views
A
Uterine tube and ovary
Uterus
Vagina
B
Clitoris
Vaginal orifice
Labium minus
C

3.41 LYMPHATIC DRAINAGE OF FEMALE PELVIS AND PERINEUM

A. Pelvic urinary system. **B.** Internal genital organs. **C.** Vulva.

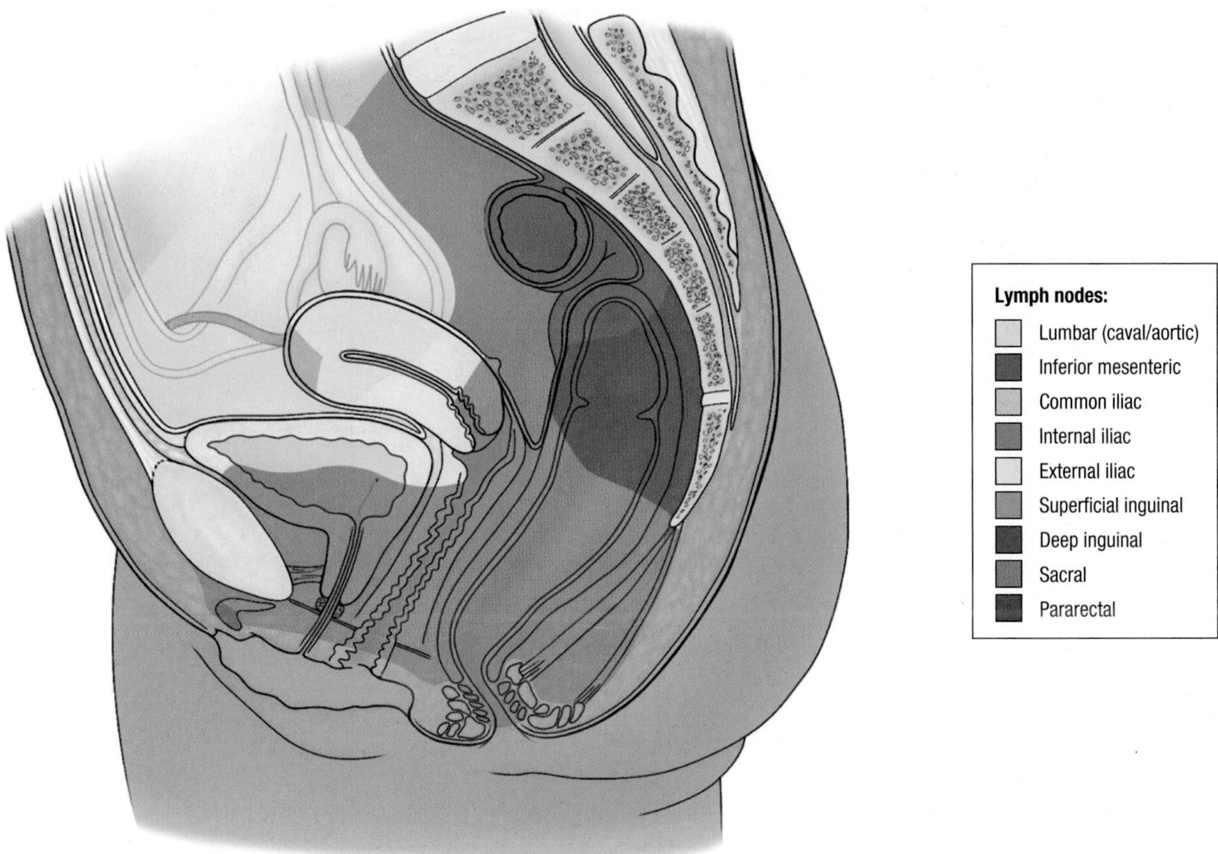
Lymph nodes:
Lumbar (caval/aortic)
Inferior mesenteric
Common iliac
Internal iliac
External iliac
Superficial inguinal
Deep inguinal
Sacral
Pararectal

3.41 *LYMPHATIC DRAINAGE OF FEMALE PELVIS AND PERINEUM (CONTINUED)*

TABLE 3.8 *LYMPHATIC DRAINAGE OF STRUCTURES OF FEMALE PELVIS AND PERINEUM*

Lymph Node Group	Structures Typically Draining to Lymph Node Group
Lumbar	Gonads and associated structures (along ovarian vessels), ovary, uterine tube (except isthmus and intra-uterine parts), fundus of uterus, common iliac nodes
Inferior mesenteric	Superiormost rectum, sigmoid colon, descending colon, pararectal nodes
Common iliac	External and internal iliac lymph nodes
Internal iliac	Inferior pelvic structures, deep perineal structures, sacral nodes, base of bladder, inferior pelvic ureter, anal canal (above pectinate line), inferior rectum, middle and upper vagina, cervix, body of uterus, sacral nodes
External iliac	Anterosuperior pelvic structures, deep inguinal nodes, superior bladder, superior pelvic ureter, upper vagina, cervix, lower body of uterus
Superficial inguinal	Lower limb, superficial drainage of inferolateral quadrant of trunk, including anterior abdominal wall inferior to umbilicus, gluteal region, superolateral uterus (near attachment of round ligament), skin of perineum including vulva, ostium of vagina (inferior to hymen), prepuce of clitoris, peri-anal skin, anal canal inferior to pectinate line
Deep inguinal	Glans of clitoris, superficial inguinal nodes
Sacral	Postero-inferior pelvic structures, inferior rectum, inferior vagina
Pararectal	Superior rectum

3.42 INNERVATION OF FEMALE PELVIC VISCERA

- Pelvic splanchnic nerves (S2–S4) supply parasympathetic motor fibers to the uterus and vagina (and vasodilator fibers to the erectile tissue of the clitoris and bulb of the vestibule; not shown).
- Presynaptic sympathetic fibers pass through the lumbar splanchnic nerves to synapse in prevertebral ganglia; the postsynaptic fibers travel through the superior and inferior hypogastric plexuses to reach the pelvic viscera.
- Visceral afferent fibers conducting pain from intraperitoneal viscera travel with the sympathetic fibers to the T12–L2 spinal ganglia. Visceral afferent fibers conducting pain from subperitoneal viscera travel with parasympathetic fibers to the S2–S4 spinal ganglia.
- Somatic sensation from the opening of the vagina also passes to the S2–S4 spinal ganglia via the pudendal nerve.
- Muscular contractions of the uterus are hormonally induced.

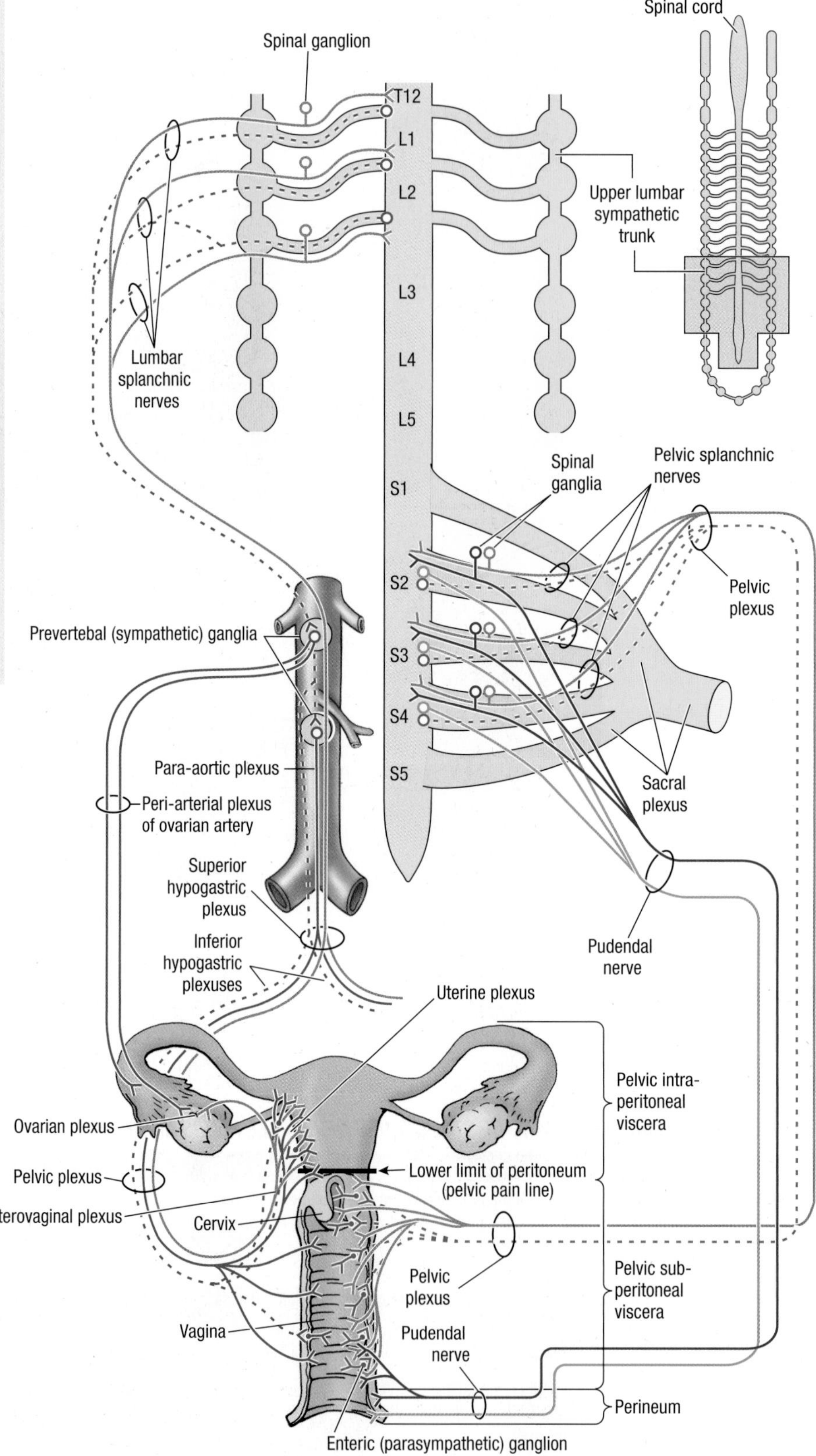

Spinal cord
Spinal ganglion
T12
L1
L2
L3
L4
L5
S1
S2
S3
S4
S5
Upper lumbar sympathetic trunk
Lumbar splanchnic nerves
Spinal ganglia
Pelvic splanchnic nerves
Pelvic plexus
Prevertebal (sympathetic) ganglia
Para-aortic plexus
Peri-arterial plexus of ovarian artery
Superior hypogastric plexus
Inferior hypogastric plexuses
Sacral plexus
Pudendal nerve
Uterine plexus
Pelvic intra-peritoneal viscera
Ovarian plexus
Pelvic plexus
Lower limit of peritoneum (pelvic pain line)
Uterovaginal plexus
Cervix
Pelvic plexus
Pelvic sub-peritoneal viscera
Vagina
Pudendal nerve
Perineum
Enteric (parasympathetic) ganglion
Innervation:
Presynaptic sympathetic
Postsynaptic sympathetic
Presynaptic parasympathetic
Postsynaptic parasympathetic
Visceral afferent running with sympathetic and parasympathetic fibers
Somatic sensory
Somatic motor

Anterior View

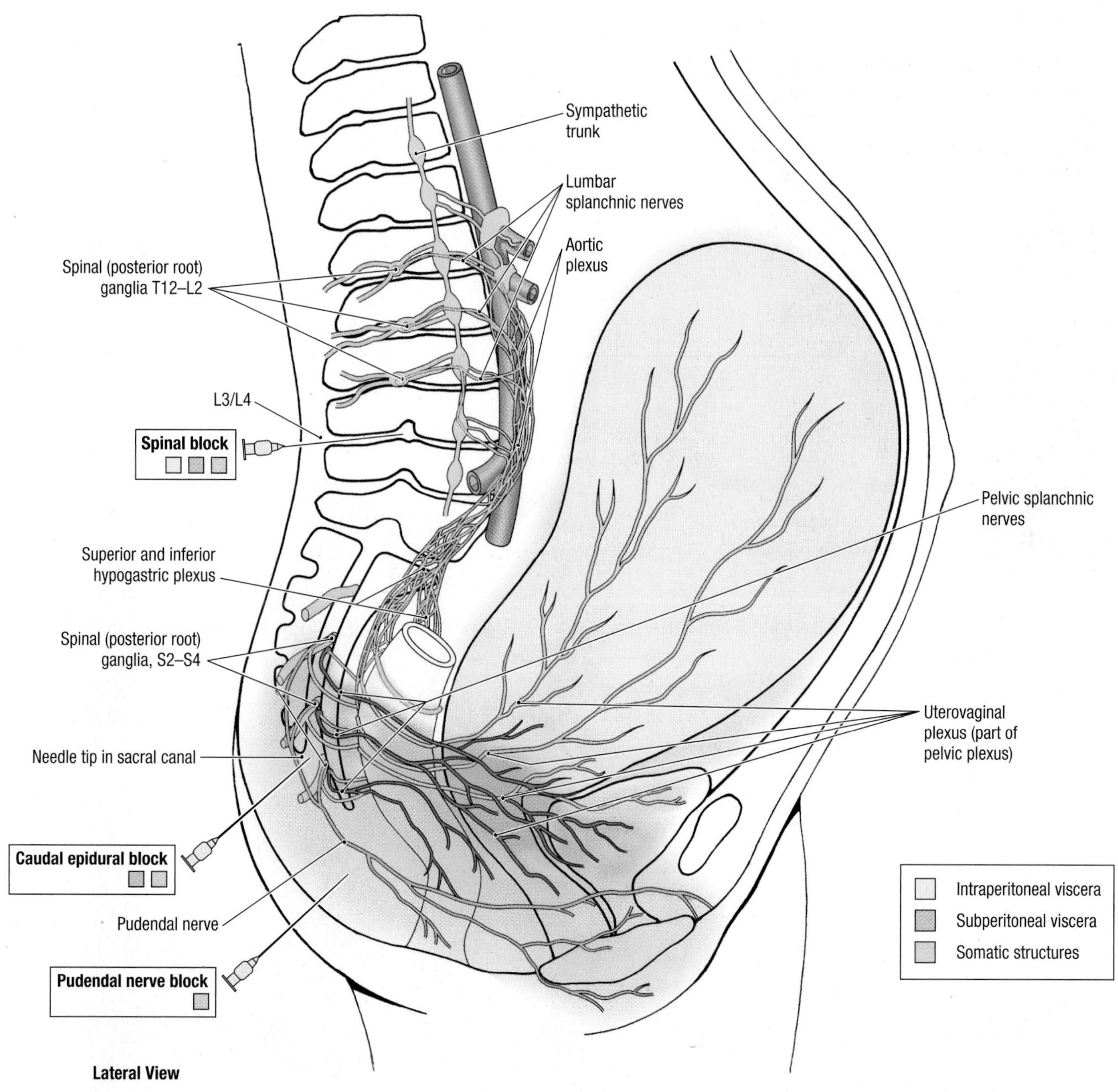
Sympathetic trunk
Lumbar splanchnic nerves
Aortic plexus
Spinal (posterior root) ganglia T12–L2
L3/L4
Spinal block
Superior and inferior hypogastric plexus
Spinal (posterior root) ganglia, S2–S4
Needle tip in sacral canal
Caudal epidural block
Pudendal nerve
Pudendal nerve block
Pelvic splanchnic nerves
Uterovaginal plexus (part of pelvic plexus)
Intraperitoneal viscera
Subperitoneal viscera
Somatic structures

Lateral View

3.43 INNERVATION OF PELVIC VISCERA DURING PREGNANCY; NERVE BLOCKS

- A **spinal block**, in which the anesthetic agent is introduced with a needle into the spinal subarachnoid space at the L3–L4 vertebral level produces complete anesthesia inferior to approximately the waist level. The perineum, pelvic floor, and birth canal are anesthetized, and motor and sensory functions of the entire lower limbs, as well as sensation of uterine contractions, are temporarily eliminated.
- With the **caudal epidural block**, the anesthetic agent is administered using an in-dwelling catheter in the sacral canal. The entire birth canal, pelvic floor, and most of the perineum are anesthetized, but the lower limbs are not usually affected. The mother is aware of her uterine contractions.
- A **pudendal nerve block** is a peripheral nerve block that provides local anesthesia over the S2–S4 dermatomes (most of the perineum) and the inferior quarter of the vagina. It does not block pain from the superior birth canal (uterine cervix and superior vagina), so the mother is able to feel uterine contractions.

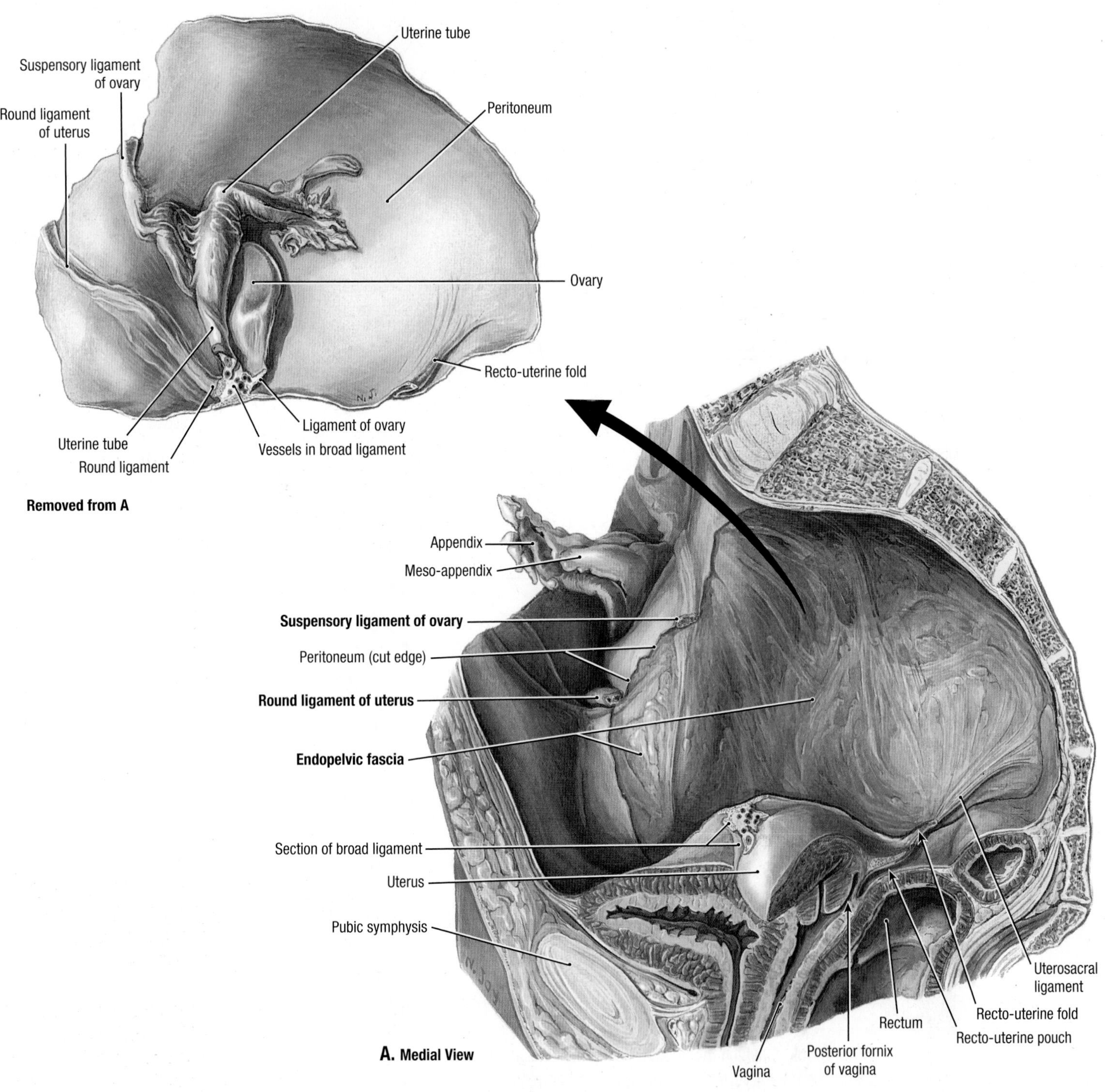

Uterine tube
Suspensory ligament of ovary
Round ligament of uterus
Peritoneum
Ovary
Recto-uterine fold
Ligament of ovary
Vessels in broad ligament
Uterine tube
Round ligament
Removed from A
Appendix
Meso-appendix
Suspensory ligament of ovary
Peritoneum (cut edge)
Round ligament of uterus
Endopelvic fascia
Section of broad ligament
Uterus
Pubic symphysis
Uterosacral ligament
Recto-uterine fold
Rectum
Recto-uterine pouch
Posterior fornix of vagina
Vagina
A. Medial View

3.44 SERIAL DISSECTION OF AUTONOMIC NERVES OF FEMALE PELVIS

A. Broad ligament and peritoneum of the lateral wall of the pelvic cavity have been removed to expose the endopelvic fascia.

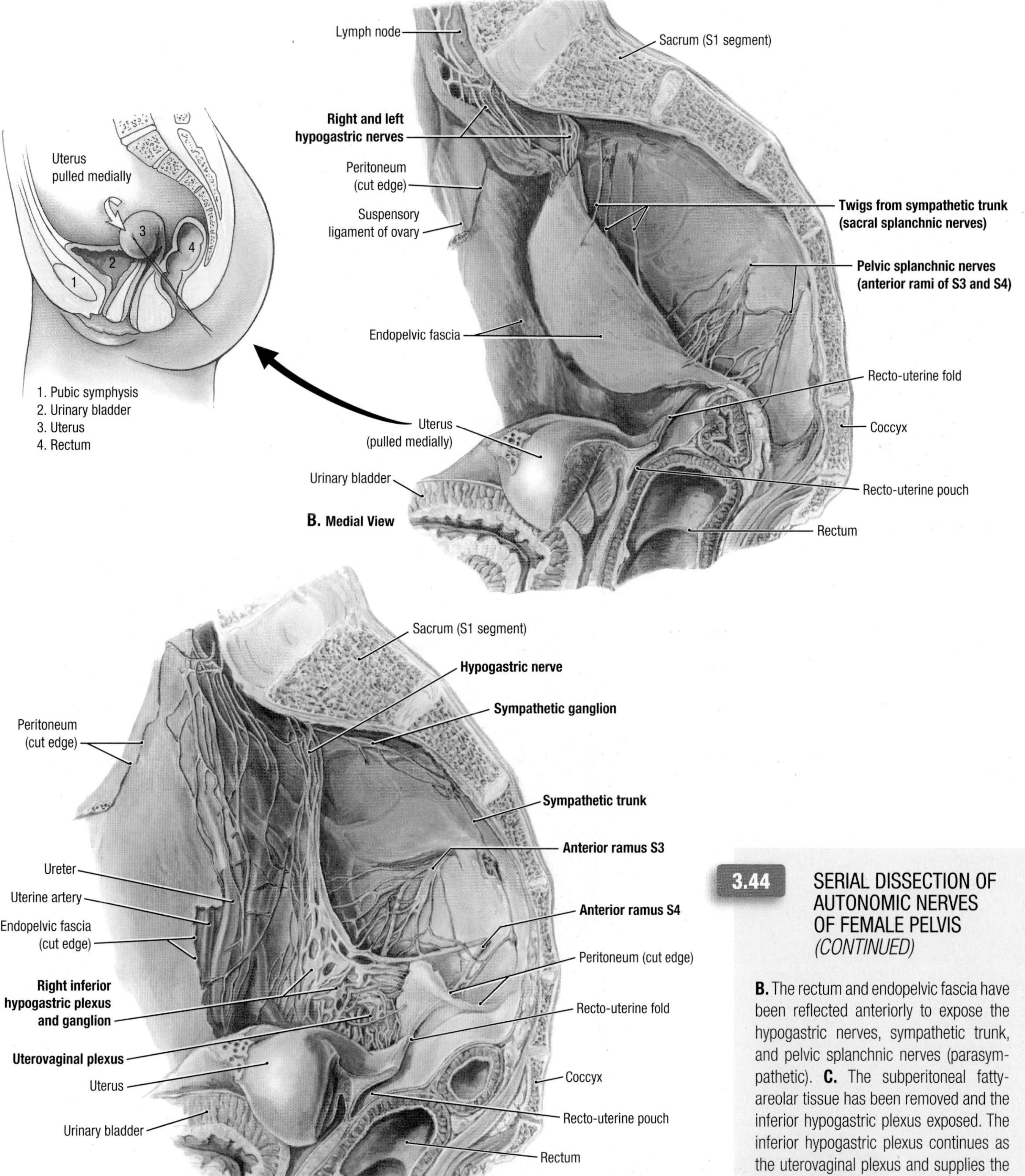
Uterus
pulled medially
1
2
3
4
1. Pubic symphysis
2. Urinary bladder
3. Uterus
4. Rectum
Lymph node
Sacrum (S1 segment)
Right and left
hypogastric nerves
Peritoneum
(cut edge)
Suspensory
ligament of ovary
Twigs from sympathetic trunk
(sacral splanchnic nerves)
Pelvic splanchnic nerves
(anterior rami of S3 and S4)
Endopelvic fascia
Recto-uterine fold
Uterus
(pulled medially)
Coccyx
Urinary bladder
Recto-uterine pouch
Rectum
Sacrum (S1 segment)
Hypogastric nerve
Sympathetic ganglion
Peritoneum
(cut edge)
Sympathetic trunk
Anterior ramus S3
Ureter
Uterine artery
Endopelvic fascia
(cut edge)
Anterior ramus S4
Peritoneum (cut edge)
Right inferior
hypogastric plexus
and ganglion
Recto-uterine fold
Uterovaginal plexus
Uterus
Coccyx
Urinary bladder
Recto-uterine pouch
Rectum

B. Medial View

C. Medial View

3.44 SERIAL DISSECTION OF AUTONOMIC NERVES OF FEMALE PELVIS *(CONTINUED)*

B. The rectum and endopelvic fascia have been reflected anteriorly to expose the hypogastric nerves, sympathetic trunk, and pelvic splanchnic nerves (parasympathetic). **C.** The subperitoneal fatty-areolar tissue has been removed and the inferior hypogastric plexus exposed. The inferior hypogastric plexus continues as the uterovaginal plexus and supplies the uterus, uterine tubes, vagina, urethra, greater vestibular glands, erectile tissue of the clitoris, and bulb of the vestibule.

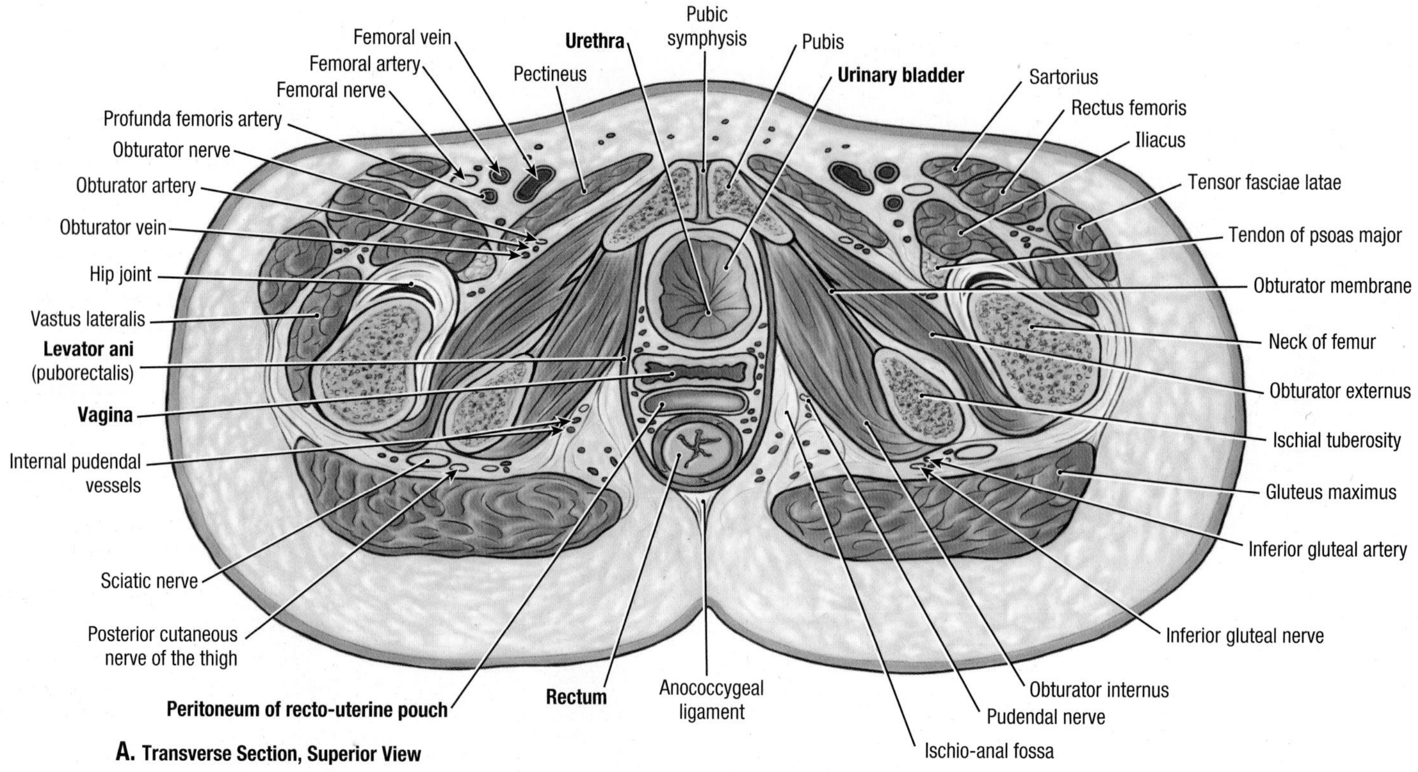

Femoral vein
Femoral artery
Femoral nerve
Profunda femoris artery
Obturator nerve
Obturator artery
Obturator vein
Hip joint
Vastus lateralis
Levator ani (puborectalis)
Vagina
Internal pudendal vessels
Sciatic nerve
Posterior cutaneous nerve of the thigh
Peritoneum of recto-uterine pouch
Urethra
Pectineus
Pubic symphysis
Pubis
Urinary bladder
Sartorius
Rectus femoris
Iliacus
Tensor fasciae latae
Tendon of psoas major
Obturator membrane
Neck of femur
Obturator externus
Ischial tuberosity
Gluteus maximus
Inferior gluteal artery
Inferior gluteal nerve
Obturator internus
Pudendal nerve
Ischio-anal fossa
Rectum
Anococcygeal ligament

A. Transverse Section, Superior View

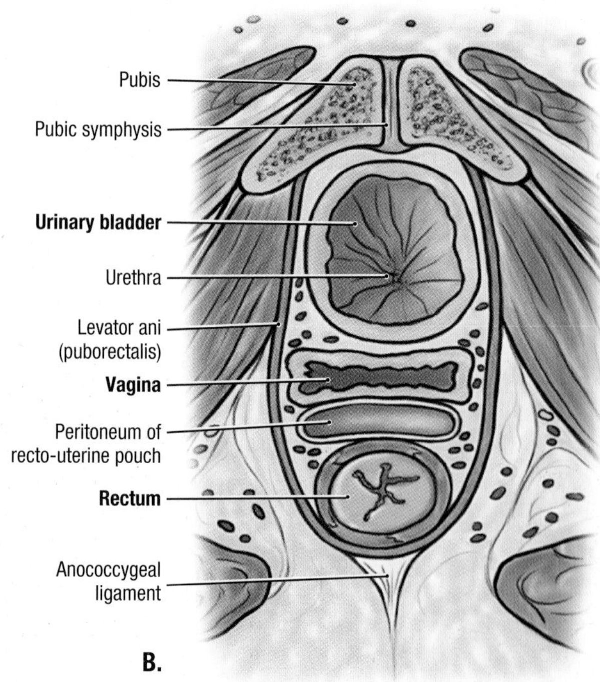

Pubis
Pubic symphysis
Urinary bladder
Urethra
Levator ani (puborectalis)
Vagina
Peritoneum of recto-uterine pouch
Rectum
Anococcygeal ligament

B.

3.45 TRANSVERSE SECTION THROUGH FEMALE PELVIS

A. Transverse section through the ischial tuberosities. **B.** Enlargement of central part of section including the bladder, vagina, rectum, and recto-uterine pouch.

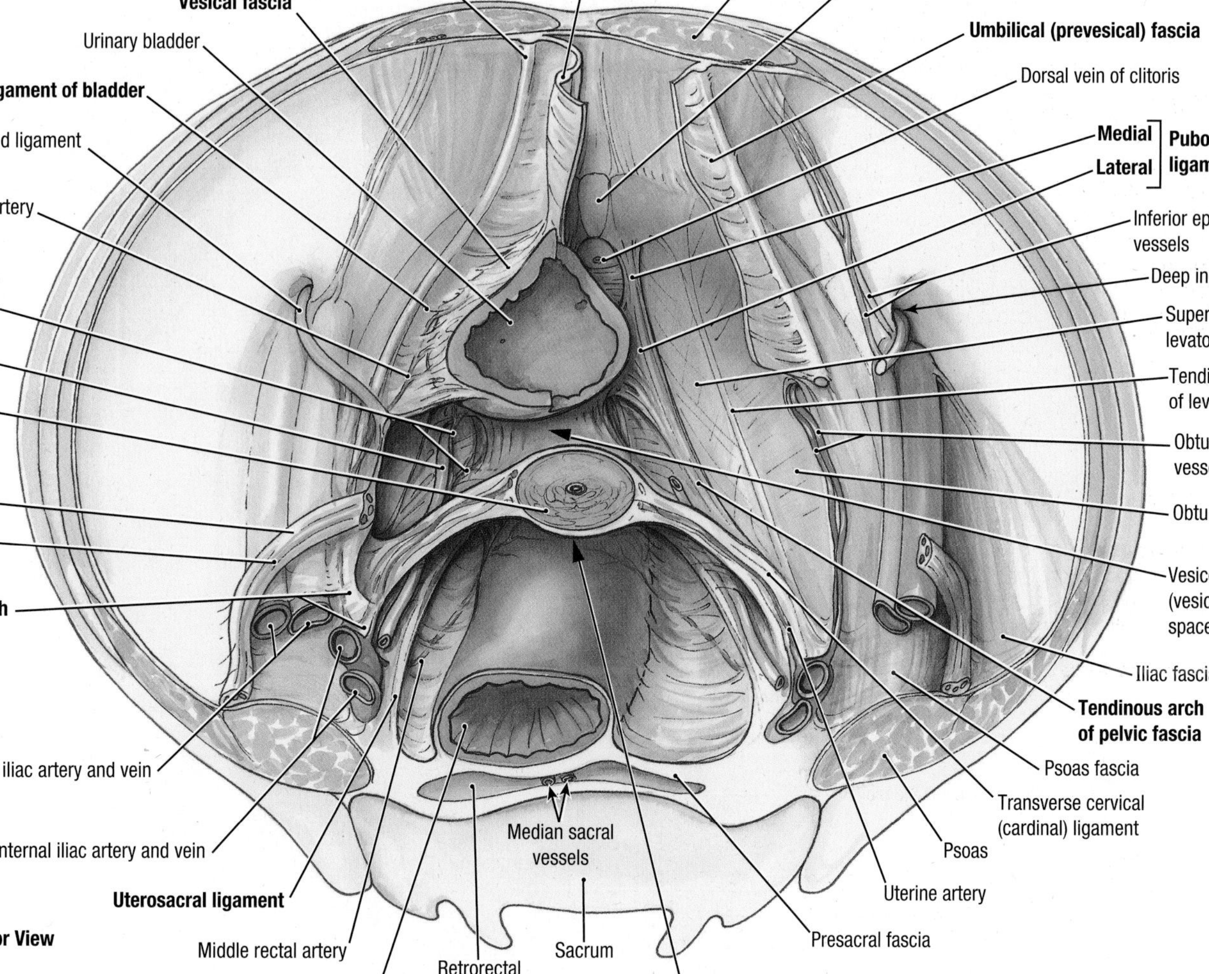

Median umbilical ligament
Medial umbilical ligament
Rectus abdominis
Pubic symphysis
Vesical fascia
Urinary bladder
Umbilical (prevesical) fascia
Lateral ligament of bladder
Dorsal vein of clitoris
Round ligament
Medial
Lateral
Pubovesical ligaments
Superior vesical artery
Inferior epigastric vessels
Inferior vesical and vaginal arteries within paracolpium
Deep inguinal ring
Superior fascia of levator ani
Ureter
Tendinous arch of levator ani
Cervix
Obturator vessels
Suspensory ligament of ovary
Obturator fascia
Ovarian artery
Vesicocervical (vesicovaginal) space
Hypogastric sheath
Iliac fascia
Tendinous arch of pelvic fascia
External iliac artery and vein
Psoas fascia
Transverse cervical (cardinal) ligament
Internal iliac artery and vein
Median sacral vessels
Psoas
Uterosacral ligament
Uterine artery
Middle rectal artery
Sacrum
Presacral fascia
Rectum
Retrorectal (presacral) space
Rectovaginal space
Tendinous arch of pelvic fascia

A. Superior View

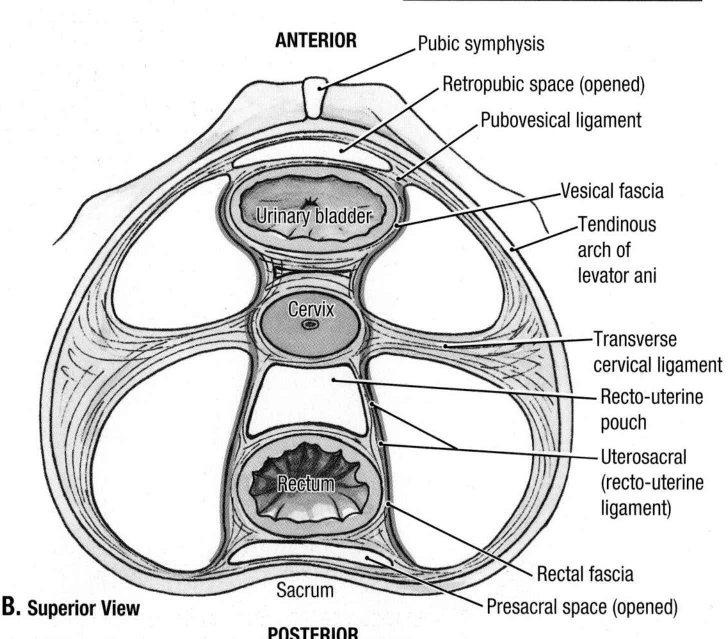
ANTERIOR
Pubic symphysis
Retropubic space (opened)
Pubovesical ligament
Vesical fascia
Urinary bladder
Tendinous arch of levator ani
Cervix
Transverse cervical ligament
Recto-uterine pouch
Uterosacral (recto-uterine ligament)
Rectum
Rectal fascia
Sacrum
Presacral space (opened)
POSTERIOR

B. Superior View

3.46 PELVIC FASCIA AND SUPPORTING MECHANISM OF CERVIX AND UPPER VAGINA

A. Greater and lesser pelvis demonstrating pelvic viscera and endopelvic fascia. **B.** Schematic illustration of fascial ligaments and areolar spaces at level of tendinous arch of pelvic fascia.

- Note the parietal pelvic fascia covering the obturator internus and levator ani muscles and the visceral pelvic fascia surrounding the pelvic organs. These membranous fasciae are continuous where the organs penetrate the pelvic floor, forming a tendinous arch of pelvic fascia bilaterally.
- The endopelvic fascia lies between, and is continuous with, both visceral and parietal layers of pelvic fascia. The loose, areolar portions of the endopelvic fascia have been removed; the fibrous, condensed portions remain. Note the condensation of this fascia into the hypogastric sheath, containing the vessels to the pelvic viscera, the ureters, and (in the male) the ductus deferens.
- Observe the ligamentous extensions of the hypogastric sheath: the lateral ligament of the urinary bladder, the transverse cervical ligament at the base of the broad ligament, and a less prominent lamina posteriorly containing the middle rectal vessels.

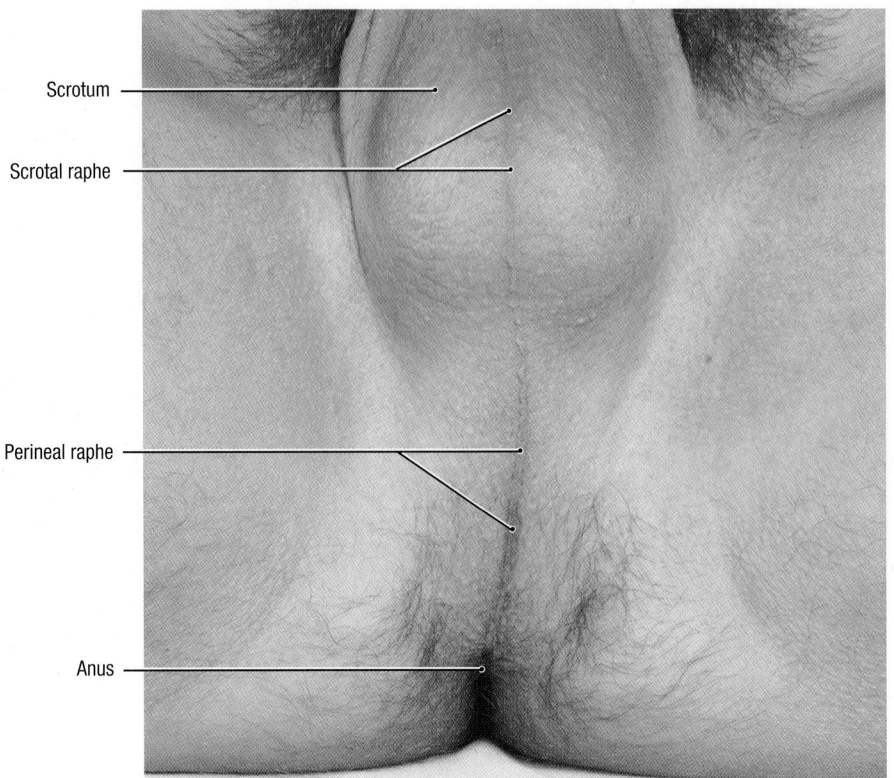
Scrotum
Scrotal raphe
Perineal raphe
Anus

A. **Inferior View**

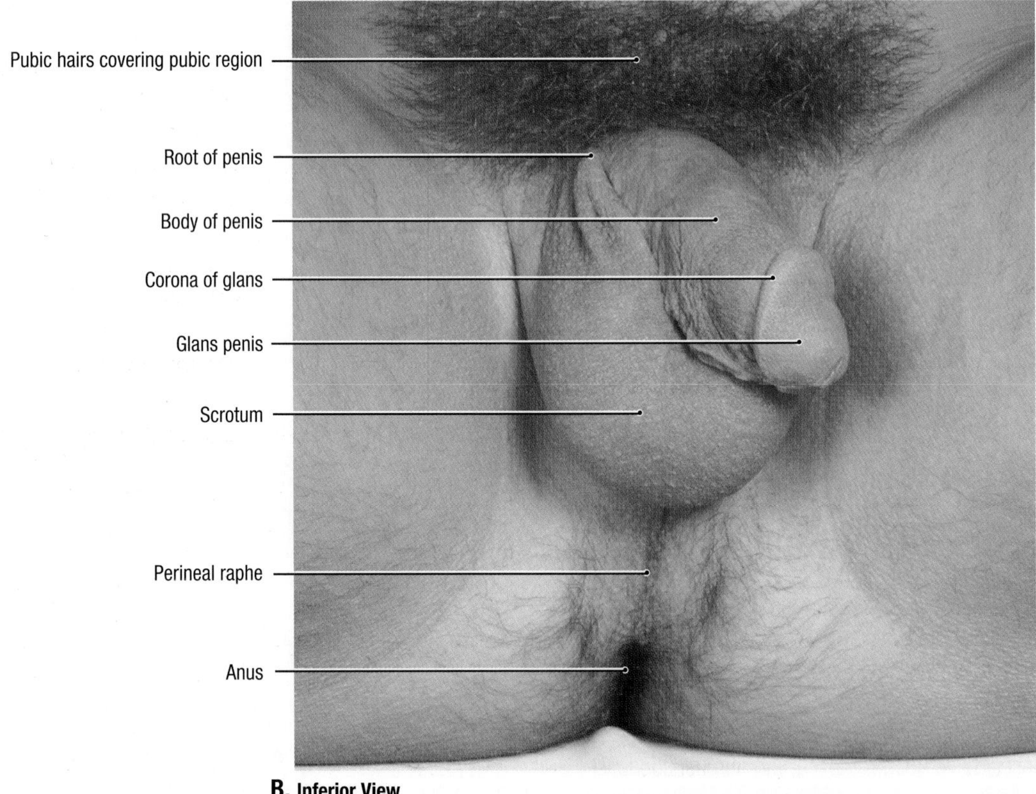
Pubic hairs covering pubic region
Root of penis
Body of penis
Corona of glans
Glans penis
Scrotum
Perineal raphe
Anus

B. **Inferior View**

3.47 SURFACE ANATOMY OF MALE PERINEUM

A. Scrotum and anal region. **B.** Penis, scrotum, and anal region.

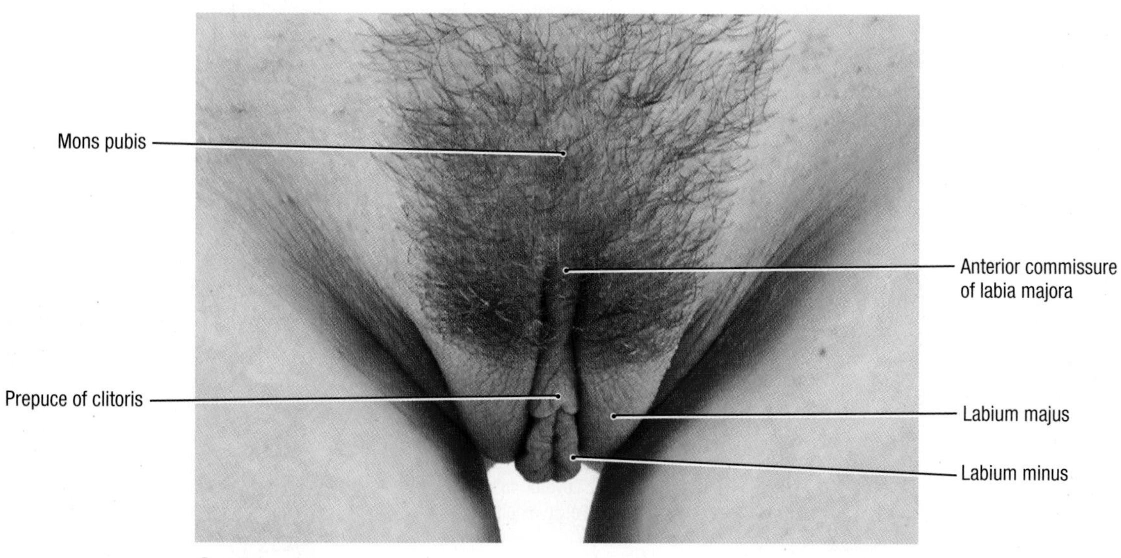
Mons pubis
Anterior commissure of labia majora
Prepuce of clitoris
Labium majus
Labium minus

A. Anterior View

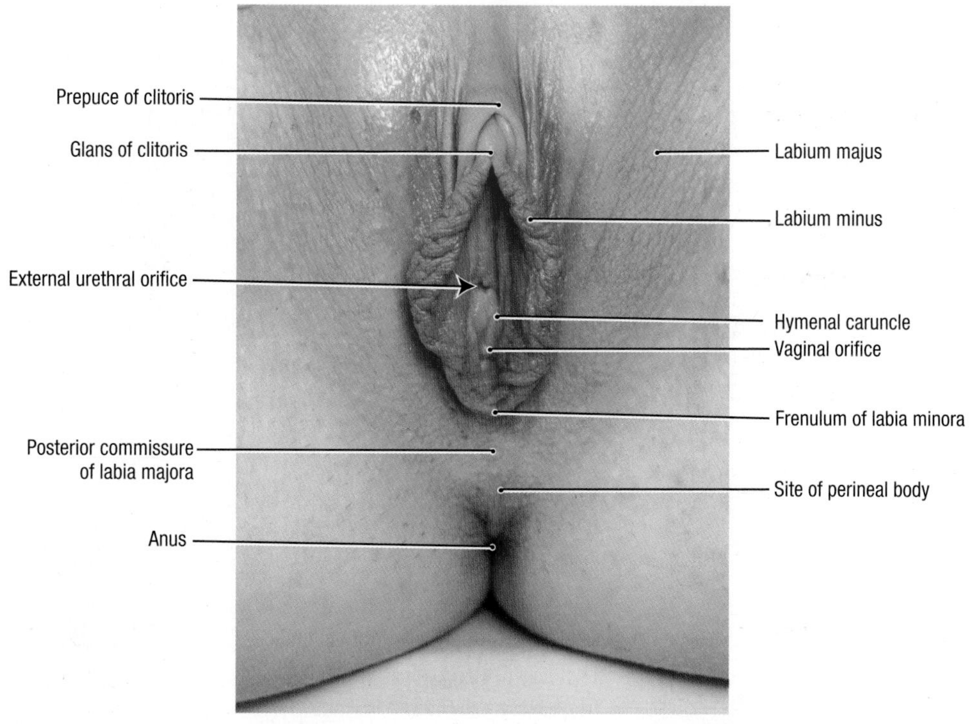
Prepuce of clitoris
Glans of clitoris
Labium majus
Labium minus
External urethral orifice
Hymenal caruncle
Vaginal orifice
Frenulum of labia minora
Posterior commissure of labia majora
Site of perineal body
Anus

B. Antero-inferior View (Lithotomy Position)

3.48 SURFACE ANATOMY OF THE FEMALE PERINEUM

A. External genitalia (pudendum; vulva), standing position. **B.** Vestibule of vagina and the external urethral and vaginal orifices opening into it (recumbent position).

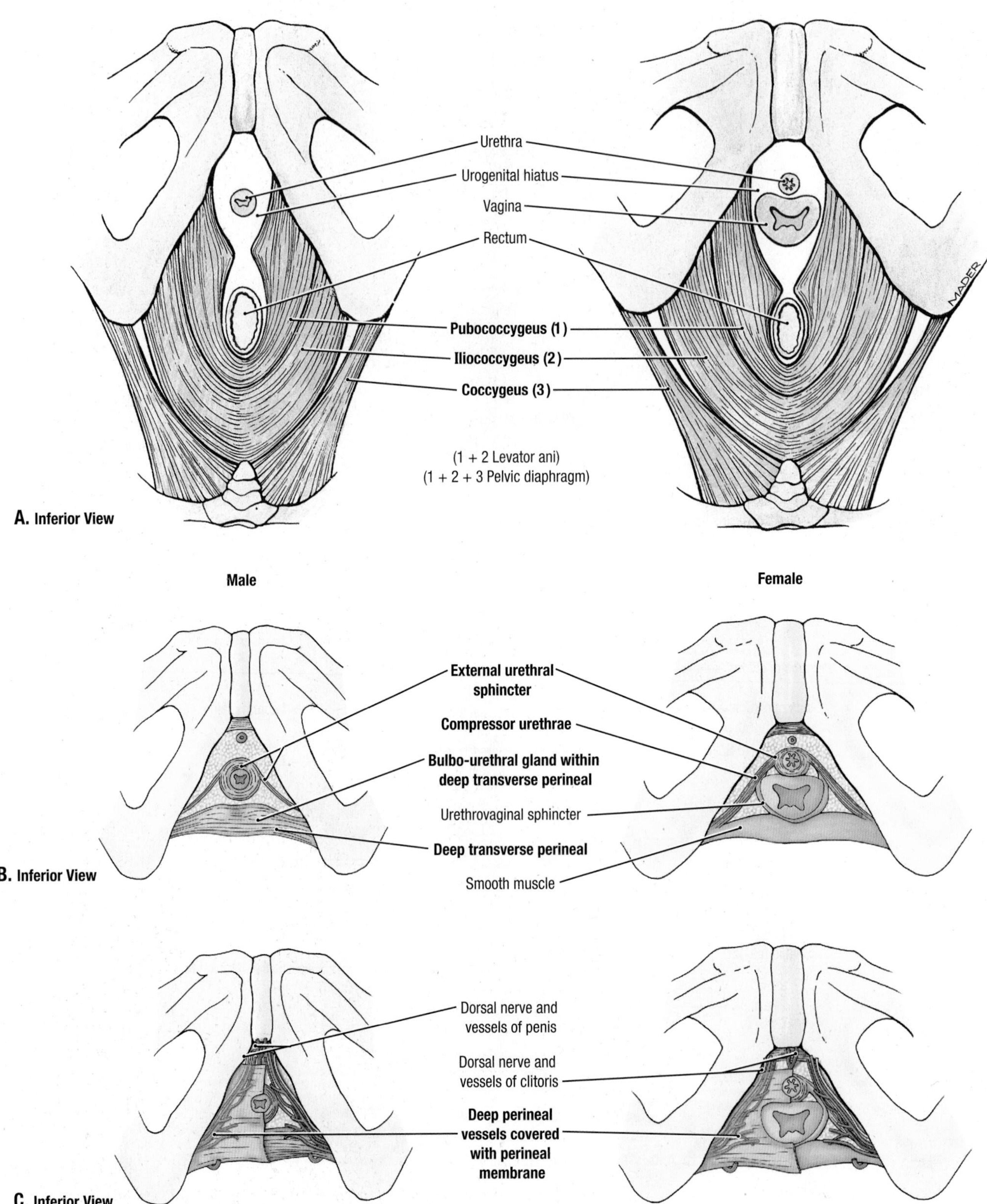

Urethra
Urogenital hiatus
Vagina
Rectum
MADER
Pubococcygeus (1)
Iliococcygeus (2)
Coccygeus (3)
(1 + 2 Levator ani)
(1 + 2 + 3 Pelvic diaphragm)
A. Inferior View
Male
Female
External urethral sphincter
Compressor urethrae
Bulbo-urethral gland within deep transverse perineal
Urethrovaginal sphincter
Deep transverse perineal
Smooth muscle
B. Inferior View
Dorsal nerve and vessels of penis
Dorsal nerve and vessels of clitoris
Deep perineal vessels covered with perineal membrane
C. Inferior View

3.49 MALE AND FEMALE PERINEAL COMPARTMENTS

A.–F. Sequential demonstration of structures of the perineal compartments, from deep to superficial. **A.–C.** Deep perineal compartment (superior to perineal membrane). **A.** Pelvic diaphragm. **B.** Muscles of deep perineal compartment. **C.** Deep perineal vessels and nerves, covered by perineal membrane on right side.

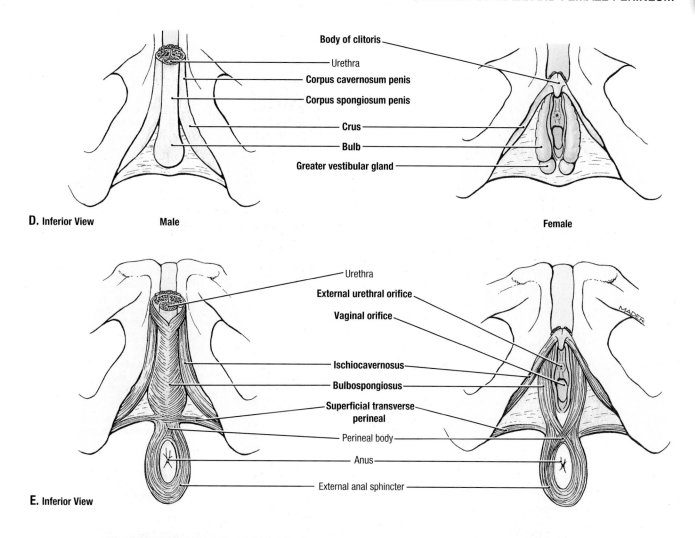

Body of clitoris
Urethra
Corpus cavernosum penis
Corpus spongiosum penis
Crus
Bulb
Greater vestibular gland

D. Inferior View — Male — Female

Urethra
External urethral orifice
Vaginal orifice
Ischiocavernosus
Bulbospongiosus
Superficial transverse perineal
Perineal body
Anus
External anal sphincter

E. Inferior View

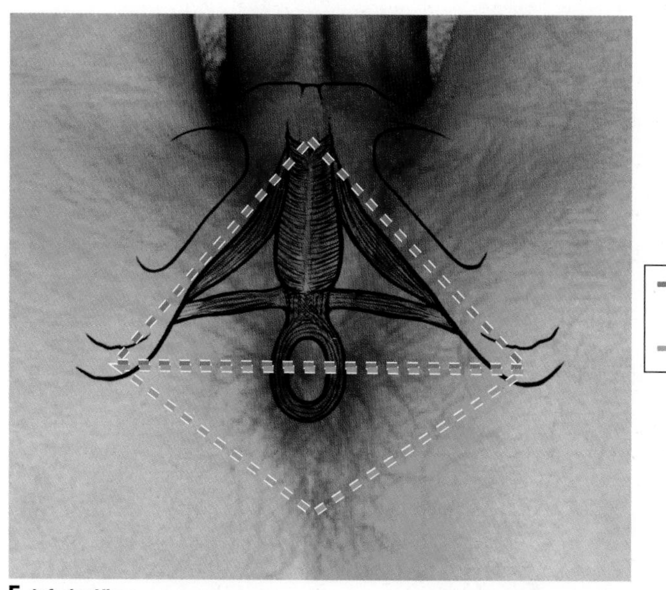

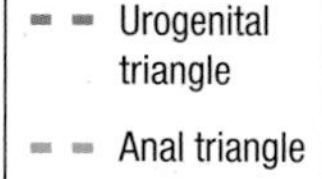
Urogenital triangle
Anal triangle

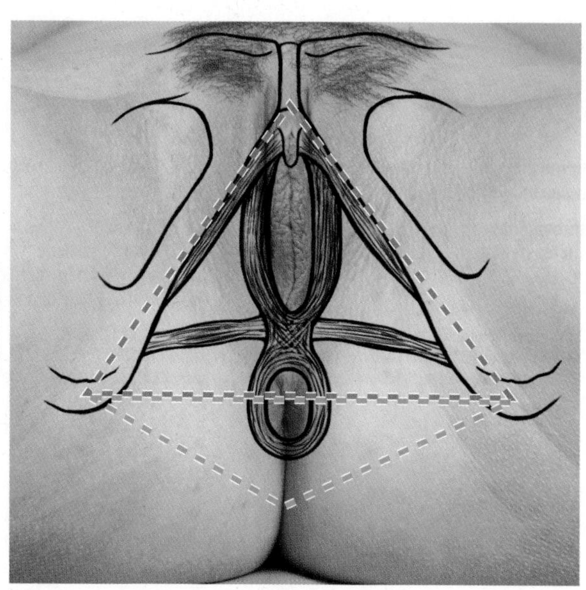

F. Inferior View

3.49 MALE AND FEMALE PERINEAL COMPARTMENTS *(CONTINUED)*

D.–F. Superficial perineal compartment (inferior to perineal membrane). **D.** Erectile bodies. **E.** Muscles of superficial perineal compartment. **F.** Superficial muscles imposed on surface anatomy of perineum.

TABLE 3.9 MUSCLES OF PERINEUM

Muscle	Origin	Course and Insertion	Innervation	Main Action
External anal sphincter	Skin and fascia surrounding anus; coccyx via anococcygeal ligament	Passes around lateral aspects of anal canal; insertion into perineal body	Inferior anal (rectal) nerve, a branch of pudendal nerve (S2–S4)	Constricts anal canal during peristalsis, resisting defecation; supports and fixes perineal body and pelvic floor
Bulbospongiosus	*Male:* median raphe on ventral surface of bulb of penis; perineal body	*Male:* surrounds lateral aspects of bulb of penis and most proximal part of body of penis, inserting into perineal membrane, dorsal aspect of corpora spongiosum and cavernosa, and fascia of bulb of penis	Muscular (deep) branch of perineal nerve, a branch of the pudendal nerve (S2–S4)	*Male:* supports and fixes perineal body/pelvic floor; compresses bulb of penis to expel last drops of urine/semen; assists erection by compressing outflow via deep perineal vein and by pushing blood from bulb into body of penis
	Female: perineal body	*Female:* passes on each side of lower vagina, enclosing bulb and greater vestibular gland; inserts onto pubic arch and fascia of corpora cavernosa of clitoris		*Female:* supports and fixes perineal body/pelvic floor; "sphincter" of vagina; assists in erection of clitoris (and perhaps bulb of vestibule); compresses greater vestibular gland
Ischiocavernosus	Internal surface of ischiopubic ramus and ischial tuberosity	Embraces crus of penis or clitoris, inserting onto the inferior and medial aspects of the crus and to the perineal membrane medial to the crus		Maintains erection of penis or clitoris by compressing outflow veins and pushing blood from the root of penis or clitoris into the body of penis or clitoris
Superficial transverse perineal	Internal surface of ischiopubic ramus and ischial tuberosity	Passes along inferior aspect of posterior border of perineal membrane to perineal body		Supports and fixes perineal body (pelvic floor) to support abdominopelvic viscera and resist increased intra-abdominal pressure
Deep transverse perineal (male only)		Passes along superior aspect of posterior border of perineal membrane to perineal body, and external anal sphincter	Muscular (deep) branch of perineal nerve	
Smooth muscle (female only)	Ischiopubic rami	Passes to lateral wall of urethra and vagina	Autonomic nerves	Quantity of smooth muscle increases with age; function uncertain
External urethral sphincter		Surrounds urethra superior to perineal membrane; in males, also ascends anterior aspect of prostate	Dorsal nerve of penis or clitoris, terminal branch of pudendal nerve (S2–S4)	Compresses urethra to maintain urinary continence
Compressor urethrae (females only)	Internal surface of ischiopubic ramus	Continuous with external urethral sphincter		Compresses urethra; with pelvic diaphragm; assists in elongation of urethra
Urethrovaginal sphincter (females only)	Anterior side of urethra	Continuous with compressor urethrae; extends posteriorly on lateral wall of urethra and vagina to interdigitate with fibers from opposite side of perineal body		Compresses urethra and vagina

Oelrich TM. The urethral sphincter muscle in the male. *Am J Anat* 1980;158:229–246.
Oelrich TM. The striated urogenital sphincter muscle in the female. *Anat Rec* 1983;205:223–232.
Mirilas P, Skandalakis JE. Urogenital diaphragm: an erroneous concept casting its shadow over the sphincter urethrae and deep perineal space. *J Am Coll Surg* 2004;198:279–290.
DeLancey JO. Correlative study of paraurethral anatomy. *Obstet Gynecol* 1986;68:91–97.

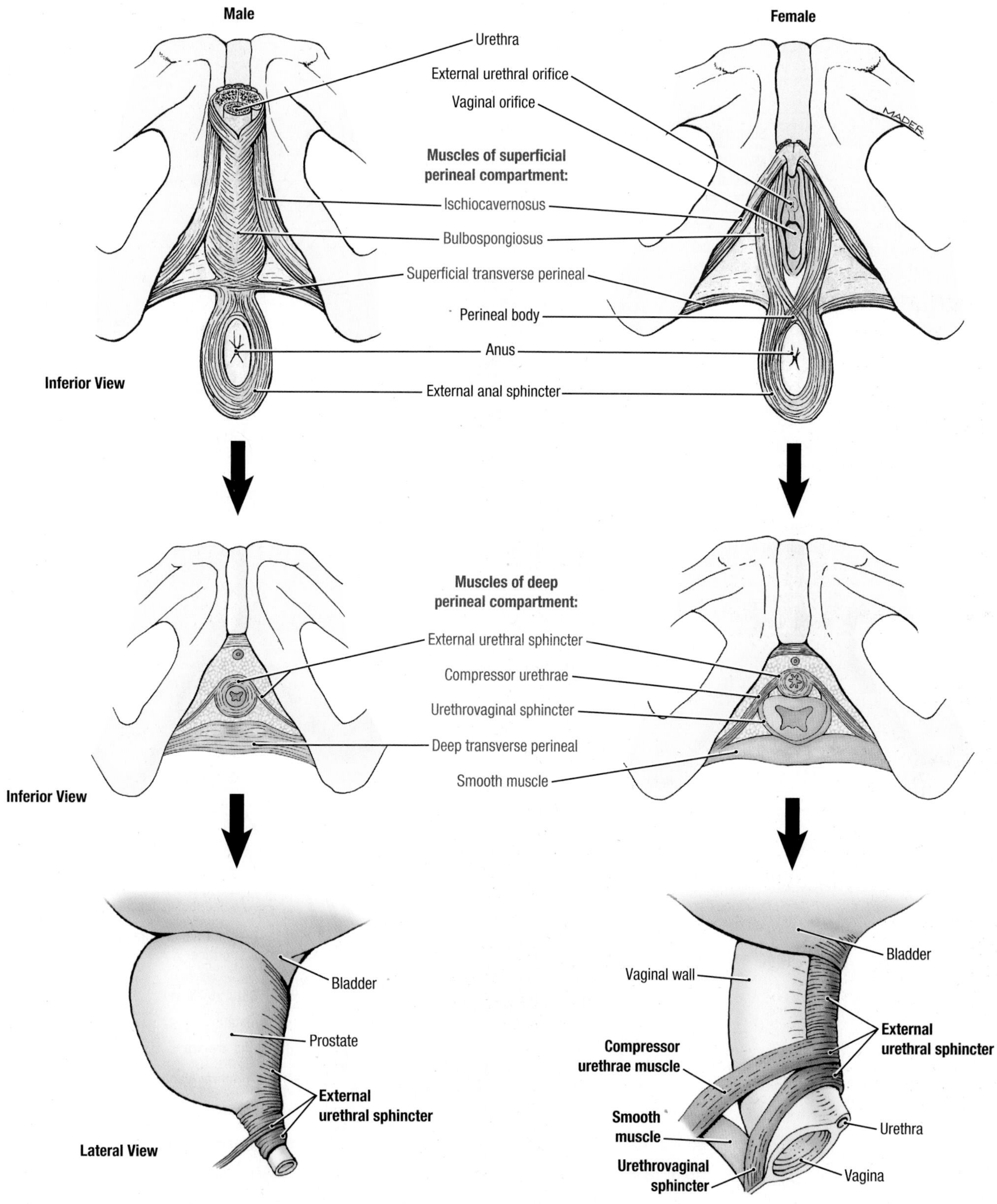
Male
Female
Urethra
External urethral orifice
Vaginal orifice
Muscles of superficial perineal compartment:
Ischiocavernosus
Bulbospongiosus
Superficial transverse perineal
Perineal body
Anus
External anal sphincter
Inferior View
Muscles of deep perineal compartment:
External urethral sphincter
Compressor urethrae
Urethrovaginal sphincter
Deep transverse perineal
Smooth muscle
Inferior View
Bladder
Prostate
External urethral sphincter
Lateral View
Bladder
Vaginal wall
External urethral sphincter
Compressor urethrae muscle
Smooth muscle
Urethrovaginal sphincter
Urethra
Vagina

3.50 MUSCLES OF PERINEUM

A potential subcutaneous perineal space (pouch) lies between the membranous layer of the subcutaneous tissue of the perineum and the perineal fascia (investing fascia of the superficial perineal muscles). The superficial perineal compartment (pouch) is an enclosed compartment bounded inferiorly by the perineal fascia and superiorly by the perineal membrane. The deep compartment is bounded inferiorly by the perineal membrane and continues superiorly to the (inferior investing fascia of the) pelvic diaphragm (Oelich, 1980, 1983; DeLancy 1986; Mirilus, 2004).

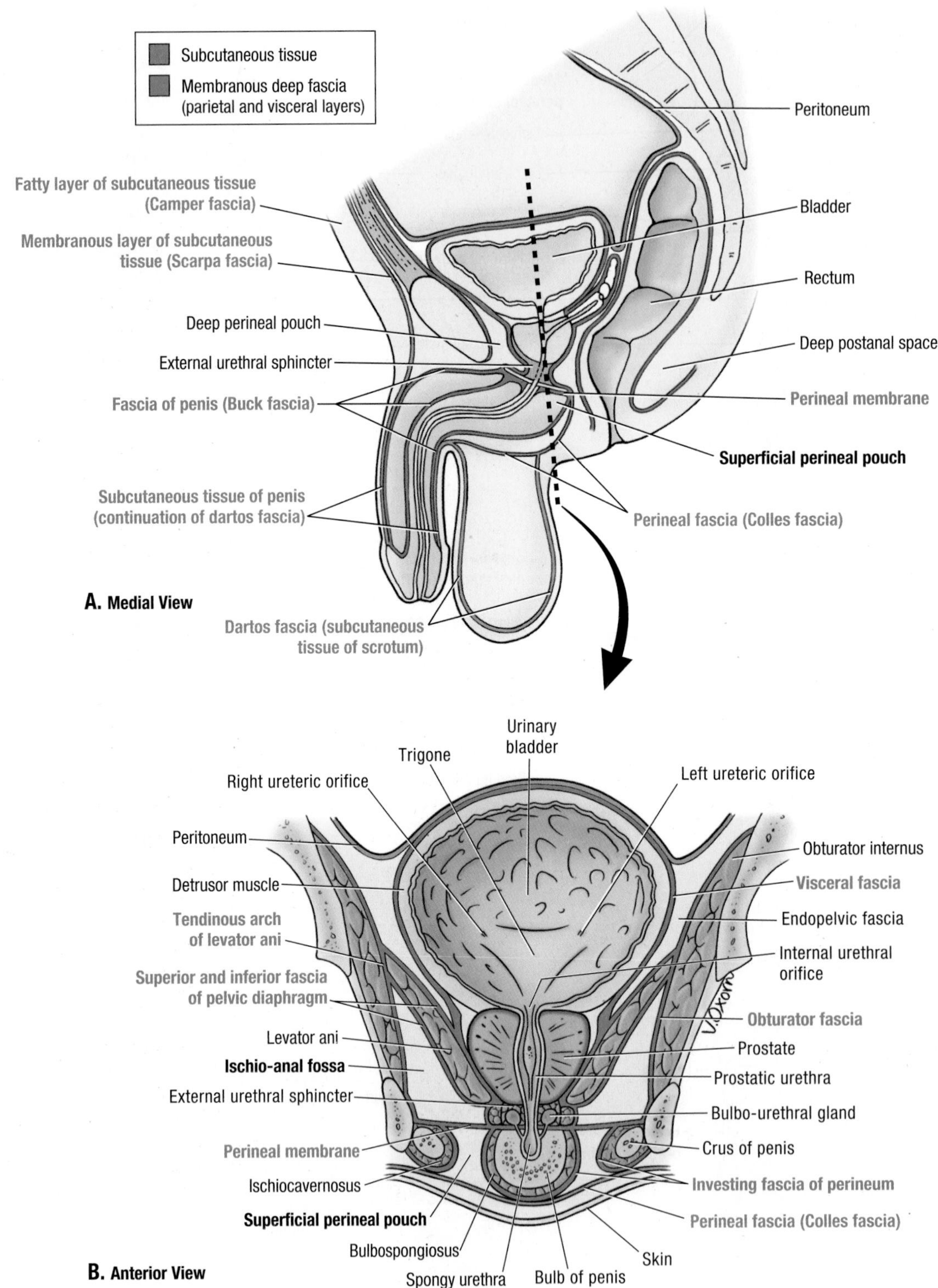

Subcutaneous tissue
Membranous deep fascia (parietal and visceral layers)
Peritoneum
Fatty layer of subcutaneous tissue (Camper fascia)
Bladder
Membranous layer of subcutaneous tissue (Scarpa fascia)
Rectum
Deep perineal pouch
Deep postanal space
External urethral sphincter
Perineal membrane
Fascia of penis (Buck fascia)
Superficial perineal pouch
Subcutaneous tissue of penis (continuation of dartos fascia)
Perineal fascia (Colles fascia)
A. Medial View
Dartos fascia (subcutaneous tissue of scrotum)
Urinary bladder
Trigone
Right ureteric orifice
Left ureteric orifice
Peritoneum
Obturator internus
Detrusor muscle
Visceral fascia
Tendinous arch of levator ani
Endopelvic fascia
Internal urethral orifice
Superior and inferior fascia of pelvic diaphragm
Obturator fascia
Levator ani
Prostate
Ischio-anal fossa
Prostatic urethra
External urethral sphincter
Bulbo-urethral gland
Perineal membrane
Crus of penis
Ischiocavernosus
Investing fascia of perineum
Superficial perineal pouch
Perineal fascia (Colles fascia)
Bulbospongiosus
Skin
B. Anterior View
Spongy urethra
Bulb of penis

3.51 PERINEAL FASCIA AND PERINEAL COMPARTMENTS

A. Fascia of male perineum, median section. **B.** Compartments of male perineum, coronal section.

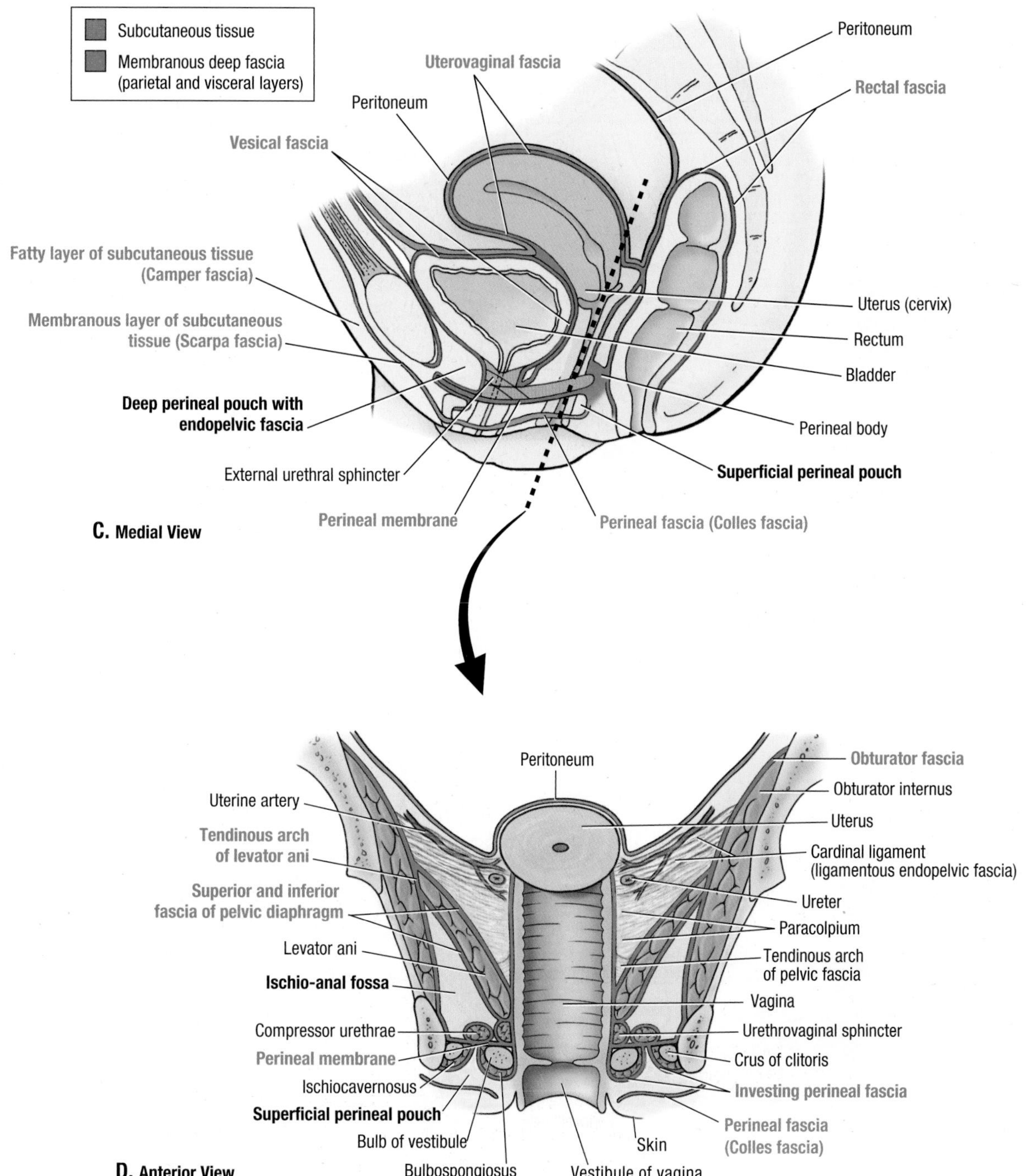
Subcutaneous tissue
Membranous deep fascia (parietal and visceral layers)
Uterovaginal fascia
Peritoneum
Rectal fascia
Peritoneum
Vesical fascia
Fatty layer of subcutaneous tissue (Camper fascia)
Membranous layer of subcutaneous tissue (Scarpa fascia)
Deep perineal pouch with endopelvic fascia
External urethral sphincter
Perineal membrane
Uterus (cervix)
Rectum
Bladder
Perineal body
Superficial perineal pouch
Perineal fascia (Colles fascia)
C. Medial View
Peritoneum
Uterine artery
Tendinous arch of levator ani
Superior and inferior fascia of pelvic diaphragm
Levator ani
Ischio-anal fossa
Compressor urethrae
Perineal membrane
Ischiocavernosus
Superficial perineal pouch
Bulb of vestibule
Bulbospongiosus
Vestibule of vagina
Skin
Obturator fascia
Obturator internus
Uterus
Cardinal ligament (ligamentous endopelvic fascia)
Ureter
Paracolpium
Tendinous arch of pelvic fascia
Vagina
Urethrovaginal sphincter
Crus of clitoris
Investing perineal fascia
Perineal fascia (Colles fascia)
D. Anterior View

3.51 PERINEAL FASCIA AND PERINEAL COMPARTMENTS *(CONTINUED)*

C. Fascia of female perineum, median section. **D.** Compartments of female perineum, coronal section. Tendinous arch of levator ani = thickening of obturator fascia providing origin for levator ani; tendinous arch of pelvic fascia = thickening where somatic and parietal membranous pelvic fascias merge.

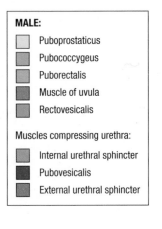

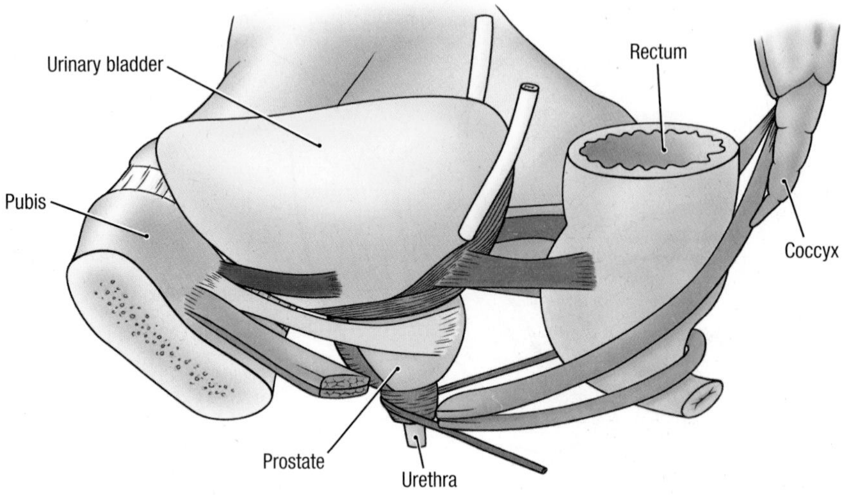
Urinary bladder
Rectum
Pubis
Coccyx
Prostate
Urethra

MALE:

- Puboprostaticus
- Pubococcygeus
- Puborectalis
- Muscle of uvula
- Rectovesicalis

Muscles compressing urethra:

- Internal urethral sphincter
- Pubovesicalis
- External urethral sphincter

A. **Left Lateral View, Male**

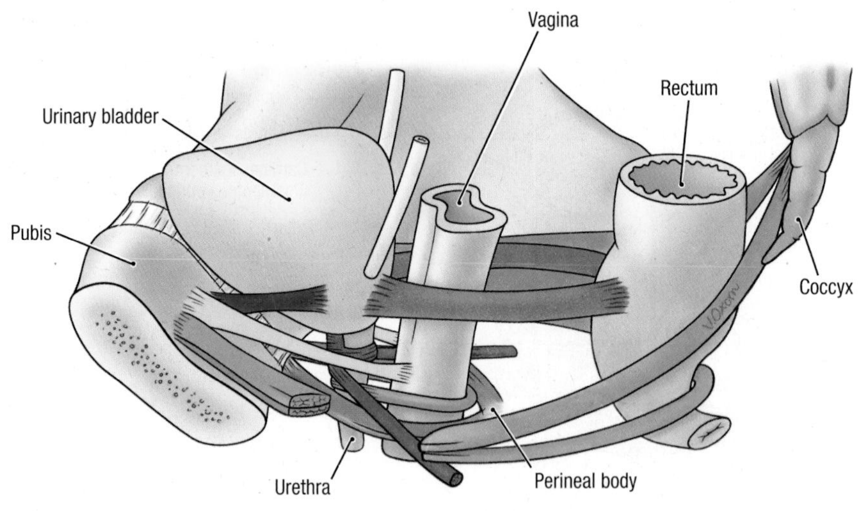
Vagina
Rectum
Urinary bladder
Pubis
Coccyx
Urethra
Perineal body

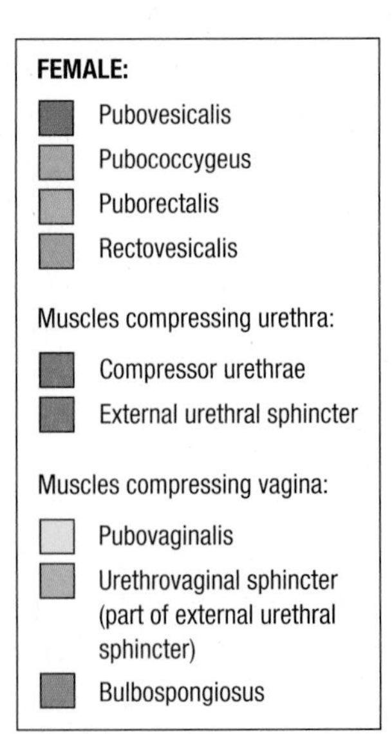
FEMALE:
Pubovesicalis
Pubococcygeus
Puborectalis
Rectovesicalis
Muscles compressing urethra:
Compressor urethrae
External urethral sphincter
Muscles compressing vagina:
Pubovaginalis
Urethrovaginal sphincter (part of external urethral sphincter)
Bulbospongiosus

B. **Left Lateral View, Female**

3.52 SUPPORTING AND COMPRESSOR/SPHINCTERIC MUSCLES OF PELVIS

A. Male. **B.** Female.

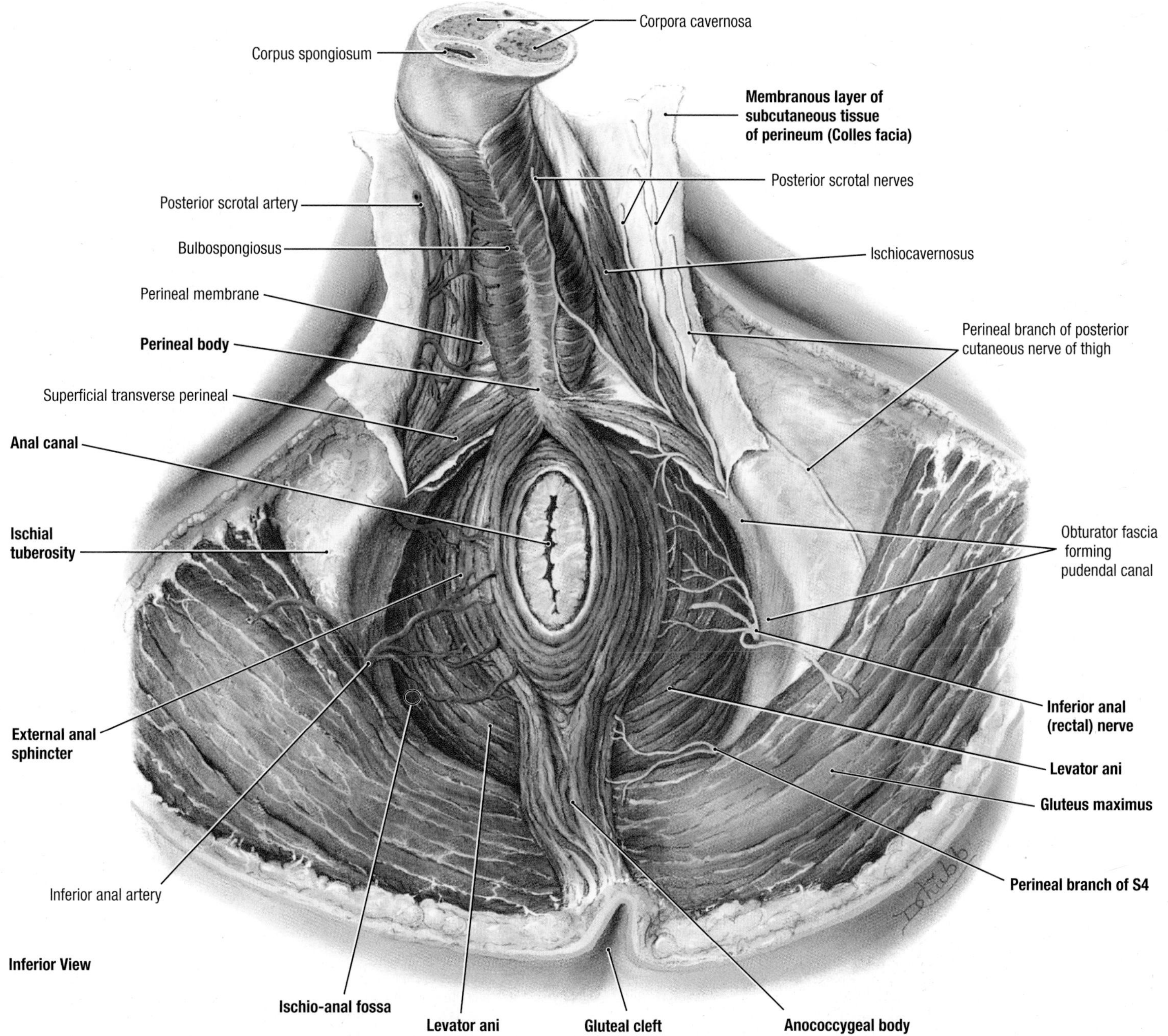
Corpora cavernosa
Corpus spongiosum
Membranous layer of subcutaneous tissue of perineum (Colles facia)
Posterior scrotal nerves
Posterior scrotal artery
Bulbospongiosus
Ischiocavernosus
Perineal membrane
Perineal branch of posterior cutaneous nerve of thigh
Perineal body
Superficial transverse perineal
Anal canal
Ischial tuberosity
Obturator fascia forming pudendal canal
Inferior anal (rectal) nerve
External anal sphincter
Levator ani
Gluteus maximus
Perineal branch of S4
Inferior anal artery
Inferior View
Ischio-anal fossa
Levator ani
Gluteal cleft
Anococcygeal body

3.53 DISSECTION OF MALE PERINEUM I

Superficial dissection.

- The membranous layer of subcutaneous tissue of the perineum was incised and reflected, opening the subcutaneous perineal compartment (pouch) in which the cutaneous nerves course.
- The perineal membrane is exposed between the three paired muscles of the superficial compartment; although not evident here, the muscles are individually ensheathed with investing fascia.
- The anal canal is surrounded by the external anal sphincter. The superficial fibers of the sphincter anchor the anal canal anteriorly to the perineal body and posteriorly, via the anococcygeal body (ligament), to the coccyx and skin of the gluteal cleft.
- Ischio-anal (ischiorectal) fossae, from which fat bodies have been removed, lie on each side of the external anal sphincter. The fossae are also bound medially and superiorly by the levator ani, laterally by the ischial tuberosities and obturator internus fascia, and posteriorly by the gluteus maximus overlying the sacrotuberous ligaments. An anterior recess of each ischio-anal fossa extends superior to the perineal membrane.
- In the lateral wall of the fossa, the inferior anal (rectal) nerve emerges from the pudendal canal and, with the perineal branch of S4, supplies the voluntary external anal sphincter and perianal skin; most cutaneous twigs have been removed.

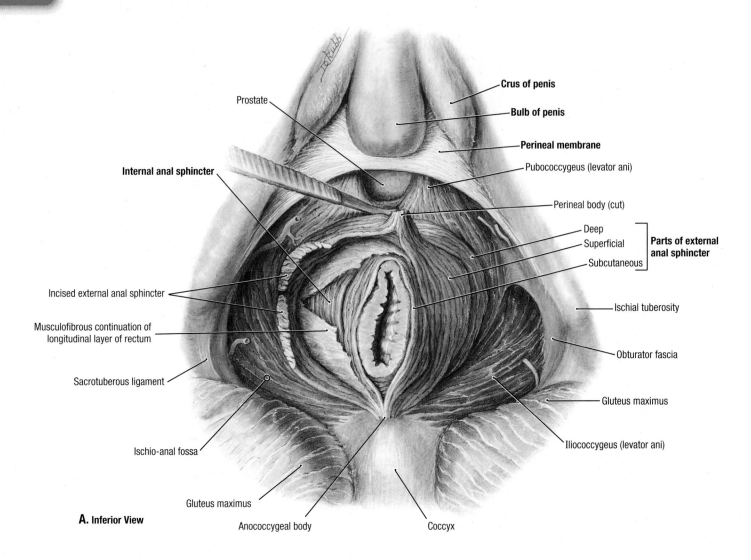

Crus of penis
Prostate
Bulb of penis
Perineal membrane
Internal anal sphincter
Pubococcygeus (levator ani)
Perineal body (cut)
Deep
Superficial
Subcutaneous
Parts of external anal sphincter
Incised external anal sphincter
Ischial tuberosity
Musculofibrous continuation of longitudinal layer of rectum
Obturator fascia
Sacrotuberous ligament
Gluteus maximus
Iliococcygeus (levator ani)
Ischio-anal fossa
Gluteus maximus
Anococcygeal body
Coccyx

A. Inferior View

3.54 DISSECTION OF THE MALE PERINEUM II

A. The superficial perineal muscles have been removed, revealing the roots of the erectile bodies (crura and bulb) of the penis, attached to the ischiopubic rami and perineal membrane. On the left side, the superficial and deep parts of the external anal sphincter were incised and reflected; the underlying musculofibrous continuation of the outer longitudinal layer of the muscular layer of the rectum is cut to reveal thickening of the inner circular layer that comprises the internal anal sphincter. **B. Rupture of the spongy urethra** in the bulb of the penis results in **extravasation** (abnormal passage) **of urine** into the subcutaneous perineal compartment. The attachments of the membranous layer of subcutaneous tissue determine the direction and restrictions of flow of the extravasated urine. Urine and blood may pass deep to the continuations of the membranous layer in the scrotum, penis, and inferior abdominal wall. The urine cannot pass laterally and inferiorly into the thighs because the membranous layer fuses with the fascia lata (deep fascia of the thigh), nor posteriorly into the anal triangle due to continuity with the perineal membrane and perineal body.

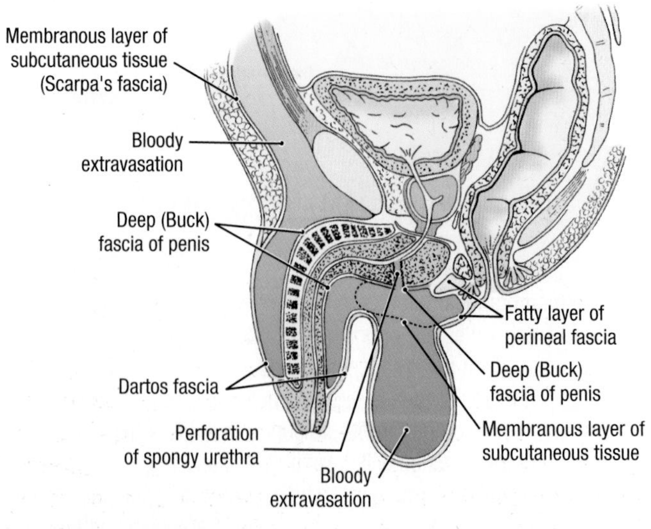
Membranous layer of subcutaneous tissue (Scarpa's fascia)
Bloody extravasation
Deep (Buck) fascia of penis
Fatty layer of perineal fascia
Deep (Buck) fascia of penis
Dartos fascia
Membranous layer of subcutaneous tissue
Perforation of spongy urethra
Bloody extravasation

B. Medial view (from left)

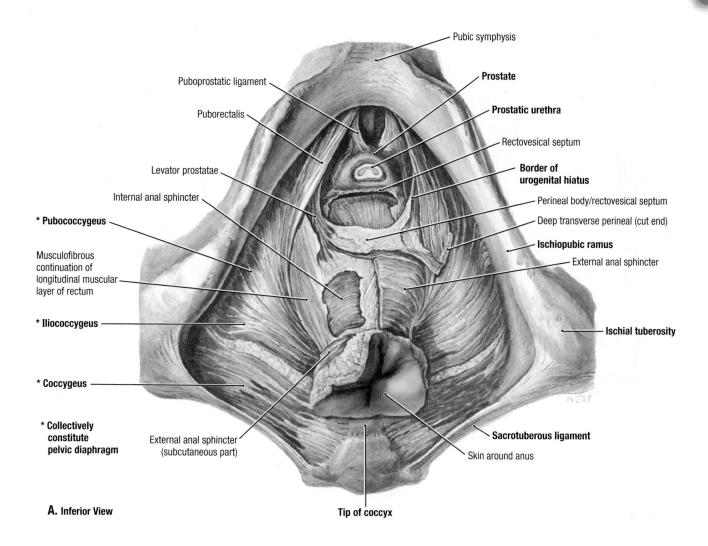

Pubic symphysis
Puboprostatic ligament
Prostate
Puborectalis
Prostatic urethra
Rectovesical septum
Levator prostatae
Border of urogenital hiatus
Internal anal sphincter
Perineal body/rectovesical septum
* Pubococcygeus
Deep transverse perineal (cut end)
Ischiopubic ramus
Musculofibrous continuation of longitudinal muscular layer of rectum
External anal sphincter
* Iliococcygeus
Ischial tuberosity
* Coccygeus
* Collectively constitute pelvic diaphragm
External anal sphincter (subcutaneous part)
Sacrotuberous ligament
Skin around anus
Tip of coccyx

A. Inferior View

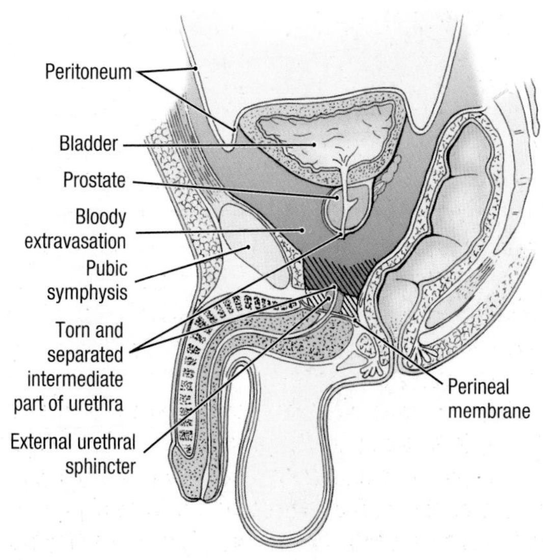
Peritoneum
Bladder
Prostate
Bloody extravasation
Pubic symphysis
Torn and separated intermediate part of urethra
External urethral sphincter
Perineal membrane

B. Medial View (from left)

3.55 DISSECTION OF THE MALE PERINEUM III

A. The perineal membrane and structures superficial to it have been removed. The prostatic urethra, base of the prostate, and rectum are visible through the urogenital hiatus of the pelvic diaphragm. The osseofibrous boundaries are demonstrated. **B. Rupture of the intermediate part of the urethra** results in extravasation of urine and blood into the deep perineal compartment. The fluid may pass superiorly through the urogenital hiatus and distribute extraperitoneally around the prostate and bladder.

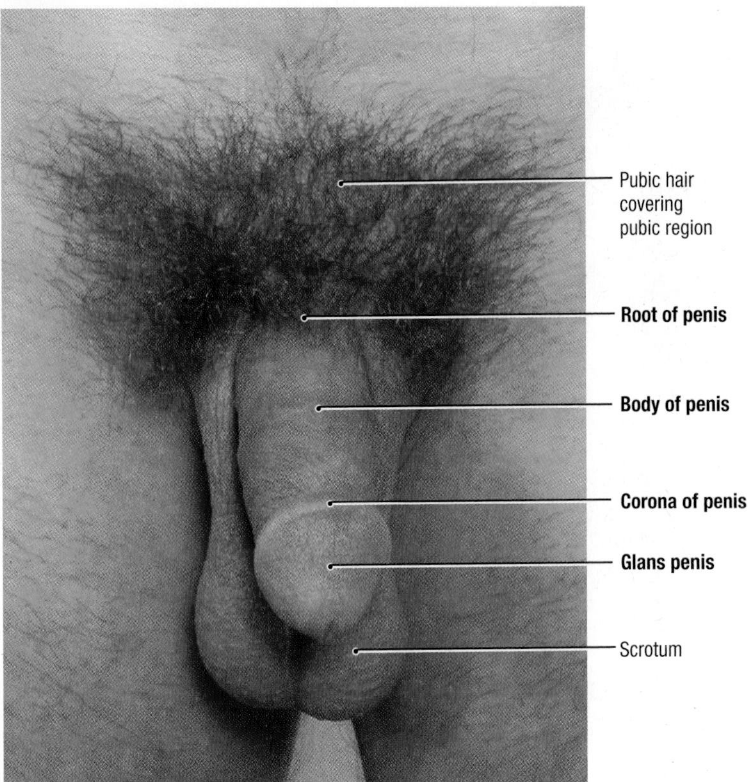

Pubic hair covering pubic region
Root of penis
Body of penis
Corona of penis
Glans penis
Scrotum

A. Anterior View

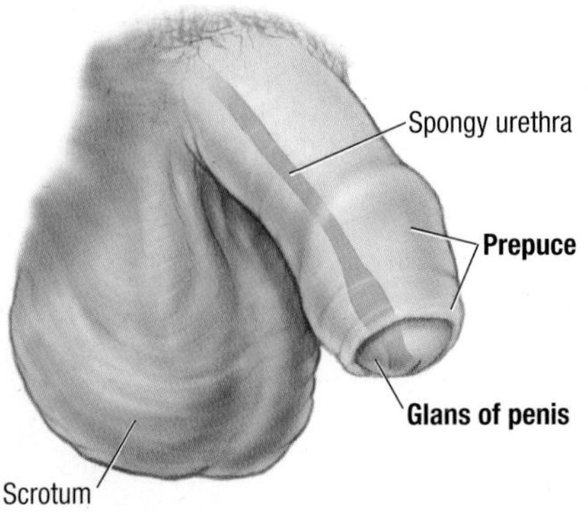

Spongy urethra
Prepuce
Glans of penis
Scrotum

B. Right Anterolateral View

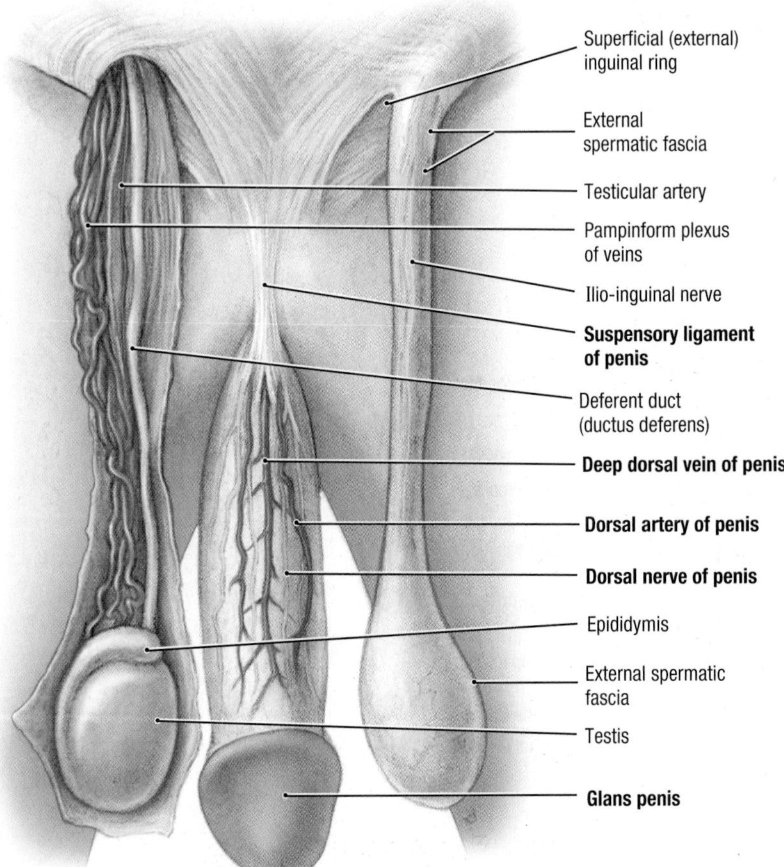

Superficial (external) inguinal ring
External spermatic fascia
Testicular artery
Pampinform plexus of veins
Ilio-inguinal nerve
Suspensory ligament of penis
Deferent duct (ductus deferens)
Deep dorsal vein of penis
Dorsal artery of penis
Dorsal nerve of penis
Epididymis
External spermatic fascia
Testis
Glans penis

C. Anterior View

3.56 GLANS, PREPUCE, AND NEUROVASCULAR BUNDLE OF PENIS

A. Surface anatomy, penis circumcised. **B.** Uncircumcised penis. **C.** Vessels and nerves of penis and contents of spermatic cord.

In **C:**

- The superficial and deep fasciae covering the penis are removed to expose the midline deep dorsal vein and the bilateral dorsal arteries and nerves of the penis. The triangular suspensory ligament of the penis attaches to the region of the pubic symphysis and blends with the deep fascia of the penis.
- On the specimen's left, the spermatic cord passes through the external inguinal ring and picks up a covering of external spermatic fascia from the margins of the superficial inguinal ring.
- On the specimen's right, the coverings of the spermatic cord and testis are incised and reflected, and the contents of the cord are separated.

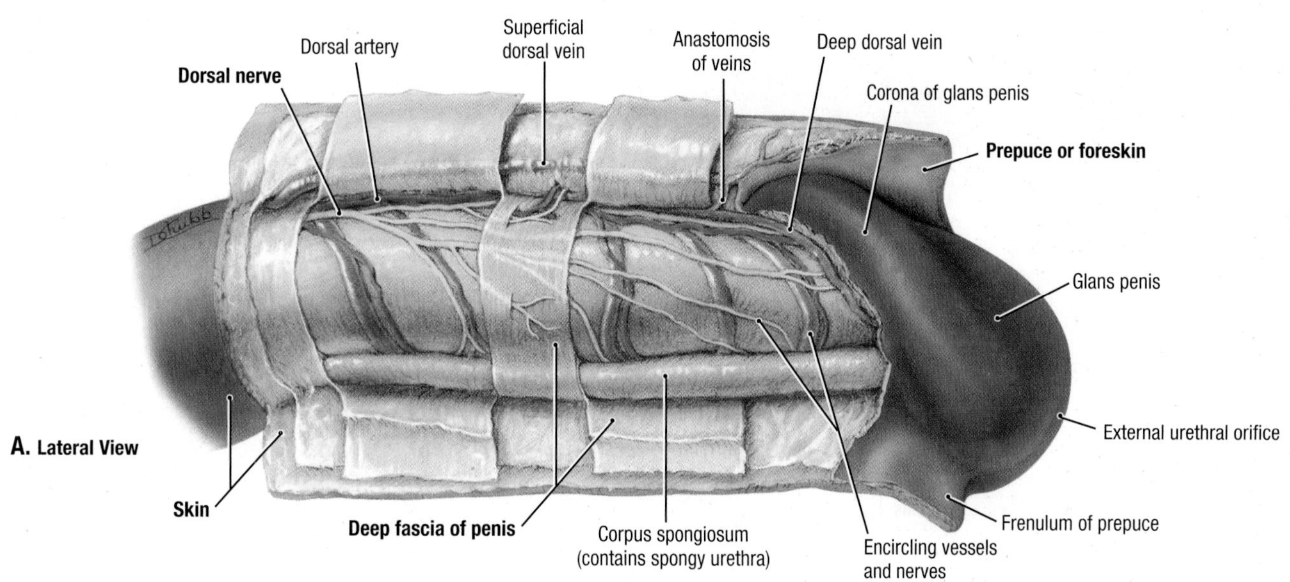
Dorsal nerve
Dorsal artery
Superficial dorsal vein
Anastomosis of veins
Deep dorsal vein
Corona of glans penis
Prepuce or foreskin
Glans penis
External urethral orifice
A. Lateral View
Skin
Deep fascia of penis
Corpus spongiosum (contains spongy urethra)
Encircling vessels and nerves
Frenulum of prepuce

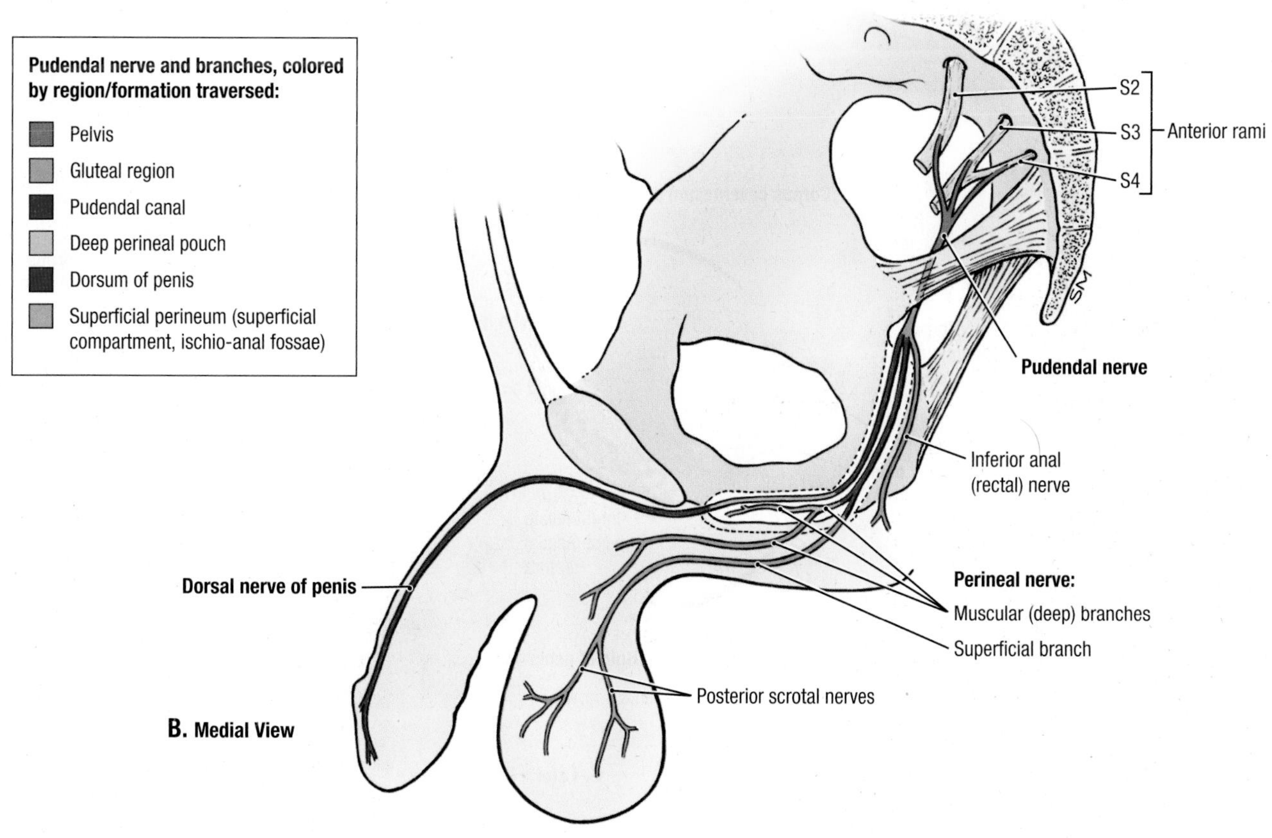
Pudendal nerve and branches, colored by region/formation traversed:
Pelvis
Gluteal region
Pudendal canal
Deep perineal pouch
Dorsum of penis
Superficial perineum (superficial compartment, ischio-anal fossae)
S2
S3
S4
Anterior rami
Pudendal nerve
Inferior anal (rectal) nerve
Dorsal nerve of penis
Perineal nerve:
Muscular (deep) branches
Superficial branch
Posterior scrotal nerves
B. Medial View

3.57 LAYERS AND NERVES OF PENIS

A. Dissection. The skin, subcutaneous tissue, and deep fascia of the penis and prepuce are reflected separately. **B.** Distribution of pudendal nerve, right hemipelvis. Five regions transversed by the nerve are demonstrated.

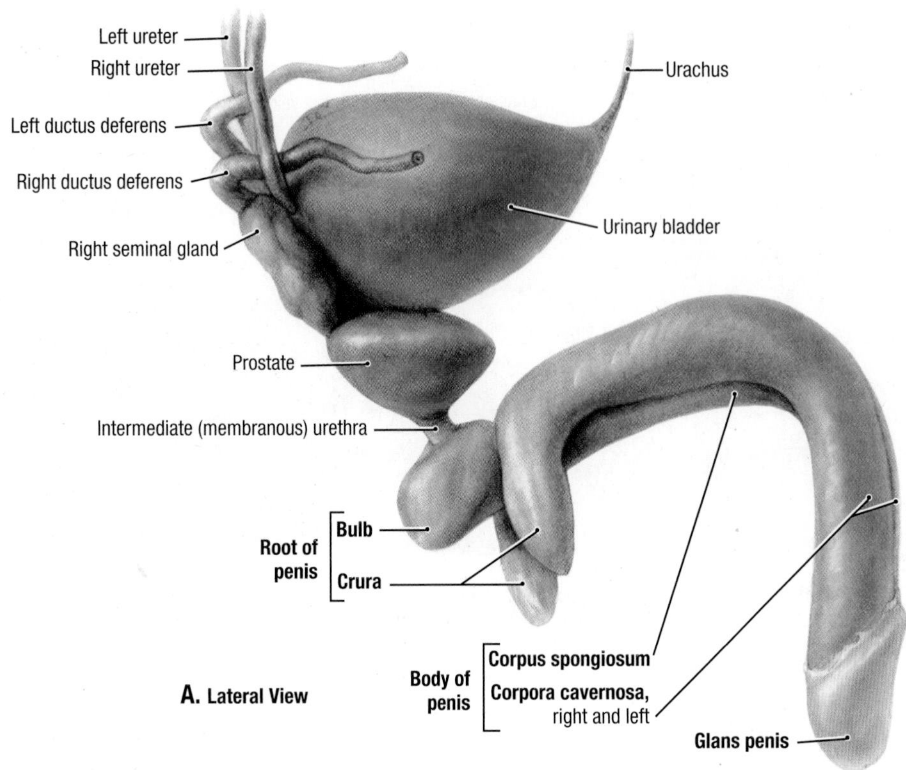
Left ureter
Right ureter
Urachus
Left ductus deferens
Right ductus deferens
Urinary bladder
Right seminal gland
Prostate
Intermediate (membranous) urethra
Root of penis
Bulb
Crura
Body of penis
Corpus spongiosum
Corpora cavernosa, right and left
Glans penis

A. Lateral View

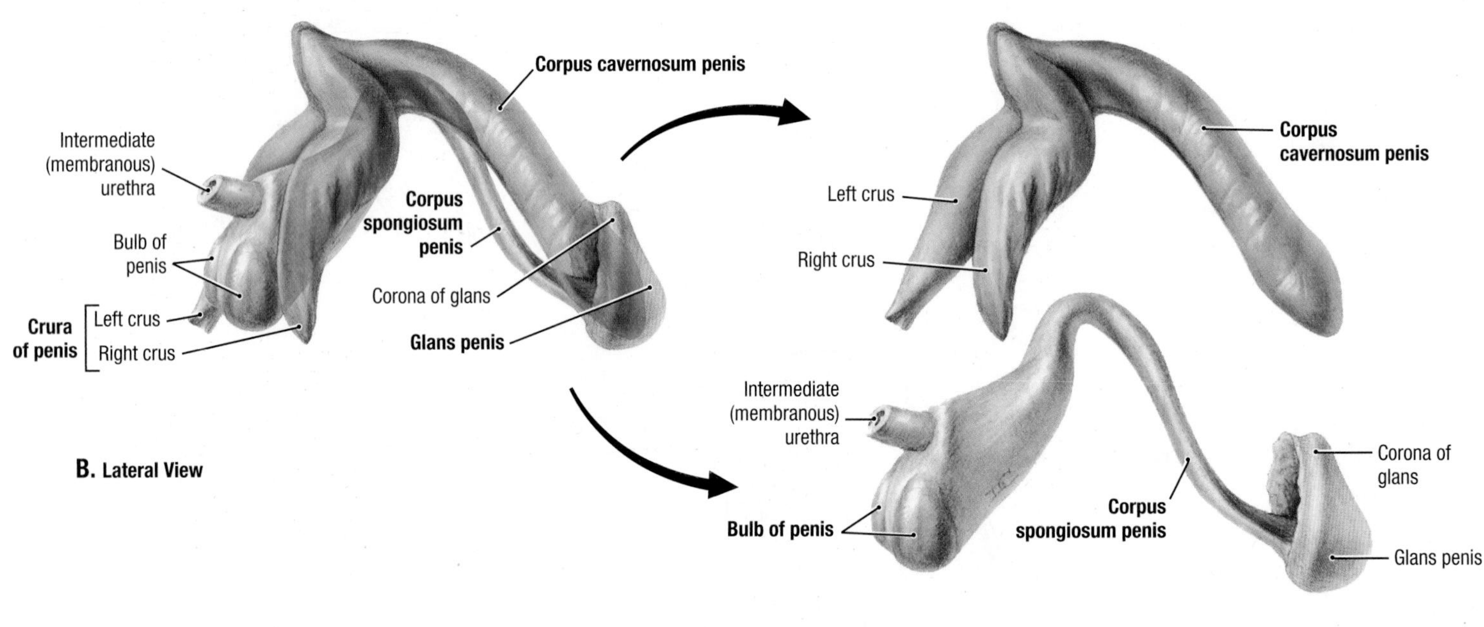
Corpus cavernosum penis
Intermediate (membranous) urethra
Bulb of penis
Crura of penis
Left crus
Right crus
Corpus spongiosum penis
Corona of glans
Glans penis
Corpus cavernosum penis
Left crus
Right crus
Intermediate (membranous) urethra
Corona of glans
Corpus spongiosum penis
Bulb of penis
Glans penis

B. Lateral View

C. Lateral View

3.58 MALE UROGENITAL SYSTEM, ERECTILE BODIES

A. Pelvic components of genital and urinary tracts and erectile bodies of perineum. **B.** Dissection of male erectile bodies (corpora cavernosa and corpus spongiosum). **C.** Corpus spongiosum and corpora cavernosa, separated. The corpora cavernosa are bent where the penis is suspended by the suspensory ligament of the penis from the pubic symphysis. The corpus spongiosum extends posteriorly as the bulb of the penis and terminates anteriorly as the glans.

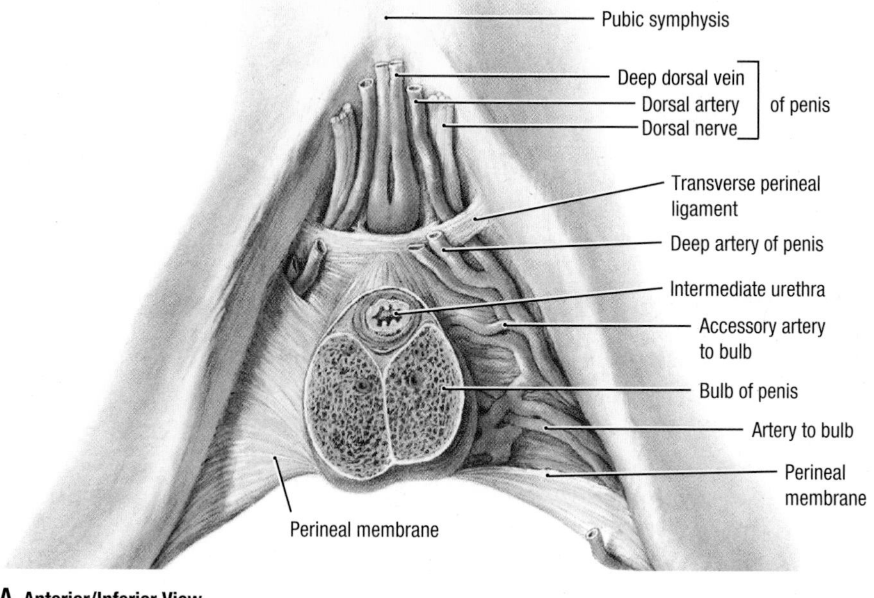
Pubic symphysis
Deep dorsal vein
Dorsal artery
Dorsal nerve
of penis
Transverse perineal ligament
Deep artery of penis
Intermediate urethra
Accessory artery to bulb
Bulb of penis
Artery to bulb
Perineal membrane
Perineal membrane

A. Anterior/Inferior View

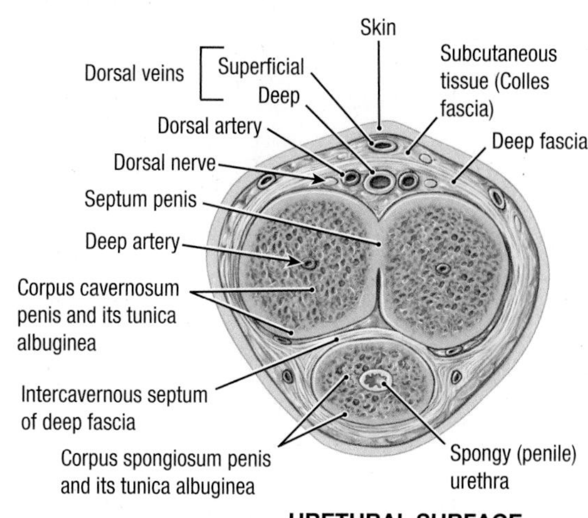
DORSUM
Skin
Dorsal veins
Superficial
Deep
Subcutaneous tissue (Colles fascia)
Dorsal artery
Deep fascia
Dorsal nerve
Septum penis
Deep artery
Corpus cavernosum penis and its tunica albuginea
Intercavernous septum of deep fascia
Corpus spongiosum penis and its tunica albuginea
Spongy (penile) urethra
URETHRAL SURFACE

C. Transverse Section

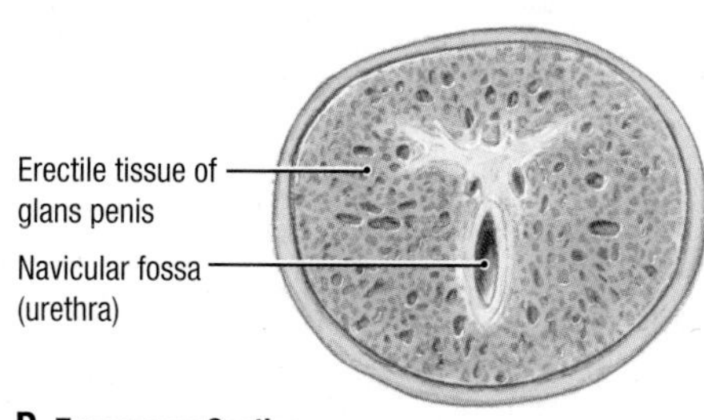
Erectile tissue of glans penis
Navicular fossa (urethra)

D. Transverse Section

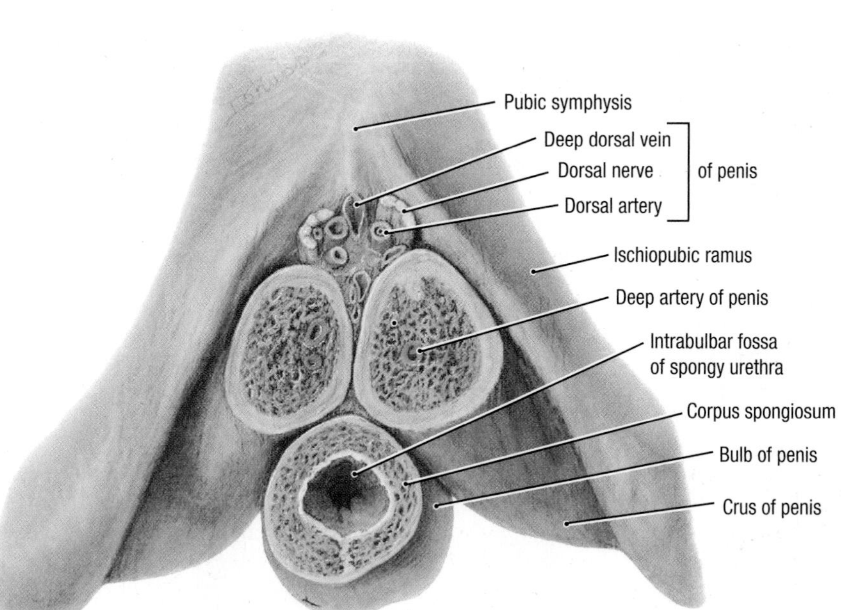
Pubic symphysis
Deep dorsal vein
Dorsal nerve
Dorsal artery
of penis
Ischiopubic ramus
Deep artery of penis
Intrabulbar fossa of spongy urethra
Corpus spongiosum
Bulb of penis
Crus of penis

B. Anterior View

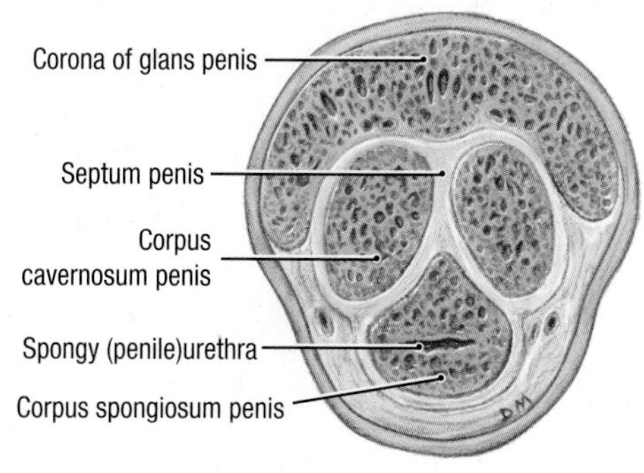
Corona of glans penis
Septum penis
Corpus cavernosum penis
Spongy (penile)urethra
Corpus spongiosum penis

E. Transverse Section

3.59 CROSS SECTIONS OF PENIS

A. Transverse section through bulb of penis with crura removed. The bulb is cut posterior to the entry of the intermediate urethra. On the left side, the perineal membrane is partially removed, opening the deep perineal compartment. **B.** The crura and bulb of penis have been sectioned obliquely. The spongy urethra is dilated within the bulb of the penis. **C.** Transverse section through body of penis. **D.** Transverse section through the proximal part of the glans penis. **E.** Transverse section through the distal part of the glans penis.

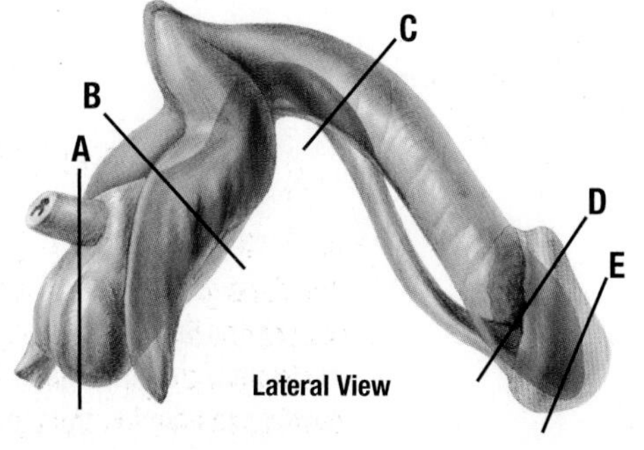
A
B
C
D
E
Lateral View

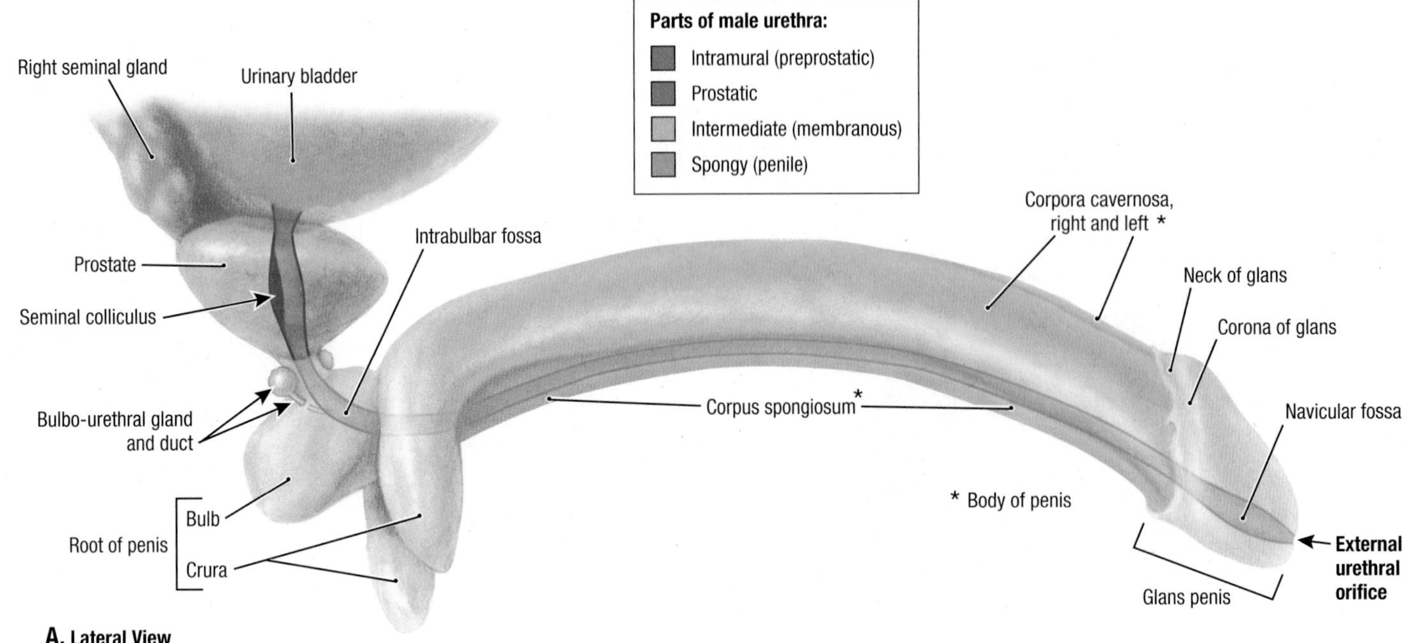
Parts of male urethra:
Intramural (preprostatic)
Prostatic
Intermediate (membranous)
Spongy (penile)
Right seminal gland
Urinary bladder
Prostate
Seminal colliculus
Intrabulbar fossa
Bulbo-urethral gland and duct
Root of penis
Bulb
Crura
Corpora cavernosa, right and left *
Neck of glans
Corona of glans
Corpus spongiosum*
Navicular fossa
* Body of penis
External urethral orifice
Glans penis

A. Lateral View

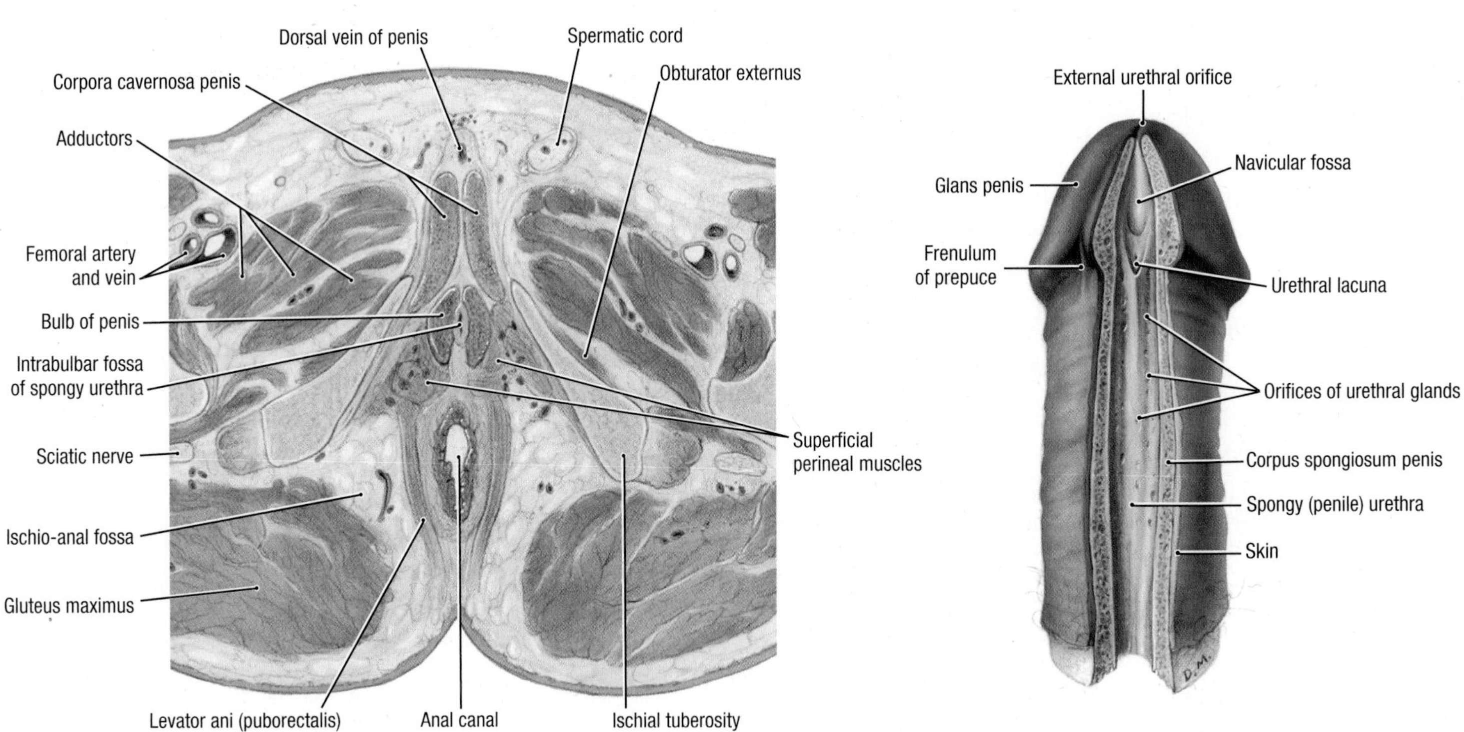
Dorsal vein of penis
Spermatic cord
Obturator externus
Corpora cavernosa penis
Adductors
Femoral artery and vein
Bulb of penis
Intrabulbar fossa of spongy urethra
Sciatic nerve
Ischio-anal fossa
Gluteus maximus
Superficial perineal muscles
Levator ani (puborectalis)
Anal canal
Ischial tuberosity
External urethral orifice
Glans penis
Navicular fossa
Frenulum of prepuce
Urethral lacuna
Orifices of urethral glands
Corpus spongiosum penis
Spongy (penile) urethra
Skin

B. Transverse Section, Inferior View

C. Urethal Aspect of Distal Penis

3.60 URETHRA

A. Urethra and related structures. **B.** Transverse section of body passing through the bulb of the penis. **C.** Spongy urethra, interior. A longitudinal incision was made on the urethral surface of the penis and carried through the floor of the urethra, allowing a view of the dorsal surface of the interior of the urethra.

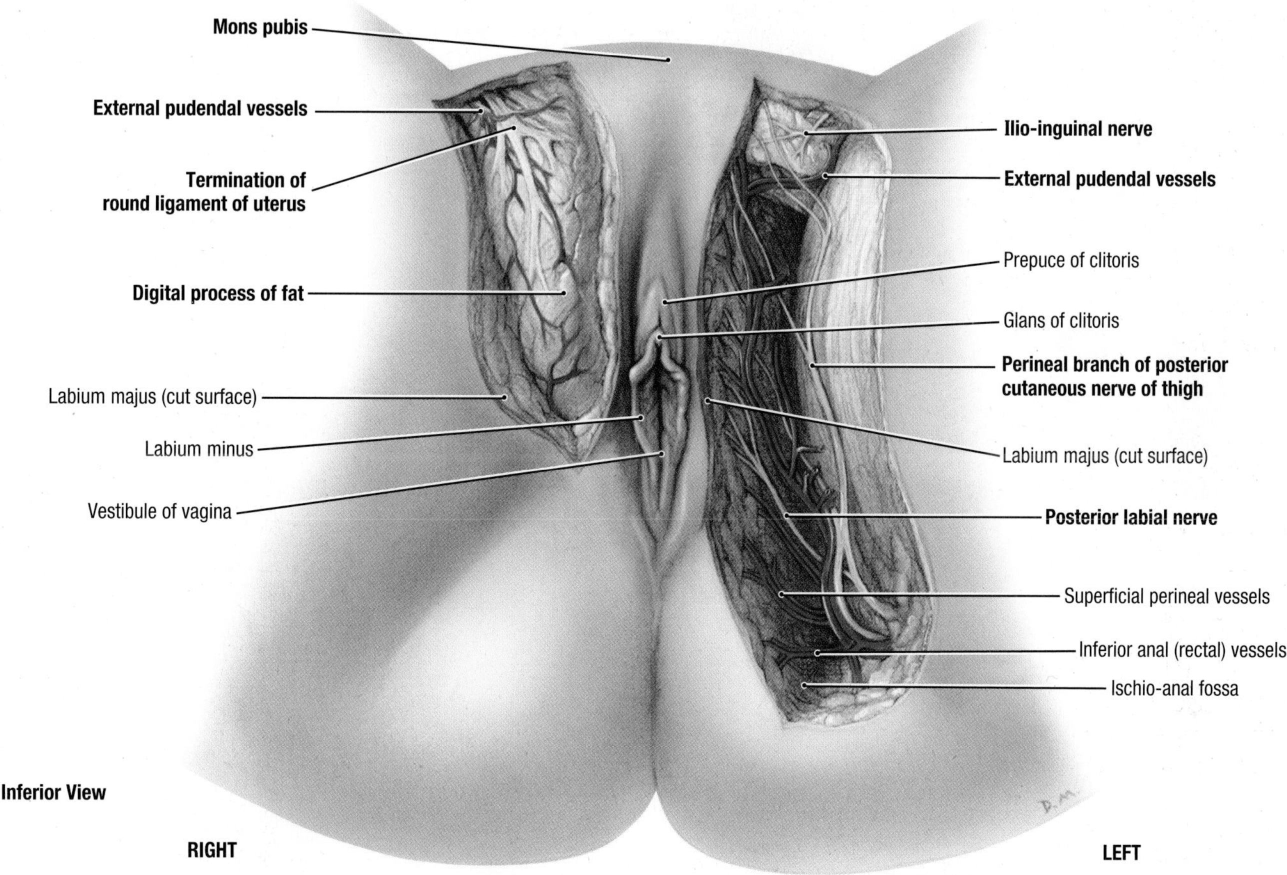
Mons pubis
External pudendal vessels
Termination of round ligament of uterus
Digital process of fat
Labium majus (cut surface)
Labium minus
Vestibule of vagina
Ilio-inguinal nerve
External pudendal vessels
Prepuce of clitoris
Glans of clitoris
Perineal branch of posterior cutaneous nerve of thigh
Labium majus (cut surface)
Posterior labial nerve
Superficial perineal vessels
Inferior anal (rectal) vessels
Ischio-anal fossa
Inferior View
RIGHT
LEFT

3.61 FEMALE PERINEUM I

Superficial dissection.

On the right side of the specimen:

- A long digital process of fat lies deep to the fatty subcutaneous tissue and descends into the labium majus.
- The round ligament of the uterus ends as a branching band of fascia that spreads out superficial to the fatty digital process.

On the left side of the specimen:

- Most of the fatty digital process is removed.
- The mons pubis is the rounded fatty prominence anterior to the pubic symphysis and bodies of the pubic bones.
- The posterior labial vessels and nerves (S2, S3) are joined by the perineal branch of the posterior cutaneous nerve of thigh (S1, S2, S3) and run anterior to the mons pubis. At the mons pubis, the vessels anastomose with the external pudendal vessels, and the nerves overlap in supply with the ilio-inguinal nerve (L1).

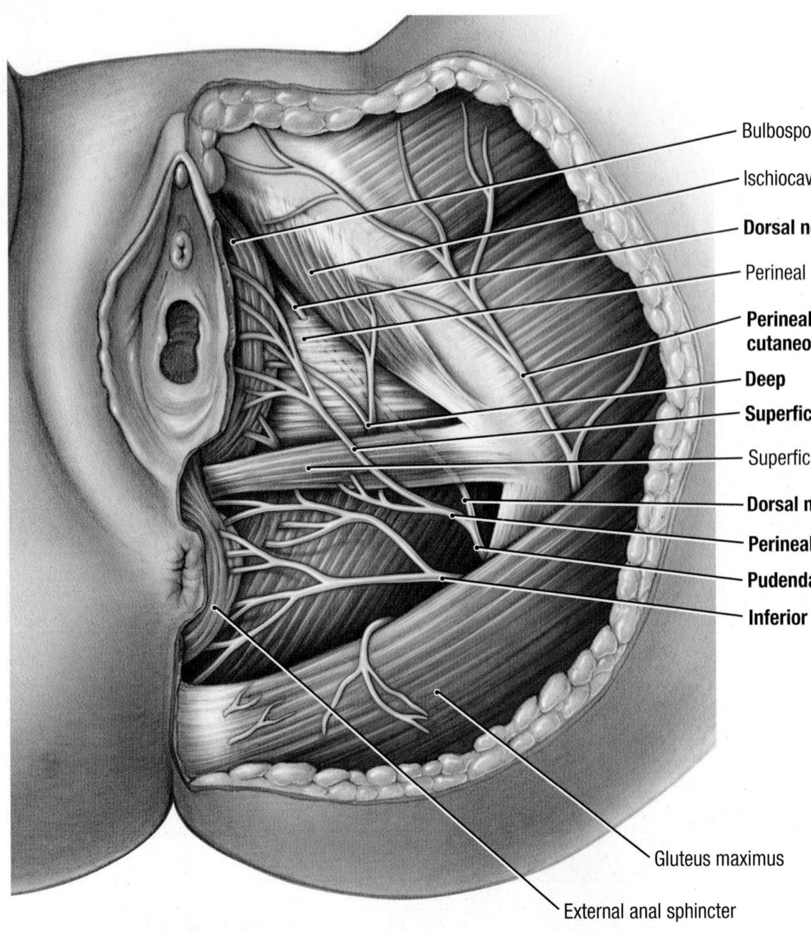
Bulbospongiosus
Ischiocavernosus
Dorsal nerve of clitoris
Perineal membrane
Perineal branch of posterior cutaneous nerve of thigh
Deep
Superficial
Branches of perineal nerve
Superficial transverse perineal
Dorsal nerve of clitoris
Perineal nerve
Pudendal nerve
Inferior anal (rectal) nerve
Gluteus maximus
External anal sphincter

A. Inferior View

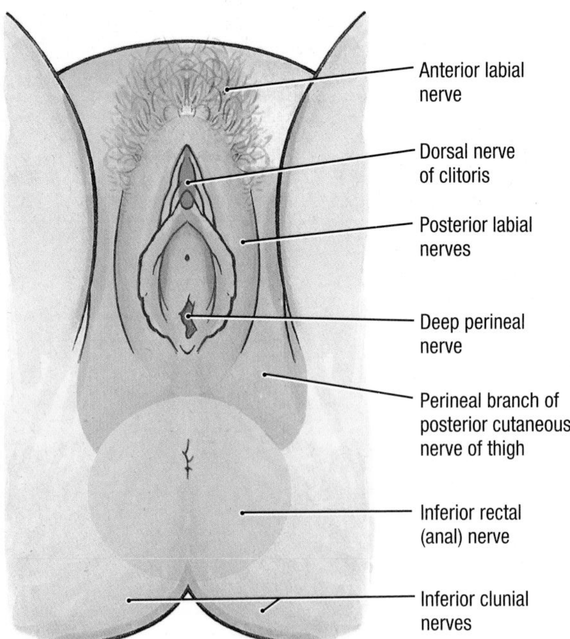
Anterior labial nerve
Dorsal nerve of clitoris
Posterior labial nerves
Deep perineal nerve
Perineal branch of posterior cutaneous nerve of thigh
Inferior rectal (anal) nerve
Inferior clunial nerves

B. Inferior View

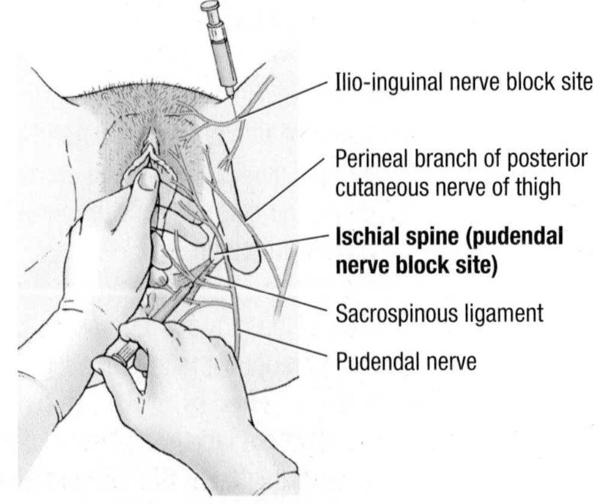
Ilio-inguinal nerve block site
Perineal branch of posterior cutaneous nerve of thigh
Ischial spine (pudendal nerve block site)
Sacrospinous ligament
Pudendal nerve

C. Inferior View

3.62 INNERVATION OF THE FEMALE PERINEUM

A. and B. The anterior aspect of the perineum is supplied by anterior labial nerves, derived from the ilio-inguinal nerve and genital branch of the genitofemoral nerve. The pudendal nerve is the main nerve of the perineum. Posterior labial nerves, derived from the superficial perineal nerve, supply most of the vulva. The deep perineal nerve supplies the orifice of the vagina and superficial perineal muscles; and the dorsal nerve of the clitoris supplies deep perineal muscles and sensations to the clitoris. The inferior anal (rectal) nerve, also from the pudendal nerve, innervates the external anal sphincter and the perianal skin. The lateral perineum is supplied by the perineal branch of the posterior cutaneous nerve of the thigh. **C.** To relieve the pain experienced during childbirth, **pudendal nerve block anesthesia** may be performed by injecting a local anesthetic agent into the tissue surrounding the pudendal nerve, near the ischial spine. A pudendal nerve block does not abolish sensations from the anterior and lateral parts of the perineum. Therefore, **an anesthetic block of the ilio-inguinal and/or perineal branch of the posterior cutaneous nerve of the thigh** may also need to be performed.

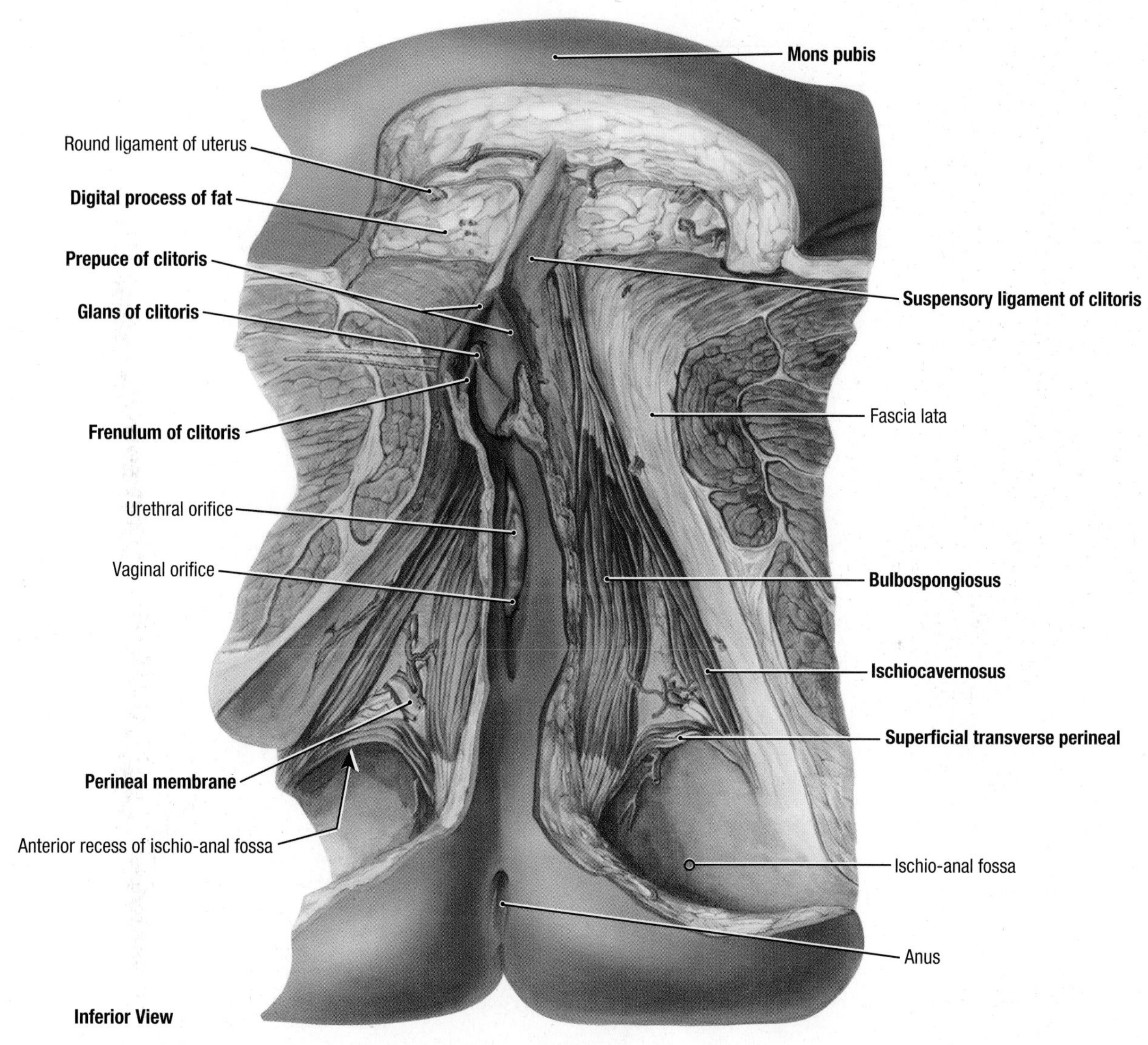
Mons pubis
Round ligament of uterus
Digital process of fat
Prepuce of clitoris
Glans of clitoris
Suspensory ligament of clitoris
Fascia lata
Frenulum of clitoris
Urethral orifice
Vaginal orifice
Bulbospongiosus
Ischiocavernosus
Superficial transverse perineal
Perineal membrane
Anterior recess of ischio-anal fossa
Ischio-anal fossa
Anus
Inferior View

3.63 FEMALE PERINEUM II

- Note the thickness of the subcutaneous fatty tissue of the mons pubis and the encapsulated digital process of fat deep to this. The suspensory ligament of the clitoris descends from the linea alba.
- Anteriorly, each labium minus forms two laminae or folds: the lateral laminae of the labia pass on each side of the glans clitoris and unite, forming a hood that partially or completely covers the glans, the prepuce (foreskin) of the clitoris. The medial laminae of the labia merge posterior to the glans, forming the frenulum of the clitoris.
- There are three muscles on each side: bulbospongiosus, ischiocavernosus, and superficial transverse perineal; the perineal membrane is visible between them.
- The bulbospongiosus muscle overlies the bulb of the vestibule and the great vestibular gland. In the male, the muscles of the two sides are united by a median raphe; in the female, the orifice of the vagina separates the right from the left.

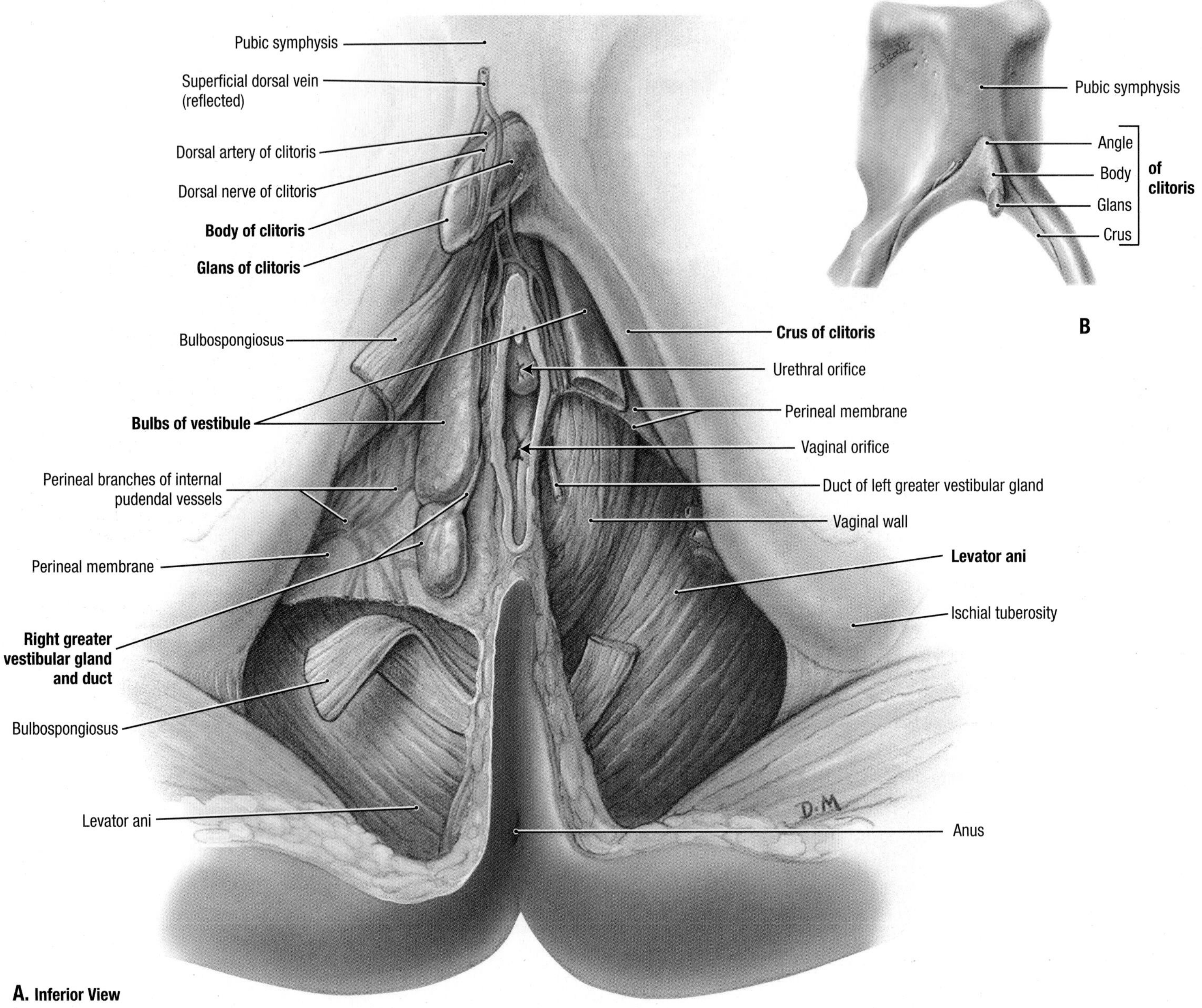
Pubic symphysis
Superficial dorsal vein (reflected)
Dorsal artery of clitoris
Dorsal nerve of clitoris
Body of clitoris
Glans of clitoris
Bulbospongiosus
Bulbs of vestibule
Perineal branches of internal pudendal vessels
Perineal membrane
Right greater vestibular gland and duct
Bulbospongiosus
Levator ani
Crus of clitoris
Urethral orifice
Perineal membrane
Vaginal orifice
Duct of left greater vestibular gland
Vaginal wall
Levator ani
Ischial tuberosity
Anus
D.M
A. Inferior View
Pubic symphysis
Angle
Body
Glans
Crus
of clitoris
B

3.64 FEMALE PERINEUM III

A. Deeper dissection. **B.** Clitoris.

In **A:**

- The bulbospongiosus muscle is reflected on the right side and mostly removed on the left side; the posterior portion of the bulb of the vestibule and the greater vestibular gland have been removed on the left side.
- The glans and body of the clitoris is displaced to the right so that the distribution of the dorsal vessels and nerve of the clitoris can be seen.
- Homologues of the bulb of the penis, the bulbs of the vestibule exist as two masses of elongated erectile tissue that lie along the sides of the vaginal orifice; veins connect the bulbs of the vestibule to the glans of the clitoris.
- On the specimen's right side, the greater vestibular gland is situated at the posterior end of the bulb; both structures are covered by bulbospongiosus muscle.
- On the specimen's left side, the bulb, gland, and perineal membrane are cut away, thereby revealing the external aspect of the vaginal wall.

In **B:**

- The body of the clitoris, composed of two crura (corpora cavernosa), is capped by the glans.

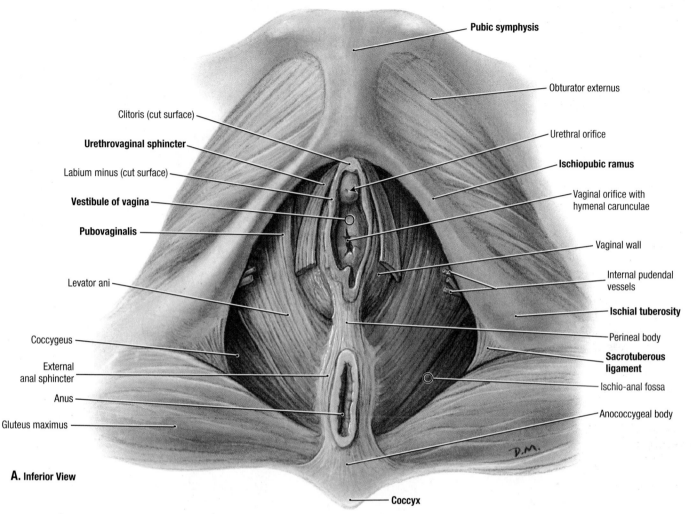

Pubic symphysis
Obturator externus
Clitoris (cut surface)
Urethrovaginal sphincter
Urethral orifice
Ischiopubic ramus
Labium minus (cut surface)
Vestibule of vagina
Vaginal orifice with hymenal caruncluae
Pubovaginalis
Vaginal wall
Levator ani
Internal pudendal vessels
Ischial tuberosity
Perineal body
Coccygeus
Sacrotuberous ligament
External anal sphincter
Ischio-anal fossa
Anus
Anococcygeal body
Gluteus maximus
Coccyx

A. Inferior View

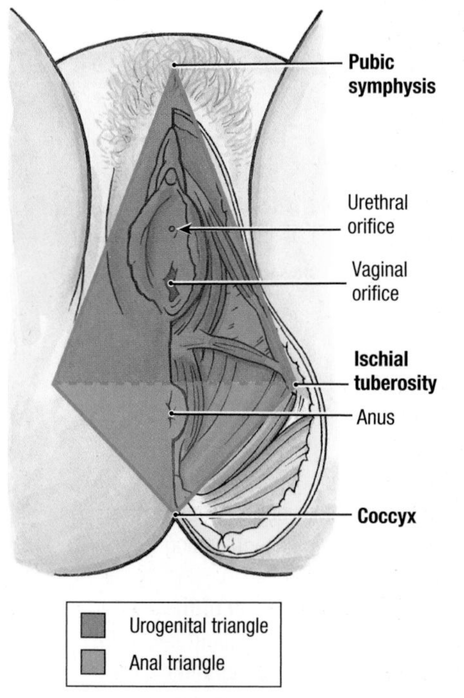
Pubic symphysis
Urethral orifice
Vaginal orifice
Ischial tuberosity
Anus
Coccyx
Urogenital triangle
Anal triangle

B. Inferior View

3.65 FEMALE PERINEUM IV

A. Deep perineal compartment. The perineal membrane and smooth muscle corresponding in position to the deep transverse perineal muscle in the male have been removed.

- The most anterior and medial part of the levator ani muscle, the pubovaginalis, passes posterior to the vaginal orifice.
- The urethrovaginal sphincter, part of the external urethral sphincter of the female, rests on the urethra and straddles the vagina.
- The labia minora (cut short here) bound the vestibule of the vagina.

A. and B. The osseoligamentous boundaries of the diamond-shaped perineum are the pubic symphysis, ischiopubic rami, ischial tuberosities, sacrotuberous ligaments, and coccyx. For descriptive purposes, a transverse line connecting the ischial tuberosities subdivides the diamond into urogenital and anal triangles.

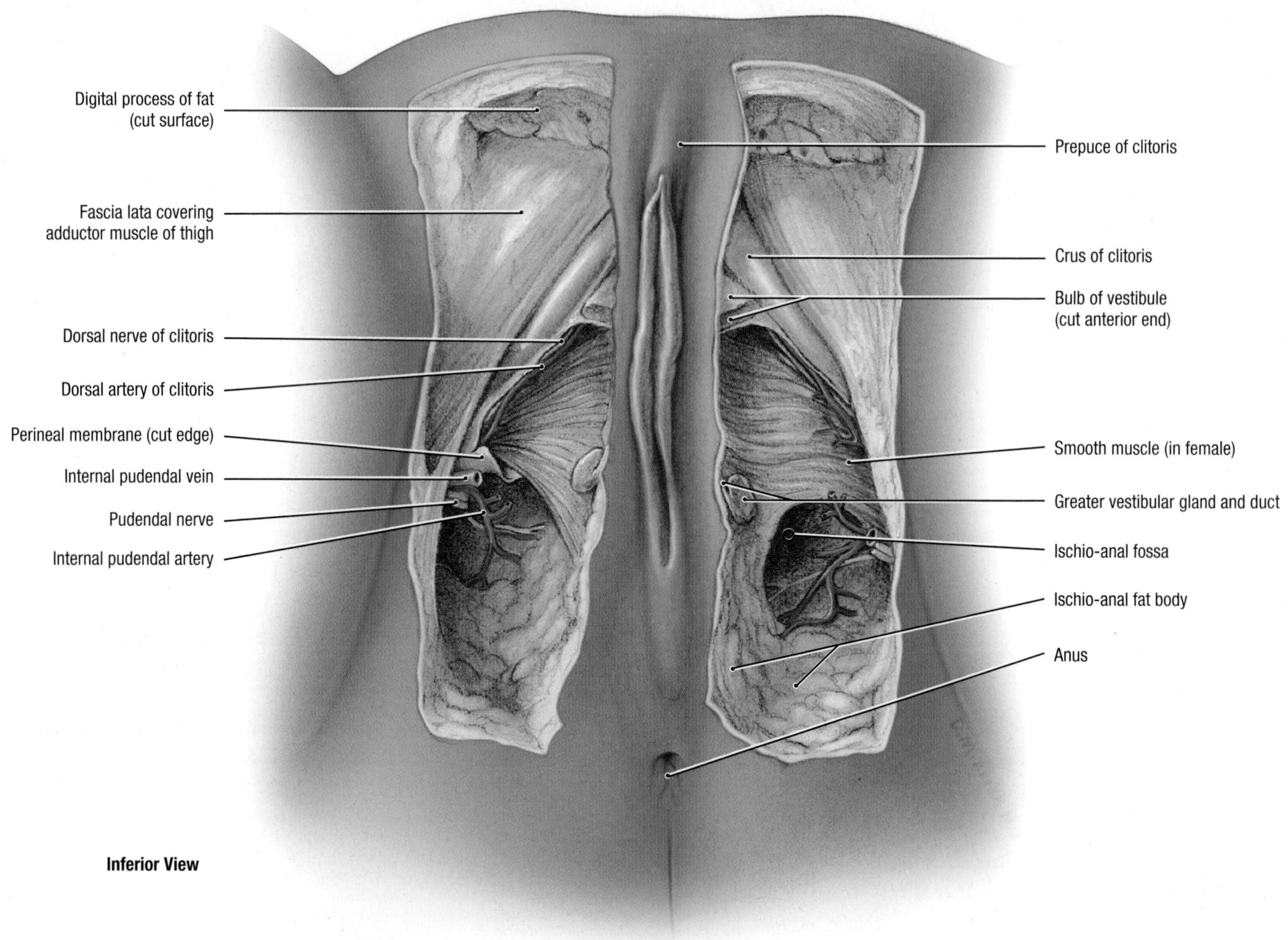
Digital process of fat (cut surface)
Fascia lata covering adductor muscle of thigh
Dorsal nerve of clitoris
Dorsal artery of clitoris
Perineal membrane (cut edge)
Internal pudendal vein
Pudendal nerve
Internal pudendal artery
Prepuce of clitoris
Crus of clitoris
Bulb of vestibule (cut anterior end)
Smooth muscle (in female)
Greater vestibular gland and duct
Ischio-anal fossa
Ischio-anal fat body
Anus
Inferior View

3.66 FEMALE PERINEUM V

This is a different dissection than the previous series, with the vulva undissected centrally but the perineum dissected deeply on each side. Although most of the perineal membrane and bulbs of the vestibule have been removed, the greater vestibular glands (structures of the superficial perineal compartment) have been left in place. The development and extent of the smooth muscle layer corresponding in position to the voluntary deep transverse perineal muscles of the male are highly variable, being relatively extensive in this case, blending centrally with voluntary fibers of the external urethral sphincter and the perineal body.

The greater vestibular glands are usually not palpable, but are so when infected. Occlusion of the vestibular gland duct can predispose the individual to **infection of the vestibular gland.** The gland is the site or origin of most **vulvar adenocarcinomas** (cancers). **Bartholinitis**, inflammation of the greater vestibular (Bartholin) glands, may result from a number of pathogenic organisms. Infected glands may enlarge to a diameter of 4 to 5 cm and impinge on the wall of the rectum. Occlusion of the vestibular gland duct without infection can result in the accumulation of mucin (**Bartholin cyst**).

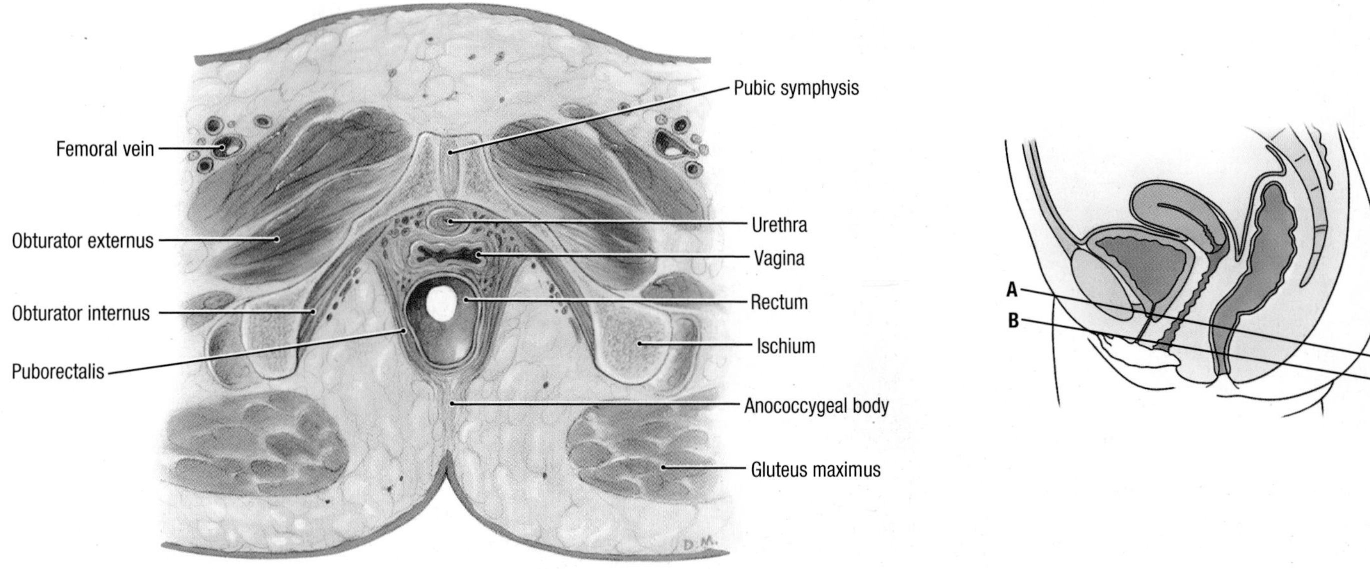
Pubic symphysis
Femoral vein
Urethra
Obturator externus
Vagina
Obturator internus
Rectum
Puborectalis
Ischium
Anococcygeal body
Gluteus maximus
A
B

A. **Transverse Section**

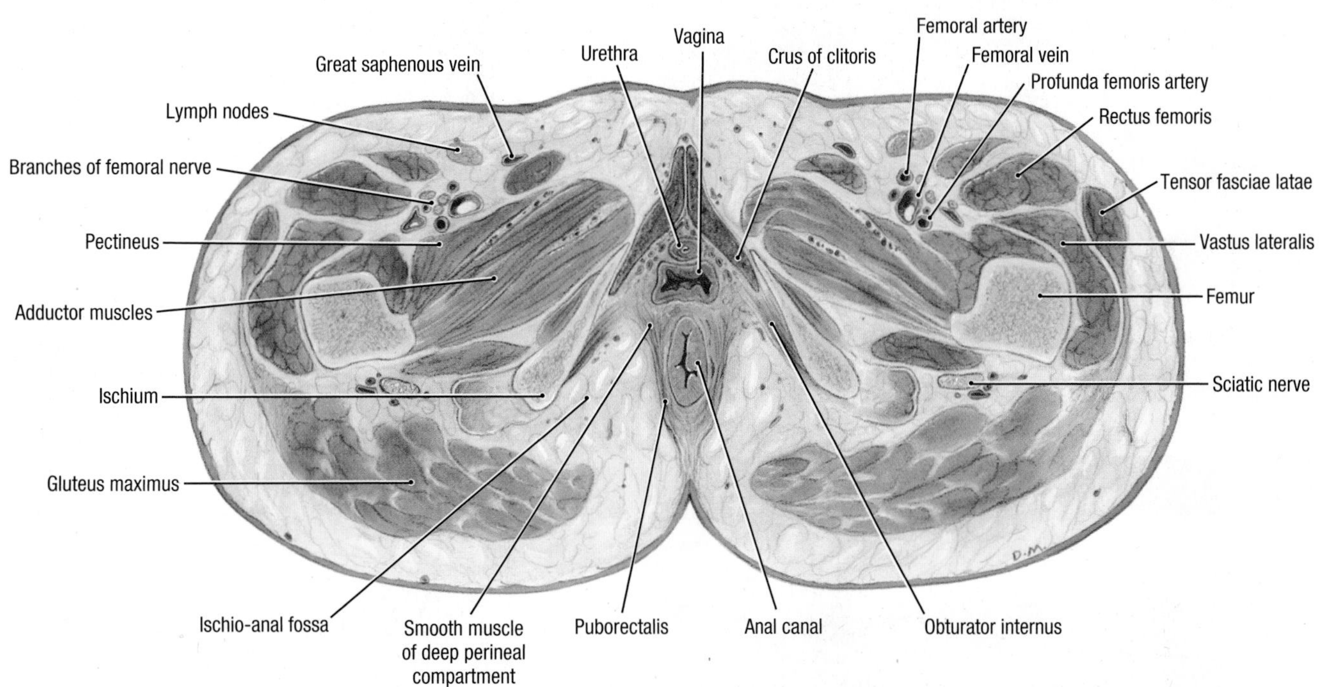
Vagina
Femoral artery
Urethra
Crus of clitoris
Femoral vein
Great saphenous vein
Profunda femoris artery
Lymph nodes
Rectus femoris
Branches of femoral nerve
Tensor fasciae latae
Pectineus
Vastus lateralis
Adductor muscles
Femur
Ischium
Sciatic nerve
Gluteus maximus
Ischio-anal fossa
Smooth muscle of deep perineal compartment
Puborectalis
Anal canal
Obturator internus

B. **Transverse Section**

3.67 FEMALE PERINEUM V

A. Section through vagina and urethra at base of urinary bladder. **B.** Section through vagina, urethra, and crura of clitoris.

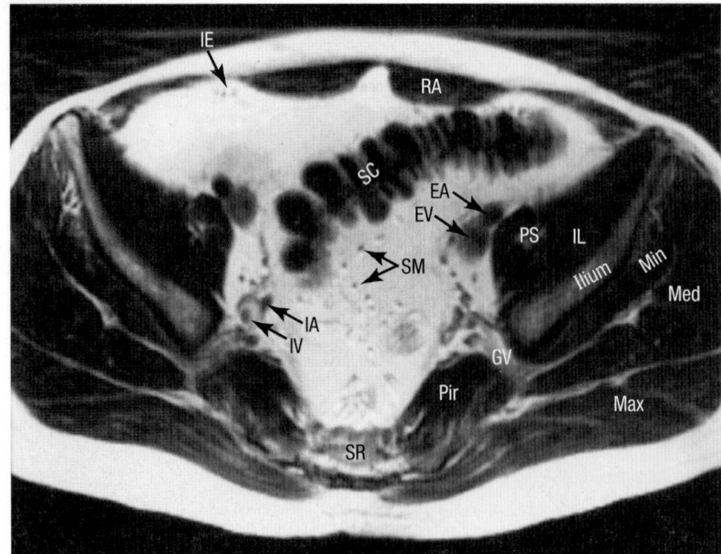
IE
RA
SC
EA
EV
SM
PS
IL
Ilium
Min
Med
IA
IV
GV
Pir
Max
SR

A

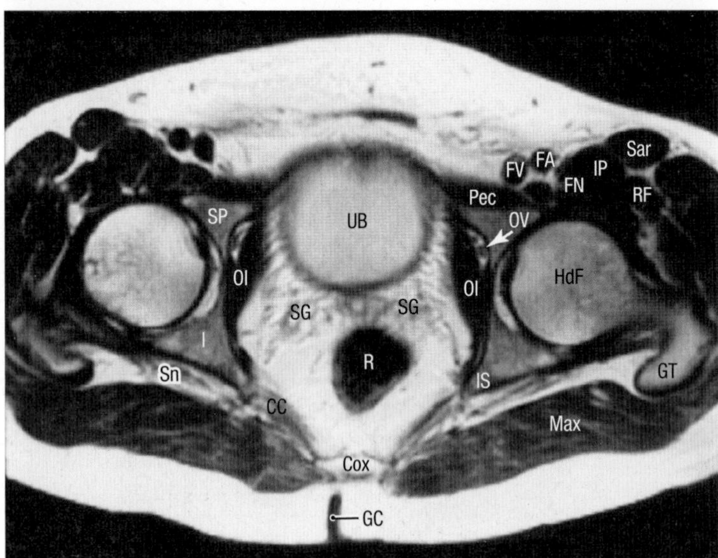
FV
FA
IP
Sar
FN
RF
Pec
SP
UB
OV
OI
OI
HdF
SG
SG
I
R
Sn
IS
GT
CC
Max
Cox
GC

B

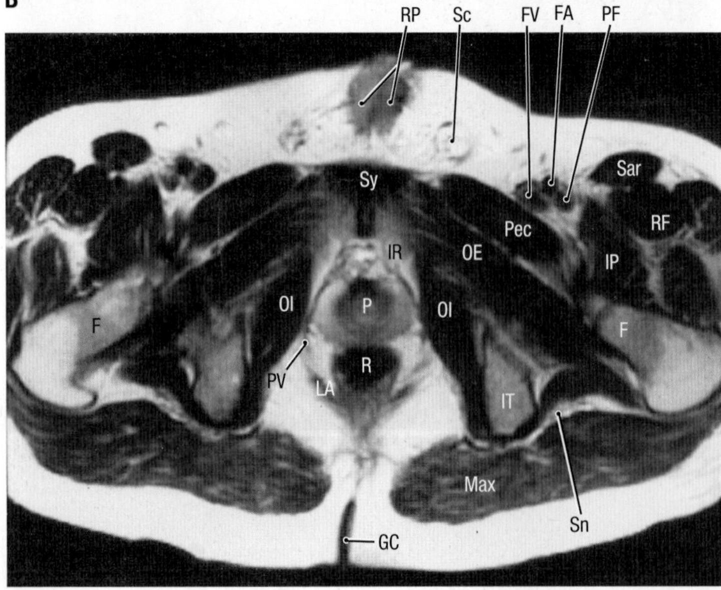
RP
Sc
FV
FA
PF
Sy
Sar
Pec
RF
IR
OE
IP
OI
P
OI
F
F
PV
LA
R
IT
Max
Sn
GC

C

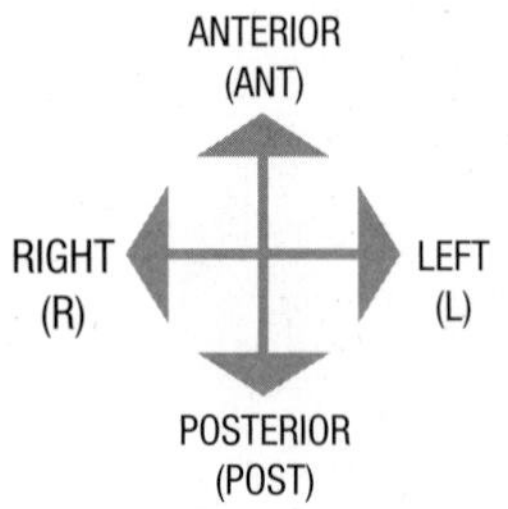
ANTERIOR
(ANT)
RIGHT
(R)
LEFT
(L)
POSTERIOR
(POST)

A	**Anus**	**LA**	**Levator ani**
Ad	Adductor muscles	Max	Gluteus maximus
Bi	Biceps femoris tendon	Med	Gluteus medius
Bu	**Bulb of penis**	Min	Gluteus minimus
Cav	**Corpus cavernosum penis**	OE	Obturator externus
CC	Coccygeus	OI	Obturator internus
Cox	Coccyx	OV	Obturator vessels and nerve
Cr	**Crus of penis**		
DD	Ductus deferens	**P**	**Prostate**
DVP	Dorsal vein of penis	**PB**	**Perineal body**
EA	External iliac artery	Pec	Pectineus
EAS	External anal sphincter	PF	Profunda femoris artery
EV	External iliac vein	Pir	Piriformis
F	Femur	**PR**	**Puborectalis**
FA	Femoral artery	PS	Psoas
FN	Femoral nerve	PV	Pudenal vessels and nerves
FV	Femoral vein	QF	Quadratus femoris
GC	Gluteal cleft	**R**	**Rectum**
GSV	Great saphenous vein	RA	Rectus abdominis
GT	Greater trochanter	RF	Rectus femoris
GV	Superior gluteal vein	**RP**	**Root of penis**
HdF	Head of femur	Sar	Sartorius
I	Body of ischium	Sc	Spermatic cord
IA	Internal iliac artery	SC	Sigmoid colon
IAF	**Ischio-anal fossa (pararectal fat)**	**SG**	**Seminal gland**
		SM	Sigmoidal vessels in mesentery of sigmoid colon
IC	**Ischiocavernosus**		
IE	Inferior epigastric vessels	Sn	Sciatic nerve
IL	Iliacus	SP	Superior ramus of pubis
IP	Iliopsoas	SR	Sacrum
IPR	Ischiopubic ramus	Sy	Pubic symphysis
IR	Inferior pubic ramus	**U**	**Urethra**
IS	Ischial spine	**UB**	**Urinary bladder**
IT	Ischial tuberosity	VI	Vastus intermedius
IV	Internal iliac vein		

(Organs/structures of male pelvis and perineum are in boldface)

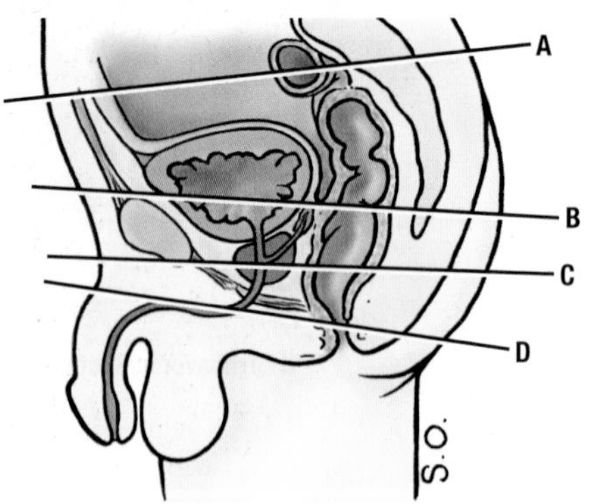
A
B
C
D
S.O.

3.68 TRANSVERSE (AXIAL) MRIs AND SECTIONAL SPECIMEN OF MALE PELVIS AND PERINEUM, INFERIOR VIEWS

A.–D. MRIs. **E.** Anatomical section.

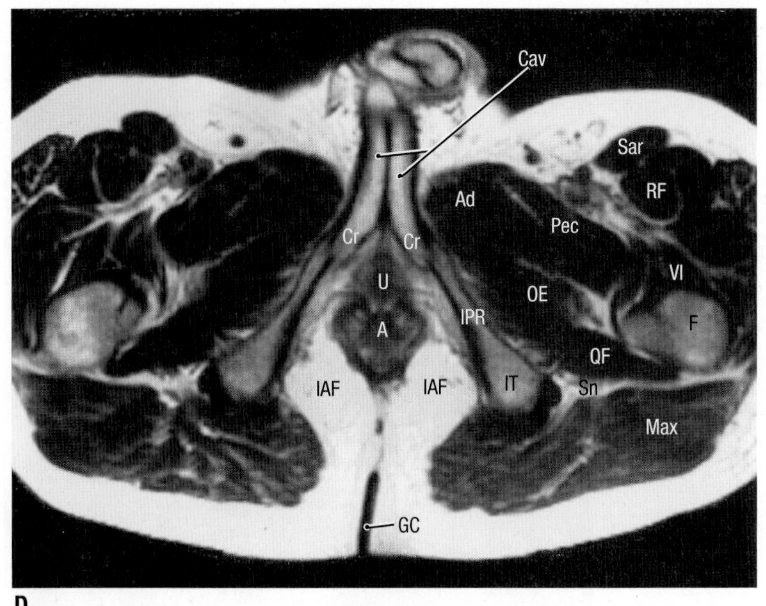
Cav
Sar
Ad
RF
Pec
Cr
Cr
VI
U
OE
A
IPR
F
QF
IAF
IAF
IT
Sn
Max
GC

D

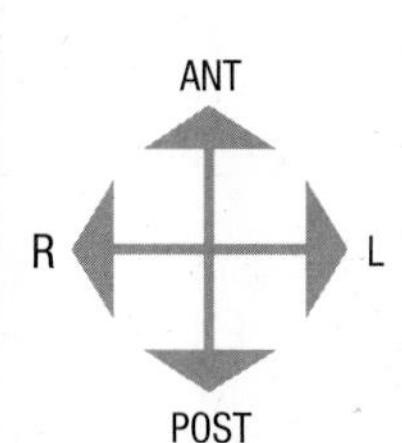
ANT
R
L
POST

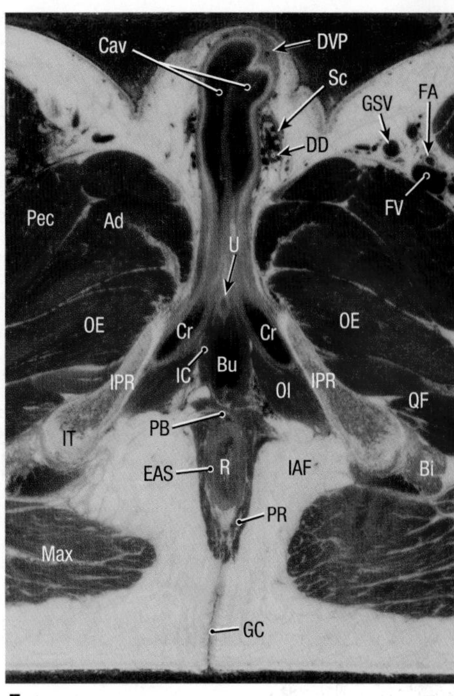
Cav
DVP
Sc
GSV
FA
DD
FV
Pec
Ad
U
OE
Cr
Cr
OE
IC
Bu
IPR
OI
IPR
QF
PB
IT
EAS
R
IAF
Bi
PR
Max
GC

E

3.68 TRANSVERSE (AXIAL) MRIs AND SECTIONAL SPECIMEN OF MALE PELVIS AND PERINEUM, INFERIOR VIEWS *(CONTINUED)*

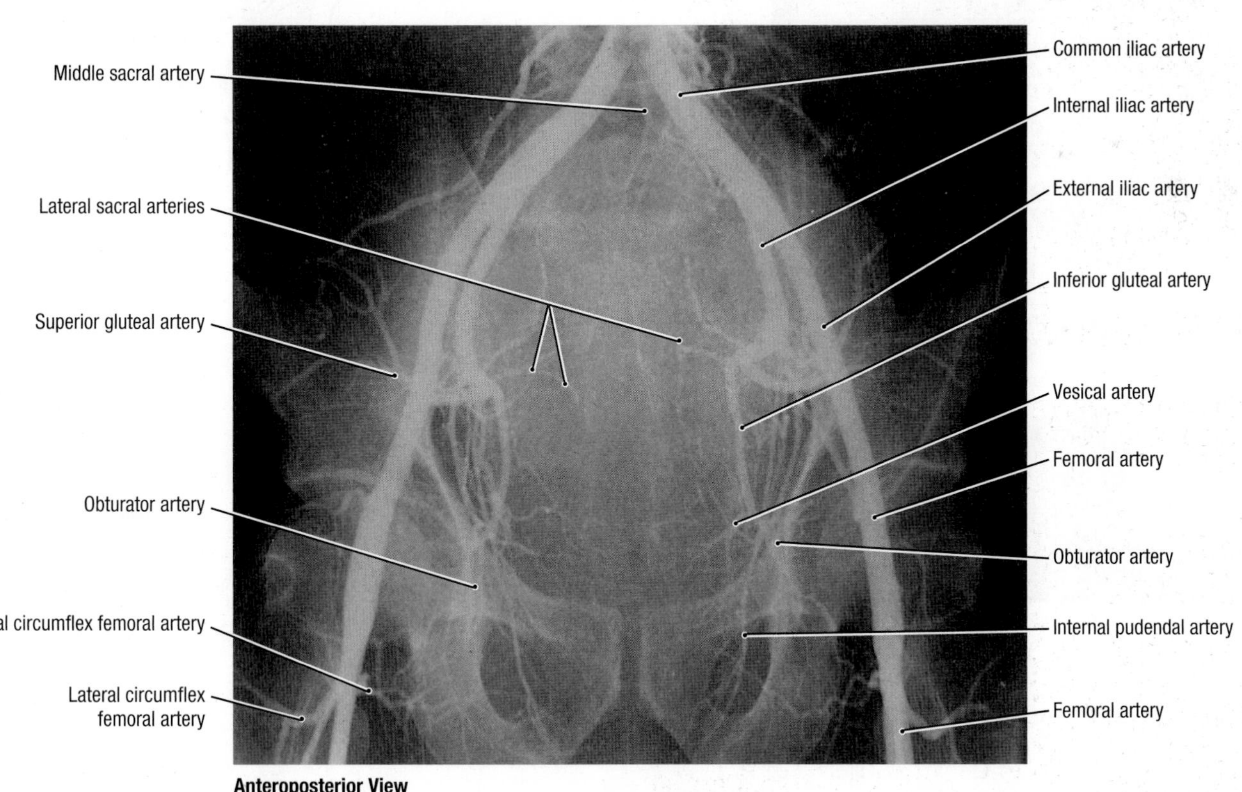
Middle sacral artery
Common iliac artery
Internal iliac artery
Lateral sacral arteries
External iliac artery
Inferior gluteal artery
Superior gluteal artery
Vesical artery
Femoral artery
Obturator artery
Obturator artery
Internal pudendal artery
Medial circumflex femoral artery
Lateral circumflex femoral artery
Femoral artery

Anteroposterior View

3.69 PELVIC ANGIOGRAPHY

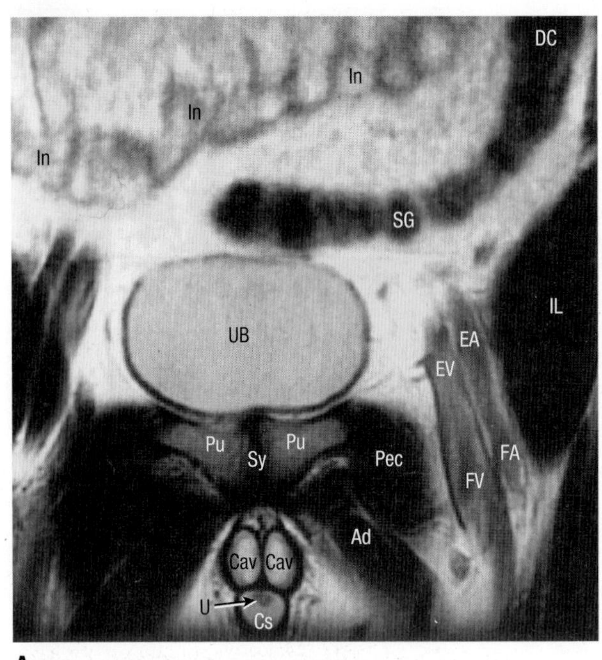

DC
In
In
In
SG
UB
EA
EV
IL
Pu
Pu
Sy
Pec
FA
FV
Ad
Cav
Cav
U
Cs

A

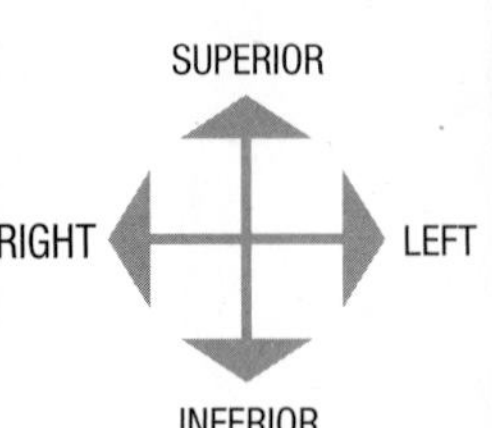

SUPERIOR
RIGHT
LEFT
INFERIOR

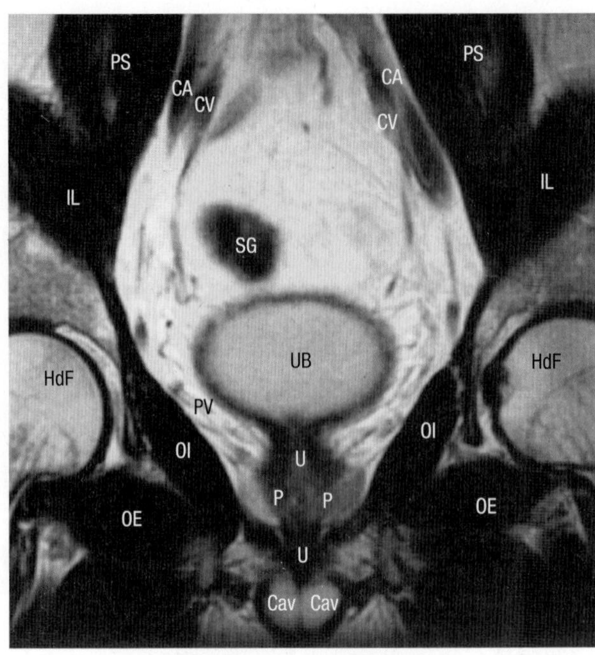

PS
PS
CA
CV
CA
CV
IL
IL
SG
HdF
UB
HdF
PV
OI
OI
U
P
P
OE
OE
U
Cav
Cav

B

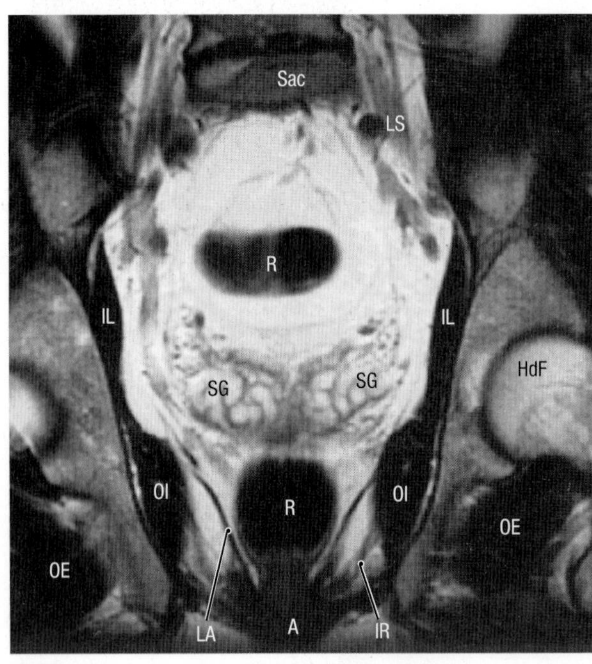

Sac
LS
R
IL
IL
HdF
SG
SG
OI
OI
R
OE
OE
LA
A
IR

C

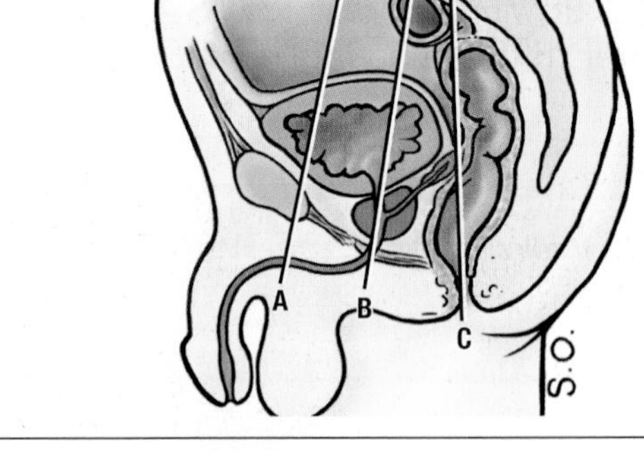

A
B
C
S.O.

A	**Anus**	LS	Lumbosacral trunk
Ad	Adductors	OE	Obturator externus
CA	Common iliac artery	**OI**	**Obturator internus**
Cav	**Corpus cavernosum penis**	**P**	**Prostate**
Cs	**Corpus spongiosum penis**	Pec	Pectineus
CV	Common iliac vein	PS	Psoas
DC	Descending colon	Pu	Pubic bone
EA	External iliac artery	**PV**	**Pelvic vessels and nerves**
EV	External iliac vein	**R**	**Rectum**
FA	Femoral artery	**Sac**	**Sacrum**
FV	Femoral vein	SC	Sigmoid colon
HdF	Head of femur	**SG**	**Seminal gland**
IL	Iliacus	**Sy**	**Pubic symphysis**
In	Small intestine	**U**	**Urethra**
IR	**Inferior rectal nerve and vessels**	**UB**	**Urinary bladder**
LA	**Levator ani**		

3.70 CORONAL MRIs OF MALE PELVIS AND PERINEUM, ANTERIOR VIEWS

MALE

FEMALE

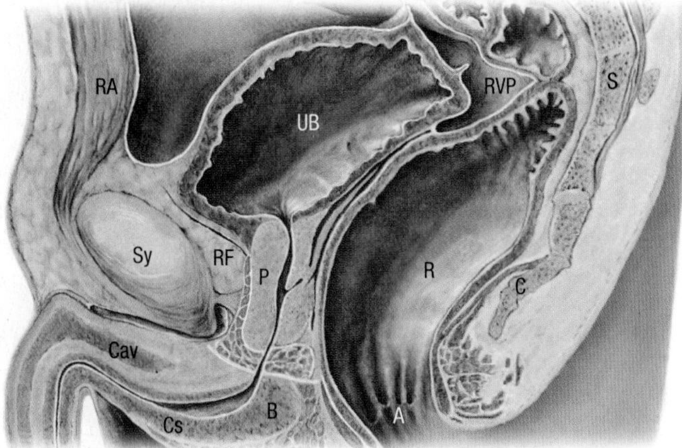
RA
UB
RVP
S
Sy
RF
P
R
C
Cav
Cs
B
A

Median Section, Male

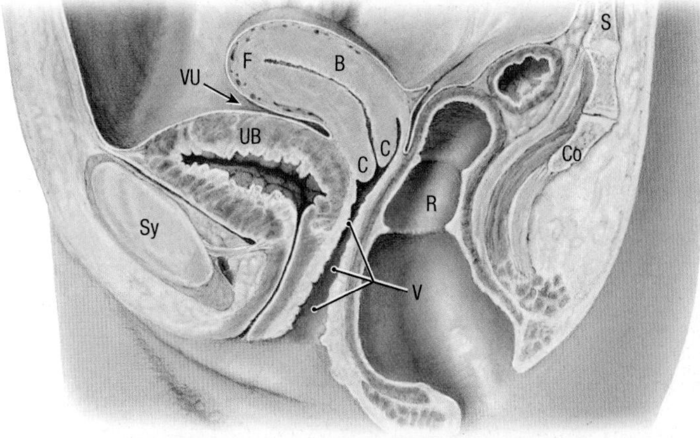
S
VU
F
B
UB
C
C
Co
R
Sy
V

Median Section, Female

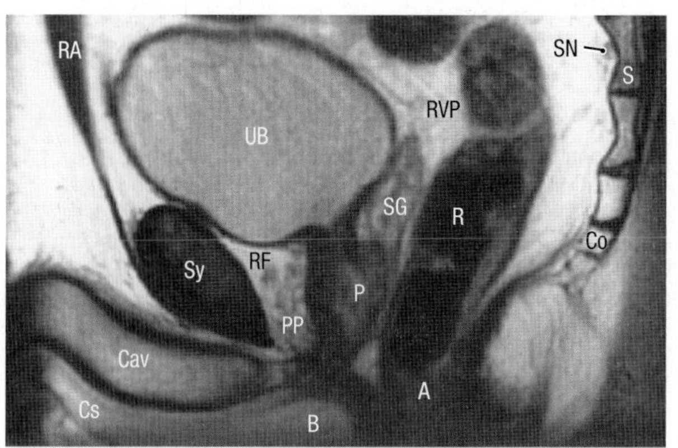
RA
SN
S
RVP
UB
SG
R
Co
Sy
RF
P
PP
Cav
A
Cs
B

Median MRI Scan, Male

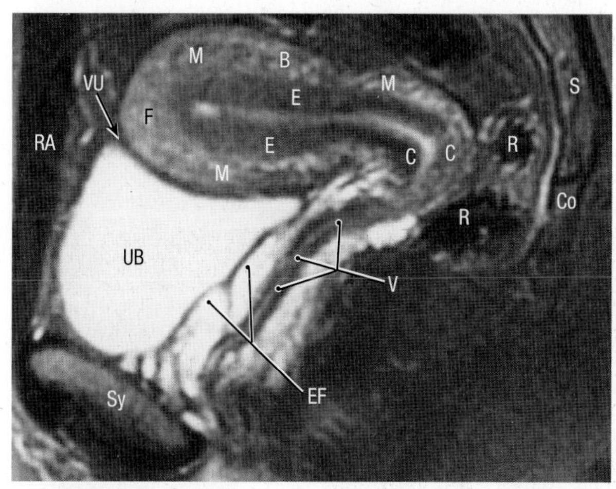
M
B
VU
E
M
S
F
RA
E
C
C
R
M
Co
R
UB
V
EF
Sy

Median MRI Scan, Female

Male:

A	Anus
B	Bulb of penis
Co	Coccyx
Cav	Corpus cavernosum penis
Cs	Corpus spongiosum penis
P	Prostate
PP	Prostatic venous plexus
R	Rectum
RA	Rectus abdominis
RF	Retropubic fat
RVP	Rectovesical pouch
S	Sacrum
SG	Seminal gland
SN	Sacral nerves
Sy	Pubic symphysis
UB	Urinary bladder

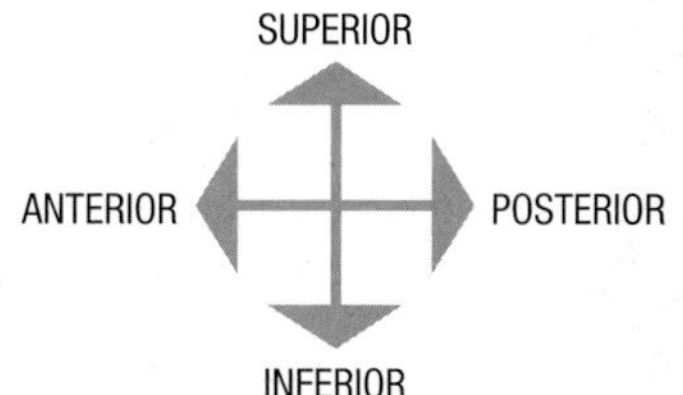
SUPERIOR
ANTERIOR
POSTERIOR
INFERIOR

Female:

B	Body of uterus
C	Cervix of uterus
Co	Coccyx
E	Endometrium
EF	Endopelvic fascia
F	Fundus of uterus
M	Myometrium
R	Rectum
RA	Rectus abdominis
S	Sacrum
Sy	Pubic symphysis
UB	Urinary bladder
V	Vagina
VU	Vesico-uterine pouch

3.71 MEDIAN MRIs OF MALE AND FEMALE PELVIS AND PERINEUM

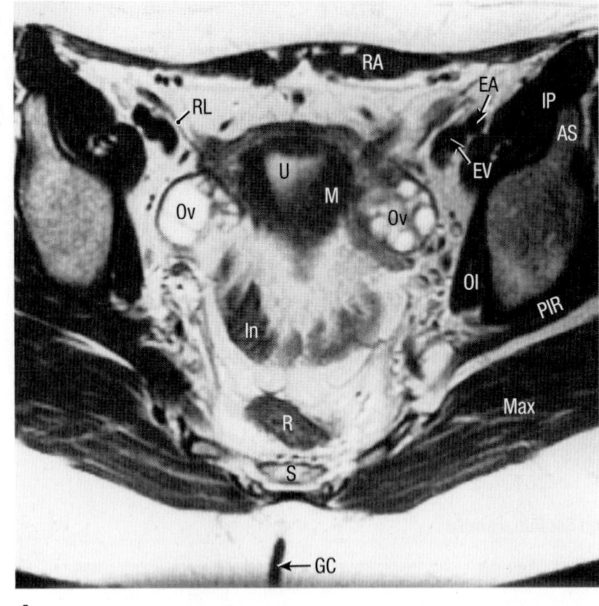
RA
RL
EA
IP
AS
EV
U
M
Ov
Ov
OI
PIR
In
Max
R
S
GC

A

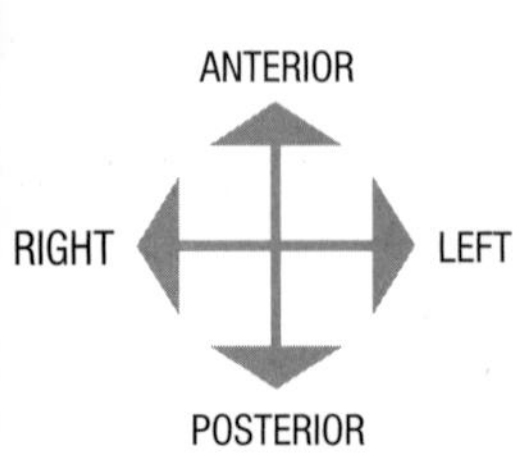
ANTERIOR
RIGHT
LEFT
POSTERIOR

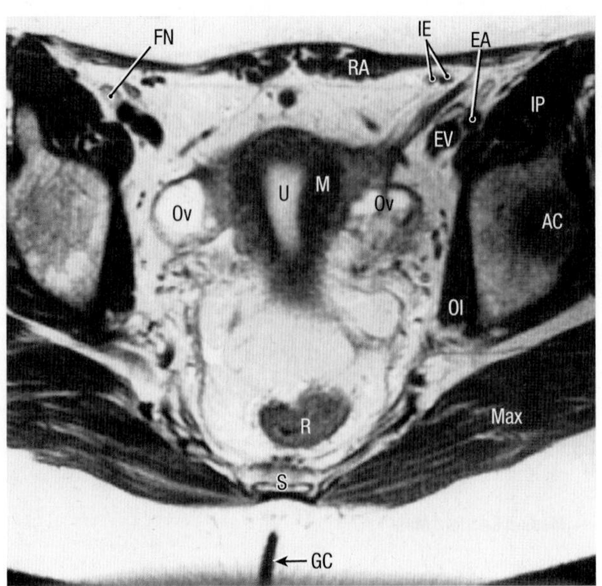
FN
IE
EA
RA
IP
EV
U
M
Ov
Ov
AC
OI
Max
R
S
GC

B

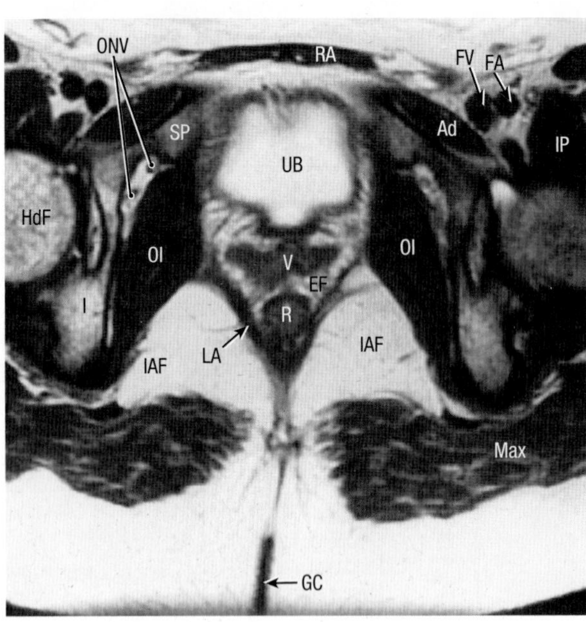
ONV
RA
FV
FA
SP
Ad
IP
UB
HdF
OI
OI
V
EF
R
I
LA
IAF
IAF
Max
GC

C

A	**Anus**	**M**	**Myometrium**
AC	Acetabulum	Max	Gluteus maximus
Ad	Adductor muscles	OE	Obturator externus
AS	Anterior superior iliac spine	**OI**	**Obturator internus**
BC	Body of clitoris	**Ov**	**Ovary**
CC	Crus of clitoris	ONV	Obturator nerve and vessels
EA	External iliac artery	Pd	Pudendal nerve and vessels
EF	Endopelvic fascia	Pec	Pectineus
EV	External iliac vein	PIR	Piriformis
FA	Femoral artery	**Pm**	**Perineal membrane**
FN	Femoral nerve	**Pu**	**Pubic bone**
FV	Femoral vein	QF	Quadratus femoris
GC	Gluteal cleft	**R**	**Rectum**
HdF	Head of femur	RA	Rectus abdominis
I	Ilium	**RF**	**Recto-uterine fold**
IAF	**Ischio-anal fossa**	**RL**	**Round ligament**
IE	Inferior epigastric vessels	**S**	**Sacrum**
In	Intestine	SP	Superior ramus of pubis
IP	Iliopsoas	Sy	Pubic symphysis
IPR	Ischiopubic ramus	**U**	**Uterus**
IT	Ischial tuberosity	**UB**	**Urinary bladder**
LA	**Levator ani**	**Ur**	**Urethra**
Lin	Linea alba	**V**	**Vagina**
LM	**Labia majus**	**Ve**	**Vestibule**

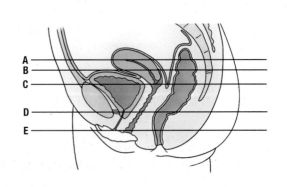

3.72 TRANSVERSE (AXIAL) MRIs AND SECTIONAL SPECIMENS OF FEMALE PELVIS AND PERINEUM, INFERIOR VIEWS

A.–C. MRIs.

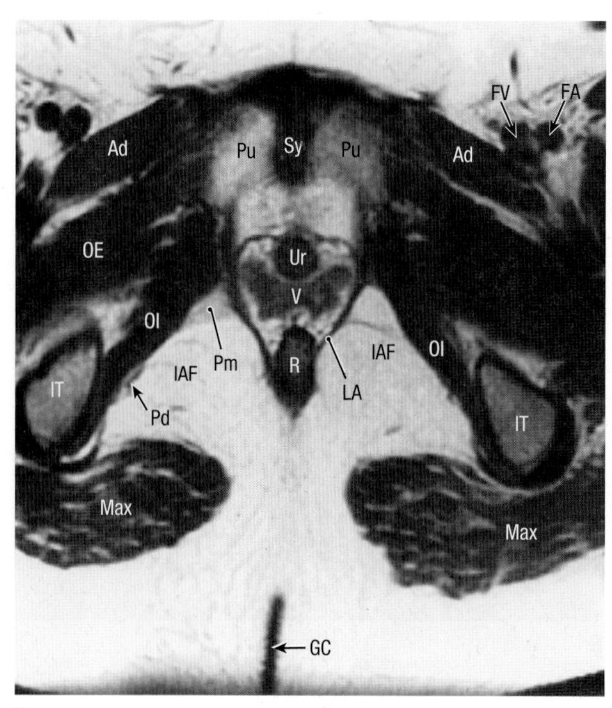
FV
FA
Ad
Pu
Sy
Pu
Ad
OE
Ur
V
OI
Pm
R
IAF
OI
IAF
LA
IT
Pd
IT
Max
Max
GC
D

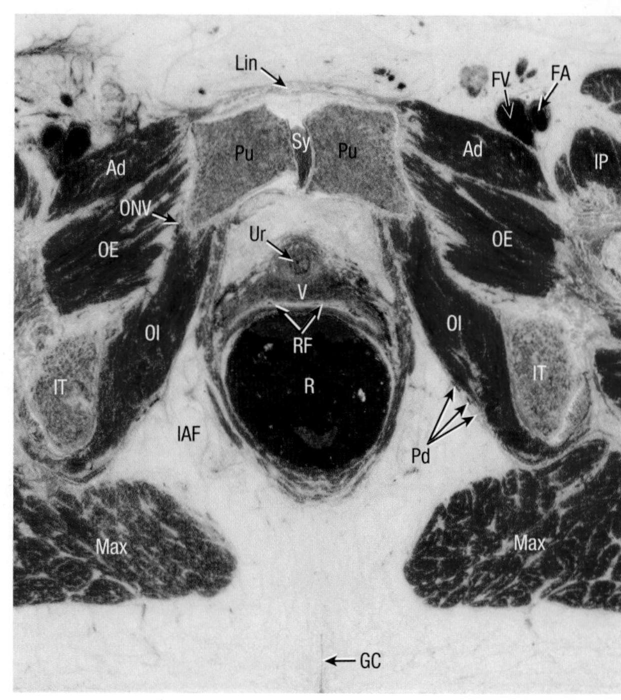
Lin
FV
FA
Ad
Pu
Sy
Pu
Ad
IP
ONV
OE
Ur
OE
V
OI
RF
OI
IT
R
IT
IAF
Pd
Max
Max
GC
E

ANTERIOR
RIGHT
LEFT
POSTERIOR

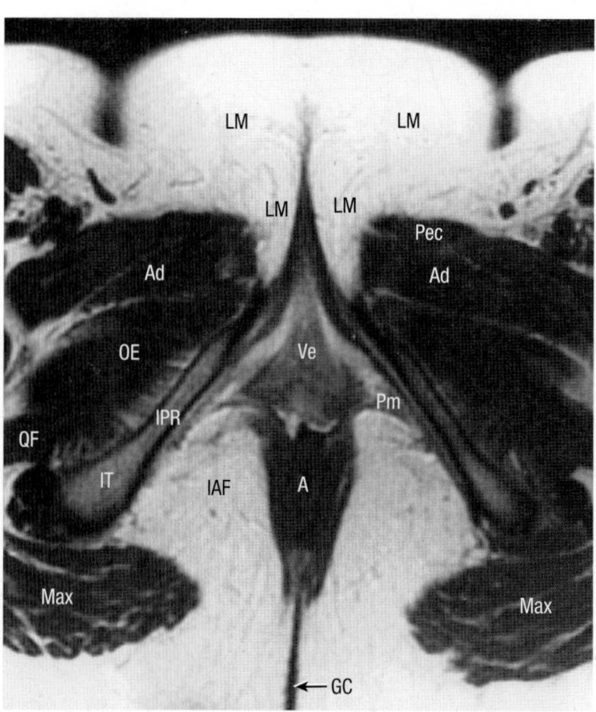
LM
LM
LM
LM
Pec
Ad
Ad
OE
Ve
Pm
IPR
QF
IT
IAF
A
Max
Max
GC
F

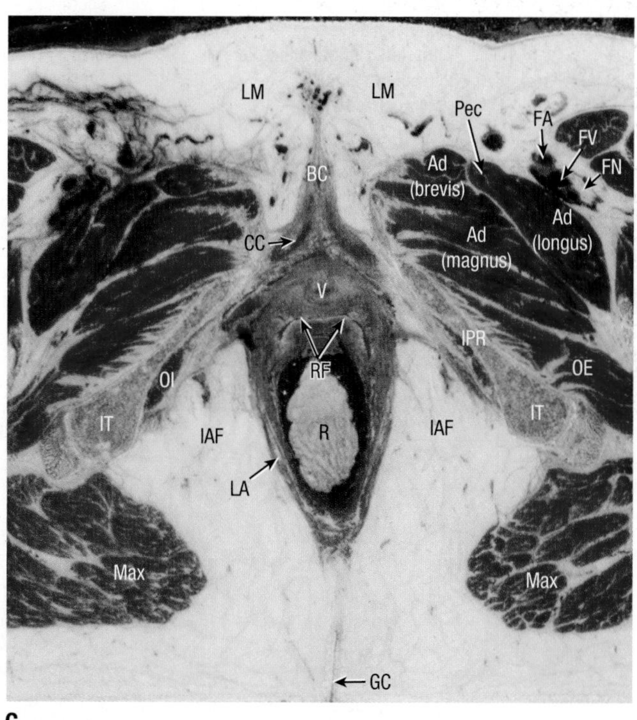
LM
LM
Pec
FA
FV
FN
BC
Ad (brevis)
Ad (longus)
CC
Ad (magnus)
V
IPR
OE
OI
RF
IT
IAF
R
IAF
IT
LA
Max
Max
GC
G

3.72 TRANSVERSE (AXIAL) MRIs AND SECTIONAL SPECIMENS OF FEMALE PELVIS AND PERINEUM, INFERIOR VIEWS *(CONTINUED)*

D. and F. MRIs. **E. and G.** Anatomical sections.

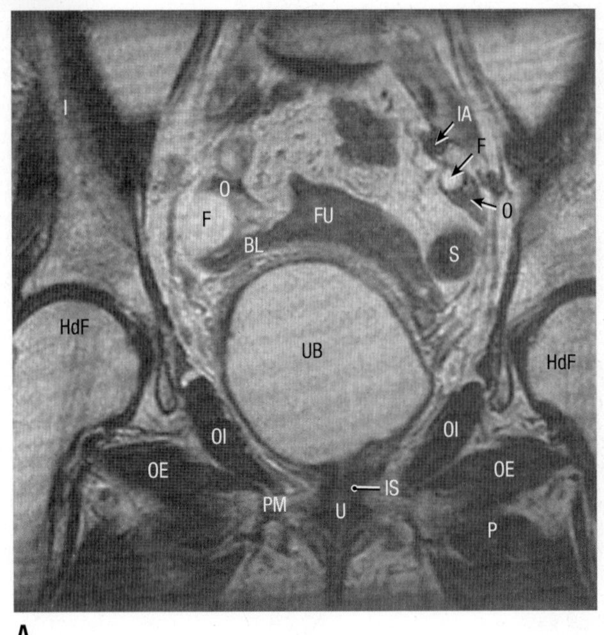
I
IA
F
O
F
O
FU
BL
S
HdF
UB
HdF
OI
OI
OE
OE
IS
PM
U
P

A

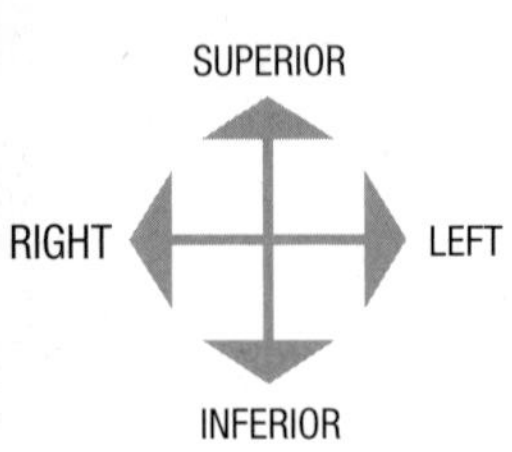
SUPERIOR
RIGHT
LEFT
INFERIOR

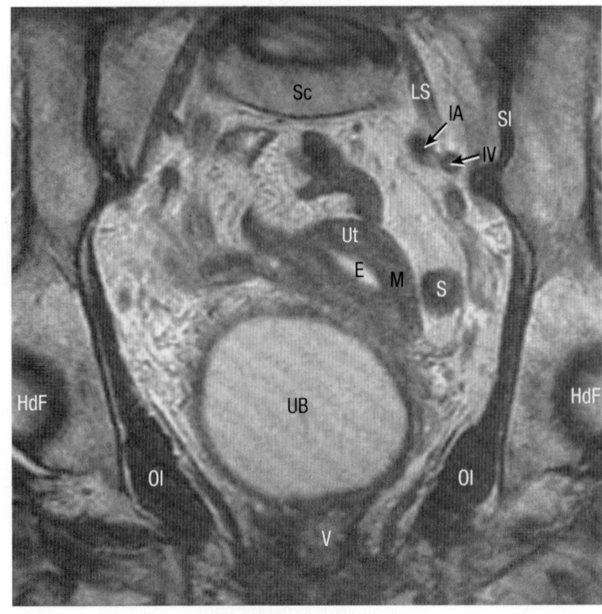
Sc
LS
IA
SI
IV
Ut
E
M
S
HdF
UB
HdF
OI
OI
V

B

BL	**Broad ligament**	OE	Obturator externus
E	**Endometrium**	**OI**	**Obturator internus**
F	**Ovarian follicle**	P	Pectineus
FU	**Fundus of uterus**	**PM**	**Perineal membrane**
HdF	Head of femur	**S**	**Sigmoid colon**
I	Ilium	**Sc**	**Sacrum**
IA	Internal iliac artery	SI	Sacro-iliac joint
IV	Internal iliac vein	**U**	**Urethra**
IS	**Internal urethral sphincter**	**UB**	**Urinary bladder**
LS	Lumbosacral trunk	**Ut**	**Uterus**
M	**Myometrium**	**V**	**Vagina**
O	**Ovary**		

A B

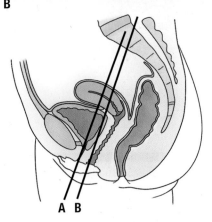

3.73 CORONAL MRIs OF FEMALE PELVIS AND PERINEUM, ANTERIOR VIEWS

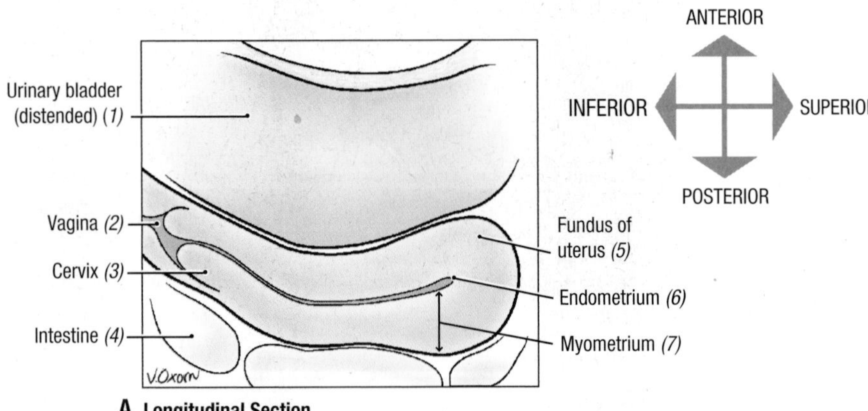
Urinary bladder (distended) (1)
Vagina (2)
Cervix (3)
Intestine (4)
Fundus of uterus (5)
Endometrium (6)
Myometrium (7)
V.Oxorn
ANTERIOR
INFERIOR
SUPERIOR
POSTERIOR

A. **Longitudinal Section**

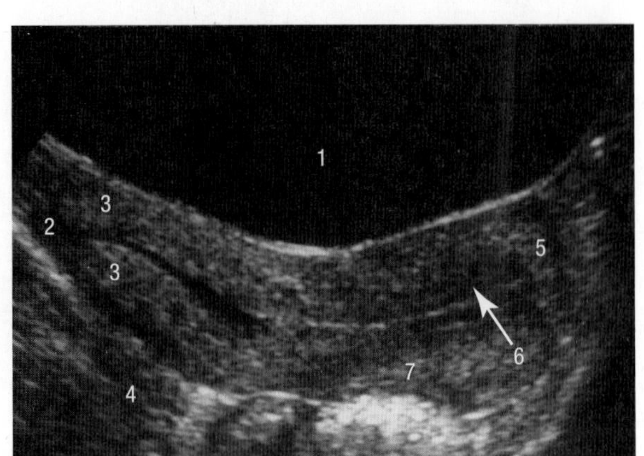
1
2
3
3
4
5
6
7

Longitudinal US Section

3.74 ULTRASOUND SCANS OF FEMALE PELVIS

A. Median (transabdominal) ultrasound scan and orientation drawing (numbers in parentheses correspond to labels on the ultrasound scan).

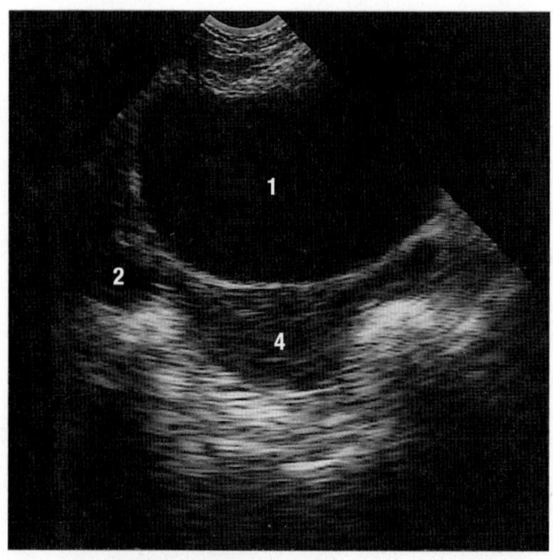
1
2
4

B. Transverse (Axial) Scan

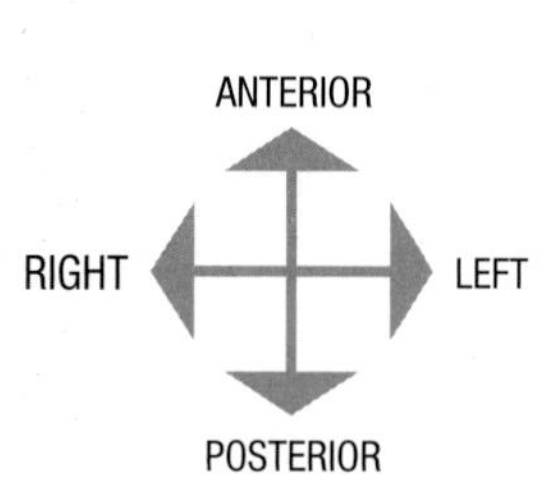
ANTERIOR
RIGHT
LEFT
POSTERIOR

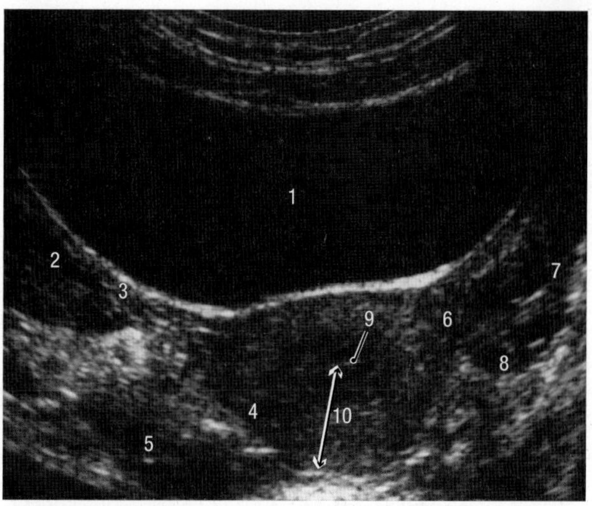
1
2
3
4
5
6
7
8
9
10

C. Transverse (Axial) Scan

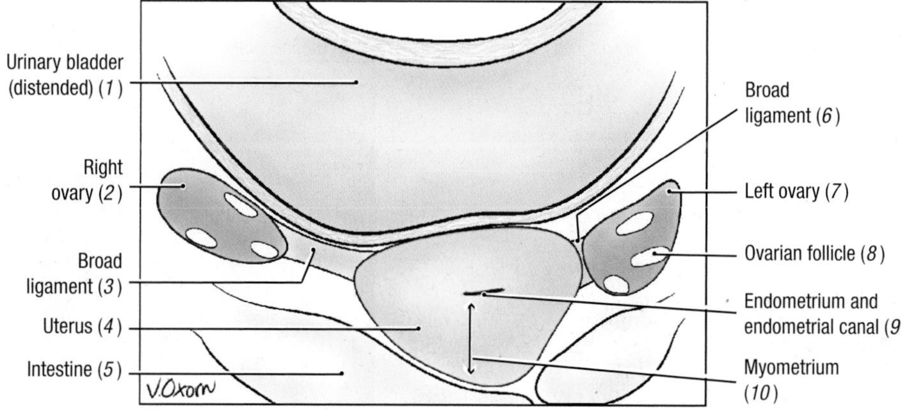
Urinary bladder (distended) (1)
Right ovary (2)
Broad ligament (3)
Uterus (4)
Intestine (5)
Broad ligament (6)
Left ovary (7)
Ovarian follicle (8)
Endometrium and endometrial canal (9)
Myometrium (10)
V.Oxorn

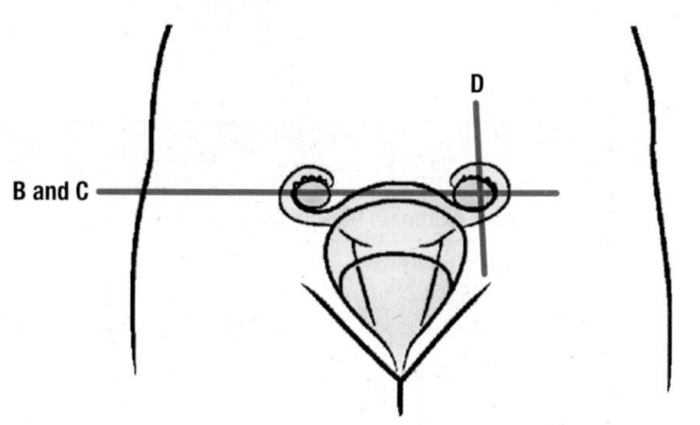
D
B and C

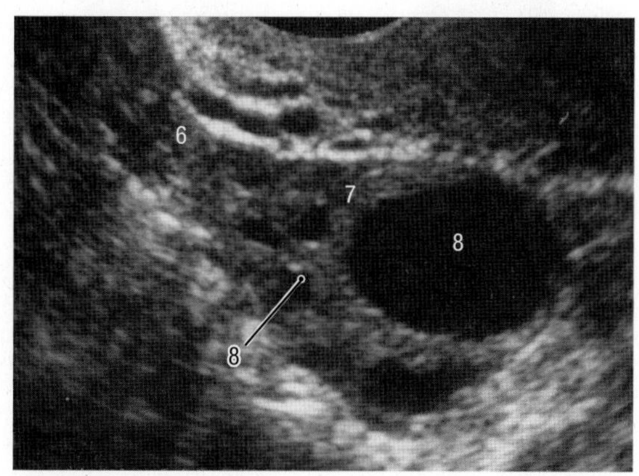
6
7
8
8

D. Sagittal Scan

3.74 ULTRASOUND SCANS OF FEMALE PELVIS *(CONTINUED)*

B. and C. Transabdominal axial (transverse) scan through uterus and ovaries. **Transabdominal US scanning** requires a fully distended urinary bladder to displace the bowel loops from the pelvis and to provide an acoustical window through which to observe pelvic anatomy.

D. Transvaginal sagittal scan of left ovary (numbers in parentheses correspond to labels on the ultrasound scans). **Transvaginal and transrectal ultrasonography** enables the placing of the probe closer to the structures of interest, allowing increased resolution.

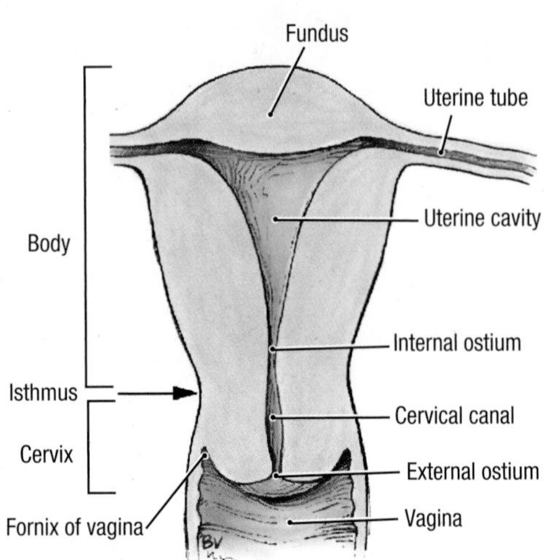
Fundus
Uterine tube
Body
Uterine cavity
Internal ostium
Isthmus
Cervical canal
Cervix
External ostium
Fornix of vagina
Vagina

A. Coronal Section

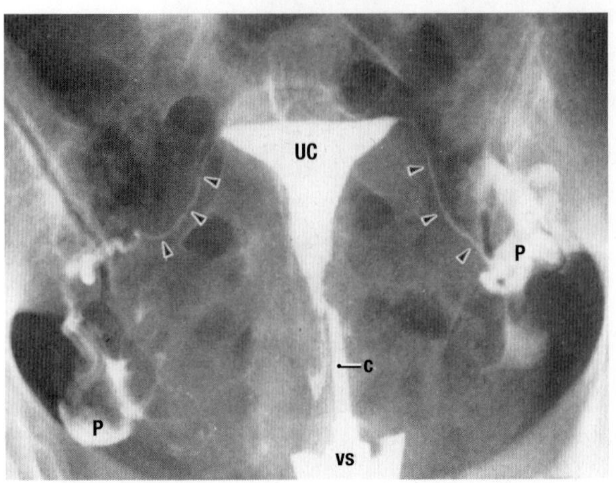
UC
P
P
C
VS

B. Hysterosalpingogram of Normal Uterus, Anteroposterior View

KEY for B:

UC	Uterine cavity	P	Pararectal fossae	VS	Vaginal speculum
▲▲	Uterine tubes	C	Catheter in cervical canal		

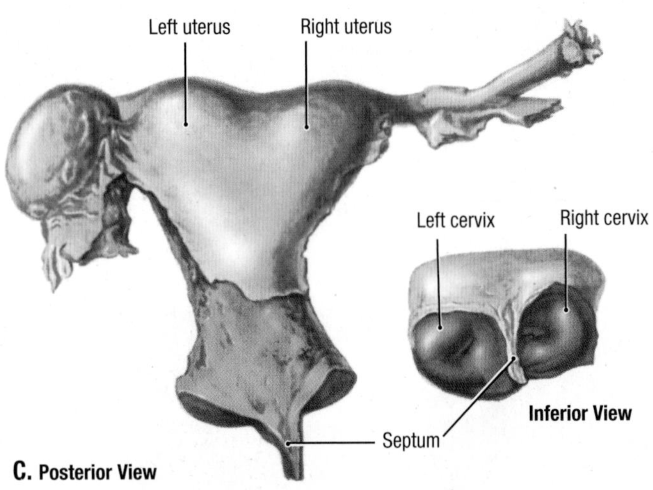
Left uterus
Right uterus
Left cervix
Right cervix
Inferior View
Septum

C. Posterior View

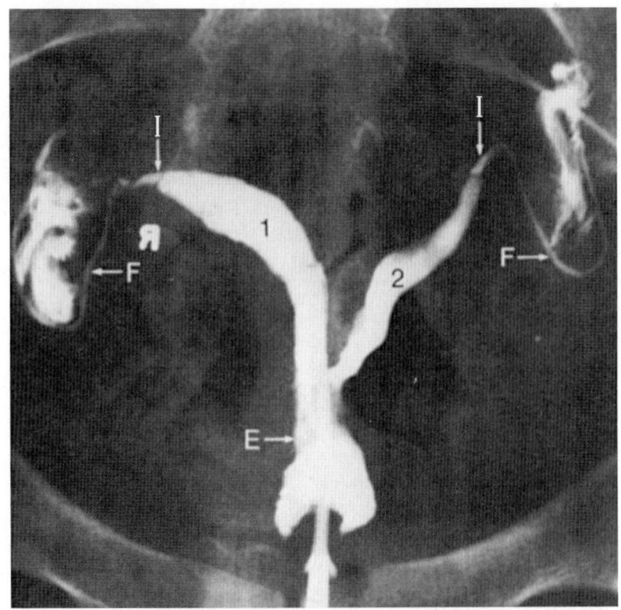
I
I
1
2
F
F
E

D. Hysterosalpingogram of Bicornate Uterus, Anteroposterior View

KEY for D:

1 and 2	Uterine cavities	F	Uterine tubes
E	Cervical canal	I	Isthmus of uterine tubes

3.75 RADIOGRAPH OF UTERUS AND UTERINE TUBES (HYSTEROSALPINGOGRAM)

A. Coronal section of uterus. **B.** During *hysterosalpingography*, radiopaque material is injected into the uterus through external os of the uterus. If normal, contrast medium travels through the triangular uterine cavity (UC) and uterine tubes (*arrowheads*) and passes into the pararectal fossae *(P)* of the peritoneal cavity. The female genital tract is in direct communication with the peritoneal cavity and is, therefore, a potential pathway for the spread of an infection from the vagina and uterus. **C.** Illustration of duplicated uterus. **D.** Hysterosalpingogram of a bicornate ("two-horned") uterus.

CHAPTER 4

Back

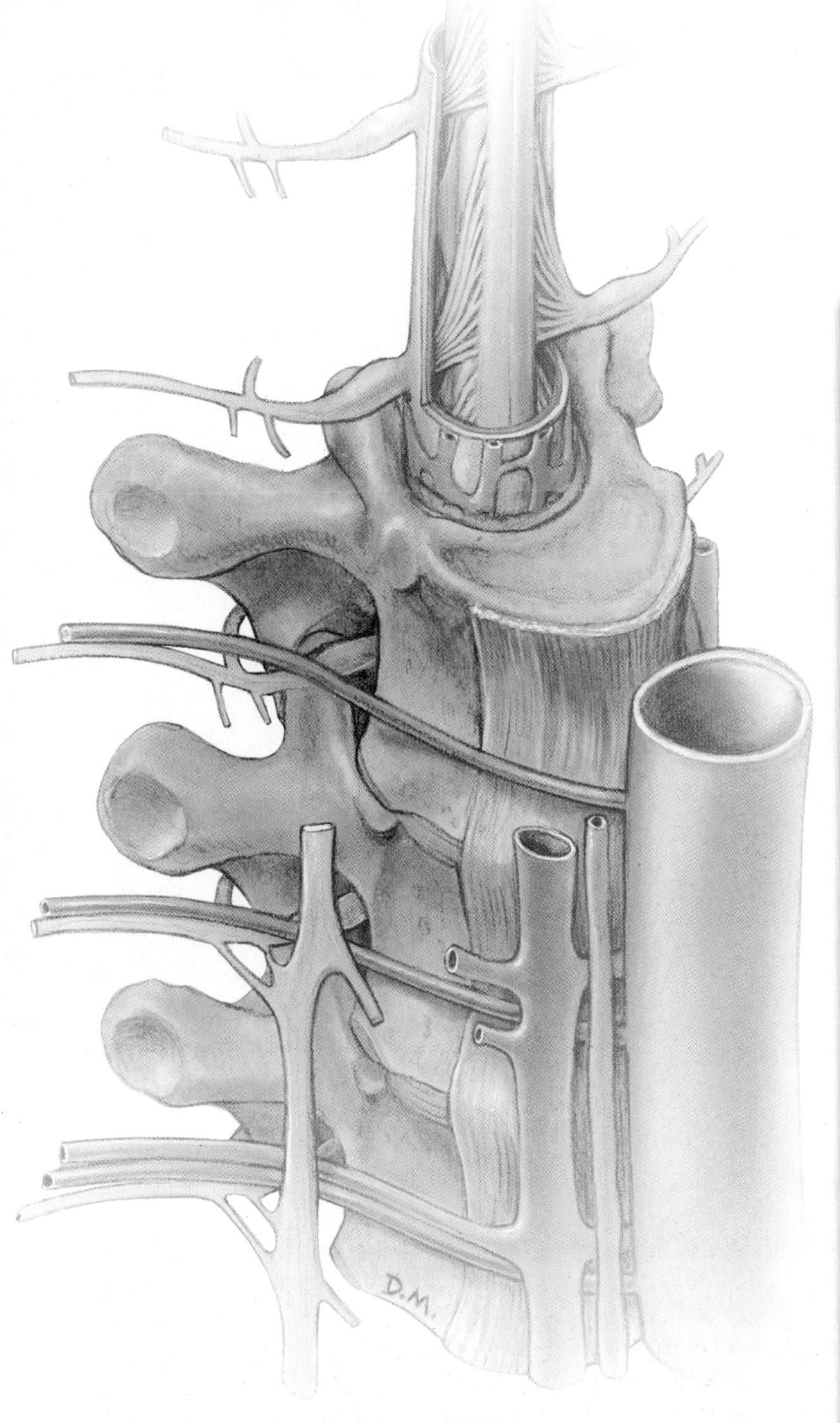
D.M.

Overview of Vertebral Column	290
Cervical Spine	298
Craniovertebral Joints	302
Thoracic Spine	304
Lumbar Spine	306
Ligaments and Intervertebral Discs	308
Bones, Joints, and Ligaments of Pelvic Girdle	313
Anomalies of Vertebrae	320
Muscles of Back	322
Suboccipital Region	332
Spinal Cord and Meninges	336
Vertebral Venous Plexuses	344
Components of Spinal Nerves	345
Dermatomes and Myotomes	348
Autonomic Nerves	350
Imaging of Vertebral Column	354

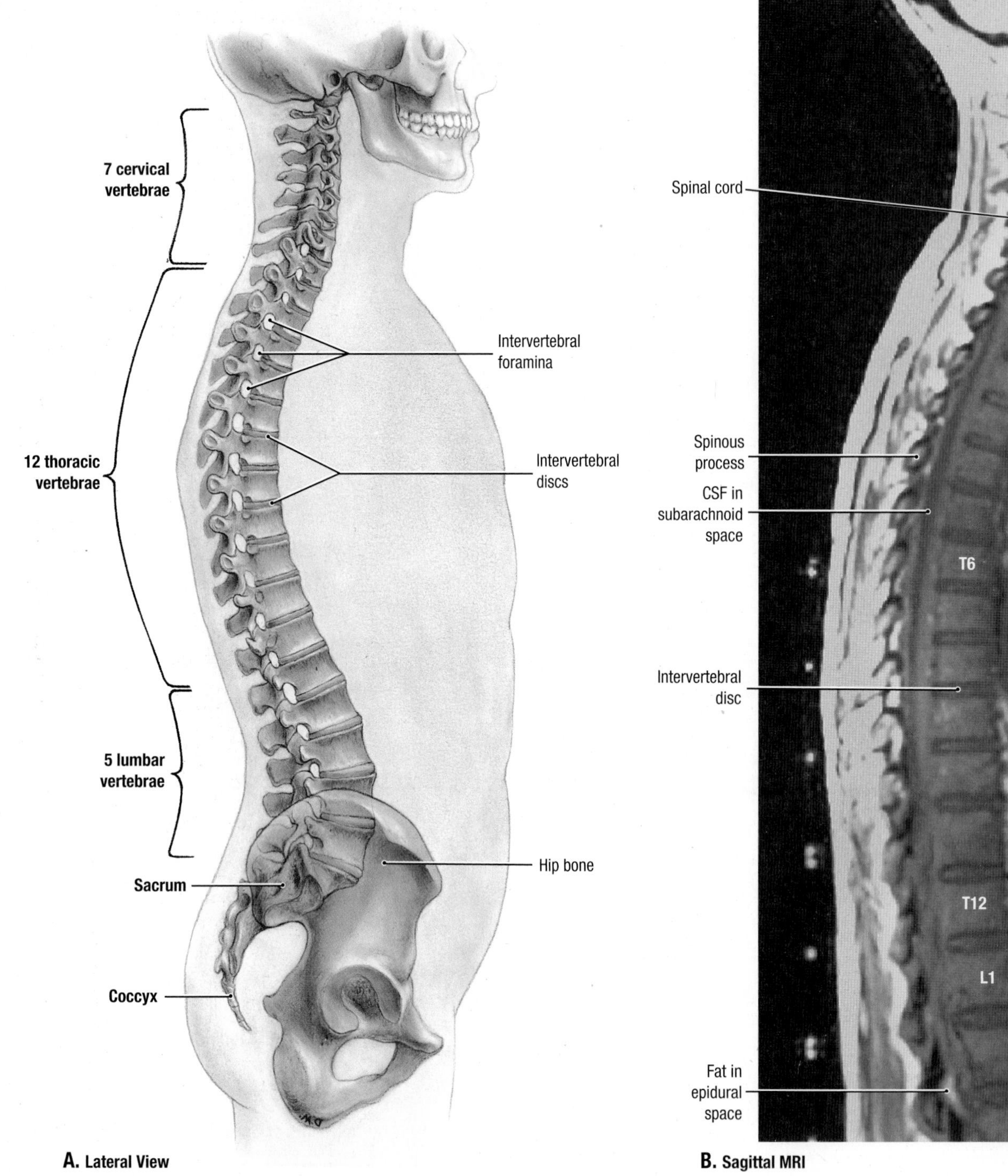
7 cervical vertebrae
12 thoracic vertebrae
5 lumbar vertebrae
Sacrum
Coccyx
Intervertebral foramina
Intervertebral discs
Hip bone
Spinal cord
Spinous process
CSF in subarachnoid space
Intervertebral disc
Fat in epidural space
C2
C7
T1
T6
T12
L1

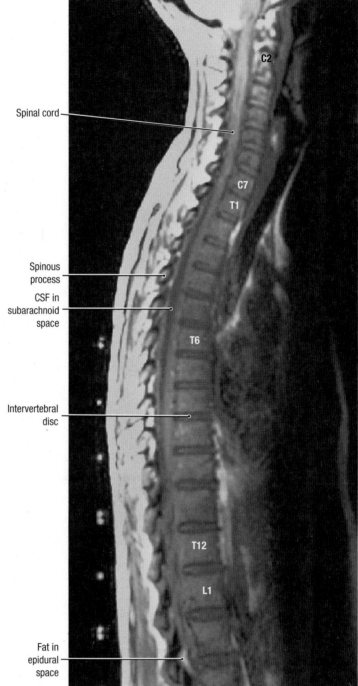

A. Lateral View

B. Sagittal MRI

4.1 OVERVIEW OF VERTEBRAL COLUMN

A. Vertebral column showing articulation with skull and hip bone. **B.** Sagittal MRI, lateral view.

- The vertebral column usually consists of 24 separate (presacral) vertebrae, 5 fused vertebrae in the sacrum, and variably 4 fused or separate coccygeal vertebrae. Of the 24 separate vertebrae, 12 support ribs (thoracic), 7 are in the neck (cervical), and 5 are in the lumbar region (lumbar).
- Vertebrae contributing to the posterior walls of the thoracic and pelvic cavities are concave anteriorly; elsewhere (in the cervical and lumbar regions) they are convex anteriorly.
- The spinal nerves exit the vertebral (spinal) canal via the intervertebral (IV) foramina. There are 8 cervical, 12 thoracic, 5 lumbar, 5 sacral, and 1 to 2 coccygeal spinal nerves.
- Note the size and shape of the vertebral bodies, the direction of the spinous processes, cerebrospinal fluid (CSF) in the subarachnoid space, and the spinal cord in the vertebral canal (in **B**).

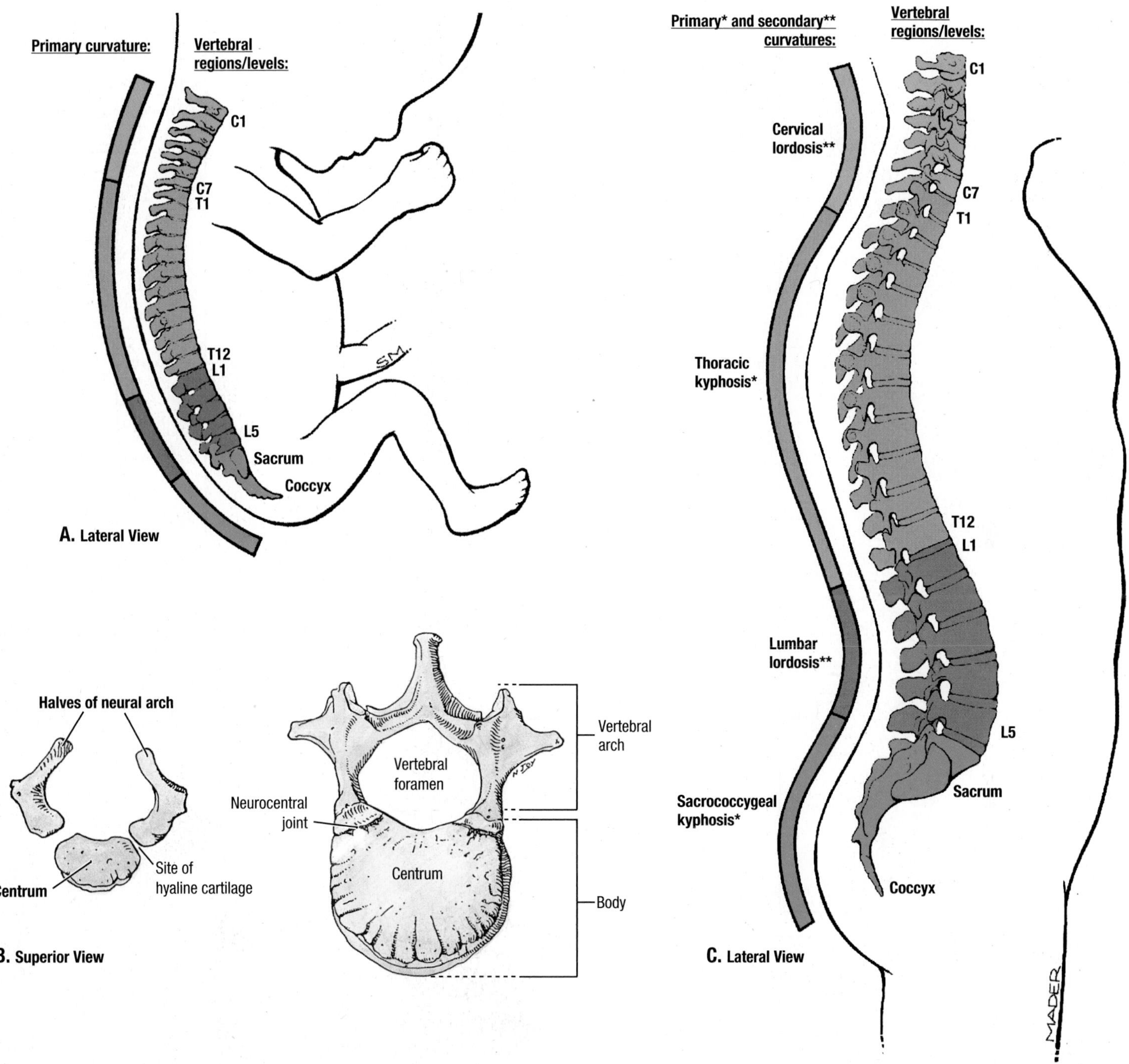
Primary curvature:
Vertebral regions/levels:
C1
C7
T1
T12
L1
L5
Sacrum
Coccyx
A. Lateral View
Halves of neural arch
Centrum
Site of hyaline cartilage
B. Superior View
Neurocentral joint
Vertebral foramen
Centrum
Vertebral arch
Body
Primary* and secondary** curvatures:
Vertebral regions/levels:
Cervical lordosis**
Thoracic kyphosis*
Lumbar lordosis**
Sacrococcygeal kyphosis*
C1
C7
T1
T12
L1
L5
Sacrum
Coccyx
C. Lateral View

4.2 CURVATURES OF VERTEBRAL COLUMN

A. Fetus. Note the C-shaped curvature of the fetal spine, which is concave anteriorly over its entire length. **B.** Development of the vertebrae. At birth, a vertebra consists of three bony parts (two halves of the neural arch and the centrum) united by hyaline cartilage. At age 2, the halves of each neural arch begin to fuse, proceeding from the lumbar to the cervical region; at approximately age 7, the arches begin to fuse to the centrum, proceeding from the cervical to lumbar regions. **C.** Adult. The four curvatures of the adult vertebral column include the cervical lordosis, which is convex anteriorly and lies between vertebrae C1 and T2; the thoracic kyphosis, which is concave anteriorly, between vertebrae T2 and T12; the lumbar lordosis, convex anteriorly and lying between T12 and the lumbosacral joint; and the sacrococcygeal kyphosis, concave anteriorly and spanning from the lumbosacral joint to the tip of the coccyx. The anteriorly concave thoracic kyphosis and sacrococcygeal kyphosis are primary curves, and the anteriorly convex cervical lordosis and lumbar lordosis are secondary curves that develop after birth. The cervical lordosis develops when the child begins to hold the head up, and the lumbar kyphosis develops when the child begins to walk.

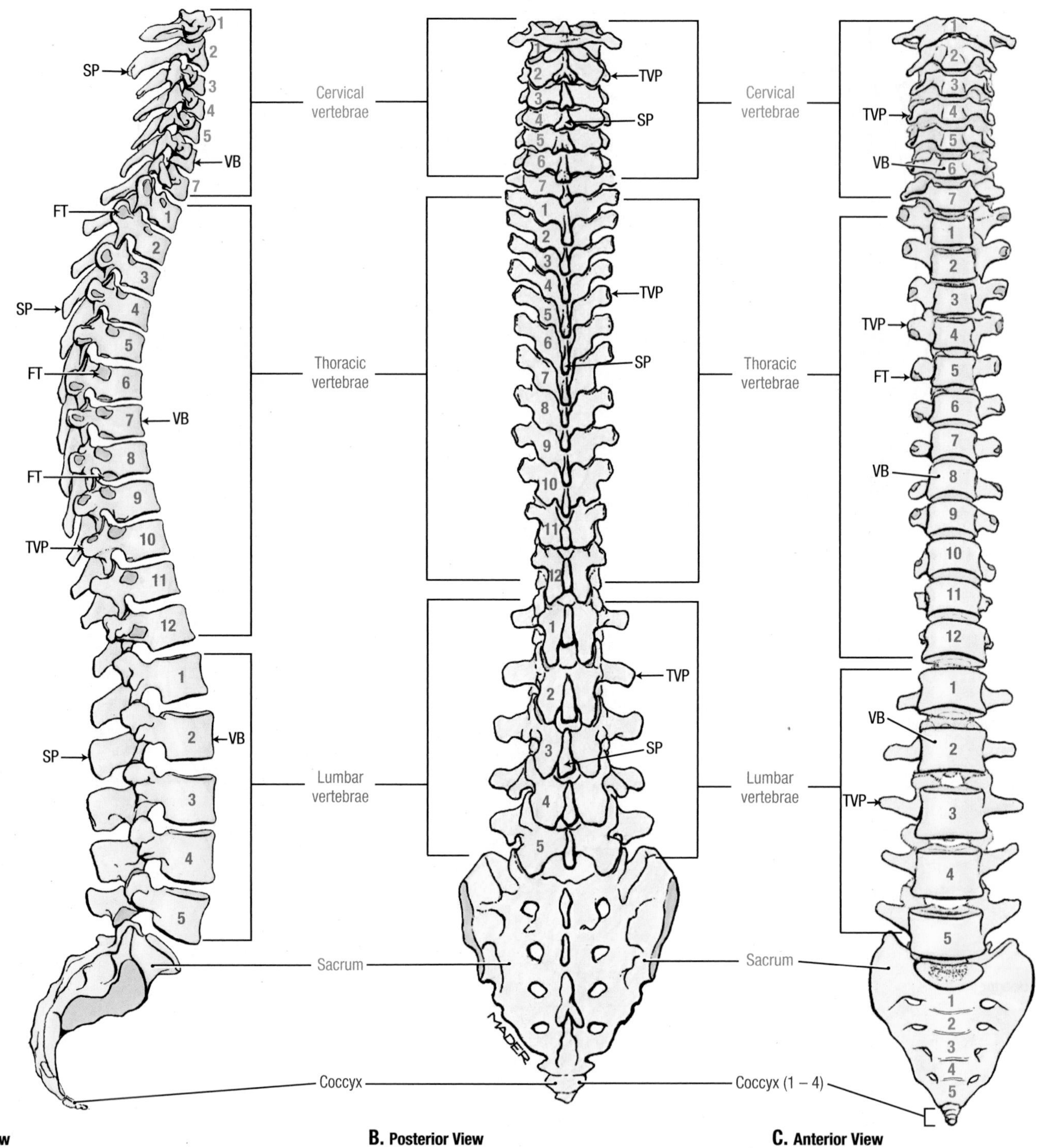

SP
VB
FT
SP
FT
VB
FT
TVP
SP
VB
Cervical vertebrae
Thoracic vertebrae
Lumbar vertebrae
Sacrum
Coccyx
TVP
SP
TVP
SP
TVP
SP
MADER
Cervical vertebrae
Thoracic vertebrae
Lumbar vertebrae
Sacrum
Coccyx (1 – 4)
TVP
VB
TVP
FT
VB
VB
TVP

A. Lateral View **B.** Posterior View **C.** Anterior View

4.3 THREE VIEWS OF VERTEBRAL COLUMN

- The vertebral bodies (*VB*) vary in size and shape.
- Transverse processes (*TVP*) in the cervical region are directed laterally, inferiorly, and anteriorly. In the thoracic region, the vertebrae have facets for articulation with the ribs (FT); the TVPs are directed laterally, posteriorly, and superiorly; and are stout. In the lumbar region, the TVPs point laterally and are long and slender.
- Generally, spinous processes (*SP*) are bifid in Caucasians in the cervical region, long and spinelike in the thoracic region, and stout and oblong in the lumbar region. The cervical and thoracic SPs often overlap the adjacent, inferior vertebrae.

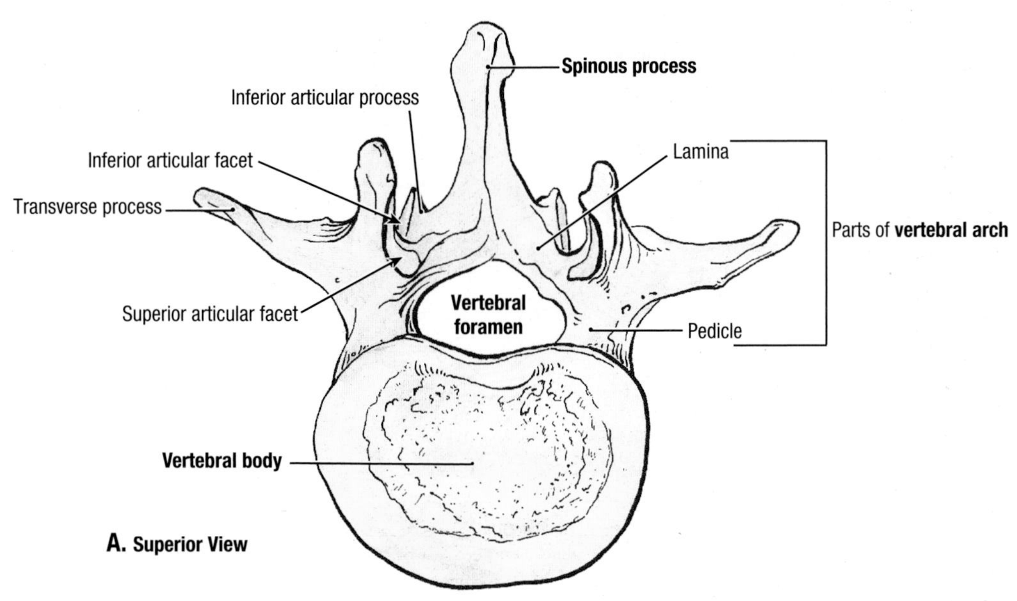
Spinous process
Inferior articular process
Inferior articular facet
Lamina
Transverse process
Parts of vertebral arch
Superior articular facet
Vertebral foramen
Pedicle
Vertebral body
A. Superior View

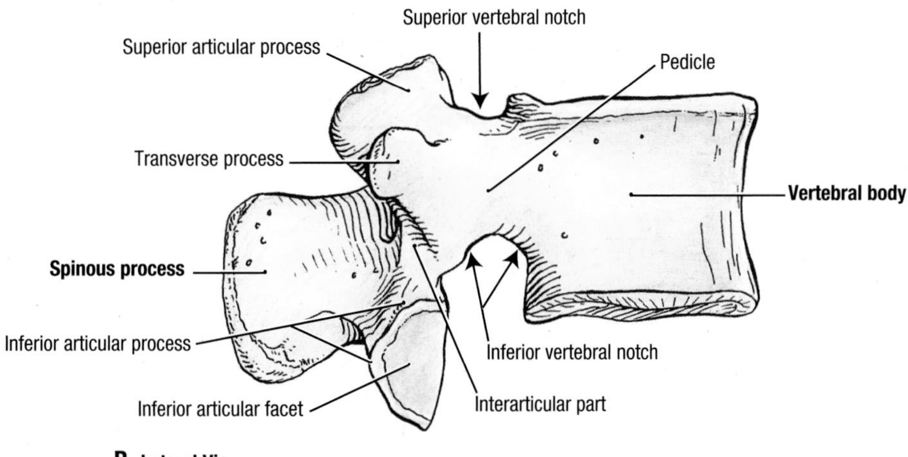
Superior vertebral notch
Superior articular process
Pedicle
Transverse process
Vertebral body
Spinous process
Inferior articular process
Inferior vertebral notch
Inferior articular facet
Interarticular part
B. Lateral View

4.4 TYPICAL VERTEBRA

A typical vertebra (e.g., the 2nd lumbar vertebra) consists of the following parts:

- A vertebral body, situated anteriorly, functions to support weight.
- The vertebral arch consists of two columnar pedicles, one on each side, which arise from the body, and two flat plates called laminae that unite posteriorly in the midline. The vertebral foramen is enclosed by the vertebral body and arch. Collectively, the vertebral foramina constitute the vertebral canal, in which the spinal cord lies. The function of a vertebral arch is to protect the spinal cord.
- Three processes, two transverse and one spinous, provide attachment for muscles and are the levers that help move the vertebrae.
- Four articular processes, two superior and two inferior, each have an articular facet. The articular processes project superiorly and inferiorly from the vertebral arch and come into apposition with the articular facet of the corresponding processes of the vertebrae above and below. The direction of the articular facets determines the nature of the movement between adjacent vertebrae.

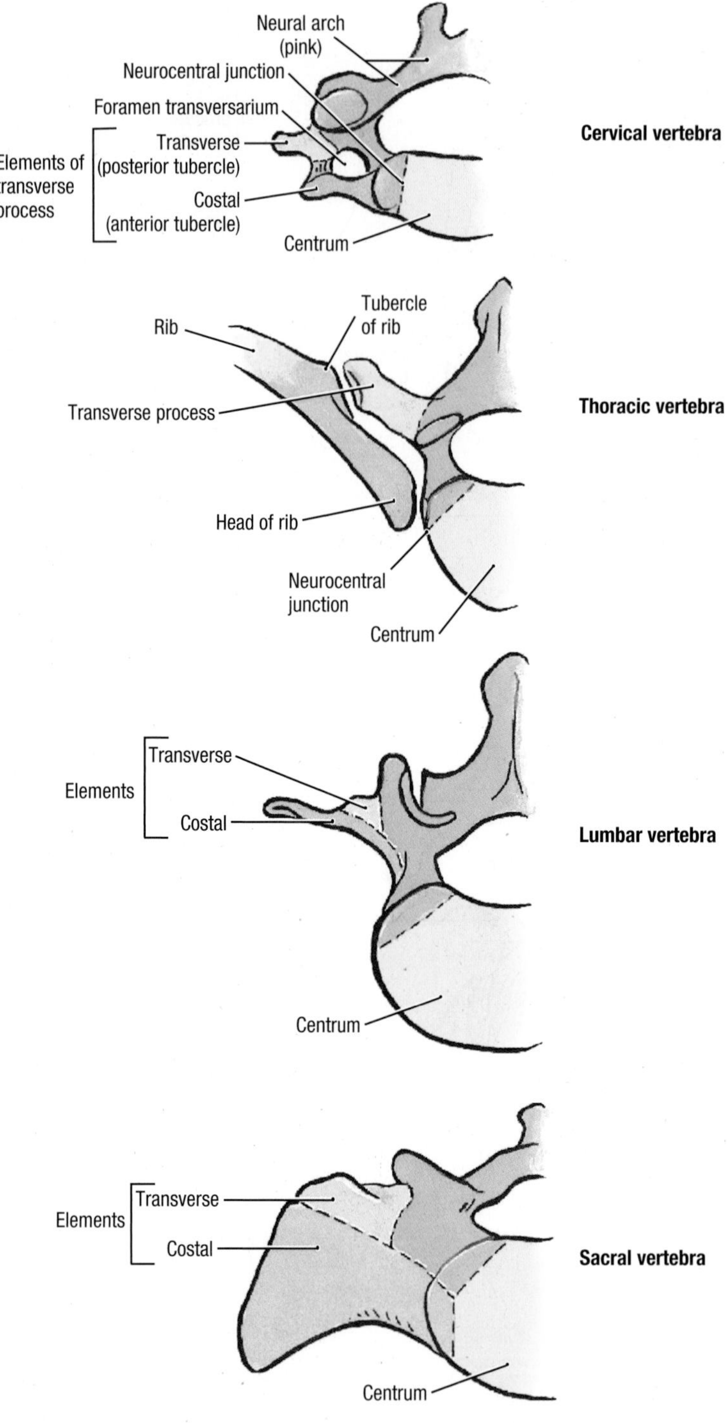
Neural arch
(pink)
Neurocentral junction
Foramen transversarium
Elements of transverse process
Transverse
(posterior tubercle)
Costal
(anterior tubercle)
Centrum
Cervical vertebra
Rib
Tubercle of rib
Transverse process
Head of rib
Neurocentral junction
Centrum
Thoracic vertebra
Elements
Transverse
Costal
Centrum
Lumbar vertebra
Elements
Transverse
Costal
Centrum
Sacral vertebra

Superior Views

4.5 HOMOLOGOUS PARTS OF VERTEBRAE

A rib is a free costal element in the thoracic region; in the cervical and lumbar regions, it is represented by the anterior part of a transverse process, and in the sacrum, by the anterior part of the lateral mass. The heads of the ribs (thoracic region) articulate with the sides of the vertebral bodies posterior to the neurocentral junction and the tubercles of the ribs articulate with the transverse processes of the vertebrae.

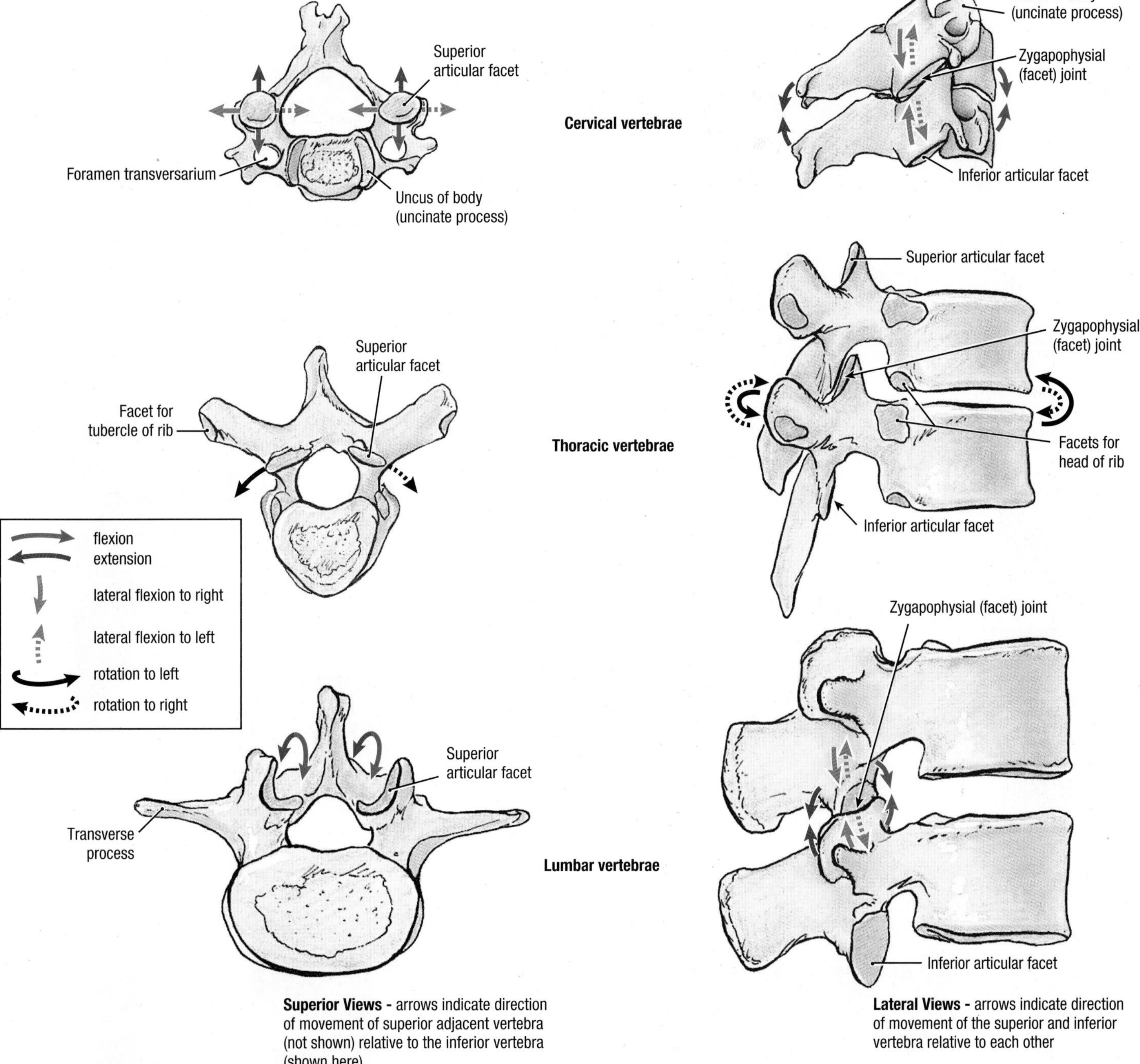
Superior articular facet
Foramen transversarium
Uncus of body (uncinate process)
Cervical vertebrae
Uncus of body (uncinate process)
Zygapophysial (facet) joint
Inferior articular facet
Superior articular facet
Facet for tubercle of rib
Thoracic vertebrae
Superior articular facet
Zygapophysial (facet) joint
Facets for head of rib
Inferior articular facet
flexion
extension
lateral flexion to right
lateral flexion to left
rotation to left
rotation to right
Zygapophysial (facet) joint
Superior articular facet
Transverse process
Lumbar vertebrae
Inferior articular facet

Superior Views - arrows indicate direction of movement of superior adjacent vertebra (not shown) relative to the inferior vertebra (shown here)

Lateral Views - arrows indicate direction of movement of the superior and inferior vertebra relative to each other

4.6 VERTEBRAL FEATURES AND MOVEMENTS

Direction of movement is indicated by *arrows.*

- In the thoracic and lumbar regions, the articular processes/facets lie posterior to the vertebral bodies and in the cervical region posterolateral to the bodies. Superior articular facets in the cervical region face mainly superiorly, in the thoracic region, mainly posteriorly, and in the lumbar region, mainly medially. The change in direction is gradual from cervical to thoracic but abrupt from thoracic to lumbar.
- Although movements between adjacent vertebrae are relatively small, especially in the thoracic region, the summation of all the small movements produces a considerable range of movement of the vertebral column as a whole.
- Movements of the vertebral column are freer (have greater range of motion) in the cervical and lumbar regions than in the thoracic region. Lateral bending is freest in the cervical and lumbar regions; flexion of the vertebral column is greatest in the cervical region; extension is most marked in the lumbar region, but the interlocking articular processes prevent rotation.
- The thoracic region is most stable because of the external support gained from the articulations of the ribs and costal cartilages with the sternum. The direction of the articular facets permits rotation, but flexion, extension, and lateral bending are severely restricted.

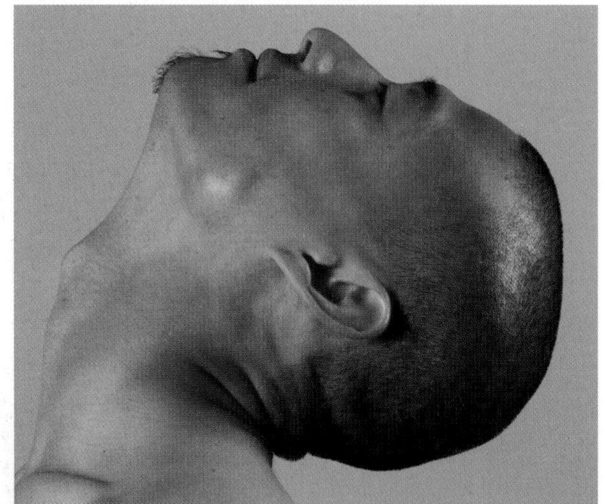

A. Lateral View

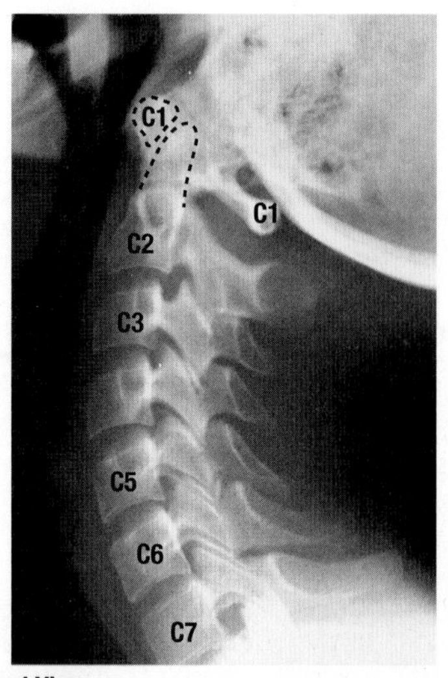
C1
C1
C2
C3
C5
C6
C7

B. Lateral View

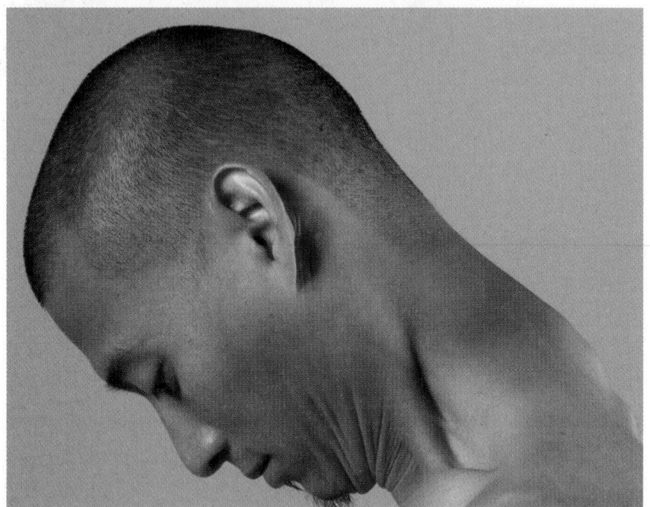

C. Lateral View

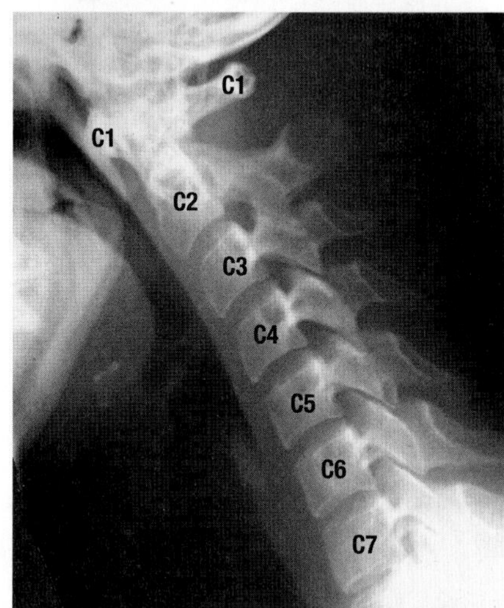
C1
C1
C2
C3
C4
C5
C6
C7

D. Lateral View

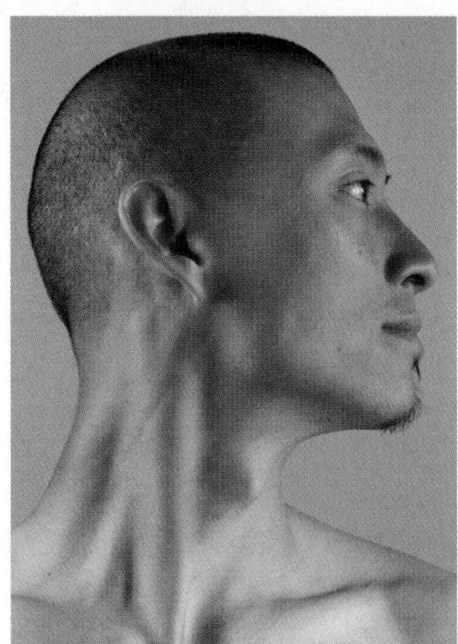

E. Anterior View

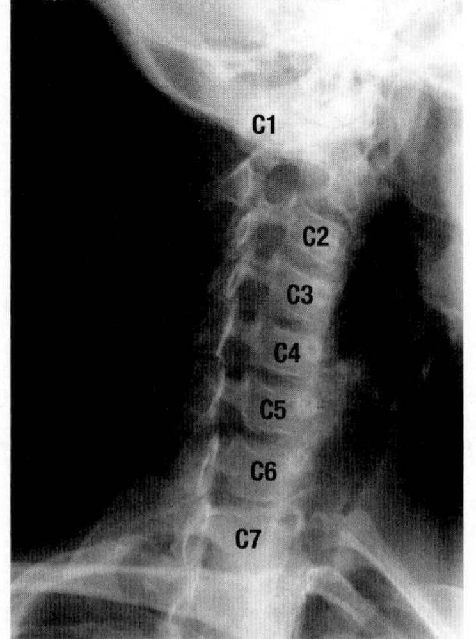
C1
C2
C3
C4
C5
C6
C7

F. Oblique View

4.7 SURFACE ANATOMY WITH RADIOGRAPHIC CORRELATION OF SELECTED MOVEMENTS OF THE CERVICAL SPINE

A. Extension of the neck. **B.** Radiograph of the extended cervical spine. **C.** Flexion of the neck. **D.** Radiograph of the flexed cervical spine. **E.** Head turned (rotated) to left. **F.** Radiograph of cervical spine rotated to left.

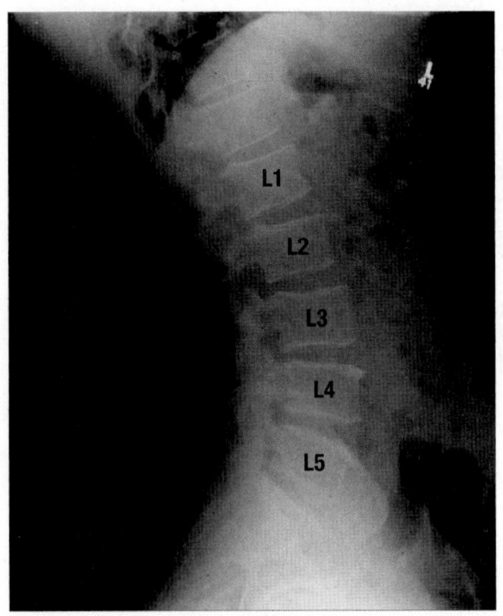
L1
L2
L3
L4
L5
A. Lateral View

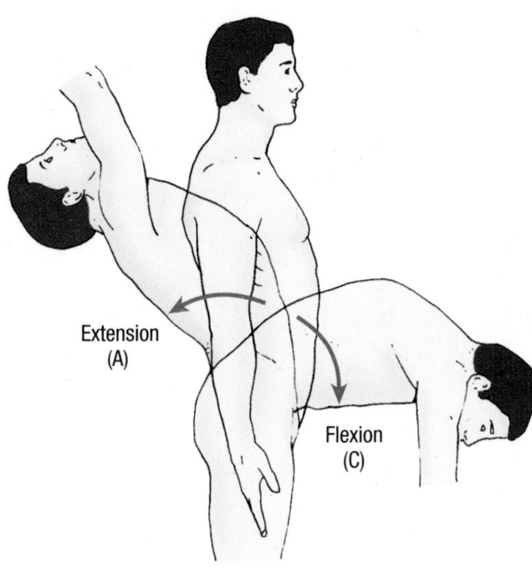
Extension
(A)
Flexion
(C)
B. Lateral View

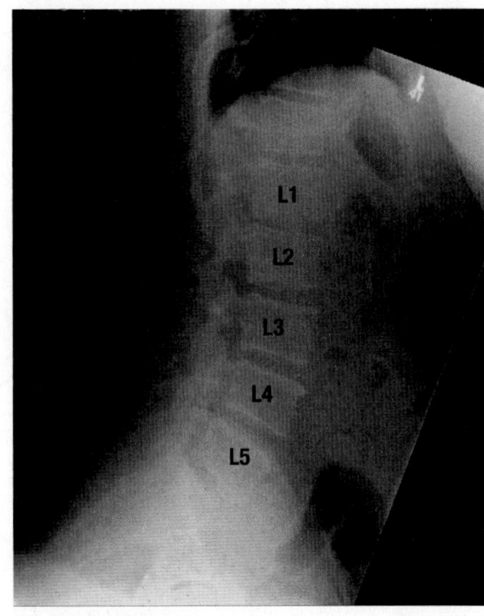
L1
L2
L3
L4
L5
C. Lateral View

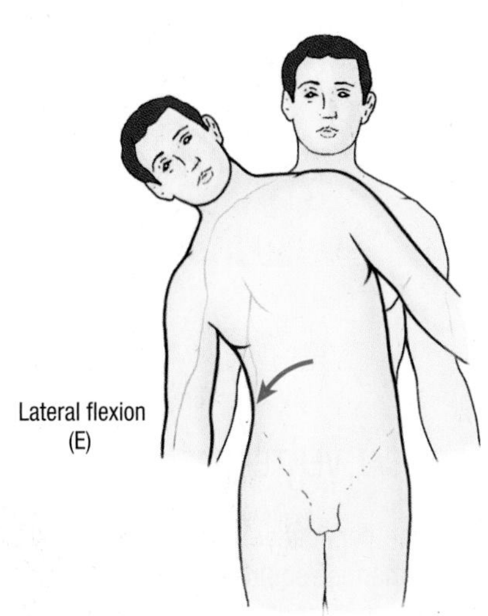
Lateral flexion
(E)
D. Anterior View

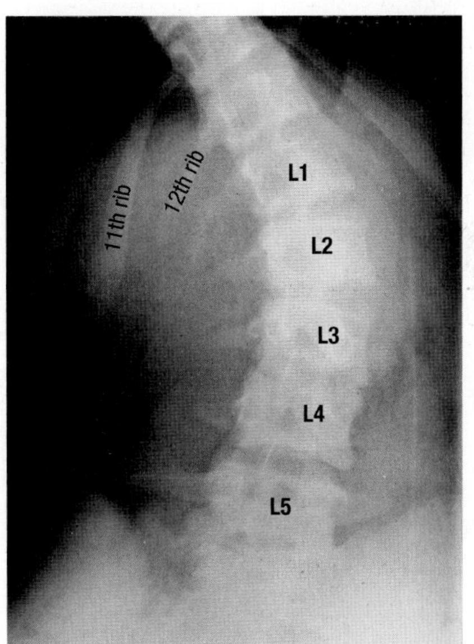
11th rib
12th rib
L1
L2
L3
L4
L5
E. Anteroposterior View

4.8 SURFACE ANATOMY WITH RADIOGRAPHIC CORRELATION OF SELECTED MOVEMENTS OF THE LUMBAR SPINE

A. Radiograph of the extended lumbar spine. **B.** Flexion and extension of the trunk. **C.** Radiograph of the flexed lumbar spine. **D.** Lateral flexion (side flexion) of the trunk. **E.** Radiograph of the lumbar spine during lateral bending.

The range of movement of the vertebral column is limited by the thickness, elasticity, and compressibility of the IV discs; shape and orientation of the zygapophysial joints; tension of the joint capsules of the zygapophysial joints; resistance of the ligaments and back muscles; connection to thoracic (rib) cage and bulk of surrounding tissue.

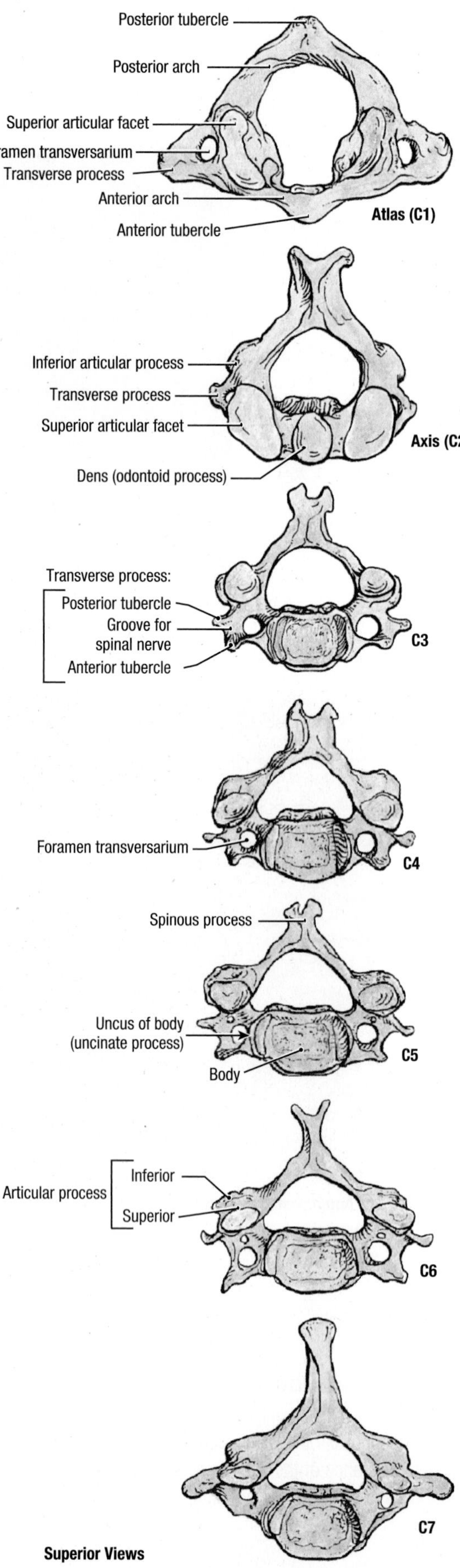
Posterior tubercle
Posterior arch
Superior articular facet
Foramen transversarium
Transverse process
Anterior arch
Anterior tubercle
Atlas (C1)
Inferior articular process
Transverse process
Superior articular facet
Axis (C2)
Dens (odontoid process)
Transverse process:
Posterior tubercle
Groove for spinal nerve
Anterior tubercle
C3
Foramen transversarium
C4
Spinous process
Uncus of body (uncinate process)
Body
C5
Articular process
Inferior
Superior
C6
C7
Superior Views

TABLE 4.1 TYPICAL CERVICAL VERTEBRAE (C3–C7)[a]

Part	Distinctive Characteristics
Body	Small and wider from side to side than anteroposteriorly; superior surface is concave with an uncus of body (uncinate process bilaterally); inferior surface is convex
Vertebral foramen	Large and triangular
Transverse processes	Foramina transversaria small or absent in vertebra C7; vertebral arteries and accompanying venous and sympathetic plexuses pass through foramina, except C7 foramina, which transmits only small accessory vertebral veins; anterior and posterior tubercles separated by groove for spinal nerve
Articular processes	Superior articular facets directed superoposteriorly; inferior articular facets directed infero-anteriorly; obliquely placed facets are most nearly horizontal in this region
Spinous process	Short (C3–C5) and bifid, only in Caucasians (C3–C5); process of C6 is long but that of C7 is longer; C7 is called "vertebra prominens"

[a]C1 and C2 vertebrae are atypical.

4.9 CERVICAL VERTEBRAE

The bodies of the cervical vertebrae can be dislocated in neck injuries with less force than is required to fracture them. Because of the large vertebral canal in the cervical region, slight dislocation can occur without damaging the spinal cord. When a cervical vertebra is severely dislocated, it injures the spinal cord. If the dislocation does not result in "facet jumping" with locking of the displaced articular processes, the cervical vertebrae may self-reduce ("slip back into place") so that a radiograph may not indicate that the cord has been injured. MRI may reveal the resulting soft tissue damage.

Aging of the IV disc combined with the changing shape of the vertebrae results in an increase in compressive forces at the periphery of the vertebral bodies, where the disc attaches. In response **osteophytes** (bony spurs) commonly develop around the margins of the vertebral body, especially along the outer attachment of the IV disc. Similarly, as altered mechanics place greater stresses on the zygapophysial joints, osteophytes develop along the attachments of the joint capsules, especially those of the superior articular process.

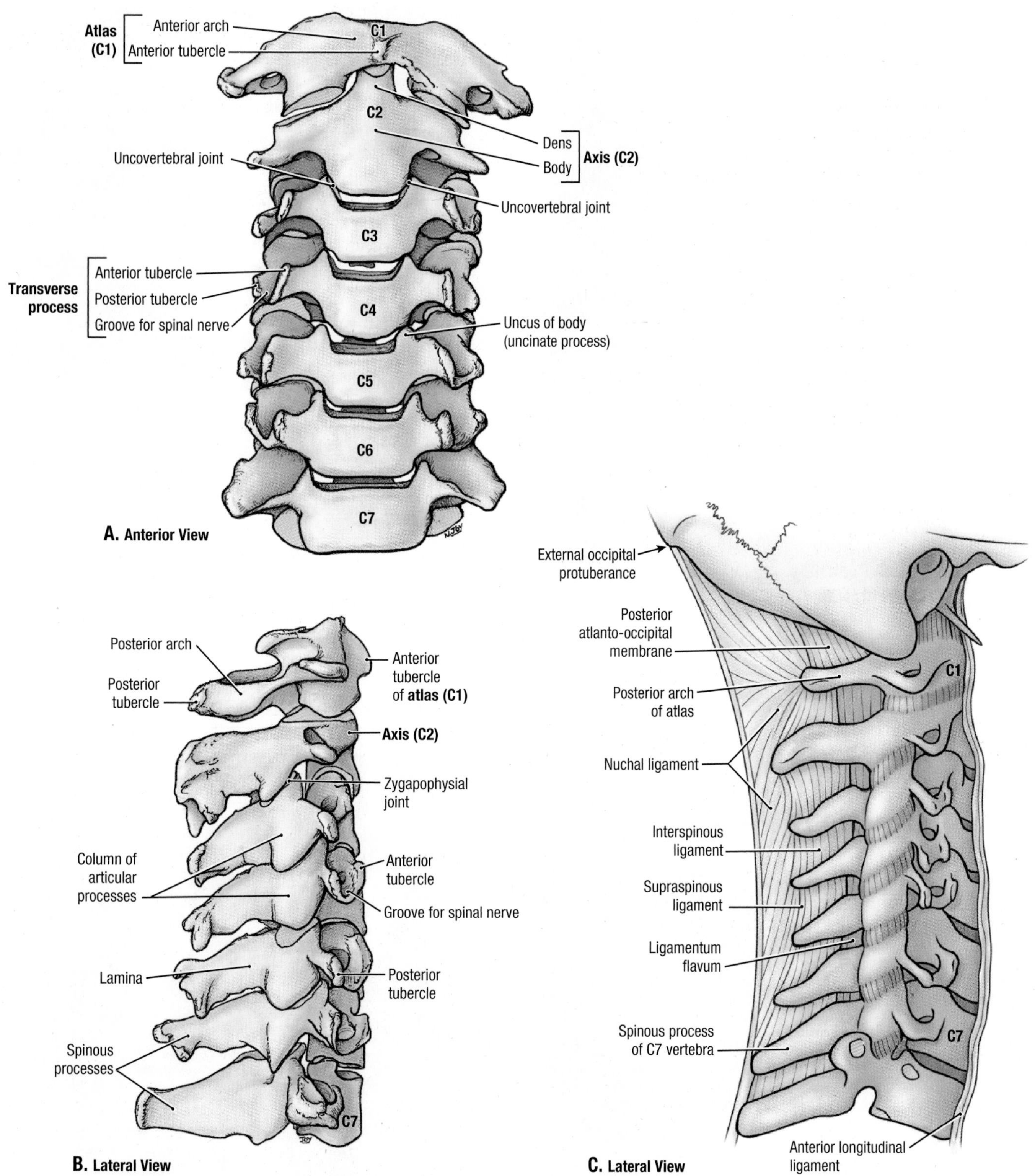
Atlas (C1)
Anterior arch
Anterior tubercle
C1
C2
Dens
Body
Axis (C2)
Uncovertebral joint
Uncovertebral joint
C3
Transverse process
Anterior tubercle
Posterior tubercle
Groove for spinal nerve
C4
Uncus of body (uncinate process)
C5
C6
C7
A. Anterior View
Posterior arch
Posterior tubercle
Anterior tubercle of atlas (C1)
Axis (C2)
Zygapophysial joint
Column of articular processes
Anterior tubercle
Groove for spinal nerve
Lamina
Posterior tubercle
Spinous processes
C7
B. Lateral View
External occipital protuberance
Posterior atlanto-occipital membrane
C1
Posterior arch of atlas
Nuchal ligament
Interspinous ligament
Supraspinous ligament
Ligamentum flavum
Spinous process of C7 vertebra
C7
Anterior longitudinal ligament
C. Lateral View

4.10 CERVICAL SPINE

A. and B. Articulated cervical vertebrae. **C.** Ligaments.

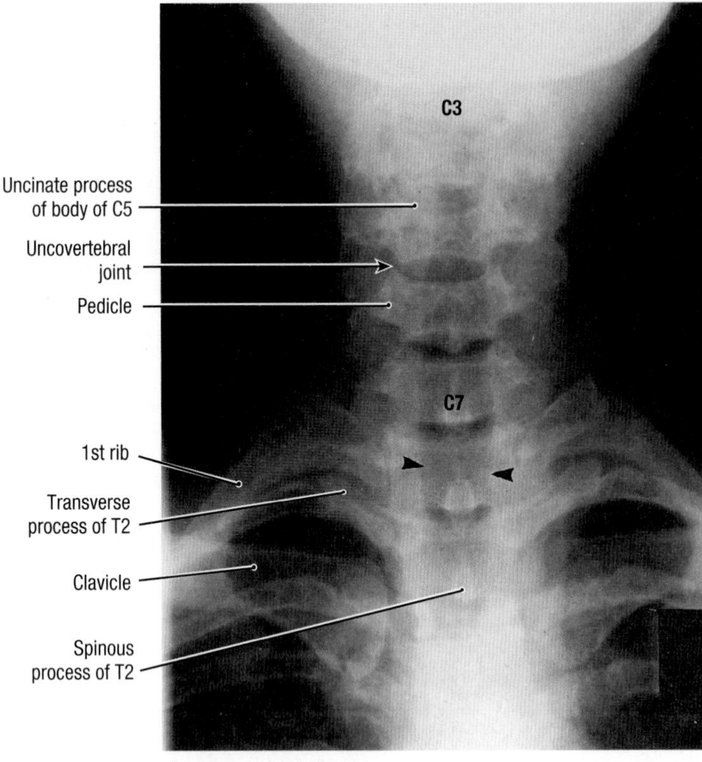
C3
Uncinate process of body of C5
Uncovertebral joint
Pedicle
C7
1st rib
Transverse process of T2
Clavicle
Spinous process of T2

A. **Anteroposterior View**

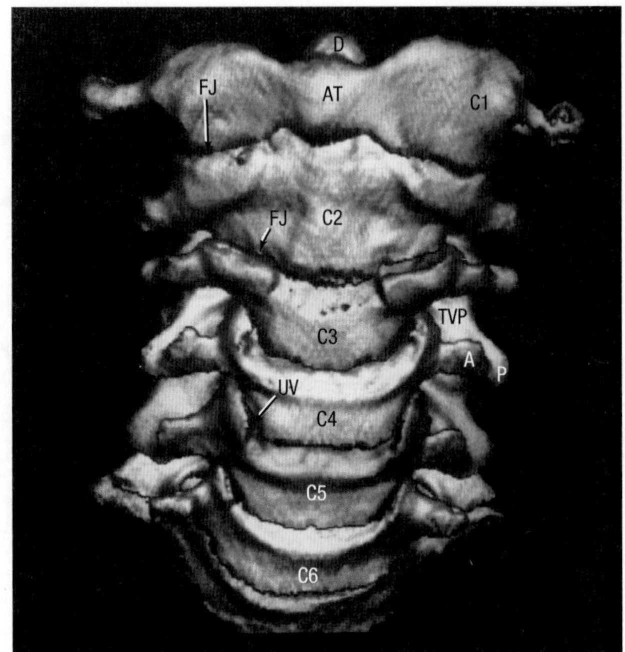
D
FJ
AT
C1
FJ
C2
TVP
C3
A
P
UV
C4
C5
C6

C. **Anterior View**

A	Anterior tubercle of transverse process	PA	Posterior arch of C1
AA	Anterior arch of C1	PT	Posterior tubercle of C1
AT	Anterior tubercle of C1	SF	Superior articular facet of C1
C1-C7	Vertebrae	SP	Spinous process
D	Dens (odontoid) process of C2	T	Foramen transversarium
FJ	Zygapophysial (facet) joint	TVP	Transverse process
La	Lamina	UV	Uncovertebral joint
P	Posterior tubercle of transverse process	VC	Vertebral canal

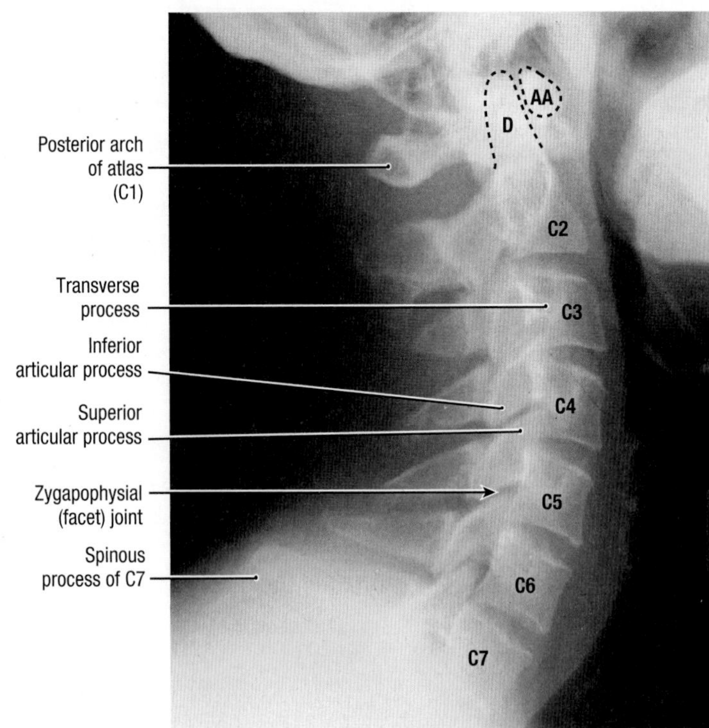
AA
D
Posterior arch of atlas (C1)
C2
Transverse process
C3
Inferior articular process
C4
Superior articular process
Zygapophysial (facet) joint
C5
Spinous process of C7
C6
C7

B. **Lateral View**

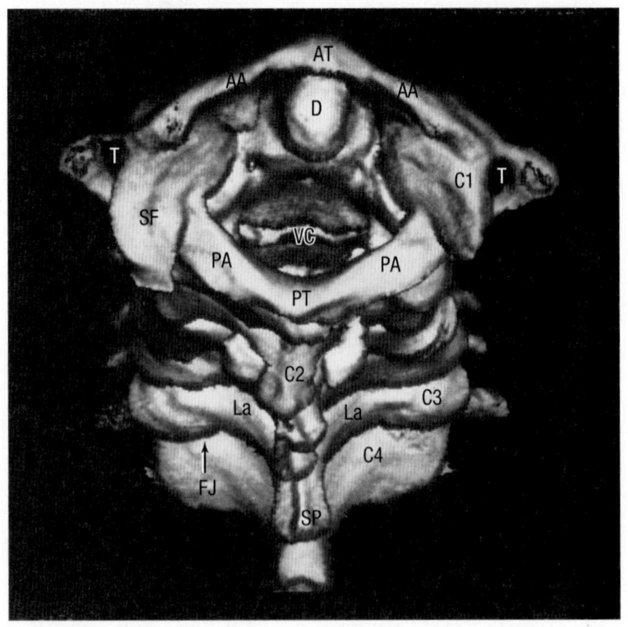
AT
AA
AA
D
T
C1
T
SF
VC
PA
PA
PT
C2
La
La
C3
C4
FJ
SP

D. **Posterior View**

4.11 IMAGING OF THE CERVICAL SPINE

A. and B. Radiographs. The arrowheads demarcate the margins of the *(black)* column of air in the trachea.
C. and D. Three-dimensional (3D) reconstructed computed tomographic (CT) images.

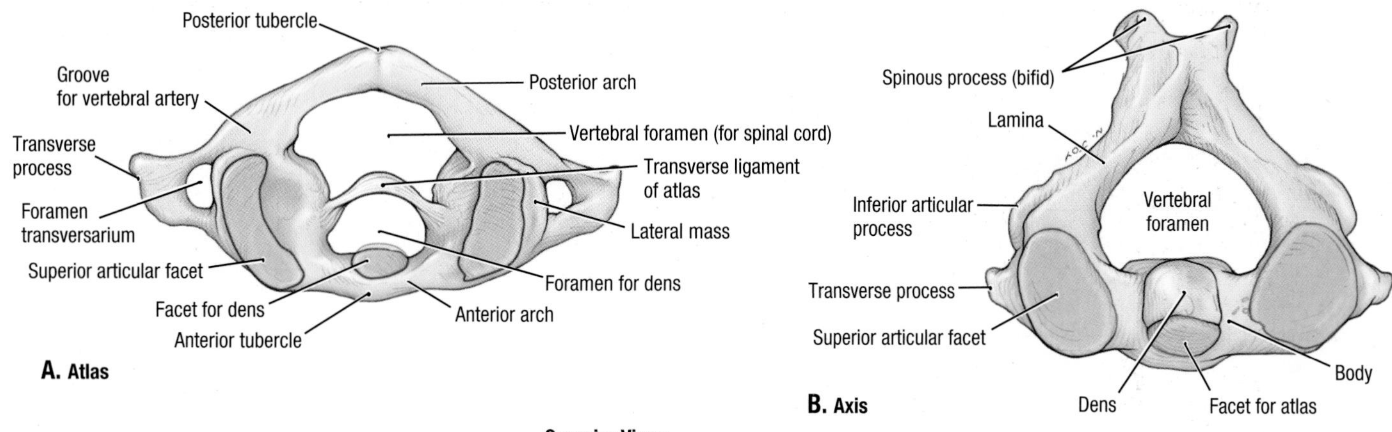
Posterior tubercle
Groove for vertebral artery
Posterior arch
Vertebral foramen (for spinal cord)
Transverse process
Transverse ligament of atlas
Foramen transversarium
Lateral mass
Superior articular facet
Foramen for dens
Facet for dens
Anterior arch
Anterior tubercle
A. Atlas
Spinous process (bifid)
Lamina
Inferior articular process
Vertebral foramen
Transverse process
Superior articular facet
Body
B. Axis
Dens
Facet for atlas
Superior Views

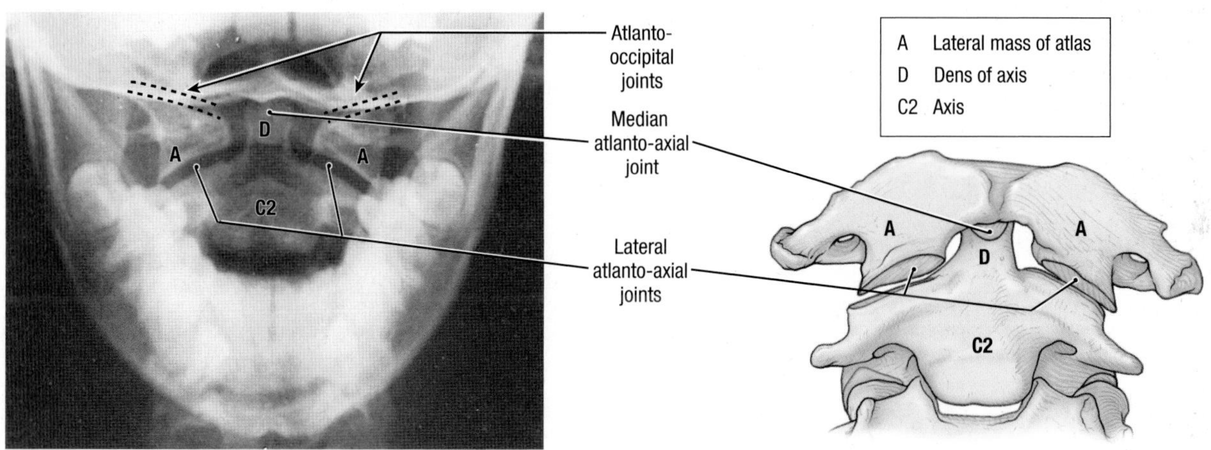
Atlanto-occipital joints
Median atlanto-axial joint
Lateral atlanto-axial joints
A
D
C2
A Lateral mass of atlas
D Dens of axis
C2 Axis
C. Anteroposterior View

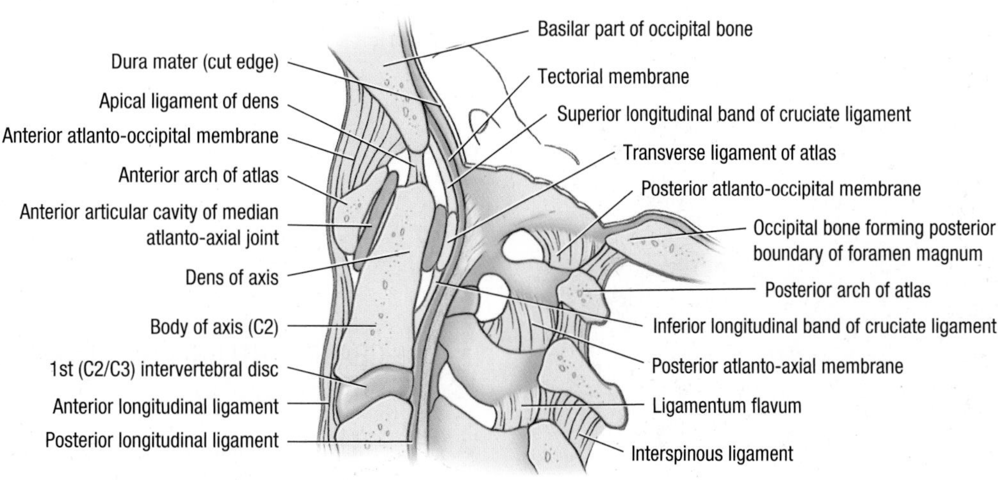
Basilar part of occipital bone
Dura mater (cut edge)
Tectorial membrane
Apical ligament of dens
Superior longitudinal band of cruciate ligament
Anterior atlanto-occipital membrane
Transverse ligament of atlas
Anterior arch of atlas
Posterior atlanto-occipital membrane
Anterior articular cavity of median atlanto-axial joint
Occipital bone forming posterior boundary of foramen magnum
Dens of axis
Posterior arch of atlas
Body of axis (C2)
Inferior longitudinal band of cruciate ligament
1st (C2/C3) intervertebral disc
Posterior atlanto-axial membrane
Anterior longitudinal ligament
Ligamentum flavum
Posterior longitudinal ligament
Interspinous ligament
E. Median Section

4.12 ATLAS AND AXIS AND THE ATLANTO-AXIAL JOINT

A. Atlas. **B.** Axis. **C.** Radiograph taken through the open mouth. **D.** Articulated atlas and axis. **E.** Median section with ligaments.

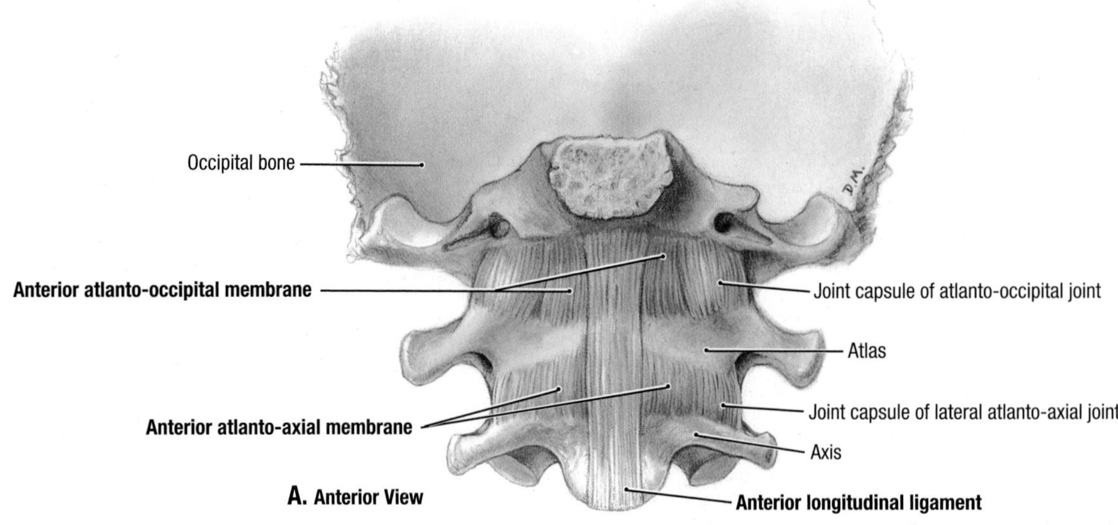
Occipital bone
Anterior atlanto-occipital membrane
Joint capsule of atlanto-occipital joint
Atlas
Joint capsule of lateral atlanto-axial joint
Anterior atlanto-axial membrane
Axis
Anterior longitudinal ligament

A. Anterior View

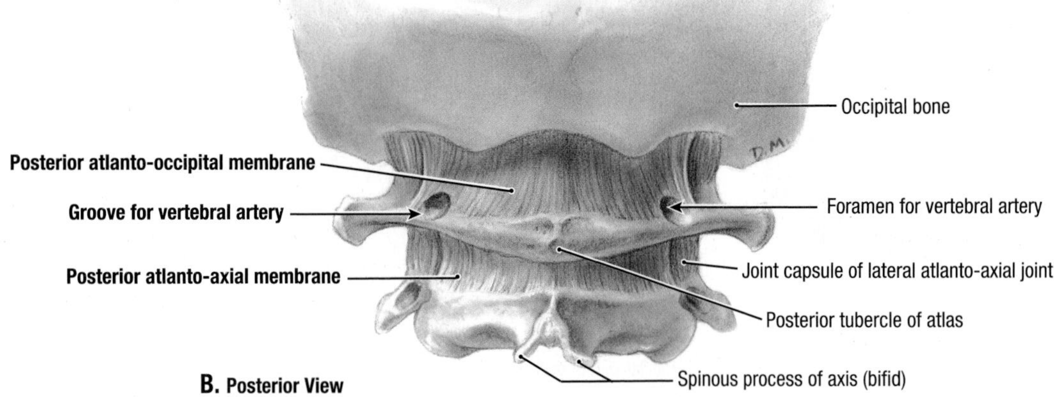
Occipital bone
Posterior atlanto-occipital membrane
Groove for vertebral artery
Foramen for vertebral artery
Posterior atlanto-axial membrane
Joint capsule of lateral atlanto-axial joint
Posterior tubercle of atlas
Spinous process of axis (bifid)

B. Posterior View

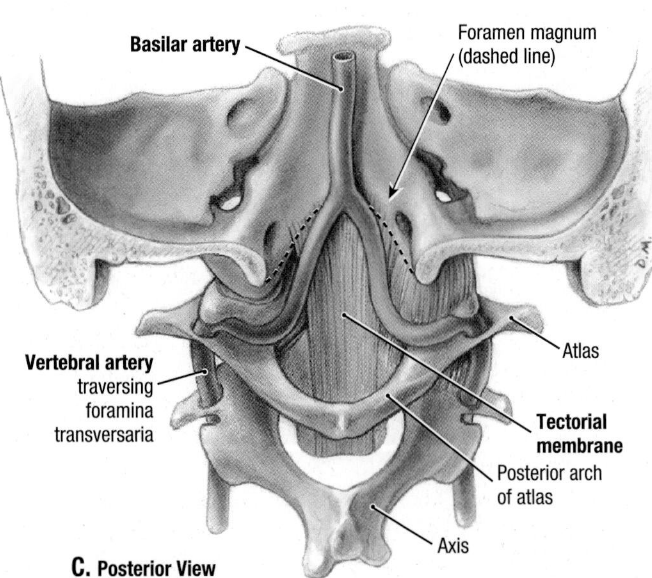
Basilar artery
Foramen magnum
(dashed line)
Atlas
Vertebral artery
traversing
foramina
transversaria
Tectorial
membrane
Posterior arch
of atlas
Axis

C. Posterior View

4.13 CRANIOVERTEBRAL JOINTS AND VERTEBRAL ARTERY

A. Anterior atlanto-axial and atlanto-occipital membranes. The anterior longitudinal ligament ascends to blend with, and form a central thickening in, the anterior atlanto-axial and atlanto-occipital membranes. **B.** Posterior atlanto-axial and atlanto-occipital membranes. Inferior to the axis (C2 vertebra), ligamenta flava occur in this position. **C.** Tectorial membrane and vertebral artery. The tectorial membrane is a superior continuation of the posterior longitudinal ligament superior to the body of the axis. After coursing through the foramina transversaria of vertebrae C6–C1, the vertebral arteries turn medially, grooving the superior aspect of the posterior arch of the atlas and piercing the posterior atlanto-occipital membrane (**B**). The right and left vertebral arteries traverse the foramen magnum and merge intracranially, forming the basilar artery.

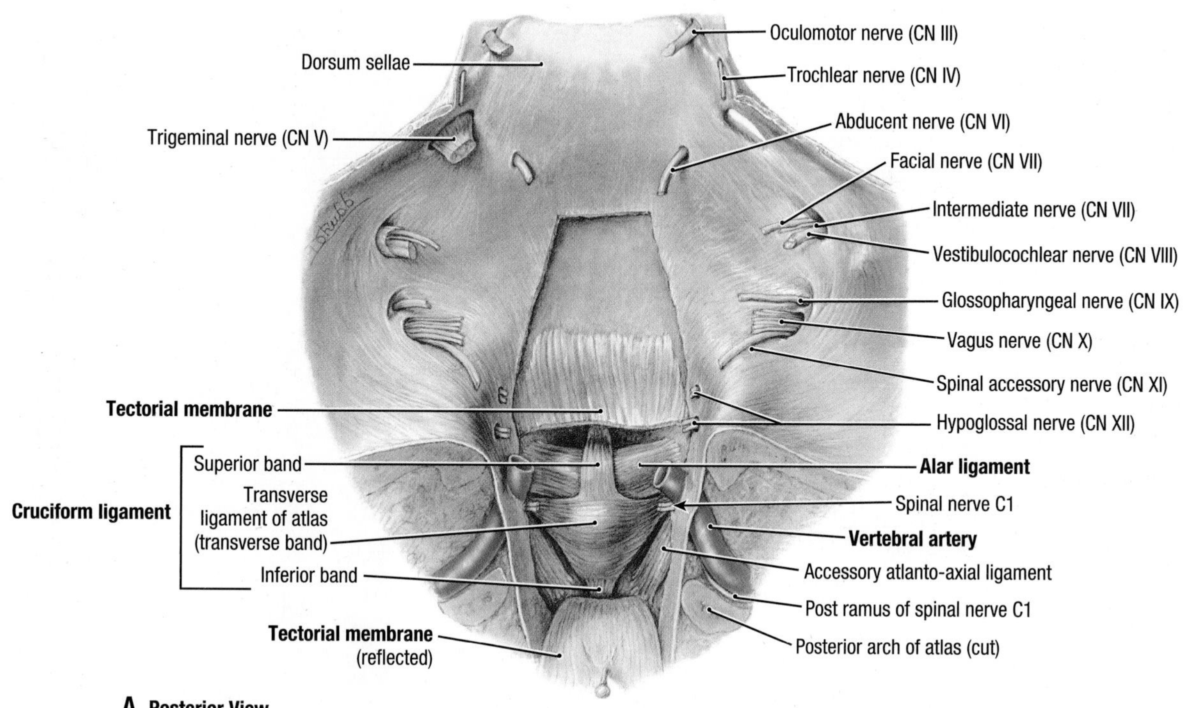
Dorsum sellae
Trigeminal nerve (CN V)
Oculomotor nerve (CN III)
Trochlear nerve (CN IV)
Abducent nerve (CN VI)
Facial nerve (CN VII)
Intermediate nerve (CN VII)
Vestibulocochlear nerve (CN VIII)
Glossopharyngeal nerve (CN IX)
Vagus nerve (CN X)
Spinal accessory nerve (CN XI)
Hypoglossal nerve (CN XII)
Tectorial membrane
Cruciform ligament
Superior band
Transverse ligament of atlas (transverse band)
Inferior band
Alar ligament
Spinal nerve C1
Vertebral artery
Accessory atlanto-axial ligament
Post ramus of spinal nerve C1
Posterior arch of atlas (cut)
Tectorial membrane (reflected)

A. Posterior View

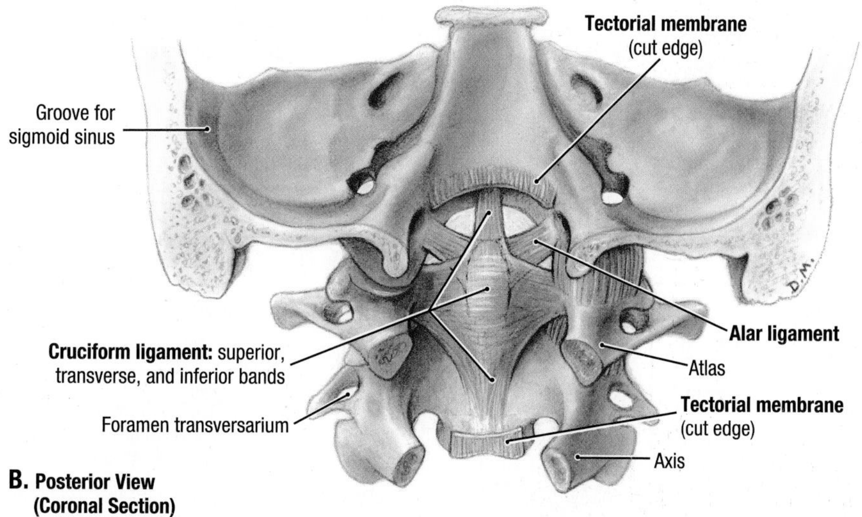
Tectorial membrane (cut edge)
Groove for sigmoid sinus
Cruciform ligament: superior, transverse, and inferior bands
Foramen transversarium
Alar ligament
Atlas
Tectorial membrane (cut edge)
Axis

B. Posterior View (Coronal Section)

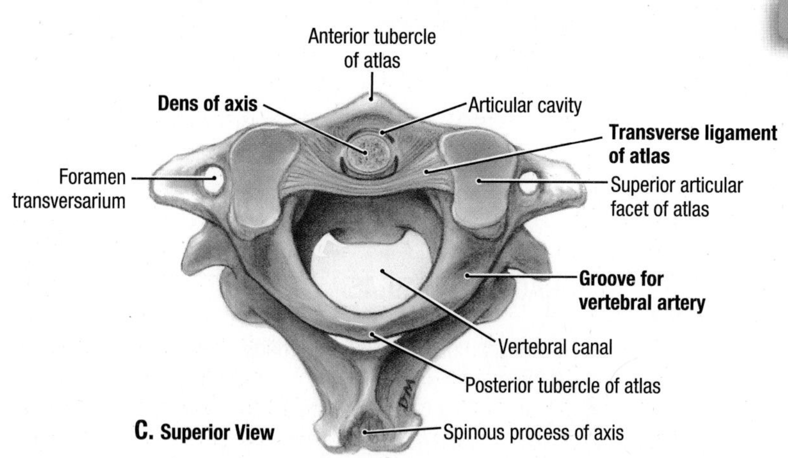
Anterior tubercle of atlas
Dens of axis
Articular cavity
Transverse ligament of atlas
Foramen transversarium
Superior articular facet of atlas
Groove for vertebral artery
Vertebral canal
Posterior tubercle of atlas
Spinous process of axis

C. Superior View

4.14 LIGAMENTS OF ATLANTO-OCCIPITAL AND ATLANTO-AXIAL JOINTS

A. Cranial nerves and dura mater of posterior cranial fossa with dura mater and tentorial membrane incised and removed to reveal the medial atlanto-axial joint. **B.** The alar ligaments serve as check ligaments for the rotary movements of the atlanto-axial joints. **B. and C.** The transverse ligament of the atlas, the transverse band of the cruciform ligament, provides the posterior wall of a socket that receives the dens of the axis, forming a pivot joint.

Fracture of atlas. The atlas is a bony ring, with two wedge-shaped lateral masses, connected by relatively thin anterior and posterior arches and the transverse ligament of the atlas (see Figs. 4.12A & C). Vertical forces (e.g., striking the head on bottom of pool) may force the lateral masses apart fracturing one or both of the anterior or posterior arches. If the force is sufficient, rupture of the transverse ligament of the atlas will also occur.

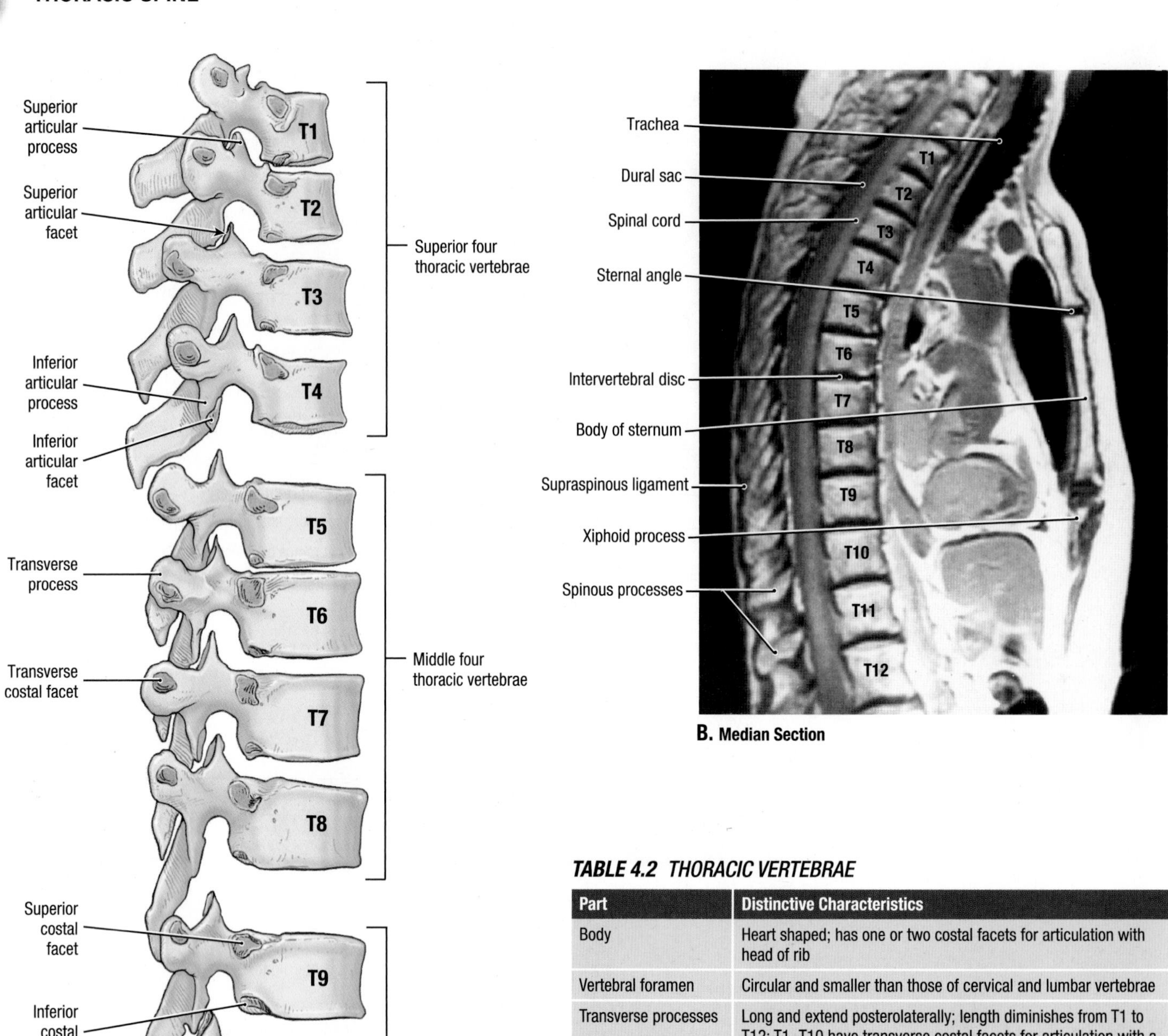

Superior articular process
Superior articular facet
Inferior articular process
Inferior articular facet
Transverse process
Transverse costal facet
Superior costal facet
Inferior costal facet
Spinous process
Processes
Mammillary
Accessory
Transverse
T1
T2
T3
T4
T5
T6
T7
T8
T9
T10
T11
T12
Superior four thoracic vertebrae
Middle four thoracic vertebrae
Inferior four thoracic vertebrae
Trachea
Dural sac
Spinal cord
Sternal angle
Intervertebral disc
Body of sternum
Supraspinous ligament
Xiphoid process
Spinous processes

A. Lateral View

B. Median Section

TABLE 4.2 THORACIC VERTEBRAE

Part	Distinctive Characteristics
Body	Heart shaped; has one or two costal facets for articulation with head of rib
Vertebral foramen	Circular and smaller than those of cervical and lumbar vertebrae
Transverse processes	Long and extend posterolaterally; length diminishes from T1 to T12; T1–T10 have transverse costal facets for articulation with a tubercle of ribs 1–10 (ribs 11 and 12 have no tubercle and do not articulate with a transverse process)
Articular processes	Superior articular facets directed posteriorly and slightly laterally; inferior articular facets directed anteriorly and slightly medially
Spinous process	Long and slopes postero-inferiorly; tip extends to level of vertebral body below

4.15 THORACIC VERTEBRAE

A. Features. **B.** MRI scan of thoracic spine, median section.

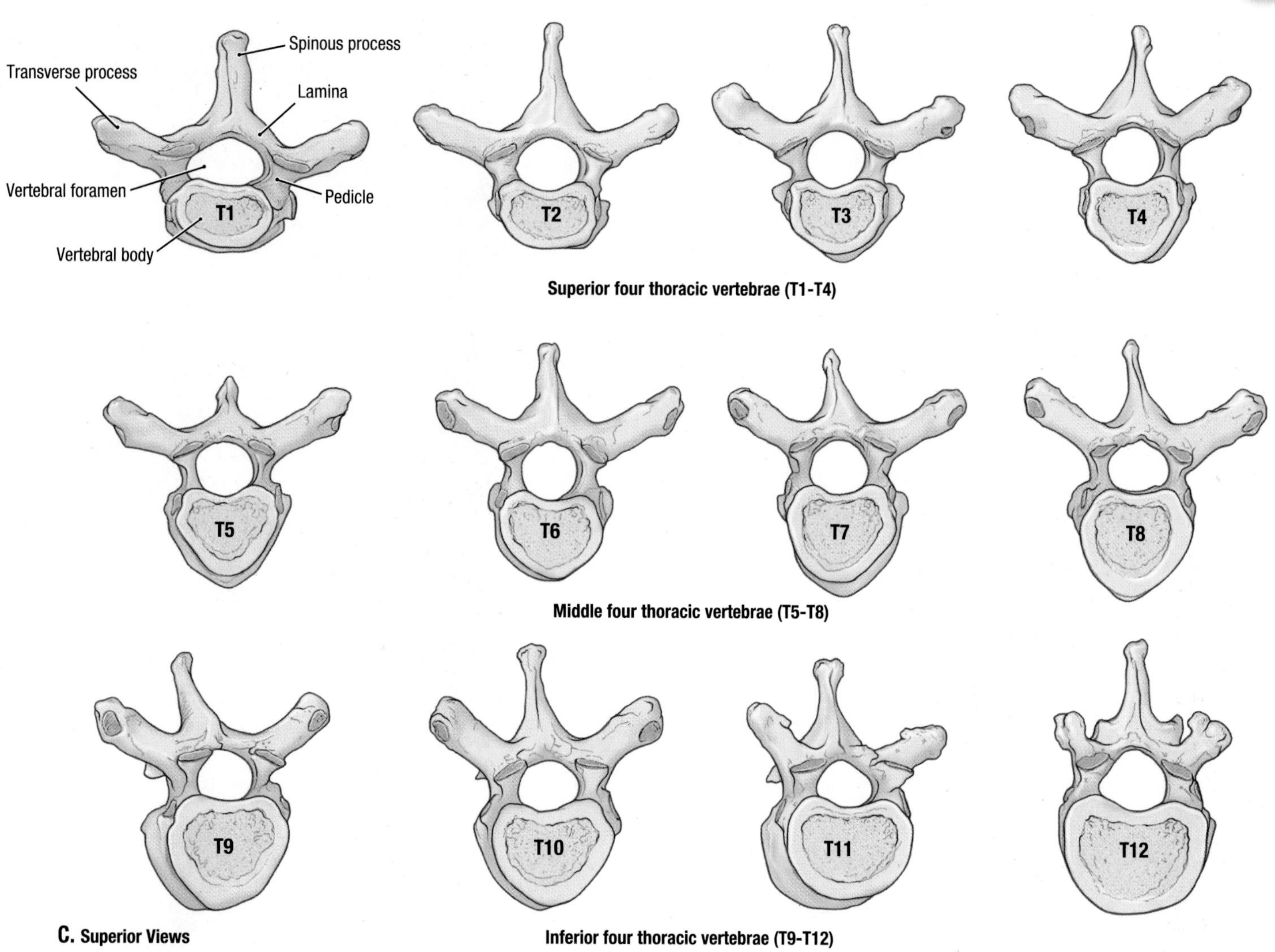

Transverse process
Spinous process
Lamina
Vertebral foramen
Pedicle
Vertebral body
T1 T2 T3 T4

Superior four thoracic vertebrae (T1-T4)

T5 T6 T7 T8

Middle four thoracic vertebrae (T5-T8)

T9 T10 T11 T12

C. Superior Views

Inferior four thoracic vertebrae (T9-T12)

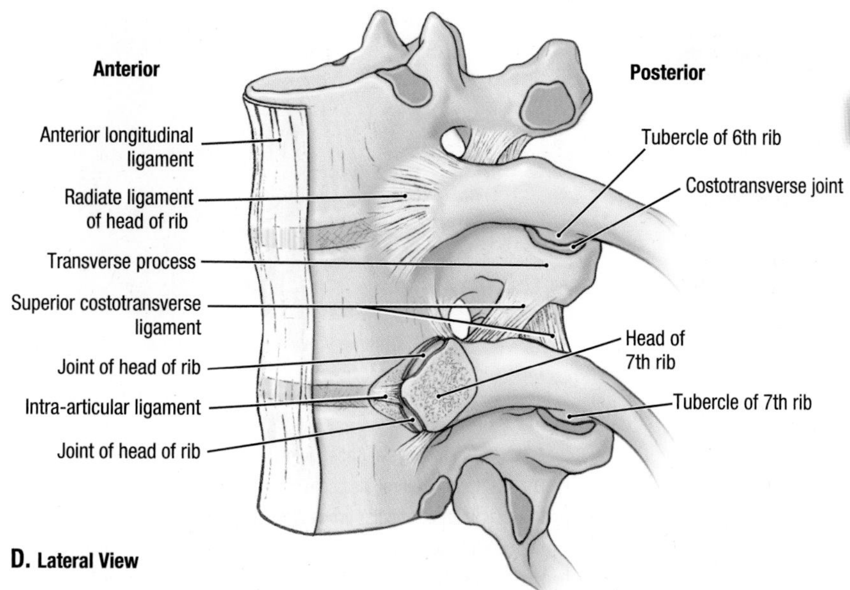
Anterior
Posterior
Anterior longitudinal ligament
Radiate ligament of head of rib
Transverse process
Superior costotransverse ligament
Joint of head of rib
Intra-articular ligament
Joint of head of rib
Tubercle of 6th rib
Costotransverse joint
Head of 7th rib
Tubercle of 7th rib

D. Lateral View

4.15 THORACIC VERTEBRAE (*CONTINUED*)

C. Comparative anatomy. The vertebral bodies increase in size as the vertebral column descends, each bearing an increasing amount of weight transferred by the vertebra above. **Fracture of thoracic vertebrae**. Although the characteristics of the superior aspect of vertebra T12 are distinctly thoracic, its inferior aspect has lumbar characteristics for articulation with vertebra L1. The abrupt transition allowing primarily rotational movements with vertebra T11 while disallowing rotational movements with vertebral L1 makes vertebra T12 especially susceptible to fracture. **D.** Intra- and extra-articular ligaments of the costovertebral articulations. Typically, the head of each rib articulates with the bodies of two adjacent vertebrae and the IV disc between them, and the tubercle of the rib articulates with the transverse process of the inferior vertebra.

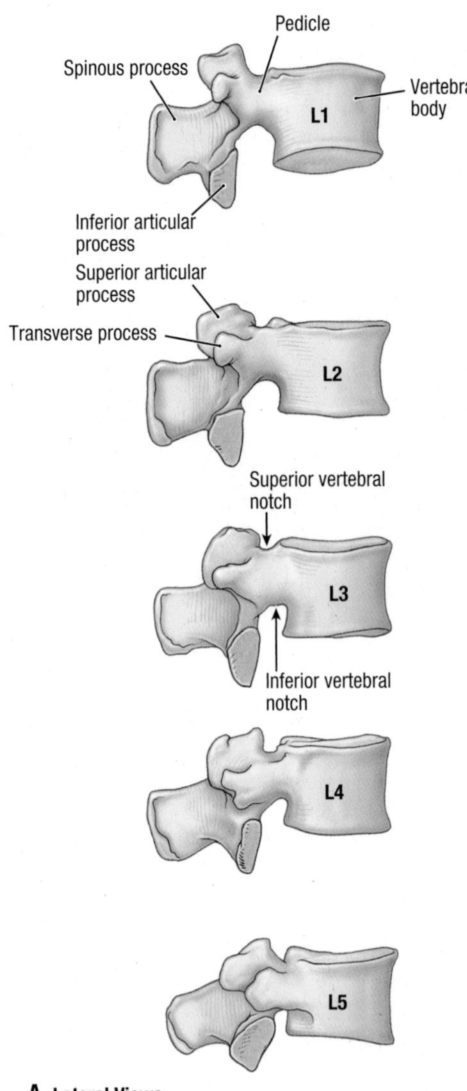
Pedicle
Spinous process
Vertebral body
L1
Inferior articular process
Superior articular process
Transverse process
L2
Superior vertebral notch
L3
Inferior vertebral notch
L4
L5

A. Lateral Views

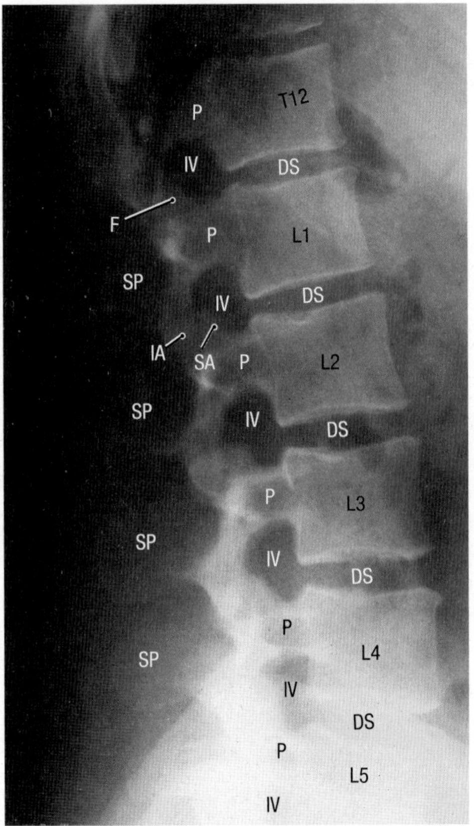
T12
P
IV
DS
F
L1
SP
IA
SA
L2
L3
L4
L5

B. Lateral View

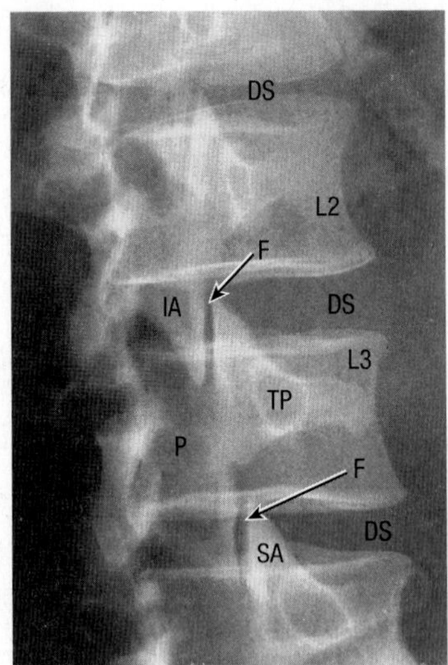
DS
L2
F
IA
L3
TP
P
SA

C. Oblique View

TABLE 4.3 LUMBAR VERTEBRAE

Part	Distinctive Characteristics
Body	Massive; kidney shaped when viewed superiorly
Vertebral	Triangular; larger than in thoracic vertebrae and foramen smaller than in cervical vertebrae
Transverse	Long and slender; accessory process on posterior surface of base of each transverse process
Articular processes	Superior articular facets directed posteromedially (or medially); inferior articular facets directed anterolaterally (or laterally); mammillary process on posterior surface of each superior articular process
Spinous process	Short and sturdy; thick, broad, and rectangular

Key for B, C and D

F	Zygapophysial (facet) joint	P	Pedicle
DS	Intervertebral disc space	SA	Superior articular process
IA	Inferior articular process	SP	Spinous process
IV	Intervertebral foramen	T12–L5	Vertebral bodies
L	Lamina	TP	Transverse process

4.16 LUMBAR VERTEBRAE

A, E, and F. Features. **B, C, and D.** Radiographs **G.** Laminectomy. A **laminectomy** is the surgical excision of one or more spinous processes and their supporting laminae in a particular region of the vertebral column (number 1 in **G.**). The term is also commonly used to denote the removal of most of the vertebral arch by transecting the pedicles (number 2 in **G.**). Laminectomies provide access to the vertebral canal to relieve pressure on the spinal cord or nerve roots, commonly caused by a tumor or herniated IV disc.

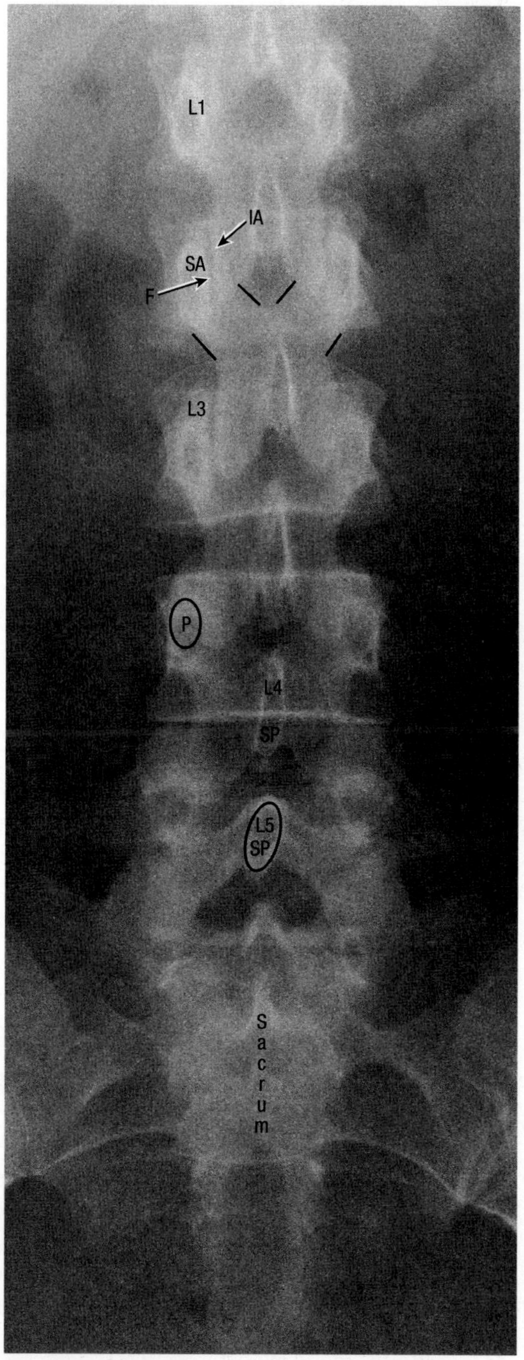

L1
IA
SA
F
L3
P
L4
SP
L5
SP
Sacrum

D. Superior View

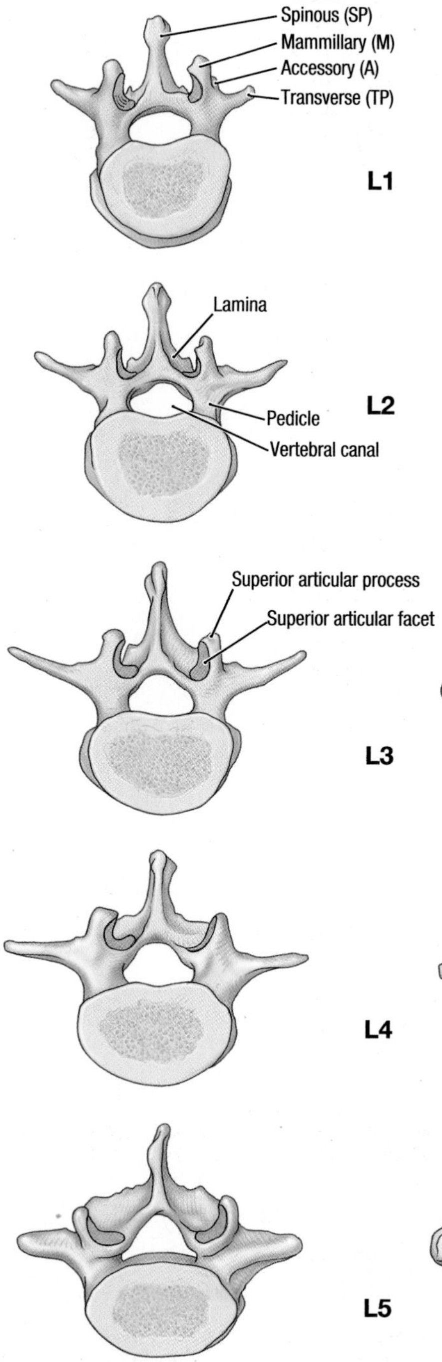

Process:
Spinous (SP)
Mammillary (M)
Accessory (A)
Transverse (TP)
L1
Lamina
Pedicle
Vertebral canal
L2
Superior articular process
Superior articular facet
L3
L4
L5

E. Superior View

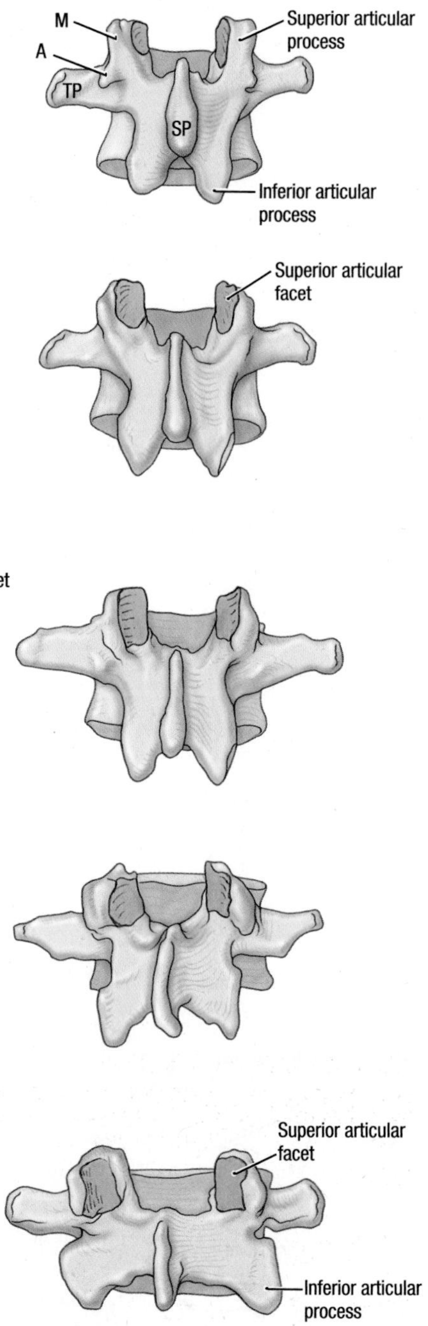

M
A
TP
SP
Superior articular process
Inferior articular process
Superior articular facet
Superior articular facet
Inferior articular process

F. Posterior View

4.16 LUMBAR VERTEBRAE (*CONTINUED*)

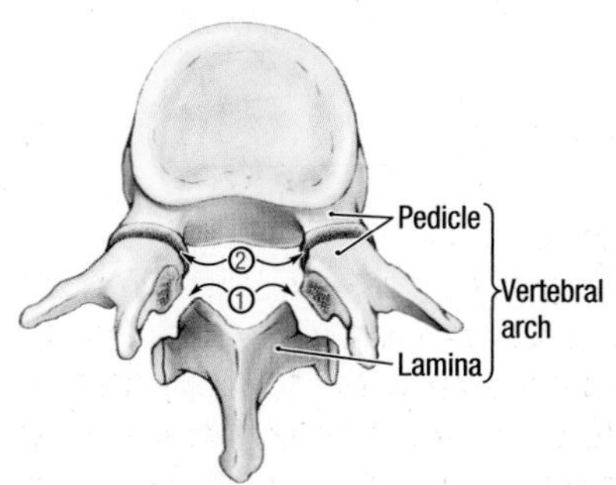
Pedicle
Vertebral arch
Lamina
2
1

G. Superior View, Sites of Laminectomy (1 and 2)

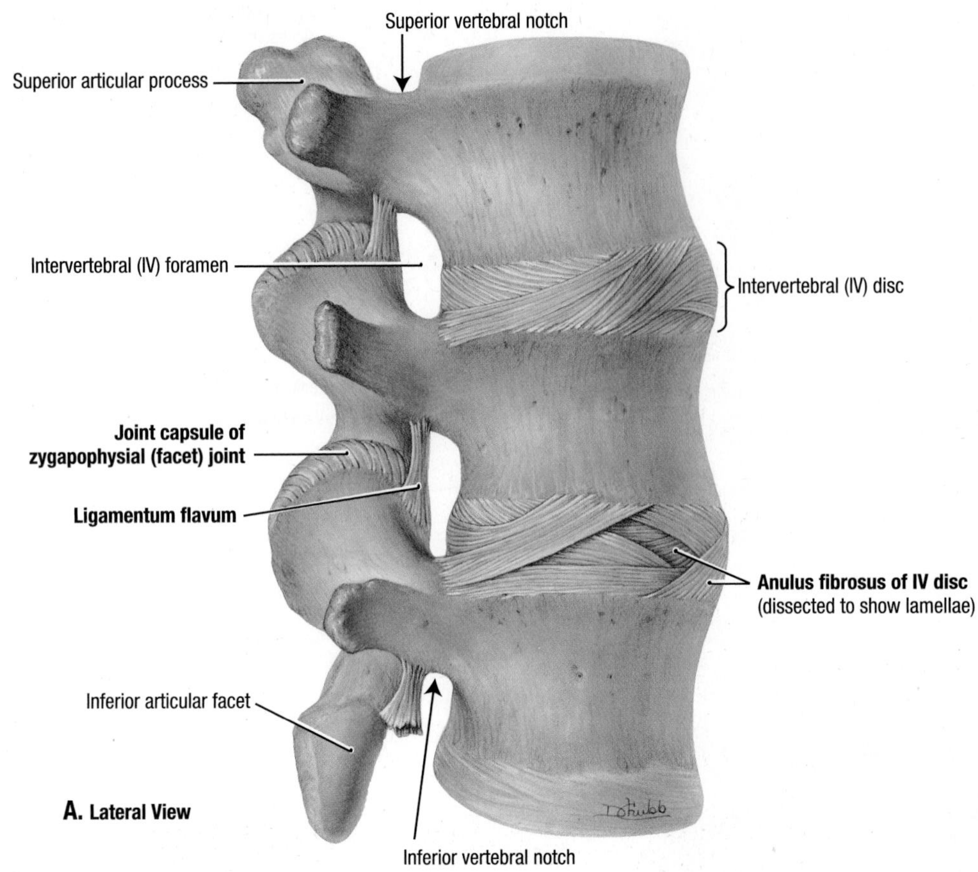
Superior vertebral notch
Superior articular process
Intervertebral (IV) foramen
Intervertebral (IV) disc
Joint capsule of zygapophysial (facet) joint
Ligamentum flavum
Anulus fibrosus of IV disc
(dissected to show lamellae)
Inferior articular facet
Inferior vertebral notch

A. Lateral View

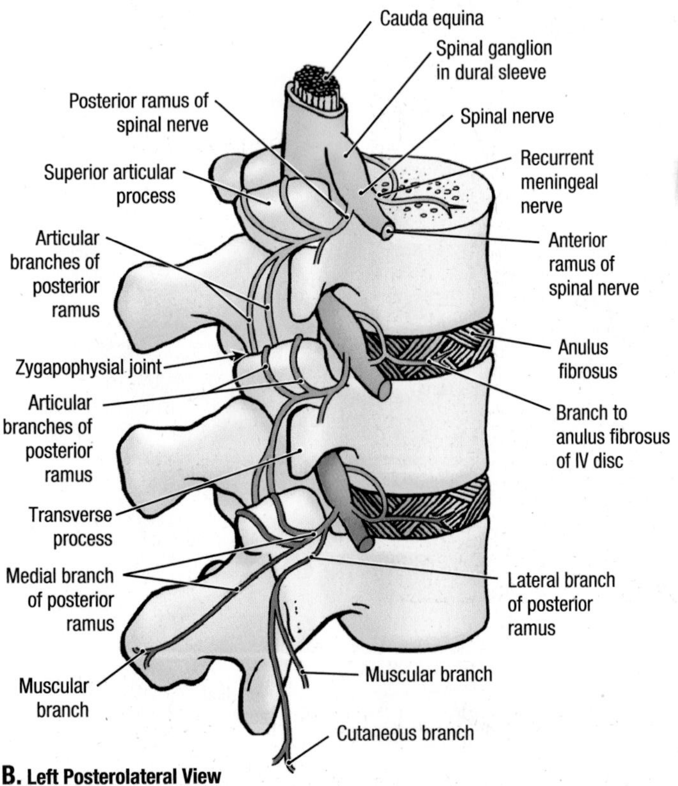
Cauda equina
Spinal ganglion in dural sleeve
Posterior ramus of spinal nerve
Spinal nerve
Superior articular process
Recurrent meningeal nerve
Articular branches of posterior ramus
Anterior ramus of spinal nerve
Zygapophysial joint
Anulus fibrosus
Articular branches of posterior ramus
Branch to anulus fibrosus of IV disc
Transverse process
Medial branch of posterior ramus
Lateral branch of posterior ramus
Muscular branch
Muscular branch
Cutaneous branch

B. Left Posterolateral View

4.17 STRUCTURE AND INNERVATION OF INTERVERTEBRAL DISCS AND ZYGAPOPHYSIAL JOINTS

A. Intervertebral discs and intervertebral foramen. Sections have been removed from the superficial layers of the anulus fibrosus of the inferior IV disc to show the change in direction of the fibers in the concentric layers of the anulus. Note that the IV discs form the inferior half of the anterior boundary of the IV foramen. **B.** Innervation of zygapophysial joints and the anulus fibrosus of IV discs.

When the **zygapophysial joints are injured** or develop osteophytes during aging (osteoarthritis), the related spinal nerves are affected. This causes pain along the distribution pattern of the dermatomes and spasm in the muscles derived from the associated myotomes (a myotome consists of all the muscles or parts of muscles receiving innervation from one spinal nerve). Denervation of lumbar zygapophysial joints is a procedure that may be used for treatment of back pain caused by disease of these joints. The nerves are sectioned near the joints or are destroyed by radiofrequency percutaneous rhizolysis (root dissolution). The denervation process is directed at the articular branches of two adjacent posterior rami of the spinal nerves because each joint receives innervation from both the nerve exiting that level and the superjacent nerve.

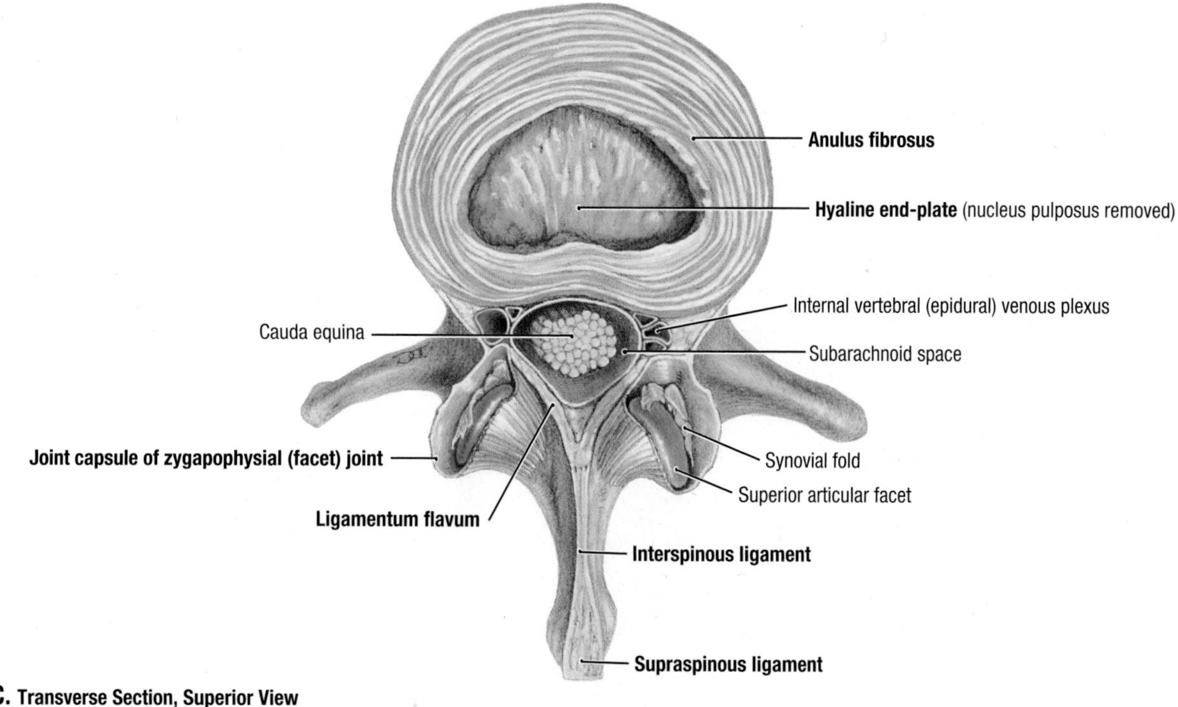
Anulus fibrosus
Hyaline end-plate (nucleus pulposus removed)
Internal vertebral (epidural) venous plexus
Cauda equina
Subarachnoid space
Joint capsule of zygapophysial (facet) joint
Synovial fold
Superior articular facet
Ligamentum flavum
Interspinous ligament
Supraspinous ligament

C. Transverse Section, Superior View

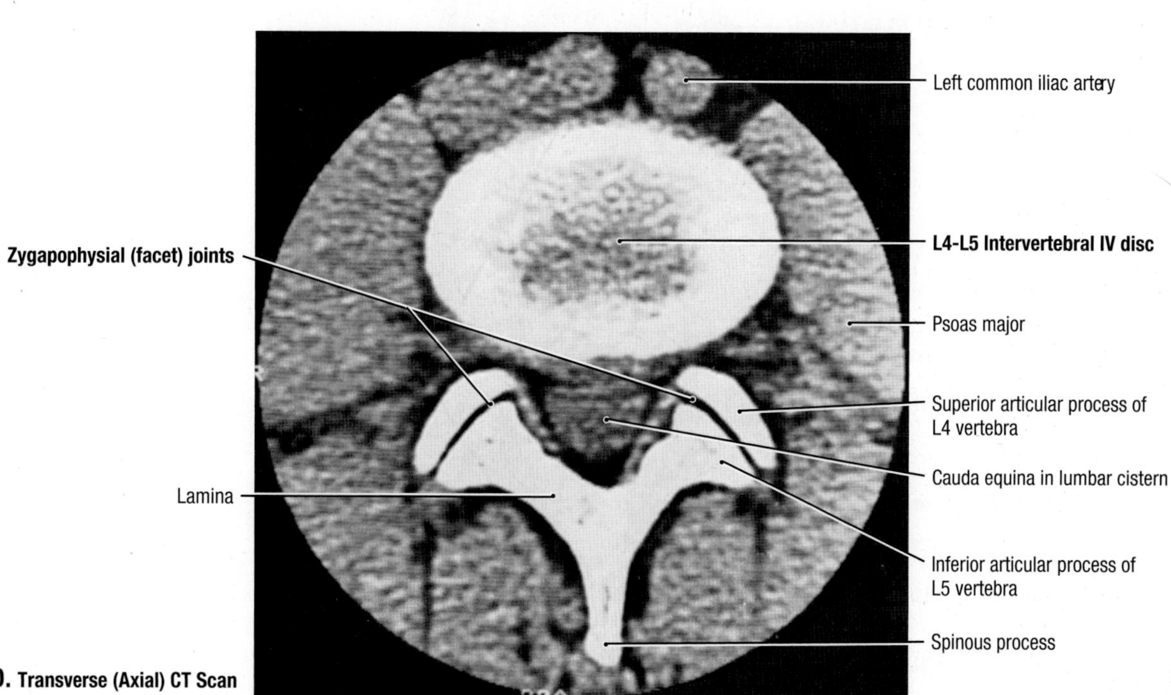
Left common iliac artery
Zygapophysial (facet) joints
L4-L5 Intervertebral IV disc
Psoas major
Superior articular process of L4 vertebra
Cauda equina in lumbar cistern
Lamina
Inferior articular process of L5 vertebra
Spinous process

D. Transverse (Axial) CT Scan

4.17 STRUCTURE AND INNERVATION OF INTERVERTEBRAL DISCS AND ZYGAPOPHYSIAL JOINTS (*CONTINUED*)

C. Transverse section. The nucleus pulposus has been removed, and the cartilaginous epiphysial plate exposed. There are fewer rings of the anulus fibrosus posteriorly, and consequently, this portion of the annulus fibrosus is thinner. The ligamentum flavum, interspinous, and supraspinous ligaments are continuous. **D.** CT image of L4/L5 IV disc.

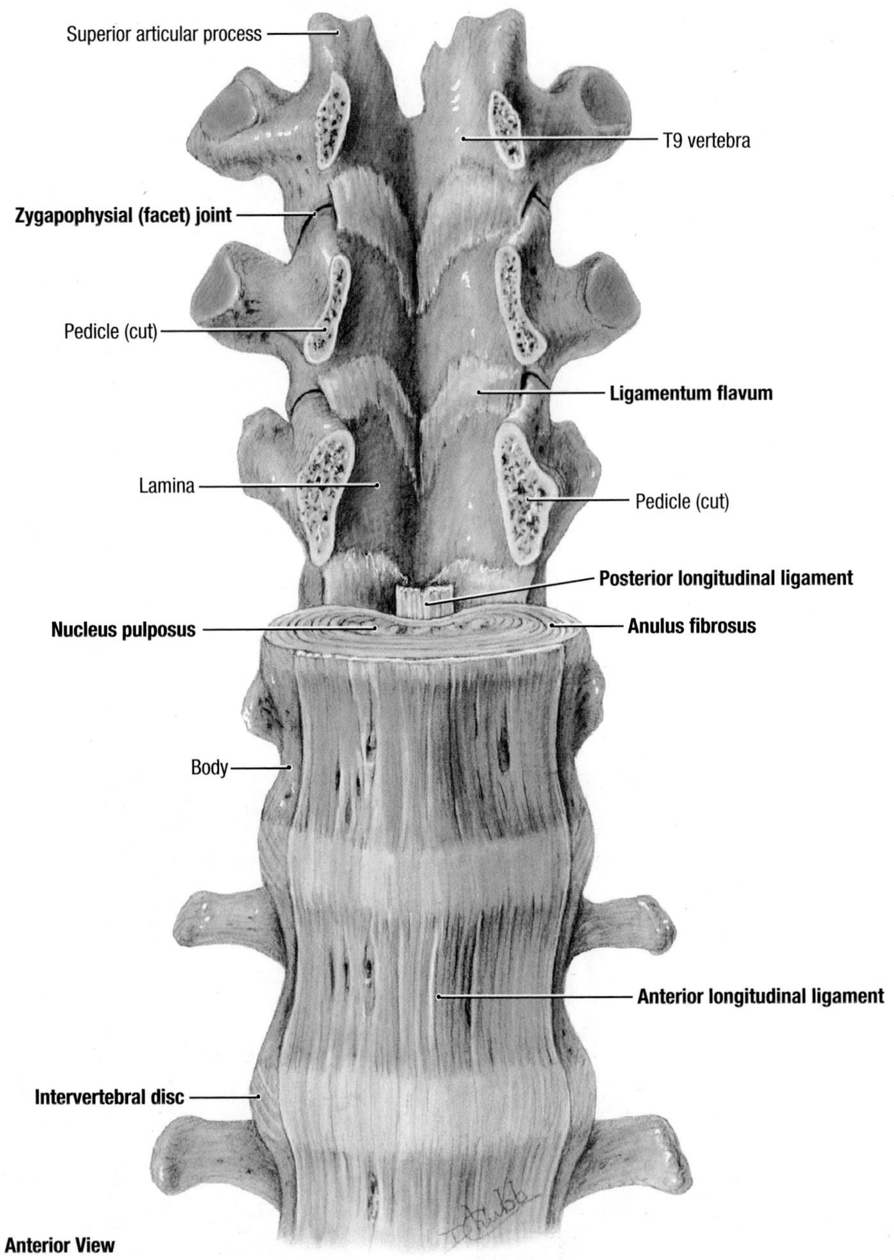

Superior articular process
T9 vertebra
Zygapophysial (facet) joint
Pedicle (cut)
Ligamentum flavum
Lamina
Pedicle (cut)
Posterior longitudinal ligament
Nucleus pulposus
Anulus fibrosus
Body
Anterior longitudinal ligament
Intervertebral disc

A. **Anterior View**

4.18 INTERVERTEBRAL DISCS: LIGAMENTS AND MOVEMENTS

A. Anterior longitudinal ligament and ligamenta flava. The pedicles of vertebrae T9 to T11 were sawed through, and the posterior aspect of the bodies is shown in **B.**

B. Posterior longitudinal ligament. **C.** IV disc during loading and movement.

- The anterior and posterior longitudinal ligaments are ligaments of the vertebral bodies; the ligamenta flava are ligaments of the vertebral arches.
- The anterior longitudinal ligament consists of broad, strong, fibrous bands, thickened centrally, that are attached to the IV discs and vertebral bodies anteriorly and are perforated by the foramina for arteries and veins passing to and from the vertebral bodies.
- The ligamenta flava, composed of elastic fibers, extend between adjacent laminae; right and left ligaments converge in the median plane. They extend laterally to the articular processes, where they blend with the joint capsule of the zygapophysial joints.

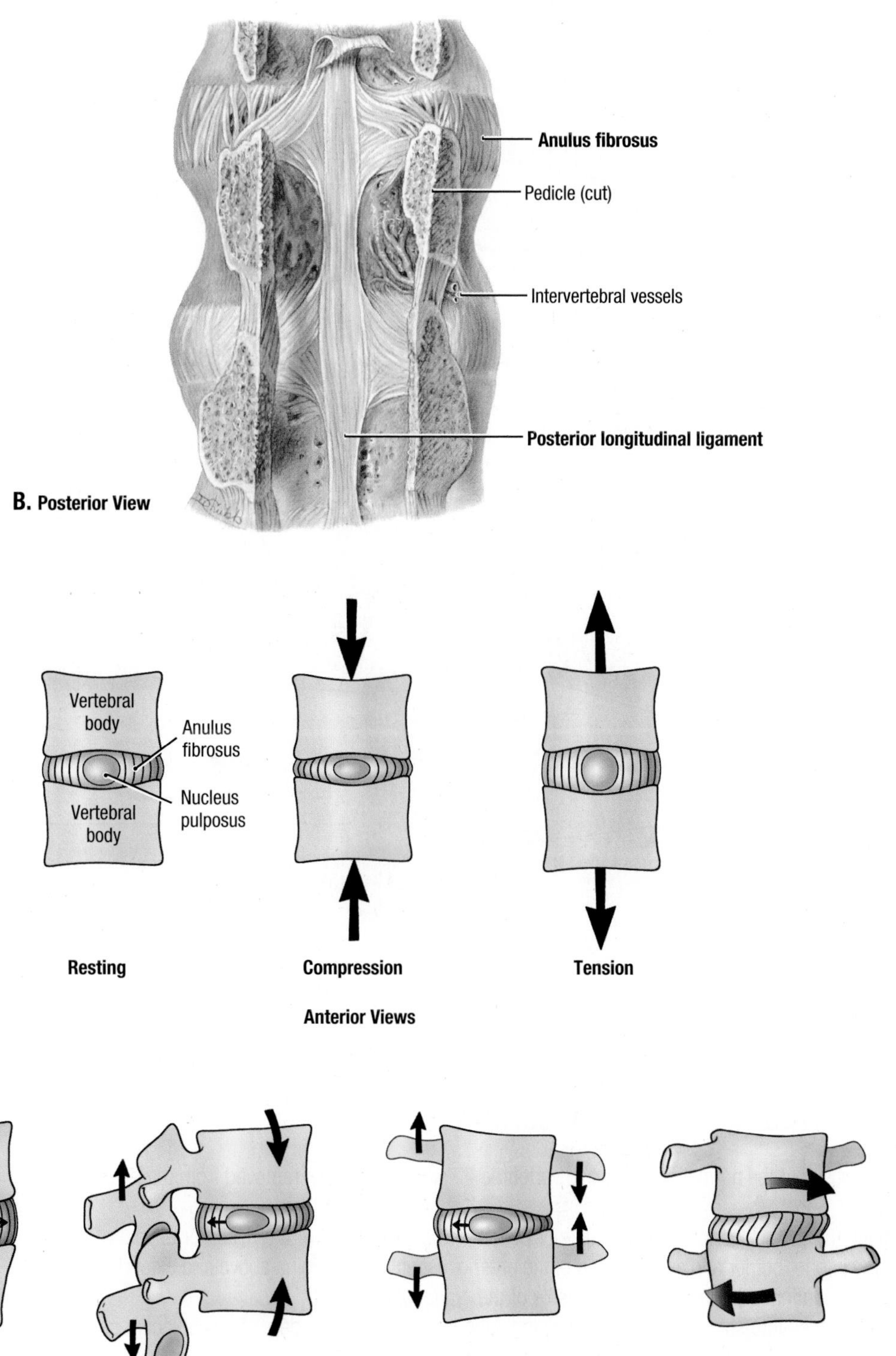
Anulus fibrosus
Pedicle (cut)
Intervertebral vessels
Posterior longitudinal ligament
B. Posterior View
Vertebral body
Anulus fibrosus
Nucleus pulposus
Vertebral body
Resting
Compression
Tension
Anterior Views
C.
Extension
Flexion
Lateral flexion
Rotation (torsion)
Lateral Views
Anterior Views

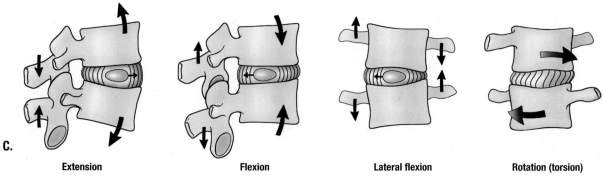

4.18 INTERVERTEBRAL DISCS: LIGAMENTS AND MOVEMENTS (*CONTINUED*)

- The posterior longitudinal ligament is a narrow band passing from disc to disc, spanning the posterior surfaces of the vertebral bodies (in **B**). The ligament is diamond shaped posterior to each IV disc, where it exchanges fibers with the anulus fibrosus; the ligament extends to the sacrum inferiorly and becomes the tectorial membrane cranially.
- The movement or loading of the IV disc changes its shape and the position of the nucleus pulposus. Flexion and extension movements cause compression and tension simultaneously.

Anterior longitudinal ligament
Posterior longitudinal ligament
L1
Ligamentum flavum
Nucleus pulposus protruding posteriorly
L2
Interspinous ligament
Cavity for **nucleus pulposus**
Intervertebral foramen
Anulus fibrosus
Hyaline plate
L3
Supraspinous ligament
Spinal nerve
Nucleus pulposus protruding into vertebral bodies
Anterior and posterior nerve roots
Bursa
Canal for basivertebral vein
Dura mater
L4
Median Section

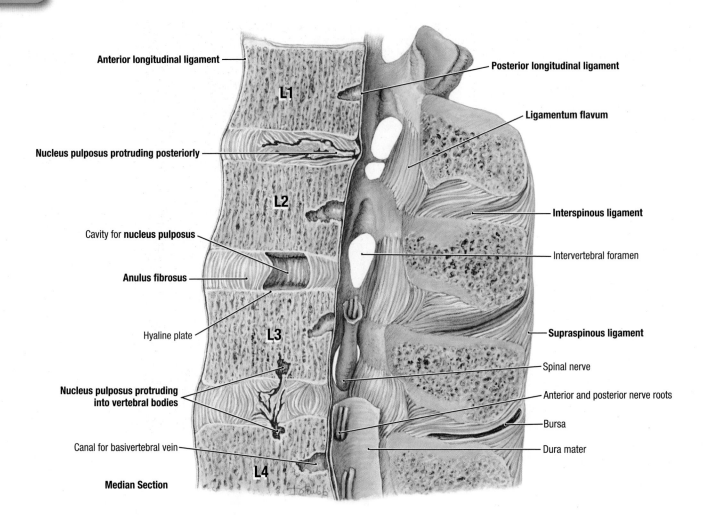

4.19 LUMBAR REGION OF VERTEBRAL COLUMN

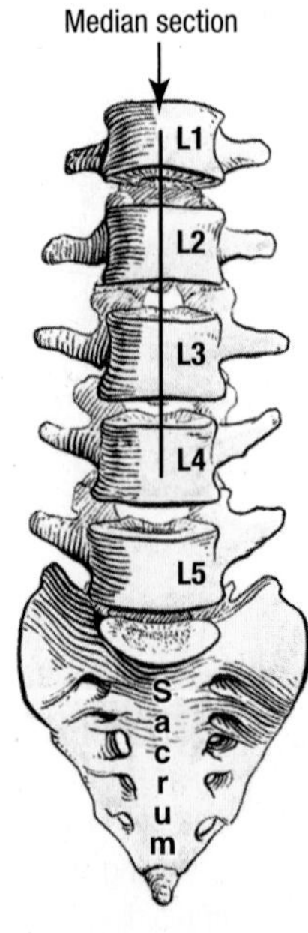
Median section
L1
L2
L3
L4
L5
Sacrum

The nucleus pulposus of the normal disc between vertebrae L2 and L3 has been removed from the enclosing anulus fibrosus.

- The ligamentum flavum extends from the superior border and adjacent part of the posterior aspect of one lamina to the inferior border and adjacent part of the anterior aspect of the lamina above and extends laterally to become continuous with the fibrous capsule of the zygapophysial joint.
- The obliquely placed interspinous ligament unites the superior and inferior borders of two adjacent spines.
- The bursa between L3 and L4 spines is presumably the result of habitual hyperextension, which brings the lumbar spines into contact.

The nucleus pulposus of the disc between L1 and L2 has herniated posteriorly through the anulus. **Herniation** or **protrusion of the gelatinous nucleus pulposus** into or through the anulus fibrosus is a well-recognized cause of low back and lower limb pain. If degeneration of the posterior longitudinal ligament and wearing of the anulus fibrosus has occurred, the nucleus pulposus may herniate into the vertebral canal and compress the spinal cord or nerve roots of spinal nerves in the cauda equina. Herniations usually occur posterolaterally, where the anulus is relatively thin and does not receive support from either the posterior or anterior longitudinal ligaments.

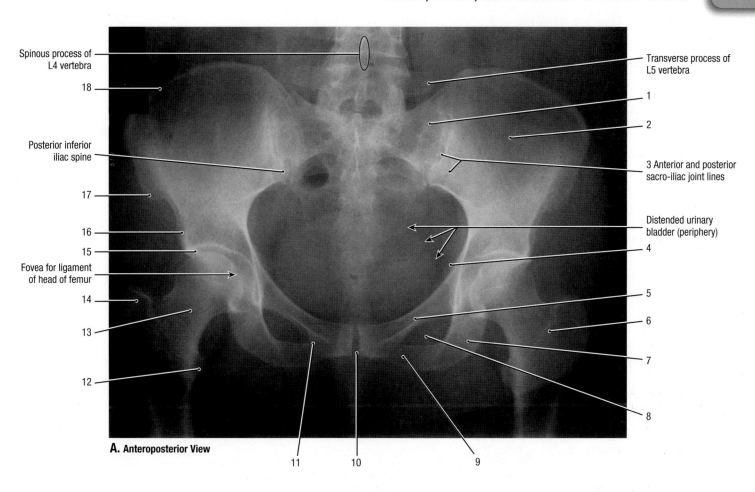

Spinous process of L4 vertebra
18
Posterior inferior iliac spine
17
16
15
Fovea for ligament of head of femur
14
13
12
Transverse process of L5 vertebra
1
2
3 Anterior and posterior sacro-iliac joint lines
Distended urinary bladder (periphery)
4
5
6
7
8
11
10
9

A. **Anteroposterior View**

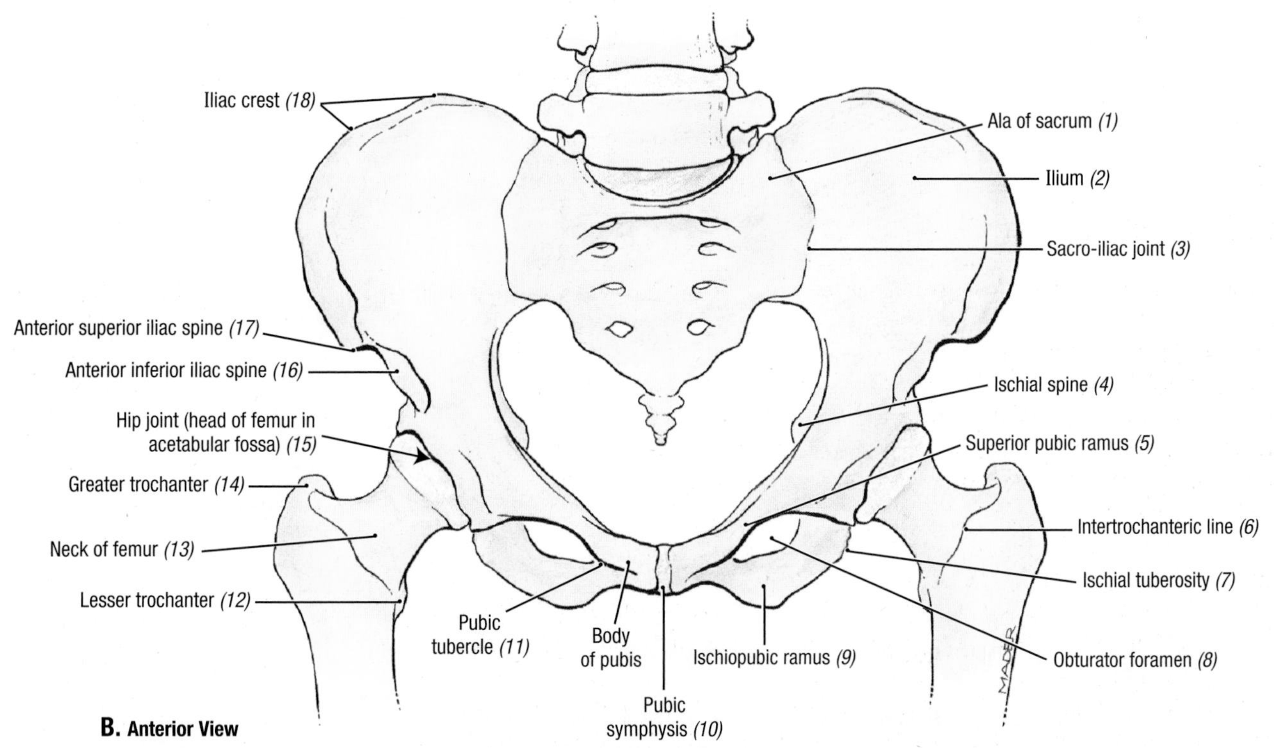
Iliac crest *(18)*
Ala of sacrum *(1)*
Ilium *(2)*
Sacro-iliac joint *(3)*
Anterior superior iliac spine *(17)*
Anterior inferior iliac spine *(16)*
Ischial spine *(4)*
Hip joint (head of femur in acetabular fossa) *(15)*
Superior pubic ramus *(5)*
Greater trochanter *(14)*
Intertrochanteric line *(6)*
Neck of femur *(13)*
Ischial tuberosity *(7)*
Lesser trochanter *(12)*
Pubic tubercle *(11)*
Body of pubis
Ischiopubic ramus *(9)*
Obturator foramen *(8)*
Pubic symphysis *(10)*
MADER

B. **Anterior View**

4.20 PELVIS

A. Radiograph of pelvis. **B.** Bony pelvis with articulated femora.

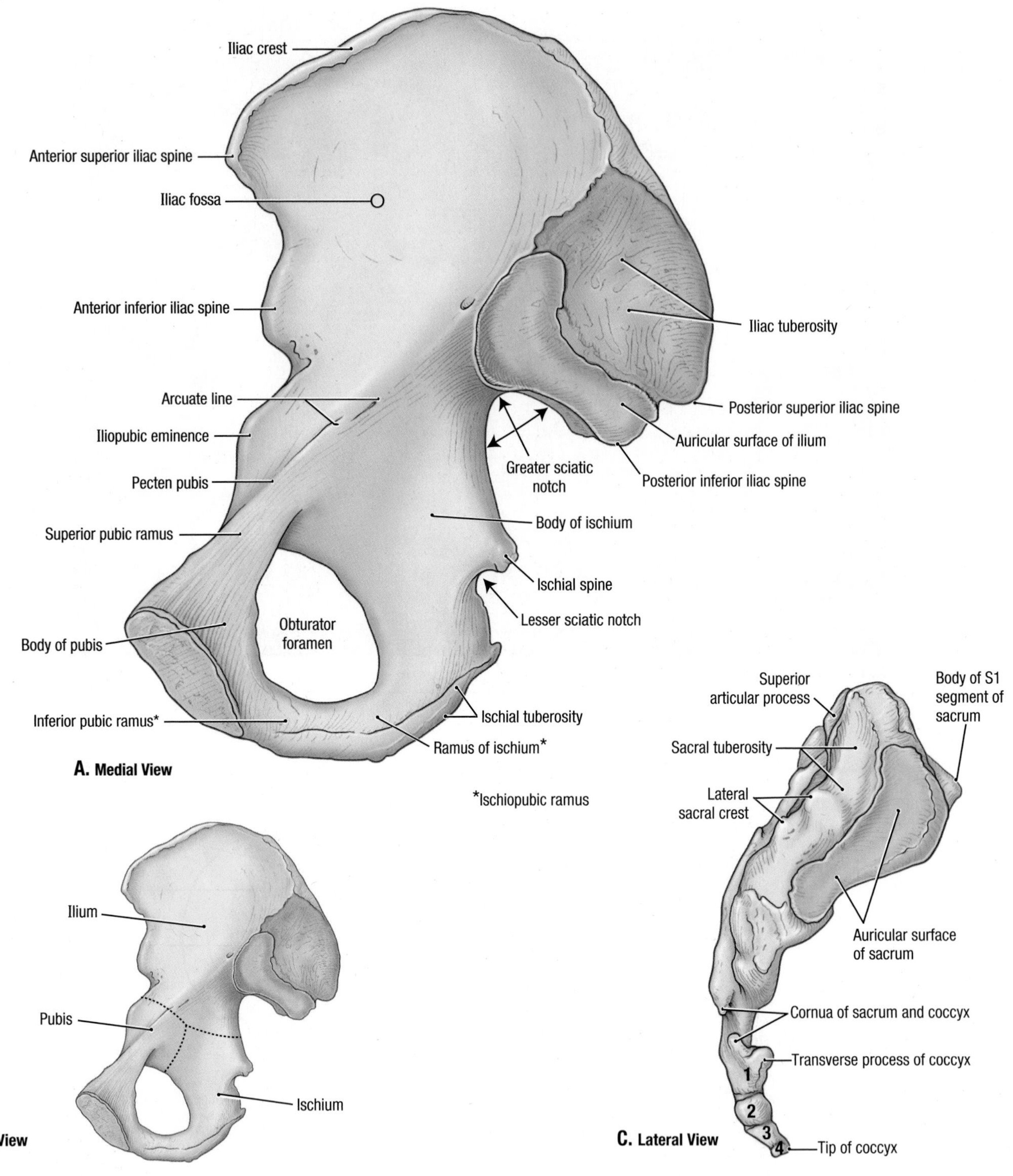

Iliac crest
Anterior superior iliac spine
Iliac fossa
Anterior inferior iliac spine
Iliac tuberosity
Arcuate line
Posterior superior iliac spine
Iliopubic eminence
Auricular surface of ilium
Greater sciatic notch
Pecten pubis
Posterior inferior iliac spine
Body of ischium
Superior pubic ramus
Ischial spine
Lesser sciatic notch
Obturator foramen
Body of pubis
Ischial tuberosity
Inferior pubic ramus*
Ramus of ischium*
A. Medial View
*Ischiopubic ramus
Superior articular process
Body of S1 segment of sacrum
Sacral tuberosity
Lateral sacral crest
Auricular surface of sacrum
Ilium
Pubis
Ischium
Cornua of sacrum and coccyx
Transverse process of coccyx
1
2
3
4
Tip of coccyx
B. Medial View
C. Lateral View

4.21 HIP BONE, SACRUM, AND COCCYX

A. Features of hip bone. **B.** Ilium, ischium, and pubis. **C.** Sacrum and coccyx. Vertebral column is fused to the sacrum.

- Each hip bone consists of three bones: ilium, ischium, and pubis.
- Anterosuperiorly, the auricular, ear-shaped surface of the sacrum articulates with the auricular surface of the ilium; the sacral and iliac tuberosities are for the attachment of the posterior sacro-iliac and interosseous sacro-iliac ligaments.

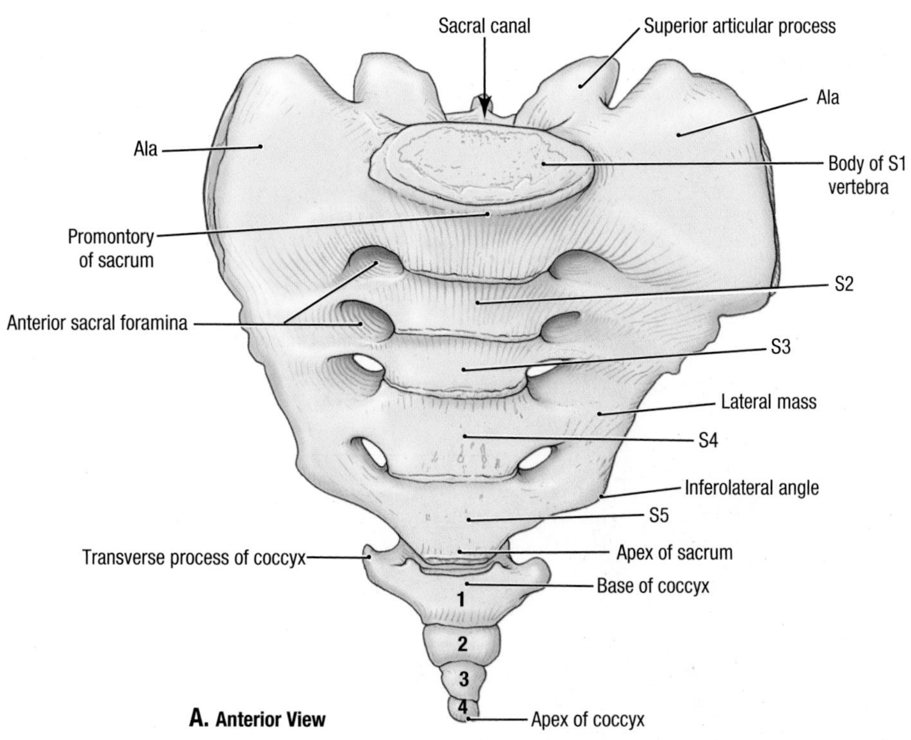
Sacral canal
Superior articular process
Ala
Ala
Body of S1 vertebra
Promontory of sacrum
S2
Anterior sacral foramina
S3
Lateral mass
S4
Inferolateral angle
S5
Transverse process of coccyx
Apex of sacrum
Base of coccyx
1
2
3
4
Apex of coccyx

A. Anterior View

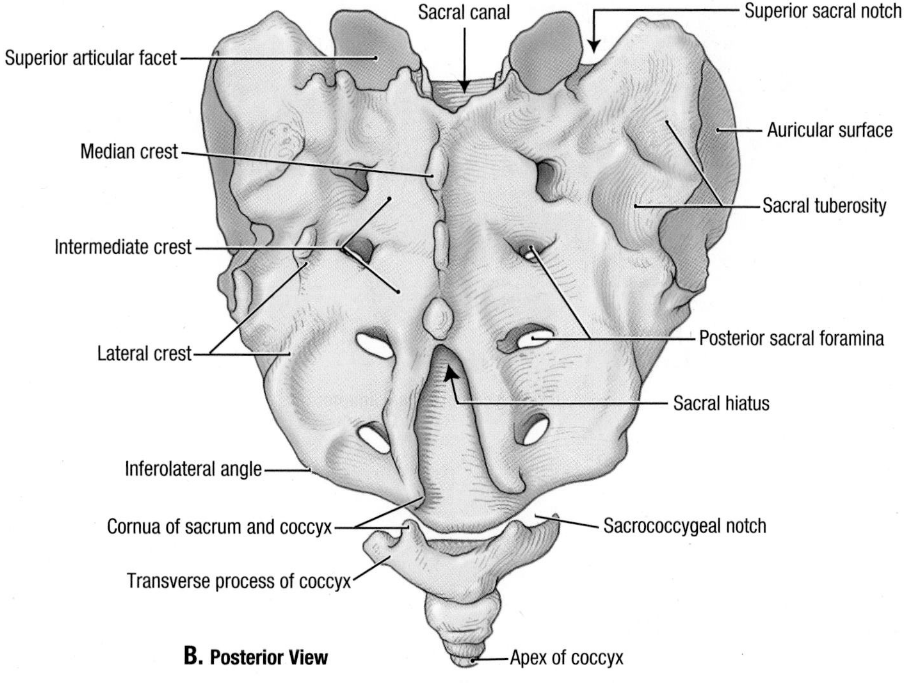
Sacral canal
Superior sacral notch
Superior articular facet
Auricular surface
Median crest
Sacral tuberosity
Intermediate crest
Lateral crest
Posterior sacral foramina
Sacral hiatus
Inferolateral angle
Cornua of sacrum and coccyx
Sacrococcygeal notch
Transverse process of coccyx
Apex of coccyx

B. Posterior View

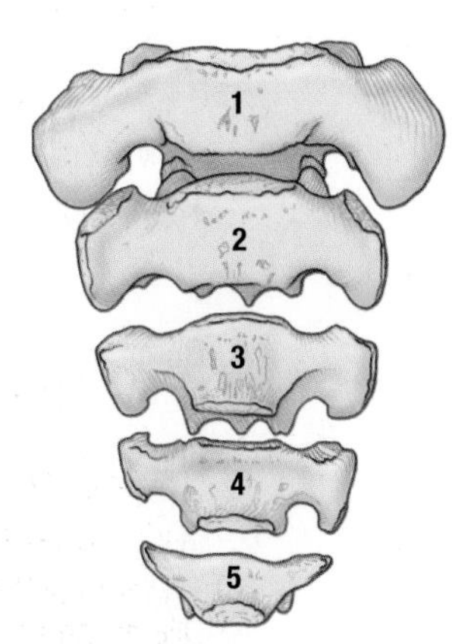
1
2
3
4
5

C. Anterior View

4.22 SACRUM AND COCCYX

A. Pelvic (anterior) surface. **B.** Dorsal (posterior surface). **C.** Sacrum in youth.

- In **A,** the bodies of the five sacral vertebrae are demarcated in the mature sacrum by four transverse lines ending laterally in four pairs of anterior sacral foramina. The coccyx has four vertebrae (segments)—the first having a pair of transverse processes and a pair of cornua (horns).
- The costal (lateral) elements of the coccygeal vertebrae begin to fuse around puberty. The bodies begin to fuse from inferior to superior at about the 17th to 18th year, with fusion usually completed by the 23rd year.

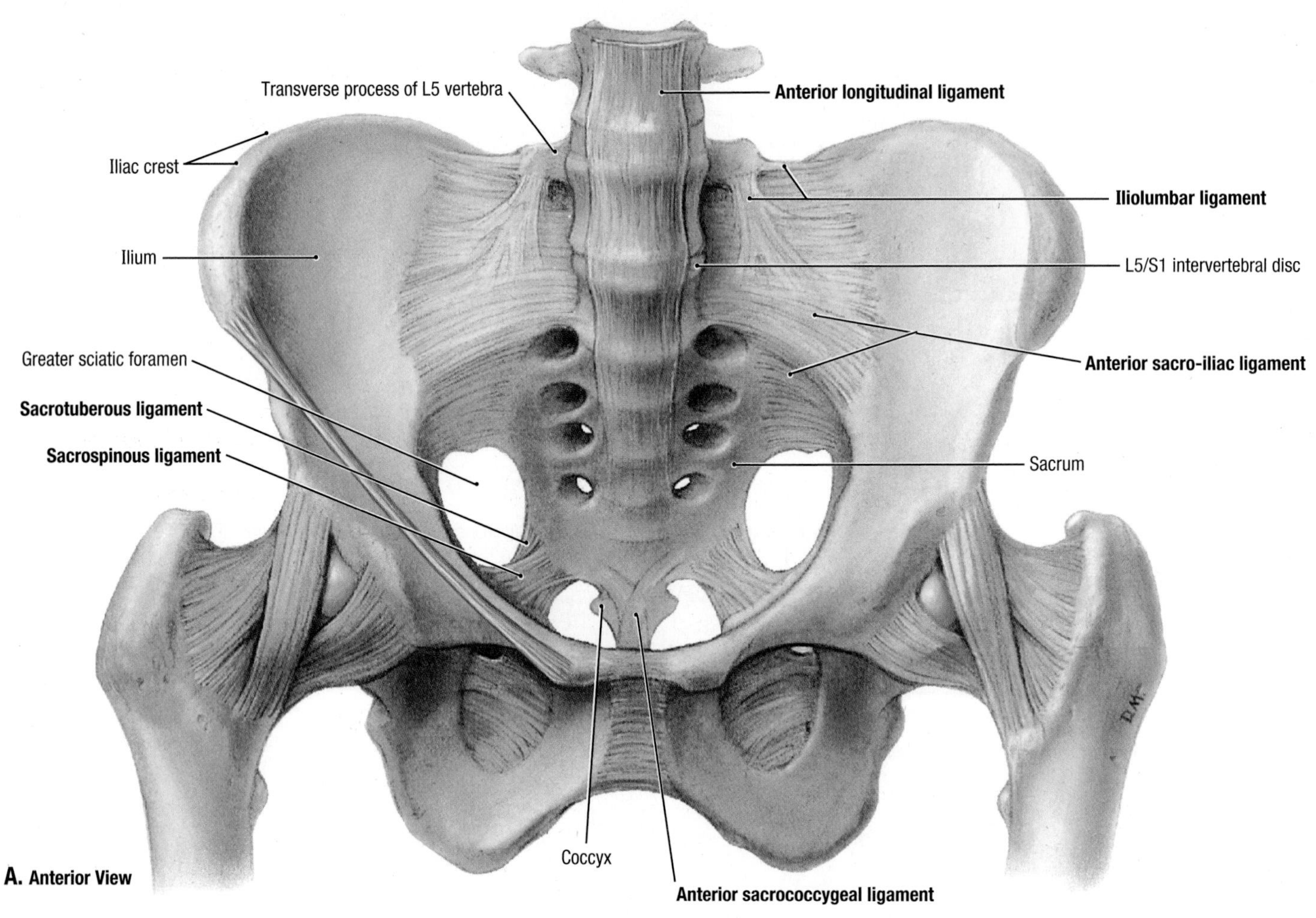
Transverse process of L5 vertebra
Anterior longitudinal ligament
Iliac crest
Iliolumbar ligament
Ilium
L5/S1 intervertebral disc
Greater sciatic foramen
Anterior sacro-iliac ligament
Sacrotuberous ligament
Sacrospinous ligament
Sacrum
Coccyx
Anterior sacrococcygeal ligament

A. Anterior View

4.23 LUMBAR AND PELVIC LIGAMENTS

- The anterior sacro-iliac ligament is part of the fibrous capsule of the sacro-iliac joint anteriorly and spans between the lateral aspect of the sacrum and the ilium, anterior to the auricular surfaces.

During **pregnancy,** the pelvic joints and ligaments relax**,** and pelvic movements increase. The sacro-iliac interlocking mechanism is less effective because the relaxation permits greater rotation of the pelvis and contributes to the lordotic posture often assumed during pregnancy with the change in the center of gravity. Relaxation of the sacro-iliac joints and pubic symphysis permits as much as 10% to 15% increase in diameters (mostly transverse), facilitating passage of the fetus through the pelvic canal. The coccyx is also allowed to move posteriorly.

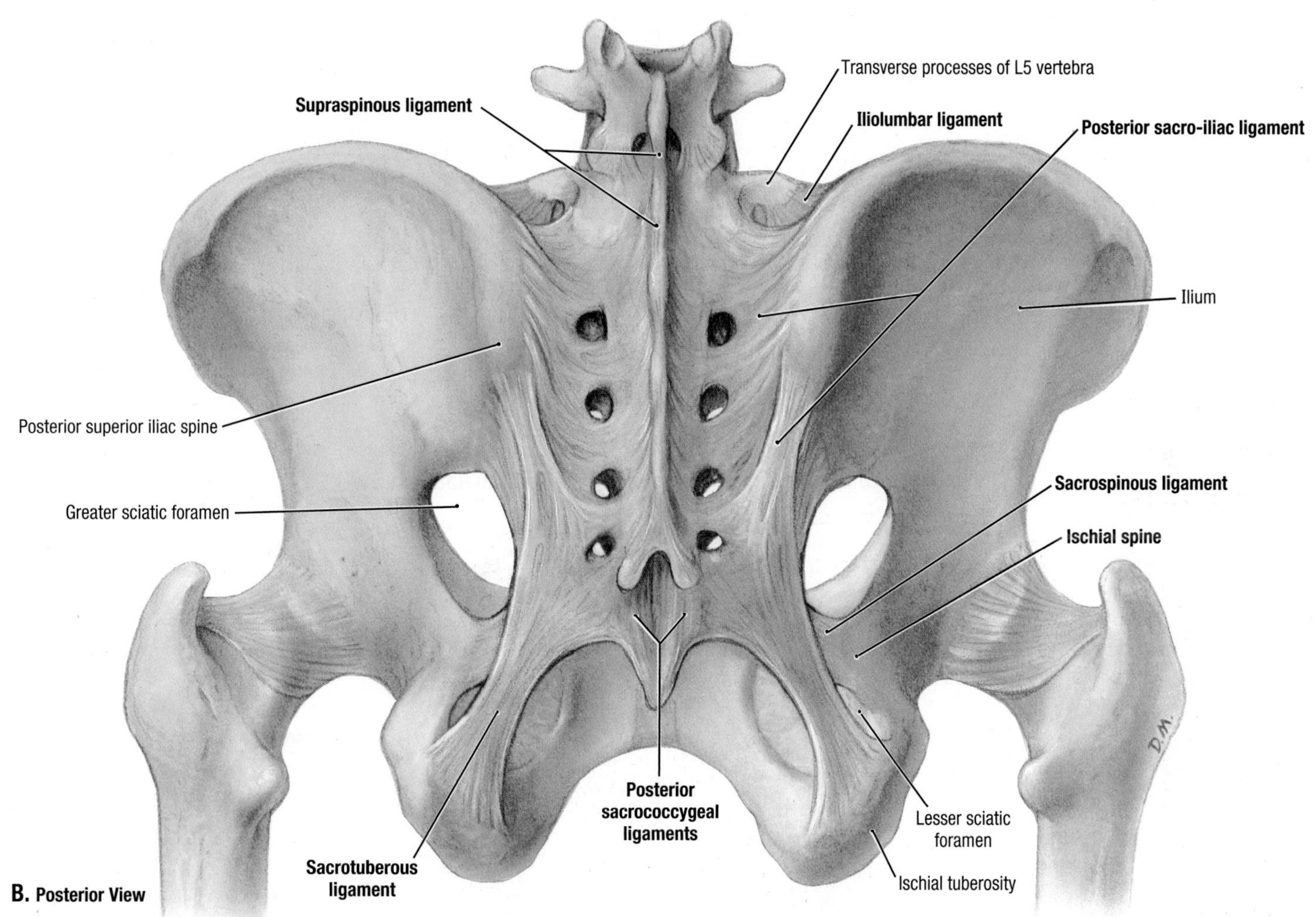
Transverse processes of L5 vertebra
Supraspinous ligament
Iliolumbar ligament
Posterior sacro-iliac ligament
Ilium
Posterior superior iliac spine
Sacrospinous ligament
Greater sciatic foramen
Ischial spine
Posterior sacrococcygeal ligaments
Lesser sciatic foramen
Sacrotuberous ligament
Ischial tuberosity
D.M.

B. Posterior View

4.23 LUMBAR AND PELVIC LIGAMENTS (*CONTINUED*)

- The sacrotuberous ligaments attach the sacrum, ilium, and coccyx to the ischial tuberosity; the sacrospinous ligaments unite the sacrum and coccyx to the ischial spine. The sacrotuberous and sacrospinous ligaments convert the sciatic notches of the hip bones into greater and lesser sciatic foramina.
- The fibers of the posterior sacro-iliac ligament vary in obliquity; the superior fibers are shorter and lie between the ilium and superior part of the sacrum; the longer, obliquely oriented inferior fibers span between the posterior superior iliac spine and the inferior part of the sacrum, also blending with the sacrotuberous ligament.
- The interosseous sacro-iliac ligament lies deep to the posterior sacro-iliac ligament (see Fig. 4.24).
- The iliolumbar ligaments unite the ilia and transverse processes of L5; the lumbosacral portions of the ligaments descend to the alae of the sacrum and blend with the anterior sacro-iliac ligaments.

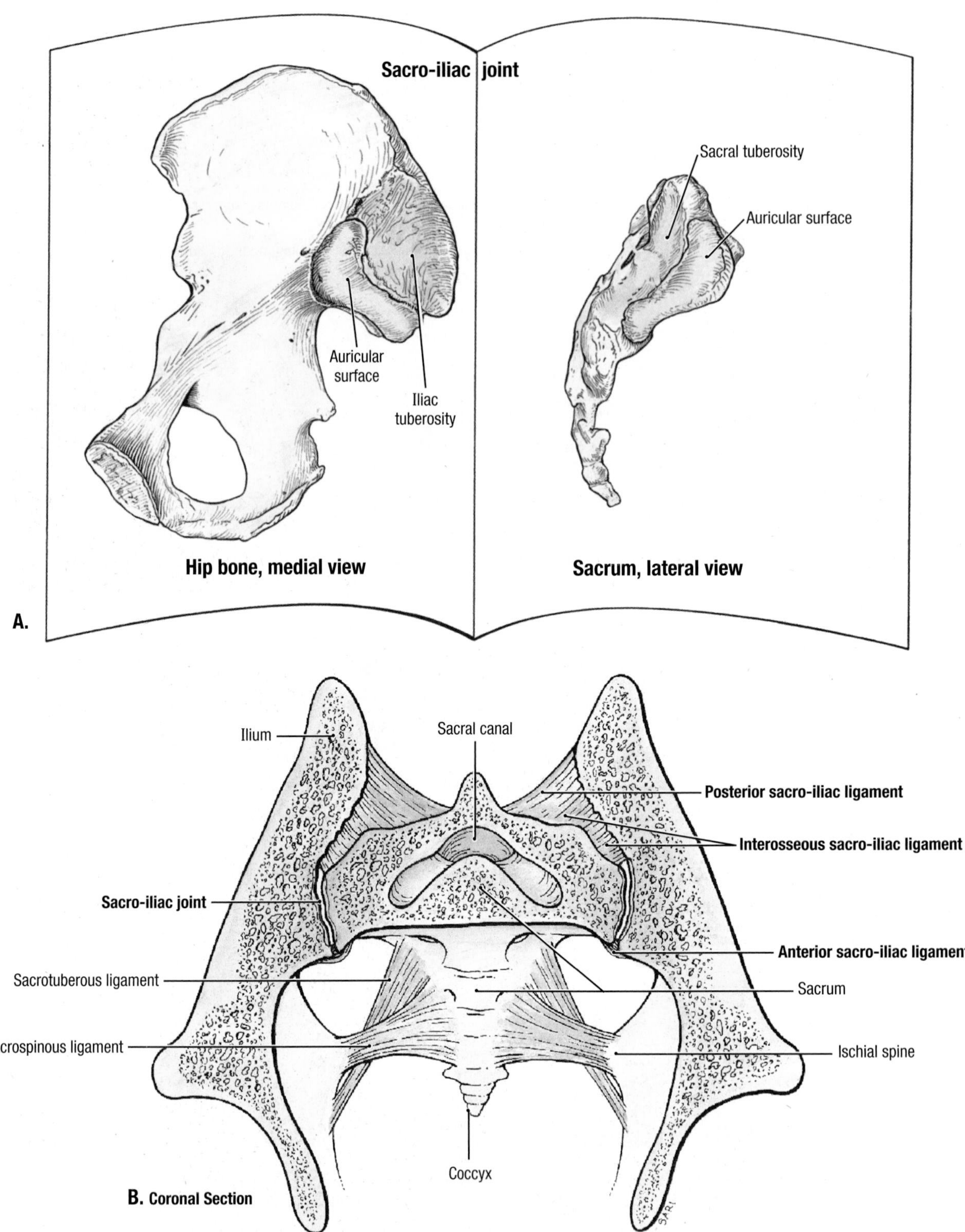
Sacro-iliac joint
Sacral tuberosity
Auricular surface
Auricular surface
Iliac tuberosity
Hip bone, medial view
Sacrum, lateral view
A.
Ilium
Sacral canal
Posterior sacro-iliac ligament
Interosseous sacro-iliac ligament
Sacro-iliac joint
Anterior sacro-iliac ligament
Sacrotuberous ligament
Sacrum
Sacrospinous ligament
Ischial spine
Coccyx
B. Coronal Section

4.24 ARTICULAR SURFACES OF SACRO-ILIAC JOINT AND LIGAMENTS

A. Articular surfaces. Note the auricular surface (articular area, *blue*) of the sacrum and hip bone and the roughened areas superior and posterior to the auricular areas (*orange*) for the attachment of the interosseous sacro-iliac ligament. **B.** Sacro-iliac ligaments. Note the sacro-iliac joints and the strong interosseous sacro-iliac ligament that lies inferior and anterior to the posterior sacro-iliac ligament. The interosseous sacro-iliac ligament consists of short fibers connecting the sacral tuberosity to the iliac tuberosity. The sacrum is suspended from the ilia by the posterior and interosseous sacro-iliac ligaments.

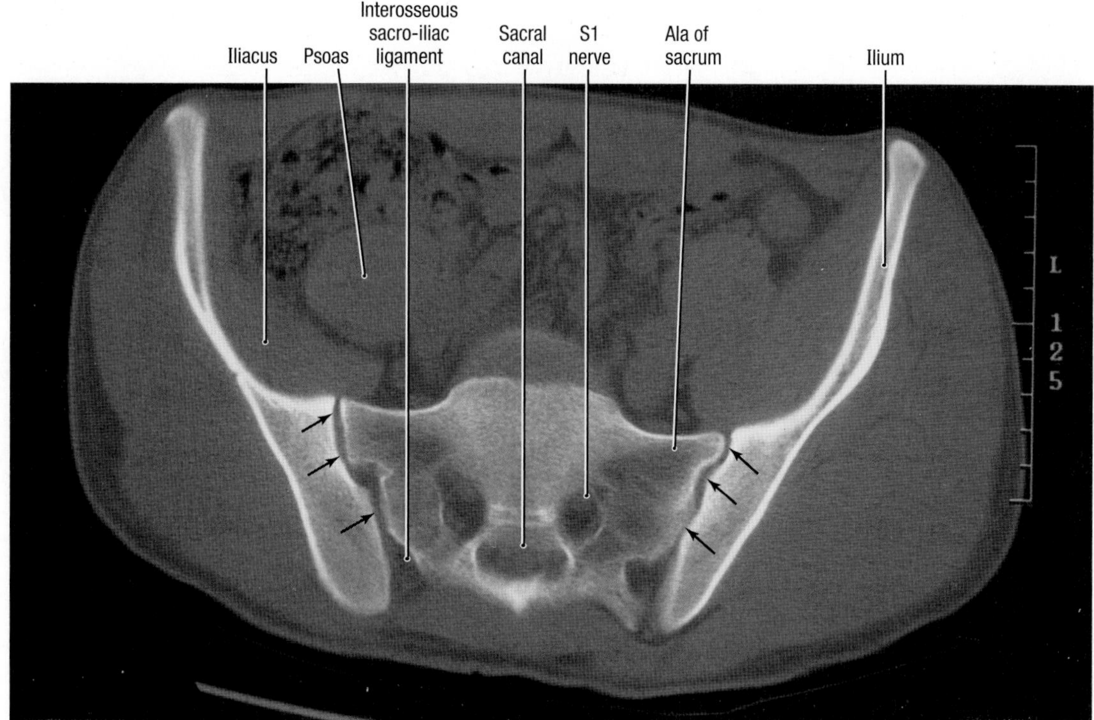
Iliacus
Psoas
Interosseous sacro-iliac ligament
Sacral canal
S1 nerve
Ala of sacrum
Ilium

A. Transverse (axial) CT Scan

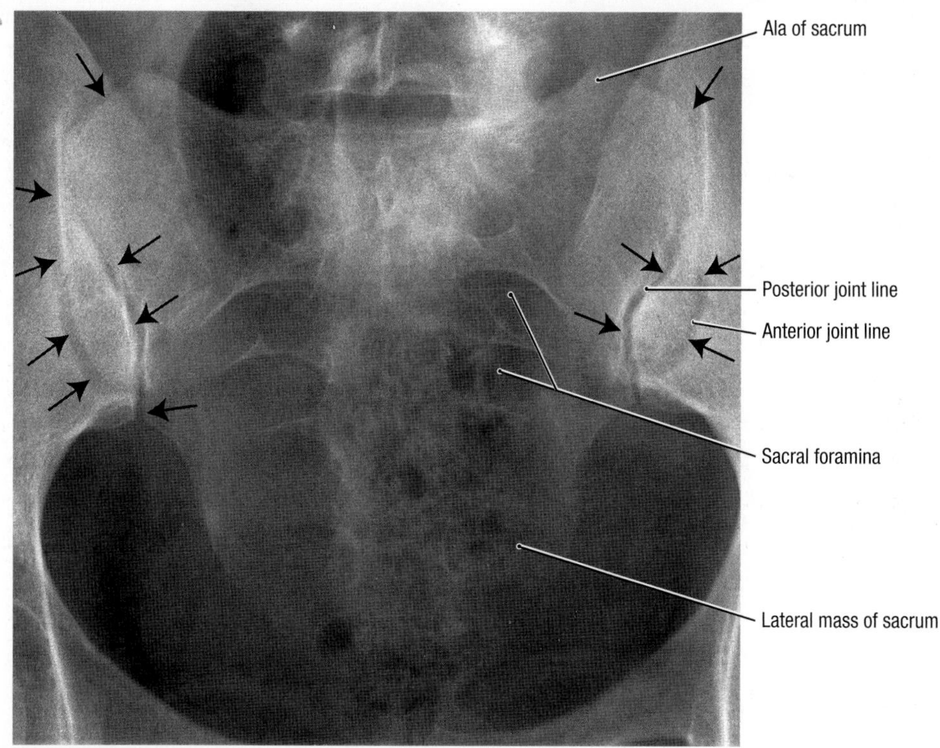
Ala of sacrum
Posterior joint line
Anterior joint line
Sacral foramina
Lateral mass of sacrum

B. Anteroposterior View

4.25 IMAGING OF SACRO-ILIAC JOINT

A. CT scan. The sacro-iliac joint is indicated by *arrows*. Note that the articular surfaces of the ilium and sacrum have irregular shapes that result in partial interlocking of the bones. The sacro-iliac joint is oblique, with the anterior aspect of the joint situated lateral to the posterior aspect of the joint. **B.** Radiograph. Due to the oblique placement of the sacro-iliac joints, the anterior and posterior joint lines appear separately.

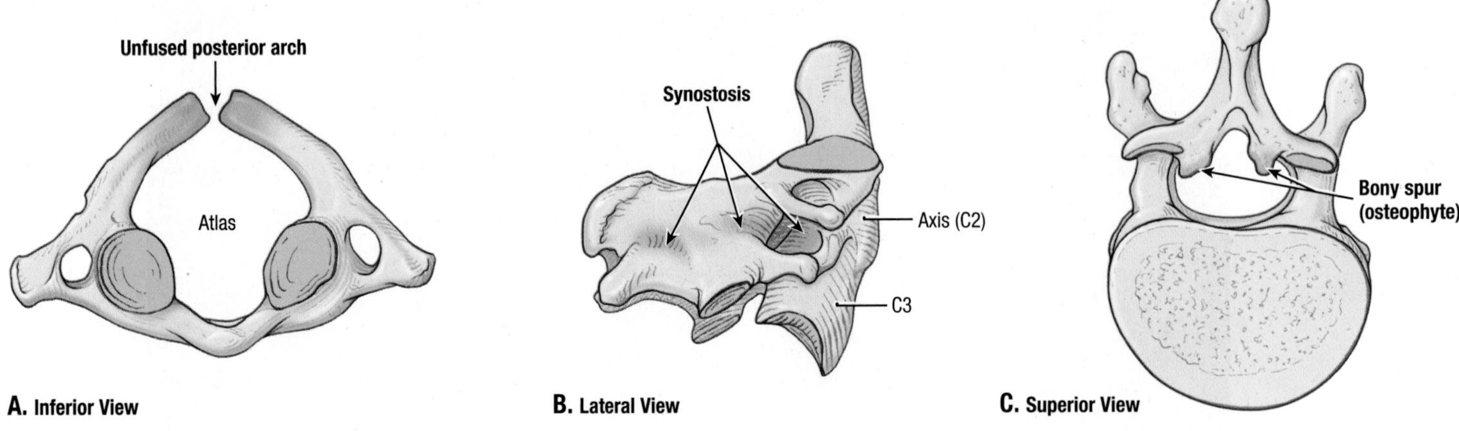
Unfused posterior arch
Atlas
A. Inferior View
Synostosis
Axis (C2)
C3
B. Lateral View
Bony spur
(osteophyte)
C. Superior View

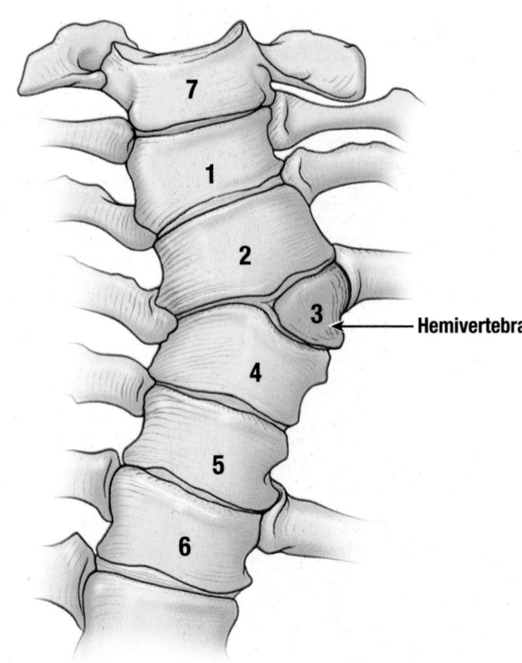
7
1
2
3
Hemivertebra
4
5
6
D. Anterior View

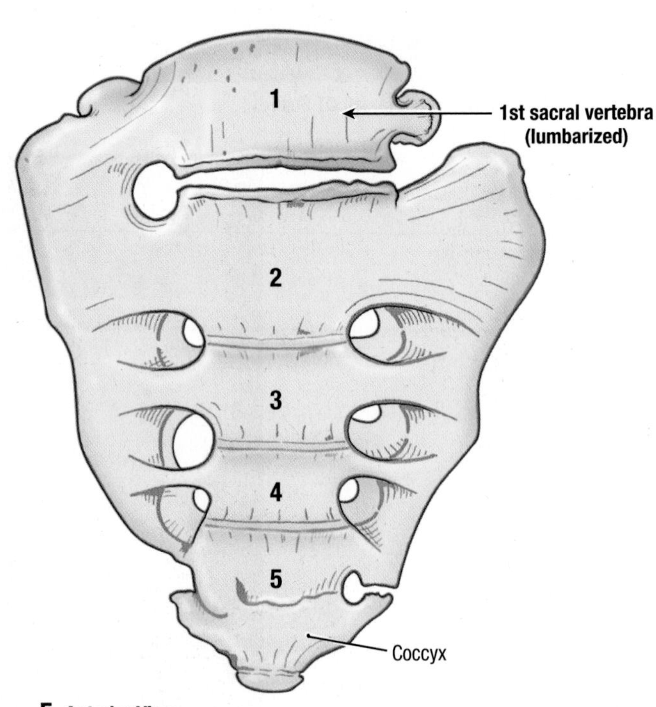
1
1st sacral vertebra
(lumbarized)
2
3
4
5
Coccyx
E. Anterior View

4.26 ANOMALIES OF VERTEBRAE

A. Unfused posterior arch of the atlas. The centrum fused to the right and left halves of the neural arch, but the arch did not fuse in the midline posteriorly. **B. Synostosis (fusion) of vertebrae C2 (axis) and C3. C. Bony spurs.** Sharp bony spurs may grow from the laminae inferiorly into the ligamenta flava, thereby reducing the lengths of the functional portions of these ligaments. When the vertebral column is flexed, the ligaments may be torn. **D. Hemivertebra.** The entire right half of vertebra T3 and the corresponding rib are absent. The left lamina and the spine are fused with those of T4, and the left IV foramen is reduced in size. Observe the associated scoliosis (lateral curvature of the spine). **E. Transitional lumbosacral vertebra.** Here, the 1st sacral vertebra is partly free (lumbarized). Not uncommonly, the 5th lumbar vertebra may be partly fused to the sacrum (sacralized).

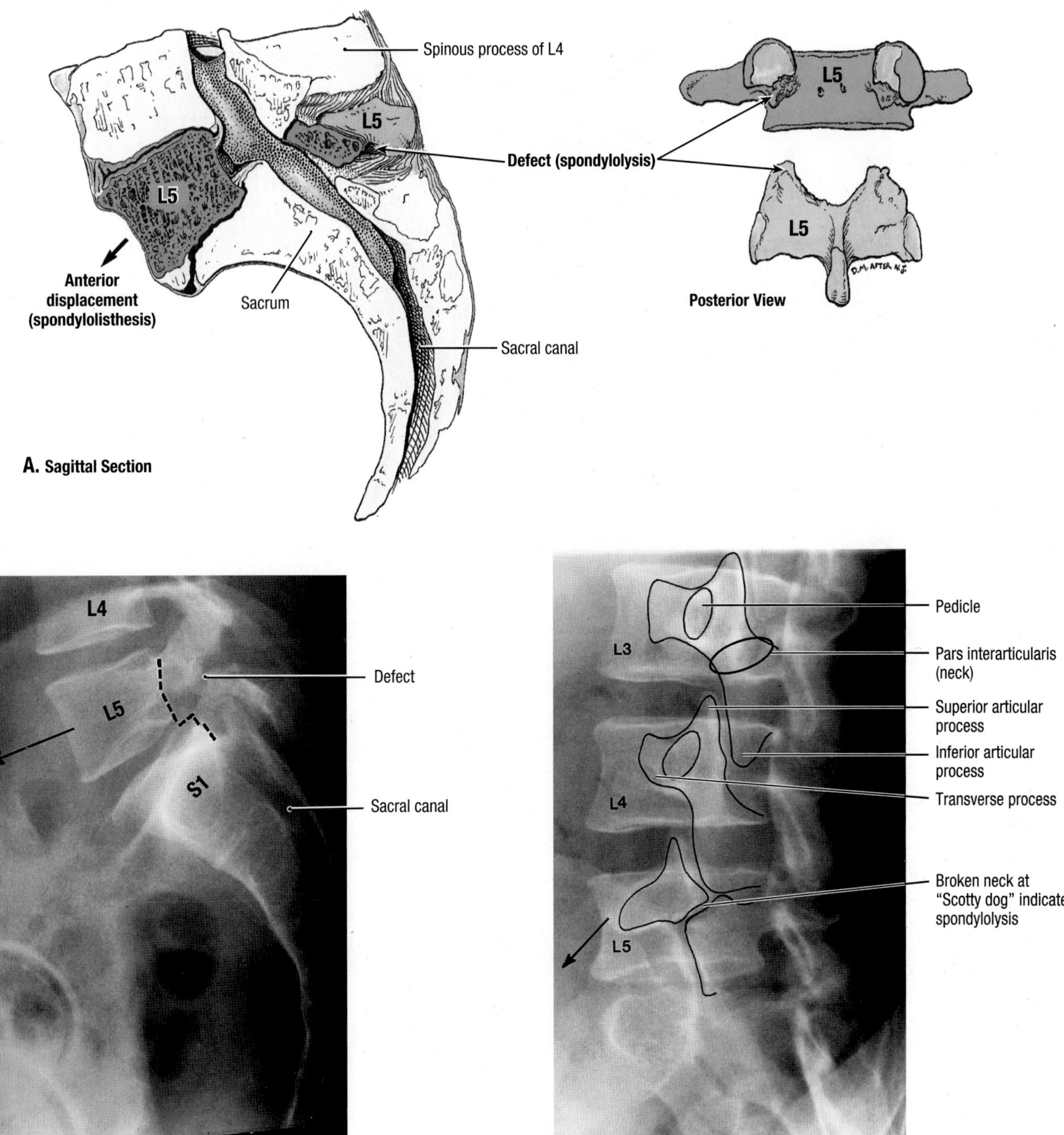
Spinous process of L4
L5
L5
Defect (spondylolysis)
Anterior displacement (spondylolisthesis)
Sacrum
Sacral canal
L5
L5
Posterior View
A. Sagittal Section
L4
L5
S1
Defect
Sacral canal
B. Lateral View
L3
L4
L5
Pedicle
Pars interarticularis (neck)
Superior articular process
Inferior articular process
Transverse process
Broken neck at "Scotty dog" indicates spondylolysis
C. Oblique View

4.27 SPONDYLOLYSIS AND SPONDYLOLISTHESIS

A. Articulated and isolated spondylolytic L5 vertebra. The vertebra has an oblique defect (spondylolysis) through the interarticular part (pars interarticularis). The interarticular part is the region of the lamina of a lumbar vertebra between the superior and inferior articular processes. The defect may be traumatic or congenital in origin. Also, the vertebral body of L5 has slipped anteriorly (spondylolisthesis). **B and C.** Radiographs. In **B,** the *dotted line* following the posterior vertebral margins of L5 and the sacrum shows the anterior displacement of L5 (*arrow*)**.** In **C**, note the superimposed outline of a dog: the neck is the transverse process, the eye is the pedicle, and the ear is the superior articular process. The lucent (dark) cleft across the "neck" of the dog is the **spondylolysis**; the anterior displacement (*arrow*) is the **spondylolisthesis**.

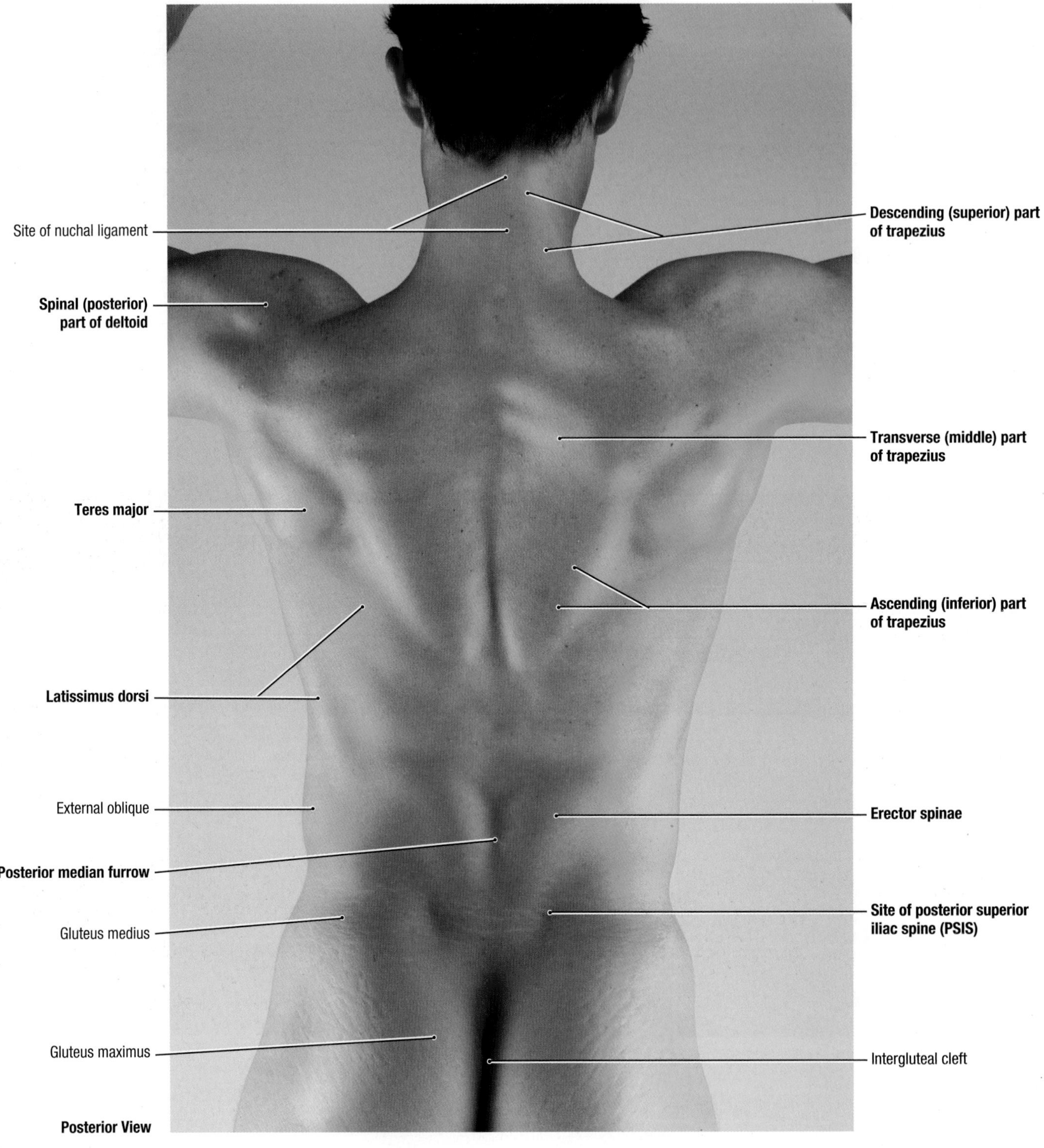

Site of nuchal ligament
Descending (superior) part of trapezius
Spinal (posterior) part of deltoid
Transverse (middle) part of trapezius
Teres major
Ascending (inferior) part of trapezius
Latissimus dorsi
External oblique
Erector spinae
Posterior median furrow
Site of posterior superior iliac spine (PSIS)
Gluteus medius
Gluteus maximus
Intergluteal cleft
Posterior View

4.28 SURFACE ANATOMY OF BACK

- The arms are abducted, so the scapulae have rotated superiorly on the thoracic wall.
- The latissimus dorsi and teres major muscles form the posterior axillary fold.
- The trapezius muscle has three parts: descending, transverse, and ascending.
- Note the deep median furrow that separates the longitudinal bulges formed by the contracted erector spinae group of muscles;
- Dimples (depressions) indicate the site of the posterior superior iliac spines, which usually lie at the level of the sacro-iliac joints.

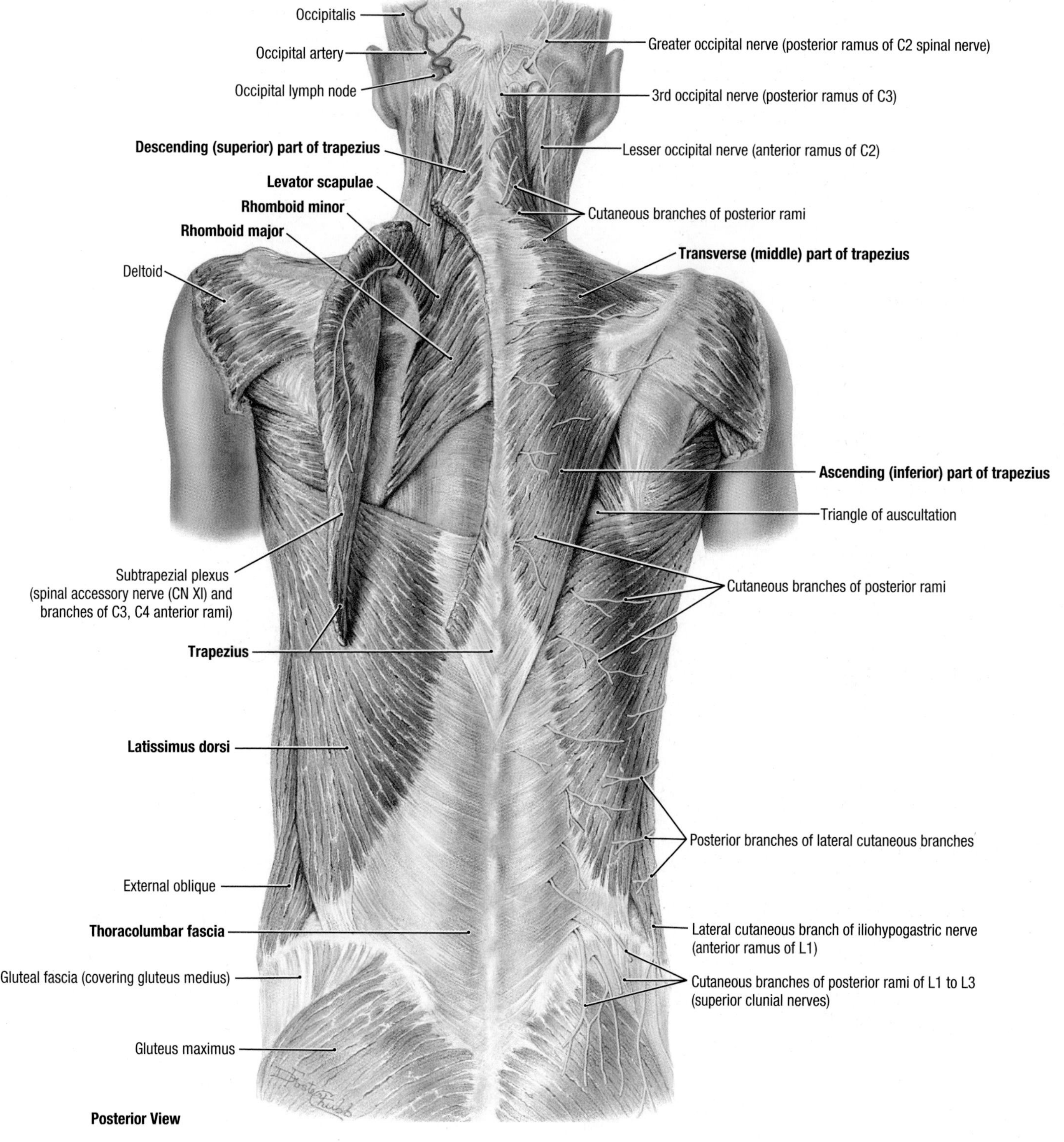
Occipitalis
Occipital artery
Occipital lymph node
Descending (superior) part of trapezius
Levator scapulae
Rhomboid minor
Rhomboid major
Deltoid
Greater occipital nerve (posterior ramus of C2 spinal nerve)
3rd occipital nerve (posterior ramus of C3)
Lesser occipital nerve (anterior ramus of C2)
Cutaneous branches of posterior rami
Transverse (middle) part of trapezius
Ascending (inferior) part of trapezius
Triangle of auscultation
Subtrapezial plexus (spinal accessory nerve (CN XI) and branches of C3, C4 anterior rami)
Cutaneous branches of posterior rami
Trapezius
Latissimus dorsi
Posterior branches of lateral cutaneous branches
External oblique
Thoracolumbar fascia
Lateral cutaneous branch of iliohypogastric nerve (anterior ramus of L1)
Gluteal fascia (covering gluteus medius)
Cutaneous branches of posterior rami of L1 to L3 (superior clunial nerves)
Gluteus maximus
Posterior View

4.29 SUPERFICIAL MUSCLES OF BACK

On the *left,* the trapezius muscle is reflected. Observe two layers: the trapezius and latissimus dorsi muscles, and the levator scapulae and rhomboids minor and major. These axio-appendicular muscles help attach the upper limb to the trunk.

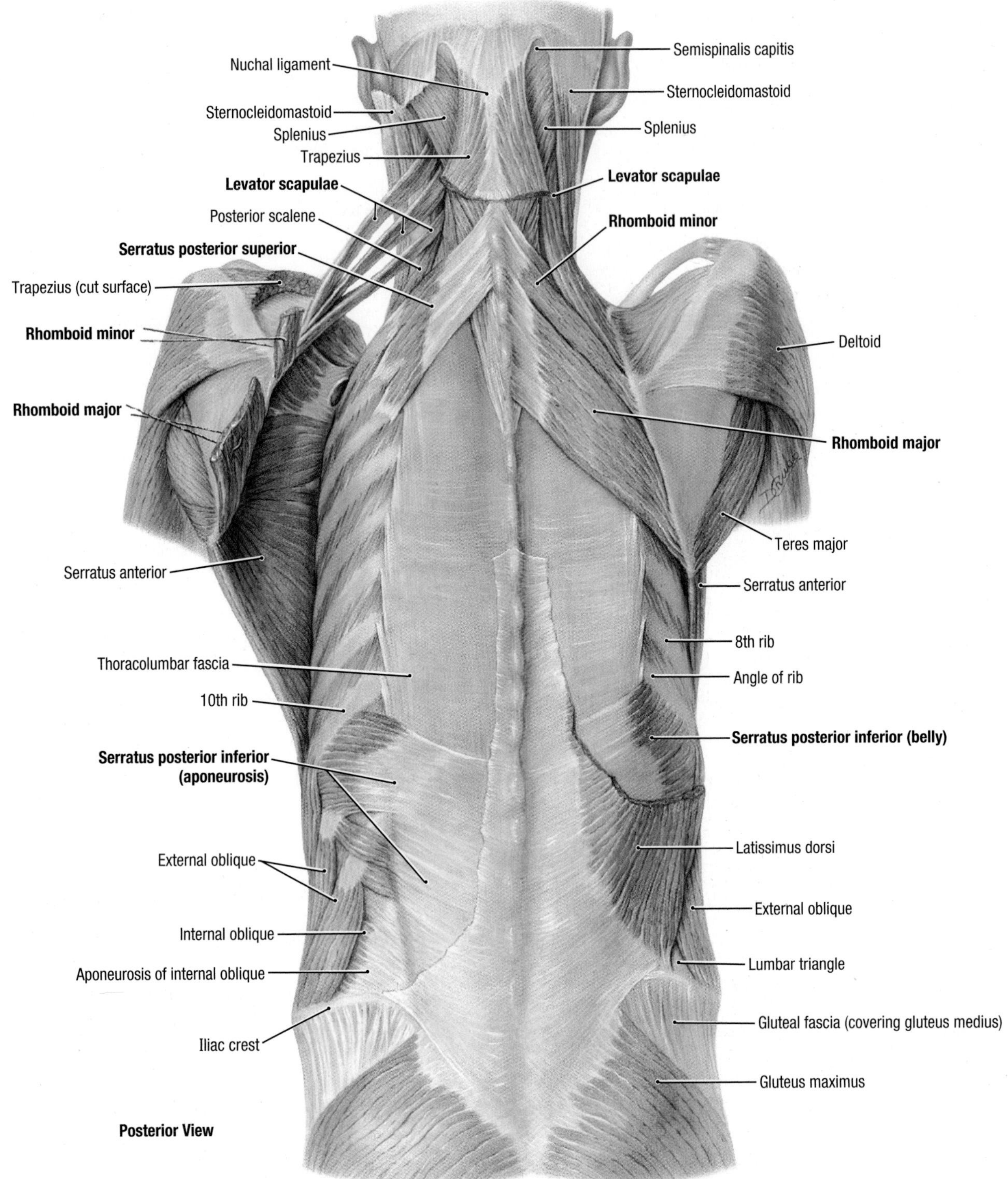

Nuchal ligament
Sternocleidomastoid
Splenius
Trapezius
Levator scapulae
Posterior scalene
Serratus posterior superior
Trapezius (cut surface)
Rhomboid minor
Rhomboid major
Serratus anterior
Thoracolumbar fascia
10th rib
Serratus posterior inferior (aponeurosis)
External oblique
Internal oblique
Aponeurosis of internal oblique
Iliac crest
Posterior View
Semispinalis capitis
Sternocleidomastoid
Splenius
Levator scapulae
Rhomboid minor
Deltoid
Rhomboid major
Teres major
Serratus anterior
8th rib
Angle of rib
Serratus posterior inferior (belly)
Latissimus dorsi
External oblique
Lumbar triangle
Gluteal fascia (covering gluteus medius)
Gluteus maximus

4.30 INTERMEDIATE MUSCLES OF BACK

The trapezius and latissimus dorsi muscles are largely cut away on both sides. On the *left*, the rhomboid muscles have been severed, allowing the vertebral border of the scapula to be raised from the thoracic wall. The serratus posterior superior and inferior form the intermediate layer of muscles, passing from the vertebral spines to the ribs; the two muscles slope in opposite directions and are muscles of respiration. The thoracolumbar fascia extends laterally to the angles of the ribs, becoming thin superiorly and passing deep to the serratus posterior superior muscle. The fascia gives attachment to the latissimus dorsi and serratus posterior inferior muscles (see Fig. 4.35).

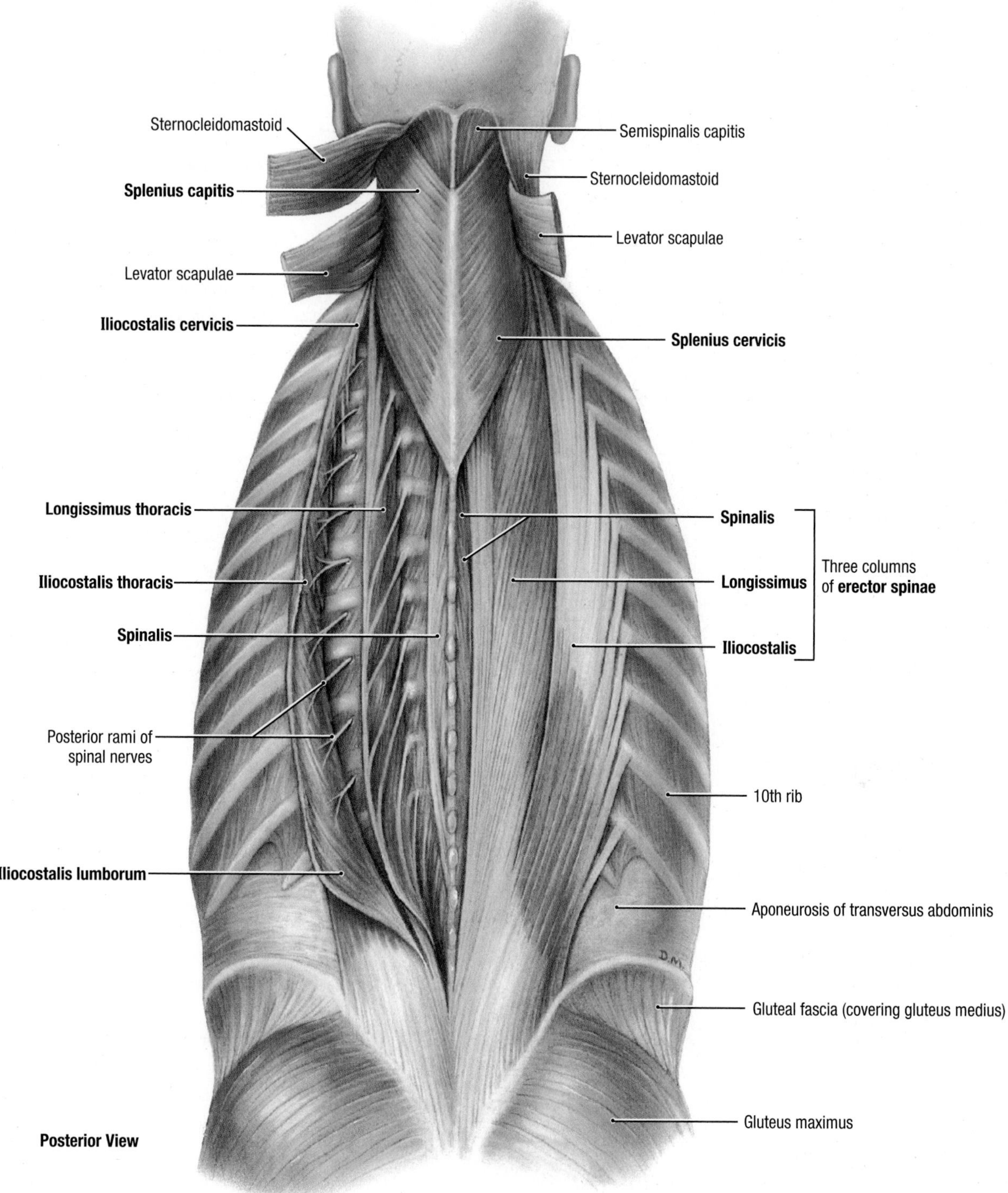
Sternocleidomastoid
Semispinalis capitis
Sternocleidomastoid
Splenius capitis
Levator scapulae
Levator scapulae
Iliocostalis cervicis
Splenius cervicis
Longissimus thoracis
Spinalis
Iliocostalis thoracis
Longissimus
Three columns of erector spinae
Spinalis
Iliocostalis
Posterior rami of spinal nerves
10th rib
Iliocostalis lumborum
Aponeurosis of transversus abdominis
Gluteal fascia (covering gluteus medius)
Gluteus maximus
Posterior View

4.31 DEEP MUSCLES OF BACK: SPLENIUS AND ERECTOR SPINAE

On the *right* of the body, the erector spinae muscles are in situ, lying between the spinous processes medially and the angles of the ribs laterally. The erector spinae are split into three longitudinal columns: iliocostalis laterally, longissimus in the middle, and spinalis medially. On the *left,* the longissimus muscle is pulled laterally to show the insertion into the transverse processes and ribs; not shown here are its extensions to the neck and head, longissimus cervicis and capitis.

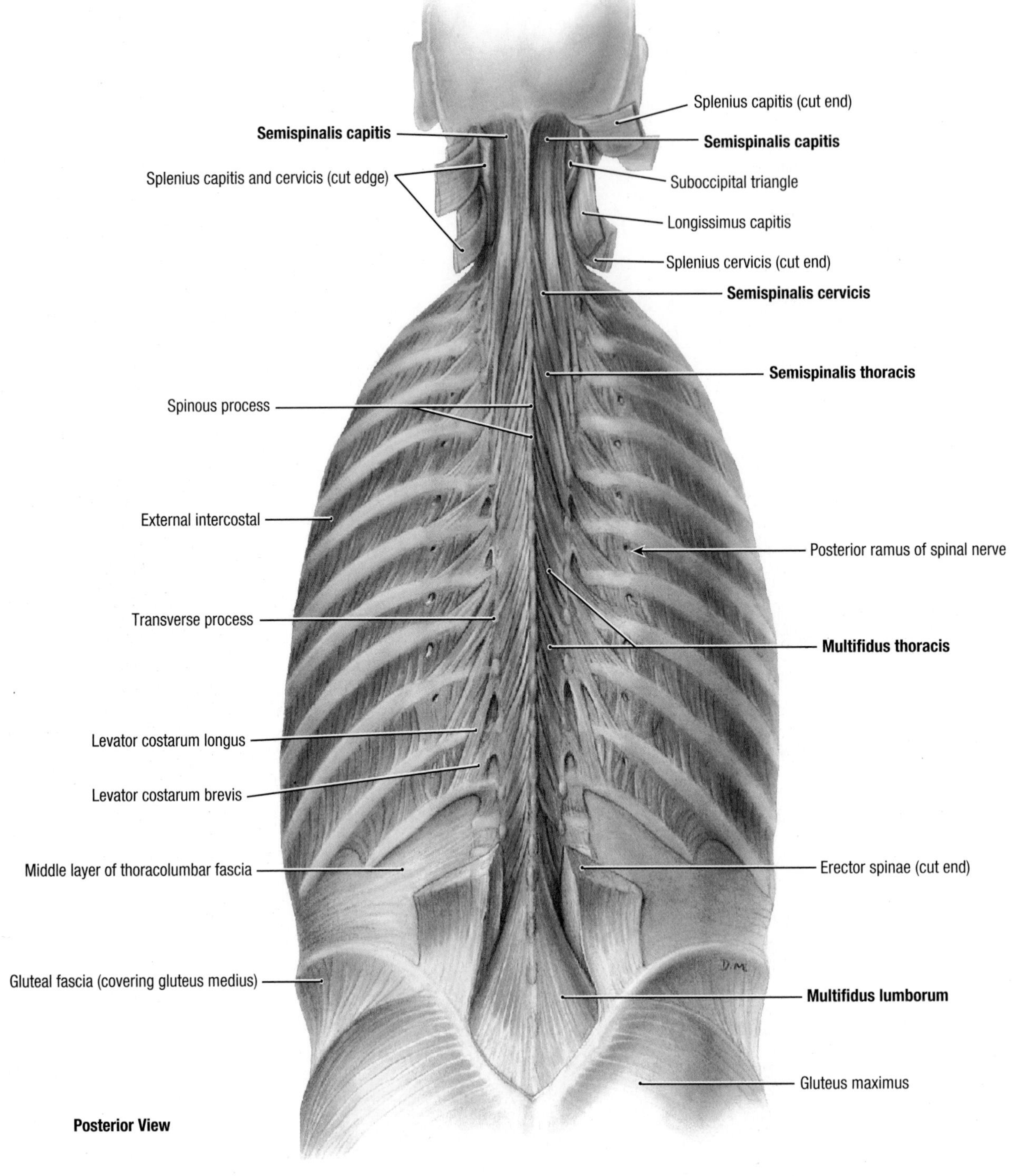
Semispinalis capitis
Splenius capitis and cervicis (cut edge)
Splenius capitis (cut end)
Semispinalis capitis
Suboccipital triangle
Longissimus capitis
Splenius cervicis (cut end)
Semispinalis cervicis
Semispinalis thoracis
Spinous process
External intercostal
Posterior ramus of spinal nerve
Transverse process
Multifidus thoracis
Levator costarum longus
Levator costarum brevis
Middle layer of thoracolumbar fascia
Erector spinae (cut end)
Gluteal fascia (covering gluteus medius)
Multifidus lumborum
Gluteus maximus
Posterior View

4.32 DEEP MUSCLES OF BACK: SEMISPINALIS AND MULTIFIDUS

- The semispinalis, multifidus, and rotatores muscles constitute the transverso spinalis group of deep muscles. In general, their bundles pass obliquely in a superomedial direction, from transverse processes to spinous processes in successively deeper layers. The bundles of semispinalis span approximately five interspaces, those of multifidus, approximately three, and those of rotatores, one or two.
- The semispinalis (thoracis, cervicis, and capitis) muscles span the lower thoracic region to the skull.
- The multifidus muscle extends from the sacrum to the spine of the axis. In the lumbosacral region it emerges from the aponeurosis of the erector spinae, and extends from the sacrum, and mammillary processes of the lumbar vertebrae, to insert into spinous processes approximately three segments higher.

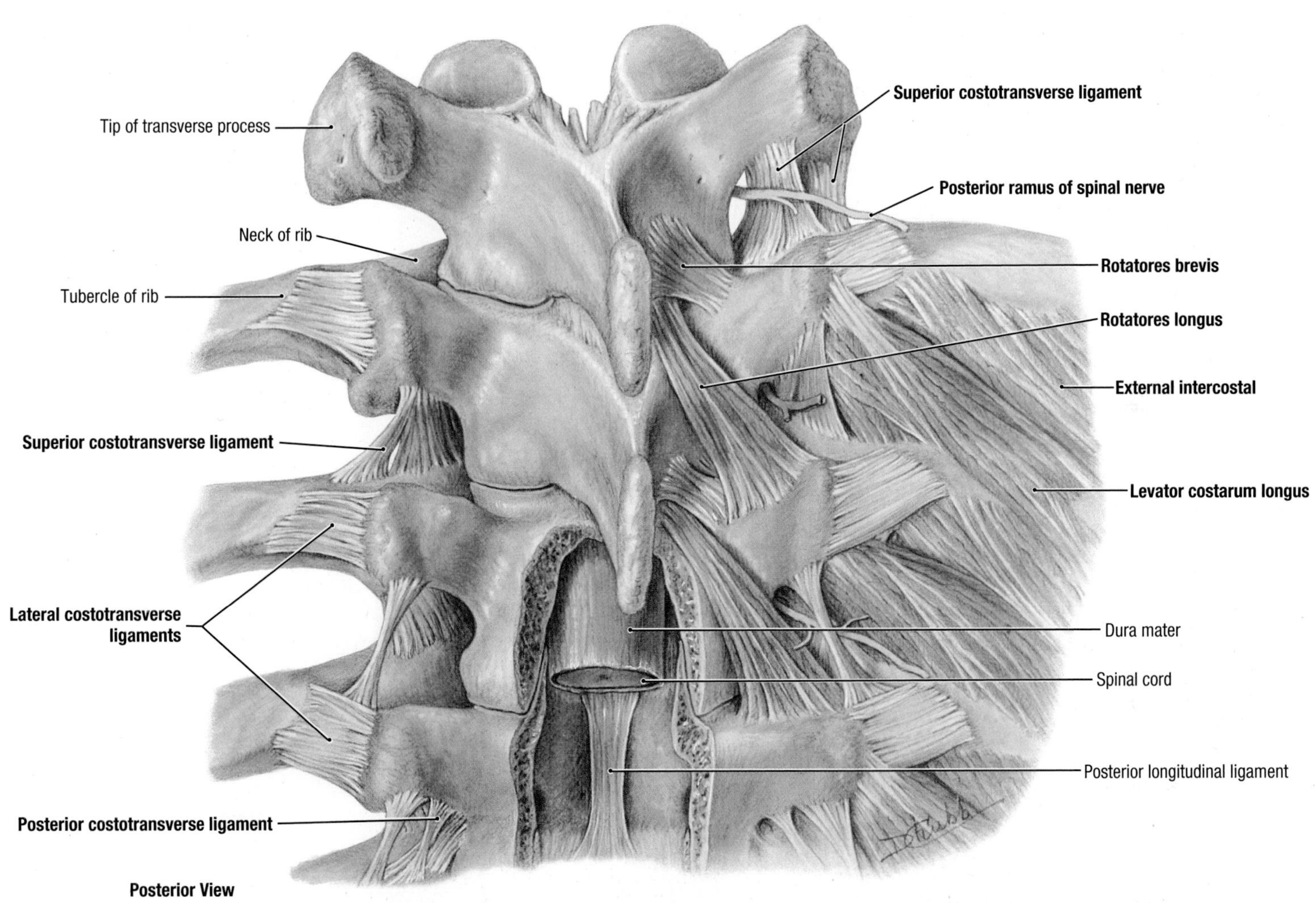
Tip of transverse process
Superior costotransverse ligament
Posterior ramus of spinal nerve
Neck of rib
Rotatores brevis
Tubercle of rib
Rotatores longus
External intercostal
Superior costotransverse ligament
Levator costarum longus
Lateral costotransverse ligaments
Dura mater
Spinal cord
Posterior longitudinal ligament
Posterior costotransverse ligament
Posterior View

4.33 ROTATORES AND COSTOTRANSVERSE LIGAMENTS

- Of the three layers of transversospinalis, or oblique muscles of the back (semispinalis, multifidus, rotatores), the rotatores are the deepest and shortest. They pass from the root of one transverse process superomedially to the junction of the transverse process and lamina of the vertebra above. Rotatores longus span two vertebrae.
- The levatores costarum pass from the tip of one transverse process inferiorly to the rib below; some span two ribs.
- The superior costotransverse ligament splits laterally into two sheets, between which lie the levatores costarum and external intercostal muscles; the posterior ramus passes posterior to this ligament.
- The lateral costotransverse ligament is strong and joins the tubercle of the rib to the tip of the transverse process. It forms the posterior aspect of the joint capsule of the costotransverse joint.

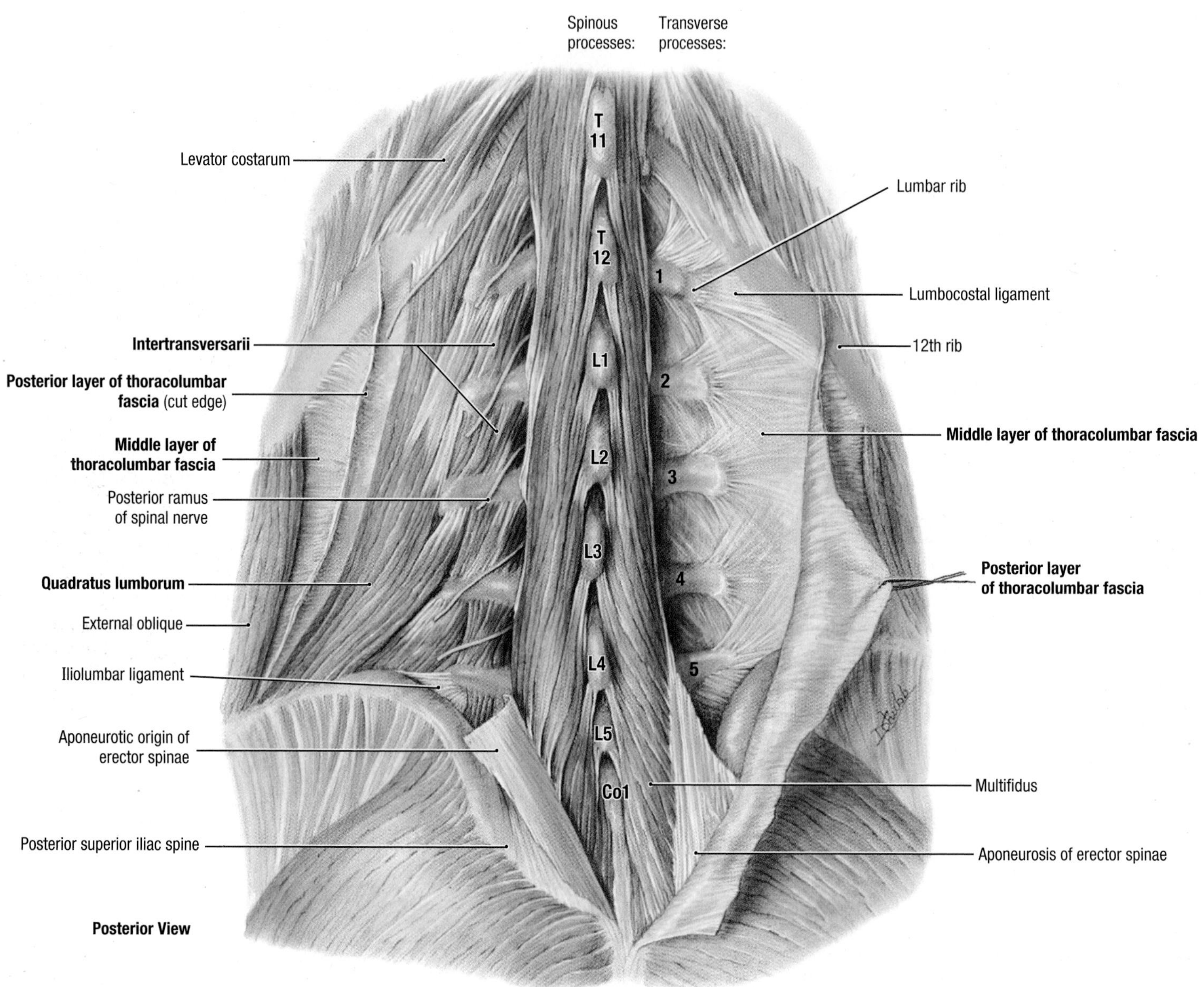
Spinous processes:
Transverse processes:
T 11
T 12
L1
L2
L3
L4
L5
Co1
1
2
3
4
5
Levator costarum
Lumbar rib
Lumbocostal ligament
Intertransversarii
12th rib
Posterior layer of thoracolumbar fascia (cut edge)
Middle layer of thoracolumbar fascia
Middle layer of thoracolumbar fascia
Posterior ramus of spinal nerve
Quadratus lumborum
Posterior layer of thoracolumbar fascia
External oblique
Iliolumbar ligament
Aponeurotic origin of erector spinae
Multifidus
Posterior superior iliac spine
Aponeurosis of erector spinae
Posterior View

4.34 BACK: MULTIFIDUS, QUADRATUS LUMBORUM, AND THORACOLUMBAR FASCIA

Right: After removal of erector spinae at the L1 level, the middle layer of thoracolumbar fascia extends from the tip of each lumbar transverse process in a fan-shaped manner. A short lumbar rib is present at the level of L1. *Left:* After removal of the posterior and middle layers of thoracolumbar fascia, the lateral border of the quadratus lumborum muscle is oblique, and the medial border is in continuity with the intertransversarii.

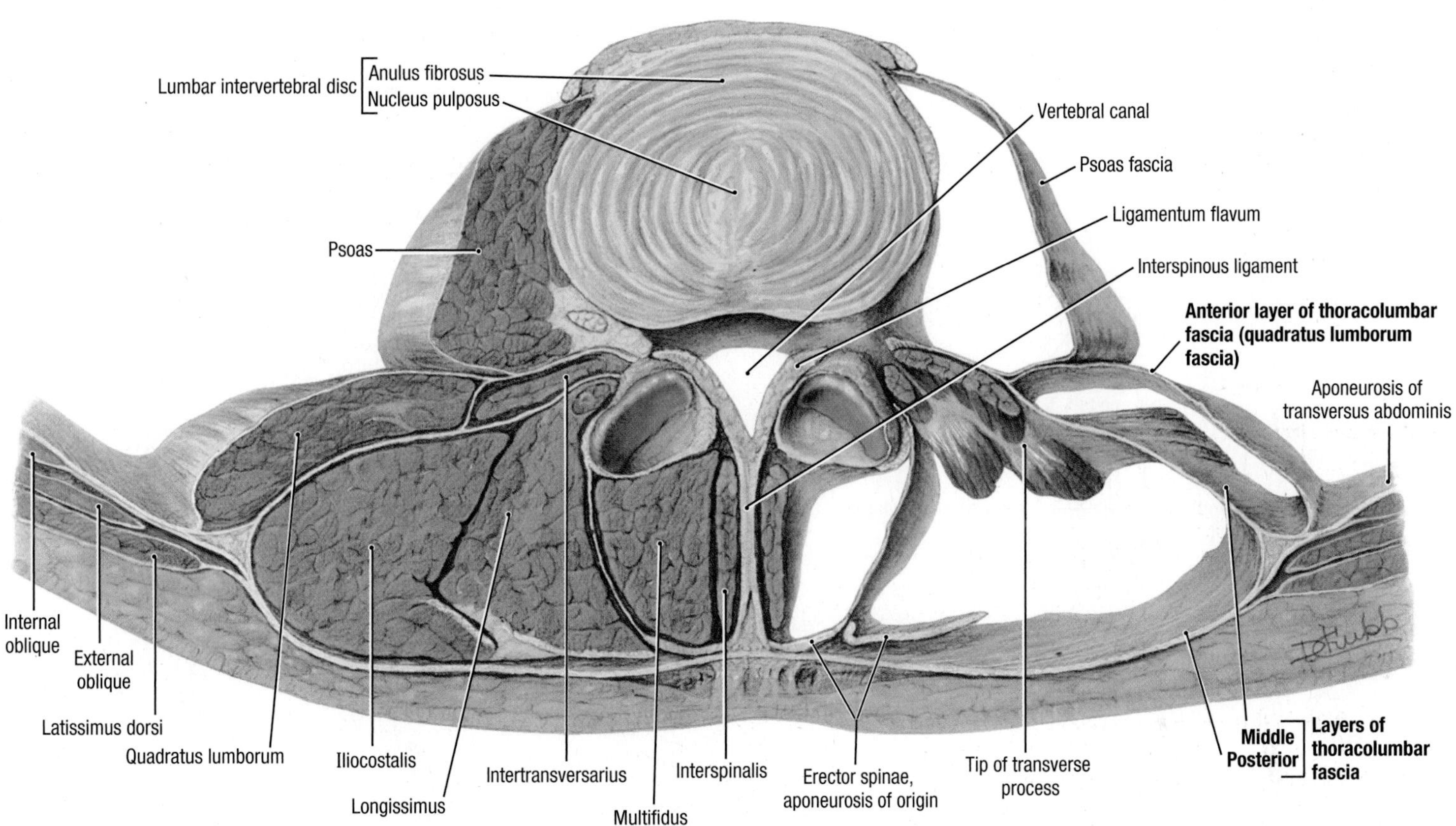
Lumbar intervertebral disc
Anulus fibrosus
Nucleus pulposus
Vertebral canal
Psoas fascia
Ligamentum flavum
Psoas
Interspinous ligament
Anterior layer of thoracolumbar fascia (quadratus lumborum fascia)
Aponeurosis of transversus abdominis
Internal oblique
External oblique
Latissimus dorsi
Quadratus lumborum
Iliocostalis
Longissimus
Intertransversarius
Multifidus
Interspinalis
Erector spinae, aponeurosis of origin
Tip of transverse process
Middle
Posterior
Layers of thoracolumbar fascia

Transverse Section (Dissected), Superior View

4.35 TRANSVERSE SECTION OF BACK MUSCLES AND THORACOLUMBAR FASCIA

- On the *left,* the muscles are seen in their fascial sheaths or compartments; on the *right,* the muscles have been removed from their sheaths.
- The deep back muscles extend from the pelvis to the cranium and are enclosed in fascia. This fascia attaches medially to the nuchal ligament, the tips of the spinous processes, the supraspinous ligament, and the median crest of the sacrum. The lateral attachment of the fascia is to the cervical transverse processes, the angles of the ribs, and the aponeurosis of transversus abdominis. The thoracic and lumbar parts of the fascia are named thoracolumbar fascia.
- The aponeurosis of transversus abdominis and posterior aponeurosis of internal oblique muscles split into two strong sheets, the middle and posterior layers of thoracolumbar fascia. The anterior layer of thoracolumbar fascia is the deep fascia of the quadratus lumborum (quadratus lumborum fascia). The posterior layer of the thoracolumbar fascia provides proximal attachment for the latissimus dorsi muscle and, at a higher level, the serratus posterior inferior muscle.

Back strain is a common back problem that usually results from extreme movements of the vertebral column, such as extension or rotation. Back strain refers to some stretching or microscopic tearing of muscle fibers and/or ligaments of the back. The muscles usually involved are those producing movements of the lumbar IV joints.

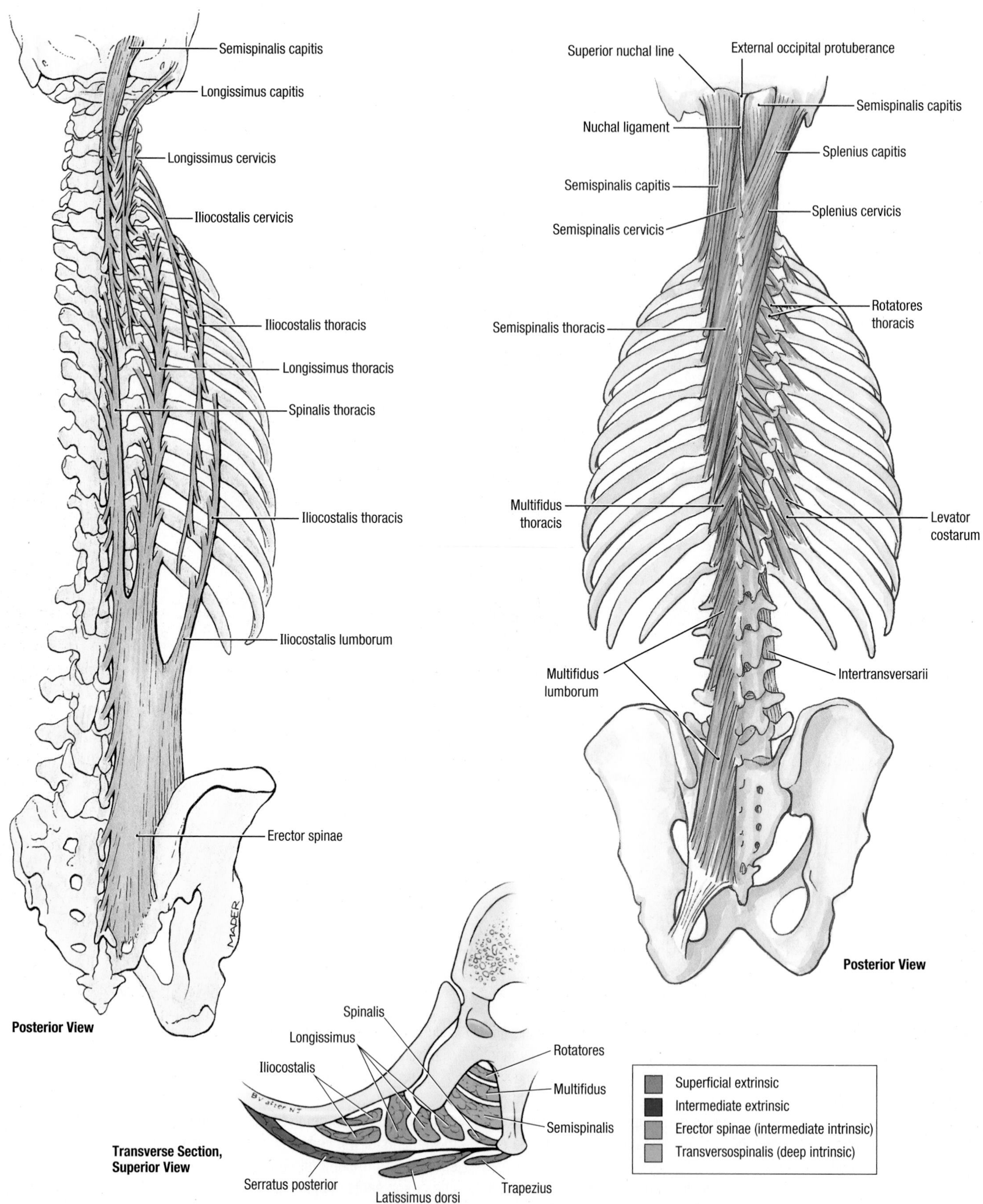

Semispinalis capitis
Longissimus capitis
Longissimus cervicis
Iliocostalis cervicis
Iliocostalis thoracis
Longissimus thoracis
Spinalis thoracis
Iliocostalis thoracis
Iliocostalis lumborum
Erector spinae
MADER
Posterior View
Superior nuchal line
External occipital protuberance
Semispinalis capitis
Nuchal ligament
Splenius capitis
Semispinalis capitis
Splenius cervicis
Semispinalis cervicis
Rotatores thoracis
Semispinalis thoracis
Multifidus thoracis
Levator costarum
Multifidus lumborum
Intertransversarii
Posterior View
Spinalis
Longissimus
Iliocostalis
Rotatores
Multifidus
Semispinalis
Serratus posterior
Latissimus dorsi
Trapezius
Transverse Section, Superior View
Superficial extrinsic
Intermediate extrinsic
Erector spinae (intermediate intrinsic)
Transversospinalis (deep intrinsic)

4.36 OVERVIEW OF DEEP BACK MUSCLES

TABLE 4.4 INTRINSIC BACK MUSCLES[a]

Muscles	Caudal (Inferior) Attachment	Rostral (Superior) Attachment	Nerve Supply[b]	Main Actions
Superficial layer				
Splenius	Nuchal ligament and spinous processes of C7–T6 vertebrae	*Splenius capitis:* fibers run superolaterally to mastoid process of temporal bone and lateral third of superior nuchal line of occipital bone *Splenius cervicis:* posterior tubercles of transverse processes of C1–C3/C4 vertebrae	Posterior rami of spinal nerves	*Acting unilaterally*: laterally flex neck and rotate head to side of active muscles; *Acting bilaterally*: extend head and neck
Intermediate layer				
Erector spinae	Arises by a broad tendon from posterior part of iliac crest, posterior surface of sacrum, sacral and inferior lumbar spinous processes, and supraspinous ligament	*Iliocostalis (lumborum, thoracis, and cervicis):* fibers run superiorly to angles of lower ribs and cervical transverse processes *Longissimus (thoracis, cervicis, and capitis):* fibers run superiorly to ribs between tubercles and angles to transverse processes in thoracic and cervical regions, and to mastoid process of temporal bone *Spinalis (thoracis, cervicis, and capitis):* fibers run superiorly to spinous processes in the upper thoracic region and to skull		*Acting unilaterally:* laterally bend vertebral column to side of active muscles *Acting bilaterally:* extend vertebral column and head; as back is flexed, control movement by gradually lengthening their fibers
Deep layer				
Transversospinalis	*Semispinalis:* arises from thoracic and cervical transverse processes *Multifidus:* arises from sacrum and ilium, transverse processes of T1–L5, and articular processes of C4–C7 *Rotatores:* arise from transverse processes of vertebrae; best developed in thoracic region	*Semispinalis: thoracis, cervicis, and capitis:* fibers run superomedially and attach to occipital bone and spinous processes in thoracic and cervical regions, spanning four to six segments *Multifidus (lumborum, thoracis, and cervicis):* fibers pass superomedially to spinous processes, spanning two to four segments *Rotatores (thoracis and cervicis):* Pass superomedially and attach to junction of lamina and transverse process of vertebra of origin or into spinous process above their origin, spanning one to two segments		**Extension** *Semispinalis:* extends head and thoracic and cervical regions of vertebral column and rotates them contralaterally *Multifidus:* stabilizes vertebrae during local movement of vertebral column *Rotatores:* Stabilize vertebrae and assist with local extension and rotary movements of vertebral column; may function as organ of proprioception
Minor deep layer				
Interspinales	Superior surfaces of spinous processes of cervical and lumbar vertebrae	Inferior surfaces of spinous processes of vertebrae superior to vertebrae of origin	Posterior rami of spinal nerves	Aid in extension and rotation of vertebral column
Intertransversarii	Transverse processes of cervical and lumbar vertebrae	Transverse processes of adjacent vertebrae	Posterior and anterior rami of spinal nerves	Aid in lateral flexion of vertebral column *Acting bilaterally:* stabilize vertebral column
Levatores costarum	**Medial attachment:** Tips of transverse processes of C7 and T1–T11 vertebrae	**Lateral attachment:** Pass inferolaterally and insert on rib between its tubercle and angle	Posterior rami of C8–T11 spinal nerves	Elevate ribs, assisting inspiration Assist with lateral flexion of vertebral column

[a]See figures on opposite page.
[b]Most back muscles are innervated by posterior rami of spinal nerves, but a few are innervated by anterior rami. Intertransversarii of cervical region are supplied by anterior rami.

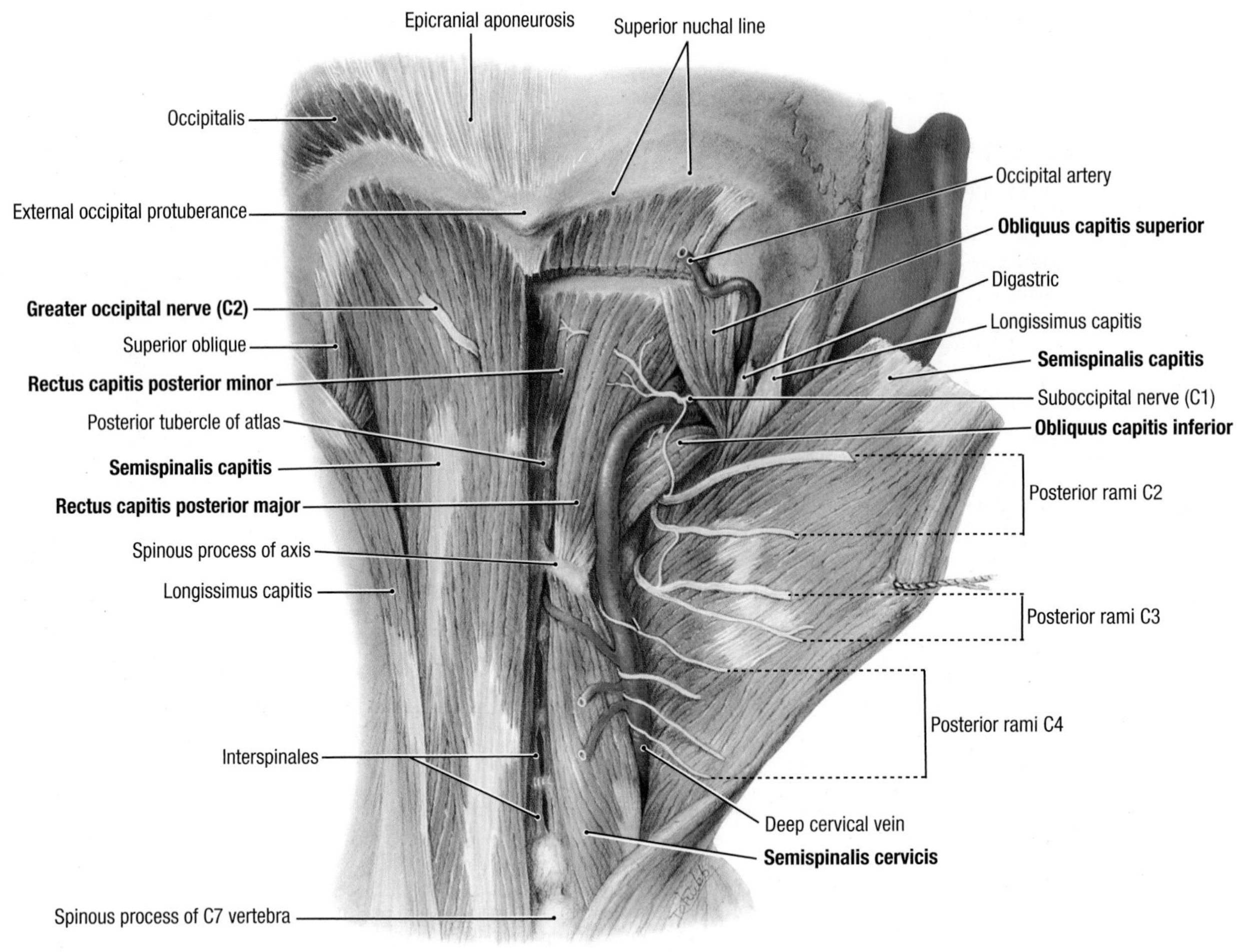
Epicranial aponeurosis
Superior nuchal line
Occipitalis
External occipital protuberance
Occipital artery
Obliquus capitis superior
Digastric
Greater occipital nerve (C2)
Longissimus capitis
Superior oblique
Semispinalis capitis
Rectus capitis posterior minor
Suboccipital nerve (C1)
Posterior tubercle of atlas
Obliquus capitis inferior
Semispinalis capitis
Posterior rami C2
Rectus capitis posterior major
Spinous process of axis
Longissimus capitis
Posterior rami C3
Posterior rami C4
Interspinales
Deep cervical vein
Semispinalis cervicis
Spinous process of C7 vertebra

Posterior View

4.37 SUBOCCIPITAL REGION I

The trapezius, sternocleidomastoid, and splenius muscles are removed. The right semispinalis capitis muscle is cut and reflected laterally.

- The semispinalis capitis, the great extensor muscle of the head and neck, forms the posterior wall of the suboccipital region. It is pierced by the greater occipital nerve (posterior ramus of C2) and has free medial and lateral borders at this level.
- The greater occipital nerve, when followed caudally, leads to the inferior border of the obliquus capitis inferior muscle, around which it turns. Following the inferior border of the obliquus capitis inferior muscle medially from the nerve leads to the spinous process of the axis; followed laterally, this leads to the transverse process of the atlas.
- Five muscles (all paired) are attached to the spinous process of the axis: obliquus capitis inferior, rectus capitis posterior major, semispinalis cervicis, multifidus, and interspinalis; the latter two are largely concealed by the semispinalis cervicis.

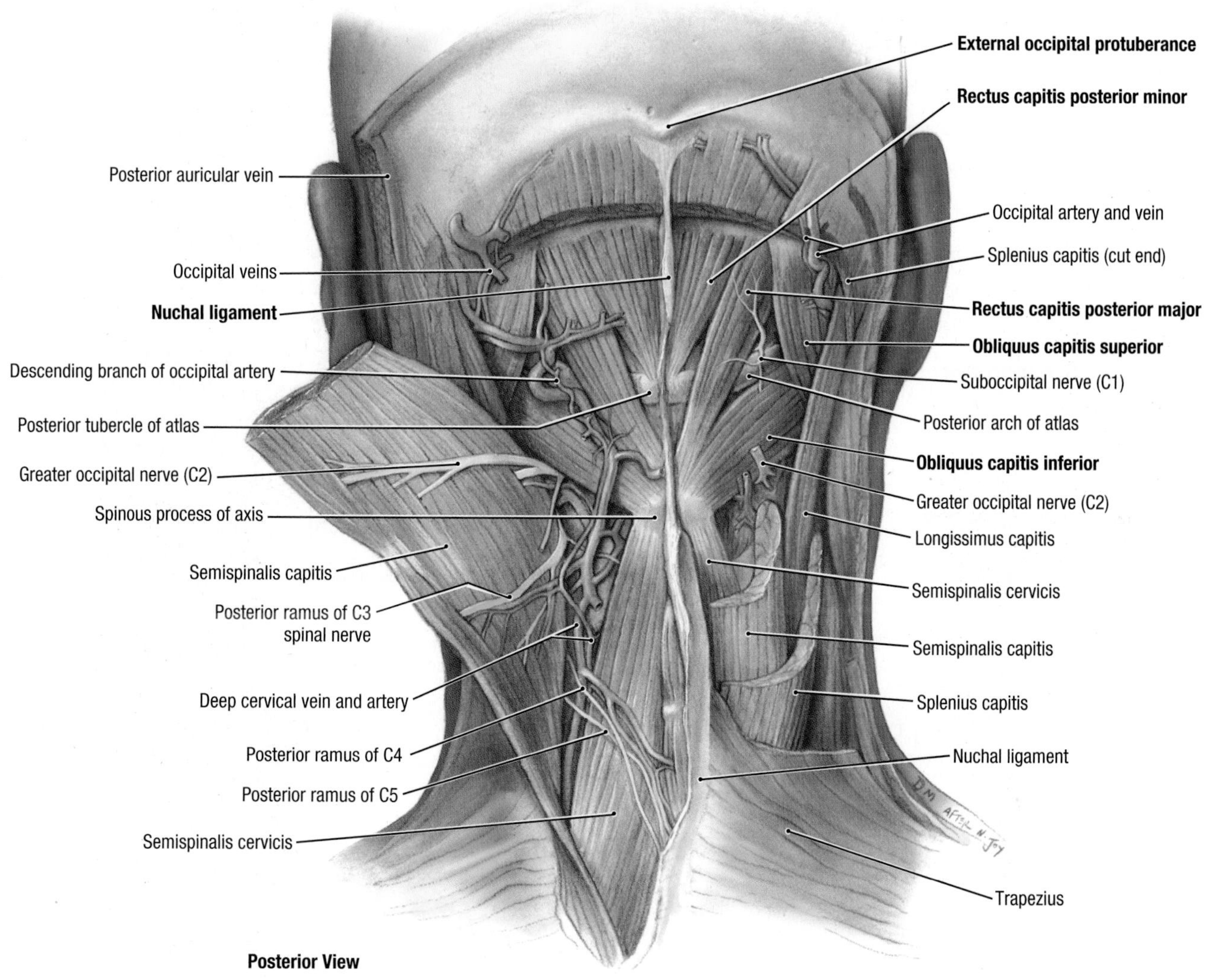
External occipital protuberance
Rectus capitis posterior minor
Posterior auricular vein
Occipital artery and vein
Splenius capitis (cut end)
Occipital veins
Nuchal ligament
Rectus capitis posterior major
Obliquus capitis superior
Descending branch of occipital artery
Suboccipital nerve (C1)
Posterior tubercle of atlas
Posterior arch of atlas
Obliquus capitis inferior
Greater occipital nerve (C2)
Greater occipital nerve (C2)
Spinous process of axis
Longissimus capitis
Semispinalis capitis
Semispinalis cervicis
Posterior ramus of C3 spinal nerve
Semispinalis capitis
Deep cervical vein and artery
Splenius capitis
Posterior ramus of C4
Nuchal ligament
Posterior ramus of C5
Semispinalis cervicis
Trapezius
Posterior View

4.38 SUBOCCIPITAL REGION II

The semispinalis capitis is reflected on the *left* and removed on the *right* side of the body; neck is flexed.

- The suboccipital region contains four pairs of structures: two straight muscles, the rectus capitis posterior major and minor; two oblique muscles, the obliquus capitis superior and obliquus capitis inferior; two nerves (posterior rami), C1 suboccipital (motor) and C2 greater occipital (sensory); and two arteries, the occipital and vertebral.
- The nuchal ligament, which represents the cervical part of the supraspinous ligament, is a median, thin, fibrous partition attached to the spinous processes of cervical vertebrae and the external occipital protuberance.
- The suboccipital triangle is bounded by three muscles: obliquus capitis superior and inferior and rectus capitis posterior major.
- The suboccipital nerve (posterior ramus of C1) supplies the three muscles bounding the suboccipital triangle and also the rectus capitis minor muscle and communicates with the greater occipital nerve.
- The occipital veins along with the suboccipital nerve (posterior ramus of C1) emerge through the suboccipital triangle to join the deep cervical vein.
- The posterior arch of the atlas forms the floor of the suboccipital triangle.

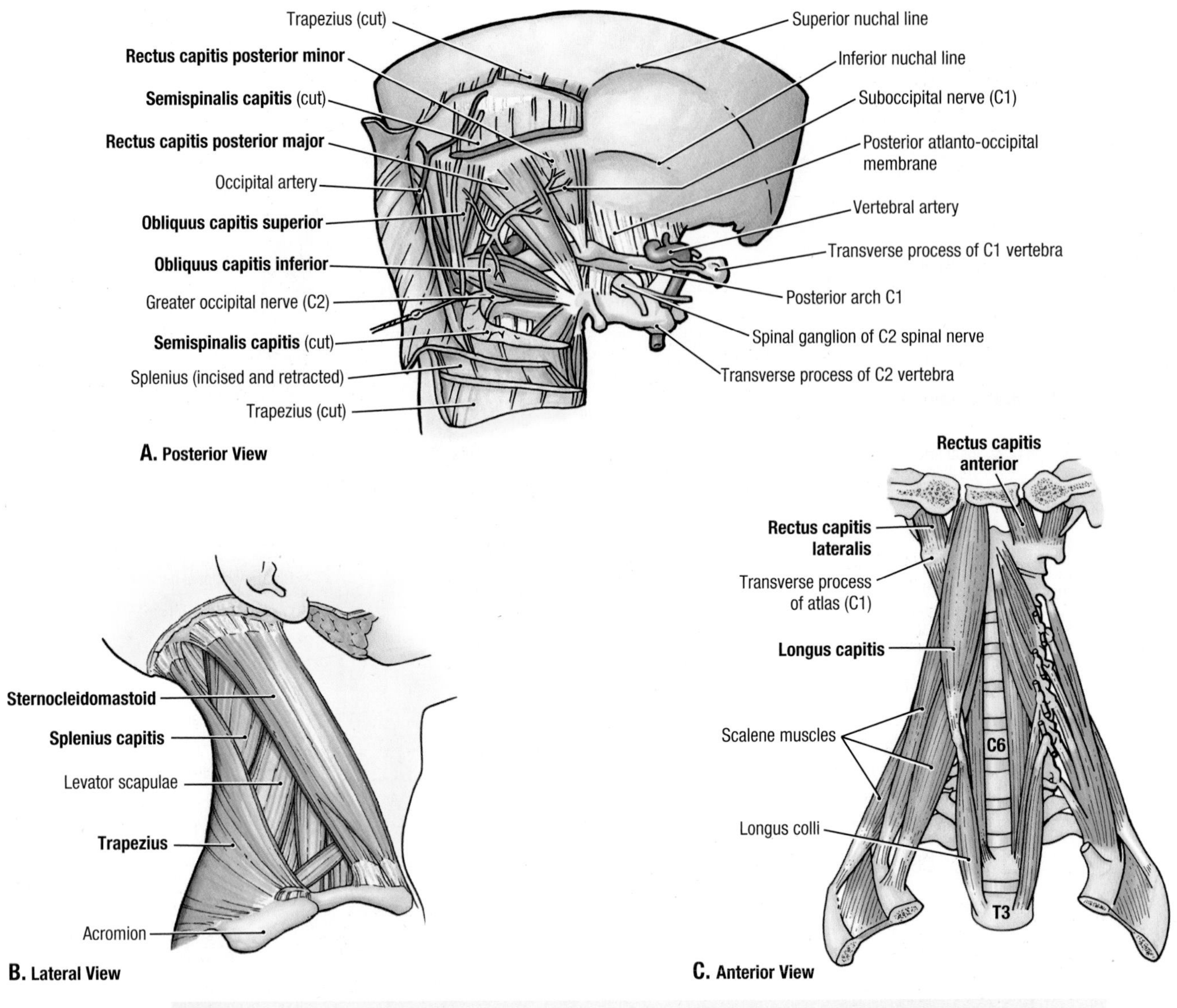

Trapezius (cut)
Rectus capitis posterior minor
Semispinalis capitis (cut)
Rectus capitis posterior major
Occipital artery
Obliquus capitis superior
Obliquus capitis inferior
Greater occipital nerve (C2)
Semispinalis capitis (cut)
Splenius (incised and retracted)
Trapezius (cut)
Superior nuchal line
Inferior nuchal line
Suboccipital nerve (C1)
Posterior atlanto-occipital membrane
Vertebral artery
Transverse process of C1 vertebra
Posterior arch C1
Spinal ganglion of C2 spinal nerve
Transverse process of C2 vertebra
A. Posterior View
Sternocleidomastoid
Splenius capitis
Levator scapulae
Trapezius
Acromion
B. Lateral View
Rectus capitis anterior
Rectus capitis lateralis
Transverse process of atlas (C1)
Longus capitis
Scalene muscles
C6
Longus colli
T3
C. Anterior View

4.39 MUSCLES OF BASE OF SKULL

A. Suboccipital region. **B.** Lateral cervical region. **C.** Prevertebral muscles.

TABLE 4.5 MUSCLES OF ATLANTO-OCCIPITAL AND ATLANTO-AXIAL JOINTS

Movements of Atlanto-Occipital Joints

Flexion	Extension	Lateral Bending
Longus capitis Rectus capitis anterior Anterior fibers of sternocleidomastoid	Rectus capitis posterior major and minor Obliquus capitis superior Semispinalis capitis Splenius capitis Longissimus capitis Trapezius	Sternocleidomastoid Longissimus capitis Rectus capitis lateralis Splenius capitis

Rotation of Atlanto-Axial Joints[a]

Ipsilateral[b]	Contralateral
Obliquus capitis inferior Rectus capitis posterior, major and minor Longissimus capitis Splenius capitis	Sternocleidomastoid Semispinalis capitis

[a]Rotation is the specialized movement at these joints. Movement of one joint involves the other.
[b]Same side to which head is rotated.

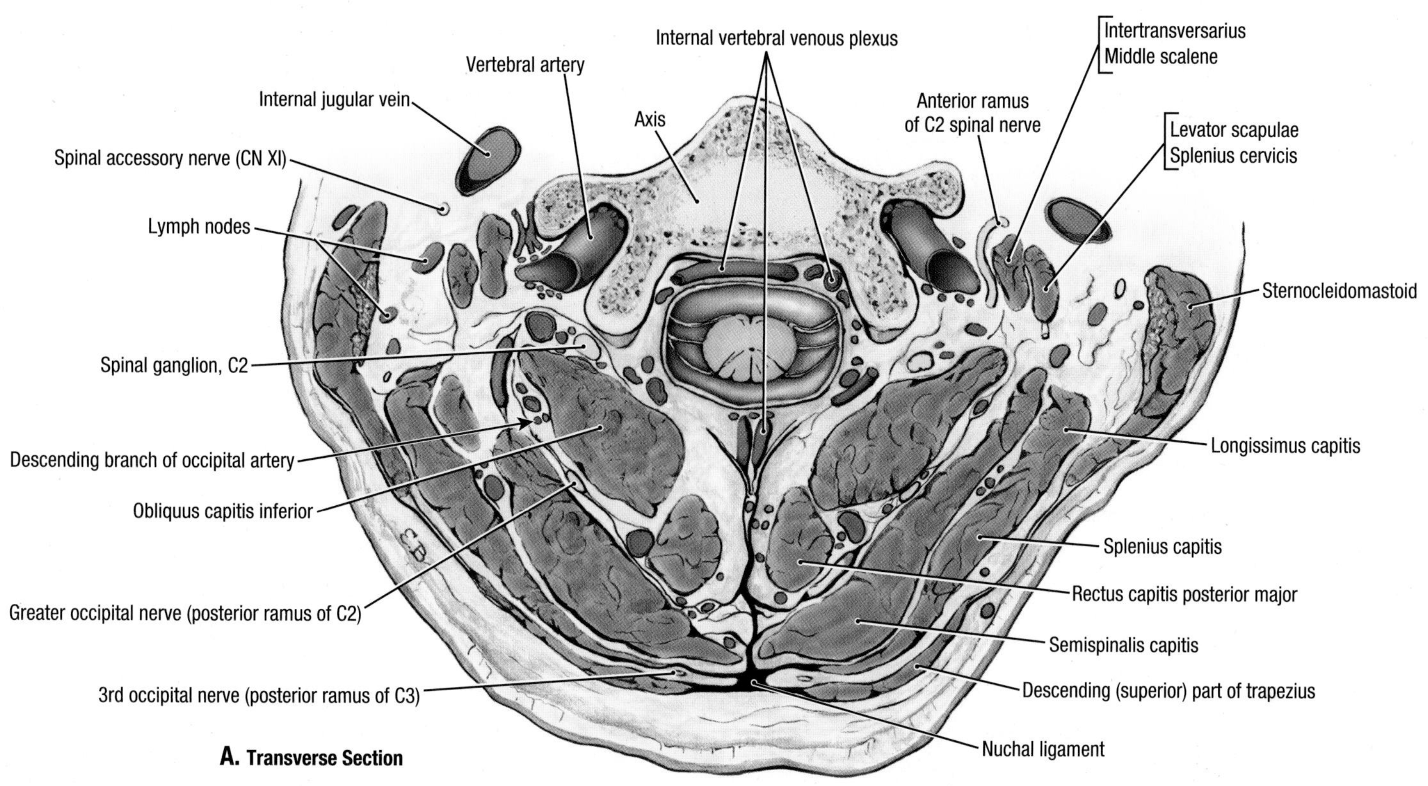
Internal vertebral venous plexus
Vertebral artery
Internal jugular vein
Axis
Spinal accessory nerve (CN XI)
Lymph nodes
Spinal ganglion, C2
Descending branch of occipital artery
Obliquus capitis inferior
Greater occipital nerve (posterior ramus of C2)
3rd occipital nerve (posterior ramus of C3)
Intertransversarius
Middle scalene
Anterior ramus
of C2 spinal nerve
Levator scapulae
Splenius cervicis
Sternocleidomastoid
Longissimus capitis
Splenius capitis
Rectus capitis posterior major
Semispinalis capitis
Descending (superior) part of trapezius
Nuchal ligament

A. **Transverse Section**

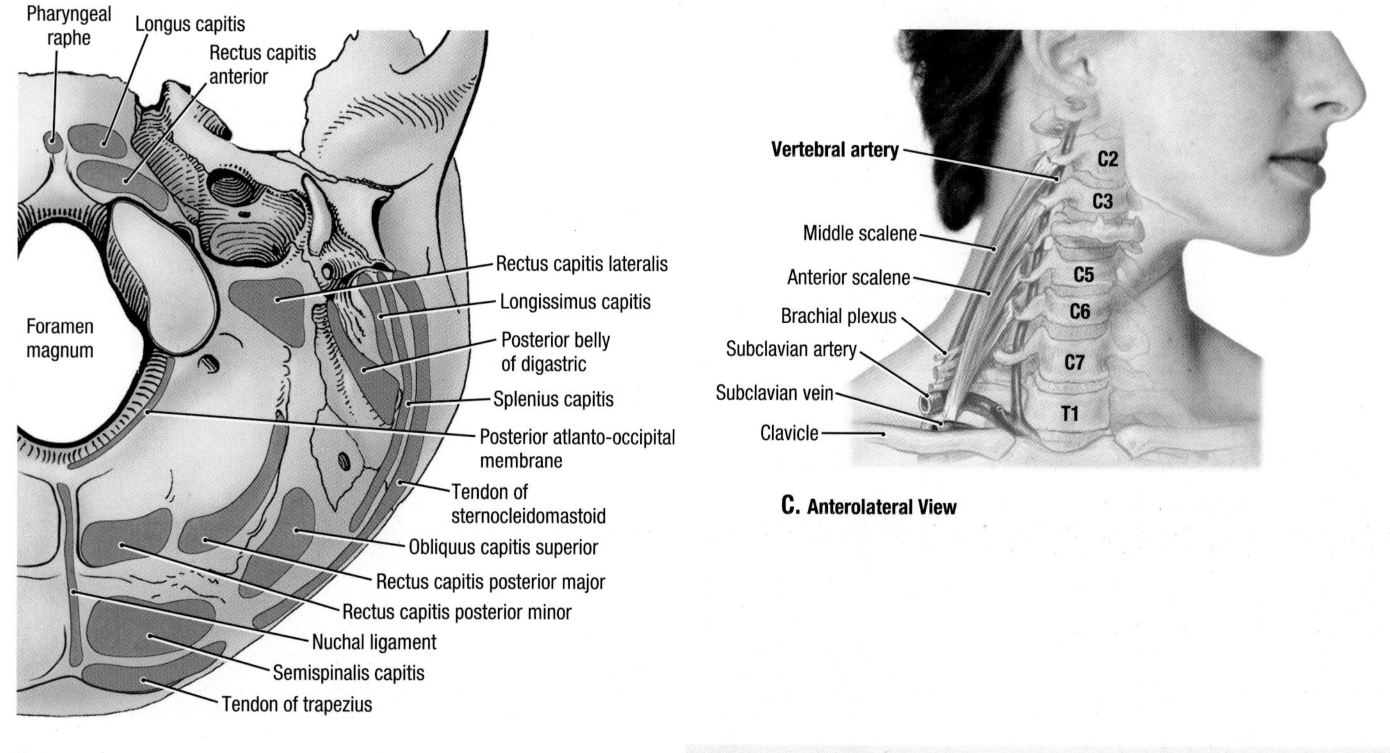
Pharyngeal
raphe
Longus capitis
Rectus capitis
anterior
Foramen
magnum
Rectus capitis lateralis
Longissimus capitis
Posterior belly
of digastric
Splenius capitis
Posterior atlanto-occipital
membrane
Tendon of
sternocleidomastoid
Obliquus capitis superior
Rectus capitis posterior major
Rectus capitis posterior minor
Nuchal ligament
Semispinalis capitis
Tendon of trapezius
Vertebral artery
Middle scalene
Anterior scalene
Brachial plexus
Subclavian artery
Subclavian vein
Clavicle
C2
C3
C5
C6
C7
T1

B. **Inferior View**

C. **Anterolateral View**

4.40 NUCHAL REGION

A. Transverse section at the level of the axis. **B.** Muscle attachments on the inferior aspect of the skull. **C.** Vertebral artery.

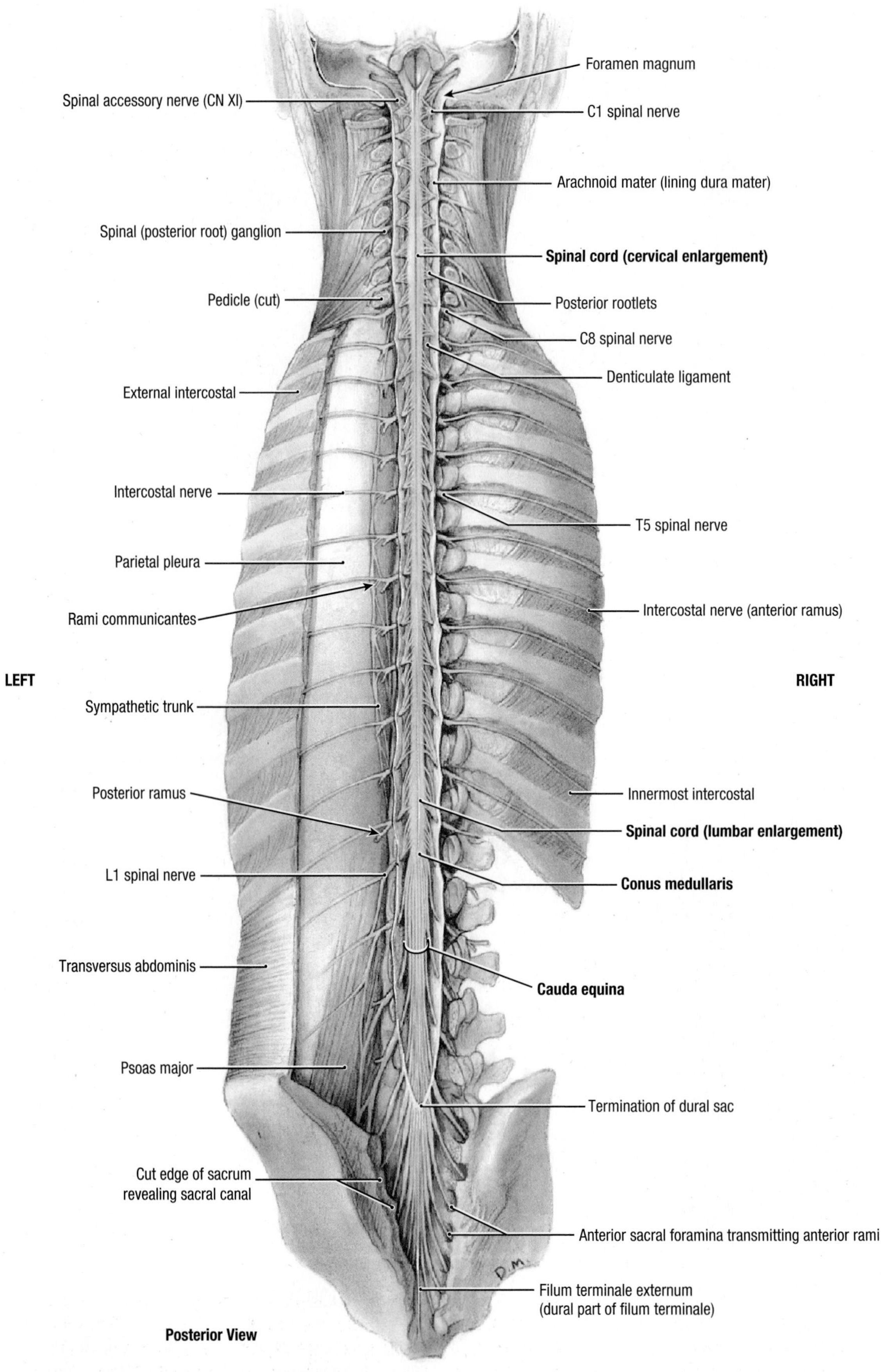
Foramen magnum
Spinal accessory nerve (CN XI)
C1 spinal nerve
Arachnoid mater (lining dura mater)
Spinal (posterior root) ganglion
Spinal cord (cervical enlargement)
Pedicle (cut)
Posterior rootlets
C8 spinal nerve
Denticulate ligament
External intercostal
Intercostal nerve
T5 spinal nerve
Parietal pleura
Rami communicantes
Intercostal nerve (anterior ramus)
LEFT
RIGHT
Sympathetic trunk
Posterior ramus
Innermost intercostal
Spinal cord (lumbar enlargement)
L1 spinal nerve
Conus medullaris
Transversus abdominis
Cauda equina
Psoas major
Termination of dural sac
Cut edge of sacrum revealing sacral canal
Anterior sacral foramina transmitting anterior rami
D.M.
Filum terminale externum (dural part of filum terminale)
Posterior View

4.41 SPINAL CORD IN SITU

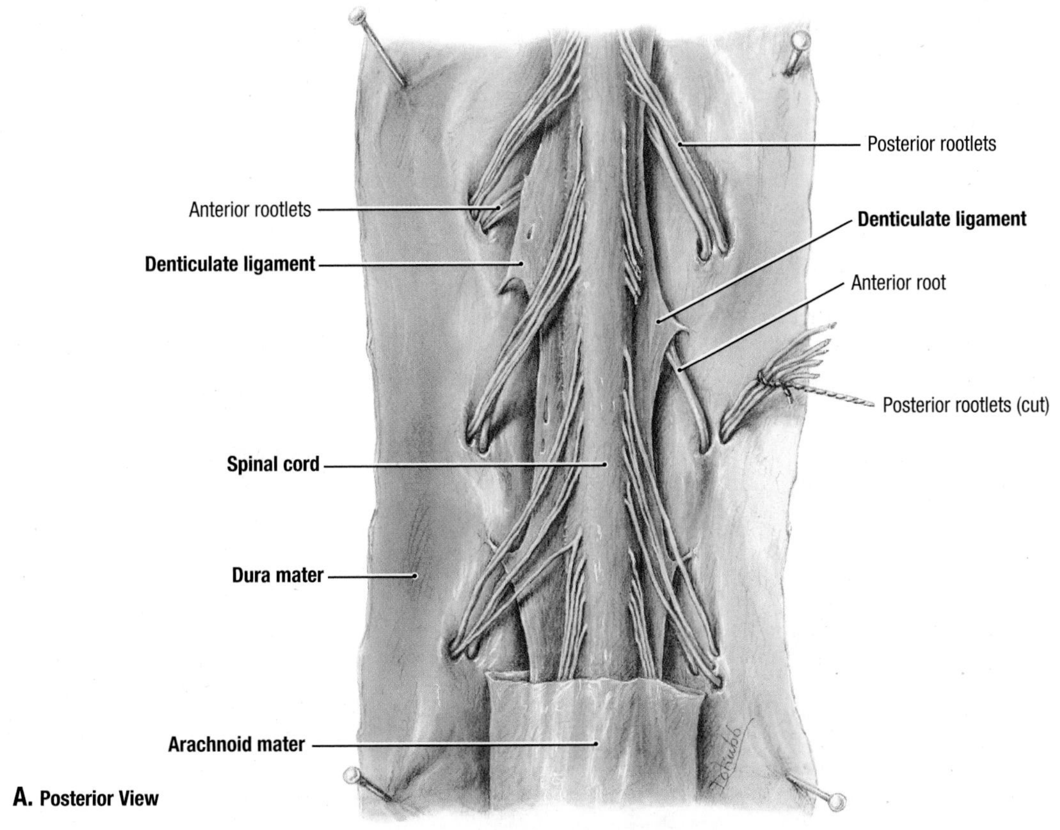
Posterior rootlets
Anterior rootlets
Denticulate ligament
Denticulate ligament
Anterior root
Posterior rootlets (cut)
Spinal cord
Dura mater
Arachnoid mater

A. **Posterior View**

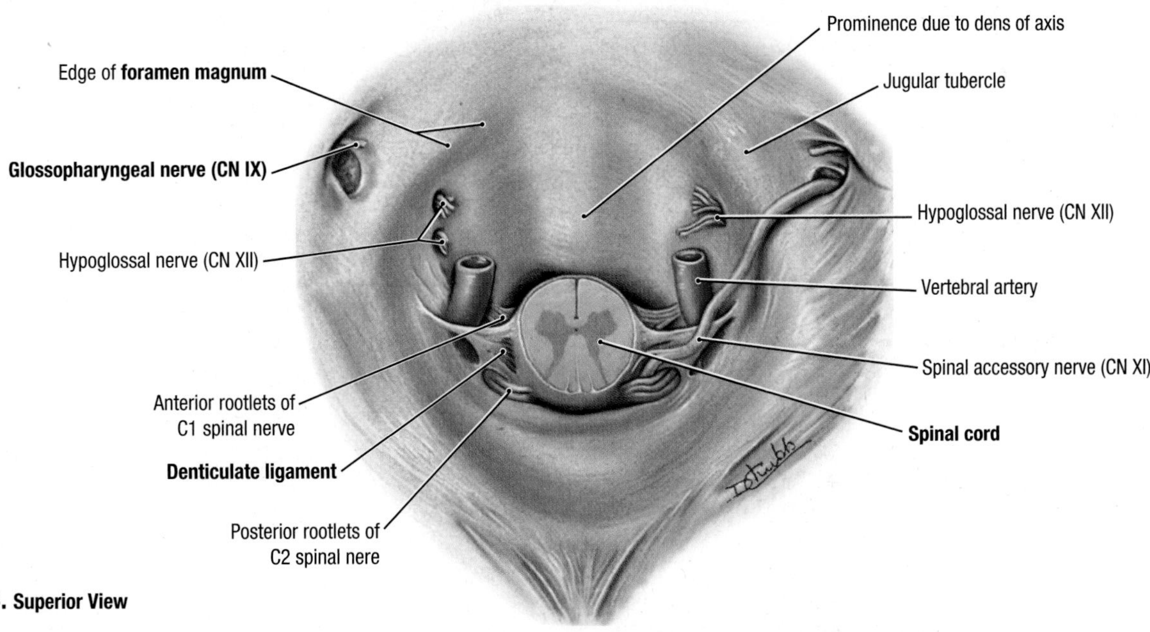
Prominence due to dens of axis
Edge of foramen magnum
Jugular tubercle
Glossopharyngeal nerve (CN IX)
Hypoglossal nerve (CN XII)
Hypoglossal nerve (CN XII)
Vertebral artery
Spinal accessory nerve (CN XI)
Anterior rootlets of C1 spinal nerve
Spinal cord
Denticulate ligament
Posterior rootlets of C2 spinal nere

B. **Superior View**

4.42 SPINAL CORD AND MENINGES

A. Dural sac cut open. The denticulate ligament anchors the cord to the dural sac between successive nerve roots by means of strong, toothlike processes. The anterior nerve roots (rootlets) lie anterior to the denticulate ligament, and the posterior nerve roots (rootlets) lie posterior to the ligament. **B.** Structures of vertebral canal seen through foramen magnum. The spinal cord, vertebral arteries, spinal accessory nerve (CN XI), and most superior part of the denticulate ligament pass through the foramen magnum within the meninges.

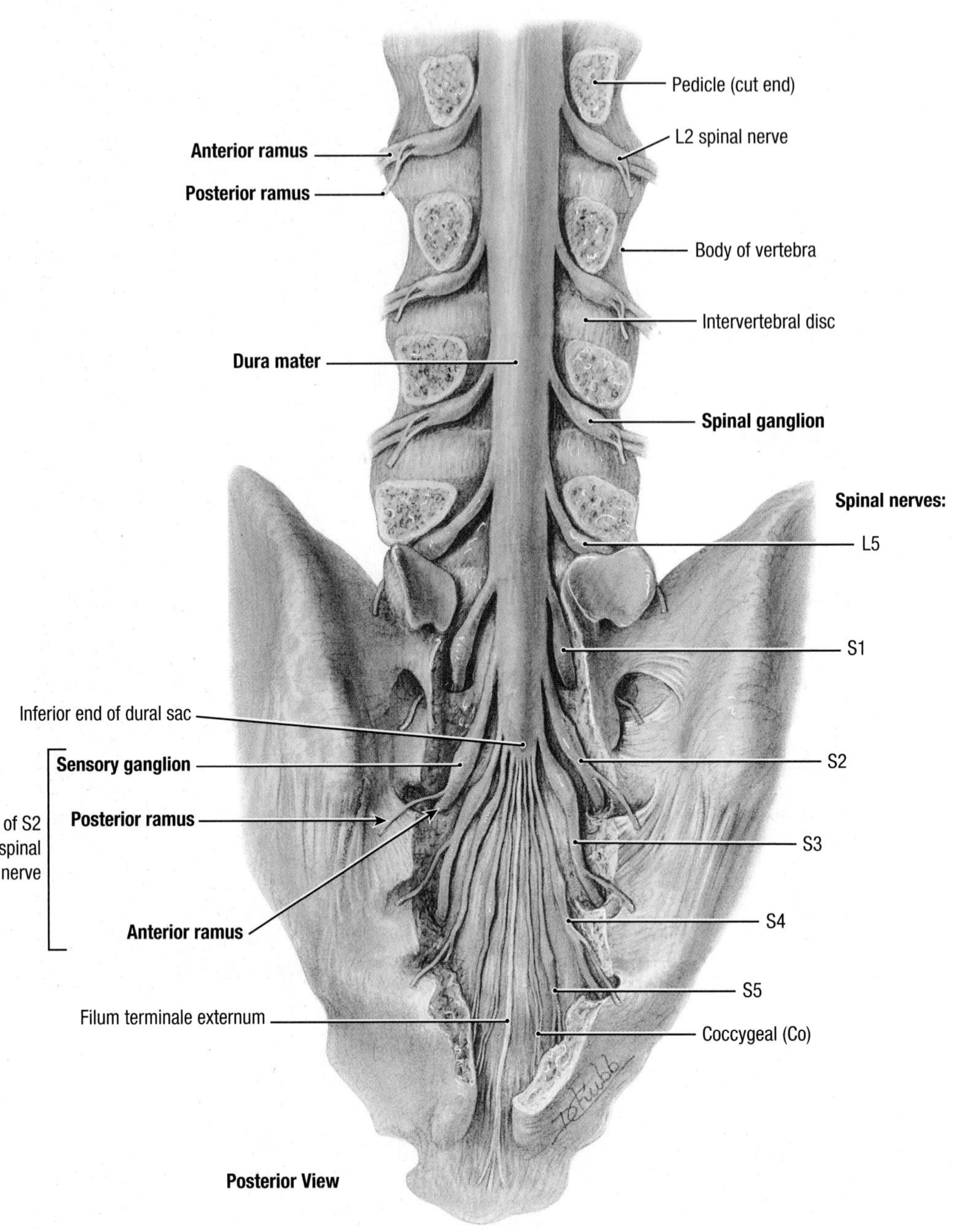
Pedicle (cut end)
L2 spinal nerve
Anterior ramus
Posterior ramus
Body of vertebra
Intervertebral disc
Dura mater
Spinal ganglion
Spinal nerves:
L5
S1
Inferior end of dural sac
Sensory ganglion
of S2 spinal nerve
Posterior ramus
S2
S3
Anterior ramus
S4
S5
Filum terminale externum
Coccygeal (Co)
Posterior View

4.43 INFERIOR END OF DURAL SAC I

The posterior parts of the lumbar vertebrae and sacrum were removed.

- The inferior limit of the dural sac is at the level of the posterior superior iliac spine (body of 2nd sacral vertebra); the dura continues as the filum terminale externum.
- The lumbar spinal ganglia are in the IV foramina, and the sacral spinal ganglia are somewhat asymmetrically placed within the sacral canal.
- The posterior rami are smaller than the anterior rami.

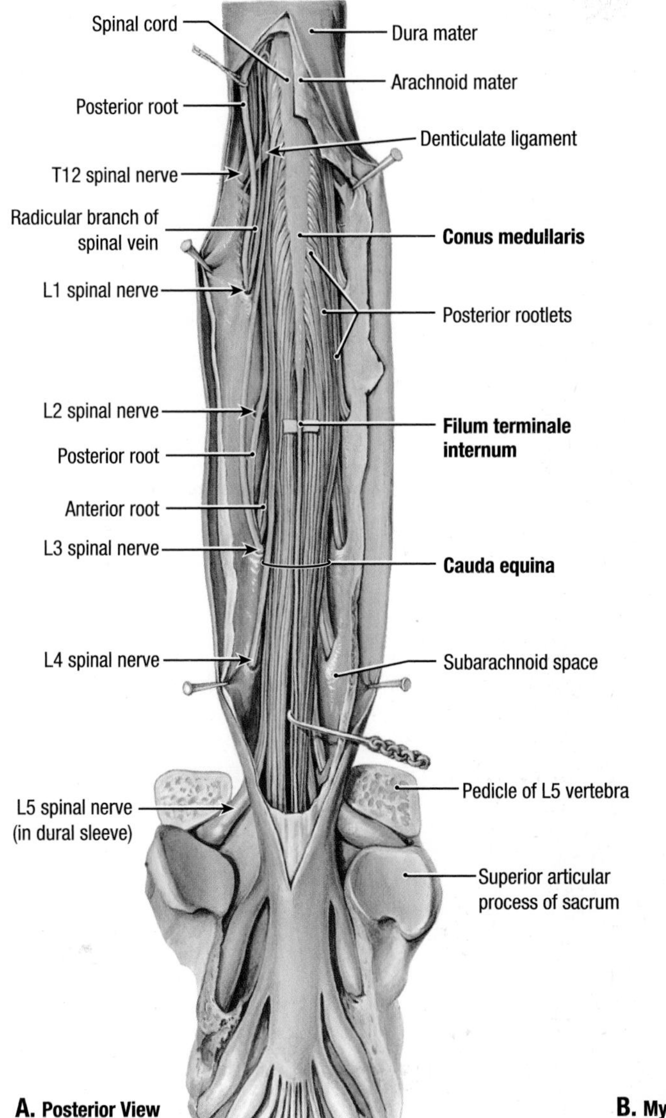
Spinal cord
Dura mater
Arachnoid mater
Posterior root
Denticulate ligament
T12 spinal nerve
Radicular branch of spinal vein
Conus medullaris
L1 spinal nerve
Posterior rootlets
L2 spinal nerve
Filum terminale internum
Posterior root
Anterior root
L3 spinal nerve
Cauda equina
L4 spinal nerve
Subarachnoid space
Pedicle of L5 vertebra
L5 spinal nerve (in dural sleeve)
Superior articular process of sacrum

A. Posterior View

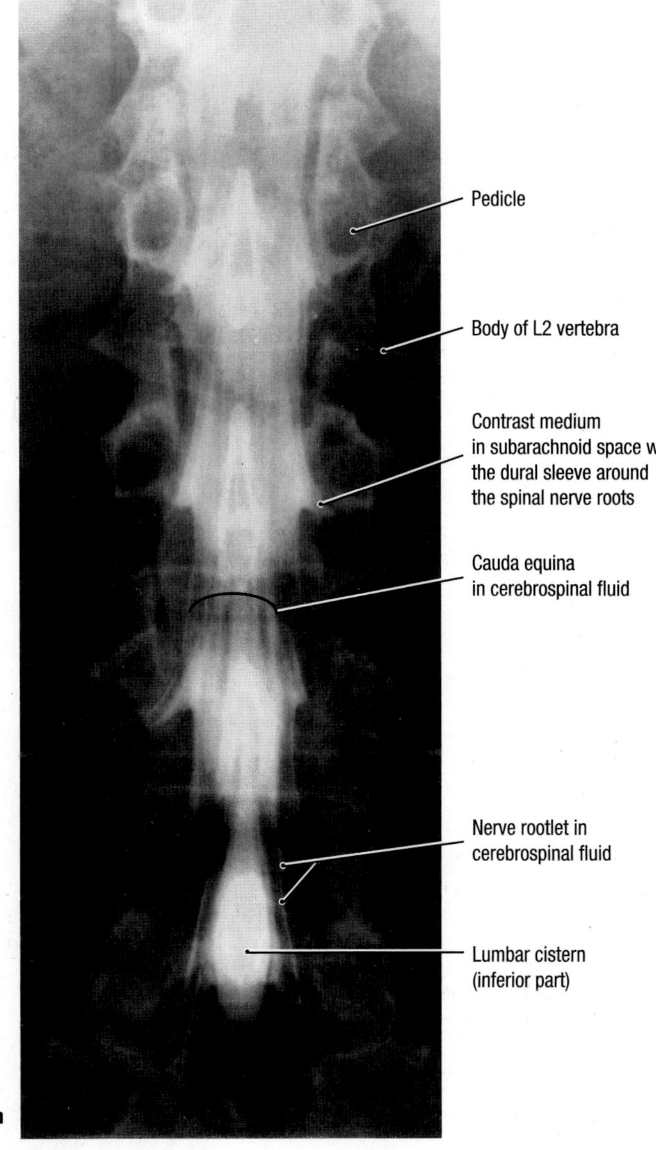
Pedicle
Body of L2 vertebra
Contrast medium in subarachnoid space within the dural sleeve around the spinal nerve roots
Cauda equina in cerebrospinal fluid
Nerve rootlet in cerebrospinal fluid
Lumbar cistern (inferior part)

B. Myelogram

4.44 INFERIOR END OF DURAL SAC II

A. Inferior dural sac and lumbar cistern of subarachnoid space, opened. **B.** Myelogram of the lumbar region of the vertebral column. Contrast medium was injected into the subarachnoid space. **C.** Termination of spinal cord, in situ, sagittal section.

- The conus medullaris, or conical lower end of the spinal cord, continues as a glistening thread, the filum terminale internum, which descends with the posterior and anterior nerve roots; these constitute the cauda equina.
- In the adult, the spinal cord usually ends at the level of the disc between vertebrae L1 and L2. Variations: 95% of cords end within the limits of the bodies of L1 and L2, whereas 3% end posterior to the inferior half of T12, and 2% posterior to L3.
- The subarachnoid space usually ends at the level of the disc between S1 and S2, but it can be more inferior.

To obtain a **sample of CSF from the lumbar cistern**, a lumbar puncture needle, fitted with a stylet, is inserted into the subarachnoid space. Flexion of the vertebral column facilitates insertion of the needle by stretching the ligamenta flava and spreading the laminae and spinous processes apart. The needle is inserted in the midline between the spinous processes of the L3 and L4 (or the L4 and L5) vertebrae. At these levels in adults, there is little danger of damaging the spinal cord.

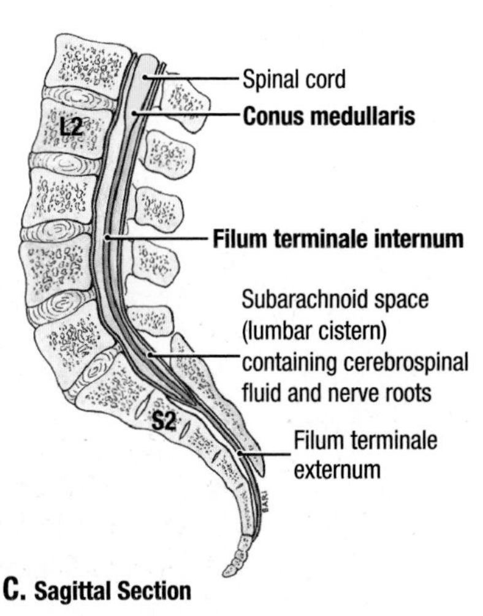
L2
Spinal cord
Conus medullaris
Filum terminale internum
Subarachnoid space (lumbar cistern) containing cerebrospinal fluid and nerve roots
S2
Filum terminale externum

C. Sagittal Section

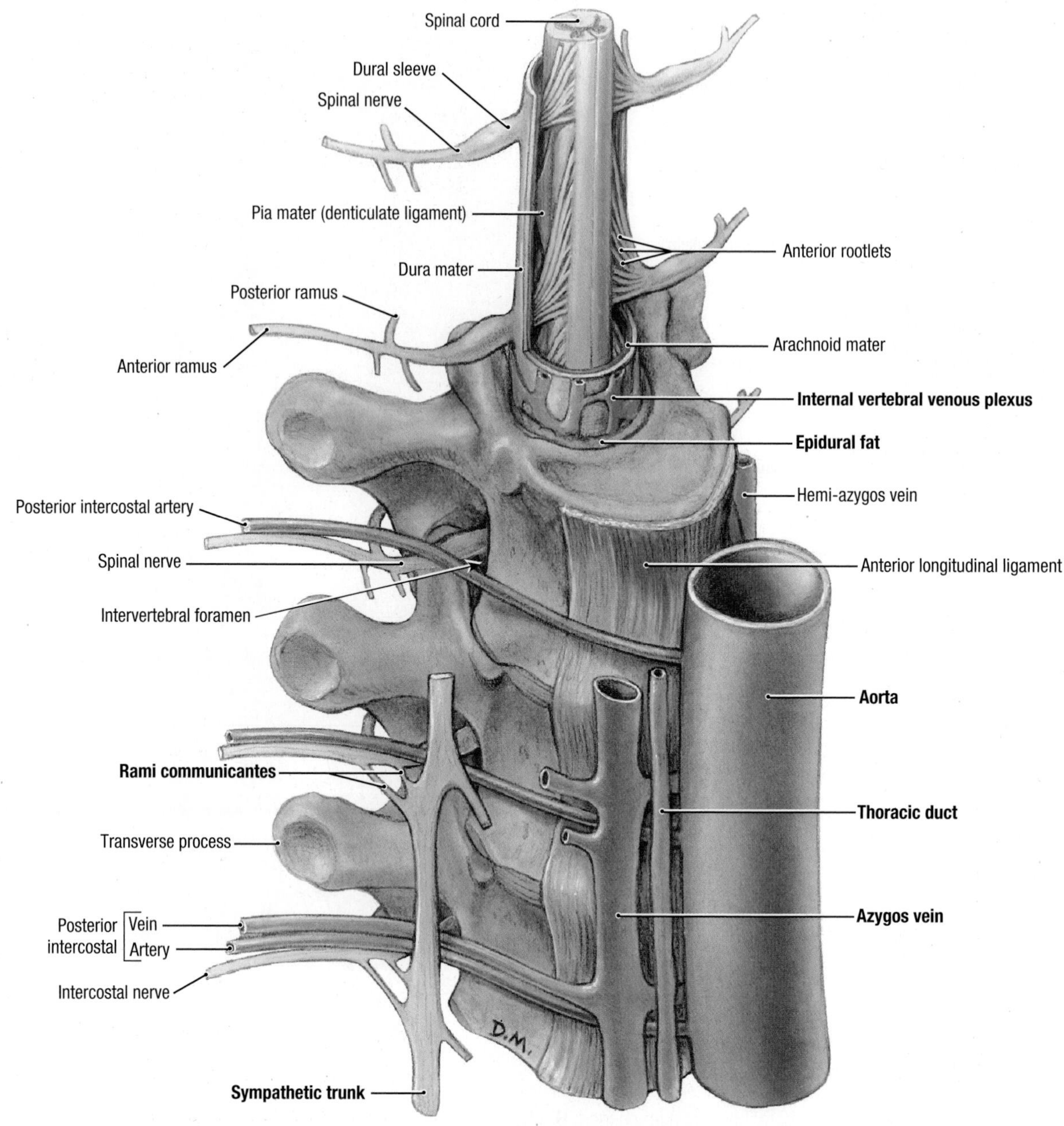

Spinal cord
Dural sleeve
Spinal nerve
Pia mater (denticulate ligament)
Dura mater
Anterior rootlets
Posterior ramus
Anterior ramus
Arachnoid mater
Internal vertebral venous plexus
Epidural fat
Hemi-azygos vein
Posterior intercostal artery
Spinal nerve
Anterior longitudinal ligament
Intervertebral foramen
Aorta
Rami communicantes
Thoracic duct
Transverse process
Posterior intercostal
Vein
Artery
Azygos vein
Intercostal nerve
D.M.
Sympathetic trunk

Right Anterolateral View

4.45 SPINAL CORD AND PREVERTEBRAL STRUCTURES

The vertebrae have been removed superiorly to expose the spinal cord and meninges.

- The aorta descends to the left of the midline, with the thoracic duct and azygos vein to its right.
- Typically, the azygos vein is on the right side of the vertebral bodies, and the hemi-azygos vein is on the left.
- The thoracic sympathetic trunk and ganglia lie lateral to the thoracic vertebrae; the rami communicantes connect the sympathetic ganglia with the spinal nerve.
- A sleeve of dura mater surrounds the spinal nerves and blends with the sheath (epineurium) of the spinal nerve.
- The dura mater is separated from the walls of the vertebral canal by epidural fat and the internal vertebral venous plexus.

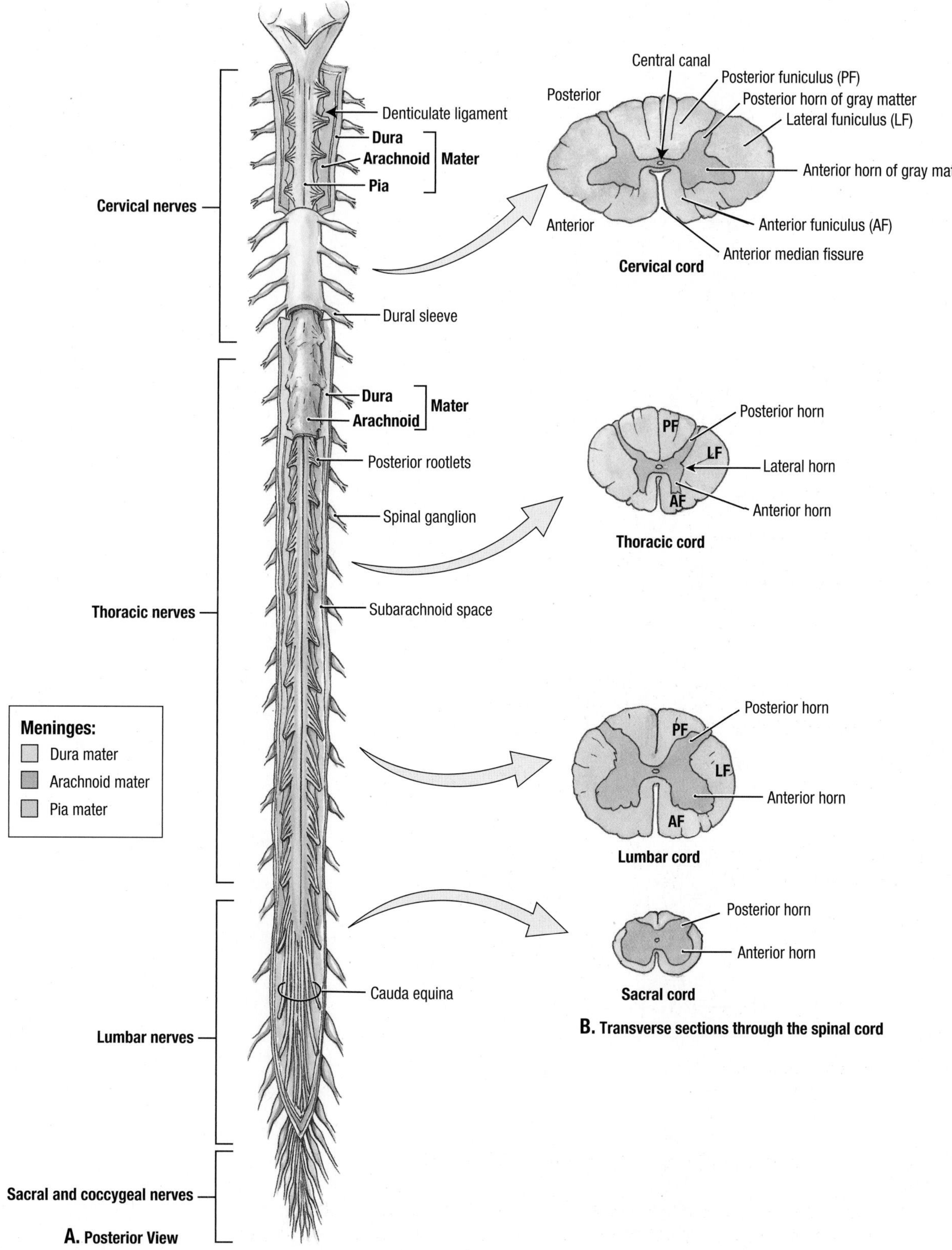
Denticulate ligament
Dura
Arachnoid
Pia
Mater
Cervical nerves
Dural sleeve
Dura
Arachnoid
Mater
Posterior rootlets
Spinal ganglion
Thoracic nerves
Subarachnoid space
Meninges:
Dura mater
Arachnoid mater
Pia mater
Lumbar nerves
Cauda equina
Sacral and coccygeal nerves
Central canal
Posterior funiculus (PF)
Posterior
Posterior horn of gray matter
Lateral funiculus (LF)
Anterior horn of gray matter
Anterior
Anterior funiculus (AF)
Anterior median fissure
Cervical cord
PF
LF
AF
Posterior horn
Lateral horn
Anterior horn
Thoracic cord
Posterior horn
PF
LF
Anterior horn
AF
Lumbar cord
Posterior horn
Anterior horn
Sacral cord

A. Posterior View

B. Transverse sections through the spinal cord

4.46 ISOLATED SPINAL CORD AND SPINAL NERVE ROOTS WITH COVERINGS AND REGIONAL SECTIONS

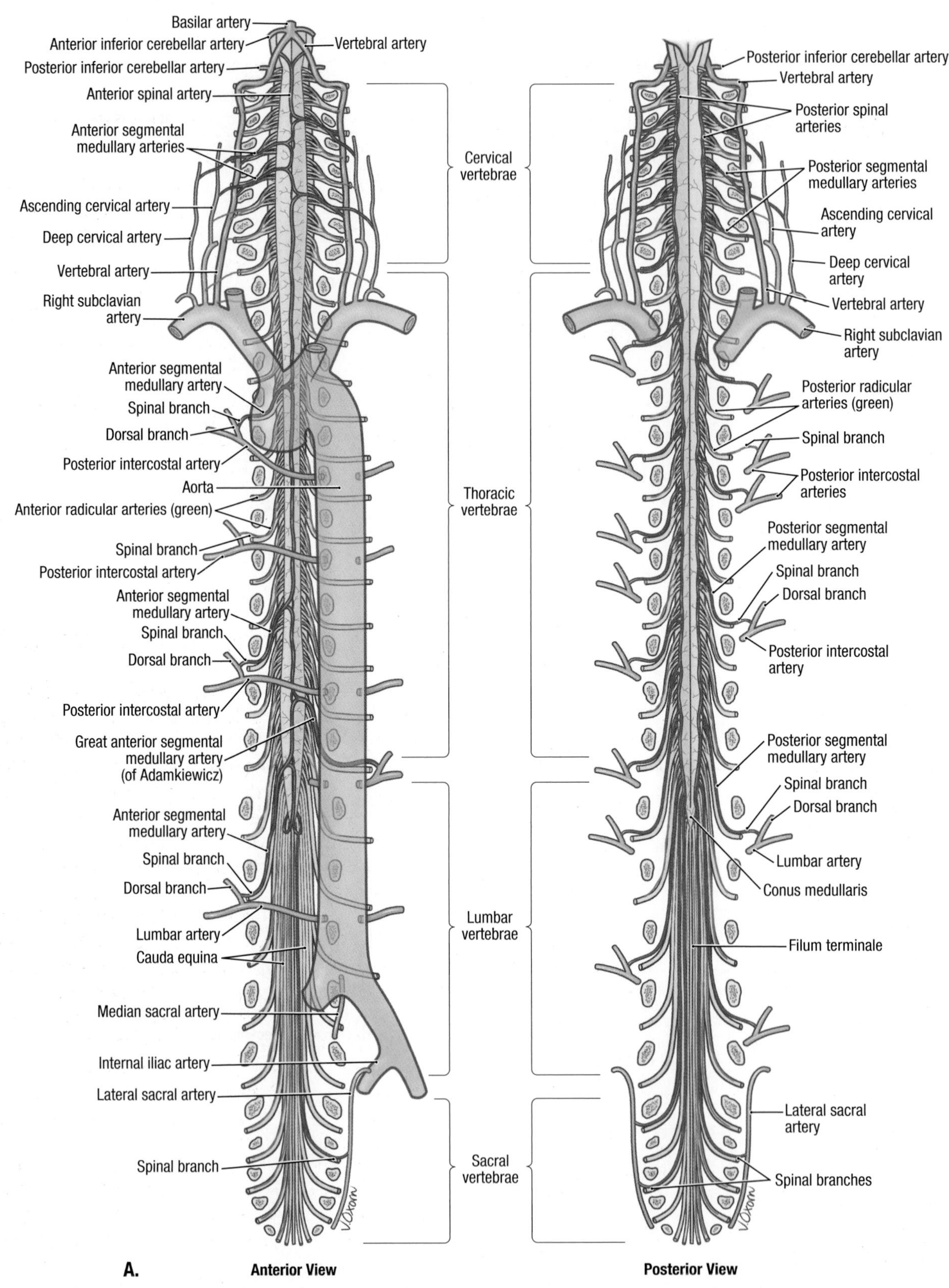
Basilar artery
Anterior inferior cerebellar artery
Vertebral artery
Posterior inferior cerebellar artery
Anterior spinal artery
Anterior segmental medullary arteries
Ascending cervical artery
Deep cervical artery
Vertebral artery
Right subclavian artery
Anterior segmental medullary artery
Spinal branch
Dorsal branch
Posterior intercostal artery
Aorta
Anterior radicular arteries (green)
Spinal branch
Posterior intercostal artery
Anterior segmental medullary artery
Spinal branch
Dorsal branch
Posterior intercostal artery
Great anterior segmental medullary artery (of Adamkiewicz)
Anterior segmental medullary artery
Spinal branch
Dorsal branch
Lumbar artery
Cauda equina
Median sacral artery
Internal iliac artery
Lateral sacral artery
Spinal branch
Cervical vertebrae
Thoracic vertebrae
Lumbar vertebrae
Sacral vertebrae
Posterior inferior cerebellar artery
Vertebral artery
Posterior spinal arteries
Posterior segmental medullary arteries
Ascending cervical artery
Deep cervical artery
Vertebral artery
Right subclavian artery
Posterior radicular arteries (green)
Spinal branch
Posterior intercostal arteries
Posterior segmental medullary artery
Spinal branch
Dorsal branch
Posterior intercostal artery
Posterior segmental medullary artery
Spinal branch
Dorsal branch
Lumbar artery
Conus medullaris
Filum terminale
Lateral sacral artery
Spinal branches
A.
Anterior View
Posterior View

4.47 BLOOD SUPPLY OF SPINAL CORD

A. Arteries of spinal cord. The segmental reinforcements of blood supply from the segmental medullary arteries are important in supplying blood to the anterior and posterior spinal arteries. Fractures, dislocations, and fracture-dislocations may interfere with the blood supply to the spinal cord from the spinal and medullary arteries.

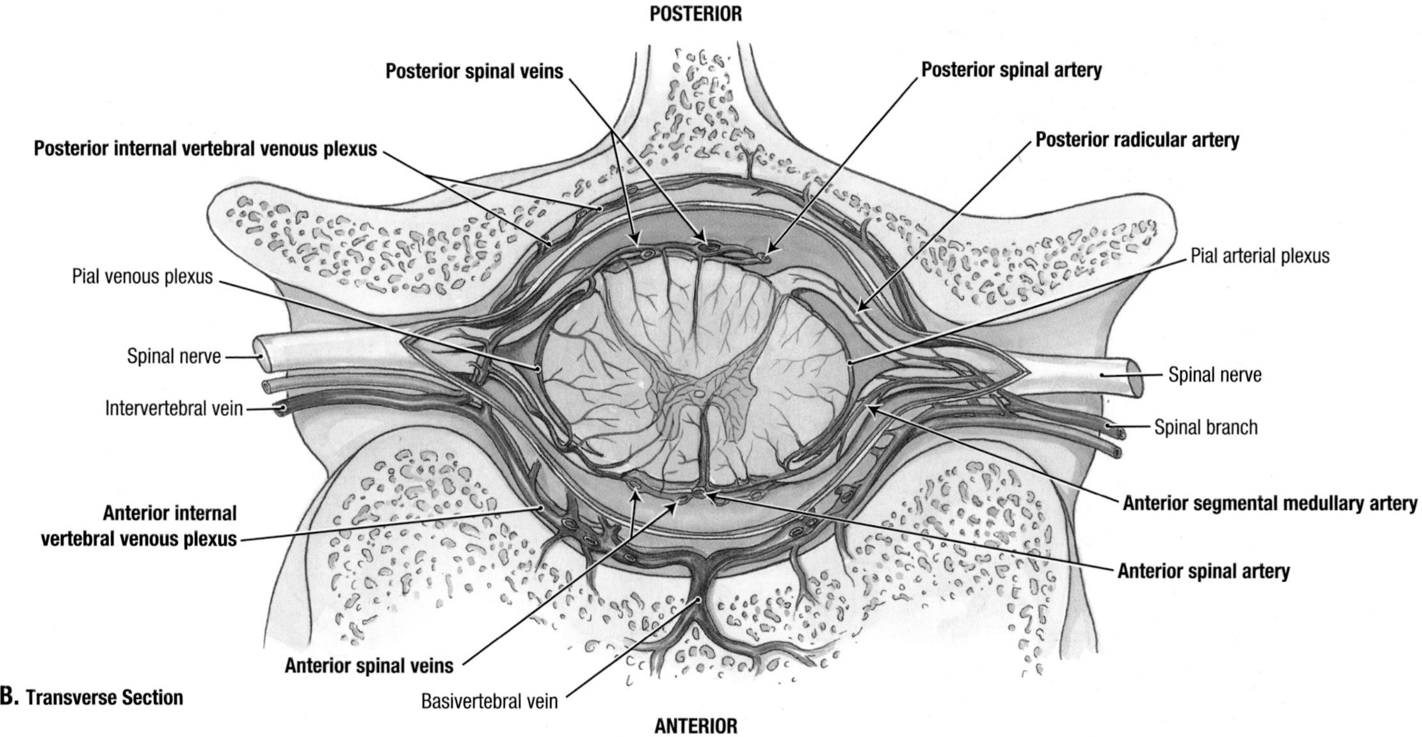
POSTERIOR
Posterior spinal veins
Posterior spinal artery
Posterior internal vertebral venous plexus
Posterior radicular artery
Pial venous plexus
Pial arterial plexus
Spinal nerve
Intervertebral vein
Spinal nerve
Spinal branch
Anterior segmental medullary artery
Anterior internal vertebral venous plexus
Anterior spinal artery
Anterior spinal veins
Basivertebral vein
ANTERIOR

B. **Transverse Section**

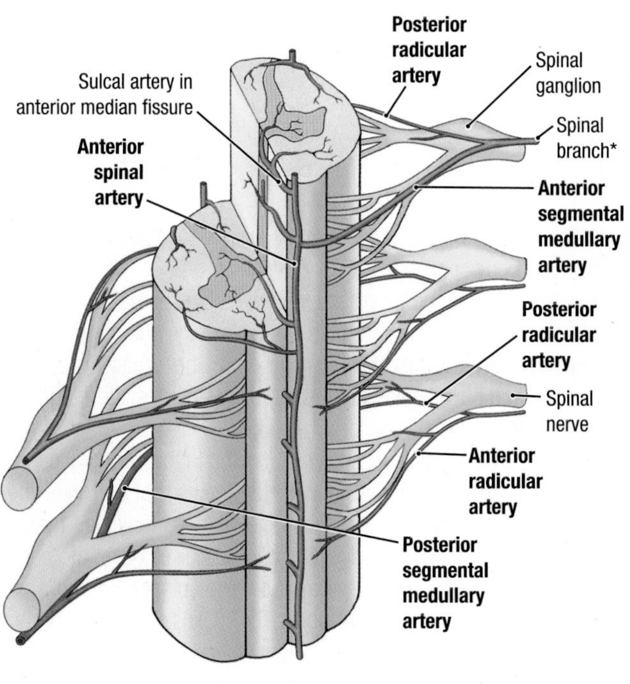
Posterior radicular artery
Spinal ganglion
Sulcal artery in anterior median fissure
Spinal branch*
Anterior spinal artery
Anterior segmental medullary artery
Posterior radicular artery
Spinal nerve
Anterior radicular artery
Posterior segmental medullary artery

* Spinal branches arise from the vertebral, intercostal, lumbar, or sacral artery, depending on level of spinal cord.

C. **Anterolateral View**

4.47 BLOOD SUPPLY OF SPINAL CORD (*CONTINUED*)

B. Arterial supply and venous drainage. **C.** Segmental medullary and radicular arteries. Three longitudinal arteries supply the spinal cord: an anterior spinal artery, formed by the union of branches of vertebral arteries, and paired posterior spinal arteries, each of which is a branch of either the vertebral artery or the posterior inferior cerebellar artery.

- The spinal arteries run longitudinally from the medulla oblongata of the brainstem to the conus medullaris of the spinal cord. By themselves, the anterior and posterior spinal arteries supply only the short superior part of the spinal cord. The circulation to much of the spinal cord depends on segmental medullary and radicular arteries.
- The anterior and posterior segmental medullary arteries enter the IV foramen to unite with the spinal arteries to supply blood to the spinal cord. The great anterior segmental medullary artery (Adamkiewicz artery) occurs on the left side in 65% of people. It reinforces the circulation to two thirds of the spinal cord.
- Posterior and anterior roots of the spinal nerves and their coverings are supplied by posterior and anterior radicular arteries, which run along the nerve roots. These vessels do not reach the posterior or anterior spinal arteries.
- The 3 anterior and 3 posterior spinal veins are arranged longitudinally; they communicate freely with each other and are drained by up to 12 anterior and posterior medullary and radicular veins. The veins draining the spinal cord join the internal vertebral plexus in the epidural space.

Ischemia. Deficiency of blood supply (ischemia) of the spinal cord affects its function and can lead to muscle weakness and paralysis. The spinal cord may also suffer circulatory impairment if the segmental medullary arteries, particularly the great anterior segmental medullary artery (of Adamkiewicz), are narrowed by obstructive arterial disease or aortic clamping during surgery.

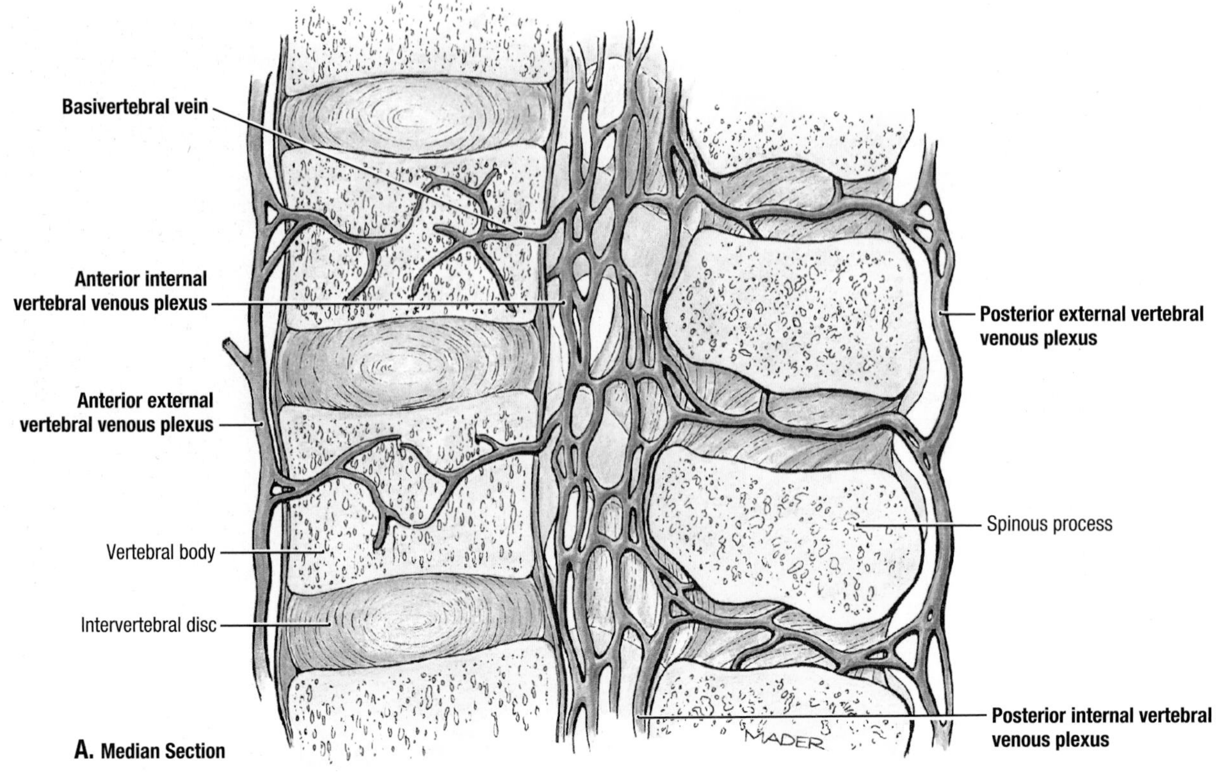

Basivertebral vein
Anterior internal vertebral venous plexus
Anterior external vertebral venous plexus
Vertebral body
Intervertebral disc
Posterior external vertebral venous plexus
Spinous process
Posterior internal vertebral venous plexus
MADER

A. Median Section

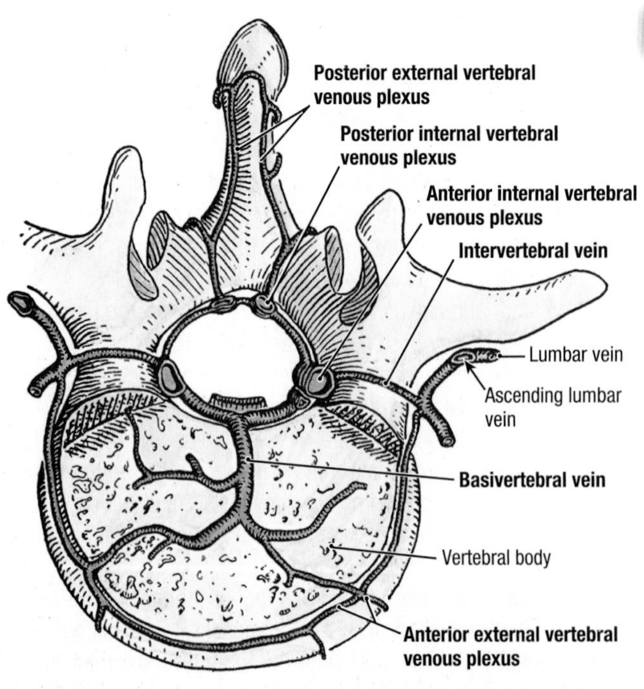

Posterior external vertebral venous plexus
Posterior internal vertebral venous plexus
Anterior internal vertebral venous plexus
Intervertebral vein
Lumbar vein
Ascending lumbar vein
Basivertebral vein
Vertebral body
Anterior external vertebral venous plexus

B. Superior View

4.48 VERTEBRAL VENOUS PLEXUSES

A. Median section of lumbar spine. **B.** Superior view of lumbar vertebra with the vertebral body sectioned transversely.

- There are internal and external vertebral venous plexuses, communicating with each other and with both systemic veins and the portal system. **Infection and tumors can spread** from the areas drained by the systemic and portal veins to the vertebral venous system and lodge in the vertebrae, spinal cord, brain, or skull.
- The internal vertebral venous plexus, located in the vertebral canal, consists of a plexus of thin-walled, valveless veins that surround the dura mater. Cranially, the internal venous plexus communicates through the foramen magnum with the occipital and basilar sinuses; at each spinal segment, the plexus receives veins from the spinal cord and a basivertebral vein from the vertebral body. The plexus is drained by IV veins that pass through the intervertebral and sacral foramina to the vertebral, intercostal, lumbar, and lateral sacral veins.
- The anterior external vertebral venous plexus is formed by veins that course through the body of each vertebra. Veins that pass through the ligamenta flava form the posterior external vertebral venous plexus. In the cervical region, these plexuses communicate with the occipital and deep cervical veins. In the thoracic, lumbar, and pelvic regions, the azygos (or hemi-azygos), ascending lumbar, and lateral sacral veins, respectively, further link segment to segment.

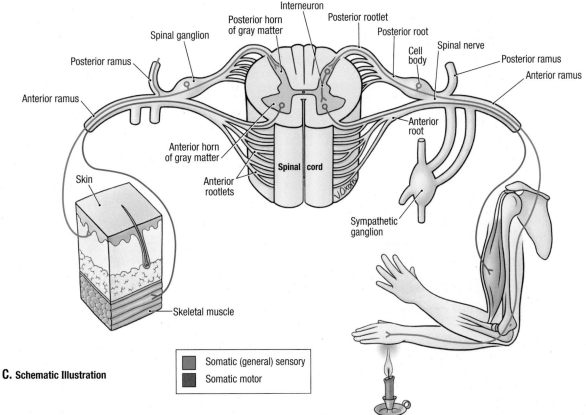

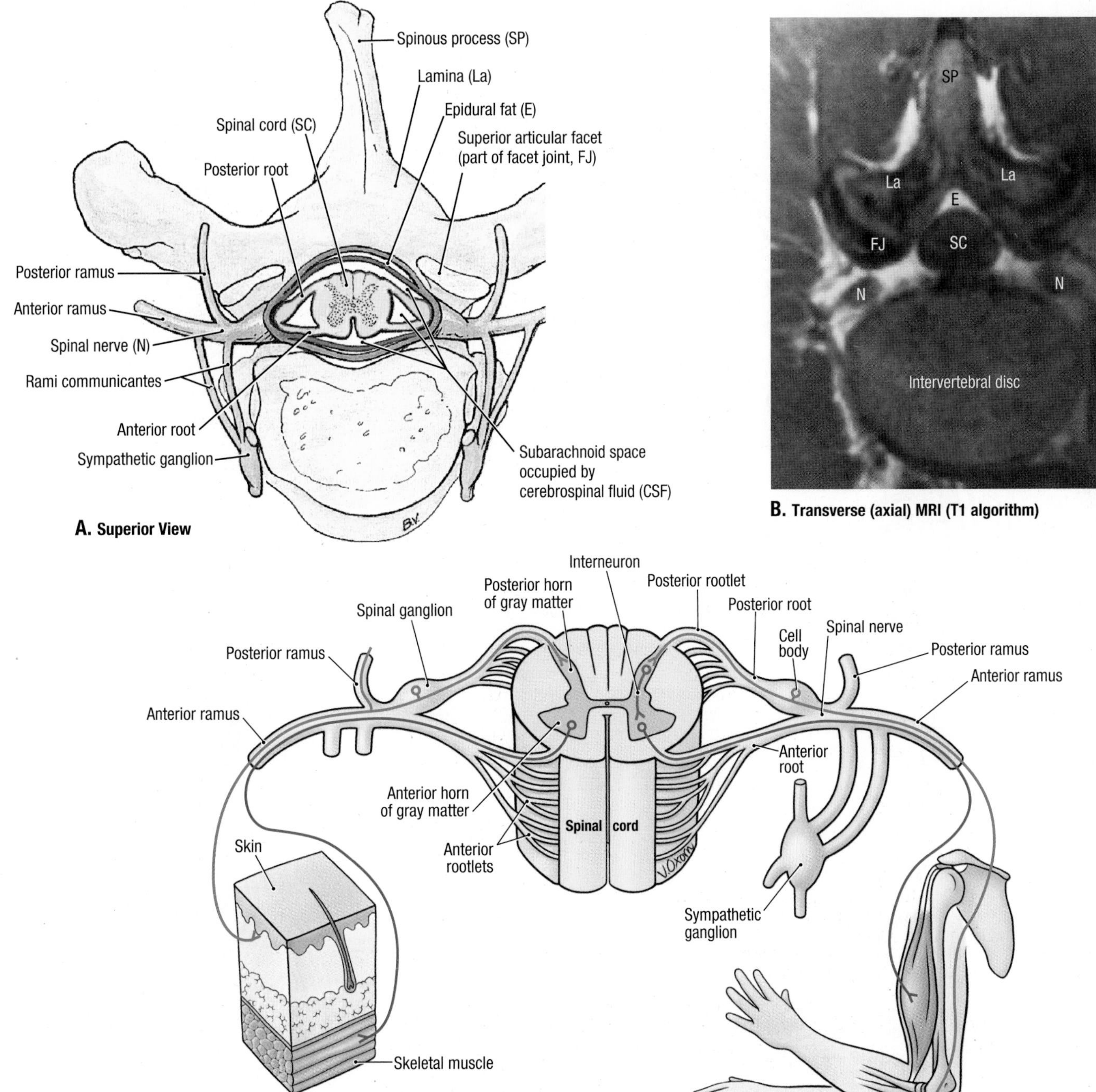
Spinous process (SP)
Lamina (La)
Epidural fat (E)
Spinal cord (SC)
Superior articular facet (part of facet joint, FJ)
Posterior root
Posterior ramus
Anterior ramus
Spinal nerve (N)
Rami communicantes
Anterior root
Sympathetic ganglion
Subarachnoid space occupied by cerebrospinal fluid (CSF)
A. Superior View
SP
La
La
E
FJ
SC
N
N
Intervertebral disc
B. Transverse (axial) MRI (T1 algorithm)
Interneuron
Posterior horn of gray matter
Posterior rootlet
Posterior root
Spinal ganglion
Cell body
Spinal nerve
Posterior ramus
Posterior ramus
Anterior ramus
Anterior ramus
Anterior root
Anterior horn of gray matter
Skin
Anterior rootlets
Spinal cord
Sympathetic ganglion
Skeletal muscle
C. Schematic Illustration
Somatic (general) sensory
Somatic motor

4.49 OVERVIEW OF SOMATIC NERVOUS SYSTEM

A. Spinal cord in situ in vertebral canal. **B.** Axial (transverse) MRI of lumbar spine. **C.** Components of typical spinal nerve. The somatic nervous system, or voluntary nervous system, composed of somatic parts of the CNS and PNS, provides general sensory and motor innervation to all parts of the body (G. *soma*), except the viscera in the body cavities, smooth muscle, and glands. The somatic (general) sensory fibers transmit sensations of touch, pain, temperature, and position from sensory receptors. The somatic motor fibers permit voluntary and reflexive movement by causing contraction of skeletal muscles, such as occurs when one touches a candle flame.

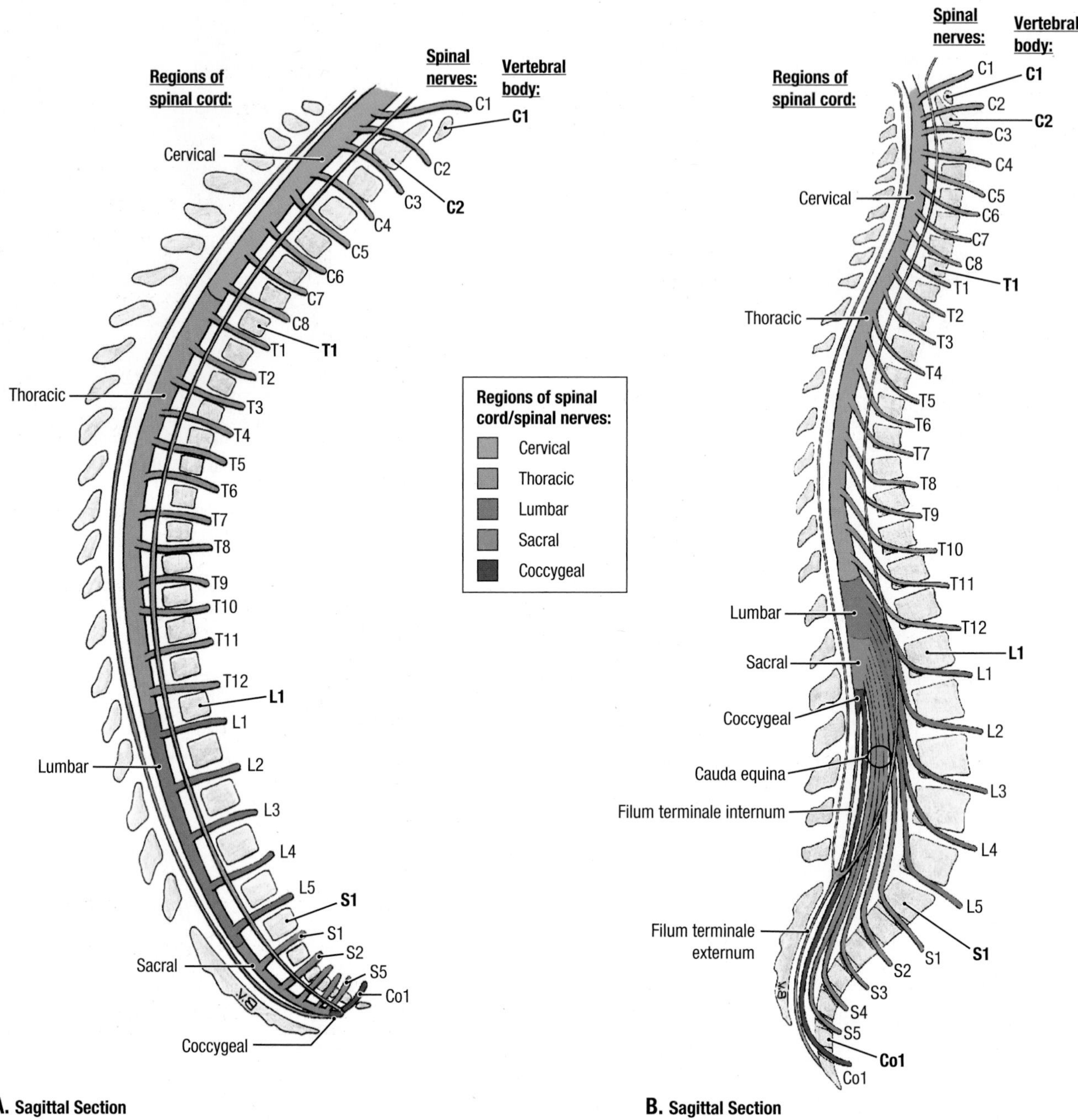
Regions of spinal cord:
Spinal nerves:
Vertebral body:
Cervical
Thoracic
Lumbar
Sacral
Coccygeal
C1
C2
C3
C4
C5
C6
C7
C8
T1
T2
T3
T4
T5
T6
T7
T8
T9
T10
T11
T12
L1
L2
L3
L4
L5
S1
S2
S3
S4
S5
Co1
Regions of spinal cord/spinal nerves:
Cervical
Thoracic
Lumbar
Sacral
Coccygeal
Cauda equina
Filum terminale internum
Filum terminale externum

A. Sagittal Section

B. Sagittal Section

4.50 SPINAL CORD AND SPINAL NERVES

A. Spinal cord at 12 weeks gestation. **B.** Spinal cord of an adult.

- Early in development, the spinal cord and vertebral (spinal) canal are nearly equal in length. The canal grows longer, so spinal nerves have an increasingly longer course to reach the IV foramen at the correct level for their exit. The spinal cord of adults terminates between vertebral bodies L1–L2. The remaining spinal nerves, seeking their IV foramen of exit, form the cauda equina.
- All 31 pairs of spinal nerves—8 cervical (C), 12 thoracic (T), 5 lumbar (L), 5 sacral (S), and 1 coccygeal (Co)—arise from the spinal cord and exit through the IV foramina in the vertebral column.

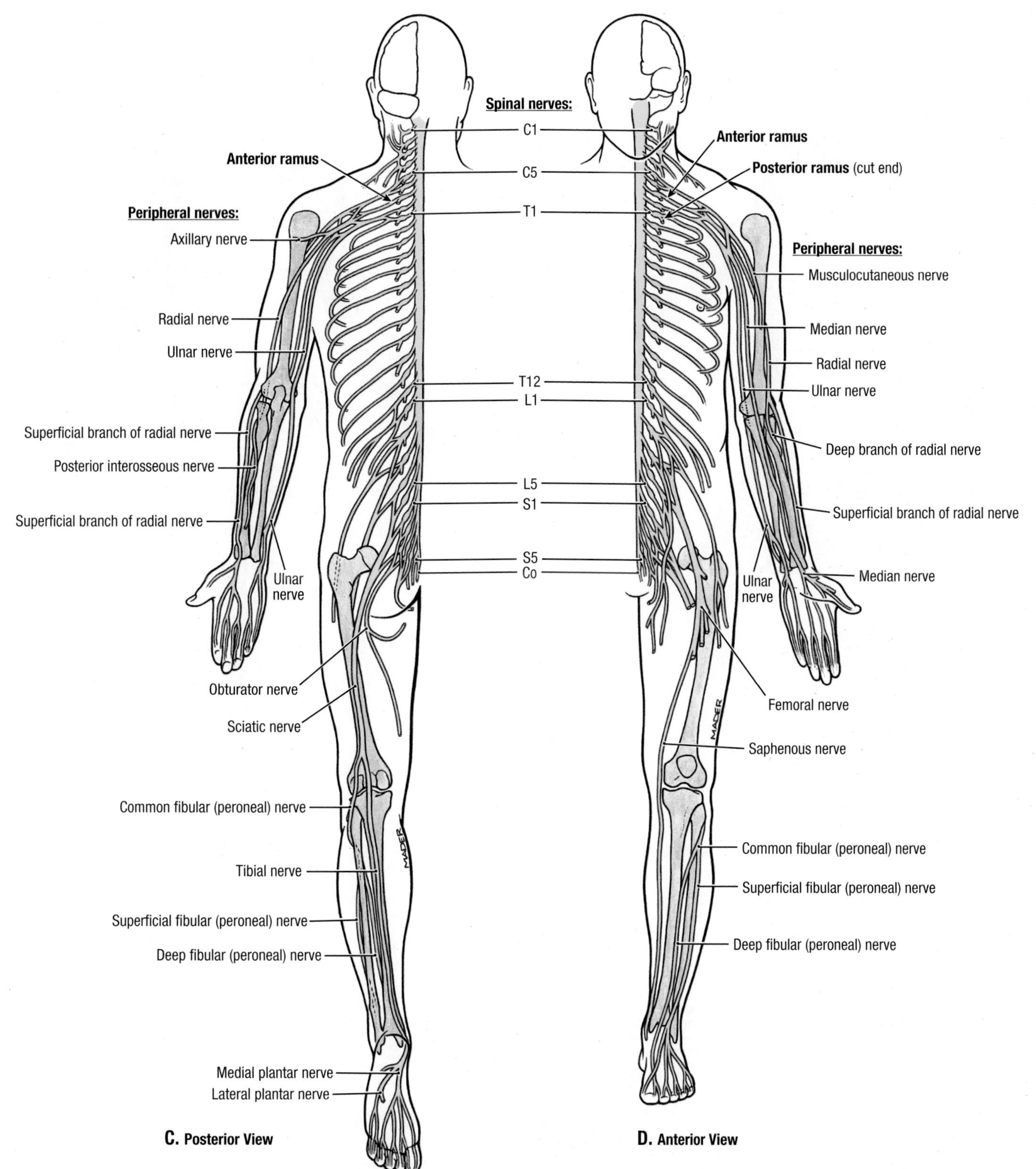
Spinal nerves:
C1
C5
T1
T12
L1
L5
S1
S5
Co
Anterior ramus
Peripheral nerves:
Axillary nerve
Radial nerve
Ulnar nerve
Superficial branch of radial nerve
Posterior interosseous nerve
Superficial branch of radial nerve
Ulnar nerve
Obturator nerve
Sciatic nerve
Common fibular (peroneal) nerve
Tibial nerve
Superficial fibular (peroneal) nerve
Deep fibular (peroneal) nerve
Medial plantar nerve
Lateral plantar nerve
Anterior ramus
Posterior ramus (cut end)
Peripheral nerves:
Musculocutaneous nerve
Median nerve
Radial nerve
Ulnar nerve
Deep branch of radial nerve
Superficial branch of radial nerve
Median nerve
Ulnar nerve
Femoral nerve
Saphenous nerve
Common fibular (peroneal) nerve
Superficial fibular (peroneal) nerve
Deep fibular (peroneal) nerve
MADER

C. Posterior View

D. Anterior View

4.50 SPINAL CORD AND SPINAL NERVES (*CONTINUED*)

C. and D. Peripheral nerves.

- The anterior rami supply nerve fibers to the anterior and lateral regions of the trunk and upper and lower limbs.
- The posterior rami supply nerve fibers to synovial joints of the vertebral column, deep muscles of the back, and overlying skin.

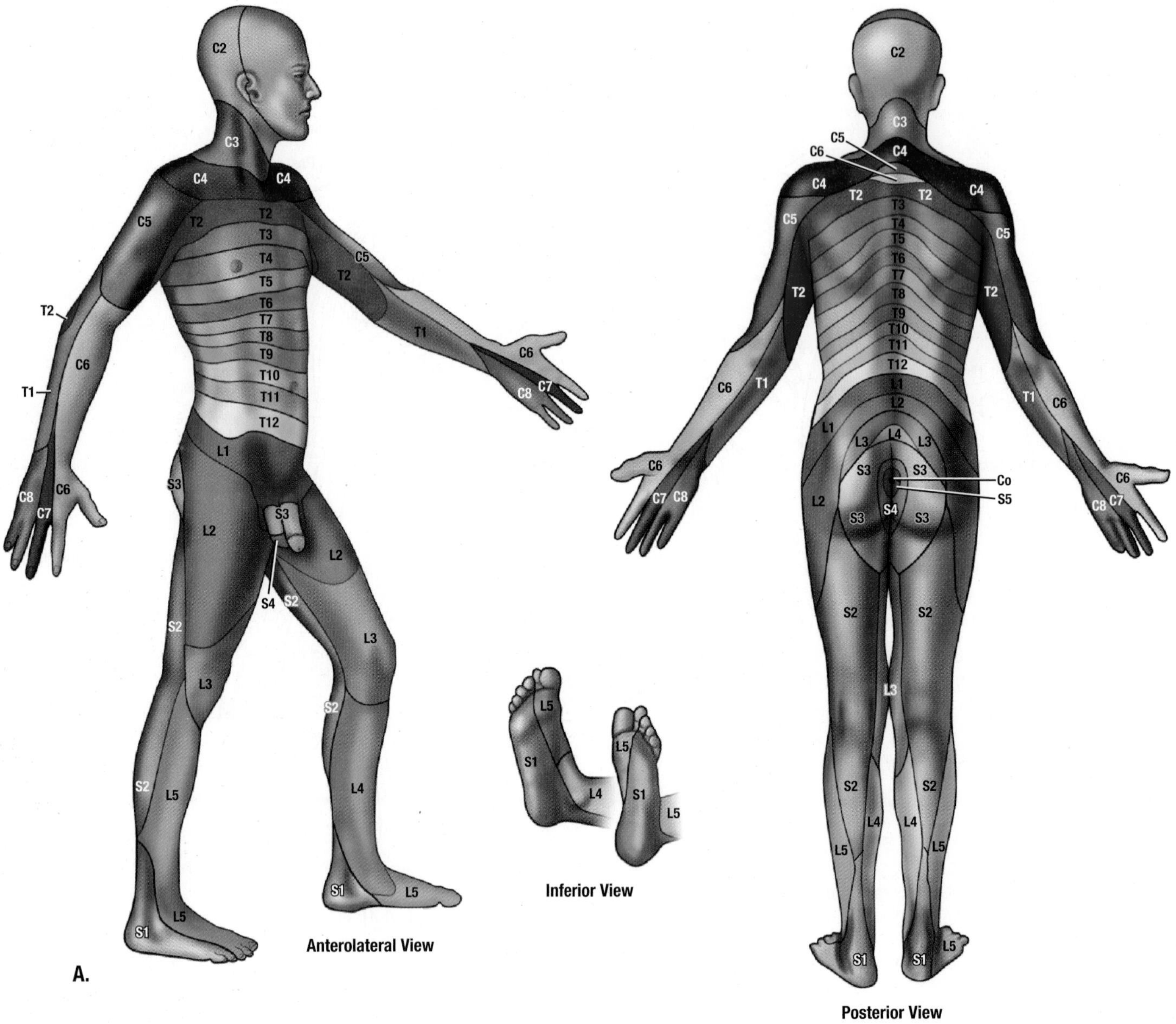

A.

Anterolateral View

Inferior View

Posterior View

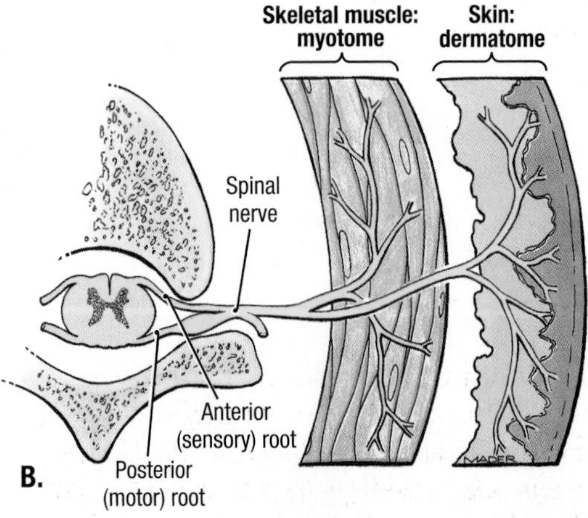
Skeletal muscle: myotome
Skin: dermatome
Spinal nerve
Anterior (sensory) root
Posterior (motor) root

B.

4.51 DERMATOMES

A.–C. Dermatome map (Foerster, 1933). The Keegan and Garrett (1948) dermatome map is not included here. The two schemes are similar in the trunk but differ in the limbs, where both are presented. **B.** Schematic illustration of a dermatome and myotome. The unilateral area of skin innervated by the general sensory fibers of a single spinal nerve is called a dermatome. From clinical studies of lesions in the posterior roots or spinal nerves, dermatome maps have been devised that indicate the typical patterns of innervation of the skin by specific spinal nerves.

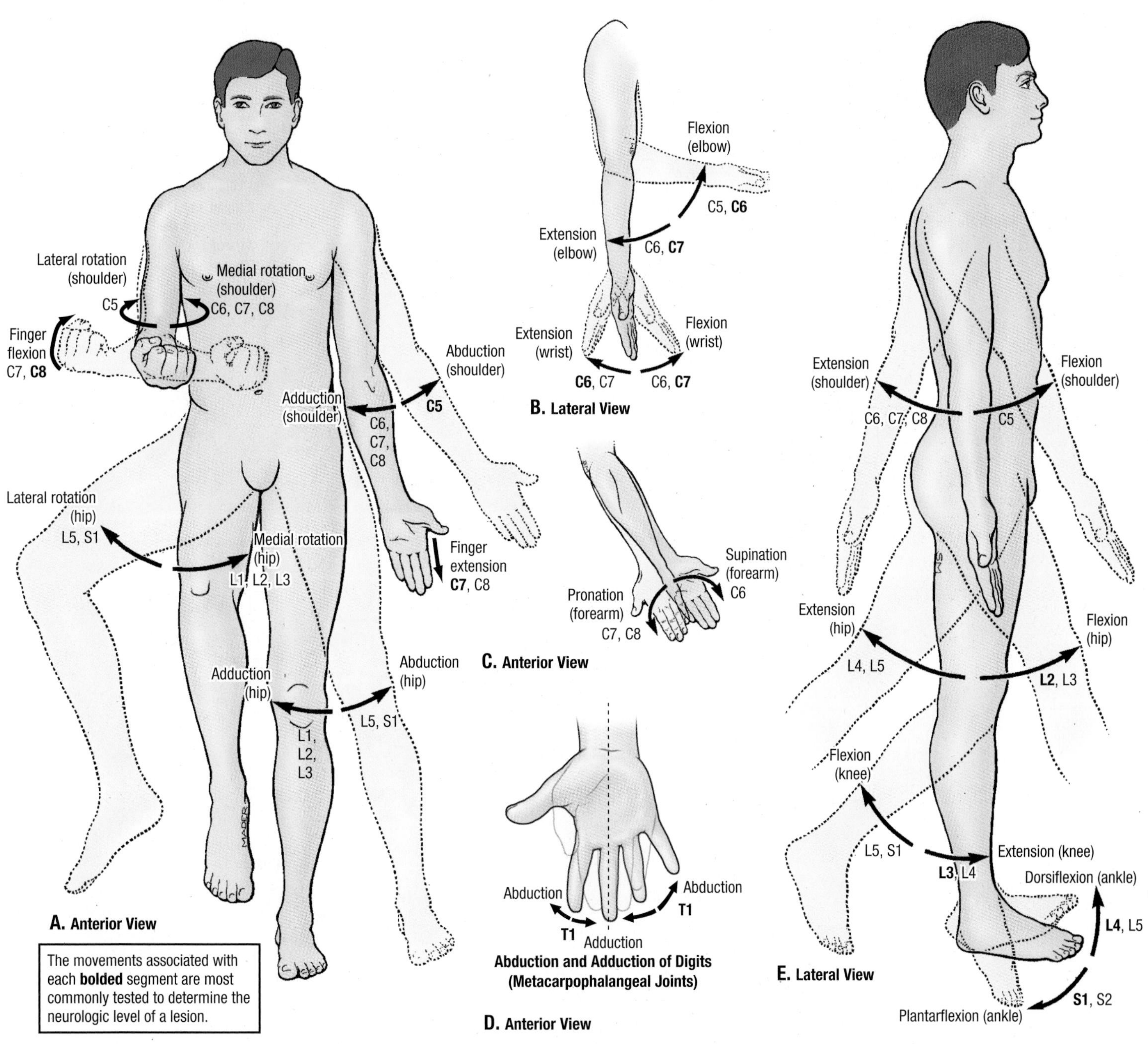
Lateral rotation
(shoulder)
C5
Medial rotation
(shoulder)
C6, C7, C8
Finger
flexion
C7, **C8**
Abduction
(shoulder)
C5
Adduction
(shoulder)
C6,
C7,
C8
Lateral rotation
(hip)
L5, S1
Medial rotation
(hip)
L1, L2, L3
Finger
extension
C7, C8
Abduction
(hip)
Adduction
(hip)
L5, S1
L1,
L2,
L3
Flexion
(elbow)
C5, **C6**
Extension
(elbow)
C6, **C7**
Extension
(wrist)
Flexion
(wrist)
C6, C7
C6, **C7**
Supination
(forearm)
C6
Pronation
(forearm)
C7, C8
Abduction
Abduction
T1
T1
Adduction
Extension
(shoulder)
Flexion
(shoulder)
C6, C7, C8
C5
Extension
(hip)
Flexion
(hip)
L4, L5
L2, L3
Flexion
(knee)
L5, S1
Extension (knee)
L3, L4
Dorsiflexion (ankle)
L4, L5
S1, S2
Plantarflexion (ankle)
The movements associated with each **bolded** segment are most commonly tested to determine the neurologic level of a lesion.

A. **Anterior View**

B. **Lateral View**

C. **Anterior View**

Abduction and Adduction of Digits (Metacarpophalangeal Joints)

D. **Anterior View**

E. **Lateral View**

4.52 MYOTOMES

Somatic motor (general somatic efferent) fibers transmit impulses to skeletal (voluntary) muscles. The unilateral muscle mass receiving innervation from the somatic motor fibers conveyed by a single spinal nerve is a myotome. Each skeletal muscle is innervated by the somatic motor fibers of several spinal nerves; therefore, the muscle myotome will consist of several segments. The muscle myotomes have been grouped by joint movement to facilitate clinical testing. The intrinsic muscles of the hand constitute a single myotome—T1.

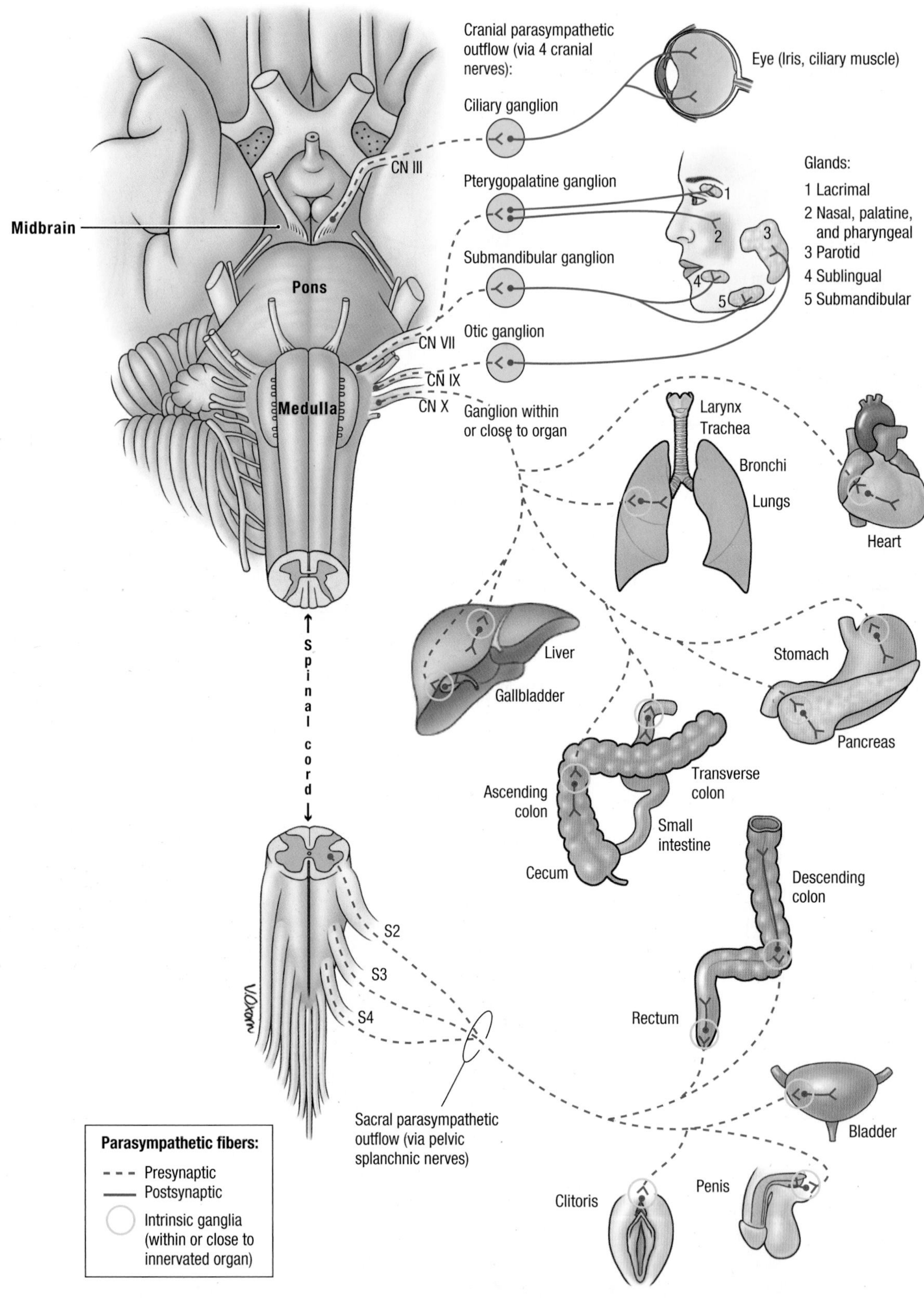
Cranial parasympathetic outflow (via 4 cranial nerves):
Eye (Iris, ciliary muscle)
Ciliary ganglion
CN III
Midbrain
Pterygopalatine ganglion
Glands:
1 Lacrimal
2 Nasal, palatine, and pharyngeal
3 Parotid
4 Sublingual
5 Submandibular
Submandibular ganglion
Pons
Otic ganglion
CN VII
CN IX
CN X
Medulla
Ganglion within or close to organ
Larynx
Trachea
Bronchi
Lungs
Heart
Spinal cord
Liver
Gallbladder
Stomach
Pancreas
Transverse colon
Ascending colon
Small intestine
Cecum
Descending colon
S2
S3
S4
Rectum
Bladder
Sacral parasympathetic outflow (via pelvic splanchnic nerves)
Parasympathetic fibers:
Presynaptic
Postsynaptic
Intrinsic ganglia (within or close to innervated organ)
Clitoris
Penis

4.53 DISTRIBUTION OF PARASYMPATHETIC NERVE FIBERS

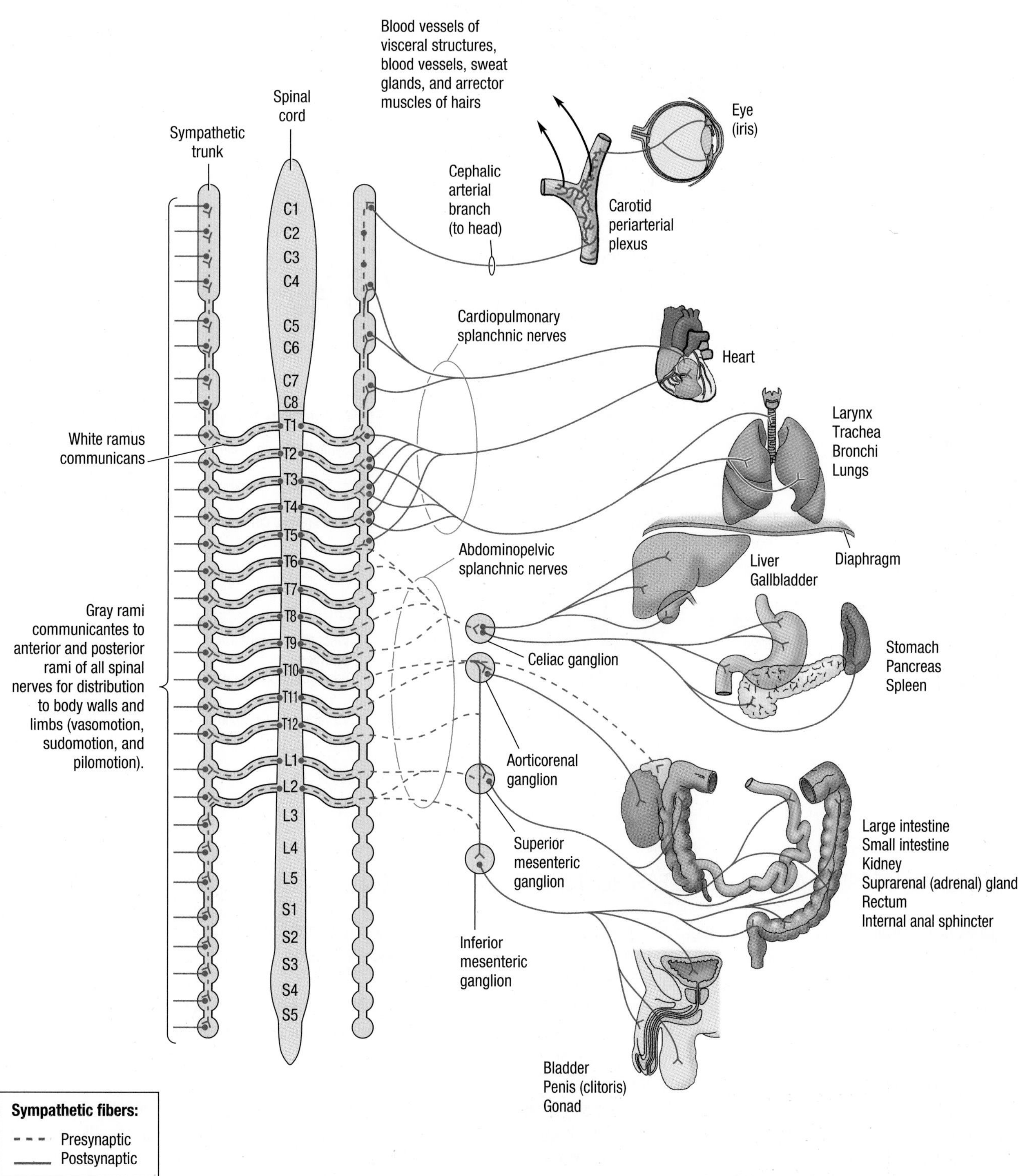
Blood vessels of visceral structures, blood vessels, sweat glands, and arrector muscles of hairs
Spinal cord
Sympathetic trunk
Eye (iris)
Cephalic arterial branch (to head)
Carotid periarterial plexus
C1
C2
C3
C4
C5
C6
C7
C8
T1
T2
T3
T4
T5
T6
T7
T8
T9
T10
T11
T12
L1
L2
L3
L4
L5
S1
S2
S3
S4
S5
Cardiopulmonary splanchnic nerves
Heart
White ramus communicans
Larynx
Trachea
Bronchi
Lungs
Diaphragm
Abdominopelvic splanchnic nerves
Liver
Gallbladder
Gray rami communicantes to anterior and posterior rami of all spinal nerves for distribution to body walls and limbs (vasomotion, sudomotion, and pilomotion).
Celiac ganglion
Stomach
Pancreas
Spleen
Aorticorenal ganglion
Superior mesenteric ganglion
Large intestine
Small intestine
Kidney
Suprarenal (adrenal) gland
Rectum
Internal anal sphincter
Inferior mesenteric ganglion
Bladder
Penis (clitoris)
Gonad
Sympathetic fibers:
Presynaptic
Postsynaptic

4.54 DISTRIBUTION OF SYMPATHETIC NERVE FIBERS

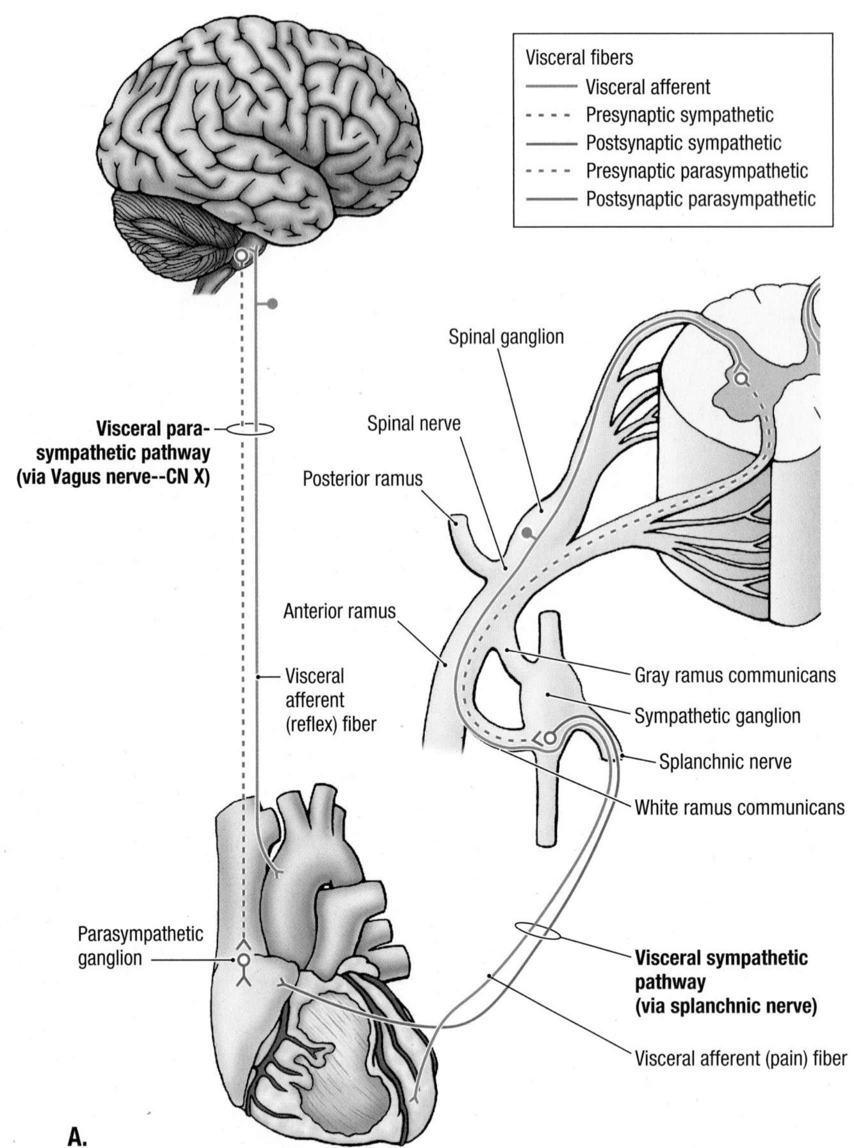
Visceral fibers
Visceral afferent
Presynaptic sympathetic
Postsynaptic sympathetic
Presynaptic parasympathetic
Postsynaptic parasympathetic
Spinal ganglion
Spinal nerve
Posterior ramus
Visceral para-sympathetic pathway (via Vagus nerve--CN X)
Anterior ramus
Visceral afferent (reflex) fiber
Gray ramus communicans
Sympathetic ganglion
Splanchnic nerve
White ramus communicans
Parasympathetic ganglion
Visceral sympathetic pathway (via splanchnic nerve)
Visceral afferent (pain) fiber
A.

4.55 VISCERAL AFFERENT AND VISCERAL EFFERENT (MOTOR) INNERVATION

A. Schematic illustration. Visceral afferent fibers have important relationships to the CNS, both anatomically and functionally. We are usually unaware of the sensory input of these fibers, which provides information about the condition of the body's internal environment. This information is integrated in the CNS, often triggering visceral or somatic reflexes or both. Visceral reflexes regulate blood pressure and chemistry by altering such functions as heart and respiratory rates and vascular resistance. Visceral sensation that reaches a conscious level is generally categorized as pain that is usually poorly localized and may be perceived as hunger or nausea. However, adequate stimulation may elicit true pain. Most visceral/reflex (unconscious) sensation and some pain travel in visceral afferent fibers that accompany the parasympathetic fibers retrograde. Most visceral pain impulses (from the heart and most organs of the peritoneal cavity) travel along visceral afferent fibers accompanying sympathetic fibers.

Visceral efferent (motor) innervation. The efferent nerve fibers and ganglia of the ANS are organized into two systems or divisions.

1. Sympathetic (thoracolumbar) division. In general, the effects of sympathetic stimulation are catabolic (preparing the body for "flight or fight").
2. Parasympathetic (craniosacral) division. In general, the effects of parasympathetic stimulation are anabolic (promoting normal function and conserving energy).

Conduction of impulses from the CNS to the effector organ involves a series of two neurons in both sympathetic and parasympathetic systems. The cell body of the presynaptic (preganglionic) neuron (first neuron) is located in the gray matter of the CNS. Its fiber (axon) synapses on the cell body of a postsynaptic (postganglionic) neuron, the second neuron in the series. The cell bodies of such second neurons are located in autonomic ganglia outside the CNS, and the postsynaptic fibers terminate on the effector organ (smooth muscle, modified cardiac muscle, or glands).

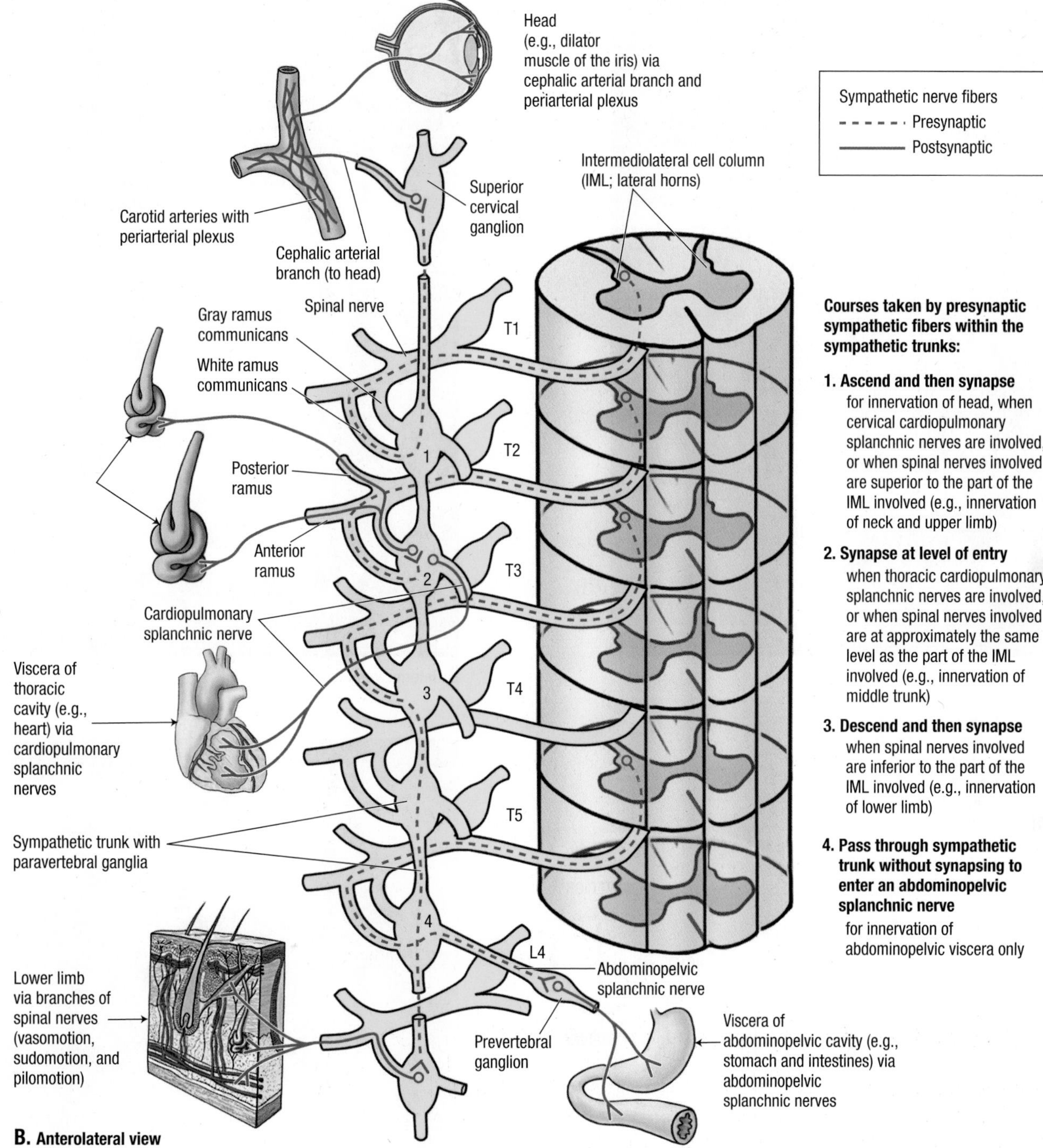
Head
(e.g., dilator
muscle of the iris) via
cephalic arterial branch and
periarterial plexus
Sympathetic nerve fibers
Presynaptic
Postsynaptic
Intermediolateral cell column
(IML; lateral horns)
Superior
cervical
ganglion
Carotid arteries with
periarterial plexus
Cephalic arterial
branch (to head)
Spinal nerve
Gray ramus
communicans
White ramus
communicans
T1
T2
T3
T4
T5
L4
1
2
3
4
Posterior
ramus
Anterior
ramus
Cardiopulmonary
splanchnic nerve
Viscera of
thoracic
cavity (e.g.,
heart) via
cardiopulmonary
splanchnic
nerves
Sympathetic trunk with
paravertebral ganglia
Lower limb
via branches of
spinal nerves
(vasomotion,
sudomotion, and
pilomotion)
Abdominopelvic
splanchnic nerve
Prevertebral
ganglion
Viscera of
abdominopelvic cavity (e.g.,
stomach and intestines) via
abdominopelvic
splanchnic nerves
Courses taken by presynaptic
sympathetic fibers within the
sympathetic trunks:
1. Ascend and then synapse
for innervation of head, when
cervical cardiopulmonary
splanchnic nerves are involved,
or when spinal nerves involved
are superior to the part of the
IML involved (e.g., innervation
of neck and upper limb)
2. Synapse at level of entry
when thoracic cardiopulmonary
splanchnic nerves are involved,
or when spinal nerves involved
are at approximately the same
level as the part of the IML
involved (e.g., innervation of
middle trunk)
3. Descend and then synapse
when spinal nerves involved
are inferior to the part of the
IML involved (e.g., innervation
of lower limb)
4. Pass through sympathetic
trunk without synapsing to
enter an abdominopelvic
splanchnic nerve
for innervation of
abdominopelvic viscera only

B. Anterolateral view

4.55 VISCERAL AFFERENT AND VISCERAL EFFERENT (MOTOR) INNERVATION (*CONTINUED*)

B. Courses taken by sympathetic motor fibers. Presynaptic fibers all follow the same course until they reach the sympathetic trunks. In the sympathetic trunks, they follow one of four possible courses. Fibers involved in providing sympathetic innervation to the body wall and limbs or viscera above the level of the diaphragm follow paths 1 to 3. They synapse in the paravertebral ganglia of the sympathetic trunks. Fibers involved in innervating abdominopelvic viscera follow path 4 to prevertebral ganglion via abdominopelvic splanchnic nerves. Postsynaptic fibers usually don't ascend or descend within the sympathetic trunks, exiting at the level of synapse.

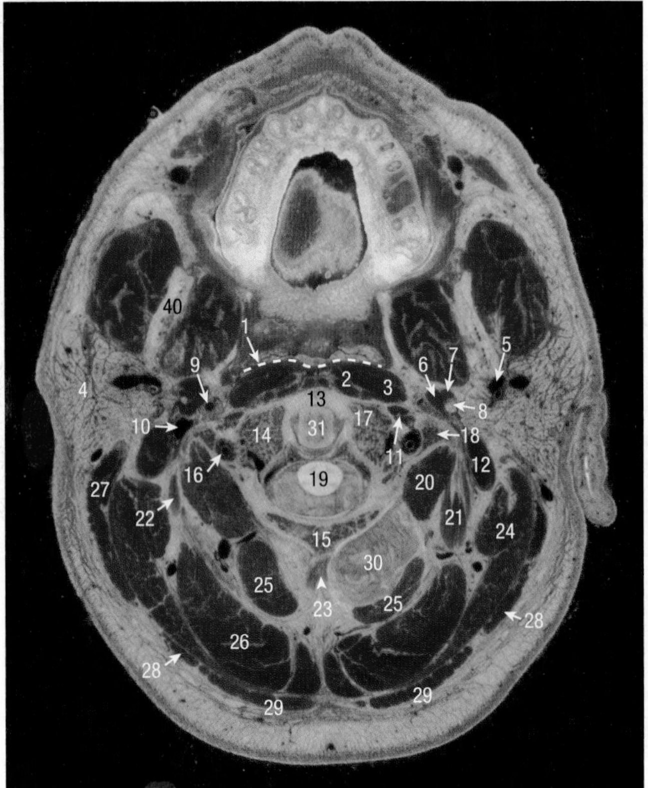
40
1
9
2
3
6
7
5
4
13
8
10
14
31
17
18
11
12
16
19
20
27
22
21
24
15
30
25
23
25
28
26
28
29
29

A. Inferior View

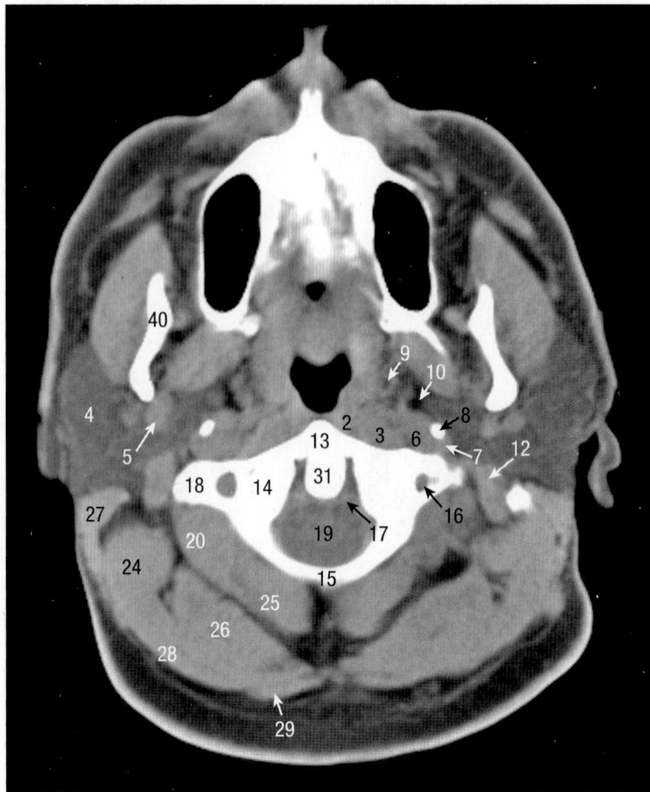
40
9
10
4
2
8
13
3
6
5
7
12
31
18
14
16
17
27
19
20
24
15
25
26
28
29

B. Inferior View

1	Site of retropharyngeal space
2	Longus colli
3	Longus capitis
4	Parotid gland
5	Retromandibular vein
6	Stylopharyngeus
7	Styloglossus
8	Stylohyoid muscle and ligament/process
9	Internal carotid artery
10	Internal jugular vein
11	Rectus capitis lateralis
12	Posterior belly of digastric
13	Anterior arch of atlas (C1 vertebra)
14	Lateral mass of atlas (C1)
15	Posterior arch of atlas (C1)
16	Vertebral artery
17	Transverse ligament of atlas (C1)
18	Transverse process of atlas (C1)
19	Spinal cord
20	Rectus capitis posterior major
21	Obliquus capitis inferior
22	Obliquus capitis superior
23	Spinous process of atlas (C1)
24	Longissimus capitis
25	Rectus capitis posterior minor
26	Semispinalis capitis
27	Sternocleidomastoid
28	Splenius capitis
29	Trapezius
30	Fatty mass
31	Dens of axis (C2 vertebra)
32	Anterior tubercle of atlas (C1)
33	Inferior articular facet of atlas (C1)
34	Foramen magnum
35	Foramen transversarium
36	Posterior tubercle of atlas (C1)
37	Mastoid process
38	Occipital bone of skull
39	External occipital protuberance
40	Ramus of mandible

ANTERIOR

RIGHT LEFT

POSTERIOR

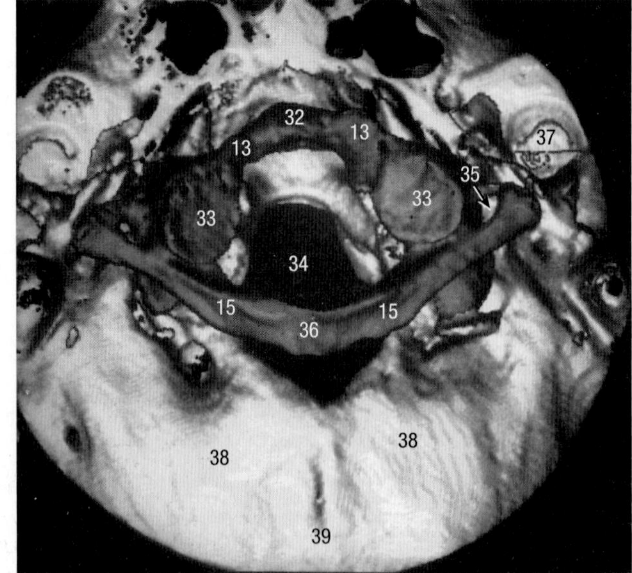
32
13
13
37
35
33
33
34
15
15
36
38
38
39

C. Postero-inferior View

4.56 IMAGING OF SUPERIOR NUCHAL REGION AT LEVEL OF ATLAS

A. Transverse section of specimen. **B.** Transverse computed tomographic (CT) scan. **C.** Three-dimensional (3D) CT of the base of the skull and atlas.

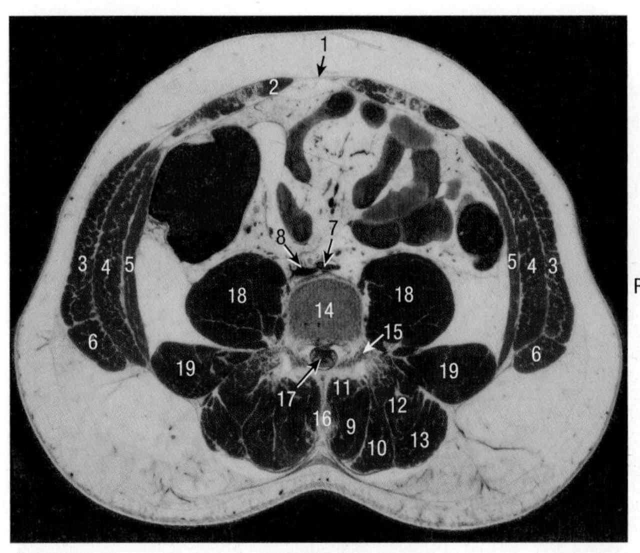

A. Inferior View

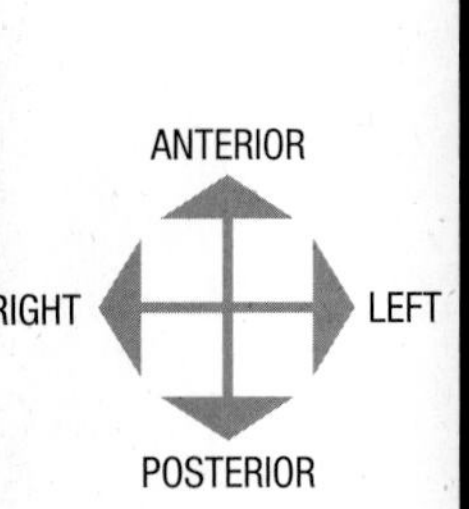
ANTERIOR
RIGHT
LEFT
POSTERIOR

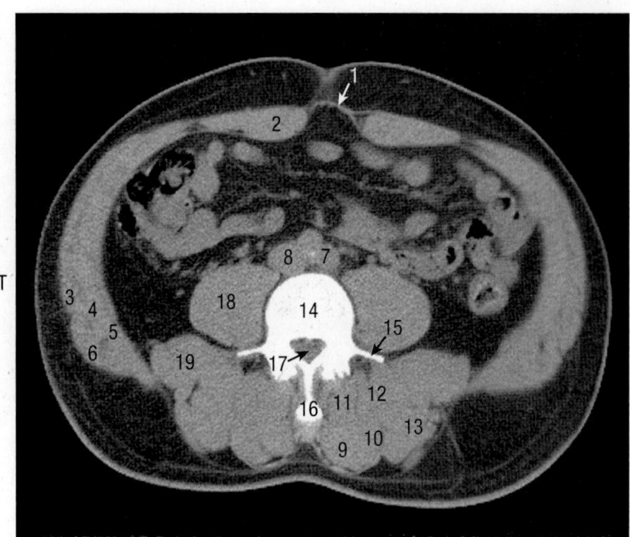

B. Inferior View

1	Linea alba	6	Latissimus dorsi	11	Multifidus	16	Spinous process		
2	Rectus abdominis	7	Descending aorta	12	Rotatores	17	Cauda equina		
3	External oblique	8	Inferior vena cava	13	Iliocostalis	18	Psoas major		
4	Internal oblique	9	Spinalis	14	4th lumbar vertebra	19	Quadratus lumborum		
5	Transversus abdominis	10	Longissimus	15	Transverse process				

4.57 IMAGING OF LUMBAR SPINE AT L4

A. Transverse section of specimen. **B.** Transverse computed tomographic (CT) scan.

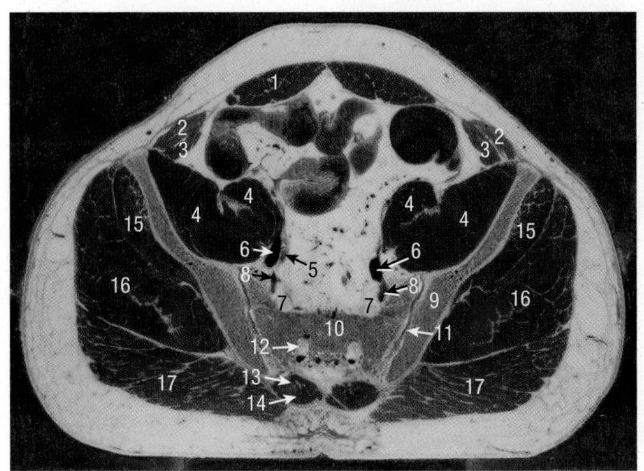

A. Inferior View

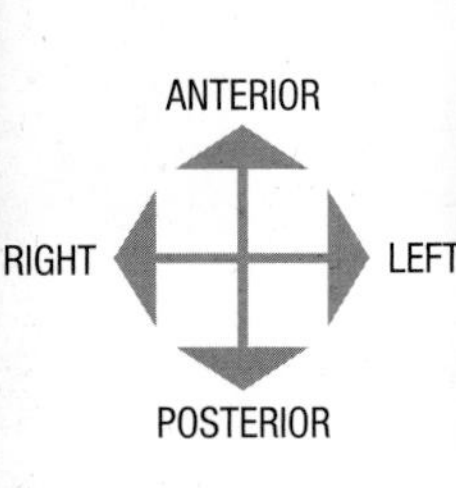
ANTERIOR
RIGHT
LEFT
POSTERIOR

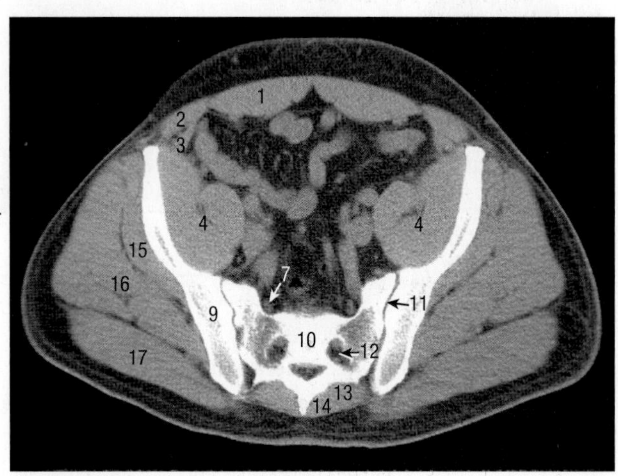

B. Inferior View

1	Rectus abdominis	6	Internal iliac vein	10	2nd sacral vertebra	14	Erector spinae
2	External oblique	7	Anterior rami	11	Sacro-iliac joint	15	Gluteus minimis
3	Internal oblique	8	Superior gluteal vessels	12	Sacral nerve root	16	Gluteus medius
4	Iliopsoas	9	Body of ilium	13	Multifidus	17	Gluteus maximus
5	Internal iliac artery						

4.58 IMAGING OF SACRO-ILIAC JOINT

A. Transverse section of specimen. **B.** Transverse computed tomographic (CT) scan.

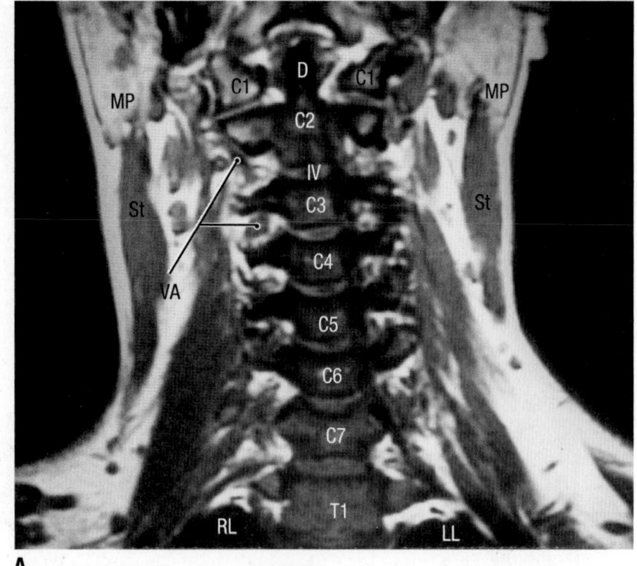
D
C1
C1
MP
MP
C2
IV
C3
St
St
C4
VA
C5
C6
C7
T1
RL
LL
A.

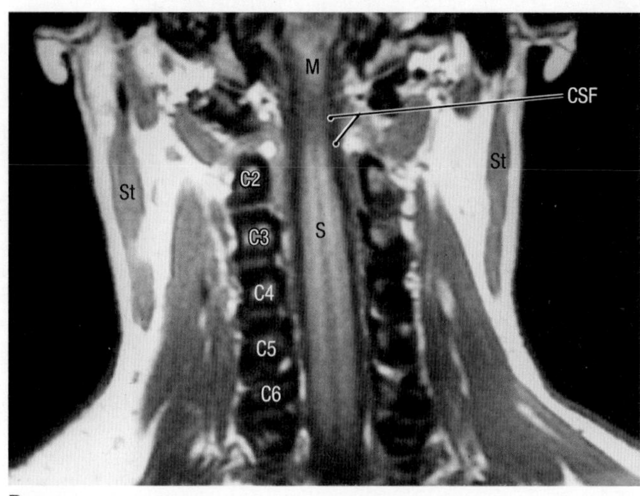
M
CSF
St
St
C2
C3
S
C4
C5
C6
B.

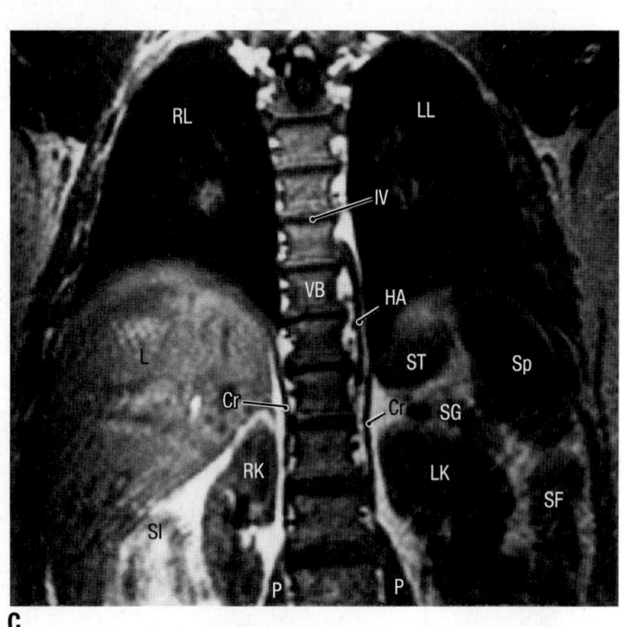
RL
LL
IV
VB
HA
L
ST
Sp
Cr
Cr
SG
RK
LK
SF
SI
P
P
C.

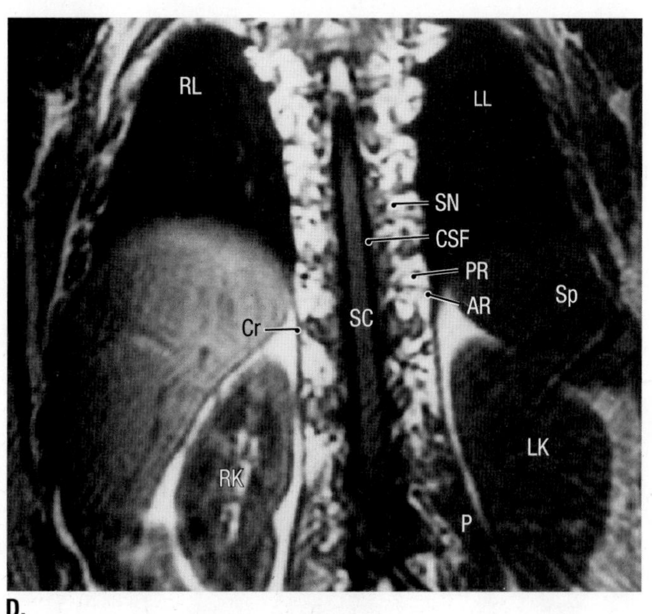
RL
LL
SN
CSF
PR
AR
Sp
Cr
SC
LK
RK
P
D.

AR Anterior ramus	LL Left lung	SG Suprarenal gland
C1-T1 Vertebrae	M Medulla oblongata	SI Small intestine
Cr Crus of diaphragm	MP Mastoid process	SN Spinal nerve
CSF Cerebrospinal fluid in subarachnoid space	P Psoas muscle	Sp Spleen
D Dens (odontoid) process of C2	PR Posterior ramus	St Sternocleidomastoid
HA Hemi-azygos vein	RK Right kidney	ST Stomach
IV Intervertebral disc	RL Right lung	VA Vertebral artery
L Liver	S Spinal cord	
LK Left kidney	SF Splenic flexure	

4.59 CORONAL MRI SCANS OF CERVICAL AND THORACIC SPINE

A. and **B.** Cervical spine. **C.** and **D.** Thoracic spine.

CHAPTER 5

Lower Limb

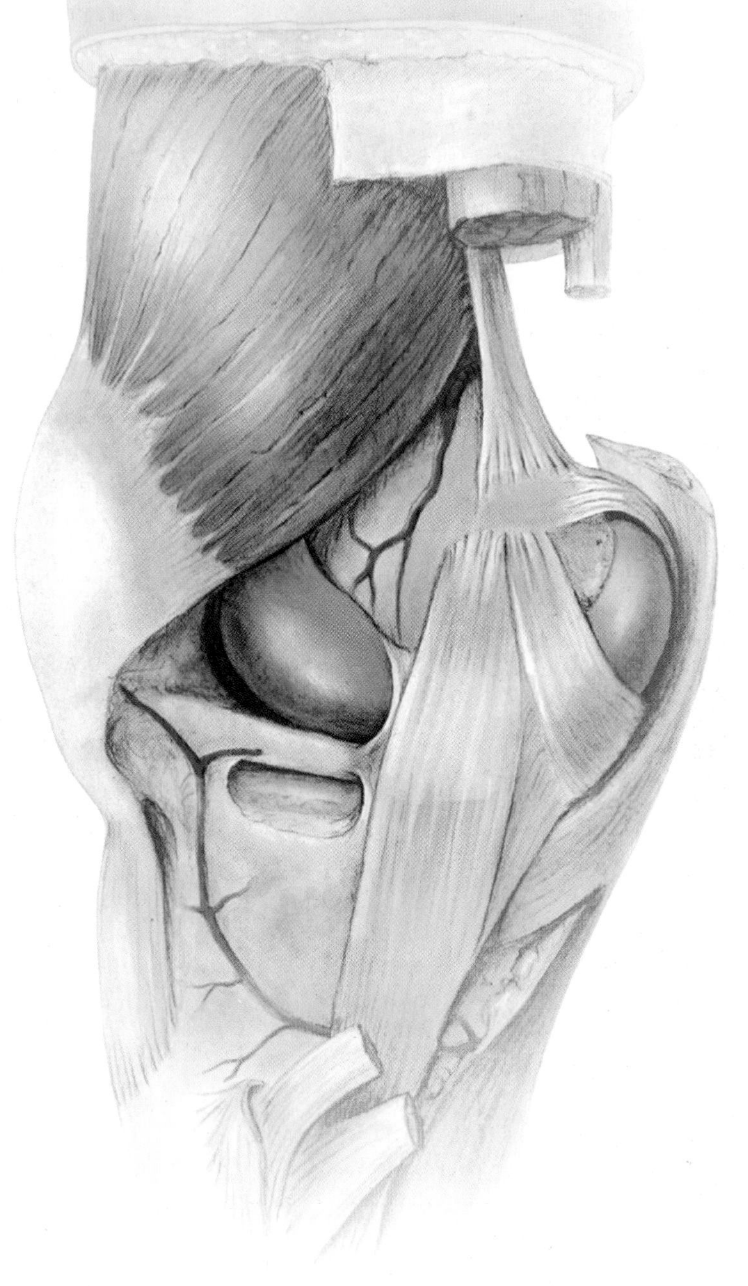

Systemic Overview of Lower Limb	358
Bones	358
Nerves	362
Blood Vessels	370
Lymphatics	374
Musculofascial Compartments	376
Retro-Inguinal Passage and Femoral Triangle	378
Anterior and Medial Compartments of Thigh	382
Lateral Thigh	389
Bones and Muscle Attachments of Thigh	390
Gluteal Region and Posterior Compartment of Thigh	392
Hip Joint	402
Knee Region	410
Knee Joint	416
Anterior and Lateral Compartments of Leg, Dorsum of Foot	430
Posterior Compartment of Leg	440
Tibiofibular Joints	450
Sole of Foot	451
Ankle, Subtalar, and Foot Joints	456
Arches of Foot	474
Bony Anomalies	475
Imaging and Sectional Anatomy	476

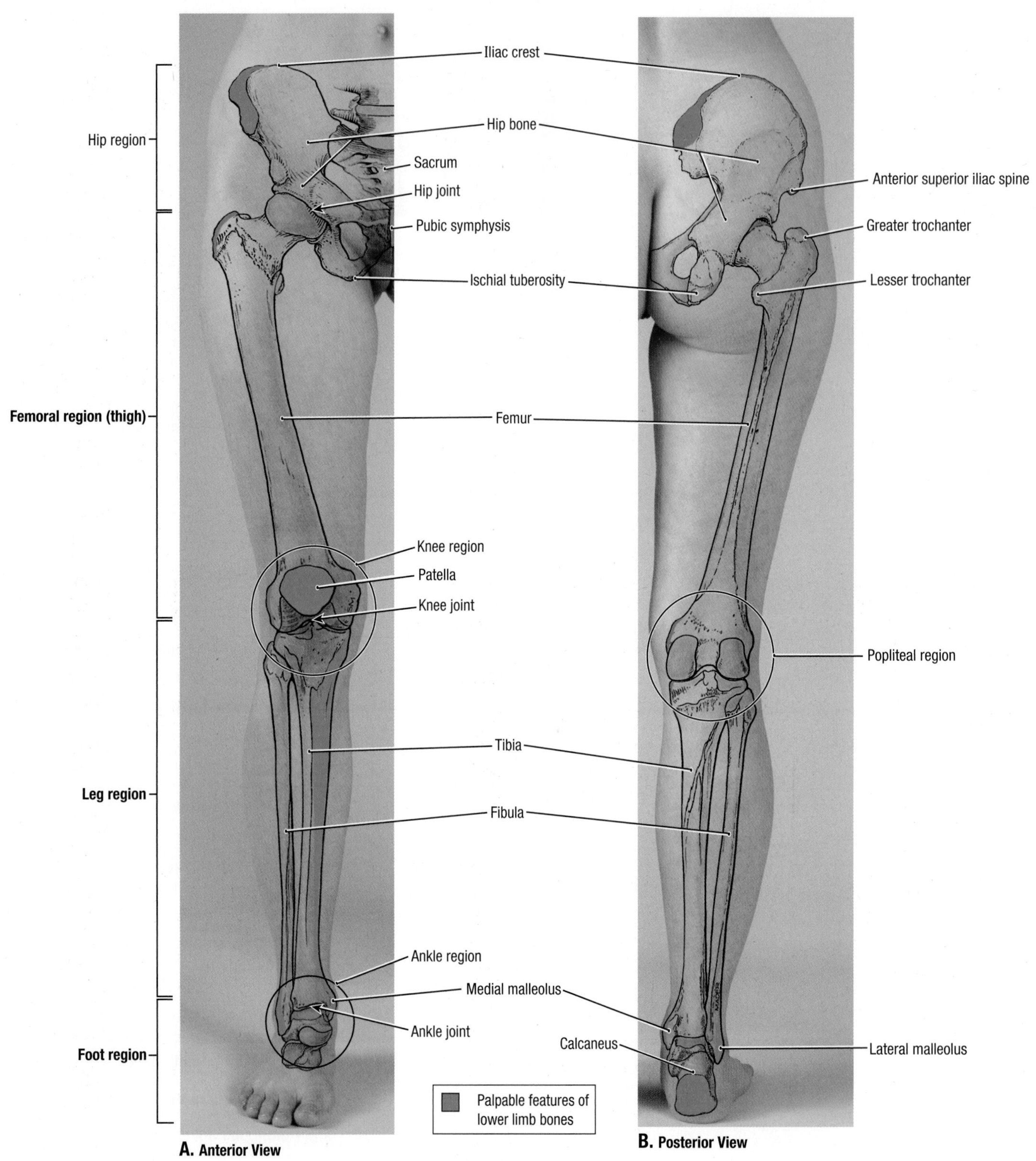
Hip region
Femoral region (thigh)
Leg region
Foot region
Iliac crest
Hip bone
Sacrum
Hip joint
Pubic symphysis
Ischial tuberosity
Femur
Knee region
Patella
Knee joint
Tibia
Fibula
Ankle region
Medial malleolus
Ankle joint
Anterior superior iliac spine
Greater trochanter
Lesser trochanter
Popliteal region
Calcaneus
Lateral malleolus
Palpable features of lower limb bones
A. Anterior View
B. Posterior View

5.1 REGIONS, BONES, AND MAJOR JOINTS OF LOWER LIMB

The hip bones meet anteriorly at the pubic symphysis and articulate with the sacrum posteriorly. The femur articulates with the hip bone proximally and the tibia distally. The tibia and fibula are the bones of the leg that join the foot at the ankle.

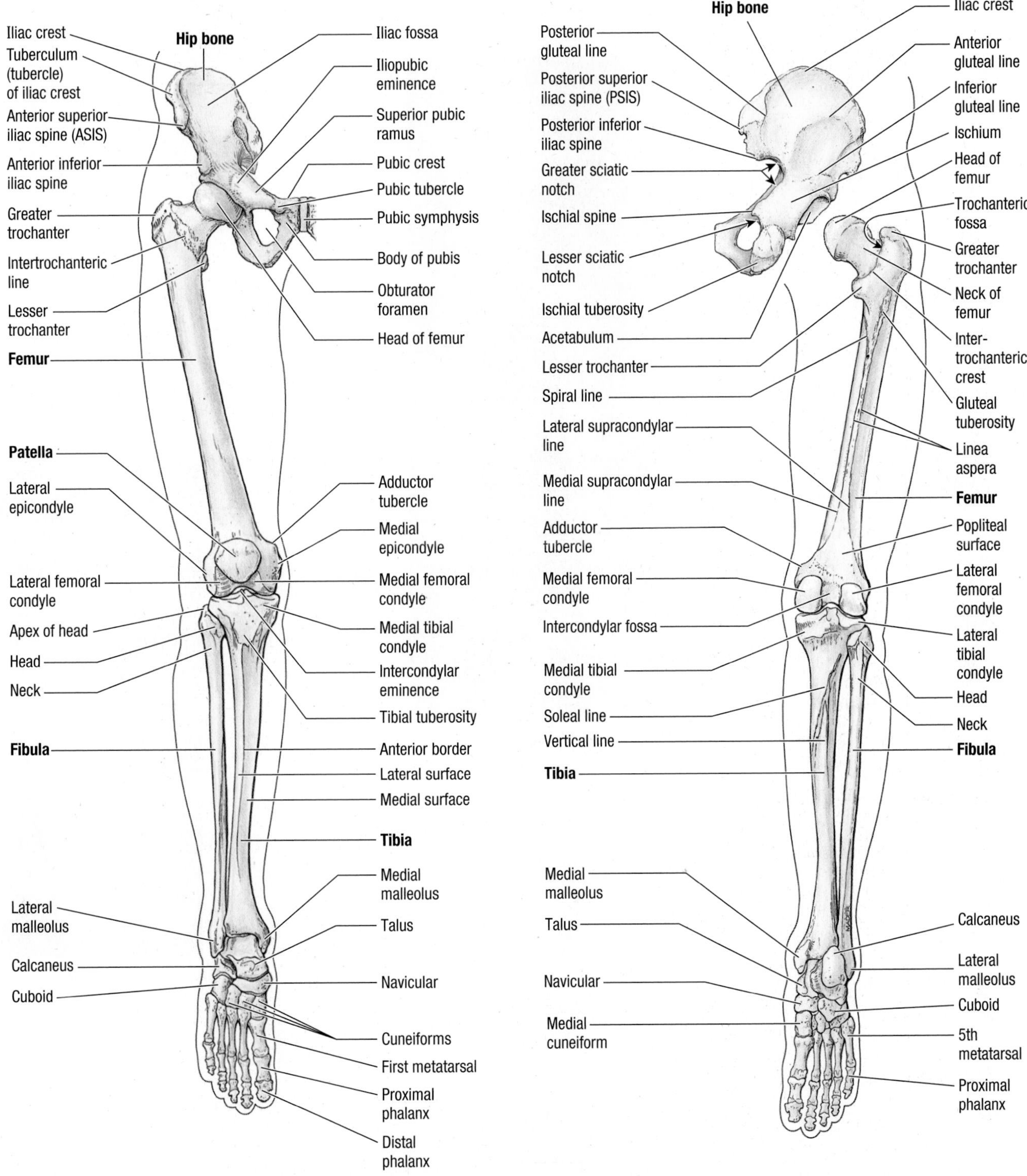
Hip bone
Iliac crest
Tuberculum (tubercle) of iliac crest
Anterior superior iliac spine (ASIS)
Anterior inferior iliac spine
Greater trochanter
Intertrochanteric line
Lesser trochanter
Femur
Patella
Lateral epicondyle
Lateral femoral condyle
Apex of head
Head
Neck
Fibula
Lateral malleolus
Calcaneus
Cuboid
Iliac fossa
Iliopubic eminence
Superior pubic ramus
Pubic crest
Pubic tubercle
Pubic symphysis
Body of pubis
Obturator foramen
Head of femur
Adductor tubercle
Medial epicondyle
Medial femoral condyle
Medial tibial condyle
Intercondylar eminence
Tibial tuberosity
Anterior border
Lateral surface
Medial surface
Tibia
Medial malleolus
Talus
Navicular
Cuneiforms
First metatarsal
Proximal phalanx
Distal phalanx
A. Anterior View
Hip bone
Posterior gluteal line
Posterior superior iliac spine (PSIS)
Posterior inferior iliac spine
Greater sciatic notch
Ischial spine
Lesser sciatic notch
Ischial tuberosity
Acetabulum
Lesser trochanter
Spiral line
Lateral supracondylar line
Medial supracondylar line
Adductor tubercle
Medial femoral condyle
Intercondylar fossa
Medial tibial condyle
Soleal line
Vertical line
Tibia
Medial malleolus
Talus
Navicular
Medial cuneiform
Iliac crest
Anterior gluteal line
Inferior gluteal line
Ischium
Head of femur
Trochanteric fossa
Greater trochanter
Neck of femur
Inter-trochanteric crest
Gluteal tuberosity
Linea aspera
Femur
Popliteal surface
Lateral femoral condyle
Lateral tibial condyle
Head
Neck
Fibula
Calcaneus
Lateral malleolus
Cuboid
5th metatarsal
Proximal phalanx
B. Posterior View

5.2 FEATURES OF BONES OF LOWER LIMB

The foot is in full plantar flexion. The hip joint is disarticulated in **B** to demonstrate the acetabulum of the hip bone and the entire head of the femur.

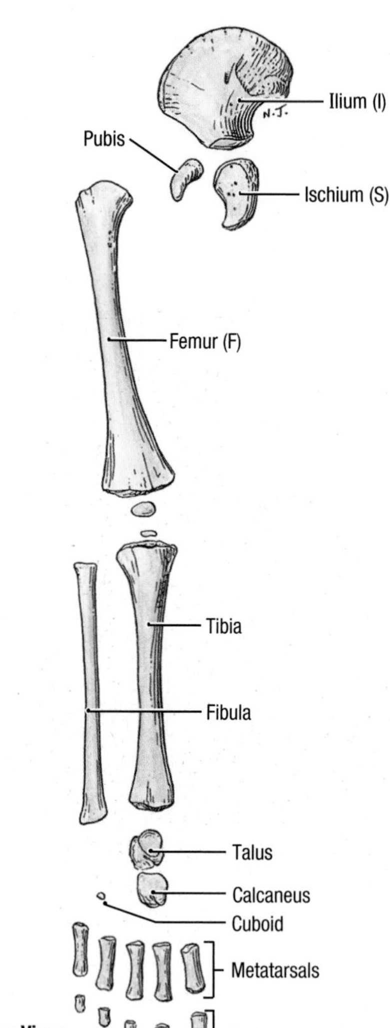
Ilium (I)
Pubis
Ischium (S)
Femur (F)
Tibia
Fibula
Talus
Calcaneus
Cuboid
Metatarsals
Phalanges
A. Anterior View

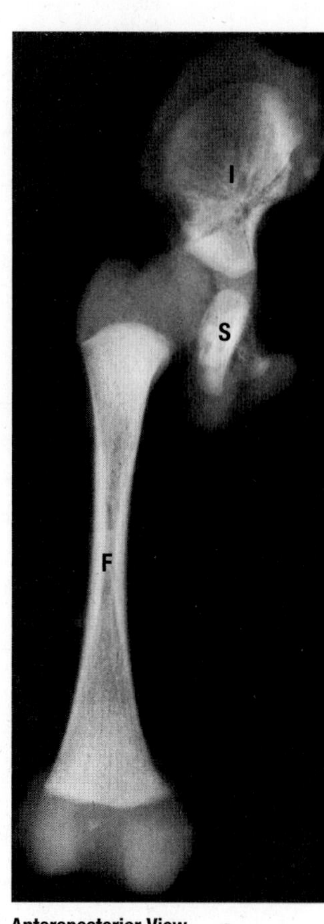
I
S
F
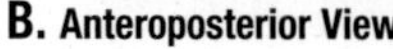
B. Anteroposterior View

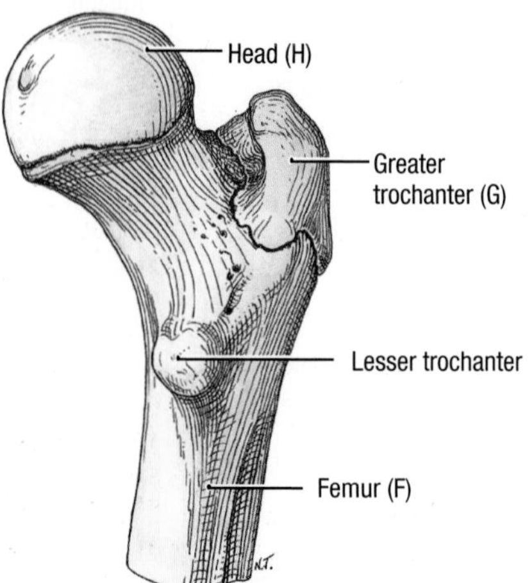
Head (H)
Greater trochanter (G)
Lesser trochanter
Femur (F)
C. Posterior View

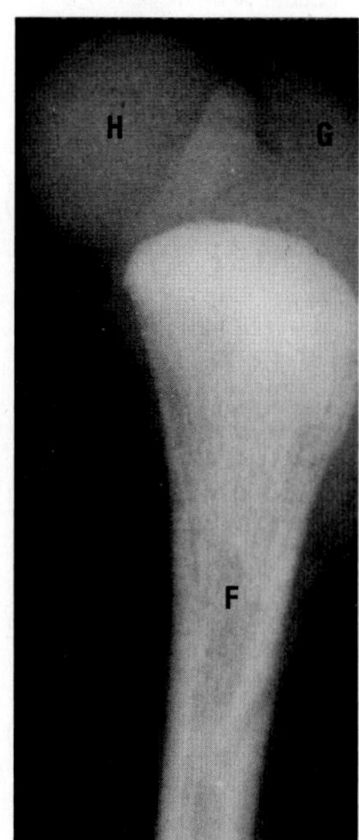
H
G
F
D. Anteroposterior View

5.3 POSTNATAL LOWER LIMB DEVELOPMENT

A. Bones of lower limb at birth. The hip bone can be divided into three primary parts: ilium, ischium, and pubis. The diaphyses (bodies) of the long bones are well ossified. Some epiphyses (growth plates) and tarsal bones have begun to ossify, including the distal epiphysis of the femur and proximal epiphysis of the tibia, calcaneus, talus, and cuboid. **B. and D.** Anteroposterior radiographs of postmortem specimens of newborns show the bony (*white*) and cartilaginous *(gray)* components of the femur and hip bone. **C.** Epiphyses at proximal end of femur. The epiphysis of the head of the femur begins to ossify during the 1st year, that of the greater trochanter before the 5th year, and that of the lesser trochanter before the 14th year. These usually fuse completely with the body (shaft) before the end of the 18th year.

Dislocated epiphysis of femoral head. In older children and adolescents (10 to 17 years of age), the epiphysis of the femoral head may slip away from the femoral neck because of weakness of the epiphyseal plate. This injury may be caused by acute trauma or repetitive microtraumas that place increased shearing stress on the epiphysis, especially with abduction and lateral rotation.

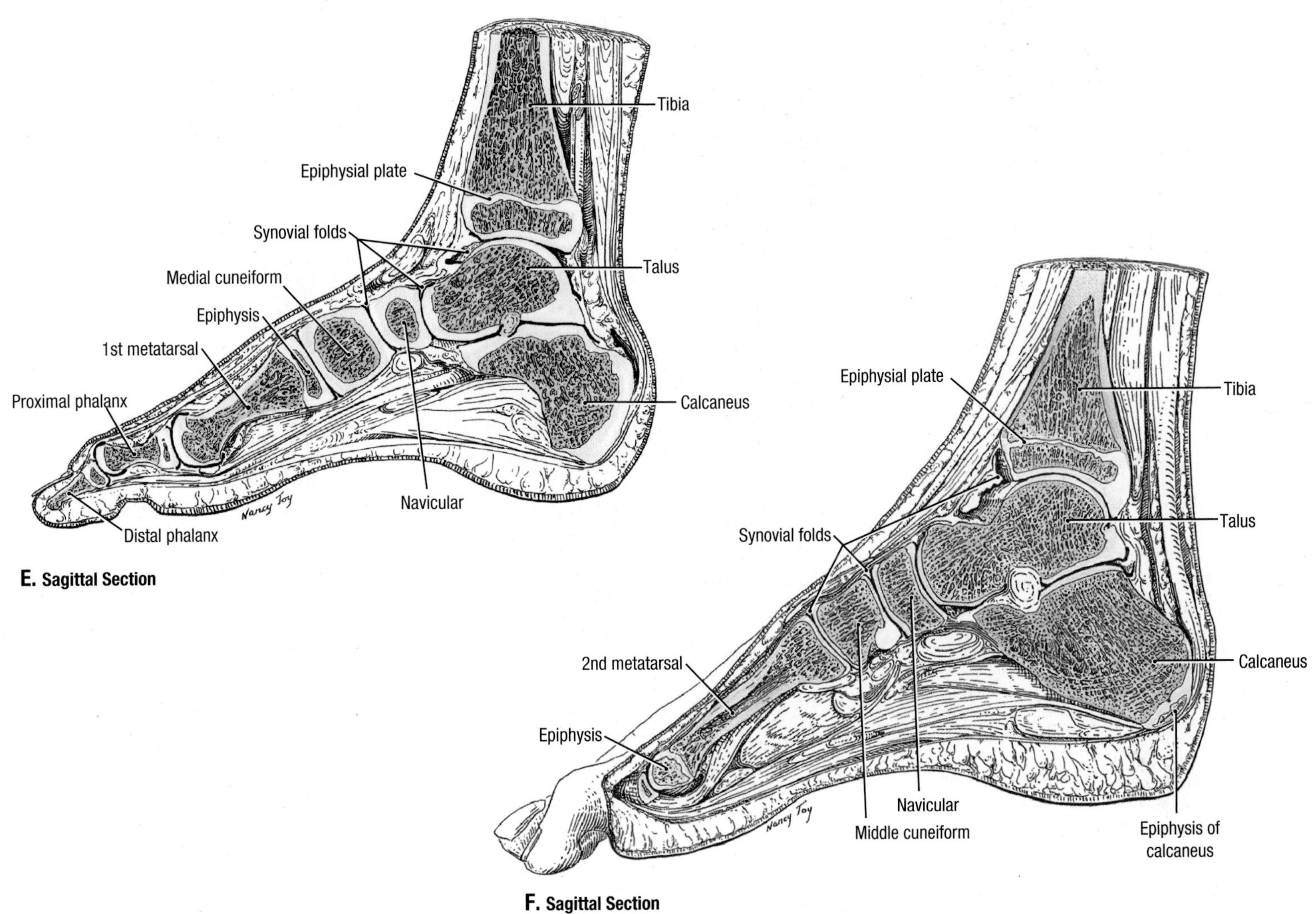
Tibia
Epiphysial plate
Synovial folds
Talus
Medial cuneiform
Epiphysis
1st metatarsal
Proximal phalanx
Calcaneus
Navicular
Distal phalanx
Epiphysial plate
Tibia
Synovial folds
Talus
2nd metatarsal
Calcaneus
Epiphysis
Navicular
Middle cuneiform
Epiphysis of calcaneus

E. **Sagittal Section**

F. **Sagittal Section**

5.3 POSTNATAL LOWER LIMB DEVELOPMENT (*CONTINUED*)

E. Foot of child age 4. **F.** Foot of child age 10.

- In the foot of the younger child **(E),** epiphyses of long bones (tibia, metatarsals, and phalanges) ossify like short bones, with the ossification centers being enveloped in cartilage. Ossification has already extended to the surface of the larger tarsal bones.
- In the foot of the older child **(F),** ossification has spread to the dorsal and plantar surfaces of all tarsal bones in view, and cartilage persists on the articular surfaces only.
- The traction epiphysis of the calcaneus for the calcaneal tendon and plantar aponeurosis begins to ossify from the ages of 6 to 10 years.
- The first metatarsal bone is similar to a phalanx in that its epiphysis is at the base instead of the head, as in the second and other metatarsal bones.
- The tuberosity of the calcaneus and the sesamoid bones of the first and the heads of the second to fifth metatarsals (here the second) support the longitudinal arch of the foot; the medial part of the longitudinal arch is higher and more mobile than the lateral.

Fractures involving epiphysial plates. The primary ossification center for the superior end of the tibia appears shortly after birth and joins the shaft of the tibia during adolescence (usually 16 to 18 years of age). Tibial fractures in children are more serious if they involve the epiphysial plates because continued normal growth of bone may be jeopardized. Disruption of the epiphysial plate at the tibial tuberosity may cause inflammation of the tuberosity and chronic recurring pain during adolescence (Osgood-Schlatter disease), especially in young athletes.

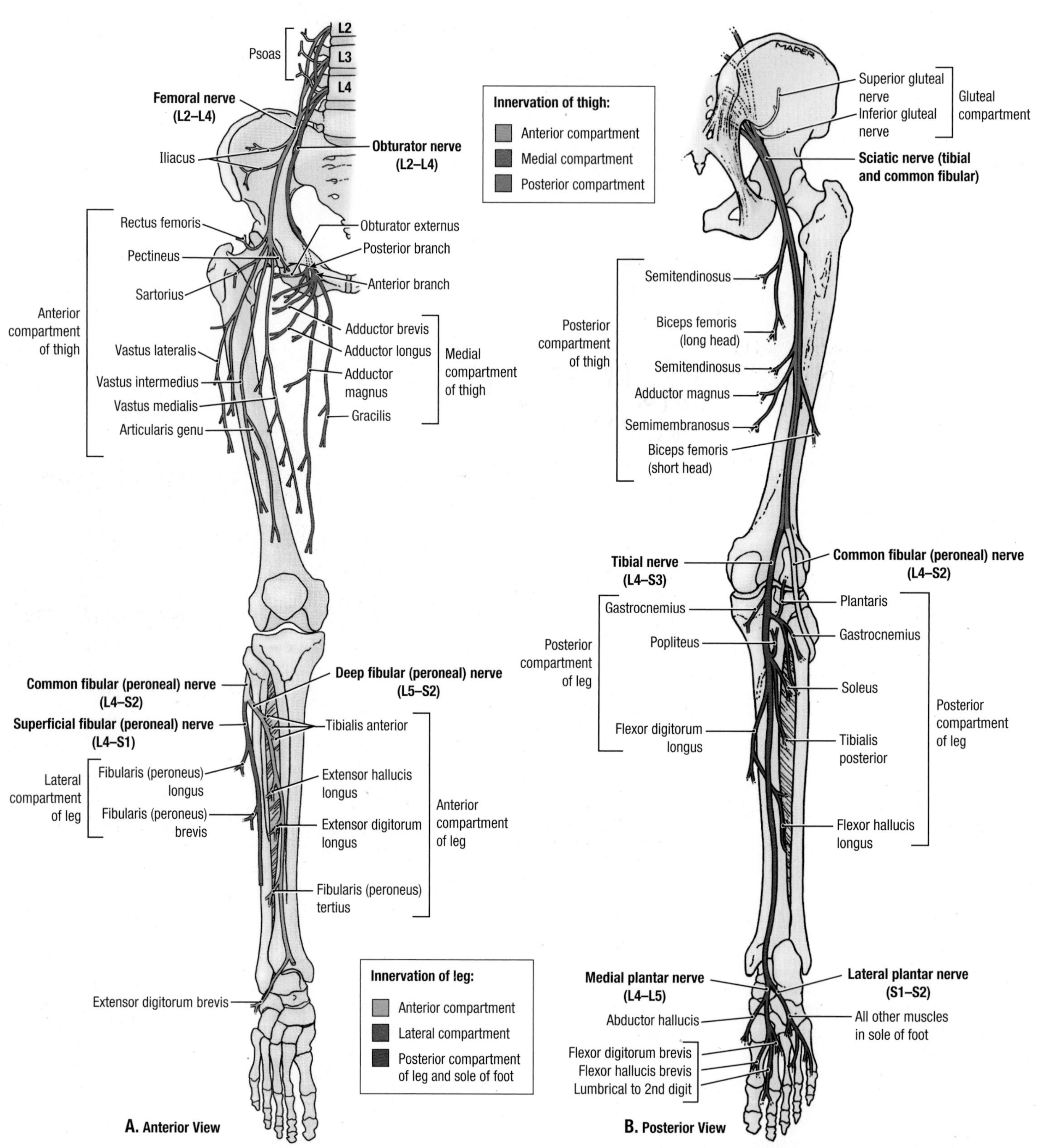
Psoas
L2
L3
L4
Femoral nerve (L2–L4)
Iliacus
Obturator nerve (L2–L4)
Innervation of thigh:
Anterior compartment
Medial compartment
Posterior compartment
Rectus femoris
Pectineus
Sartorius
Anterior compartment of thigh
Vastus lateralis
Vastus intermedius
Vastus medialis
Articularis genu
Obturator externus
Posterior branch
Anterior branch
Adductor brevis
Adductor longus
Adductor magnus
Gracilis
Medial compartment of thigh
Common fibular (peroneal) nerve (L4–S2)
Superficial fibular (peroneal) nerve (L4–S1)
Deep fibular (peroneal) nerve (L5–S2)
Tibialis anterior
Lateral compartment of leg
Fibularis (peroneus) longus
Fibularis (peroneus) brevis
Extensor hallucis longus
Extensor digitorum longus
Fibularis (peroneus) tertius
Anterior compartment of leg
Extensor digitorum brevis
Innervation of leg:
Anterior compartment
Lateral compartment
Posterior compartment of leg and sole of foot
Superior gluteal nerve
Inferior gluteal nerve
Gluteal compartment
Sciatic nerve (tibial and common fibular)
Semitendinosus
Biceps femoris (long head)
Semitendinosus
Adductor magnus
Semimembranosus
Biceps femoris (short head)
Posterior compartment of thigh
Tibial nerve (L4–S3)
Common fibular (peroneal) nerve (L4–S2)
Gastrocnemius
Popliteus
Flexor digitorum longus
Posterior compartment of leg
Plantaris
Gastrocnemius
Soleus
Tibialis posterior
Flexor hallucis longus
Posterior compartment of leg
Medial plantar nerve (L4–L5)
Lateral plantar nerve (S1–S2)
Abductor hallucis
All other muscles in sole of foot
Flexor digitorum brevis
Flexor hallucis brevis
Lumbrical to 2nd digit

A. Anterior View

B. Posterior View

5.4 OVERVIEW OF MOTOR INNERVATION OF LOWER LIMB

TABLE 5.1 MOTOR NERVES OF LOWER LIMB

Nerve	Origin	Course	Distribution
Femoral	Lumbar plexus (L2–L4)	Passes deep to midpoint of inguinal ligament, lateral to femoral vessels, dividing into muscular and cutaneous branches in femoral triangle	Anterior thigh muscles
Obturator		Traverses lesser pelvis to enter thigh via obturator foramen and then divides; its anterior branch descends between adductor longus and adductor brevis; its posterior branch descends between adductor brevis and adductor magnus	*Anterior branch:* adductor longus, adductor brevis, gracilis, and pectineus; *Posterior branch:* obturator externus and adductor magnus
Sciatic	Sacral plexus (L4–S3)	Enters gluteal region through greater sciatic foramen, usually passing inferior to piriformis, descends in posterior compartment of thigh, bifurcating at apex of popliteal fossa into tibial and common fibular (peroneal) nerves	Muscles of posterior thigh, leg and sole and dorsum of foot
Tibial	Sciatic nerve	Terminal branch of sciatic nerve arising at apex of popliteal fossa; descends through popliteal fossa with popliteal vessels, continuing in deep posterior compartment of leg with posterior tibial vessels; bifurcates into medial and lateral plantar nerves	Hamstring muscles of posterior compartment of thigh, muscles of posterior compartment of leg, and sole of foot
Common fibular (peroneal)		Terminal branch of sciatic nerve arising at apex of popliteal fossa; follows medial border of biceps femoris and its tendon to wind around neck of fibula deep to fibularis longus, where it bifurcates into superficial and deep fibular nerves	Short head of biceps femoris, muscles of anterior and lateral compartments of leg, and dorsum of foot
Superficial fibular (peroneal)	Common fibular nerve	Arises deep to fibularis longus on neck of fibula and descends in lateral compartment of the leg; pierces crural fascia in distal third of leg to become cutaneous	Muscles of lateral compartment of leg
Deep fibular (peroneal)		Arises deep to fibularis longus on neck of fibula; passes through extensor digitorum longus into anterior compartment, descending on interosseous membrane; crosses ankle joint and enters dorsum of foot	Muscles of anterior compartment of leg and dorsum of foot

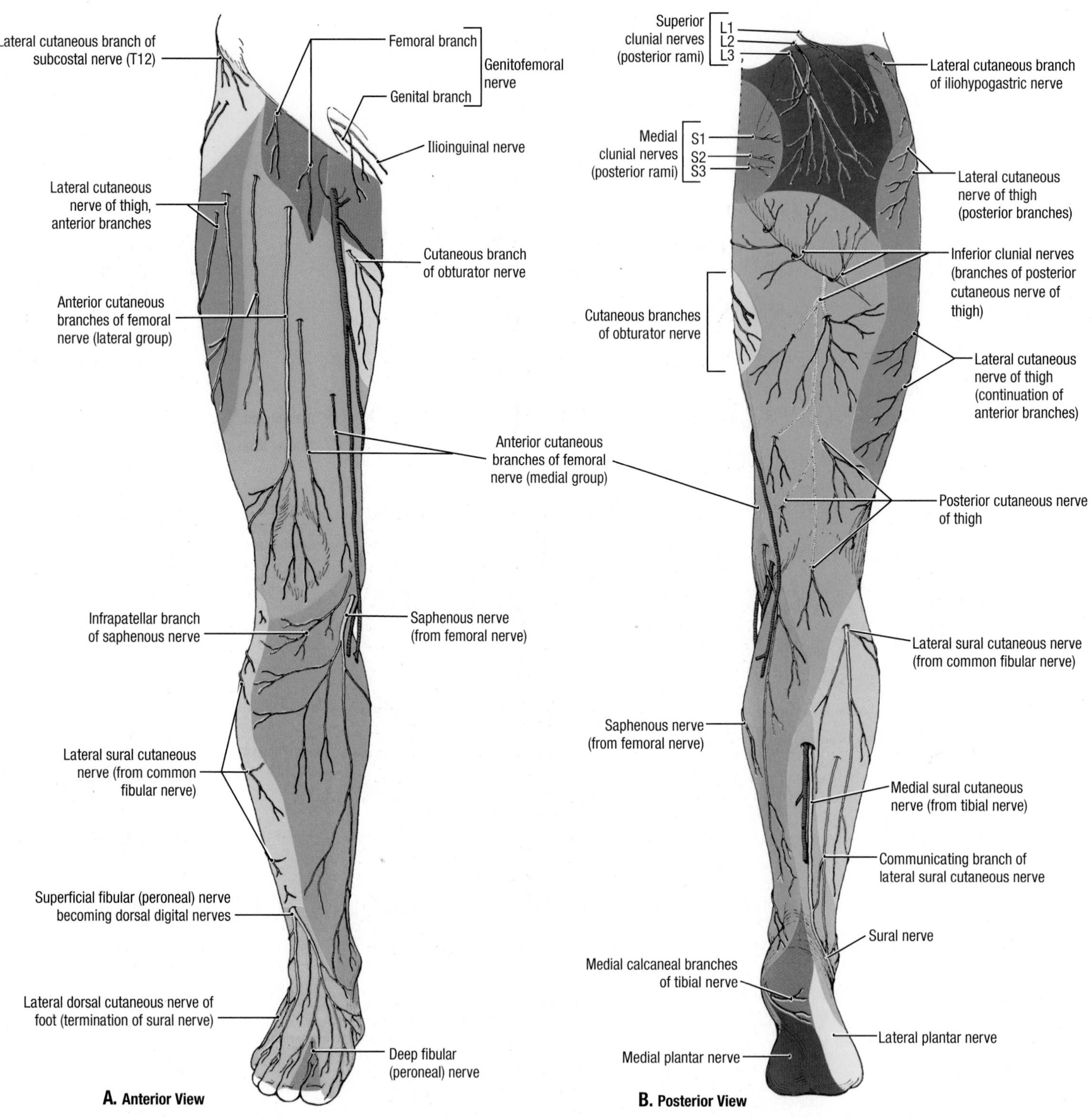
Lateral cutaneous branch of subcostal nerve (T12)
Femoral branch
Genital branch
Genitofemoral nerve
Ilioinguinal nerve
Lateral cutaneous nerve of thigh, anterior branches
Cutaneous branch of obturator nerve
Anterior cutaneous branches of femoral nerve (lateral group)
Anterior cutaneous branches of femoral nerve (medial group)
Infrapatellar branch of saphenous nerve
Saphenous nerve (from femoral nerve)
Lateral sural cutaneous nerve (from common fibular nerve)
Superficial fibular (peroneal) nerve becoming dorsal digital nerves
Lateral dorsal cutaneous nerve of foot (termination of sural nerve)
Deep fibular (peroneal) nerve
A. Anterior View
Superior clunial nerves (posterior rami)
L1
L2
L3
Lateral cutaneous branch of iliohypogastric nerve
Medial clunial nerves (posterior rami)
S1
S2
S3
Lateral cutaneous nerve of thigh (posterior branches)
Inferior clunial nerves (branches of posterior cutaneous nerve of thigh)
Cutaneous branches of obturator nerve
Lateral cutaneous nerve of thigh (continuation of anterior branches)
Posterior cutaneous nerve of thigh
Lateral sural cutaneous nerve (from common fibular nerve)
Saphenous nerve (from femoral nerve)
Medial sural cutaneous nerve (from tibial nerve)
Communicating branch of lateral sural cutaneous nerve
Sural nerve
Medial calcaneal branches of tibial nerve
Lateral plantar nerve
Medial plantar nerve
B. Posterior View

5.5 CUTANEOUS NERVES OF LOWER LIMB

Cutaneous nerves in the subcutaneous tissue supply the skin of the lower limb. The cutaneous innervation of the lower limb reflects both the original segmental innervation of the skin via separate spinal nerves in its dermatomal pattern (Fig. 5.8) and the result of plexus formation of segmental peripheral nerves. In **B,** the medial sural cutaneous nerve (*sural* is Latin for calf) is joined between the popliteal fossa and posterior aspect of the ankle by a communicating branch of the lateral sural cutaneous nerve to form the sural nerve. The level of the junction is variable and is low in this specimen.

TABLE 5.2 CUTANEOUS NERVES OF LOWER LIMB

Nerve	Origin (Contributing Spinal Nerves)	Course	Distribution to Skin of Lower Limb
Subcostal (lateral cutaneous branch)	T12 anterior ramus	Descends over iliac crest	Hip region inferior to anterior part of iliac crest and anterior to greater trochanter
Iliohypogastric	Lumbar plexus (L1; occasionally T12)	Parallels iliac crest	Lateral cutaneous branch supplies superolateral quadrant of buttock
Ilio-inguinal	Lumbar plexus (L1; occasionally T12)	Passes through inguinal canal	Inguinal fold; femoral branch supplies skin over medial femoral triangle
Genitofemoral	Lumbar plexus (L1–L2)	Descends anterior surface of psoas major	Femoral branch supplies skin over lateral part of femoral triangle; genital branch supplies anterior scrotumor labia majora
Lateral cutaneous nerve of thigh	Lumbar plexus (L2–L3)	Passes deep to inguinal ligament, 2–3 cm medial to anterior superior iliac spine	Skin on anterior and lateral aspects of thigh
Anterior cutaneous branches	Lumbar plexus via femoral nerve (L2–L4)	Arise in femoral triangle; pierce fascia lata along the path of sartorius muscle	Skin of anterior and medial aspects of thigh
Cutaneous branch of obturator nerve	Lumbar plexus via obturator nerve (L2–L4)	Following its descent between adductors longus and brevis, obturator nerve pierces fascia lata to reach the skin of thigh	Skin of middle part of medial thigh
Posterior cutaneous nerve of thigh	Sacral plexus (S1–S3)	Enters gluteal region via greater sciatic foramen deep to gluteus maximus; then descends deep to fascia lata; terminal branches pierce fascia lata	Supply skin of posterior thigh and popliteal fossa
Saphenous nerve	Lumbar plexus via femoral nerve (L3–L4)	Traverses adductor canal but does not pass through adductor hiatus	Skin on medial side of leg and foot
Superficial fibular nerve	Common fibular nerve (L4–S1)	After supplying fibular muscles, perforates deep fascia of leg	Skin of anterolateral leg and dorsum of foot
Deep fibular nerve	Common fibular nerve (L5)	After supplying muscles on dorsum of foot, pierces deep fascia superior to heads of 1st and 2nd metatarsals	Skin of web between great and 2nd toes
Sural nerve	Tibial and common fibular nerves (S1–S2)	Medial sural cutaneous branch of tibial nerve and lateral sural cutaneous branch of common fibular nerve merge at varying levels on posterior leg	Skin of posterolateral leg and lateral margin of foot
Medial plantar nerve	Tibial nerve (L4–L5)	Passes between first and second layers of plantar muscles	Skin of medial side of sole, and plantar aspect, sides, and nail beds of medial 3½ toes
Lateral plantar nerve	Tibial nerve (S1–S2)	Passes between first and second layers of plantar muscles	Skin of lateral sole, and plantar aspect, sides, and nail beds of lateral 1½ toes
Calcaneal nerves	Tibial and sural nerves (S1–S2)	Branches over calcaneal tuberosity	Skin of heel
Superior clunial nerves	L1–L3 posterior rami	Course laterally/inferiorly in subcutaneous tissue	Skin overlying superior and central parts of buttock
Medial clunial nerves	S1–S3 posterior rami	From dorsal sacral foramina; enter overlying subcutaneous tissue	Skin of medial buttock and intergluteal cleft
Inferior clunial nerves	Posterior cutaneous nerve of thigh (S2-S3)	Arise deep to gluteus maximus; emerge from beneath inferior border of muscle	Skin of inferior buttock (overlying gluteal fold)

TABLE 5.3 NERVE LESIONS

Nerve Injury	Injury Description	Impairments	Clinical Aspects
Femoral nerve	Trauma at femoral triangle Pelvic fracture	Flexion of thigh is weakened Extension of leg is lost Sensory loss on anterior thigh and medial leg	Loss of knee jerk reflex Anesthesia on anterior thigh
Obturator nerve	Anterior hip dislocation Radical retropubic prostatectomy	Adduction of thigh is lost Sensory loss on medial thigh	
Superior gluteal nerve	Surgery Posterior hip dislocation Poliomyelitis	Gluteus medius and minimus function is lost Ability to pull contralateral pelvis up to level and abduction of thigh are lost	Gluteus medius limp or "waddling gait" Positive Trendelenburg sign Contralateral
Inferior gluteal nerve	Surgery Posterior hip dislocation	Gluteus maximus function is lost Ability to rise from a seated position, climb stairs or incline, or jump is lost	Patient will lean the body trunk backward at heel strike
Common fibular nerve	Blow to lateral aspect of leg Fracture of neck of fibula	Eversion of foot is lost Dorsiflexion of foot is lost Extension of toes is lost Sensory loss on anterolateral leg and dorsum of foot	Patient will present with foot plantar flexed ("foot drop") and inverted Patient cannot stand on heels "Foot slap"
Tibial nerve at popliteal fossa	Trauma at popliteal fossa	Inversion of foot is weakened Plantar flexion of foot is lost Sensory loss on sole of foot	Patient will present with foot dorsiflexed and everted Patient cannot stand on toes

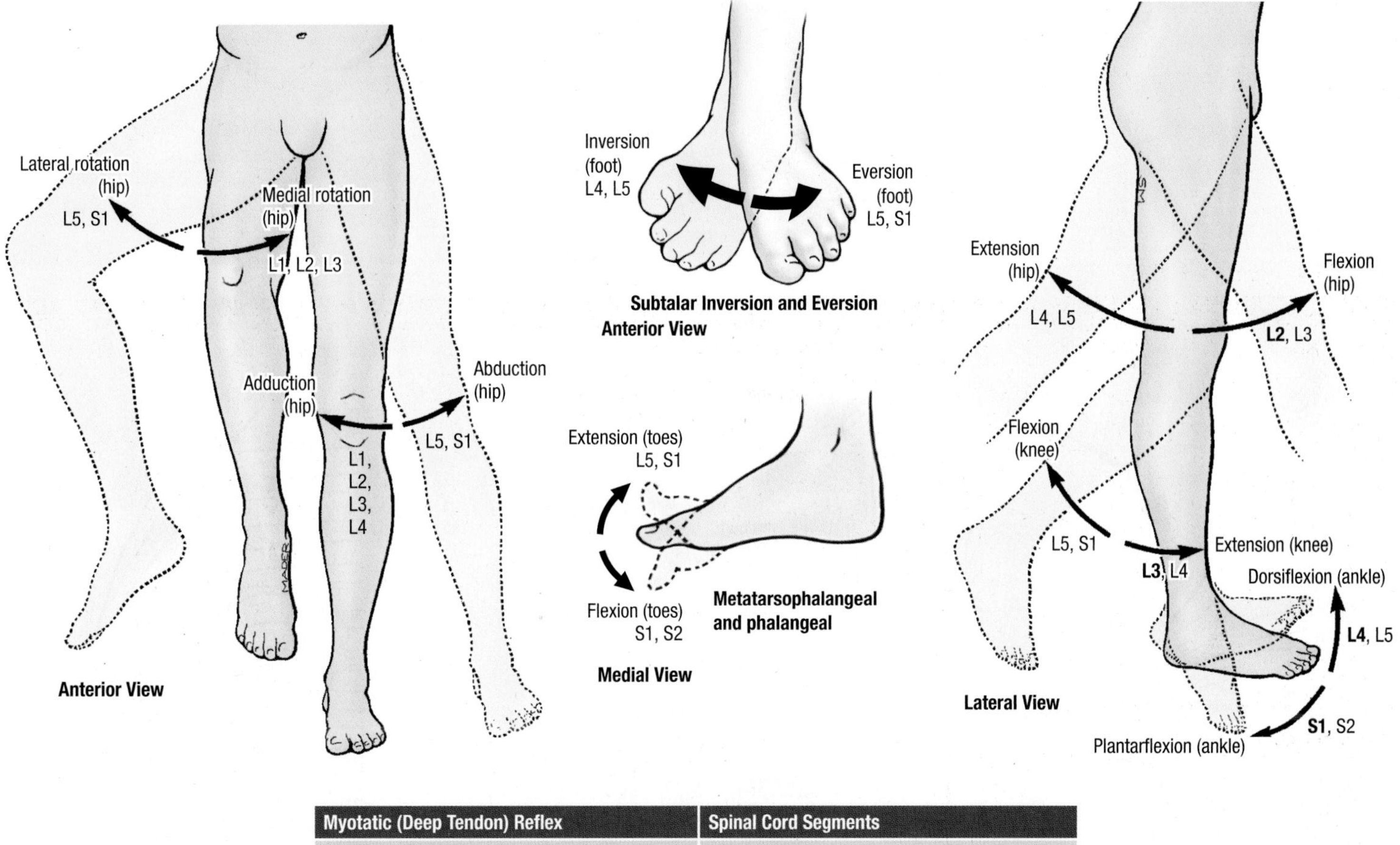
Lateral rotation (hip)
L5, S1
Medial rotation (hip)
L1, L2, L3
Adduction (hip)
L1, L2, L3, L4
Abduction (hip)
L5, S1
Anterior View
Inversion (foot) L4, L5
Eversion (foot) L5, S1
Subtalar Inversion and Eversion
Anterior View
Extension (toes) L5, S1
Flexion (toes) S1, S2
Metatarsophalangeal and phalangeal
Medial View
Extension (hip)
L4, L5
Flexion (hip)
L2, L3
Flexion (knee)
L5, S1
Extension (knee)
L3, L4
Dorsiflexion (ankle)
L4, L5
S1, S2
Plantarflexion (ankle)
Lateral View

Myotatic (Deep Tendon) Reflex	Spinal Cord Segments
Quadriceps (knee joint)	L3/L4
Calcaneal (Achilles; ankle jerk)	S1/S2

5.6 MYOTOMES AND DEEP TENDON REFLEXES

A. Myotomes. Somatic motor (general somatic efferent) fibers transmit impulses to skeletal (voluntary) muscles. The unilateral muscle mass receiving innervation from the somatic motor fibers conveyed by a single spinal nerve is a myotome. Each skeletal muscle is usually innervated by the somatic motor fibers of several spinal nerves; therefore, the muscle myotome will consist of several segments. The muscle myotomes have been grouped by joint movement to facilitate clinical testing.

B. Myotactic (deep tendon) reflexes. A myotatic (stretch) reflex is an involuntary contraction of a muscle in response to being stretched. Deep tendon reflexes (e.g., "knee jerk") are monosynaptic stretch reflexes that are elicited by briskly tapping the tendon with a reflex hammer. Each tendon reflex is mediated by specific spinal nerves. Stretch reflexes control muscle tone (e.g., in antigravity, muscles that keep the body upright against gravity).

TABLE 5.4 NERVE ROOT (ANTERIOR RAMUS) LESIONS

Compressed Nerve Root	Dermatome Affected	Muscles Affected	Movement Weakness/Deficit	Nerve and Reflex Involved
L4	L4: medial surface of leg; big toe	Quadriceps	Extension of knee	Femoral nerve ↓ Knee jerk
L5	L5: lateral surface of leg; dorsum of foot	Tibialis anterior Extensor hallucis longus Extensor digitorum longus	Dorsiflexion of ankle (patient cannot stand on heels) Extension of toes	Common fibular nerve No reflex loss
S1	S1: posterior surface of lower limb; little toe	Gastrocnemius Soleus	Plantar flexion of ankle (patient cannot stand on toes) Flexion of toes	Tibial nerve ↓ Ankle jerk

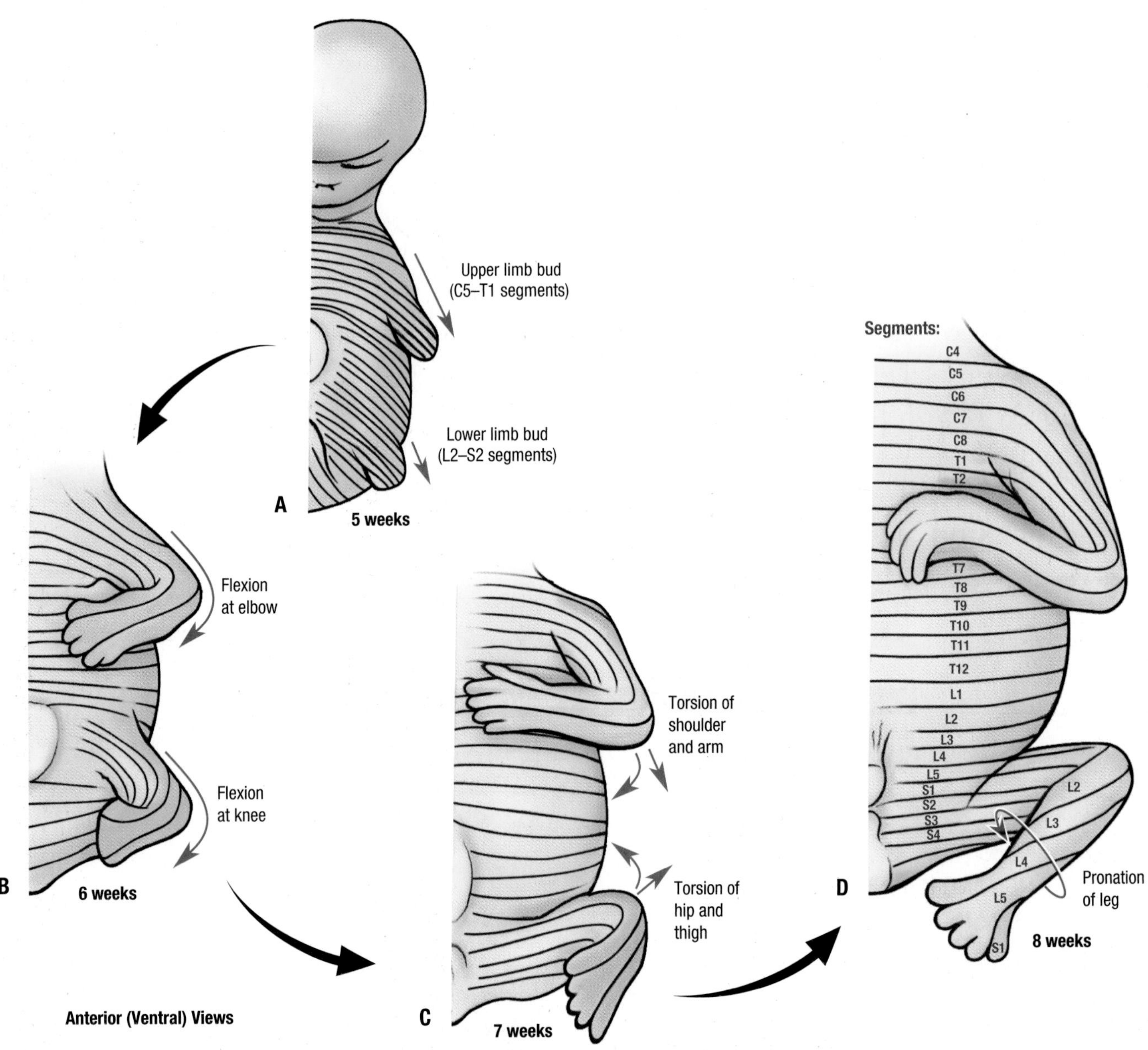
Upper limb bud
(C5–T1 segments)
Lower limb bud
(L2–S2 segments)
A
5 weeks
Flexion
at elbow
Flexion
at knee
B
6 weeks
Anterior (Ventral) Views
Torsion of
shoulder
and arm
Torsion of
hip and
thigh
C
7 weeks
Segments:
C4
C5
C6
C7
C8
T1
T2
T7
T8
T9
T10
T11
T12
L1
L2
L3
L4
L5
S1
S2
S3
S4
L2
L3
L4
L5
S1
Pronation
of leg
D
8 weeks

5.7 ROTATION OF LIMBS DURING DEVELOPMENT; EFFECT ON LOWER LIMB DERMATOME PATTERN

A. During early development, the trunk is divided into segments (metameres) that correspond to, and receive innervation from, the corresponding spinal cord segments. During the 4th week of development, the upper limb buds appear as elevations of the C5 to T1 segments of the ventrolateral body wall. Following the cranial-to-caudal pattern of development the lower limb buds appear about a week later (5th week). The lower limb buds grow laterally from broader bases formed by the L2 to S2 segments.

B. The distal ends of the limb buds flatten into paddlelike hand plates and foot plates that are elongated in the craniocaudal axis. Initially, both the thumb and the great toe are on the cranial sides of the developing hand and foot, directed superiorly, with the palms and soles directed anteriorly. Where gaps develop between the precursors of the long bones (future elbow and knee joints), flexures occur. At first, the limbs bend anteriorly, so that the elbow and knee are directed laterally, causing the palm and sole to be directed medially (toward the trunk).

C. By the end of the 7th week, the proximal parts of the upper and lower limbs undergo a 90-degree torsion around their long axes, but in opposite directions, so that the elbow becomes directed caudally and posteriorly and the knee cranially and anteriorly.

D. In the lower limb, the torsion of the proximal limb is accompanied by a permanent pronation (twisting) of the leg, so that the foot becomes oriented with the great toe on the medial side.

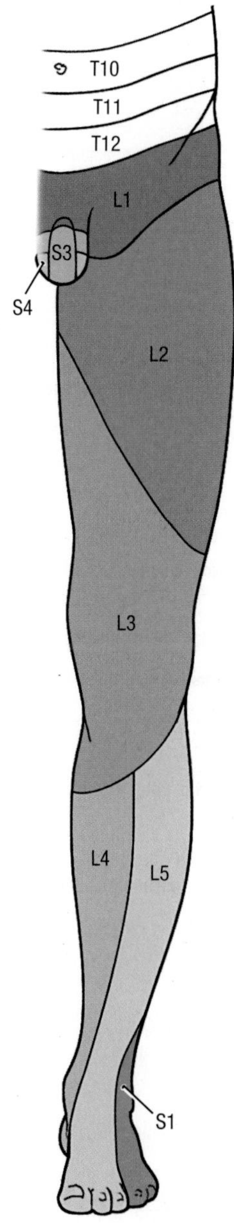
T10
T11
T12
L1
S3
S4
L2
L3
L4
L5
S1

A. Anterior View

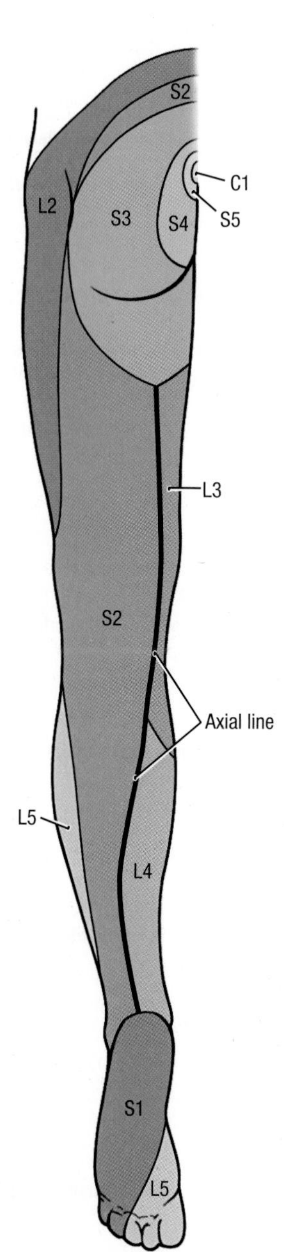
S2
C1
L2
S3
S4
S5
L3
S2
Axial line
L5
L4
S1
L5

B. Posterior View

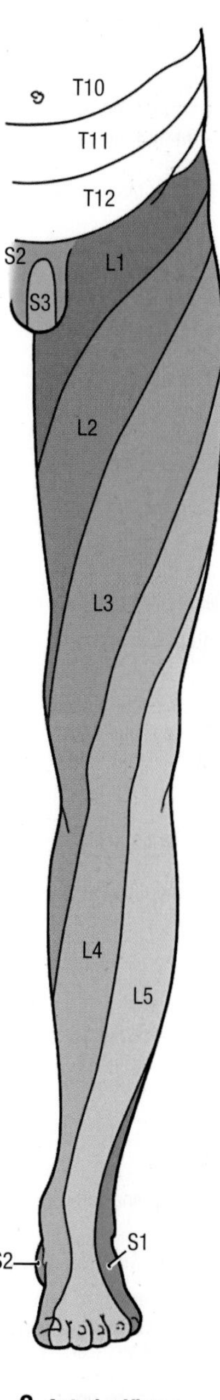
T10
T11
T12
S2
L1
S3
L2
L3
L4
L5
S2
S1

C. Anterior View

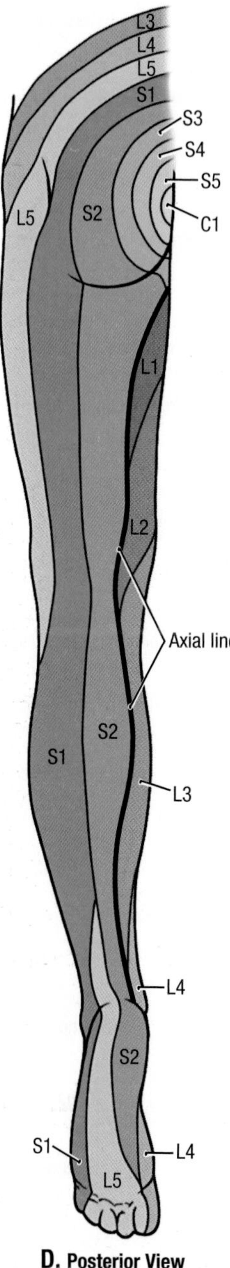
L3
L4
L5
S1
S3
S4
S5
L5
S2
C1
L1
L2
Axial line
S2
S1
L3
L4
S2
S1
L4
L5

D. Posterior View

5.8 DERMATOMES OF LOWER LIMB

The dermatomal, or segmental, pattern of distribution of sensory nerve fibers persists despite the merging of spinal nerves in plexus formation during development. Two different dermatome maps are commonly used. **A. and B.** The dermatome pattern of the lower limb according to Foerster (1933) is preferred by many because of its correlation with clinical findings. **C. and D.** The dermatome pattern of the lower limb according to Keegan and Garrett (1948) is preferred by others for its aesthetic uniformity and obvious correlation with development. Although depicted as distinct zones, adjacent dermatomes overlap considerably, except along the axial line.

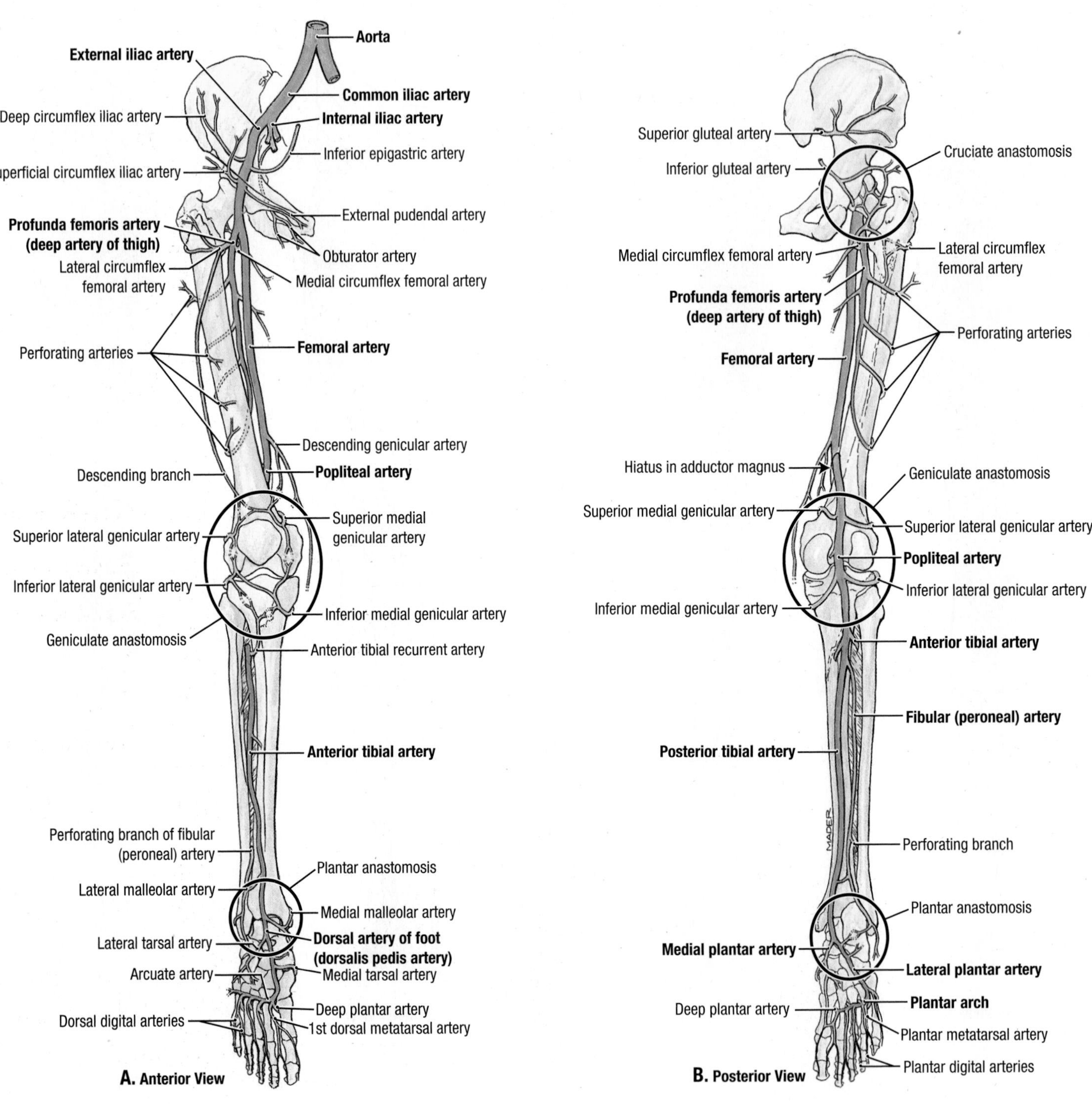
Aorta
External iliac artery
Common iliac artery
Deep circumflex iliac artery
Internal iliac artery
Inferior epigastric artery
Superficial circumflex iliac artery
External pudendal artery
Profunda femoris artery (deep artery of thigh)
Obturator artery
Lateral circumflex femoral artery
Medial circumflex femoral artery
Perforating arteries
Femoral artery
Descending genicular artery
Descending branch
Popliteal artery
Superior medial genicular artery
Superior lateral genicular artery
Inferior lateral genicular artery
Inferior medial genicular artery
Geniculate anastomosis
Anterior tibial recurrent artery
Anterior tibial artery
Perforating branch of fibular (peroneal) artery
Plantar anastomosis
Lateral malleolar artery
Medial malleolar artery
Lateral tarsal artery
Dorsal artery of foot (dorsalis pedis artery)
Arcuate artery
Medial tarsal artery
Deep plantar artery
Dorsal digital arteries
1st dorsal metatarsal artery
A. Anterior View
Superior gluteal artery
Cruciate anastomosis
Inferior gluteal artery
Medial circumflex femoral artery
Lateral circumflex femoral artery
Profunda femoris artery (deep artery of thigh)
Perforating arteries
Femoral artery
Hiatus in adductor magnus
Geniculate anastomosis
Superior medial genicular artery
Superior lateral genicular artery
Popliteal artery
Inferior lateral genicular artery
Inferior medial genicular artery
Anterior tibial artery
Fibular (peroneal) artery
Posterior tibial artery
MADER
Perforating branch
Plantar anastomosis
Medial plantar artery
Lateral plantar artery
Plantar arch
Deep plantar artery
Plantar metatarsal artery
Plantar digital arteries
B. Posterior View

5.9 OVERVIEW OF ARTERIES OF LOWER LIMB

The arteries often anastomose or communicate to form networks to ensure blood supply distal to the joint throughout the range of movement (cruciate, geniculate and plantar anastomoses). If a main channel is slowly occluded, the smaller alternate channels can usually increase in size, providing a **collateral circulation** that ensures the blood supply to structures distal to the blockage.

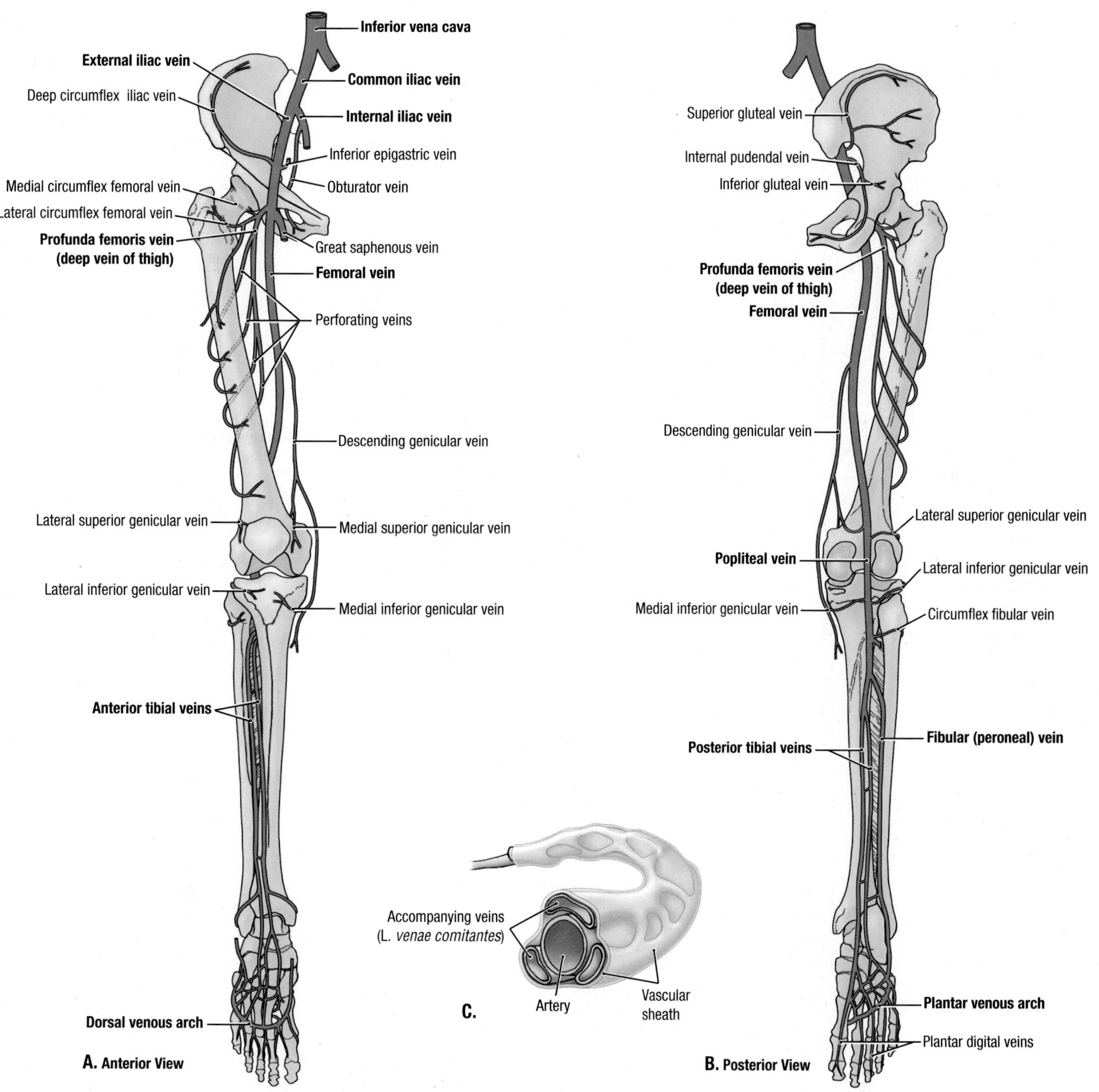
Inferior vena cava
External iliac vein
Common iliac vein
Deep circumflex iliac vein
Internal iliac vein
Inferior epigastric vein
Medial circumflex femoral vein
Obturator vein
Lateral circumflex femoral vein
Profunda femoris vein
(deep vein of thigh)
Great saphenous vein
Femoral vein
Perforating veins
Descending genicular vein
Lateral superior genicular vein
Medial superior genicular vein
Lateral inferior genicular vein
Medial inferior genicular vein
Anterior tibial veins
Dorsal venous arch
A. Anterior View
Superior gluteal vein
Internal pudendal vein
Inferior gluteal vein
Profunda femoris vein
(deep vein of thigh)
Femoral vein
Descending genicular vein
Lateral superior genicular vein
Popliteal vein
Lateral inferior genicular vein
Medial inferior genicular vein
Circumflex fibular vein
Posterior tibial veins
Fibular (peroneal) vein
Plantar venous arch
Plantar digital veins
B. Posterior View
Accompanying veins
(L. venae comitantes)
Artery
Vascular
sheath
C.

5.10 DEEP VEINS OF LOWER LIMB

A. and B. Deep veins lie internal to the deep fascia. Although only the anterior and posterior tibial veins are depicted as paired structures in this schematic illustration, typically in the limbs deep veins occur as multiple, generally parallel, continually interanastomosing accompanying veins (L., venae comitantes) surrounding and sharing the name of the artery they accompany. **C.** Accompanying veins.

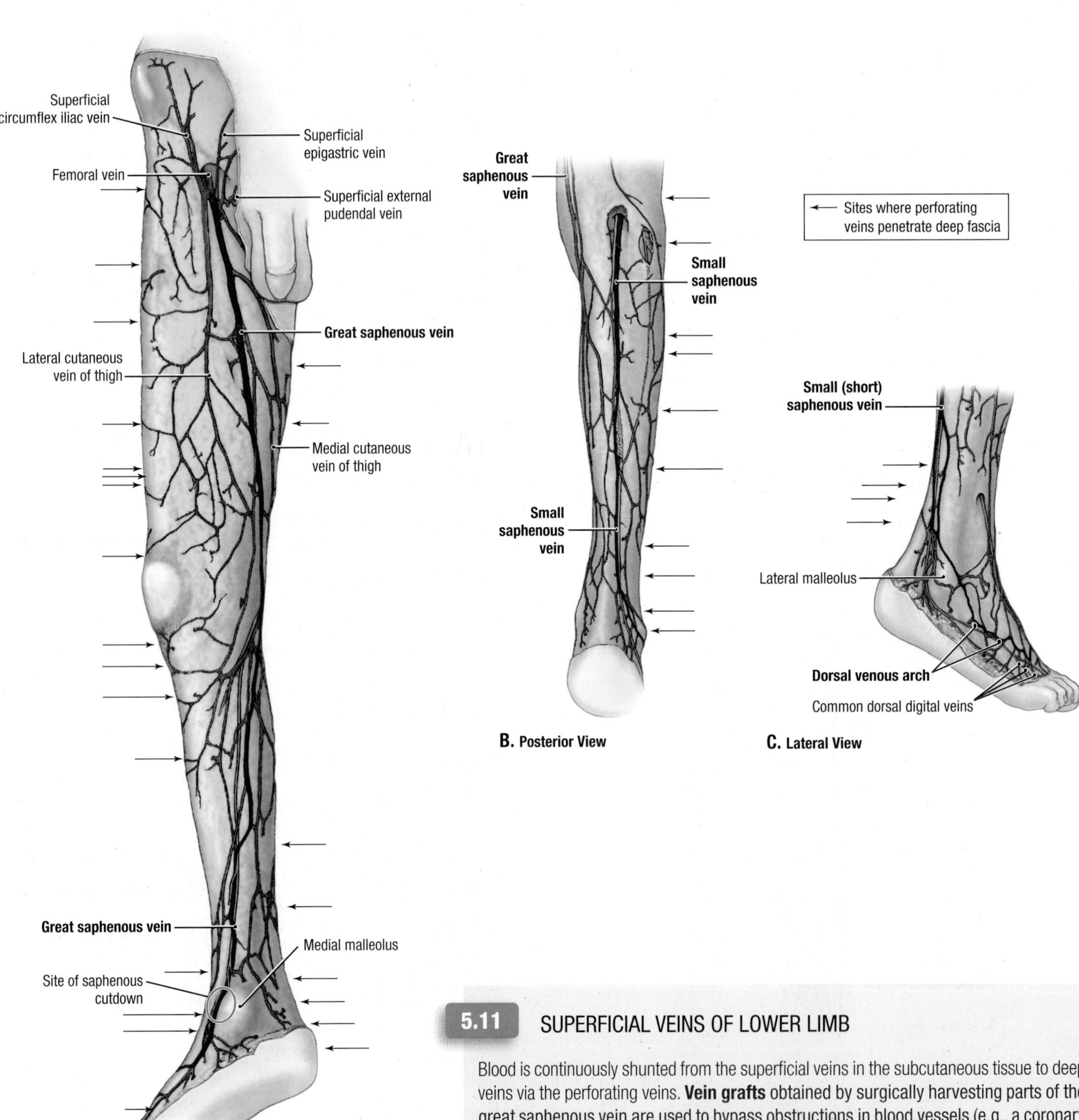
Superficial circumflex iliac vein
Femoral vein
Superficial epigastric vein
Superficial external pudendal vein
Great saphenous vein
Lateral cutaneous vein of thigh
Medial cutaneous vein of thigh
Great saphenous vein
Medial malleolus
Site of saphenous cutdown
Great saphenous vein
Small saphenous vein
Small saphenous vein
Sites where perforating veins penetrate deep fascia
Small (short) saphenous vein
Lateral malleolus
Dorsal venous arch
Common dorsal digital veins

A. Anteromedial View

B. Posterior View

C. Lateral View

5.11 SUPERFICIAL VEINS OF LOWER LIMB

Blood is continuously shunted from the superficial veins in the subcutaneous tissue to deep veins via the perforating veins. **Vein grafts** obtained by surgically harvesting parts of the great saphenous vein are used to bypass obstructions in blood vessels (e.g., a coronary artery). When used as a bypass, the vein is reversed so that the valves do not obstruct blood flow. Because there are so many anastomosing leg veins, removal of the great saphenous vein rarely affects circulation seriously, provided the deep veins are intact.

Saphenous cut down. The great saphenous vein can be located by making a skin incision anterior to the medial malleolus. This procedure is used to insert a cannula for prolonged administration of blood, electrolytes, drugs etc.

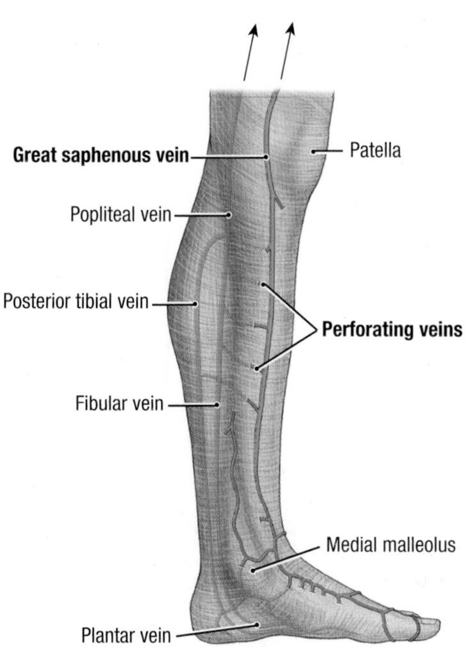
Great saphenous vein
Patella
Popliteal vein
Posterior tibial vein
Perforating veins
Fibular vein
Medial malleolus
Plantar vein

A. Medial View

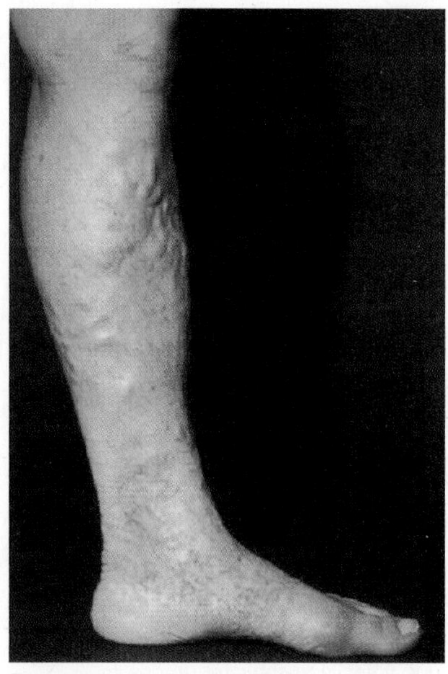

B. Medial View, Varicose Veins

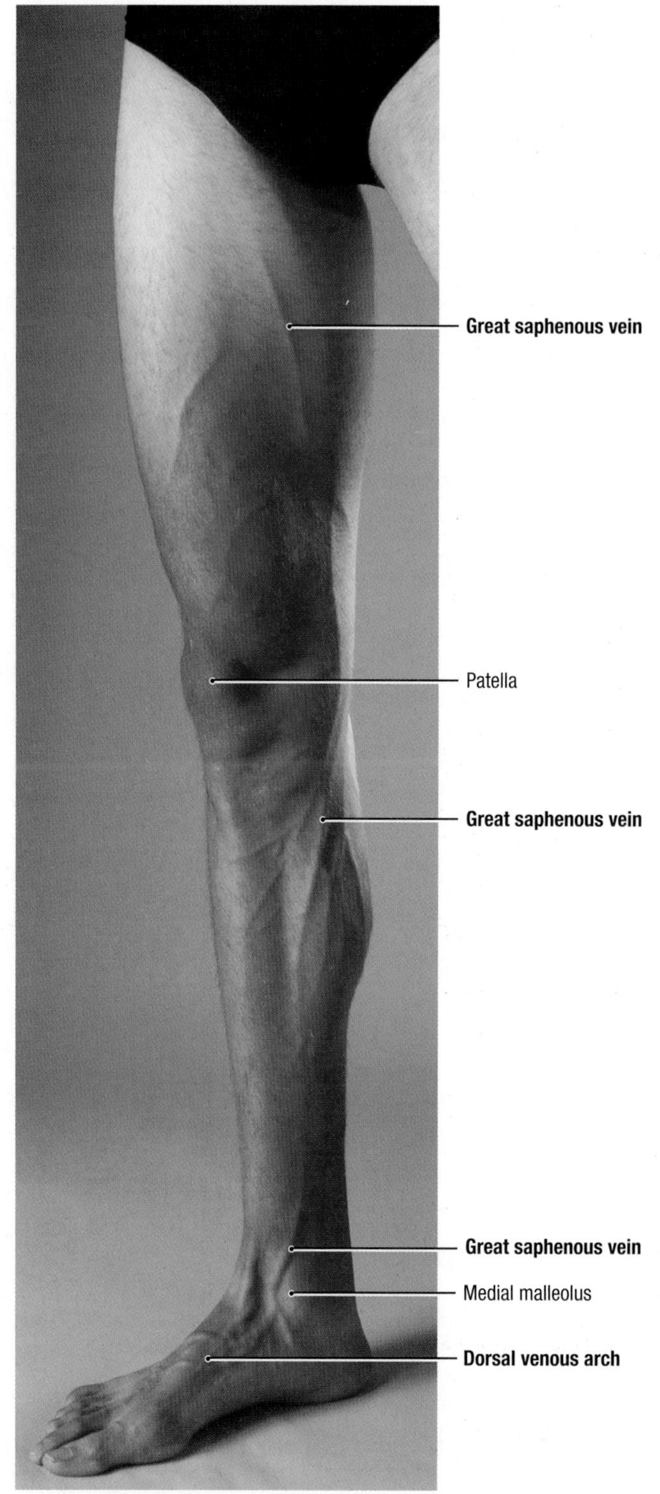
Great saphenous vein
Patella
Great saphenous vein
Great saphenous vein
Medial malleolus
Dorsal venous arch

C. Anteromedial View, Normal Veins

5.12 DRAINAGE AND SURFACE ANATOMY OF SUPERFICIAL VEINS OF LOWER LIMB

A. Schematic diagram of drainage of superficial veins. Blood is shunted from the superficial veins (e.g., great saphenous vein) to the deep veins (e.g., fibular and posterior tibial veins) via perforating veins that penetrate the deep fascia. Muscular compression of deep veins assists return of blood to the heart against gravity. **B. Varicose veins** form when either the deep fascia or the valves of the perforating veins are incompetent. This allows the muscular compression that normally propels blood toward the heart to push blood from the deep to the superficial veins. Consequently, superficial veins become enlarged and tortuous. **C.** Normal veins, distended following exercise.

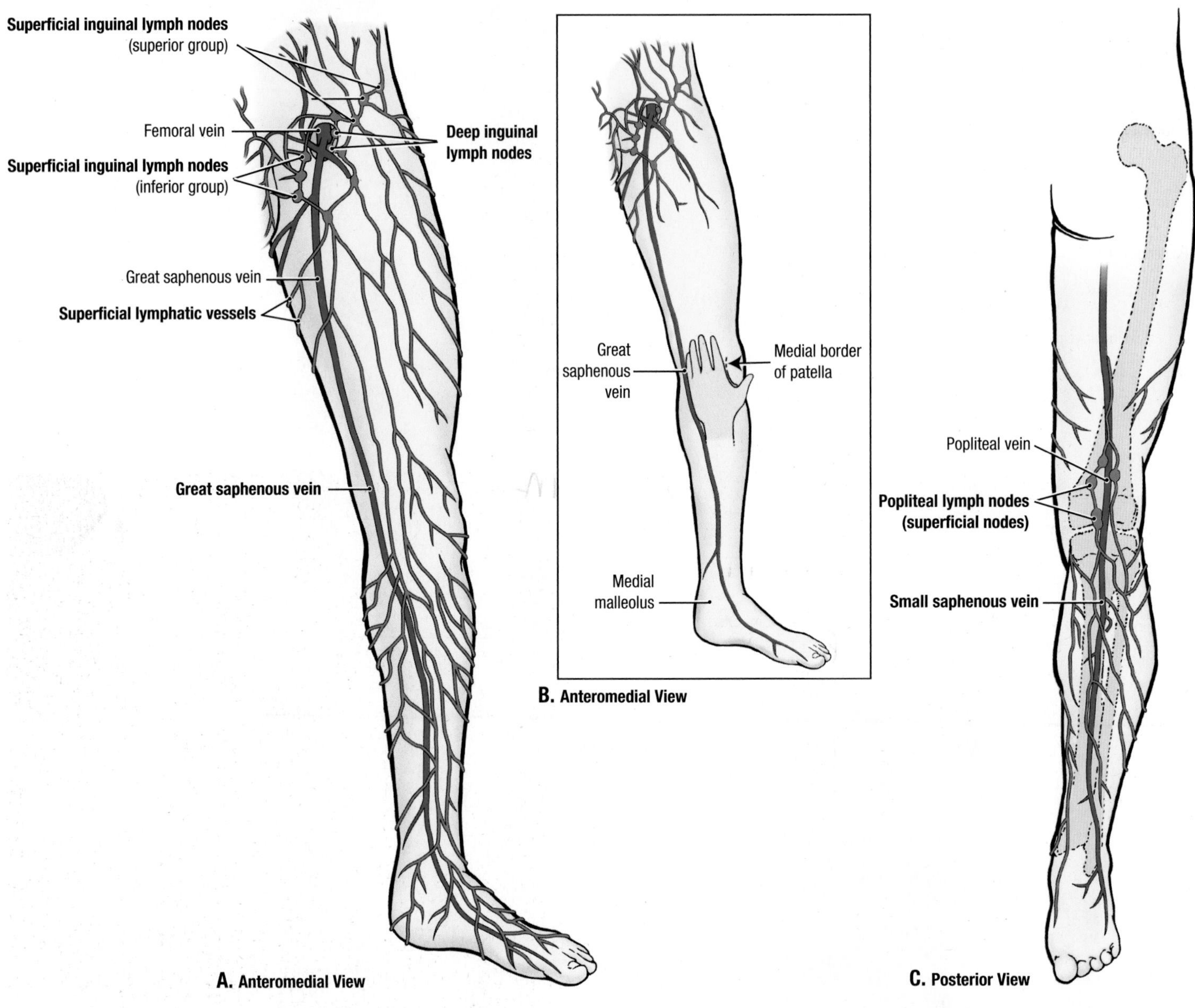

Superficial inguinal lymph nodes
(superior group)
Femoral vein
Deep inguinal
lymph nodes
Superficial inguinal lymph nodes
(inferior group)
Great saphenous vein
Superficial lymphatic vessels
Great saphenous vein
A. Anteromedial View
Great
saphenous
vein
Medial border
of patella
Medial
malleolus
B. Anteromedial View
Popliteal vein
Popliteal lymph nodes
(superficial nodes)
Small saphenous vein
C. Posterior View

5.13 SUPERFICIAL LYMPHATIC DRAINAGE OF LOWER LIMB

The superficial lymphatic vessels converge on and accompany the saphenous veins and their tributaries in the superficial fascia. The lymphatic vessels along the great saphenous vein drain into the superficial inguinal lymph nodes; those along the small saphenous vein drain into the popliteal lymph nodes. Lymph from the superficial inguinal nodes drains to the deep inguinal and external iliac nodes. Lymph from the popliteal nodes ascends through deep lymphatic vessels accompanying the deep blood vessels to the deep inguinal nodes. In **B,** note that the great saphenous vein lies anterior to the medial malleolus and a hand's breadth posterior to the medial border of the patella. **Lymph nodes enlarge** when diseased. Abrasions and minor sepsis, caused by pathogenic micro-organisms or their toxins in the blood or other tissues, may produce slight enlargement of the superficial inguinal nodes (lymphadenopathy) in otherwise healthy people. Malignancies (e.g., of the external genitalia and uterus) and perineal abscesses also result in enlargement of these nodes.

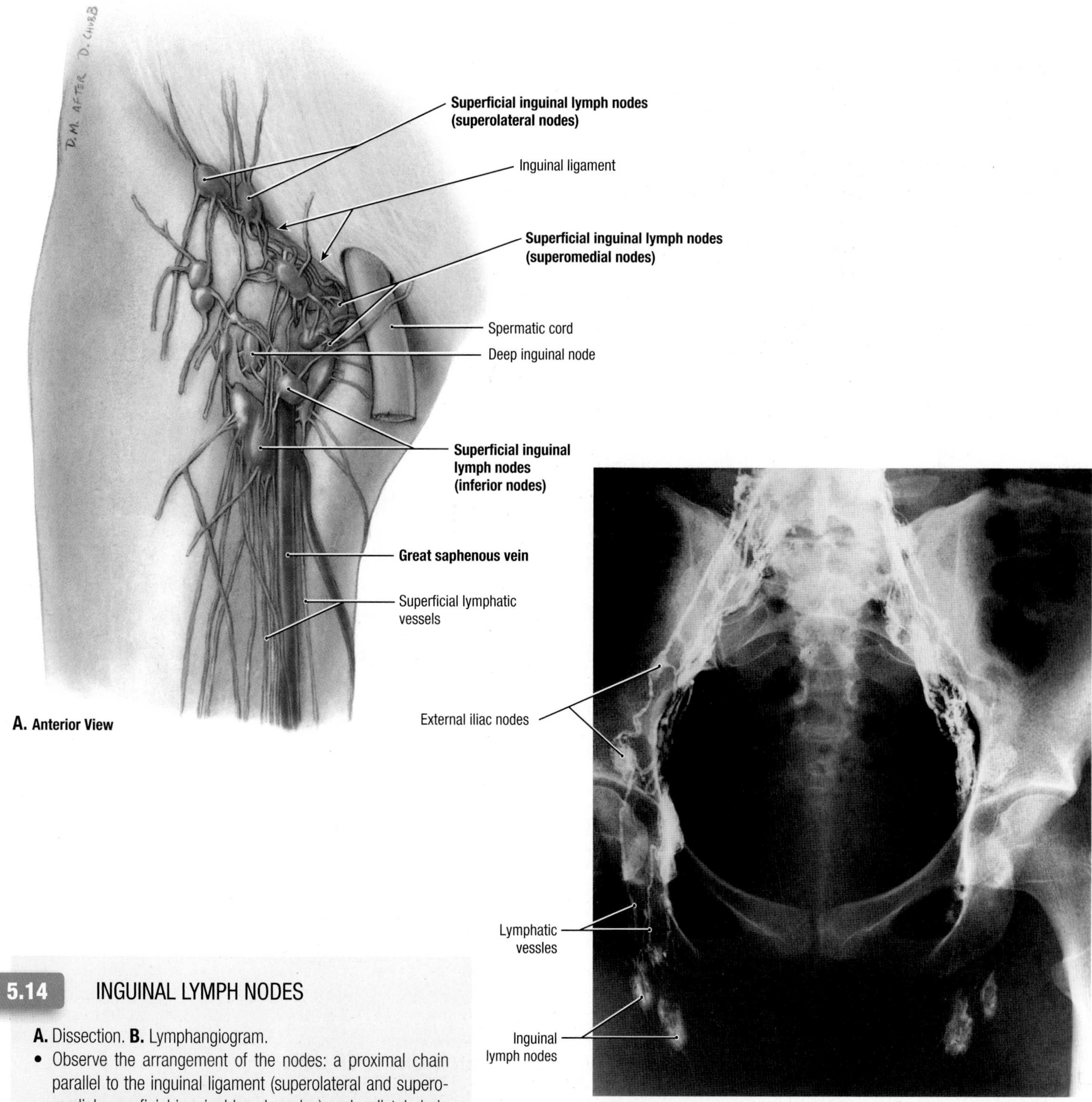
D.M. AFTER D. CHUBB
Superficial inguinal lymph nodes (superolateral nodes)
Inguinal ligament
Superficial inguinal lymph nodes (superomedial nodes)
Spermatic cord
Deep inguinal node
Superficial inguinal lymph nodes (inferior nodes)
Great saphenous vein
Superficial lymphatic vessels
External iliac nodes
Lymphatic vessles
Inguinal lymph nodes

A. Anterior View

B. Anteroposterior View

5.14 INGUINAL LYMPH NODES

A. Dissection. **B.** Lymphangiogram.

- Observe the arrangement of the nodes: a proximal chain parallel to the inguinal ligament (superolateral and superomedial superficial inguinal lymph nodes) and a distal chain on the sides of the great saphenous vein (inferior superficial inguinal lymph nodes). Efferent vessels leave these nodes and pass deep to the inguinal ligament to enter the deep inguinal and external iliac nodes. Some of the lymphatic vessels traverse the femoral canal, and others ascend alongside the femoral artery and vein, some inside the femoral sheath, and some outside it.
- Note the anastomosis between the lymph vessels.

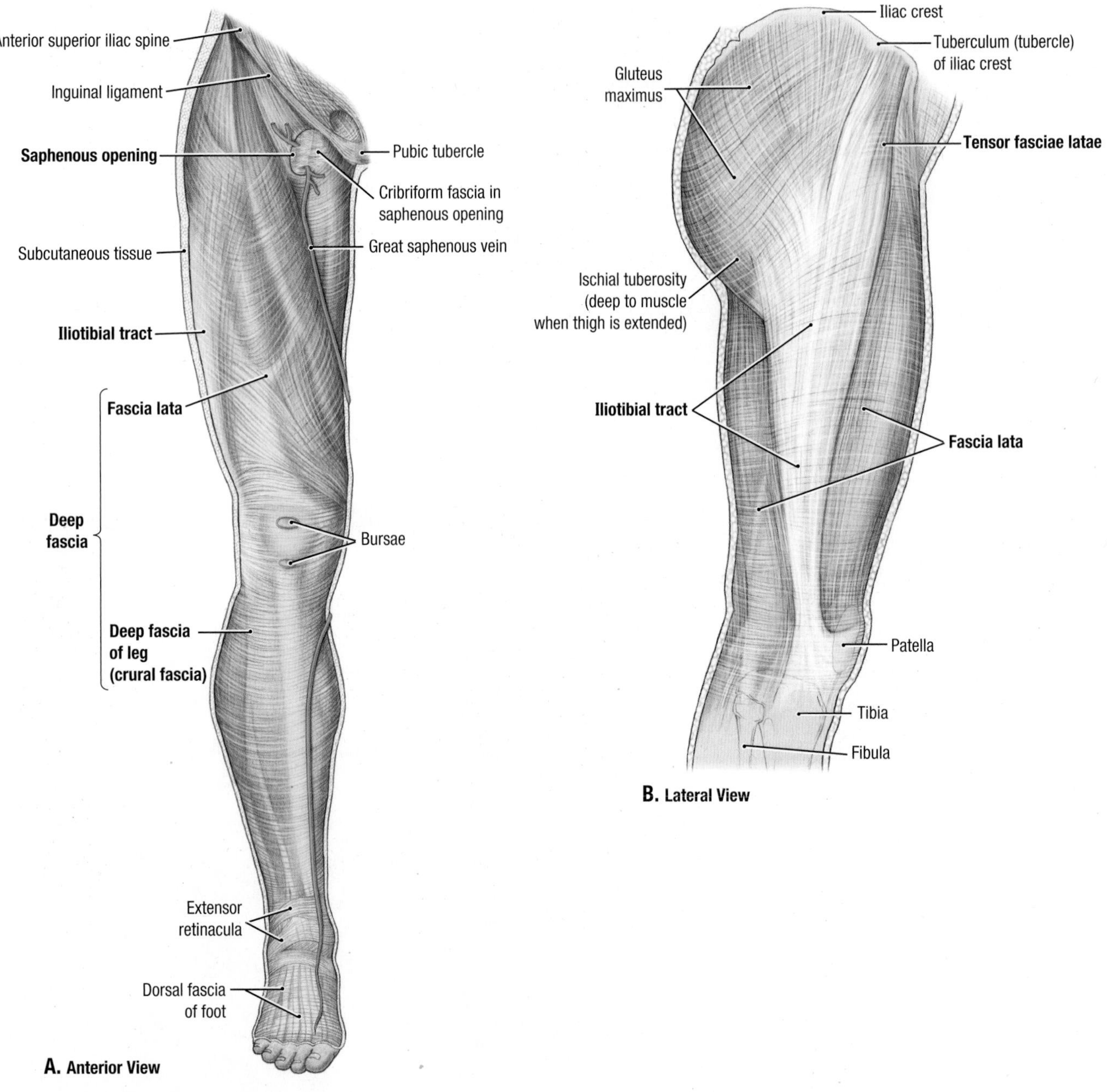
Anterior superior iliac spine
Inguinal ligament
Saphenous opening
Pubic tubercle
Cribriform fascia in saphenous opening
Great saphenous vein
Subcutaneous tissue
Iliotibial tract
Fascia lata
Deep fascia
Bursae
Deep fascia of leg (crural fascia)
Extensor retinacula
Dorsal fascia of foot
A. Anterior View
Iliac crest
Tuberculum (tubercle) of iliac crest
Gluteus maximus
Tensor fasciae latae
Ischial tuberosity (deep to muscle when thigh is extended)
Iliotibial tract
Fascia lata
Patella
Tibia
Fibula
B. Lateral View

5.15 FASCIA AND MUSCULOFASCIAL COMPARTMENTS OF LOWER LIMB

A. Anterior skin and subcutaneous tissue have been removed to reveal the deep fascia of the thigh (fascia lata) and leg (crural fascia). **B.** Lateral skin and subcutaneous tissue have been removed to reveal the fascia lata. The fascia lata is thick laterally and forms the iliotibial tract. The iliotibial tract serves as a common aponeurosis for the gluteus maximus and tensor fasciae latae muscles.

One of the most common causes of lateral knee pain in endurance athletes (e.g., runners, cyclers, hikers) is **iliotibial tract (band) syndrome (ITBS)**. Friction of the IT tract against the lateral epicondyle of the femur with flexion and extension of the knee (e.g., during running) may result in the inflammation of the IT tract over the lateral aspect of the knee or its attachment to the dorsolateral tubercle (Gerdy tubercle). ITBS may also occur in the hip region, especially in older individuals.

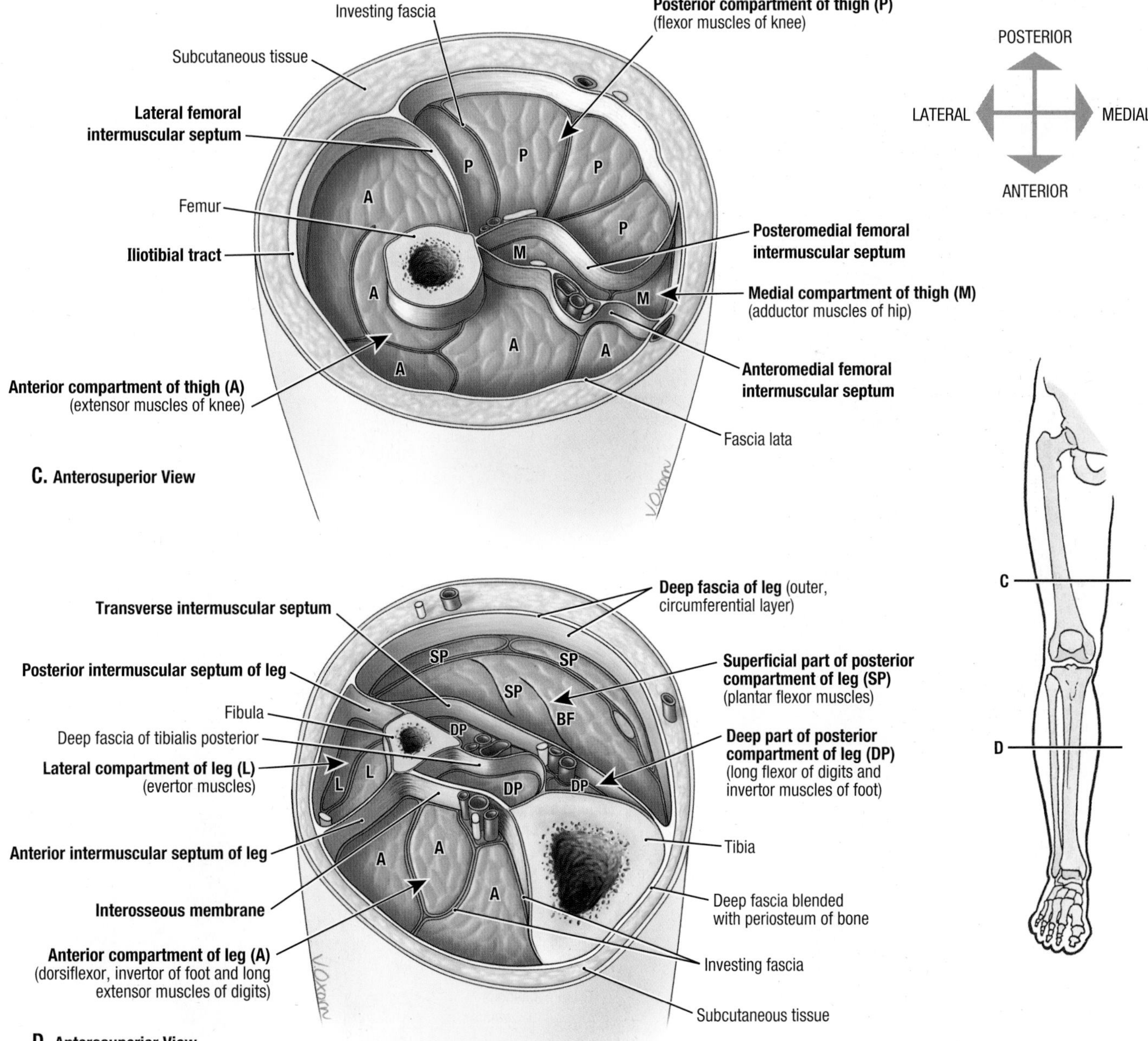
Investing fascia
Posterior compartment of thigh (P)
(flexor muscles of knee)
POSTERIOR
LATERAL
MEDIAL
ANTERIOR
Subcutaneous tissue
Lateral femoral intermuscular septum
Femur
Iliotibial tract
Posteromedial femoral intermuscular septum
Medial compartment of thigh (M)
(adductor muscles of hip)
Anteromedial femoral intermuscular septum
Anterior compartment of thigh (A)
(extensor muscles of knee)
Fascia lata
P
A
M
C
D
Transverse intermuscular septum
Deep fascia of leg (outer, circumferential layer)
Posterior intermuscular septum of leg
Superficial part of posterior compartment of leg (SP)
(plantar flexor muscles)
Fibula
Deep fascia of tibialis posterior
Deep part of posterior compartment of leg (DP)
(long flexor of digits and invertor muscles of foot)
Lateral compartment of leg (L)
(evertor muscles)
Anterior intermuscular septum of leg
Tibia
Interosseous membrane
Deep fascia blended with periosteum of bone
Anterior compartment of leg (A)
(dorsiflexor, invertor of foot and long extensor muscles of digits)
Investing fascia
Subcutaneous tissue
SP
DP
BF
L

C. Anterosuperior View

D. Anterosuperior View

5.15 FASCIA AND MUSCULOFASCIAL COMPARTMENTS OF LOWER LIMB (*CONTINUED*)

C. and D. The fascial compartments of the thigh **(C)** and leg **(D)** are demonstrated in transverse section. The fascial compartments contain muscles that generally perform common functions and share common innervation, and contain the spread of infection. While both thigh and leg have anterior and posterior compartments, the thigh also includes a medial compartment and the leg a lateral compartment. Trauma to muscles and/or vessels in the compartments may produce hemorrhage, edema, and inflammation of the muscles. Because the septa, deep fascia, and bony attachments firmly bound the compartments, increased volume resulting from these processes raises intracompartmental pressure. In **compartment syndromes,** structures within or distal to the compressed area become ischemic and may become permanently injured (e.g., compression of capillary beds results in denervation and consequent paralysis of muscles). A **fasciotomy** (incision of bounding fascia or septum) may be performed to relieve the pressure in the compartment and restore circulation.

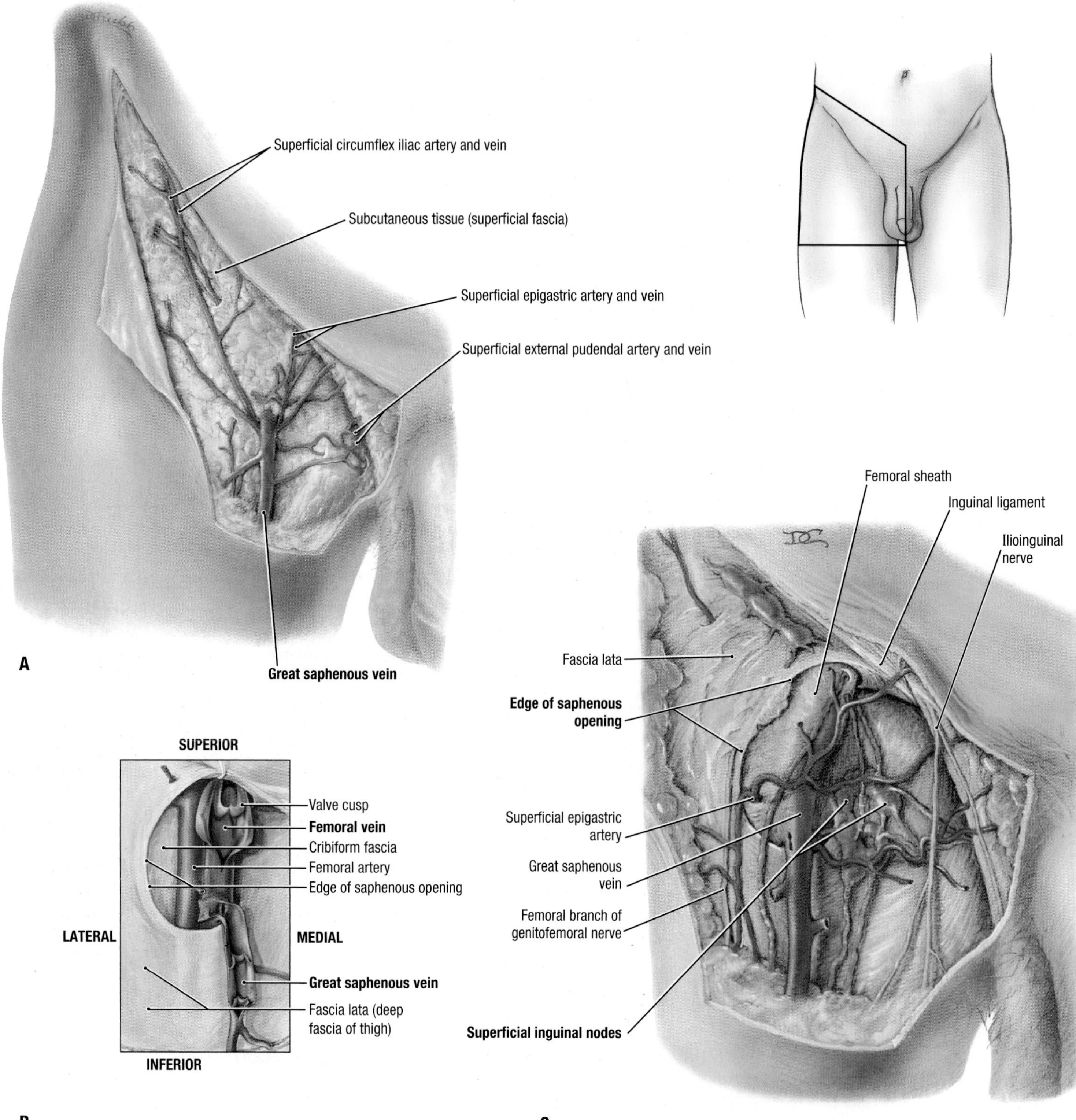
Superficial circumflex iliac artery and vein
Subcutaneous tissue (superficial fascia)
Superficial epigastric artery and vein
Superficial external pudendal artery and vein
A
Great saphenous vein
SUPERIOR
Valve cusp
Femoral vein
Cribiform fascia
Femoral artery
Edge of saphenous opening
LATERAL
MEDIAL
Great saphenous vein
Fascia lata (deep fascia of thigh)
INFERIOR
B
Femoral sheath
Inguinal ligament
Ilioinguinal nerve
Fascia lata
Edge of saphenous opening
Superficial epigastric artery
Great saphenous vein
Femoral branch of genitofemoral nerve
Superficial inguinal nodes
C

5.16 SUPERFICIAL INGUINAL VESSELS AND SAPHENOUS OPENING

A. Superficial inguinal vessels. The arteries are branches of the femoral artery, and the veins are tributaries of the great saphenous vein. **B.** Valves of the proximal part of femoral and great saphenous veins. **C.** Saphenous opening.

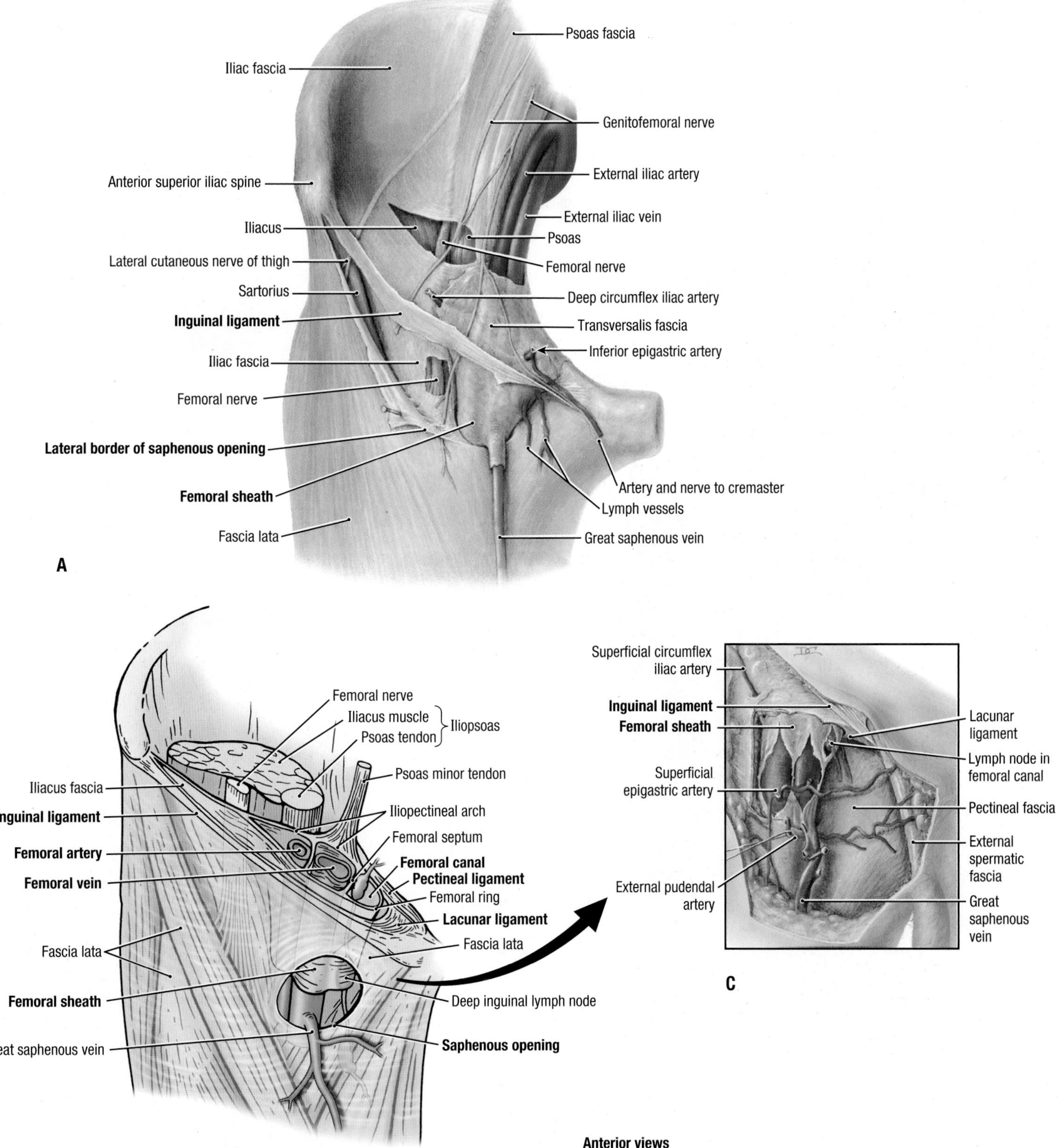
Psoas fascia
Iliac fascia
Genitofemoral nerve
Anterior superior iliac spine
External iliac artery
External iliac vein
Iliacus
Psoas
Lateral cutaneous nerve of thigh
Femoral nerve
Sartorius
Deep circumflex iliac artery
Inguinal ligament
Transversalis fascia
Inferior epigastric artery
Iliac fascia
Femoral nerve
Lateral border of saphenous opening
Femoral sheath
Artery and nerve to cremaster
Lymph vessels
Fascia lata
Great saphenous vein
A
Femoral nerve
Iliacus muscle
Psoas tendon
Iliopsoas
Psoas minor tendon
Iliacus fascia
Inguinal ligament
Iliopectineal arch
Femoral septum
Femoral artery
Femoral canal
Femoral vein
Pectineal ligament
Femoral ring
Lacunar ligament
Fascia lata
Fascia lata
Femoral sheath
Deep inguinal lymph node
Great saphenous vein
Saphenous opening
B
Superficial circumflex iliac artery
Inguinal ligament
Femoral sheath
Lacunar ligament
Lymph node in femoral canal
Superficial epigastric artery
Pectineal fascia
External spermatic fascia
External pudendal artery
Great saphenous vein
C
Anterior views

5.17 FEMORAL SHEATH AND INGUINAL LIGAMENT

A. Dissection. **B.** Schematic illustration. The femoral sheath contains the femoral artery, vein, and lymph vessels, but the femoral nerve, lying posterior to the iliacus fascia, is outside the femoral sheath. **C.** Femoral sheath and femoral ring. The three compartments of the femoral sheath are the lateral for the femoral artery; intermediate for the femoral vein; and medial for the femoral canal. The base of the femoral canal is formed by the small (about 1 cm wide) proximal opening at its abdominal end, the femoral ring. This opening is closed by extraperitoneal fatty tissue.

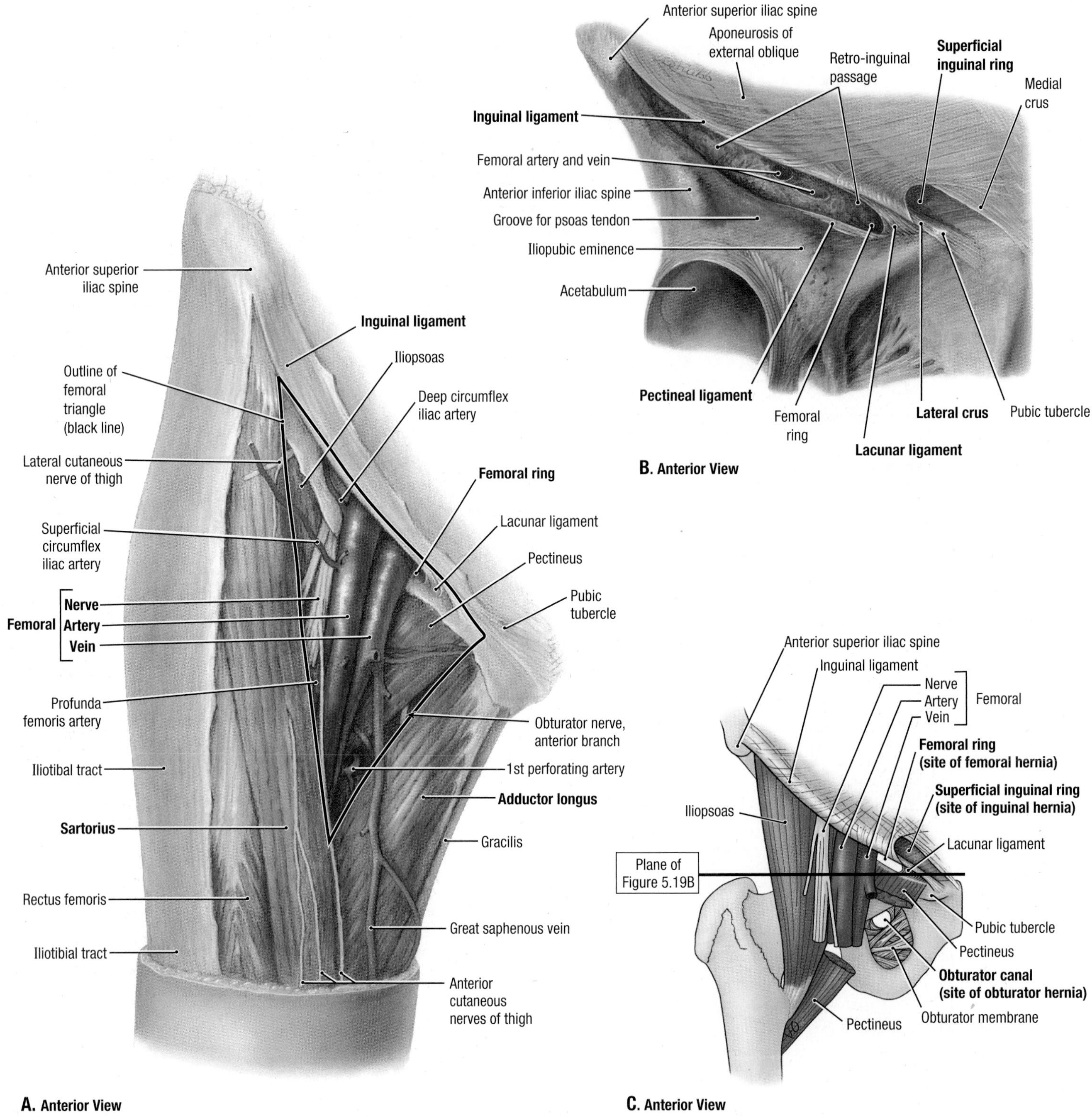
Anterior superior iliac spine
Inguinal ligament
Iliopsoas
Outline of femoral triangle (black line)
Deep circumflex iliac artery
Lateral cutaneous nerve of thigh
Femoral ring
Lacunar ligament
Superficial circumflex iliac artery
Pectineus
Pubic tubercle
Femoral
Nerve
Artery
Vein
Profunda femoris artery
Obturator nerve, anterior branch
Iliotibal tract
1st perforating artery
Adductor longus
Sartorius
Gracilis
Rectus femoris
Great saphenous vein
Iliotibial tract
Anterior cutaneous nerves of thigh
A. Anterior View
Anterior superior iliac spine
Aponeurosis of external oblique
Retro-inguinal passage
Superficial inguinal ring
Medial crus
Inguinal ligament
Femoral artery and vein
Anterior inferior iliac spine
Groove for psoas tendon
Iliopubic eminence
Acetabulum
Pectineal ligament
Femoral ring
Lateral crus
Pubic tubercle
Lacunar ligament
B. Anterior View
Anterior superior iliac spine
Inguinal ligament
Nerve
Artery
Vein
Femoral
Femoral ring (site of femoral hernia)
Superficial inguinal ring (site of inguinal hernia)
Iliopsoas
Lacunar ligament
Plane of Figure 5.19B
Pubic tubercle
Pectineus
Obturator canal (site of obturator hernia)
Pectineus
Obturator membrane
C. Anterior View

5.18 STRUCTURES PASSING TO/FROM FEMORAL TRIANGLE VIA RETRO-INGUINAL PASSAGE

A. Dissection. The boundaries of the femoral triangle are the inguinal ligament superiorly (base of triangle), the medial border of the sartorius (lateral side), and the lateral border of the adductor longus (medial side). The point at which the lateral and medial sides converge inferiorly forms the apex. The femoral triangle is bisected by the femoral vessels. **B.** Retro-inguinal passage between the inguinal ligament anteriorly and the bony pelvis posteriorly. **C.** The iliopsoas muscle, the femoral nerve, artery, and vein, and the lymphatic vessels draining the inguinal nodes pass deep to the inguinal ligament to enter the anterior thigh or return to the trunk. Three potential sites for **hernia formation** are indicated. **Pulsations of the femoral artery** can be felt distal to the inguinal ligament, midway between the anterior superior iliac spine and the pubic tubercle.

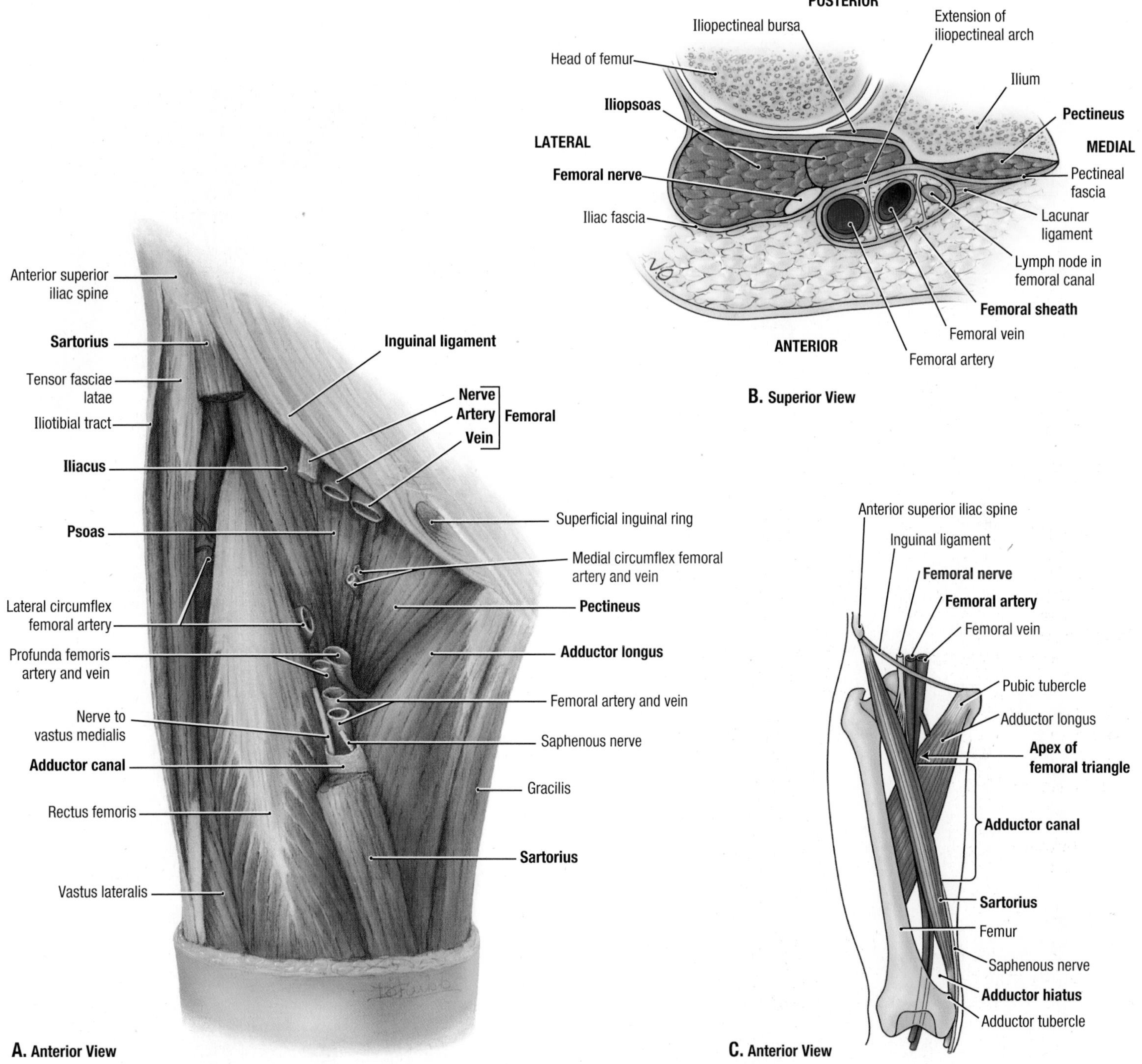
POSTERIOR
Iliopectineal bursa
Extension of iliopectineal arch
Head of femur
Ilium
Iliopsoas
Pectineus
LATERAL
MEDIAL
Femoral nerve
Pectineal fascia
Iliac fascia
Lacunar ligament
Lymph node in femoral canal
Femoral sheath
Femoral vein
ANTERIOR
Femoral artery
B. Superior View
Anterior superior iliac spine
Sartorius
Inguinal ligament
Tensor fasciae latae
Nerve
Artery
Vein
Femoral
Iliotibial tract
Iliacus
Superficial inguinal ring
Psoas
Medial circumflex femoral artery and vein
Pectineus
Lateral circumflex femoral artery
Profunda femoris artery and vein
Adductor longus
Femoral artery and vein
Nerve to vastus medialis
Saphenous nerve
Adductor canal
Gracilis
Rectus femoris
Sartorius
Vastus lateralis
A. Anterior View
Anterior superior iliac spine
Inguinal ligament
Femoral nerve
Femoral artery
Femoral vein
Pubic tubercle
Adductor longus
Apex of femoral triangle
Adductor canal
Sartorius
Femur
Saphenous nerve
Adductor hiatus
Adductor tubercle
C. Anterior View

5.19 FLOOR OF FEMORAL CANAL AND RETRO-INGUINAL PASSAGE

A. Dissection. Portions of the sartorius muscle, femoral vessels, and femoral nerve have been removed revealing the floor of the femoral triangle, formed by the iliopsoas laterally and the pectineus medially. At the apex of the triangle the femoral vessels, saphenous nerve, and the nerve to the vastus medialis pass deep to the sartorius into the adductor (subsartorial) canal. **B.** Transverse section of the femoral triangle at the level of head of femur. (Level of section is indicated in Fig. 5.18 **C.**) The iliopsoas and femoral nerve traverse the retro-inguinal passage and femoral triangle in a fascial sheath separate from the femoral vessels, which are contained within the femoral sheath. **C.** Schematic illustration of course of femoral vessels. The adductor canal extends from the apex of the femoral triangle to the adductor hiatus, by which the vessels enter and leave the popliteal fossa.

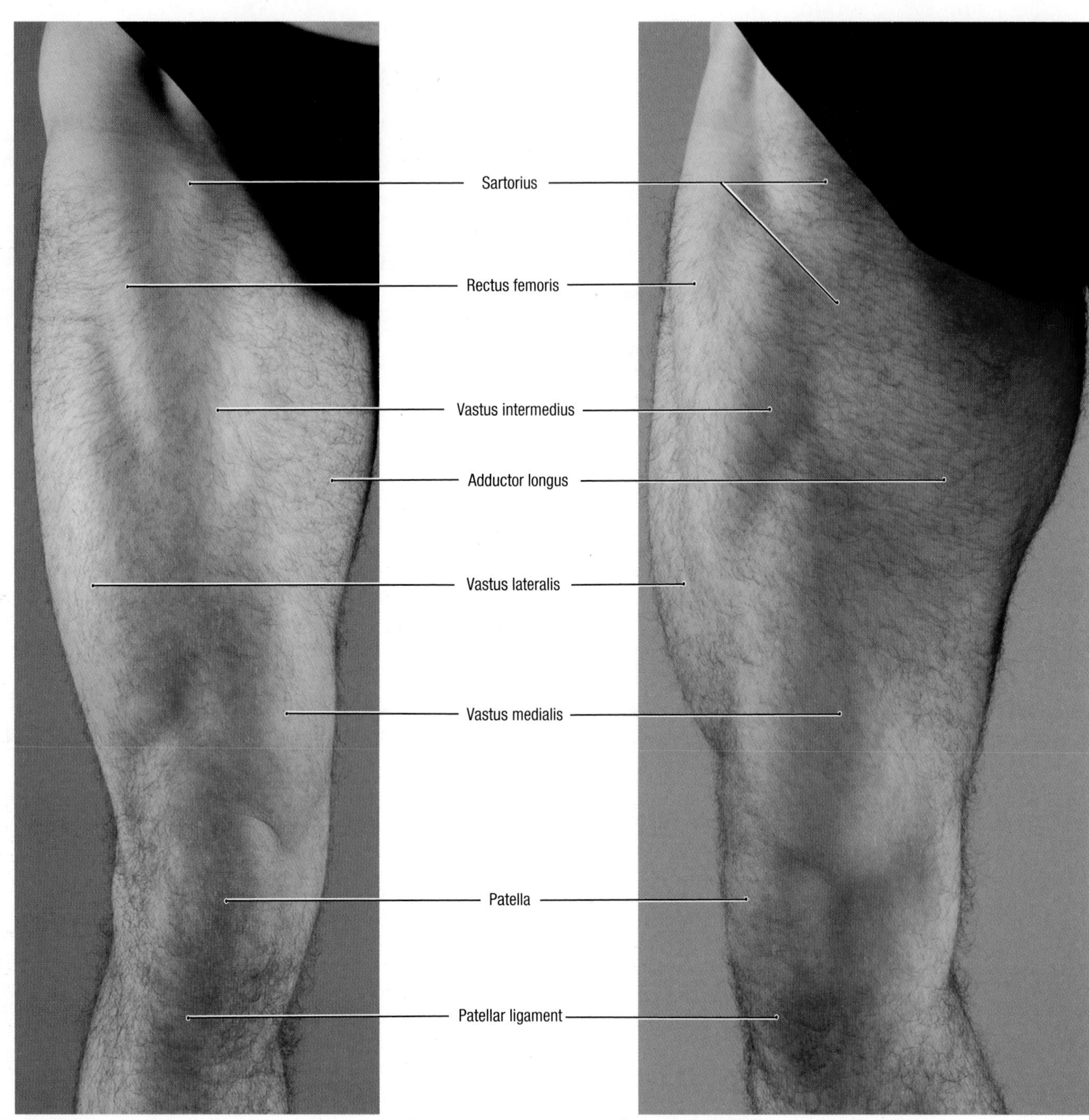
Sartorius
Rectus femoris
Vastus intermedius
Adductor longus
Vastus lateralis
Vastus medialis
Patella
Patellar ligament
A. Anterior View
B. Anteromedial View

5.20 SURFACE ANATOMY OF ANTERIOR AND MEDIAL ASPECTS OF THIGH

Patellar tendinitis (jumper's knee) is caused by continuous overloading of the knee extensor mechanism, resulting in microtears of the tendon. The most vulnerable site is where the patellar ligament (tendon) attaches to the patella. This overuse injury can result in degeneration and tearing of the tendon.

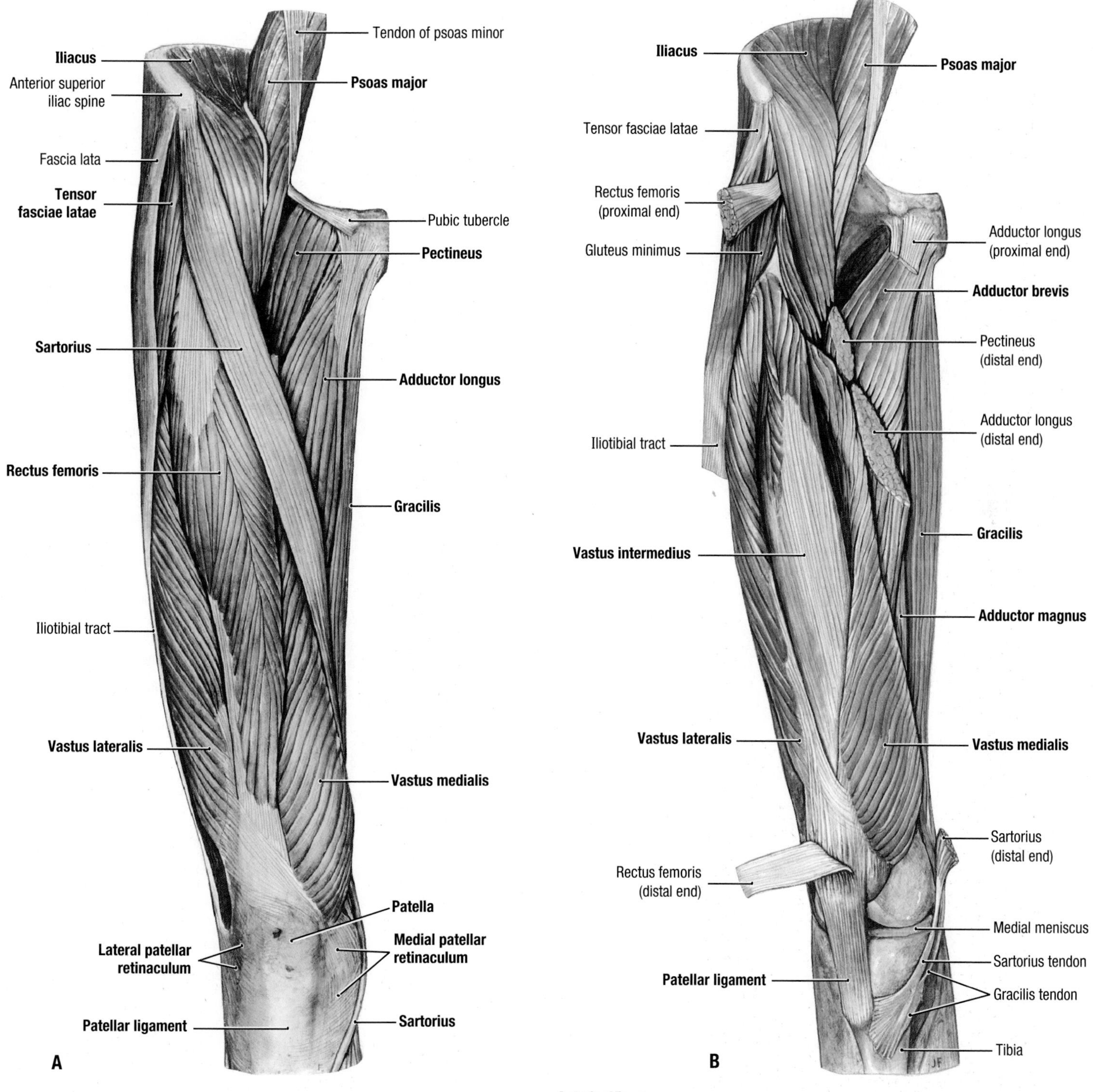
Tendon of psoas minor
Iliacus
Anterior superior iliac spine
Psoas major
Fascia lata
Tensor fasciae latae
Pubic tubercle
Pectineus
Sartorius
Adductor longus
Rectus femoris
Gracilis
Iliotibial tract
Vastus lateralis
Vastus medialis
Patella
Lateral patellar retinaculum
Medial patellar retinaculum
Patellar ligament
Sartorius
A
Iliacus
Psoas major
Tensor fasciae latae
Rectus femoris (proximal end)
Adductor longus (proximal end)
Gluteus minimus
Adductor brevis
Pectineus (distal end)
Adductor longus (distal end)
Iliotibial tract
Gracilis
Vastus intermedius
Adductor magnus
Vastus lateralis
Vastus medialis
Sartorius (distal end)
Rectus femoris (distal end)
Medial meniscus
Sartorius tendon
Patellar ligament
Gracilis tendon
Tibia
B
Anterior Views

5.21 ANTERIOR AND MEDIAL THIGH MUSCLES, SUPERFICIAL AND DEEP DISSECTIONS

A. Superficial dissection. **B.** Deep dissection. The central portions of the muscle bellies of the sartorius, rectus femoris, pectineus, and adductor longus muscles have been removed. **Weakness of the vastus medialis or vastus lateralis,** resulting from arthritis or trauma to the knee joint, for example, can result in abnormal patellar movement and loss of joint stability.

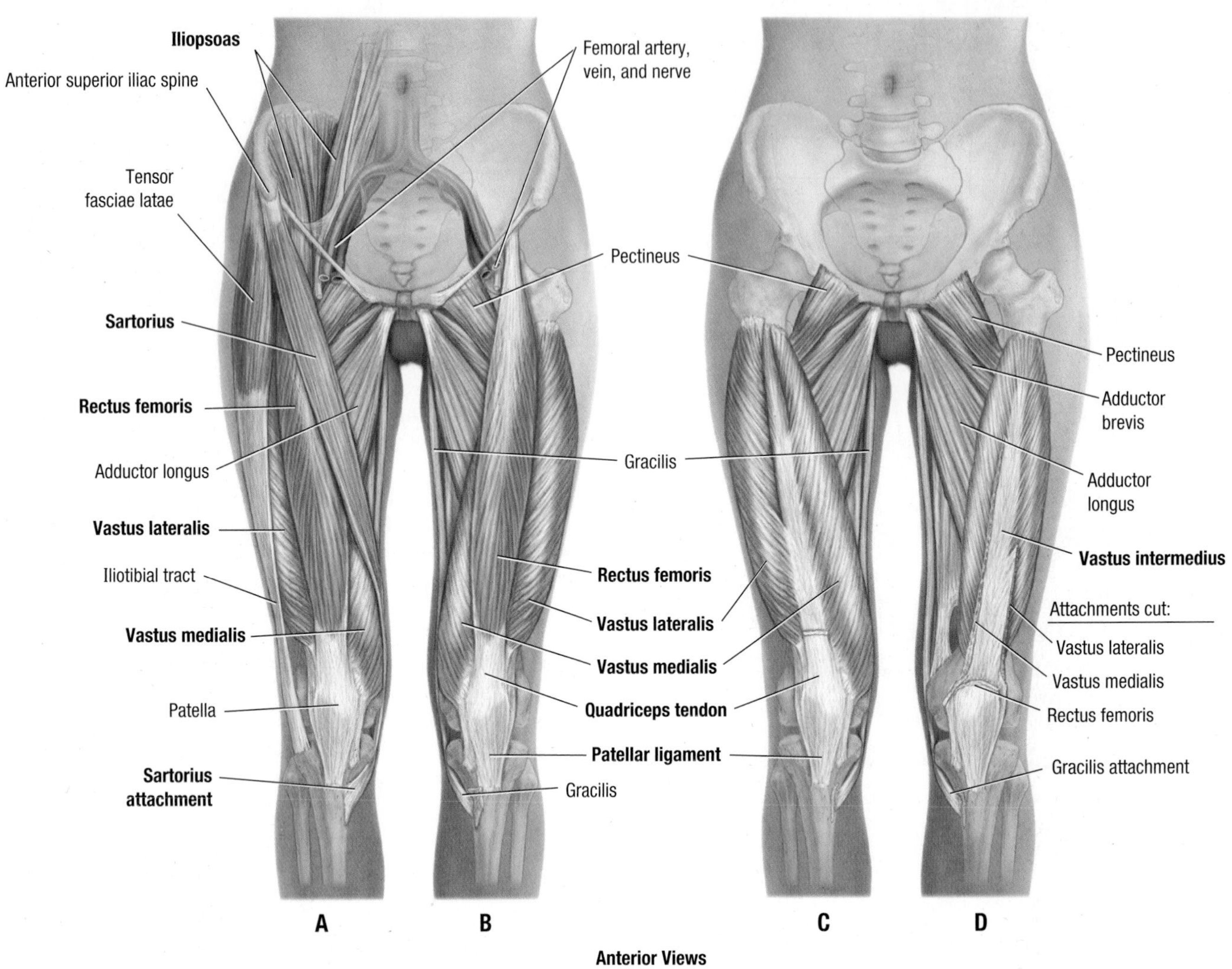

Iliopsoas
Anterior superior iliac spine
Femoral artery, vein, and nerve
Tensor fasciae latae
Pectineus
Sartorius
Rectus femoris
Adductor longus
Vastus lateralis
Iliotibial tract
Vastus medialis
Patella
Sartorius attachment
Gracilis
Rectus femoris
Vastus lateralis
Vastus medialis
Quadriceps tendon
Patellar ligament
Gracilis
Pectineus
Adductor brevis
Adductor longus
Vastus intermedius
Attachments cut:
Vastus lateralis
Vastus medialis
Rectus femoris
Gracilis attachment
A
B
C
D
Anterior Views

5.22 ANTERIOR AND MEDIAL THIGH MUSCLES, SCHEMATIC ILLUSTRATIONS

A.–D. Sequential views from superficial to deep.

A "hip pointer," which is a **contusion of the iliac crest,** usually occurs at its anterior part (e.g., where the sartorius attaches to the anterior superior iliac spine). This is one of the most common injuries to the hip region, usually occurring in association with collision sports. Contusions cause bleeding from ruptured capillaries and infiltration of blood into the muscles, tendons, and other soft tissues. The term hip pointer may also refer to avulsion of bony muscle attachments, for example, of the sartorius or rectus femoris from the anterior superior or inferior iliac spines or of the iliopsoas from the lesser trochanter of the femur. However, these injuries should be called **avulsion fractures.**

A person with a **paralyzed quadriceps** cannot extend the leg against resistance and usually presses on the distal end of the thigh during walking to prevent inadvertent flexion of the knee joint.

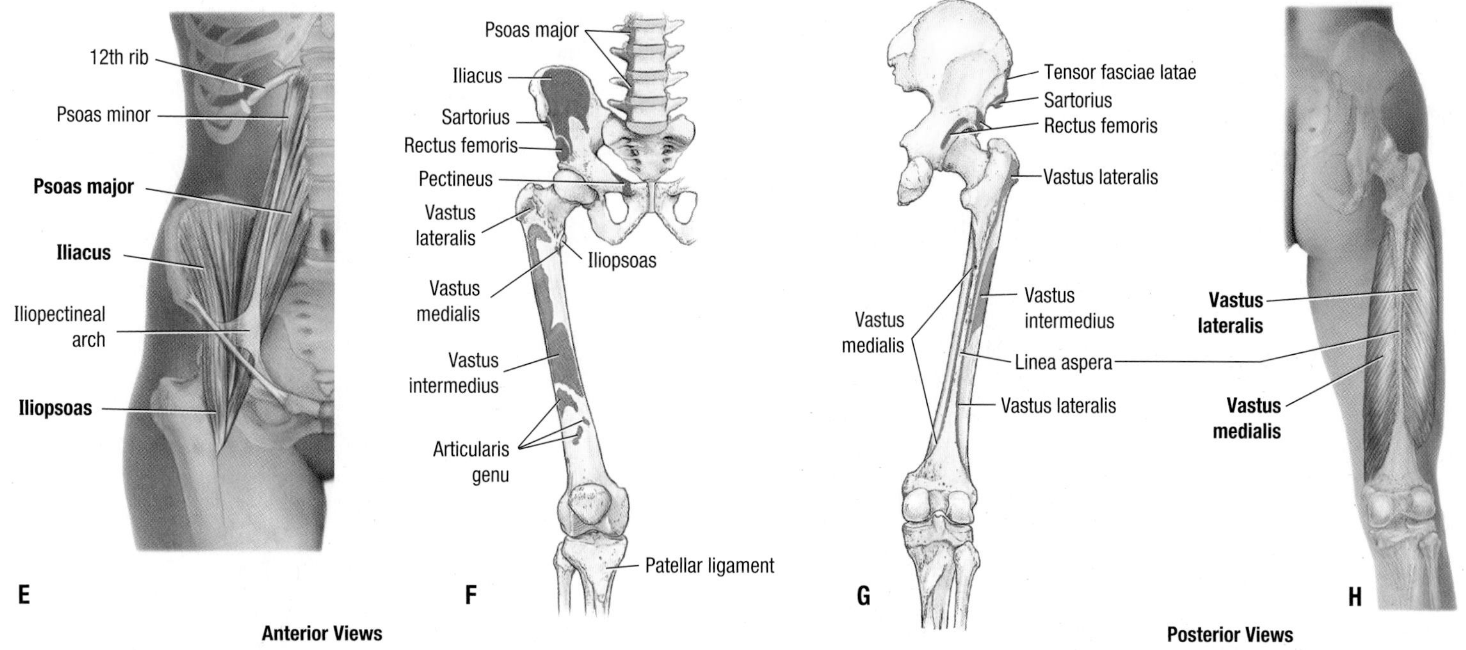
12th rib
Psoas minor
Psoas major
Iliacus
Iliopectineal arch
Iliopsoas
E
Psoas major
Iliacus
Sartorius
Rectus femoris
Pectineus
Vastus lateralis
Iliopsoas
Vastus medialis
Vastus intermedius
Articularis genu
Patellar ligament
F
Anterior Views
Tensor fasciae latae
Sartorius
Rectus femoris
Vastus lateralis
Vastus intermedius
Vastus medialis
Linea aspera
Vastus lateralis
G
Vastus lateralis
Vastus medialis
H
Posterior Views

5.22 ANTERIOR AND MEDIAL THIGH MUSCLES, SCHEMATIC ILLUSTRATIONS (*CONTINUED)*

E. Iliopsoas. **F. and G.** Attachments of anterior muscles of thigh. **H.** Posterior attachment of vastus medialis and lateralis.

TABLE 5.5 MUSCLES OF ANTERIOR THIGH

Muscle	Proximal Attachment[a]	Distal Attachment[a]	Innervation[b]	Main Actions
Iliopsoas				
Psoas major	Lateral aspects of T12–L5 vertebrae and IV discs; transverse processes of all lumbar vertebrae	Lesser trochanter of femur	Anterior rami of lumbar nerves (**L1, L2,** and L3)	Flexes and stabilizes[c] hip joint
Iliacus	Iliac crest, iliac fossa, ala of sacrum and anterior sacro-iliac ligaments	Tendon of psoas major, lesser trochanter, and femur distal to it	Femoral nerve (L2 and L3)	
Tensor fasciae latae	Anterior superior iliac spine and anterior part of iliac crest	Iliotibial tract that attaches to lateral condyle of tibia	Superior gluteal (L4 and L5)	Abducts, medially rotates, and flexes hip joint; helps to keep knee extended; steadies trunk on thigh
Sartorius	Anterior superior iliac spine and superior part of notch inferior to it	Superior part of medial surface of tibia	Femoral nerve (L2 and L3)	Flexes, abducts, and laterally rotates hip joint; flexes knee joint[d]
Quadriceps femoris				
Rectus femoris	Anterior inferior iliac spine and ilium superior to acetabulum	Base of patella and by patellar ligament to tibial tuberosity; medial and lateral vasti also attach to tibia and patella via aponeuroses (medial and lateral patellar retinacula)	Femoral nerve (L2, **L3,** and **L4**)	Extends knee joint; rectus femoris also steadies hip joint and helps iliopsoas to flex hip joint
Vastus lateralis	Greater trochanter and lateral lip of linea aspera of femur			
Vastus medialis	Intertrochanteric line and medial lip of linea aspera of femur			
Vastus intermedius	Anterior and lateral surfaces of body of femur			

[a]See also Figure 5.22 for muscle attachments.
[b]Numbers indicate spinal cord segmental innervation of nerves (e.g., L1, L2, and L3 indicate that nerves supplying psoas major are derived from first three lumbar segments of the spinal cord; boldface type [**L1, L2**] indicates main segmental innervation). Damage to one or more of these spinal cord segments or to motor nerve roots arising from these segments results in paralysis of the muscles concerned.
[c]Psoas major is also a postural muscle that helps control deviation of trunk and is active during standing.
[d]Four actions of sartorius (L. sartor, tailor) produce the once-common cross-legged sitting position used by tailors—hence the name.

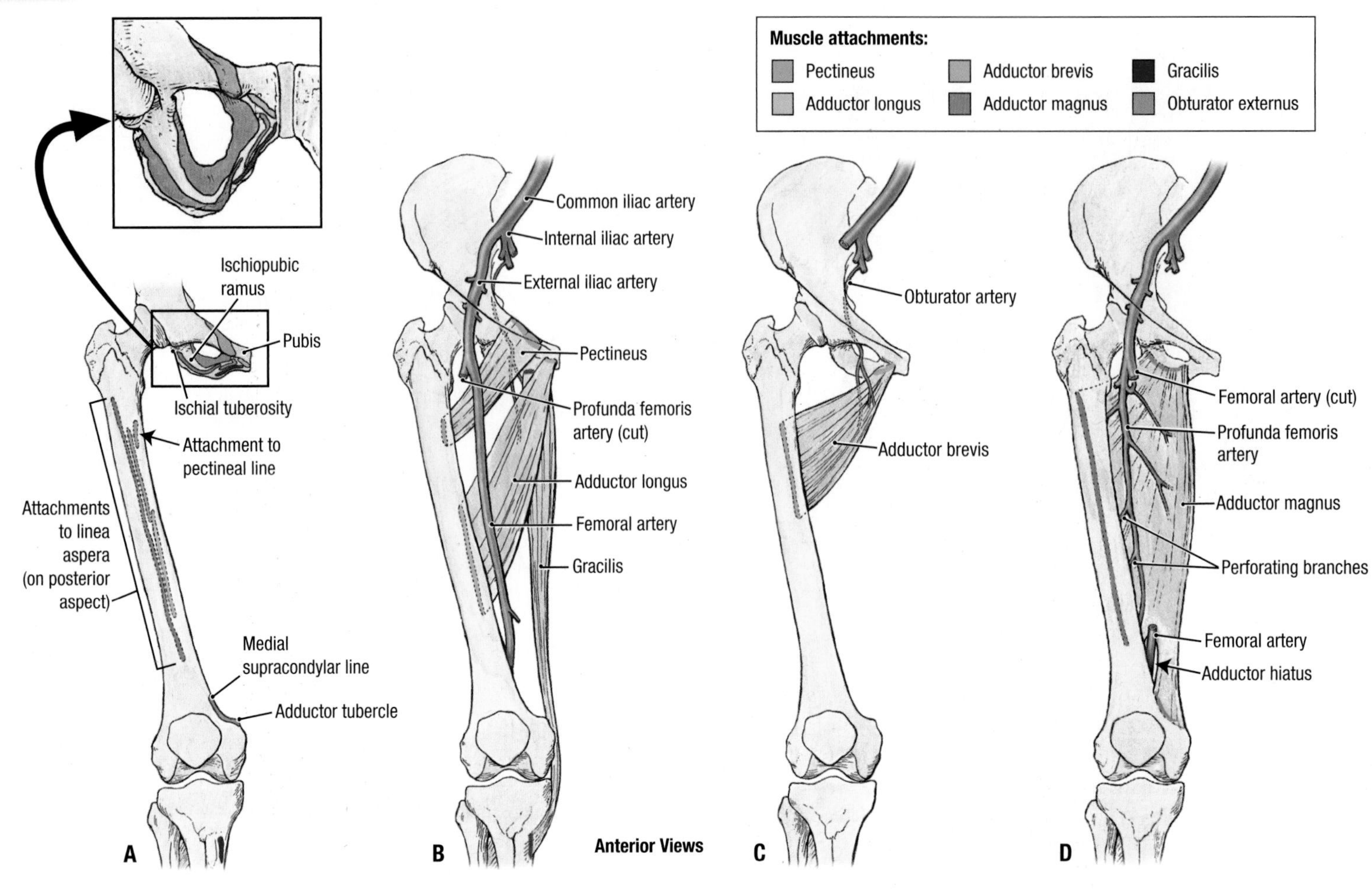

Muscle attachments:
Pectineus
Adductor brevis
Gracilis
Adductor longus
Adductor magnus
Obturator externus
Ischiopubic ramus
Pubis
Ischial tuberosity
Attachment to pectineal line
Attachments to linea aspera (on posterior aspect)
Medial supracondylar line
Adductor tubercle
Common iliac artery
Internal iliac artery
External iliac artery
Pectineus
Profunda femoris artery (cut)
Adductor longus
Femoral artery
Gracilis
Obturator artery
Adductor brevis
Femoral artery (cut)
Profunda femoris artery
Adductor magnus
Perforating branches
Femoral artery
Adductor hiatus
A
B
Anterior Views
C
D

5.23 ATTACHMENTS OF MUSCLES OF MEDIAL ASPECT OF THIGH

A. Overview of attachments. **B.** Pectineus, adductor longus, and gracilis. **C.** Adductor brevis. **D.** Adductor magnus.

TABLE 5.6 MUSCLES OF MEDIAL THIGH

Muscle	Proximal Attachment	Distal Attachment[a]	Innervation[b]	Main Actions
Pectineus	Superior pubic ramus	Pectineal line of femur, just inferior to lesser trochanter	Femoral nerve (**L2** and L3) may receive a branch from obturator nerve	Adducts and flexes hip joint; assists with medial rotation of hip joint
Adductor longus	Body of pubis inferior to pubic crest	Middle third of linea aspera of femur	Obturator nerve, anterior branch (L2, **L3**, and L4)	Adducts hip joint
Adductor brevis	Body of pubis and inferior pubic ramus	Pectineal line and proximal part of linea aspera of femur	Obturator nerve (L2, **L3**, and L4)	Adducts hip joint and, to some extent, flexes it
Adductor magnus	Inferior pubic ramus, ramus of ischium (adductor part), and ischial tuberosity	Gluteal tuberosity, linea aspera, medial supracondylar line (adductor part), and adductor tubercle of femur (hamstring part)	*Adductor part:* obturator nerve (L2, **L3**, and **L4**) *Hamstring part:* tibial part of sciatic nerve **(L4)**	Adducts hip joint; its adductor part also flexes hip joint, and its hamstring part extends it
Gracilis	Body of pubis and inferior pubic ramus	Superior part of medial surface of tibia	Obturator nerve (**L2** and L3)	Adducts hip joint, flexes knee joint, and helps rotate it medially
Obturator externus	Margins of obturator foramen and obturator membrane	Trochanteric fossa of femur	Obturator nerve (L3 and **L4)**	Laterally rotates hip joint; steadies head of femur in acetabulum

Collectively, the first five muscles listed are the adductors of the thigh, but their actions are more complex (e.g., they act as flexors of the hip joint during flexion of the knee joint and are active during walking).
[a]See Figure 5.22 for muscle attachments.
[b]See Table 5.1 for explanation of segmental innervation.

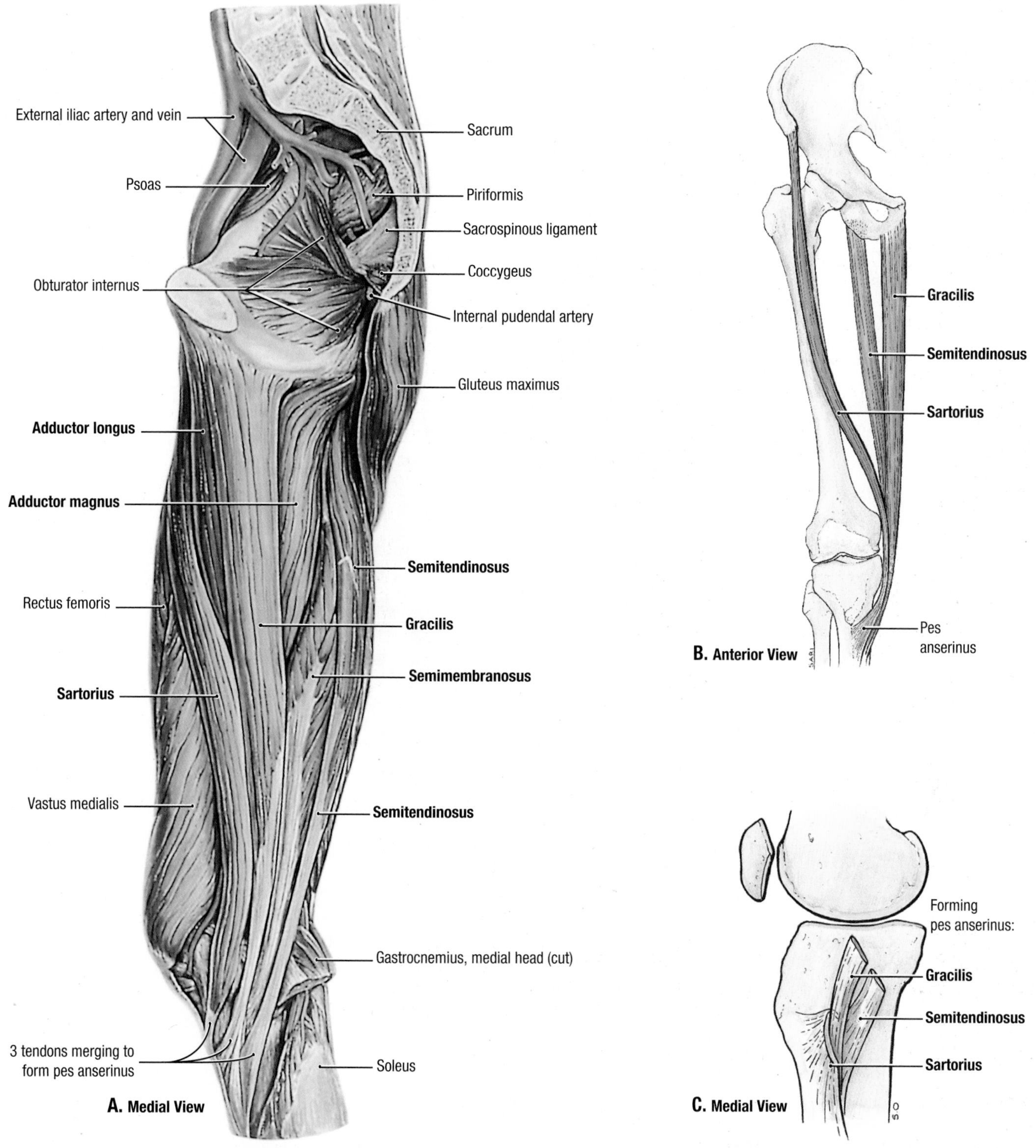
External iliac artery and vein
Psoas
Obturator internus
Adductor longus
Adductor magnus
Rectus femoris
Sartorius
Vastus medialis
3 tendons merging to form pes anserinus
Sacrum
Piriformis
Sacrospinous ligament
Coccygeus
Internal pudendal artery
Gluteus maximus
Semitendinosus
Gracilis
Semimembranosus
Semitendinosus
Gastrocnemius, medial head (cut)
Soleus
A. Medial View
Gracilis
Semitendinosus
Sartorius
Pes anserinus
B. Anterior View
Forming pes anserinus:
Gracilis
Semitendinosus
Sartorius
C. Medial View

5.24 MUSCLES OF MEDIAL ASPECT OF THIGH

A. Dissection. **B.** Muscular tripod. The sartorius, gracilis, and semitendinosus muscles form an inverted tripod arising from three different components of the hip bone. These muscles course within three different compartments, perform three different functions, and are innervated by three different nerves yet share a common distal attachment. **C.** Distal attachment of sartorius, gracilis, and semitendinosus muscles. All three tendons become thin and aponeurotic and are collectively referred to as the pes anserinus. The gracilis is a relatively weak member of the adductor group and hence can be removed without noticeable loss of its actions on the leg. Surgeons often **transplant the gracilis**, or part of it, with its nerve and blood vessels to replace a damaged muscle in the hand, for example.

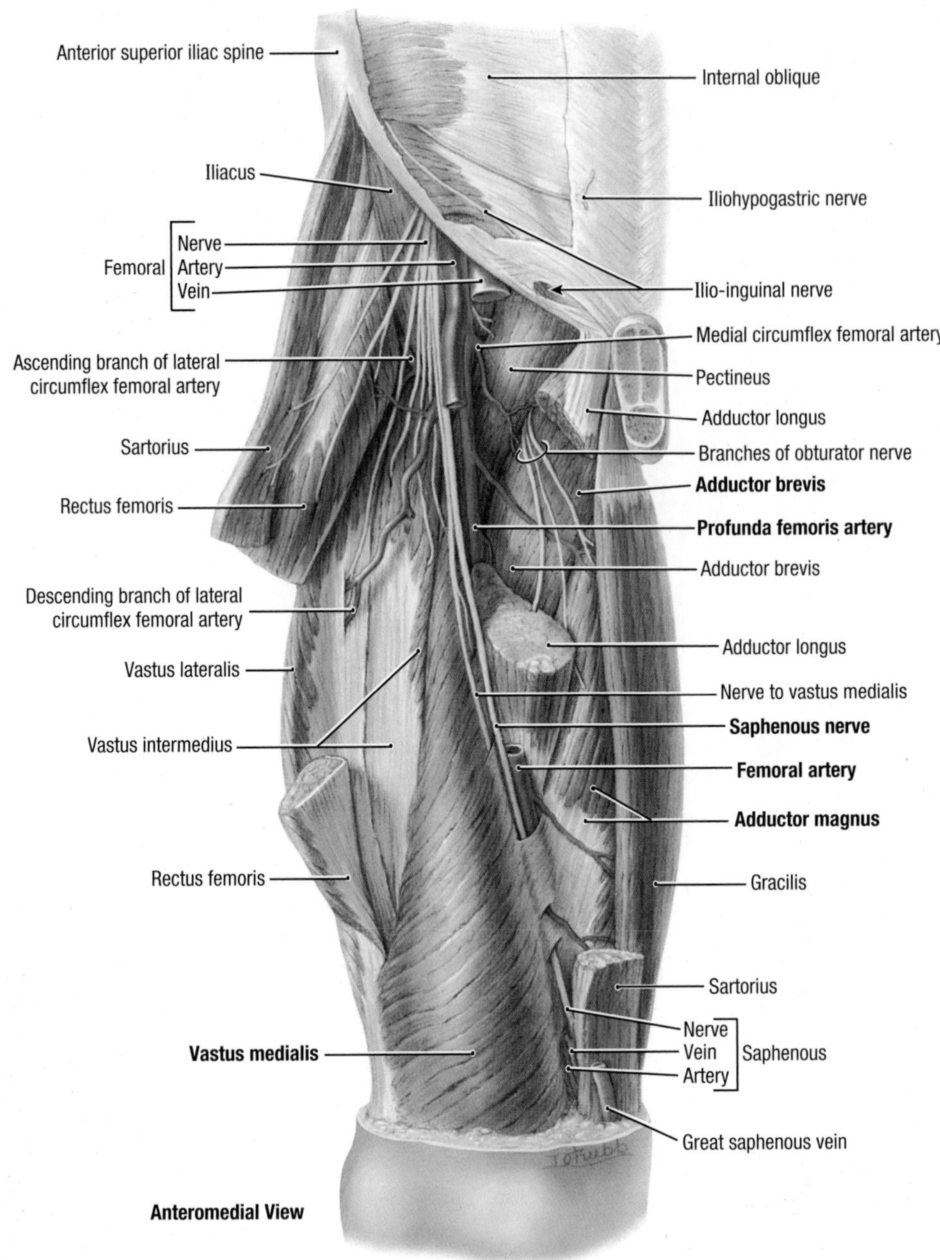
Anterior superior iliac spine
Internal oblique
Iliacus
Iliohypogastric nerve
Femoral
Nerve
Artery
Vein
Ilio-inguinal nerve
Medial circumflex femoral artery
Ascending branch of lateral circumflex femoral artery
Pectineus
Adductor longus
Sartorius
Branches of obturator nerve
Adductor brevis
Rectus femoris
Profunda femoris artery
Adductor brevis
Descending branch of lateral circumflex femoral artery
Adductor longus
Vastus lateralis
Nerve to vastus medialis
Saphenous nerve
Vastus intermedius
Femoral artery
Adductor magnus
Rectus femoris
Gracilis
Sartorius
Nerve
Vein
Artery
Saphenous
Vastus medialis
Great saphenous vein
Anteromedial View

5.25 ANTEROMEDIAL ASPECT OF THIGH

- The limb is rotated laterally.
- The femoral nerve breaks up into several nerves on entering the thigh.
- The femoral artery lies between two motor territories: that of the obturator nerve, which is medial, and that of the femoral nerve, which is lateral. No motor nerve crosses anterior to the femoral artery, but the twig to the pectineus muscle crosses posterior to the femoral artery.
- The nerve to the vastus medialis muscle and the saphenous nerve accompany the femoral artery into the adductor canal. The saphenous nerve and artery and their anastomotic accompanying vein emerge from the canal distally between the sartorius and gracilis muscles.
- The profunda femoris artery (deep artery of thigh) is the largest branch of the femoral artery and the chief artery to the thigh. It arises from the femoral artery in the femoral triangle. In the middle third of the thigh, it is separated from the femoral artery and vein by the adductor longus. It gives off three or four perforating arteries that wrap around the posterior aspect of the femur and supply the adductor magnus, hamstring and vastus lateralis muscles.

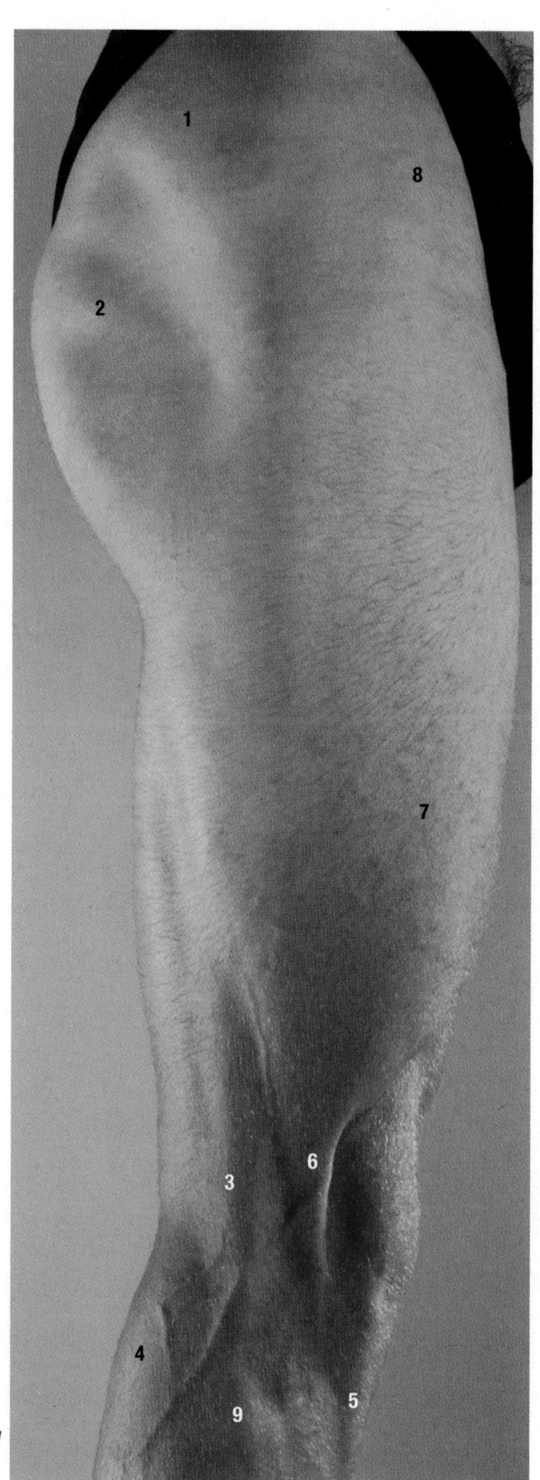
1
8
2
7
6
3
4
9
5

A. Lateral View

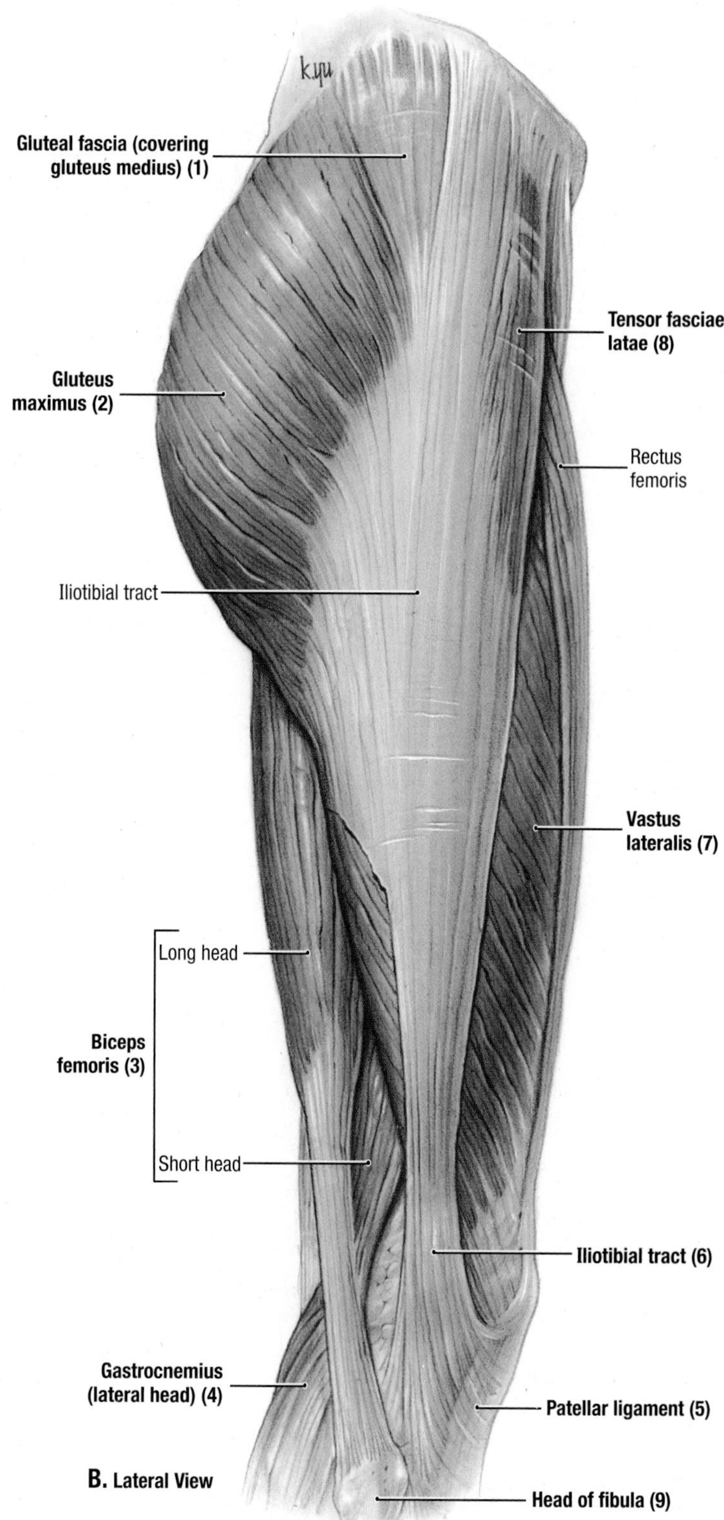
Gluteal fascia (covering gluteus medius) (1)
Tensor fasciae latae (8)
Gluteus maximus (2)
Rectus femoris
Iliotibial tract
Vastus lateralis (7)
Long head
Biceps femoris (3)
Short head
Iliotibial tract (6)
Gastrocnemius (lateral head) (4)
Patellar ligament (5)
Head of fibula (9)

B. Lateral View

5.26 LATERAL ASPECT OF THIGH

A. Surface anatomy (*numbers* refer to structures in **B**). **B.** Dissection showing the iliotibial tract, a thickening of the fascia lata, which serves as a tendon for the gluteus maximus and tensor fasciae latae. The iliotibial tract attaches to the anterolateral (Gerdy) tubercle of the lateral condyle of the tibia. The biceps femoris tendon attaches on the head of the fibula.

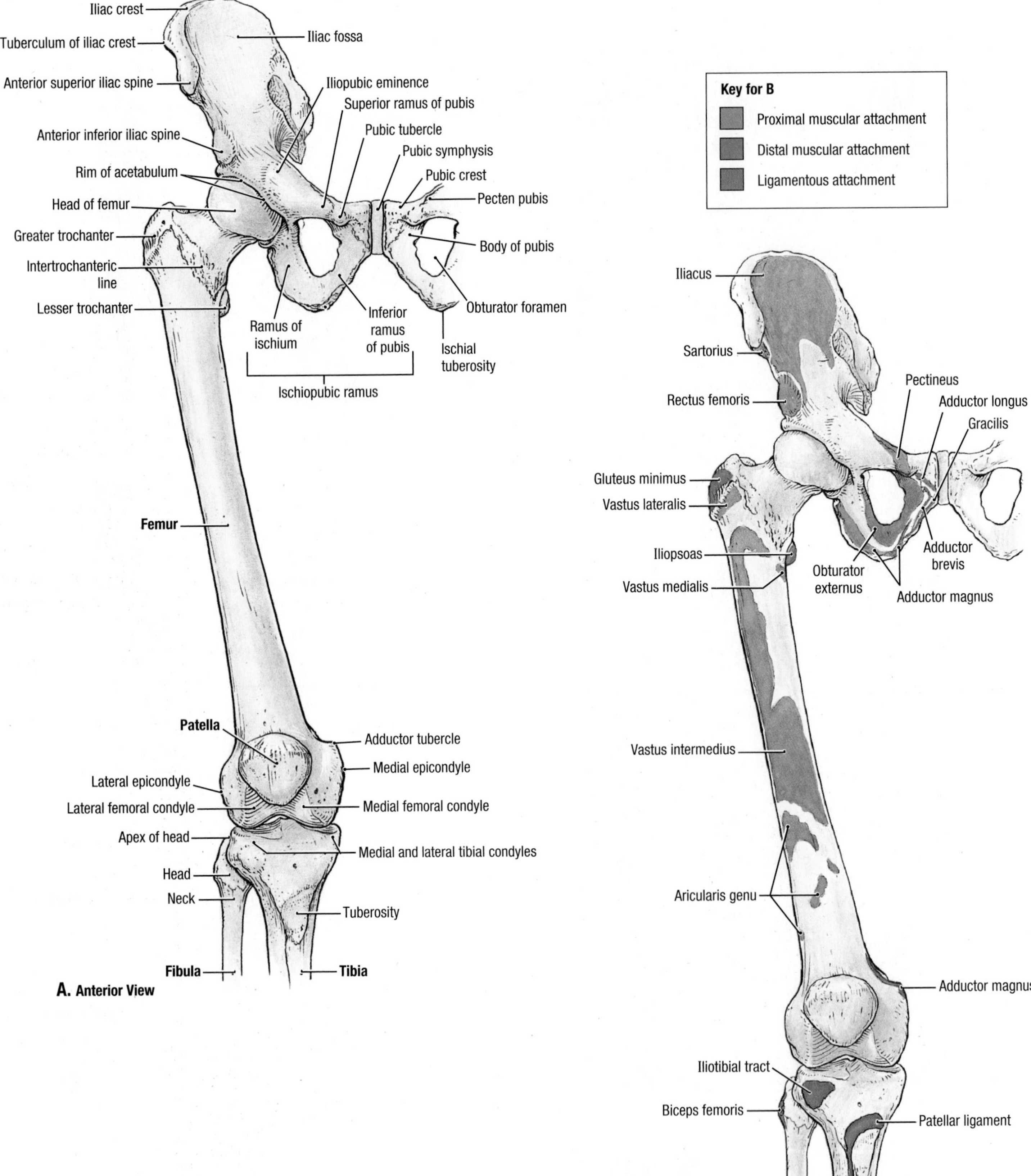
Iliac crest
Tuberculum of iliac crest
Iliac fossa
Anterior superior iliac spine
Iliopubic eminence
Superior ramus of pubis
Anterior inferior iliac spine
Pubic tubercle
Pubic symphysis
Rim of acetabulum
Pubic crest
Pecten pubis
Head of femur
Greater trochanter
Body of pubis
Intertrochanteric line
Lesser trochanter
Obturator foramen
Inferior ramus of pubis
Ramus of ischium
Ischial tuberosity
Ischiopubic ramus
Femur
Patella
Adductor tubercle
Medial epicondyle
Lateral epicondyle
Lateral femoral condyle
Medial femoral condyle
Apex of head
Medial and lateral tibial condyles
Head
Neck
Tuberosity
Fibula
Tibia
A. Anterior View
Key for B
Proximal muscular attachment
Distal muscular attachment
Ligamentous attachment
Iliacus
Sartorius
Rectus femoris
Pectineus
Adductor longus
Gracilis
Gluteus minimus
Vastus lateralis
Iliopsoas
Vastus medialis
Obturator externus
Adductor brevis
Adductor magnus
Vastus intermedius
Aricularis genu
Adductor magnus
Iliotibial tract
Biceps femoris
Patellar ligament
B. Anterior View

5.27 BONES OF THE THIGH AND PROXIMAL LEG

A. Bony features. **B.** Muscle attachment sites.

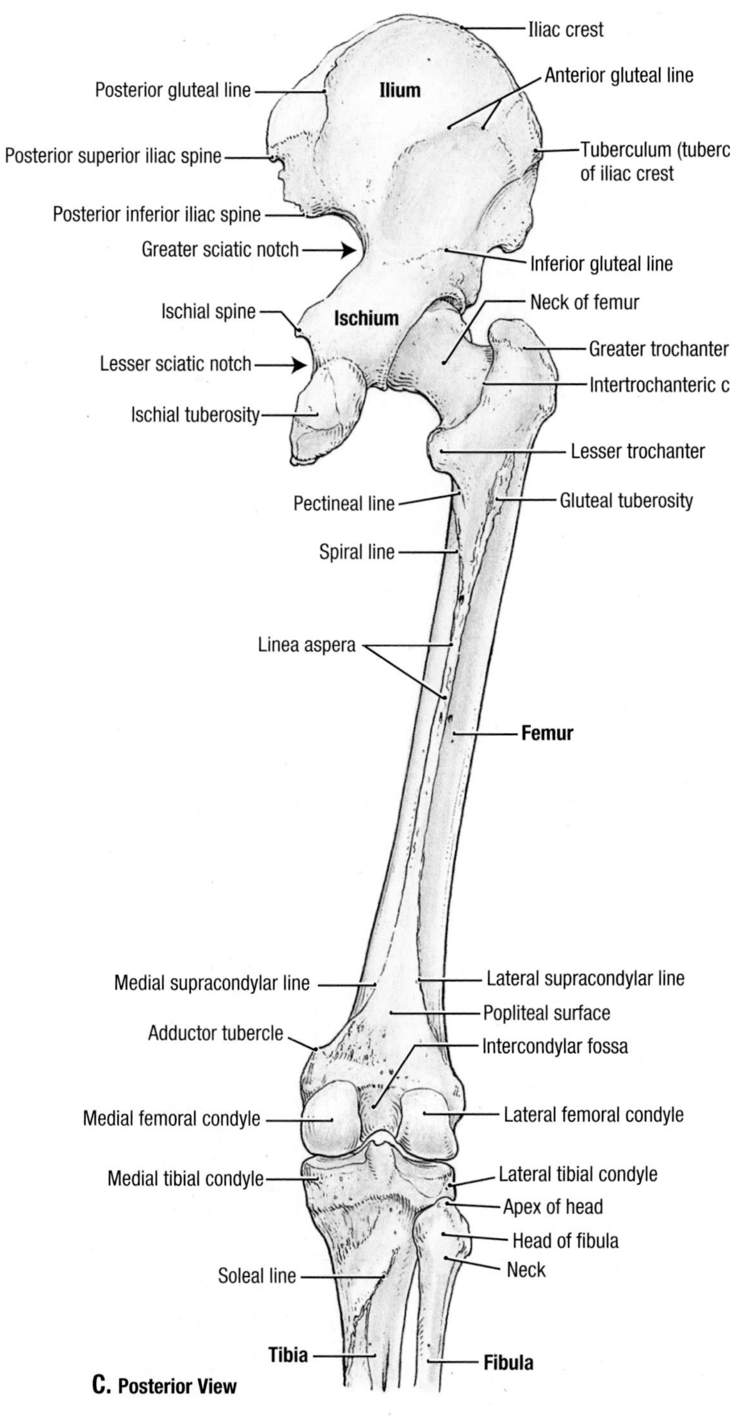
Iliac crest
Posterior gluteal line
Ilium
Anterior gluteal line
Posterior superior iliac spine
Tuberculum (tubercle) of iliac crest
Posterior inferior iliac spine
Greater sciatic notch
Inferior gluteal line
Ischial spine
Ischium
Neck of femur
Greater trochanter
Lesser sciatic notch
Intertrochanteric crest
Ischial tuberosity
Lesser trochanter
Pectineal line
Gluteal tuberosity
Spiral line
Linea aspera
Femur
Medial supracondylar line
Lateral supracondylar line
Popliteal surface
Adductor tubercle
Intercondylar fossa
Medial femoral condyle
Lateral femoral condyle
Medial tibial condyle
Lateral tibial condyle
Apex of head
Head of fibula
Neck
Soleal line
Tibia
Fibula

C. Posterior View

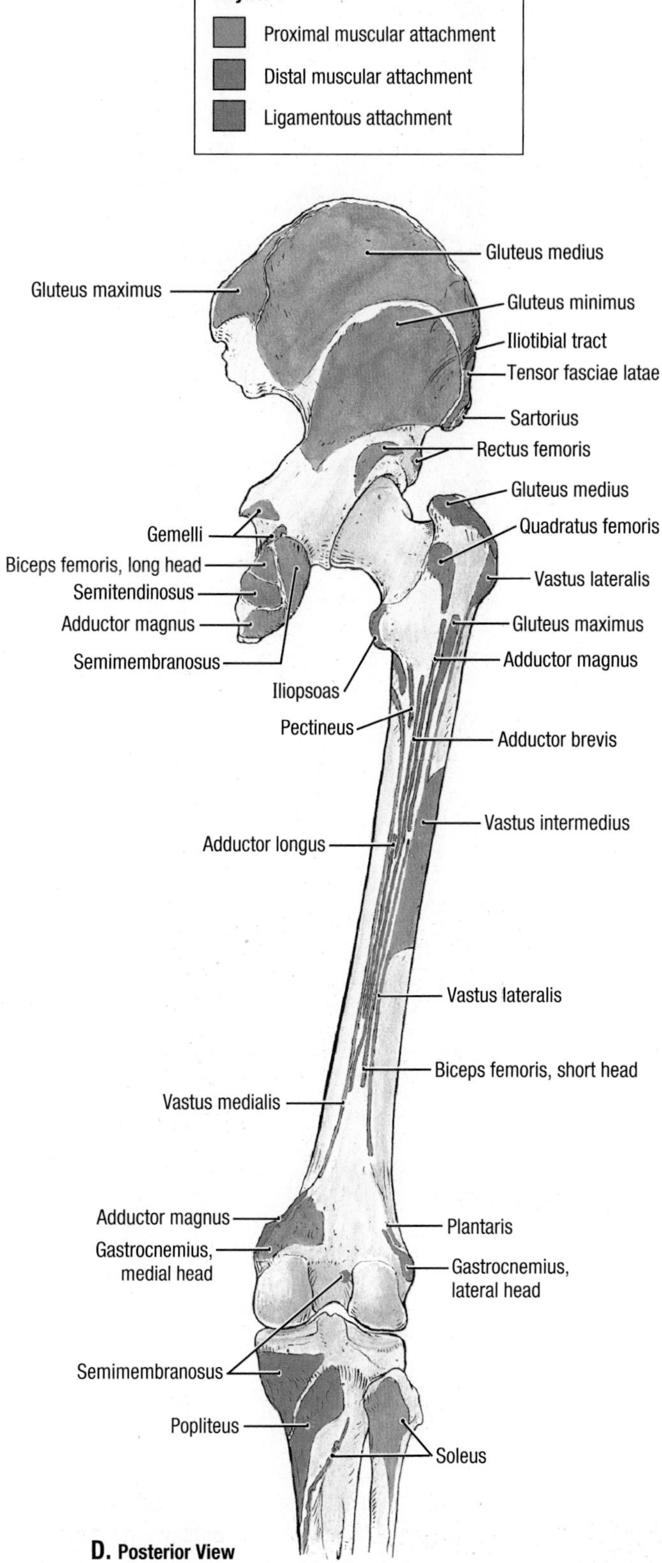
Key for D
Proximal muscular attachment
Distal muscular attachment
Ligamentous attachment
Gluteus medius
Gluteus maximus
Gluteus minimus
Iliotibial tract
Tensor fasciae latae
Sartorius
Rectus femoris
Gluteus medius
Quadratus femoris
Gemelli
Biceps femoris, long head
Vastus lateralis
Semitendinosus
Adductor magnus
Gluteus maximus
Semimembranosus
Adductor magnus
Iliopsoas
Pectineus
Adductor brevis
Vastus intermedius
Adductor longus
Vastus lateralis
Biceps femoris, short head
Vastus medialis
Adductor magnus
Plantaris
Gastrocnemius, medial head
Gastrocnemius, lateral head
Semimembranosus
Popliteus
Soleus

D. Posterior View

5.27 BONES OF THE THIGH AND PROXIMAL LEG (*CONTINUED*)

C. Bony features. **D.** Muscle attachment sites.

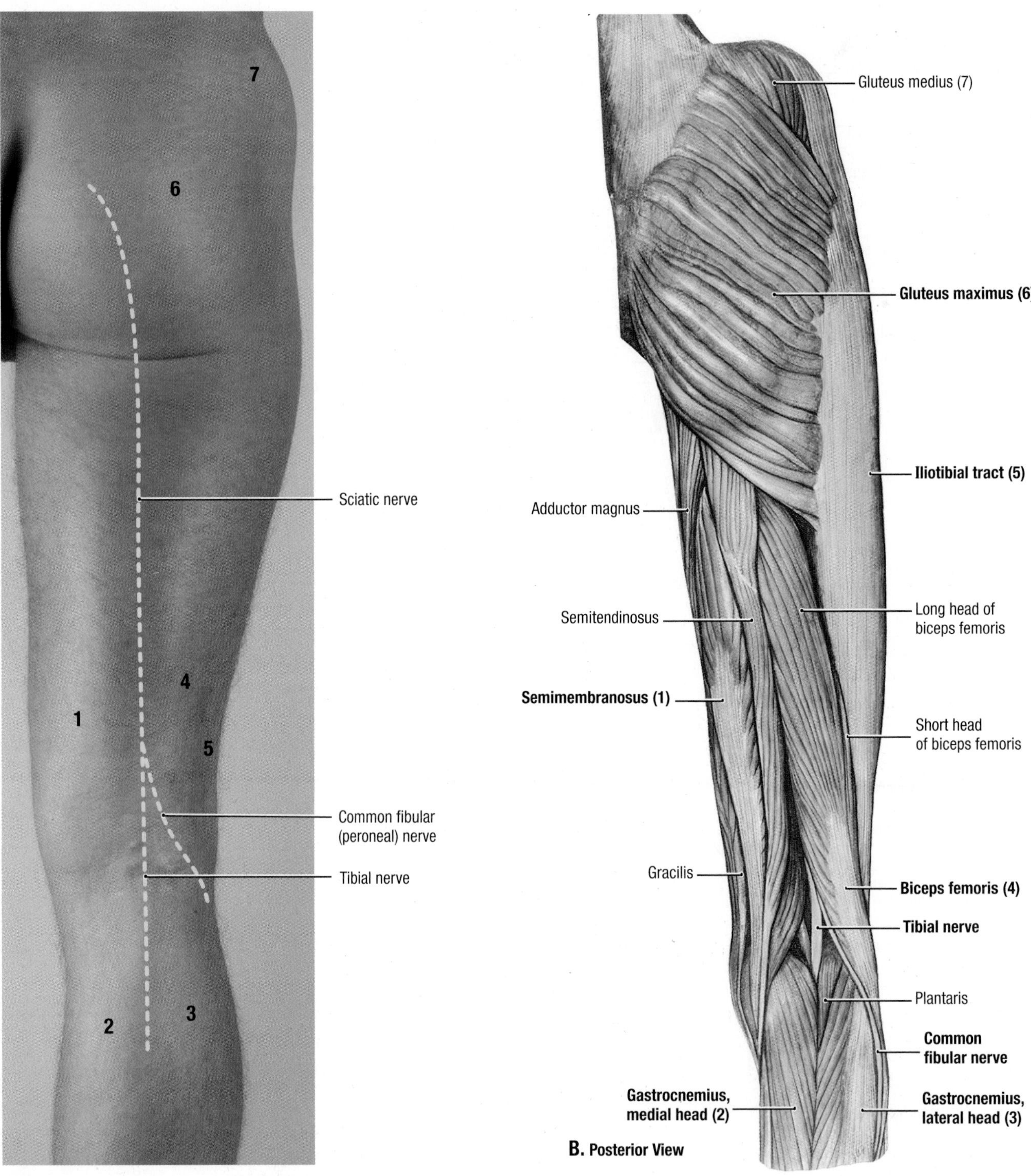

7
6
Sciatic nerve
4
1
5
Common fibular (peroneal) nerve
Tibial nerve
2
3
A. Posterior View
Gluteus medius (7)
Gluteus maximus (6)
Iliotibial tract (5)
Adductor magnus
Semitendinosus
Long head of biceps femoris
Semimembranosus (1)
Short head of biceps femoris
Gracilis
Biceps femoris (4)
Tibial nerve
Plantaris
Common fibular nerve
Gastrocnemius, medial head (2)
Gastrocnemius, lateral head (3)
B. Posterior View

5.28 MUSCLES OF THE GLUTEAL REGION AND POSTERIOR THIGH I

A. Surface anatomy (*numbers* refer to structures in **B**). **B.** Superficial dissection of muscles of gluteal region and posterior thigh (hamstring muscles consisting of semimembranosus, semitendinosus, and biceps femoris). **Hamstring strains** (pulled and/or torn hamstrings) are common in running, jumping, and quick-start sports. The muscular exertion required to excel in these sports may tear part of the proximal attachments of the hamstrings from the ischial tuberosity.

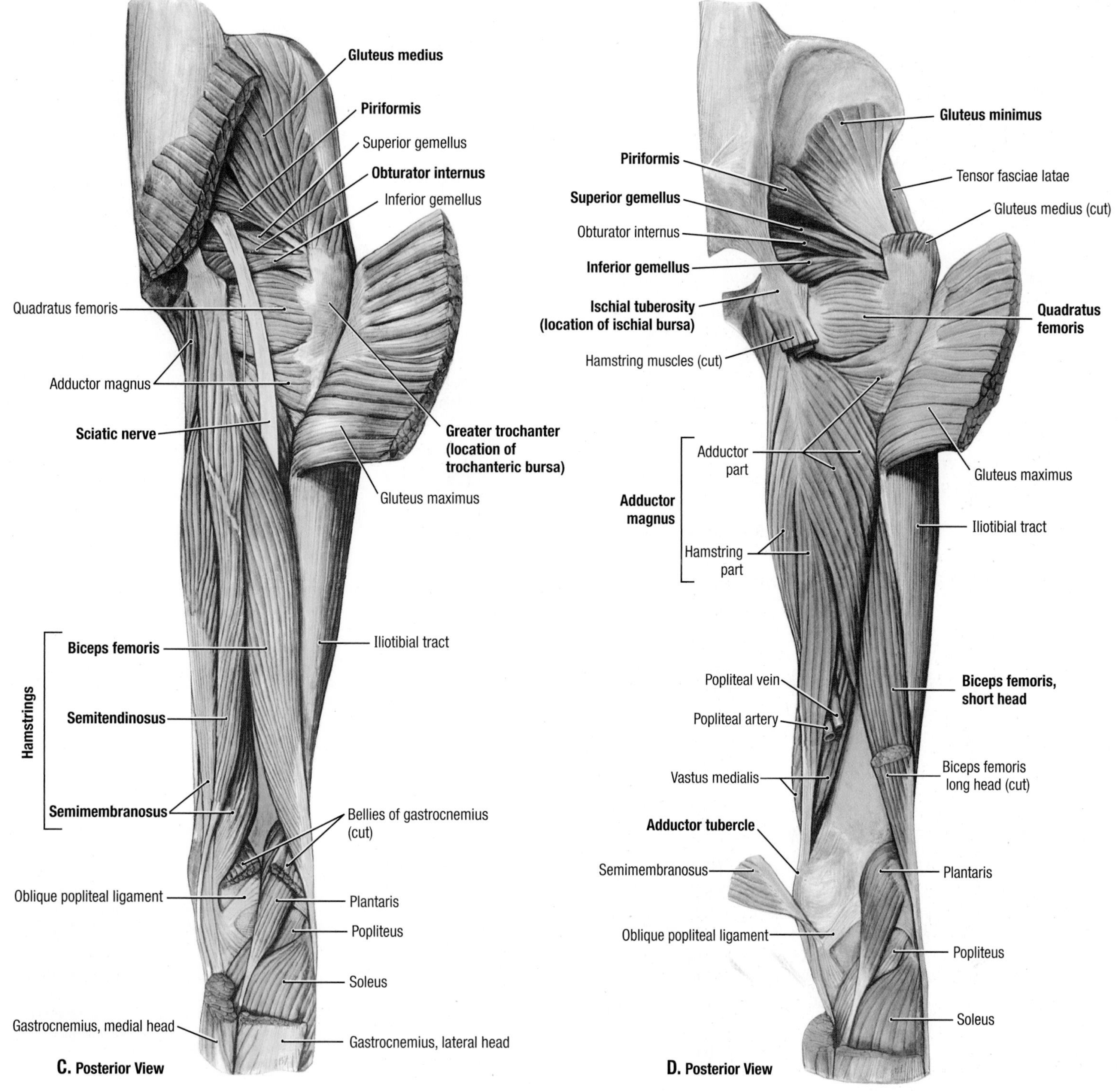
Gluteus medius
Piriformis
Superior gemellus
Obturator internus
Inferior gemellus
Quadratus femoris
Adductor magnus
Sciatic nerve
Greater trochanter (location of trochanteric bursa)
Gluteus maximus
Iliotibial tract
Hamstrings
Biceps femoris
Semitendinosus
Semimembranosus
Bellies of gastrocnemius (cut)
Oblique popliteal ligament
Plantaris
Popliteus
Soleus
Gastrocnemius, medial head
Gastrocnemius, lateral head
C. Posterior View
Gluteus minimus
Piriformis
Tensor fasciae latae
Superior gemellus
Gluteus medius (cut)
Obturator internus
Inferior gemellus
Ischial tuberosity (location of ischial bursa)
Quadratus femoris
Hamstring muscles (cut)
Adductor part
Gluteus maximus
Adductor magnus
Iliotibial tract
Hamstring part
Popliteal vein
Biceps femoris, short head
Popliteal artery
Biceps femoris long head (cut)
Vastus medialis
Adductor tubercle
Semimembranosus
Plantaris
Oblique popliteal ligament
Popliteus
Soleus
D. Posterior View

5.28 MUSCLES OF GLUTEAL REGION AND POSTERIOR THIGH (*CONTINUED*) II AND III

C. Muscles of gluteal region and posterior thigh with gluteus maximus reflected. **D.** Adductor magnus muscle. The adductor magnus has two parts: one belongs to the adductor group, innervated by the obturator nerve and the other to the hamstring group, innervated by the tibial portion of the sciatic nerve. The trochanteric bursa separates the superior fibers of the gluteus maximus from the greater trochanter of the femur and the ischial bursa separates the inferior part of the gluteus maximus from the ischial tuberosity. Diffuse deep pain in the lateral thigh region (e.g., during stair climbing) may be caused by **trochanteric bursitis.** It is characterized by point tenderness over the greater trochanter, with pain radiating along the iliotibial tract. **Ischial bursitis** results from excessive friction between the ischial bursae and ischial tuberosities (e.g., as from cycling).

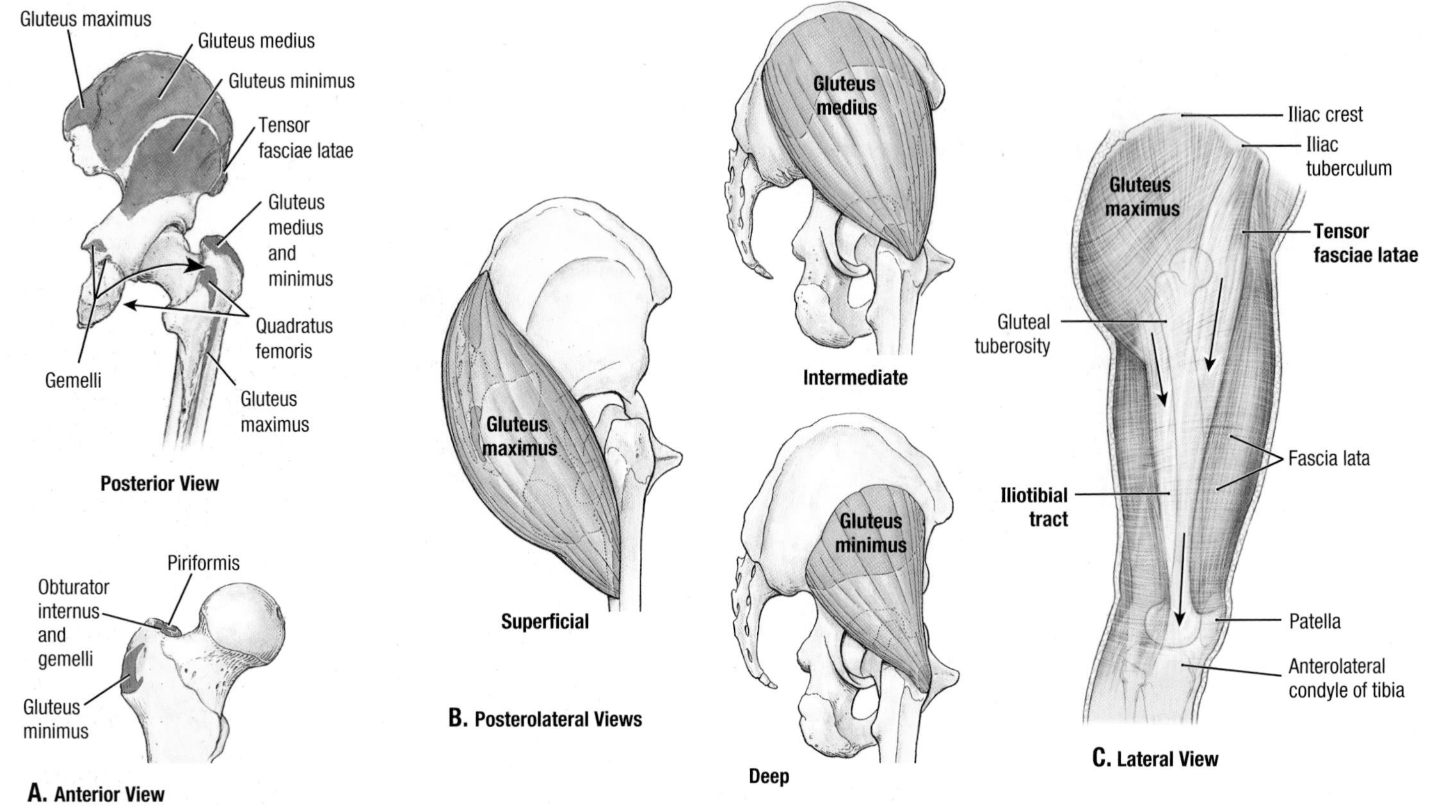
Gluteus maximus
Gluteus medius
Gluteus minimus
Tensor fasciae latae
Gluteus medius and minimus
Quadratus femoris
Gemelli
Gluteus maximus
Posterior View
Piriformis
Obturator internus and gemelli
Gluteus minimus
A. Anterior View
Gluteus maximus
Superficial
B. Posterolateral Views
Gluteus medius
Intermediate
Gluteus minimus
Deep
Iliac crest
Iliac tuberculum
Gluteus maximus
Tensor fasciae latae
Gluteal tuberosity
Fascia lata
Iliotibial tract
Patella
Anterolateral condyle of tibia
C. Lateral View

5.29 MUSCLES OF GLUTEAL REGION

A. Attachments. **B.** Relationship of gluteal muscles. **C.** Gluteus maximus and tensor fasciae latae.

TABLE 5.7 MUSCLES OF GLUTEAL REGION

Muscle	Proximal Attachment[a] (*Red*)	Distal Attachment[a] (*Blue*)	Innervation[b]	Main Actions
Gluteus maximus	Ilium posterior to posterior gluteal line, dorsal surface of sacrum and coccyx, sacrotuberous ligament	Iliotibial tract that inserts into lateral condyle of tibia; some fibers to gluteal tuberosity	Inferior gluteal nerve (L5, **S1, S2**)	Extends hip joint and assists in lateral rotation; steadies thigh and assists in raising trunk from flexed position
Gluteus medius	External surface of ilium between anterior and posterior gluteal lines; gluteal fascia	Lateral surface of greater trochanter of femur	Superior gluteal nerve (**L5,** S1)	Abducts and medially rotates hip joint[c]; keeps pelvis level when opposite leg is off ground and advances pelvis during swing phase of gait; TFL also contributes to stability of extended knee
Gluteus minimus	External surface of ilium between anterior and inferior gluteal lines	Anterior surface of greater trochanter of femur		
Tensor fasciae latae (TFL)	Anterior superior iliac spine and iliac crest	Iliotibial tract that attaches to lateral condyle (Gerdy tubercle) of tibia		
Piriformis	Anterior surface of sacrum and sacrotuberous ligament	Superior border of greater trochanter of femur	Anterior rami of S1 and S2	Laterally rotate extended hip joint and abduct flexed hip joint; steady femoral head in acetabulum
Obturator internus	Pelvic surface of obturator membrane and surrounding bones	Medial surface of greater trochanter of femur by common tendons	Nerve to obturator internus (L5, S1)	
Superior gemellus	Ischial spine			
Inferior gemellus	Ischial tuberosity			
Quadratus femoris	Lateral border of ischial tuberosity	Quadrate tubercle on intertrochanteric crest of femur	Nerve to quadratus femoris (L5, S1)	Laterally rotates hip joint,[d] steadies femoral head in acetabulum

[a]See Figure 5.22 for muscle attachments.
[b]See Table 5.1 for explanation of segmental innervation.
[c]Guteus medius and minimus: anterior fibers medially rotate hip joint and posterior fibers laterally rotate hip joint.
[d]There are six lateral rotators of the hip joint: piriformis, obturator internus, gemelli (superior and inferior), quadratus femoris, and obturator externus. These muscles also stabilize the hip joint.

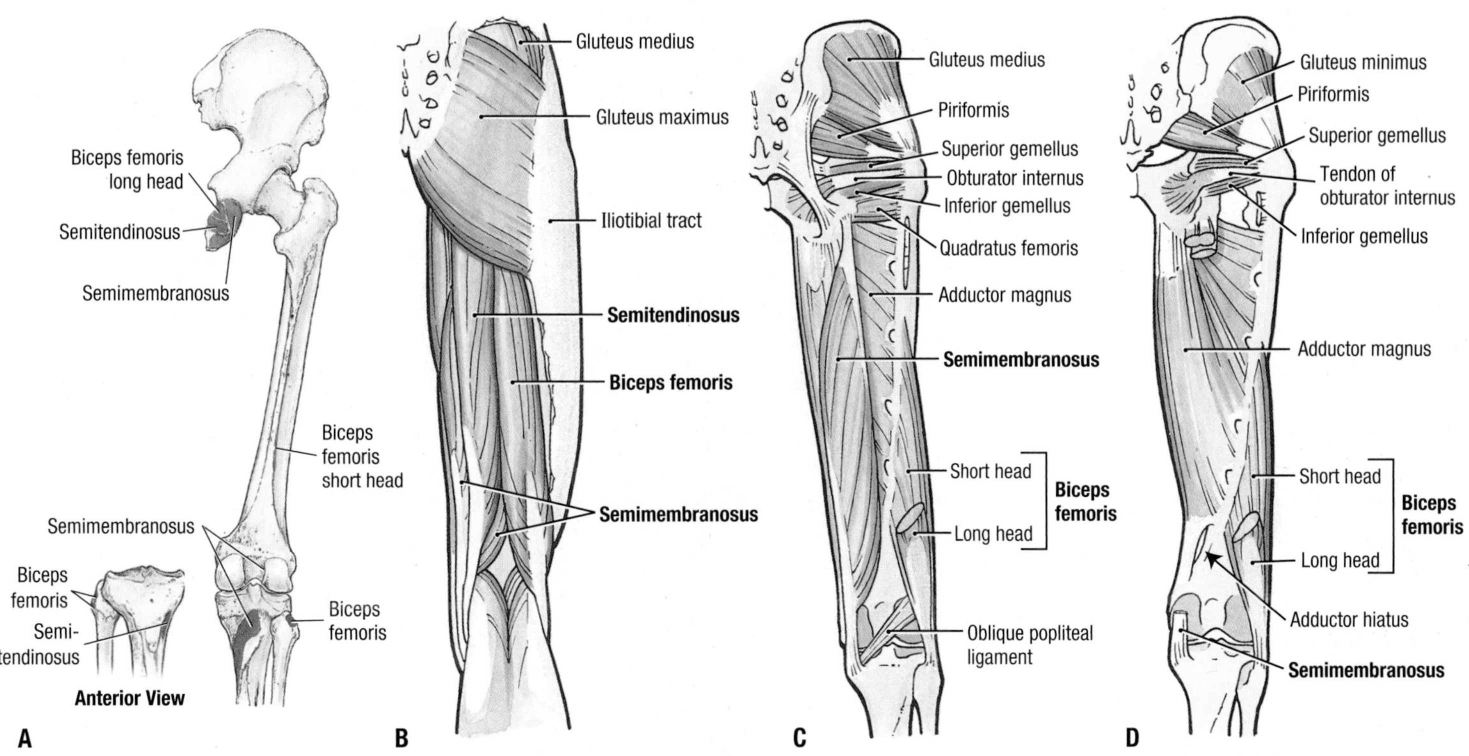
Biceps femoris long head
Semitendinosus
Semimembranosus
Biceps femoris short head
Semimembranosus
Biceps femoris
Semi-tendinosus
Biceps femoris
Anterior View
A
Gluteus medius
Gluteus maximus
Iliotibial tract
Semitendinosus
Biceps femoris
Semimembranosus
B
Gluteus medius
Piriformis
Superior gemellus
Obturator internus
Inferior gemellus
Quadratus femoris
Adductor magnus
Semimembranosus
Short head
Long head
Biceps femoris
Oblique popliteal ligament
C
Gluteus minimus
Piriformis
Superior gemellus
Tendon of obturator internus
Inferior gemellus
Adductor magnus
Short head
Long head
Biceps femoris
Adductor hiatus
Semimembranosus
D
Posterior Views

5.30 MUSCLES OF POSTERIOR THIGH

A. Attachments. **B.** Superficial layer. **C.** Intermediate layer. **D.** Deep layer.

TABLE 5.8 MUSCLES OF POSTERIOR THIGH (HAMSTRING)

Muscle[a]	Proximal Attachment[a] (*Red*)	Distal Attachment[a] (*Blue*)	Innervation[b]	Main Actions
Semitendinosus	Ischial tuberosity	Medial surface of superior part of tibia	Tibial division of sciatic nerve (L5, S1, and S2)	Extend hip joint; flex knee joint and rotate it medially; when hip and knee joints are flexed, can extend trunk
Semimembranosus		Posterior part of medial condyle of tibia; reflected attachment forms oblique popliteal ligament to lateral femoral condyle		
Biceps femoris	*Long head:* ischial tuberosity; *Short head:* linea aspera and lateral supracondylar line of femur	Lateral side of head of fibula; tendon is split at this site by fibular collateral ligament of knee	*Long head:* tibial division of sciatic nerve (L5, S1, and S2); *Short head:* common fibular (peroneal) division of sciatic nerve (L5, S1, and S2)	Flexes knee joint and rotates it laterally; extends hip joint (e.g., when initiating a walking gait)

[a]See Figure 5.22 for muscle attachments.
[b]See Table 5.1 for explanation of segmental innervation.

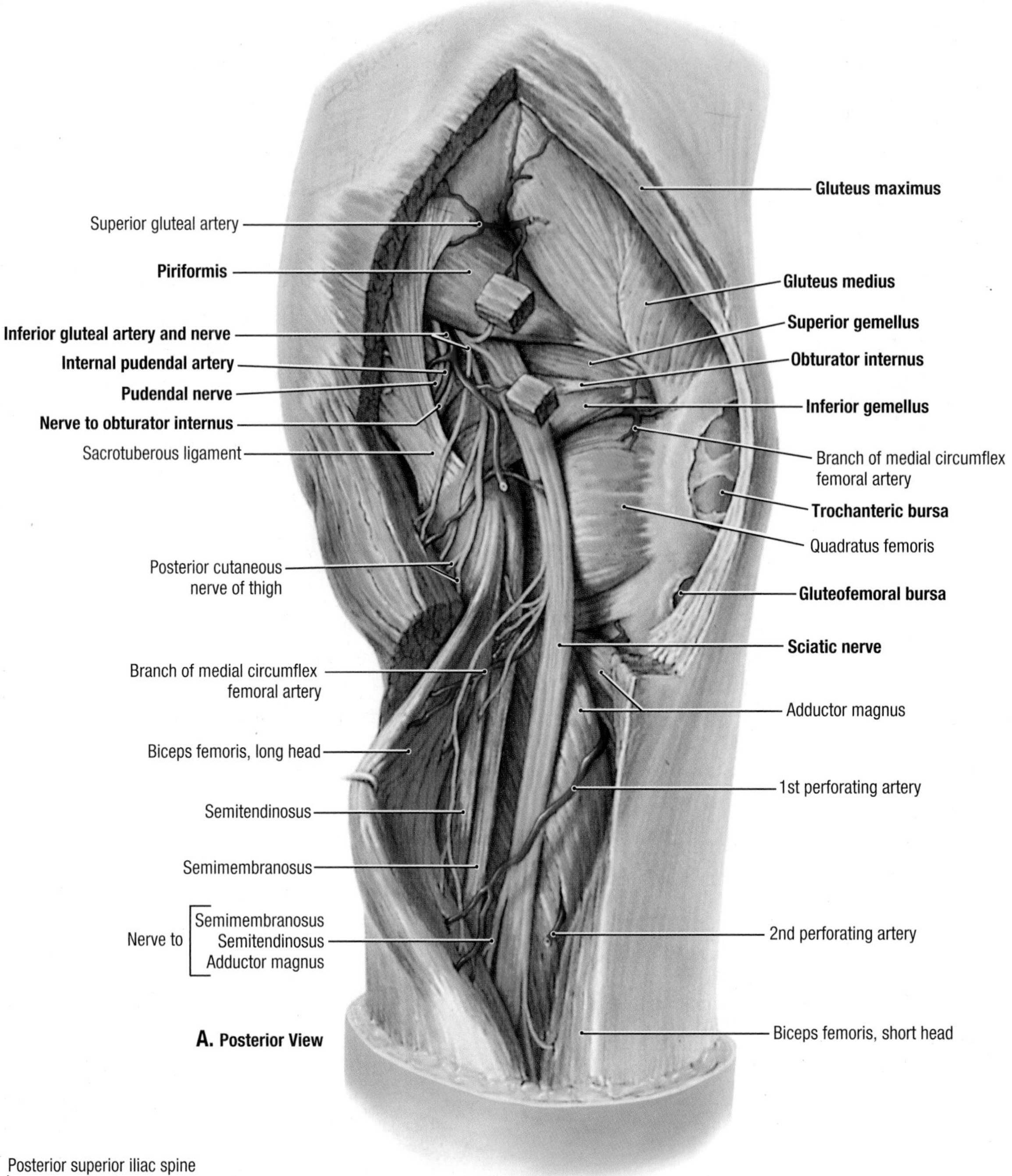

Gluteus maximus
Superior gluteal artery
Piriformis
Gluteus medius
Superior gemellus
Inferior gluteal artery and nerve
Obturator internus
Internal pudendal artery
Pudendal nerve
Inferior gemellus
Nerve to obturator internus
Sacrotuberous ligament
Branch of medial circumflex femoral artery
Trochanteric bursa
Quadratus femoris
Posterior cutaneous nerve of thigh
Gluteofemoral bursa
Sciatic nerve
Branch of medial circumflex femoral artery
Adductor magnus
Biceps femoris, long head
1st perforating artery
Semitendinosus
Semimembranosus
Nerve to Semimembranosus, Semitendinosus, Adductor magnus
2nd perforating artery
Biceps femoris, short head

A. Posterior View

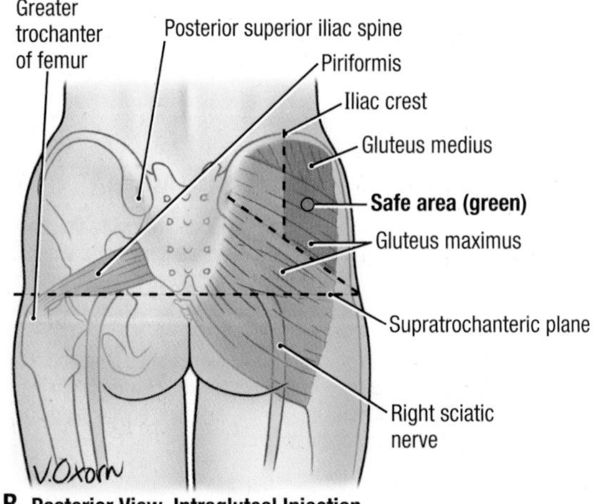
Greater trochanter of femur
Posterior superior iliac spine
Piriformis
Iliac crest
Gluteus medius
Safe area (green)
Gluteus maximus
Supratrochanteric plane
Right sciatic nerve
V.Oxorn

B. Posterior View, Intragluteal Injection

5.31 MUSCLES OF GLUTEAL REGION AND POSTERIOR THIGH IV

A. Dissection. The gluteus maximus muscle is split superiorly and inferiorly, and the middle part is excised; two cubes remain to identify its nerve. The gluteus maximus is the only muscle to cover the greater trochanter; it is aponeurotic and has underlying bursae where it glides on the trochanter (trochanteric bursa) and the aponeurosis of the vastus lateralis muscle (gluteofemoral bursa). **B. Intragluteal injection.** Injections can be made safely only into the superolateral part of the buttock to avoid injury to the sciatic and gluteal nerves. This site has a rich vascular network from the superior gluteal vessels that lie between the gluteus medius and minimus muscles.

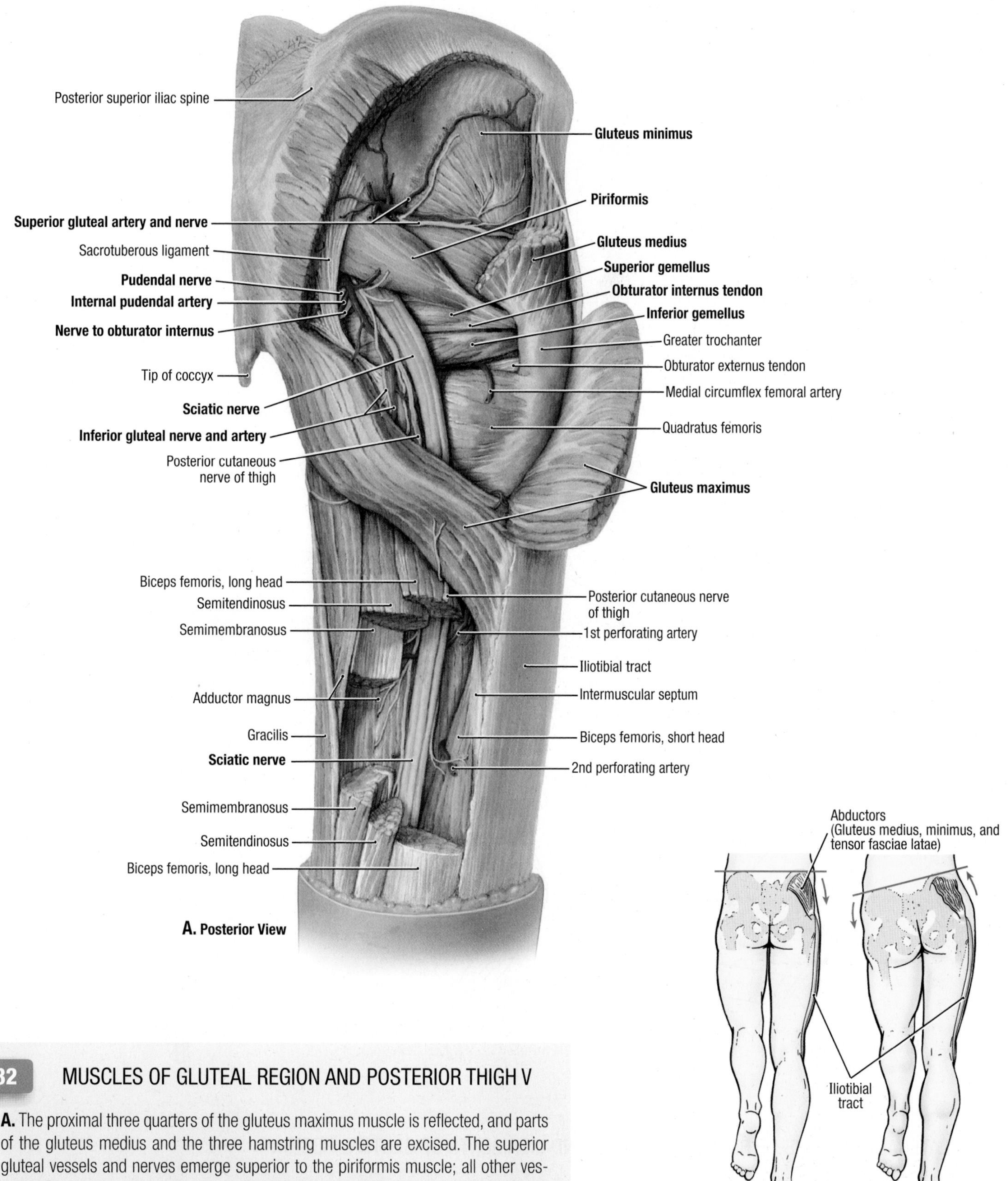
Posterior superior iliac spine
Gluteus minimus
Piriformis
Superior gluteal artery and nerve
Sacrotuberous ligament
Gluteus medius
Superior gemellus
Pudendal nerve
Obturator internus tendon
Internal pudendal artery
Inferior gemellus
Nerve to obturator internus
Greater trochanter
Obturator externus tendon
Tip of coccyx
Medial circumflex femoral artery
Sciatic nerve
Inferior gluteal nerve and artery
Quadratus femoris
Posterior cutaneous nerve of thigh
Gluteus maximus
Biceps femoris, long head
Posterior cutaneous nerve of thigh
Semitendinosus
Semimembranosus
1st perforating artery
Iliotibial tract
Adductor magnus
Intermuscular septum
Gracilis
Biceps femoris, short head
Sciatic nerve
2nd perforating artery
Semimembranosus
Semitendinosus
Biceps femoris, long head
A. Posterior View
Abductors (Gluteus medius, minimus, and tensor fasciae latae)
Iliotibial tract
B
C
Posterior Views

5.32 MUSCLES OF GLUTEAL REGION AND POSTERIOR THIGH V

A. The proximal three quarters of the gluteus maximus muscle is reflected, and parts of the gluteus medius and the three hamstring muscles are excised. The superior gluteal vessels and nerves emerge superior to the piriformis muscle; all other vessels and nerves emerge inferior to it. **B.** When the weight is borne by one limb, the muscles on the supported side fix the pelvis so that it does not sag to the unsupported side, keeping the pelvis level. **C.** When the right **abductors are paralyzed,** owing to a lesion of the right superior gluteal nerve, fixation by these muscles is lost and the pelvis tilts to the unsupported left side (positive Trendelenburg sign).

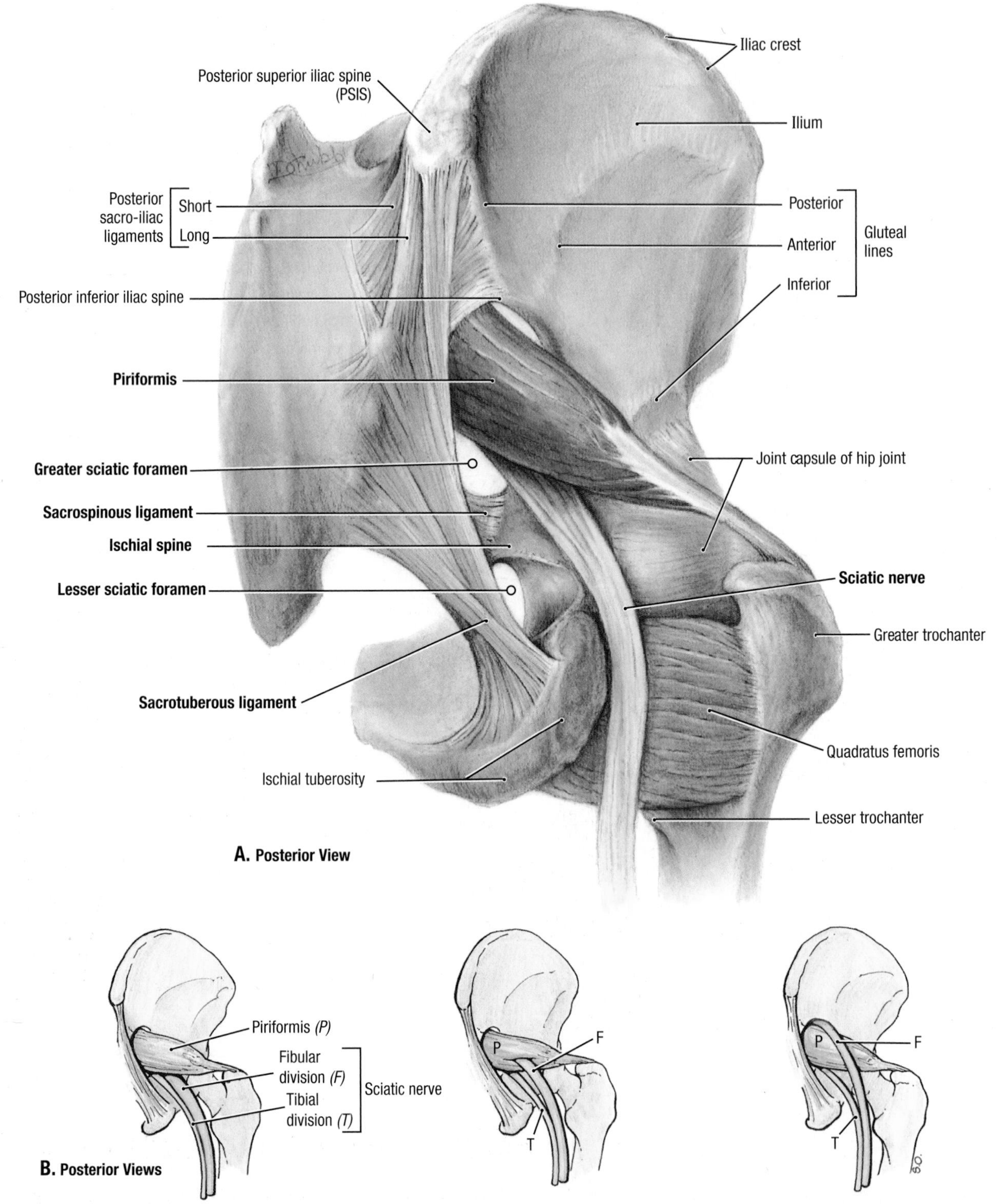
Iliac crest
Posterior superior iliac spine (PSIS)
Ilium
Posterior sacro-iliac ligaments
Short
Long
Posterior
Anterior
Inferior
Gluteal lines
Posterior inferior iliac spine
Piriformis
Greater sciatic foramen
Joint capsule of hip joint
Sacrospinous ligament
Ischial spine
Lesser sciatic foramen
Sciatic nerve
Greater trochanter
Sacrotuberous ligament
Quadratus femoris
Ischial tuberosity
Lesser trochanter
A. Posterior View
Piriformis (P)
Fibular division (F)
Tibial division (T)
Sciatic nerve
P
F
T
B. Posterior Views

5.33 LATERAL ROTATORS OF HIP, SCIATIC NERVE, AND LIGAMENTS OF GLUTEAL REGION

A. Piriformis and quadratus femoris. In the anatomical position the tip of the coccyx lies superior to the level of the ischial tuberosity and inferior to that of the ischial spine. The lateral border of the sciatic nerve lies midway between the lateral surface of the greater trochanter and the medial surface of the ischial tuberosity.

B. Relationship of sciatic nerve to piriformis muscle. Of 640 limbs studied in Dr. Grant's laboratory, in 87%, the tibial and fibular (peroneal) divisions passed inferior to the piriformis (*left*); in 12.2%, the fibular (peroneal) division passed through the piriformis (*center*); and in 0.5% the fibular (peroneal) division passed superior to the piriformis (*right*).

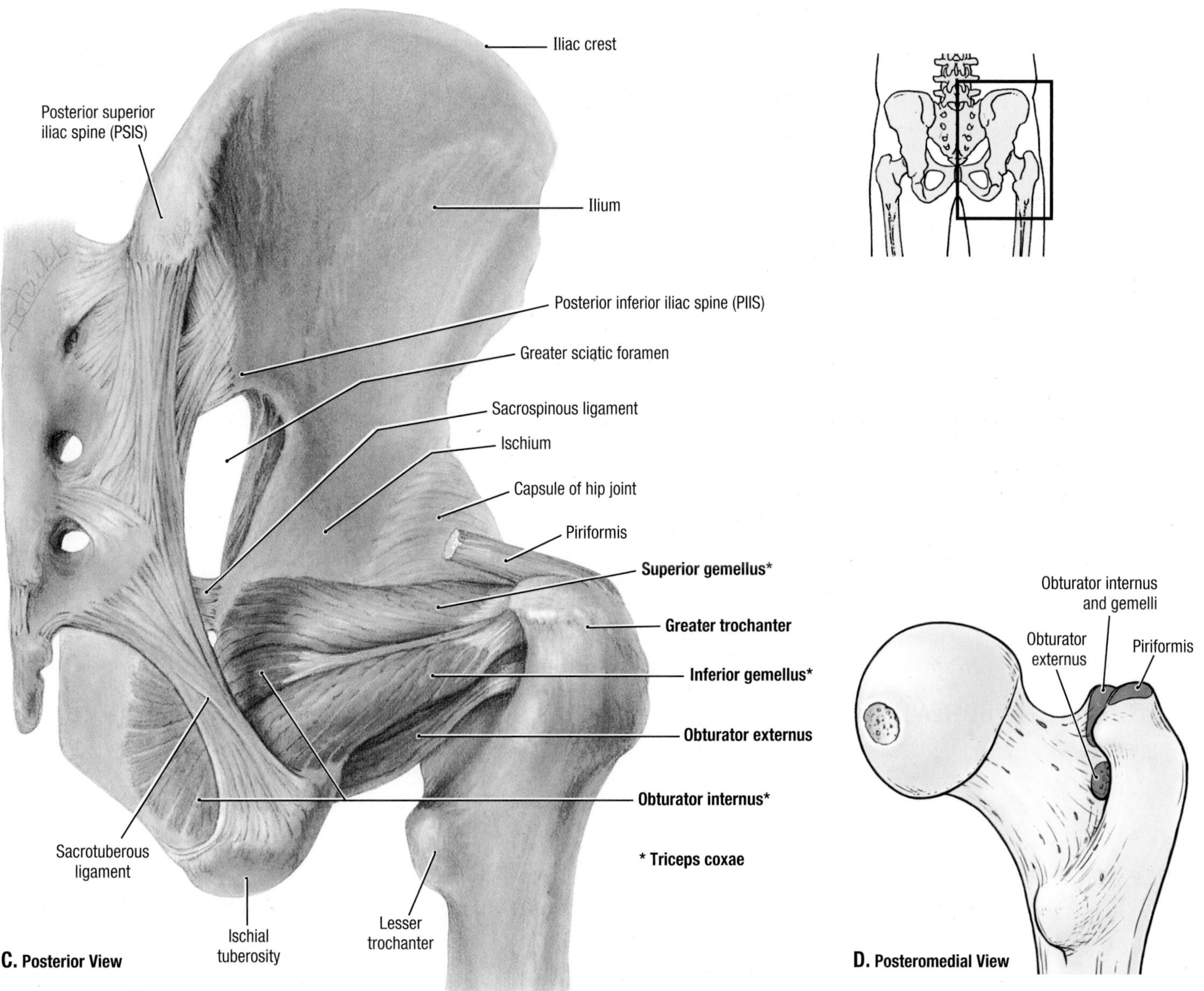
Iliac crest
Posterior superior iliac spine (PSIS)
Ilium
Posterior inferior iliac spine (PIIS)
Greater sciatic foramen
Sacrospinous ligament
Ischium
Capsule of hip joint
Piriformis
Superior gemellus*
Greater trochanter
Inferior gemellus*
Obturator externus
Obturator internus*
* Triceps coxae
Sacrotuberous ligament
Ischial tuberosity
Lesser trochanter
Obturator internus and gemelli
Obturator externus
Piriformis

C. **Posterior View**

D. **Posteromedial View**

5.33 LATERAL ROTATORS OF HIP, SCIATIC NERVE, AND LIGAMENTS OF GLUTEAL REGION (*CONTINUED*)

C. Obturator internus, obturator externus, and superior and inferior gemelli.

- The obturator internus is located partly in the pelvis, where it covers most of the lateral wall of the lesser pelvis. It leaves the pelvis through the lesser sciatic foramen, makes a right-angle turn, becomes tendinous, and receives the distal attachments of the gemelli before attaching to the medial surface of the greater trochanter (trochanteric fossa).
- The obturator externus extends from the external surface of the obturator membrane and surrounding bone of the pelvis to the posterior aspect of the greater trochanter, passing directly under the acetabulum and neck of the femur.
- **Sciatic nerve block.** Sensation conveyed by the sciatic nerve can be blocked by injecting an anesthetic agent a few centimeters inferior to the midpoint of the line joining the PSIS and the superior border of the greater trochanter. Paresthesia radiates to the foot because of anesthesia of the plantar nerves, which are terminal branches of the tibial nerve derived from the sciatic nerve.
- **Common fibular nerve compression at piriformis.** In the approximately 12% of people in whom the common fibular division of the sciatic nerve passes through the piriformis, this muscle may compress the nerve.

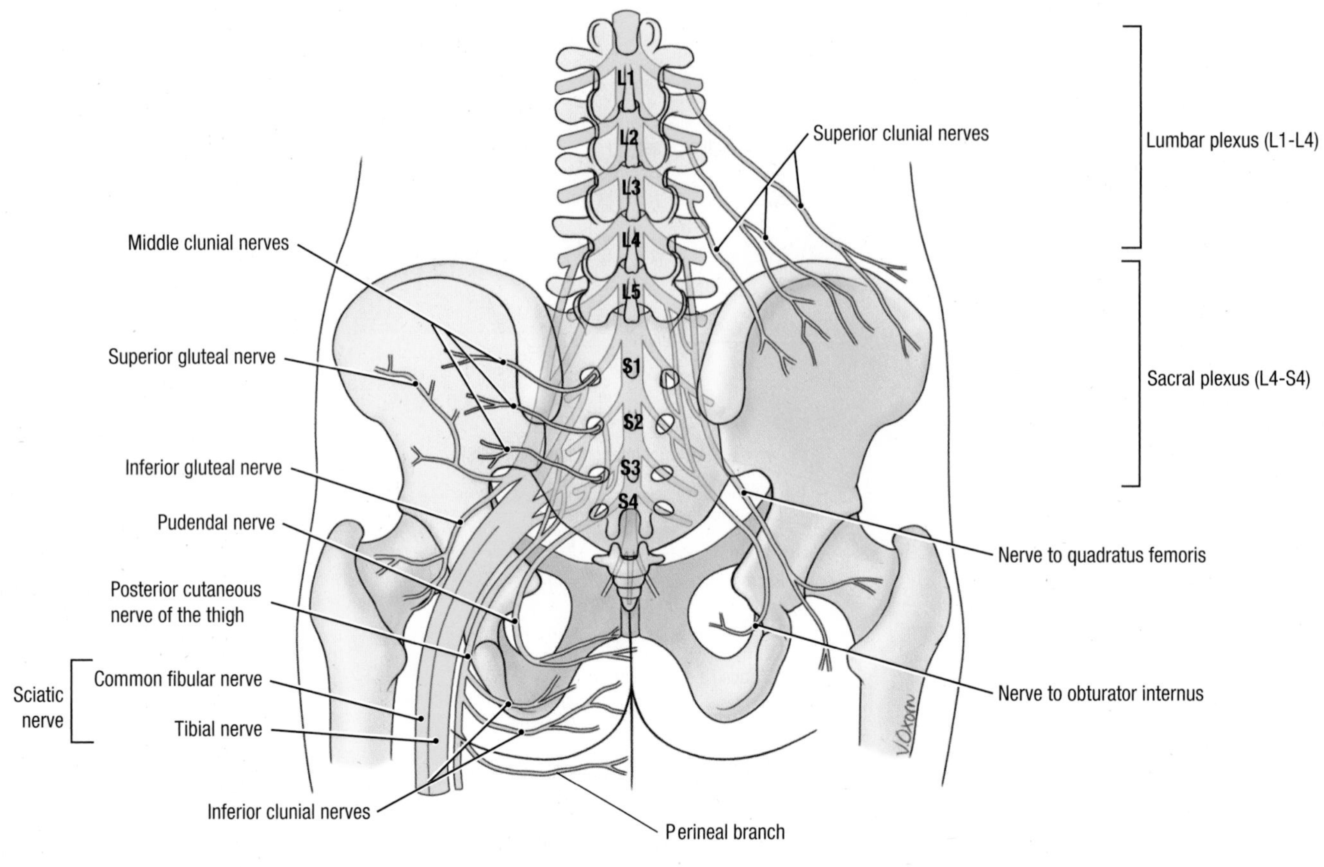
Superior clunial nerves
Lumbar plexus (L1-L4)
Sacral plexus (L4-S4)
Middle clunial nerves
Superior gluteal nerve
Inferior gluteal nerve
Pudendal nerve
Posterior cutaneous nerve of the thigh
Sciatic nerve
Common fibular nerve
Tibial nerve
Inferior clunial nerves
Perineal branch
Nerve to quadratus femoris
Nerve to obturator internus
L1
L2
L3
L4
L5
S1
S2
S3
S4
Posterior View

5.34 NERVES OF GLUTEAL REGION

TABLE 5.9 NERVES OF GLUTEAL REGION

Nerve	Origin	Course	Distribution in Gluteal Region
Clunial (superior, middle, and inferior)	*Superior:* posterior rami of L1–L3 nerves *Middle:* posterior rami of S1–S3 nerves *Inferior:* posterior cutaneous nerve of thigh	*Superior nerves* cross iliac crest; *middle nerves* exit through posterior sacral foramina and enter gluteal region; *inferior nerves* curve around inferior border of gluteus maximus	Gluteal region as far laterally as greater trochanter
Sciatic	Sacral plexus (L4–S3)	Exits pelvis via greater sciatic foramen inferior to piriformis to enter gluteal region	No muscles in gluteal region
Posterior cutaneous nerve of thigh	Sacral plexus (S1–S3)	Exits pelvis via greater sciatic foramen inferior to piriformis, emerges from inferior border of gluteus maximus coursing deep to fascia lata	Skin of buttock via inferior cluneal branches, skin over posterior thigh and popliteal fossa; skin of lateral perineum and upper medial thigh via perineal branch
Superior gluteal	Anterior rami of L4–S1 nerves	Exits pelvis via greater sciatic foramen superior to piriformis; courses between gluteus medius and minimus	Gluteus medius, gluteus minimus, and TFL
Inferior gluteal	Anterior rami of L5–S2 nerves	Exits pelvis via greater sciatic foramen inferior to piriformis, dividing into multiple branches	Gluteus maximus
Nerve to quadratus femoris	Anterior rami of L4–S1 nerves	Exits pelvis via greater sciatic foramen deep to sciatic nerve	Posterior hip joint, inferior gemellus, and quadratus femoris
Pudendal	Anterior rami of S2–S4 nerves	Exits pelvis via greater sciatic foramen inferior to piriformis; descends posterior to sacrospinous ligament; enters perineum (pudendal canal) through lesser sciatic foramen	No structures in gluteal region (supplies most of perineum)
Nerve to obturator internus	Anterior rami of L5–S2 nerves	Exits pelvis via greater sciatic foramen inferior to piriformis; descends posterior to ischial spine; enters lesser sciatic foramen and passes to obturator internus	Superior gemellus and obturator internus

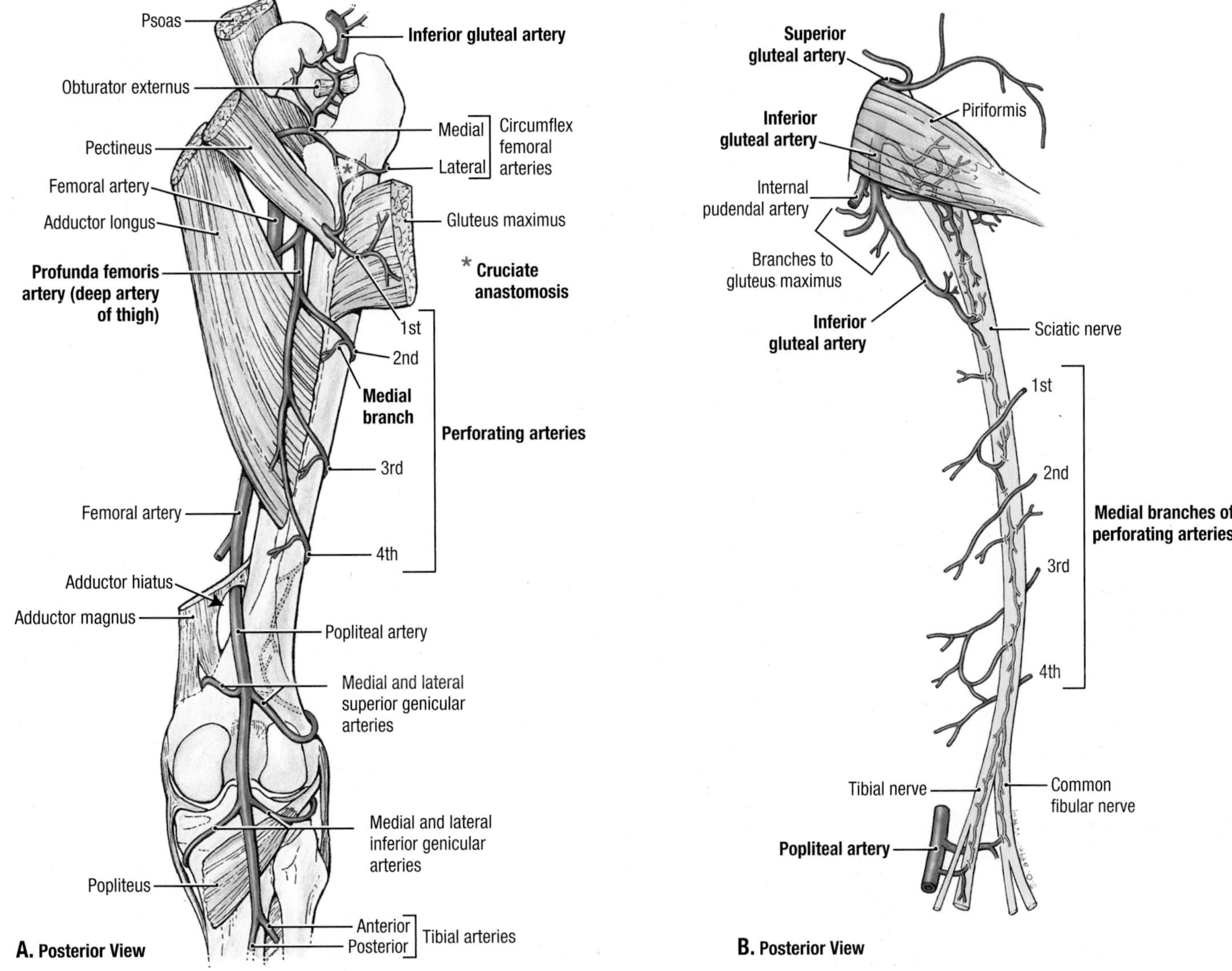
Psoas
Inferior gluteal artery
Obturator externus
Pectineus
Medial
Lateral
Circumflex femoral arteries
Femoral artery
Adductor longus
Gluteus maximus
Profunda femoris artery (deep artery of thigh)
* Cruciate anastomosis
1st
2nd
Medial branch
Perforating arteries
3rd
Femoral artery
4th
Adductor hiatus
Adductor magnus
Popliteal artery
Medial and lateral superior genicular arteries
Medial and lateral inferior genicular arteries
Popliteus
Anterior
Posterior
Tibial arteries
A. Posterior View
Superior gluteal artery
Piriformis
Inferior gluteal artery
Internal pudendal artery
Branches to gluteus maximus
Inferior gluteal artery
Sciatic nerve
1st
2nd
Medial branches of perforating arteries
3rd
4th
Tibial nerve
Common fibular nerve
Popliteal artery
B. Posterior View

5.35 ARTERIES OF GLUTEAL REGION AND POSTERIOR THIGH

TABLE 5.10 ARTERIES OF GLUTEAL REGION AND POSTERIOR THIGH

Artery	Origin	Course	Distribution
Superior gluteal	Internal iliac	Enters gluteal region through greater sciatic foramen superior to piriformis; divides into superficial and deep branches; anastomoses with inferior gluteal and medial circumflex femoral arteries	*Superficial branch:* superior gluteus maximus *Deep branch:* runs between gluteus medius and minimus, supplying both and tensor fasciae latae
Inferior gluteal		Enters gluteal region through greater sciatic foramen inferior to piriformis; descends on medial side of sciatic nerve; anastomoses with superior gluteal artery and participates in cruciate anastomosis of thigh	Inferior gluteus maximus, obturator internus, quadratus femoris, and superior parts of hamstring muscles
Internal pudendal		Enters gluteal region through greater sciatic foramen; descends posterior to ischial spine; exits gluteal region via lesser sciatic foramen to perineum	No structures in gluteal region (supplies external genitalia and muscles in perineal region)
Perforating arteries		Perforate aponeurotic portion of adductor magnus attachment and medial intermuscular septum to enter and supply muscular branches to posterior compartment; then pierce lateral intermuscular septum to enter posterolateral aspect of anterior compartment	Hamstring muscles in posterior compartment; posterior portion of vastus lateralis in anterior compartment; femur (via femoral nutrient arteries); reinforce arterial supply of sciatic nerve
Lateral circumflex femoral	Profunda femoris (may arise from femoral)	Passes laterally deep to sartorius and rectus femoris; enter gluteal region	Anterior part of gluteal region
Medial circumflex femoral		Passes medially and posteriorly between pectineus and iliopsoas; enters gluteal region	Supplies most blood to head and neck of femur; hip region

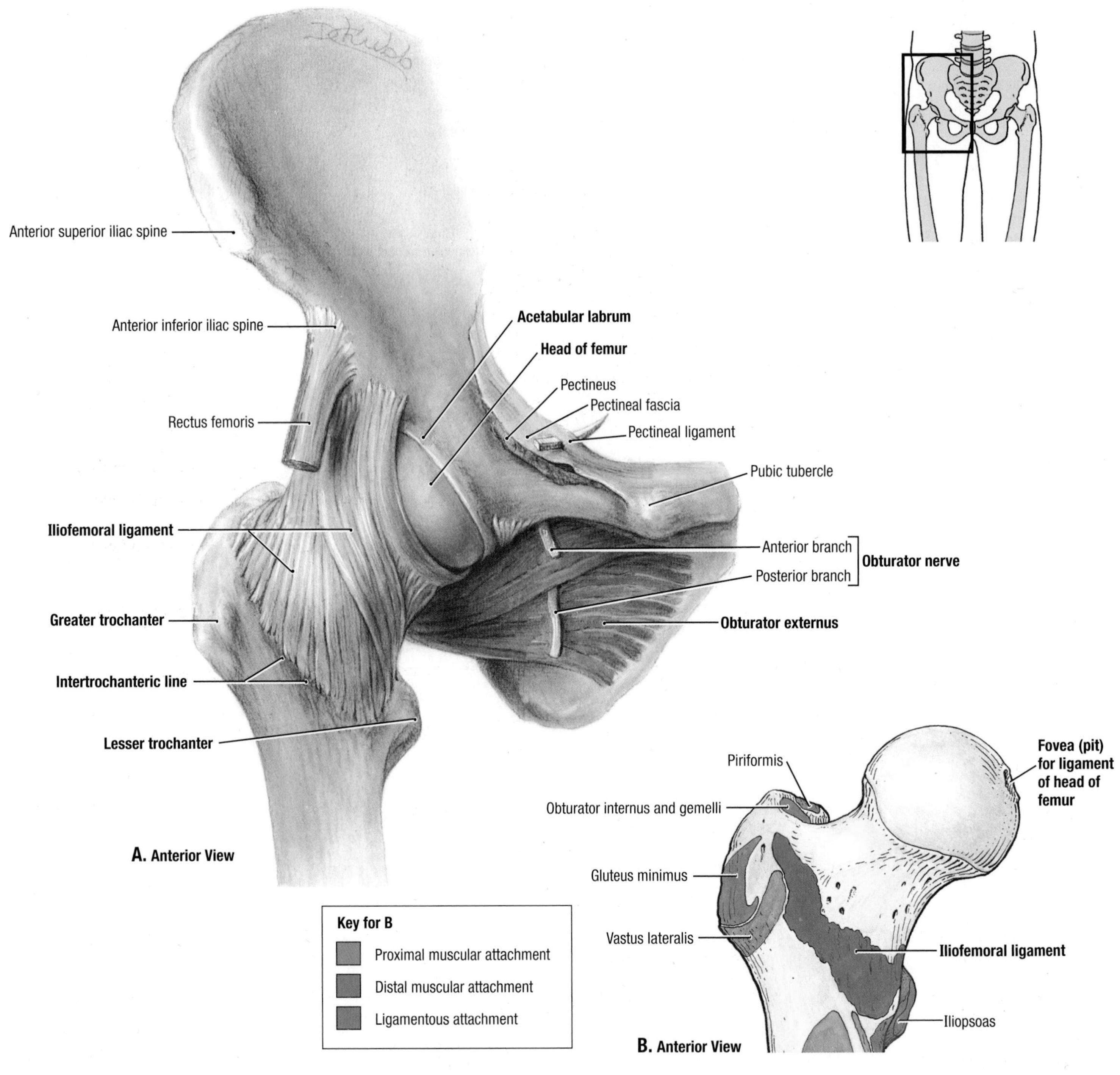

Anterior superior iliac spine
Anterior inferior iliac spine
Rectus femoris
Iliofemoral ligament
Greater trochanter
Intertrochanteric line
Lesser trochanter
Acetabular labrum
Head of femur
Pectineus
Pectineal fascia
Pectineal ligament
Pubic tubercle
Anterior branch
Posterior branch
Obturator nerve
Obturator externus
A. Anterior View
Piriformis
Obturator internus and gemelli
Gluteus minimus
Vastus lateralis
Fovea (pit) for ligament of head of femur
Iliofemoral ligament
Iliopsoas
B. Anterior View
Key for B
Proximal muscular attachment
Distal muscular attachment
Ligamentous attachment

5.36 HIP JOINT

A. Iliofemoral ligament. **B.** Muscle attachments of anterior aspect of the proximal femur. In **A:**

- The head of the femur is exposed just medial to the iliofemoral ligament and faces superiorly, medially, and anteriorly. At the site of the subtendinous bursa of psoas, the capsule is weak or (as in this specimen) partially deficient, but it is guarded by the psoas tendon.
- The iliofemoral ligament, shaped like an inverted "Y." Superiorly it is attached deep to the rectus femoris muscle; the ligament becomes tight on medial rotation of the femur.
- The pectineus muscle is thin, and its fascia blends with the pectineal ligament.

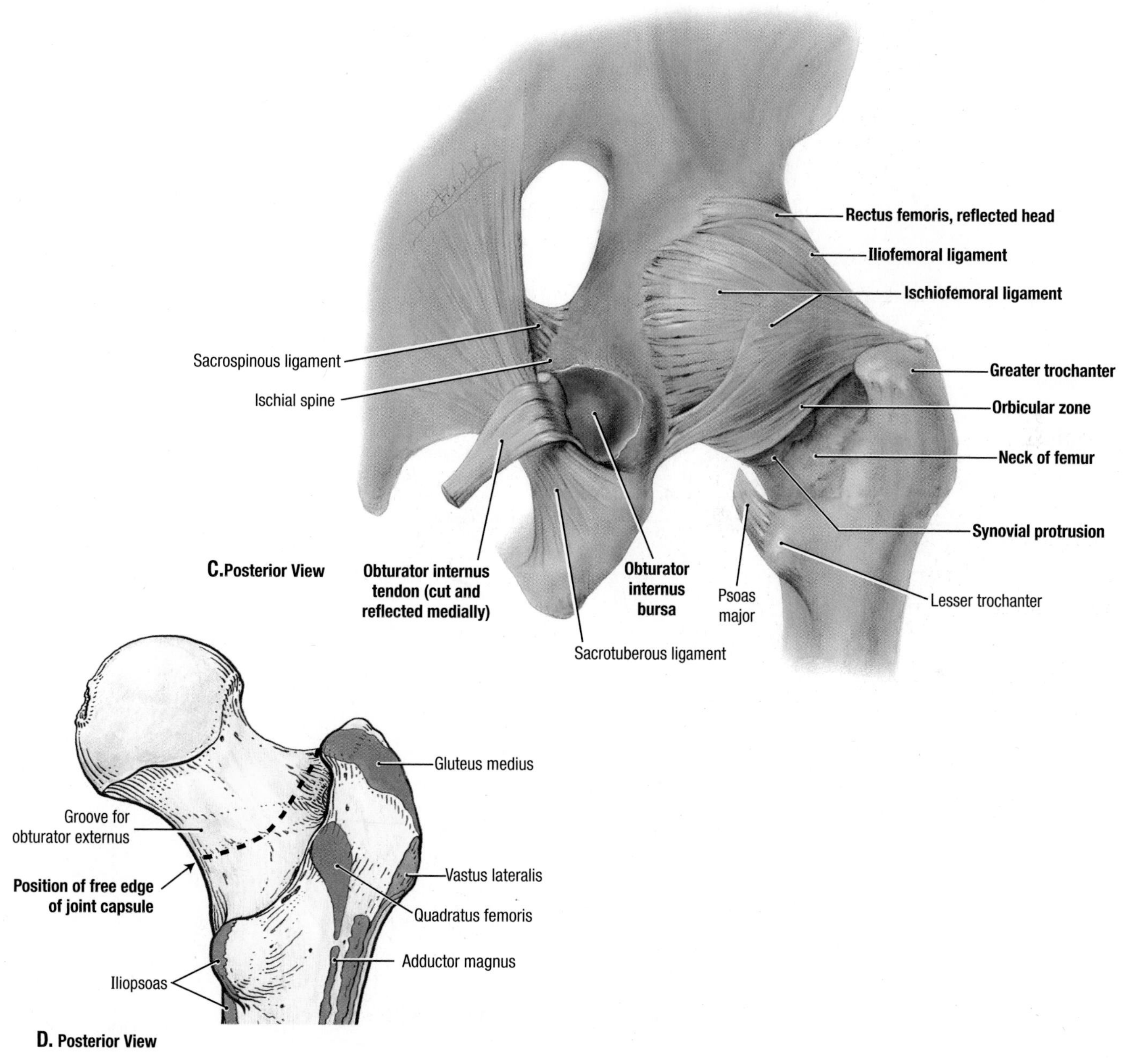
Rectus femoris, reflected head
Iliofemoral ligament
Ischiofemoral ligament
Greater trochanter
Orbicular zone
Neck of femur
Synovial protrusion
Lesser trochanter
Sacrospinous ligament
Ischial spine
C.Posterior View
Obturator internus tendon (cut and reflected medially)
Obturator internus bursa
Psoas major
Sacrotuberous ligament
Gluteus medius
Groove for obturator externus
Position of free edge of joint capsule
Vastus lateralis
Quadratus femoris
Adductor magnus
Iliopsoas
D. Posterior View

5.36 HIP JOINT (*CONTINUED*)

C. Ischiofemoral ligament. **D.** Muscle attachments onto the posterior aspect of proximal femur. In **C:**

- The fibers of the capsule spiral to become taut during extension and medial rotation of the femur.
- The synovial membrane protrudes inferior to the fibrous capsule and forms a bursa for the tendon of the obturator externus muscle. Note the large subtendinous bursa of the obturator internus at the lesser sciatic notch, where the tendon turns 90 degrees to attach to the greater trochanter.

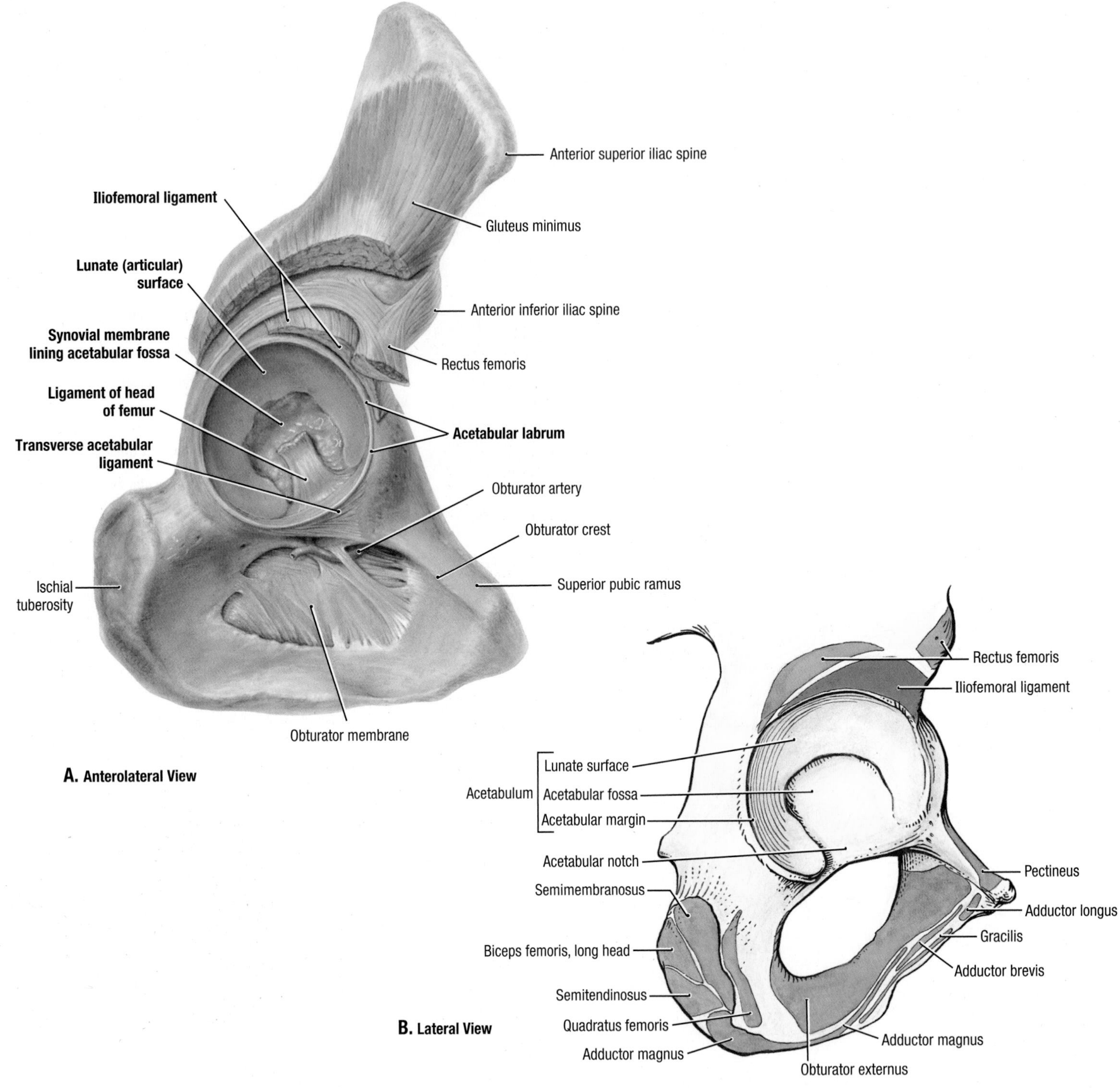

Anterior superior iliac spine
Iliofemoral ligament
Gluteus minimus
Lunate (articular) surface
Anterior inferior iliac spine
Synovial membrane lining acetabular fossa
Rectus femoris
Ligament of head of femur
Acetabular labrum
Transverse acetabular ligament
Obturator artery
Obturator crest
Ischial tuberosity
Superior pubic ramus
Obturator membrane
A. Anterolateral View
Rectus femoris
Iliofemoral ligament
Acetabulum
Lunate surface
Acetabular fossa
Acetabular margin
Acetabular notch
Semimembranosus
Pectineus
Adductor longus
Gracilis
Biceps femoris, long head
Adductor brevis
Semitendinosus
Quadratus femoris
B. Lateral View
Adductor magnus
Adductor magnus
Obturator externus

5.37 ACETABULAR REGION

A. Dissection of acetabulum. **B.** Muscle attachments of acetabular region.

In **A:**

- The transverse acetabular ligament bridges the acetabular notch.
- The acetabular labrum is attached to the acetabular rim and transverse acetabular ligament and forms a complete ring around the head of the femur.
- The ligament of the head of the femur lies between the head of the femur and the acetabulum. These fibers are attached superiorly to the pit (fovea) on the head of the femur and inferiorly to the transverse acetabular ligament and the margins of the acetabular notch. The artery of the ligament of the head of the femur passes through the acetabular notch and into the ligament of the head of the femur.

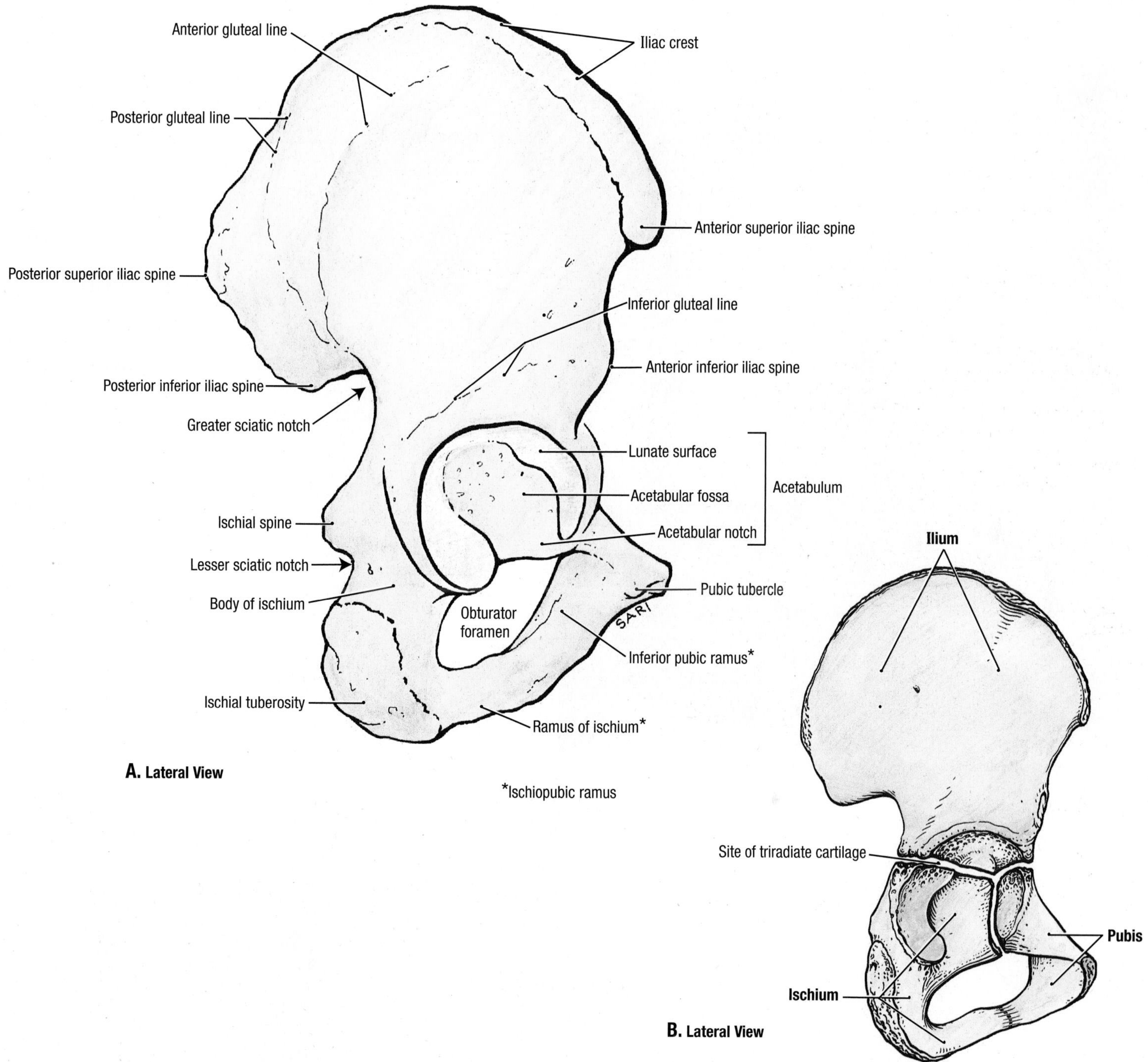
Anterior gluteal line
Iliac crest
Posterior gluteal line
Anterior superior iliac spine
Posterior superior iliac spine
Inferior gluteal line
Anterior inferior iliac spine
Posterior inferior iliac spine
Greater sciatic notch
Lunate surface
Acetabular fossa
Acetabulum
Acetabular notch
Ischial spine
Lesser sciatic notch
Pubic tubercle
Body of ischium
Obturator foramen
Inferior pubic ramus*
Ischial tuberosity
Ramus of ischium*
A. Lateral View
*Ischiopubic ramus
Ilium
Site of triradiate cartilage
Pubis
Ischium
B. Lateral View

5.38 HIP BONE

A. Features of the lateral aspect. In the anatomical position, the anterior superior iliac spine and pubic tubercle are in the same coronal plane, and the ischial spine and superior end of the pubic symphysis are in the same horizontal plane; the internal aspect of the body of the pubis faces superiorly, and the acetabulum faces inferolaterally. **B.** Hip bone in youth. The three parts of the hip bone (ilium, ischium, and pubis) meet in the acetabulum at the triradiate synchondrosis. One or more primary centers of ossification appear in the triradiate cartilage at approximately the 12th year. Secondary centers of ossification appear along the length of the iliac crest, at the anterior inferior iliac spine, the ischial tuberosity, and the pubic symphysis at about puberty; fusion is usually complete by age 23.

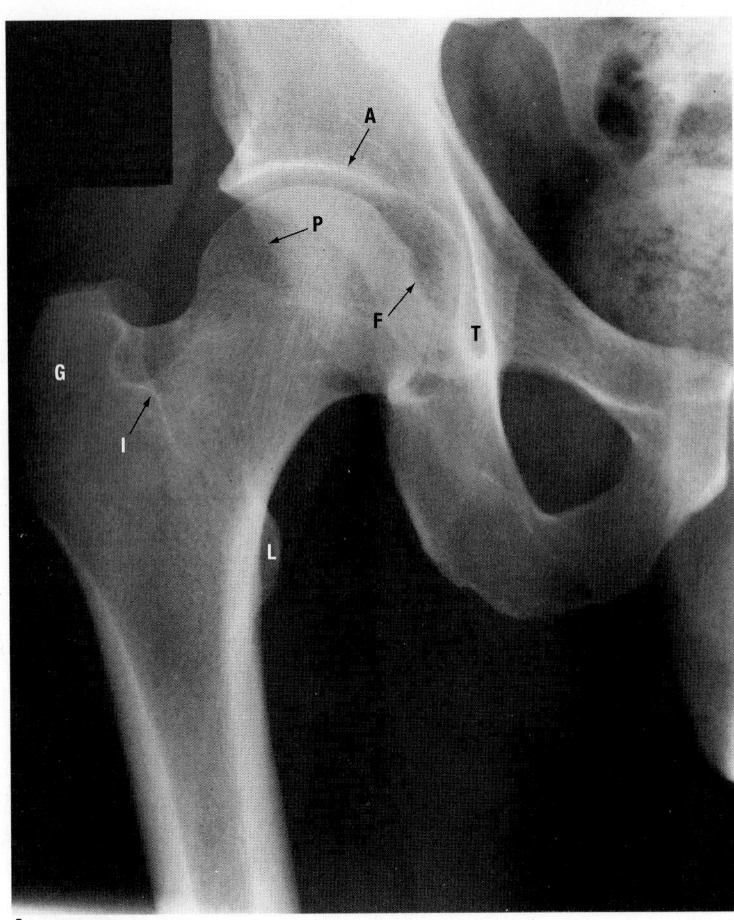
A
P
F
T
G
I
L
A. Anteroposterior View

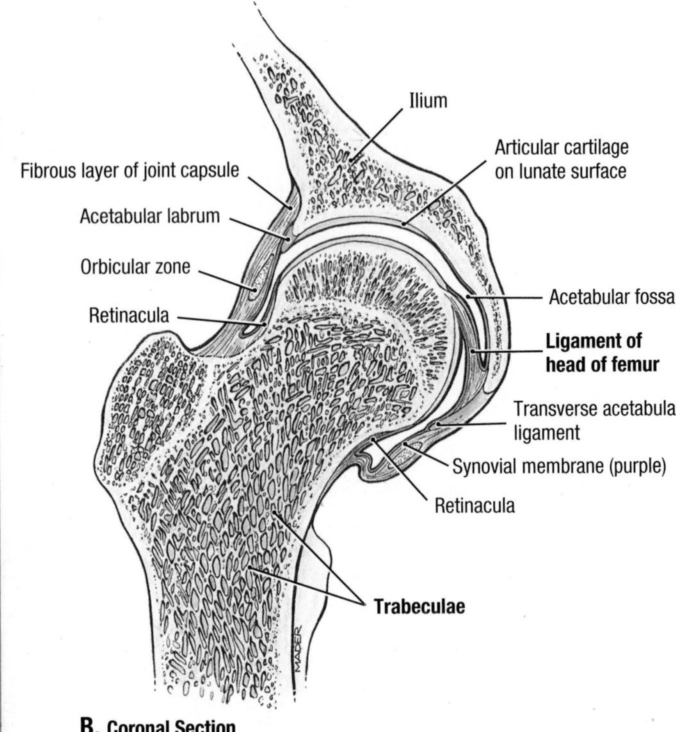
Ilium
Articular cartilage on lunate surface
Fibrous layer of joint capsule
Acetabular labrum
Orbicular zone
Retinacula
Acetabular fossa
Ligament of head of femur
Transverse acetabular ligament
Synovial membrane (purple)
Retinacula
Trabeculae
MADER
B. Coronal Section

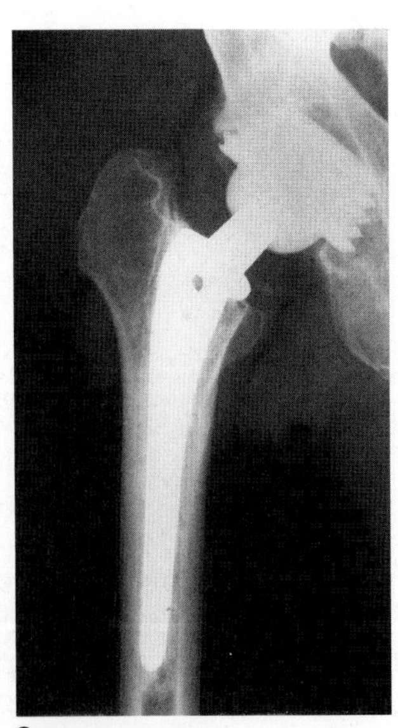
C. Hip Prosthesis

5.39 RADIOGRAPH AND CORONAL SECTION OF HIP JOINT

A. Radiograph. On the femur, note the greater (*G*) and lesser (*L*) trochanters, the intertrochanteric crest (*I*), and the pit or fovea (*F*) for the ligament of the head. On the pelvis, note the roof (*A*) and posterior rim (*P*) of the acetabulum and the "teardrop" appearance (*T*) caused by the superimposition of structures at the inferior margin of the acetabulum. **B.** Coronal section. Observe the bony trabeculae projecting into the head of the femur. The ligament of the head of the femur becomes taut during adduction of the hip joint, such as when crossing the legs. **C. Hip replacement.** The hip joint is subject to severe traumatic injury and degenerative disease. **Osteoarthritis of the hip joint**, characterized by pain, edema, limitation of motion, and erosion of articular cartilage, is a common cause of disability. During hip replacement, a metal prosthesis anchored to the femur by bone cement replaces the femoral head and neck. A plastic socket is cemented to the hip bone to replace the acetabulum. See Figure 5.41 clinical blue text.

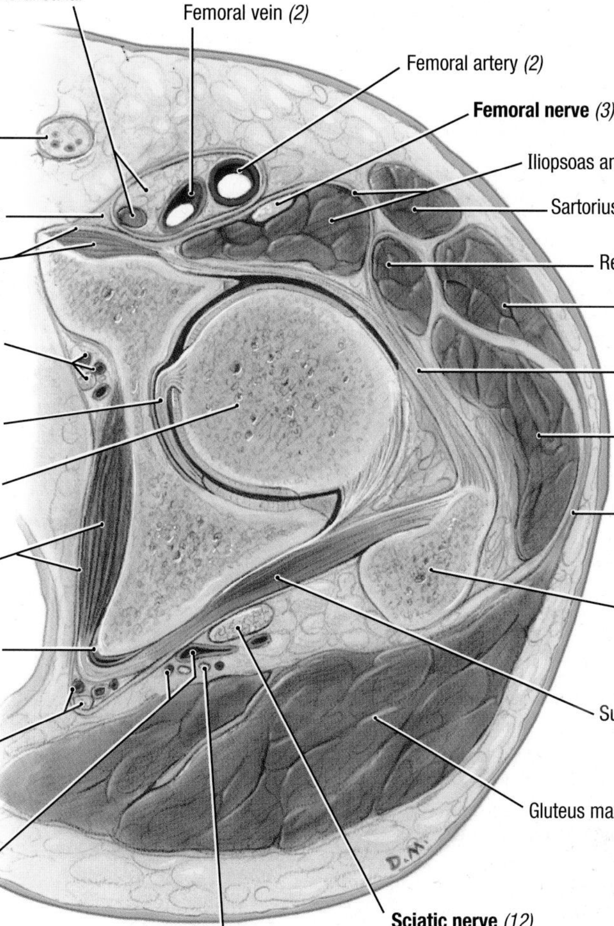

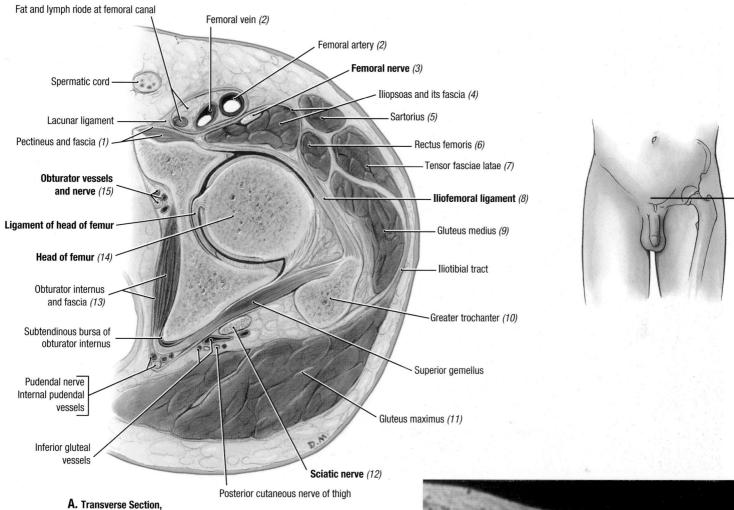

Fat and lymph node at femoral canal
Femoral vein *(2)*
Femoral artery *(2)*
Femoral nerve *(3)*
Spermatic cord
Iliopsoas and its fascia *(4)*
Lacunar ligament
Sartorius *(5)*
Pectineus and fascia *(1)*
Rectus femoris *(6)*
Tensor fasciae latae *(7)*
Obturator vessels and nerve *(15)*
Iliofemoral ligament *(8)*
Ligament of head of femur
Gluteus medius *(9)*
Head of femur *(14)*
Iliotibial tract
Obturator internus and fascia *(13)*
Greater trochanter *(10)*
Subtendinous bursa of obturator internus
Superior gemellus
Pudendal nerve
Internal pudendal vessels
Gluteus maximus *(11)*
Inferior gluteal vessels
Sciatic nerve *(12)*
Posterior cutaneous nerve of thigh

A. Transverse Section, Inferior View

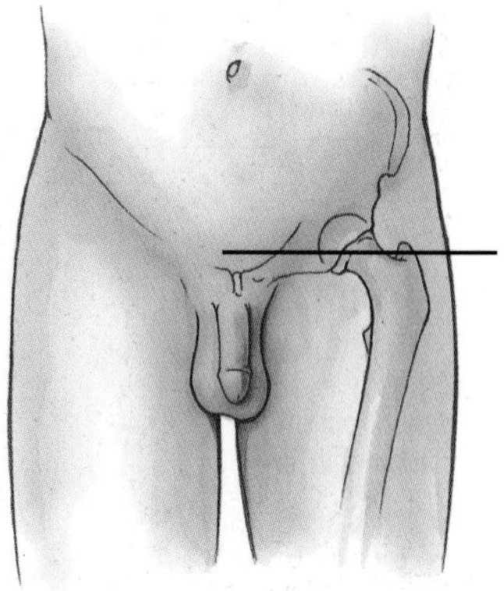

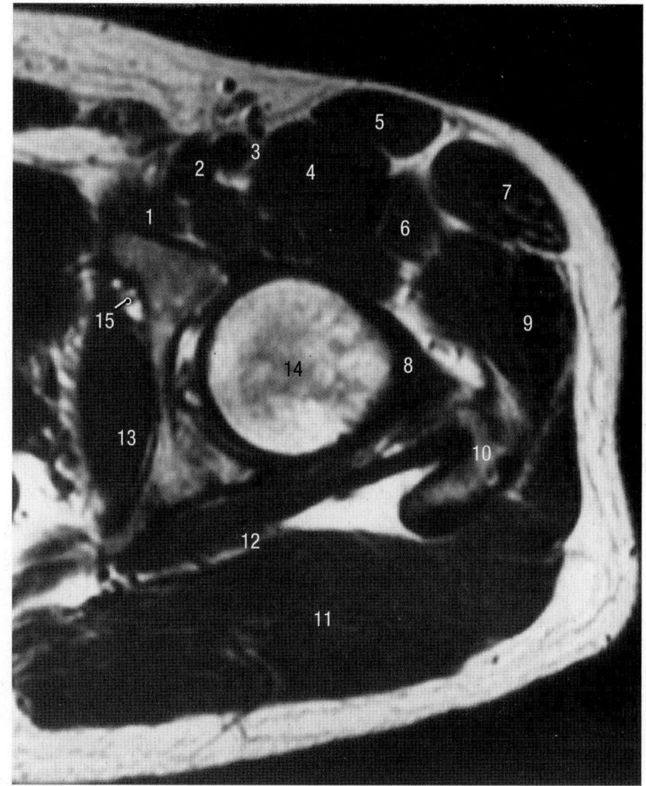

B. Transverse MRI

5.40 TRANSVERSE SECTION THROUGH THIGH AT LEVEL OF HIP JOINT

A. Transverse section. **B.** MRI (*numbers* refer to structures in **A**). In **A**:

- The fibrous capsule of the joint is thick where it forms the iliofemoral ligament and thin posterior to the subtendinous bursa of psoas and tendon.
- The femoral sheath, enclosing the femoral artery, vein, lymph node, lymph vessels, and fat, is free, except posteriorly where, between the psoas and pectineus muscles, it is attached to the capsule of the hip joint.
- The femoral vein is located at the interval between the psoas and pectineus muscles. The femoral nerve lies between the iliacus muscle and fascia.

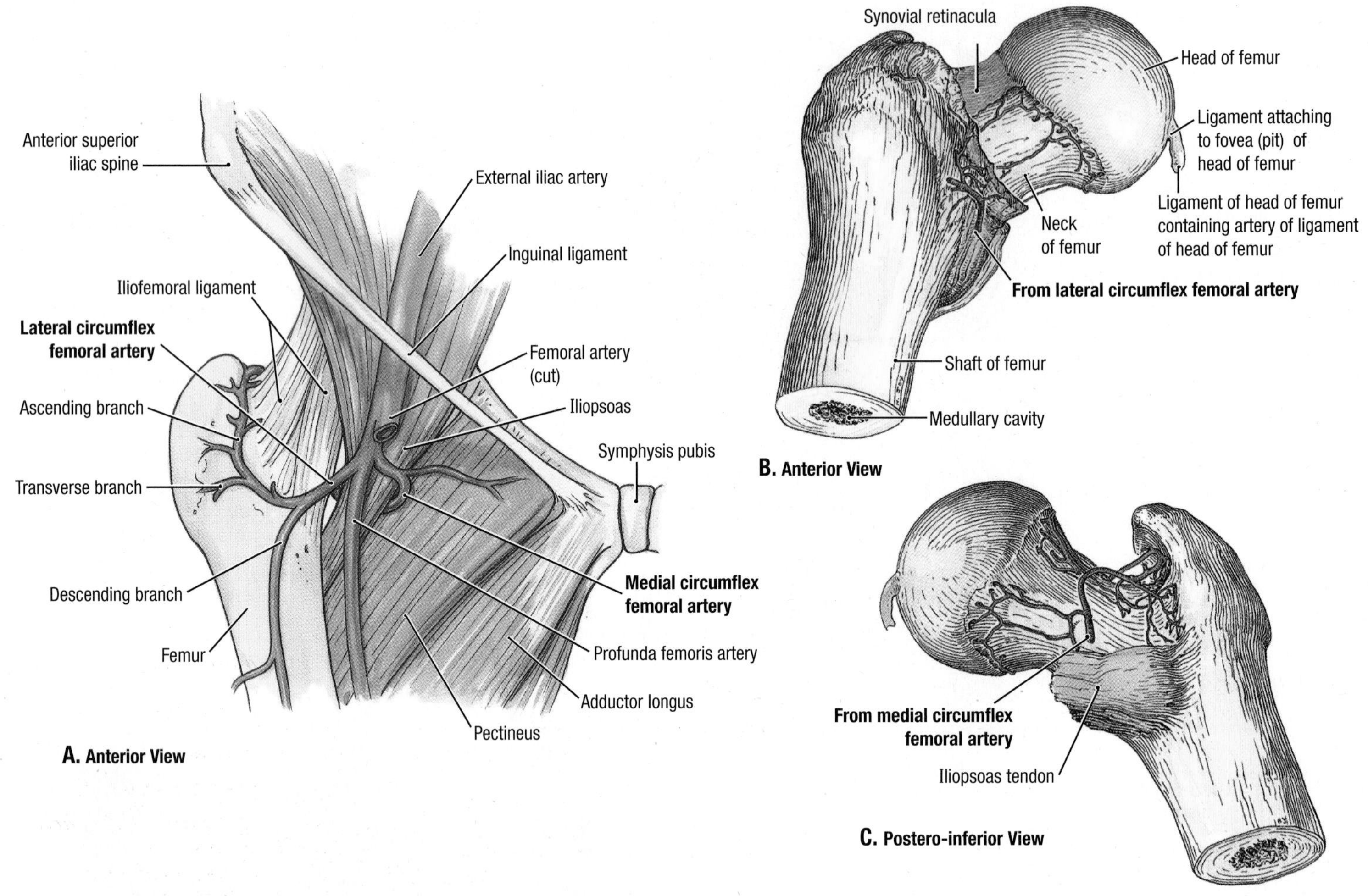
Anterior superior iliac spine
External iliac artery
Inguinal ligament
Iliofemoral ligament
Lateral circumflex femoral artery
Femoral artery (cut)
Iliopsoas
Ascending branch
Symphysis pubis
Transverse branch
Descending branch
Medial circumflex femoral artery
Femur
Profunda femoris artery
Adductor longus
Pectineus
A. Anterior View
Synovial retinacula
Head of femur
Ligament attaching to fovea (pit) of head of femur
Ligament of head of femur containing artery of ligament of head of femur
Neck of femur
From lateral circumflex femoral artery
Shaft of femur
Medullary cavity
B. Anterior View
From medial circumflex femoral artery
Iliopsoas tendon
C. Postero-inferior View

5.41 BLOOD SUPPLY TO HEAD OF FEMUR

A. Medial and lateral circumflex femoral arteries in femoral triangle. **B.** Branches of lateral circumflex femoral artery. **C.** Branches of medial circumflex femoral artery.

- Branches of the medial and lateral circumflex femoral arteries ascend on the posterosuperior and postero-inferior parts of the neck of the femur. The vessels ascend in synovial retinacula—reflections of synovial membrane along the neck of the femur. The retinacula (in **B** and **C**) have been mostly removed; thus, the vessels can be clearly visualized.
- The branches of the medial and lateral circumflex femoral arteries perforate the bone just distal to the head of the femur, where they anastomose with branches from the artery of the ligament of the head of the femur and with medullary branches located within the shaft of the femur.
- The ligament of the head of the femur usually contains the artery of the ligament of the head of the femur, a branch of the obturator artery. The artery enters the head of the femur only when the center of the ossification has extended to the pit (fovea) for the ligament of the head (12th to 14th year). When present, this anastomosis persists even in advanced age; however, in 20% of persons, it is never established.

Fractures of the femoral neck often disrupt the blood supply to the head of the femur. The medial circumflex femoral artery supplies most of the blood to the head and neck of the femur and is often torn when the femoral neck is fractured. In some cases, the blood supplied by the artery of the ligament of the head may be the only blood received by the proximal fragment of the femoral head, which may be inadequate. If the blood vessels are ruptured, the fragment of bone may receive no blood and undergo aseptic avascular necrosis.

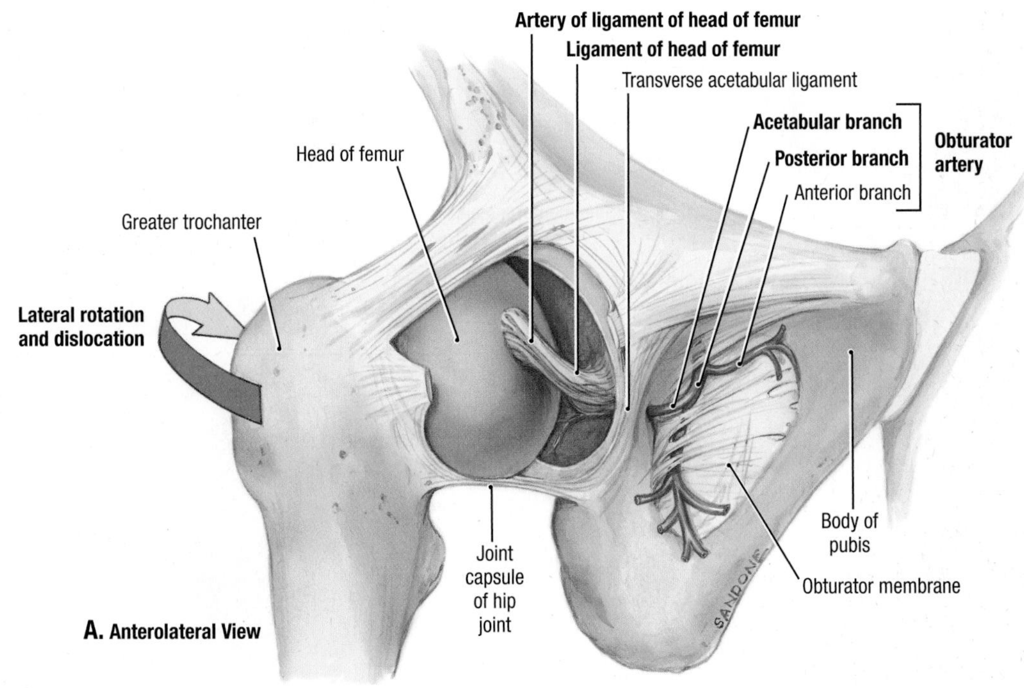
Artery of ligament of head of femur
Ligament of head of femur
Transverse acetabular ligament
Acetabular branch
Posterior branch
Anterior branch
Obturator artery
Head of femur
Greater trochanter
Lateral rotation and dislocation
Body of pubis
Obturator membrane
Joint capsule of hip joint
A. Anterolateral View

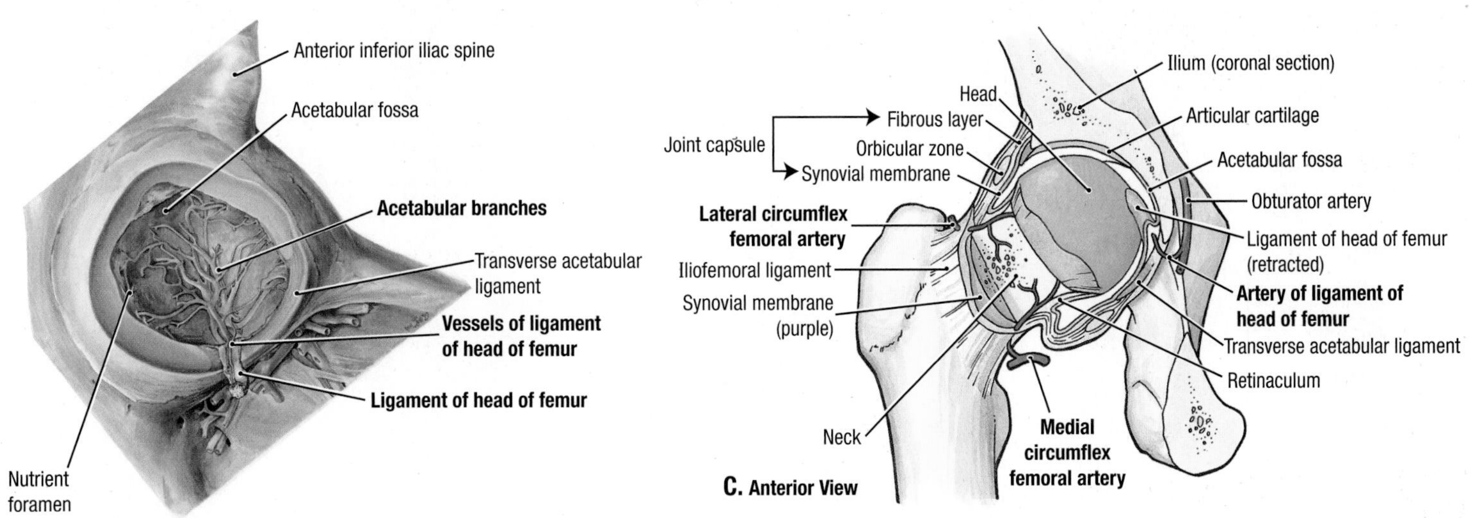
Anterior inferior iliac spine
Acetabular fossa
Acetabular branches
Transverse acetabular ligament
Vessels of ligament of head of femur
Ligament of head of femur
Nutrient foramen
B. Lateral View
Ilium (coronal section)
Head
Fibrous layer
Articular cartilage
Joint capsule
Orbicular zone
Synovial membrane
Acetabular fossa
Obturator artery
Lateral circumflex femoral artery
Ligament of head of femur (retracted)
Iliofemoral ligament
Artery of ligament of head of femur
Synovial membrane (purple)
Transverse acetabular ligament
Retinaculum
Neck
Medial circumflex femoral artery
C. Anterior View

5.42 BLOOD VESSELS OF ACETABULAR FOSSA AND LIGAMENT OF HEAD OF FEMUR

A. Obturator artery. The hip joint has been dislocated to reveal the ligament of the head of the femur. The obturator artery divides into anterior and posterior branches, and the acetabular branch arises from the posterior branch. The artery of the ligament of the head of the femur is a branch of the acetabular artery and can be seen traveling in the ligament to the head of the femur. **B.** Acetabular artery and vein. The acetabular branches (artery and vein) pass through the acetabular foramen and enter the acetabular fossa, where they diverge in the fatty areolar tissue. The branches radiate to the margin of the fossa, where they enter nutrient foramina. **C.** Blood supply of the head and neck of the femur. A section of bone has been removed from the femoral neck.

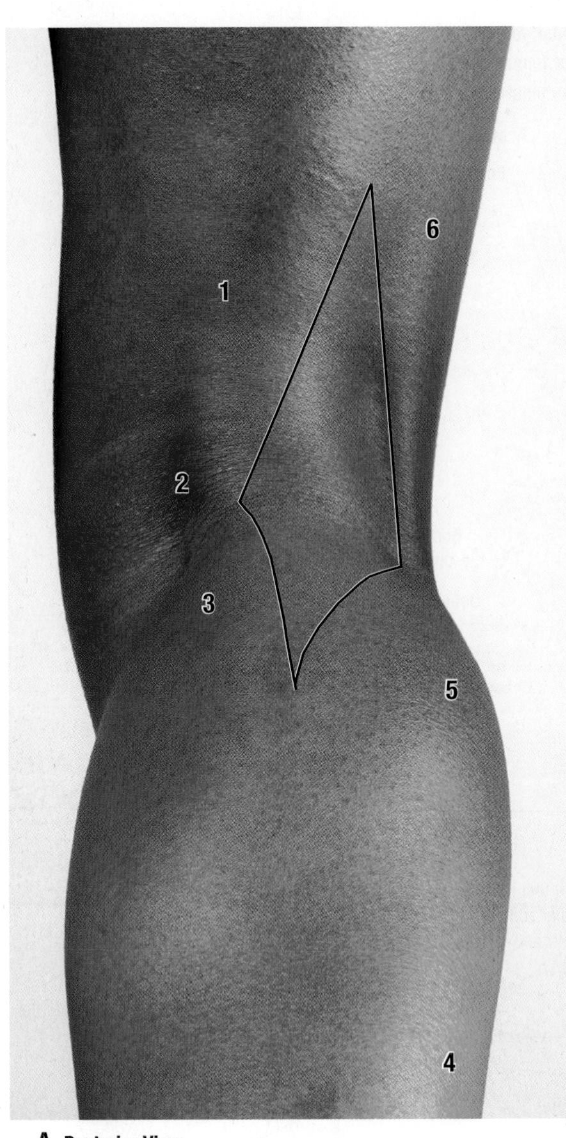
6
1
2
3
5
4

A. Posterior View

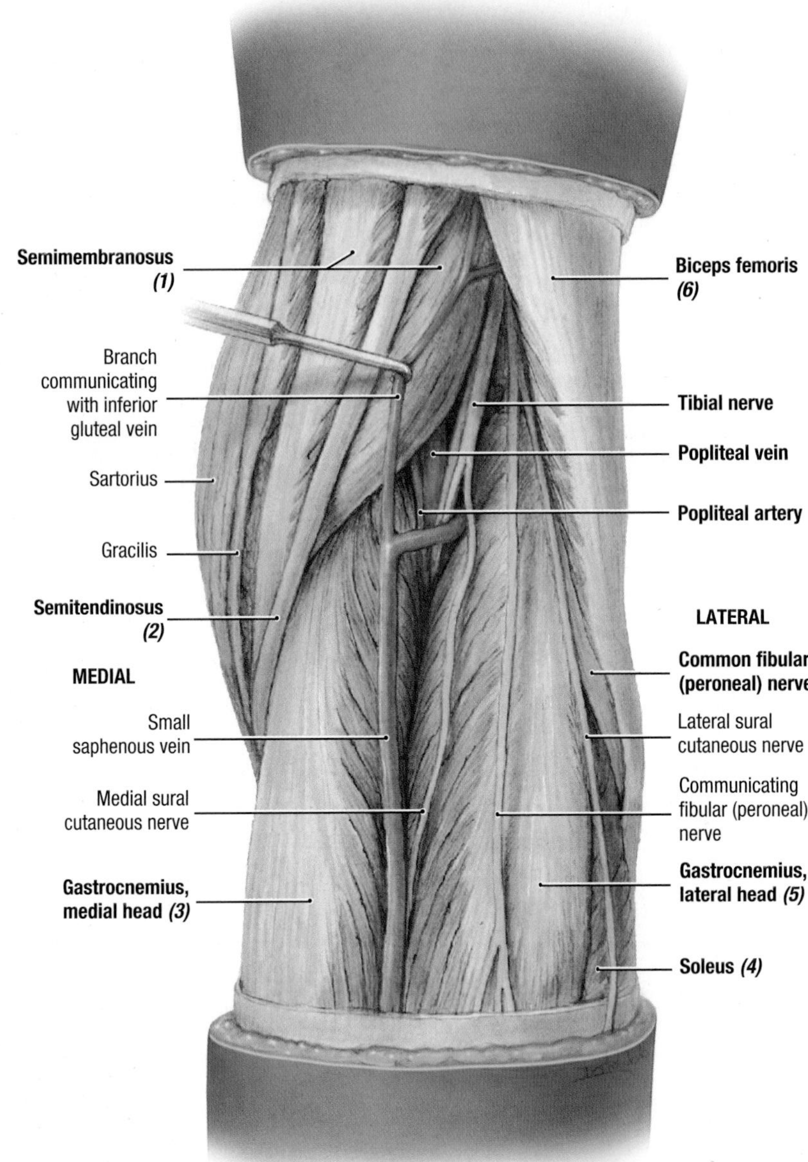
Semimembranosus (1)
Branch communicating with inferior gluteal vein
Sartorius
Gracilis
Semitendinosus (2)
MEDIAL
Small saphenous vein
Medial sural cutaneous nerve
Gastrocnemius, medial head (3)
Biceps femoris (6)
Tibial nerve
Popliteal vein
Popliteal artery
LATERAL
Common fibular (peroneal) nerve
Lateral sural cutaneous nerve
Communicating fibular (peroneal) nerve
Gastrocnemius, lateral head (5)
Soleus (4)

B. Posterior View

5.43 POPLITEAL FOSSA

A. Surface anatomy (*numbers* refer to structures in **B**). **B.** Superficial dissection.

- The two heads of the gastrocnemius muscle are embraced on the medial side by the semimembranosus muscle, which is overlaid by the semitendinosus muscle, and on the lateral side by the biceps femoris muscle.
- The small saphenous vein runs between the two heads of the gastrocnemius muscle. Deep to this vein is the medial sural cutaneous nerve, which, followed proximally, leads to the tibial nerve. The tibial nerve is superficial to the popliteal vein, which, in turn, is superficial to the popliteal artery.

Because the popliteal artery is deep in the popliteal fossa, it may be difficult to feel the **popliteal pulse.** Palpation of this pulse is commonly performed by placing the person in the prone position with the knee flexed to relax the popliteal fascia and hamstrings. The pulsations are best felt in the inferior part of the fossa. Weakening or loss of the popliteal pulse is a sign of femoral artery obstruction.

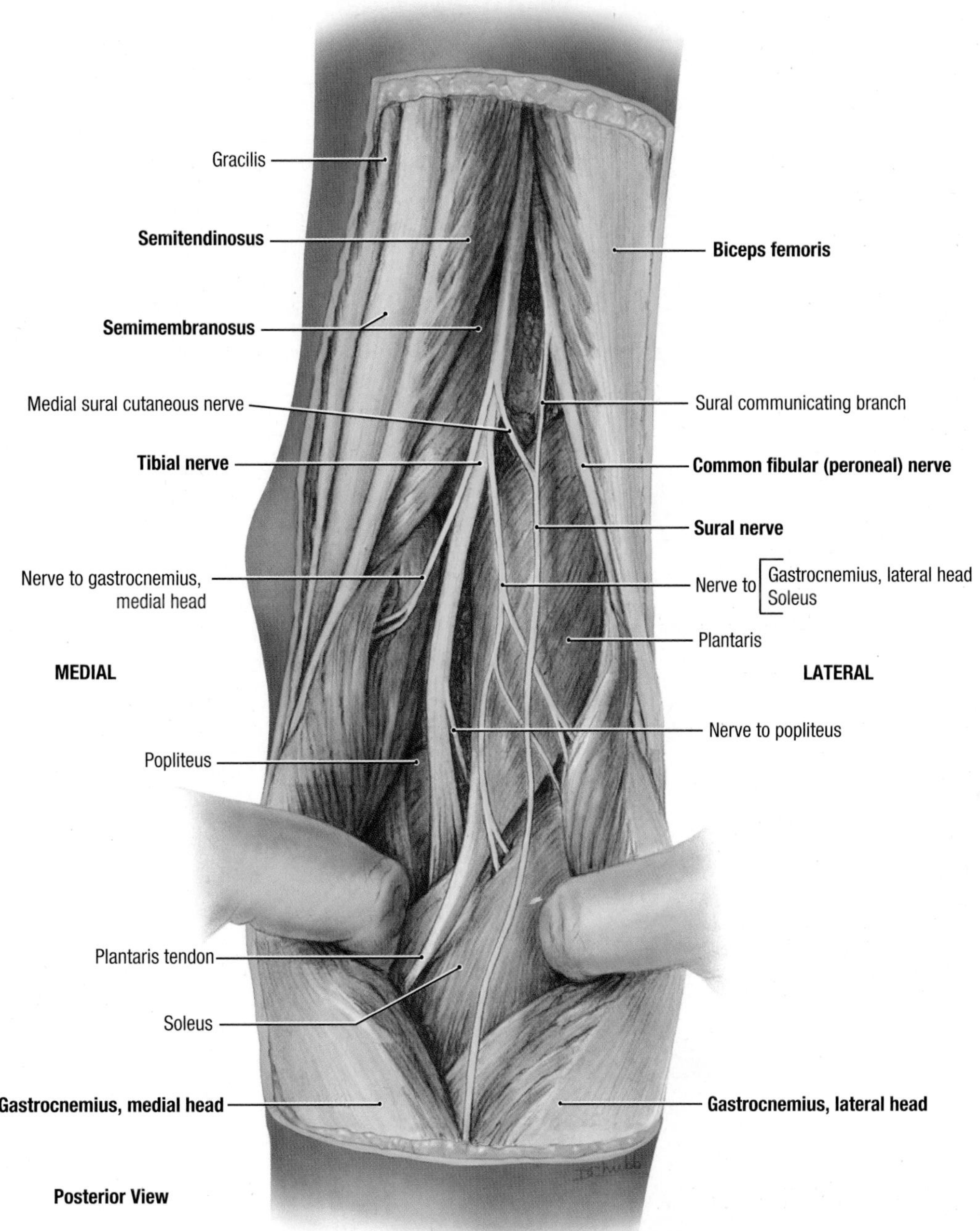
Gracilis
Semitendinosus
Biceps femoris
Semimembranosus
Medial sural cutaneous nerve
Sural communicating branch
Tibial nerve
Common fibular (peroneal) nerve
Sural nerve
Nerve to gastrocnemius, medial head
Nerve to
Gastrocnemius, lateral head
Soleus
Plantaris
MEDIAL
LATERAL
Nerve to popliteus
Popliteus
Plantaris tendon
Soleus
Gastrocnemius, medial head
Gastrocnemius, lateral head
Posterior View

5.44 NERVES OF POPLITEAL FOSSA

The two heads of the gastrocnemius muscle are separated. A cutaneous branch of the tibial nerve joins a cutaneous branch of the common fibular (peroneal) nerve to form the sural nerve. In this specimen, the junction is high; usually it is 5 to 8 cm proximal to the ankle.

All motor branches in this region emerge from the tibial nerve, one branch from its medial side and the others from its lateral side; hence, it is safer to dissect on the medial side.

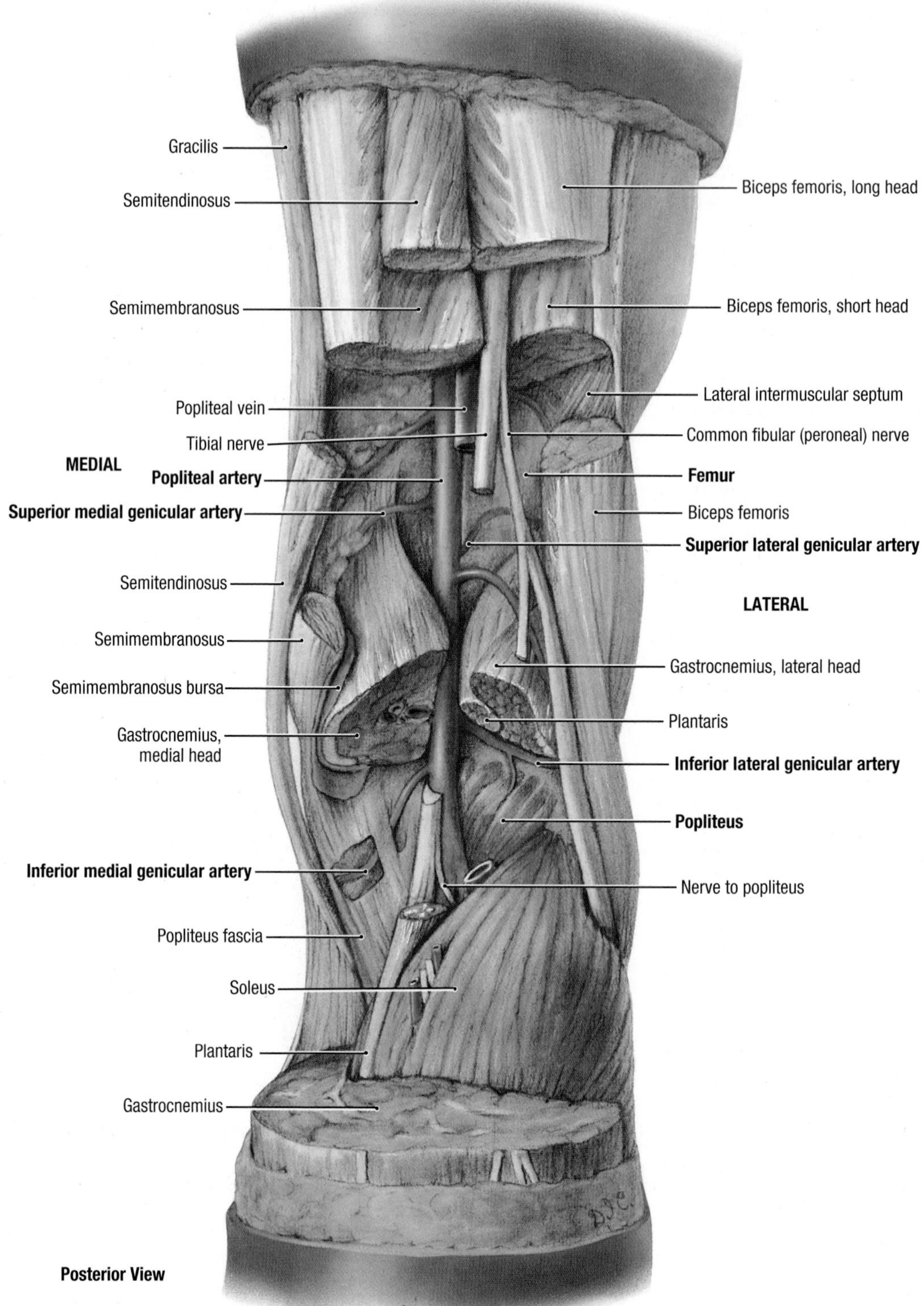
Gracilis
Semitendinosus
Semimembranosus
Popliteal vein
Tibial nerve
MEDIAL
Popliteal artery
Superior medial genicular artery
Semitendinosus
Semimembranosus
Semimembranosus bursa
Gastrocnemius, medial head
Inferior medial genicular artery
Popliteus fascia
Soleus
Plantaris
Gastrocnemius
Posterior View
Biceps femoris, long head
Biceps femoris, short head
Lateral intermuscular septum
Common fibular (peroneal) nerve
Femur
Biceps femoris
Superior lateral genicular artery
LATERAL
Gastrocnemius, lateral head
Plantaris
Inferior lateral genicular artery
Popliteus
Nerve to popliteus

5.45 DEEP DISSECTION OF POPLITEAL FOSSA

The common fibular (peroneal) nerve follows the posterior border of the biceps femoris muscle and, in this specimen, gives off two cutaneous branches. The popliteal artery lies on the floor of the popliteal fossa. The floor is formed by the femur, capsule of the knee joint, and popliteus muscle and fascia. The popliteal artery gives off genicular branches that also lie on the floor of the fossa. A **popliteal aneurysm** (abnormal dilation of all or part of the popliteal artery) usually causes edema (swelling) and pain in the popliteal fossa. If the femoral artery has to be ligated, blood can bypass the occlusion through the genicular anastomosis and reach the popliteal artery distal to the ligation.

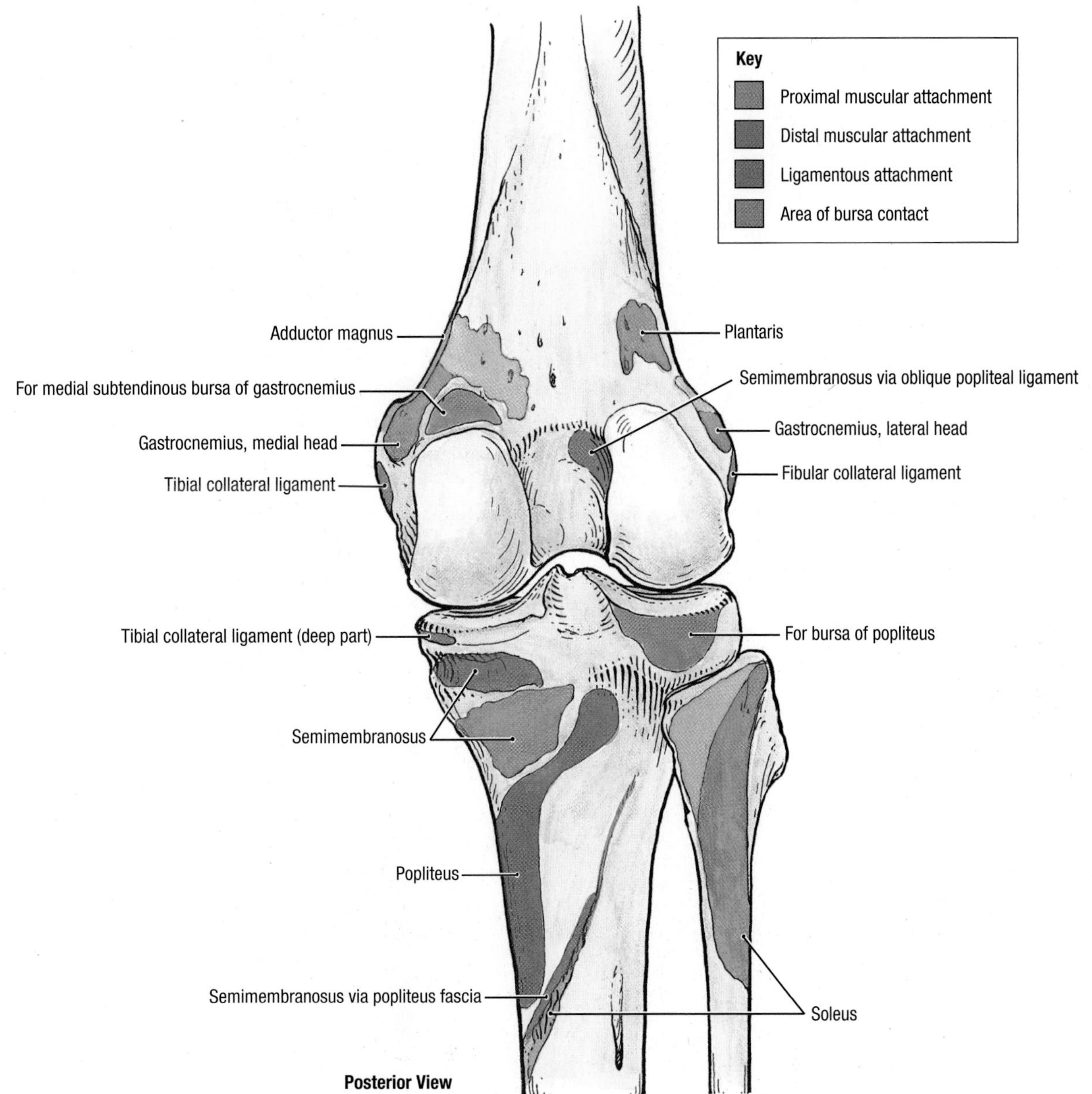
Key
Proximal muscular attachment
Distal muscular attachment
Ligamentous attachment
Area of bursa contact
Adductor magnus
Plantaris
For medial subtendinous bursa of gastrocnemius
Semimembranosus via oblique popliteal ligament
Gastrocnemius, medial head
Gastrocnemius, lateral head
Tibial collateral ligament
Fibular collateral ligament
Tibial collateral ligament (deep part)
For bursa of popliteus
Semimembranosus
Popliteus
Semimembranosus via popliteus fascia
Soleus
Posterior View

5.46 ATTACHMENT OF MUSCLES OF POPLITEAL REGION

Lighter tones are secondary attachments.

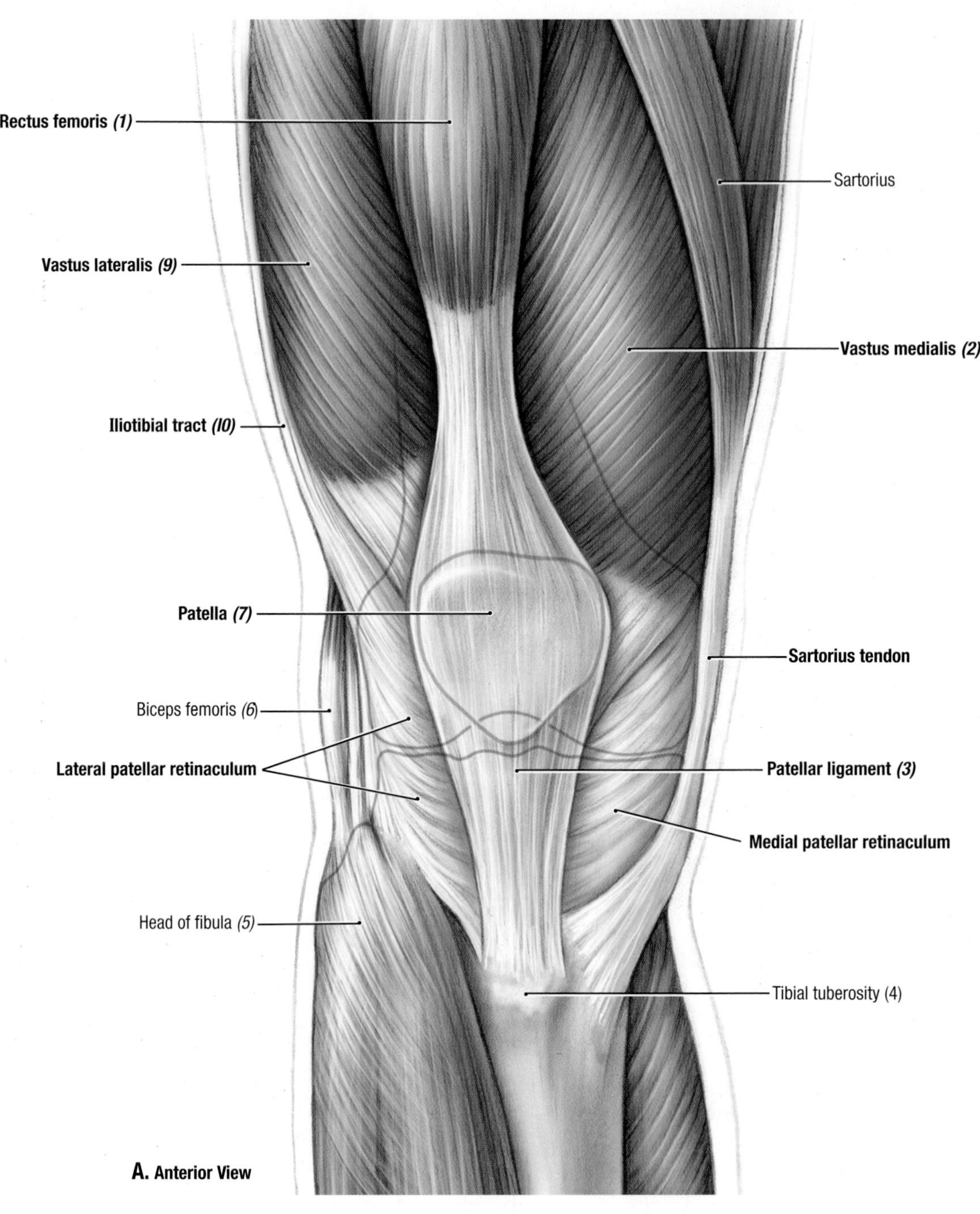
Rectus femoris (1)
Sartorius
Vastus lateralis (9)
Vastus medialis (2)
Iliotibial tract (10)
Patella (7)
Sartorius tendon
Biceps femoris (6)
Lateral patellar retinaculum
Patellar ligament (3)
Medial patellar retinaculum
Head of fibula (5)
Tibial tuberosity (4)

A. **Anterior View**

5.47 ANTERIOR ASPECT OF KNEE

A. Distal thigh and knee regions. Note that the tendons of the four parts of the quadriceps unite to form the quadriceps tendon, a broad band that attaches to the patella. The patellar ligament, a continuation of the quadriceps tendon, attaches the patella to the tibial tuberosity. The lateral and medial patellar retinacula, formed largely by continuation of the iliotibial tract, and investing fascia of the vasti muscles, maintains alignment of the patella and patellar ligament. The retinacula also form the anterolateral and anteromedial portions of the fibrous layer of the joint capsule of the knee.

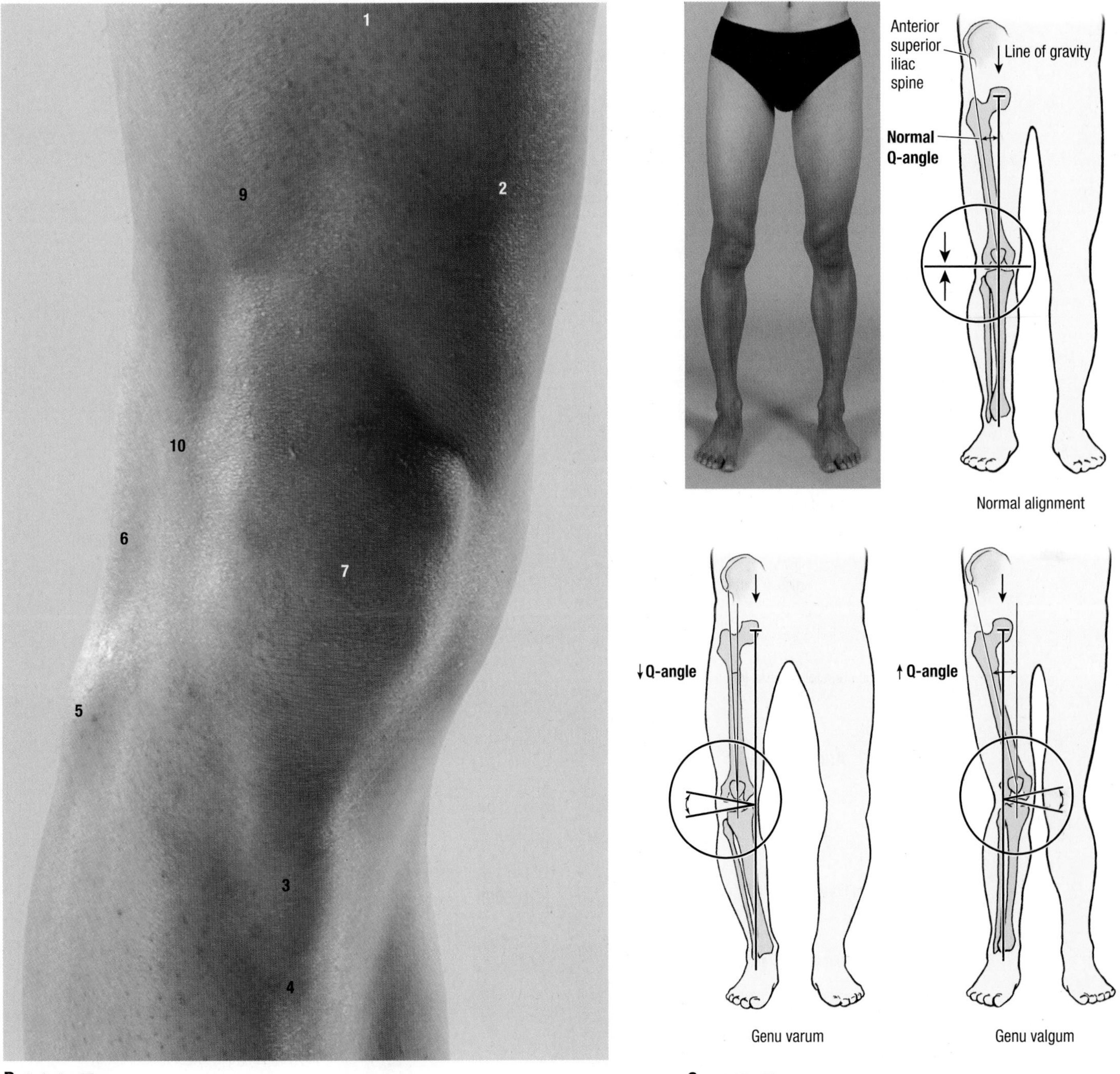
1
9
2
10
6
7
5
3
4
Anterior
superior
iliac
spine
Line of gravity
Normal
Q-angle
Normal alignment
↓Q-angle
↑Q-angle
Genu varum
Genu valgum

B. Anterior Views

C. Anterior Views

5.47 ANTERIOR ASPECT OF KNEE (*CONTINUED*)

B. Surface anatomy (numbers refer to structures in **A**). The femur is placed diagonally within the thigh, whereas the tibia is almost vertical within the leg, creating an angle at the knee between the long axes of the bones. The angle between the two bones, referred to clinically as the **Q-angle,** is assessed by drawing a line from the anterior superior iliac spine to the middle of the patella and extrapolating a second (vertical) line passing through the middle of the patella and tibial tuberosity. The Q-angle is typically greater in adult females, owing to their wider pelves. **C. Genu valgum and genu varum.** A medial angulation of the leg in relation to the thigh, in which the femur is abnormally vertical and the Q-angle is small, is a deformity called genu varum (bowleg) that causes unequal weight bearing resulting in arthrosis (destruction of knee cartilages), and an overstressed fibular collateral ligament. A lateral angulation of the leg (large Q-angle, >17 degrees) in relation to the thigh is called genu valgum (knock-knee). This results in excess stress and degeneration of the lateral structures of the knee joint.

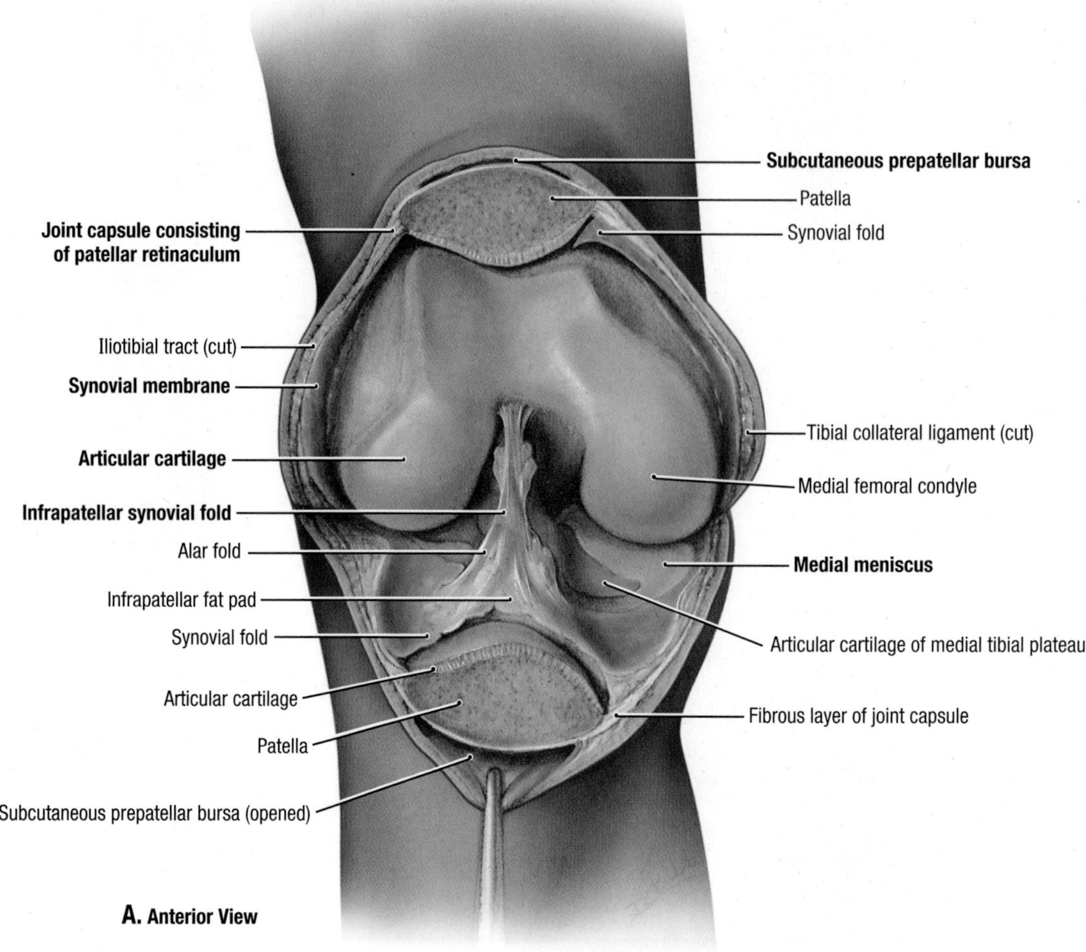
Subcutaneous prepatellar bursa
Patella
Synovial fold
Joint capsule consisting of patellar retinaculum
Iliotibial tract (cut)
Synovial membrane
Tibial collateral ligament (cut)
Articular cartilage
Medial femoral condyle
Infrapatellar synovial fold
Alar fold
Medial meniscus
Infrapatellar fat pad
Synovial fold
Articular cartilage of medial tibial plateau
Articular cartilage
Fibrous layer of joint capsule
Patella
Subcutaneous prepatellar bursa (opened)

A. **Anterior View**

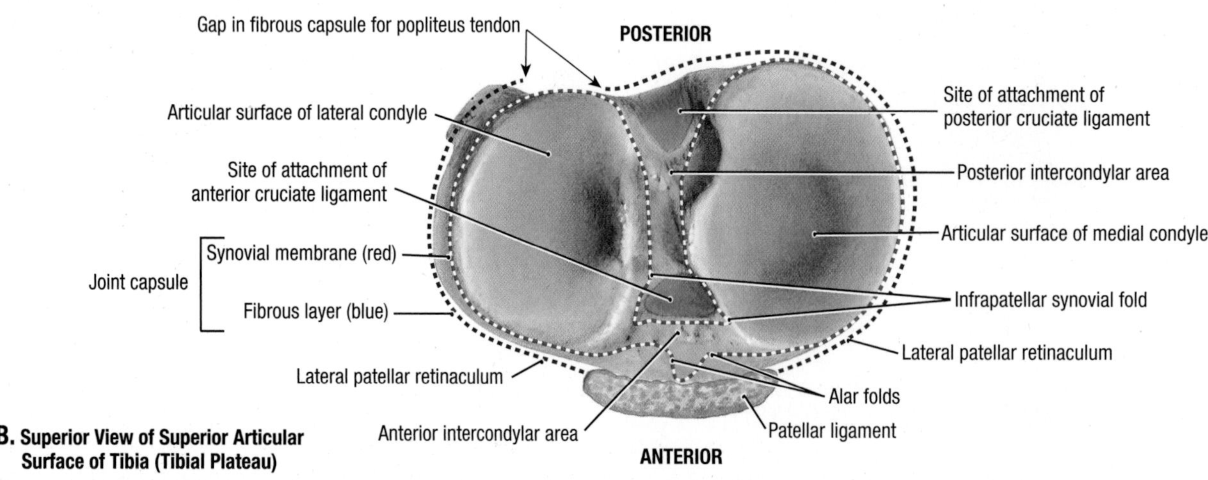
Gap in fibrous capsule for popliteus tendon
POSTERIOR
Articular surface of lateral condyle
Site of attachment of posterior cruciate ligament
Site of attachment of anterior cruciate ligament
Posterior intercondylar area
Articular surface of medial condyle
Joint capsule
Synovial membrane (red)
Fibrous layer (blue)
Infrapatellar synovial fold
Lateral patellar retinaculum
Lateral patellar retinaculum
Alar folds
Anterior intercondylar area
Patellar ligament
ANTERIOR

B. **Superior View of Superior Articular Surface of Tibia (Tibial Plateau)**

5.48 FIBROUS LAYER AND SYNOVIAL MEMBRANE OF JOINT CAPSULE

A. Dissection. **B.** Attachment of the layers of the joint capsule to the tibia. The fibrous layer (*blue dotted line*) and synovial membrane (*red dotted line*) are adjacent on each side, but they part company centrally to accommodate intercondylar and infrapatellar structures that are intracapsular (inside the fibrous layer) but extra-articular (excluded from the articular cavity by synovial membrane).

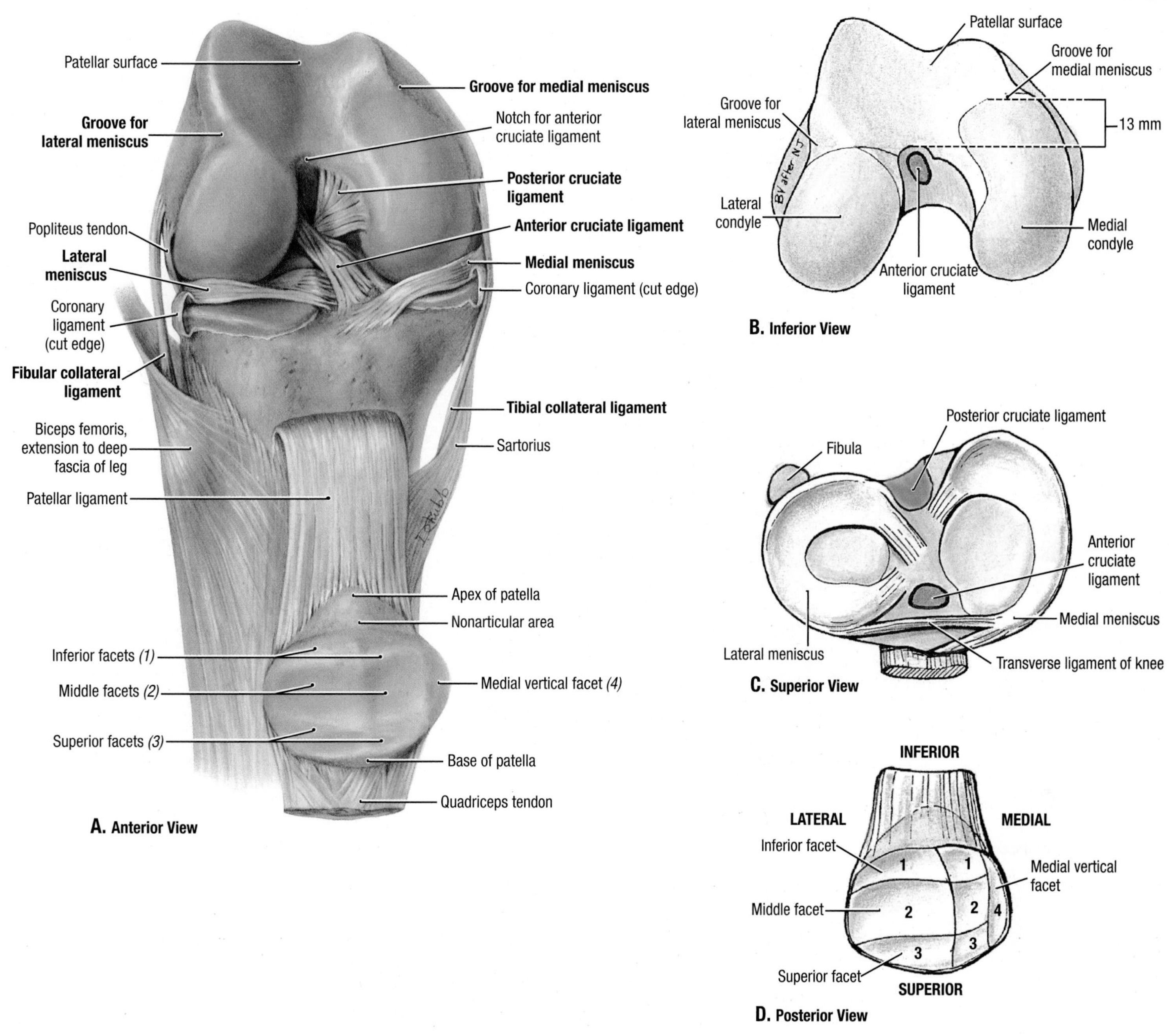
Patellar surface
Groove for medial meniscus
Groove for lateral meniscus
Notch for anterior cruciate ligament
Posterior cruciate ligament
Popliteus tendon
Anterior cruciate ligament
Lateral meniscus
Medial meniscus
Coronary ligament (cut edge)
Coronary ligament (cut edge)
Fibular collateral ligament
Tibial collateral ligament
Biceps femoris, extension to deep fascia of leg
Sartorius
Patellar ligament
Apex of patella
Nonarticular area
Inferior facets (1)
Middle facets (2)
Medial vertical facet (4)
Superior facets (3)
Base of patella
Quadriceps tendon
A. Anterior View
Patellar surface
Groove for medial meniscus
Groove for lateral meniscus
13 mm
Lateral condyle
Medial condyle
Anterior cruciate ligament
B. Inferior View
Posterior cruciate ligament
Fibula
Anterior cruciate ligament
Medial meniscus
Lateral meniscus
Transverse ligament of knee
C. Superior View
INFERIOR
LATERAL
MEDIAL
Inferior facet
Medial vertical facet
Middle facet
Superior facet
SUPERIOR
1
1
2
2
4
3
3
D. Posterior View

5.49 ARTICULAR SURFACES AND LIGAMENTS OF KNEE JOINT

A. Flexed knee joint with patella reflected. There are indentations on the sides of the femoral condyles at the junction of the patellar and tibial articular areas. The lateral tibial articular area is shorter than the medial one. The notch at the anterolateral part of the intercondylar notch is for the anterior cruciate ligament on full extension. **B.** Distal femur. **C.** Tibial plateaus. **D.** Articular surfaces of patella. The three paired facets (superior, middle, and inferior) on the posterior surface of the patella articulate with the patellar surface of the femur successively during (*1*) extension, (*2*) slight flexion, (*3*) flexion, and the most medial vertical facet on the patella (*4*) articulates during full flexion with the crescentic facet on the medial margin of the intercondylar notch of the femur. When the **patellar dislocation** occurs, it nearly always dislocates laterally. The tendency toward lateral dislocation is normally counterbalanced by the medial, more horizontal pull of the powerful vastus medialis. In addition, the more anterior projection of the lateral femoral condyle and deeper slope for the large lateral patellar facet provides a mechanical deterrent to lateral dislocation. An imbalance of the lateral pull and the mechanisms resisting it result in abnormal tracking of the patella within the patellar groove and chronic patellar pain, even if actual dislocation does not occur.

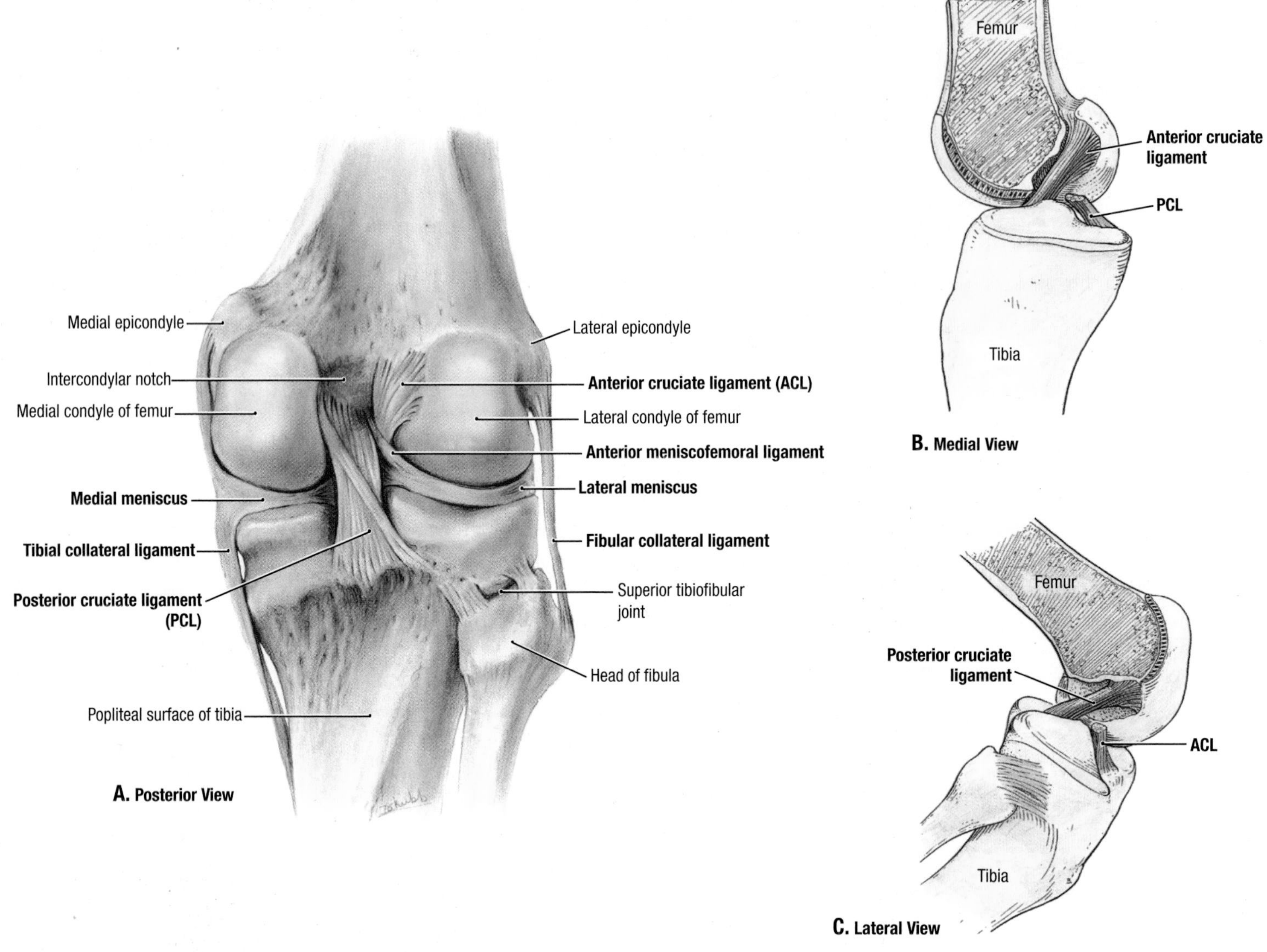
Medial epicondyle
Intercondylar notch
Medial condyle of femur
Medial meniscus
Tibial collateral ligament
Posterior cruciate ligament (PCL)
Popliteal surface of tibia
Lateral epicondyle
Anterior cruciate ligament (ACL)
Lateral condyle of femur
Anterior meniscofemoral ligament
Lateral meniscus
Fibular collateral ligament
Superior tibiofibular joint
Head of fibula
A. Posterior View
Femur
Anterior cruciate ligament
PCL
Tibia
B. Medial View
Femur
Posterior cruciate ligament
ACL
Tibia
C. Lateral View

5.50 LIGAMENTS OF KNEE JOINT

A. Posterior aspect of joint. The bandlike tibial (medial) collateral ligament is attached to the medial meniscus, and the cordlike fibular (lateral) collateral ligament is separated from the lateral meniscus by the width of the popliteus tendon (removed). The posterior cruciate ligament is joined by a cord from the lateral meniscus called the anterior meniscofemoral ligament. The posterior meniscofemoral ligament attaches to the medial condyle of the femur just posterior to the attachment of the posterior cruciate ligament. **B.** Anterior cruciate ligament (ACL). **C.** Posterior cruciate ligament (PCL). In each illustration, half the femur is sagittally sectioned and removed with the proximal part of the corresponding cruciate ligament. Note that the posterior cruciate ligament prevents the femur from sliding anteriorly on the tibia, particularly when the knee is flexed. The anterior cruciate ligament prevents the femur from sliding posteriorly on the tibia, preventing hyperextension of the knee, and limits medial rotation of the femur when the foot is on the ground (i.e., when the leg is fixed). **Injury to the knee joint** is frequently caused by a blow to the lateral side of the extended knee or excessive lateral twisting of the flexed knee, which disrupts the tibial collateral ligament and concomitantly tears and/or detaches the medial meniscus from the joint capsule. This injury is common in athletes who twist their flexed knees while running (e.g., in football and soccer). The anterior cruciate ligament, which serves as a pivot for rotary movements of the knee, is taut during flexion and may also tear subsequent to the rupture of the tibial collateral ligament.

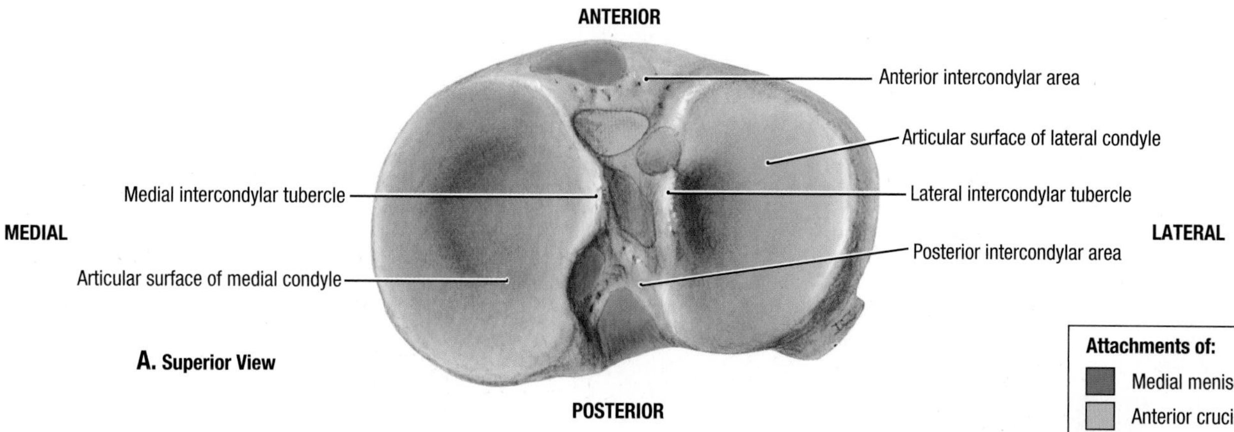

ANTERIOR

Anterior intercondylar area
Articular surface of lateral condyle
Medial intercondylar tubercle
Lateral intercondylar tubercle
MEDIAL
LATERAL
Posterior intercondylar area
Articular surface of medial condyle

A. Superior View

POSTERIOR

Attachments of:
- Medial meniscus
- Anterior cruciate ligament
- Lateral meniscus
- Posterior cruciate ligament

Patellar ligament
Coronary ligament
Anterior cruciate ligament
Iliotibial tract
Medial meniscus
Lateral meniscus
Bursa in tibial collateral ligament
Fibular collateral ligament
Popliteus tendon
Fibula
Coronary ligament
Posterior meniscofemoral ligament
Posterior cruciate ligament

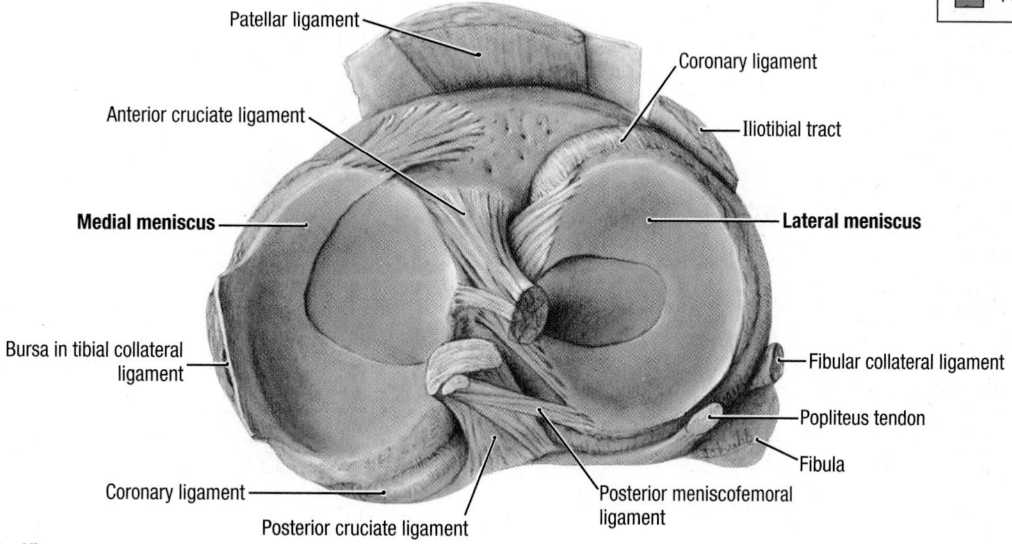

B. Superior View

5.51 CRUCIATE LIGAMENTS AND MENISCI

A. Attachments sites on tibia. **B.** Menisci in situ.

- The lateral tibial condyle is flatter, shorter from anterior to posterior, and more circular. The medial condyle is concave, longer from anterior to posterior, and more oval.
- The menisci conform to the shapes of the surfaces on which they rest. Because the horns of the lateral meniscus are attached close together and its coronary ligament is slack, this meniscus can slide anteriorly and posteriorly on the (flat) condyle; because the horns of the medial meniscus are attached further apart, its movements on the (concave) condyle are restricted.

Arthroscopy is an endoscopic examination that allows visualization of the interior of the knee joint cavity with minimal disruption of tissue. The arthroscope and one (or more) additional canula(e) are inserted through tiny incisions, known as portals. The second canula is for passage of specialized tools (e.g., manipulative probes or forceps) or equipment for trimming, shaping, or removing damaged tissue. This technique allows removal of torn menisci, loose bodies in the joint such as bone chips, and debridement (the excision of devitalized articular cartilaginous material in advanced cases of arthritis). Ligament repair or replacement may also be performed using an arthroscope.

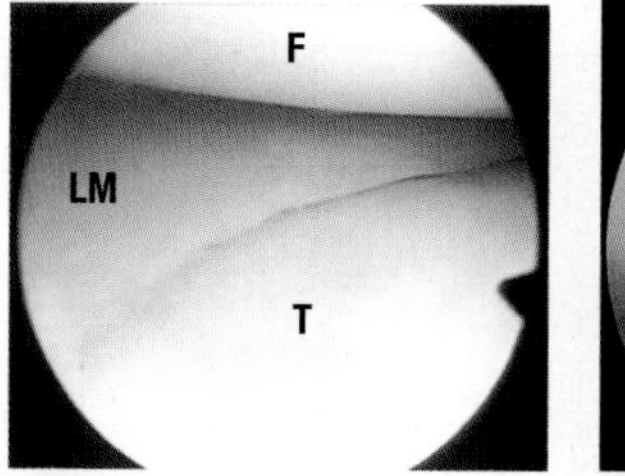
F
LM
T
Normal lateral meniscus

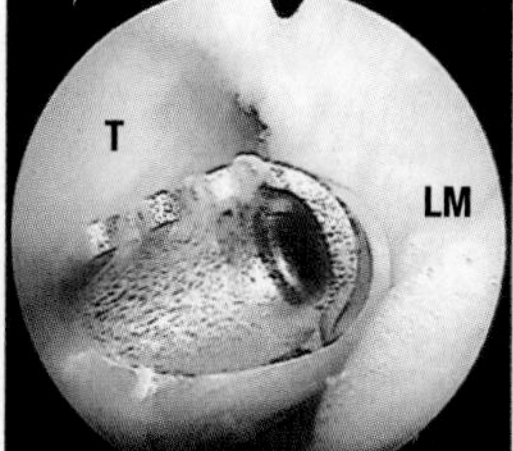
T
LM
Trimming torn lateral meniscus

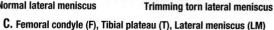

C. Femoral condyle (F), Tibial plateau (T), Lateral meniscus (LM)

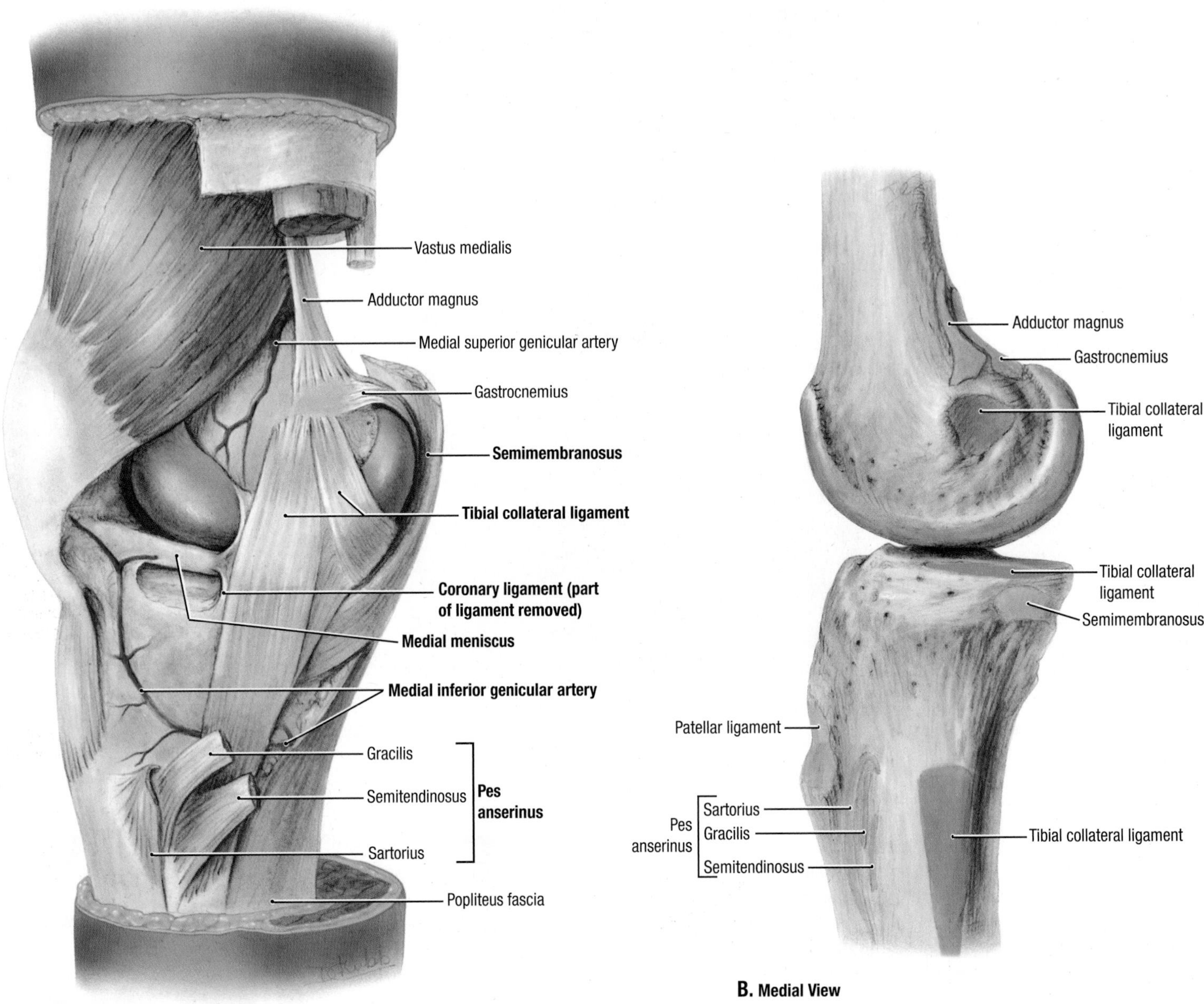

Vastus medialis
Adductor magnus
Medial superior genicular artery
Gastrocnemius
Semimembranosus
Tibial collateral ligament
Coronary ligament (part of ligament removed)
Medial meniscus
Medial inferior genicular artery
Gracilis
Semitendinosus
Sartorius
Pes anserinus
Popliteus fascia
A. Medial View
Adductor magnus
Gastrocnemius
Tibial collateral ligament
Tibial collateral ligament
Semimembranosus
Patellar ligament
Pes anserinus
Sartorius
Gracilis
Semitendinosus
Tibial collateral ligament
B. Medial View

5.52 MEDIAL ASPECT OF KNEE

A. Dissection. The bandlike part of the tibial collateral ligament attaches to the medial epicondyle of the femur, bridges superficial to the insertion of the semimembranosus muscle, and crosses the medial inferior genicular artery. Distally, the ligament is crossed by the three tendons forming the pes anserinus (sartorius, gracilis, and semitendinosus). **B.** Bones, showing muscle and ligament attachment sites.

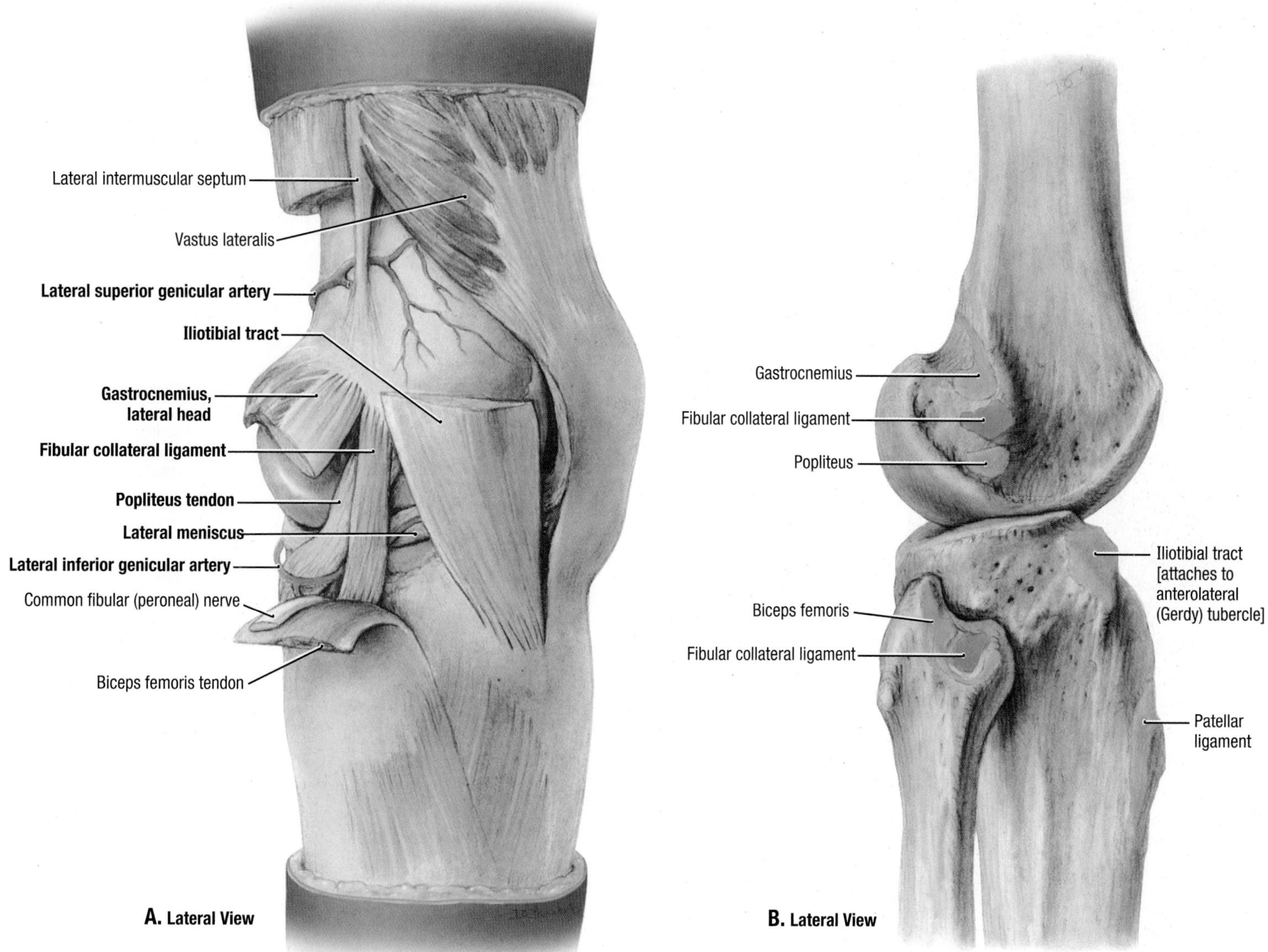
Lateral intermuscular septum
Vastus lateralis
Lateral superior genicular artery
Iliotibial tract
Gastrocnemius, lateral head
Fibular collateral ligament
Popliteus tendon
Lateral meniscus
Lateral inferior genicular artery
Common fibular (peroneal) nerve
Biceps femoris tendon
A. Lateral View
Gastrocnemius
Fibular collateral ligament
Popliteus
Iliotibial tract [attaches to anterolateral (Gerdy) tubercle]
Biceps femoris
Fibular collateral ligament
Patellar ligament
B. Lateral View

5.53 LATERAL ASPECT OF KNEE

A. Dissection. **B.** Bones, showing muscle and ligament attachments. Three structures arise from the lateral epicondyle and are uncovered by reflecting the biceps muscle: the gastrocnemius muscle is posterosuperior; the popliteus muscle is antero-inferior; and the fibular collateral ligament is in between, crossing superficial to the popliteus muscle. The lateral inferior genicular artery courses along the lateral meniscus.

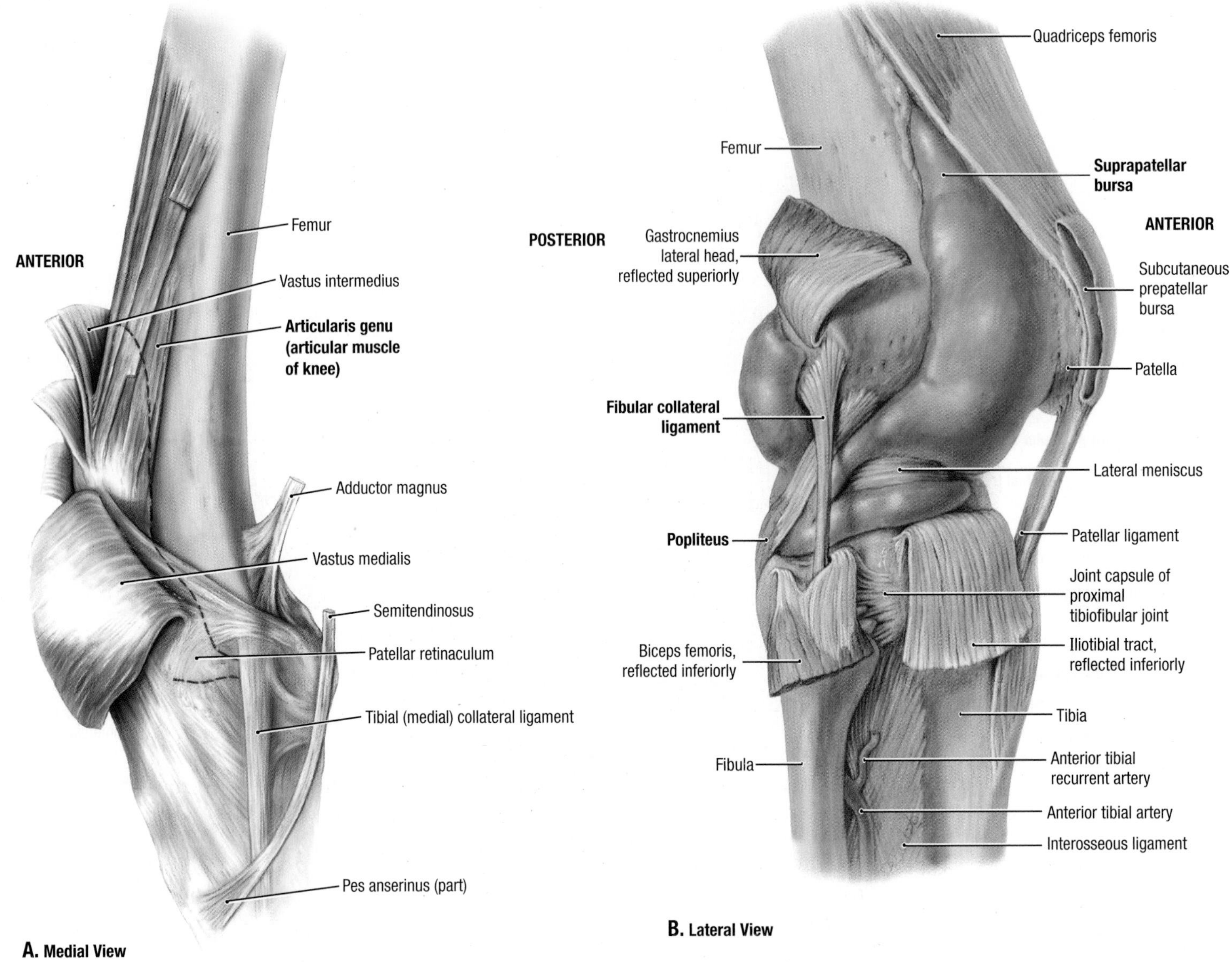
ANTERIOR
Femur
Vastus intermedius
Articularis genu (articular muscle of knee)
Adductor magnus
Vastus medialis
Semitendinosus
Patellar retinaculum
Tibial (medial) collateral ligament
Pes anserinus (part)
POSTERIOR
Quadriceps femoris
Femur
Suprapatellar bursa
ANTERIOR
Gastrocnemius lateral head, reflected superiorly
Subcutaneous prepatellar bursa
Patella
Fibular collateral ligament
Lateral meniscus
Popliteus
Patellar ligament
Joint capsule of proximal tibiofibular joint
Biceps femoris, reflected inferiorly
Iliotibial tract, reflected inferiorly
Tibia
Fibula
Anterior tibial recurrent artery
Anterior tibial artery
Interosseous ligament

A. Medial View

B. Lateral View

5.54 ARTICULARIS GENU AND BURSAE OF KNEE REGION

A. Articularis genu (articular muscle of the knee). This muscle lies deep to the vastus intermedius muscle and consists of fibers arising from the anterior surface of the femur proximally and attaching into the synovial membrane distally. The articularis genu pulls the synovial membrane of the suprapatellar bursa (*dotted line*) superiorly during extension of the knee so that it will not be caught between the patella and femur within the knee joint. **B.** Lateral aspect of knee. Latex was injected into the articular cavity and fixed with acetic acid. The distended synovial membrane was exposed and cleaned. The gastrocnemius muscle was reflected proximally, and the biceps femoris muscle and the iliotibial tract were reflected distally. The extent of the synovial capsule: superiorly, it rises superior to the patella, where it rests on a layer of fat that allows it to glide freely with movements of the joint; this superior part is called the suprapatellar bursa; posteriorly, it rises as high as the origin of the gastrocnemius muscle; laterally, it curves inferior to the lateral femoral epicondyle, where the popliteus tendon and fibular collateral ligament are attached; and inferiorly, it bulges inferior to the lateral meniscus, overlapping the tibia (the coronary ligament is removed to show this). **Prepatellar bursitis** (housemaid's knee) is usually a friction bursitis caused by friction between the skin and the patella. The suprapatellar bursa communicates with the articular cavity of the knee joint; consequently, abrasions or penetrating wounds superior to the patella may result in **suprapatellar bursitis** caused by bacteria entering the bursa from the torn skin. The infection may spread to the knee joint. **C.** Posterior aspect of knee.

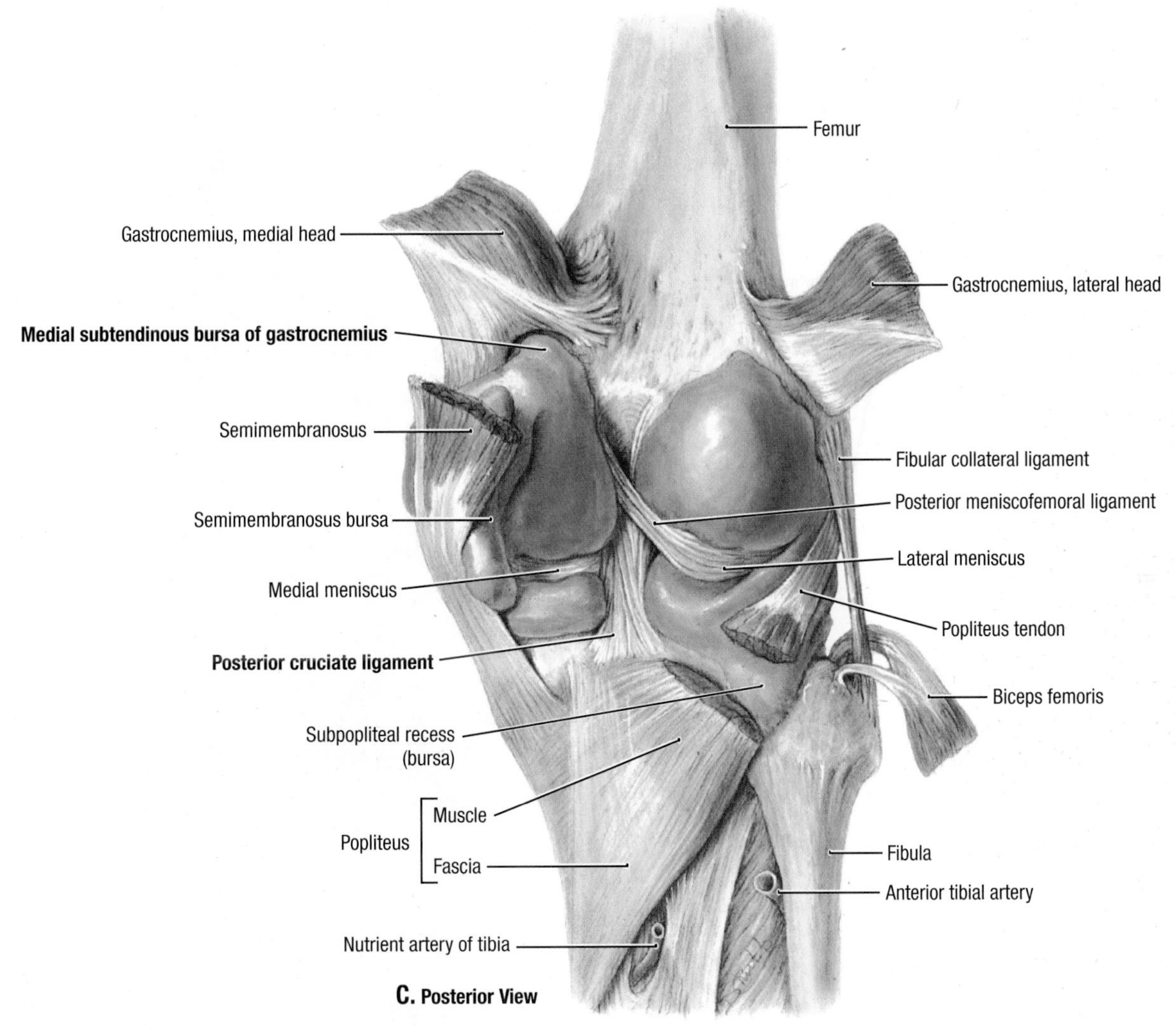
Femur
Gastrocnemius, medial head
Gastrocnemius, lateral head
Medial subtendinous bursa of gastrocnemius
Semimembranosus
Fibular collateral ligament
Semimembranosus bursa
Posterior meniscofemoral ligament
Lateral meniscus
Medial meniscus
Popliteus tendon
Posterior cruciate ligament
Biceps femoris
Subpopliteal recess (bursa)
Popliteus
Muscle
Fascia
Fibula
Anterior tibial artery
Nutrient artery of tibia

C. Posterior View

5.54 ARTICULARIS GENU AND BURSAE OF KNEE REGION (*CONTINUED*), DISTENDED KNEE JOINT

TABLE 5.11 BURSAE AROUND KNEE

Bursa	Location	Structural Features or Functions
Suprapatellar	Located between femur and tendon of quadriceps femoris	Held in position by articular muscle of knee; communicates freely with synovial cavity of knee joint
Popliteus	Located between tendon of popliteus and lateral condyle of tibia	Opens into synovial cavity of knee joint, inferior to lateral meniscus
Anserine	Separates tendons of sartorius, gracilis, and semitendinosus from tibia and tibial collateral ligament	Area where tendons of these muscles attach to tibia (pes anserinus) resembles the foot of a goose (L. *pes,* foot; L. *anser,* goose)
Medial subtendinous bursa of gastrocnemius	Lies deep to proximal attachment of tendon of medial head of gastrocnemius	Extension of synovial cavity of knee joint
Semimembranosus	Located between medial head of gastrocnemius and semimembranosus tendon	Related to the distal attachment of semimembranosus
Subcutaneous prepatellar	Lies between skin and anterior surface of patella	Allows free movement of skin over patella during movements of leg
Subcutaneous infrapatellar	Located between skin and tibial tuberosity	Helps knee to withstand pressure when kneeling
Deep infrapatellar	Lies between patellar ligament and anterior surface of tibia	Separated from knee joint by infrapatellar fat pad

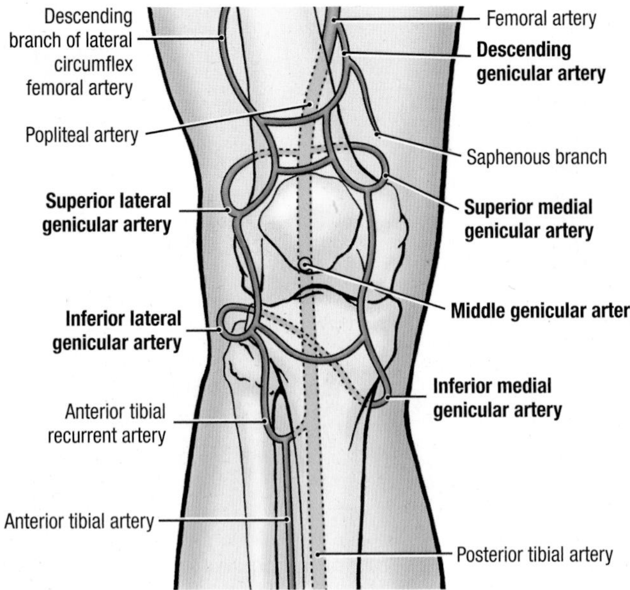
Descending branch of lateral circumflex femoral artery
Femoral artery
Descending genicular artery
Popliteal artery
Saphenous branch
Superior lateral genicular artery
Superior medial genicular artery
Middle genicular artery
Inferior lateral genicular artery
Inferior medial genicular artery
Anterior tibial recurrent artery
Anterior tibial artery
Posterior tibial artery

A. Anterior View

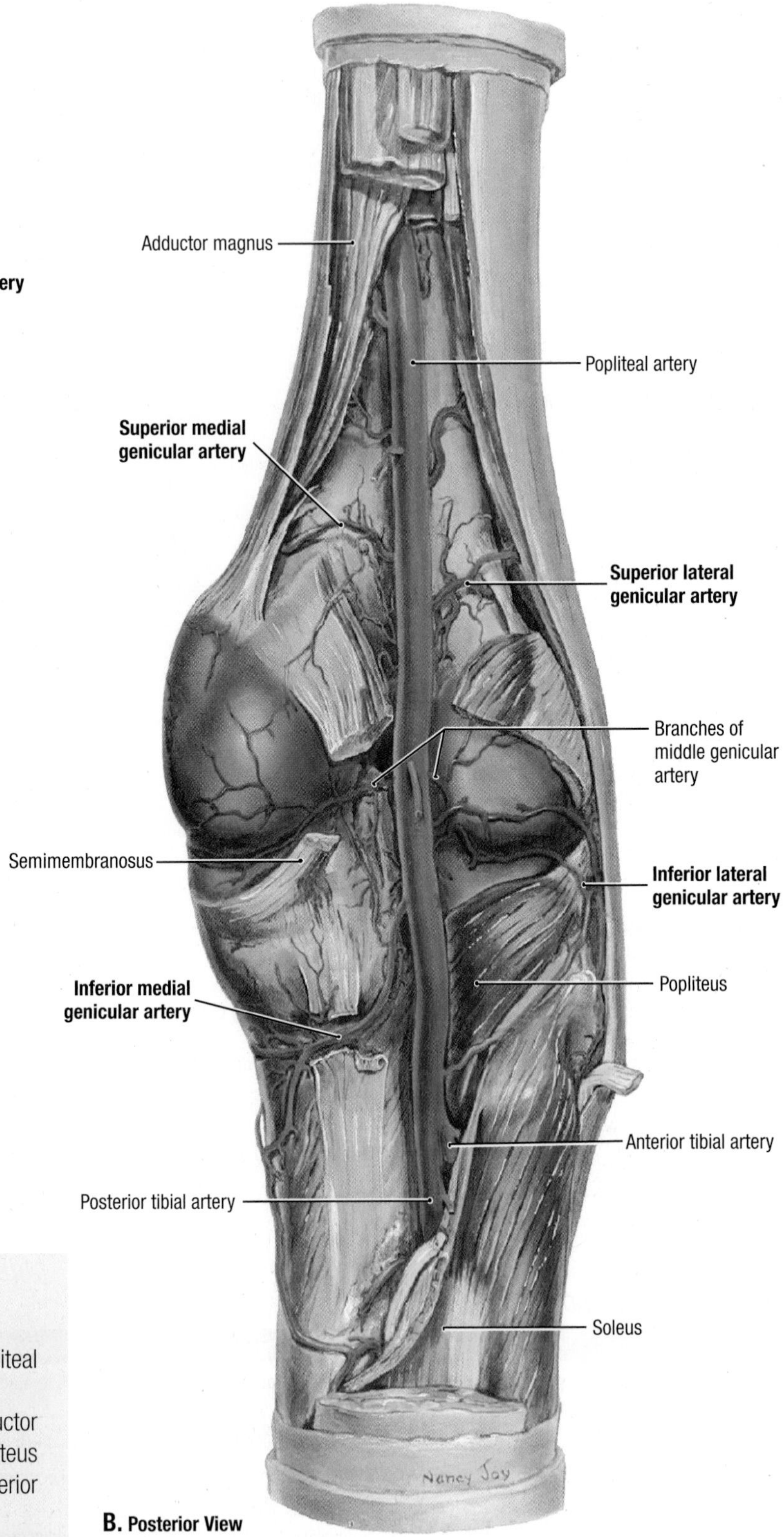

Adductor magnus
Popliteal artery
Superior medial genicular artery
Superior lateral genicular artery
Branches of middle genicular artery
Semimembranosus
Inferior lateral genicular artery
Popliteus
Inferior medial genicular artery
Anterior tibial artery
Posterior tibial artery
Soleus
Nancy Joy

B. Posterior View

5.55 ANASTOMOSES AROUND KNEE

A. Genicular anastomosis on the anterior aspect of the knee. **B.** Popliteal artery in popliteal fossa.

- The popliteal artery runs from the adductor hiatus (in the adductor magnus muscle) proximally to the inferior border of the popliteus muscle distally, where it bifurcates into the anterior and posterior tibial arteries.
- The three anterior relations of the popliteal artery include the femur (fat intervening), the joint capsule of the knee; and the popliteus muscle.
- Five genicular branches of the popliteal artery supply the capsule and ligaments of the knee joint. The genicular arteries are the superior lateral, superior medial, middle, inferior lateral, and inferior medial genicular arteries.

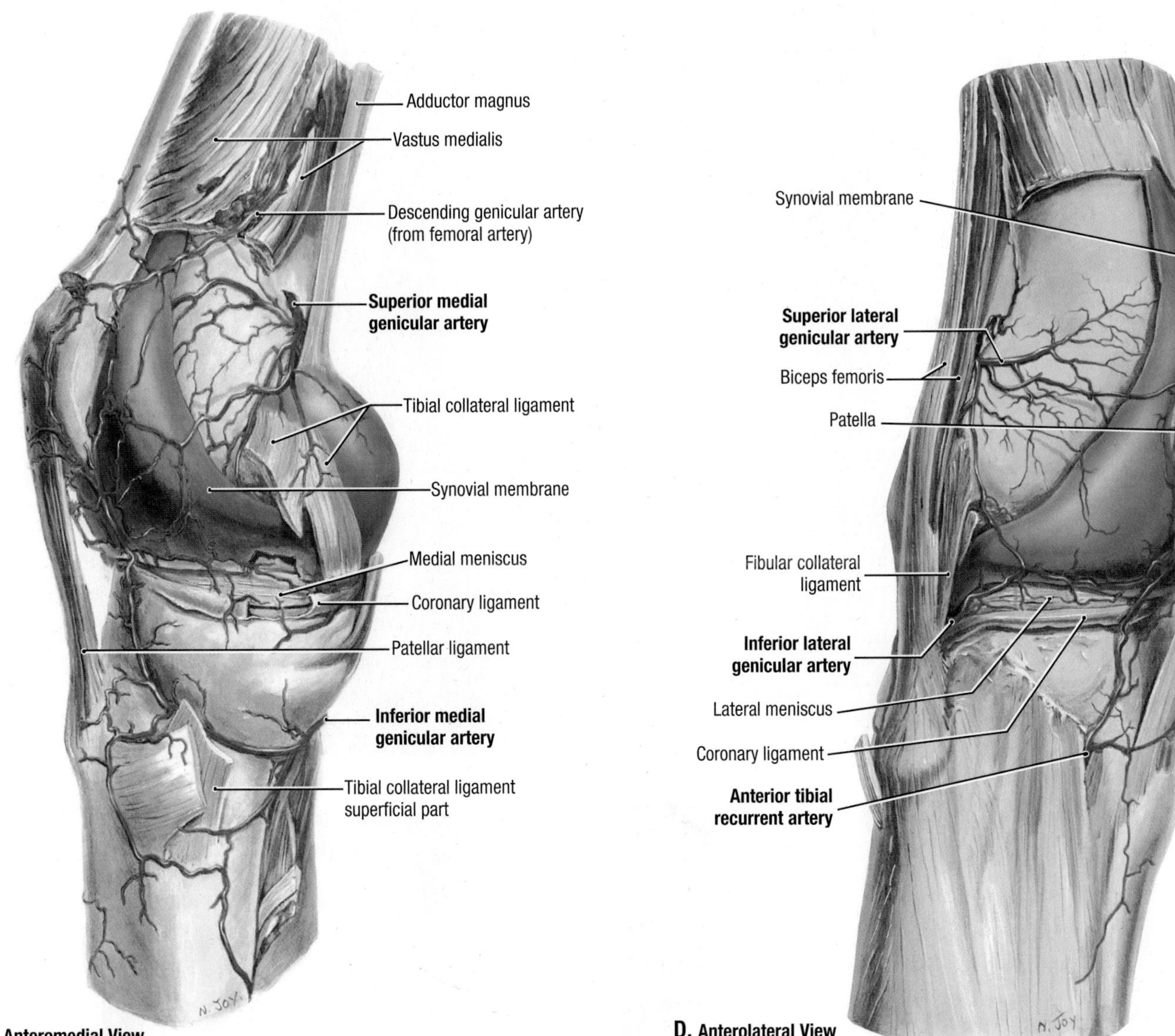
Adductor magnus
Vastus medialis
Descending genicular artery (from femoral artery)
Superior medial genicular artery
Tibial collateral ligament
Synovial membrane
Medial meniscus
Coronary ligament
Patellar ligament
Inferior medial genicular artery
Tibial collateral ligament superficial part
Synovial membrane
Superior lateral genicular artery
Biceps femoris
Patella
Fibular collateral ligament
Inferior lateral genicular artery
Lateral meniscus
Coronary ligament
Anterior tibial recurrent artery

C. Anteromedial View

D. Anterolateral View

5.55 ANASTOMOSES AROUND KNEE (*CONTINUED*)

C. Medial aspect of the knee showing superior and inferior medial genicular arteries. **D.** Lateral aspect of the knee showing superior and inferior lateral genicular arteries.

The genicular arteries participate in the formation of the periarticular genicular anastomosis, a network of vessels surrounding the knee that provides collateral circulation capable of maintaining blood supply to the leg during full knee flexion, which may kink the popliteal artery. Other contributors to this important anastomosis are the descending genicular artery, a branch of the femoral artery, superomedially; descending branch of the lateral circumflex femoral artery, superolaterally; and anterior tibial recurrent artery, a branch of the anterior tibial artery, inferolaterally.

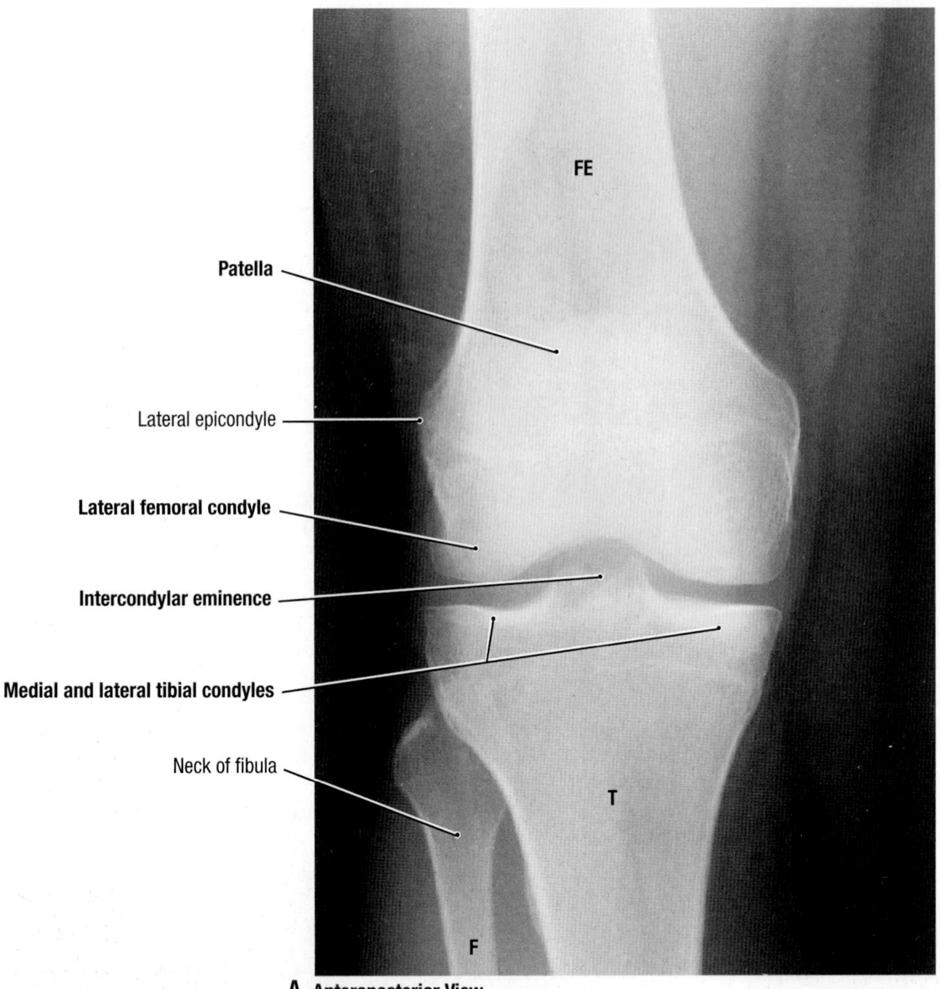
FE
Patella
Lateral epicondyle
Lateral femoral condyle
Intercondylar eminence
Medial and lateral tibial condyles
Neck of fibula
T
F

A. Anteroposterior View

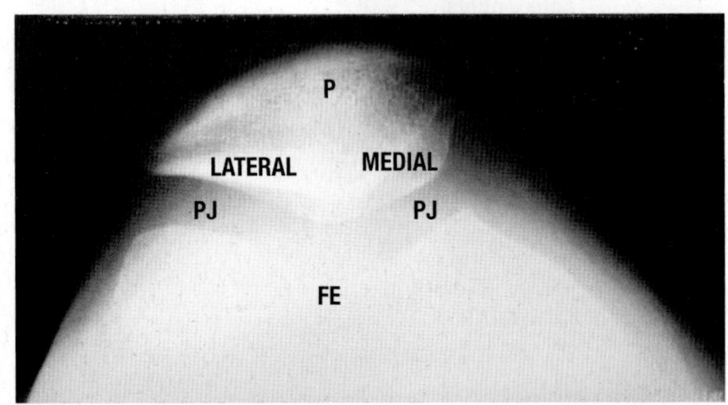
P
LATERAL
MEDIAL
PJ
PJ
FE

B. Skyline View (Knee in Flexion)

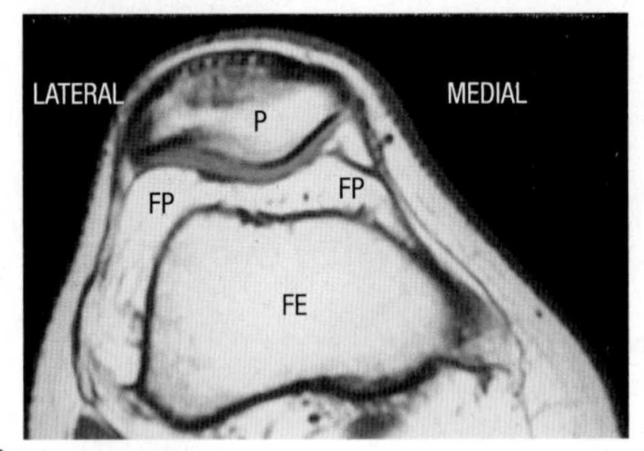
LATERAL
MEDIAL
P
FP
FP
FE

C. Transverse MRI

5.56 IMAGING OF THE KNEE AND PATELLOFEMORAL ARTICULATION

A. Anteroposterior radiograph of knee. **B.** Radiograph of patella (knee joint flexed). *FE*, femur; *FP*, fat pad; *P*, patella; *PJ*, patellofemoral joint. **C.** Transverse MRI showing the patellofemoral joint.

Pain deep to the patella often results from excessive running; hence, this type of pain is often called "runner's knee." The pain results from repetitive microtrauma caused by abnormal tracking of the patella relative to the patellar surface of the femur, a condition known as the **patellofemoral syndrome**. This syndrome may also result from a direct blow to the patella and from osteoarthritis of the patellofemoral compartment (degenerative wear and tear of articular cartilages). In some cases, strengthening of the vastus medialis corrects patellofemoral dysfunction. This muscle tends to prevent lateral dislocation of the patella resulting from the Q-angle because the vastus medialis attaches to and pulls on the medial border of the patella. Hence, weakness of the vastus medialis predisposes the individual to patellofemoral dysfunction and patellar dislocation.

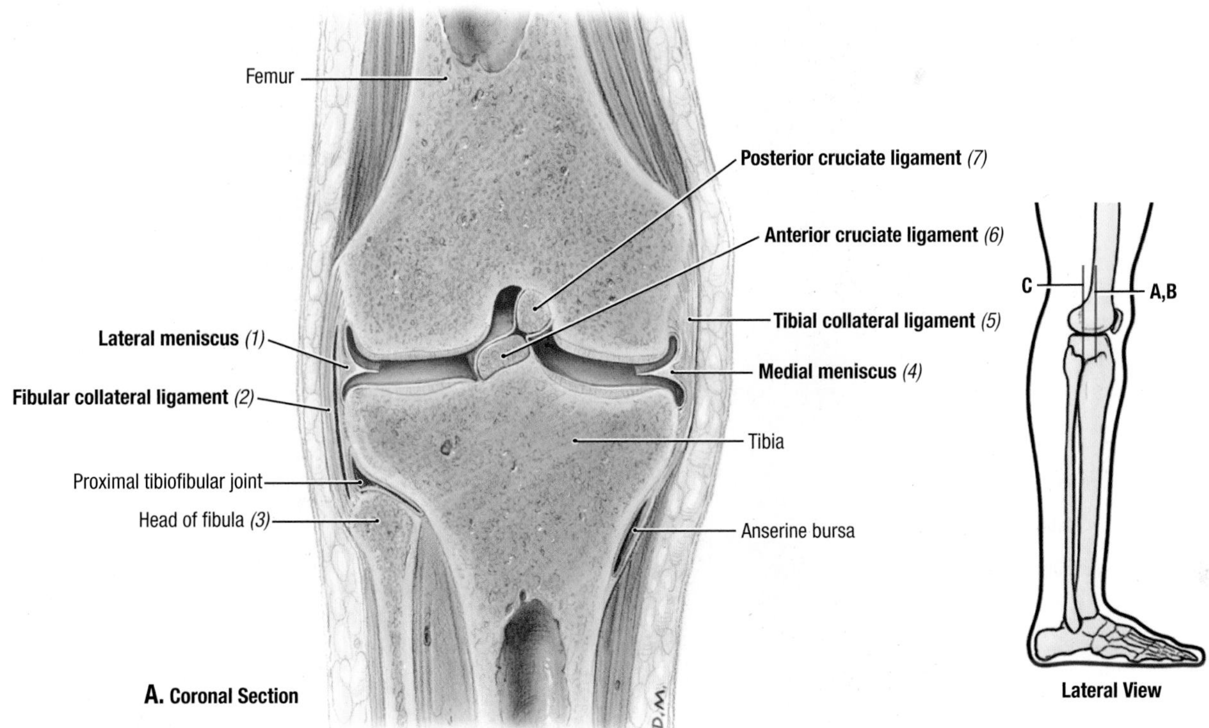
Femur
Posterior cruciate ligament (7)
Anterior cruciate ligament (6)
Lateral meniscus (1)
Tibial collateral ligament (5)
Medial meniscus (4)
Fibular collateral ligament (2)
Tibia
Proximal tibiofibular joint
Head of fibula (3)
Anserine bursa
D.M.
C
A,B
Lateral View

A. Coronal Section

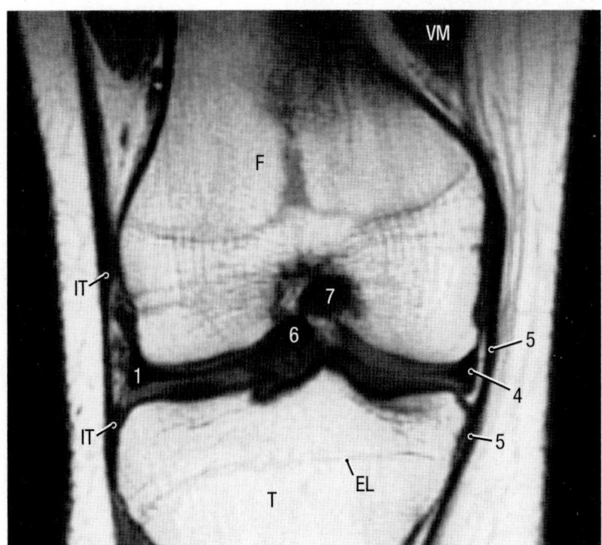
VM
F
IT
7
6
5
1
4
IT
5
EL
T

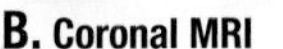

B. Coronal MRI

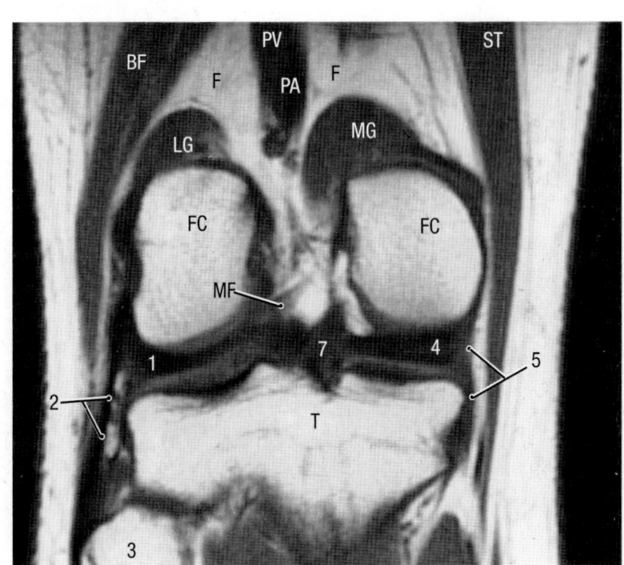
PV
ST
BF
F
PA
F
LG
MG
FC
FC
MF
7
4
5
1
2
T
3

C. Coronal MRI

5.57 CORONAL SECTION AND MRIs OF KNEE

A. Section through intercondylar notch of femur, tibia, and fibula. **B.** MRI through intercondylar notch of femur and tibia. **C.** MRI through femoral condyles tibia and fibula. *Numbers* in MRIs refer to structures in **A.** *VM*, vastus medialis; *EL*, epiphyseal line; *IT*, iliotibial tract; *FC*, femoral condyle; *BF*, biceps femoris; *ST*, semitendinosus; *LG*, lateral head of gastrocnemius; *MG*, medial head of gastrocnemius; *PV*, popliteal vein; *PA*, popliteal artery; *F*, fat in popliteal fossa; *MF*, meniscofemoral ligament.

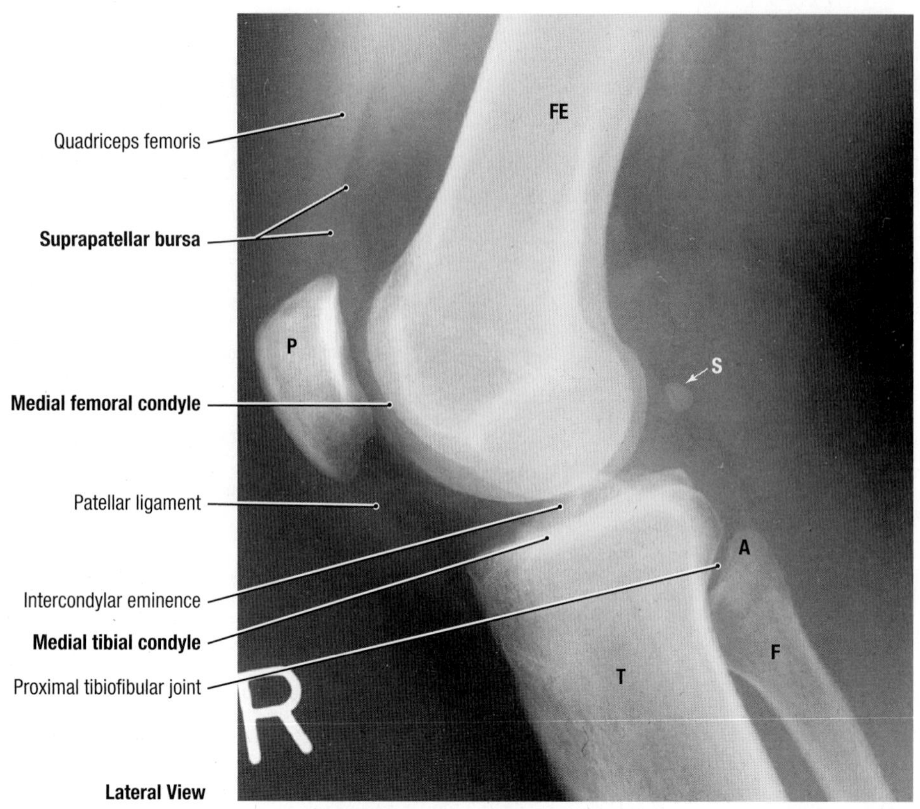
Quadriceps femoris
Suprapatellar bursa
Medial femoral condyle
Patellar ligament
Intercondylar eminence
Medial tibial condyle
Proximal tibiofibular joint
FE
P
S
A
F
T
R
Lateral View

5.58 RADIOGRAPH OF KNEE

Lateral radiograph of flexed knee. *FE*, femur; *T*, tibia; *F*, fibula; *A*, apex of fibula; *S*, fabella; *P*, patella. The fabella is an inconsistent sesamoid bone in the lateral head of gastrocnemius muscle.

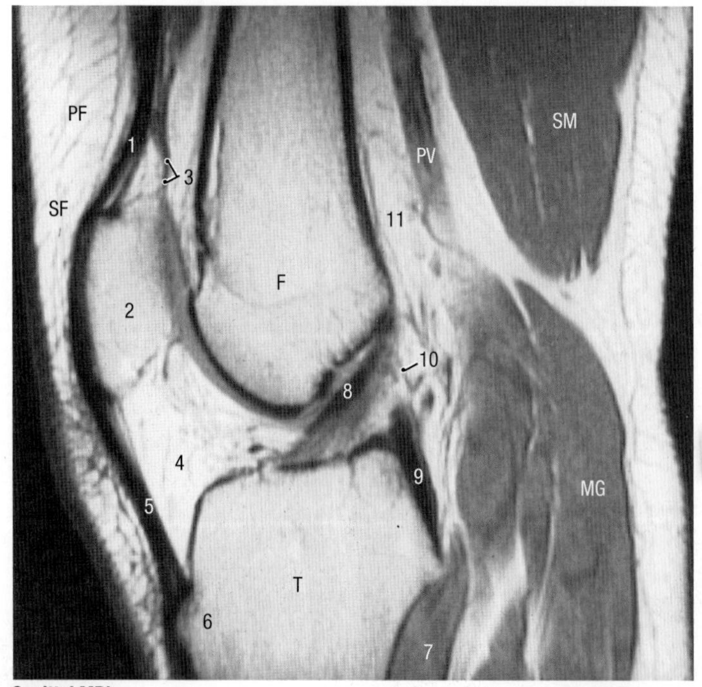
PF
SF
1
2
3
4
5
6
7
8
9
10
11
F
T
PV
SM
MG

A. Sagittal MRI

5.59 SAGITTAL SECTION AND MRIs OF KNEE

A. MRI through medial aspect of intercondylar notch of femur showing cruciate ligaments. **B.** Illustration of section through lateral aspect of intercondylar notch of femur. **C.** MRI through medial femoral and tibial condyles. *Numbers* in MRIs refer to structures in **A.** *SM*, semimembranosus; *ST*, semitendinosus; *MG*, medial head of gastrocnemius; *VM*, vastus medialis; *PF*, prefemoral fat; *SF*, suprapatellar fat; *AM*, anterior horn of medial meniscus; *PM*, posterior horn of medial meniscus; *PV*, popliteal vessels.

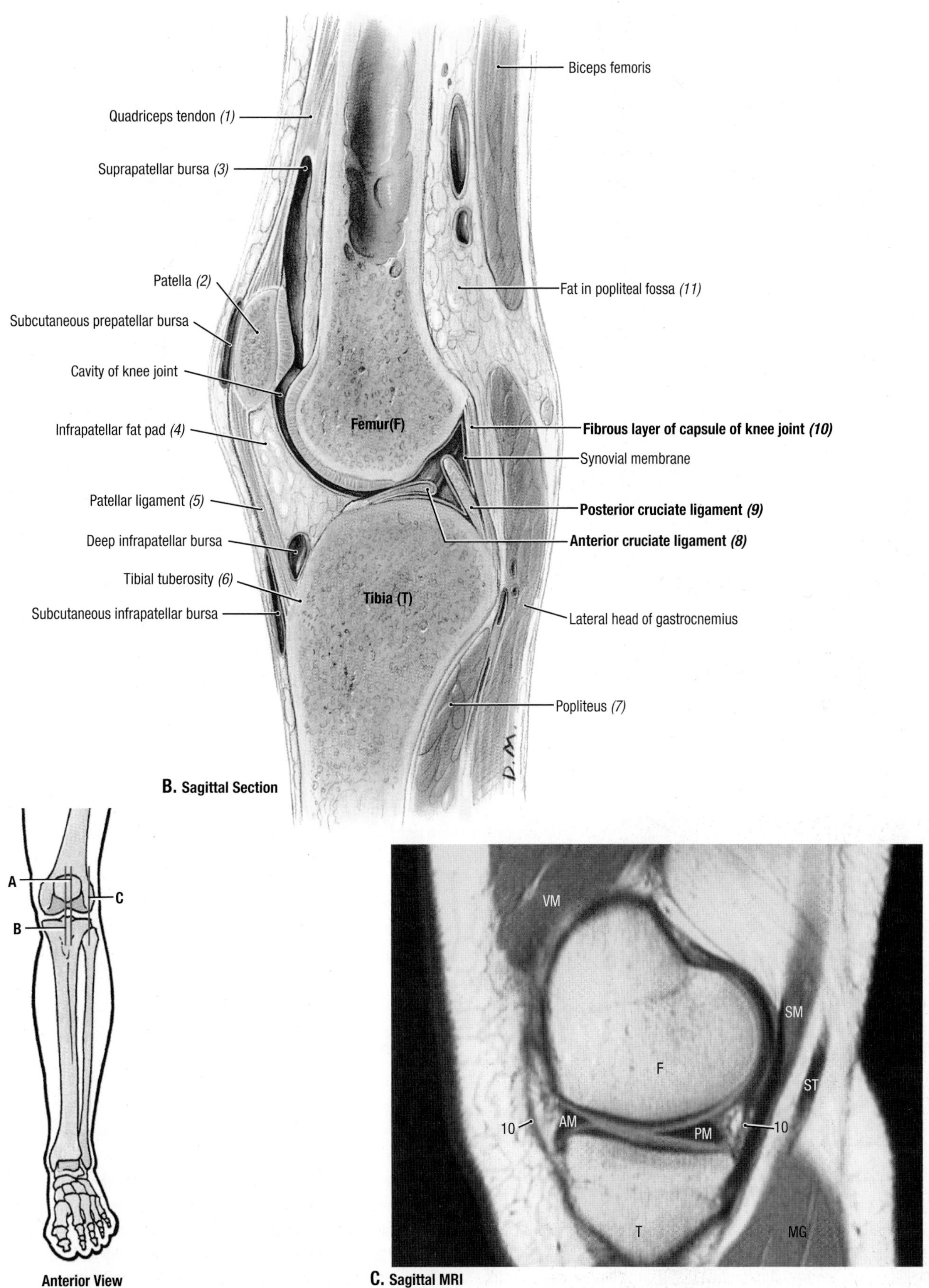
Biceps femoris
Quadriceps tendon (1)
Suprapatellar bursa (3)
Patella (2)
Subcutaneous prepatellar bursa
Cavity of knee joint
Fat in popliteal fossa (11)
Infrapatellar fat pad (4)
Femur(F)
Fibrous layer of capsule of knee joint (10)
Synovial membrane
Patellar ligament (5)
Posterior cruciate ligament (9)
Deep infrapatellar bursa
Anterior cruciate ligament (8)
Tibial tuberosity (6)
Tibia (T)
Subcutaneous infrapatellar bursa
Lateral head of gastrocnemius
Popliteus (7)
D.M.
A
B
C
VM
SM
F
ST
10
AM
PM
10
T
MG

B. Sagittal Section

Anterior View

C. Sagittal MRI

5.59 SAGITTAL SECTION AND MRIs OF KNEE (*CONTINUED*)

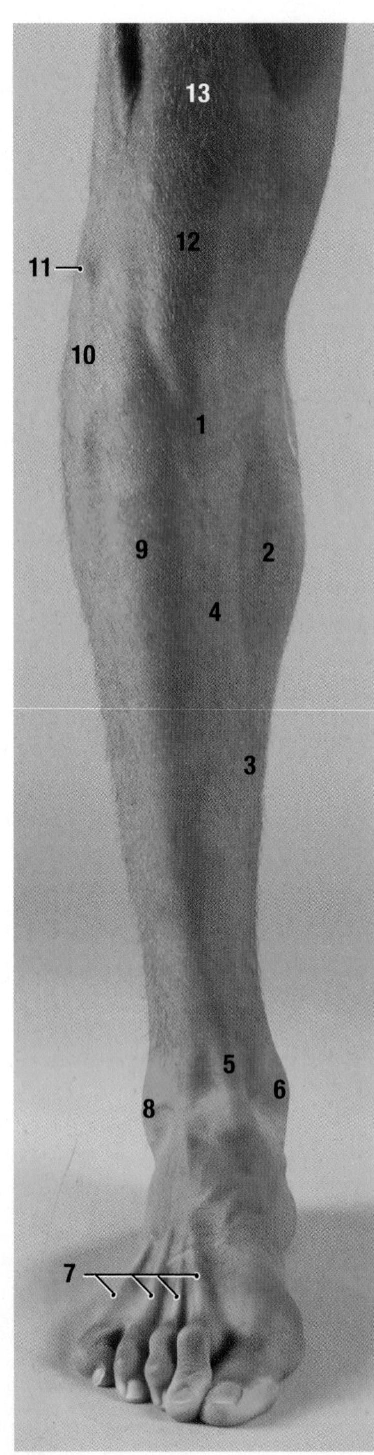
13
12
11
10
1
9
2
4
3
5
6
8
7

A. Anterior View

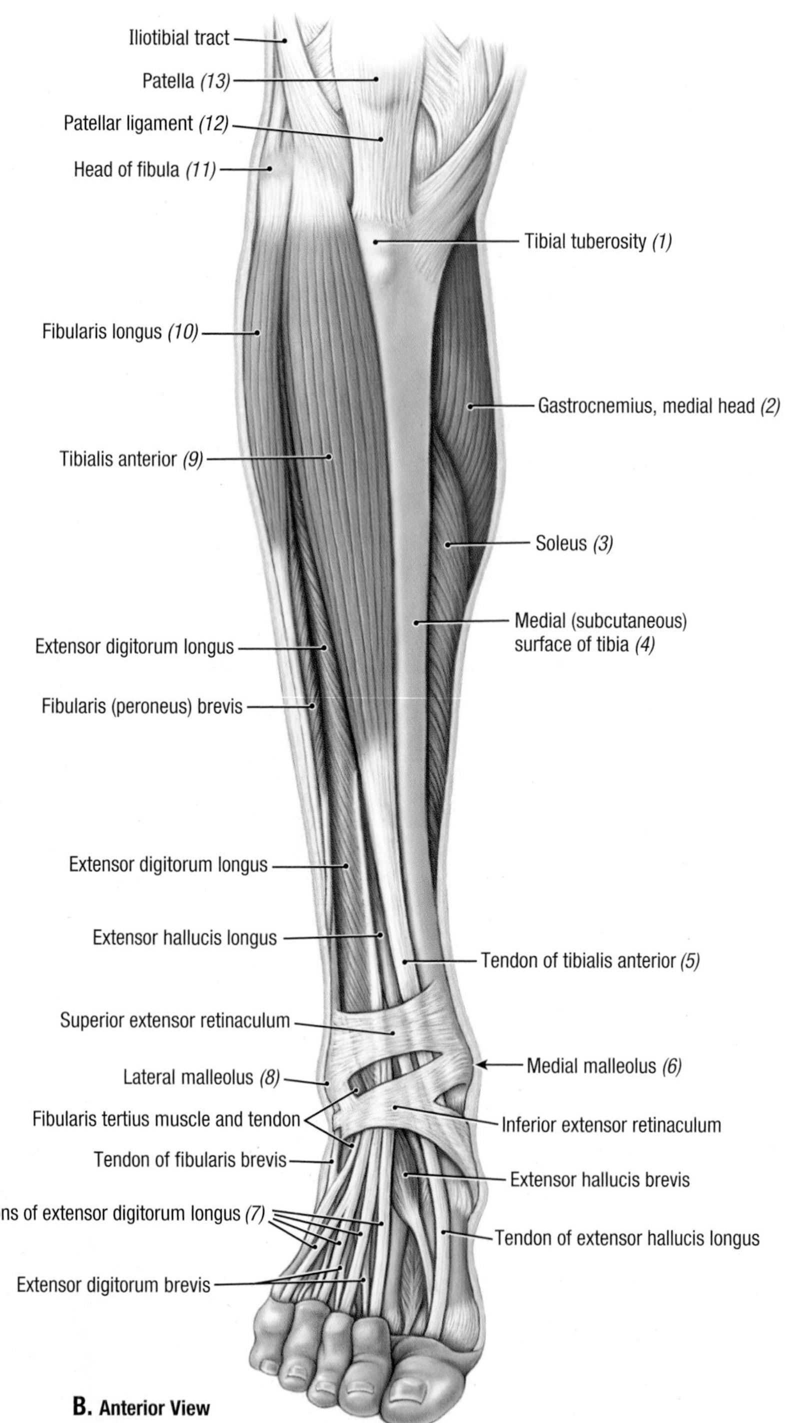
Iliotibial tract
Patella (13)
Patellar ligament (12)
Head of fibula (11)
Tibial tuberosity (1)
Fibularis longus (10)
Gastrocnemius, medial head (2)
Tibialis anterior (9)
Soleus (3)
Medial (subcutaneous) surface of tibia (4)
Extensor digitorum longus
Fibularis (peroneus) brevis
Extensor digitorum longus
Extensor hallucis longus
Tendon of tibialis anterior (5)
Superior extensor retinaculum
Medial malleolus (6)
Lateral malleolus (8)
Fibularis tertius muscle and tendon
Inferior extensor retinaculum
Tendon of fibularis brevis
Extensor hallucis brevis
Tendons of extensor digitorum longus (7)
Tendon of extensor hallucis longus
Extensor digitorum brevis

B. Anterior View

5.60 ANTERIOR LEG—SUPERFICIAL MUSCLES

A. Surface anatomy (*numbers* refer to structures labeled in **B**). **B.** Dissection. The muscles of the anterior compartment are ankle dorsiflexors/toe extensors. They are active in walking as they concentrically contract to raise the forefoot to clear the ground during the swing phase of the gait cycle and eccentrically contract to lower the forefoot to the ground after the heel strike of the stance phase.

Shin splints, edema, and pain in the area of the distal third of the tibia, result from repetitive microtrauma of the anterior compartment muscles, especially the tibialis anterior. This produces a mild form of **anterior compartment syndrome**. The pain commonly occurs during traumatic injury or athletic overexertion of the muscles. Edema and muscle-tendon inflammation causes swelling that reduces blood flow to the muscles. The swollen ischemic muscles are painful and tender to pressure.

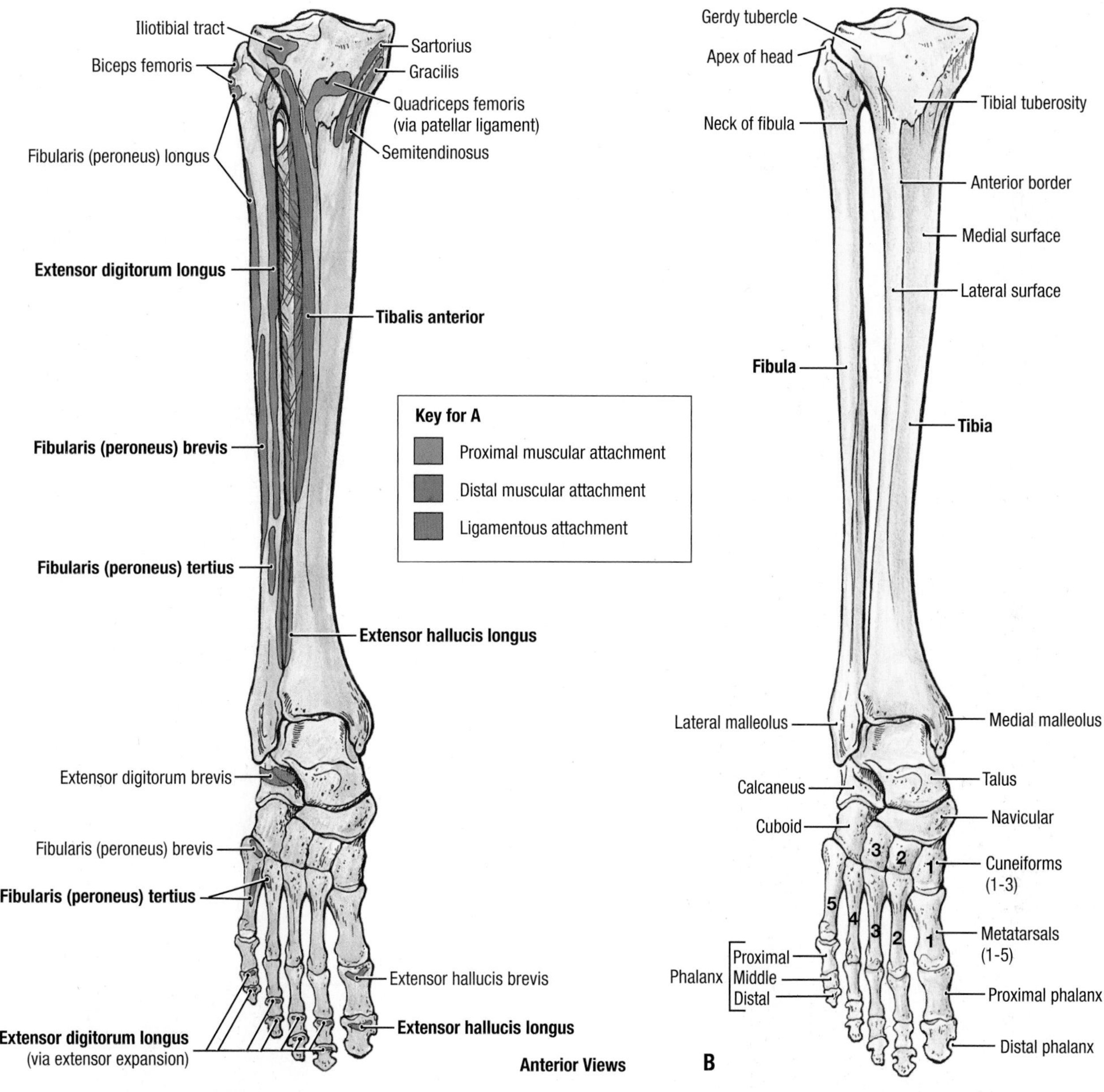
Iliotibial tract
Biceps femoris
Fibularis (peroneus) longus
Sartorius
Gracilis
Quadriceps femoris
(via patellar ligament)
Semitendinosus
Extensor digitorum longus
Tibalis anterior
Key for A
Proximal muscular attachment
Distal muscular attachment
Ligamentous attachment
Fibularis (peroneus) brevis
Fibularis (peroneus) tertius
Extensor hallucis longus
Extensor digitorum brevis
Fibularis (peroneus) brevis
Fibularis (peroneus) tertius
Extensor hallucis brevis
Extensor hallucis longus
Extensor digitorum longus
(via extensor expansion)
A
Anterior Views
B
Gerdy tubercle
Apex of head
Neck of fibula
Tibial tuberosity
Anterior border
Medial surface
Lateral surface
Fibula
Tibia
Lateral malleolus
Medial malleolus
Calcaneus
Talus
Cuboid
Navicular
Cuneiforms
(1-3)
Metatarsals
(1-5)
Phalanx
Proximal
Middle
Distal
Proximal phalanx
Distal phalanx

5.61 FEATURES OF BONES AND MUSCLE ATTACHMENTS: ANTERIOR LEG AND DORSUM OF FOOT

A. Attachments. **B.** Features of bones.

TABLE 5.12 MUSCLES OF ANTERIOR COMPARTMENT OF LEG

Muscle	Proximal Attachment	Distal Attachment	Innervation[a]	Main Actions
Tibialis anterior	Lateral condyle and superior half of lateral surface of tibia	Medial and inferior surfaces of medial cuneiform and base of first metatarsal	Deep fibular (peroneal) nerve (L4–L5)	Dorsiflexes ankle joint and inverts foot
Extensor hallucis longus	Middle part of anterior surface of fibula and interosseous membrane	Dorsal aspect of base of distal phalanx of great toe (hallux)		Extends great toe and dorsiflexes ankle joint
Extensor digitorum longus	Lateral condyle of tibia and superior three fourths of anterior surface of interosseous membrane	Middle and distal phalanges of lateral four digits	Deep fibular (peroneal) nerve (L5–S1)	Extends lateral four digits and dorsiflexes ankle joint
Fibularis (peroneus) tertius	Inferior third of anterior surface of fibula and interosseus membrane	Dorsum of base of fifth metatarsal		Dorsiflexes ankle joint and aids in eversion of foot

[a]See Table 5.1 for explanation of segmental innervation.

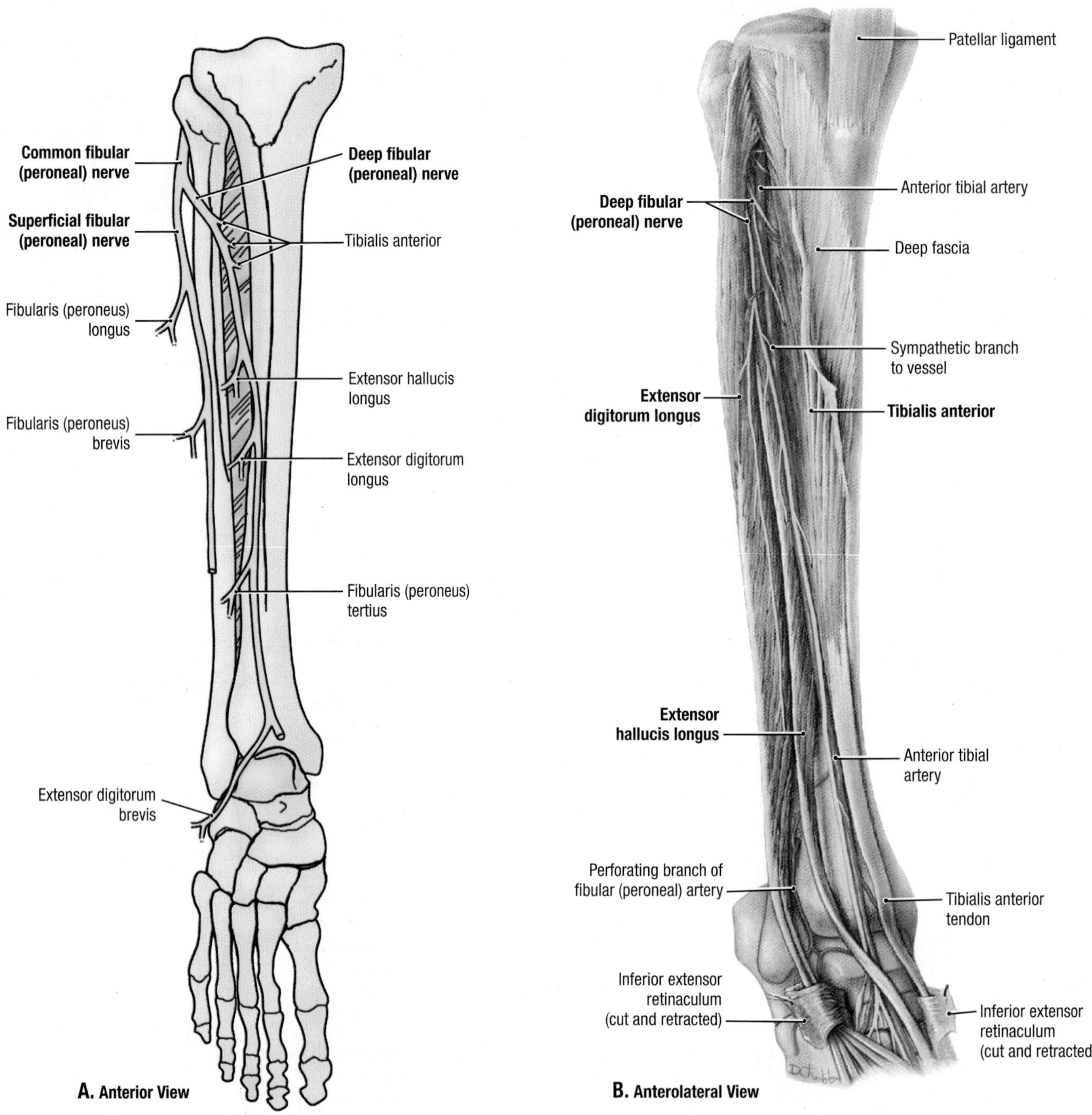
Common fibular (peroneal) nerve
Deep fibular (peroneal) nerve
Superficial fibular (peroneal) nerve
Tibialis anterior
Fibularis (peroneus) longus
Extensor hallucis longus
Fibularis (peroneus) brevis
Extensor digitorum longus
Fibularis (peroneus) tertius
Extensor digitorum brevis
A. Anterior View
Patellar ligament
Anterior tibial artery
Deep fibular (peroneal) nerve
Deep fascia
Sympathetic branch to vessel
Extensor digitorum longus
Tibialis anterior
Extensor hallucis longus
Anterior tibial artery
Perforating branch of fibular (peroneal) artery
Tibialis anterior tendon
Inferior extensor retinaculum (cut and retracted)
Inferior extensor retinaculum (cut and retracted)
B. Anterolateral View

5.62 ANTERIOR LEG—DEEP MUSCLES, NERVES, AND VESSELS

TABLE 5.13 COMMON, SUPERFICIAL, AND DEEP FIBULAR (PERONEAL) NERVES

Nerve	Origin	Course	Distribution/Structure(S) Supplied
Common fibular	Sciatic nerve	Forms as sciatic nerve bifurcates at the apex of popliteal fossa and follows medial border of biceps femoris; winds around neck of fibula, dividing into superficial and deep fibular nerves	Skin on lateral part of posterior aspect of leg via the lateral sural cutaneous nerve; lateral aspect of knee joint via its articular branch
Superficial fibular	Common fibular nerve	Arises deep to fibularis longus and descends in lateral compartment of leg; pierces crural fascia at distal third of leg to become cutaneous	Fibularis longus and brevis and skin on distal third of anterolateral surface of leg and dorsum of foot
Deep fibular	Common fibular nerve	Arises deep to fibularis longus; passes through extensor digitorum longus, descends on interosseous membrane, and continues on dorsum of foot	Anterior muscles of leg, dorsum of foot, and skin of first interdigital cleft; dorsal aspect of joints crossed via articular branches

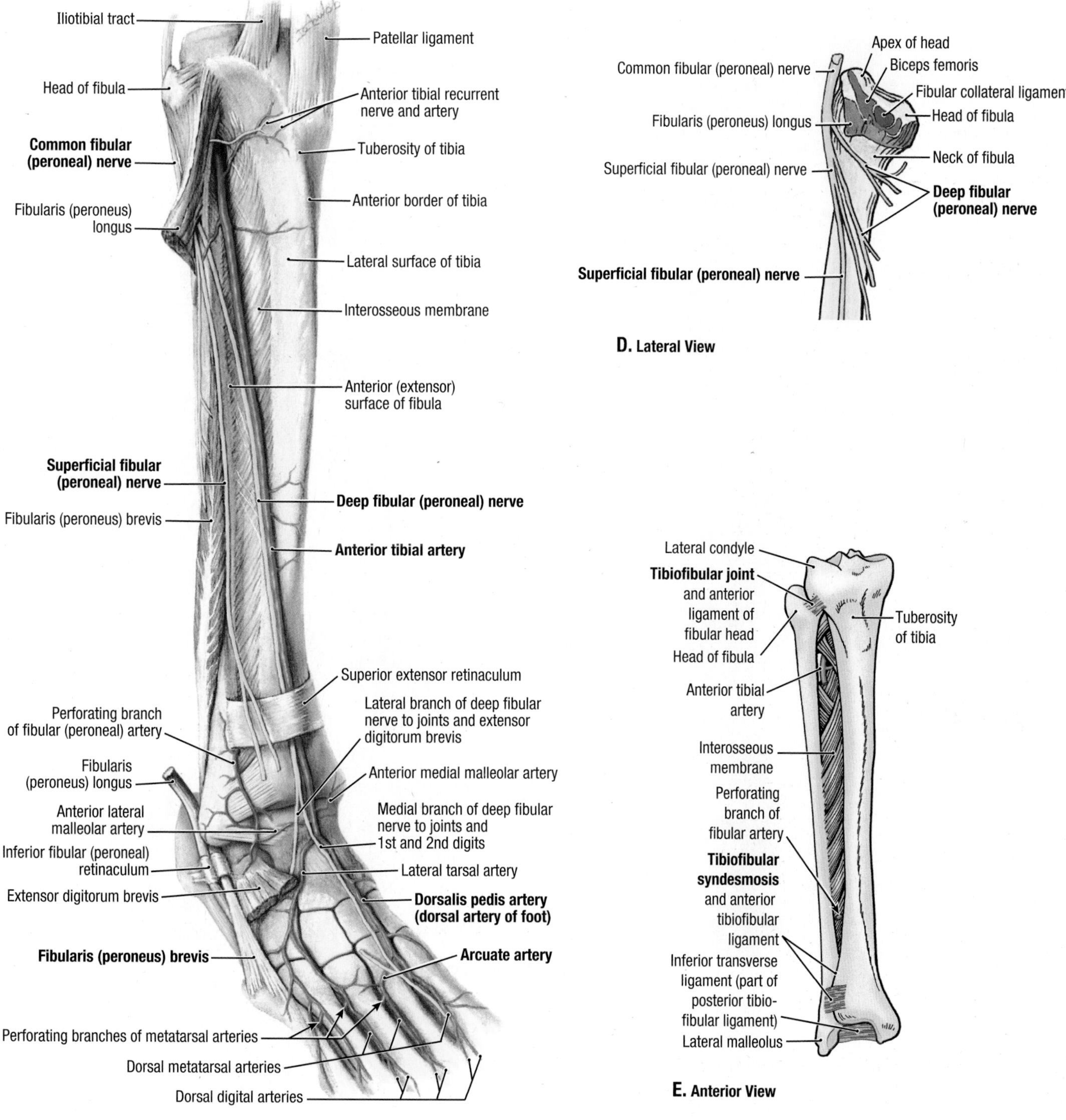
Iliotibial tract
Patellar ligament
Head of fibula
Anterior tibial recurrent nerve and artery
Common fibular (peroneal) nerve
Tuberosity of tibia
Anterior border of tibia
Fibularis (peroneus) longus
Lateral surface of tibia
Interosseous membrane
Anterior (extensor) surface of fibula
Superficial fibular (peroneal) nerve
Deep fibular (peroneal) nerve
Fibularis (peroneus) brevis
Anterior tibial artery
Superior extensor retinaculum
Perforating branch of fibular (peroneal) artery
Lateral branch of deep fibular nerve to joints and extensor digitorum brevis
Fibularis (peroneus) longus
Anterior medial malleolar artery
Anterior lateral malleolar artery
Medial branch of deep fibular nerve to joints and 1st and 2nd digits
Inferior fibular (peroneal) retinaculum
Lateral tarsal artery
Extensor digitorum brevis
Dorsalis pedis artery (dorsal artery of foot)
Fibularis (peroneus) brevis
Arcuate artery
Perforating branches of metatarsal arteries
Dorsal metatarsal arteries
Dorsal digital arteries
Common fibular (peroneal) nerve
Apex of head
Biceps femoris
Fibular collateral ligament
Head of fibula
Fibularis (peroneus) longus
Neck of fibula
Superficial fibular (peroneal) nerve
Deep fibular (peroneal) nerve
Superficial fibular (peroneal) nerve
Lateral condyle
Tibiofibular joint and anterior ligament of fibular head
Tuberosity of tibia
Head of fibula
Anterior tibial artery
Interosseous membrane
Perforating branch of fibular artery
Tibiofibular syndesmosis and anterior tibiofibular ligament
Inferior transverse ligament (part of posterior tibio-fibular ligament)
Lateral malleolus

C. Anterolateral View

D. Lateral View

E. Anterior View

5.62 ANTERIOR LEG—DEEP MUSCLES, NERVES, AND VESSELS (*CONTINUED*)

A. Overview of motor innervation. **B.** Deep dissection of the anterior compartment of the leg. The muscles are separated to display the anterior tibial artery and deep fibular nerve. **C.** Neurovascular structures. **D.** Relations of common fibular nerve and branches to the proximal fibula. **E.** Interosseous membrane.

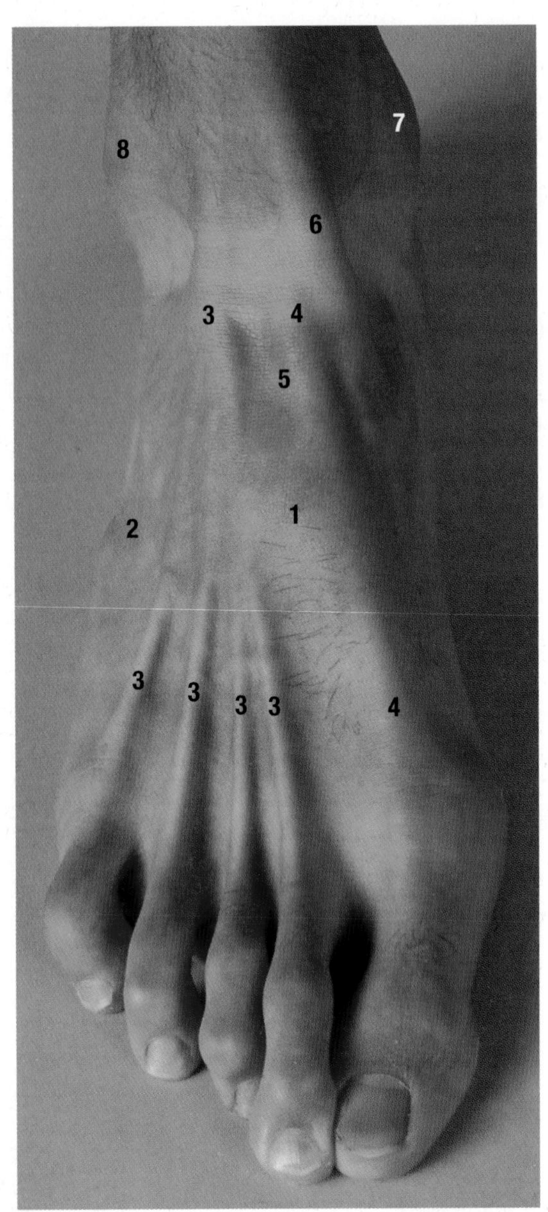

8
7
6
3
4
5
2
1
3
3
3 3
4

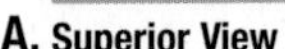

A. Superior View

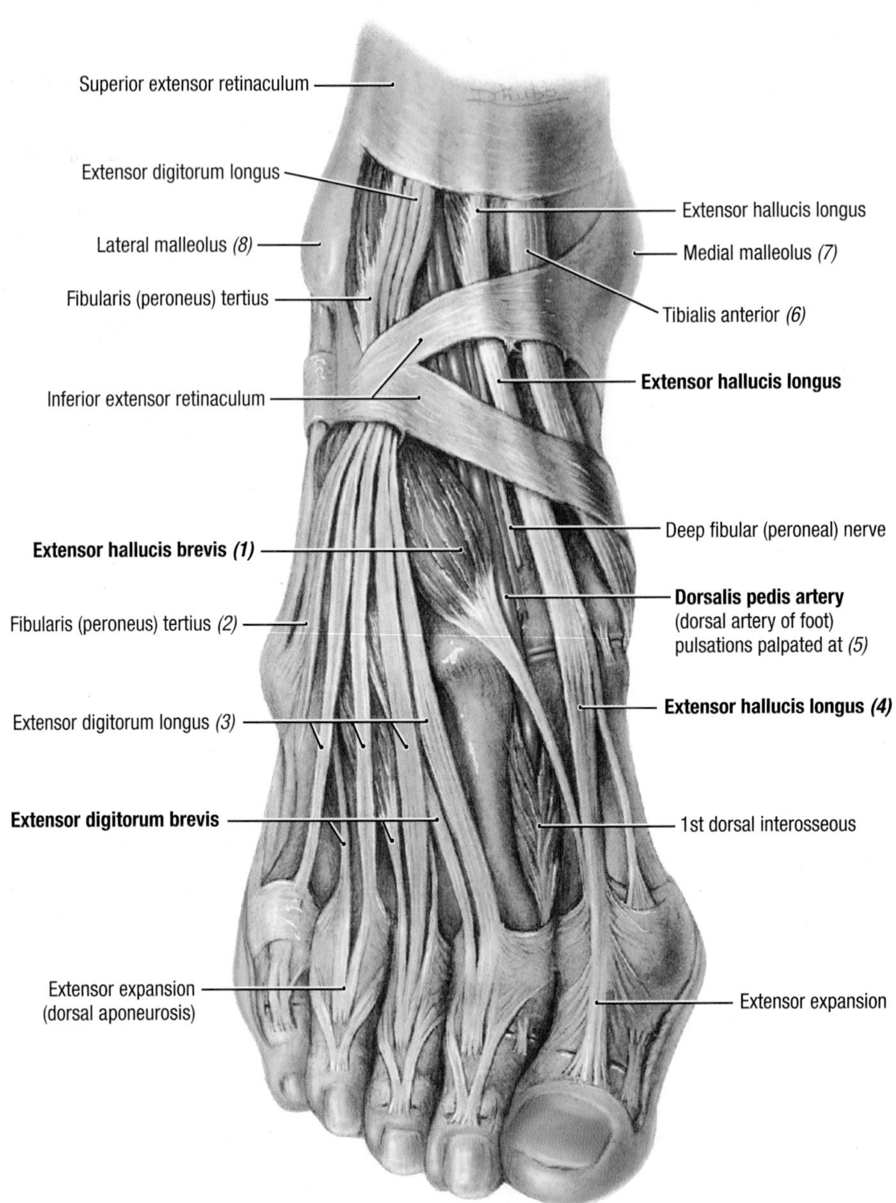

Superior extensor retinaculum
Extensor digitorum longus
Lateral malleolus (8)
Fibularis (peroneus) tertius
Inferior extensor retinaculum
Extensor hallucis brevis (1)
Fibularis (peroneus) tertius (2)
Extensor digitorum longus (3)
Extensor digitorum brevis
Extensor expansion (dorsal aponeurosis)
Extensor hallucis longus
Medial malleolus (7)
Tibialis anterior (6)
Extensor hallucis longus
Deep fibular (peroneal) nerve
Dorsalis pedis artery (dorsal artery of foot) pulsations palpated at (5)
Extensor hallucis longus (4)
1st dorsal interosseous
Extensor expansion

B. Superior View

5.63 DORSUM OF FOOT

A. Surface anatomy (*numbers* refer to structures labeled in **B**). **B.** Dissection. The dorsal vein of foot and deep fibular nerve are cut.

At the ankle, the dorsalis pedis artery (dorsal artery of foot) and deep fibular nerve lie midway between the malleoli. On the dorsum of the foot, the dorsal artery of foot is crossed by the extensor hallucis brevis muscle and disappears between the two heads of the first dorsal interosseous muscle.

Clinically, knowing the location of the belly of the extensor digitorum brevis is important for distinguishing this muscle from abnormal edema. Contusion and tearing of the muscle fibers and associated blood vessels result in a **hematoma in extensor digitorum brevis**, producing edema anteromedial to the lateral malleolus. Most people who have not seen this inflamed muscle assume they have a severely sprained ankle.

The **dorsalis pedis pulse** may be palpated with the feet slightly dorsiflexed. The pulse is usually easy to palpate because the dorsal arteries of the foot are subcutaneous and pass along a line from the extensor retinaculum to a point just lateral to the extensor hallucis longus tendon. A diminished or absent dorsalis pedis pulse usually suggests vascular insufficiency resulting from arterial disease.

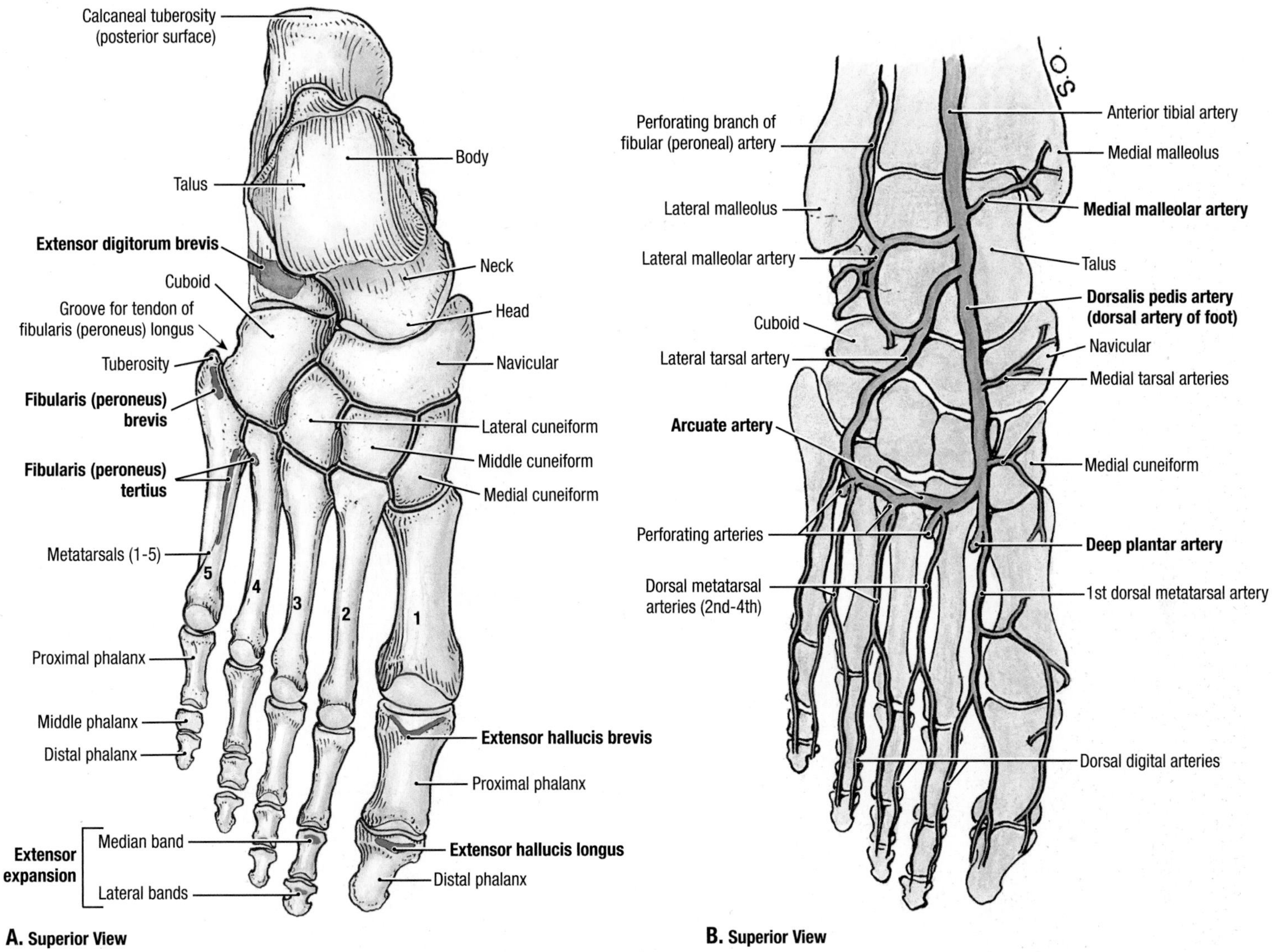
Calcaneal tuberosity (posterior surface)
Talus
Body
Extensor digitorum brevis
Cuboid
Groove for tendon of fibularis (peroneus) longus
Neck
Head
Tuberosity
Navicular
Fibularis (peroneus) brevis
Lateral cuneiform
Middle cuneiform
Fibularis (peroneus) tertius
Medial cuneiform
Metatarsals (1-5)
5
4
3
2
1
Proximal phalanx
Middle phalanx
Distal phalanx
Extensor hallucis brevis
Proximal phalanx
Extensor expansion
Median band
Lateral bands
Extensor hallucis longus
Distal phalanx
A. Superior View
Perforating branch of fibular (peroneal) artery
Anterior tibial artery
Medial malleolus
Lateral malleolus
Medial malleolar artery
Lateral malleolar artery
Talus
Cuboid
Dorsalis pedis artery (dorsal artery of foot)
Navicular
Lateral tarsal artery
Medial tarsal arteries
Arcuate artery
Medial cuneiform
Perforating arteries
Deep plantar artery
Dorsal metatarsal arteries (2nd-4th)
1st dorsal metatarsal artery
Dorsal digital arteries
B. Superior View

5.64 ATTACHMENTS OF MUSCLES AND ARTERIES OF DORSUM OF FOOT

A. Attachments. **B.** Arterial supply.

TABLE 5.14 ARTERIAL SUPPLY TO DORSUM OF FOOT

Artery	Origin	Course	Distribution
Dorsalis pedis (dorsal artery of foot)	Continuation of anterior tibial artery distal to talocrural joint	Descends anteromedially to 1st interosseous space and divides into deep plantar and arcuate arteries	Dorsal surface of foot
Lateral tarsal artery	From dorsalis pedis artery (dorsal artery of foot)	Runs an arched course laterally beneath extensor digitorum brevis to anastomose with branches of arcuate artery	
Arcuate artery		Runs laterally from 1st interosseous space across bases of lateral four metatarsals, deep to extensor tendons	
Deep plantar artery		Passes to sole of foot and joins plantar arch	Sole of foot
Metatarsal arteries 1st	From deep plantar artery	Run between metatarsals to clefts of toes where each vessel divides into two dorsal digital arteries.	Dorsal surface of foot
2nd to 4th	From arcuate artery	Perforating arteries connect to plantar arch and plantar metatarsal arteries.	
Dorsal digital arteries	From metatarsal arteries	Pass to sides of adjoining digits	Digits

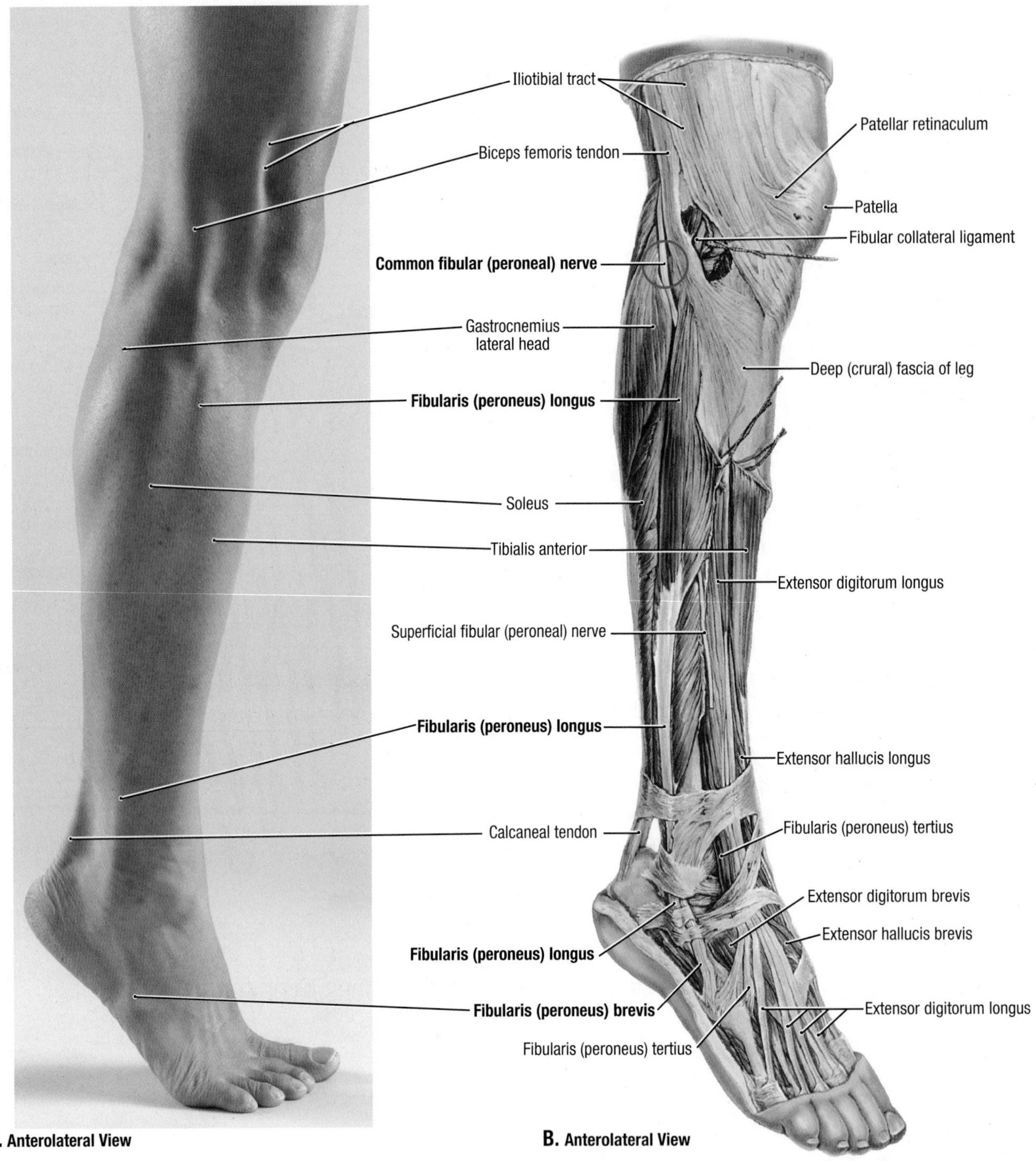
Iliotibial tract
Biceps femoris tendon
Patellar retinaculum
Patella
Fibular collateral ligament
Common fibular (peroneal) nerve
Gastrocnemius lateral head
Deep (crural) fascia of leg
Fibularis (peroneus) longus
Soleus
Tibialis anterior
Extensor digitorum longus
Superficial fibular (peroneal) nerve
Fibularis (peroneus) longus
Extensor hallucis longus
Calcaneal tendon
Fibularis (peroneus) tertius
Extensor digitorum brevis
Extensor hallucis brevis
Fibularis (peroneus) longus
Fibularis (peroneus) brevis
Extensor digitorum longus
Fibularis (peroneus) tertius

A. Anterolateral View

B. Anterolateral View

5.65 MUSCLES OF LATERAL LEG AND FOOT

A. Surface anatomy. **B.** Dissection.

- The two fibular (peroneal) muscles both attach to two thirds of the fibula, the fibularis (peroneus) longus muscle to the proximal two thirds, and the fibularis (peroneus) brevis muscle to the distal two thirds. Where they overlap, the fibularis brevis muscle lies anteriorly.
- The fibularis (peroneus) longus muscle enters the foot by hooking around the cuboid and traveling medially to the base of the first metatarsal and medial cuneiform.
- **Common fibular (peroneal) nerve lesion.** The nerve lies in contact with the neck of the fibula deep to the fibularis longus muscle, where it is vulnerable to injury (**B,** *red circle*). This injury may have serious implications because the nerve supplies the extensor and everter muscle groups, with loss of function resulting in foot-drop (inability to dorsiflex the ankle) and difficulty in everting the foot.

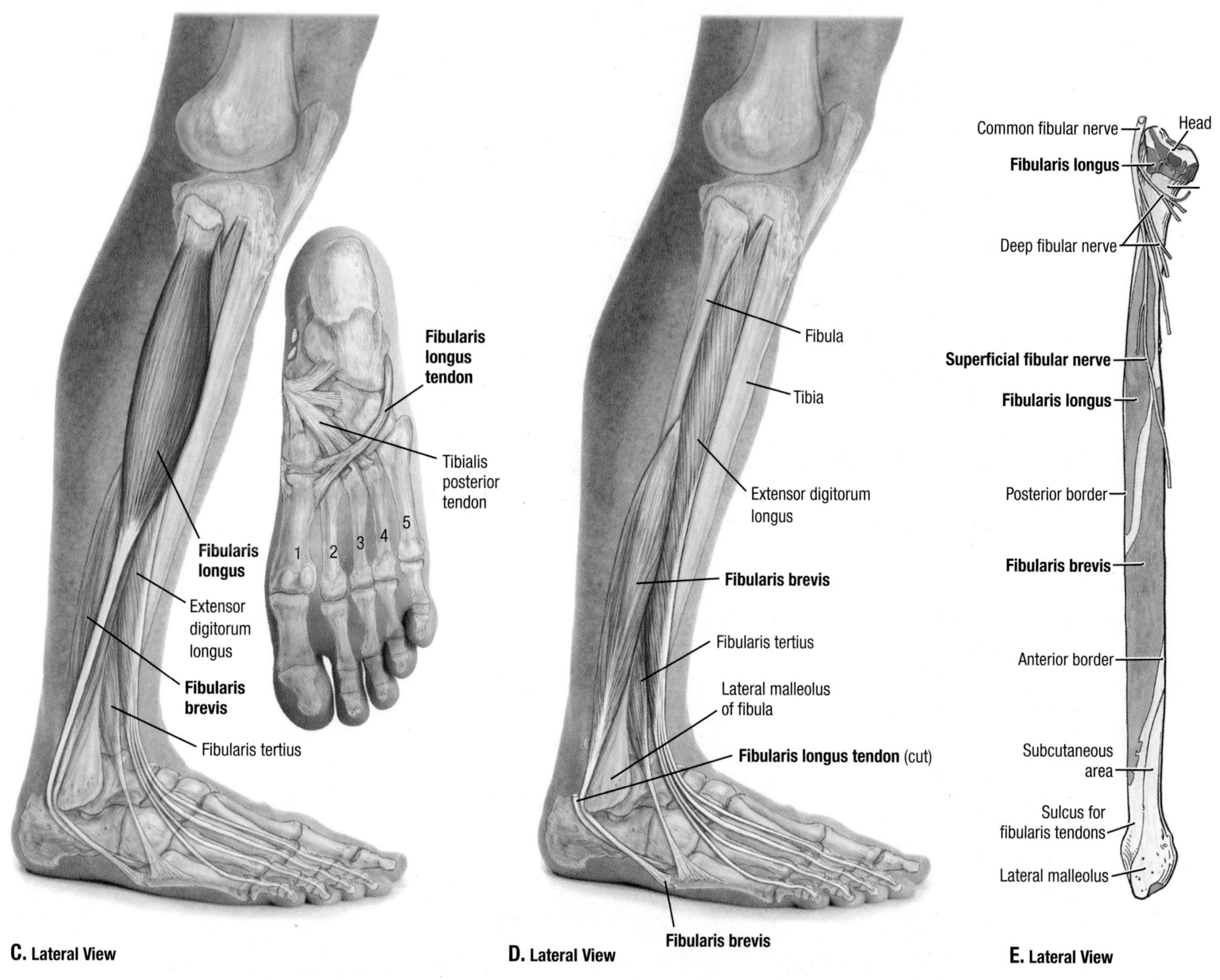
Fibularis longus tendon
Tibialis posterior tendon
1
2
3
4
5
Fibularis longus
Extensor digitorum longus
Fibularis brevis
Fibularis tertius
Fibula
Tibia
Extensor digitorum longus
Fibularis brevis
Fibularis tertius
Lateral malleolus of fibula
Fibularis longus tendon (cut)
Fibularis brevis
Common fibular nerve
Head
Fibularis longus
Deep fibular nerve
Superficial fibular nerve
Fibularis longus
Posterior border
Fibularis brevis
Anterior border
Subcutaneous area
Sulcus for fibularis tendons
Lateral malleolus

C. Lateral View

D. Lateral View

E. Lateral View

5.65 MUSCLES OF LATERAL LEG AND FOOT (*CONTINUED*)

C. Fibularis (peroneus) longus. **D.** Fibularis (peroneus) brevis. **E.** Attachments sites on fibula.

TABLE 5.15 MUSCLES OF LATERAL COMPARTMENT OF LEG

Muscle	Proximal Attachment	Distal Attachment	Innervation[a]	Main Actions
Fibularis (peroneus) longus	Head and superior two thirds of lateral surface of fibula	Base of first metatarsal and medial cuneiform	Superficial fibular (peroneal) nerve (L5, S1, and S2)	Evert foot and weakly plantar flex ankle joint
Fibularis (peroneus) brevis	Inferior two thirds of lateral surface of fibula	Dorsal surface of tuberosity on lateral side of base of fifth metatarsal		

[a]See Table 5.1 for explanation of segmental innervation

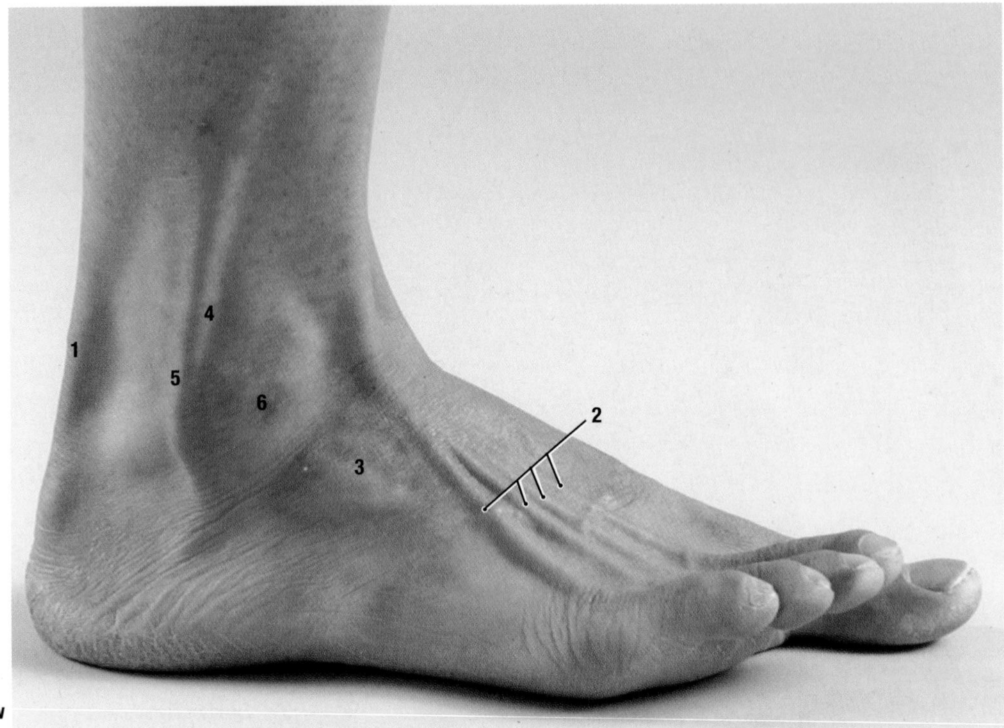
1
2
3
4
5
6

A. Lateral View

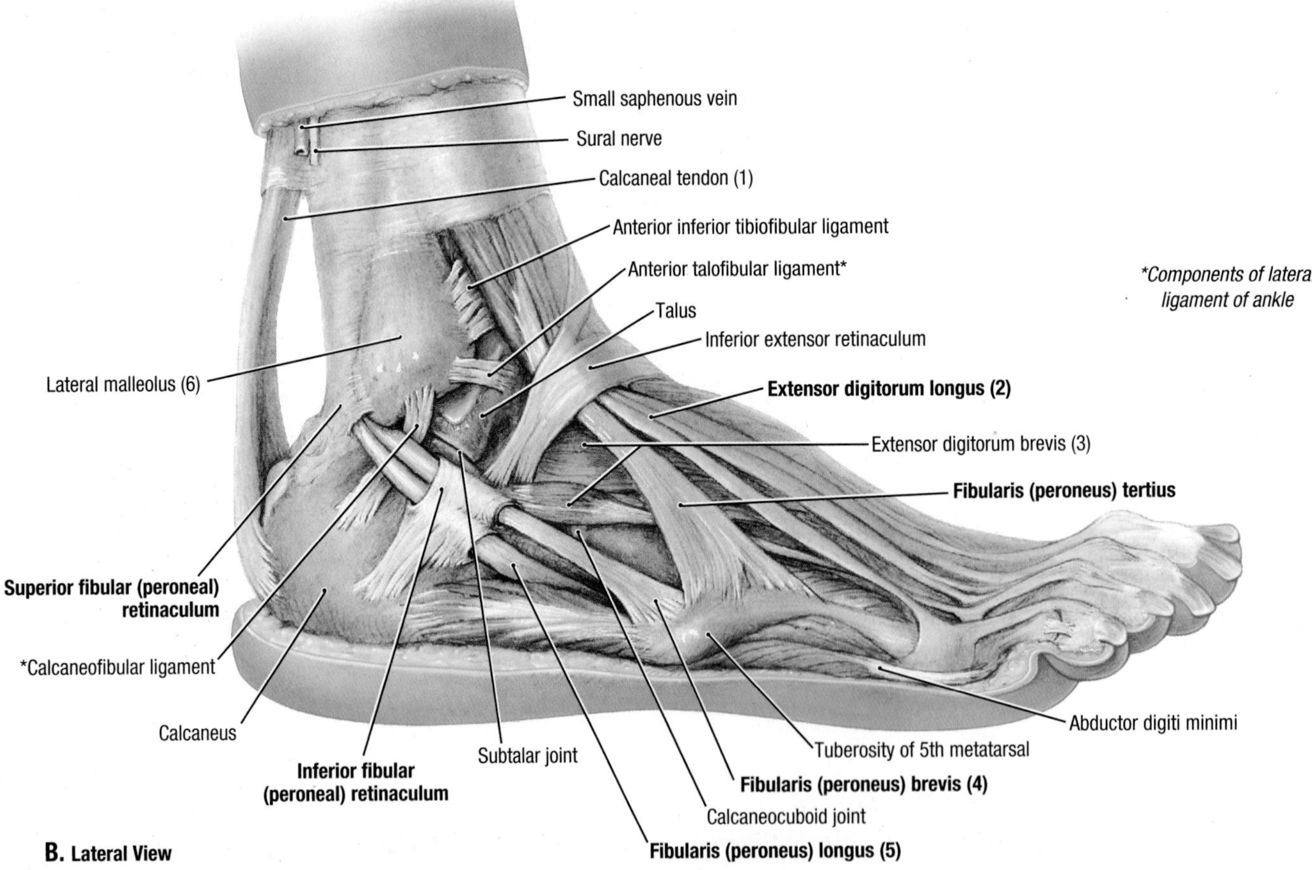
Small saphenous vein
Sural nerve
Calcaneal tendon (1)
Anterior inferior tibiofibular ligament
Anterior talofibular ligament*
Talus
Inferior extensor retinaculum
Extensor digitorum longus (2)
Extensor digitorum brevis (3)
Fibularis (peroneus) tertius
*Components of lateral ligament of ankle
Lateral malleolus (6)
Superior fibular (peroneal) retinaculum
*Calcaneofibular ligament
Calcaneus
Inferior fibular (peroneal) retinaculum
Subtalar joint
Fibularis (peroneus) longus (5)
Calcaneocuboid joint
Fibularis (peroneus) brevis (4)
Tuberosity of 5th metatarsal
Abductor digiti minimi

B. Lateral View

5.66 SYNOVIAL SHEATHS AND TENDONS AT ANKLE

A. Surface anatomy (*numbers* refer to structures labeled in **B**). **B.** Tendons at the lateral aspect of the ankle.

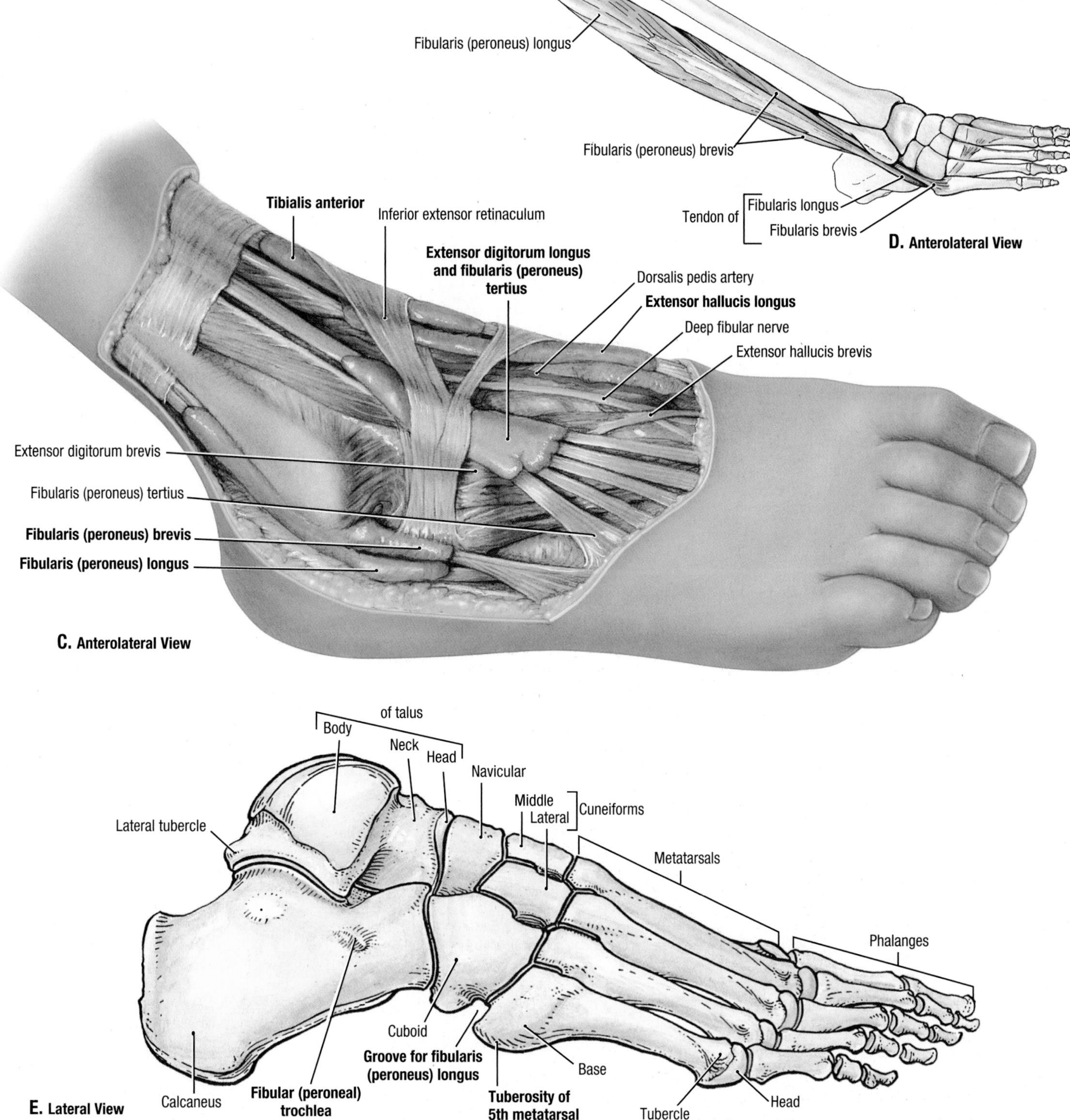
Fibularis (peroneus) longus
Fibularis (peroneus) brevis
Tendon of
Fibularis longus
Fibularis brevis
D. Anterolateral View
Tibialis anterior
Inferior extensor retinaculum
Extensor digitorum longus and fibularis (peroneus) tertius
Dorsalis pedis artery
Extensor hallucis longus
Deep fibular nerve
Extensor hallucis brevis
Extensor digitorum brevis
Fibularis (peroneus) tertius
Fibularis (peroneus) brevis
Fibularis (peroneus) longus
C. Anterolateral View
of talus
Body
Neck
Head
Navicular
Middle
Lateral
Cuneiforms
Lateral tubercle
Metatarsals
Phalanges
Cuboid
Groove for fibularis (peroneus) longus
Base
Head
E. Lateral View
Calcaneus
Fibular (peroneal) trochlea
Tuberosity of 5th metatarsal
Tubercle

5.66 SYNOVIAL SHEATHS AND TENDONS AT ANKLE (*CONTINUED*)

C. Synovial sheaths of tendons on the anterolateral aspect of the ankle. The tendons of the fibularis (peroneus) longus and fibularis (peroneus) brevis muscles are enclosed in a common synovial sheath posterior to the lateral malleolus. This sheath splits into two, one for each tendon, posterior to the fibular (peroneal) trochlea. **D.** Schematic illustration of fibularis longus and brevis. **E.** Lateral aspect of bones of foot.

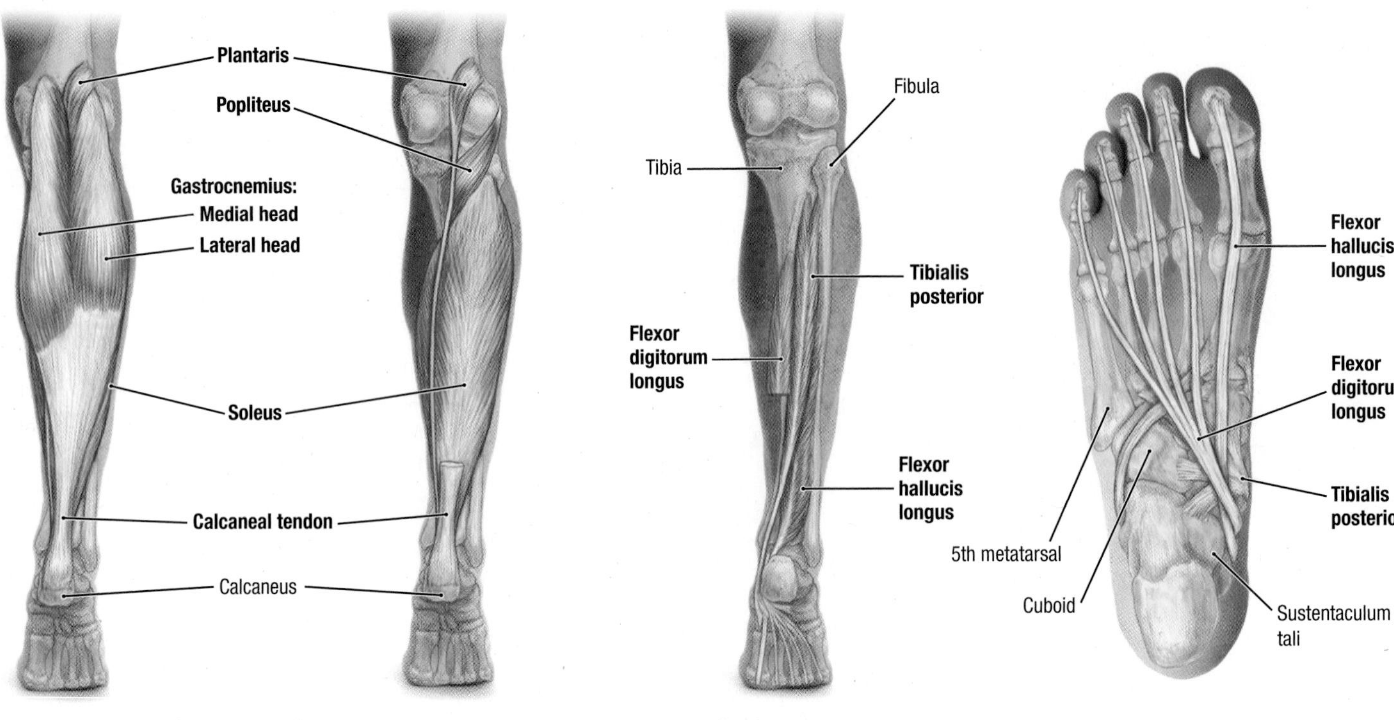
Plantaris
Popliteus
Gastrocnemius:
Medial head
Lateral head
Soleus
Calcaneal tendon
Calcaneus
Fibula
Tibia
Tibialis posterior
Flexor digitorum longus
Flexor hallucis longus
Flexor hallucis longus
Flexor digitorum longus
Tibialis posterior
5th metatarsal
Cuboid
Sustentaculum tali

5.67 MUSCLES OF POSTERIOR LEG

A. and B. Muscles of superficial compartment. **C. and D.** Muscles of deep compartment.

TABLE 5.16 MUSCLES OF POSTERIOR COMPARTMENT OF LEG

Muscle	Proximal Attachment	Distal Attachment	Innervation[a]	Main Actions
Superficial muscles				
Gastrocnemius	*Lateral head:* lateral aspect of lateral condyle of femur *Medial head:* popliteal surface of femur, superior to medial condyle	Posterior surface of calcaneus via calcaneal tendon (tendocalcaneus)	Tibial nerve (S1 and S2)	Plantar flexes ankle joint when knee joint is extended; raises heel during walking, and flexes knee joint
Soleus	Posterior aspect of head of fibula, superior fourth of posterior surface of fibula, soleal line and medial border of tibia			Plantar flexes ankle joint (independent of knee position) and steadies leg on foot
Plantaris	Inferior end of lateral supracondylar line of femur and oblique popliteal ligament			Weakly assists gastrocnemius in plantar flexing ankle joint and flexing knee joint
Deep muscles				
Popliteus	Lateral surface of lateral condyle of femur and lateral meniscus	Posterior surface of tibia, superior to soleal line	Tibial nerve (**L4,** L5, and S1)	Unlocks fully extended knee joint (laterally rotates femur 5 degrees on planted tibia); weakly flexes knee joint
Flexor hallucis longus	Inferior two thirds of posterior surface of fibula and inferior part of interosseous membrane	Base of distal phalanx of great toe (hallux)		Flexes great toe at all joints and plantar flexes ankle joint; supports medial longitudinal arch of foot
Flexor digitorum longus	Medial part of posterior surface of tibia inferior to soleal line, and by a broad tendon to fibula	Bases of distal phalanges of lateral four digits	Tibial nerve (**S2** and S3)	Flexes lateral four digits and plantar flexes ankle joint; supports longitudinal arches of foot
Tibialis posterior	Interosseous membrane, posterior surface of tibia inferior to soleal line and posterior surface of fibula	Tuberosity of navicular, cuneiform, and cuboid and bases of metatarsals 2–4	Tibial nerve (L4 and L5)	Plantar flexes ankle joint and inverts foot

[a]See Table 5.1 for explanation of segmental innervation.

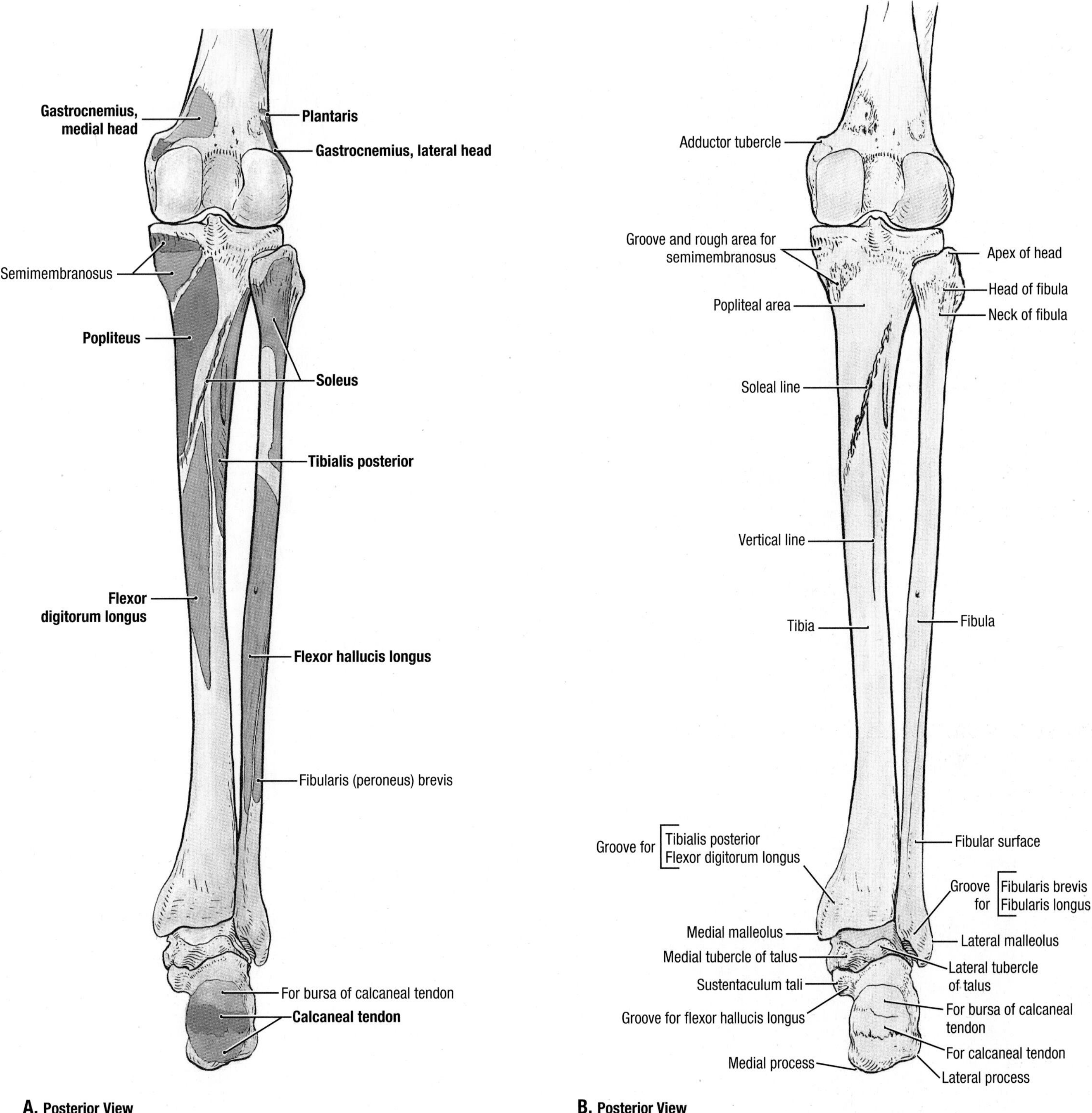
Gastrocnemius, medial head
Plantaris
Gastrocnemius, lateral head
Semimembranosus
Popliteus
Soleus
Tibialis posterior
Flexor digitorum longus
Flexor hallucis longus
Fibularis (peroneus) brevis
For bursa of calcaneal tendon
Calcaneal tendon
A. Posterior View
Adductor tubercle
Groove and rough area for semimembranosus
Apex of head
Head of fibula
Neck of fibula
Popliteal area
Soleal line
Vertical line
Tibia
Fibula
Groove for Tibialis posterior Flexor digitorum longus
Fibular surface
Groove for Fibularis brevis Fibularis longus
Medial malleolus
Lateral malleolus
Medial tubercle of talus
Lateral tubercle of talus
Sustentaculum tali
For bursa of calcaneal tendon
Groove for flexor hallucis longus
For calcaneal tendon
Medial process
Lateral process
B. Posterior View

5.68 BONES OF THE POSTERIOR LEG

A. Muscle attachments. **B.** Features of bones.

Tibial fractures. The tibial shaft is narrowest at the junction of its middle and inferior thirds, which is the most frequent site of fracture. Unfortunately, this area of the bone also has the poorest blood supply.

Fibular fractures. These commonly occur 2 to 6 cm proximal to the distal end of the lateral malleolus and are often associated with fracture/dislocations of the ankle joint, which are combined with tibial fractures. When a person slips and the foot is forced into an excessively inverted position, the ankle ligaments tear, forcibly tilting the talus against the lateral malleolus and shearing it off.

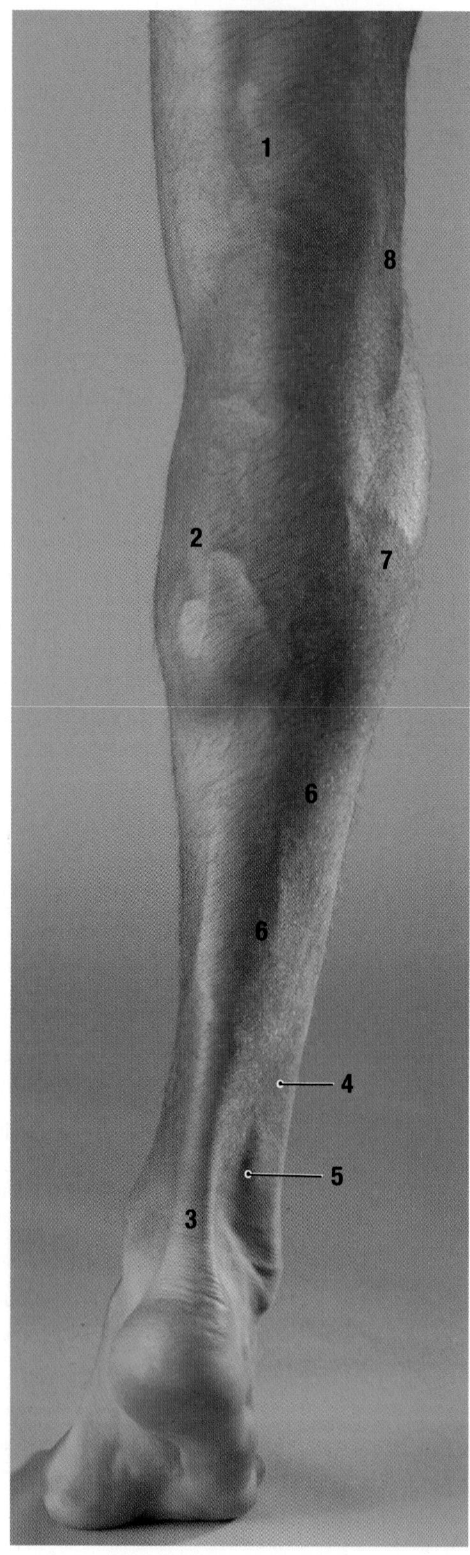
1
8
2
7
6
6
4
5
3

A. Posterior View

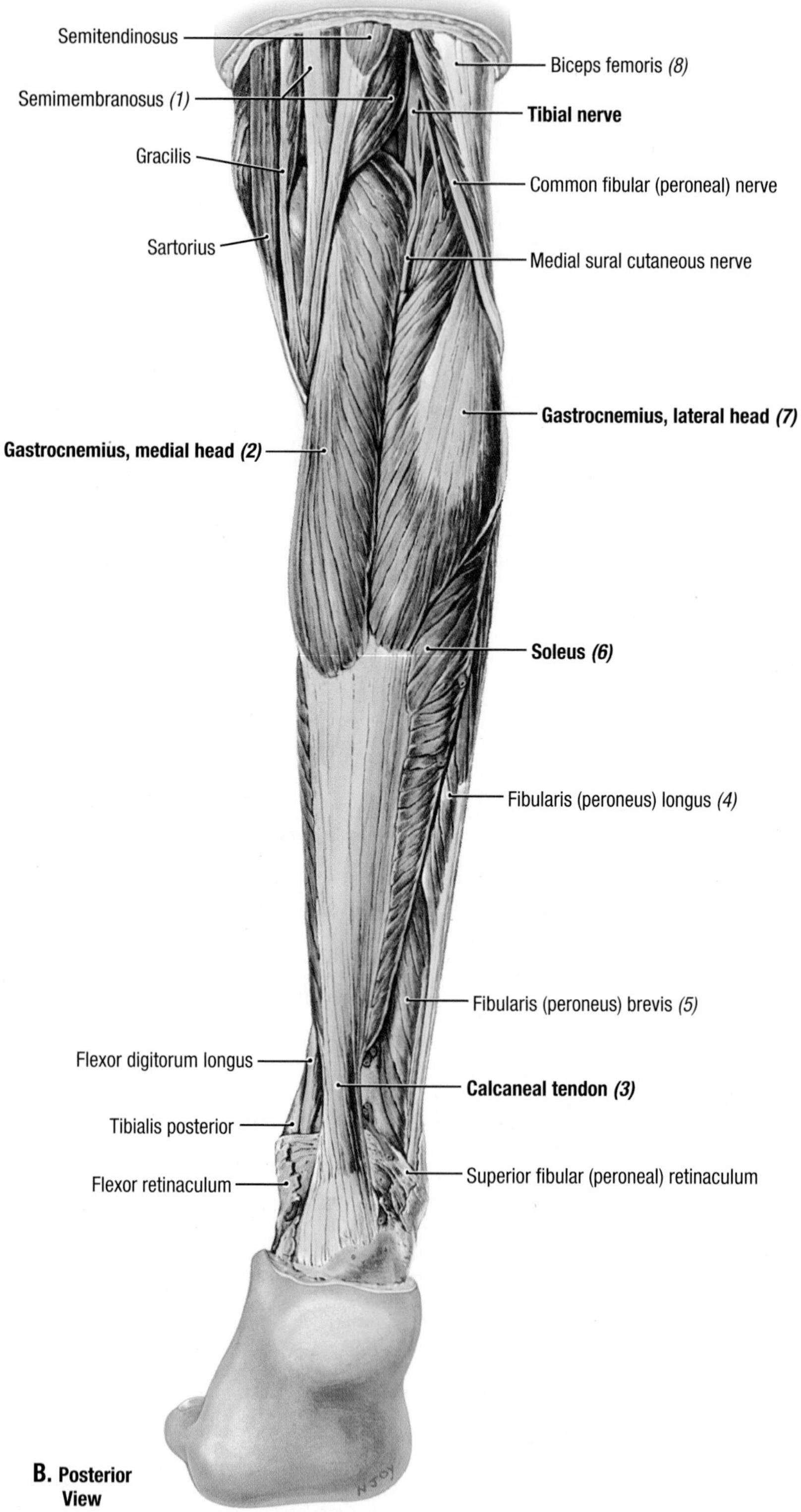

Semitendinosus

Biceps femoris *(8)*

Semimembranosus *(1)*

Tibial nerve

Gracilis

Common fibular (peroneal) nerve

Sartorius

Medial sural cutaneous nerve

Gastrocnemius, lateral head *(7)*

Gastrocnemius, medial head *(2)*

Soleus *(6)*

Fibularis (peroneus) longus *(4)*

Fibularis (peroneus) brevis *(5)*

Flexor digitorum longus

Calcaneal tendon *(3)*

Tibialis posterior

Flexor retinaculum

Superior fibular (peroneal) retinaculum

B. Posterior View

5.69 POSTERIOR LEG, SUPERFICIAL MUSCLES OF POSTERIOR COMPARTMENT

A. Surface anatomy (*numbers* refer to structures labeled in **B**). **B.** Dissection. **Gastrocnemius strain** (tennis leg) is a painful calf injury resulting from partial tearing of the medial belly of the muscle at or near its musculotendinous junction. It is caused by overstretching the muscle during simultaneous full extension of the knee joint and dorsiflexion of the ankle joint.

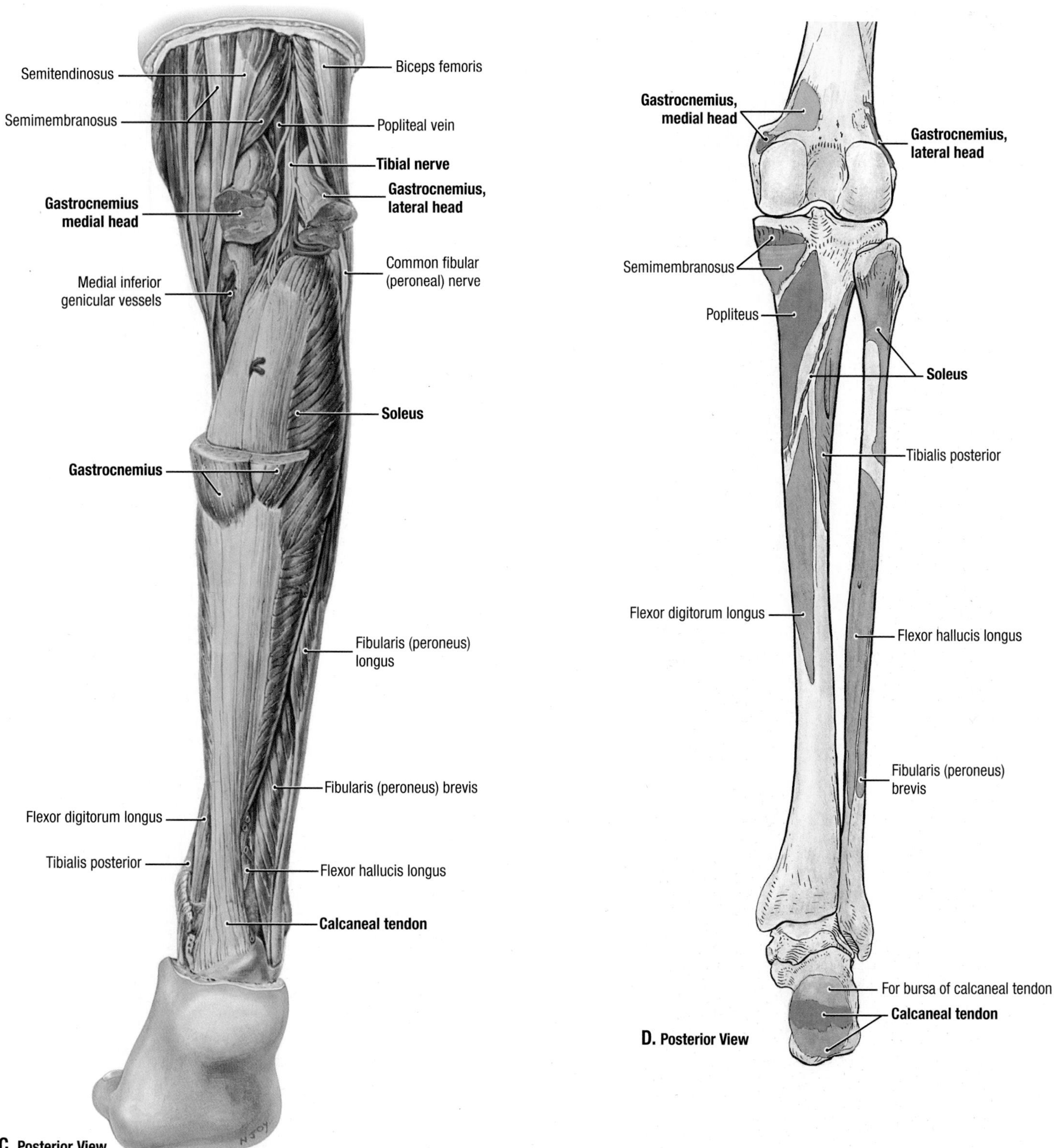
Semitendinosus
Biceps femoris
Semimembranosus
Popliteal vein
Tibial nerve
Gastrocnemius, lateral head
Gastrocnemius medial head
Common fibular (peroneal) nerve
Medial inferior genicular vessels
Soleus
Gastrocnemius
Fibularis (peroneus) longus
Fibularis (peroneus) brevis
Flexor digitorum longus
Tibialis posterior
Flexor hallucis longus
Calcaneal tendon
Gastrocnemius, medial head
Gastrocnemius, lateral head
Semimembranosus
Popliteus
Soleus
Tibialis posterior
Flexor digitorum longus
Flexor hallucis longus
Fibularis (peroneus) brevis
For bursa of calcaneal tendon
Calcaneal tendon

C. Posterior View

D. Posterior View

5.69 POSTERIOR LEG, SUPERFICIAL MUSCLES OF POSTERIOR COMPARTMENT (*CONTINUED*)

C. Dissection revealing soleus. **D.** Bones of leg showing muscle attachments. Inflammation of the calcaneal tendon due to microscopic tears of collagen fibers in the tendon, particularly just superior to its attachment to the calcaneus, results in **calcaneal tendinitis**, which causes pain during walking. **Calcaneal tendon rupture** is probably the most severe acute muscular problem of the leg. Following complete rupture of the tendon, passive dorsiflexion is excessive, and the person cannot plantar flex against resistance.

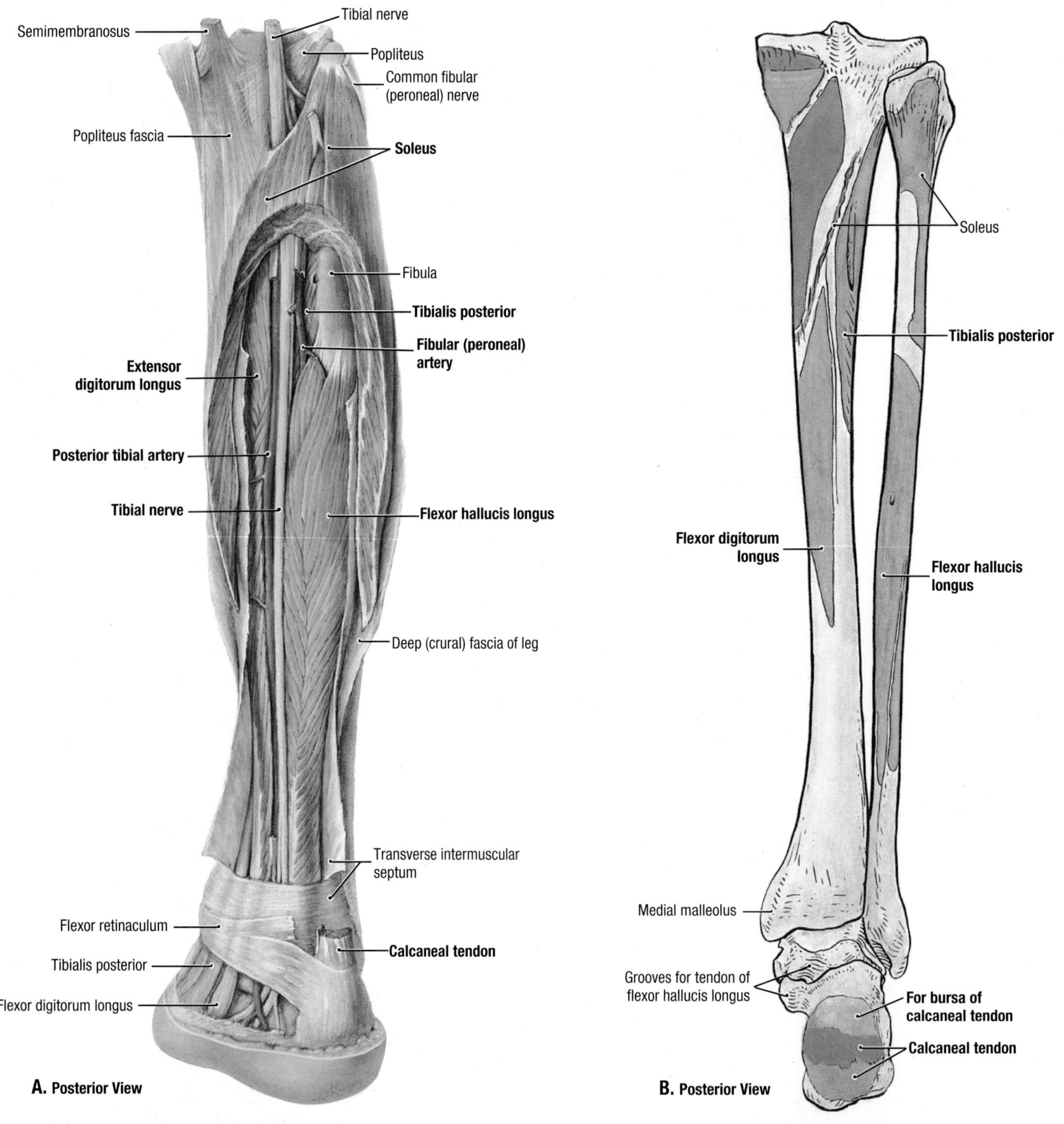
Semimembranosus
Tibial nerve
Popliteus
Common fibular (peroneal) nerve
Popliteus fascia
Soleus
Fibula
Tibialis posterior
Fibular (peroneal) artery
Extensor digitorum longus
Posterior tibial artery
Tibial nerve
Flexor hallucis longus
Deep (crural) fascia of leg
Transverse intermuscular septum
Flexor retinaculum
Calcaneal tendon
Tibialis posterior
Flexor digitorum longus
A. Posterior View
Soleus
Tibialis posterior
Flexor digitorum longus
Flexor hallucis longus
Medial malleolus
Grooves for tendon of flexor hallucis longus
For bursa of calcaneal tendon
Calcaneal tendon
B. Posterior View

5.70 POSTERIOR LEG, DEEP MUSCLES OF POSTERIOR COMPARTMENT

A. Superficial dissection. The calcaneal (Achilles) tendon is cut, the gastrocnemius muscle is removed, and only a horseshoe-shaped proximal part of the soleus muscle remains in place. **B.** Bones of leg showing muscle attachments. **Calcaneal bursitis** results from inflammation of the bursa of the calcaneal tendon located between the calcaneal tendon and the superior part of the posterior surface of the calcaneus. Calcaneal bursitis causes pain posterior to the heel and occurs commonly during long-distance running, basketball, and tennis. It is caused by excessive friction on the bursa as the calcaneal tendon continuously slides over it.

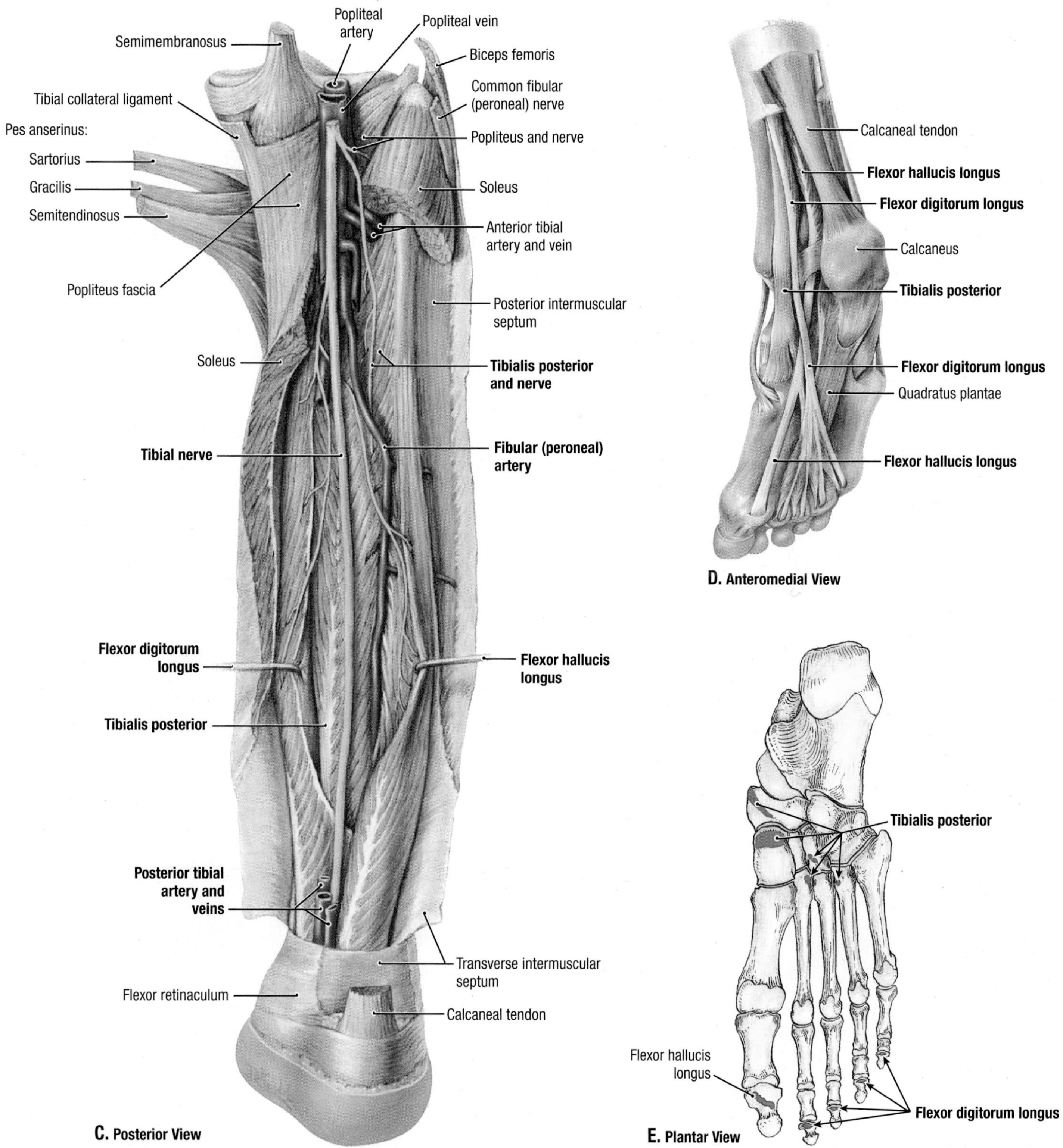
Popliteal artery
Popliteal vein
Semimembranosus
Biceps femoris
Common fibular (peroneal) nerve
Tibial collateral ligament
Pes anserinus:
Popliteus and nerve
Sartorius
Gracilis
Soleus
Semitendinosus
Anterior tibial artery and vein
Popliteus fascia
Posterior intermuscular septum
Soleus
Tibialis posterior and nerve
Tibial nerve
Fibular (peroneal) artery
Flexor digitorum longus
Flexor hallucis longus
Tibialis posterior
Posterior tibial artery and veins
Transverse intermuscular septum
Flexor retinaculum
Calcaneal tendon
C. Posterior View
Calcaneal tendon
Flexor hallucis longus
Flexor digitorum longus
Calcaneus
Tibialis posterior
Flexor digitorum longus
Quadratus plantae
Flexor hallucis longus
D. Anteromedial View
Tibialis posterior
Flexor hallucis longus
Flexor digitorum longus
E. Plantar View

5.70 POSTERIOR LEG, DEEP MUSCLES OF POSTERIOR COMPARTMENT (*CONTINUED*)

C. Deeper dissection. The flexor hallucis longus and flexor digitorum longus are pulled apart, and the posterior tibial artery is partly excised. The tibialis posterior lies deep to the two long digital flexors. **D.** Crossing of muscles (tendons) of the deep compartment superoposterior to the medial malleolus and into the sole of the foot. **E.** Bones of foot showing muscle attachments.

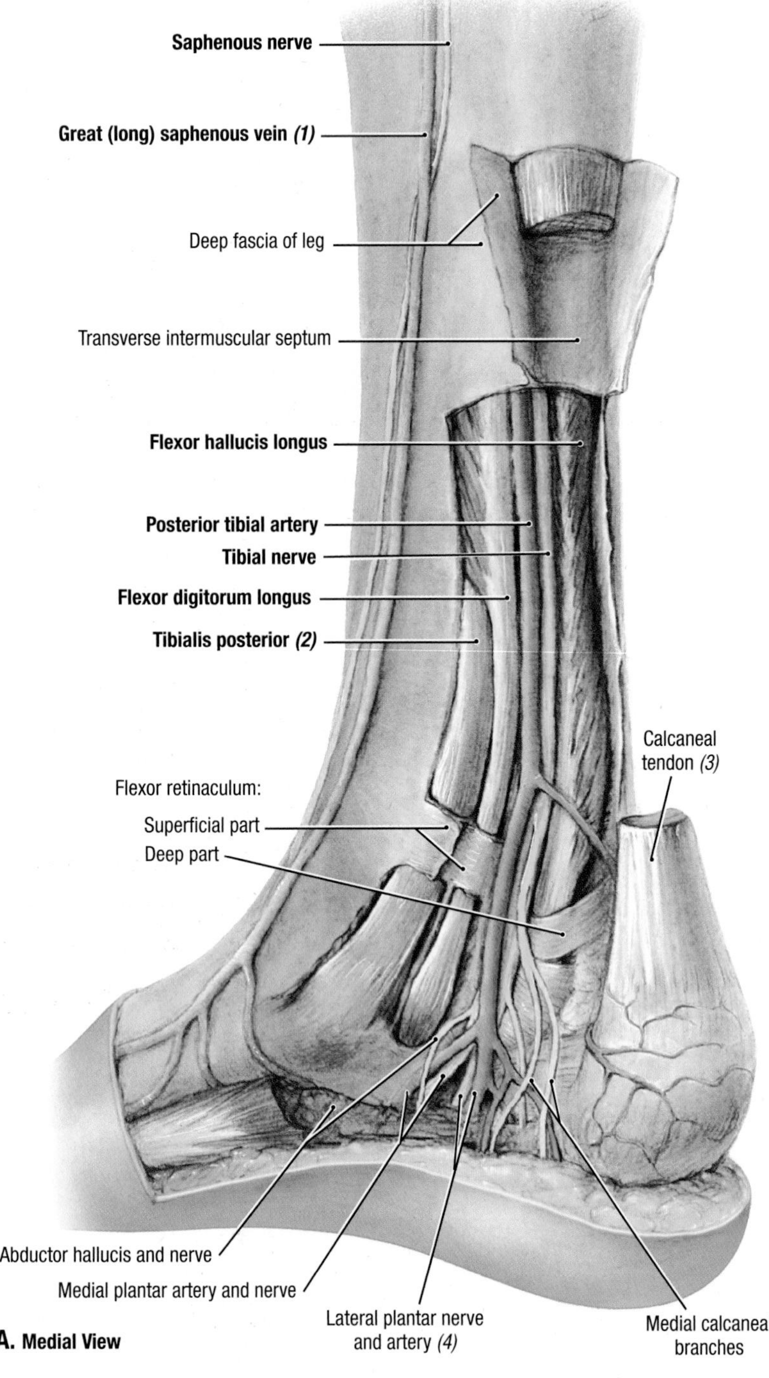
Saphenous nerve
Great (long) saphenous vein (1)
Deep fascia of leg
Transverse intermuscular septum
Flexor hallucis longus
Posterior tibial artery
Tibial nerve
Flexor digitorum longus
Tibialis posterior (2)
Calcaneal tendon (3)
Flexor retinaculum:
Superficial part
Deep part
Abductor hallucis and nerve
Medial plantar artery and nerve
Lateral plantar nerve and artery (4)
Medial calcaneal branches

A. Medial View

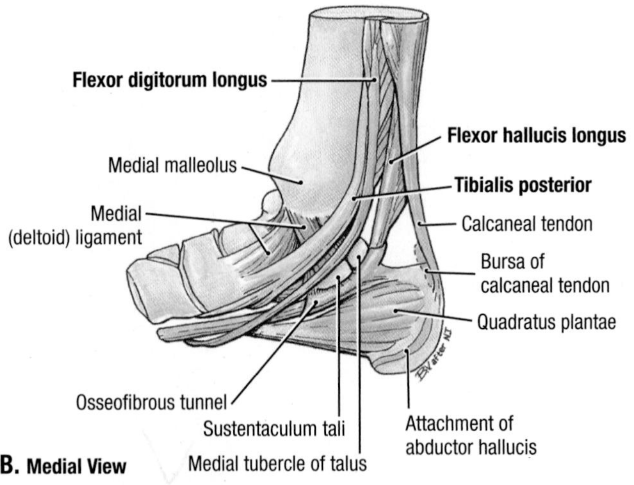
Flexor digitorum longus
Medial malleolus
Medial (deltoid) ligament
Flexor hallucis longus
Tibialis posterior
Calcaneal tendon
Bursa of calcaneal tendon
Quadratus plantae
Osseofibrous tunnel
Sustentaculum tali
Medial tubercle of talus
Attachment of abductor hallucis

B. Medial View

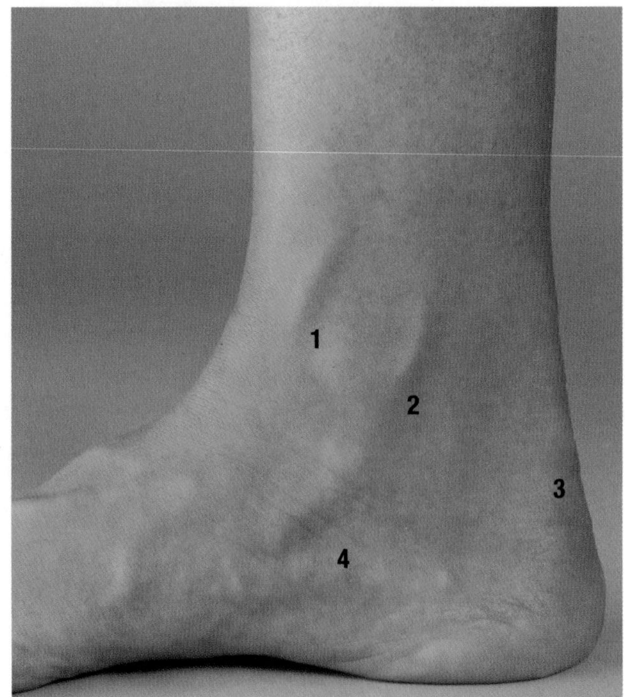
1
2
3
4

C. Medial View

5.71 MEDIAL ANKLE REGION

A. Dissection. The calcaneal tendon and posterior part of the abductor hallucis were excised. **B.** Schematic illustration of the tendons passing posterior to medial malleolus. **C.** Surface anatomy (*numbers* refer to structures labeled in **A**).

- The posterior tibial artery and the tibial nerve lie between the flexor digitorum longus and flexor hallucis longus muscles and divide into medial and lateral plantar branches.
- The tibialis posterior and flexor digitorum longus tendons occupy separate osseofibrous tunnels posterior to the medial malleolus.
- The **posterior tibial pulse** can usually be palpated between the posterior surface of the medial malleolus and the medial border of the calcaneal tendon.

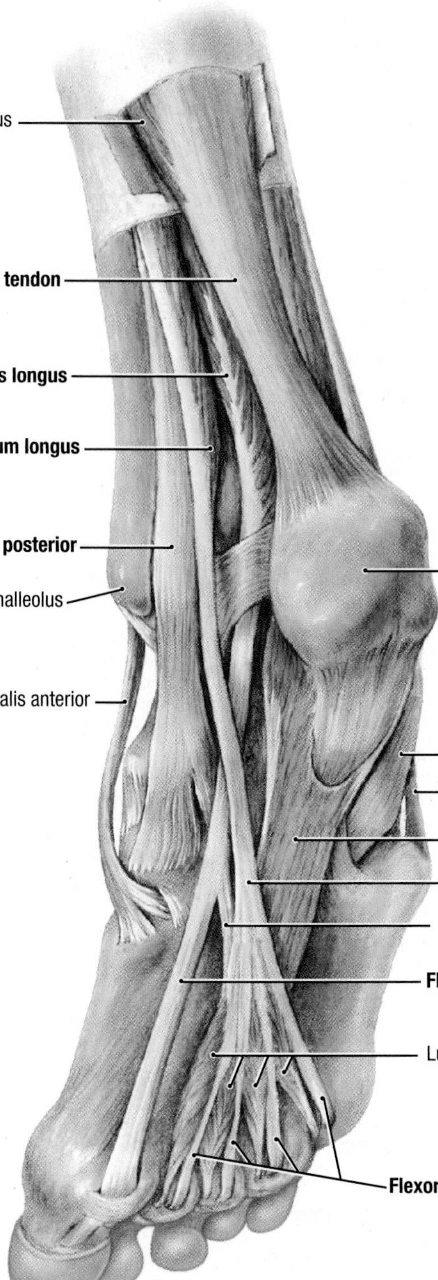

Soleus
Calcaneal tendon
Flexor hallucis longus
Flexor digitorum longus
Tibialis posterior
Medial malleolus
Tibialis anterior
Calcaneus
Fibularis (peroneus) longus
Fibularis (peroneus) brevis
Quadratus plantae
Flexor digitorum longus
Slip from flexor hallucis longus
Flexor hallucis longus
Lumbricals
Flexor digitorum longus

A. Posteromedial View

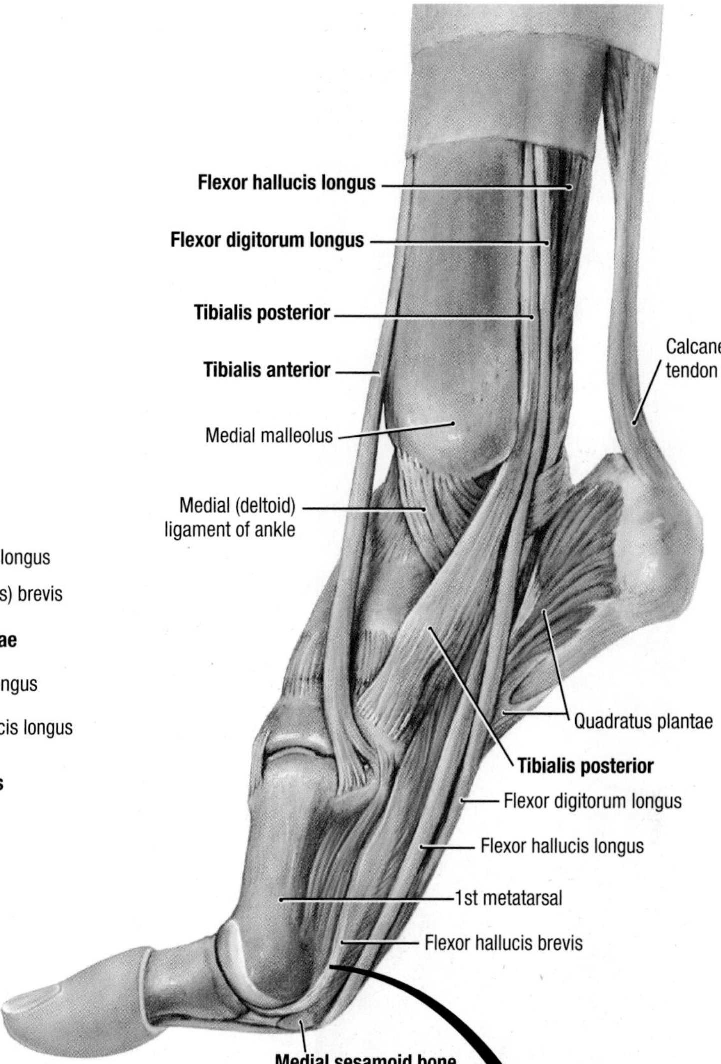

Flexor hallucis longus
Flexor digitorum longus
Tibialis posterior
Tibialis anterior
Medial malleolus
Medial (deltoid) ligament of ankle
Calcaneal tendon
Quadratus plantae
Tibialis posterior
Flexor digitorum longus
Flexor hallucis longus
1st metatarsal
Flexor hallucis brevis
Medial sesamoid bone

B. Medial View

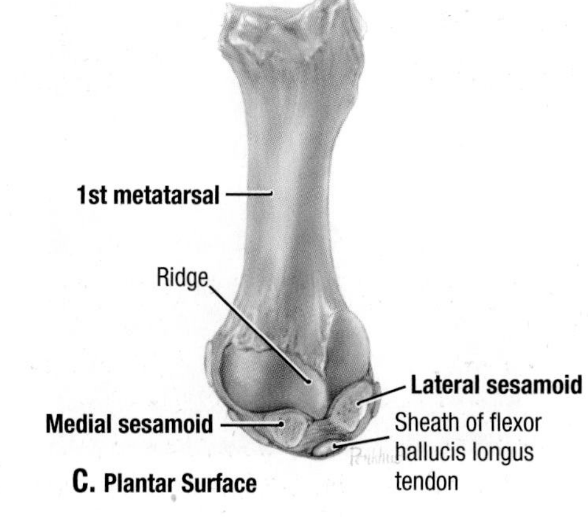
1st metatarsal
Ridge
Lateral sesamoid
Medial sesamoid
Sheath of flexor hallucis longus tendon

C. Plantar Surface

5.72 MEDIAL ANKLE AND FOOT

A. Tendons of deep compartment of the leg traced to their distal attachments in the sole of the foot. **B.** Foot raised as in walking and sesamoid bones of the great toe. The sesamoid bones of the great toe are located on each side of a bony ridge on the 1st metatarsal.

- The sesamoid bones are a "footstool" for the first metatarsal, giving it increased height.
- By inserting into the flexor digitorum longus muscle, the quadratus plantae muscle modifies the oblique pull of the flexor tendons.
- The flexor hallucis longus muscle uses three pulleys: a groove on the posterior aspect of the distal end of the tibia, a groove on the posterior aspect of the talus, and a groove inferior to the sustentaculum tali.
- The flexor digitorum longus muscle crosses superficial to the tibialis posterior, superoposterior to the medial malleolus.

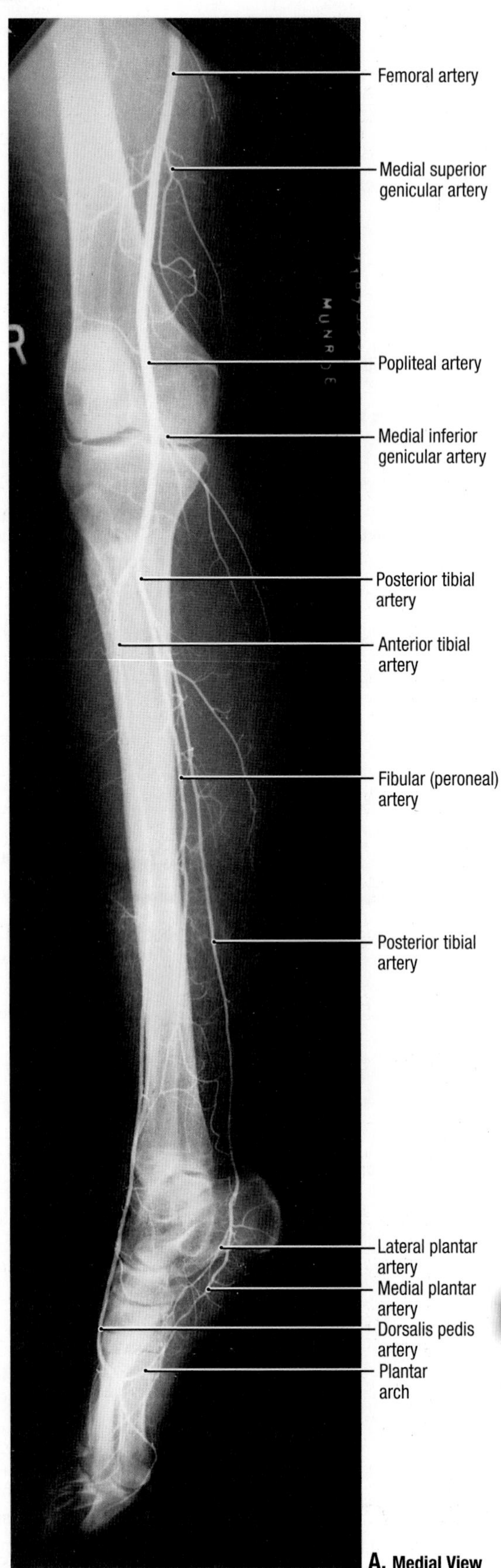

Femoral artery
Medial superior genicular artery
Popliteal artery
Medial inferior genicular artery
Posterior tibial artery
Anterior tibial artery
Fibular (peroneal) artery
Posterior tibial artery
Lateral plantar artery
Medial plantar artery
Dorsalis pedis artery
Plantar arch
R
MUNROE

A. Medial View

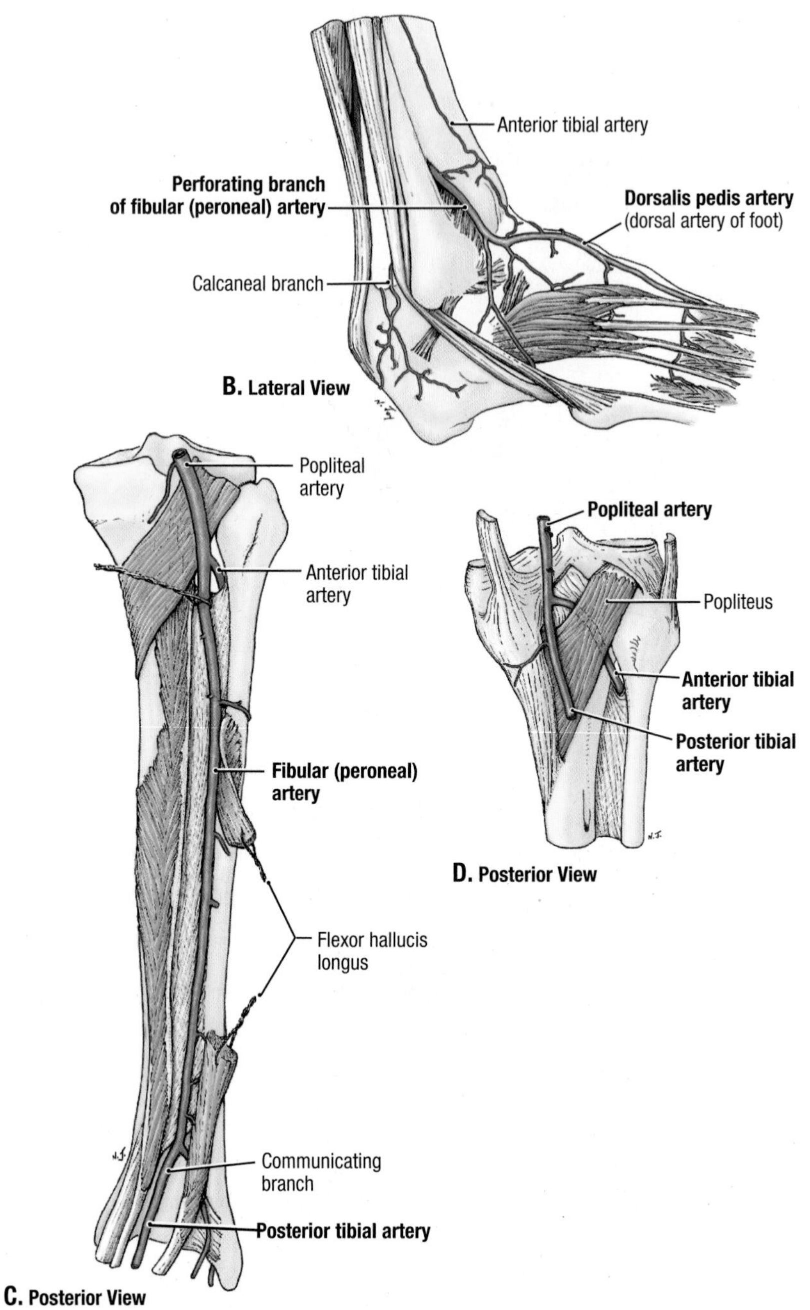

Anterior tibial artery
Perforating branch of fibular (peroneal) artery
Dorsalis pedis artery (dorsal artery of foot)
Calcaneal branch
Popliteal artery
Anterior tibial artery
Fibular (peroneal) artery
Flexor hallucis longus
Communicating branch
Posterior tibial artery
Popliteal artery
Popliteus
Anterior tibial artery
Posterior tibial artery

B. Lateral View

C. Posterior View

D. Posterior View

5.73 POPLITEAL ARTERIOGRAM AND ARTERIAL ANOMALIES

A. Popliteal arteriogram. The femoral artery becomes the popliteal artery at the adductor hiatus. The anterior tibial artery continues as the dorsalis pedis (dorsal artery of the foot). The posterior tibial artery terminates as the medial and lateral plantar arteries; its major branch is the fibular artery. **B. Anomalous dorsalis pedis artery**. The perforating branch of the fibular artery rarely continues as the dorsalis pedis artery, but when it does, the anterior tibial artery ends proximal to the ankle or is a slender vessel. **C. Absence of posterior tibial artery**. Compensatory enlargement of the fibular artery was found to occur in approximately 5% of limbs. **D. High division of popliteal artery**. Along with the anterior tibial artery descending anterior to the popliteus muscle; this anomaly was found to occur in approximately 2% of limbs.

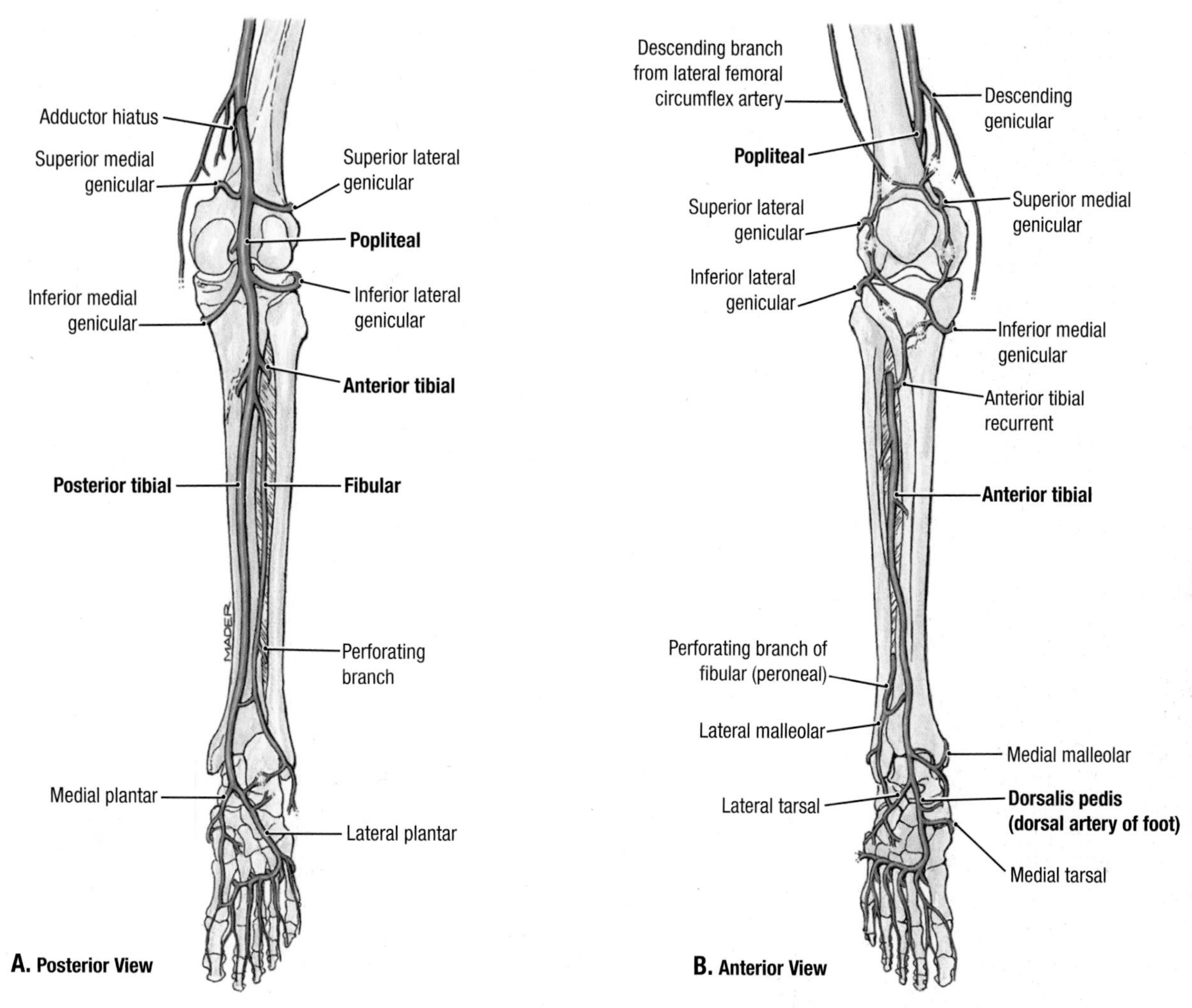
Adductor hiatus
Superior medial genicular
Superior lateral genicular
Popliteal
Inferior medial genicular
Inferior lateral genicular
Anterior tibial
Posterior tibial
Fibular
MADER
Perforating branch
Medial plantar
Lateral plantar
A. Posterior View
Descending branch from lateral femoral circumflex artery
Descending genicular
Popliteal
Superior lateral genicular
Superior medial genicular
Inferior lateral genicular
Inferior medial genicular
Anterior tibial recurrent
Anterior tibial
Perforating branch of fibular (peroneal)
Lateral malleolar
Medial malleolar
Lateral tarsal
Dorsalis pedis (dorsal artery of foot)
Medial tarsal
B. Anterior View

5.74 ARTERIAL SUPPLY OF LEG AND FOOT

TABLE 5.17 ARTERIAL SUPPLY OF LEG AND FOOT

Artery	Origin	Course	Distribution in Leg
Popliteal	Continuation of femoral artery at adductor hiatus	Passes through popliteal fossa to leg; divides into anterior and posterior tibial arteries at lower border of popliteus	Lateral and medial aspects of knee via genicular arteries
Anterior tibial	From popliteal	Passes between tibia and fibula into anterior compartment through gap superior to interosseous membrane; descends between tibialis anterior and extensor digitorum longus muscles	Anterior compartment
Dorsalis pedis (dorsal artery of foot)	Continuation of anterior tibial artery distal to talocrural joint	Descends to first interosseous space; pierces first dorsal interosseous muscle as deep plantar artery; joins deep plantar arch	Muscles on dorsum of foot
Posterior tibial	From popliteal	Passes through posterior compartment; divides into medial and lateral plantar arteries posterior to medial malleolus	Posterior and lateral compartments, nutrient artery passes to tibia
Fibular (peroneal)	From posterior tibial	Descends in posterior compartment adjacent to posterior intermuscular septum	Posterior compartment: perforating branches supply lateral compartment
Medial plantar		In foot between abductor hallucis and flexor digitorum brevis muscles	Supplies mainly muscles of great toe and skin on medial side of sole of foot
Lateral plantar		Runs anterolaterally deep to abductor hallucis and flexor digitorum brevis, and then arches medially to form deep plantar arch	Supplies lateral aspect of sole of foot

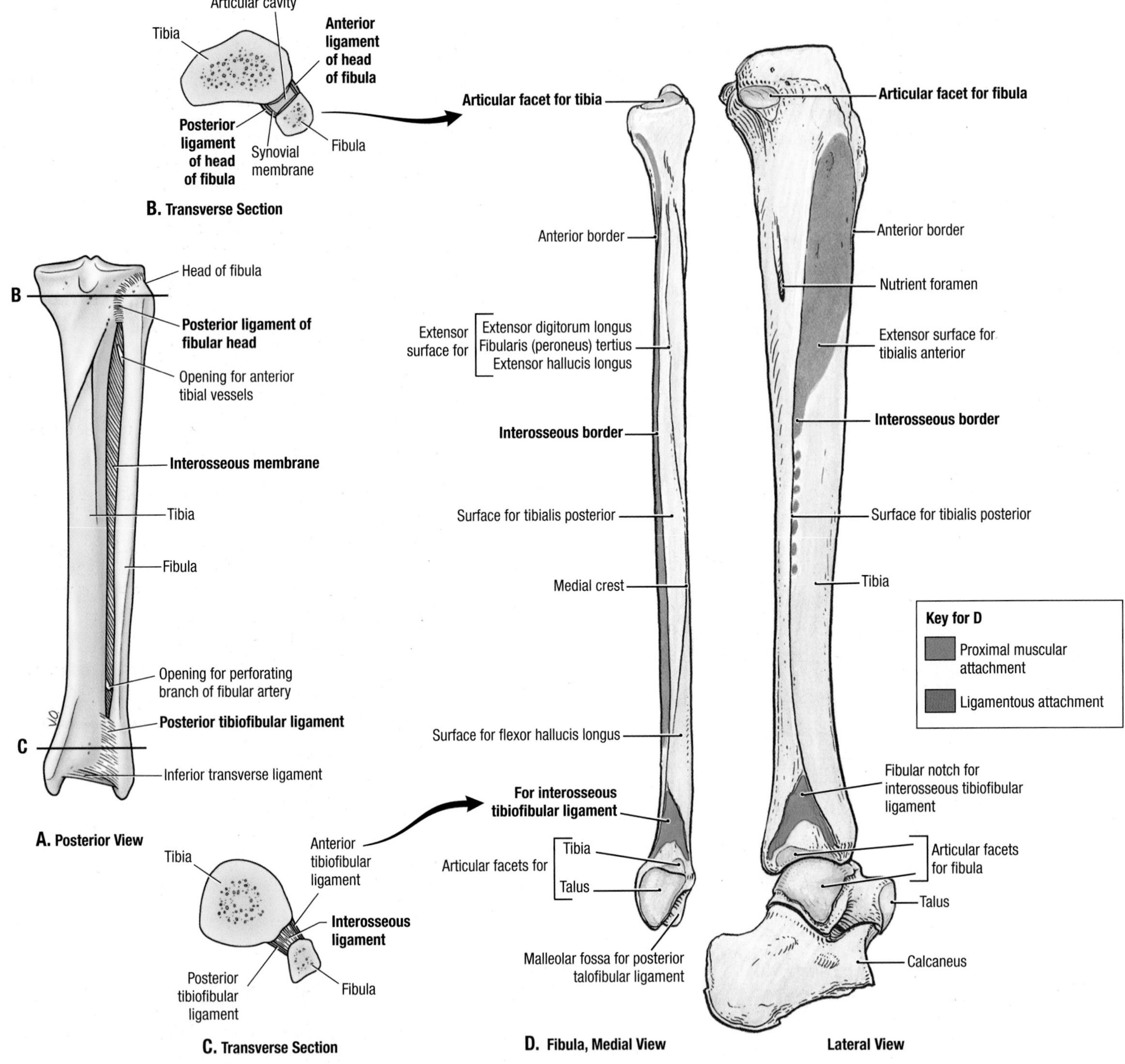

Articular cavity
Tibia
Anterior ligament of head of fibula
Posterior ligament of head of fibula
Synovial membrane
Fibula
B. Transverse Section
Head of fibula
B
Posterior ligament of fibular head
Opening for anterior tibial vessels
Interosseous membrane
Tibia
Fibula
Opening for perforating branch of fibular artery
Posterior tibiofibular ligament
C
Inferior transverse ligament
A. Posterior View
Tibia
Anterior tibiofibular ligament
Interosseous ligament
Posterior tibiofibular ligament
Fibula
C. Transverse Section
Articular facet for tibia
Anterior border
Extensor surface for
Extensor digitorum longus
Fibularis (peroneus) tertius
Extensor hallucis longus
Interosseous border
Surface for tibialis posterior
Medial crest
Surface for flexor hallucis longus
For interosseous tibiofibular ligament
Articular facets for
Tibia
Talus
Malleolar fossa for posterior talofibular ligament
D. Fibula, Medial View
Articular facet for fibula
Anterior border
Nutrient foramen
Extensor surface for tibialis anterior
Interosseous border
Surface for tibialis posterior
Tibia
Key for D
Proximal muscular attachment
Ligamentous attachment
Fibular notch for interosseous tibiofibular ligament
Articular facets for fibula
Talus
Calcaneus
Lateral View

5.75 TIBIOFIBULAR JOINT AND TIBIOFIBULAR SYNDESMOSIS

A. Overview. **B.** Tibiofibular joint. **C.** Tibiofibular syndesmosis. **D.** Tibia and fibula, disarticulated.

- The superior tibiofibular joint (proximal tibiofibular joint) is a plane type of synovial joint between the flat facet on the fibular head and a similar facet located posterolaterally on the lateral tibial condyle. The tense joint capsule surrounds the joint and attaches to the margins of the articular surfaces of the fibula and tibia.
- The tibiofibular syndesmosis is a fibrous joint. This articulation is essential for stability of the ankle joint because it keeps the lateral malleolus firmly against the lateral surface of the talus. The strong interosseous tibiofibular ligament is continuous superiorly with the interosseous membrane and forms the principal connection between the distal ends of the tibia and fibula.

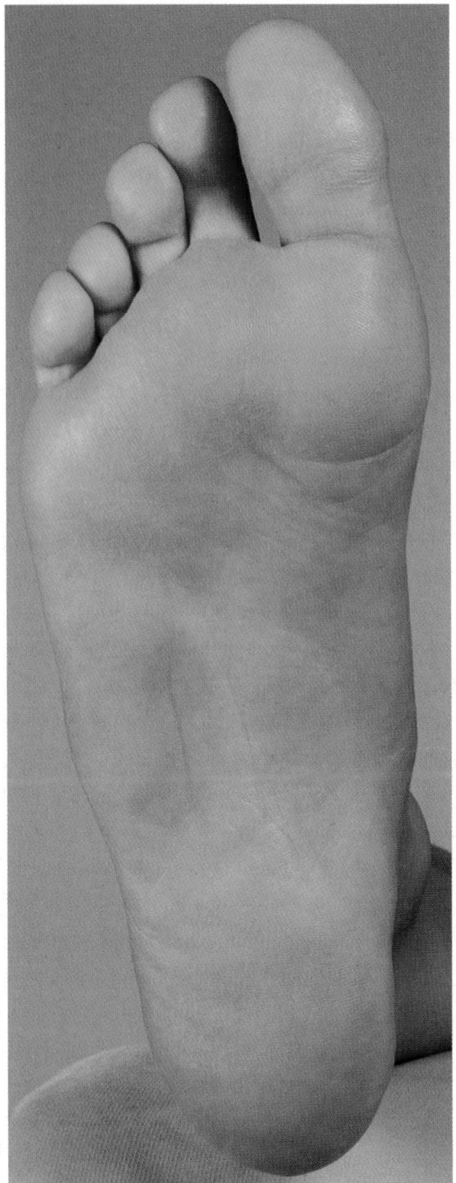

A. Plantar View

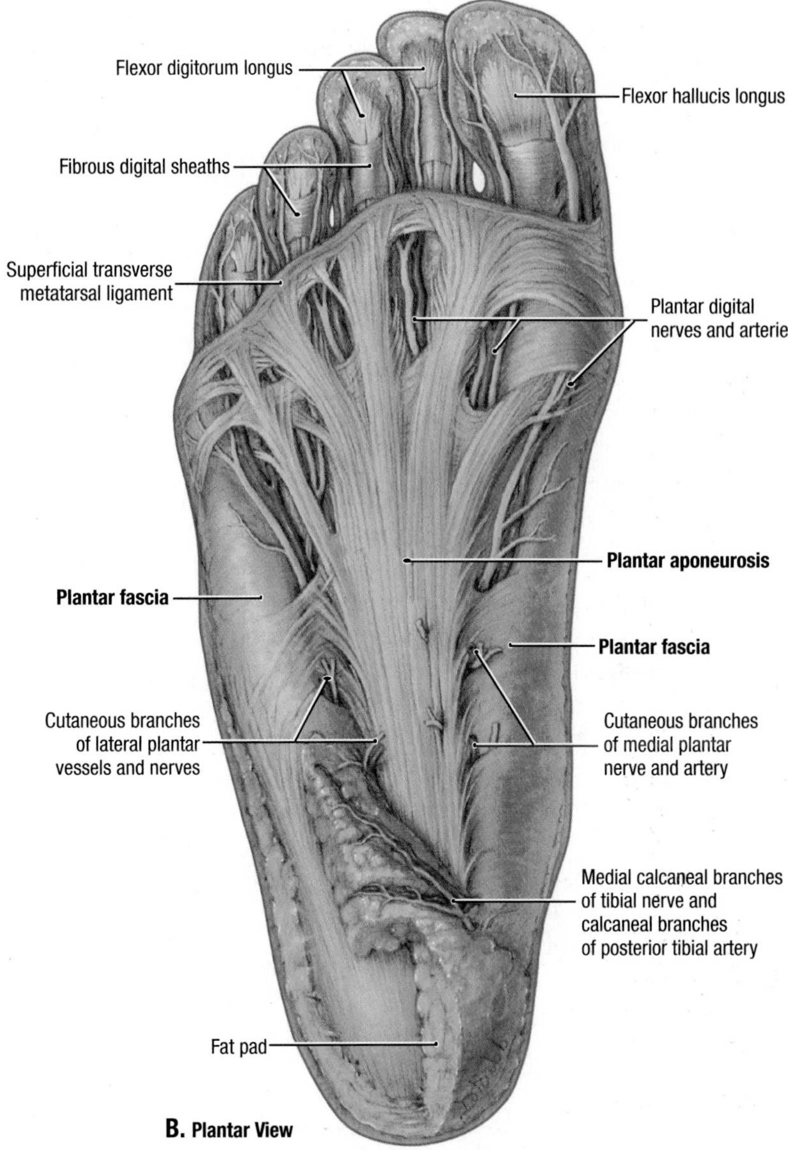
Flexor digitorum longus
Flexor hallucis longus
Fibrous digital sheaths
Superficial transverse metatarsal ligament
Plantar digital nerves and arteries
Plantar aponeurosis
Plantar fascia
Plantar fascia
Cutaneous branches of lateral plantar vessels and nerves
Cutaneous branches of medial plantar nerve and artery
Medial calcaneal branches of tibial nerve and calcaneal branches of posterior tibial artery
Fat pad

B. Plantar View

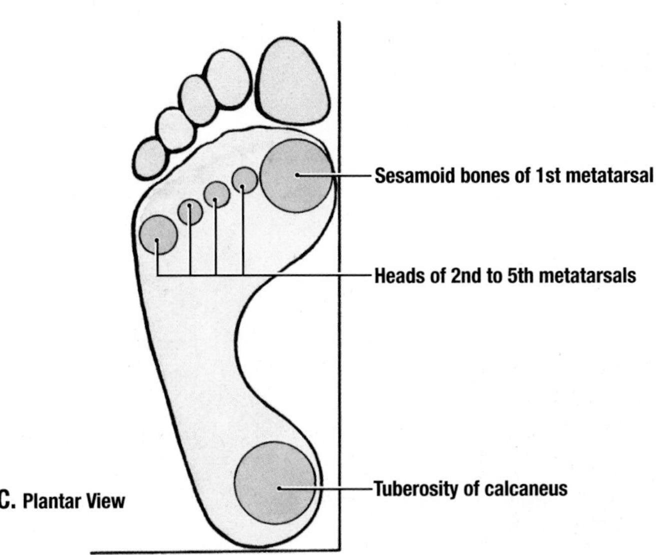
Sesamoid bones of 1st metatarsal
Heads of 2nd to 5th metatarsals
Tuberosity of calcaneus

C. Plantar View

5.76 SOLE OF FOOT, SUPERFICIAL

A. Surface anatomy. **B.** Dissection. Plantar aponeurosis and fascia, with neurovascular structures. **C.** Weight-bearing areas.

- The weight of the body is transmitted to the talus from the tibia and fibula. It is then transmitted to the tuberosity of the calcaneus, the heads of the second to fifth metatarsals, and the sesamoid bones of the first digit.

Plantar fasciitis, strain and inflammation of the plantar aponeurosis, may result from running and high-impact aerobics, especially when inappropriate footwear is worn. It causes pain on the plantar surface of the heel and on the medial aspect of the foot. Point tenderness is located at the proximal attachment of the plantar aponeurosis to the medial tubercle of the calcaneus and on the medial surface of this bone. The pain increases with passive extension of the great toe and may be further exacerbated by dorsiflexion of the ankle and/or weight bearing.

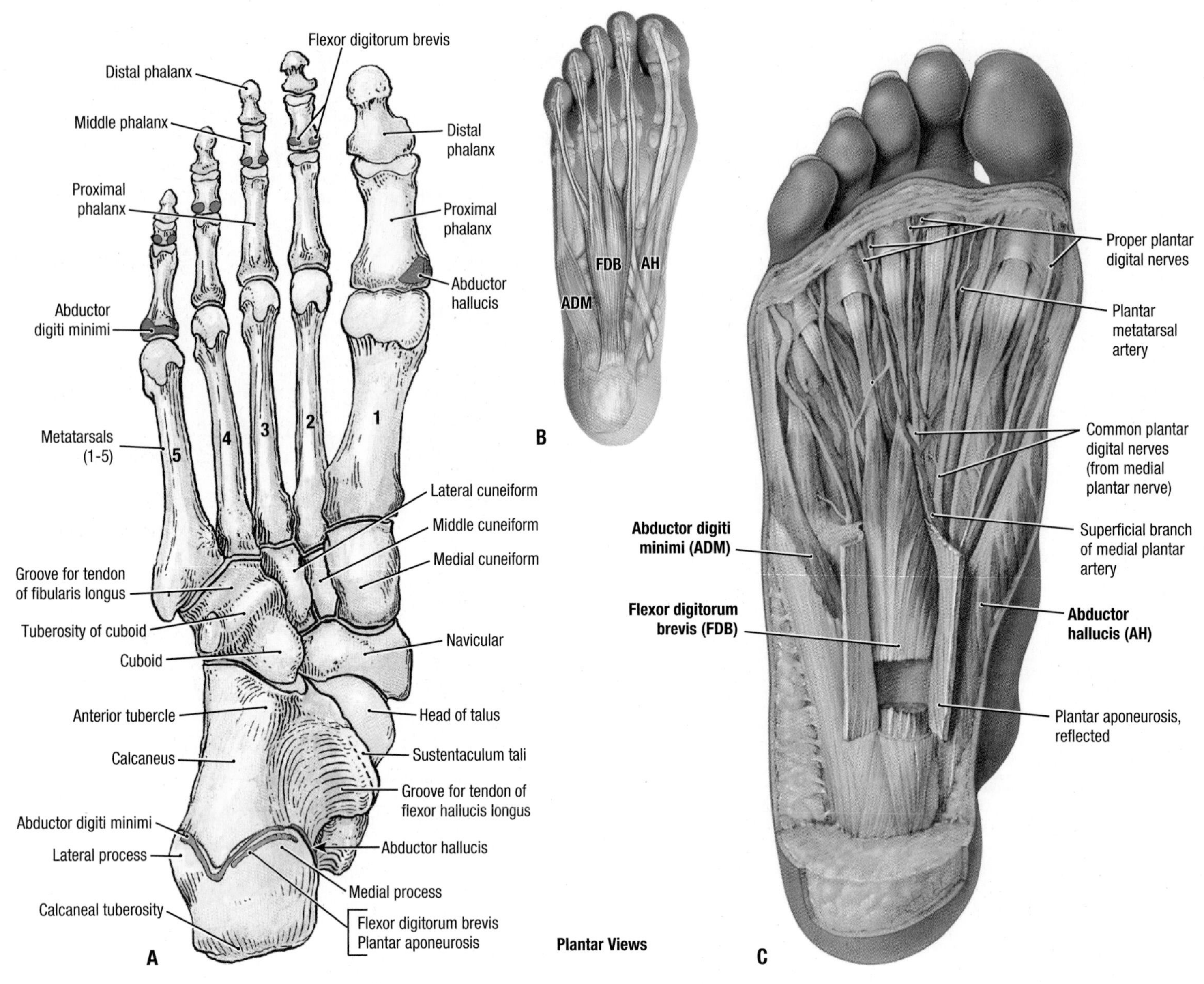
Flexor digitorum brevis
Distal phalanx
Middle phalanx
Proximal phalanx
Distal phalanx
Proximal phalanx
Abductor hallucis
Abductor digiti minimi
Metatarsals (1-5)
5
4
3
2
1
Lateral cuneiform
Middle cuneiform
Medial cuneiform
Groove for tendon of fibularis longus
Tuberosity of cuboid
Cuboid
Navicular
Anterior tubercle
Head of talus
Calcaneus
Sustentaculum tali
Groove for tendon of flexor hallucis longus
Abductor digiti minimi
Lateral process
Abductor hallucis
Medial process
Calcaneal tuberosity
Flexor digitorum brevis
Plantar aponeurosis
A
FDB
AH
ADM
B
Plantar Views
Proper plantar digital nerves
Plantar metatarsal artery
Common plantar digital nerves (from medial plantar nerve)
Abductor digiti minimi (ADM)
Superficial branch of medial plantar artery
Flexor digitorum brevis (FDB)
Abductor hallucis (AH)
Plantar aponeurosis, reflected
C

5.77 FIRST LAYER OF MUSCLES OF SOLE OF FOOT

A. Bones. **B.** Overview. **C.** Dissection. Muscles and neurovascular structures.

TABLE 5.18 MUSCLES IN SOLE OF FOOT—FIRST LAYER

Muscle	Proximal Attachment	Distal Attachment	Innervation	Actions[a]
Abductor hallucis	Medial process of tuberosity of calcaneus, flexor retinaculum, and plantar aponeurosis	Medial side of base of proximal phalanx of first digit	Medial plantar nerve (S2–S3)	Abducts and flexes first digit
Flexor digitorum brevis	Medial process of tuberosity of calcaneus, plantar aponeurosis, and intermuscular septa	Both sides of middle phalanges of lateral four digits		Flexes lateral four digits
Abductor digiti minimi	Medial and lateral processes of tuberosity of calcaneus, plantar aponeurosis, and intermuscular septa	Lateral side of base of proximal phalanx of fifth digit	Lateral plantar nerve (S2–S3)	Abducts and flexes fifth digit

[a]Although individual actions are described, the primary function of the intrinsic muscles of the foot is to act collectively to resist forces that stress (attempt to flatten) the arches of the foot.

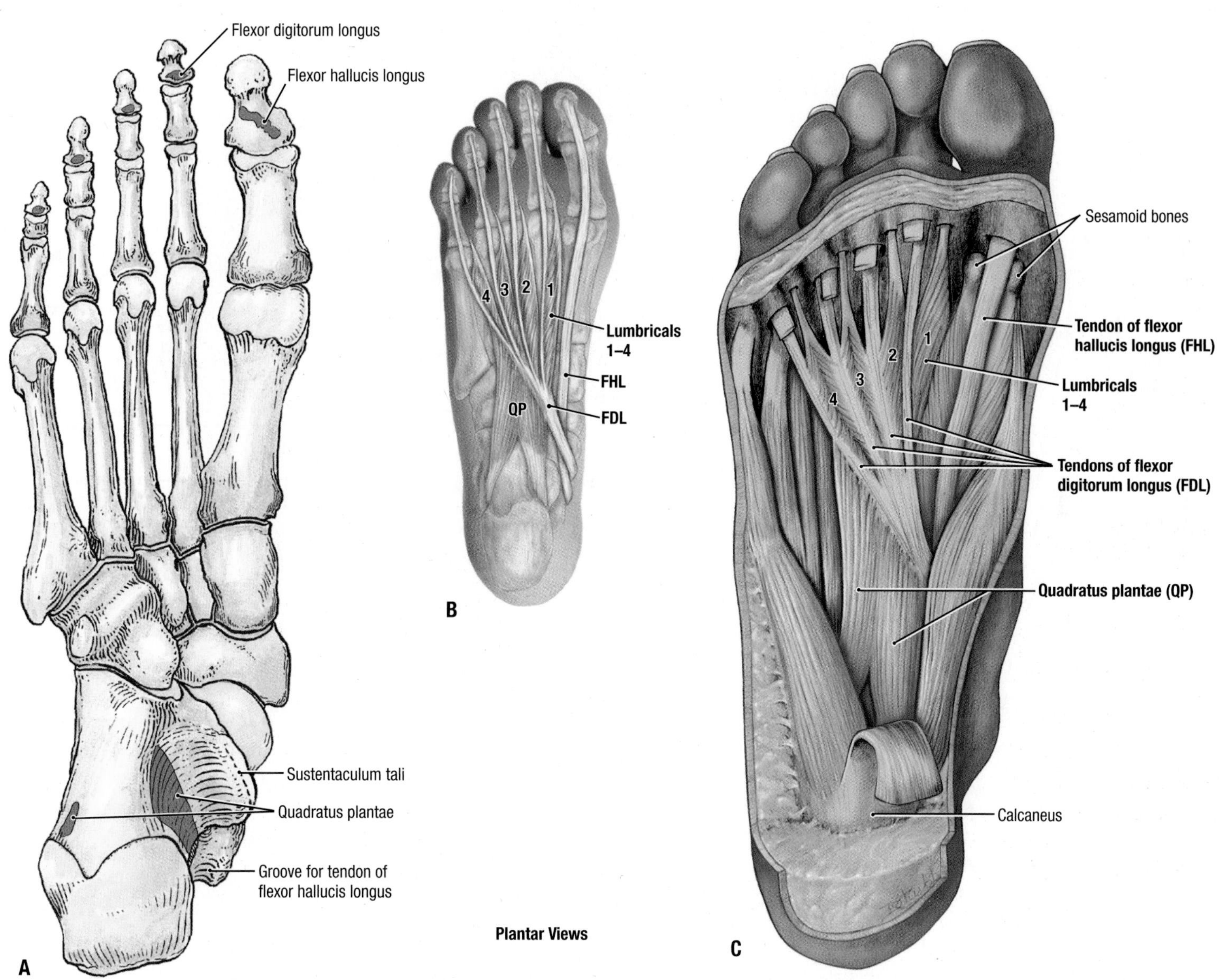
Flexor digitorum longus
Flexor hallucis longus
Sustentaculum tali
Quadratus plantae
Groove for tendon of flexor hallucis longus
A
4 3 2 1
Lumbricals 1–4
FHL
QP
FDL
B
Plantar Views
Sesamoid bones
Tendon of flexor hallucis longus (FHL)
Lumbricals 1–4
Tendons of flexor digitorum longus (FDL)
Quadratus plantae (QP)
Calcaneus
C

5.78 SECOND LAYER OF MUSCLES OF SOLE OF FOOT

A. Bony attachments. **B.** Overview. **C.** Dissection.

TABLE 5.19 MUSCLES IN SOLE OF FOOT—SECOND LAYER

Muscle	Proximal Attachment	Distal Attachment	Innervation	Actions[a]
Quadratus plantae	Medial surface and lateral margin of plantar surface of calcaneus	Posterolateral margin of tendon of flexor digitorum longus	Lateral plantar nerve (S2–S3)	Assists flexor digitorum longus in flexing lateral four digits
Lumbricals	Tendons of flexor digitorum longus	Medial aspect of extensor expansion over lateral four digits	*Medial one:* medial plantar nerve (S2–S3); *Lateral three:* lateral plantar nerve (S2–S3)	Flex proximal phalanges and extend middle and distal phalanges of lateral four digits

[a]Although individual actions are described, the primary function of the intrinsic muscles of the foot is to act collectively to resist forces that stress (attempt to flatten) the arches of the foot.

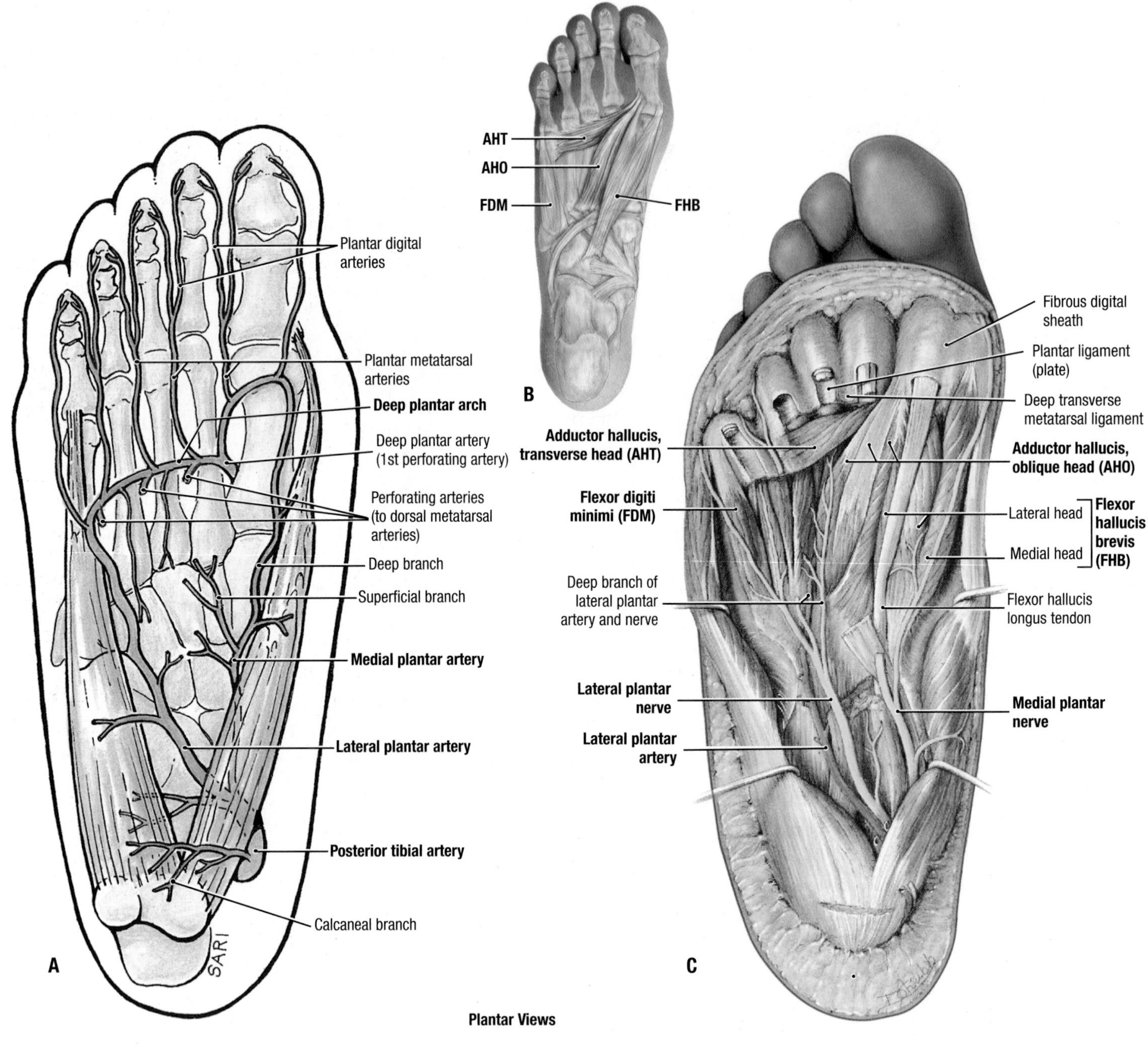
Plantar digital arteries
Plantar metatarsal arteries
Deep plantar arch
Deep plantar artery (1st perforating artery)
Perforating arteries (to dorsal metatarsal arteries)
Deep branch
Superficial branch
Medial plantar artery
Lateral plantar artery
Posterior tibial artery
Calcaneal branch
A
AHT
AHO
FDM
FHB
B
Fibrous digital sheath
Plantar ligament (plate)
Deep transverse metatarsal ligament
Adductor hallucis, transverse head (AHT)
Adductor hallucis, oblique head (AHO)
Flexor digiti minimi (FDM)
Lateral head
Medial head
Flexor hallucis brevis (FHB)
Deep branch of lateral plantar artery and nerve
Flexor hallucis longus tendon
Lateral plantar nerve
Medial plantar nerve
Lateral plantar artery
C
Plantar Views

5.79 THIRD LAYER OF MUSCLES AND ARTERIAL SUPPLY OF SOLE OF FOOT

A. Arterial supply. **B.** Overview. **C.** Dissection. Muscles and neurovascular structures.

TABLE 5.20 MUSCLES IN SOLE OF FOOT—THIRD LAYER

Muscle	Proximal Attachment	Distal Attachment	Innervation	Actions[a]
Flexor hallucis brevis	Plantar surfaces of cuboid and lateral cuneiforms	Both sides of base of proximal phalanx of first digit	Medial plantar nerve (S2–S3)	Flexes proximal phalanx of first digit
Adductor hallucis	*Oblique head:* bases of metatarsals 2–4; *Transverse head:* plantar ligaments of metatarsophalangeal joints	Tendons of both heads attach to lateral side of base of proximal phalanx of first digit	Deep branch of lateral plantar nerve (S2–S3)	Adducts first digit; assists in maintaining transverse arch of foot
Flexor digiti minimi	Base of fifth metatarsal	Base of proximal phalanx of fifth digit	Superficial branch of lateral plantar nerve (S2–S3)	Flexes proximal phalanx of fifth digit, thereby assisting with its flexion

[a]Although individual actions are described, the primary function of the intrinsic muscles of the foot is to act collectively to resist forces that stress (attempt to flatten) the arches of the foot.

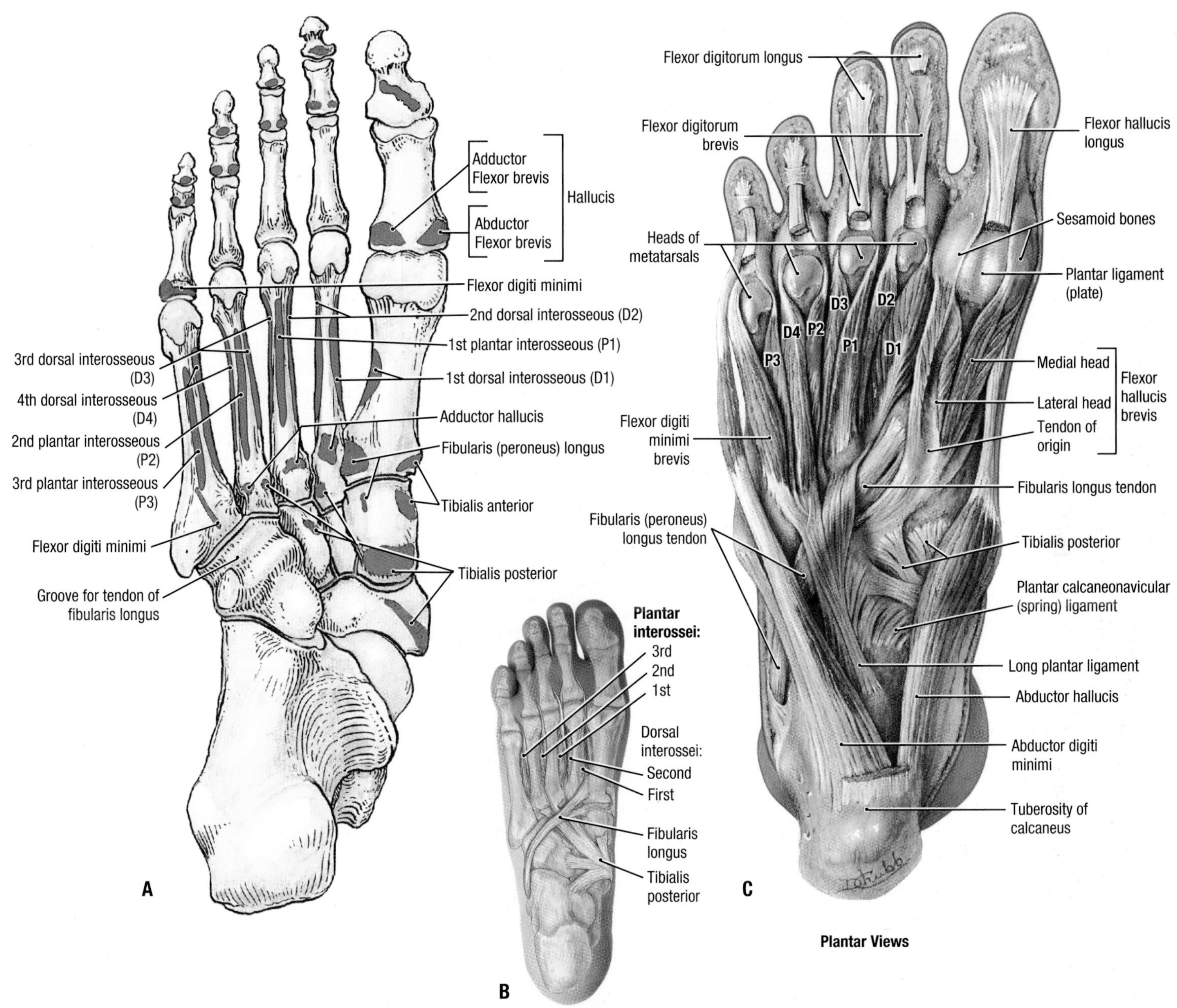
Adductor
Flexor brevis
Abductor
Flexor brevis
Hallucis
Flexor digiti minimi
2nd dorsal interosseous (D2)
1st plantar interosseous (P1)
1st dorsal interosseous (D1)
3rd dorsal interosseous (D3)
4th dorsal interosseous (D4)
2nd plantar interosseous (P2)
3rd plantar interosseous (P3)
Adductor hallucis
Fibularis (peroneus) longus
Tibialis anterior
Flexor digiti minimi
Groove for tendon of fibularis longus
Tibialis posterior
A
Plantar interossei:
3rd
2nd
1st
Dorsal interossei:
Second
First
Fibularis longus
Tibialis posterior
B
Flexor digitorum longus
Flexor digitorum brevis
Flexor hallucis longus
Sesamoid bones
Heads of metatarsals
Plantar ligament (plate)
D3
D2
D4
P2
P1
D1
P3
Medial head
Lateral head
Tendon of origin
Flexor hallucis brevis
Flexor digiti minimi brevis
Fibularis longus tendon
Fibularis (peroneus) longus tendon
Tibialis posterior
Plantar calcaneonavicular (spring) ligament
Long plantar ligament
Abductor hallucis
Abductor digiti minimi
Tuberosity of calcaneus
C
Plantar Views

5.80 FOURTH LAYER OF MUSCLES OF SOLE OF FOOT

A. Bony attachments of muscles of third and fourth layers. **B.** Overview. **C.** Dissection. Muscles and ligaments.

TABLE 5.21 MUSCLES IN SOLE OF FOOT—FOURTH LAYER

Muscle	Proximal Attachment	Distal Attachment	Innervation	Actions[a]
Plantar interossei (three muscles; P1–P3)	Plantar aspect of medial sides of shafts of metatarsals 3–5	Medial sides of bases of proximal phalanges of third to fifth digits	Lateral plantar nerve (S2–S3)	Adduct digits 3–5 and flex metatarsophalangeal joints
Dorsal interossei (four muscles; D1–D4)	Adjacent sides of shafts of metatarsals 1–5	First: medial side of proximal phalanx of second digit Second to fourth: lateral sides of second to fourth digits		Abduct digits 2–4 and flex metatarsophalangeal joints

[a]Although individual actions are described, the primary function of the intrinsic muscles of the foot is to act collectively to resist forces that stress (attempt to flatten) the arches of the foot.

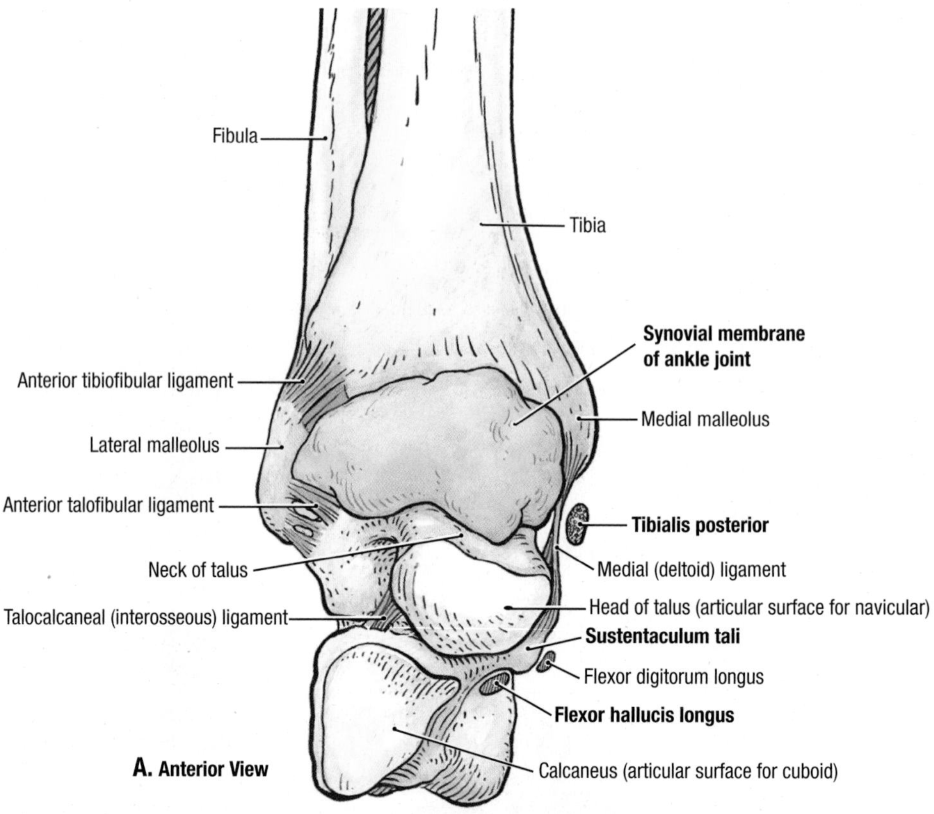
Fibula
Tibia
Synovial membrane of ankle joint
Anterior tibiofibular ligament
Medial malleolus
Lateral malleolus
Anterior talofibular ligament
Tibialis posterior
Neck of talus
Medial (deltoid) ligament
Head of talus (articular surface for navicular)
Talocalcaneal (interosseous) ligament
Sustentaculum tali
Flexor digitorum longus
Flexor hallucis longus
Calcaneus (articular surface for cuboid)

A. **Anterior View**

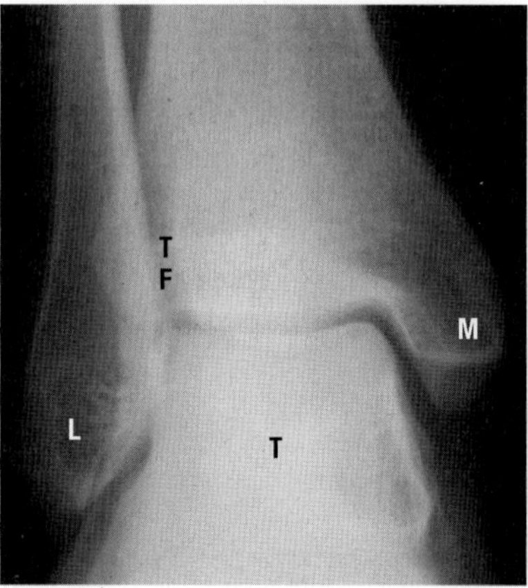
T
F
M
L
T

B. **Anteroposterior View**

5.81 JOINT CAVITY OF ANKLE JOINT

A. Ankle joint with joint cavity distended with injected latex. **B.** Radiograph of joints of ankle region. *L*, lateral malleolus; *M*, medial malleolus; *T*, talus; *TF*, tibiofibular syndesmosis.

- The anterior articular surfaces of the calcaneus and head of the talus are each convex from side to side; thus the foot can be inverted and everted at the transverse tarsal joint.
- Note the relations of the tendons to the sustentaculum tali: the flexor hallucis longus inferior to it, flexor digitorum longus along its medial aspect, and tibialis posterior superior to it and in contact with the medial (deltoid) ligament.

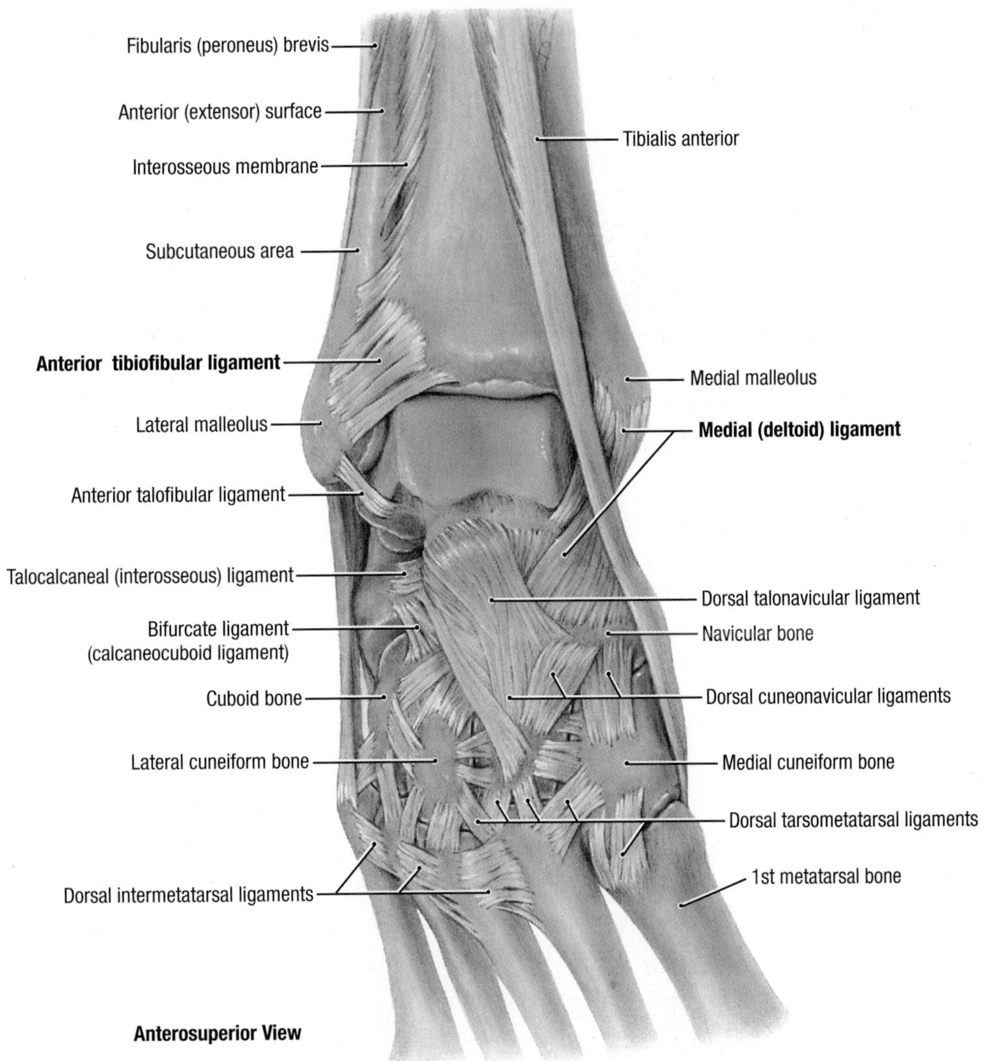
Fibularis (peroneus) brevis
Anterior (extensor) surface
Interosseous membrane
Subcutaneous area
Anterior tibiofibular ligament
Lateral malleolus
Anterior talofibular ligament
Talocalcaneal (interosseous) ligament
Bifurcate ligament
(calcaneocuboid ligament)
Cuboid bone
Lateral cuneiform bone
Dorsal intermetatarsal ligaments
Tibialis anterior
Medial malleolus
Medial (deltoid) ligament
Dorsal talonavicular ligament
Navicular bone
Dorsal cuneonavicular ligaments
Medial cuneiform bone
Dorsal tarsometatarsal ligaments
1st metatarsal bone
Anterosuperior View

5.82 ANKLE JOINT AND LIGAMENTS OF DORSUM OF FOOT

Dissection. The ankle joint is plantar flexed, and its anterior capsular fibers are removed.

- All muscles attached to the fibula except the biceps femoris pull inferiorly on the bone during contraction. The oblique fibers of the interosseous membrane and ligaments uniting the fibula to the tibia resist this inferior pull but allow the fibula to be forced superiorly during full dorsiflexion of the ankle.
- The bifurcate ligament, a Y-shaped ligament consisting of calcaneocuboid and calcaneonavicular ligaments, and the talonavicular ligament are the primary dorsal ligaments of the transverse tarsal joint.

A **Pott fracture-dislocation of the ankle** occurs when the foot is forcibly everted. This action pulls on the extremely strong medial (deltoid) ligament, often avulsing the medial malleolus and compressing the lateral malleolus against the talus, shearing off the malleolus or, more often, fracturing the fibula superior to the tibiofibular syndesmosis.

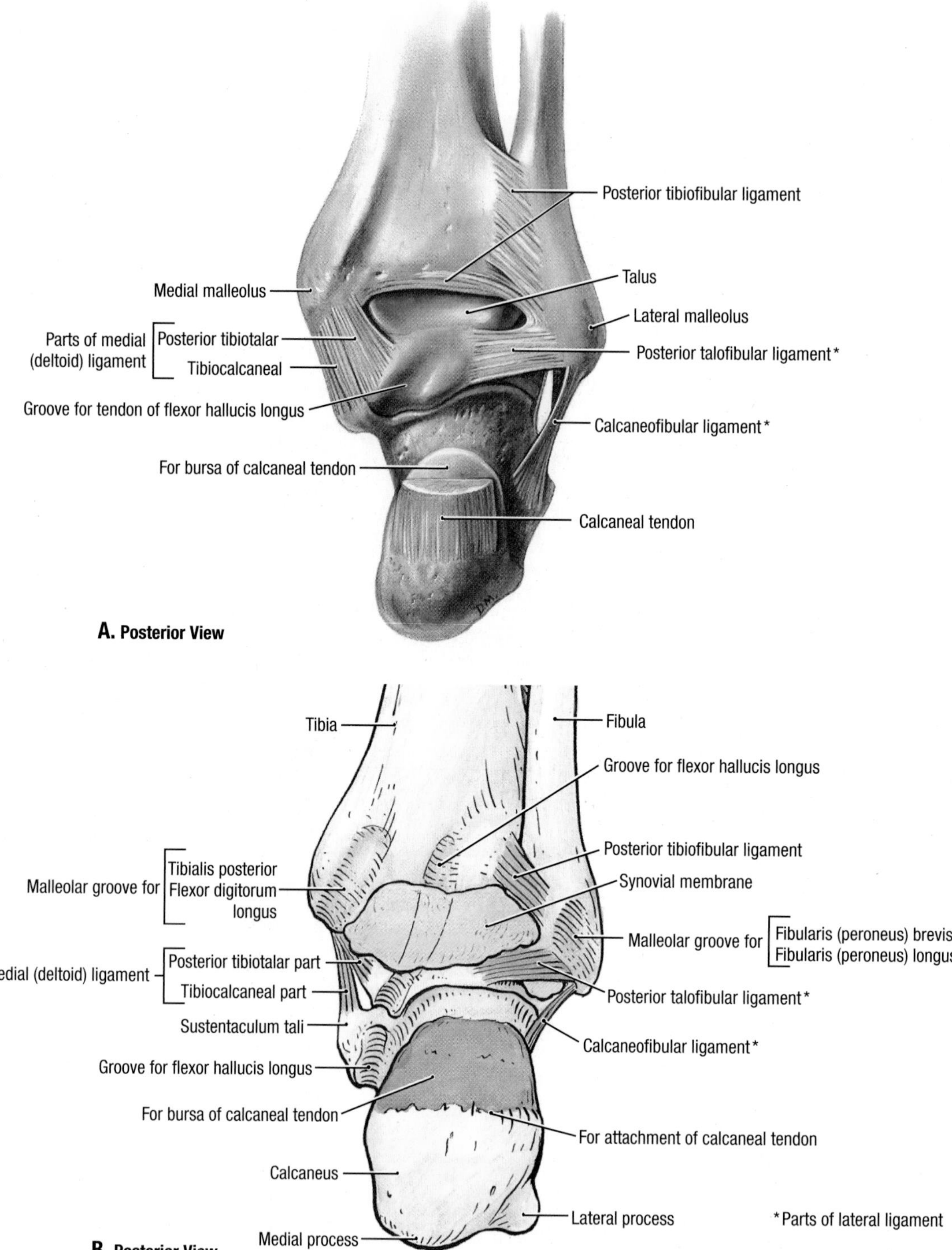
Posterior tibiofibular ligament
Talus
Medial malleolus
Lateral malleolus
Parts of medial (deltoid) ligament
Posterior tibiotalar
Tibiocalcaneal
Posterior talofibular ligament*
Groove for tendon of flexor hallucis longus
Calcaneofibular ligament*
For bursa of calcaneal tendon
Calcaneal tendon
A. Posterior View
Tibia
Fibula
Groove for flexor hallucis longus
Posterior tibiofibular ligament
Synovial membrane
Malleolar groove for
Tibialis posterior
Flexor digitorum longus
Malleolar groove for
Fibularis (peroneus) brevis
Fibularis (peroneus) longus
Medial (deltoid) ligament
Posterior tibiotalar part
Tibiocalcaneal part
Posterior talofibular ligament*
Sustentaculum tali
Calcaneofibular ligament*
Groove for flexor hallucis longus
For bursa of calcaneal tendon
For attachment of calcaneal tendon
Calcaneus
Lateral process
*Parts of lateral ligament
Medial process
B. Posterior View

5.83 POSTERIOR ASPECT OF ANKLE JOINT

A. Dissection. **B.** Ankle joint with joint cavity distended with latex. Observe the grooves for the flexor hallucis longus muscle, which crosses the middle of the ankle joint posteriorly, the two tendons posterior to the medial malleolus, and the two tendons posterior to the lateral malleolus.

- The posterior aspect of the ankle joint is strengthened by the transversely oriented posterior tibiofibular and posterior talofibular ligaments.
- The calcaneofibular ligament stabilizes the joint laterally, and the posterior tibiotalar and tibiocalcanean parts of the medial (deltoid) ligament stabilize it medially.
- The groove for the flexor hallucis tendon is between the medial and lateral tubercles of the talus and continues inferior to the sustentaculum tali.

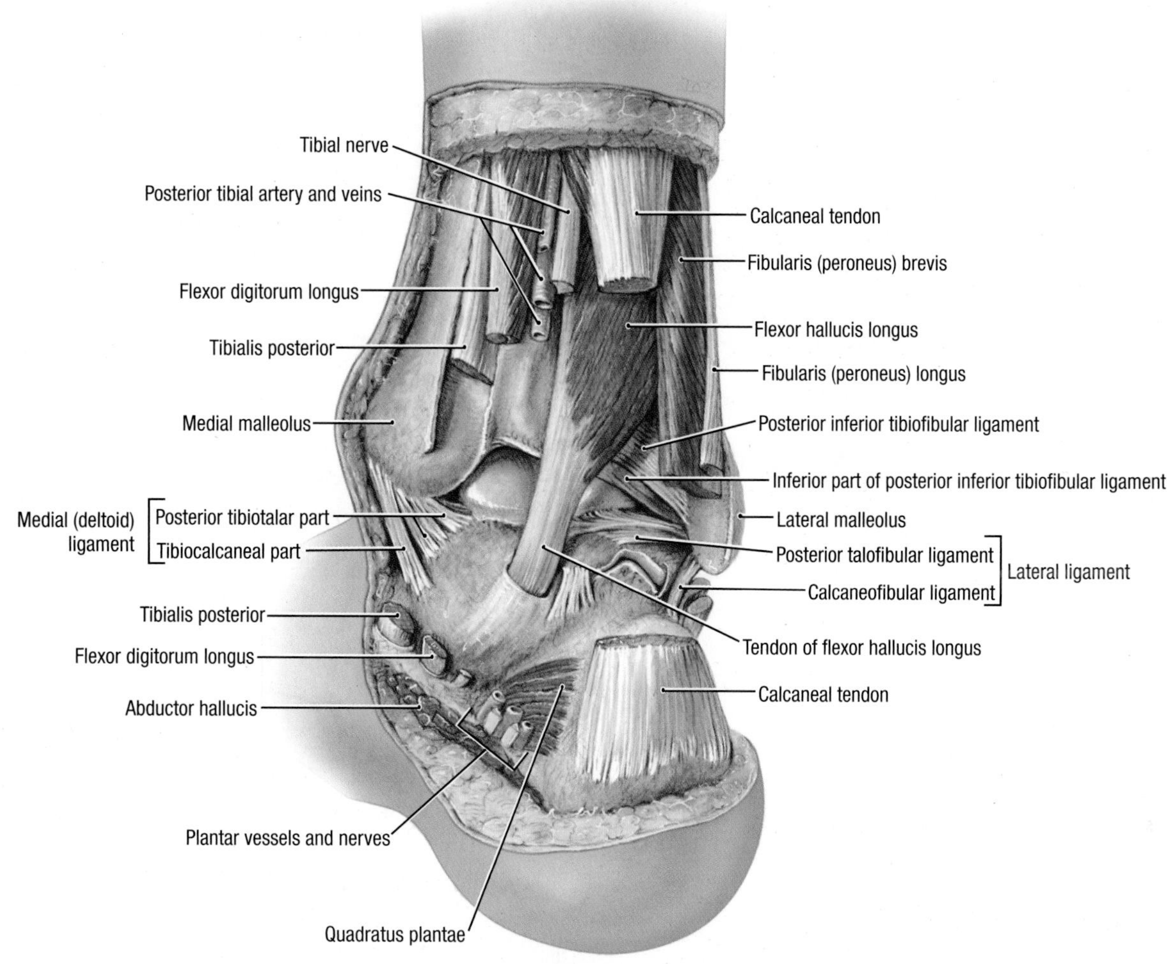
Tibial nerve
Posterior tibial artery and veins
Flexor digitorum longus
Tibialis posterior
Medial malleolus
Medial (deltoid) ligament
Posterior tibiotalar part
Tibiocalcaneal part
Tibialis posterior
Flexor digitorum longus
Abductor hallucis
Plantar vessels and nerves
Quadratus plantae
Calcaneal tendon
Fibularis (peroneus) brevis
Flexor hallucis longus
Fibularis (peroneus) longus
Posterior inferior tibiofibular ligament
Inferior part of posterior inferior tibiofibular ligament
Lateral malleolus
Posterior talofibular ligament
Calcaneofibular ligament
Lateral ligament
Tendon of flexor hallucis longus
Calcaneal tendon

Posteromedial View

5.84 POSTEROMEDIAL ANKLE

- The flexor hallucis longus muscle is midway between the medial and lateral malleoli; the tendons of the flexor digitorum and tibialis posterior are medial to it, and the tendons of the fibularis longus and brevis are lateral to it.
- The strongest parts of the ligaments of the ankle are those that prevent anterior displacement of the leg bones, namely, the posterior part of the medial ligament (posterior tibiotalar), the posterior talofibular, and calcaneofibular and tibiocalcaneal parts.

Tarsal tunnel syndrome, the entrapment and compression of the tibial nerve, occurs when there is edema and tightness in the ankle involving the synovial sheaths of the tendons of muscles in the posterior compartment of the leg. The area involved is from the medial malleolus to the calcaneus. The heel pain results from compression of the tibial nerve by the flexor retinaculum.

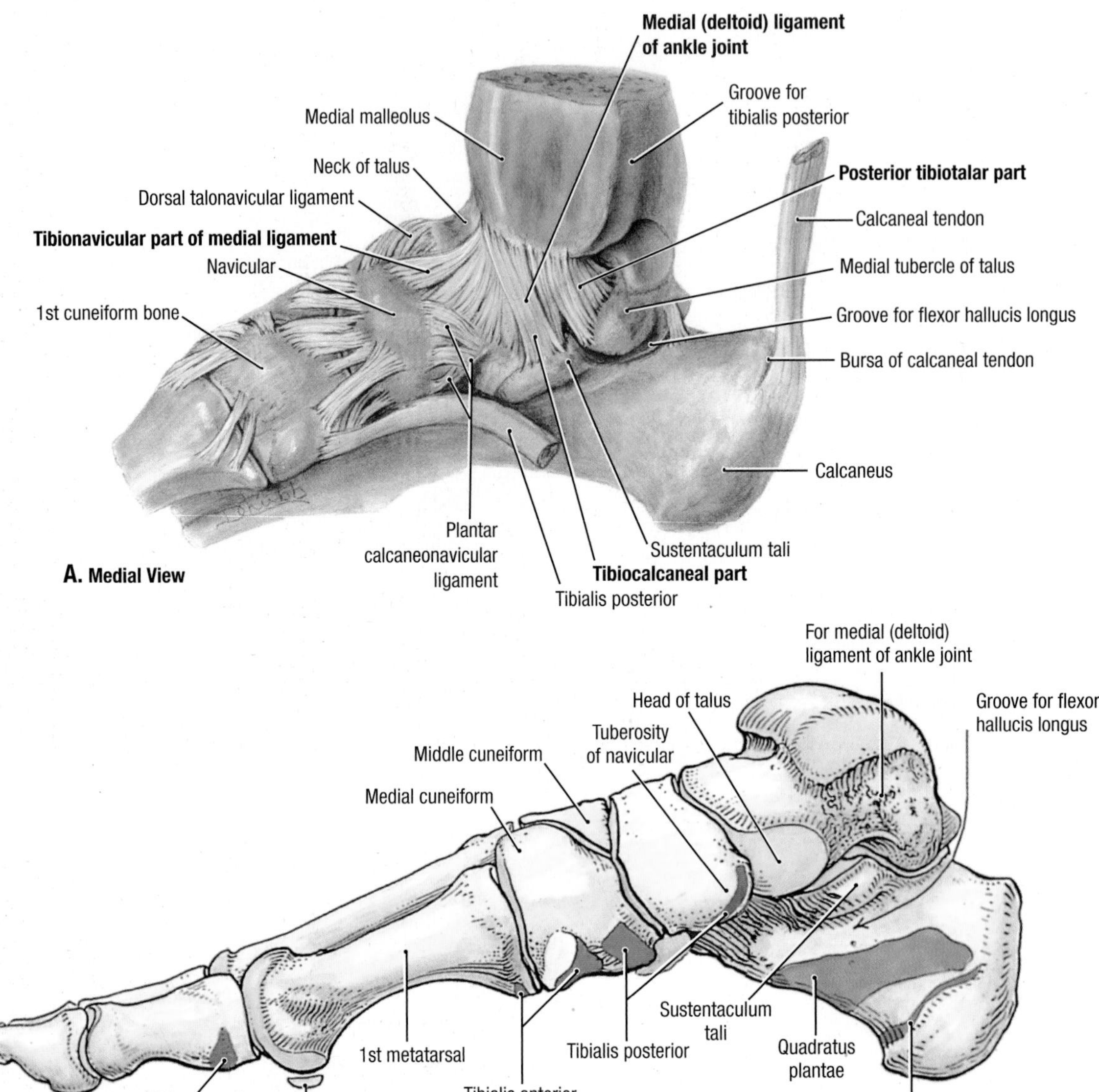

Medial (deltoid) ligament of ankle joint
Groove for tibialis posterior
Medial malleolus
Neck of talus
Dorsal talonavicular ligament
Posterior tibiotalar part
Calcaneal tendon
Tibionavicular part of medial ligament
Navicular
Medial tubercle of talus
1st cuneiform bone
Groove for flexor hallucis longus
Bursa of calcaneal tendon
Calcaneus
Plantar calcaneonavicular ligament
Sustentaculum tali
Tibiocalcaneal part
Tibialis posterior
A. Medial View
For medial (deltoid) ligament of ankle joint
Head of talus
Groove for flexor hallucis longus
Tuberosity of navicular
Middle cuneiform
Medial cuneiform
Sustentaculum tali
1st metatarsal
Tibialis posterior
Quadratus plantae
Tibialis anterior
B.
Abductor hallucis
Flexor hallucis brevis
Medial sesamoid
Abductor hallucis

5.85 MEDIAL LIGAMENTS OF ANKLE REGION

A. Dissection. **B.** Bones. The joint capsule of the ankle joint is reinforced medially by the large, strong medial (deltoid) ligament that attaches proximally to the medial malleolus and fans out from it to attach distally to the talus, calcaneus, and navicular via four adjacent and continuous parts: the tibionavicular part, the tibiocalcaneal part, and the anterior and posterior tibiotalar parts. The medial ligament stabilizes the ankle joint during eversion of the foot and prevents subluxation (partial dislocation) of the ankle joint.

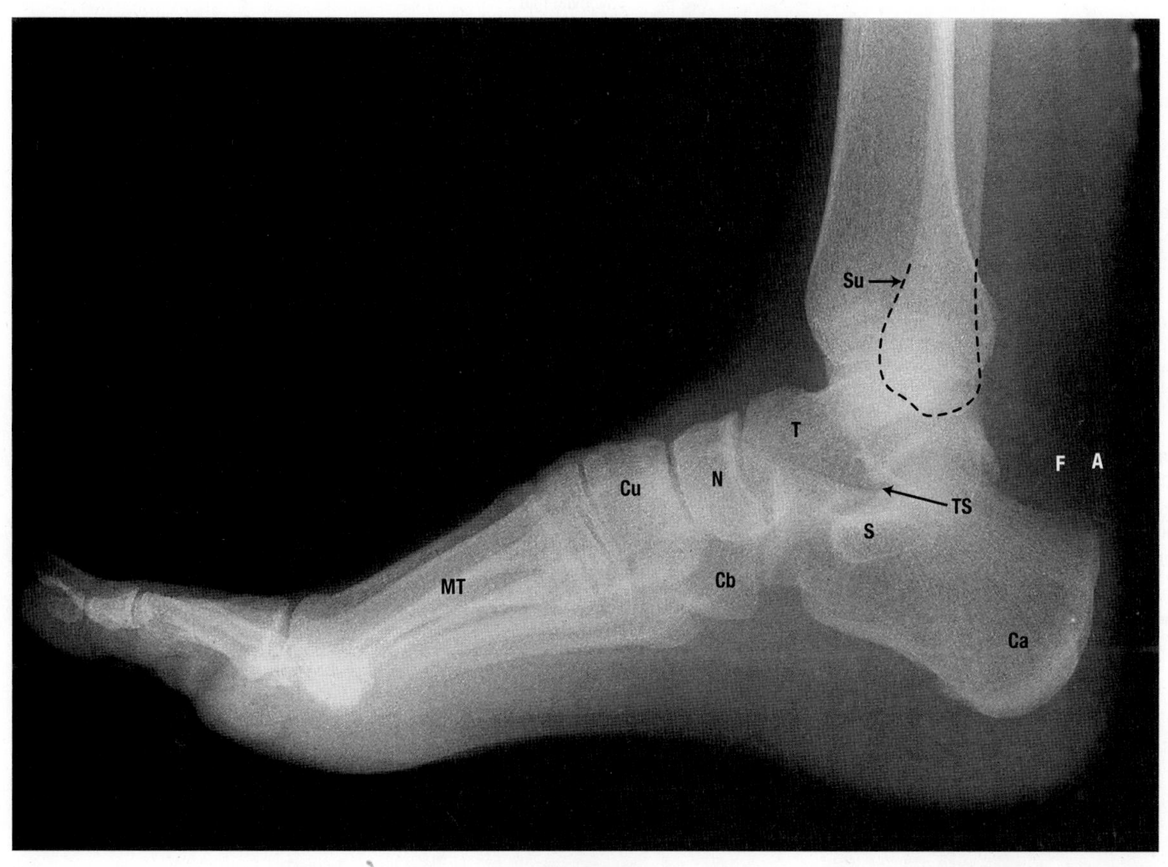
Su
T
F
A
Cu
N
TS
S
MT
Cb
Ca

A

Medial Views

A	Calcaneal (Achilles) tendon
Ca	Calcaneus
Cb	Cuboid
Cu	Cuneiforms
F	Fat
L	Lateral malleolus
MT	Metatarsal
N	Navicular
S	Sustentaculum tali
Su	Superimposed tibia and fibula
T	Talus
TS	Tarsal sinus

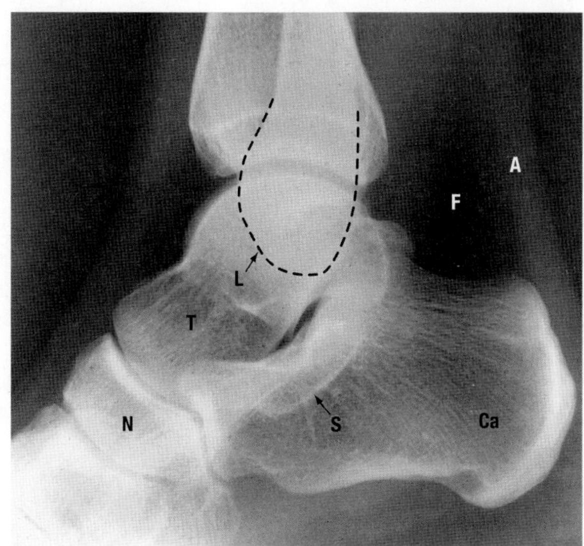
A
F
L
T
N
S
Ca

B

5.86 RADIOGRAPHS OF ANKLE AND FOOT

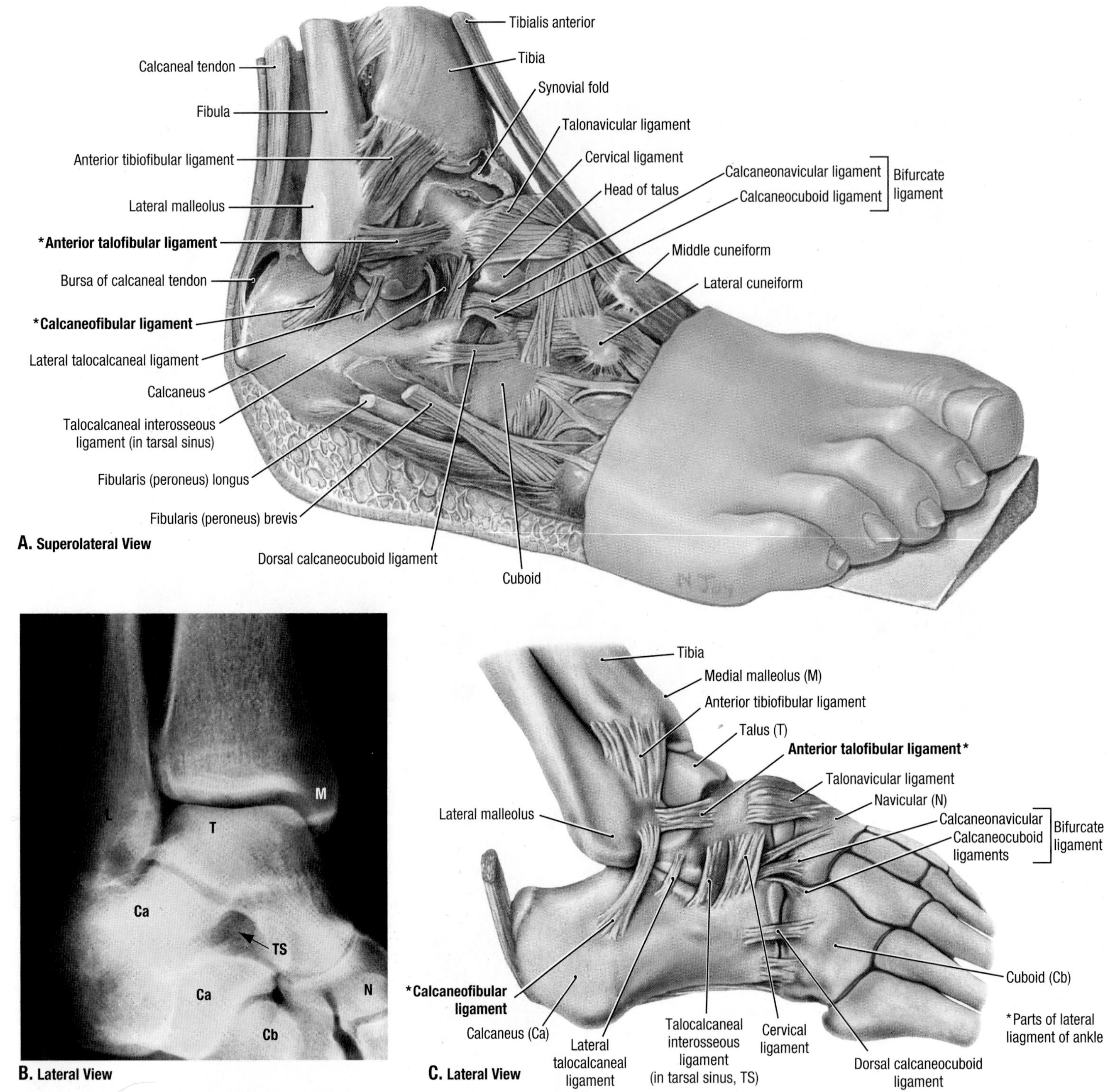

Tibialis anterior
Tibia
Calcaneal tendon
Synovial fold
Fibula
Talonavicular ligament
Anterior tibiofibular ligament
Cervical ligament
Calcaneonavicular ligament
Calcaneocuboid ligament
Bifurcate ligament
Head of talus
Lateral malleolus
*Anterior talofibular ligament
Middle cuneiform
Bursa of calcaneal tendon
Lateral cuneiform
*Calcaneofibular ligament
Lateral talocalcaneal ligament
Calcaneus
Talocalcaneal interosseous ligament (in tarsal sinus)
Fibularis (peroneus) longus
Fibularis (peroneus) brevis
A. Superolateral View
Dorsal calcaneocuboid ligament
Cuboid
M
L
T
Ca
TS
Ca
N
Cb
B. Lateral View
Tibia
Medial malleolus (M)
Anterior tibiofibular ligament
Talus (T)
Anterior talofibular ligament*
Talonavicular ligament
Navicular (N)
Lateral malleolus
Calcaneonavicular
Calcaneocuboid ligaments
Bifurcate ligament
Cuboid (Cb)
*Calcaneofibular ligament
*Parts of lateral liagment of ankle
Calcaneus (Ca)
Lateral talocalcaneal ligament
Talocalcaneal interosseous ligament (in tarsal sinus, TS)
Cervical ligament
Dorsal calcaneocuboid ligament
C. Lateral View

5.87 LATERAL LIGAMENTS OF ANKLE REGION

A. Dissection with foot inverted by underlying wedge. **B.** Lateral radiograph. **C.** Dissection. (Abbreviations refer to structures identified in **B.**)

The ankle joint is reinforced laterally by the lateral ligament of the ankle, which consists of three separate ligaments: (1) anterior talofibular ligament, a flat, weak band; (2) calcaneofibular ligament, a round cord directed posteroinferiorly; and (3) posterior talofibular ligament, a strong, medially directed horizontal ligament (see Fig. 5.83).

Ankle sprains (partial or fully torn ligaments) are common injuries. Ankle sprains nearly always result from forceful inversion of the weight-bearing plantar flexed foot. The anterior talofibular ligament is most commonly injured, resulting in instability of the ankle. The calcaneofibular is also often torn.

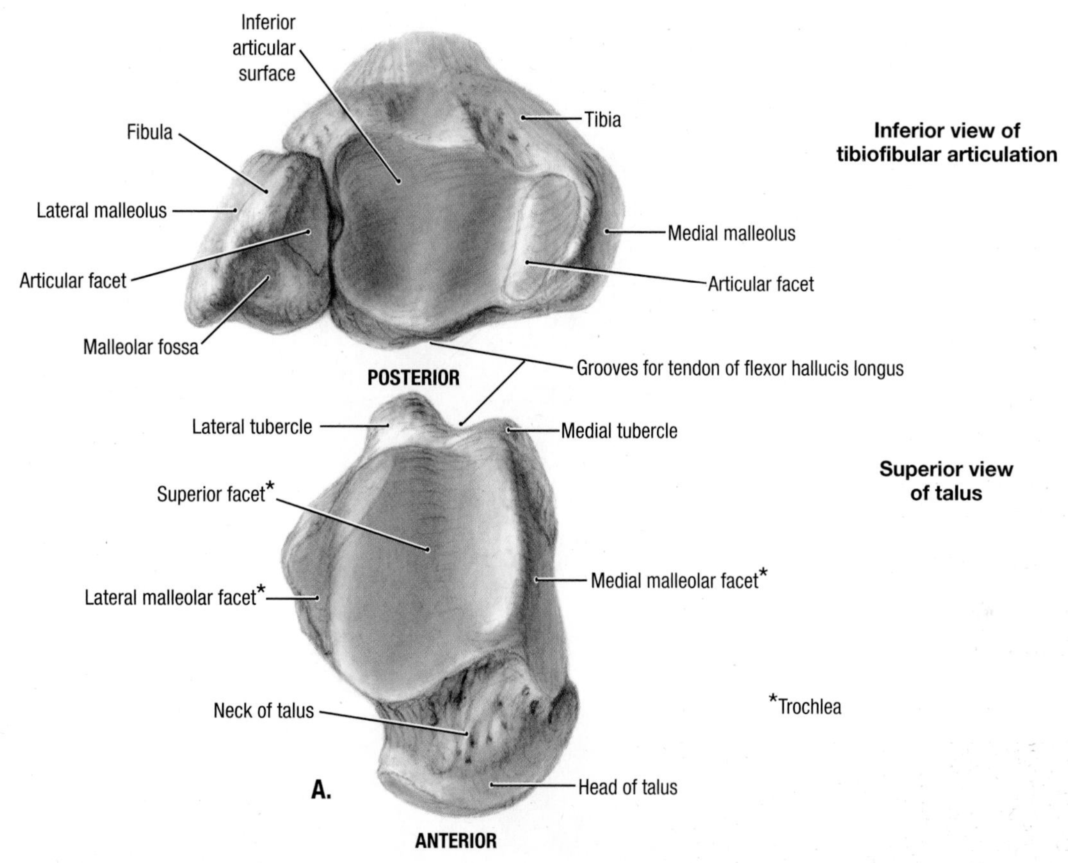
Inferior articular surface
Tibia
Fibula
Inferior view of tibiofibular articulation
Lateral malleolus
Medial malleolus
Articular facet
Articular facet
Malleolar fossa
Grooves for tendon of flexor hallucis longus
POSTERIOR
Lateral tubercle
Medial tubercle
Superior view of talus
Superior facet*
Medial malleolar facet*
Lateral malleolar facet*
Neck of talus
*Trochlea
A.
Head of talus
ANTERIOR

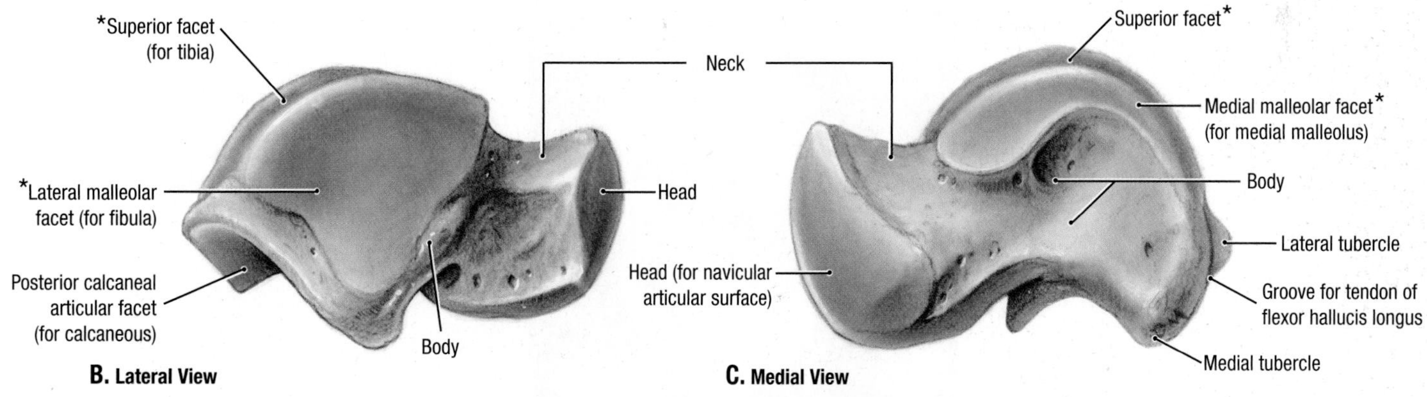
*Superior facet (for tibia)
Neck
Superior facet*
Medial malleolar facet* (for medial malleolus)
*Lateral malleolar facet (for fibula)
Head
Body
Lateral tubercle
Posterior calcaneal articular facet (for calcaneous)
Head (for navicular articular surface)
Groove for tendon of flexor hallucis longus
Body
Medial tubercle
B. Lateral View
C. Medial View

5.88 ARTICULAR SURFACES OF ANKLE JOINT

A. Superior aspect of talus separated from distal ends of tibia and fibula. The superior articular surface of the talus is broader anteriorly than posteriorly; hence the medial and lateral malleoli, which grasp the sides of the talus, tend to be forced apart in dorsiflexion. The fully dorsiflexed position is stable compared with the fully plantar flexed position. In plantar flexion, when the tibia and fibula articulate with the narrower posterior part of the superior articular surface of the talus, some side-to-side movement of the joint is allowed, accounting for the instability of the joint in this position. **B.** Lateral aspect of talus. The lateral, triangular articular area is for articulation with the lateral malleolus. **C.** Medial aspect of talus. The comma-shaped articular area is for articulation with the medial malleolus.

Fractures of the talar neck may occur during severe forceful dorsiflexion of the ankle, for example, from a motor vehicle accident. In some cases the body of the talus dislocates posteriorly.

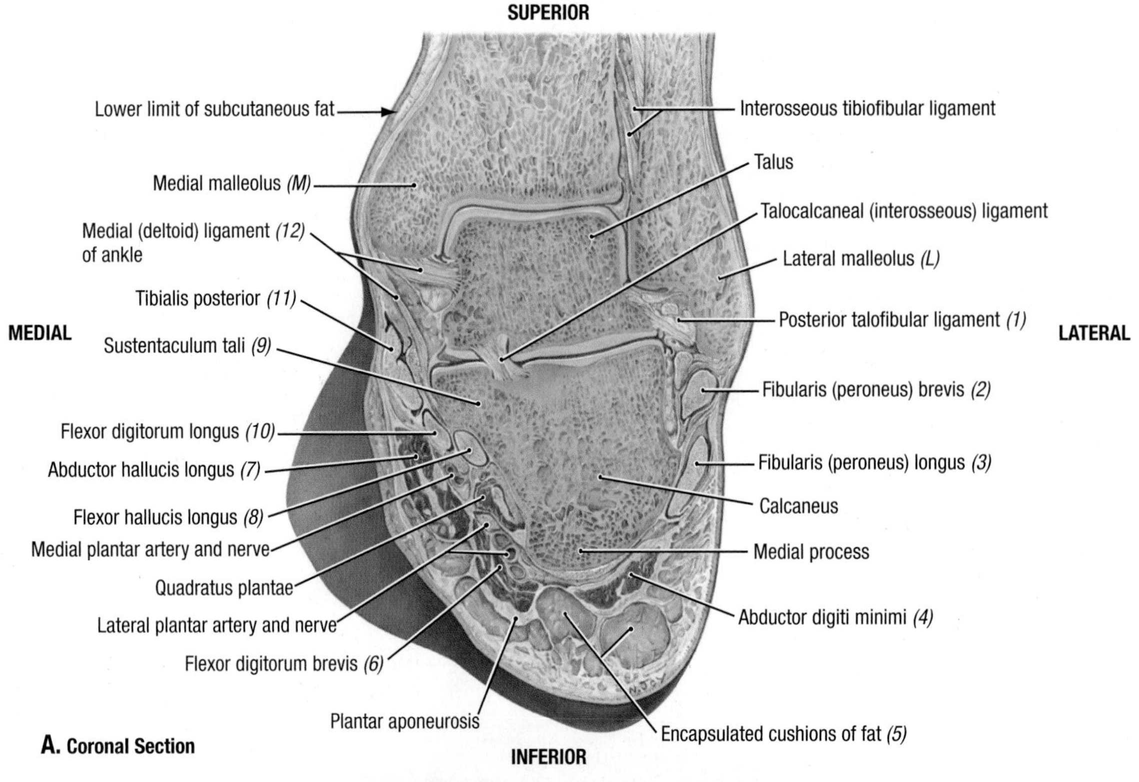
SUPERIOR
INFERIOR
MEDIAL
LATERAL
Lower limit of subcutaneous fat
Medial malleolus (M)
Medial (deltoid) ligament (12) of ankle
Tibialis posterior (11)
Sustentaculum tali (9)
Flexor digitorum longus (10)
Abductor hallucis longus (7)
Flexor hallucis longus (8)
Medial plantar artery and nerve
Quadratus plantae
Lateral plantar artery and nerve
Flexor digitorum brevis (6)
Plantar aponeurosis
Interosseous tibiofibular ligament
Talus
Talocalcaneal (interosseous) ligament
Lateral malleolus (L)
Posterior talofibular ligament (1)
Fibularis (peroneus) brevis (2)
Fibularis (peroneus) longus (3)
Calcaneus
Medial process
Abductor digiti minimi (4)
Encapsulated cushions of fat (5)

A. **Coronal Section**

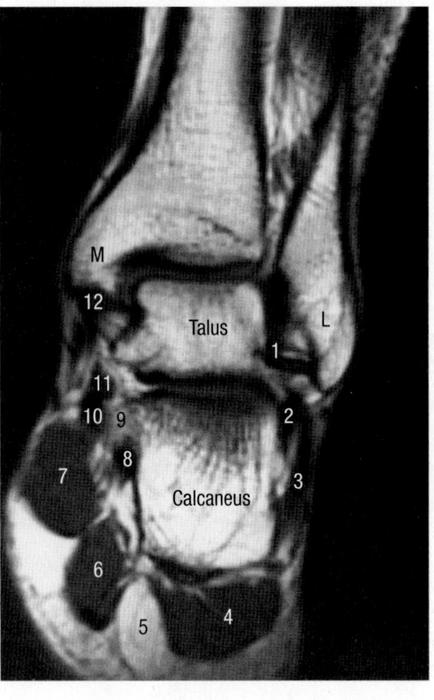
M
12
Talus
L
1
11
10
9
2
8
7
3
Calcaneus
6
4
5

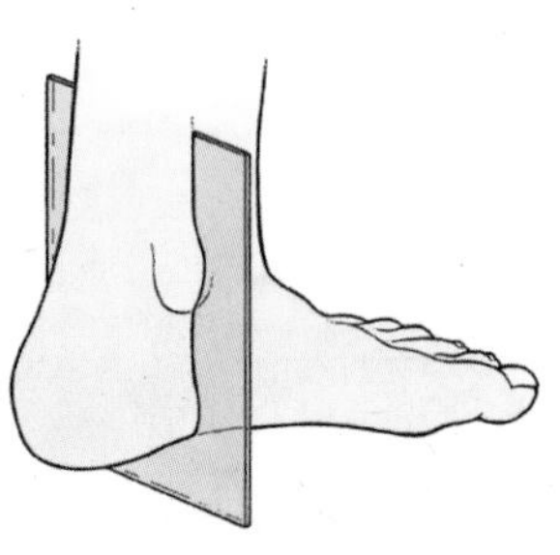

B. **Coronal MRI**

5.89 CORONAL SECTION AND MRI THROUGH ANKLE

A. Coronal section. **B.** Coronal MRI (*numbers* in **B** refer to structures labeled in **A**).

- The tibia rests on the talus, and the talus rests on the calcaneus; between the calcaneus and the skin are several encapsulated cushions of fat.
- The lateral malleolus descends farther inferiorly than the medial malleolus.
- The talocalcaneal (interosseous) ligament between the talus and calcaneus separates the subtalar, or posterior talocalcaneal joint from the talocalcaneonavicular joint.

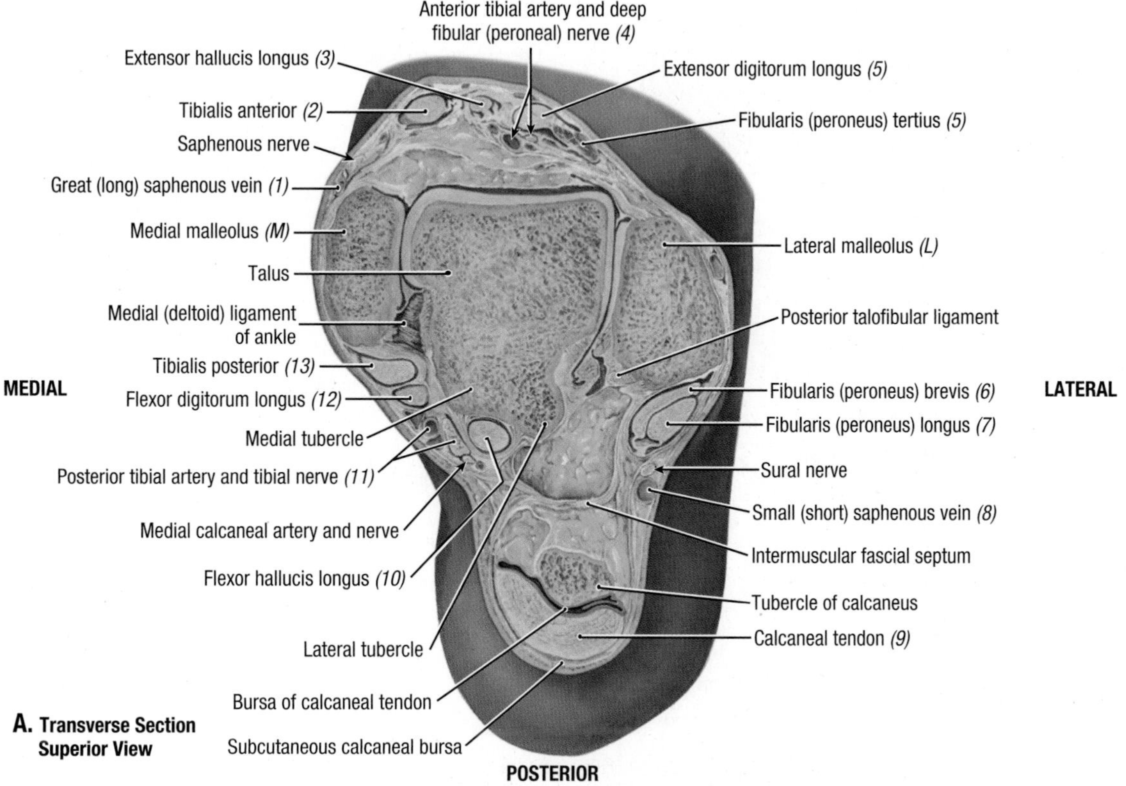
ANTERIOR
Anterior tibial artery and deep fibular (peroneal) nerve (4)
Extensor hallucis longus (3)
Extensor digitorum longus (5)
Tibialis anterior (2)
Fibularis (peroneus) tertius (5)
Saphenous nerve
Great (long) saphenous vein (1)
Medial malleolus (M)
Lateral malleolus (L)
Talus
Medial (deltoid) ligament of ankle
Posterior talofibular ligament
Tibialis posterior (13)
MEDIAL
Flexor digitorum longus (12)
Fibularis (peroneus) brevis (6)
LATERAL
Medial tubercle
Fibularis (peroneus) longus (7)
Posterior tibial artery and tibial nerve (11)
Sural nerve
Small (short) saphenous vein (8)
Medial calcaneal artery and nerve
Intermuscular fascial septum
Flexor hallucis longus (10)
Tubercle of calcaneus
Calcaneal tendon (9)
Lateral tubercle
Bursa of calcaneal tendon
Subcutaneous calcaneal bursa
POSTERIOR

A. Transverse Section Superior View

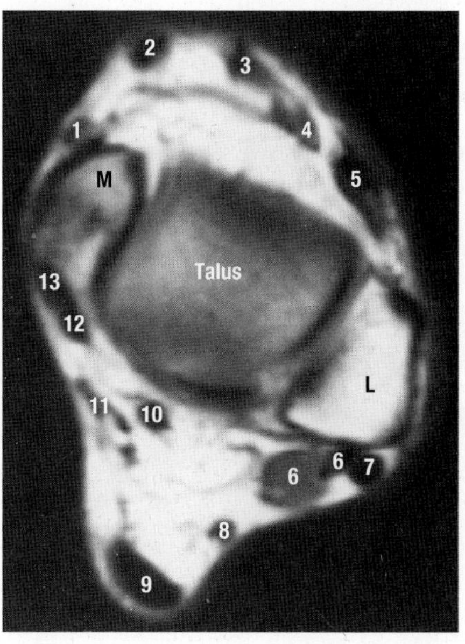
2
3
1
4
M
5
Talus
13
12
L
11
10
6
6
7
8
9

B. Transverse MRI

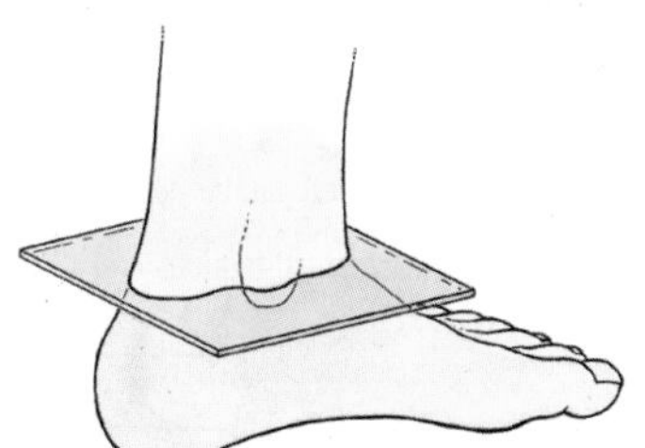

5.90 TRANSVERSE SECTION AND MRI THROUGH ANKLE

A. Transverse section. **B.** Transverse MRI (*numbers* in **B** refer to structures labeled in **A**).

- The body of the talus is wedge shaped and positioned between the malleoli, which are bound to it by the medial (deltoid) and posterior talofibular ligaments.
- The flexor hallucis longus muscle lies within its osseofibrous sheath between the medial and lateral tubercles of the talus.
- There is a small, inconstant subcutaneous bursa superficial to the calcaneal tendon and a large, constant bursa of calcaneal tendon deep to it.

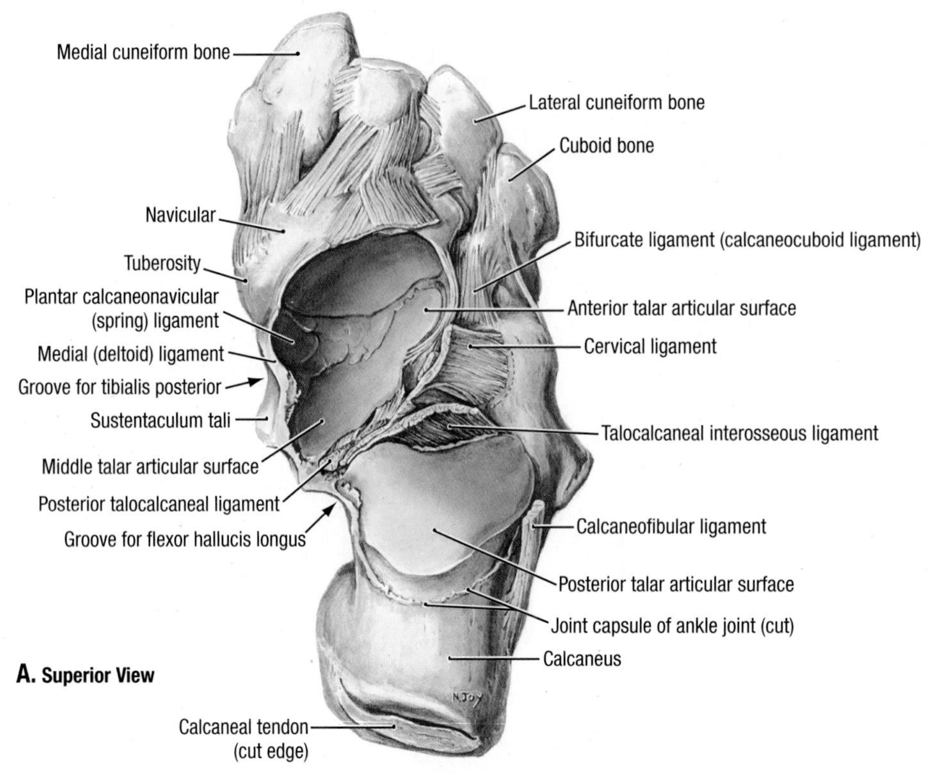
Medial cuneiform bone
Lateral cuneiform bone
Cuboid bone
Navicular
Tuberosity
Bifurcate ligament (calcaneocuboid ligament)
Plantar calcaneonavicular (spring) ligament
Anterior talar articular surface
Medial (deltoid) ligament
Cervical ligament
Groove for tibialis posterior
Sustentaculum tali
Talocalcaneal interosseous ligament
Middle talar articular surface
Posterior talocalcaneal ligament
Calcaneofibular ligament
Groove for flexor hallucis longus
Posterior talar articular surface
Joint capsule of ankle joint (cut)
Calcaneus
Calcaneal tendon (cut edge)

A. **Superior View**

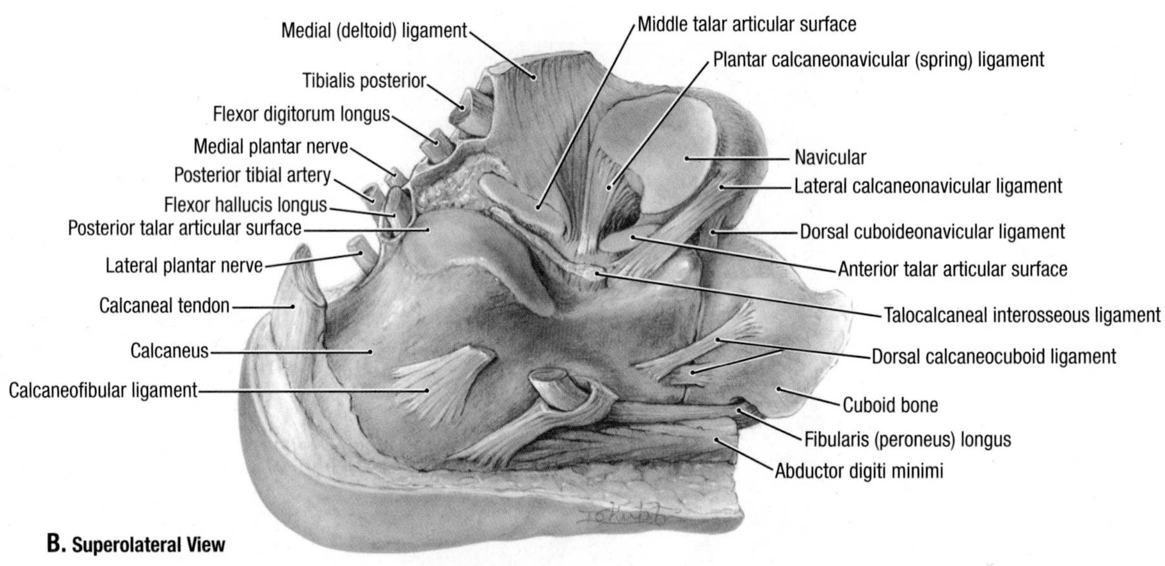
Medial (deltoid) ligament
Middle talar articular surface
Plantar calcaneonavicular (spring) ligament
Tibialis posterior
Flexor digitorum longus
Medial plantar nerve
Navicular
Posterior tibial artery
Lateral calcaneonavicular ligament
Flexor hallucis longus
Posterior talar articular surface
Dorsal cuboideonavicular ligament
Lateral plantar nerve
Anterior talar articular surface
Calcaneal tendon
Talocalcaneal interosseous ligament
Calcaneus
Dorsal calcaneocuboid ligament
Calcaneofibular ligament
Cuboid bone
Fibularis (peroneus) longus
Abductor digiti minimi

B. **Superolateral View**

5.91 JOINTS OF INVERSION AND EVERSION

The joints of inversion and eversion are the subtalar (posterior talocalcaneal) joint, talocalcaneonavicular joint, and transverse tarsal (combined calcaneocuboid and talonavicular) joint. **A.** Posterior and middle parts of foot with talus removed. **B.** Posterior part of foot with talus removed. The convex posterior talar facet is separated from the concave middle, and anterior facets by the talocalcaneal (interosseous) ligament within the tarsal sinus.

Calcaneal fractures. A hard fall onto the heel, for example, from a ladder, may fracture the calcaneous into several pieces, resulting in a comminuted fracture. A calcaneal fracture is usually disabling because it disrupts the subtalar (talocalcaneal) joint.

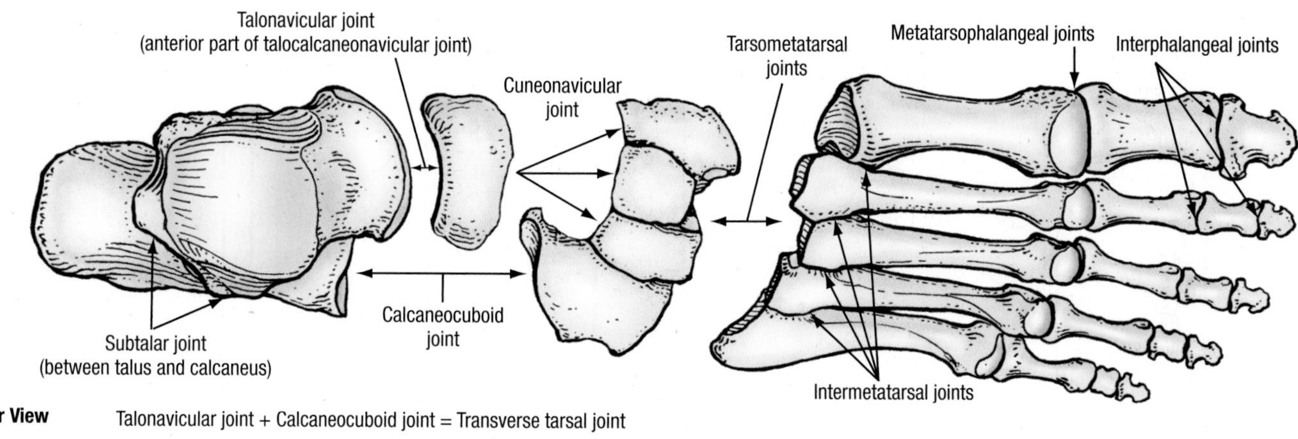
Talonavicular joint
(anterior part of talocalcaneonavicular joint)
Cuneonavicular joint
Tarsometatarsal joints
Metatarsophalangeal joints
Interphalangeal joints
Calcaneocuboid joint
Subtalar joint
(between talus and calcaneus)
Intermetatarsal joints
Superior View
Talonavicular joint + Calcaneocuboid joint = Transverse tarsal joint

5.92 JOINTS OF FOOT

TABLE 5.22 JOINTS OF FOOT

Joint	Type	Articular Surface	Joint Capsule	Ligaments	Movements
Subtalart	Synovial (plane) joint	Inferior surface of body of talus articulates with superior surface of calcaneus	Attached to margins of articular surfaces	Medial, lateral, and posterior talocalcaneal ligaments support capsule; talocalcaneal (interosseous) ligament binds bones together	Inversion and eversion of foot
Talocalcaneo-navicular	Synovial joint; talonavicular part is a pivot joint	Head of talus articulates with calcaneus and navicular bones	Incompletely encloses joint	Plantar calcaneonavicular ("spring") ligament supports head of talus	Gliding and rotary movements
Calcaneocuboid	Synovial (plane) joint	Anterior end of calcaneus articulates with posterior surface of cuboid	Encloses joint	Dorsal calcaneocuboid ligament, plantar calcaneocuboid ligament, and long plantar ligament support joint capsule	Inversion and eversion of foot
Cuneonavicular	Synovial (plane) joint	Anterior navicular articulates with posterior surface of cuneiforms	Common joint capsule	Dorsal and plantar ligaments	Limited gliding movement
Tarsometatarsal	Synovial (plane) joint	Anterior tarsal bones articulate with bases of metatarsal bones	Encloses joint	Dorsal, plantar, and interosseous ligaments	Gliding or sliding
Intermetatarsal	Synovial (plane) joint	Bases of metatarsal bones articulate with each other	Encloses each joint	Dorsal, plantar, and interosseous ligaments bind bones together	Little individual movement
Metatarsophalangeal	Synovial (condyloid) joint	Heads of metatarsal bones articulate with bases of proximal phalanges	Encloses each joint	Collateral ligaments support capsule on each side; plantar ligament supports plantar part of capsule	Flexion, extension, and some abduction, adduction and circumduction
Interphalangeal	Synovial (hinge) joint	Head of proximal or middle phalanx articulates with base of phalanx distal to it	Encloses each joint	Collateral and plantar ligaments support joints	Flexion and extension

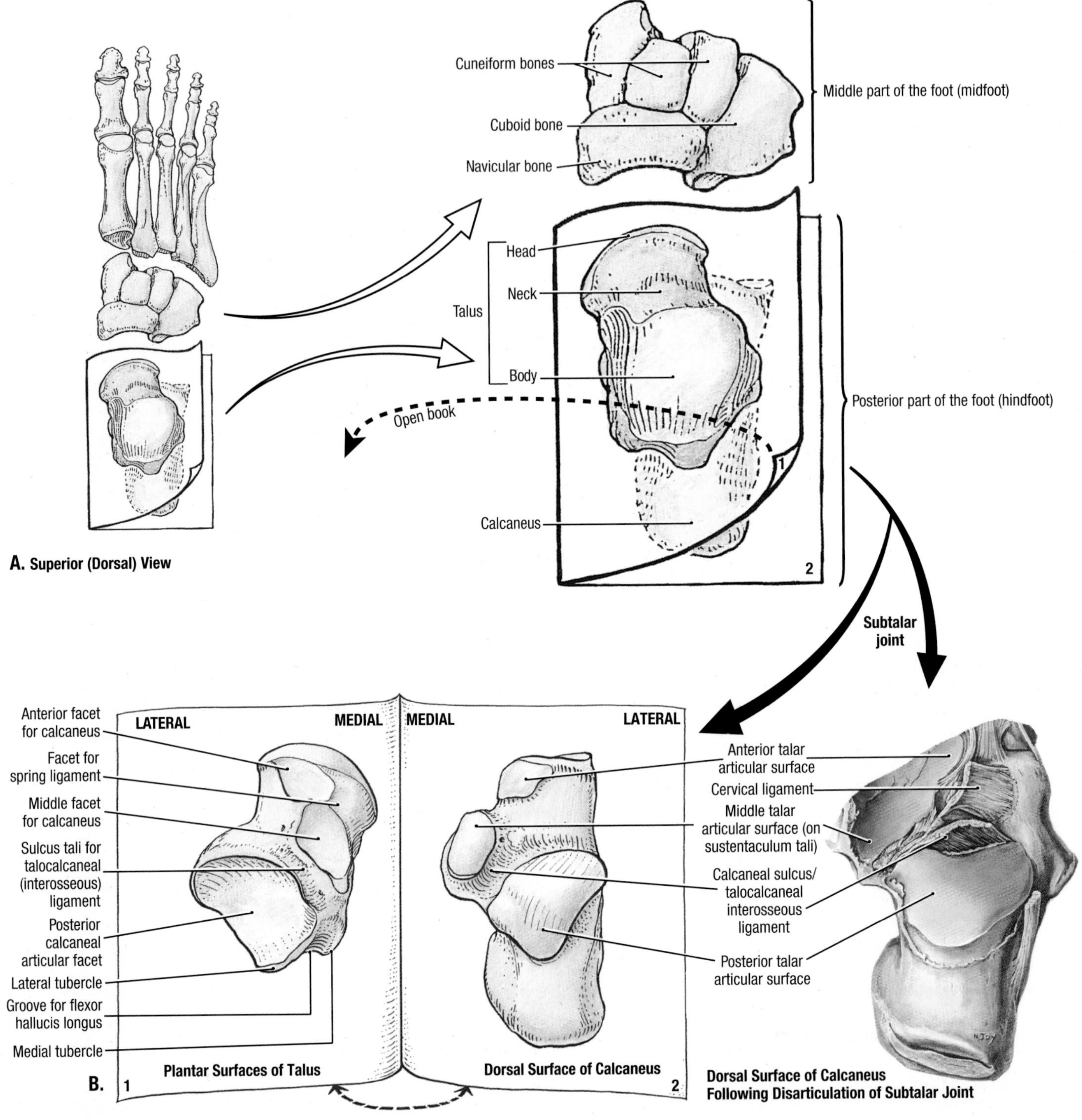

Cuneiform bones
Cuboid bone
Navicular bone
Middle part of the foot (midfoot)
Talus
Head
Neck
Body
Open book
Posterior part of the foot (hindfoot)
Calcaneus
1
2
A. Superior (Dorsal) View
Subtalar joint
Anterior facet for calcaneus
Facet for spring ligament
Middle facet for calcaneus
Sulcus tali for talocalcaneal (interosseous) ligament
Posterior calcaneal articular facet
Lateral tubercle
Groove for flexor hallucis longus
Medial tubercle
LATERAL
MEDIAL
MEDIAL
LATERAL
Anterior talar articular surface
Cervical ligament
Middle talar articular surface (on sustentaculum tali)
Calcaneal sulcus/ talocalcaneal interosseous ligament
Posterior talar articular surface
B.
1
Plantar Surfaces of Talus
Dorsal Surface of Calcaneus
2
Dorsal Surface of Calcaneus Following Disarticulation of Subtalar Joint

5.93 TALOCALCANEAL JOINT

A. Bones of foot, with "closed book" inserted in joint plane of subtalar joint. **B.** "Open book" view of the bony surfaces of talocalcaneal joints. The plantar surface of the talus and dorsal surface of the calcaneus are displayed as pages in a book.

- The joints of inversion and eversion are the subtalar (posterior talocalcaneal) joint, talocalcaneonavicular joint, and transverse tarsal (combined calcaneocuboid and talonavicular) joint.
- The talus participates in the ankle joint, of the posterior and anterior talocalcaneal joints, and of the talonavicular joint.
- The posterior and anterior talocalcaneal joints are separated from each other by the sulcus tali and calcaneal sulcus, which, when the talus and calcaneus are in articulation, become the tarsal sinus.

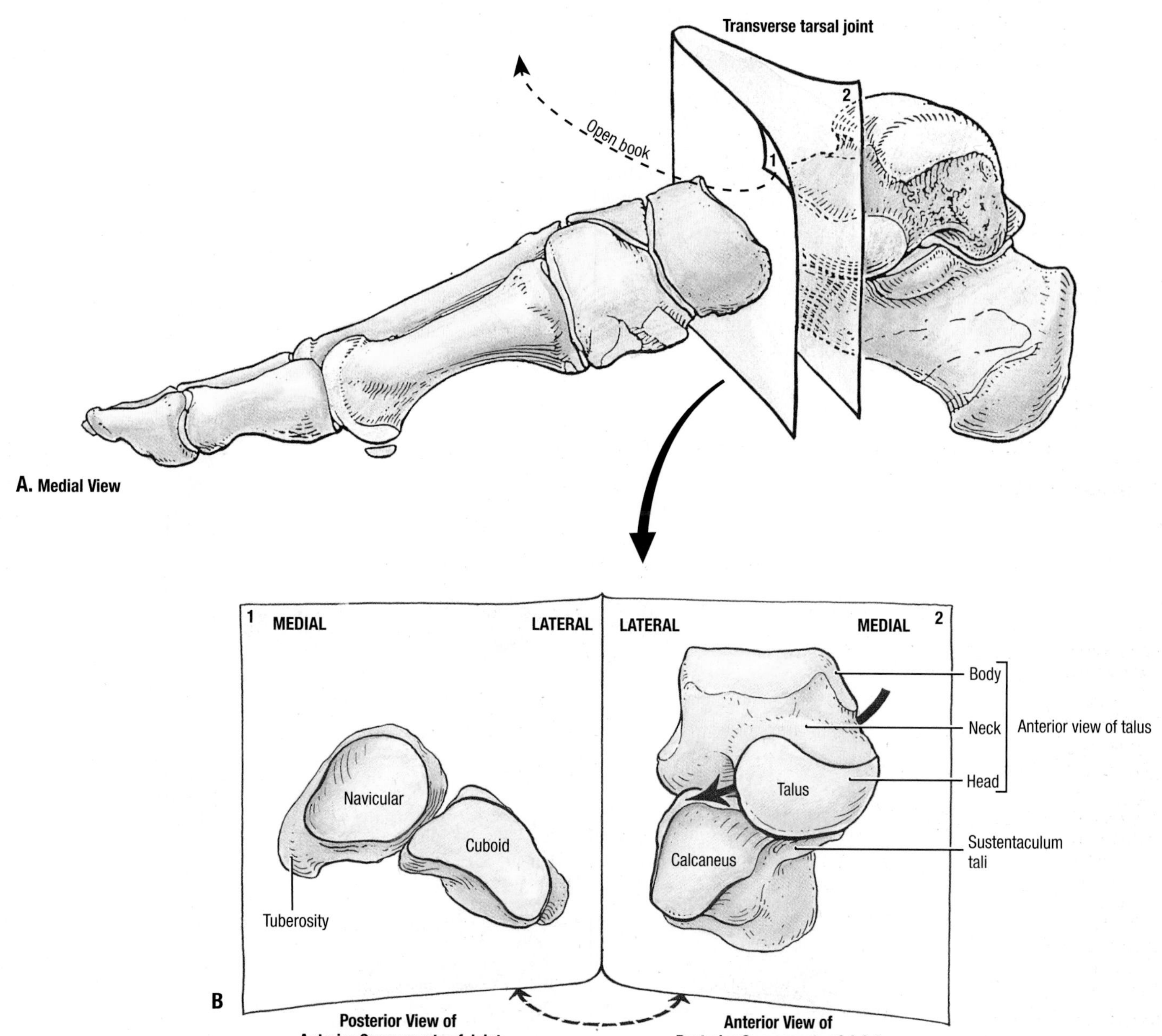
Transverse tarsal joint
Open book
2
1
A. Medial View
1 MEDIAL
LATERAL
LATERAL
MEDIAL 2
Navicular
Cuboid
Tuberosity
Body
Neck
Head
Anterior view of talus
Talus
Calcaneus
Sustentaculum tali
B
Posterior View of Anterior Components of Joint
Anterior View of Posterior Components of Joint

5.94 TRANSVERSE TARSAL JOINT

A. Bones of foot, with "closed book" inserted in joint plane of transverse tarsal joint. **B.** Articular surfaces of transverse tarsal joint. This compound joint includes the talonavicular and calcaneocuboid articulations. The posterior surfaces of the navicular and cuboid bones and the anterior surfaces of the talus and calcaneus are displayed as pages in an "open book". The *black arrow* traverses the tarsal sinus, in which the talocalcaneal (interosseous) ligament is located.

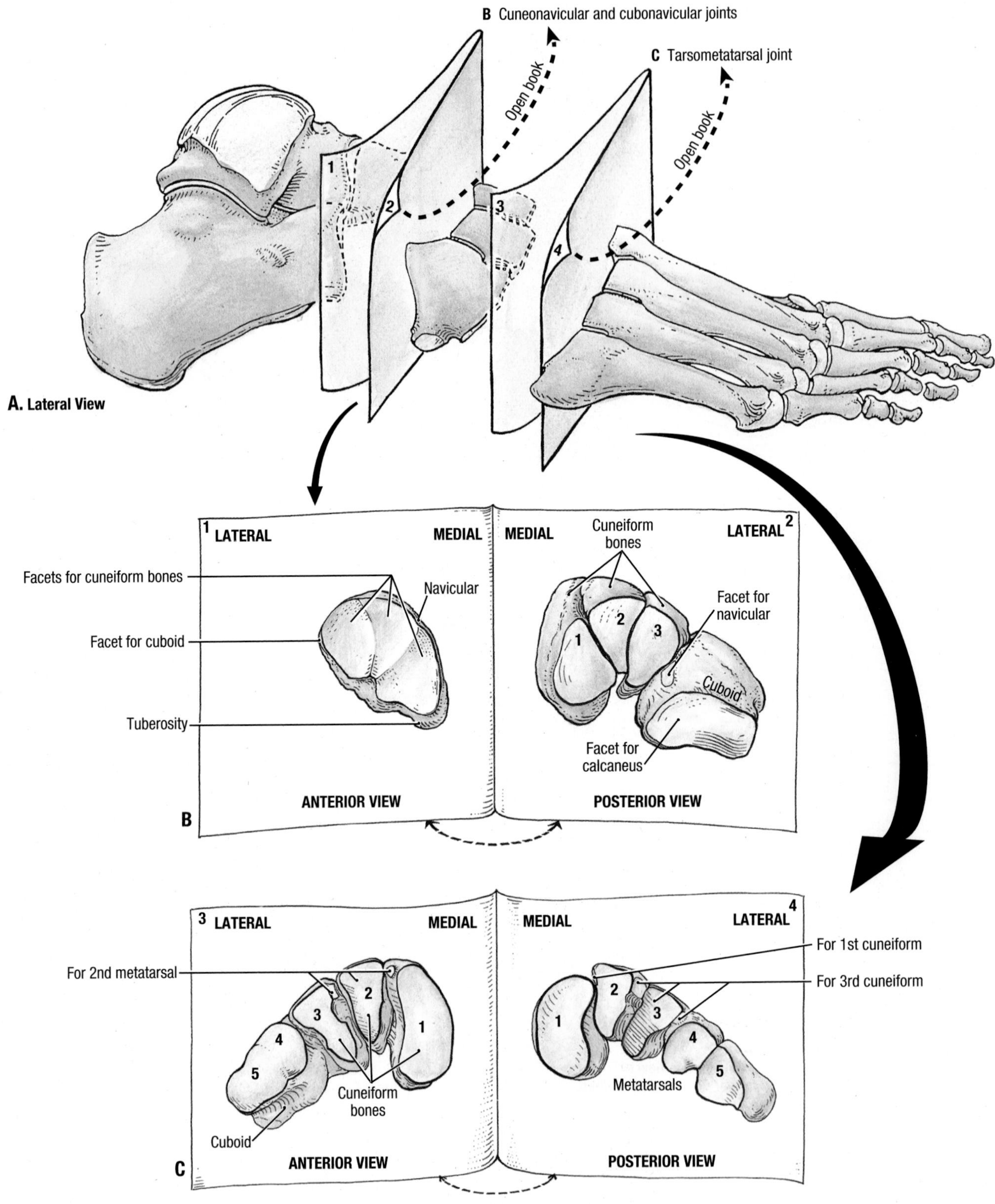

B Cuneonavicular and cubonavicular joints
C Tarsometatarsal joint
Open book
Open book
1
2
3
4
A. Lateral View
1 LATERAL
MEDIAL
MEDIAL
LATERAL 2
Cuneiform bones
Facets for cuneiform bones
Navicular
Facet for navicular
Facet for cuboid
1
2
3
Cuboid
Tuberosity
Facet for calcaneus
ANTERIOR VIEW
POSTERIOR VIEW
B
3 LATERAL
MEDIAL
MEDIAL
LATERAL 4
For 1st cuneiform
For 2nd metatarsal
For 3rd cuneiform
2
3
4
5
1
Cuneiform bones
Cuboid
Metatarsals
ANTERIOR VIEW
POSTERIOR VIEW
C

5.95 CUNEONAVICULAR, CUBONAVICULAR, AND TARSOMETATARSAL JOINTS

A. Bones of foot, with "closed book" inserted in indicated joint planes. **B.** "Open book" view of the bony surfaces of the cuneonavicular and cubonavicular joints. **C.** "Open book" view of the bony surfaces of the tarsometatarsal joints.

Metatarsal fractures (dancer's fracture) usually occur when the dancer loses balance, putting full body weight on the metatarsal. **Fatigue fractures of the metatarsals,** usually transverse, may result from prolonged walking with repeated stress on the metatarsals.

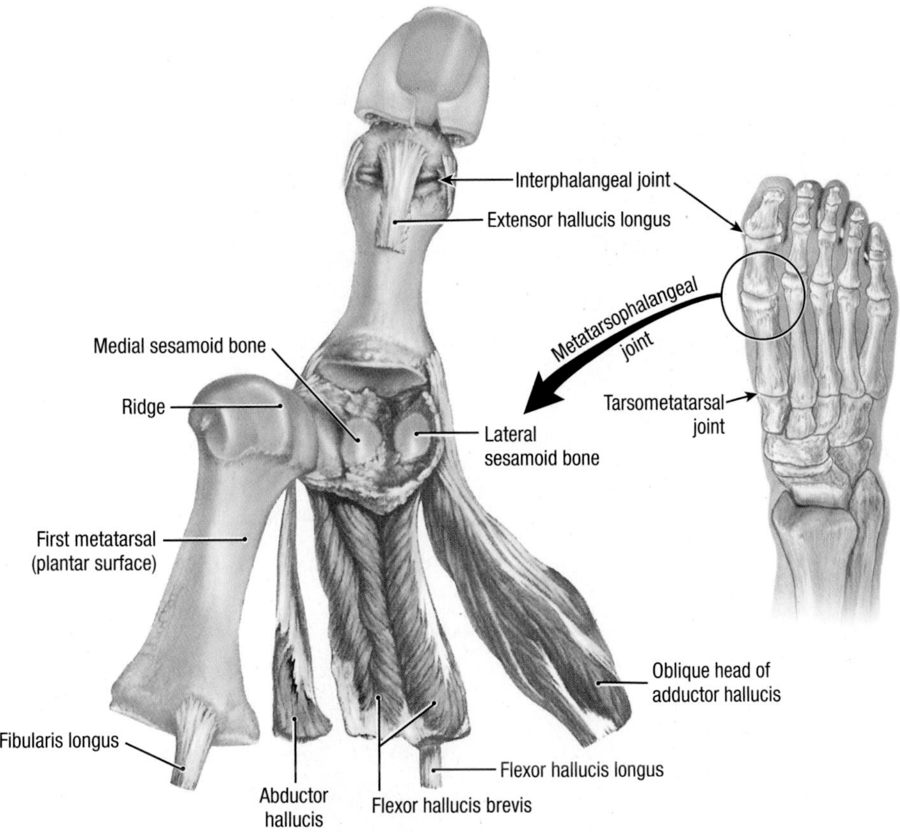
Interphalangeal joint
Extensor hallucis longus
Metatarsophalangeal joint
Medial sesamoid bone
Ridge
Lateral sesamoid bone
Tarsometatarsal joint
First metatarsal (plantar surface)
Oblique head of adductor hallucis
Fibularis longus
Flexor hallucis longus
Abductor hallucis
Flexor hallucis brevis

A. Superior View of Phalanges and Nail, Right Great Toe, Medial View of First Metetarsal

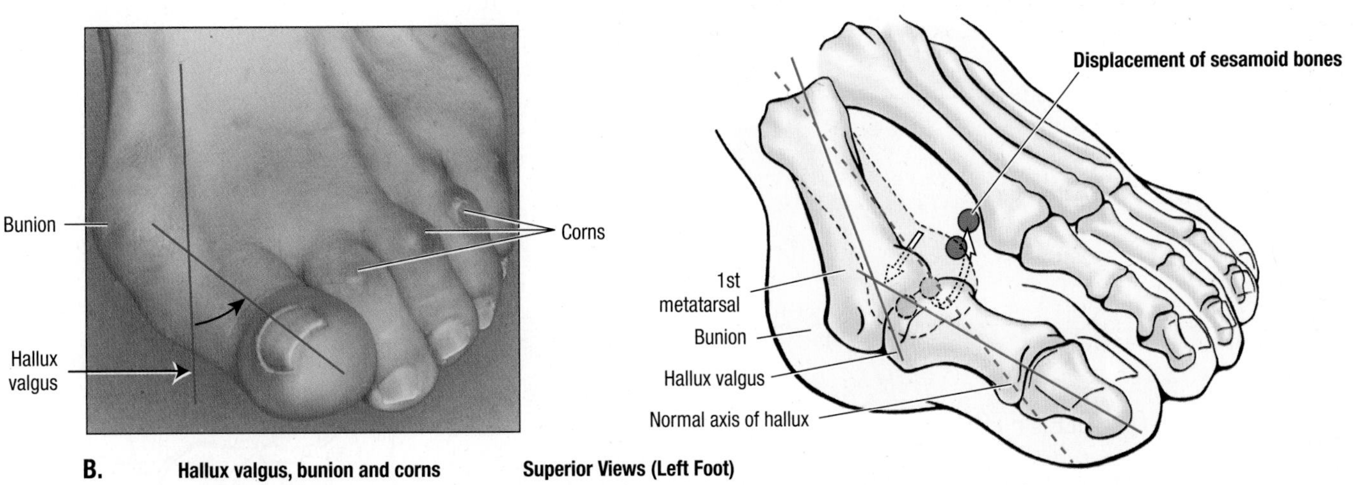
Bunion
Corns
Hallux valgus
Displacement of sesamoid bones
1st metatarsal
Bunion
Hallux valgus
Normal axis of hallux

B. **Hallux valgus, bunion and corns** **Superior Views (Left Foot)**

5.96 METATARSOPHALANGEAL JOINT OF GREAT TOE

A. First metatarsal and sesamoid bones of the right great toe. The sesamoid bones of the great toe (hallux) are bound together and located on each side of a bony ridge on the first metatarsal. **B. Hallux valgus** is a foot deformity caused by pressure from footwear and degenerative joint disease. It is characterized by lateral deviation of the base of the first metatarsal and base of the proximal phalanx of the great toe (L. *hallux*). In some people, the deviation is so great that the 1st toe overlaps the 2nd toe. These individuals are unable to move their 1st digit away from their 2nd digit because the sesamoid bones under the head of the 1st metatarsal are displaced and lie in the space between the heads of the 1st and 2nd metatarsals. In addition, a subcutaneous bursa may form owing to pressure and friction against the shoe. When tender and inflamed, the bursa is called a **bunion.**

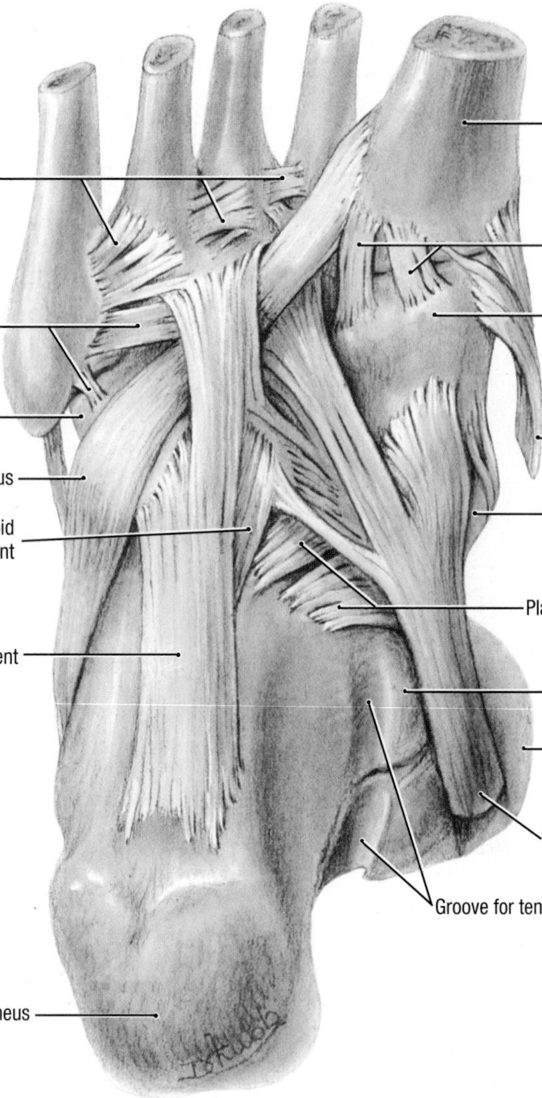

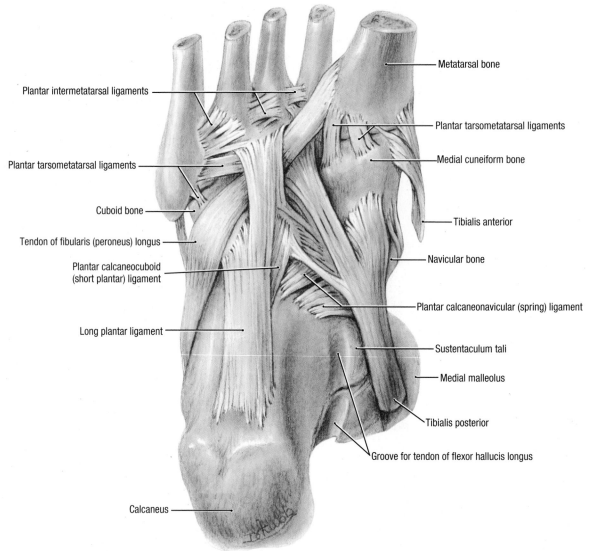

Metatarsal bone
Plantar intermetatarsal ligaments
Plantar tarsometatarsal ligaments
Medial cuneiform bone
Plantar tarsometatarsal ligaments
Cuboid bone
Tibialis anterior
Tendon of fibularis (peroneus) longus
Navicular bone
Plantar calcaneocuboid (short plantar) ligament
Plantar calcaneonavicular (spring) ligament
Long plantar ligament
Sustentaculum tali
Medial malleolus
Tibialis posterior
Groove for tendon of flexor hallucis longus
Calcaneus

A. Plantar View

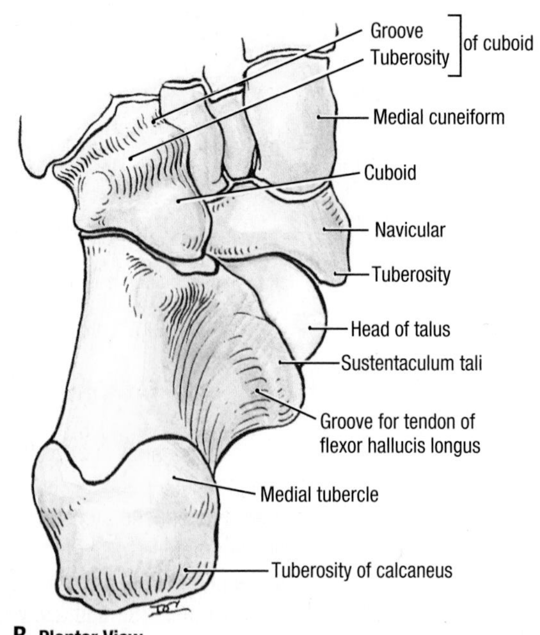
Groove
Tuberosity
of cuboid
Medial cuneiform
Cuboid
Navicular
Tuberosity
Head of talus
Sustentaculum tali
Groove for tendon of flexor hallucis longus
Medial tubercle
Tuberosity of calcaneus

B. Plantar View

5.97 LIGAMENTS OF SOLE OF FOOT

A. Dissection of superficial ligaments. **B.** Bones lying deep to ligaments of **A.**

In **A**:

- The head of the talus is exposed between the sustentaculum tali of the calcaneus and the navicular.
- Note the insertions of three long tendons: fibularis (peroneus) longus, tibialis anterior, and tibialis posterior.
- The tendon of the fibularis (peroneus) longus muscle crosses the sole of the foot in the groove anterior to the ridge of the cuboid, is bridged by some fibers of the long plantar ligament, and inserts into the base of the first metatarsal.
- Observe the slips of the tibialis posterior tendon extending to the bones anterior to the transverse tarsal joint.

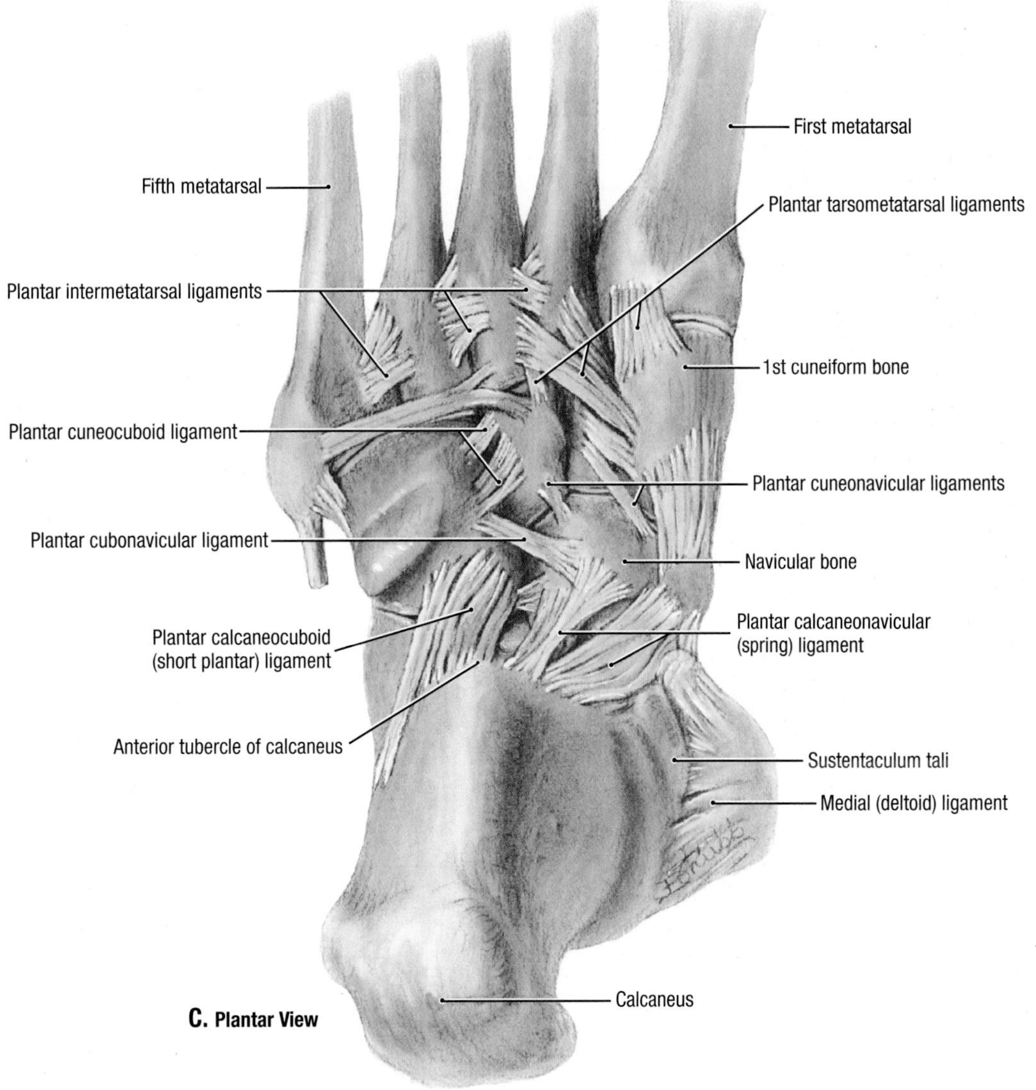
First metatarsal
Fifth metatarsal
Plantar tarsometatarsal ligaments
Plantar intermetatarsal ligaments
1st cuneiform bone
Plantar cuneocuboid ligament
Plantar cuneonavicular ligaments
Plantar cubonavicular ligament
Navicular bone
Plantar calcaneocuboid
(short plantar) ligament
Plantar calcaneonavicular
(spring) ligament
Anterior tubercle of calcaneus
Sustentaculum tali
Medial (deltoid) ligament
Calcaneus

C. Plantar View

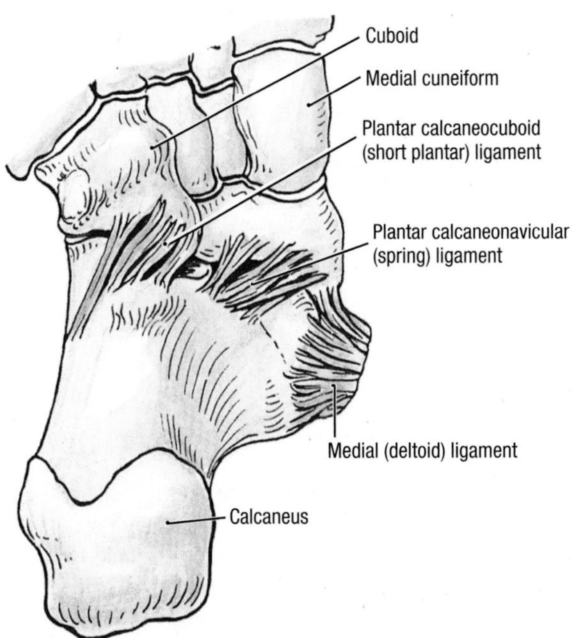
Cuboid
Medial cuneiform
Plantar calcaneocuboid
(short plantar) ligament
Plantar calcaneonavicular
(spring) ligament
Medial (deltoid) ligament
Calcaneus

D. Plantar View

5.97 LIGAMENTS OF SOLE OF FOOT (*CONTINUED*)

C. Dissection of the deep ligaments. **D.** Support for head of talus. The head of the talus is supported by the plantar calcaneonavicular ligament (spring ligament) and the tendon of the tibialis posterior.

- The plantar calcaneocuboid (short plantar) and plantar calcaneonavicular (spring) ligaments are the primary plantar ligaments of the transverse tarsal joint.
- The ligaments of the anterior foot diverge laterally and posteriorly from each side of the long axis of the third metatarsal and third cuneiform; hence a posterior thrust received by the first metatarsal, as when rising on the big toe while in walking, is transmitted directly to the navicular and talus by the first cuneiform and indirectly by the second metatarsal, second cuneiform, third metatarsal, and third cuneiform.
- A posterior thrust received by the fourth and fifth metatarsals is transmitted directly to the cuboid and calcaneus.

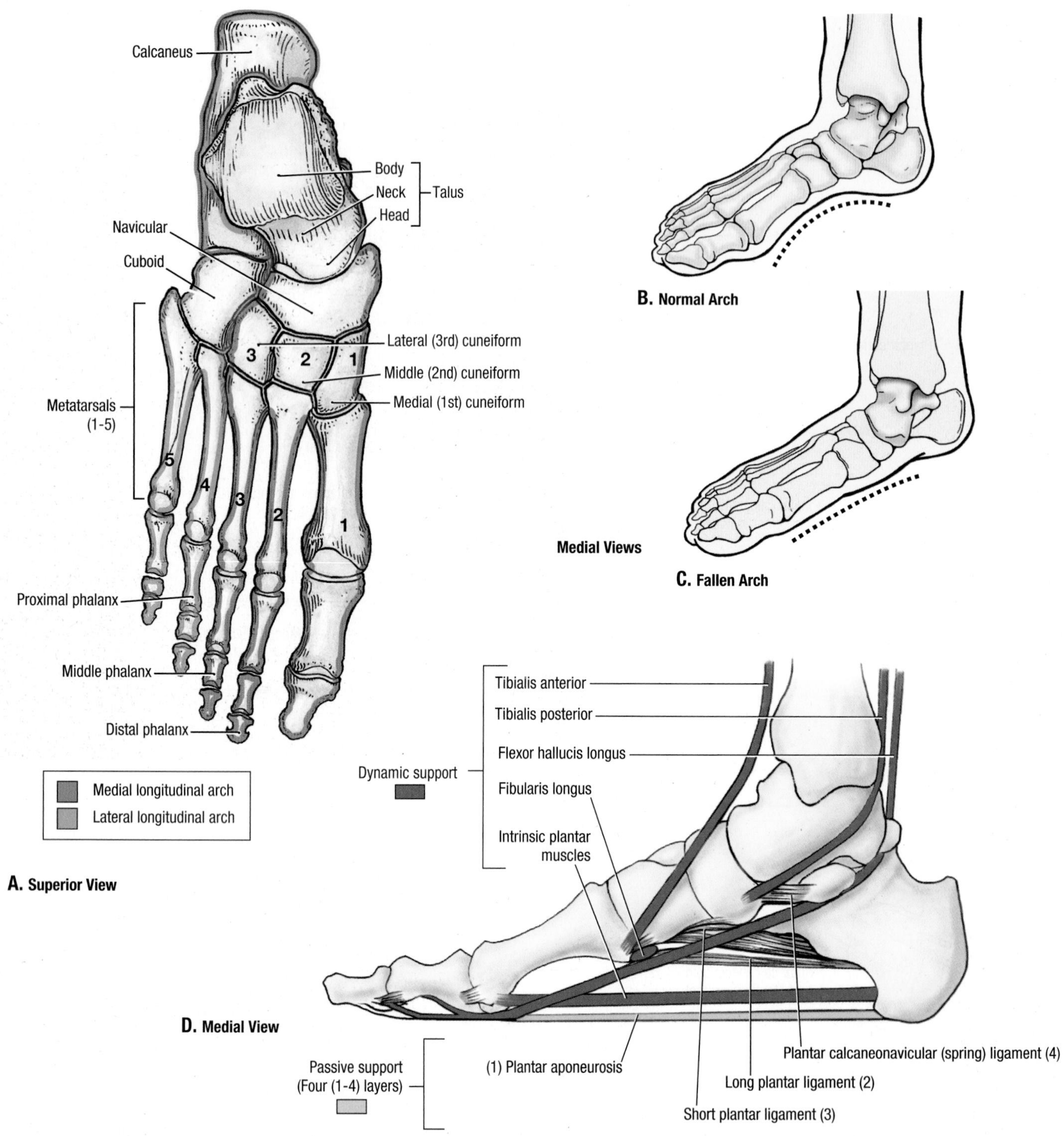

Calcaneus
Body
Neck
Head
Talus
Navicular
Cuboid
Lateral (3rd) cuneiform
Middle (2nd) cuneiform
Medial (1st) cuneiform
Metatarsals (1-5)
Proximal phalanx
Middle phalanx
Distal phalanx
Medial longitudinal arch
Lateral longitudinal arch
A. Superior View
B. Normal Arch
Medial Views
C. Fallen Arch
Dynamic support
Tibialis anterior
Tibialis posterior
Flexor hallucis longus
Fibularis longus
Intrinsic plantar muscles
D. Medial View
Passive support (Four (1-4) layers)
(1) Plantar aponeurosis
Plantar calcaneonavicular (spring) ligament (4)
Long plantar ligament (2)
Short plantar ligament (3)

5.98 ARCHES OF FOOT

A. Medial and lateral longitudinal arches. **B.** Normal arch. **C.** Fallen arch. **D.** Supports of the longitudinal arches.

Pes planus (flatfeet). Acquired flatfeet ("fallen arches") are likely to be secondary to dysfunction of the tibialis posterior due to trauma, degeneration with age, or denervation. In the absence of normal passive or dynamic support, the plantar calcaneonavicular ligament fails to support the head of the talus. Consequently, the head of the talus displaces inferomedially. As a result flattening of the medial longitudinal arch occurs **(C)** along with lateral deviation of the forefoot. Flatfeet are common in older people, particularly if they undertake much unaccustomed standing or gain weight rapidly, adding stress on the muscles and increasing strain on the ligaments supporting the arches.

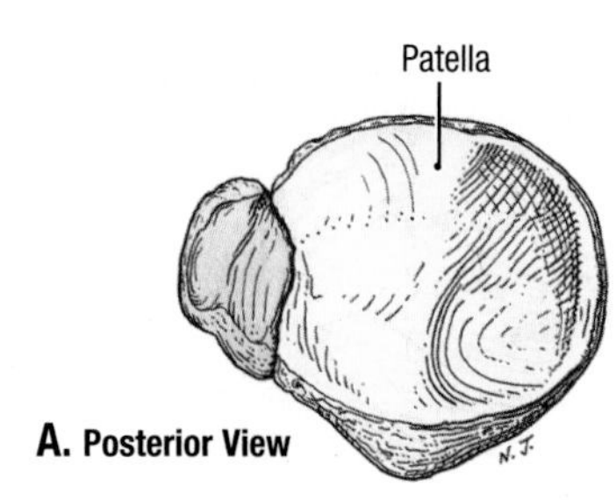
Patella

A. Posterior View

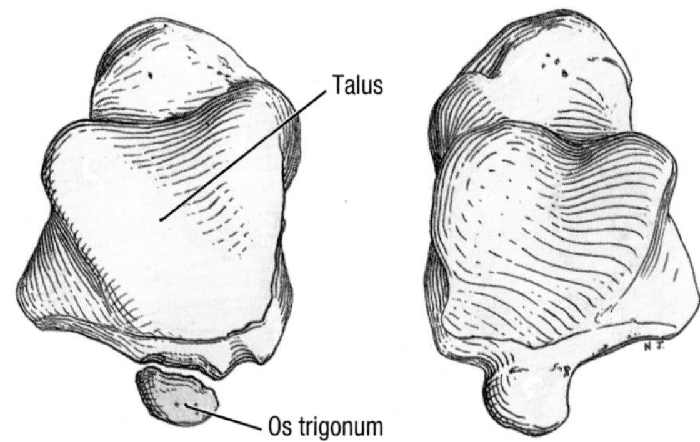
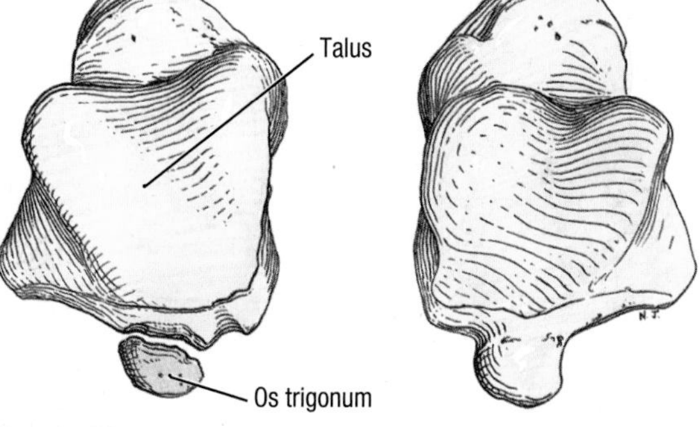
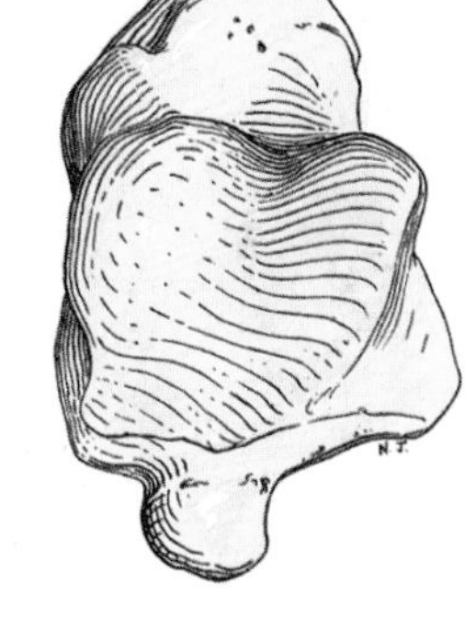
Talus
Os trigonum

B. Superior Views

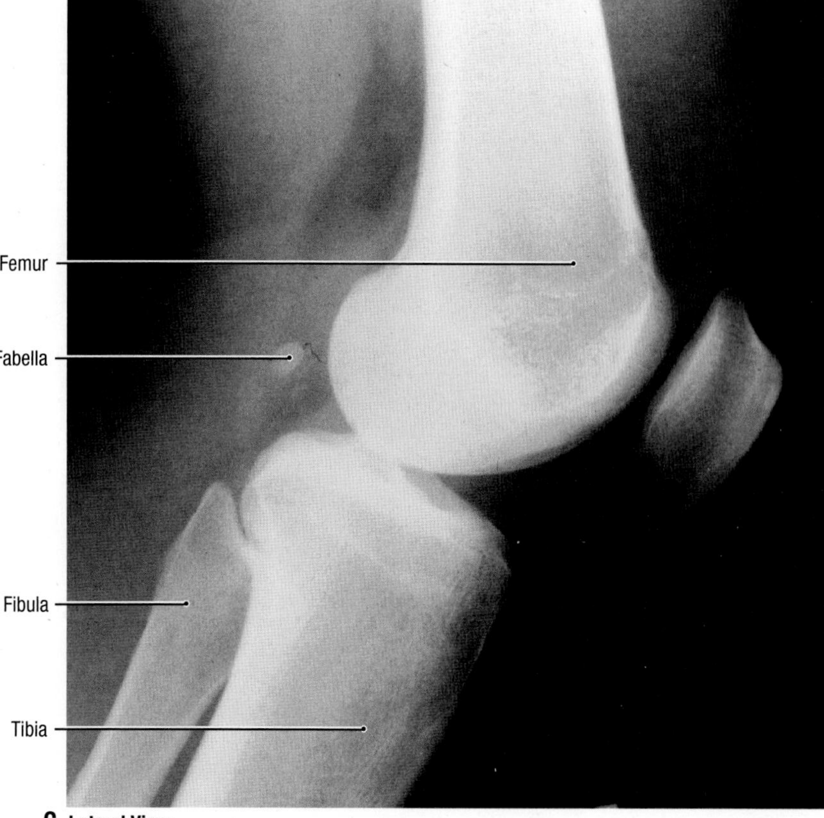
Femur
Fabella
Fibula
Tibia

C. Lateral View

Navicular
Sesamoid bone
Tendon of tibialis posterior

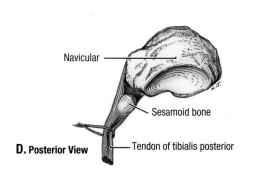

D. Posterior View

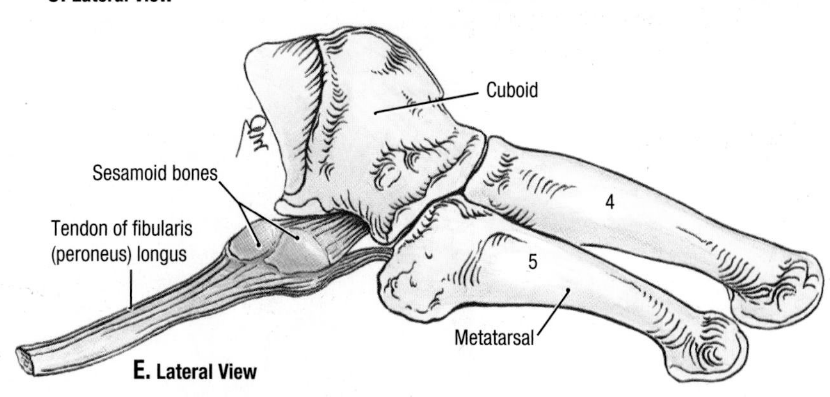
Cuboid
Sesamoid bones
Tendon of fibularis (peroneus) longus
4
5
Metatarsal

E. Lateral View

5.99 BONY ANOMALIES

A. Bipartite patella. Occasionally, the superolateral angle of the patella ossifies independently and remains discrete. **B. Os trigonum.** The lateral (posterior) tubercle of the talus has a separate center of ossification that appears from the ages of 7 to 13 years; when this fails to fuse with the body of the talus, as in the left bone of this pair, it is called an os trigonum. It was found in Dr. Grant's lab in 7.7% of 558 adult feet; 22 were paired, and 21 were unpaired. **C. Fabella.** A sesamoid bone in the lateral head of the gastrocnemius muscle was present in 21.6% of 116 limbs. **D. Sesamoid bone in the tendon of tibialis posterior.** A sesamoid bone was found in 23% of 348 adults. **E. Sesamoid bone in the tendon of fibularis (peroneus) longus.** A sesamoid bone was found in 26% of 92 specimens. In this specimen, it is bipartite, and the fibularis (peroneus) longus muscle has an additional attachment to the 5th metatarsal bone.

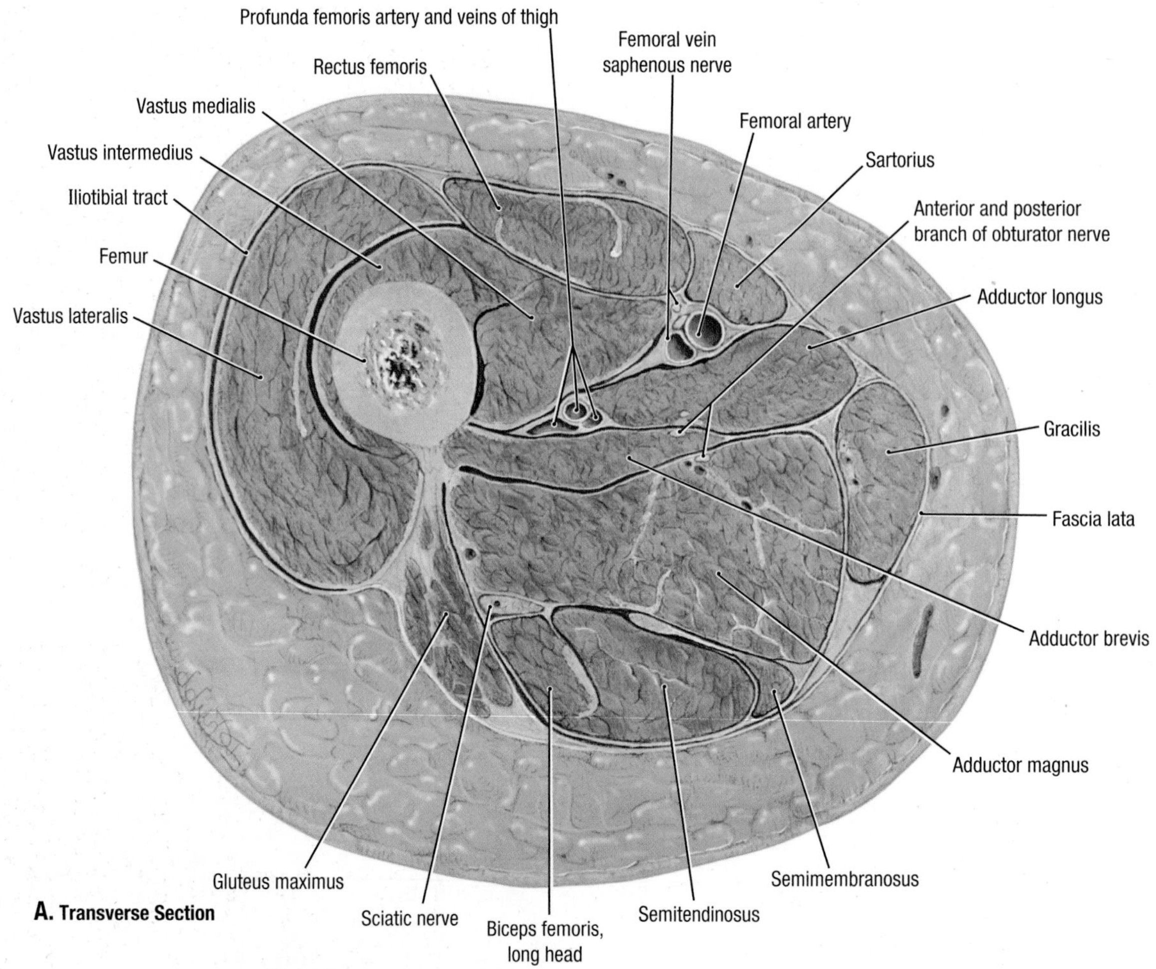

Profunda femoris artery and veins of thigh
Rectus femoris
Femoral vein
saphenous nerve
Vastus medialis
Femoral artery
Vastus intermedius
Sartorius
Iliotibial tract
Anterior and posterior
branch of obturator nerve
Femur
Adductor longus
Vastus lateralis
Gracilis
Fascia lata
Adductor brevis
Adductor magnus
Gluteus maximus
Semimembranosus
Sciatic nerve
Biceps femoris,
long head
Semitendinosus

A. Transverse Section

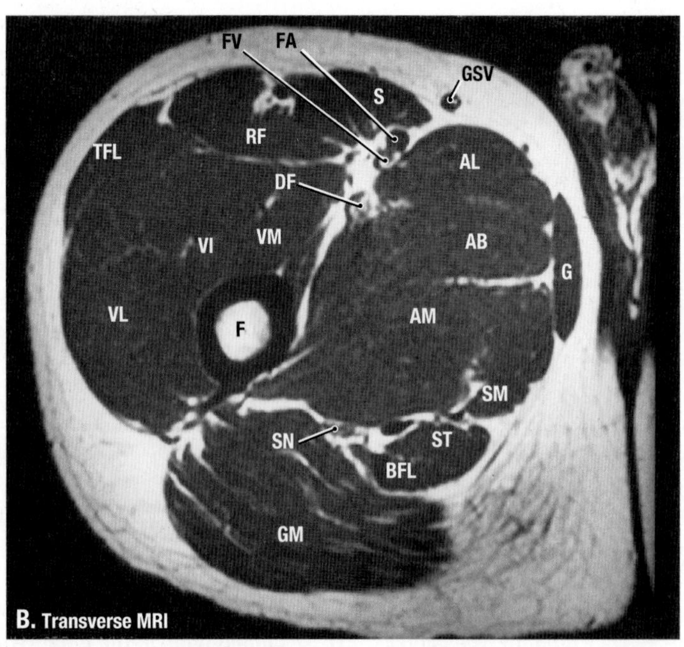

FV
FA
GSV
S
RF
TFL
AL
DF
VI
VM
AB
G
VL
F
AM
SM
SN
ST
BFL
GM

B. Transverse MRI

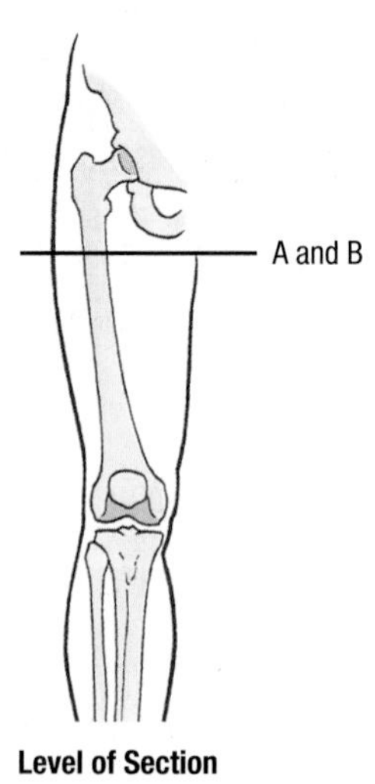

A and B

Level of Section

5.100 TRANSVERSE SECTIONS AND MRIs OF THIGH

A. Anatomical section of proximal thigh. **B.** Transverse MRI of proximal thigh.

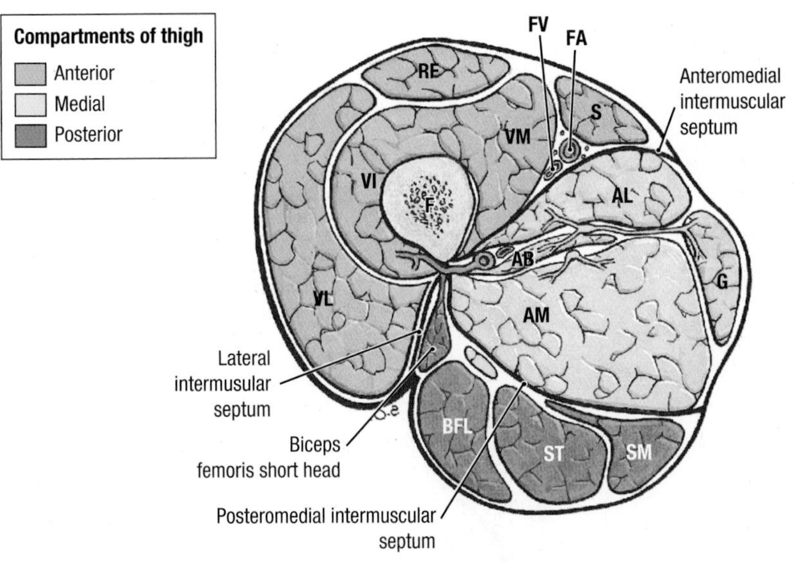
Compartments of thigh
Anterior
Medial
Posterior
FV
FA
RF
S
VM
VI
F
AL
AB
G
VL
AM
BFL
ST
SM
Anteromedial intermuscular septum
Lateral intermusular septum
Biceps femoris short head
Posteromedial intermuscular septum

C

Transverse MRI

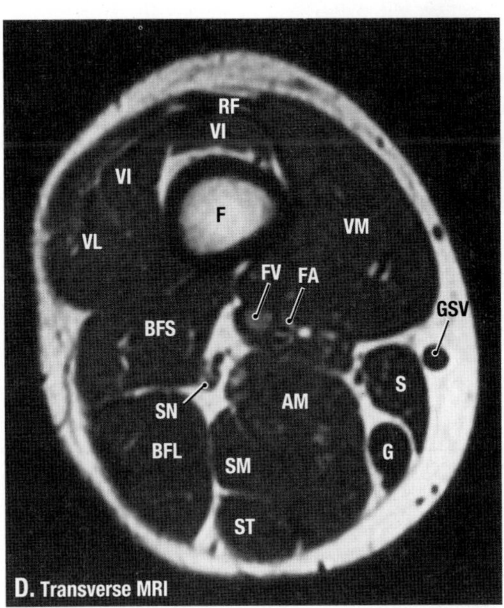
RF
VI
VI
F
VM
VL
FV
FA
GSV
BFS
SN
AM
S
BFL
SM
G
ST

D. Transverse MRI

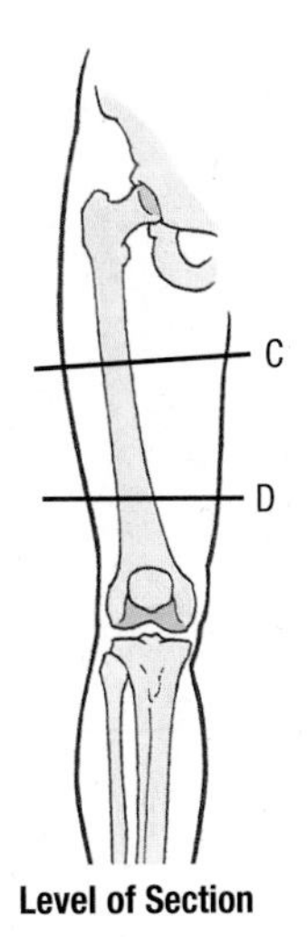
C
D

Level of Section

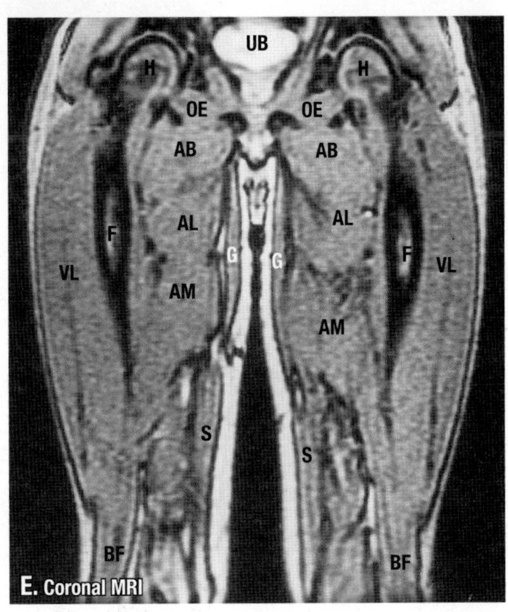
UB
H
H
OE
OE
AB
AB
AL
AL
F
F
VL
VL
G
G
AM
AM
S
S
BF
BF

E. Coronal MRI

Key	
AB	Adductor brevis
AL	Adductor longus
AM	Adductor magnus
AS	Anteromedial intermuscular septum
BF	Biceps femoris
BFL	Long head of biceps femoris
BFS	Short head of biceps femoris
F	Femur
FA	Femoral artery
FL	Fascia lata
FV	Femoral vein
G	Gracilis
GM	Gluteus maximus
GSV	Great saphenous vein
H	Head of femur
IT	Iliotibial tract
LS	Lateral intermuscular septum
OE	Obturator externus
PS	Posterior intermuscular septum
RF	Rectus femoris
S	Sartorius
SM	Semimembranosus
SN	Sciatic nerve
ST	Semitendinosus
TFL	Tensor fasciae latae
UB	Urinary bladder
VI	Vastus intermedius
VL	Vastus lateralis
VM	Vastus medialis

5.100 TRANSVERSE SECTIONS AND MRIs OF THIGH (*CONTINUED*)

C. Diagrammlatic anatomical section and transverse (axial) MRI of midthigh. **D.** Transverse (axial) MRI of distal thigh. **E.** Coronal MRI.

The thigh has three compartments, each with its own nerve supply and primary function: anterior group extends the knee and is supplied by the femoral nerve; medial group adducts the hip and is supplied by the obturator nerve; posterior group flexes the knee and is supplied by the sciatic nerve.

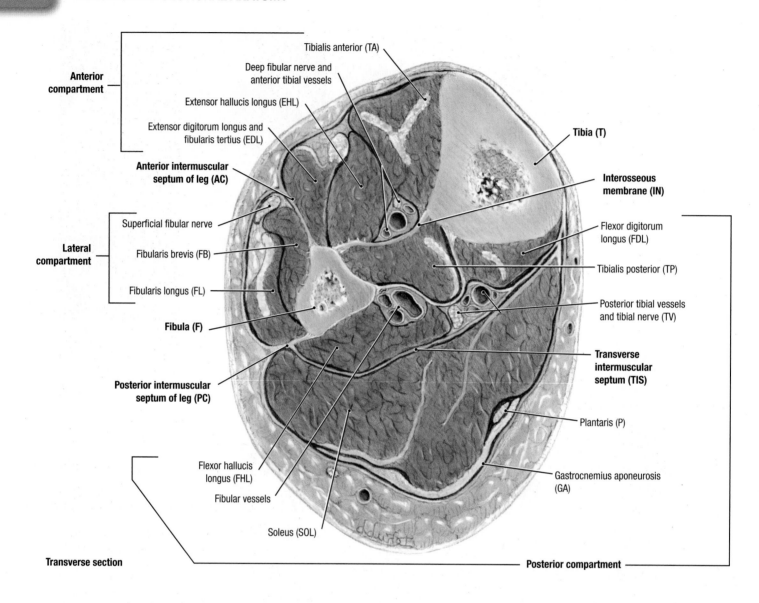

Anterior compartment
Tibialis anterior (TA)
Deep fibular nerve and anterior tibial vessels
Extensor hallucis longus (EHL)
Extensor digitorum longus and fibularis tertius (EDL)
Anterior intermuscular septum of leg (AC)
Lateral compartment
Superficial fibular nerve
Fibularis brevis (FB)
Fibularis longus (FL)
Fibula (F)
Posterior intermuscular septum of leg (PC)
Flexor hallucis longus (FHL)
Fibular vessels
Soleus (SOL)
Tibia (T)
Interosseous membrane (IN)
Flexor digitorum longus (FDL)
Tibialis posterior (TP)
Posterior tibial vessels and tibial nerve (TV)
Transverse intermuscular septum (TIS)
Plantaris (P)
Gastrocnemius aponeurosis (GA)
Posterior compartment

Transverse section

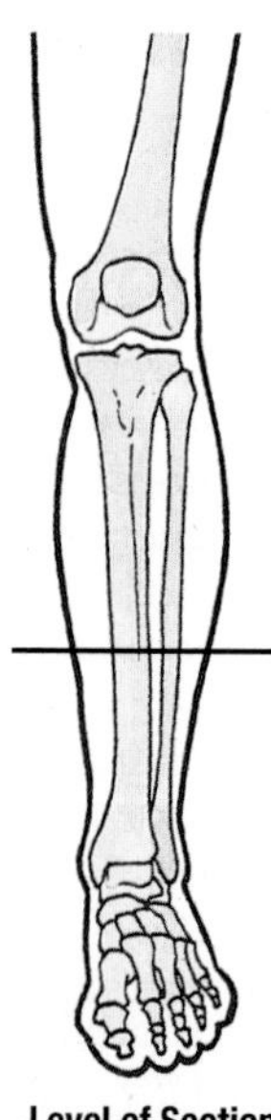
Level of Section

5.101 TRANSVERSE SECTION OF LEG

Boundaries of anterior, lateral, and posterior compartments of leg. Anterior compartment: tibia, interosseous membrane, fibula, anterior intermuscular septum, and crural fascia. Lateral compartment: fibula, anterior and posterior intermuscular septa, and the crural fascia. Posterior compartment: tibia, interosseous membrane, fibula, posterior intermuscular septum, and crural fascia. The posterior compartment is subdivided by the transverse intermuscular septum into superficial and deep subcompartments.

Compartmental infections in the leg. Because the septa and deep fascia forming the boundaries of the leg compartments are strong, the increased volume consequent to infection with suppuration (formation of pus) increases intracompartmental pressure. Inflammation within the anterior and posterior compartments spreads chiefly in a distal direction; however a purulent infection in the lateral compartment can ascend proximally into the popliteal fossa, presumably along the course of the fibular nerve. **Fasciotomy** may be necessary to relieve compartmental pressure and debride (remove by scraping) pockets of infection.

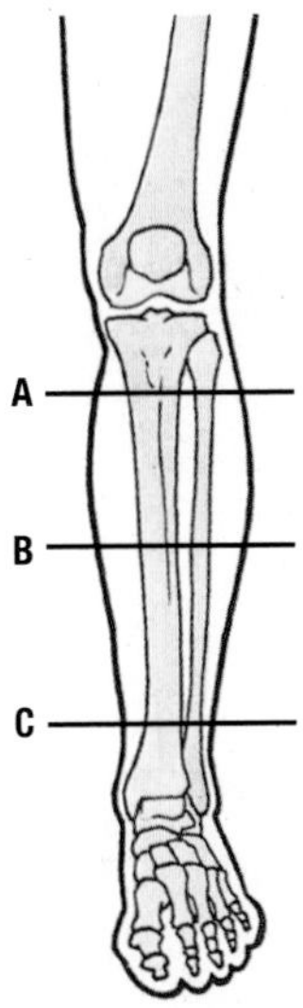
A
B
C

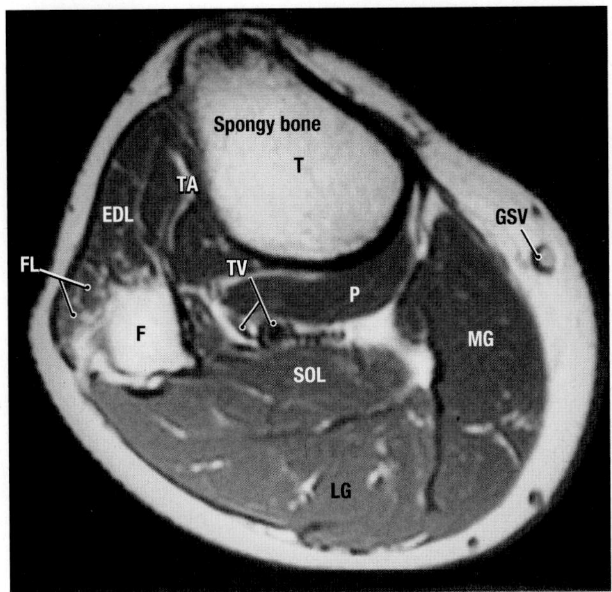
Spongy bone
T
TA
EDL
FL
TV
P
F
GSV
MG
SOL
LG

A. Transverse MRI

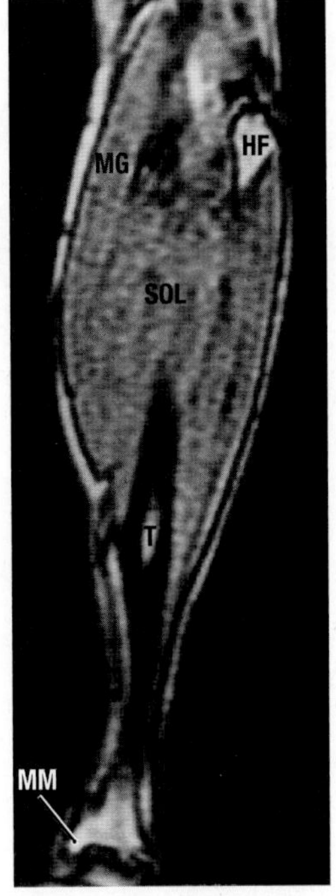
MG
HF
SOL
T
MM

D. Coronal MRI

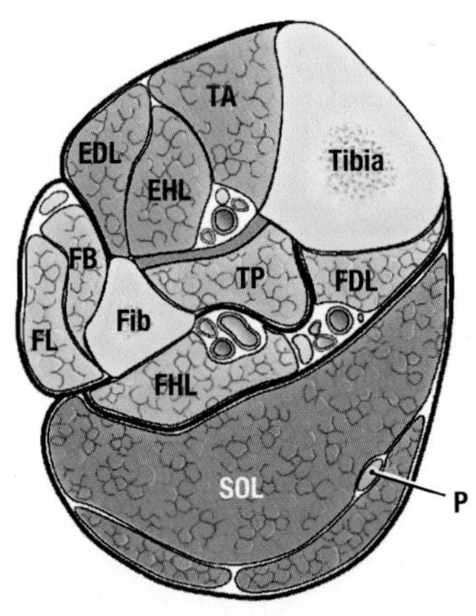
TA
EDL
Tibia
EHL
FB
TP
FDL
FL
Fib
FHL
SOL
P

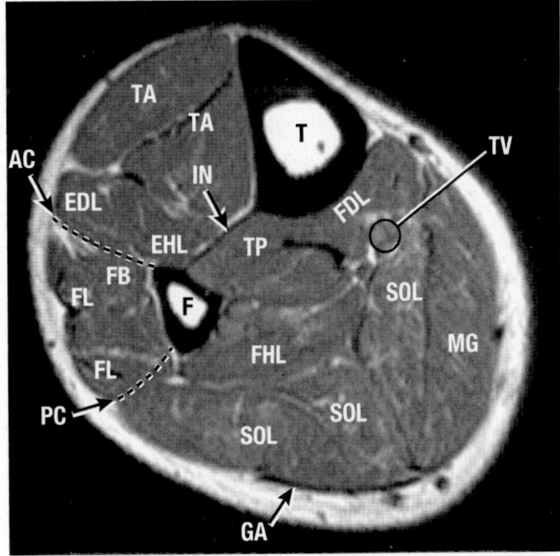
TA
TA
T
AC
IN
TV
EDL
FDL
EHL
TP
FB
FL
F
SOL
MG
FHL
FL
PC
SOL
SOL
GA

B. Transverse Section and MRI

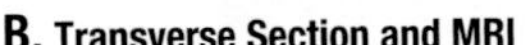

Key for B

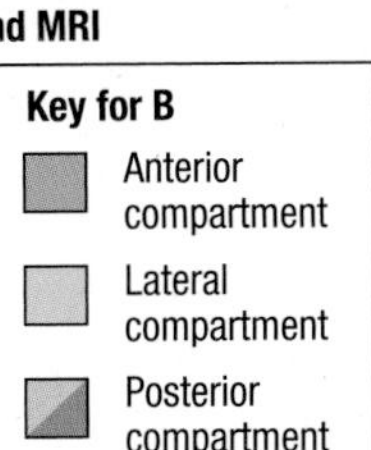

- Anterior compartment
- Lateral compartment
- Posterior compartment

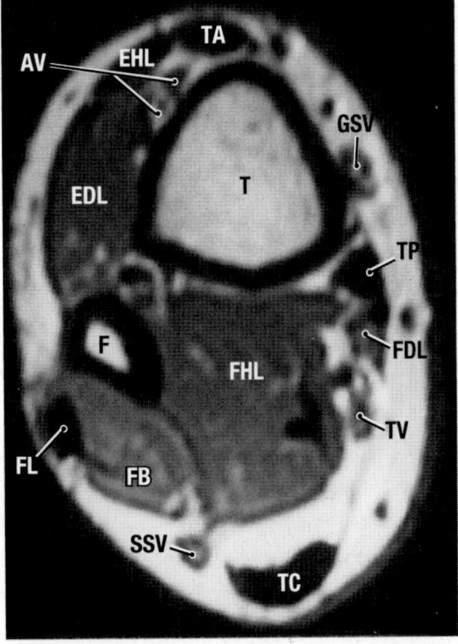
TA
AV
EHL
GSV
EDL
T
TP
F
FDL
FHL
TV
FL
FB
SSV
TC

C. Transverse MRI

Key

AC	Anterior intermuscular septum
AV	Anterior tibial vessels and deep fibular nerve
EDL	Extensor digitorum longus
EHL	Extensor hallucis longus
F	Fibula
FB	Fibularis brevis
FDL	Flexor digitorum longus
FHL	Flexor hallucis longus
FL	Fibularis longus
GA	Gastrocnemius aponeurosis
G	Gracilis
GM	Gluteus maximus
GSV	Great saphenous vein
HF	Head of fibula
IN	Interosseous membrane
LG	Lateral head of gastrocnemius
MG	Medial head of gastrocnemius
MM	Medial malleolus
P	Popliteus
PC	Posterior intermuscular septum
SOL	Soleus
SSV	Small saphenous vein
T	Tibia
TA	Tibialis anterior
Ta	Talus
TC	Calcaneal tendon
TP	Tibialis posterior
TV	Tibial nerve and posterior tibial vessels

5.102 MRIs OF LEG

A., B. and C. Transverse (axial) MRIs. **D.** Coronal MRI.

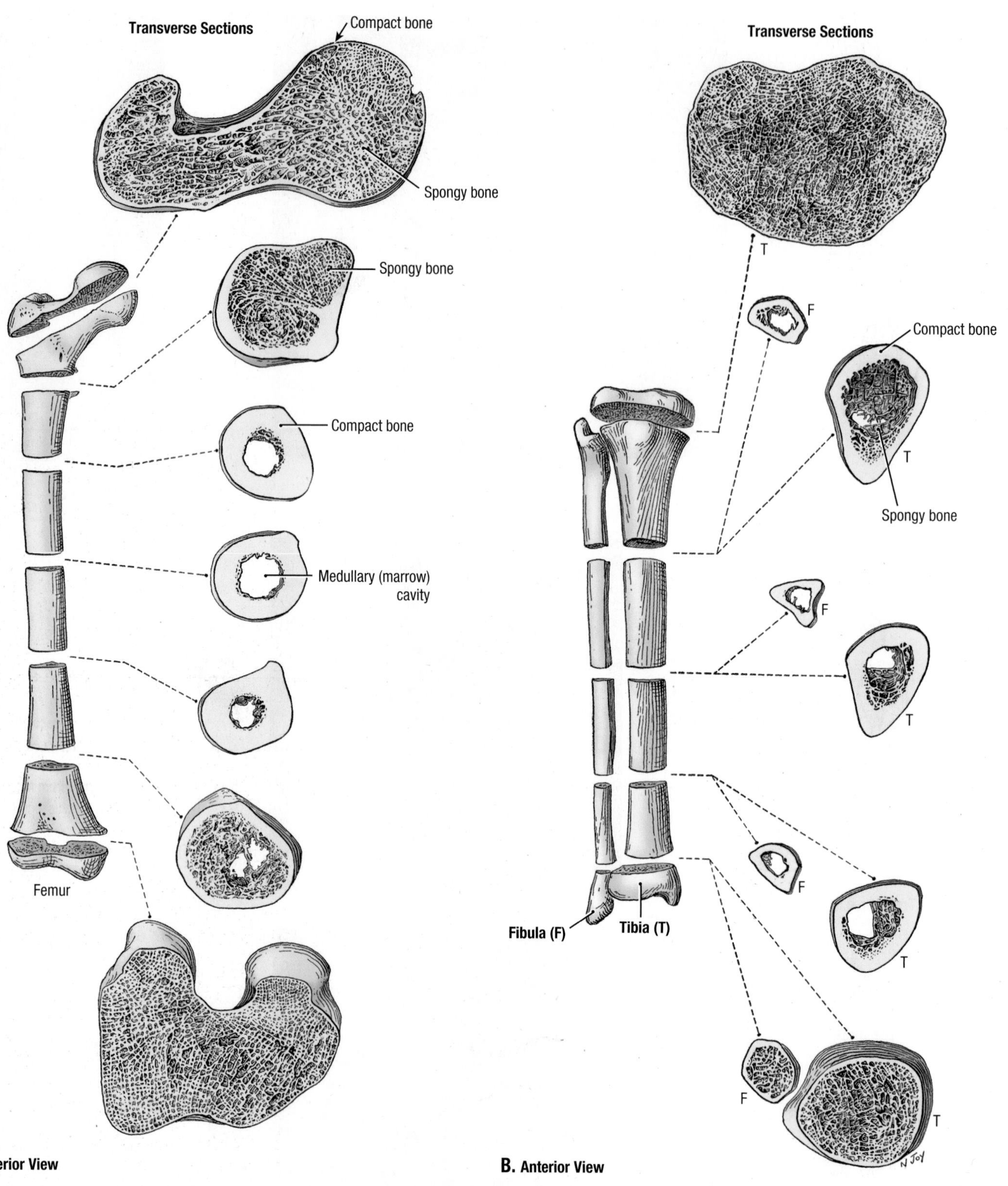
Transverse Sections
Compact bone
Spongy bone
Spongy bone
Compact bone
Medullary (marrow) cavity
Femur
A. Anterior View
Transverse Sections
T
F
Compact bone
T
Spongy bone
F
T
F
T
Fibula (F)
Tibia (T)
F
T
B. Anterior View

5.103 TRANSVERSE SECTIONS THROUGH FEMUR, TIBIA AND FIBULA

A. Femur. **B.** Tibia and fibula. Note the differences in thickness of the compact and spongy bone and in the width of the medullary (marrow) cavity. Compact and spongy bones are distinguished by the relative amount of solid matter and by the number and size of the spaces they contain. All bones have a superficial thin layer of compact bone around a central mass of spongy bone, except where the latter is replaced by the medullary (marrow) cavity. Within the medullary cavity of adult bones and between the spicules (trabeculae) of spongy bone, yellow (fatty) or red (blood cell and platelet forming) bone marrow or both are found.

CHAPTER 6

Upper Limb

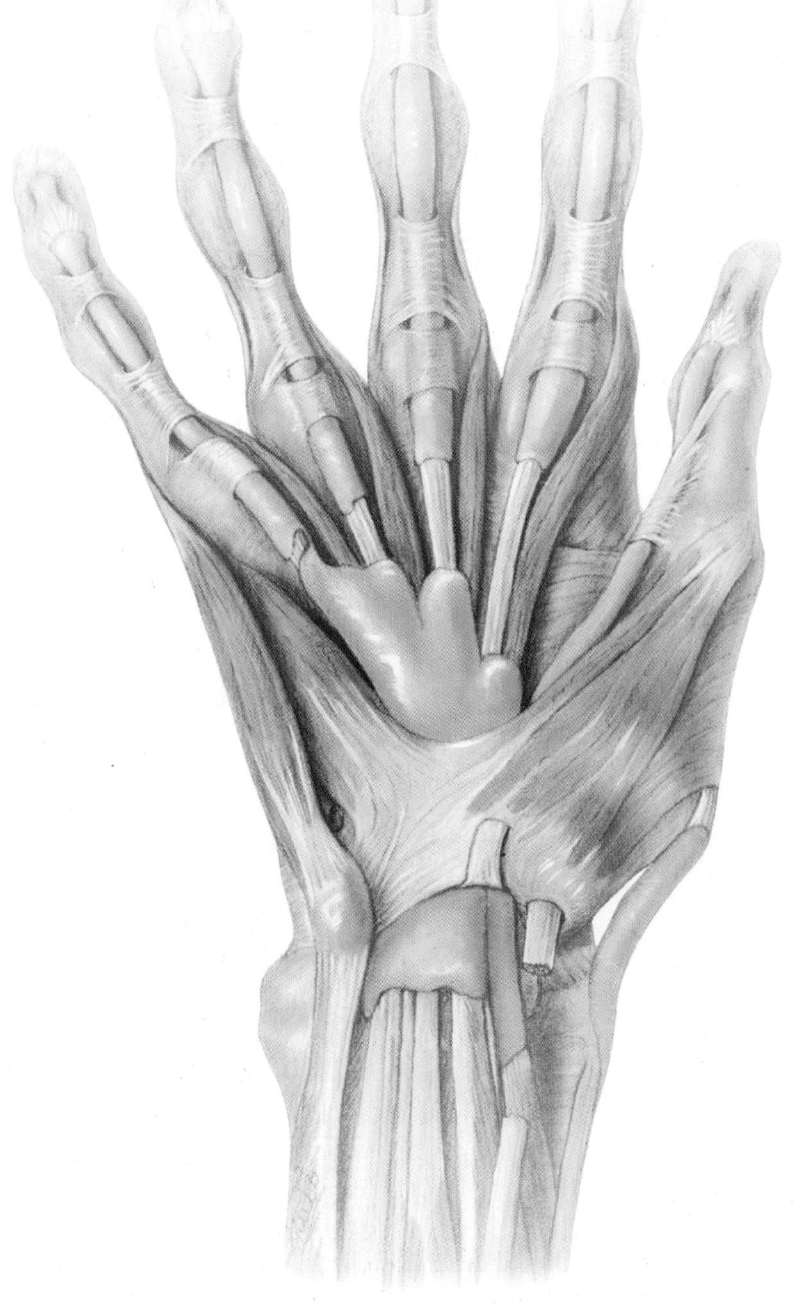

Systemic Overview of Upper Limb	
Bones	482
Nerves	488
Arteries	494
Veins and Lymphatics	496
Musculofascial Compartments	500
Pectoral Region	502
Axilla, Axillary Vessels, and Brachial Plexus	509
Scapular Region and Superficial Back	520
Arm and Rotator Cuff	524
Joints of Shoulder Region	538
Elbow Region	546
Elbow Joint	552
Anterior Aspect of Forearm	558
Anterior Aspect of Wrist and Palm of Hand	562
Posterior Aspect of Forearm	582
Posterior Aspect of Wrist and Dorsum of Hand	586
Lateral Aspect of Wrist and Hand	592
Medial Aspect of Wrist and Hand	595
Bones and Joints of Wrist and Hand	596
Function of Hand: Grips and Pinches	604
Imaging and Sectional Anatomy	605

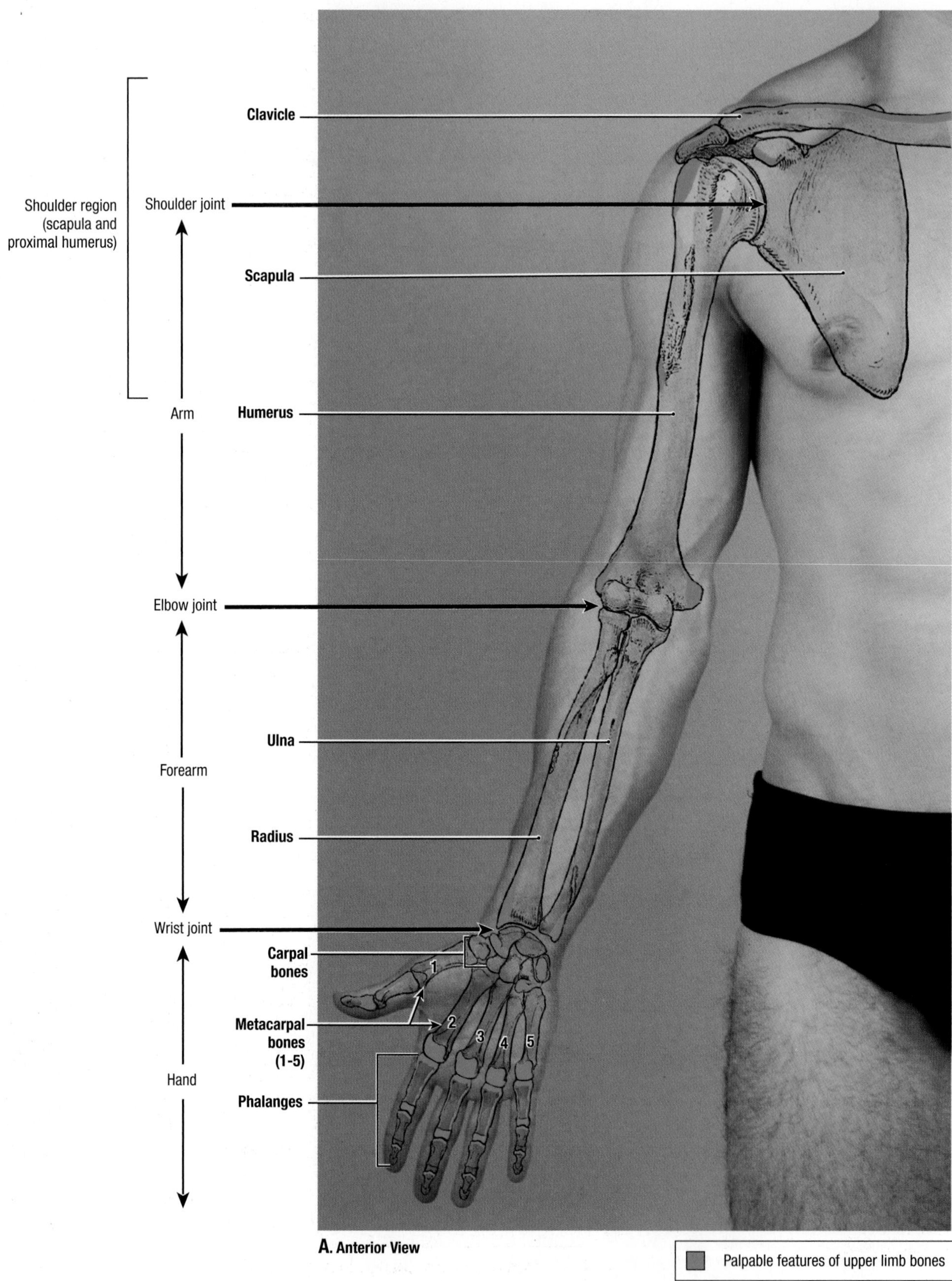
Clavicle
Shoulder region (scapula and proximal humerus)
Shoulder joint
Scapula
Arm
Humerus
Elbow joint
Ulna
Forearm
Radius
Wrist joint
Carpal bones
1
Metacarpal bones (1-5)
2
3
4
5
Hand
Phalanges
Palpable features of upper limb bones

A. Anterior View

6.1 REGIONS, BONES, AND MAJOR JOINTS OF UPPER LIMB

The joints divide the upper limb into four main regions: the shoulder, arm, forearm, and hand.

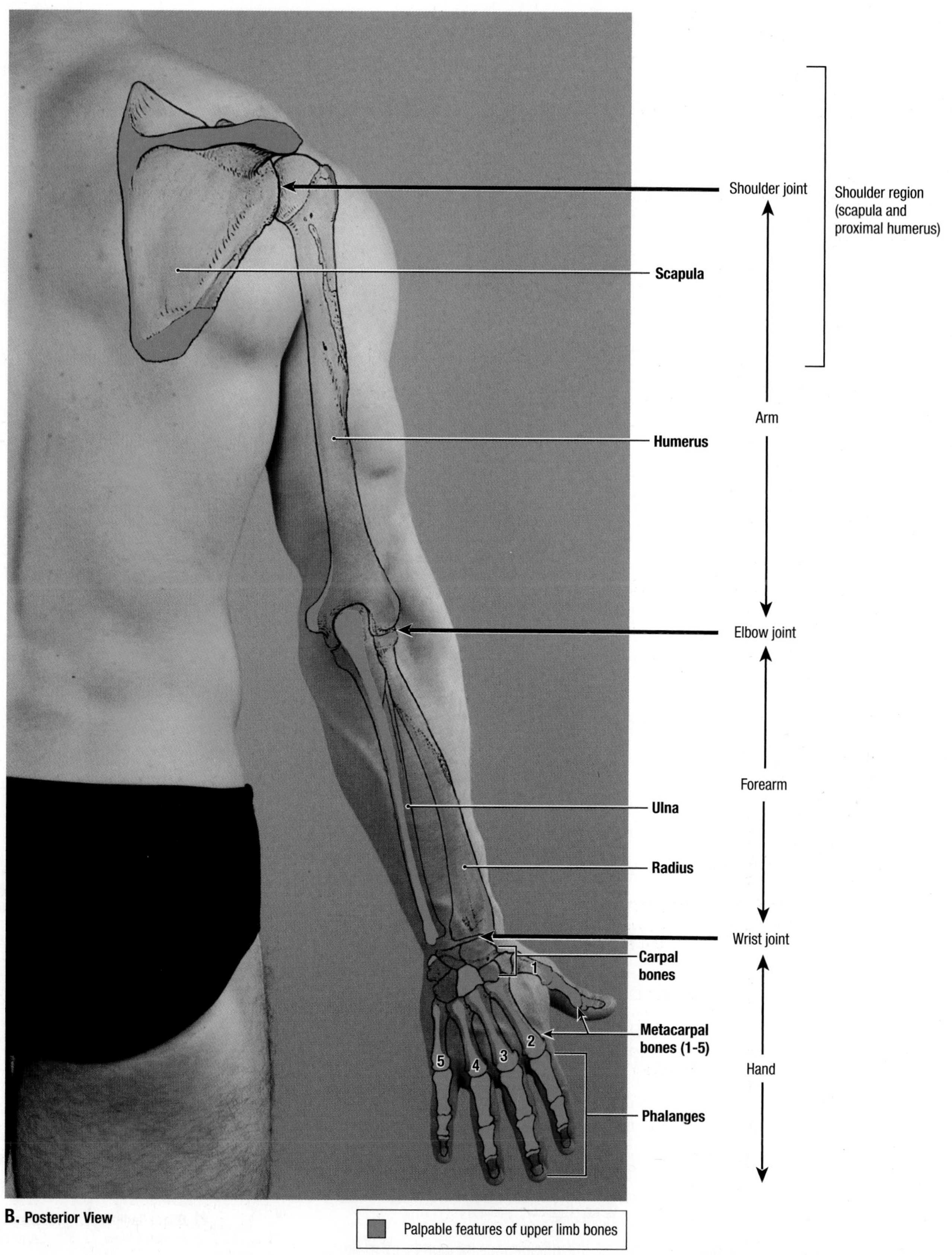
Shoulder joint
Shoulder region (scapula and proximal humerus)
Scapula
Arm
Humerus
Elbow joint
Forearm
Ulna
Radius
Wrist joint
Carpal bones
Metacarpal bones (1-5)
Hand
Phalanges
1
2
3
4
5
Palpable features of upper limb bones

B. Posterior View

6.1 REGIONS, BONES, AND MAJOR JOINTS OF UPPER LIMB *(CONTINUED)*

The pectoral (shoulder) girdle is an incomplete ring of bones formed by the right and left scapulae and clavicles and is joined medially to the manubrium of the sternum.

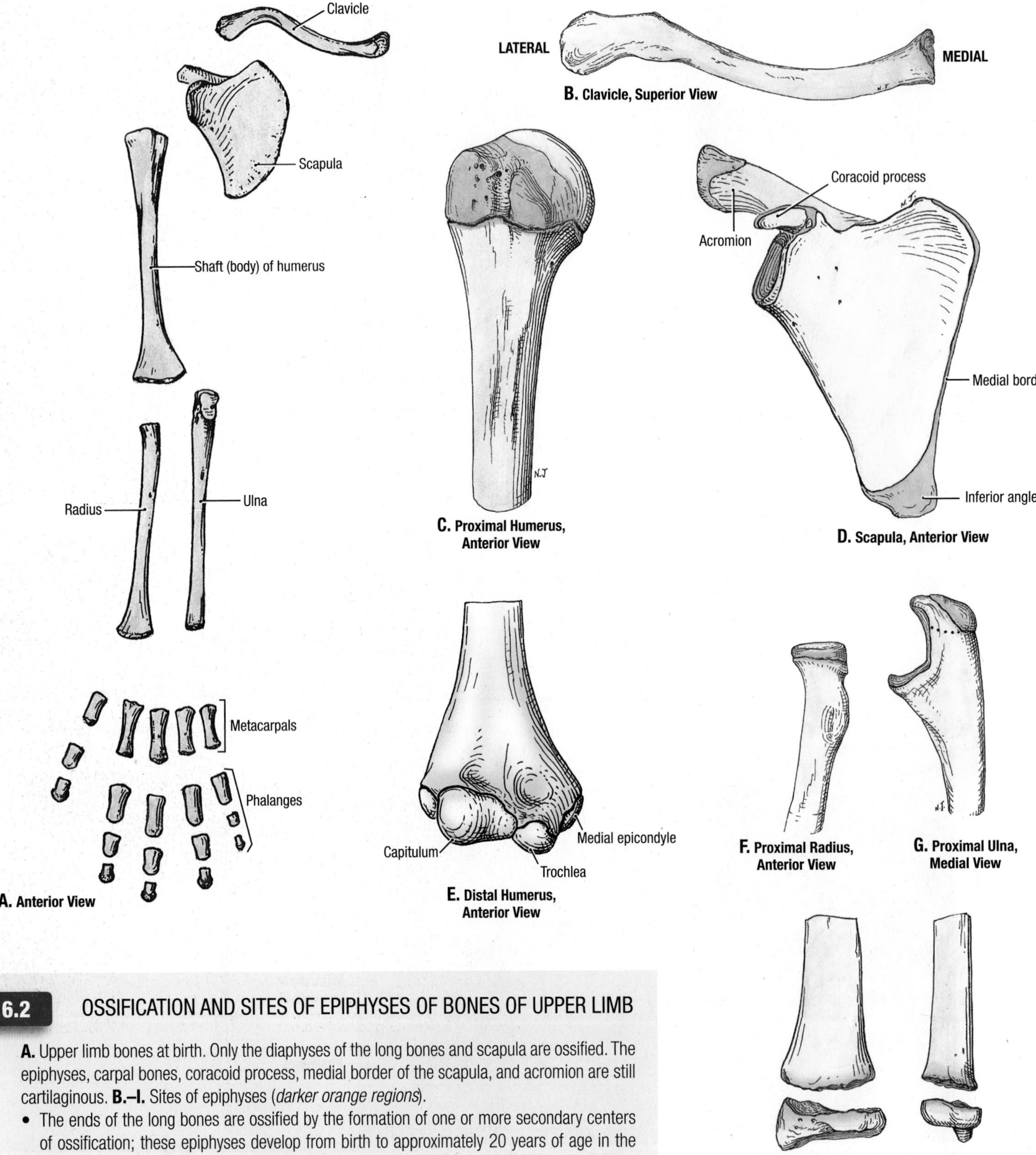

Clavicle
Scapula
Shaft (body) of humerus
Radius
Ulna
Metacarpals
Phalanges
LATERAL
MEDIAL
Coracoid process
Acromion
Medial border
Inferior angle
Capitulum
Trochlea
Medial epicondyle

A. Anterior View

B. Clavicle, Superior View

C. Proximal Humerus, Anterior View

D. Scapula, Anterior View

E. Distal Humerus, Anterior View

F. Proximal Radius, Anterior View

G. Proximal Ulna, Medial View

H. Distal Radius, Anterior View

I. Distal Ulna, Anterior View

6.2 OSSIFICATION AND SITES OF EPIPHYSES OF BONES OF UPPER LIMB

A. Upper limb bones at birth. Only the diaphyses of the long bones and scapula are ossified. The epiphyses, carpal bones, coracoid process, medial border of the scapula, and acromion are still cartilaginous. **B.–I.** Sites of epiphyses (*darker orange regions*).

- The ends of the long bones are ossified by the formation of one or more secondary centers of ossification; these epiphyses develop from birth to approximately 20 years of age in the clavicle, humerus, radius, ulna, metacarpals, and phalanges.

Epiphyses. Without knowledge of bone growth and the appearance of bones in radiographic and other diagnostic images at various ages, a displaced epiphysial plate could be mistaken for a fracture, and separation of an epiphysis could be interpreted as a displaced piece of fractured bone. Knowledge of the patient's age and the location of epiphyses can prevent these errors.

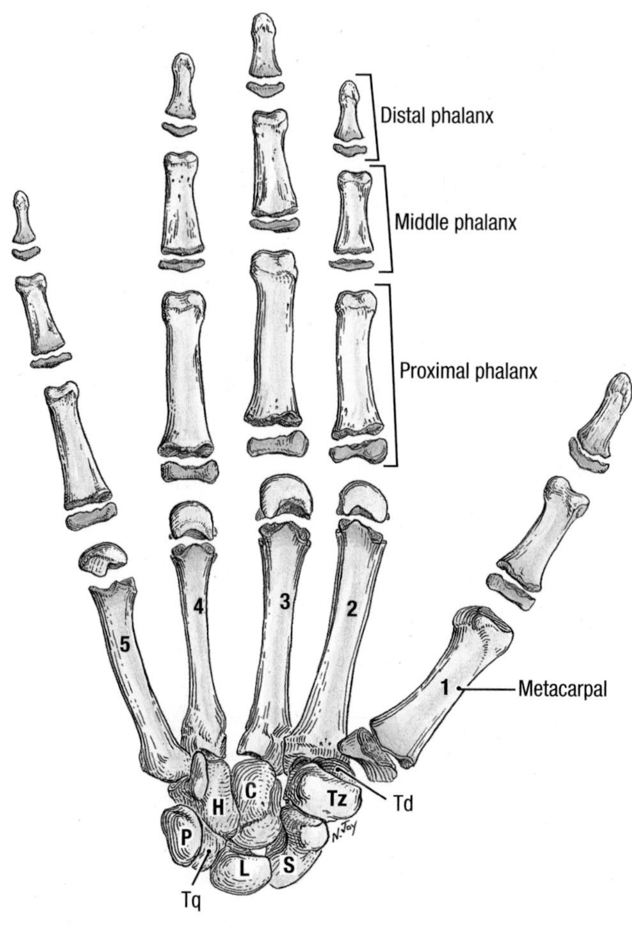
Distal phalanx
Middle phalanx
Proximal phalanx
5
4
3
2
1
Metacarpal
H
C
Tz
Td
P
L
S
Tq
N. Joy

J. Anterior View (Right Hand)

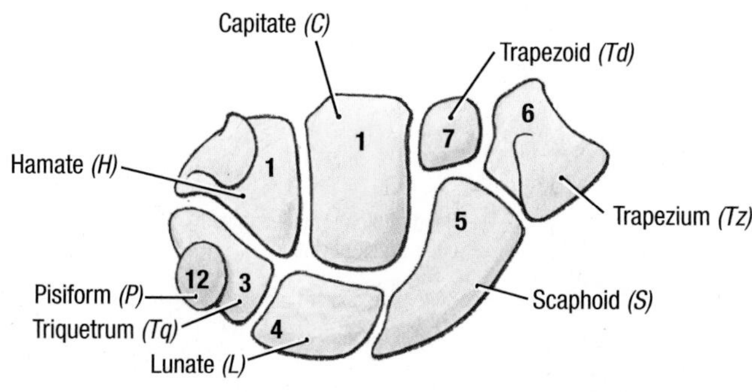
Capitate (C)
Trapezoid (Td)
Hamate (H)
Trapezium (Tz)
Pisiform (P)
Triquetrum (Tq)
Lunate (L)
Scaphoid (S)
1
1
7
6
5
12
3
4

Numbers: approximate age of ossification of carpal bones in years

K. Anterior View

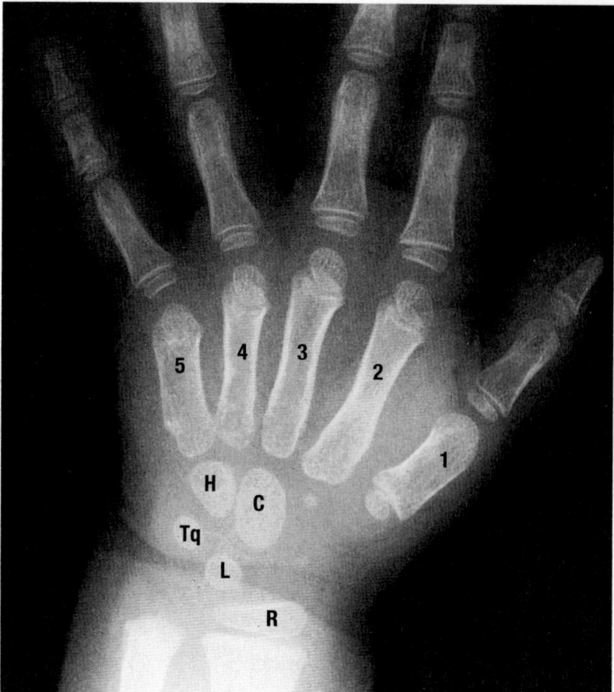
5
4
3
2
1
H
C
Tq
L
R

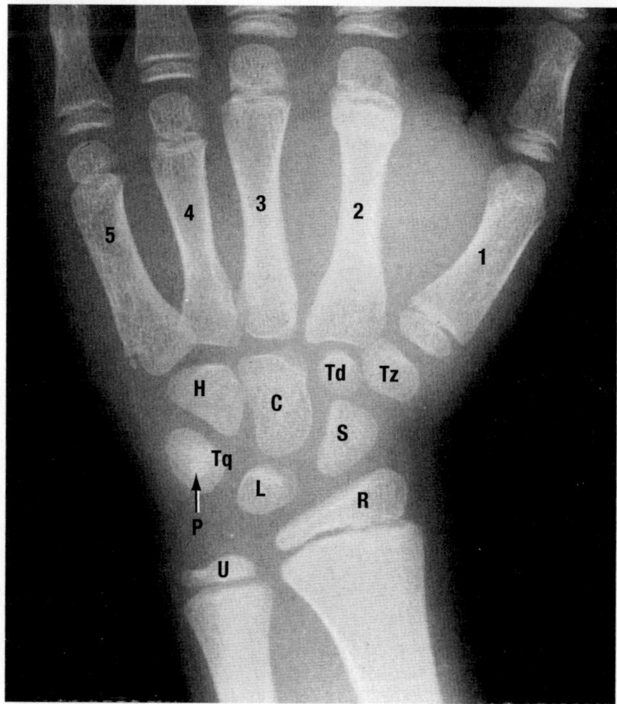
5
4
3
2
1
Td
Tz
H
C
S
Tq
L
R
P
U

L. Antero-posterior View, Right Hand

Epiphyses in radiographs appear as radiolucent lines

6.2 OSSIFICATION AND SITES OF EPIPHYSES OF BONES OF UPPER LIMB *(CONTINUED)*

J. Sequence of ossification of carpal bones. **K.** Ossification of bones of hand. Note the phalanges have a single proximal epiphysis and metacarpals 2, 3, 4, and 5 have single distal epiphyses. The 1st metacarpal behaves as a phalanx by having proximal epiphysis. Short-lived epiphyses may appear at the other ends of metacarpals 1 and/or 2. There are individual and gender differences in sequence and timing of ossification. **L.** Radiographs of stages of ossification of wrist and hand. *Top*, a $2^1/_2$-year-old child; the lunate is ossifying, and the distal radial epiphysis *(R)* is present (*C*, capitate; *H*, hamate; *Tq*, triquetrum; *L*, lunate). *Bottom*, an 11-year-old child. All carpal bones are ossified (*S*, scaphoid; *Td*, trapezoid; *Tz*, trapezium; *arrowhead*, pisiform), and the distal epiphysis of the ulna *(U)* has ossified.

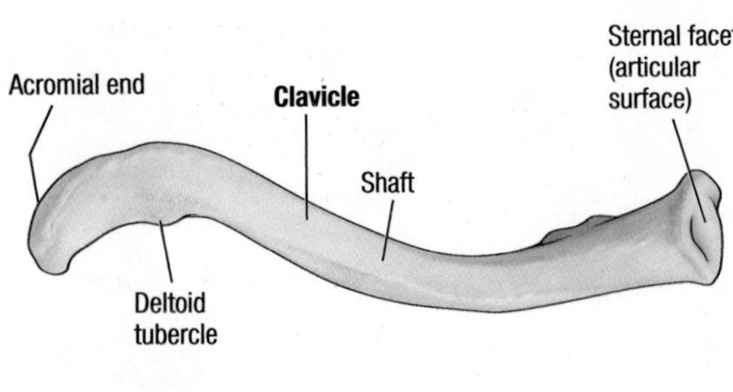
Acromial end
Clavicle
Sternal facet (articular surface)
Shaft
Deltoid tubercle

A. Superior Surface

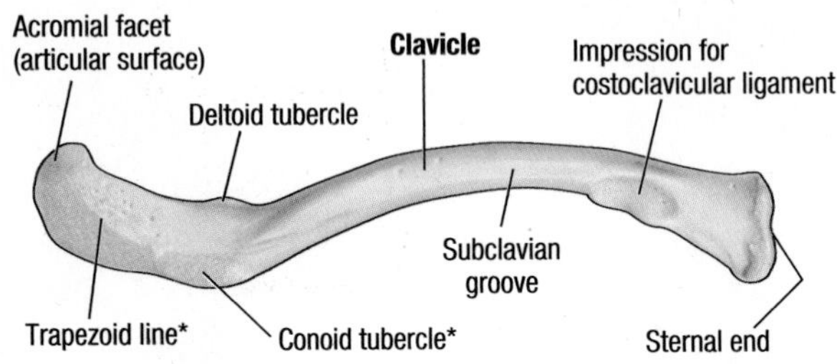
Acromial facet (articular surface)
Clavicle
Impression for costoclavicular ligament
Deltoid tubercle
Subclavian groove
Trapezoid line*
Conoid tubercle*
Sternal end

B. Inferior Surface

*Tuberosity for coracoclavicular ligament (conoid and trapezoid parts)

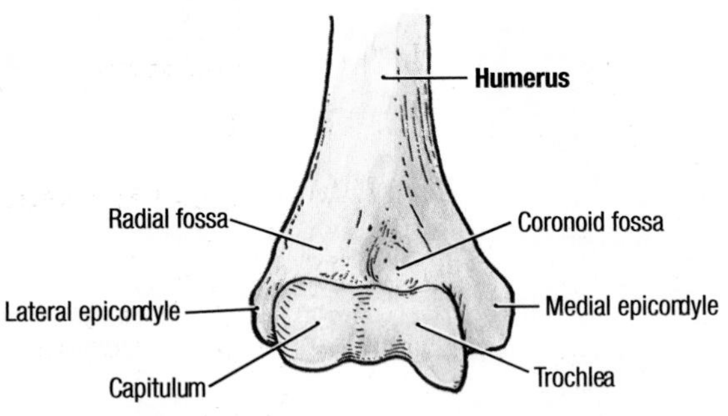
Humerus
Radial fossa
Coronoid fossa
Lateral epicondyle
Medial epicondyle
Capitulum
Trochlea

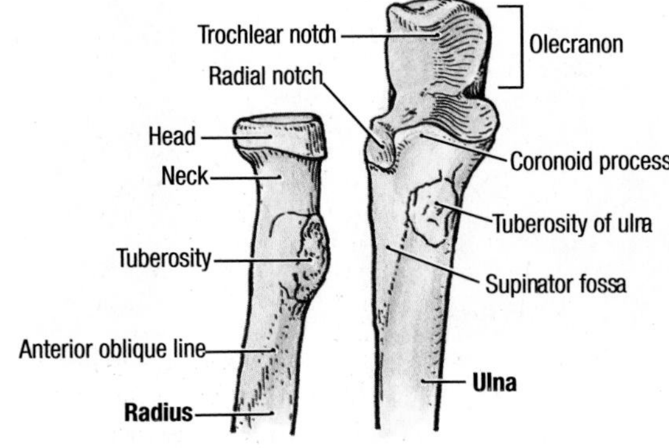
Trochlear notch
Olecranon
Radial notch
Head
Coronoid process
Neck
Tuberosity of ulna
Tuberosity
Supinator fossa
Anterior oblique line
Ulna
Radius

C. Anterior View

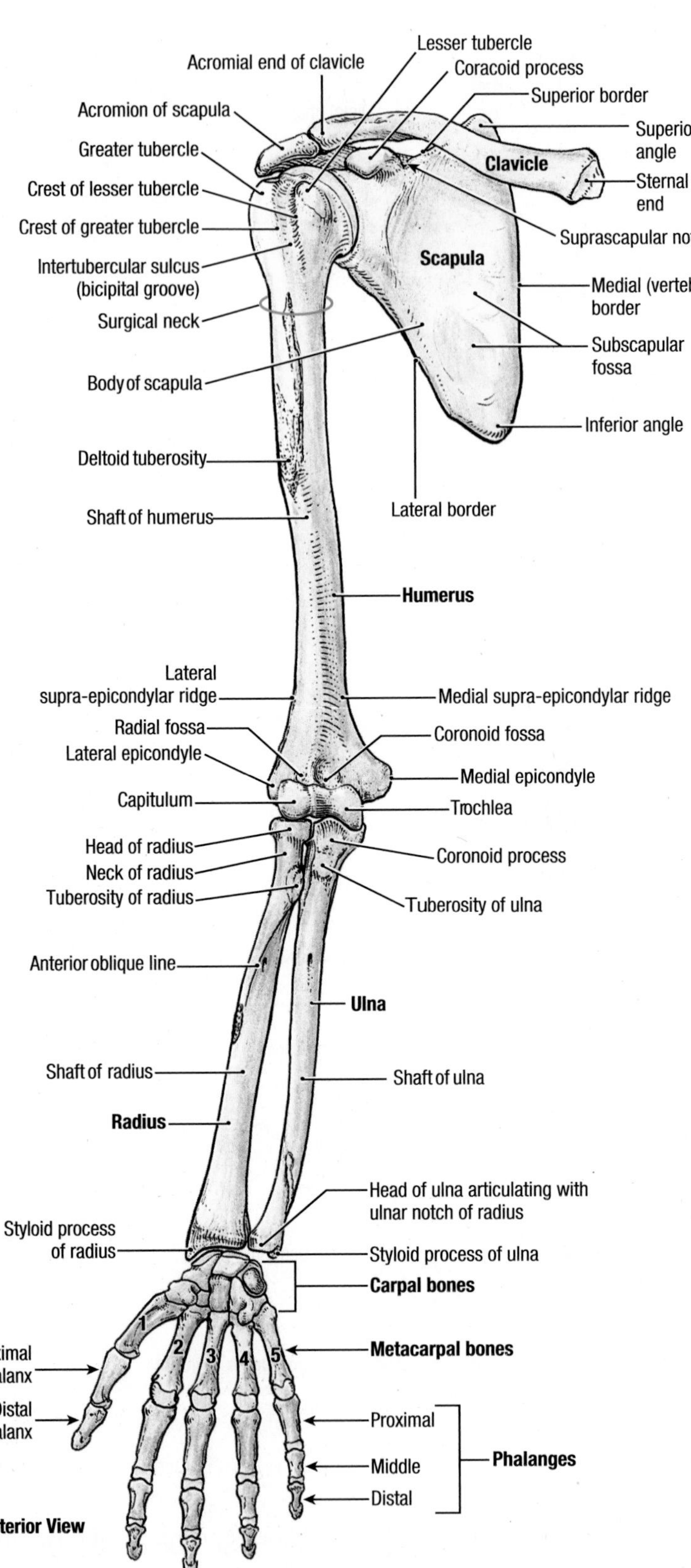
Lesser tubercle
Acromial end of clavicle
Coracoid process
Superior border
Acromion of scapula
Superior angle
Greater tubercle
Clavicle
Sternal end
Crest of lesser tubercle
Crest of greater tubercle
Suprascapular notch
Scapula
Intertubercular sulcus (bicipital groove)
Medial (vertebral) border
Surgical neck
Subscapular fossa
Body of scapula
Inferior angle
Deltoid tuberosity
Shaft of humerus
Lateral border
Humerus
Lateral supra-epicondylar ridge
Medial supra-epicondylar ridge
Radial fossa
Coronoid fossa
Lateral epicondyle
Medial epicondyle
Capitulum
Trochlea
Head of radius
Coronoid process
Neck of radius
Tuberosity of radius
Tuberosity of ulna
Anterior oblique line
Ulna
Shaft of radius
Shaft of ulna
Radius
Head of ulna articulating with ulnar notch of radius
Styloid process of radius
Styloid process of ulna
Carpal bones
1
2
3
4
5
Proximal phalanx
Metacarpal bones
Distal phalanx
Proximal
Middle
Distal
Phalanges

D. Anterior View

6.3 FEATURES OF BONES OF UPPER LIMB

A. and B. Clavicle. **C.** Anterior aspect of disarticulated distal end of humerus and proximal end of radius and ulna. **D.** Anterior aspect of articulated upper limb.

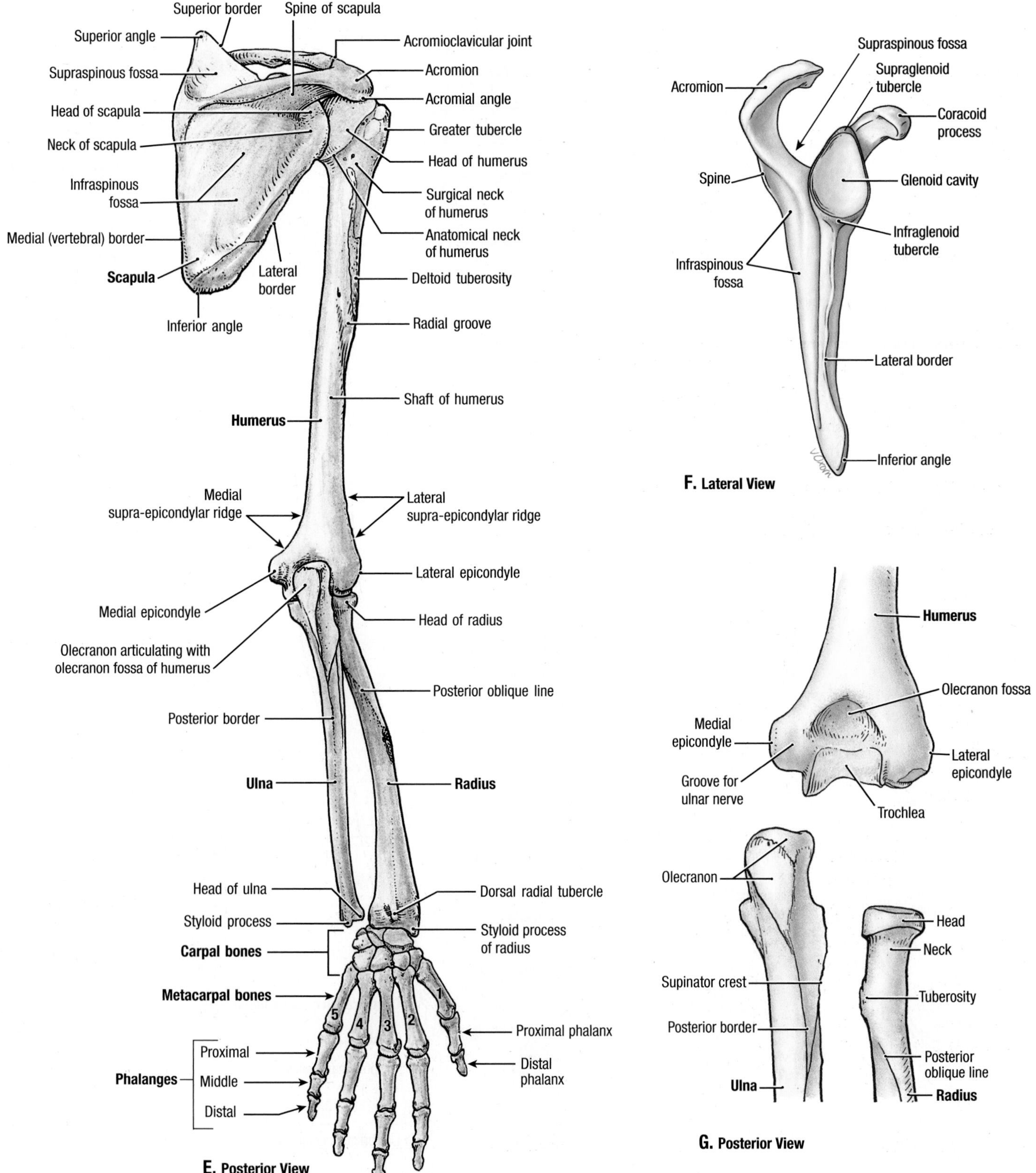
Superior border
Spine of scapula
Superior angle
Acromioclavicular joint
Supraspinous fossa
Acromion
Head of scapula
Acromial angle
Neck of scapula
Greater tubercle
Head of humerus
Infraspinous fossa
Surgical neck of humerus
Anatomical neck of humerus
Medial (vertebral) border
Scapula
Lateral border
Deltoid tuberosity
Inferior angle
Radial groove
Shaft of humerus
Humerus
Medial supra-epicondylar ridge
Lateral supra-epicondylar ridge
Lateral epicondyle
Medial epicondyle
Head of radius
Olecranon articulating with olecranon fossa of humerus
Posterior oblique line
Posterior border
Ulna
Radius
Head of ulna
Dorsal radial tubercle
Styloid process
Styloid process of radius
Carpal bones
Metacarpal bones
1
5
4
3
2
Proximal phalanx
Phalanges
Proximal
Middle
Distal
Distal phalanx
E. Posterior View
Supraspinous fossa
Supraglenoid tubercle
Acromion
Coracoid process
Spine
Glenoid cavity
Infraglenoid tubercle
Infraspinous fossa
Lateral border
Inferior angle
F. Lateral View
Humerus
Olecranon fossa
Medial epicondyle
Lateral epicondyle
Groove for ulnar nerve
Trochlea
Olecranon
Head
Neck
Supinator crest
Tuberosity
Posterior border
Posterior oblique line
Ulna
Radius
G. Posterior View

6.3 FEATURES OF BONES OF UPPER LIMB *(CONTINUED)*

E. Posterior aspect of articulated upper limb bones. **F.** Lateral aspect of scapula. **G.** Posterior aspect of disarticulated distal end of humerus and proximal ends of radius and ulna.

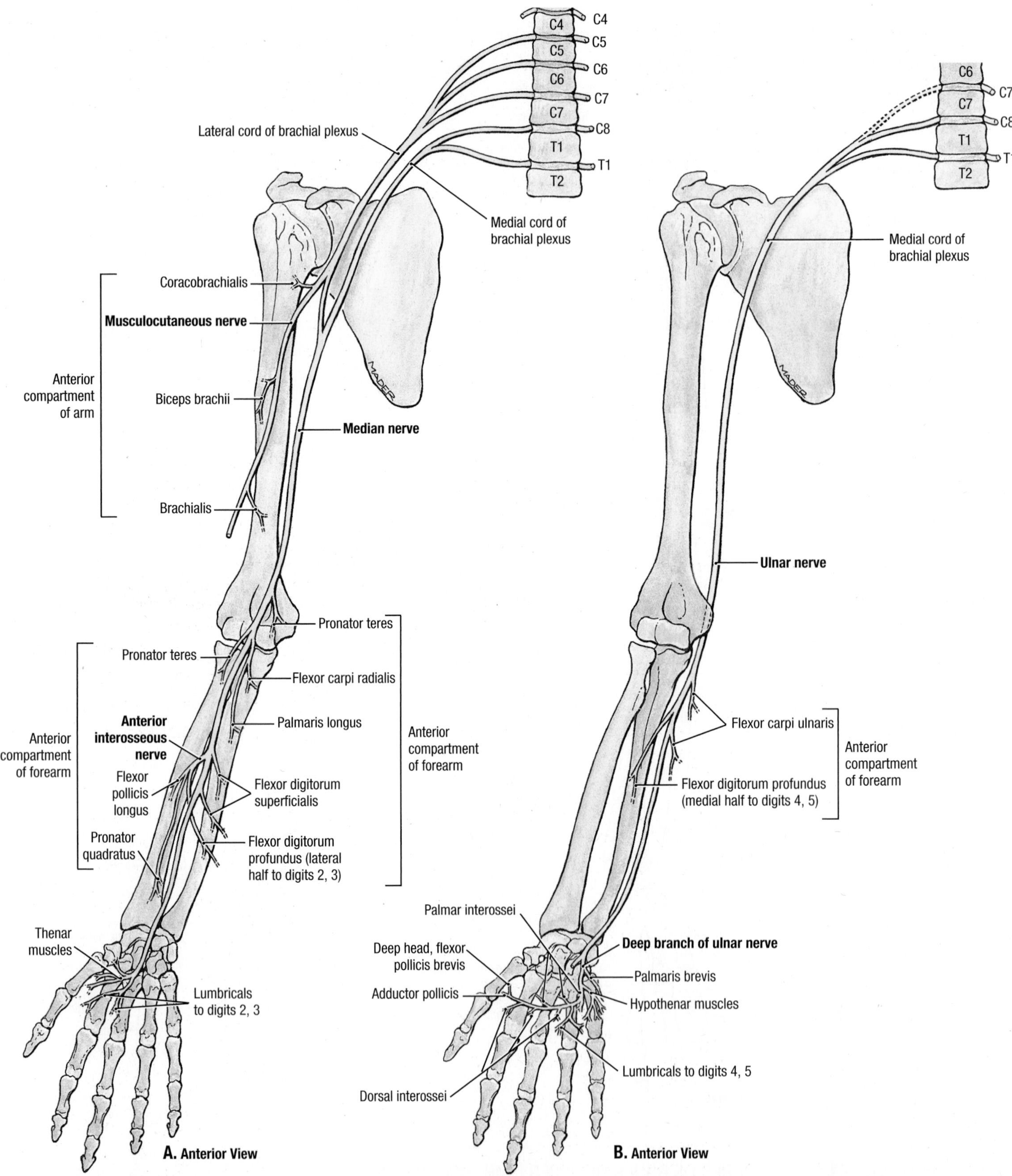
C4
C5
C6
C7
C8
T1
T2
Lateral cord of brachial plexus
Medial cord of brachial plexus
Coracobrachialis
Musculocutaneous nerve
Anterior compartment of arm
Biceps brachii
Median nerve
Brachialis
MADER
Pronator teres
Pronator teres
Flexor carpi radialis
Anterior compartment of forearm
Anterior interosseous nerve
Palmaris longus
Flexor pollicis longus
Flexor digitorum superficialis
Anterior compartment of forearm
Pronator quadratus
Flexor digitorum profundus (lateral half to digits 2, 3)
Thenar muscles
Lumbricals to digits 2, 3
A. Anterior View
C6
C7
C8
T1
T2
Medial cord of brachial plexus
Ulnar nerve
Flexor carpi ulnaris
Anterior compartment of forearm
Flexor digitorum profundus (medial half to digits 4, 5)
Palmar interossei
Deep head, flexor pollicis brevis
Deep branch of ulnar nerve
Palmaris brevis
Adductor pollicis
Hypothenar muscles
Lumbricals to digits 4, 5
Dorsal interossei
B. Anterior View

6.4 OVERVIEW OF MOTOR INNERVATION OF UPPER LIMB

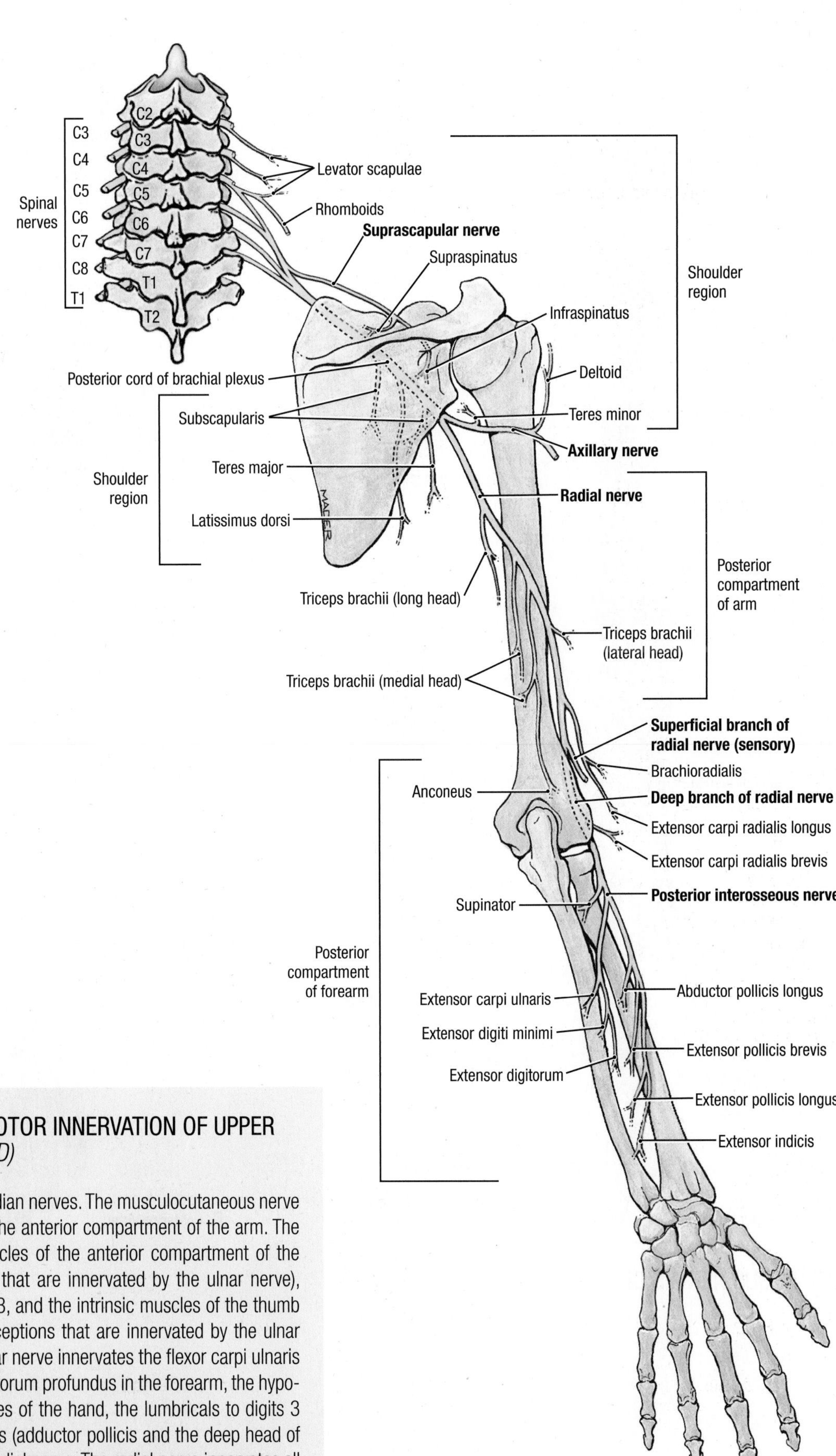
C2
C3
C4
C5
C6
C7
C8
T1
T2
Spinal nerves
Levator scapulae
Rhomboids
Suprascapular nerve
Supraspinatus
Shoulder region
Infraspinatus
Posterior cord of brachial plexus
Deltoid
Subscapularis
Teres minor
Axillary nerve
Teres major
Shoulder region
Radial nerve
Latissimus dorsi
Posterior compartment of arm
Triceps brachii (long head)
Triceps brachii (lateral head)
Triceps brachii (medial head)
Superficial branch of radial nerve (sensory)
Brachioradialis
Anconeus
Deep branch of radial nerve
Extensor carpi radialis longus
Extensor carpi radialis brevis
Supinator
Posterior interosseous nerve
Posterior compartment of forearm
Extensor carpi ulnaris
Abductor pollicis longus
Extensor digiti minimi
Extensor pollicis brevis
Extensor digitorum
Extensor pollicis longus
Extensor indicis

C. Posterior View

6.4 OVERVIEW OF MOTOR INNERVATION OF UPPER LIMB *(CONTINUED)*

A. Musculocutaneous and median nerves. The musculocutaneous nerve innervates all the muscles of the anterior compartment of the arm. The median nerve innervates muscles of the anterior compartment of the forearm (with $1^1/_2$ exceptions that are innervated by the ulnar nerve), the lumbricals to digits 2 and 3, and the intrinsic muscles of the thumb (thenar muscles) with $1^1/_2$ exceptions that are innervated by the ulnar nerve. **B.** Ulnar nerve. The ulnar nerve innervates the flexor carpi ulnaris and ulnar half of the flexor digitorum profundus in the forearm, the hypothenar and interosseus muscles of the hand, the lumbricals to digits 3 and 4, and $1^1/_2$ thenar muscles (adductor pollicis and the deep head of the flexor pollicis brevis). **C.** Radial nerve. The radial nerve innervates all muscles of the posterior compartments of the arm and forearm.

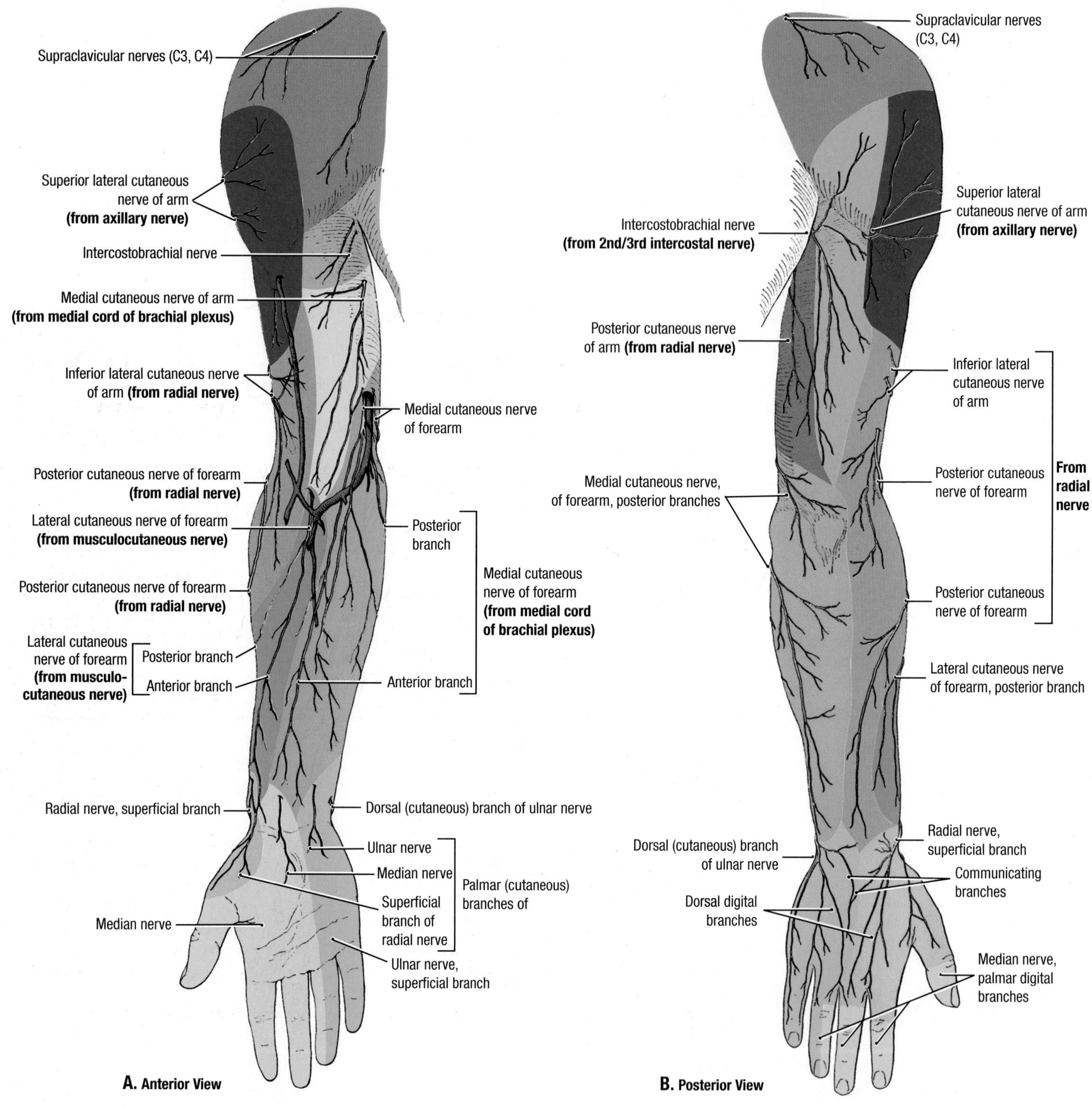
Supraclavicular nerves (C3, C4)
Superior lateral cutaneous nerve of arm **(from axillary nerve)**
Intercostobrachial nerve
Medial cutaneous nerve of arm **(from medial cord of brachial plexus)**
Inferior lateral cutaneous nerve of arm **(from radial nerve)**
Medial cutaneous nerve of forearm
Posterior cutaneous nerve of forearm **(from radial nerve)**
Lateral cutaneous nerve of forearm **(from musculocutaneous nerve)**
Posterior branch
Medial cutaneous nerve of forearm **(from medial cord of brachial plexus)**
Posterior cutaneous nerve of forearm **(from radial nerve)**
Lateral cutaneous nerve of forearm **(from musculo-cutaneous nerve)**
Posterior branch
Anterior branch
Anterior branch
Radial nerve, superficial branch
Dorsal (cutaneous) branch of ulnar nerve
Ulnar nerve
Median nerve
Superficial branch of radial nerve
Palmar (cutaneous) branches of
Median nerve
Ulnar nerve, superficial branch
A. **Anterior View**
Supraclavicular nerves (C3, C4)
Superior lateral cutaneous nerve of arm **(from axillary nerve)**
Intercostobrachial nerve **(from 2nd/3rd intercostal nerve)**
Posterior cutaneous nerve of arm **(from radial nerve)**
Inferior lateral cutaneous nerve of arm
Medial cutaneous nerve, of forearm, posterior branches
Posterior cutaneous nerve of forearm
From radial nerve
Posterior cutaneous nerve of forearm
Lateral cutaneous nerve of forearm, posterior branch
Radial nerve, superficial branch
Dorsal (cutaneous) branch of ulnar nerve
Communicating branches
Dorsal digital branches
Median nerve, palmar digital branches
B. **Posterior View**

6.5 CUTANEOUS NERVES OF UPPER LIMB

TABLE 6.1 CUTANEOUS NERVES OF UPPER LIMB[a]

Nerve	Spinal Nerve components	Source	Course/Distribution
Supraclavicular nerves	C3–C4	Cervical plexus	Pass anterior to clavicle, immediately deep to platysma, and supply the skin over the clavicle and superolateral aspect of the pectoralis major muscle
Superior lateral cutaneous nerve of arm	C5–C6	Axillary nerve (posterior cord of brachial plexus)	Emerges from posterior margin of deltoid to supply skin over lower part of this muscle and the lateral side of the midarm
Inferior lateral cutaneous nerve of arm		Radial nerve (posterior cord of brachial plexus)	Arises with the posterior cutaneous nerve of forearm; pierces lateral head of triceps brachii to supply skin over the inferolateral aspect of the arm
Posterior cutaneous nerve of arm			Arises in axilla and supplies skin on posterior surface of the arm to olecranon
Posterior cutaneous nerve of forearm	C5–C8		Arises with the inferior lateral cutaneous nerve of the arm; pierces lateral head of triceps brachii to supply skin over the posterior aspect of the arm
Superficial branch of radial nerve	C6–C7		Arises in cubital fossa; supplies lateral (radial) half of the dorsal aspect of hand and thumb, and proximal portion of the dorsal aspects of digits 2 and 3, and the lateral (radial) half of dorsal aspect of digit 4
Lateral cutaneous nerve of forearm		Musculocutaneous nerve (lateral cord of brachial plexus)	Arises between biceps brachii and brachialis muscle as continuation of musculocutaneous nerve distal to branch to brachialis; emerges in cubital fossa lateral to biceps tendon and median cubital vein; supplies skin along radial (lateral) border of forearm to base of thenar eminence
Median nerve	C6–C7 (via lateral root); C8–T1 (via medial root)	Lateral and medial cords of brachial plexus	Courses with brachial artery in arm and deep to flexor digitorum superficialis in forearm; distal to origin of palmar cutaneous branch, traverses carpal tunnel to supply skin of palmar aspect of radial $3^{1}/_{2}$ digits and adjacent palm, plus distal dorsal aspects of same, including nail beds
Ulnar nerve	(C7), C8–T1	Medial cord of brachial plexus	Courses with brachial, superior ulnar collateral, and ulnar arteries; supplies skin of palmar and dorsal aspects of medial (ulnar) $1^{1}/_{2}$ digits and palm and dorsum of hand proximal to those digits
Medial cutaneous nerve of forearm	C8–T1		Pierces deep fascia with basilic vein in midarm; divides into anterior and posterior branches supplying skin over anterior and medial surfaces of forearm to wrist
Medial cutaneous nerve of arm	C8–T2		Smallest and most medial branch of brachial plexus; communicates with intercostobrachial nerve, then descends medial to brachial artery and basilic vein to innervate skin of distal medial arm
Intercostobrachial nerve	T2	Lateral cutaneous branch of 2nd intercostal nerve	Arises distal to angle of 2nd rib; supplies skin of axilla and proximal medial arm

[a]See Table 6.16 on Lesions of nerves of upper limb at end of chapter.

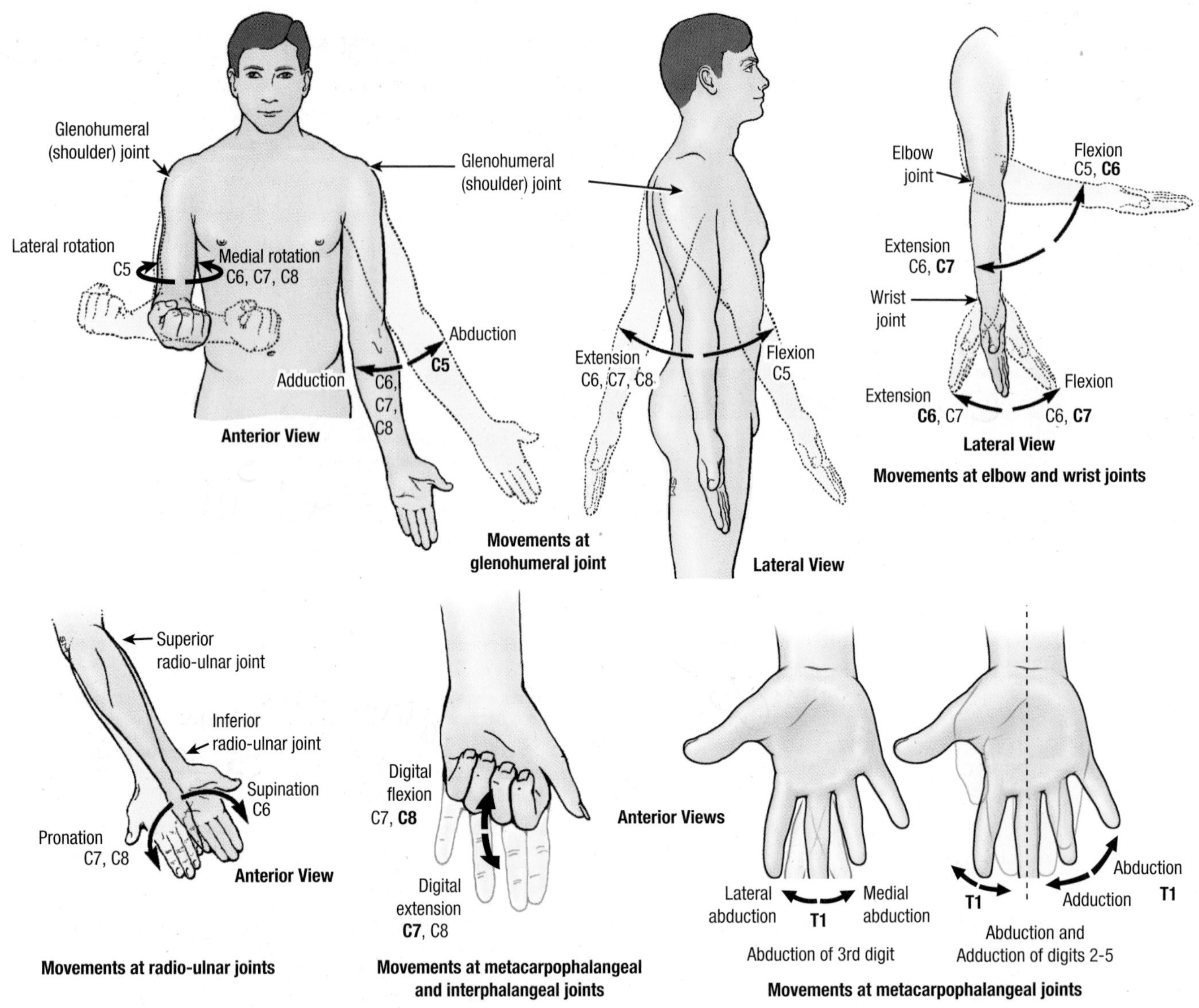
Glenohumeral (shoulder) joint
Glenohumeral (shoulder) joint
Lateral rotation C5
Medial rotation C6, C7, C8
Abduction C5
Adduction C6, C7, C8
Anterior View
Extension C6, C7, C8
Flexion C5
Movements at glenohumeral joint
Lateral View
Elbow joint
Flexion C5, C6
Extension C6, C7
Wrist joint
Extension C6, C7
Flexion C6, C7
Lateral View
Movements at elbow and wrist joints
Superior radio-ulnar joint
Inferior radio-ulnar joint
Supination C6
Pronation C7, C8
Anterior View
Movements at radio-ulnar joints
Digital flexion C7, C8
Digital extension C7, C8
Movements at metacarpophalangeal and interphalangeal joints
Anterior Views
Lateral abduction
T1
Medial abduction
Abduction of 3rd digit
T1
Abduction
Adduction
T1
Abduction and Adduction of digits 2-5
Movements at metacarpophalangeal joints

6.6 MYOTOMES AND MYOTATIC (DEEP TENDON STRETCH) REFLEXES

Myotomes. Somatic motor (general somatic efferent) fibers transmit impulses to skeletal (voluntary) muscles. The unilateral muscle mass receiving information from the somatic motor fibers conveyed by a single spinal nerve is a myotome. The movements associated with each bolded segment in Table 6.2 are most commonly tested to determine the neurologic level of a lesion.

Myotatic reflexes. A myotatic reflex (deep tendon or stretch reflex) is an involuntary contraction of a muscle in response to sudden stretching. Myotatic reflexes are elicited by briskly tapping the tendon with a reflex hammer. Each tendon reflex is mediated by specific spinal nerves. Stretch reflexes control muscle tone.

TABLE 6.2 CLINICAL MANIFESTATIONS OF NERVE ROOT COMPRESSION: UPPER LIMB (UL)

Herniated Disc Between	Compressed Nerve Roots	Dermatomes Affected	Muscles Affected	Movement Weakness	Nerve and Myotatic Reflex Involved
C4 and C5	**C5**	C5 Shoulder Lateral surface UL	Deltoid	Abduction of shoulder	Axillary nerve ↓ Biceps jerk
C5 and C6	**C6**	C6 Thumb	Biceps Brachialis Brachioradialis	Flexion of elbow Supination/pronation of forearm	Musculocutaneous nerve ↓ Biceps jerk ↓ Brachioradialis jerk
C6 and C7	**C7**	C7 Posterior surface UL Middle and index fingers	Triceps Wrist extensors	Extension of elbow Extension of wrist	Radial nerve ↓ Triceps reflex

TABLE 6.3 DERMATOMES OF UPPER LIMB

Spinal Segment/Nerve(s)	Description of Dermatome(s)
C3, C4	Region at base of neck extending laterally over shoulder
C5	Lateral aspect of arm (i.e., superior aspect of abducted arm)
C6	Lateral forearm and thumb
C7	Middle and ring fingers (or middle 3 fingers) and center of posterior aspect of forearm
C8	Little finger, medial side of hand and forearm (i.e., inferior aspect of abducted arm)
T1	Medial aspect of forearm and inferior arm
T2	Medial aspect of superior arm and skin of axilla[a]

[a]Not indicated on the Keegan and Garrett dermatome map. However, pain experienced during a heart attack, considered to be mediated by T1 and T2, is commonly described as "radiating down the medial side of the left arm").

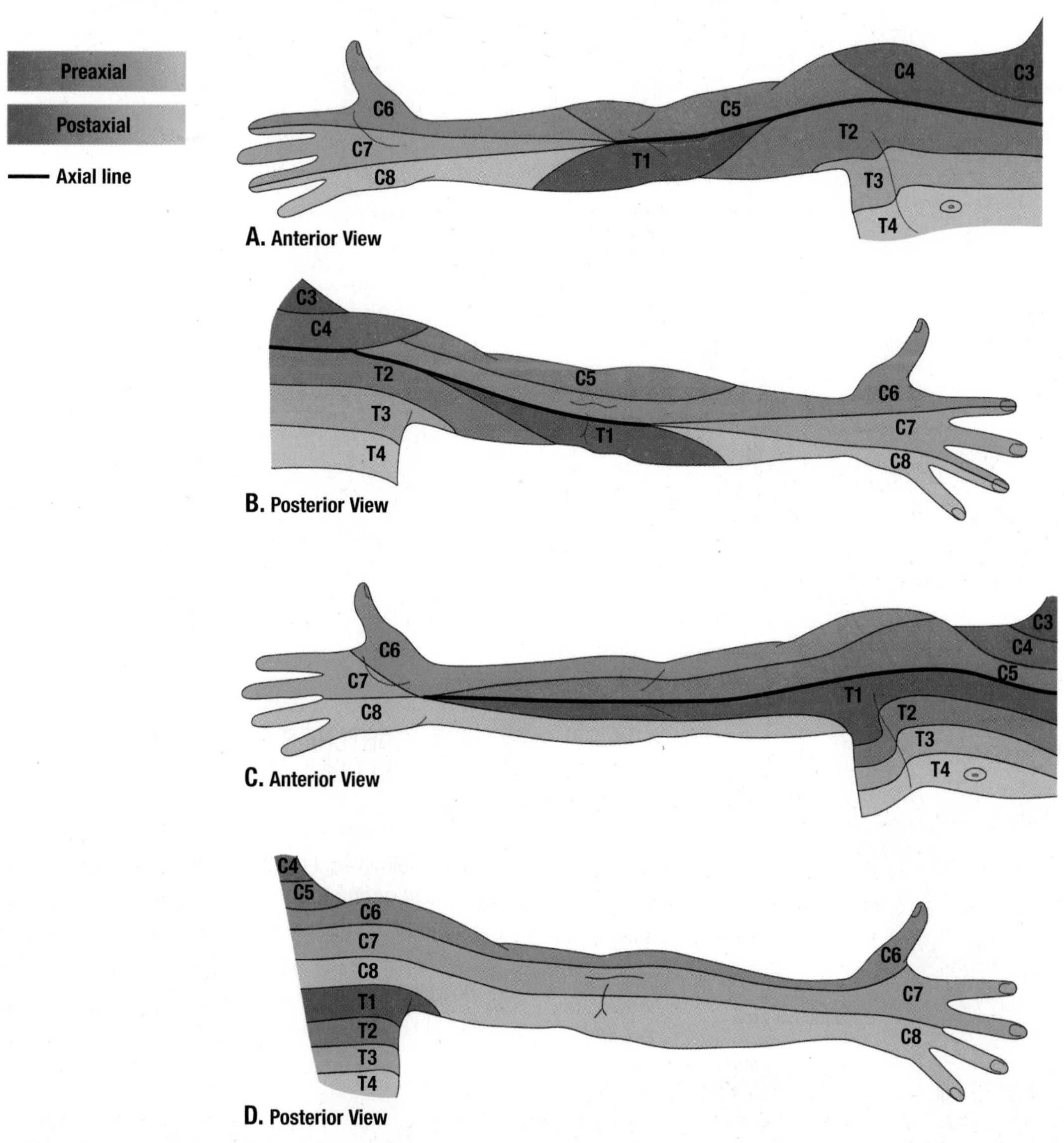
Preaxial
Postaxial
Axial line
C3
C4
C5
C6
C7
C8
T1
T2
T3
T4
A. Anterior View
B. Posterior View
C. Anterior View
D. Posterior View

6.7 DERMATOMES OF UPPER LIMB

The dermatomal or segmental pattern of distribution of sensory nerve fibers persists despite the merging of spinal nerves in plexus formation during development. Two different dermatome maps are commonly used. **A.** and **B.** The dermatome pattern of the upper limb according to Foerster (1933) is preferred by many because of its correlation with clinical findings. In the Foerster schema, dermatomes C6–T1 are displaced from the trunk to limbs. **C.** and **D.** The dermatome pattern of the upper limb according to Keegan and Garrett (1948) is preferred by others for its correlation with development. Although depicted as distinct zones, adjacent dermatomes overlap considerably except along the axial line.

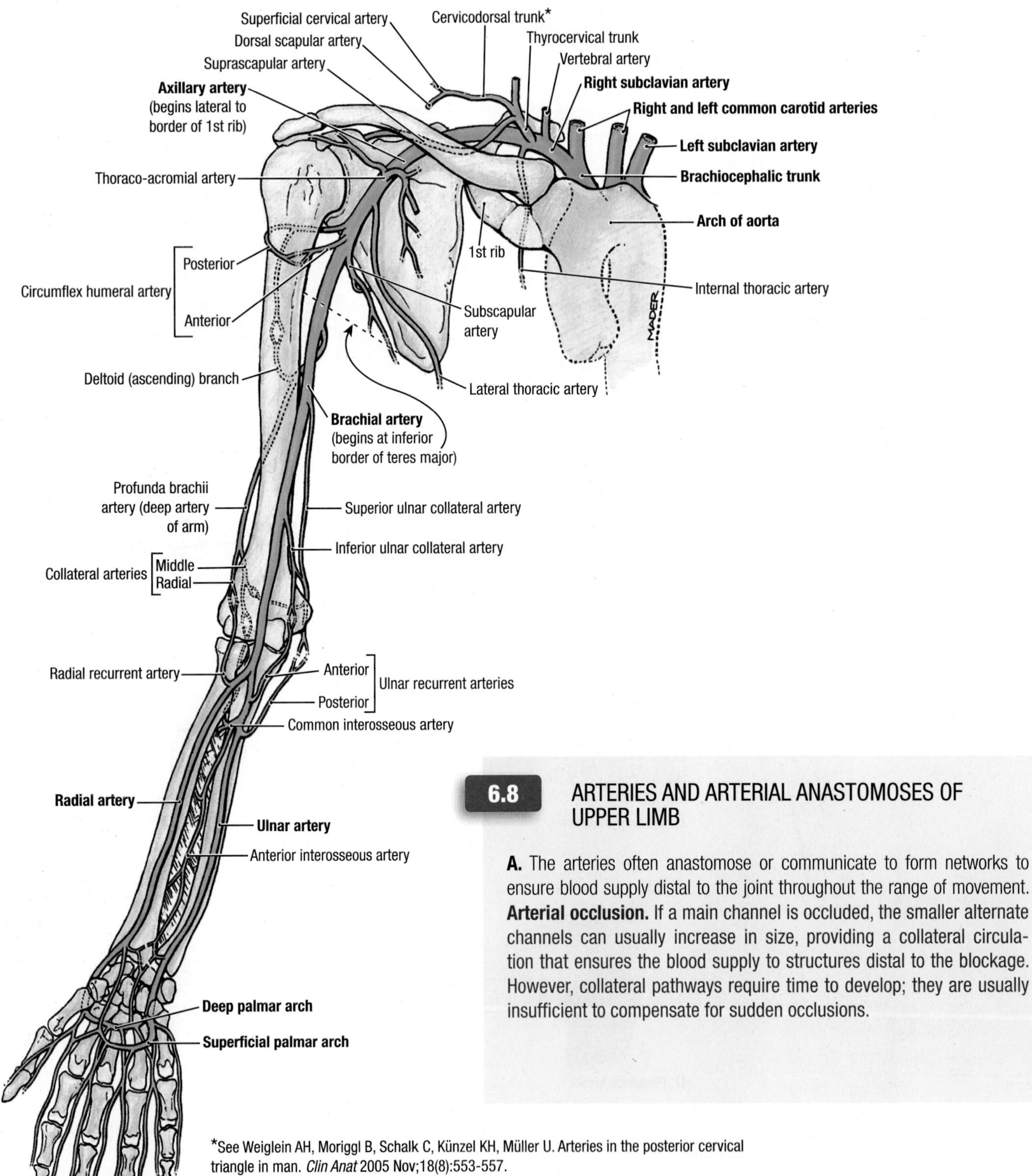
Superficial cervical artery
Cervicodorsal trunk*
Thyrocervical trunk
Dorsal scapular artery
Vertebral artery
Suprascapular artery
Right subclavian artery
Axillary artery
(begins lateral to border of 1st rib)
Right and left common carotid arteries
Left subclavian artery
Thoraco-acromial artery
Brachiocephalic trunk
Arch of aorta
1st rib
Posterior
Circumflex humeral artery
Anterior
Internal thoracic artery
Subscapular artery
Deltoid (ascending) branch
Lateral thoracic artery
Brachial artery
(begins at inferior border of teres major)
Profunda brachii artery (deep artery of arm)
Superior ulnar collateral artery
Inferior ulnar collateral artery
Collateral arteries
Middle
Radial
Radial recurrent artery
Anterior
Ulnar recurrent arteries
Posterior
Common interosseous artery
Radial artery
Ulnar artery
Anterior interosseous artery
Deep palmar arch
Superficial palmar arch
MADER

A. Anterior View

6.8 ARTERIES AND ARTERIAL ANASTOMOSES OF UPPER LIMB

A. The arteries often anastomose or communicate to form networks to ensure blood supply distal to the joint throughout the range of movement. **Arterial occlusion.** If a main channel is occluded, the smaller alternate channels can usually increase in size, providing a collateral circulation that ensures the blood supply to structures distal to the blockage. However, collateral pathways require time to develop; they are usually insufficient to compensate for sudden occlusions.

*See Weiglein AH, Moriggl B, Schalk C, Künzel KH, Müller U. Arteries in the posterior cervical triangle in man. *Clin Anat* 2005 Nov;18(8):553-557.

Dorsal scapular artery
Levator scapulae
Rhomboid minor
Suprascapular artery
Anastomoses with intercostal arteries
Axillary artery
Subscapular artery
Circumflex scapular artery
Thoracodorsal artery
Brachial artery
Teres major

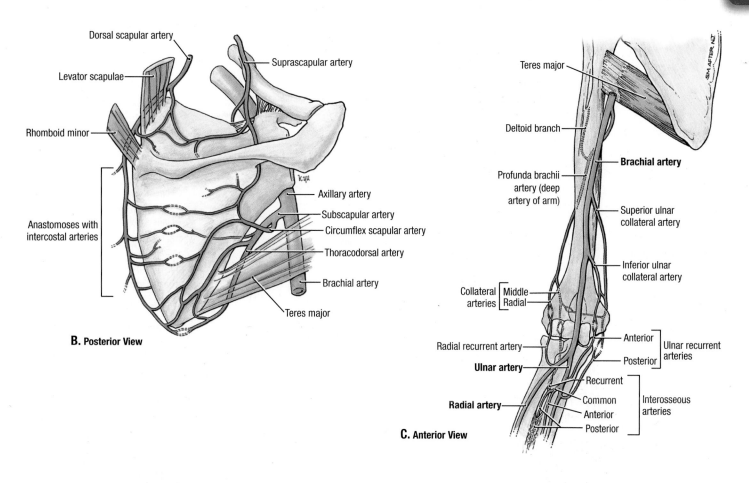

B. **Posterior View**

Teres major
Deltoid branch
Brachial artery
Profunda brachii artery (deep artery of arm)
Superior ulnar collateral artery
Inferior ulnar collateral artery
Collateral arteries: Middle, Radial
Radial recurrent artery
Ulnar artery
Radial artery
Ulnar recurrent arteries: Anterior, Posterior
Interosseous arteries: Recurrent, Common, Anterior, Posterior

C. **Anterior View**

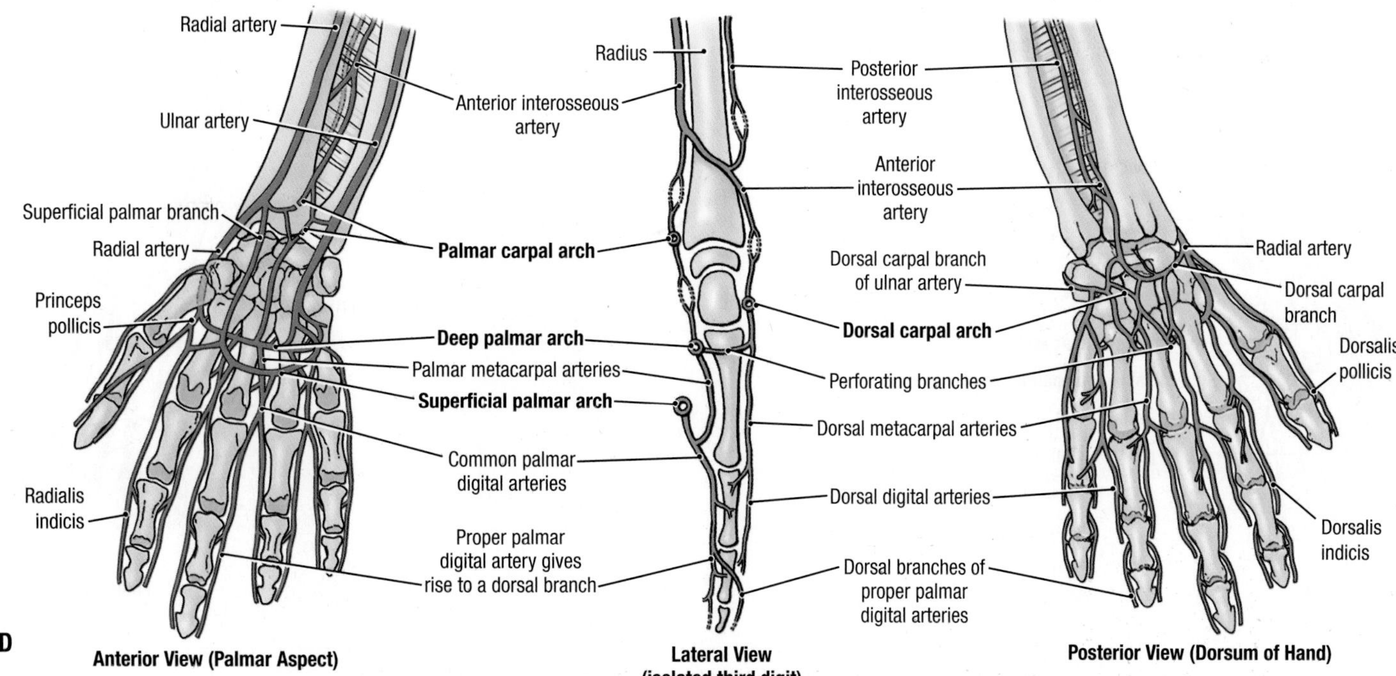
Radial artery
Ulnar artery
Anterior interosseous artery
Superficial palmar branch
Radial artery
Princeps pollicis
Palmar carpal arch
Deep palmar arch
Palmar metacarpal arteries
Superficial palmar arch
Common palmar digital arteries
Radialis indicis
Proper palmar digital artery gives rise to a dorsal branch
Radius
Posterior interosseous artery
Anterior interosseous artery
Dorsal carpal branch of ulnar artery
Dorsal carpal arch
Perforating branches
Dorsal metacarpal arteries
Dorsal digital arteries
Dorsal branches of proper palmar digital arteries
Radial artery
Dorsal carpal branch
Dorsalis pollicis
Dorsalis indicis
D
Anterior View (Palmar Aspect)
Lateral View (isolated third digit)
Posterior View (Dorsum of Hand)

6.8 ARTERIES AND ARTERIAL ANASTOMOSES OF UPPER LIMB *(CONTINUED)*

B. Scapular anastomoses. **C.** Anastomoses of the elbow. **D.** Anastomoses of the hand. Joints receive blood from articular arteries that arise from vessels around joints.

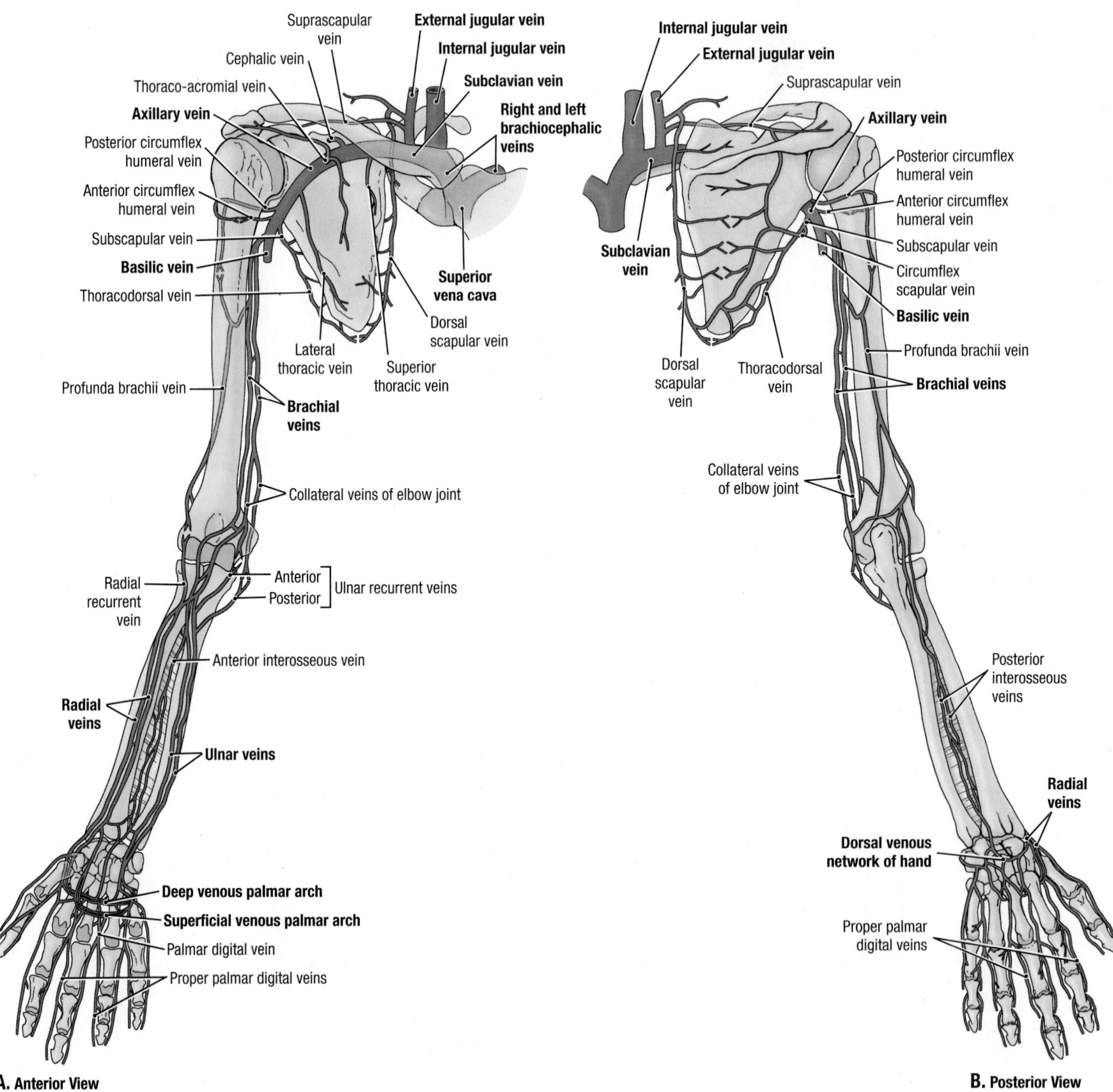
Suprascapular vein
External jugular vein
Internal jugular vein
Cephalic vein
Thoraco-acromial vein
Subclavian vein
Axillary vein
Right and left brachiocephalic veins
Posterior circumflex humeral vein
Anterior circumflex humeral vein
Subscapular vein
Basilic vein
Superior vena cava
Thoracodorsal vein
Dorsal scapular vein
Lateral thoracic vein
Superior thoracic vein
Profunda brachii vein
Brachial veins
Collateral veins of elbow joint
Radial recurrent vein
Anterior
Posterior
Ulnar recurrent veins
Anterior interosseous vein
Radial veins
Ulnar veins
Deep venous palmar arch
Superficial venous palmar arch
Palmar digital vein
Proper palmar digital veins
A. Anterior View
Internal jugular vein
External jugular vein
Suprascapular vein
Axillary vein
Posterior circumflex humeral vein
Anterior circumflex humeral vein
Subclavian vein
Subscapular vein
Circumflex scapular vein
Basilic vein
Profunda brachii vein
Dorsal scapular vein
Thoracodorsal vein
Brachial veins
Collateral veins of elbow joint
Posterior interosseous veins
Radial veins
Dorsal venous network of hand
Proper palmar digital veins
B. Posterior View

6.9 OVERVIEW OF DEEP VEINS OF UPPER LIMB

Deep veins lie internal to the deep fascia and occur as paired, continually interanastomosing "accompanying veins" (L., *venae comitantes*) surrounding and sharing the name of the artery they accompany.

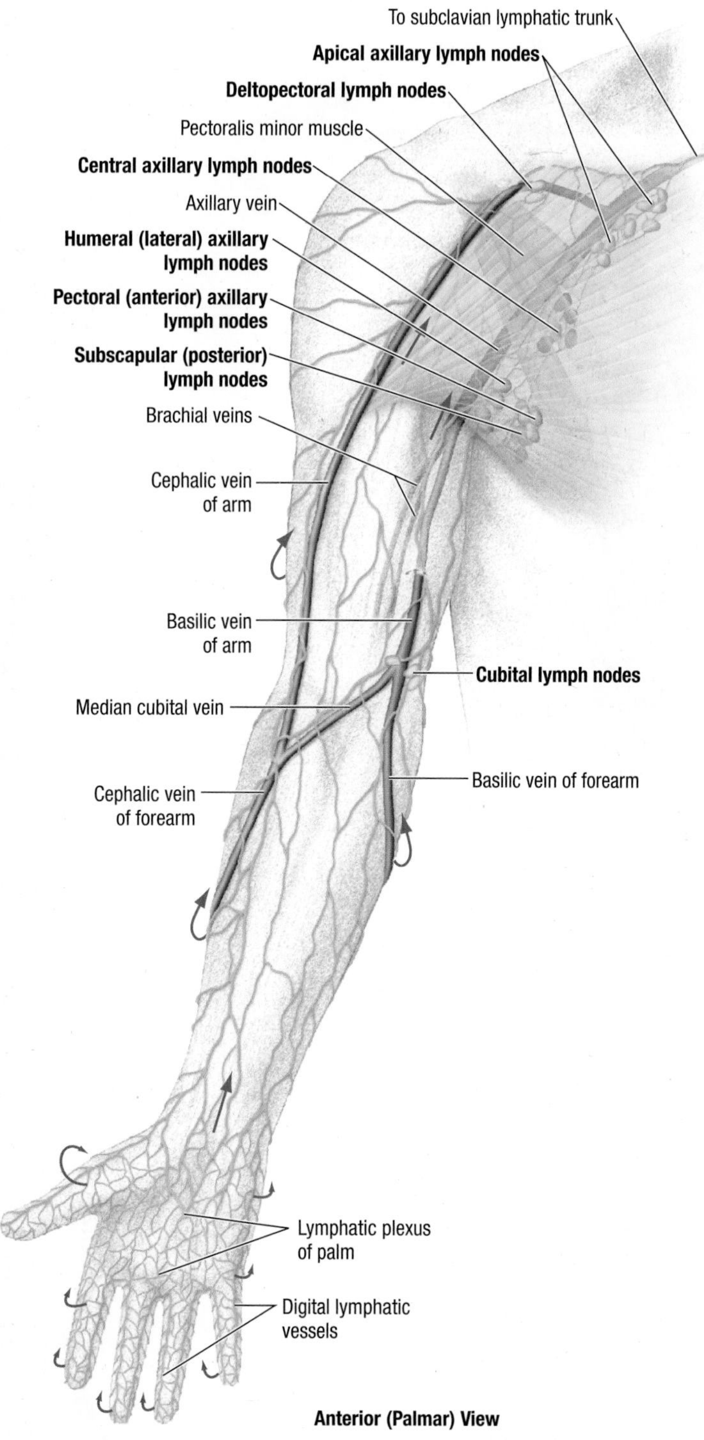
To subclavian lymphatic trunk
Apical axillary lymph nodes
Deltopectoral lymph nodes
Pectoralis minor muscle
Central axillary lymph nodes
Axillary vein
Humeral (lateral) axillary lymph nodes
Pectoral (anterior) axillary lymph nodes
Subscapular (posterior) lymph nodes
Brachial veins
Cephalic vein of arm
Basilic vein of arm
Cubital lymph nodes
Median cubital vein
Basilic vein of forearm
Cephalic vein of forearm
Lymphatic plexus of palm
Digital lymphatic vessels
Anterior (Palmar) View

6.10 SUPERFICIAL VENOUS AND LYMPHATIC DRAINAGE OF UPPER LIMB

Superficial lymphatic vessels arise from lymphatic plexuses in the digits, palm, and dorsum of the hand and ascend with the superficial veins of the upper limb. The superficial lymphatic vessels ascend through the forearm and arm, converging toward the cephalic and especially to the basilic vein to reach the axillary lymph nodes. Some lymph passes through the cubital nodes at the elbow and the deltopectoral (infraclavicular) nodes at the shoulder. Deep lymphatic vessels accompany the neurovascular bundles of the upper limb and end primarily in the humeral (lateral) and central axillary lymph nodes.

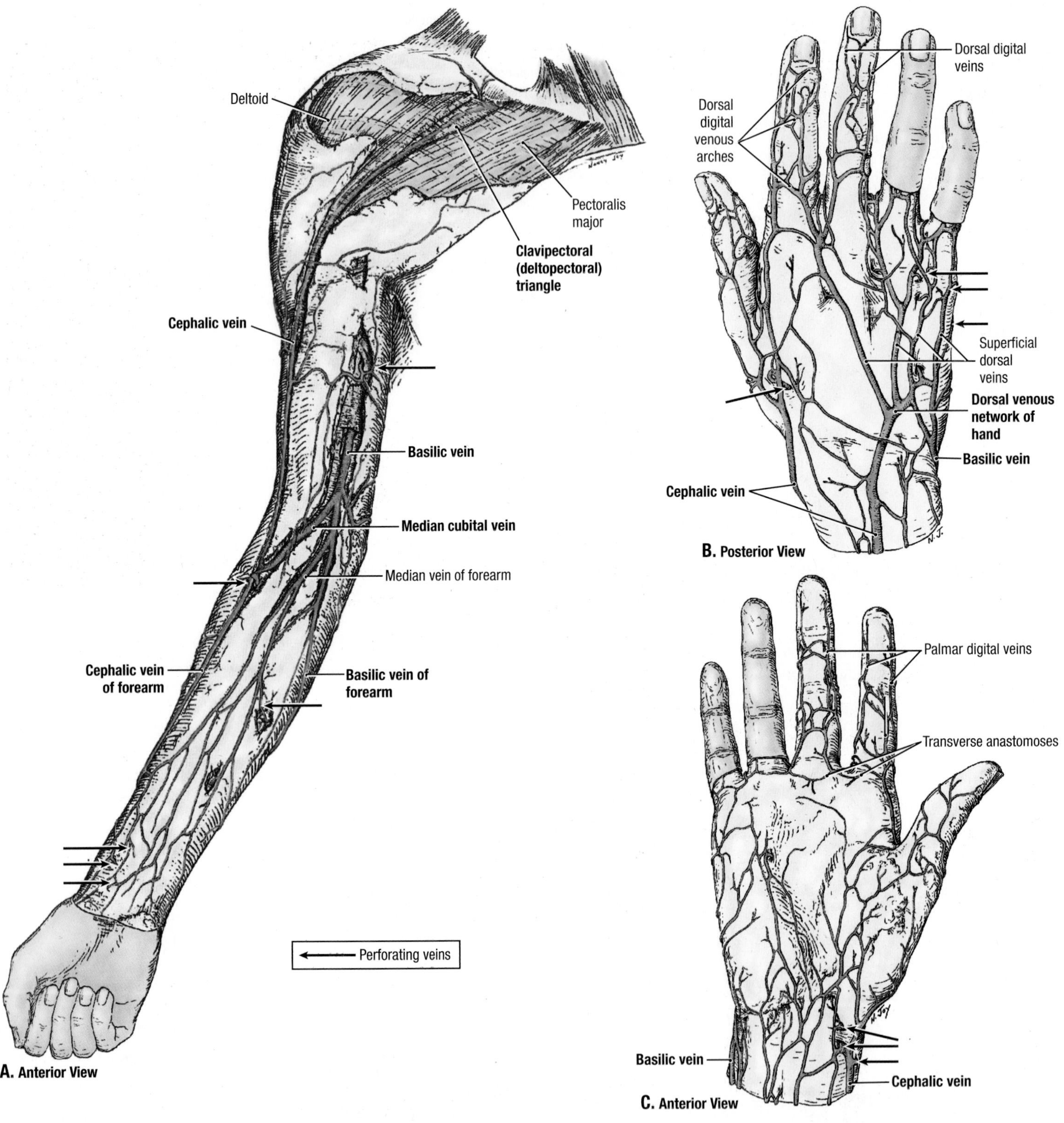
Deltoid
Pectoralis major
Clavipectoral (deltopectoral) triangle
Cephalic vein
Basilic vein
Median cubital vein
Median vein of forearm
Cephalic vein of forearm
Basilic vein of forearm
Perforating veins
A. Anterior View
Dorsal digital veins
Dorsal digital venous arches
Superficial dorsal veins
Dorsal venous network of hand
Basilic vein
Cephalic vein
B. Posterior View
Palmar digital veins
Transverse anastomoses
Basilic vein
Cephalic vein
C. Anterior View

6.11 SUPERFICIAL VENOUS DRAINAGE OF UPPER LIMB

A. Forearm, arm, and pectoral region. **B.** Dorsal surface of hand. **C.** Palmar surface of hand. The *arrows* indicate where perforating veins penetrate the deep fascia. Blood is continuously shunted from these superficial veins in the subcutaneous tissue to deep veins via the perforating veins.

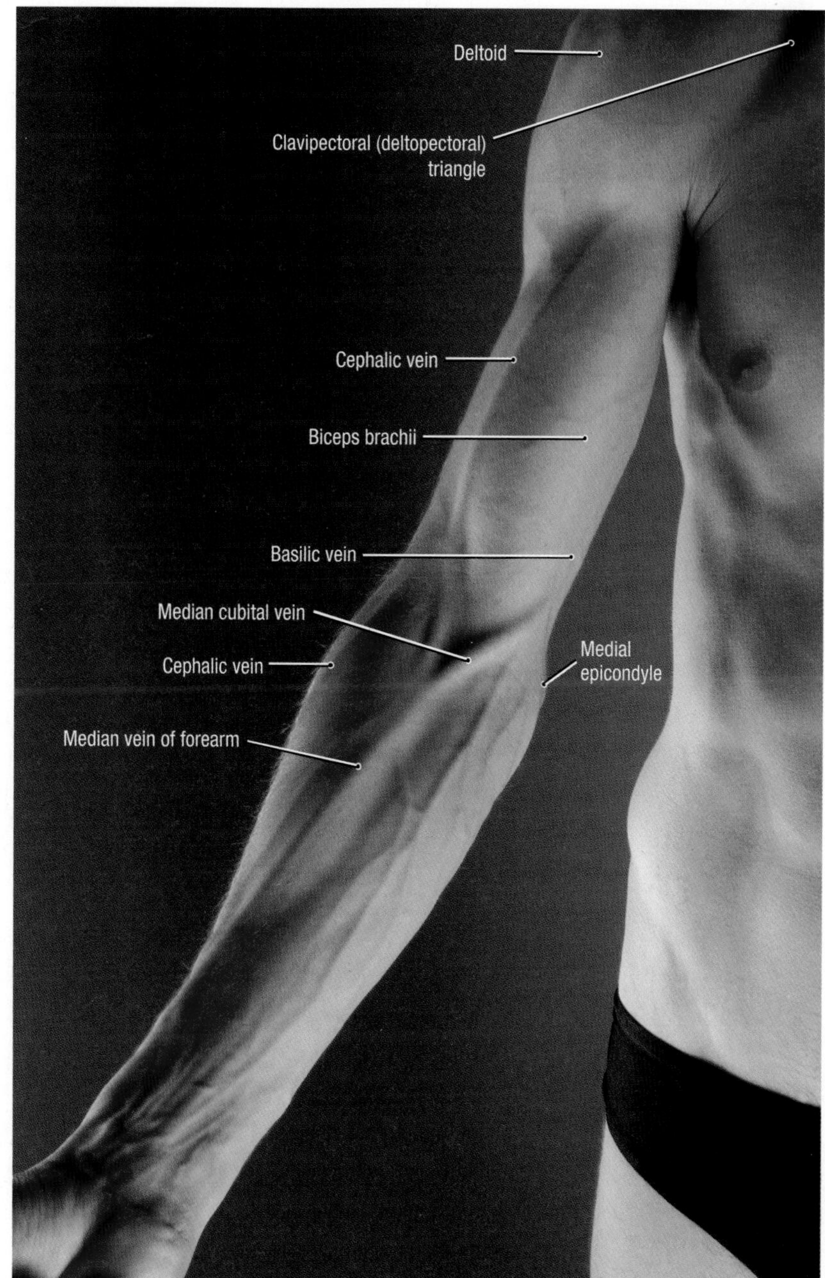
Deltoid
Clavipectoral (deltopectoral) triangle
Cephalic vein
Biceps brachii
Basilic vein
Median cubital vein
Cephalic vein
Medial epicondyle
Median vein of forearm

D. **Anterior View**

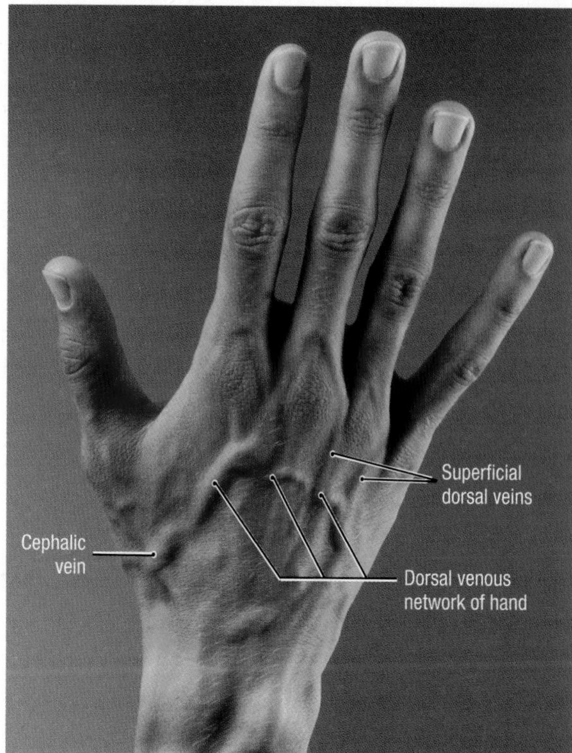
Superficial dorsal veins
Cephalic vein
Dorsal venous network of hand

E. **Posterior View**

6.11 SUPERFICIAL VENOUS DRAINAGE OF UPPER LIMB *(CONTINUED)*

D. Surface anatomy of veins of forearm and arm. **E.** Surface anatomy of veins of the dorsal surface of hand.

Because of the prominence and accessibility of the superficial veins, they are commonly used for **venipuncture** (puncture of a vein to draw blood or inject a solution). By applying a tourniquet to the arm, the venous return is occluded, and the veins distend and usually are visible and/or palpable. Once a vein is punctured, the tourniquet is removed so that when the needle is removed the vein will not bleed extensively. The median cubital vein is commonly used for venipuncture. The veins forming the dorsal venous network of the hand and the cephalic and basilic veins arising from it are commonly used for long-term introduction of fluids **(intravenous feeding)**. The cubital veins are also a site for the **introduction of cardiac catheters** to secure blood samples from the great vessels and chambers of the heart.

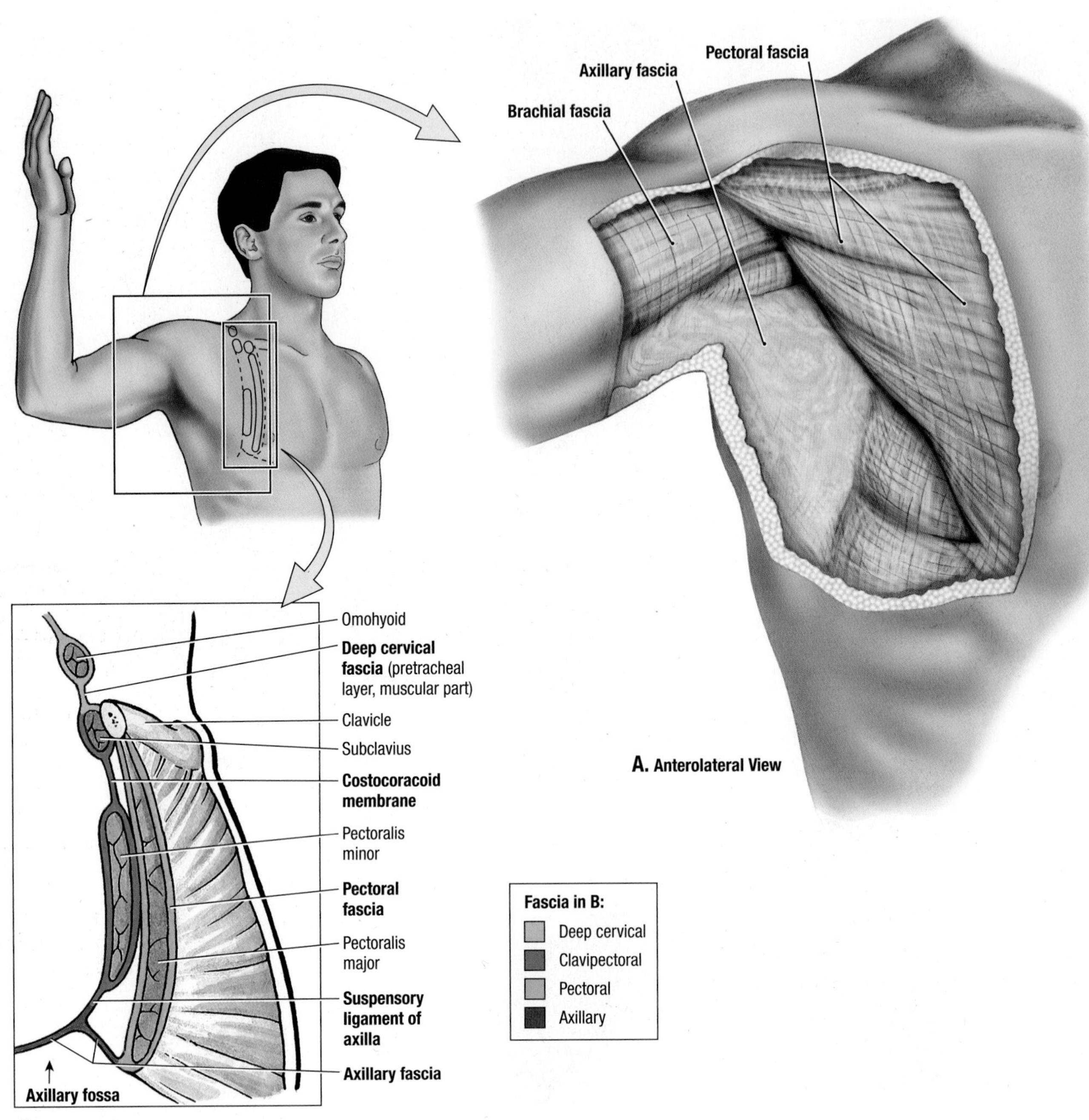
Pectoral fascia
Axillary fascia
Brachial fascia
A. Anterolateral View
Omohyoid
Deep cervical fascia (pretracheal layer, muscular part)
Clavicle
Subclavius
Costocoracoid membrane
Pectoralis minor
Pectoral fascia
Pectoralis major
Suspensory ligament of axilla
Axillary fascia
Axillary fossa
B. Sagittal Section
Fascia in B:
Deep cervical
Clavipectoral
Pectoral
Axillary

6.12 DEEP FASCIA OF UPPER LIMB—AXILLARY AND CLAVIPECTORAL FASCIA

A. Axillary fascia. The axillary fascia forms the floor of the axillary fossa and is continuous with the pectoral fascia covering the pectoralis major muscle and the brachial fascia of the arm. **B.** Clavipectoral fascia. The clavipectoral fascia extends from the axillary fascia to enclose the pectoralis minor and subclavius muscles and then attaches to the clavicle. The part of the clavipectoral fascia superior to the pectoralis minor is the costocoracoid membrane, and the part of the clavipectoral fascia inferior to the pectoralis minor is the suspensory ligament of the axilla. The suspensory ligament of the axilla, an extension of the axillary fascia, supports the axillary fascia and pulls the axillary fascia and the skin inferior to it superiorly when the arm is abducted, forming the axillary fossa or "armpit."

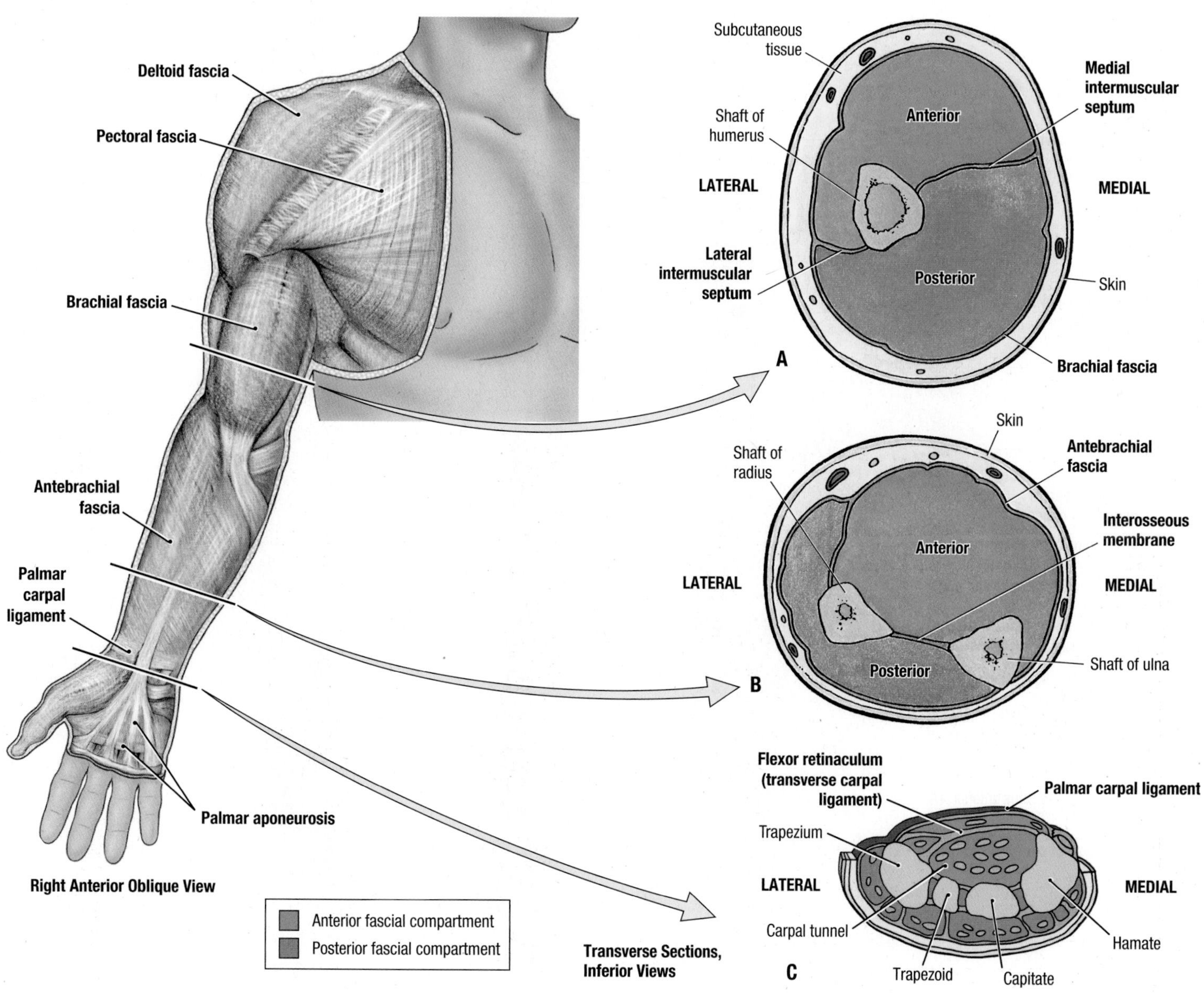
Deltoid fascia
Pectoral fascia
Brachial fascia
Antebrachial fascia
Palmar carpal ligament
Palmar aponeurosis
Right Anterior Oblique View
Anterior fascial compartment
Posterior fascial compartment
Transverse Sections, Inferior Views
Subcutaneous tissue
Shaft of humerus
LATERAL
Lateral intermuscular septum
Anterior
Posterior
Medial intermuscular septum
MEDIAL
Skin
Brachial fascia
A
Skin
Shaft of radius
Antebrachial fascia
Interosseous membrane
LATERAL
Anterior
MEDIAL
Posterior
Shaft of ulna
B
Flexor retinaculum (transverse carpal ligament)
Palmar carpal ligament
Trapezium
LATERAL
MEDIAL
Carpal tunnel
Hamate
Trapezoid
Capitate
C

6.13 DEEP FASCIA OF UPPER LIMB, BRACHIAL AND ANTEBRACHIAL FASCIA

A. Brachial fascia. The brachial fascia is the deep fascia of the arm and is continuous superiorly with the pectoral and axillary layers of fascia. Medial and lateral intermuscular septa extend from the deep aspect of the brachial fascia to the humerus, dividing the arm into anterior and posterior musculofascial compartments. **B.** Antebrachial fascia. The antebrachial fascia surrounds the forearm and is continuous with the brachial fascia and deep fascia of the hand. The interosseous membrane separates the forearm into anterior and posterior musculofascial compartments. Distally the fascia thickens to form the palmar carpal ligament, which is continuous with the flexor retinaculum and dorsally with the extensor expansion. The deep fascia of the hand is continuous with the antebrachial fascia, and on the palmar surface of the hand it thickens to form the palmar aponeurosis. **C.** Flexor retinaculum (transverse carpal ligament). The flexor retinaculum extends between the medial and lateral carpal bones to form the carpal tunnel.

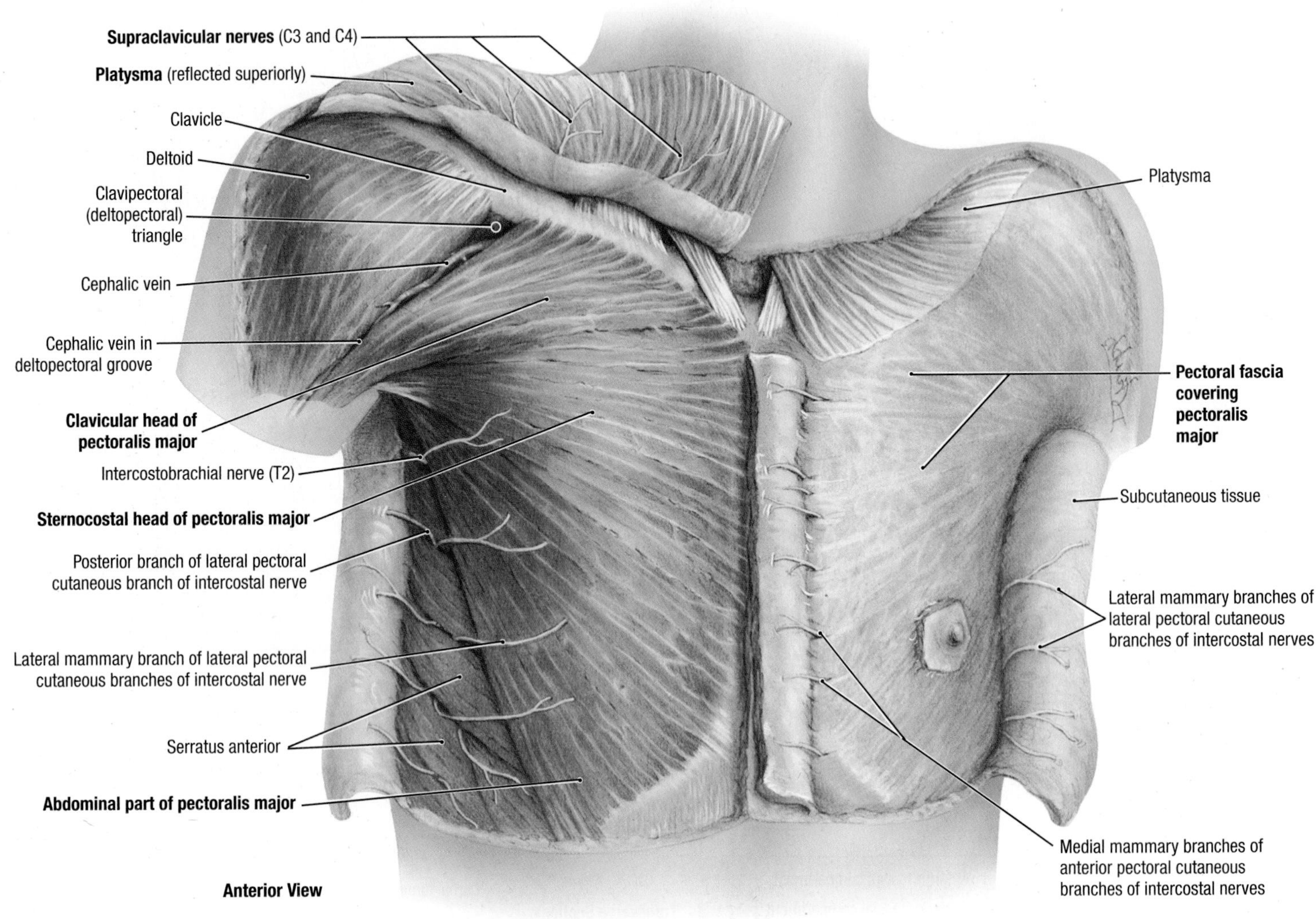
Supraclavicular nerves (C3 and C4)
Platysma (reflected superiorly)
Clavicle
Deltoid
Clavipectoral (deltopectoral) triangle
Cephalic vein
Cephalic vein in deltopectoral groove
Clavicular head of pectoralis major
Intercostobrachial nerve (T2)
Sternocostal head of pectoralis major
Posterior branch of lateral pectoral cutaneous branch of intercostal nerve
Lateral mammary branch of lateral pectoral cutaneous branches of intercostal nerve
Serratus anterior
Abdominal part of pectoralis major
Anterior View
Platysma
Pectoral fascia covering pectoralis major
Subcutaneous tissue
Lateral mammary branches of lateral pectoral cutaneous branches of intercostal nerves
Medial mammary branches of anterior pectoral cutaneous branches of intercostal nerves

6.14 SUPERFICIAL DISSECTION, MALE PECTORAL REGION

- The platysma muscle, which usually descends to the 2nd or 3rd rib, is cut short on the right side and, together with the supraclavicular nerves, is reflected on the left side.
- The exposed intermuscular bony strip of the clavicle is subcutaneous and subplatysmal.
- The cephalic vein passes deeply to join the axillary vein in the clavipectoral (deltopectoral) triangle.
- The cutaneous innervation of the pectoral region by the supraclavicular nerves (C3 and C4) and upper thoracic nerves (T2–T6); the brachial plexus (C5–T1) does not supply cutaneous branches to the pectoral region.

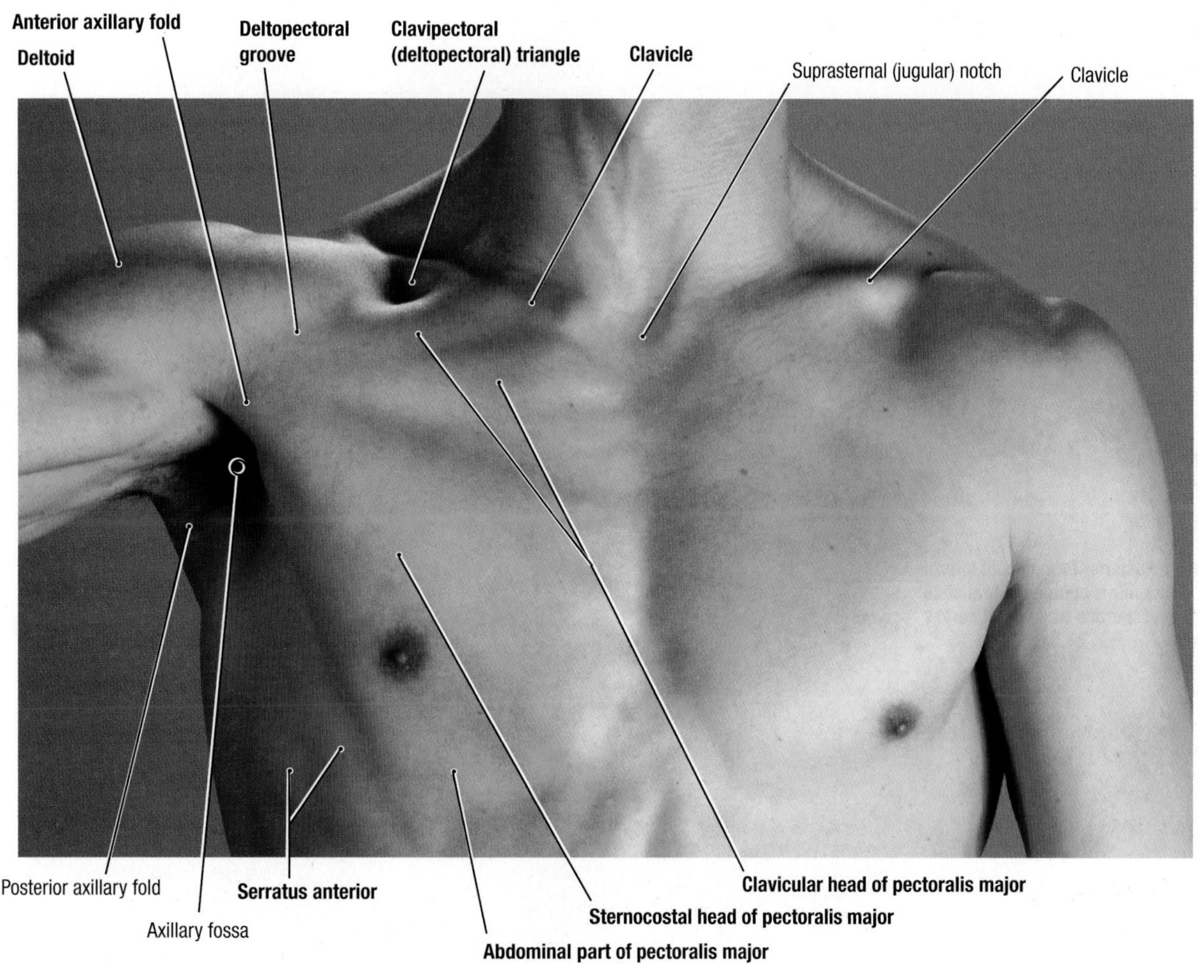
Anterior axillary fold
Deltoid
Deltopectoral groove
Clavipectoral (deltopectoral) triangle
Clavicle
Suprasternal (jugular) notch
Clavicle
Posterior axillary fold
Axillary fossa
Serratus anterior
Clavicular head of pectoralis major
Sternocostal head of pectoralis major
Abdominal part of pectoralis major

6.15 SURFACE ANATOMY, MALE PECTORAL REGION

The clavipectoral (deltopectoral) triangle is the depressed area just inferior to the lateral part of the clavicle, bounded by the clavicle superiorly, the deltoid laterally, and the clavicular head of pectoralis major medially. The clavipectoral triangle and the intermuscular deltopectoral groove extending from its inferior apex demarcate an "internervous plane" (plane not crossed by motor nerves) for an **anterior or deltopectoral surgical incision** to approach to the axilla, shoulder joint, or proximal humerus.

When the arm is abducted and then adducted against resistance, the two heads of the pectoralis major are visible and palpable. As this muscle extends from the thoracic wall to the arm, it forms the anterior axillary fold. Digitations of the serratus anterior appear inferolateral to the pectoralis major. The coracoid process of the scapula is covered by the anterior part of deltoid; however, the tip of the process can be felt on deep palpation in the clavipectoral triangle. The deltoid forms the contour of the shoulder.

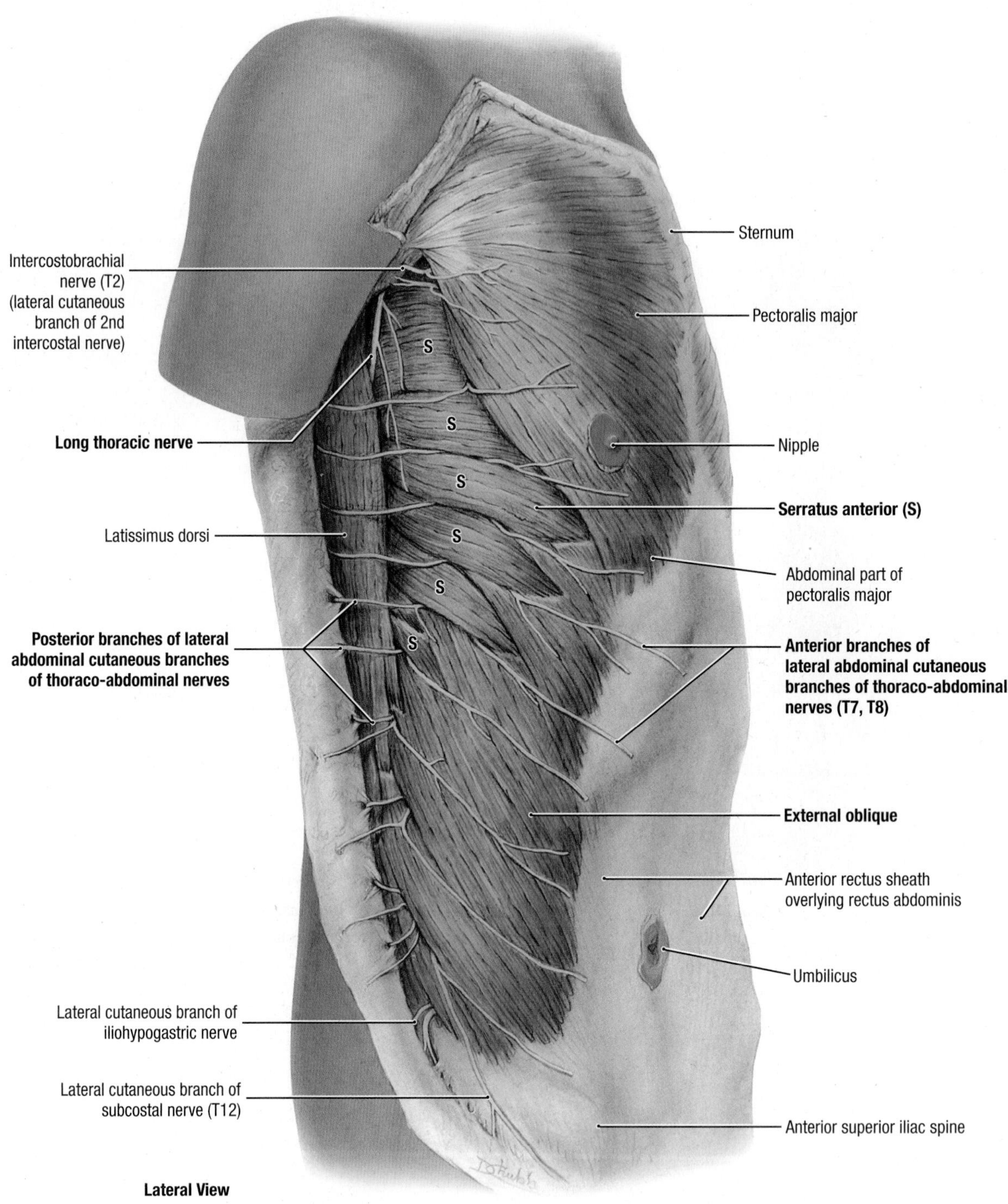

Sternum
Intercostobrachial nerve (T2) (lateral cutaneous branch of 2nd intercostal nerve)
Pectoralis major
S
S
S
S
S
S
Long thoracic nerve
Nipple
Serratus anterior (S)
Latissimus dorsi
Abdominal part of pectoralis major
Posterior branches of lateral abdominal cutaneous branches of thoraco-abdominal nerves
Anterior branches of lateral abdominal cutaneous branches of thoraco-abdominal nerves (T7, T8)
External oblique
Anterior rectus sheath overlying rectus abdominis
Umbilicus
Lateral cutaneous branch of iliohypogastric nerve
Lateral cutaneous branch of subcostal nerve (T12)
Anterior superior iliac spine
Lateral View

6.16 SUPERFICIAL DISSECTION OF TRUNK

- The slips of the serratus anterior interdigitate with the external oblique.
- The long thoracic nerve (nerve to serratus anterior) lies on the lateral (superficial) aspect of the serratus anterior; this nerve is vulnerable to damage from **stab wounds** and during surgery (e.g., radical mastectomy).
- The anterior and posterior branches of the lateral thoracic and abdominal cutaneous branches of intercostal and thoraco-abdominal nerves are dissected.

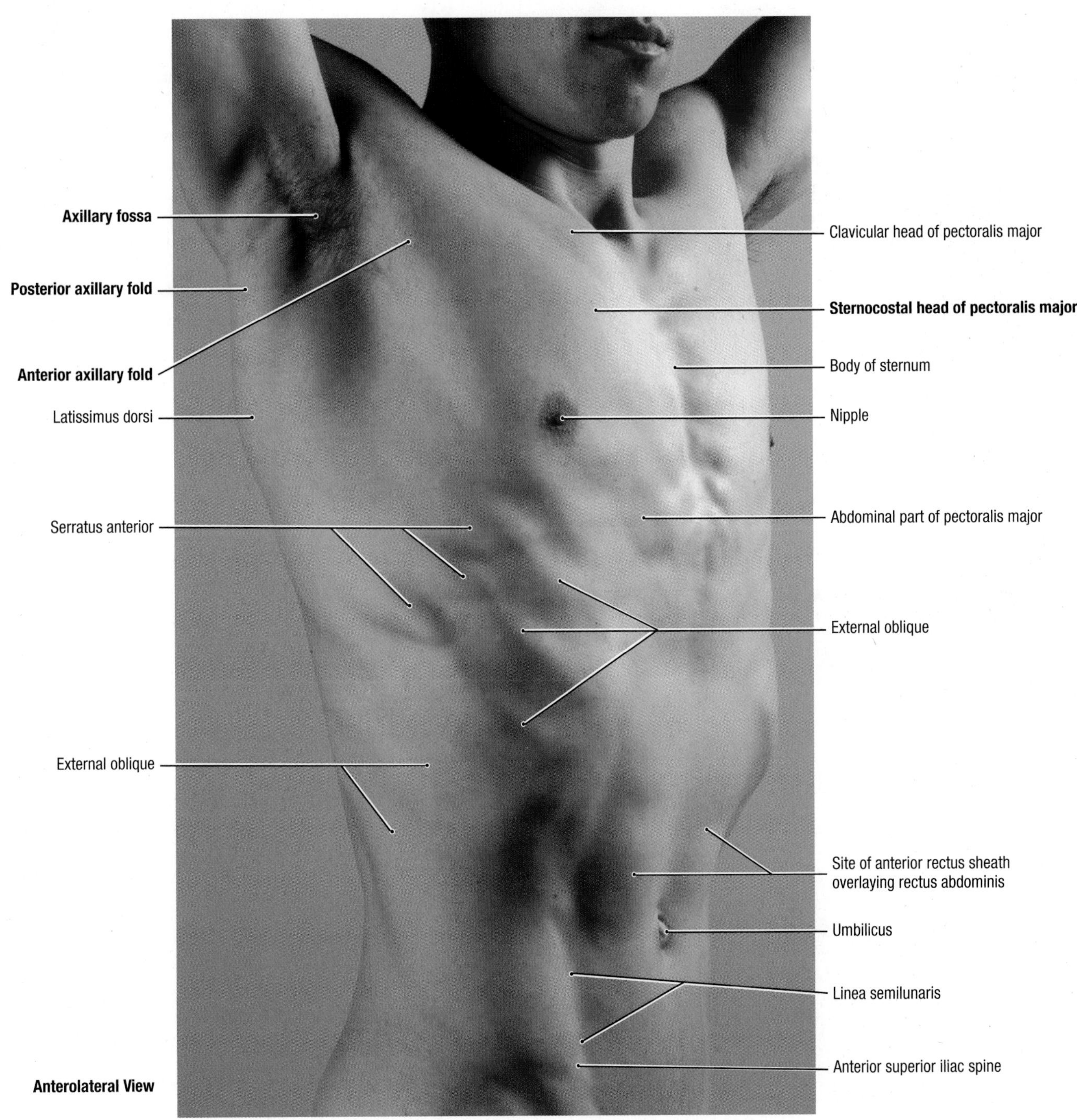
Axillary fossa
Posterior axillary fold
Anterior axillary fold
Latissimus dorsi
Serratus anterior
External oblique
Anterolateral View
Clavicular head of pectoralis major
Sternocostal head of pectoralis major
Body of sternum
Nipple
Abdominal part of pectoralis major
External oblique
Site of anterior rectus sheath overlaying rectus abdominis
Umbilicus
Linea semilunaris
Anterior superior iliac spine

6.17 SURFACE ANATOMY OF ANTEROLATERAL ASPECT OF TRUNK

When the arm is abducted and then adducted against resistance, the sternocostal part of the pectoralis major can be seen and palpated. If the anterior axillary fold bounding the axilla is grasped between the fingers and thumb, the inferior border of the sternocostal head of the pectoralis major can be felt. Several digitations of the serratus anterior are visible inferior to the anterior axillary fold. The posterior axillary fold is composed of skin and muscular tissue (latissimus dorsi and teres major) bounding the axilla posteriorly.

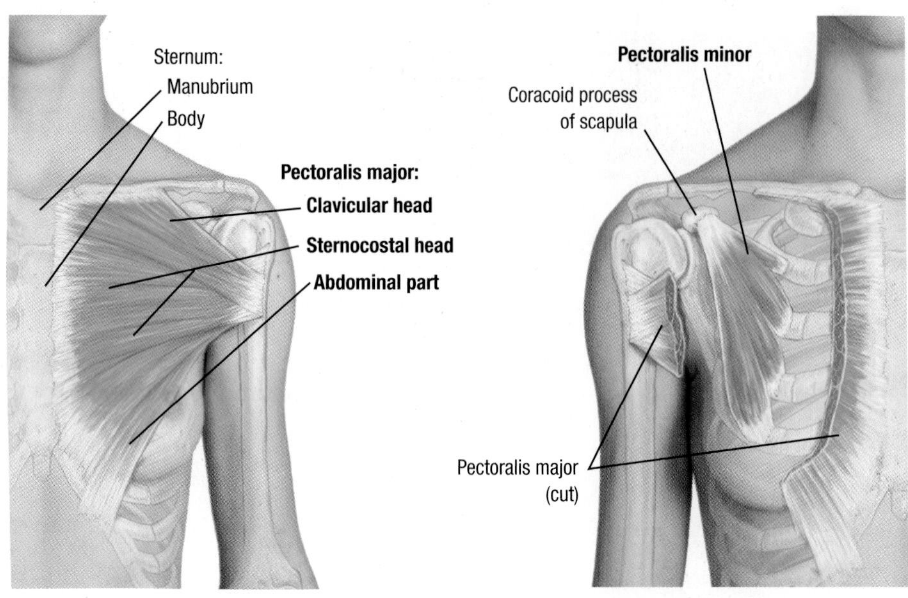
Sternum:
Manubrium
Body
Pectoralis major:
Clavicular head
Sternocostal head
Abdominal part
A. Anterior View
Pectoralis minor
Coracoid process of scapula
Pectoralis major (cut)
B. Anterior View
Clavicle
Subclavius
C. Anterior View

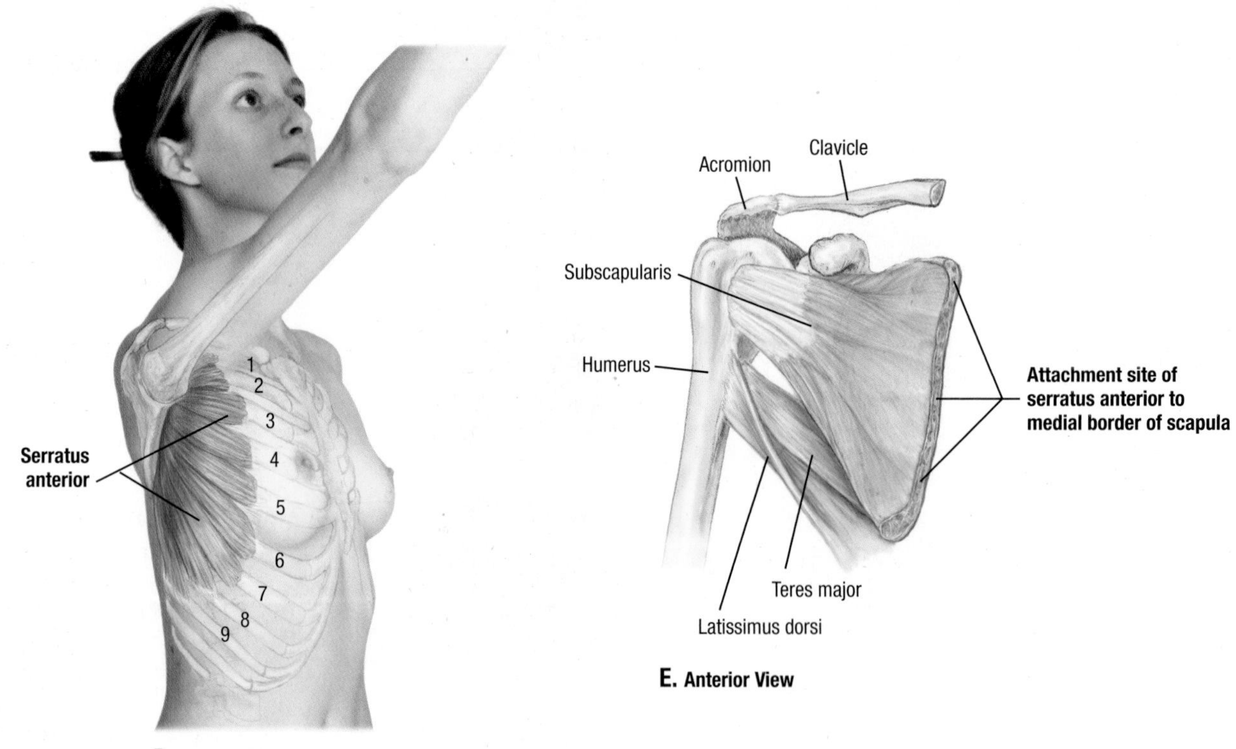
Serratus anterior
1
2
3
4
5
6
7
8
9
D. Lateral View
Acromion
Clavicle
Subscapularis
Humerus
Attachment site of serratus anterior to medial border of scapula
Teres major
Latissimus dorsi
E. Anterior View

6.18 PECTORALIS MAJOR AND MINOR AND SERRATUS ANTERIOR

A. Pectoralis major. **B.** Pectoralis minor. **C.** Subclavius. **D. and E.** Serratus anterior and its scapular attachment.

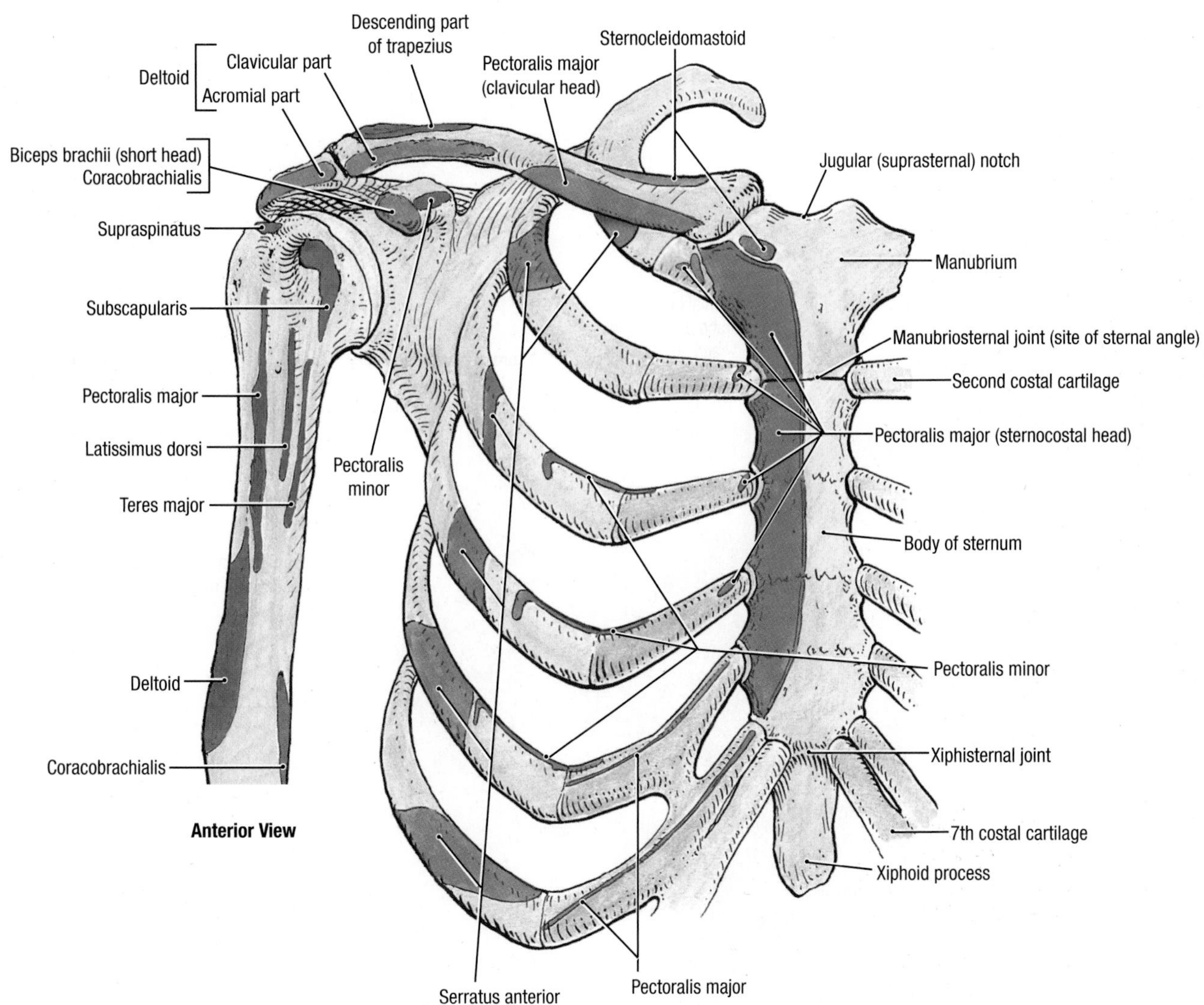
Descending part of trapezius
Sternocleidomastoid
Deltoid
Clavicular part
Acromial part
Pectoralis major (clavicular head)
Biceps brachii (short head)
Coracobrachialis
Jugular (suprasternal) notch
Supraspinatus
Manubrium
Subscapularis
Manubriosternal joint (site of sternal angle)
Second costal cartilage
Pectoralis major
Pectoralis major (sternocostal head)
Latissimus dorsi
Pectoralis minor
Teres major
Body of sternum
Pectoralis minor
Deltoid
Xiphisternal joint
Coracobrachialis
7th costal cartilage
Anterior View
Xiphoid process
Serratus anterior
Pectoralis major

6.19 ANTERIOR ATTACHMENTS OF ANTERIOR AND POSTERIOR AXIO-APPENDICULAR AND SCAPULOHUMERAL MUSCLES

TABLE 6.4 ANTERIOR AXIO-APPENDICULAR MUSCLES

Muscle	Proximal Attachment (*red*)	Distal Attachment (*blue*)	Innervation[a]	Main Actions
Pectoralis major	*Clavicular head:* anterior surface of medial half of clavicle *Sternocostal head:* anterior surface of sternum, superior six costal cartilages *Abdominal part:* aponeurosis of external oblique muscle	Crest of greater tubercle of intertubercular sulcus (lateral lip of bicipital groove)	Lateral and medial pectoral nerves; clavicular head (C5 and **C6**), sternocostal head (**C7**, **C8**, and T1)	Adducts and medially rotates humerus at shoulder joint; draws scapula anteriorly and inferiorly Acting alone: clavicular head flexes shoulder joint, and sternocostal head extends it from the flexed position
Pectoralis minor	3rd to 5th ribs near their costal cartilages	Medial border and superior surface of coracoid process of scapula	Medial pectoral nerve (C8 and T1)	Stabilizes scapula by drawing it inferiorly and anteriorly against thoracic wall
Subclavius	Junction of 1st rib and its costal cartilage	Inferior surface of middle third of clavicle	Nerve to subclavius (**C5** and C6)	Anchors and depresses clavicle at sternoclavicular joint
Serratus anterior	External surfaces of lateral parts of 1st to 8th–9th ribs	Anterior surface of medial border of scapula (see Fig. 6.18E.)	Long thoracic nerve (C5, **C6**, and **C7**)	Protracts scapula and holds it against thoracic wall; rotates scapula

[a]Numbers indicate spinal cord segmental innervation (e.g., C5 and C6 indicate that nerves supplying the clavicular head of pectoralis major are derived from 5th and 6th cervical segments of spinal cord). Boldface numbers indicate the main segmental innervation. Damage to these segments or to motor nerve roots arising from them results in paralysis of the muscles concerned.

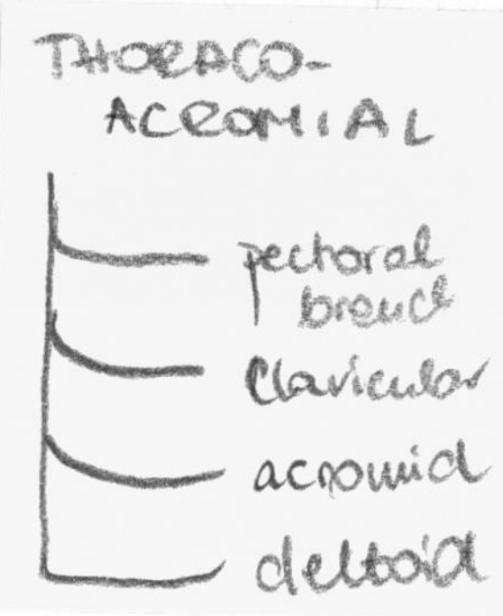
THORACO-
ACROMIAL
pectoral branch
Clavicular
acromial
deltoid

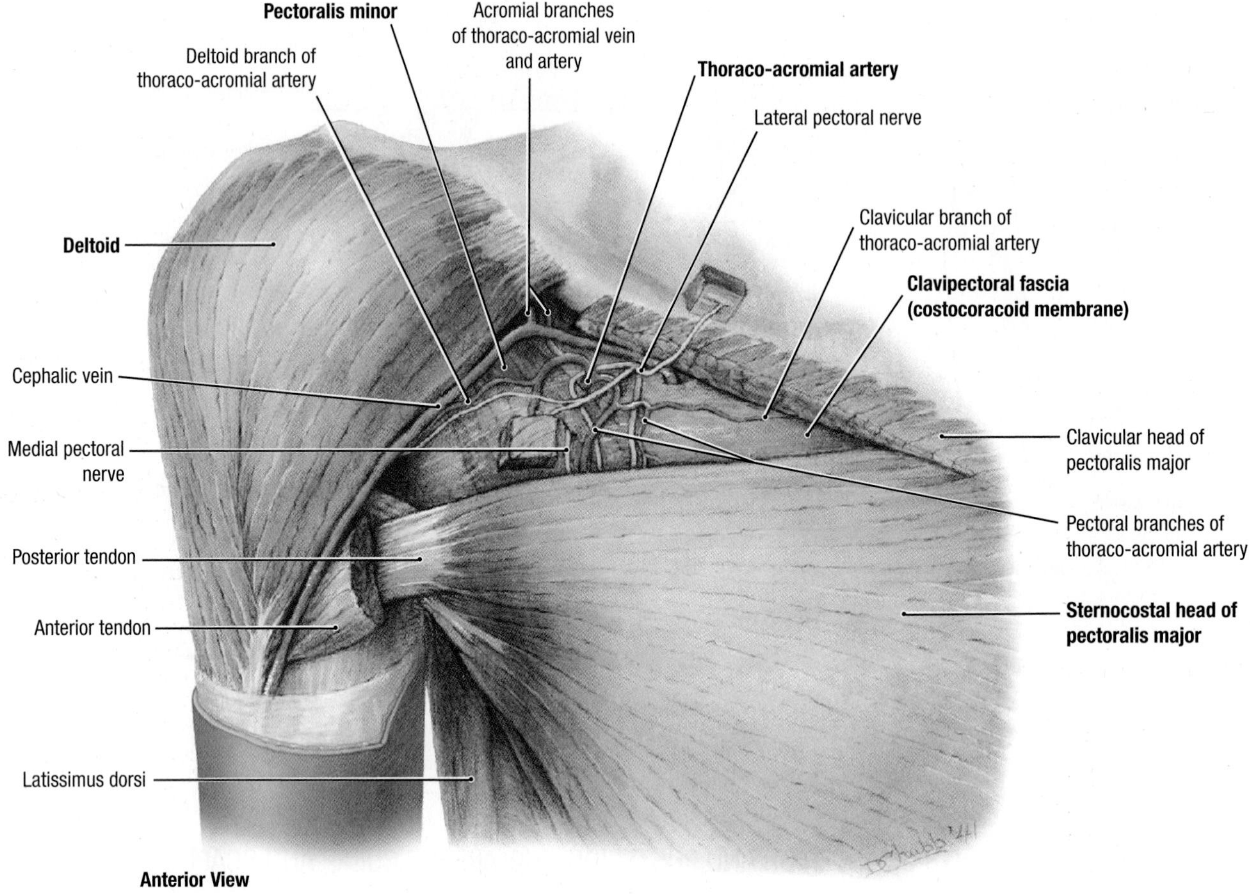
Pectoralis minor
Acromial branches of thoraco-acromial vein and artery
Deltoid branch of thoraco-acromial artery
Thoraco-acromial artery
Lateral pectoral nerve
Clavicular branch of thoraco-acromial artery
Deltoid
Clavipectoral fascia (costocoracoid membrane)
Cephalic vein
Clavicular head of pectoralis major
Medial pectoral nerve
Pectoral branches of thoraco-acromial artery
Posterior tendon
Sternocostal head of pectoralis major
Anterior tendon
Latissimus dorsi
Anterior View

6.20 ANTERIOR WALL OF AXILLA AND CLAVIPECTORAL FASCIA

A. Anterior wall of axilla. The clavicular head of the pectoralis major is excised, except for two cubes of muscle that remain to identify the branches of the lateral pectoral nerve.

- The clavipectoral fascia superior to the pectoralis minor (costocoracoid membrane) is pierced by the cephalic vein, the lateral pectoral nerve, and the thoraco-acromial vessels.
- The pectoralis minor and clavipectoral fascia are pierced by the medial pectoral nerve.
- Observe the insertion of the pectoralis major from deep to superficial: inferior part of the sternocostal head, superior part of the sternocostal head (posterior tendon), and clavicular head (anterior tendon)

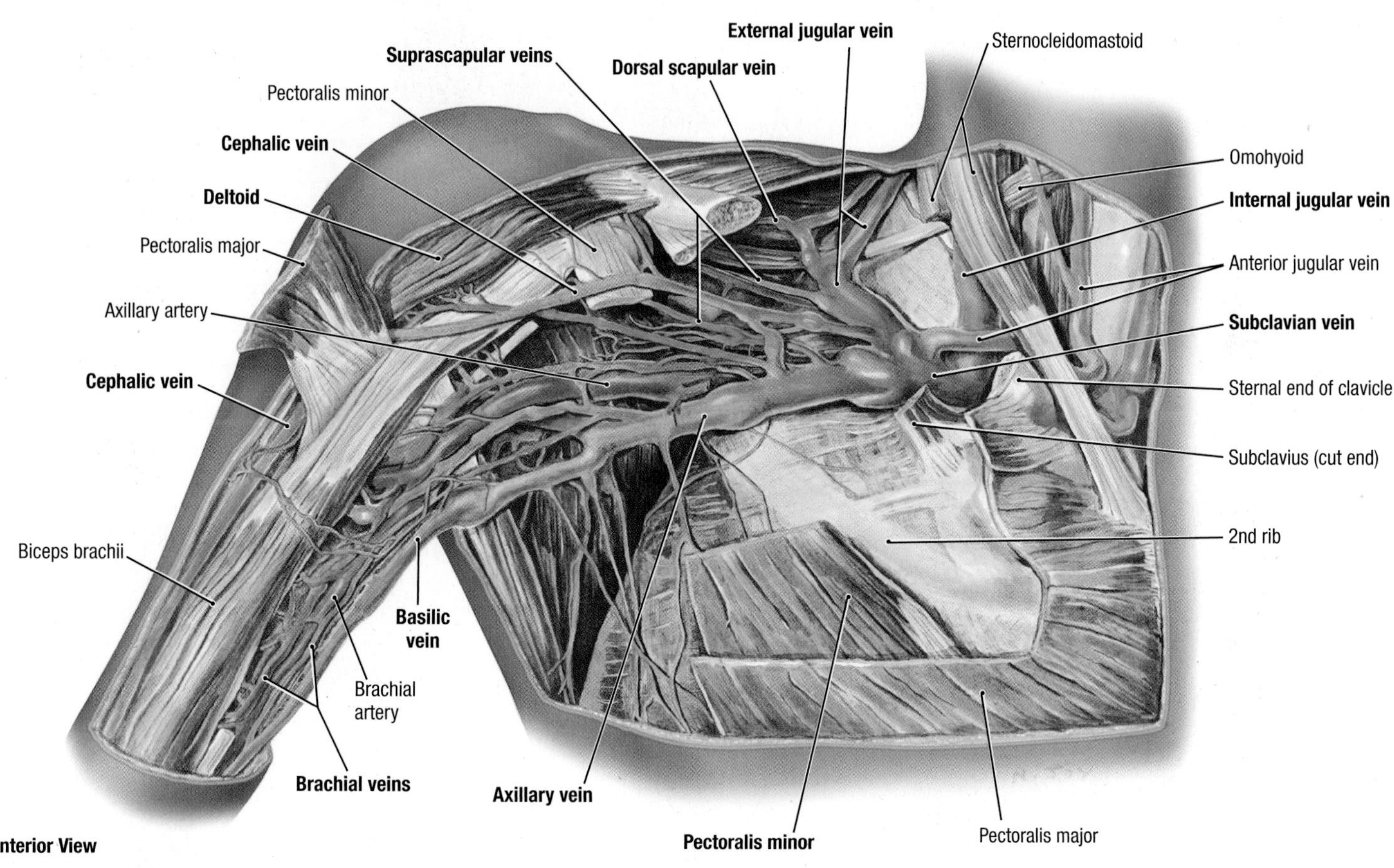
External jugular vein
Sternocleidomastoid
Suprascapular veins
Dorsal scapular vein
Pectoralis minor
Cephalic vein
Omohyoid
Deltoid
Internal jugular vein
Pectoralis major
Anterior jugular vein
Axillary artery
Subclavian vein
Cephalic vein
Sternal end of clavicle
Subclavius (cut end)
2nd rib
Biceps brachii
Basilic vein
Brachial artery
Brachial veins
Axillary vein
Pectoralis minor
Pectoralis major
Anterior View

6.21 VEINS OF AXILLA

- The basilic vein joins the brachial veins to become the axillary vein near the inferior border of teres major, the axillary vein becomes the subclavian vein at the lateral border of the 1st rib, and the subclavian joins the internal jugular to become the brachiocephalic vein posterior to the sternal end of the clavicle.
- Numerous valves, enlargements in the vein, are shown.
- The cephalic vein in this specimen bifurcates to end in the axillary and external jugular veins.

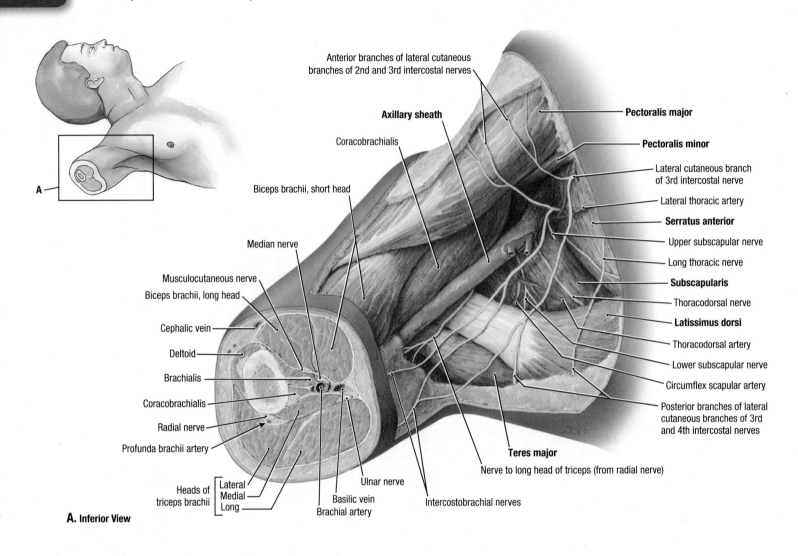

A
Anterior branches of lateral cutaneous branches of 2nd and 3rd intercostal nerves
Axillary sheath
Coracobrachialis
Biceps brachii, short head
Median nerve
Musculocutaneous nerve
Biceps brachii, long head
Cephalic vein
Deltoid
Brachialis
Coracobrachialis
Radial nerve
Profunda brachii artery
Heads of triceps brachii: Lateral, Medial, Long
Ulnar nerve
Basilic vein
Brachial artery
Intercostobrachial nerves
Nerve to long head of triceps (from radial nerve)
Teres major
Pectoralis major
Pectoralis minor
Lateral cutaneous branch of 3rd intercostal nerve
Lateral thoracic artery
Serratus anterior
Upper subscapular nerve
Long thoracic nerve
Subscapularis
Thoracodorsal nerve
Latissimus dorsi
Thoracodorsal artery
Lower subscapular nerve
Circumflex scapular artery
Posterior branches of lateral cutaneous branches of 3rd and 4th intercostal nerves

A. Inferior View

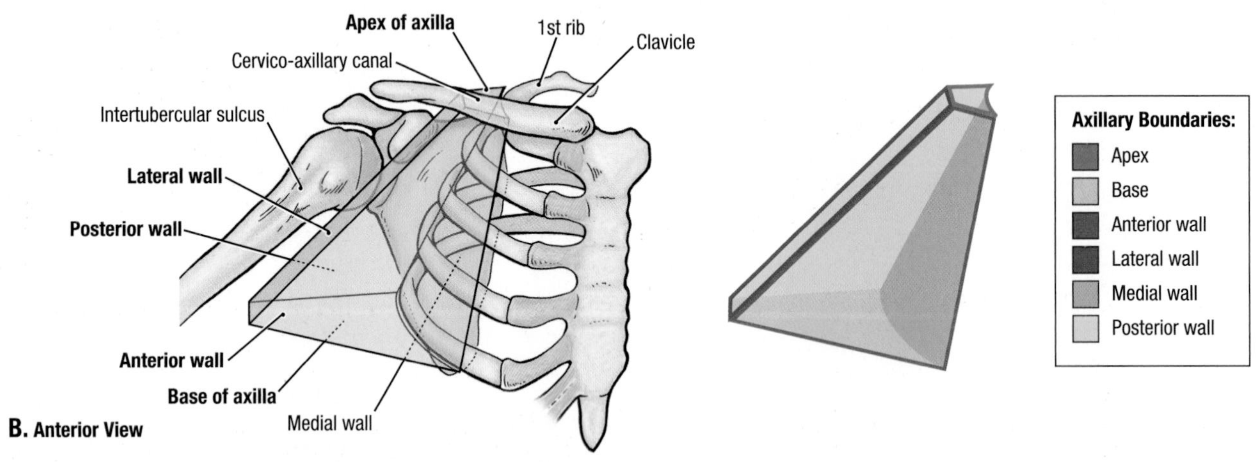
Apex of axilla
1st rib
Clavicle
Cervico-axillary canal
Intertubercular sulcus
Lateral wall
Posterior wall
Anterior wall
Base of axilla
Medial wall
Axillary Boundaries:
Apex
Base
Anterior wall
Lateral wall
Medial wall
Posterior wall

B. Anterior View

6.22 WALLS AND CONTENTS OF THE AXILLA

A. Dissection. **B.** Location and walls of axilla, schematic diagram.

- The walls of the axilla are anterior (formed by the pectoralis major, pectoralis minor, and subclavius muscles), posterior (formed by subscapularis, latissimus dorsi, and teres major muscles), medial (formed by the serratus anterior muscle), and lateral (formed by the intertubercular sulcus [bicipital groove] of the humerus [concealed by the biceps and coracobrachialis muscles]).
- The axillary sheath surrounds the nerves and vessels (neurovascular bundle) of the upper limb.

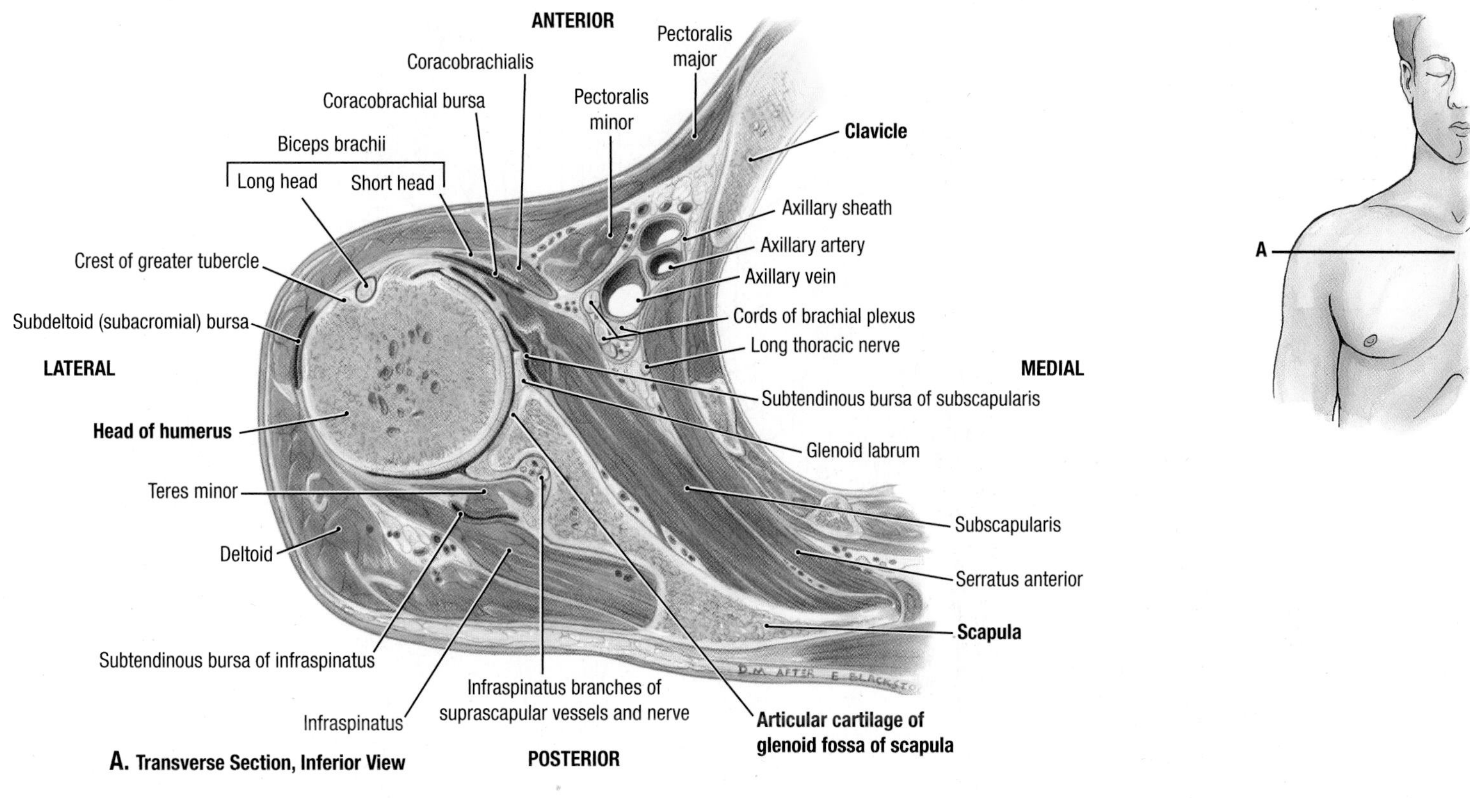
ANTERIOR
Pectoralis major
Coracobrachialis
Coracobrachial bursa
Pectoralis minor
Clavicle
Biceps brachii
Long head
Short head
Axillary sheath
Axillary artery
Crest of greater tubercle
Axillary vein
Cords of brachial plexus
Subdeltoid (subacromial) bursa
Long thoracic nerve
LATERAL
MEDIAL
Subtendinous bursa of subscapularis
Head of humerus
Glenoid labrum
Teres minor
Subscapularis
Deltoid
Serratus anterior
Scapula
Subtendinous bursa of infraspinatus
Infraspinatus branches of suprascapular vessels and nerve
Infraspinatus
Articular cartilage of glenoid fossa of scapula
POSTERIOR
A
A. Transverse Section, Inferior View

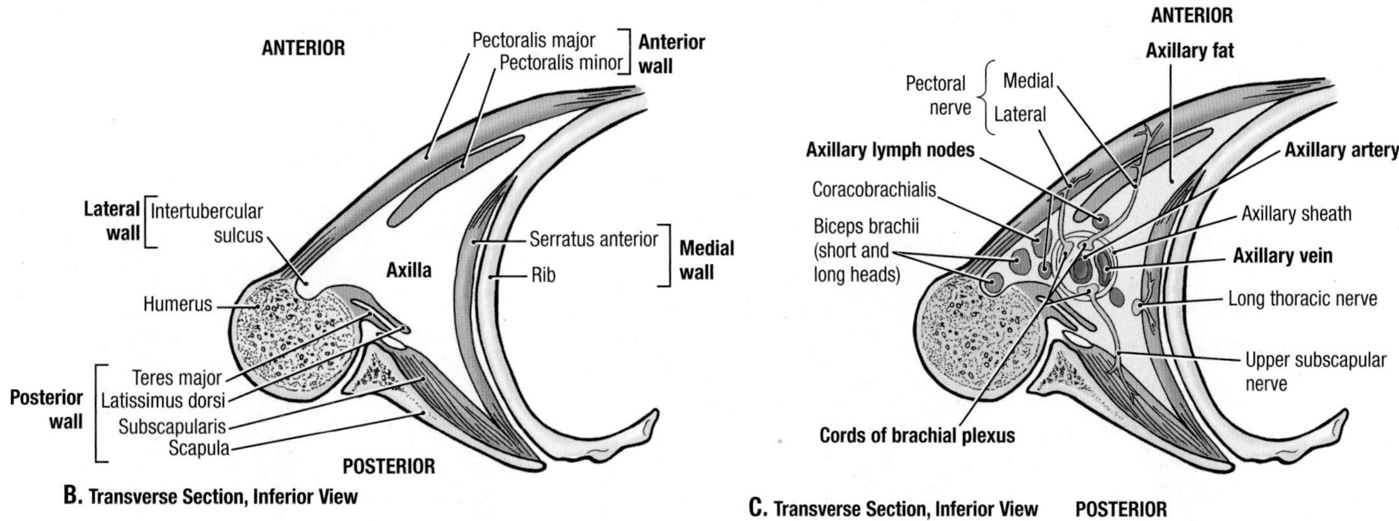
ANTERIOR
Pectoralis major
Pectoralis minor
Anterior wall
Lateral wall
Intertubercular sulcus
Serratus anterior
Rib
Medial wall
Axilla
Humerus
Posterior wall
Teres major
Latissimus dorsi
Subscapularis
Scapula
POSTERIOR
ANTERIOR
Axillary fat
Pectoral nerve
Medial
Lateral
Axillary lymph nodes
Axillary artery
Coracobrachialis
Axillary sheath
Biceps brachii (short and long heads)
Axillary vein
Long thoracic nerve
Upper subscapular nerve
Cords of brachial plexus
POSTERIOR
B. Transverse Section, Inferior View

C. Transverse Section, Inferior View

6.23 TRANSVERSE SECTIONS THROUGH SHOULDER JOINT AND AXILLA

A. Anatomical section. **B.** Walls of axilla, schematic illustration. **C.** Walls and contents of axilla, schematic illustration.

- The intertubercular sulcus (bicipital groove) containing the tendon of the long head of the biceps brachii muscle is directed anteriorly; the short head of the biceps muscle and the coracobrachialis and pectoralis minor muscles are sectioned just inferior to their attachments to the coracoid process.
- The small glenoid cavity is deepened by the glenoid labrum.
- Bursae include the subdeltoid (subacromial) bursa, between the deltoid and greater tubercle; the subtendinous bursa of subscapularis, between the subscapularis tendon and scapula; and coracobrachial bursa, between the coracobrachialis and subscapularis.
- The axillary sheath encloses the axillary artery and vein and the three cords of the brachial plexus to form a neurovascular bundle, surrounded by axillary fat.

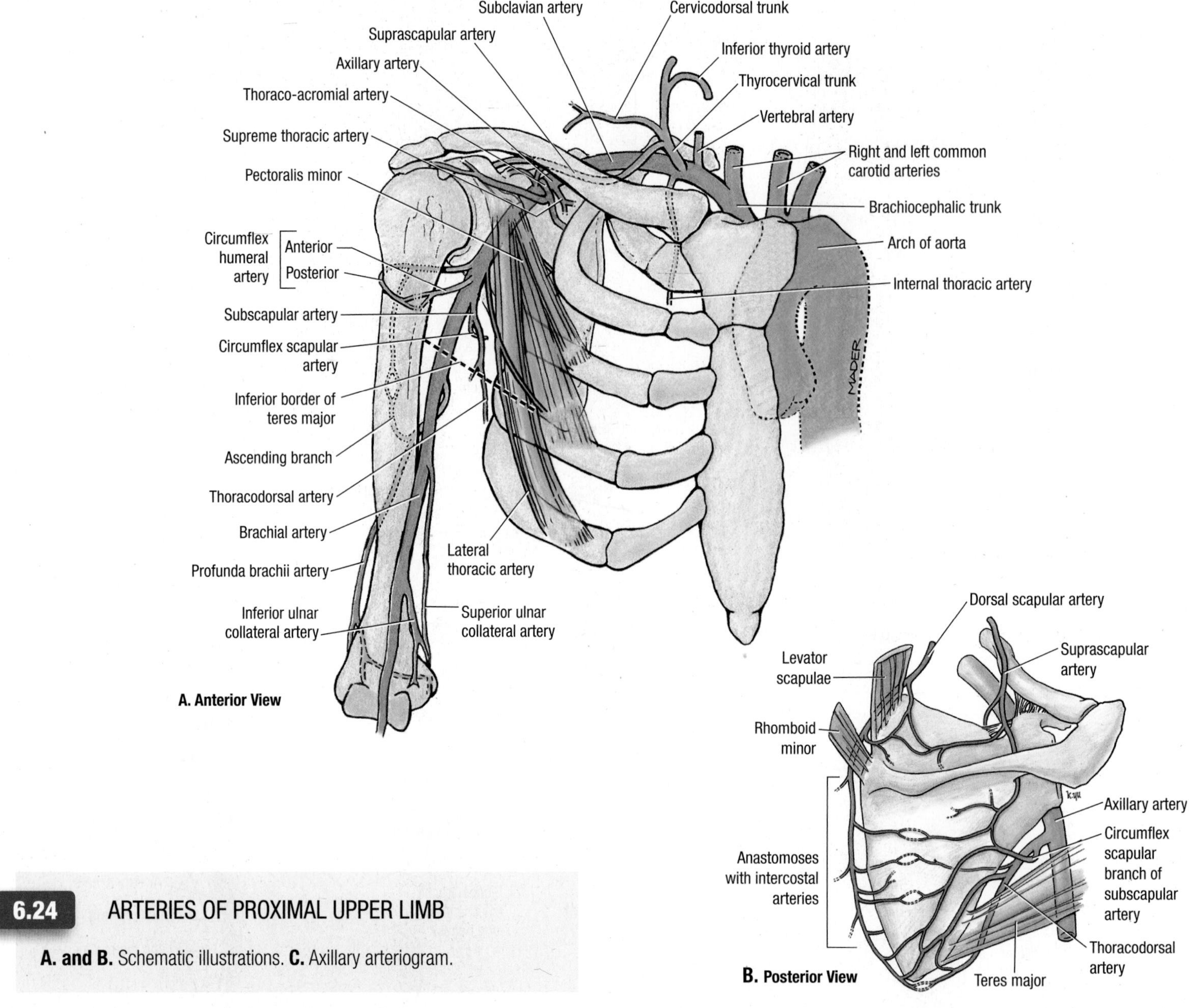
Subclavian artery
Cervicodorsal trunk
Suprascapular artery
Inferior thyroid artery
Axillary artery
Thyrocervical trunk
Thoraco-acromial artery
Vertebral artery
Supreme thoracic artery
Right and left common carotid arteries
Pectoralis minor
Brachiocephalic trunk
Circumflex humeral artery
Anterior
Posterior
Arch of aorta
Internal thoracic artery
Subscapular artery
Circumflex scapular artery
Inferior border of teres major
Ascending branch
Thoracodorsal artery
Brachial artery
Profunda brachii artery
Lateral thoracic artery
Inferior ulnar collateral artery
Superior ulnar collateral artery
A. Anterior View
Dorsal scapular artery
Levator scapulae
Suprascapular artery
Rhomboid minor
Axillary artery
Circumflex scapular branch of subscapular artery
Anastomoses with intercostal arteries
Thoracodorsal artery
Teres major
B. Posterior View

6.24 ARTERIES OF PROXIMAL UPPER LIMB

A. and B. Schematic illustrations. **C.** Axillary arteriogram.

TABLE 6.5 ARTERIES OF PROXIMAL UPPER LIMB (SHOULDER REGION AND ARM)

Artery	Origin	Course
Internal thoracic	Subclavian artery	Descends, inclining anteromedially, posterior to sternal end of clavicle and first costal cartilage; enters thorax to descend in parasternal plane; gives rise to perforating branches, anterior intercostal, musculophrenic, and superior epigastric arteries
Thyrocervical trunk		Ascends as a short, wide trunk, often giving rise to the suprascapular artery and/or cervicodorsal trunk and terminating by bifurcating into the ascending cervical and inferior thyroid arteries
Suprascapular	Cervicodorsal trunk from thyrocervical trunk (or as direct branch of subclavian artery[a])	Passes inferolaterally over anterior scalene muscle and phrenic nerve, subclavian artery and brachial plexus running laterally posterior and parallel to clavicle; next passes over transverse scapular ligament to supraspinous fossa, then lateral to scapular spine (deep to acromion) to infraspinous fossa

[a]See Weiglein AH, Moriggl B, Schalk C, et al. Arteries in the posterior cervical triangle. *Clinical Anatomy* 2005;18:533–537.

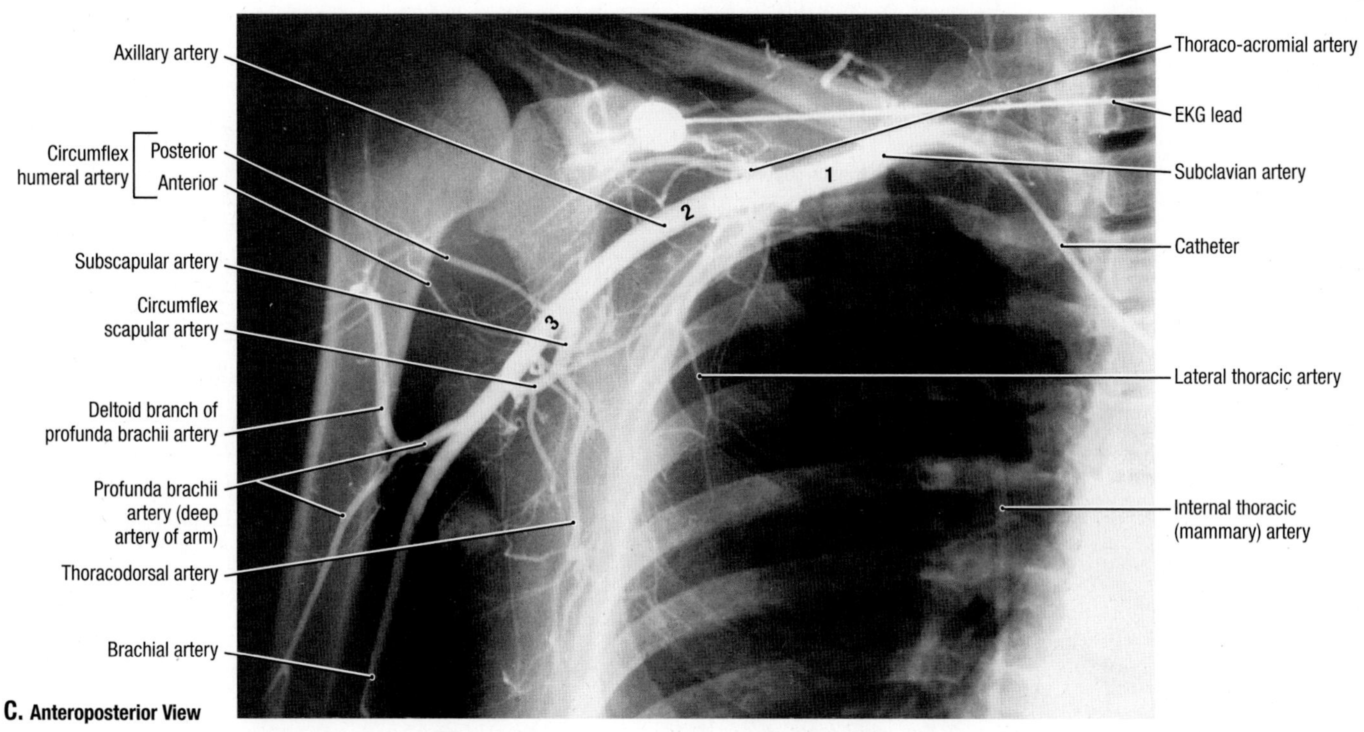
Axillary artery
Circumflex humeral artery
Posterior
Anterior
Subscapular artery
Circumflex scapular artery
Deltoid branch of profunda brachii artery
Profunda brachii artery (deep artery of arm)
Thoracodorsal artery
Brachial artery
Thoraco-acromial artery
EKG lead
Subclavian artery
Catheter
Lateral thoracic artery
Internal thoracic (mammary) artery
1
2
3

C. **Anteroposterior View**

1: First part of the axillary artery is located between the lateral border of the 1st rib and the medial border of pectoralis minor.
2: Second part of the axillary artery lies posterior to pectoralis minor.
3: Third part of the axillary artery extends from the lateral border of pectoralis minor to the inferior border of teres major, where it becomes the brachial artery.

TABLE 6.5 ARTERIES OF PROXIMAL UPPER LIMB (SHOULDER REGION AND ARM) (CONTINUED)

Artery	Origin		Course
Supreme thoracic	1st part (as only branch)	Axillary artery	Runs anteromedially along superior border of pectoralis minor; then passes between it and pectoralis major to thoracic wall; helps supply 1st and 2nd intercostal spaces and superior part of serratus anterior
Thoraco-acromial	2nd part (medial branch)	Axillary artery	Curls around superomedial border of pectoralis minor, pierces costocoracoid membrane (clavipectoral fascia), and divides into four branches: pectoral, deltoid, acromial, and clavicular
Lateral thoracic	2nd part (lateral branch)	Axillary artery	Descends along axillary border of pectoralis minor; follows it onto thoracic wall, supplying lateral aspect of breast
Circumflex humeral (anterior and posterior)	3rd part (sometimes via a common trunk)	Axillary artery	Encircle surgical neck of humerus, anastomosing with each other laterally; larger posterior branch traverses quadrangular space
Subscapular	3rd part (largest branch)	Axillary artery	Descends from level of inferior border of subscapularis along lateral border of scapula, dividing within 2–3 cm into terminal branches, the circumflex scapular and thoracodorsal arteries
Circumflex scapular	Subscapular artery	Brachial artery	Curves around lateral border of scapula to enter infraspinous fossa, anastomosing with subscapular artery
Thoracodorsal	Near its origin	Brachial artery	Continuation of subscapular artery; accompanies thoracodorsal nerve to enter latissimus dorsi
Profunda brachii (deep brachial) artery	Near middle of arm	Brachial artery	Accompanies radial nerve through radial groove of humerus, supplying posterior compartment of arm and participating in peri-articular arterial anastomosis around elbow joint
Superior ulnar collateral	Inferior to teres major	Brachial artery	Accompanies ulnar nerve to posterior aspect of elbsow; anastomoses with posterior ulnar recurrent artery
Inferior ulnar collateral	Superior to medial epicondyle of humerus	Brachial artery	Passes anterior to medial epicondyle of humerus to anastomose with anterior ulnar collateral artery around elbow joint

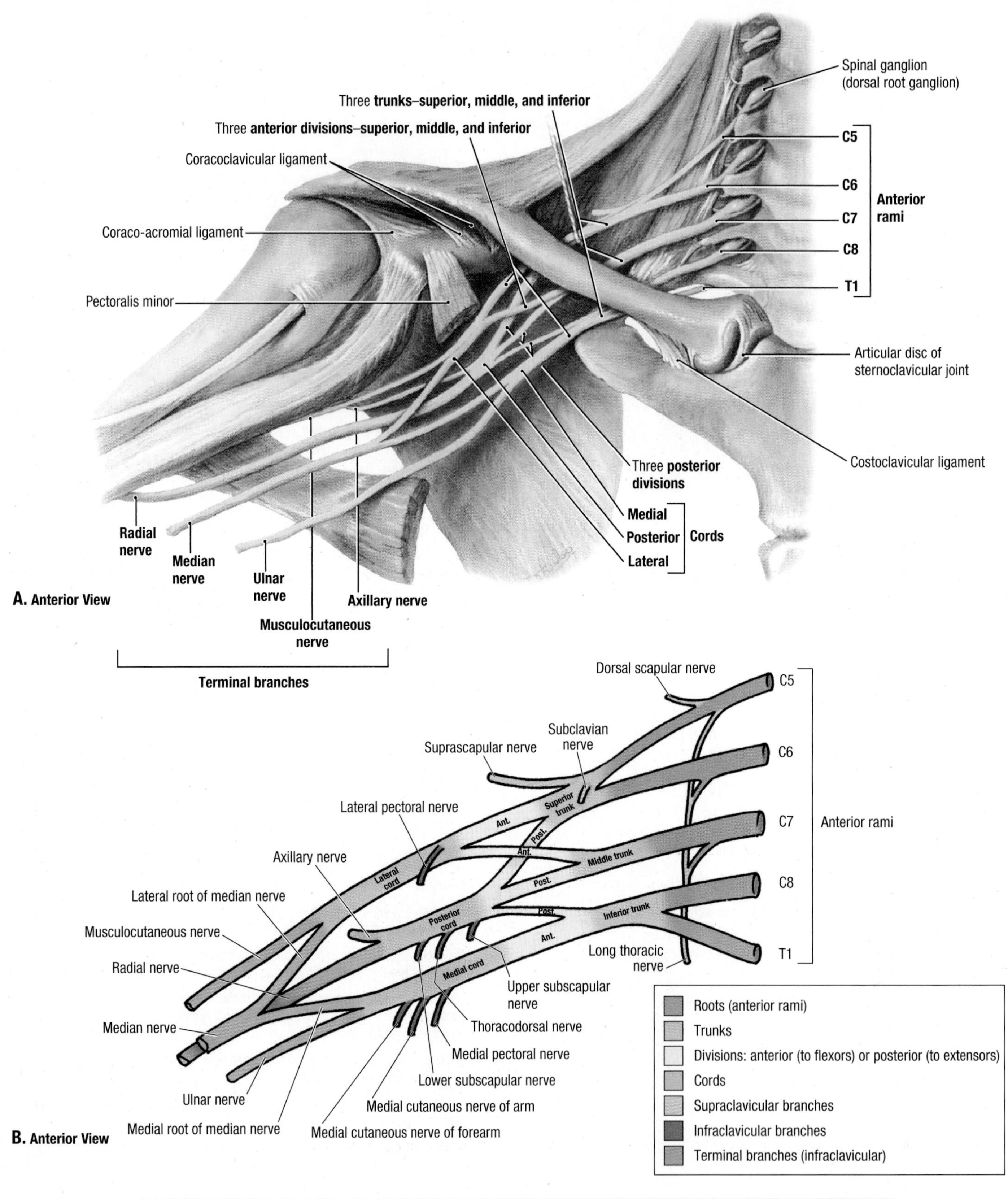

Spinal ganglion (dorsal root ganglion)
Three trunks–superior, middle, and inferior
Three anterior divisions–superior, middle, and inferior
Coracoclavicular ligament
C5
C6
C7
C8
T1
Anterior rami
Coraco-acromial ligament
Pectoralis minor
Articular disc of sternoclavicular joint
Costoclavicular ligament
Three posterior divisions
Medial
Posterior
Lateral
Cords
Radial nerve
Median nerve
Ulnar nerve
Axillary nerve
Musculocutaneous nerve
A. Anterior View
Terminal branches
Dorsal scapular nerve
Subclavian nerve
Suprascapular nerve
Lateral pectoral nerve
Superior trunk
Ant.
Post.
Middle trunk
Axillary nerve
Lateral cord
Lateral root of median nerve
Posterior cord
Inferior trunk
Musculocutaneous nerve
Long thoracic nerve
Radial nerve
Medial cord
Upper subscapular nerve
Median nerve
Thoracodorsal nerve
Medial pectoral nerve
Lower subscapular nerve
Ulnar nerve
Medial cutaneous nerve of arm
Medial root of median nerve
Medial cutaneous nerve of forearm
B. Anterior View
Roots (anterior rami)
Trunks
Divisions: anterior (to flexors) or posterior (to extensors)
Cords
Supraclavicular branches
Infraclavicular branches
Terminal branches (infraclavicular)

6.25 BRACHIAL PLEXUS

A. Dissection. **B.** Schematic illustration.

TABLE 6.6 *BRACHIAL PLEXUS*

Nerve	Origin	Course	Distribution/Structure(s) Supplied
Supraclavicular Branches			
Dorsal scapular	Anterior ramus of C5 with a frequent contribution from C4	Pierces scalenus medius, descends on deep surface of rhomboids	Rhomboids and occasionally supplies levator scapulae
Long thoracic	Anterior rami of C5–C7	Descends posterior to C8 and T1 rami and passes distally on external surface of serratus anterior	Serratus anterior
Subclavian	Superior trunk receiving fibers from C5 and C6 and often C4	Descends posterior to clavicle and anterior to brachial plexus and subclavian artery	Subclavius and sternoclavicular joint
Suprascapular	Superior trunk receiving fibers from C5 and C6 and often C4	Passes laterally across posterior triangle of neck, through suprascapular notch deep to superior transverse scapular ligament	Supraspinatus, infraspinatus, and glenohumeral (shoulder) joint
Infraclavicular branches			
Lateral pectoral	Lateral cord receiving fibers from C5–C7	Pierces clavipectoral fascia to reach deep surface of pectoral muscles	Primarily pectoralis major but sends a loop to medial pectoral nerve that innervates pectoralis minor
Musculocutaneous	Lateral cord receiving fibers from C5–C7	Pierces coracobrachialis and descends between biceps brachii and brachialis	Coracobrachialis, biceps brachii, and brachialis; continues as lateral cutaneous nerve of forearm
Median	Lateral root of median nerve is a terminal branch of lateral cord (C6, C7); medial root of median nerve is a terminal branch of medial cord (C8, T1)	Lateral and medial roots merge to form median nerve lateral to axillary artery; crosses anterior to brachial artery to lie medial to artery in cubital fossa	Flexor muscles in forearm (except flexor carpi ulnaris, ulnar half of flexor digitorum profundus), 3½ thenar and lateral 2 lumbrical muscles in hand, and skin of palm and 3½ digits lateral to a line bisecting 4th digit and the dorsum of the distal halves of these digits
Medial pectoral	Medial cord receiving fibers from C8, T1	Passes between axillary artery and vein and enters deep surface of pectoralis minor	Pectoralis minor and part of pectoralis major
Medial cutaneous nerve of arm	Medial cord receiving fibers from C8, T1	Runs along the medial side of axillary vein and communicates with intercostobrachial nerve	Skin on medial side of arm
Medial cutaneous nerve of forearm	Medial cord receiving fibers from C8, T1	Runs between axillary artery and vein	Skin over medial side of forearm
Ulnar	Terminal branch of medial cord receiving fibers from C8, T1 and often C7	Passes down medial aspect of arm and runs posterior to medial epicondyle to enter forearm	Innervates 1½ flexor muscles in forearm (see Median nerve), 1½ thenar, 2 medial lumbricals, and all interossei muscles in hand, and skin of hand medial to a line bisecting 4th digit (ring finger) anteriorly and posteriorly
Upper subscapular	Branch of posterior cord receiving fibers from C5	Passes posteriorly and enters subscapularis	Superior portion of subscapularis
Thoracodorsal	Branch of posterior cord receiving fibers from C6 to C8	Arises between upper and lower subscapular nerves and runs inferolaterally to latissimus dorsi	Latissimus dorsi
Lower subscapular	Branch of posterior cord receiving fibers from C6	Passes inferolaterally, deep to subscapular artery and vein, to subscapularis and teres major	Inferior portion of subscapularis and teres major
Axillary	Terminal branch of posterior cord receiving fibers from C5 and C6	Passes to posterior aspect of arm through quadrangular space[a] with posterior circumflex humeral artery and then winds around surgical neck of humerus; gives rise to lateral cutaneous nerve of arm	Teres minor and deltoid, glenohumeral (shoulder) joint, and skin of superolateral arm
Radial	Terminal branch of posterior cord receiving fibers from C5 to T1	Descends posterior to axillary artery; enters radial groove to pass between long and medial heads of triceps brachii	Triceps brachii, anconeus, brachioradialis, and extensor muscles of forearm; supplies skin on posterior aspect of arm and forearm and dorsum of hand lateral to axial line of digit 4

[a]Quadrangular space is bounded superiorly by subscapularis and teres minor, inferiorly by teres major, medially by long head of triceps brachii, and laterally by humerus.

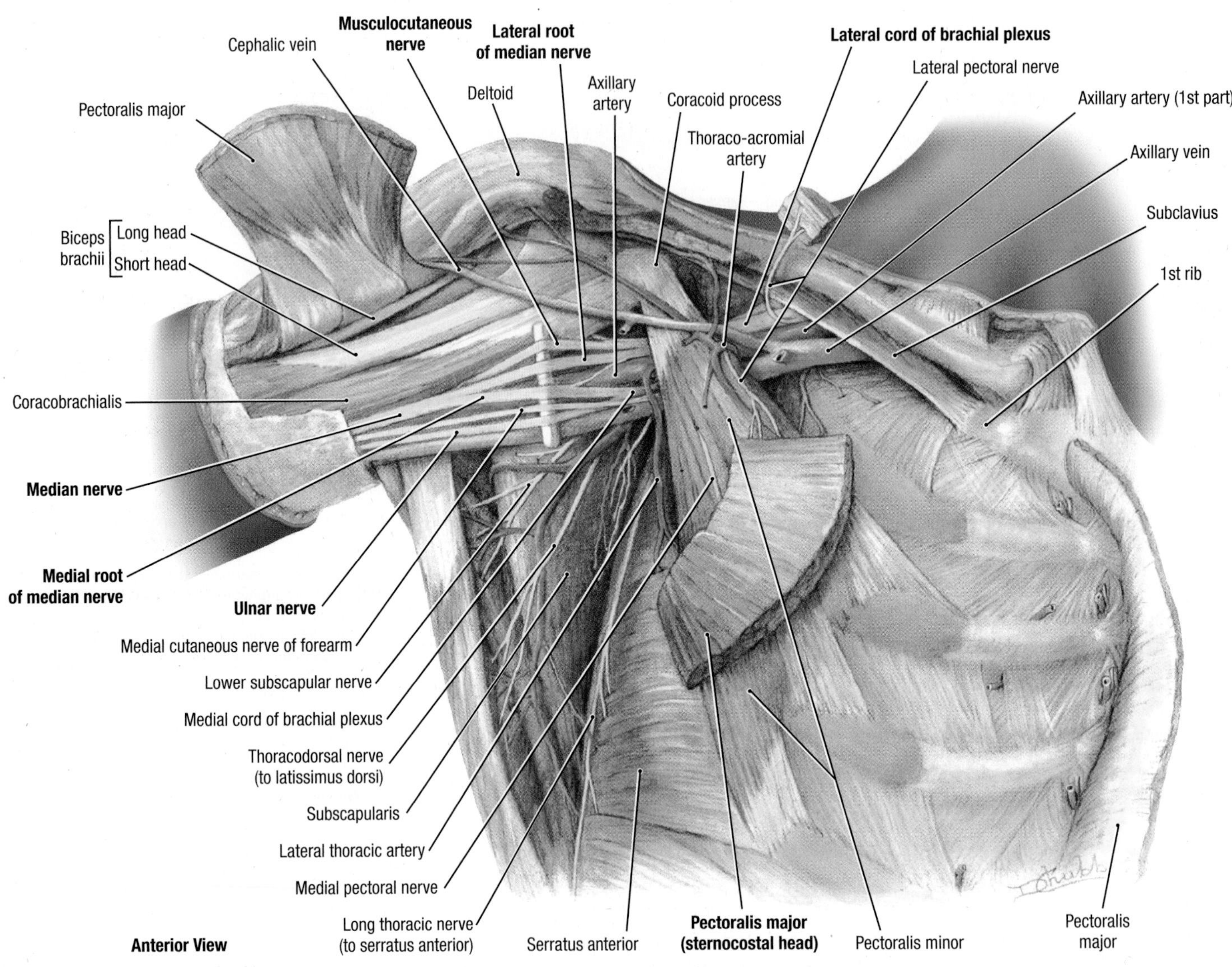
Cephalic vein
Musculocutaneous nerve
Lateral root of median nerve
Lateral cord of brachial plexus
Lateral pectoral nerve
Deltoid
Axillary artery
Coracoid process
Axillary artery (1st part)
Pectoralis major
Thoraco-acromial artery
Axillary vein
Subclavius
Biceps brachii
Long head
Short head
1st rib
Coracobrachialis
Median nerve
Medial root of median nerve
Ulnar nerve
Medial cutaneous nerve of forearm
Lower subscapular nerve
Medial cord of brachial plexus
Thoracodorsal nerve (to latissimus dorsi)
Subscapularis
Lateral thoracic artery
Medial pectoral nerve
Anterior View
Long thoracic nerve (to serratus anterior)
Serratus anterior
Pectoralis major (sternocostal head)
Pectoralis minor
Pectoralis major

6.26 STRUCTURES OF AXILLA: DEEP DISSECTION I

- The pectoralis major muscle is reflected, and the clavipectoral fascia is removed; the cube of muscle superior to the clavicle is cut from the clavicular head of the pectoralis major muscle.
- The subclavius and pectoralis minor are the two deep muscles of the anterior wall.
- The 2nd part axillary artery passes posterior to the pectoralis minor muscle, a fingerbreadth from the tip of the coracoid process; the axillary vein lies anterior and then medial to the axillary artery.
- The median nerve, followed proximally, leads by its lateral root to the lateral cord and musculocutaneous nerve and by its medial root to the medial cord and ulnar nerve. These four nerves and the medial cutaneous nerve of the forearm are derived from the anterior divisions of the brachial plexus and are raised on a stick. The lateral root of the median nerve may occur as several strands.
- The musculocutaneous nerve enters the flexor compartment of the arm by piercing the coracobrachialis muscle.

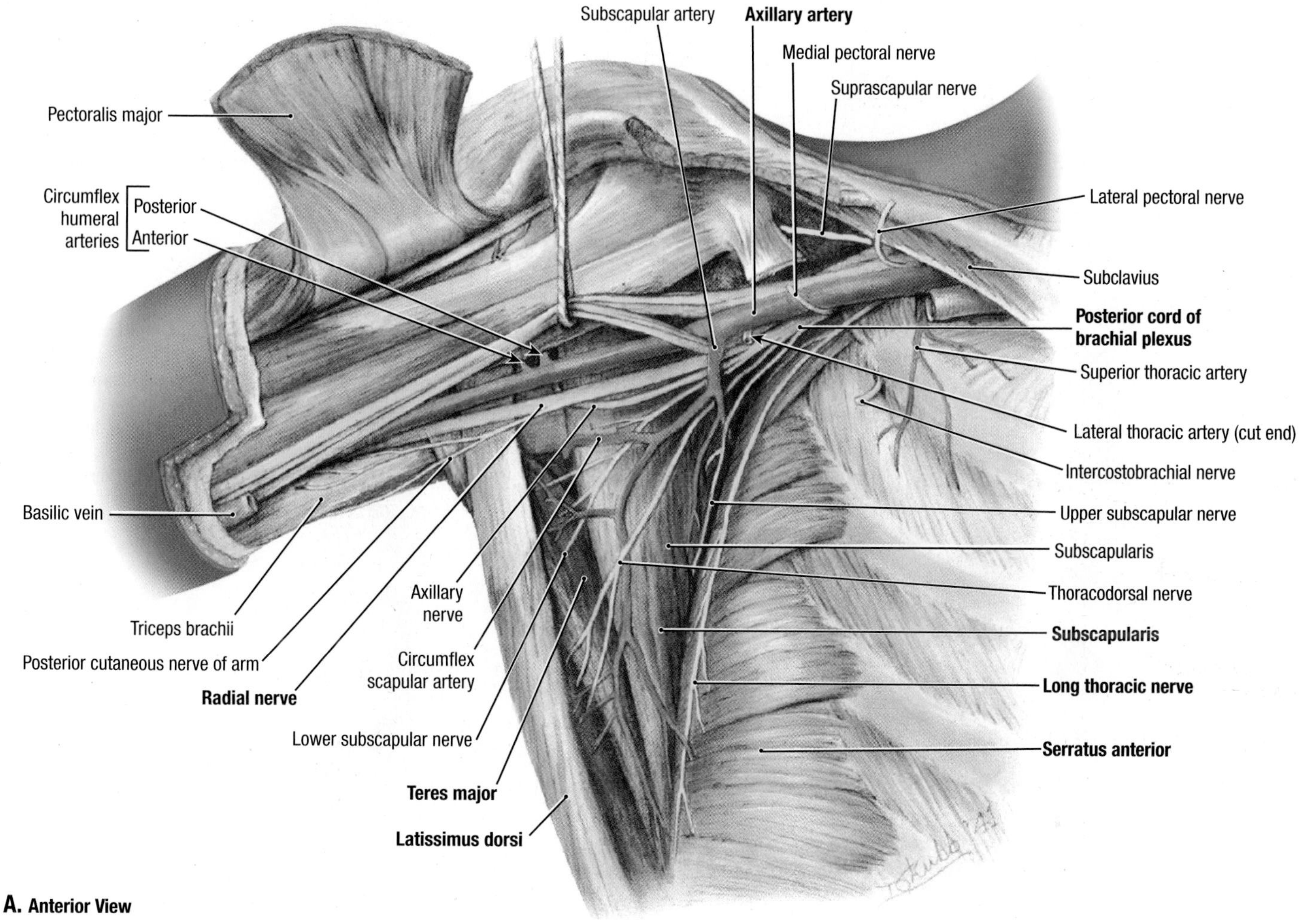

Subscapular artery
Axillary artery
Medial pectoral nerve
Suprascapular nerve
Pectoralis major
Circumflex humeral arteries: Posterior, Anterior
Lateral pectoral nerve
Subclavius
Posterior cord of brachial plexus
Superior thoracic artery
Lateral thoracic artery (cut end)
Intercostobrachial nerve
Basilic vein
Upper subscapular nerve
Subscapularis
Thoracodorsal nerve
Axillary nerve
Subscapularis
Triceps brachii
Posterior cutaneous nerve of arm
Circumflex scapular artery
Long thoracic nerve
Radial nerve
Lower subscapular nerve
Serratus anterior
Teres major
Latissimus dorsi

A. Anterior View

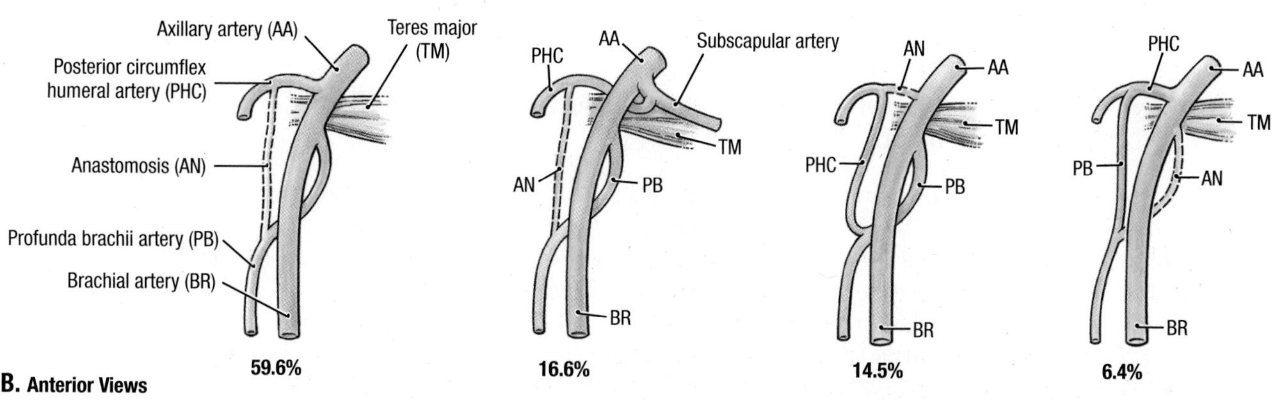
Axillary artery (AA)
Teres major (TM)
Posterior circumflex humeral artery (PHC)
Anastomosis (AN)
Profunda brachii artery (PB)
Brachial artery (BR)
59.6%
PHC
AA
Subscapular artery
TM
AN
PB
BR
16.6%
AN
AA
TM
PHC
PB
BR
14.5%
PHC
AA
TM
PB
AN
BR
6.4%

B. Anterior Views

6.27 POSTERIOR AND MEDIAL WALLS OF AXILLA: DEEP DISSECTION II

A. Dissection. The pectoralis minor muscle is excised, the lateral and medial cords of the brachial plexus are retracted, and the axillary vein is removed. **B.** Variations of the posterior circumflex humeral artery and profunda brachii artery. Percentages are based on 235 specimens dissected in Dr. Grant's laboratory.

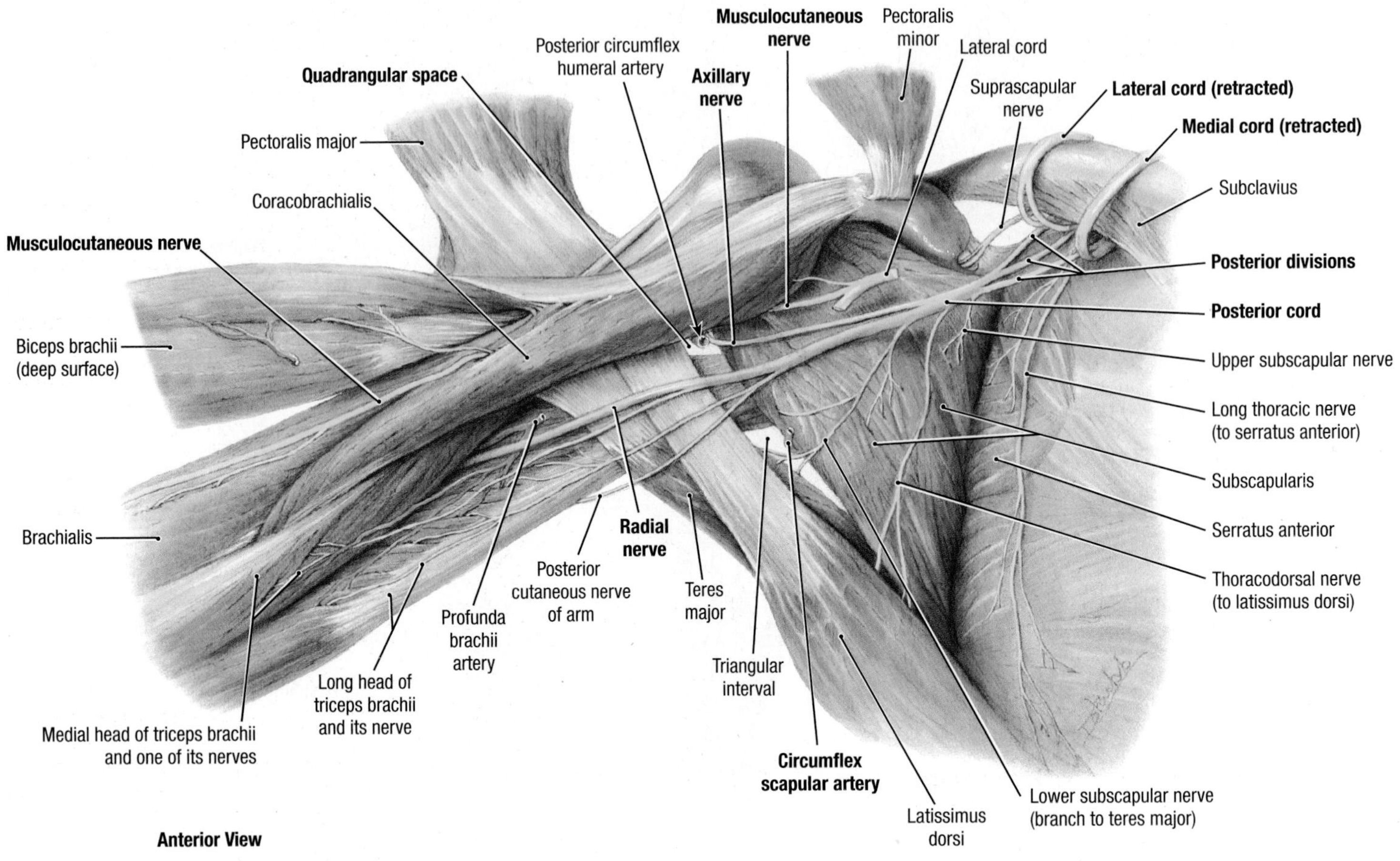
Musculocutaneous nerve
Pectoralis minor
Posterior circumflex humeral artery
Lateral cord
Quadrangular space
Axillary nerve
Suprascapular nerve
Lateral cord (retracted)
Medial cord (retracted)
Pectoralis major
Subclavius
Coracobrachialis
Musculocutaneous nerve
Posterior divisions
Posterior cord
Biceps brachii (deep surface)
Upper subscapular nerve
Long thoracic nerve (to serratus anterior)
Subscapularis
Brachialis
Radial nerve
Serratus anterior
Posterior cutaneous nerve of arm
Teres major
Thoracodorsal nerve (to latissimus dorsi)
Profunda brachii artery
Long head of triceps brachii and its nerve
Triangular interval
Medial head of triceps brachii and one of its nerves
Circumflex scapular artery
Lower subscapular nerve (branch to teres major)
Latissimus dorsi
Anterior View

6.28 POSTERIOR WALL OF AXILLA, MUSCULOCUTANEOUS NERVE, AND POSTERIOR CORD: DEEP DISSECTION III

- The pectoralis major and minor muscles are reflected laterally, the lateral and medial cords of the brachial plexus are reflected superiorly, and the arteries, veins, and median and ulnar nerves are removed.
- Coracobrachialis arises with the short head of the biceps brachii muscle from the tip of the coracoid process and attaches halfway down the medial aspect of the humerus.
- The musculocutaneous nerve pierces the coracobrachialis muscle and supplies it, the biceps, and the brachialis before becoming the lateral cutaneous nerve of the forearm.
- The posterior cord of the plexus is formed by the union of the three posterior divisions; it supplies the three muscles of the posterior wall of the axilla and then bifurcates into the radial and axillary nerves.
- In the axilla, the radial nerve gives off the nerve to the long head of the triceps brachii muscle and a cutaneous branch; in this specimen, it also gives off a branch to the medial head of the triceps. It then enters the radial groove of the humerus with the profunda brachii (deep brachial) artery.
- The axillary nerve passes through the quadrangular space along with the posterior circumflex humeral artery. The borders of the quadrangular space are superiorly, the lateral border of the scapula; inferiorly, the teres major; laterally, the humerus (surgical neck); and medially, the long head of triceps brachii. The circumflex scapular artery traverses the triangular interval.

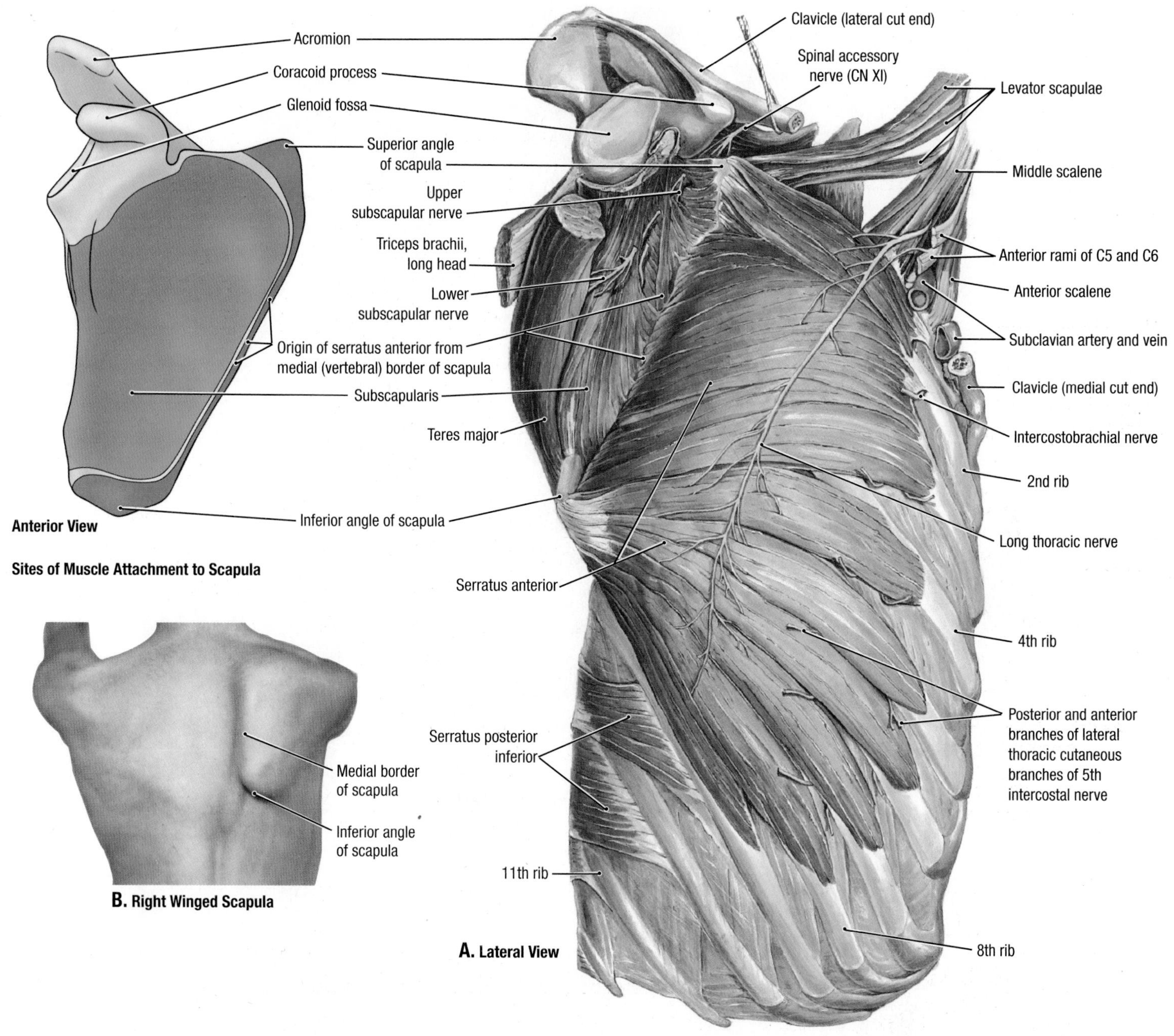
Acromion
Coracoid process
Glenoid fossa
Superior angle of scapula
Upper subscapular nerve
Triceps brachii, long head
Lower subscapular nerve
Origin of serratus anterior from medial (vertebral) border of scapula
Subscapularis
Teres major
Inferior angle of scapula
Anterior View
Sites of Muscle Attachment to Scapula
Clavicle (lateral cut end)
Spinal accessory nerve (CN XI)
Levator scapulae
Middle scalene
Anterior rami of C5 and C6
Anterior scalene
Subclavian artery and vein
Clavicle (medial cut end)
Intercostobrachial nerve
2nd rib
Long thoracic nerve
Serratus anterior
4th rib
Posterior and anterior branches of lateral thoracic cutaneous branches of 5th intercostal nerve
Serratus posterior inferior
11th rib
8th rib
Medial border of scapula
Inferior angle of scapula

B. Right Winged Scapula

A. Lateral View

6.29 SERRATUS ANTERIOR AND SUBSCAPULARIS

A. The serratus anterior muscle, which forms the medial wall of the axilla, has a fleshy belly extending from the superior 8 or 9 ribs in the midclavicular line *(right)* to the medial border of the scapula *(left)*.

- The fibers of the serratus anterior muscle from the 1st rib and the tendinous arch between the 1st and 2nd ribs (see Table 6.4) converge on the superior angle of the scapula; those from the 2nd and 3rd ribs diverge to spread thinly along the medial border; and the remainder (from the 4th to 9th ribs), which form the bulk of the muscle, converge on the inferior angle via a tendinous insertion.
- The long thoracic nerve to serratus anterior arises from spinal nerves C5, C6, and C7 and courses externally along most of the muscle's length.

Winged scapula (**B**). When the serratus anterior is paralyzed because of injury to the long thoracic nerve, the medial border of the scapula moves laterally and posteriorly, away from the thoracic wall. When the arm is abducted, the medial border and the inferior angle of the scapula pull away from the posterior thoracic wall, a deformation known as a winged scapula. In addition, the arm cannot be abducted above the horizontal position because the serratus anterior is unable to rotate the glenoid cavity superiorly.

- The trunks of the brachial plexus and the subclavian artery emerge between the anterior and middle scalene muscles; the subclavian vein is separated from the artery by the anterior scalene muscle.

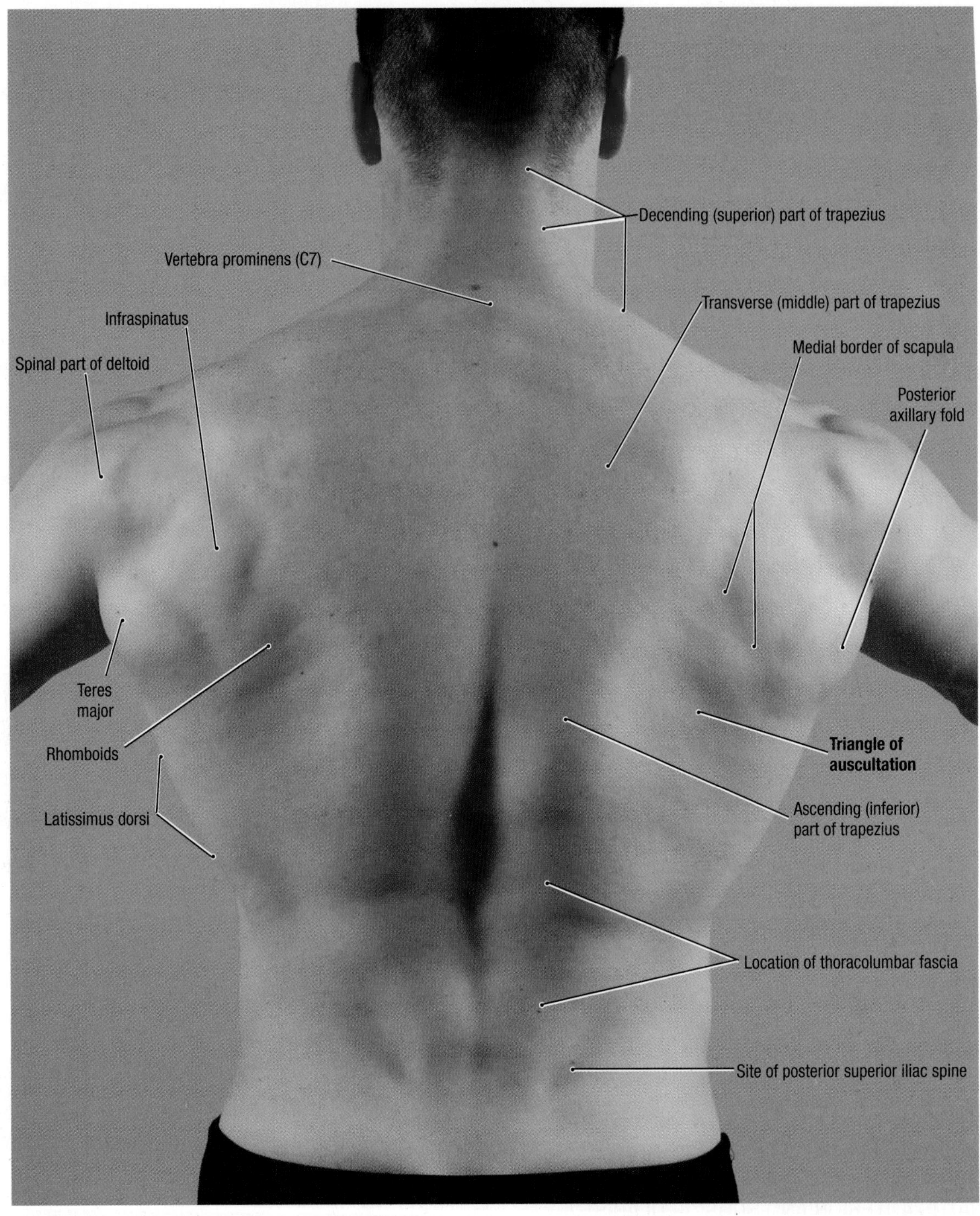

Decending (superior) part of trapezius
Vertebra prominens (C7)
Transverse (middle) part of trapezius
Infraspinatus
Medial border of scapula
Spinal part of deltoid
Posterior axillary fold
Teres major
Rhomboids
Triangle of auscultation
Latissimus dorsi
Ascending (inferior) part of trapezius
Location of thoracolumbar fascia
Site of posterior superior iliac spine

Posterior View

6.30 SURFACE ANATOMY OF SUPERFICIAL BACK

The superior border of the latissimus dorsi and a part of the rhomboid major are overlapped by the trapezius. The area formed by the superior border of latissimus dorsi, the medial border of the scapula, and the inferolateral border of the trapezius is called the **triangle of auscultation**. This gap in the thick back musculature is a good place to examine posterior segments of the lungs with a stethoscope. When the scapulae are drawn anteriorly by folding the arms across the thorax and the trunk is flexed, the auscultatory triangle enlarges. The teres major forms a raised oval area on the inferolateral third of the posterior aspect of the scapula when the arm is adducted against resistance. The posterior axillary fold is formed by the teres major and the tendon of the latissimus dorsi.

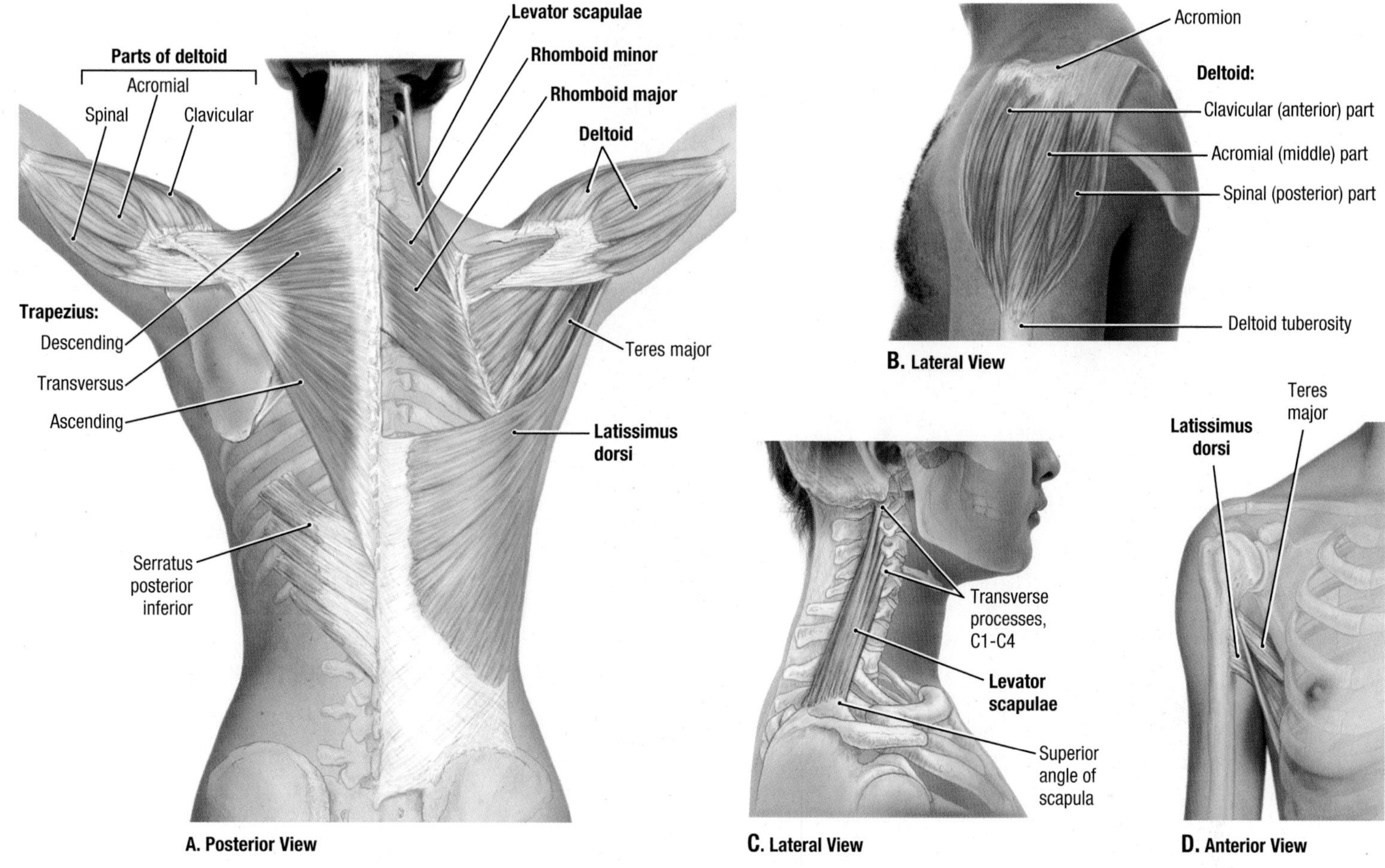
Parts of deltoid
Acromial
Spinal
Clavicular
Levator scapulae
Rhomboid minor
Rhomboid major
Deltoid
Trapezius:
Descending
Transversus
Ascending
Teres major
Latissimus dorsi
Serratus posterior inferior
A. Posterior View
Acromion
Deltoid:
Clavicular (anterior) part
Acromial (middle) part
Spinal (posterior) part
Deltoid tuberosity
B. Lateral View
Transverse processes, C1-C4
Levator scapulae
Superior angle of scapula
C. Lateral View
Teres major
Latissimus dorsi
D. Anterior View

6.31 SUPERFICIAL BACK AND DELTOID MUSCLES

TABLE 6.7 SUPERFICIAL BACK (POSTERIOR AXIO-APPENDICULAR) AND DELTOID MUSCLES

Muscle	Proximal Attachment	Distal Attachment	Innervation	Main Actions
Trapezius	Medial third of superior nuchal line; external occipital protuberance, nuchal ligament, and spinous processes of C7–T12 vertebrae	Lateral third of clavicle, acromion, and spine of scapula	Spinal accessory nerve (CN XI—motor) and cervical nerves (C3–C4—sensory)	Elevates, retracts, and rotates scapula; *descending part* elevates, *transverse part* retracts, and *ascending part* depresses scapula; descending and ascending part act together in superior rotation of scapula
Latissimus dorsi	Spinous processes of inferior six thoracic vertebrae, thoracolumbar fascia, iliac crest, and inferior three or four ribs	Intertubercular sulcus (bicipital groove) of humerus	Thoracodorsal nerve (**C6, C7**, C8)	Extends, adducts, and medially rotates shoulder joint; elevates body toward arms during climbing
Levator scapulae	Posterior tubercles of transverse processes of C1–C4 vertebrae	Superior part of medial border of scapula	Dorsal scapular (C5) and cervical (C3–C4) nerves	Elevates scapula and tilts its glenoid cavity inferiorly by rotating scapula
Rhomboid minor and major	*Minor:* Inferior part of nuchal ligament and spinous processes of C7 and T1 vertebrae *Major:* spinous processes of T2–T5 vertebrae	Medial border of scapula from level of spine to inferior angle	Dorsal scapular nerve (C4–**C5**)	Retract scapula and rotate it to depress glenoid cavity; fix scapula to thoracic wall
Deltoid	Lateral third of clavicle *(clavicular part)*, acromion *(acromial part)*, and spine *(spinal part)* of scapula	Deltoid tuberosity of humerus	Axillary nerve (**C5**–C6)	*Clavicular (anterior) part:* flexes and medially rotates shoulder joint; *acromial (middle) part:* abducts shoulder joint; *spinal (posterior) part:* extends and laterally rotates shoulder joint

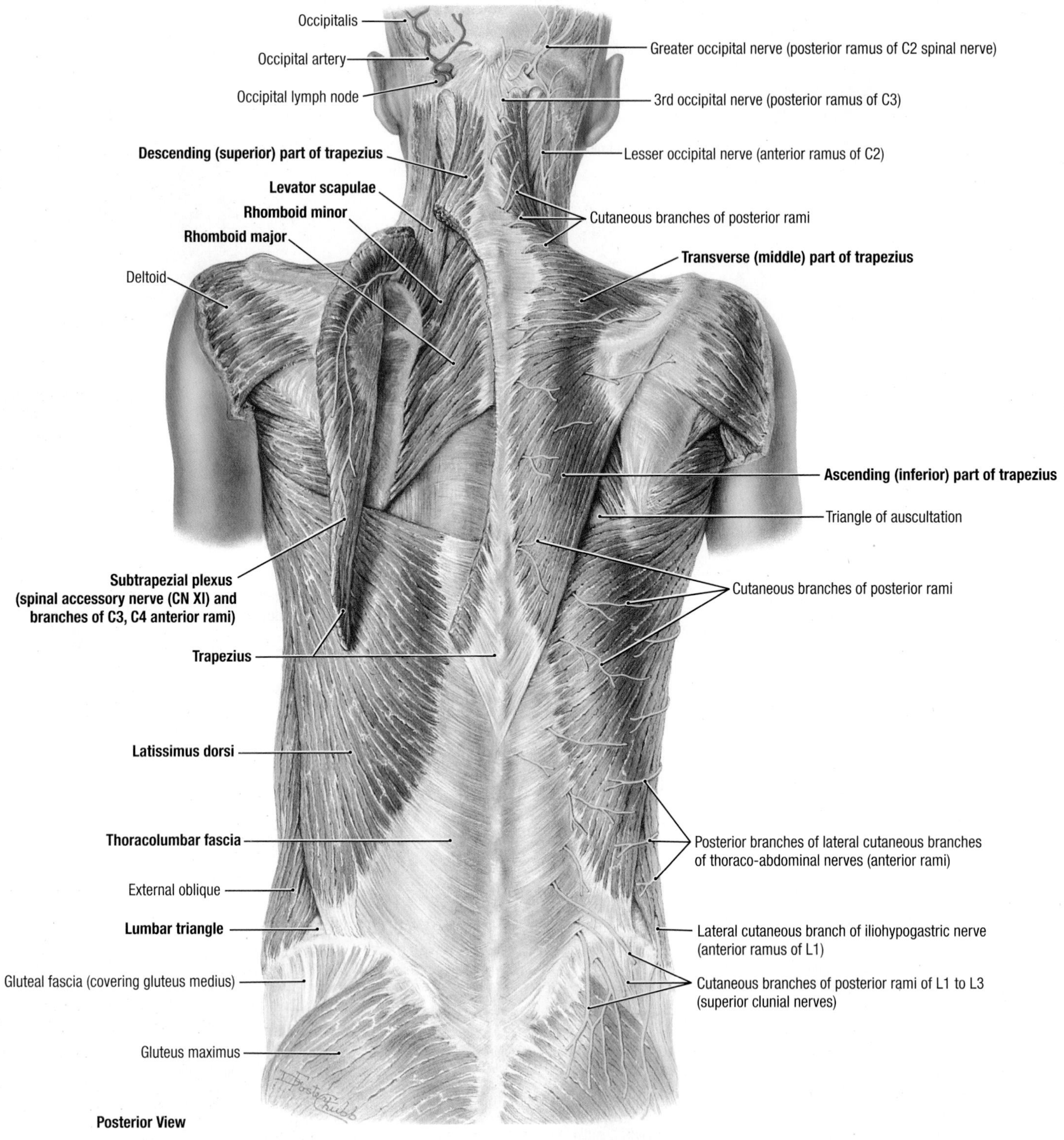
Occipitalis
Occipital artery
Occipital lymph node
Descending (superior) part of trapezius
Levator scapulae
Rhomboid minor
Rhomboid major
Deltoid
Greater occipital nerve (posterior ramus of C2 spinal nerve)
3rd occipital nerve (posterior ramus of C3)
Lesser occipital nerve (anterior ramus of C2)
Cutaneous branches of posterior rami
Transverse (middle) part of trapezius
Ascending (inferior) part of trapezius
Triangle of auscultation
Cutaneous branches of posterior rami
Subtrapezial plexus (spinal accessory nerve (CN XI) and branches of C3, C4 anterior rami)
Trapezius
Latissimus dorsi
Thoracolumbar fascia
External oblique
Lumbar triangle
Gluteal fascia (covering gluteus medius)
Gluteus maximus
Posterior branches of lateral cutaneous branches of thoraco-abdominal nerves (anterior rami)
Lateral cutaneous branch of iliohypogastric nerve (anterior ramus of L1)
Cutaneous branches of posterior rami of L1 to L3 (superior clunial nerves)
Posterior View

6.32 CUTANEOUS NERVES OF SUPERFICIAL BACK AND POSTERIOR AXIO-APPENDICULAR MUSCLES

The trapezius muscle is cut and reflected on the left side. A superficial or first muscle layer consists of the trapezius and latissimus dorsi muscles, and a second layer of the levator scapulae and rhomboids. Cutaneous branches of posterior rami penetrate but do not supply the superficial muscles.

TABLE 6.8 MOVEMENTS OF SCAPULA

Boldface indicates prime movers. In the *middle* and *right columns* the *dotted outlines* represent the starting position for each movement.

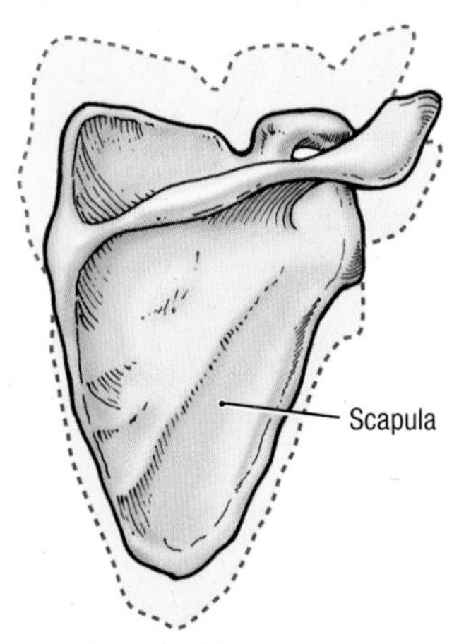
Scapula

Posterior View
Elevation (red)
Depression (green)

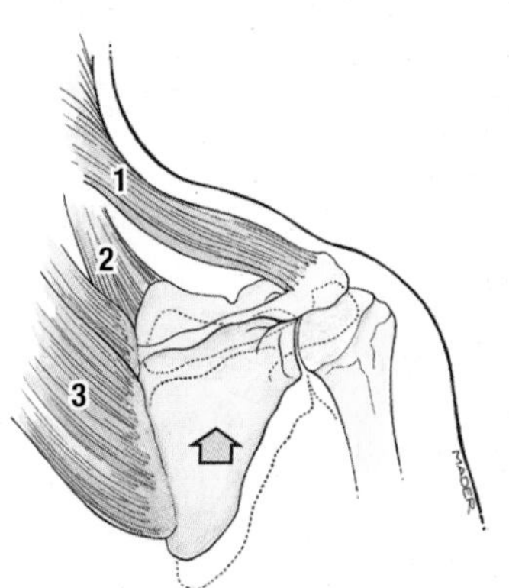
1
2
3

Posterior View

Elevation:
Trapezius, descending part (1)
Levator scapulae (2)
Rhomboids (3)

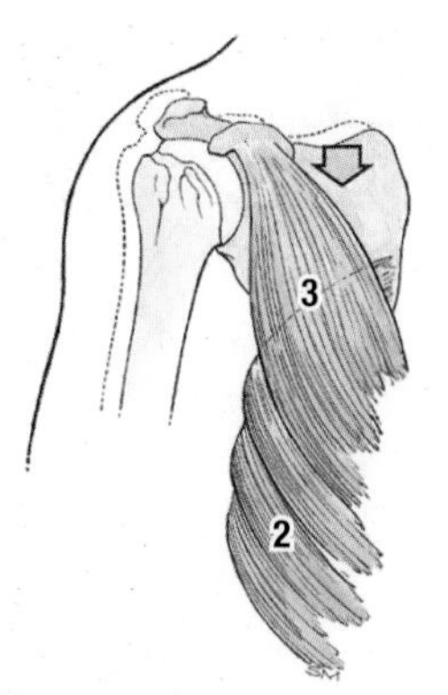
3
2

Anterior View

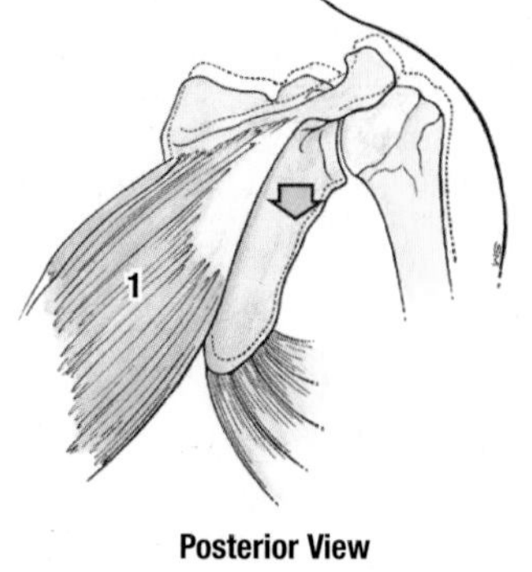
1

Posterior View

Depression:
Trapezius, ascending part (1)
Serratus anterior, inferior part (2)
Pectoralis minor (3)

Also: Gravity, Latissimus dorsi, Inferior part of sternocostal head of pectoralis major

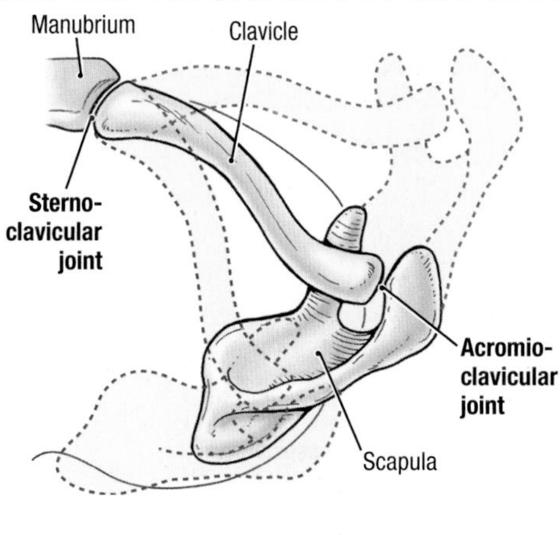
Manubrium
Clavicle
Sterno-clavicular joint
Acromio-clavicular joint
Scapula

Protraction (red)
Retraction (green)

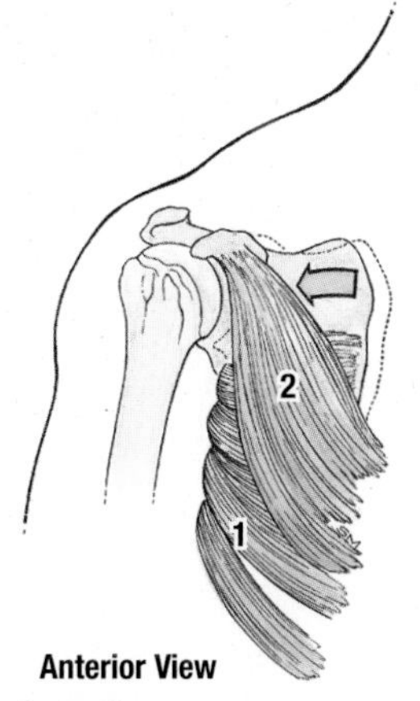
2
1

Anterior View

Protraction:
Serratus anterior (1)
Pectoralis minor (2)
Also: Pectoralis major

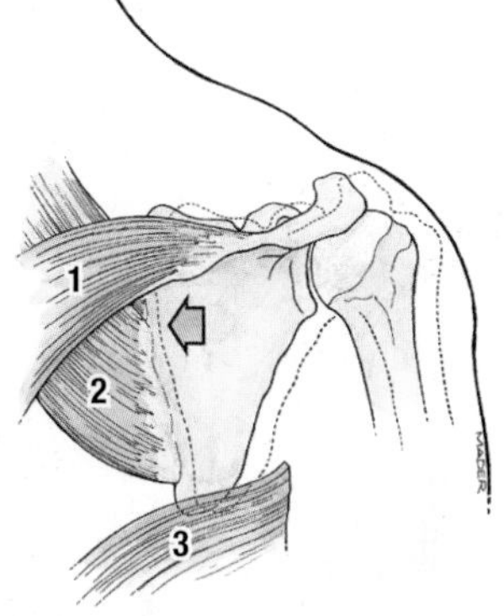
1
2
3

Posterior View

Retraction:
Trapezius, transverse part (1)
Rhomboids (2)
Latissimus dorsi (3)

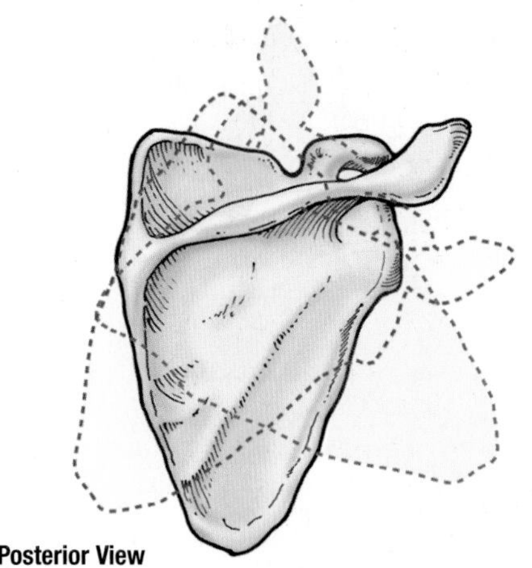

Posterior View

Upward rotation (red)
Downward rotation (green)

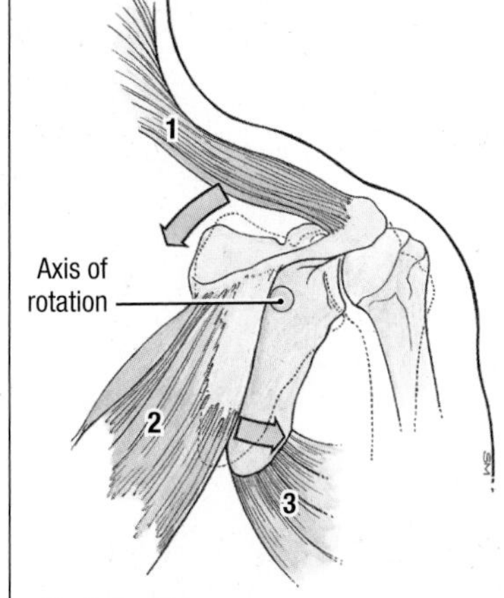
1
Axis of rotation
2
3

Posterior View

Upward rotation
Trapezius, descending part (1)
Trapezius, ascending part (2)
Serratus anterior, inferior part (3)

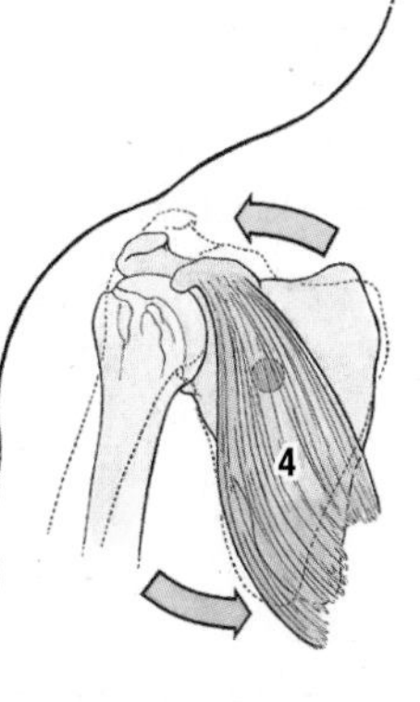
4

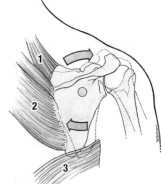

Anterior View

Posterior View

Downward rotation
Levator scapulae (1)
Rhomboids (2)
Latissimus dorsi (3)
Pectoralis minor (4)

Also: Gravity, Inferior part of sternocostal head of pectoralis major

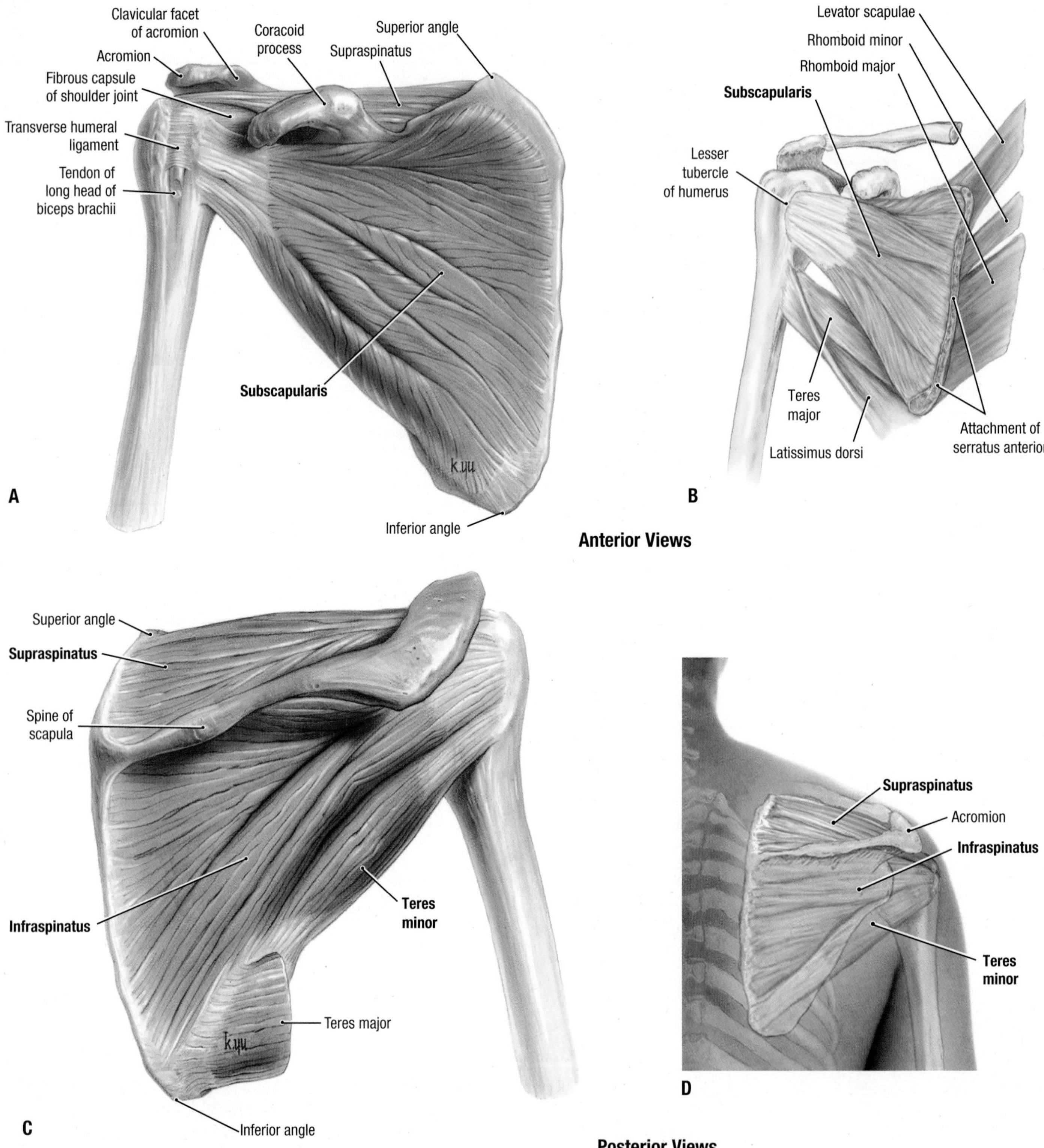
Clavicular facet of acromion
Acromion
Coracoid process
Superior angle
Supraspinatus
Fibrous capsule of shoulder joint
Transverse humeral ligament
Tendon of long head of biceps brachii
Subscapularis
Inferior angle
A
Levator scapulae
Rhomboid minor
Rhomboid major
Subscapularis
Lesser tubercle of humerus
Teres major
Latissimus dorsi
Attachment of serratus anterior
B
Anterior Views
Superior angle
Supraspinatus
Spine of scapula
Infraspinatus
Teres minor
Teres major
Inferior angle
C
Supraspinatus
Acromion
Infraspinatus
Teres minor
D
Posterior Views

6.33 ROTATOR CUFF

A. and B. Subscapularis. **C. and D.** Supraspinatus, infraspinatus, and teres minor.

Four of the scapulohumeral muscles—supraspinatus, infraspinatus, teres minor, and subscapularis—are called rotator cuff muscles because they form a musculotendinous rotator cuff around the glenohumeral joint. All except the supraspinatus are rotators of the humerus.

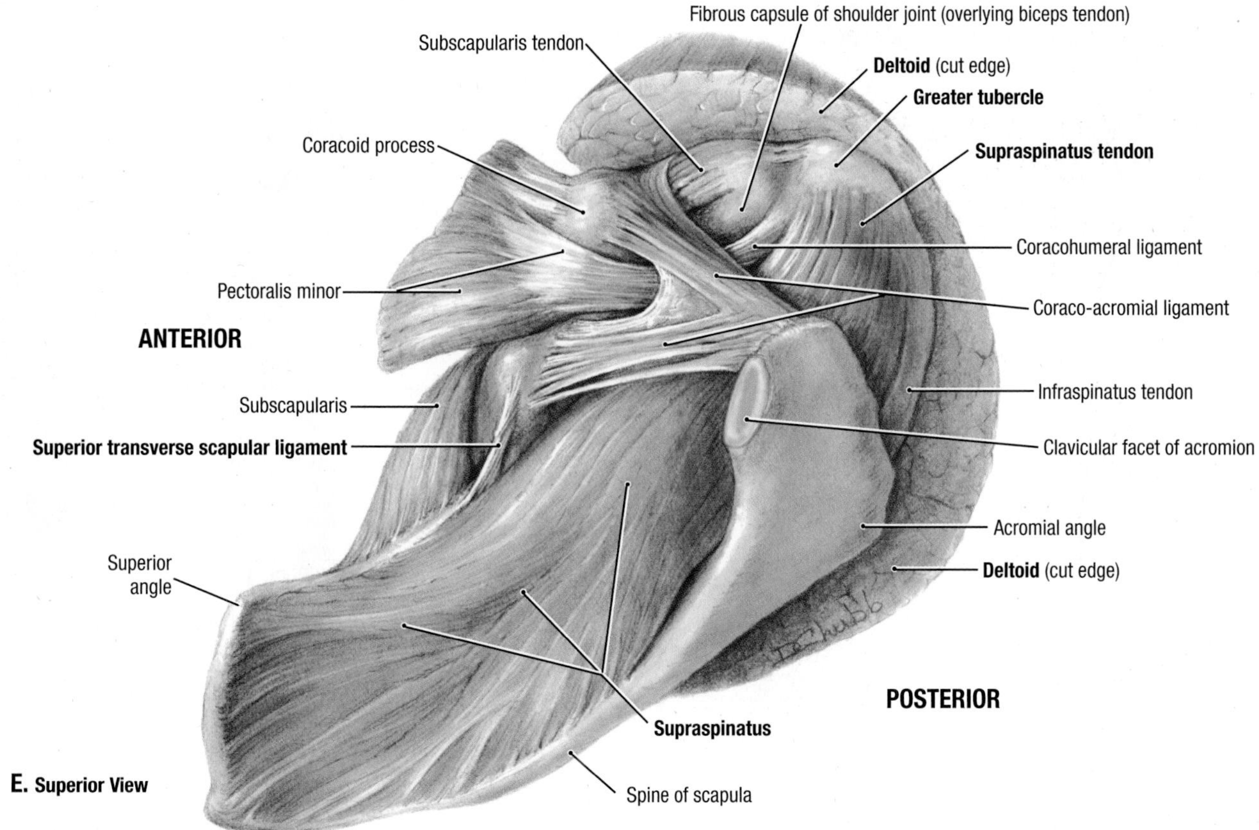
Fibrous capsule of shoulder joint (overlying biceps tendon)
Subscapularis tendon
Deltoid (cut edge)
Greater tubercle
Supraspinatus tendon
Coracoid process
Coracohumeral ligament
Pectoralis minor
Coraco-acromial ligament
ANTERIOR
Infraspinatus tendon
Subscapularis
Superior transverse scapular ligament
Clavicular facet of acromion
Acromial angle
Superior angle
Deltoid (cut edge)
POSTERIOR
Supraspinatus
Spine of scapula

E. **Superior View**

6.33 ROTATOR CUFF *(CONTINUED)*

E. Supraspinatus.

The supraspinatus, also part of the rotator cuff, initiates and assists the deltoid in abducting the shoulder joint. The tendons of the rotator cuff muscles blend with and reinforce the joint capsule of the glenohumeral joint, protecting the joint and giving it stability.

Injury or disease may damage the rotator cuff, producing instability of the glenohumeral joint. **Rupture or tear of the supraspinatus tendon** is the most common injury of the rotator cuff. **Degenerative tendinitis of the rotator cuff** is common, especially in older people.

TABLE 6.9 SCAPULOHUMERAL MUSCLES

Muscle	Proximal Attachment	Distal Attachment	Innervation	Main Actions
Supraspinatus (S)	Supraspinous fossa of scapula	Superior facet on greater tubercle of humerus	Suprascapular nerve (C4, **C5**, and C6)	Initiates abduction at shoulder joint and acts with rotator cuff muscles[a]
Infraspinatus (I)	Infraspinous fossa of scapula	Middle facet on greater tubercle of humerus	Suprascapular nerve (**C5** and C6)	Laterally rotates shoulder joint; helps to hold humeral head in glenoid cavity of scapula
Teres minor (T)	Superior part of lateral border of scapula	Inferior facet on greater tubercle of humerus	Axillary nerve (**C5** and C6)	
Subscapularis(S)	Subscapular fossa	Lesser tubercle of humerus	Upper and lower subscapular nerves (C5, **C6**, and C7)	Medially rotates shoulder joint and adducts it; helps to hold humeral head in glenoid cavity
Teres major[b]	Posterior surface of inferior angle of scapula	Crest of lesser tubercle (medial lip of bicipital groove) of humerus	Lower subscapular nerve (**C6** and C7)	Adducts and medially rotates shoulder joint

[a]Collectively, the supraspinatus, infraspinatus, teres minor, and subscapularis muscles are referred to as the rotator cuff muscles or "SITS" muscles. They function together during all movements of the shoulder joint to hold the head of the humerus in the glenoid cavity of scapula.
[b]Not a rotator cuff muscle.

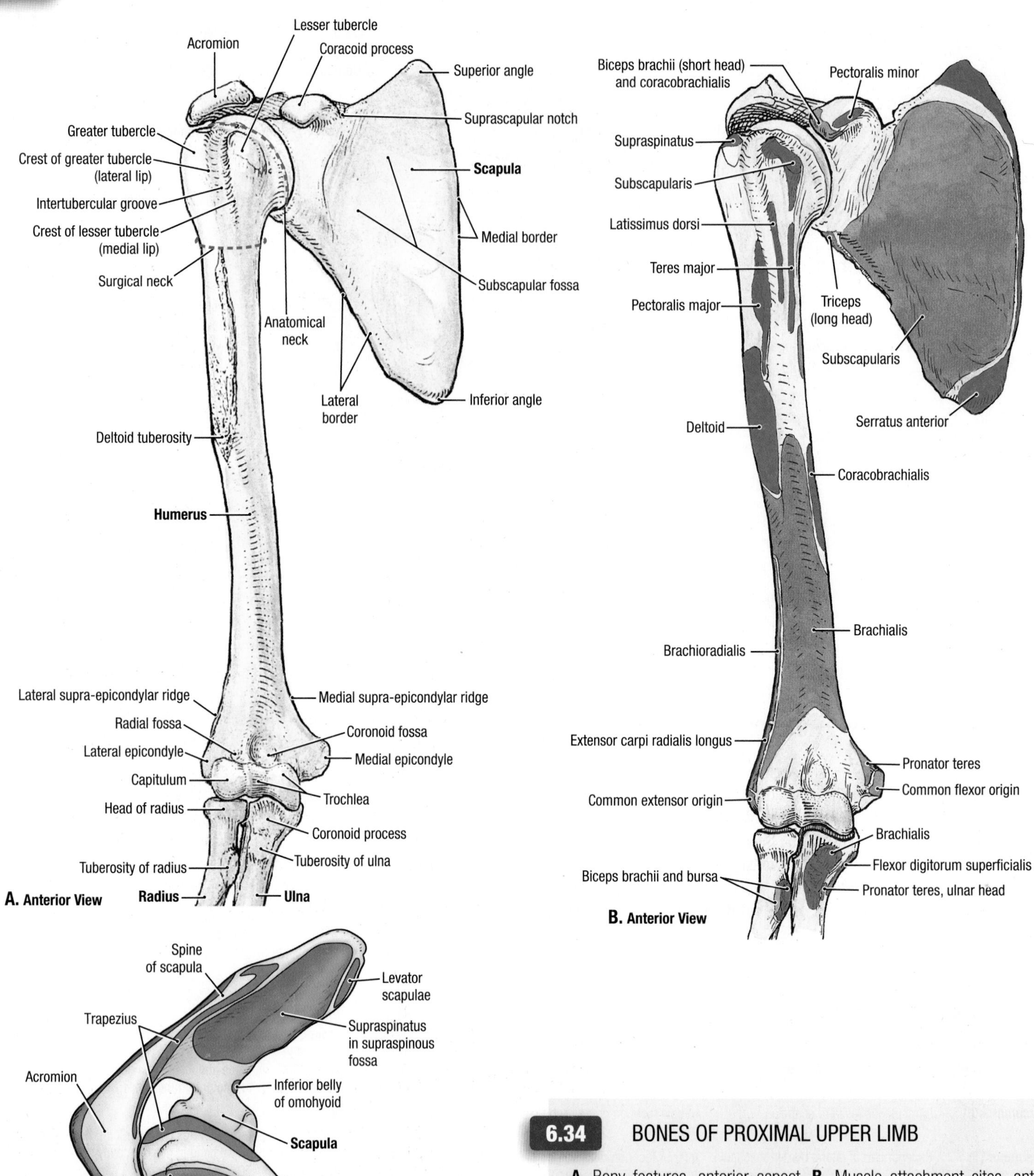

Lesser tubercle
Acromion
Coracoid process
Superior angle
Greater tubercle
Suprascapular notch
Crest of greater tubercle (lateral lip)
Scapula
Intertubercular groove
Crest of lesser tubercle (medial lip)
Medial border
Surgical neck
Subscapular fossa
Anatomical neck
Lateral border
Inferior angle
Deltoid tuberosity
Humerus
Lateral supra-epicondylar ridge
Medial supra-epicondylar ridge
Radial fossa
Coronoid fossa
Lateral epicondyle
Medial epicondyle
Capitulum
Trochlea
Head of radius
Coronoid process
Tuberosity of radius
Tuberosity of ulna
A. Anterior View
Radius
Ulna
Biceps brachii (short head) and coracobrachialis
Pectoralis minor
Supraspinatus
Subscapularis
Latissimus dorsi
Teres major
Pectoralis major
Triceps (long head)
Subscapularis
Serratus anterior
Deltoid
Coracobrachialis
Brachialis
Brachioradialis
Extensor carpi radialis longus
Pronator teres
Common flexor origin
Common extensor origin
Brachialis
Flexor digitorum superficialis
Biceps brachii and bursa
Pronator teres, ulnar head
B. Anterior View
Spine of scapula
Levator scapulae
Trapezius
Supraspinatus in supraspinous fossa
Acromion
Inferior belly of omohyoid
Scapula
Clavicle
Deltoid
Sternocleidomastoid (SCM)
Coracobrachialis and short head of biceps brachii
Coracoid process
C. Superior View
Pectoralis major

6.34 BONES OF PROXIMAL UPPER LIMB

A. Bony features, anterior aspect. **B.** Muscle attachment sites, anterior aspect. **C.** Muscle attachment sites, clavicle and scapula. **Fractures of the clavicle** are common, often caused by indirect force transmitted from an outstretched hand through the bones of the forearm and arm to the shoulder during a fall. A fracture may also result from a fall directly on the shoulder. The weakest part of the clavicle is at the junction of its middle and lateral thirds.

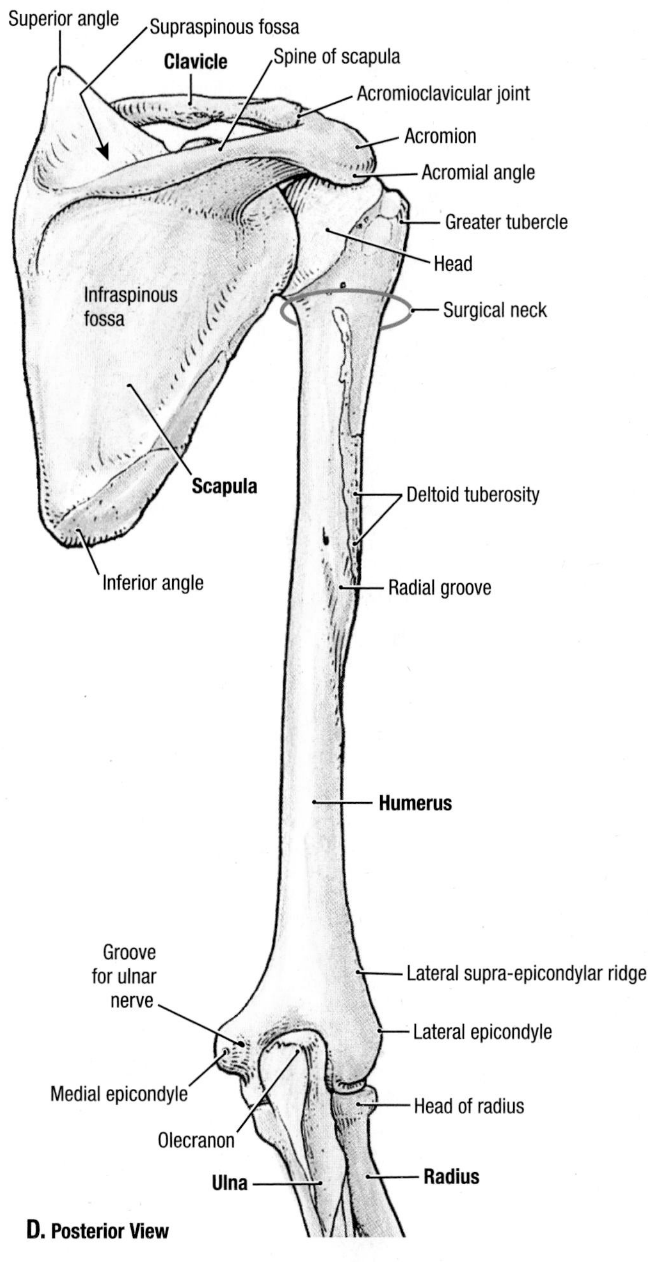
Superior angle
Supraspinous fossa
Clavicle
Spine of scapula
Acromioclavicular joint
Acromion
Acromial angle
Greater tubercle
Head
Infraspinous fossa
Surgical neck
Scapula
Deltoid tuberosity
Inferior angle
Radial groove
Humerus
Groove for ulnar nerve
Lateral supra-epicondylar ridge
Lateral epicondyle
Medial epicondyle
Head of radius
Olecranon
Ulna
Radius
D. Posterior View

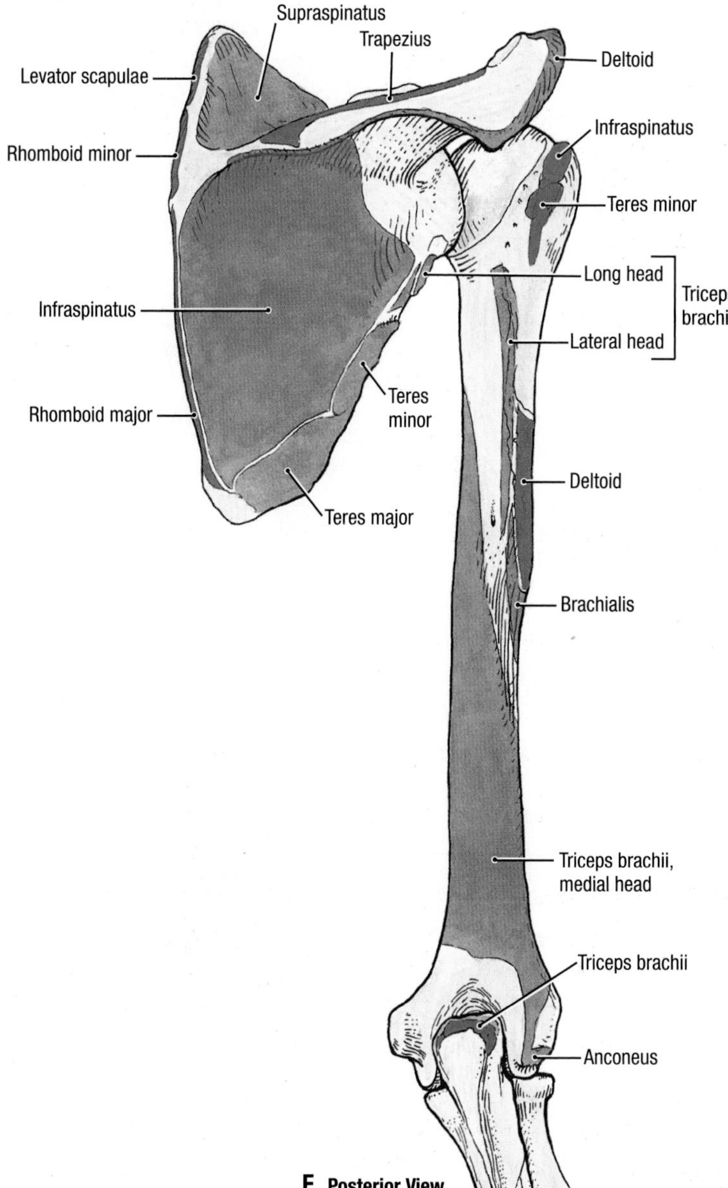
Supraspinatus
Trapezius
Levator scapulae
Deltoid
Infraspinatus
Rhomboid minor
Teres minor
Long head
Triceps brachii
Lateral head
Infraspinatus
Teres minor
Rhomboid major
Deltoid
Teres major
Brachialis
Triceps brachii, medial head
Triceps brachii
Anconeus
E. Posterior View

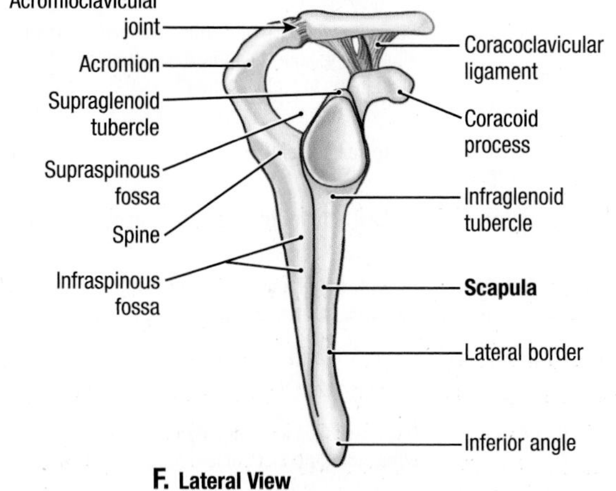
Acromioclavicular joint
Acromion
Coracoclavicular ligament
Supraglenoid tubercle
Coracoid process
Supraspinous fossa
Infraglenoid tubercle
Spine
Infraspinous fossa
Scapula
Lateral border
Inferior angle
F. Lateral View

6.34 BONES OF PROXIMAL UPPER LIMB *(CONTINUED)*

D. Bony features, posterior aspect. **E.** Muscle attachment sites, posterior aspect. **Fractures of the surgical neck of the humerus** are especially common in elderly people with **osteoporosis** (degeneration of bone). Even a low energy fall on the hand, with the force being transmitted up the forearm bones of the extended limb, may result in a fracture. **Transverse fractures of the shaft of humerus** frequently result from a direct blow to the arm. Fracture of the distal part of the humerus, near the supra-epicondylar ridges, is a **supra-epicondylar (supracondylar) fracture.**

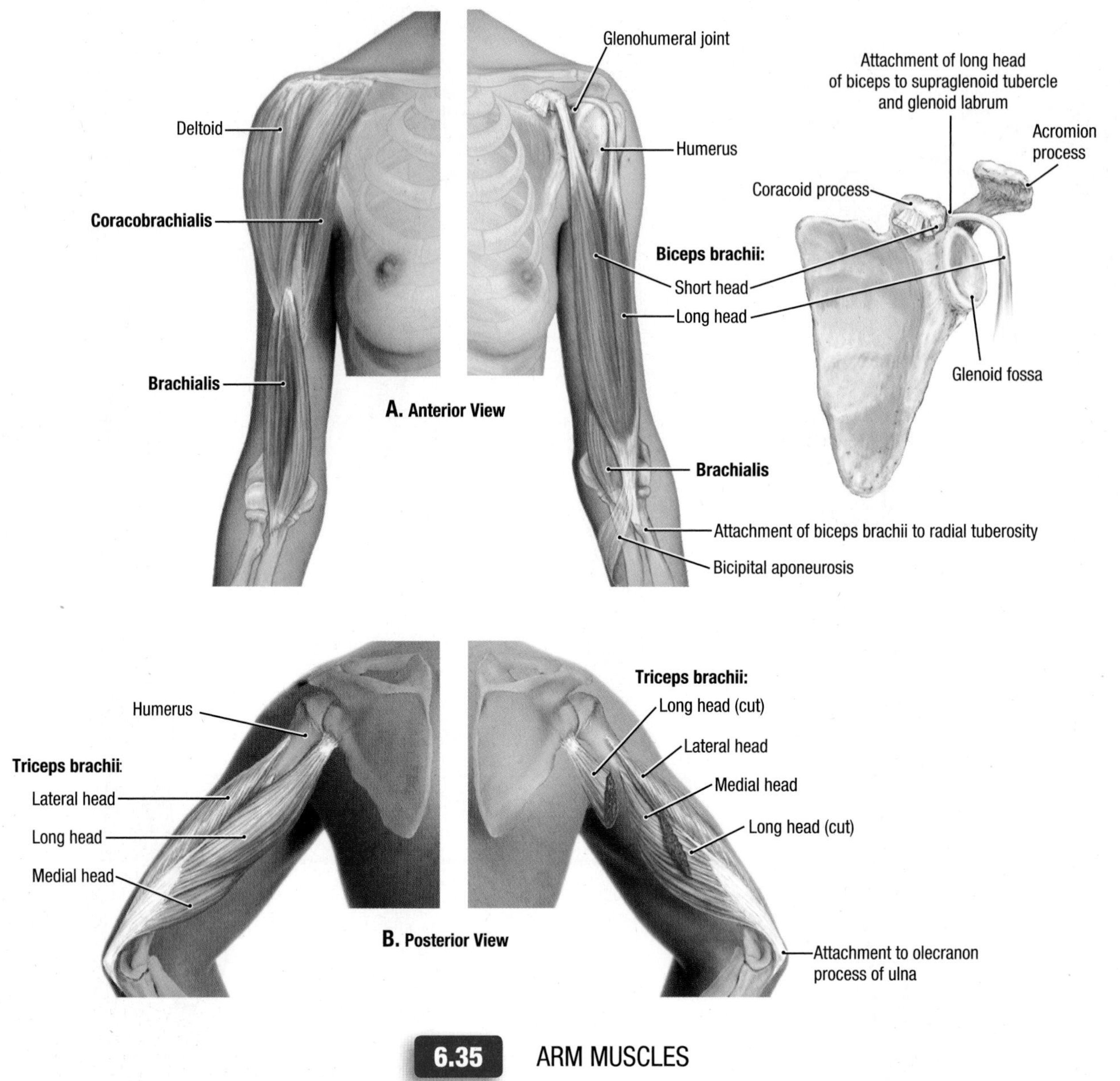
Deltoid
Coracobrachialis
Brachialis
Glenohumeral joint
Humerus
Biceps brachii:
Short head
Long head
Brachialis
Attachment of biceps brachii to radial tuberosity
Bicipital aponeurosis
Attachment of long head of biceps to supraglenoid tubercle and glenoid labrum
Acromion process
Coracoid process
Glenoid fossa
A. Anterior View
Humerus
Triceps brachii:
Lateral head
Long head
Medial head
Triceps brachii:
Long head (cut)
Lateral head
Medial head
Long head (cut)
Attachment to olecranon process of ulna
B. Posterior View

6.35 ARM MUSCLES

TABLE 6.10 ARM MUSCLES

Muscle	Proximal Attachment	Distal Attachment	Innervation	Main Actions
Biceps brachii	*Short head:* tip of coracoid process of scapula *Long head:* supraglenoid tubercle of scapula and glenoid labrum	Tuberosity of radius and fascia of forearm through bicipital aponeurosis	Musculocutaneous nerve (C5, **C6**, C7)	Supinates forearm and, when forearm is supine, flexes elbow joint; short head flexes shoulder joint; long head helps to stabilize should joint during abduction.
Brachialis	Distal half of anterior surface of humerus	Coronoid process and tuberosity of ulna	Musculocutaneous nerve (C5–C7) and radial (C5–C7)	Flexes elbow joint in all positions
Coracobrachialis	Tip of coracoid process of scapula	Middle third of medial surface of humerus	Musculocutaneous nerve (C5, **C6**, C7)	Assists with flexion and adduction of shoulder joint
Triceps brachii	*Long head:* infraglenoid tubercle of scapula *Lateral head:* posterior surface of humerus, superior to radial groove *Medial head:* posterior surface of humerus, inferior to radial groove	Proximal end of olecranon of ulna and fascia of forearm	Radial nerve (C6, **C7**, **C8**)	Extends the elbow joint; long head steadies head of humerus when shoulder joint is abducted
Anconeus	Lateral epicondyle of humerus	Lateral surface of olecranon and superior part of posterior surface of ulna	Radial nerve (C7–T1)	Assists triceps in extending elbow joint; stabilizes elbow joint; abducts ulna during pronation

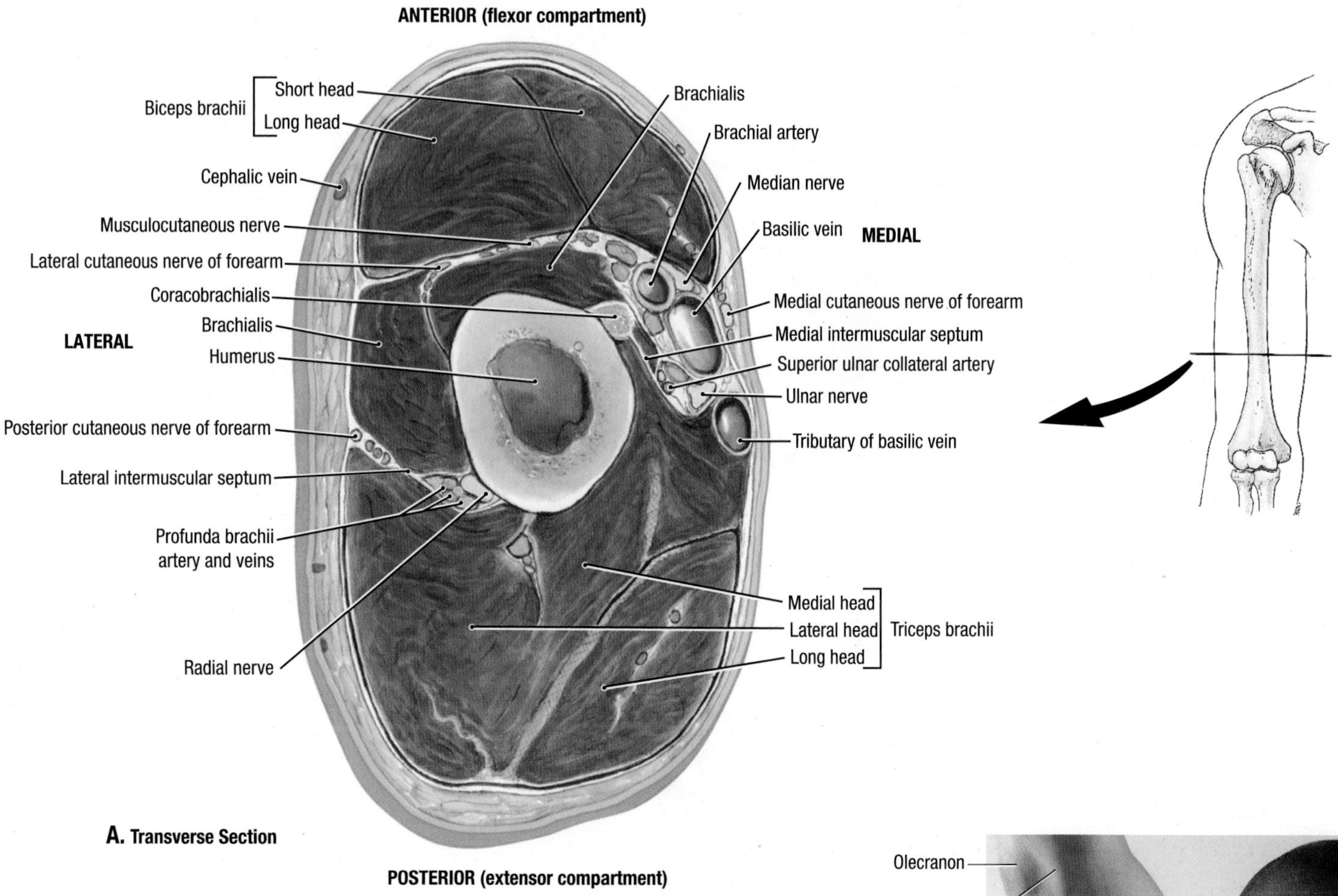

ANTERIOR (flexor compartment)

Biceps brachii
Short head
Long head
Brachialis
Brachial artery
Median nerve
Basilic vein
MEDIAL
Cephalic vein
Musculocutaneous nerve
Lateral cutaneous nerve of forearm
Coracobrachialis
Brachialis
LATERAL
Humerus
Medial cutaneous nerve of forearm
Medial intermuscular septum
Superior ulnar collateral artery
Ulnar nerve
Tributary of basilic vein
Posterior cutaneous nerve of forearm
Lateral intermuscular septum
Profunda brachii artery and veins
Radial nerve
Triceps brachii
Medial head
Lateral head
Long head

A. Transverse Section

POSTERIOR (extensor compartment)

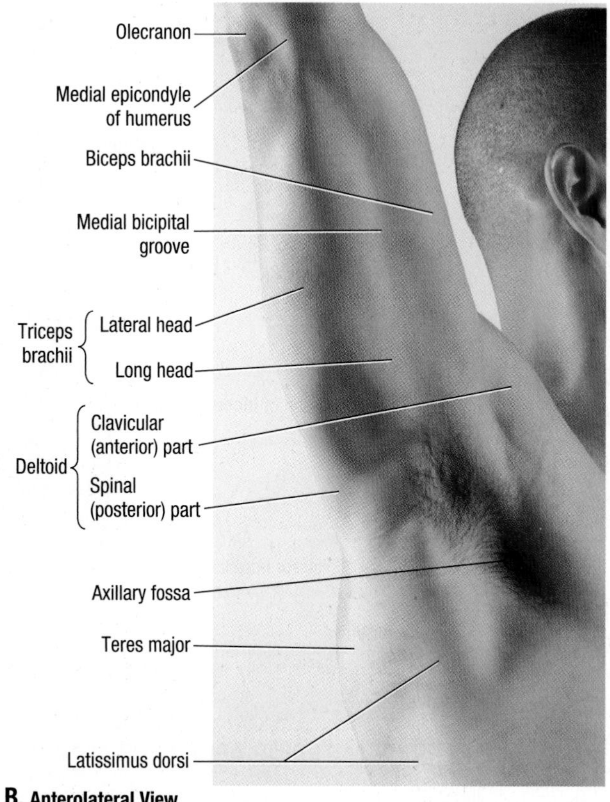
Olecranon
Medial epicondyle of humerus
Biceps brachii
Medial bicipital groove
Triceps brachii
Lateral head
Long head
Deltoid
Clavicular (anterior) part
Spinal (posterior) part
Axillary fossa
Teres major
Latissimus dorsi

B. Anterolateral View

6.36 ANTERIOR AND POSTERIOR COMPARTMENTS OF ARM

A. Anatomical section. **B.** Surface anatomy.

- Three muscles, the biceps, brachialis, and coracobrachialis, lie in the anterior compartment of the arm; the triceps brachii lies in the posterior compartment.
- The medial and lateral intermuscular septum separates these two muscle groups.
- The radial nerve and profunda brachii artery and veins serving the posterior compartment lie in contact with the radial groove of the humerus.
- The musculocutaneous nerve serving the anterior compartment lies in the plane between the biceps and the brachialis muscles.
- The median nerve crosses to the medial side of the brachial artery.
- The ulnar nerve passes posteriorly onto the medial side of the triceps muscle.
- The basilic vein (appearing here as two vessels) has pierced the deep fascia.

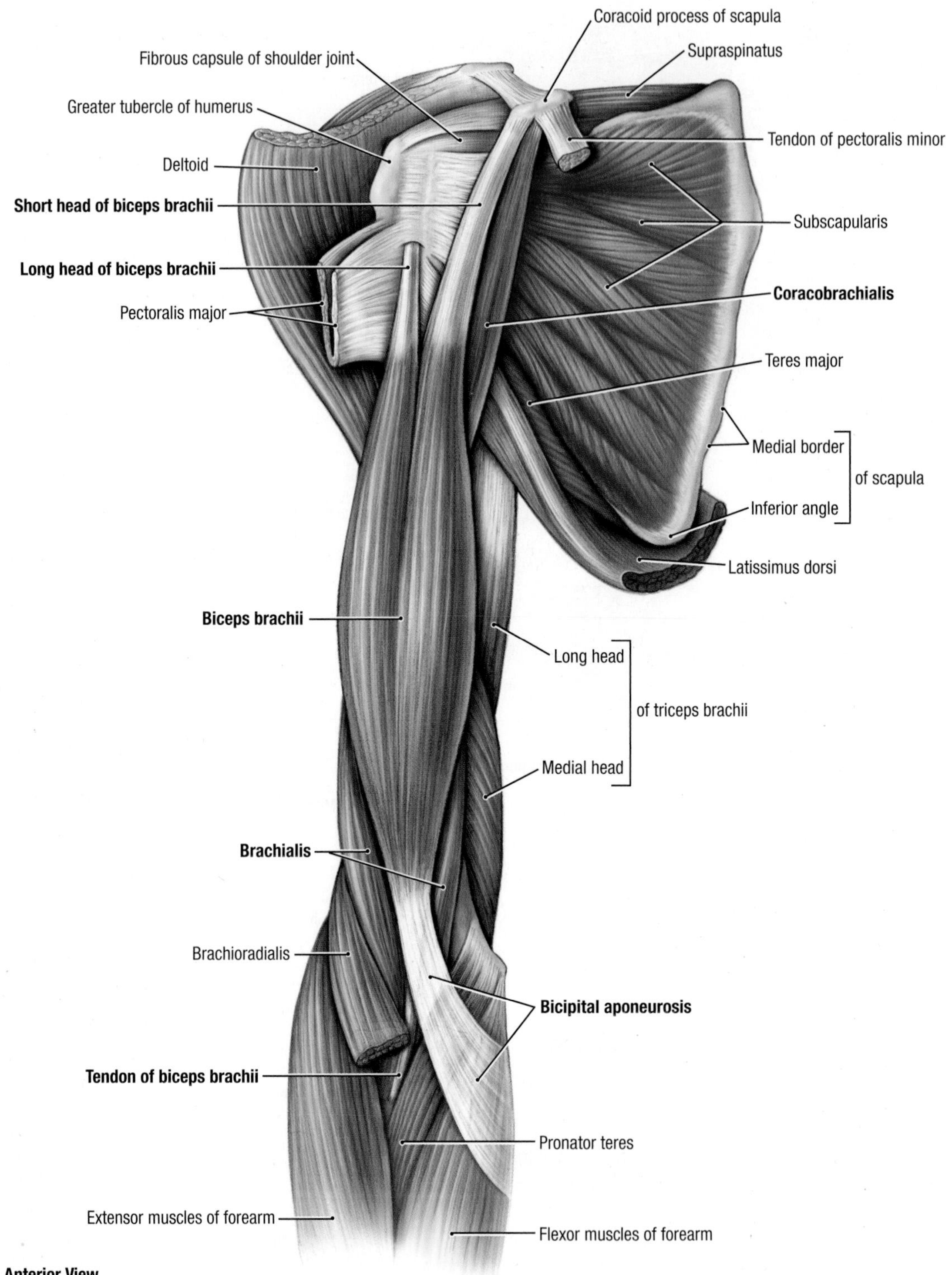
Coracoid process of scapula
Supraspinatus
Fibrous capsule of shoulder joint
Greater tubercle of humerus
Tendon of pectoralis minor
Deltoid
Short head of biceps brachii
Subscapularis
Long head of biceps brachii
Coracobrachialis
Pectoralis major
Teres major
Medial border
of scapula
Inferior angle
Latissimus dorsi
Biceps brachii
Long head
of triceps brachii
Medial head
Brachialis
Brachioradialis
Bicipital aponeurosis
Tendon of biceps brachii
Pronator teres
Extensor muscles of forearm
Flexor muscles of forearm

A. Anterior View

6.37 MUSCLES OF ANTERIOR ASPECT OF ARM I

- The biceps brachii has two heads: a long head and a short head.
- When the elbow joint is flexed approximately 90° the biceps is a flexor from the supinated position of the forearm but a very powerful supinator from the pronated position.
- A triangular membranous band, the bicipital aponeurosis, runs from the biceps tendon across the cubital fossa and merges with the antebrachial (deep) fascia covering the flexor muscles on the medial side of the forearm.

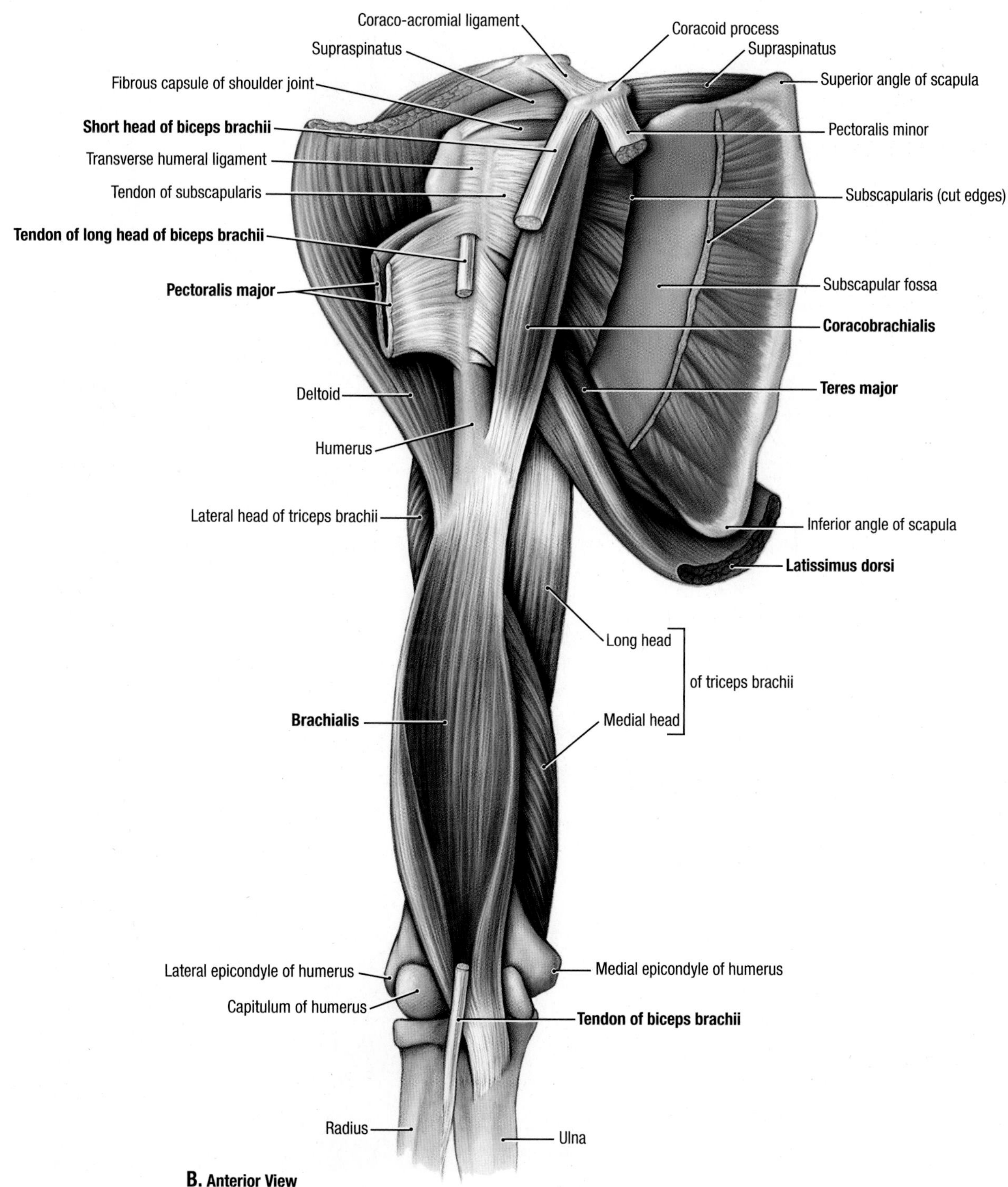
Coraco-acromial ligament
Coracoid process
Supraspinatus
Supraspinatus
Superior angle of scapula
Fibrous capsule of shoulder joint
Short head of biceps brachii
Pectoralis minor
Transverse humeral ligament
Tendon of subscapularis
Subscapularis (cut edges)
Tendon of long head of biceps brachii
Subscapular fossa
Pectoralis major
Coracobrachialis
Teres major
Deltoid
Humerus
Lateral head of triceps brachii
Inferior angle of scapula
Latissimus dorsi
Long head
of triceps brachii
Medial head
Brachialis
Lateral epicondyle of humerus
Medial epicondyle of humerus
Capitulum of humerus
Tendon of biceps brachii
Radius
Ulna

B. Anterior View

6.37 MUSCLES OF ANTERIOR ASPECT OF ARM II

- The brachialis, a flattened fusiform muscle, lies posterior (deep) to the biceps and produces the greatest amount of flexion force.
- The coracobrachialis, an elongated muscle in the superomedial part of the arm, is pierced by the musculocutaneous nerve. It helps flex and adduct the arm.
- **Rupture of the tendon of the long head of the biceps** usually results from wear and tear of an inflamed tendon **(biceps tendinitis)**. Normally, the tendon is torn from its attachment to the supraglenoid tubercle of the scapula. The detached muscle belly forms a ball near the center of the distal part of the anterior aspect of the arm.

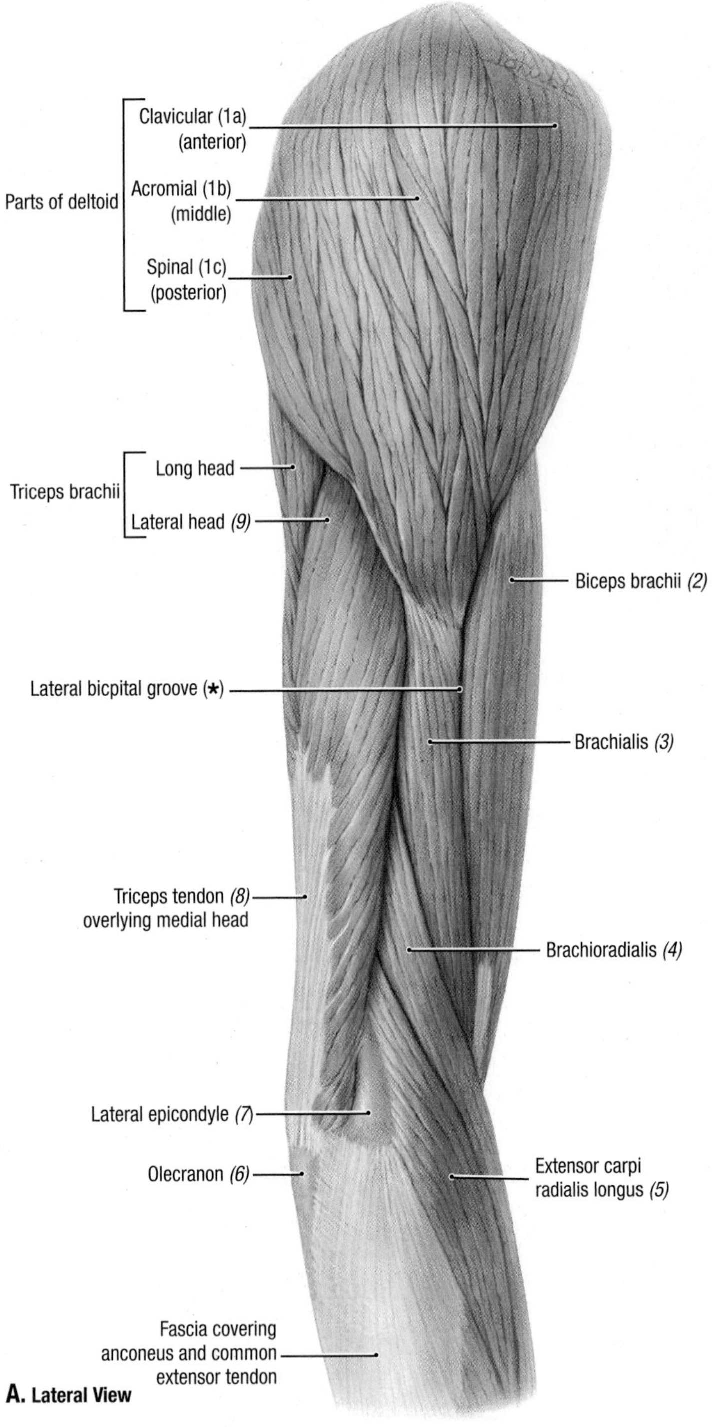

Parts of deltoid
Clavicular (1a) (anterior)
Acromial (1b) (middle)
Spinal (1c) (posterior)

Triceps brachii
Long head
Lateral head *(9)*

Biceps brachii *(2)*

Lateral bicpital groove (★)

Brachialis *(3)*

Triceps tendon *(8)* overlying medial head

Brachioradialis *(4)*

Lateral epicondyle *(7)*

Olecranon *(6)*

Extensor carpi radialis longus *(5)*

Fascia covering anconeus and common extensor tendon

A. Lateral View

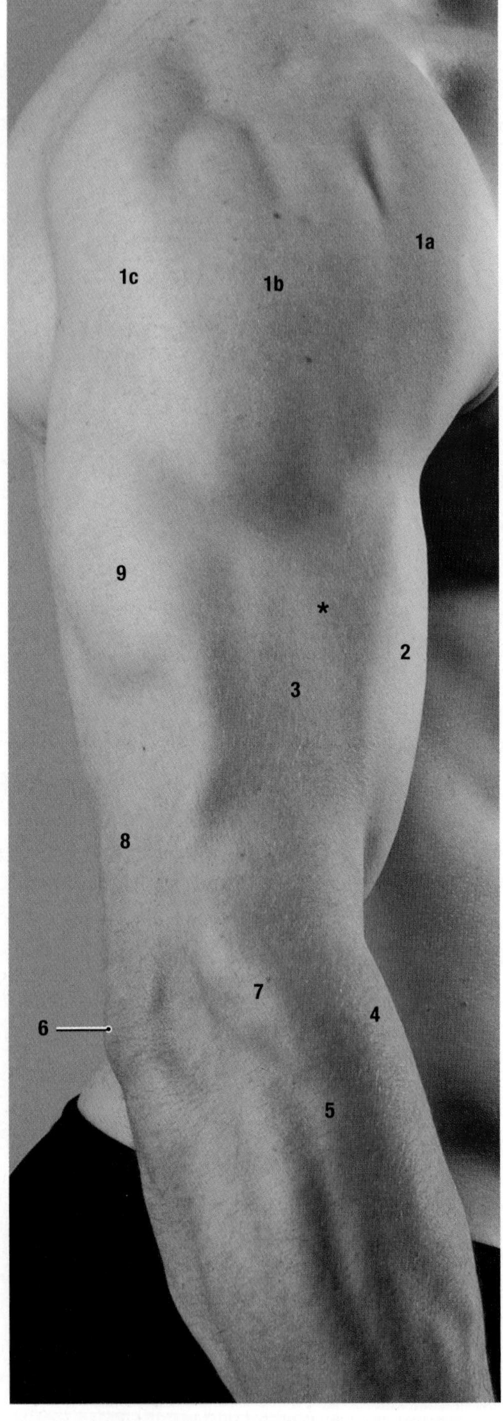
1a
1c
1b
9
*
2
3
8
7
6
4
5

B. Lateral View

6.38 LATERAL ASPECT OF ARM

A. Dissection (*numbers* in parentheses refer to structures in **B**). **B.** Surface anatomy.

Atrophy of the deltoid occurs when the axillary nerve (C5 and C6) is severely damaged (e.g., as might occur when the surgical neck of the humerus is fractured). As the deltoid atrophies, the rounded contour of the shoulder disappears. This gives the shoulder a flattened appearance and produces a slight hollow inferior to the acromion. A loss of sensation may occur over the lateral side of the proximal part of the arm, the area supplied by the superior lateral cutaneous nerve of the arm. To test the deltoid (or the function of the axillary nerve) the shoulder joint is abducted against resistance, starting from approximately 15°. Supraspinatus initiates abduction at the shoulder joint.

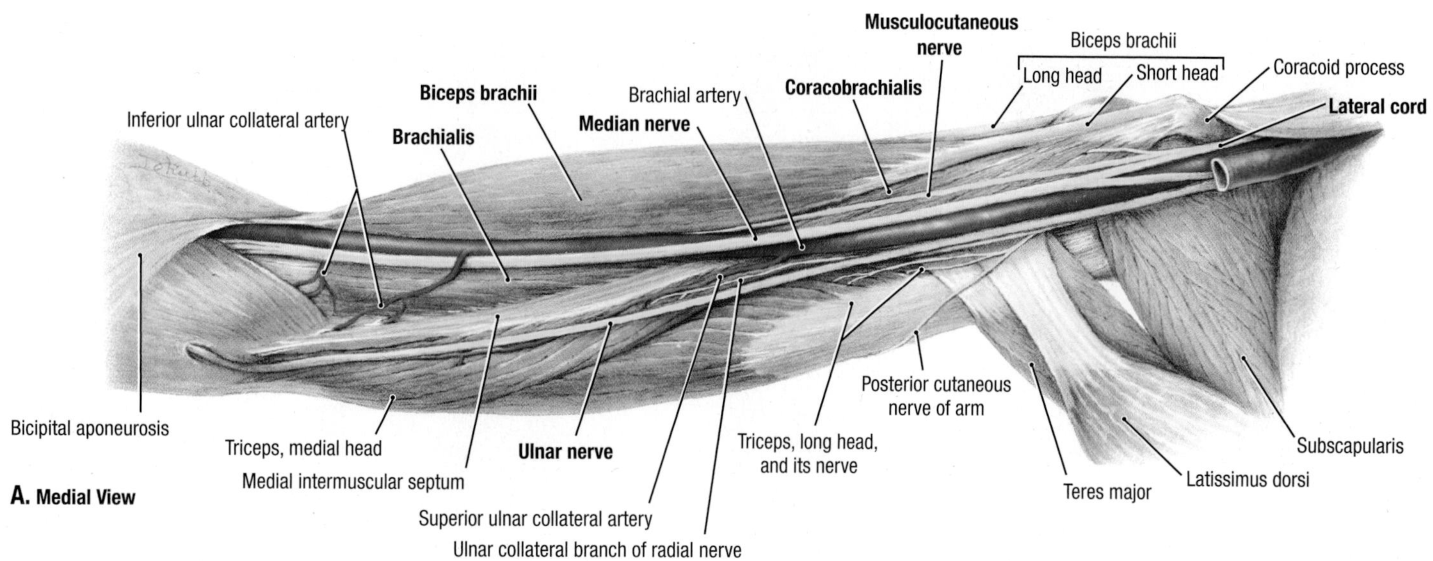
Musculocutaneous nerve
Biceps brachii
Long head
Short head
Coracoid process
Lateral cord
Coracobrachialis
Brachial artery
Median nerve
Biceps brachii
Brachialis
Inferior ulnar collateral artery
Bicipital aponeurosis
Triceps, medial head
Medial intermuscular septum
Ulnar nerve
Superior ulnar collateral artery
Ulnar collateral branch of radial nerve
Triceps, long head, and its nerve
Posterior cutaneous nerve of arm
Teres major
Latissimus dorsi
Subscapularis

A. Medial View

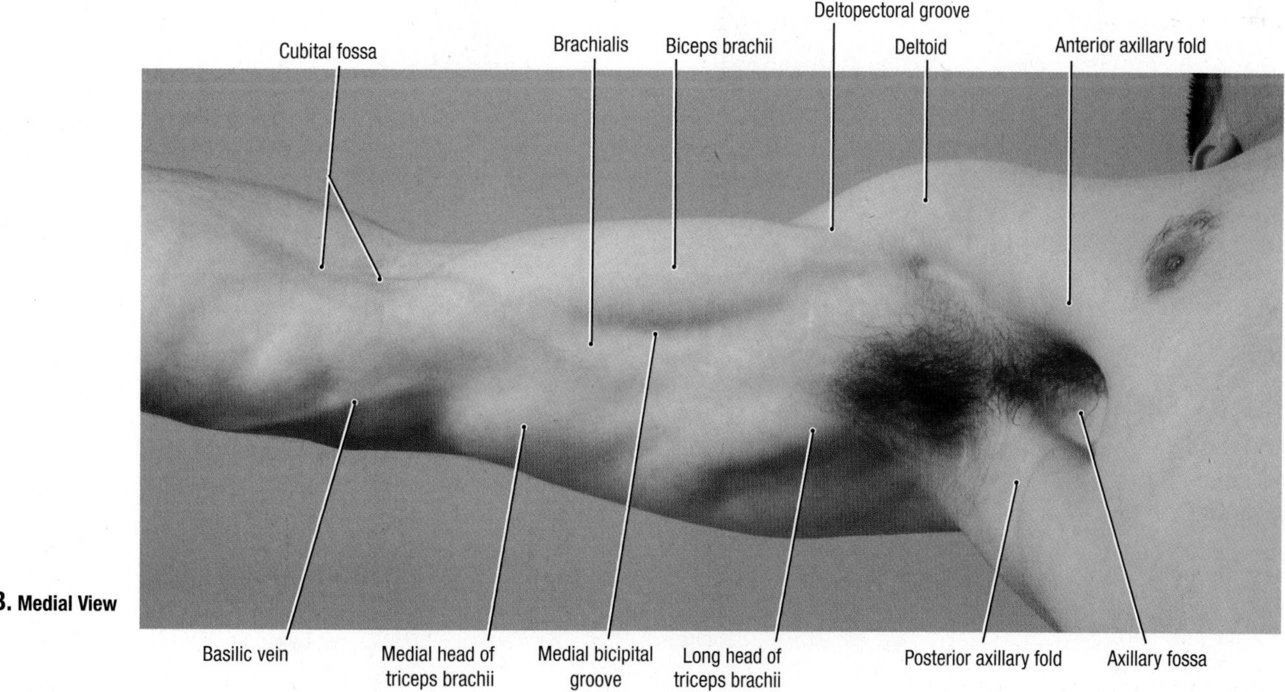
Deltopectoral groove
Cubital fossa
Brachialis
Biceps brachii
Deltoid
Anterior axillary fold
Basilic vein
Medial head of triceps brachii
Medial bicipital groove
Long head of triceps brachii
Posterior axillary fold
Axillary fossa

B. Medial View

6.39 MEDIAL ASPECT OF ARM

A. Dissection. **B.** Surface anatomy.

- The axillary artery passes just inferior to the tip of the coracoid process and courses posterior to the coracobrachialis. At the inferior border of the teres major, the axillary artery changes names to become the brachial artery and continues distally on the anterior aspect of the brachialis.
- Although collateral pathways confer some protection against gradual temporary and partial occlusion, sudden complete **occlusion or laceration of the brachial artery** creates a surgical emergency because paralysis of muscles results from ischemia within a few hours.
- The median nerve lies adjacent to the axillary and brachial arteries and then crosses the artery from lateral to medial.
- Proximally, the ulnar nerve is adjacent to the medial side of the artery, passes posterior to the medial intermuscular septum, and descends on the medial head of triceps to pass posterior to the medial epicondyle; here, the ulnar nerve is palpable.
- The superior ulnar collateral artery and ulnar collateral branch of the radial nerve (to medial head of the triceps) accompany the ulnar nerve in the arm.

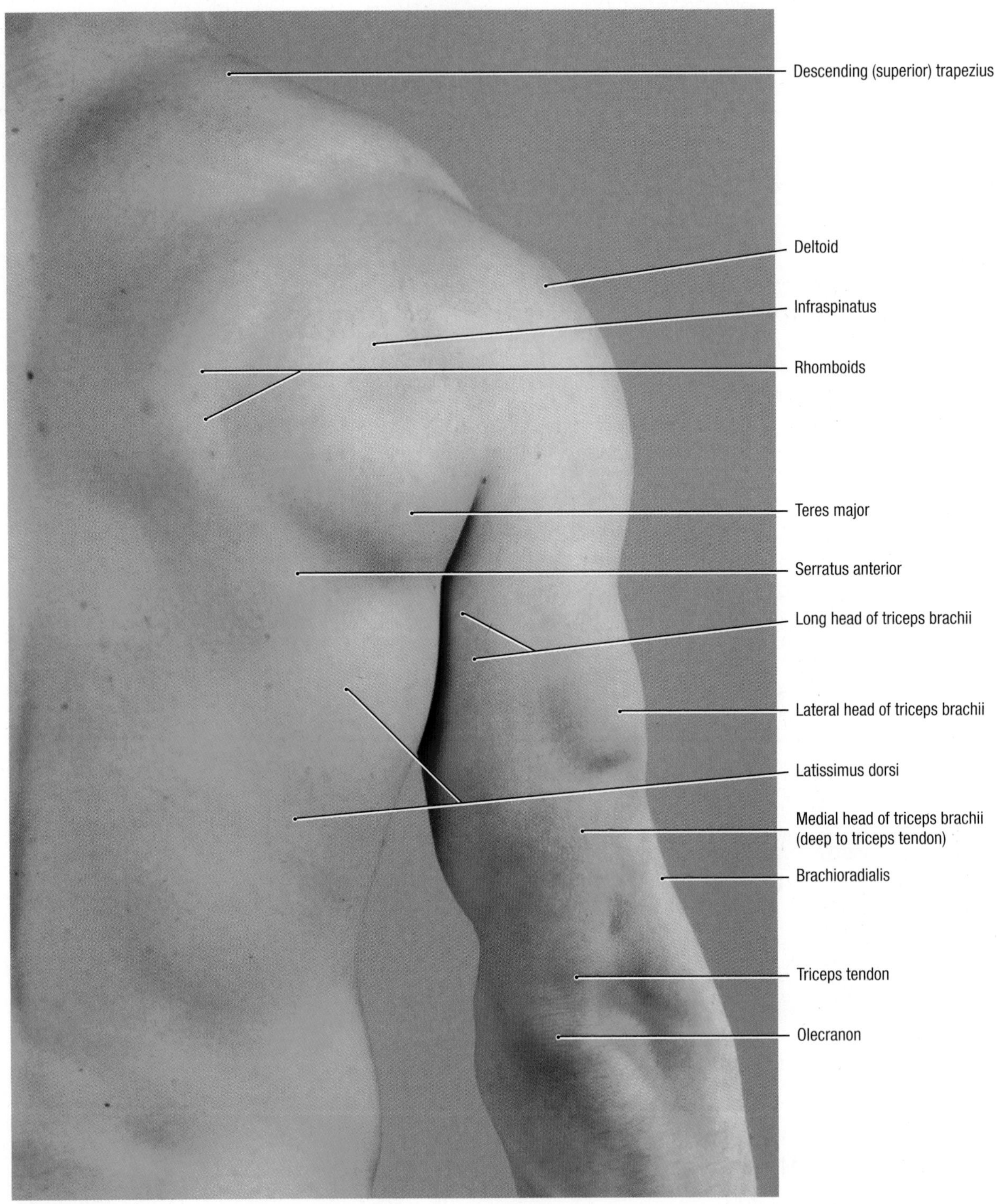
Descending (superior) trapezius
Deltoid
Infraspinatus
Rhomboids
Teres major
Serratus anterior
Long head of triceps brachii
Lateral head of triceps brachii
Latissimus dorsi
Medial head of triceps brachii (deep to triceps tendon)
Brachioradialis
Triceps tendon
Olecranon

Posterior View

6.40 SURFACE ANATOMY OF SCAPULAR REGION AND POSTERIOR ASPECT OF ARM

The three heads of the triceps form a bulge on the posterior aspect of the arm and are identifiable in a lean individual when the elbow joint is extended from the flexed position against resistance.

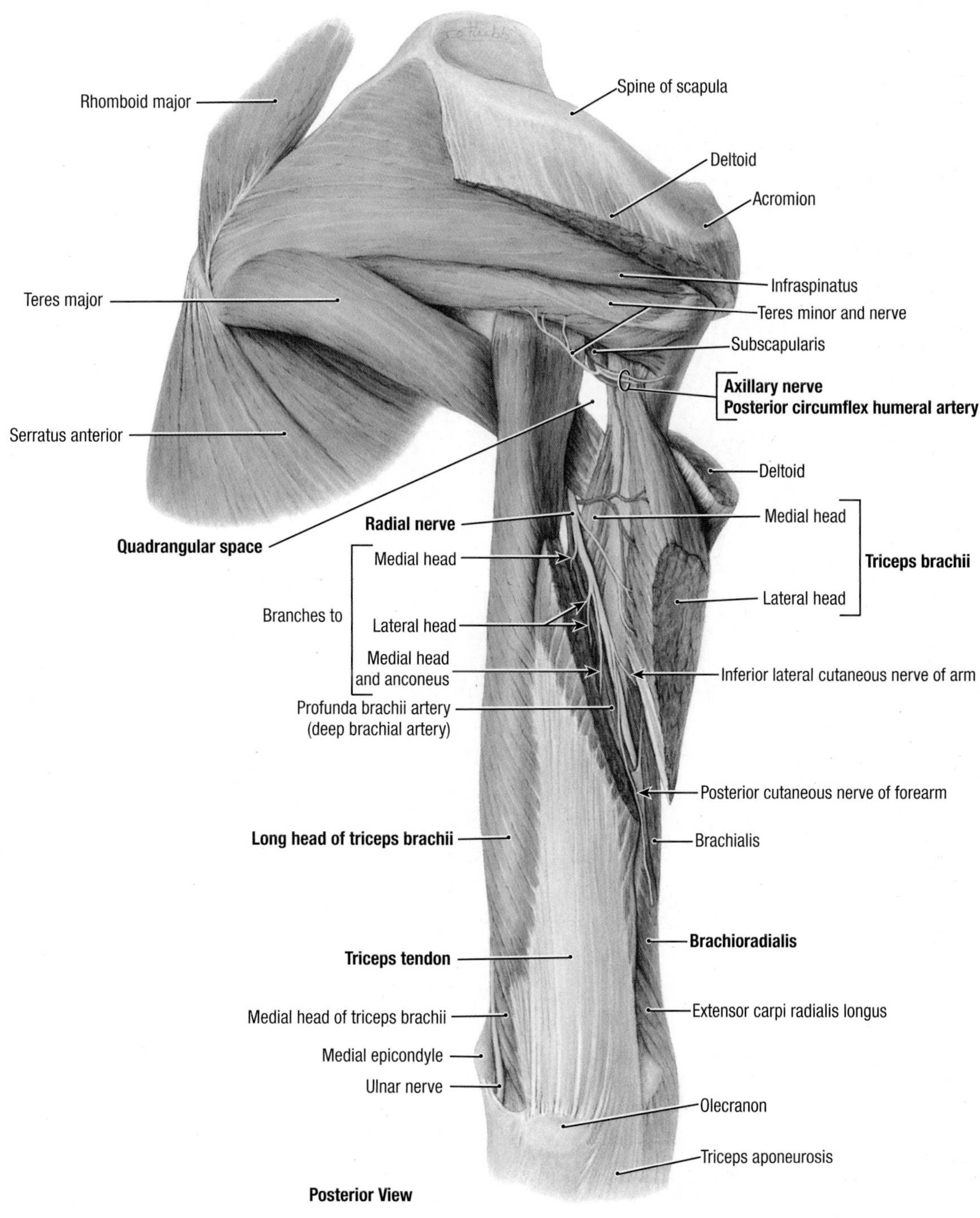
Rhomboid major
Spine of scapula
Deltoid
Acromion
Teres major
Infraspinatus
Teres minor and nerve
Subscapularis
Axillary nerve
Posterior circumflex humeral artery
Serratus anterior
Deltoid
Radial nerve
Medial head
Quadrangular space
Medial head
Triceps brachii
Lateral head
Branches to
Lateral head
Medial head and anconeus
Inferior lateral cutaneous nerve of arm
Profunda brachii artery (deep brachial artery)
Posterior cutaneous nerve of forearm
Long head of triceps brachii
Brachialis
Brachioradialis
Triceps tendon
Medial head of triceps brachii
Extensor carpi radialis longus
Medial epicondyle
Ulnar nerve
Olecranon
Triceps aponeurosis
Posterior View

6.41 TRICEPS BRACHII AND RELATED NERVES

- The lateral head is reflected laterally, and the medial head is attached to the deep surface of the triceps tendon, which attaches to the olecranon.
- The radial nerve and deep brachial artery pass between the proximal attachments of the long and medial heads of the triceps brachii in the middle third of the arm, directly contacting the radial groove of the humerus.
- **Midarm fracture.** The middle third of the arm is a common site for fractures of the humerus, often with associated **radial nerve trauma.** When the radial nerve is injured in the radial groove, the triceps brachii muscle typically is only weakened because only the medial head is affected. However, the muscles in the posterior compartment of the forearm, supplied by more distal branches of the radial nerve, are paralyzed. The characteristic clinical sign of radial nerve injury is **wrist drop** (inability to extend the wrist joint and fingers at the metacarpophalangeal joints).
- The axillary nerve passes through the quadrangular space along with the posterior humeral circumflex artery.
- The ulnar nerve follows the medial border of the triceps then passes posterior to the medial epicondyle.

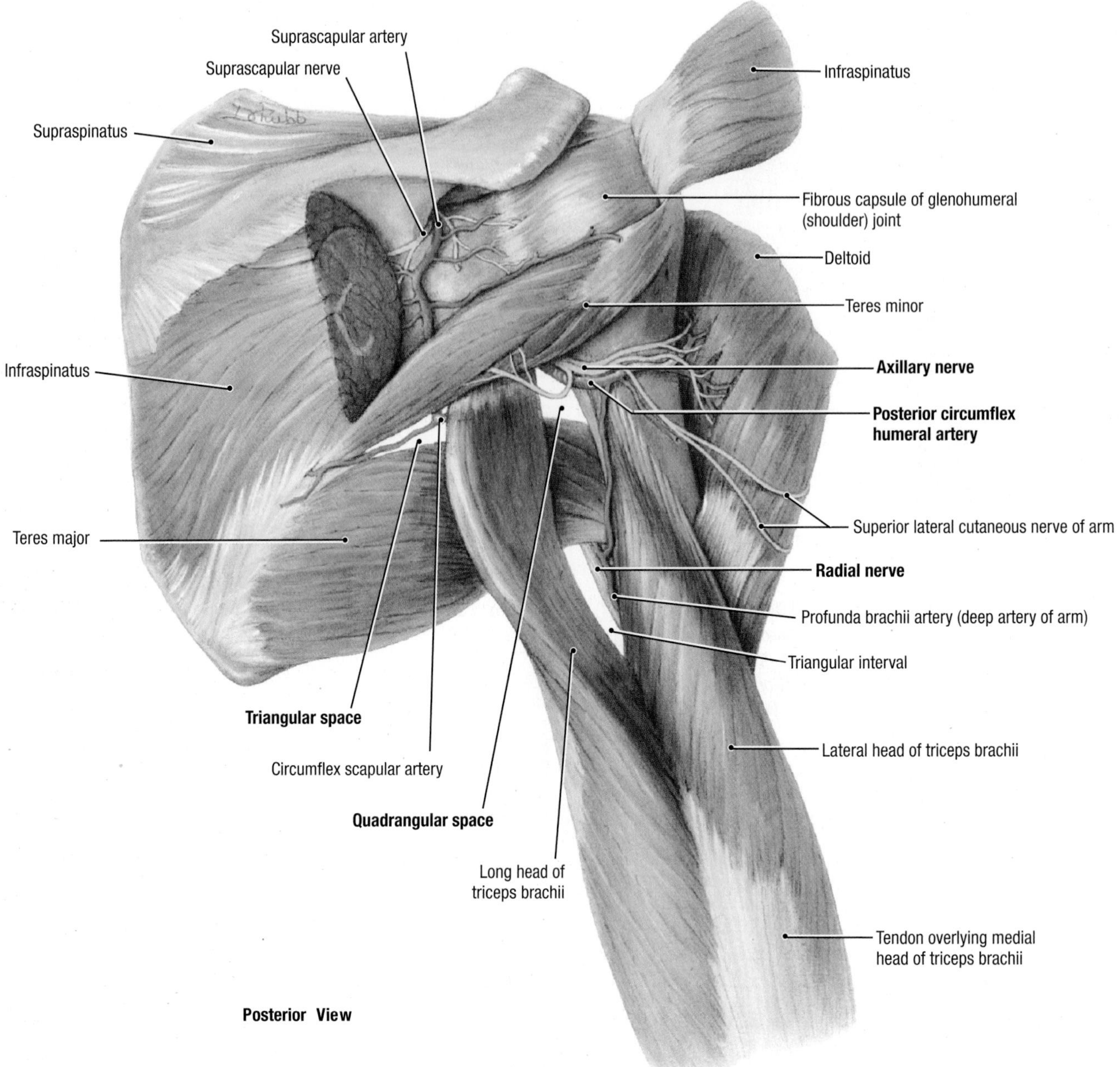
Suprascapular artery
Suprascapular nerve
Supraspinatus
Infraspinatus
Fibrous capsule of glenohumeral (shoulder) joint
Deltoid
Teres minor
Infraspinatus
Axillary nerve
Posterior circumflex humeral artery
Superior lateral cutaneous nerve of arm
Teres major
Radial nerve
Profunda brachii artery (deep artery of arm)
Triangular interval
Triangular space
Lateral head of triceps brachii
Circumflex scapular artery
Quadrangular space
Long head of triceps brachii
Tendon overlying medial head of triceps brachii
Posterior View

6.42 DORSAL SCAPULAR AND SUBDELTOID REGIONS

- The infraspinatus muscle, aided by the teres minor and spinal (posterior) fibers of the deltoid muscle, rotates the shoulder joint laterally.
- The long head of the triceps muscle passes between the teres minor (a lateral rotator) and teres major (a medial rotator).
- The long head of the triceps muscle separates the quadrangular space from the triangular interval.
- Regarding the distribution of the suprascapular and axillary nerves, each comes from C5 and C6; each supplies two muscles—the suprascapular nerve innervates the supraspinatus and infraspinatus, and the axillary nerve innervates the teres minor and deltoid muscles. Both nerves supply the shoulder joint, but only the axillary nerve has a cutaneous branch.
- **Axillary nerve injury** may occur when the glenohumeral (shoulder) joint dislocates because of its close relation to the inferior part of the joint capsule of this joint. The subglenoid displacement of the head of the humerus into the quadrangular space may damage the axillary nerve. Axillary nerve injury is indicated by paralysis of the deltoid and sensory loss over the lateral side of the proximal part of the arm.

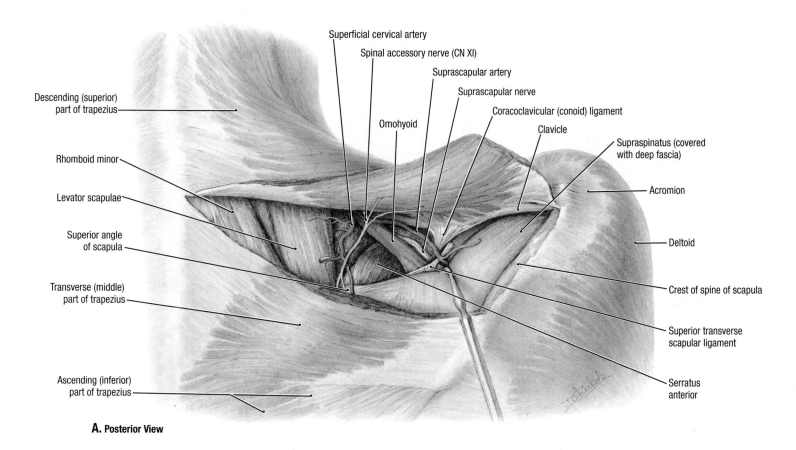

Superficial cervical artery
Spinal accessory nerve (CN XI)
Suprascapular artery
Suprascapular nerve
Coracoclavicular (conoid) ligament
Omohyoid
Clavicle
Descending (superior) part of trapezius
Rhomboid minor
Levator scapulae
Superior angle of scapula
Transverse (middle) part of trapezius
Ascending (inferior) part of trapezius
Supraspinatus (covered with deep fascia)
Acromion
Deltoid
Crest of spine of scapula
Superior transverse scapular ligament
Serratus anterior

A. **Posterior View**

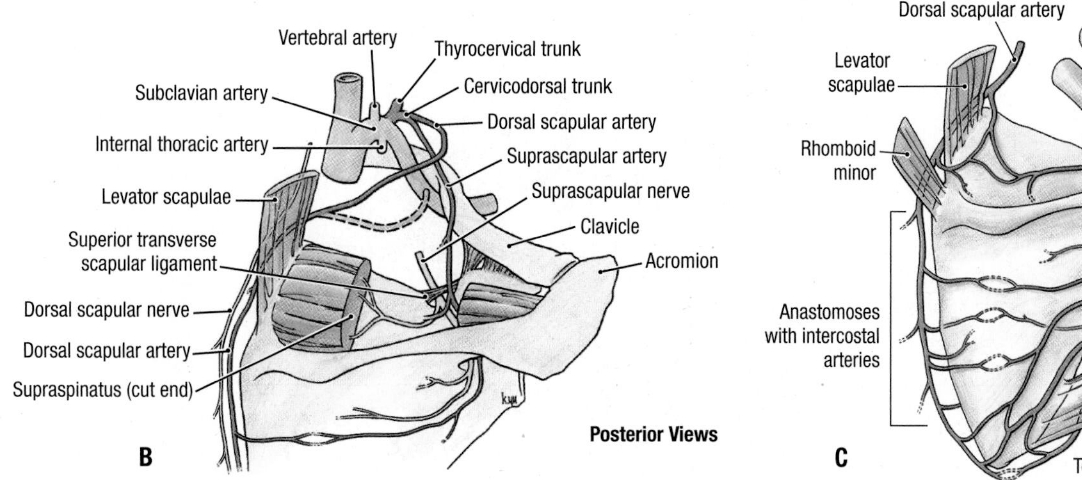
Vertebral artery
Thyrocervical trunk
Subclavian artery
Cervicodorsal trunk
Dorsal scapular artery
Internal thoracic artery
Suprascapular artery
Levator scapulae
Suprascapular nerve
Clavicle
Superior transverse scapular ligament
Acromion
Dorsal scapular nerve
Dorsal scapular artery
Supraspinatus (cut end)
B

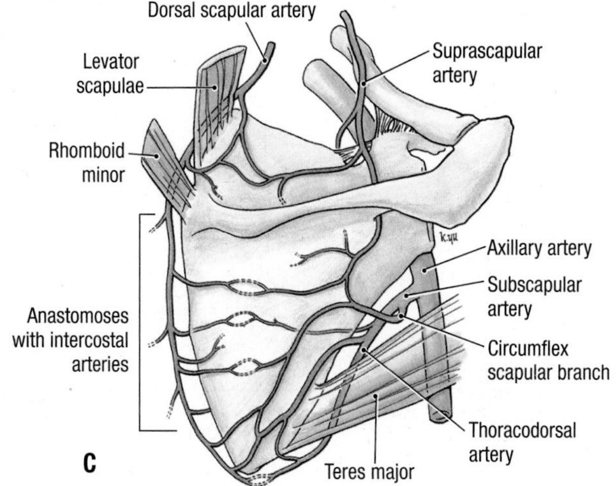
Dorsal scapular artery
Levator scapulae
Suprascapular artery
Rhomboid minor
Axillary artery
Subscapular artery
Anastomoses with intercostal arteries
Circumflex scapular branch
Thoracodorsal artery
Teres major
C

Posterior Views

6.43 SUPRASCAPULAR REGION

A. Dissection. At the level of the superior angle of the scapula, the transverse part of the trapezius muscle is reflected. **B.** Suprascapular and dorsal scapular arteries. **C.** Scapular anastomosis.

Several arteries join to form anastomoses on the anterior and posterior surfaces of the scapula. The importance of the collateral circulation made possible by these anastomoses becomes apparent when **ligation of a lacerated subclavian or axillary artery** is necessary or there is occlusion of these vessels. The direction of blood flow in the subscapular artery is then reversed, enabling blood to reach the third part of the axillary artery. In contrast to a sudden occlusion, slow occlusion of an artery often enables sufficient lateral circulation to develop, preventing **ischemia** (deficiency of blood).

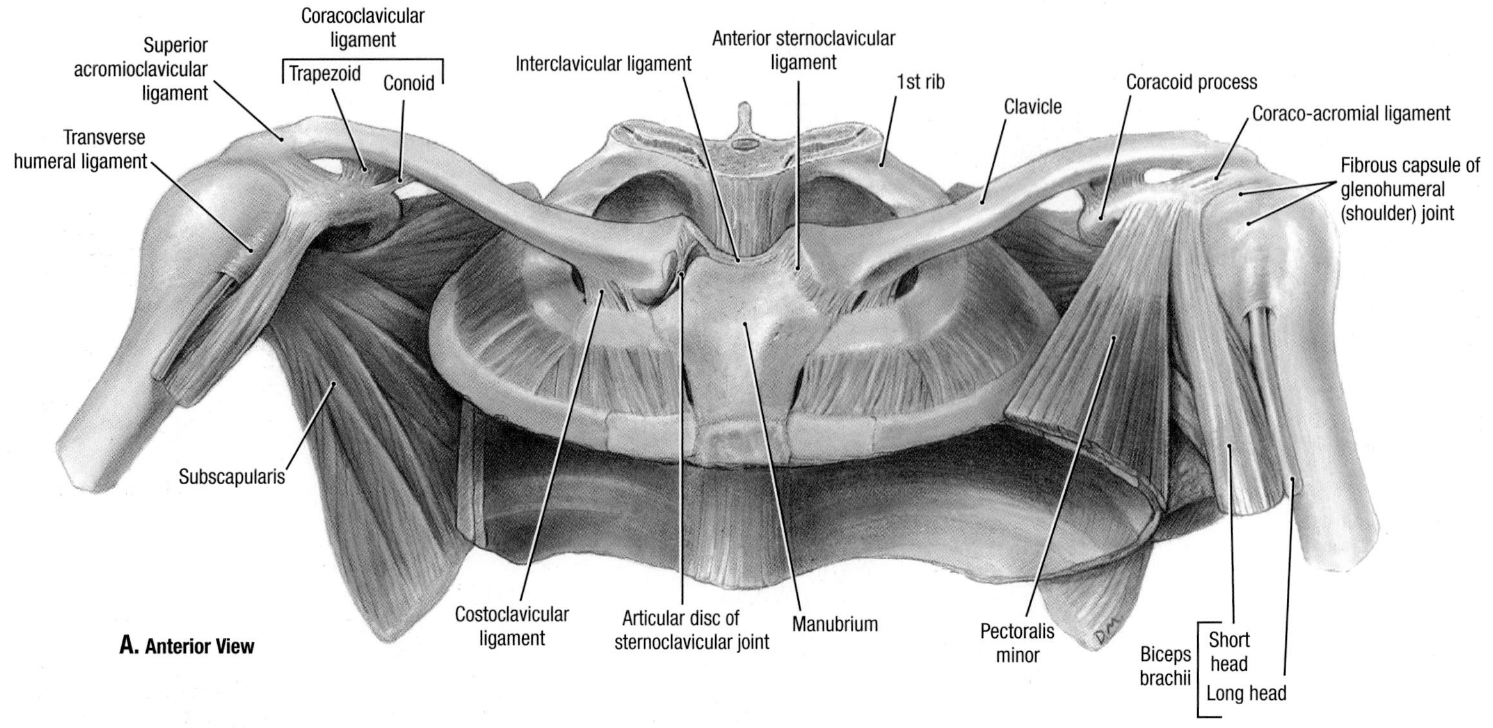

Coracoclavicular ligament
Trapezoid
Conoid
Superior acromioclavicular ligament
Transverse humeral ligament
Interclavicular ligament
Anterior sternoclavicular ligament
1st rib
Clavicle
Coracoid process
Coraco-acromial ligament
Fibrous capsule of glenohumeral (shoulder) joint
Subscapularis
Costoclavicular ligament
Articular disc of sternoclavicular joint
Manubrium
Pectoralis minor
Biceps brachii
Short head
Long head
A. Anterior View

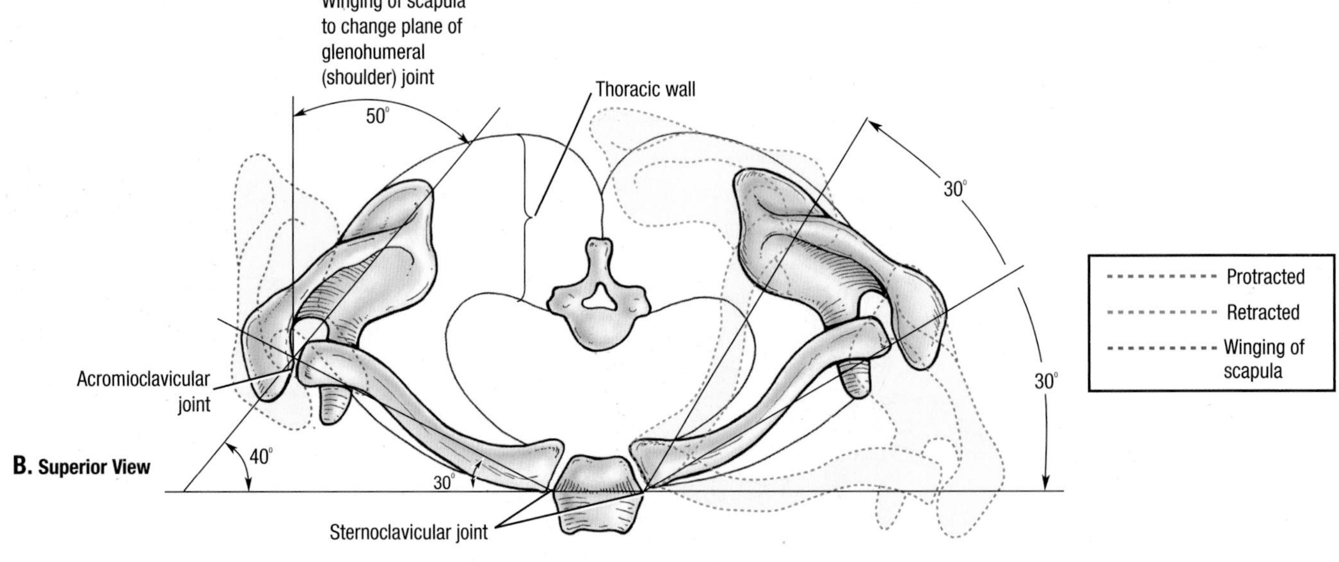

Winging of scapula to change plane of glenohumeral (shoulder) joint
50°
Thoracic wall
30°
30°
Protracted
Retracted
Winging of scapula
Acromioclavicular joint
40°
30°
B. Superior View
Sternoclavicular joint

6.44 PECTORAL GIRDLE

A. Dissection. **B.** Clavicular movements at the sternoclavicular and acromioclavicular joints during rotation, protraction, and retraction of the scapula on the thoracic wall *(left side)* and winging of the scapula *(right side)*.

- The shoulder region includes the sternoclavicular, acromioclavicular, and shoulder (glenohumeral) joints; the mobility of the clavicle is essential to the movement of the upper limb.
- The sternoclavicular joint is the only joint connecting the upper limb (appendicular skeleton) to the trunk (axial skeleton). The articular disc of the sternoclavicular joint divides the joint cavity into two parts and attaches superiorly to the clavicle and inferiorly to the first costal cartilage; the disc resists superior and medial displacement of the clavicle.

Paralysis of serratus anterior. In **B,** note that when the serratus anterior is paralyzed because of injury to the long thoracic nerve, the medial border of the scapula moves laterally and posteriorly away from the thoracic wall, giving the scapula the appearance of a wing **(winged scapula).** See Clinical Comment for Figure 6.29.

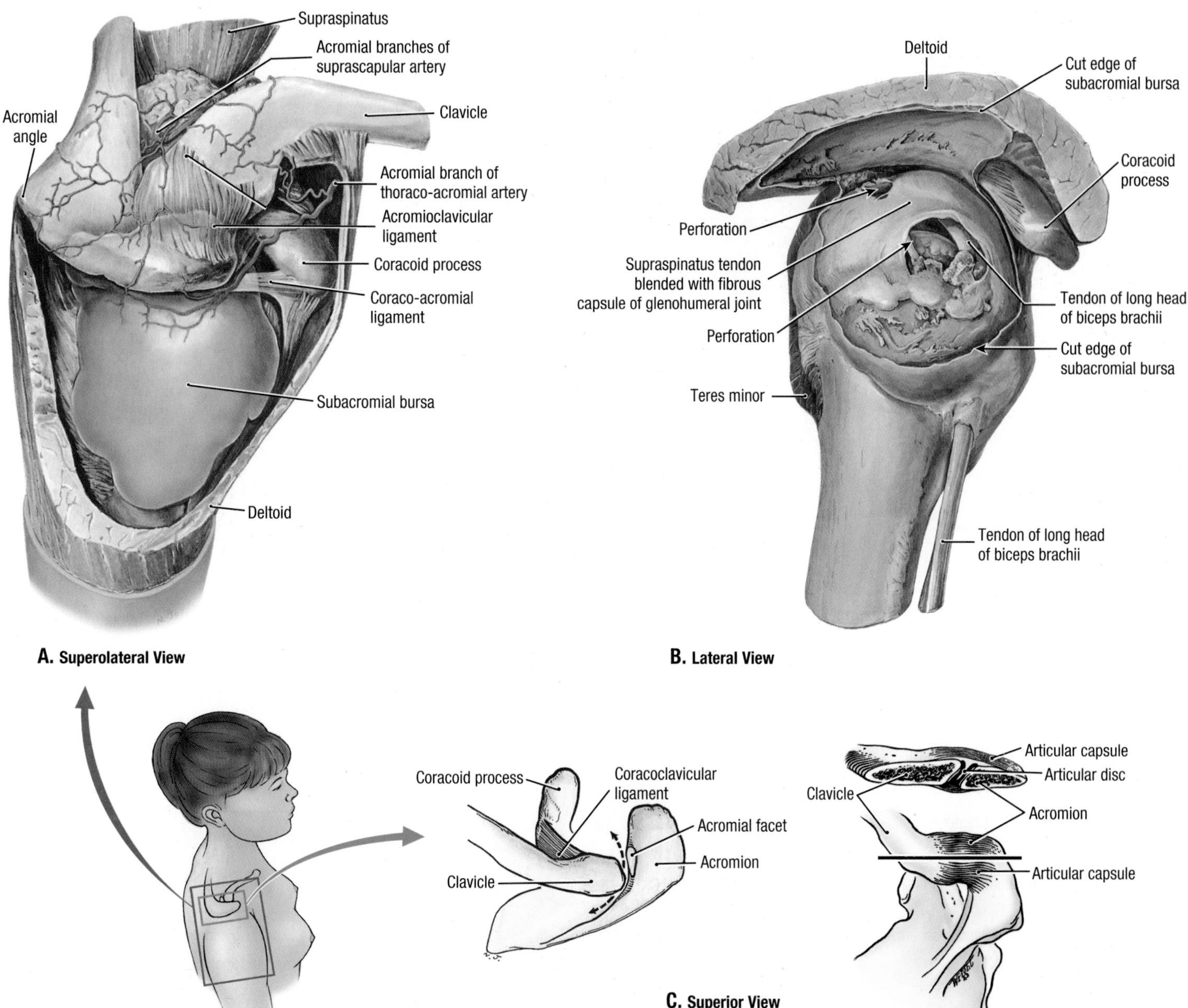
Supraspinatus
Acromial branches of suprascapular artery
Acromial angle
Clavicle
Acromial branch of thoraco-acromial artery
Acromioclavicular ligament
Coracoid process
Coraco-acromial ligament
Subacromial bursa
Deltoid
A. Superolateral View
Deltoid
Cut edge of subacromial bursa
Coracoid process
Perforation
Supraspinatus tendon blended with fibrous capsule of glenohumeral joint
Perforation
Tendon of long head of biceps brachii
Cut edge of subacromial bursa
Teres minor
Tendon of long head of biceps brachii
B. Lateral View
Coracoid process
Coracoclavicular ligament
Acromial facet
Acromion
Clavicle
Articular capsule
Articular disc
Clavicle
Acromion
Articular capsule
C. Superior View

6.45 SUBACROMIAL BURSA AND ACROMIOCLAVICULAR JOINT

A. Subacromial bursa. The bursa has been injected with purple latex. **B.** Acromioclavicular joint. **C. Attrition of supraspinatus tendon.** As a result of wearing away of the supraspinatus tendon and underlying capsule, the subacromial bursa and shoulder joint come into communication. The intracapsular part of the tendon of the long head of biceps muscle becomes frayed, leaving it adherent to the intertubercular groove. Of 95 dissecting room subjects in Dr. Grant's lab, none of the 18 younger than 50 years of age had a perforation, but 4 of the 19 who were 50 to 60 years and 23 of the 57 older than 60 years had perforations. The perforation was bilateral in 11 subjects and unilateral in 14.

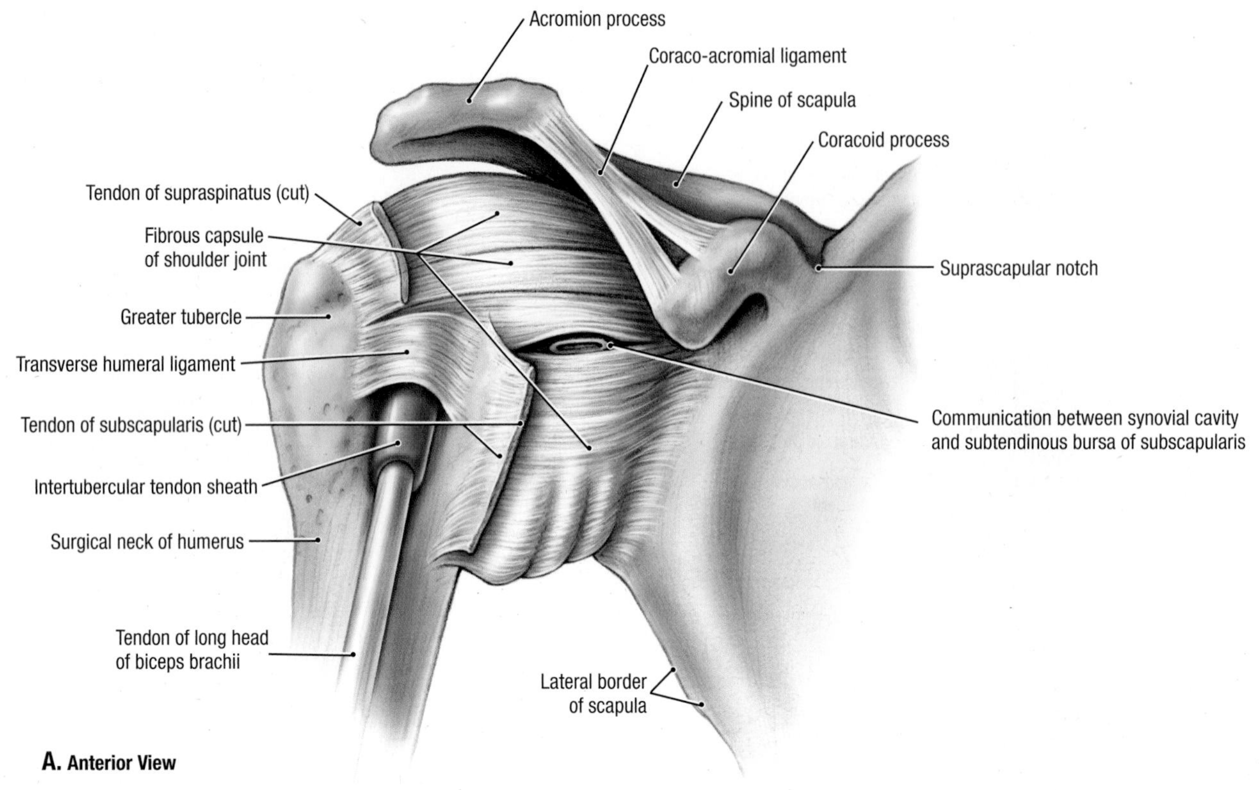
Acromion process
Coraco-acromial ligament
Spine of scapula
Coracoid process
Tendon of supraspinatus (cut)
Fibrous capsule of shoulder joint
Suprascapular notch
Greater tubercle
Transverse humeral ligament
Tendon of subscapularis (cut)
Communication between synovial cavity and subtendinous bursa of subscapularis
Intertubercular tendon sheath
Surgical neck of humerus
Tendon of long head of biceps brachii
Lateral border of scapula

A. **Anterior View**

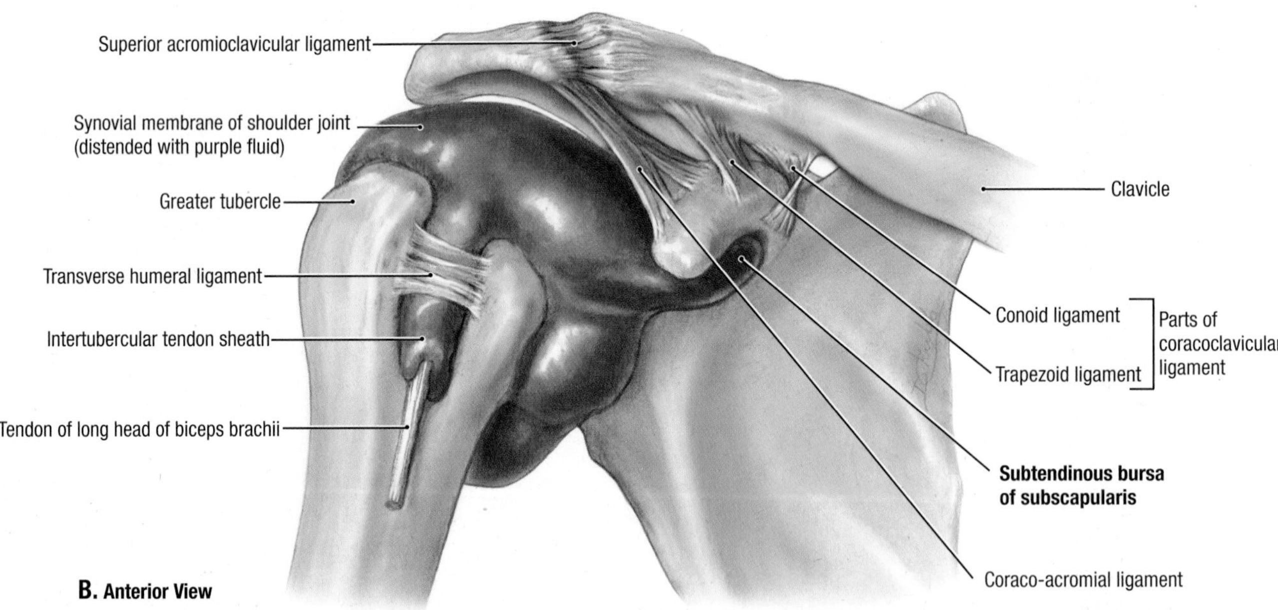
Superior acromioclavicular ligament
Synovial membrane of shoulder joint (distended with purple fluid)
Greater tubercle
Clavicle
Transverse humeral ligament
Conoid ligament
Trapezoid ligament
Parts of coracoclavicular ligament
Intertubercular tendon sheath
Tendon of long head of biceps brachii
Subtendinous bursa of subscapularis
Coraco-acromial ligament

B. **Anterior View**

6.46 LIGAMENTS AND ARTICULAR CAPSULE OF GLENOHUMERAL (SHOULDER) JOINT

A. Fibrous capsule.

- The loose fibrous capsule is attached to the margin of the glenoid cavity and to the anatomical neck of the humerus.
- The strong coracoclavicular ligament provides stability to the acromioclavicular joint and prevents the scapula from being driven medially and the acromion from being driven inferior to the clavicle.
- The coraco-acromial ligament prevents superior displacement of the head of the humerus.

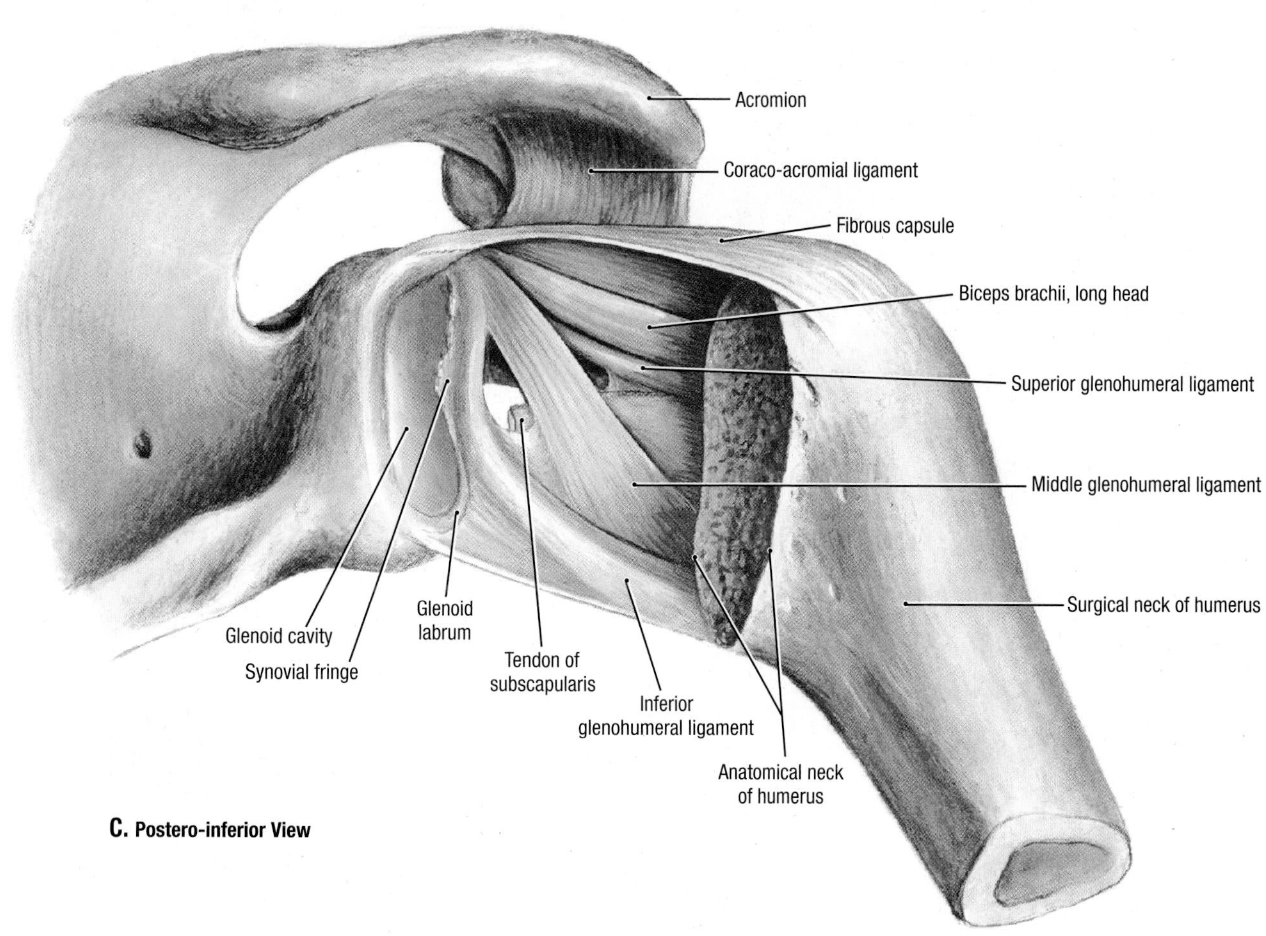
Acromion
Coraco-acromial ligament
Fibrous capsule
Biceps brachii, long head
Superior glenohumeral ligament
Middle glenohumeral ligament
Surgical neck of humerus
Glenoid cavity
Synovial fringe
Glenoid labrum
Tendon of subscapularis
Inferior glenohumeral ligament
Anatomical neck of humerus

C. Postero-inferior View

6.46 LIGAMENTS AND ARTICULAR CAPSULE OF GLENOHUMERAL (SHOULDER) JOINT *(CONTINUED)*

B. Synovial membrane of joint capsule. The synovial membrane lines the fibrous capsule and has two prolongations: (1) where it forms a synovial sheath for the tendon of the long head of the biceps muscle in its osseofibrous tunnel and (2) inferior to the coracoid process, where it forms a bursa between the subscapularis tendon and margin of the glenoid cavity—the subtendinous bursa of the subscapularis. **C.** Glenohumeral ligaments viewed from the interior of the shoulder joint.

- The joint is exposed from the posterior aspect by cutting away the thinner postero-inferior part of the capsule and sawing off the head of the humerus.
- The glenohumeral ligaments are visible from within the joint but are not easily seen externally.
- The glenohumeral ligaments and tendon of the long head of biceps brachii muscle converge on the supraglenoid tubercle.
- The slender superior glenohumeral ligament lies parallel to the tendon of the long head of biceps brachii. The middle ligament is free medially because the subtendinous bursa of subscapularis communicates with the joint cavity, usually there is only a single site of communication. In this individual there are openings on both sides of the ligament.

Because of its freedom of movement and instability, the glenohumeral joint is commonly dislocated by direct or indirect injury. Most **dislocations of the humeral head** occur in the downward (inferior) direction but are described clinically as anterior or (more rarely) posterior dislocations, indicating whether the humeral head has descended anterior or posterior to the infraglenoid tubercle and the long head of triceps. Anterior dislocation of the glenohumeral joint occurs most often in young adults, particularly athletes. It is usually caused by excessive extension and lateral rotation of the humerus.

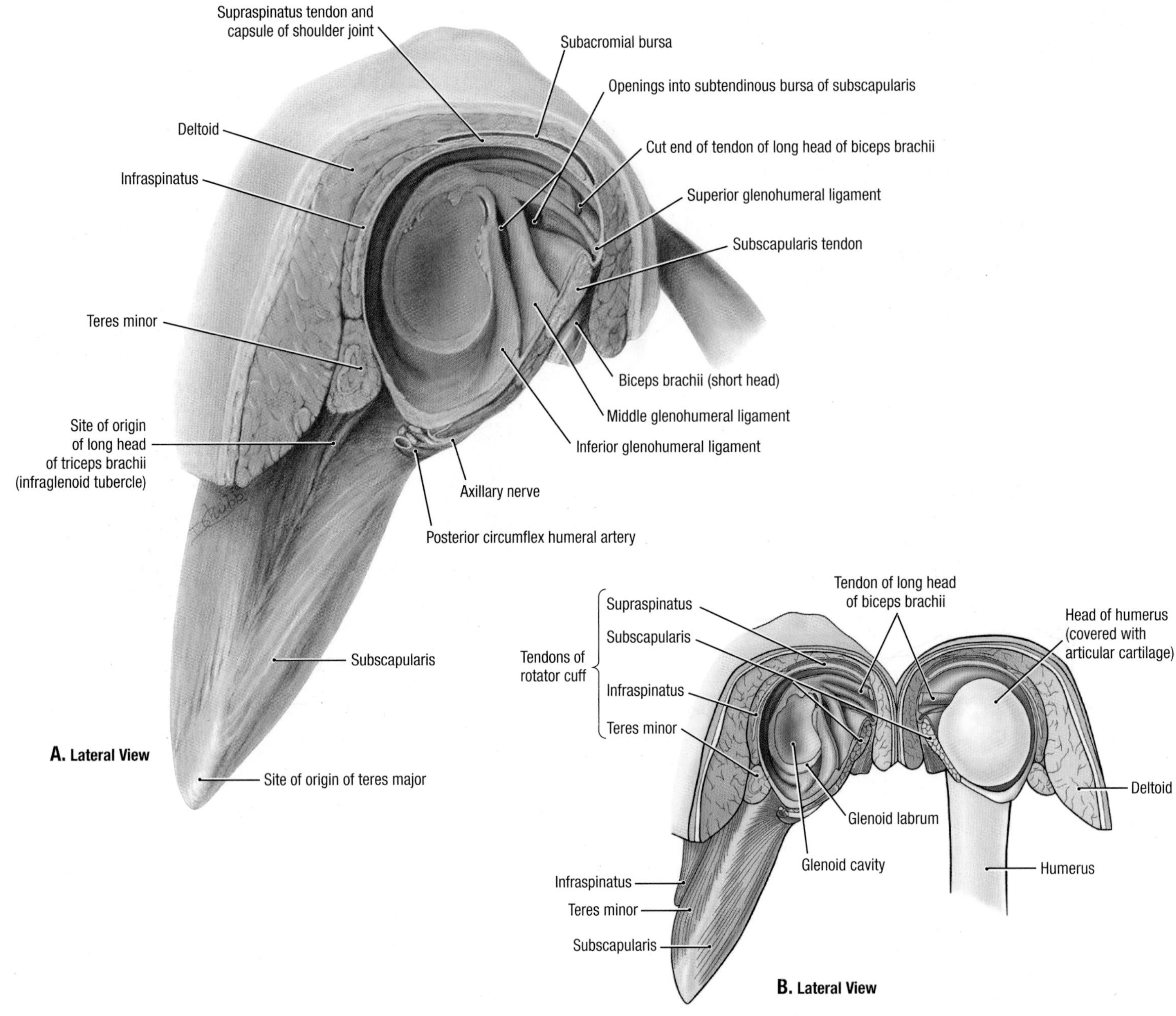

Supraspinatus tendon and capsule of shoulder joint
Subacromial bursa
Openings into subtendinous bursa of subscapularis
Deltoid
Cut end of tendon of long head of biceps brachii
Infraspinatus
Superior glenohumeral ligament
Subscapularis tendon
Teres minor
Biceps brachii (short head)
Middle glenohumeral ligament
Site of origin of long head of triceps brachii (infraglenoid tubercle)
Inferior glenohumeral ligament
Axillary nerve
Posterior circumflex humeral artery
Subscapularis
A. Lateral View
Site of origin of teres major
Tendons of rotator cuff
Supraspinatus
Subscapularis
Infraspinatus
Teres minor
Tendon of long head of biceps brachii
Head of humerus (covered with articular cartilage)
Deltoid
Glenoid labrum
Glenoid cavity
Humerus
Infraspinatus
Teres minor
Subscapularis
B. Lateral View

6.47 INTERIOR OF GLENOHUMERAL (SHOULDER) JOINT AND RELATIONSHIP OF ROTATOR CUFF

A. Dissection. **B.** Schematic illustration.

- The fibrous capsule of the joint is thickened anteriorly by the three glenohumeral ligaments.
- The subacromial bursa is between the acromion and deltoid superiorly and the tendon of supraspinatus inferiorly.
- The four short rotator cuff muscles (supraspinatus, infraspinatus, teres minor, and subscapularis) cross the joint and blend with the capsule.
- The axillary nerve and posterior circumflex humeral artery are in contact with the capsule inferiorly and may be injured when the glenohumeral joint dislocates.
- Inflammation and calcification of the subacromial bursa result in pain, tenderness, and limitation of movement of the glenohumeral joint. This condition is also known as **calcific scapulohumeral bursitis.** Deposition of calcium in the supraspinatus tendon may irritate the overlying subacromial bursa, producing an inflammatory reaction, **subacromial bursitis.**

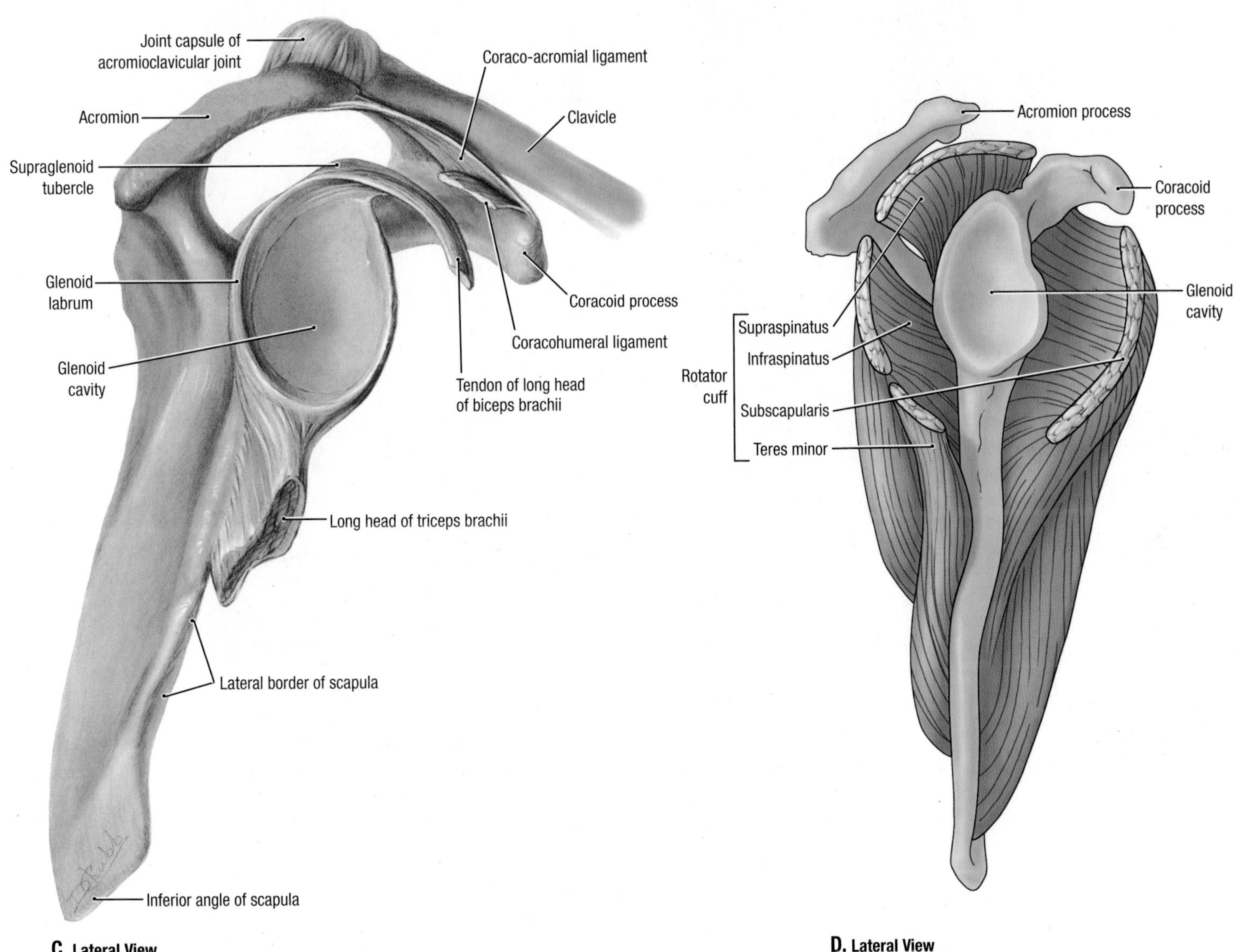
Joint capsule of acromioclavicular joint
Acromion
Supraglenoid tubercle
Glenoid labrum
Glenoid cavity
Coraco-acromial ligament
Clavicle
Coracoid process
Coracohumeral ligament
Tendon of long head of biceps brachii
Long head of triceps brachii
Lateral border of scapula
Inferior angle of scapula
Acromion process
Coracoid process
Glenoid cavity
Rotator cuff
Supraspinatus
Infraspinatus
Subscapularis
Teres minor

C. Lateral View

D. Lateral View

6.47 INTERIOR OF GLENOHUMERAL (SHOULDER) JOINT AND RELATIONSHIP OF ROTATOR CUFF *(CONTINUED)*

C. Dissection. **D.** Schematic illustration of the rotator cuff muscles and their relationship to the glenoid cavity.

- The coraco-acromial arch (coracoid process, coraco-acromial ligament, and acromion) prevents superior displacement of the head of the humerus.
- The long head of the triceps brachii muscle arises just inferior to the glenoid cavity; the long head of biceps just superior to it.
- The main function of the musculotendinous rotator cuff is to hold the large head of the humerus in the smaller and shallow glenoid cavity of the scapula, both during the relaxed state (by tonic contraction) and during active abduction.

Tearing of the fibrocartilaginous glenoid labrum commonly occurs in the athletes who throw (e.g., a baseball) and in those who have shoulder instability and subluxation (partial dislocation) of the glenohumeral joint. The tear often results from sudden contraction of the biceps or forceful subluxation of the humeral head over the glenoid labrum. Usually a tear occurs in the anterosuperior part of the labrum.

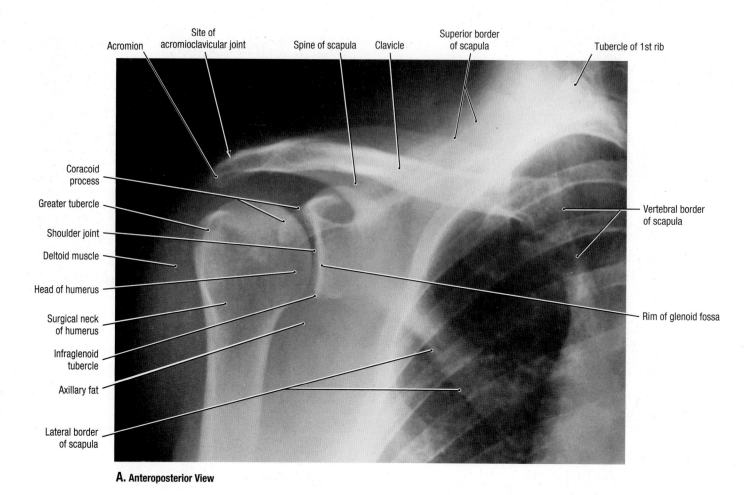

Acromion
Site of acromioclavicular joint
Spine of scapula
Clavicle
Superior border of scapula
Tubercle of 1st rib
Coracoid process
Greater tubercle
Shoulder joint
Deltoid muscle
Head of humerus
Surgical neck of humerus
Infraglenoid tubercle
Axillary fat
Lateral border of scapula
Vertebral border of scapula
Rim of glenoid fossa

A. Anteroposterior View

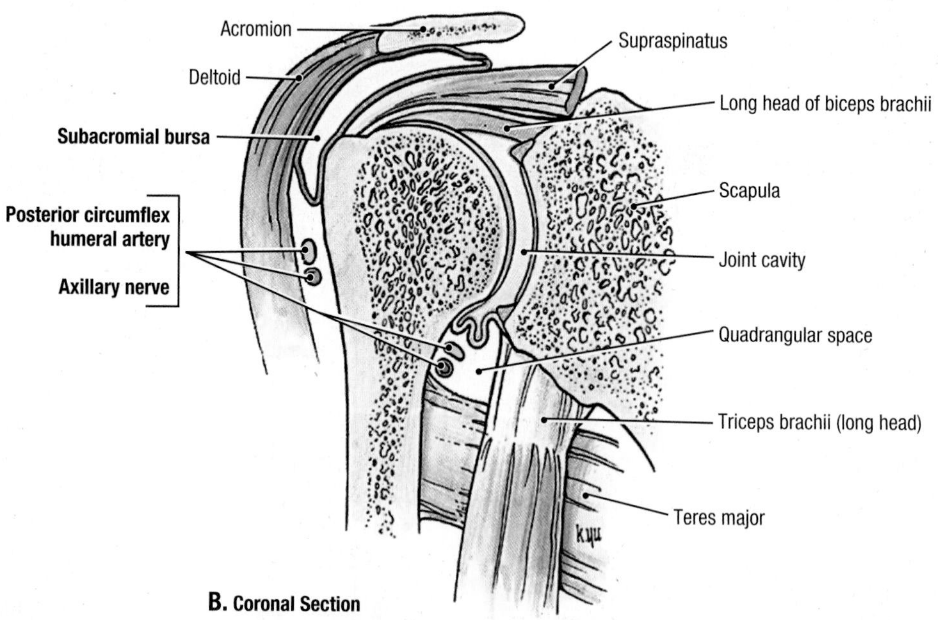
Acromion
Deltoid
Subacromial bursa
Posterior circumflex humeral artery
Axillary nerve
Supraspinatus
Long head of biceps brachii
Scapula
Joint cavity
Quadrangular space
Triceps brachii (long head)
Teres major

B. Coronal Section

6.48 IMAGING OF GLENOHUMERAL (SHOULDER) JOINT

A. Radiograph. **B.** Sectioned joint to show location of subacromial bursa and joint cavity.

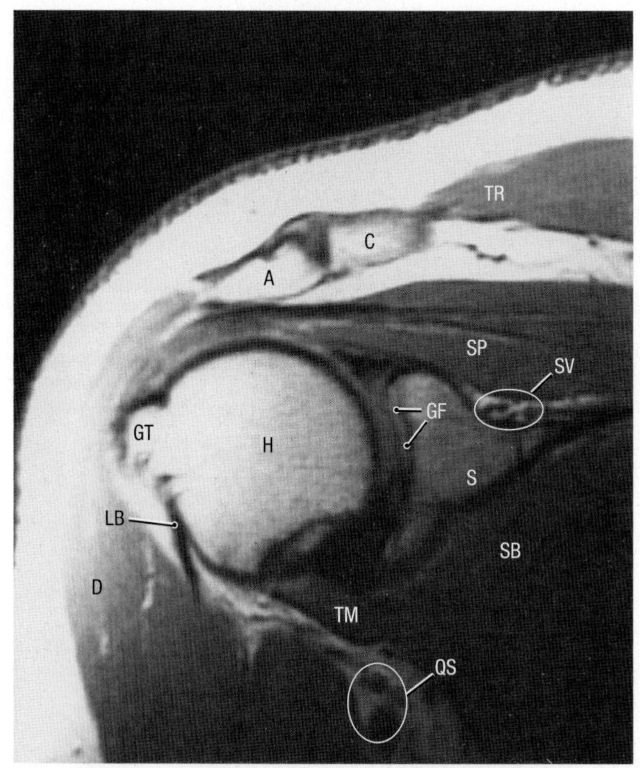
TR
C
A
SP
SV
GF
GT
H
S
LB
SB
D
TM
QS

C. Coronal MRI

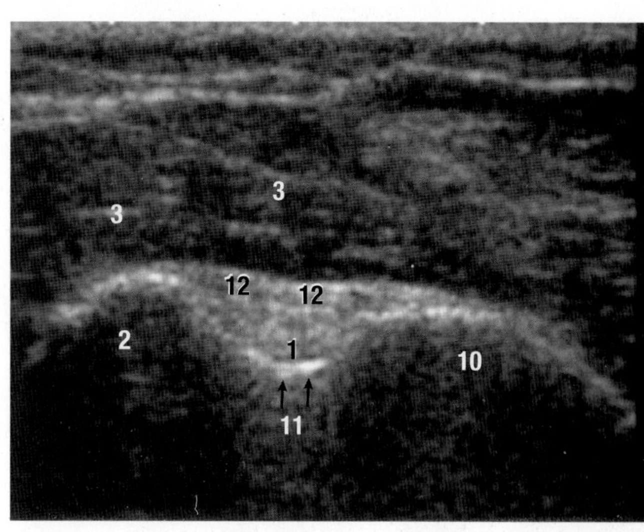
3
3
12
12
2
1
10
11

D. Transverse Scan

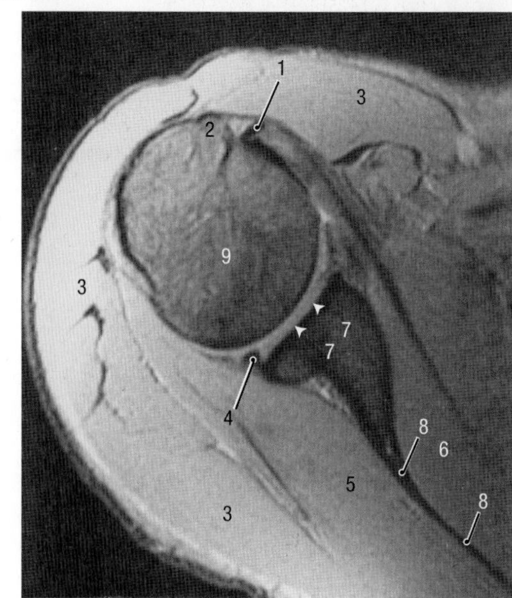
1
3
2
9
3
7
7
4
8
6
5
8
3

E. Transverse MRI

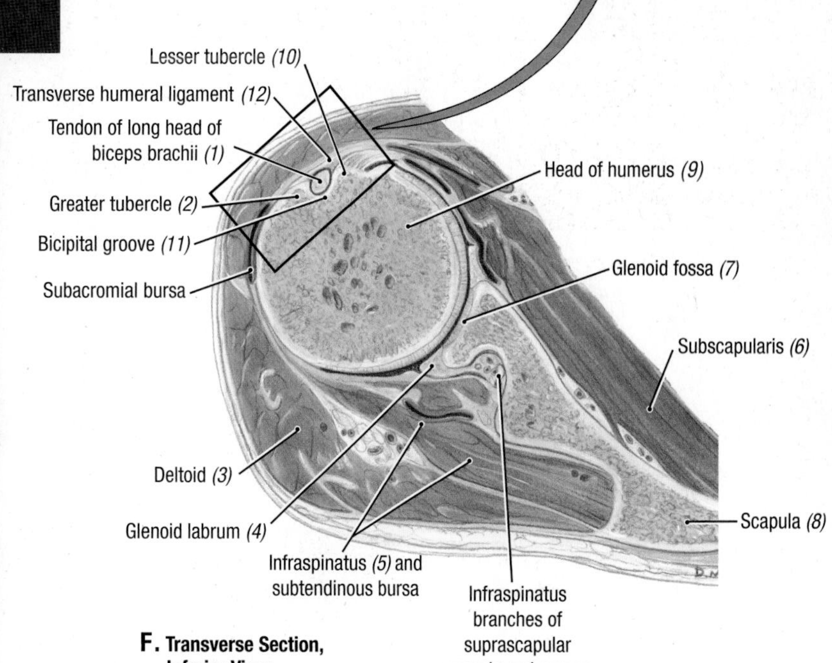
Lesser tubercle (10)
Transverse humeral ligament (12)
Tendon of long head of biceps brachii (1)
Head of humerus (9)
Greater tubercle (2)
Bicipital groove (11)
Glenoid fossa (7)
Subacromial bursa
Subscapularis (6)
Deltoid (3)
Scapula (8)
Glenoid labrum (4)
Infraspinatus (5) and subtendinous bursa
Infraspinatus branches of suprascapular vessels and nerves

F. Transverse Section, Inferior View

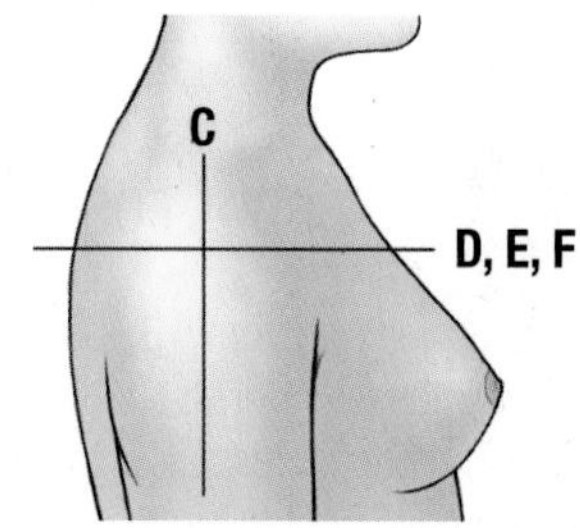
C
D, E, F

6.48 IMAGING OF GLENOHUMERAL (SHOULDER) JOINT *(CONTINUED)*

C. Coronal MRI. *A,* acromion; *C,* clavicle; *D,* deltoid; *GF,* glenoid cavity; *GT,* crest of greater tubercle; *H,* head of humerus; *LB,* long head of biceps brachii; *QS,* quadrangular space; *S,* scapula; *SB,* subscapularis; *SP,* supraspinatus; *SV,* suprascapular vessels and nerve; *TM,* teres minor; *TR,* trapezius. **D.** Transverse ultrasound scan of area indicated in **F. E.** Transverse MRI. **F.** Transverse section (*numbers* in **F** refer to structures labeled in **D** and **E**).

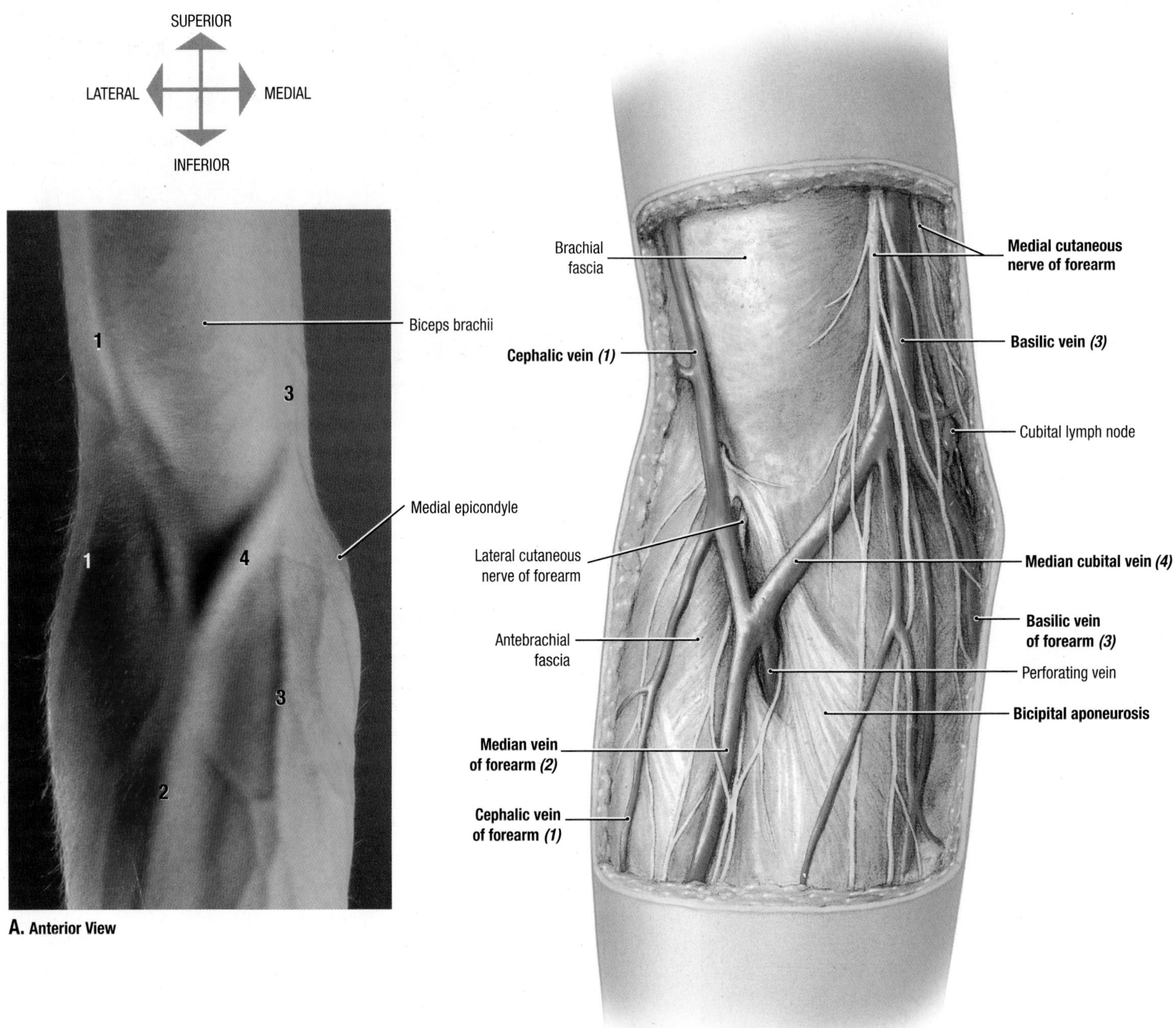
SUPERIOR
LATERAL
MEDIAL
INFERIOR
Biceps brachii
1
3
Medial epicondyle
1
4
3
2
Brachial fascia
Cephalic vein (1)
Lateral cutaneous nerve of forearm
Antebrachial fascia
Median vein of forearm (2)
Cephalic vein of forearm (1)
Medial cutaneous nerve of forearm
Basilic vein (3)
Cubital lymph node
Median cubital vein (4)
Basilic vein of forearm (3)
Perforating vein
Bicipital aponeurosis

A. Anterior View

B. Anterior View

6.49 CUBITAL FOSSA: SURFACE ANATOMY AND SUPERFICIAL DISSECTION

A. Surface anatomy. **B.** Cutaneous nerves and superficial veins (*numbers* in parentheses refer to structures in **A**).

- The cubital fossa is a triangular space (compartment) inferior to the elbow crease, roofed by deep fascia.
- In the forearm, the superficial veins (cephalic, median, basilic, and their connecting veins) make a variable, M-shaped pattern.
- The cephalic and basilic veins occupy the bicipital grooves, one on each side of the biceps brachii. In the lateral bicipital groove, the lateral cutaneous nerve of the forearm appears just superior to the elbow crease; in the medial bicipital groove, the medial cutaneous nerve of the forearm becomes cutaneous at approximately the midpoint of the arm.
- The cubital fossa is the common site for **sampling and transfusion of blood and intravenous injections** because of the prominence and accessibility of veins. Usually, the median cubital vein or basilic vein is selected.

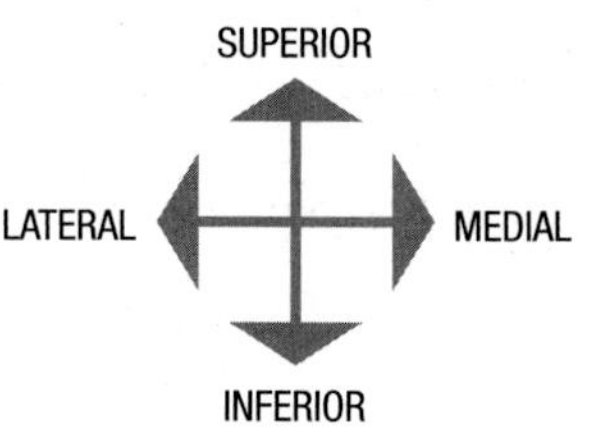
SUPERIOR
LATERAL
MEDIAL
INFERIOR

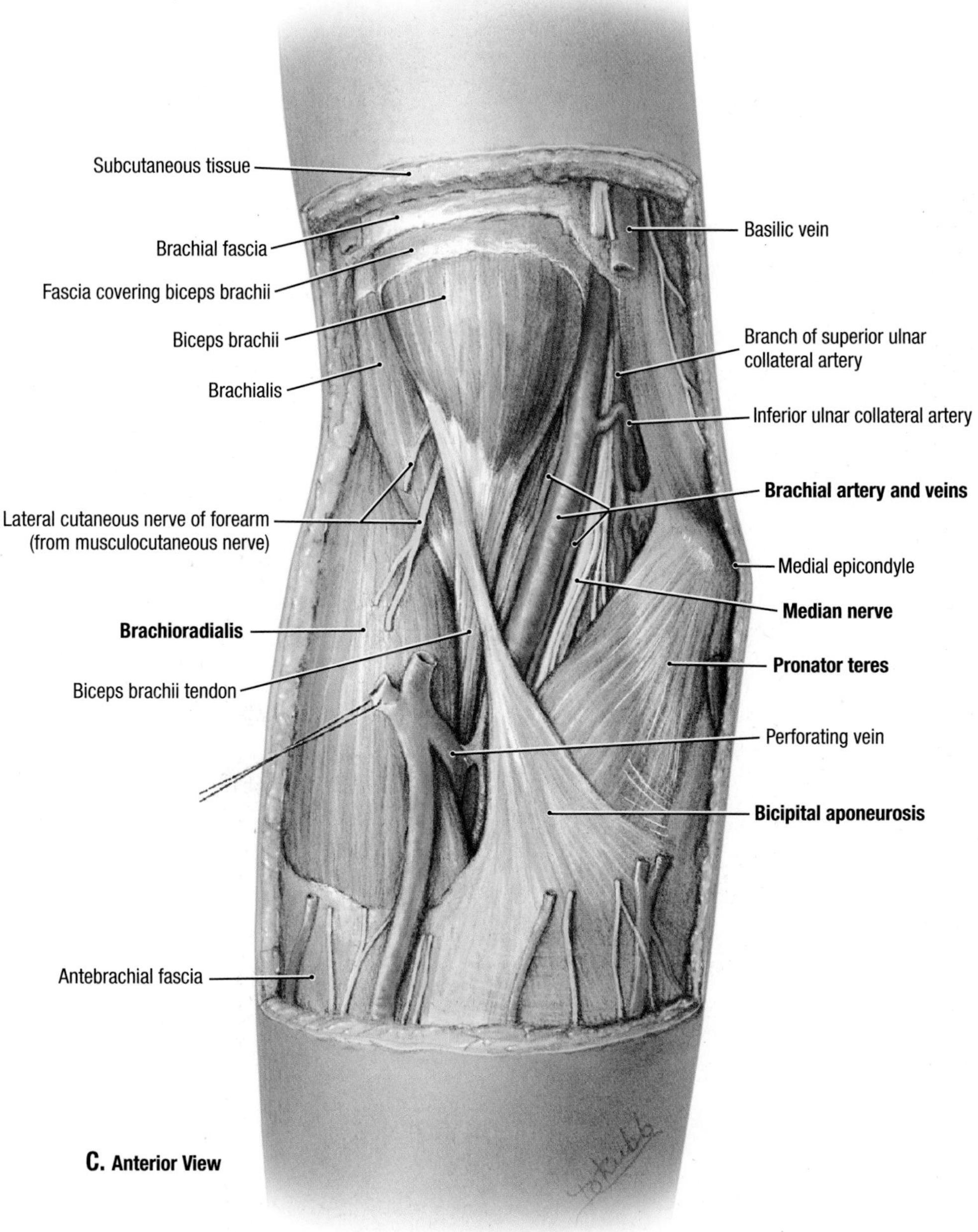

Subcutaneous tissue
Brachial fascia
Fascia covering biceps brachii
Biceps brachii
Brachialis
Lateral cutaneous nerve of forearm (from musculocutaneous nerve)
Brachioradialis
Biceps brachii tendon
Antebrachial fascia
Basilic vein
Branch of superior ulnar collateral artery
Inferior ulnar collateral artery
Brachial artery and veins
Medial epicondyle
Median nerve
Pronator teres
Perforating vein
Bicipital aponeurosis

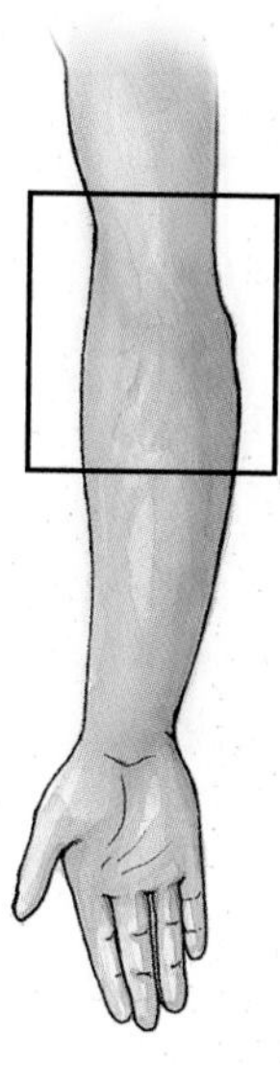

C. Anterior View

6.49 CUBITAL FOSSA: DEEP DISSECTION I

C. Boundaries and contents of the cubital fossa.

- The cubital fossa is bound laterally by the brachioradialis and medially by the pronator teres and superiorly by a line joining the medial and lateral epicondyles.
- The three chief contents of the cubital fossa are the biceps brachii tendon, brachial artery, and median nerve.
- The biceps brachii tendon, on approaching its insertion, rotates through 90°, and the bicipital aponeurosis extends medially from the proximal part of the tendon.
- A fracture of the distal part of the humerus, near the supra-epicondylar ridges, is called a **supra-epicondylar (supracondylar) fracture.** The distal bone fragment may be displaced anteriorly or posteriorly. Any of the nerves or branches of the brachial vessels related to the humerus may be injured by a displaced bone fragment.

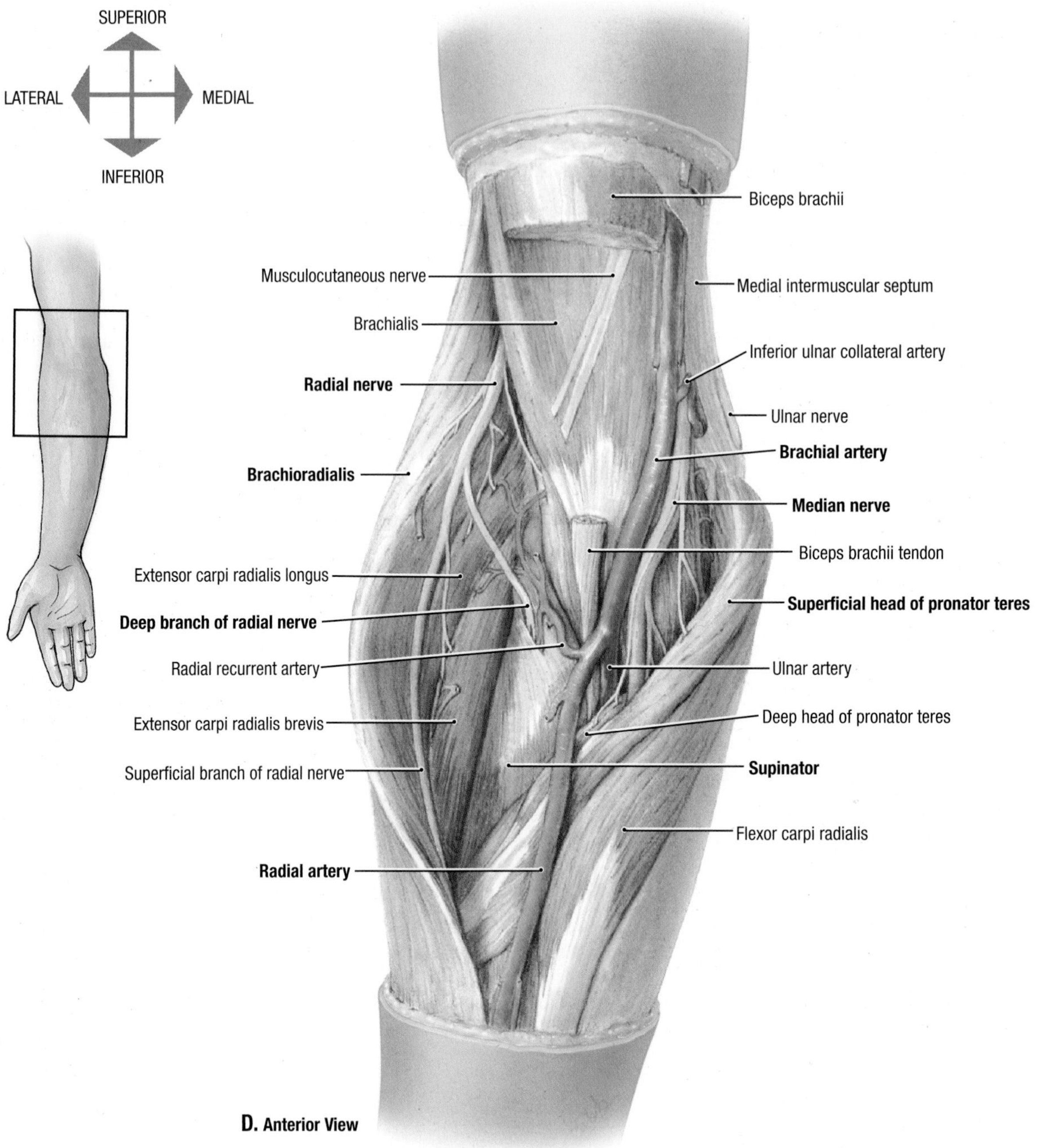
SUPERIOR
LATERAL
MEDIAL
INFERIOR
Biceps brachii
Musculocutaneous nerve
Medial intermuscular septum
Brachialis
Inferior ulnar collateral artery
Radial nerve
Ulnar nerve
Brachial artery
Brachioradialis
Median nerve
Biceps brachii tendon
Extensor carpi radialis longus
Superficial head of pronator teres
Deep branch of radial nerve
Radial recurrent artery
Ulnar artery
Deep head of pronator teres
Extensor carpi radialis brevis
Superficial branch of radial nerve
Supinator
Flexor carpi radialis
Radial artery

D. Anterior View

6.49 CUBITAL FOSSA: DEEP DISSECTION II

D. Floor of the cubital fossa.

- Part of the biceps brachii muscle is excised, and the cubital fossa is opened widely, exposing the brachialis and supinator muscles in the floor of the fossa.
- The deep branch of the radial nerve pierces the supinator.
- The brachial artery lies between the biceps tendon and median nerve and divides into two branches, the ulnar and radial arteries.
- The median nerve supplies the flexor muscles. With the exception of the twig to the deep head of pronator teres, its motor branches arise from its medial side.
- The radial nerve supplies the extensor muscles. With the exception of the twig to brachioradialis, its motor branches arise from its lateral side. In this specimen, the radial nerve has been displaced laterally, so here its lateral branches appear to run medially.

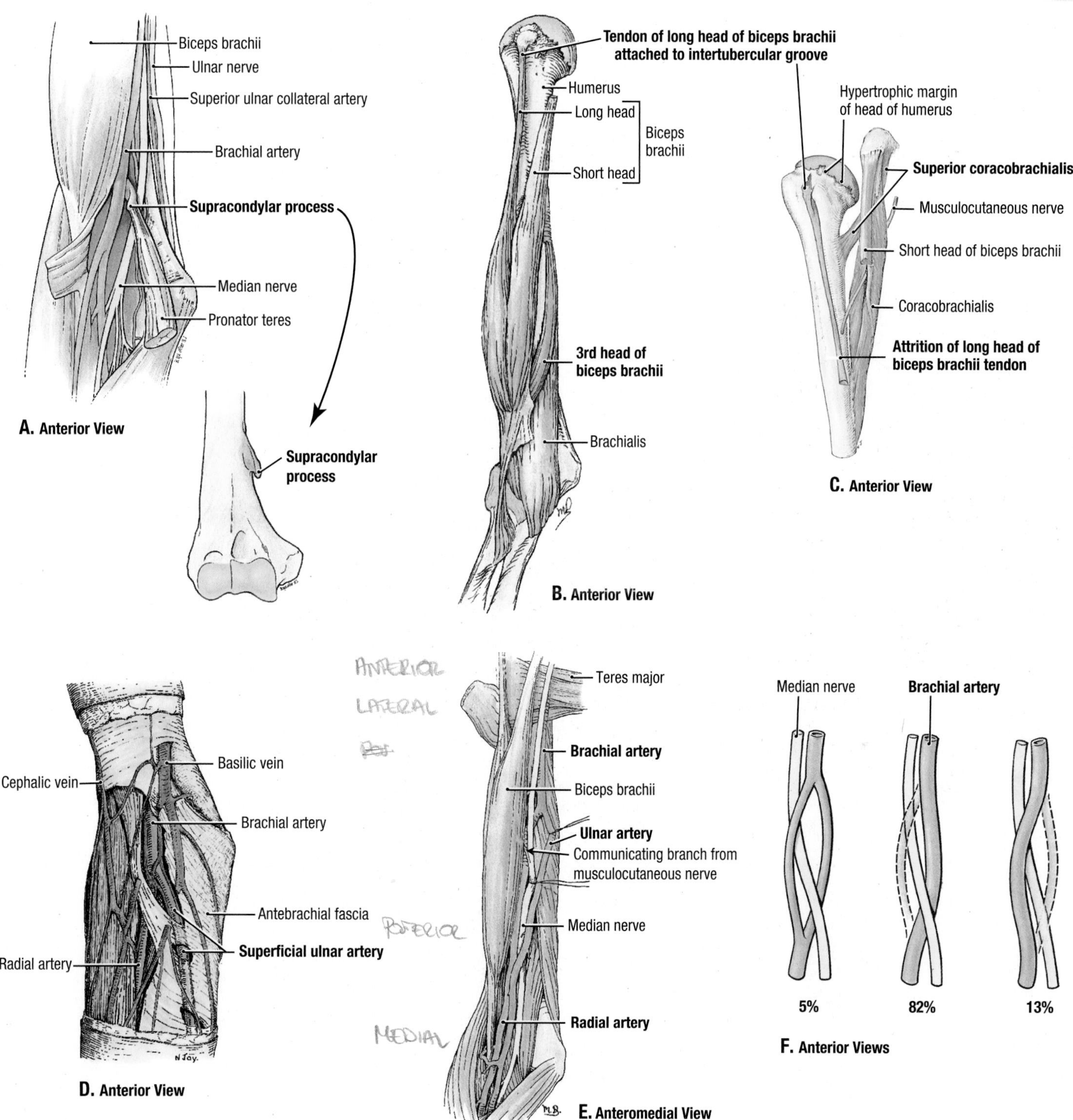
Biceps brachii
Ulnar nerve
Superior ulnar collateral artery
Brachial artery
Supracondylar process
Median nerve
Pronator teres
A. Anterior View
Supracondylar process
Tendon of long head of biceps brachii attached to intertubercular groove
Humerus
Long head
Short head
Biceps brachii
3rd head of biceps brachii
Brachialis
B. Anterior View
Hypertrophic margin of head of humerus
Superior coracobrachialis
Musculocutaneous nerve
Short head of biceps brachii
Coracobrachialis
Attrition of long head of biceps brachii tendon
C. Anterior View
Cephalic vein
Basilic vein
Brachial artery
Antebrachial fascia
Superficial ulnar artery
Radial artery
D. Anterior View
Teres major
Brachial artery
Biceps brachii
Ulnar artery
Communicating branch from musculocutaneous nerve
Median nerve
Radial artery
E. Anteromedial View
Median nerve
Brachial artery
5%
82%
13%
F. Anterior Views

6.50 ANOMALIES

A. Supracondylar process of humerus. A fibrous band, from which the pronator teres muscle arises, joins this supra-epicondylar process to the medial epicondyle. The median nerve, often accompanied by the brachial artery, passes through the foramen formed by this band. This may be a cause of nerve entrapment. **B. Third head of biceps brachii.** In this case, there is also attrition of the biceps tendon. **C.** Attrition of the tendon of the long head of biceps brachii and presence of a coracobrachialis.

D. Superficial ulnar artery. E. Anomalous division of brachial artery. In this case, the median nerve passes between the radial and ulnar arteries, which arise high in the arm. **F. Relationship of median nerve and brachial artery.** The variable relationship of these two structures can be explained developmentally. In a study of 307 limbs in Dr. Grant's lab, portions of both primitive brachial arteries persisted in 5%, the posterior in 82%, and the anterior in 13%.

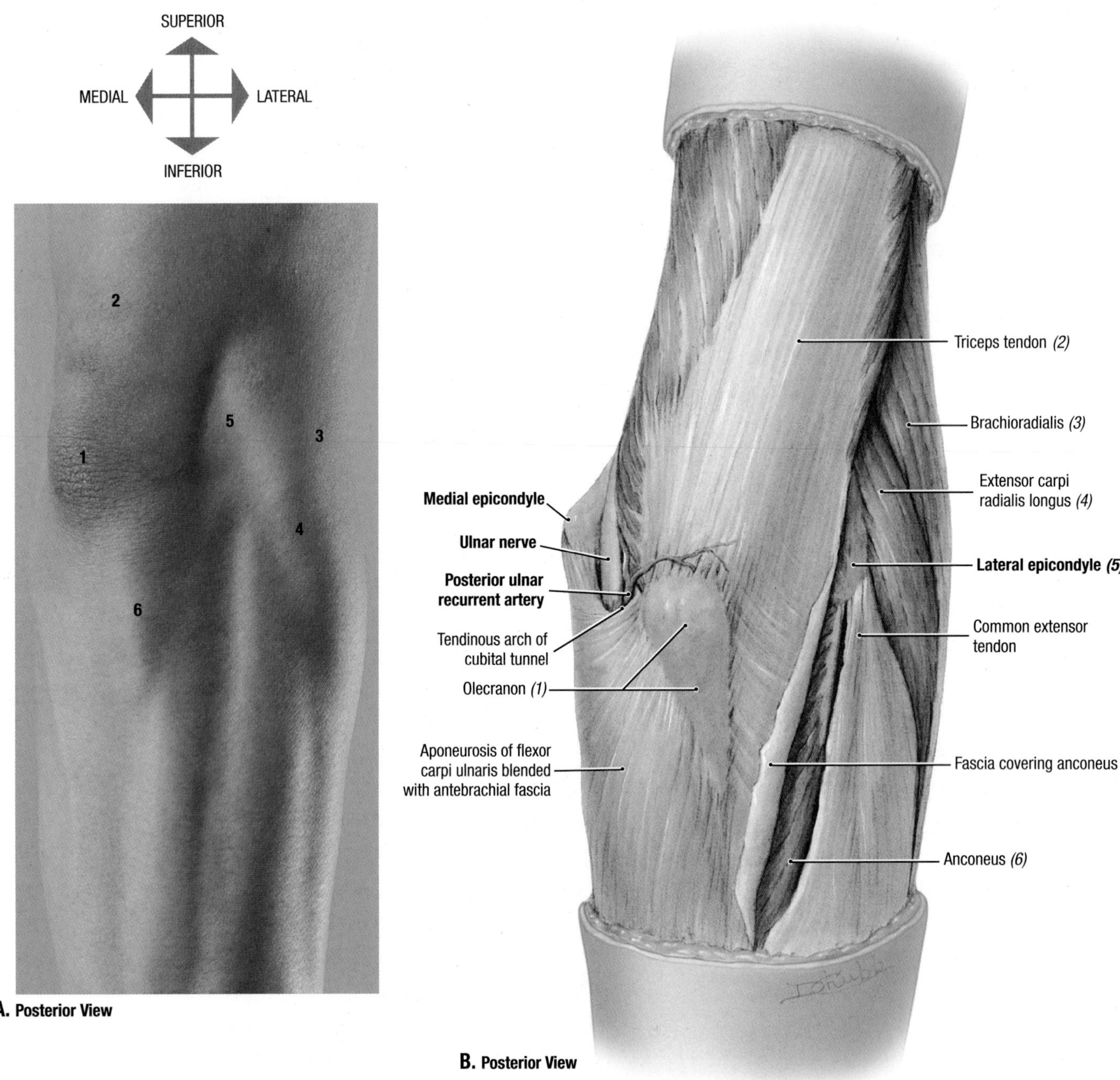
SUPERIOR
MEDIAL
LATERAL
INFERIOR
2
5
3
1
4
6
Triceps tendon (2)
Brachioradialis (3)
Extensor carpi radialis longus (4)
Medial epicondyle
Ulnar nerve
Lateral epicondyle (5)
Posterior ulnar recurrent artery
Tendinous arch of cubital tunnel
Common extensor tendon
Olecranon (1)
Aponeurosis of flexor carpi ulnaris blended with antebrachial fascia
Fascia covering anconeus
Anconeus (6)

A. Posterior View

B. Posterior View

6.51 POSTERIOR ASPECT OF ELBOW I

A. Surface anatomy. **B.** Superficial dissection (*numbers* in parentheses refer to structures in **A**).

- The triceps brachii is attached distally to the superior surface of the olecranon and, through the deep fascia covering the anconeus, into the lateral border of olecranon.
- The posterior surfaces of the medial epicondyle, lateral epicondyle, and olecranon are subcutaneous and palpable.
- The ulnar nerve, also palpable, runs subfascially posterior to the medial epicondyle; distal to this point, it disappears deep to the two heads of the flexor carpi ulnaris.

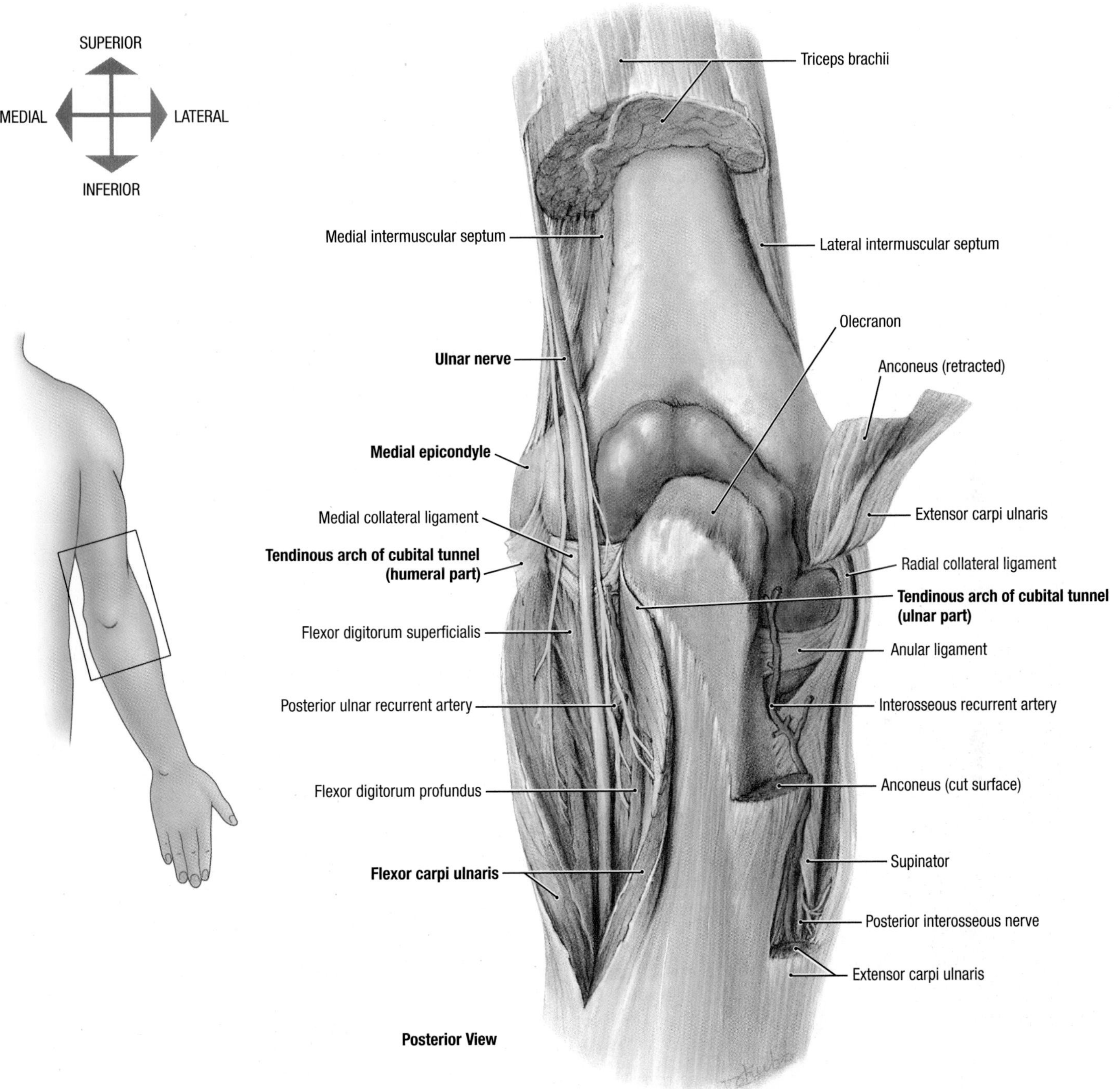
SUPERIOR
MEDIAL
LATERAL
INFERIOR
Triceps brachii
Medial intermuscular septum
Lateral intermuscular septum
Olecranon
Anconeus (retracted)
Ulnar nerve
Medial epicondyle
Medial collateral ligament
Extensor carpi ulnaris
Tendinous arch of cubital tunnel (humeral part)
Radial collateral ligament
Tendinous arch of cubital tunnel (ulnar part)
Flexor digitorum superficialis
Anular ligament
Posterior ulnar recurrent artery
Interosseous recurrent artery
Flexor digitorum profundus
Anconeus (cut surface)
Supinator
Flexor carpi ulnaris
Posterior interosseous nerve
Extensor carpi ulnaris
Posterior View

6.52 POSTERIOR ASPECT OF ELBOW II

Deep dissection. The distal portion of the triceps brachii muscle was removed.

- The ulnar nerve descends subfascially within the posterior compartment of the arm, passing posterior to the medial epicondyle in the groove for the ulnar nerve. Next it passes posterior to the ulnar collateral ligament of the elbow joint and then between the flexor carpi ulnaris and flexor digitorum profundus muscles.

Ulnar nerve injury occurs most commonly where the nerve passes posterior to the medial epicondyle of the humerus. The injury results when the medial part of the elbow hits a hard surface, fracturing the medial epicondyle. The ulnar nerve may be compressed in the cubital tunnel, resulting in **cubital tunnel syndrome.** The cubital tunnel is formed by the tendinous arch joining the humeral and ulnar heads of attachment of the flexor carpi ulnaris muscle. Ulnar nerve injury can result in extensive motor and sensory loss to the hand.

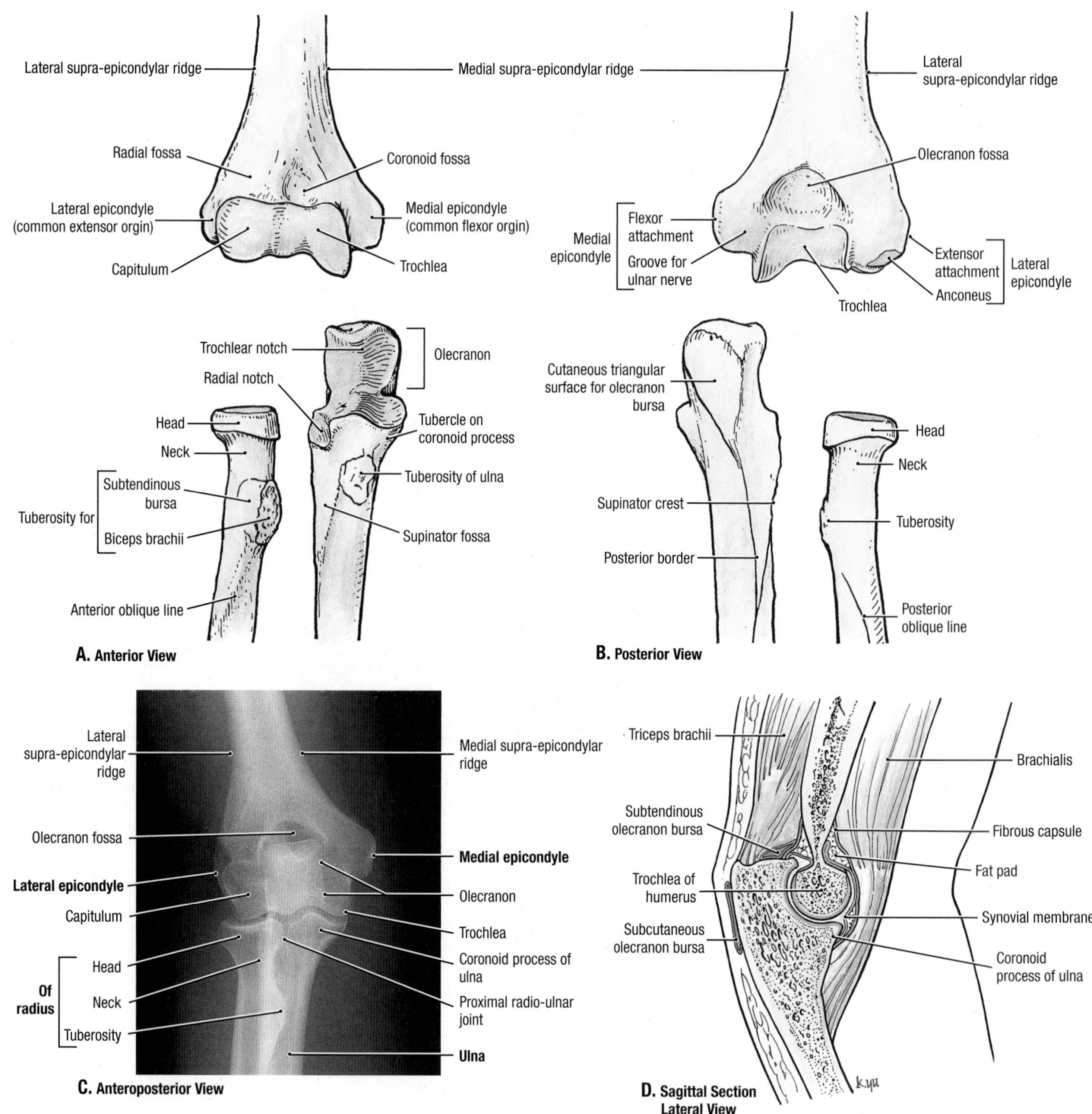
Lateral supra-epicondylar ridge
Medial supra-epicondylar ridge
Radial fossa
Coronoid fossa
Lateral epicondyle (common extensor orgin)
Medial epicondyle (common flexor orgin)
Capitulum
Trochlea
Lateral supra-epicondylar ridge
Olecranon fossa
Medial epicondyle
Flexor attachment
Groove for ulnar nerve
Extensor attachment
Anconeus
Lateral epicondyle
Trochlea
Trochlear notch
Radial notch
Olecranon
Head
Neck
Tubercle on coronoid process
Tuberosity of ulna
Tuberosity for
Subtendinous bursa
Biceps brachii
Supinator fossa
Anterior oblique line
A. Anterior View
Cutaneous triangular surface for olecranon bursa
Head
Neck
Supinator crest
Tuberosity
Posterior border
Posterior oblique line
B. Posterior View
Lateral supra-epicondylar ridge
Medial supra-epicondylar ridge
Olecranon fossa
Medial epicondyle
Lateral epicondyle
Olecranon
Capitulum
Trochlea
Of radius
Head
Coronoid process of ulna
Neck
Proximal radio-ulnar joint
Tuberosity
Ulna
C. Anteroposterior View
Triceps brachii
Brachialis
Subtendinous olecranon bursa
Fibrous capsule
Fat pad
Trochlea of humerus
Synovial membrane
Subcutaneous olecranon bursa
Coronoid process of ulna
D. Sagittal Section Lateral View

6.53 BONES AND IMAGING OF ELBOW REGION

A. Anterior bony features. **B.** Posterior bony features. **C.** Radiograph of elbow joint. **D.** Section of humero-ulnar joint.

The subcutaneous olecranon bursa is exposed to injury during falls on the elbow and to infection from abrasions of the skin covering the olecranon. Repeated excessive pressure and friction produces a friction **subcutaneous olecranon bursitis** (e.g., "student's elbow").

Subtendinous olecranon bursitis results from excessive friction between the triceps tendon and the olecranon. For example, it may occur due to repeated flexion-extension of the forearm during certain assembly-line jobs. The pain is severe during flexion of the forearm because of pressure exerted on the inflamed subtendinous olecranon bursa by the triceps tendon.

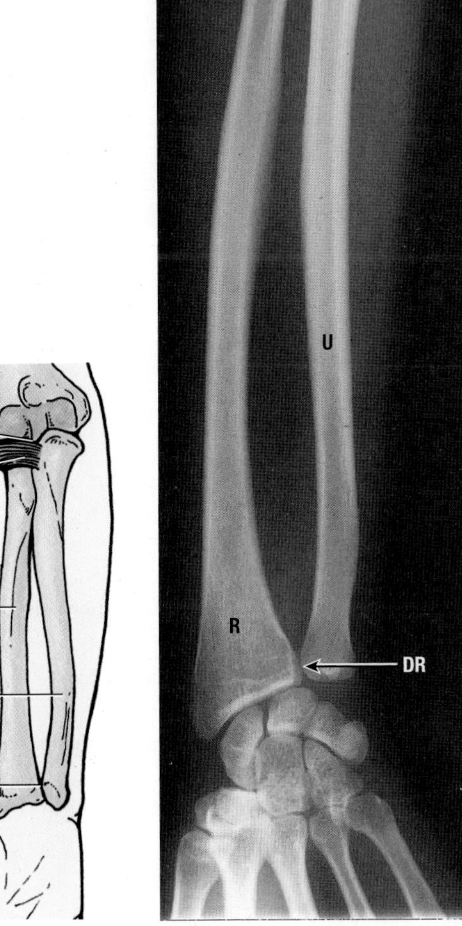
Proximal radio-ulnar joint (PR)
Anular ligament of radius
Radius (R)
Ulna (U)
Distal radio-ulnar joint (DR)
PR
U
R
U
R
DR

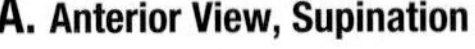

A. Anterior View, Supination

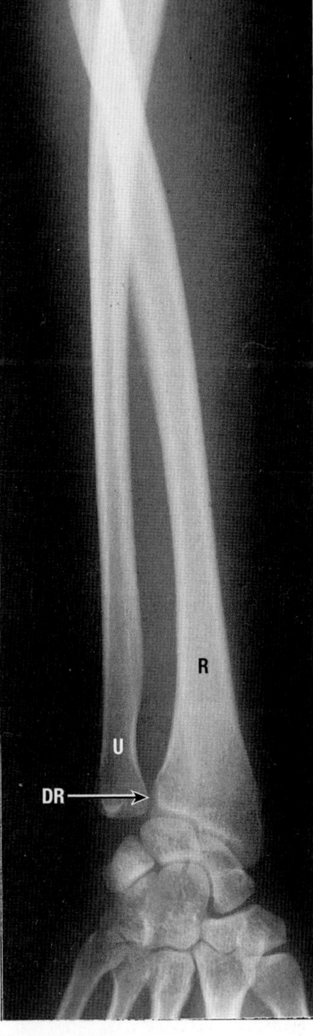
R
U
R
U
DR

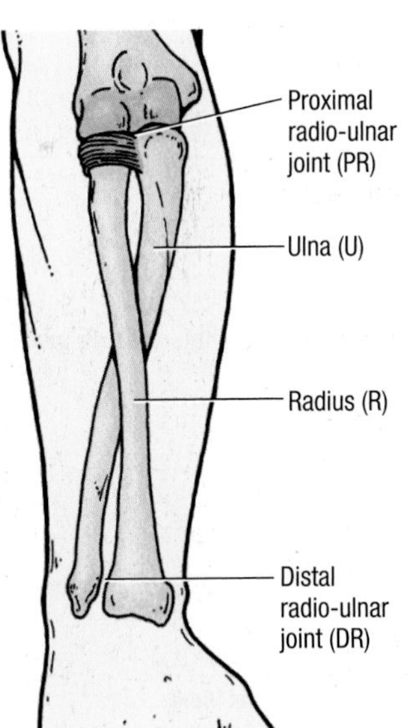
Proximal radio-ulnar joint (PR)
Ulna (U)
Radius (R)
Distal radio-ulnar joint (DR)

B. Anterior View, Pronation

6.54 SUPINATION AND PRONATION AT SUPERIOR, MIDDLE, AND INFERIOR RADIO-ULNAR JOINTS

A. Radiograph of forearm in supination. **B.** Radiograph of forearm in pronation. The radius crosses the ulna when the forearm is pronated. The superior and inferior radio-ulnar joints are synovial joints; the middle radio-ulnar joint is a syndesmosis (fibrous joint) in which the interosseous ligament connects the forearm bones.

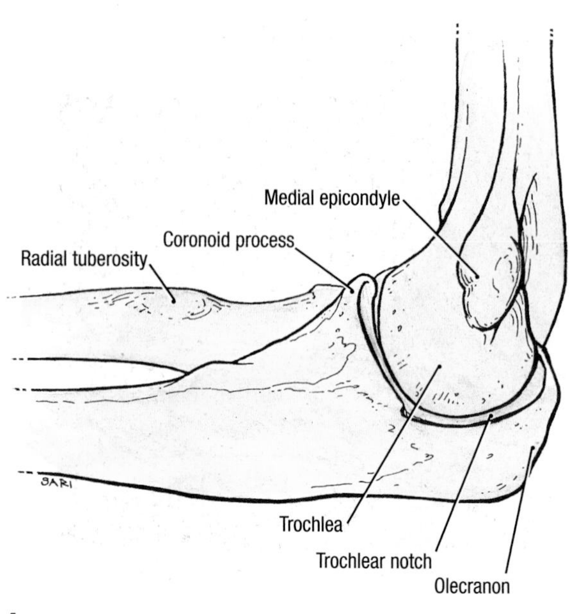
Medial epicondyle
Coronoid process
Radial tuberosity
Trochlea
Trochlear notch
Olecranon

A. **Medial View**

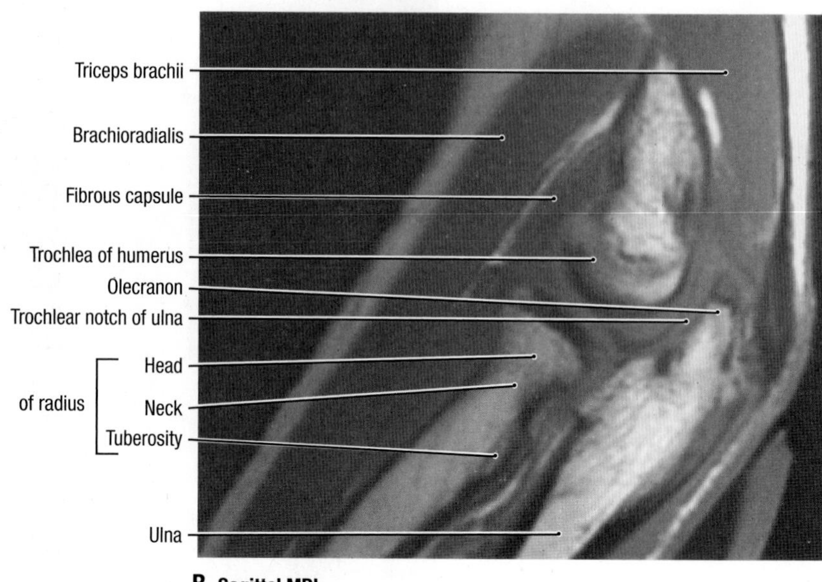
Triceps brachii
Brachioradialis
Fibrous capsule
Trochlea of humerus
Olecranon
Trochlear notch of ulna
Head
Neck
Tuberosity
of radius
Ulna

B. **Sagittal MRI**

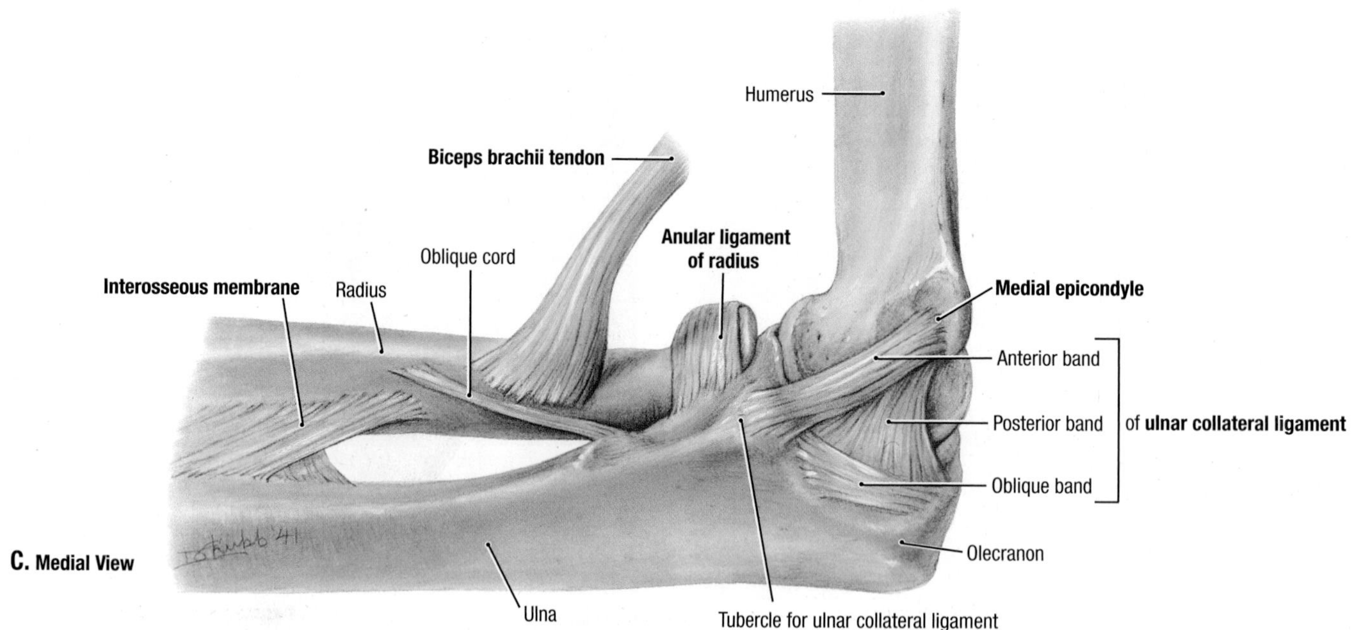
Humerus
Biceps brachii tendon
Anular ligament of radius
Oblique cord
Interosseous membrane
Radius
Medial epicondyle
Anterior band
Posterior band
Oblique band
of ulnar collateral ligament
Olecranon
Ulna
Tubercle for ulnar collateral ligament

C. **Medial View**

6.55 MEDIAL ASPECT OF BONES AND LIGAMENTS OF ELBOW REGION

A. Bony features. **B.** MRI of elbow joint. **C.** Ligaments. The anterior band of the ulnar (medial) collateral ligament is a strong, round cord that is taut when the elbow joint is extended. The posterior band is a weak fan that is taut in flexion of the joint.

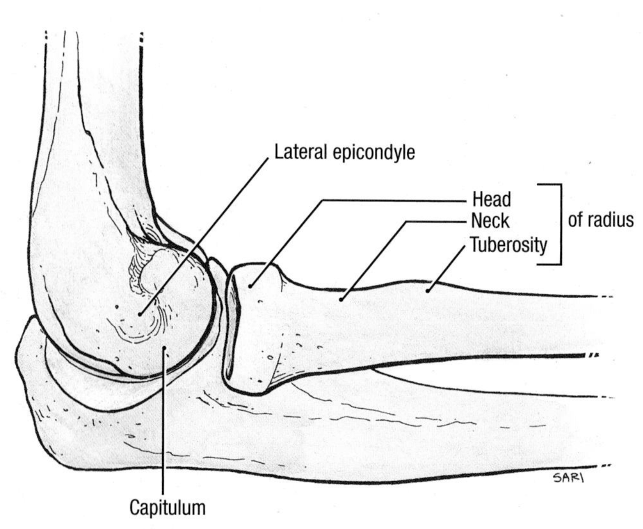
Lateral epicondyle
Head
Neck
Tuberosity
of radius
Capitulum
SARI

A. Lateral View

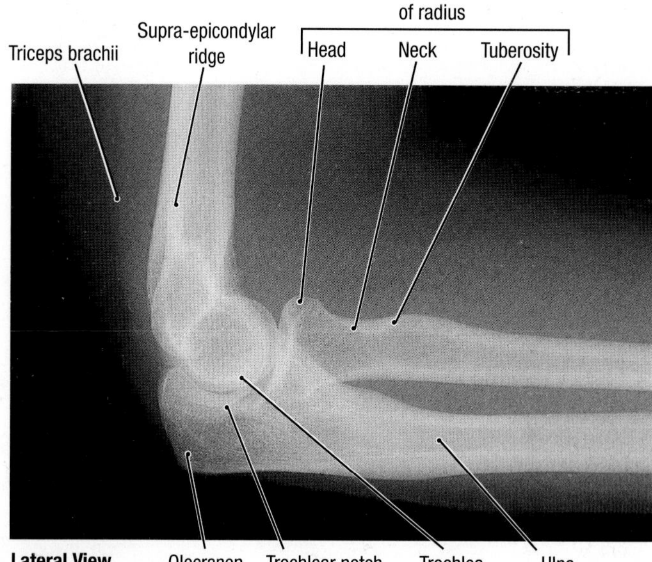
Triceps brachii
Supra-epicondylar ridge
of radius
Head
Neck
Tuberosity
Olecranon
Trochlear notch
Trochlea
Ulna

B. Lateral View

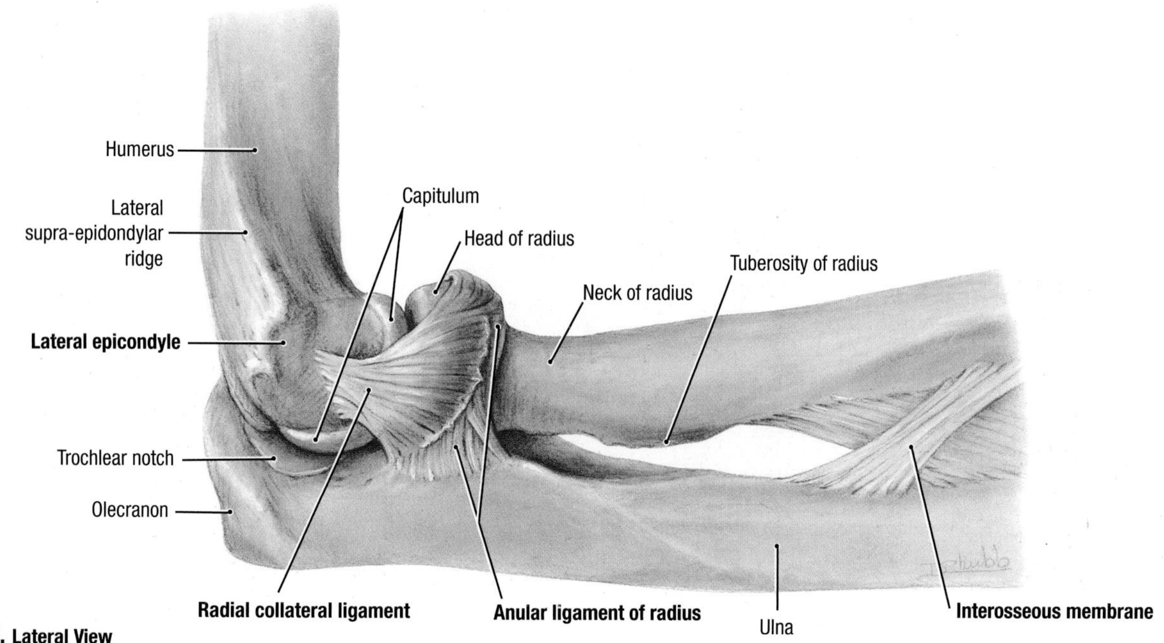
Humerus
Lateral supra-epidondylar ridge
Lateral epicondyle
Trochlear notch
Olecranon
Capitulum
Head of radius
Neck of radius
Tuberosity of radius
Radial collateral ligament
Anular ligament of radius
Ulna
Interosseous membrane

C. Lateral View

6.56 LATERAL ASPECT OF BONES AND LIGAMENTS OF ELBOW REGION

A. Bony features. **B.** Lateral radiograph. **C.** Ligaments. The fan-shaped radial (lateral) collateral ligament is primarily attached to the anular ligament of the radius; superficial fibers of the lateral ligament blend with the fibrous capsule and continue onto the radius.

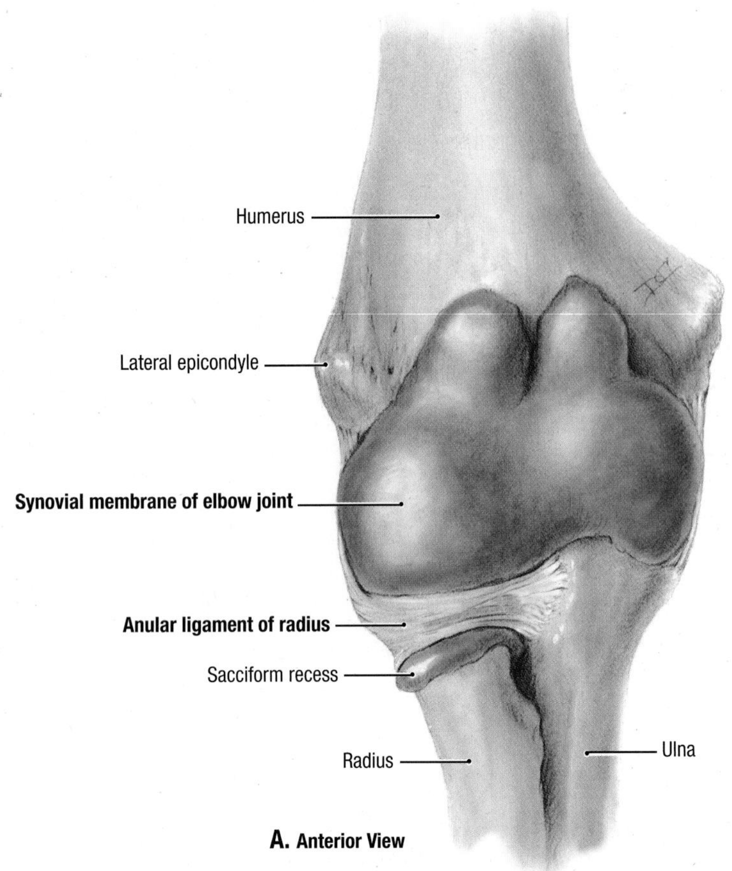
Humerus
Lateral epicondyle
Synovial membrane of elbow joint
Anular ligament of radius
Sacciform recess
Radius
Ulna
A. Anterior View

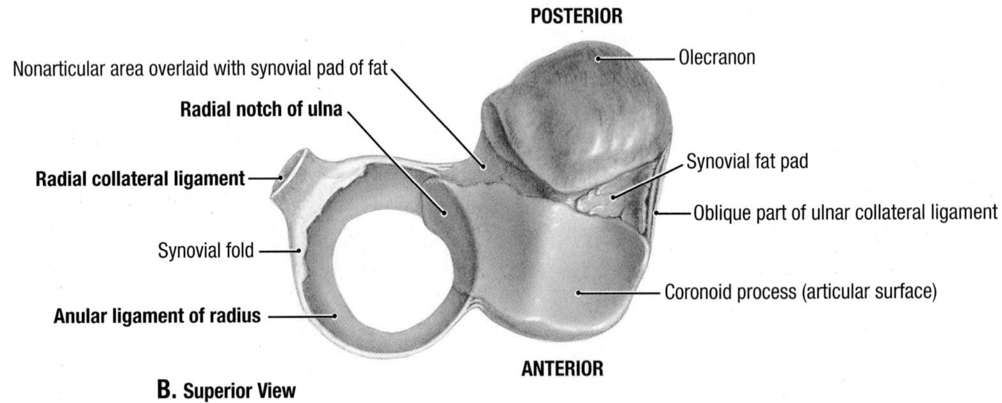
POSTERIOR
Nonarticular area overlaid with synovial pad of fat
Olecranon
Radial notch of ulna
Radial collateral ligament
Synovial fat pad
Oblique part of ulnar collateral ligament
Synovial fold
Coronoid process (articular surface)
Anular ligament of radius
ANTERIOR
B. Superior View

6.57 SYNOVIAL CAPSULE OF ELBOW JOINT AND ANULAR LIGAMENT

A. Synovial capsule of elbow and proximal radio-ulnar joints. The cavity of the elbow was injected with purple fluid (wax). The fibrous capsule was removed, and the synovial membrane remains. **B.** Anular ligament.

- The anular ligament secures the head of the radius to the radial notch of the ulna and with it forms a tapering columnar socket (i.e., wide superiorly, narrow inferiorly).
- The anular ligament is bound to the humerus by the radial collateral ligament of the elbow.

A common childhood injury is **subluxation and dislocation of the head of the radius** after traction on a pronated forearm (e.g., when lifting a child onto a bus). The sudden pulling of the upper limb tears or stretches the distal attachment of the less tapering anular ligament of a child. The radial head then moves distally, partially out of the anular ligament. The proximal part of the torn ligament may become trapped between the head of the radius and the capitulum of the humerus. The source of pain is the pinched anular ligament.

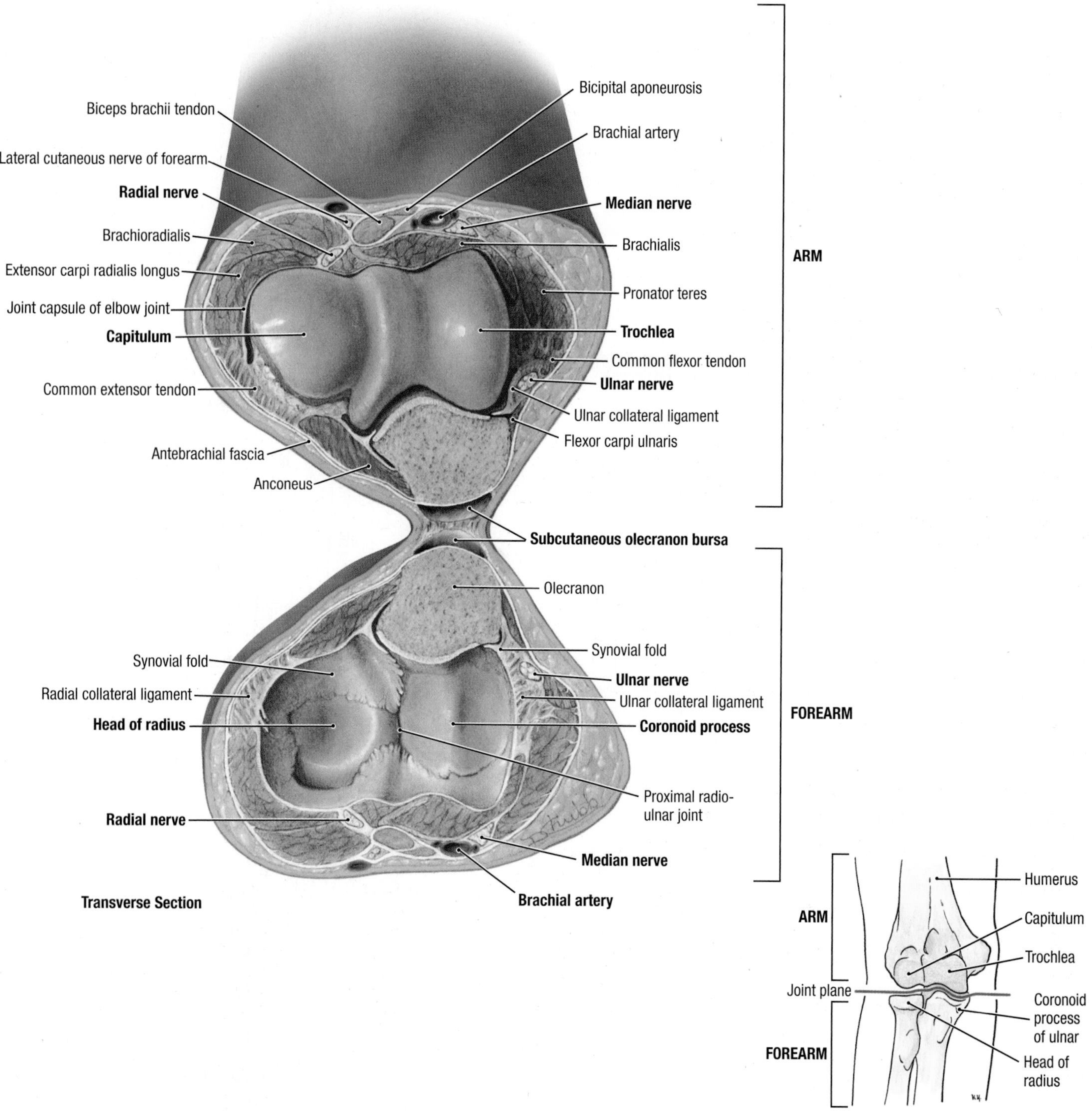
Biceps brachii tendon
Bicipital aponeurosis
Brachial artery
Lateral cutaneous nerve of forearm
Radial nerve
Median nerve
Brachioradialis
Brachialis
Extensor carpi radialis longus
Pronator teres
Joint capsule of elbow joint
Capitulum
Trochlea
Common flexor tendon
Common extensor tendon
Ulnar nerve
Ulnar collateral ligament
Flexor carpi ulnaris
Antebrachial fascia
Anconeus
ARM
Subcutaneous olecranon bursa
Olecranon
Synovial fold
Synovial fold
Ulnar nerve
Radial collateral ligament
Ulnar collateral ligament
Head of radius
Coronoid process
FOREARM
Proximal radio-ulnar joint
Radial nerve
Median nerve
Brachial artery
Transverse Section
Humerus
ARM
Capitulum
Trochlea
Joint plane
Coronoid process of ulnar
FOREARM
Head of radius

6.58 ARTICULAR SURFACES OF ELBOW JOINT

The tissue surrounding the condyles of the humerus has been sectioned in a transverse plane, followed by disarticulation of the elbow joint, revealing the articular surfaces. Compare the forearm (inferior) component with Figure 6.57B.

- Synovial folds containing fat overlie the periphery of the head of the radius and the nonarticular indentations on the trochlear notch of the ulna.
- The radial nerve is in contact with the joint capsule, the ulnar nerve is in contact with the ulnar collateral ligament, and the median nerve is separated from the joint capsule by the brachialis muscle.

TABLE 6.11 ARTERIES OF FOREARM

Radial artery
Origin: In cubital fossa, as smaller terminal branch of brachial artery
Course/Distribution: Runs distally under brachioradialis, lateral to flexor carpi radialis, defining boundary between the flexor and extensor compartments and supplying the radial aspect of both. Gives rise to a superficial palmar branch near the radiocarpal joint; it then transverses the anatomical snuff box to pass between the heads of the 1st dorsal interosseous muscle joining the deep branch of the ulnar artery to form the deep palmar arch
Ulnar artery
Origin: In cubital fossa, as larger terminal branch of brachial artery
Course/Distribution: Passes distally between 2nd and 3rd layers of forearm flexor muscles, supplying ulnar aspect of flexor compartment; passes superficial to flexor retinaculum at wrist, continuing as the superficial palmar arch (with superficial branch of radial) after its deep palmar branch joins the deep palmar arch
Radial recurrent artery
Origin: In cubital fossa, as 1st (lateral) branch of radial artery
Course/Distribution: Courses proximally, superficial to supinator, passing between brachioradialis and brachialis to anastomose with radial collateral artery
Anterior and posterior ulnar recurrent arteries
Origin: In and immediately distal to cubital fossa, as 1st and 2nd medial branches of ulnar artery
Course/Distribution: Course proximally to anastomose with the inferior and superior ulnar collateral arteries, respectively, forming collateral pathways anterior and posterior to the medial epicondyle of the humerus
Common interosseous artery
Origin: Immediately distal to the cubital fossa, as 1st lateral branch of ulnar artery
Course/Distribution: Terminates almost immediately, dividing into anterior and posterior interosseous arteries
Anterior and posterior interosseous arteries
Origin: Distal to radial tubercle, as terminal branches of common interosseous
Course/Distribution: Pass to opposite sides of interosseous membrane; anterior artery runs on interosseous membrane; posterior artery runs between superficial and deep layers of extensor muscles as primary artery of compartment
Interosseous recurrent artery
Origin: Initial part of posterior interosseous artery
Course/Distribution: Courses proximally between lateral epicondyle and olecranon, deep to anconeus, to anastomose with middle collateral artery

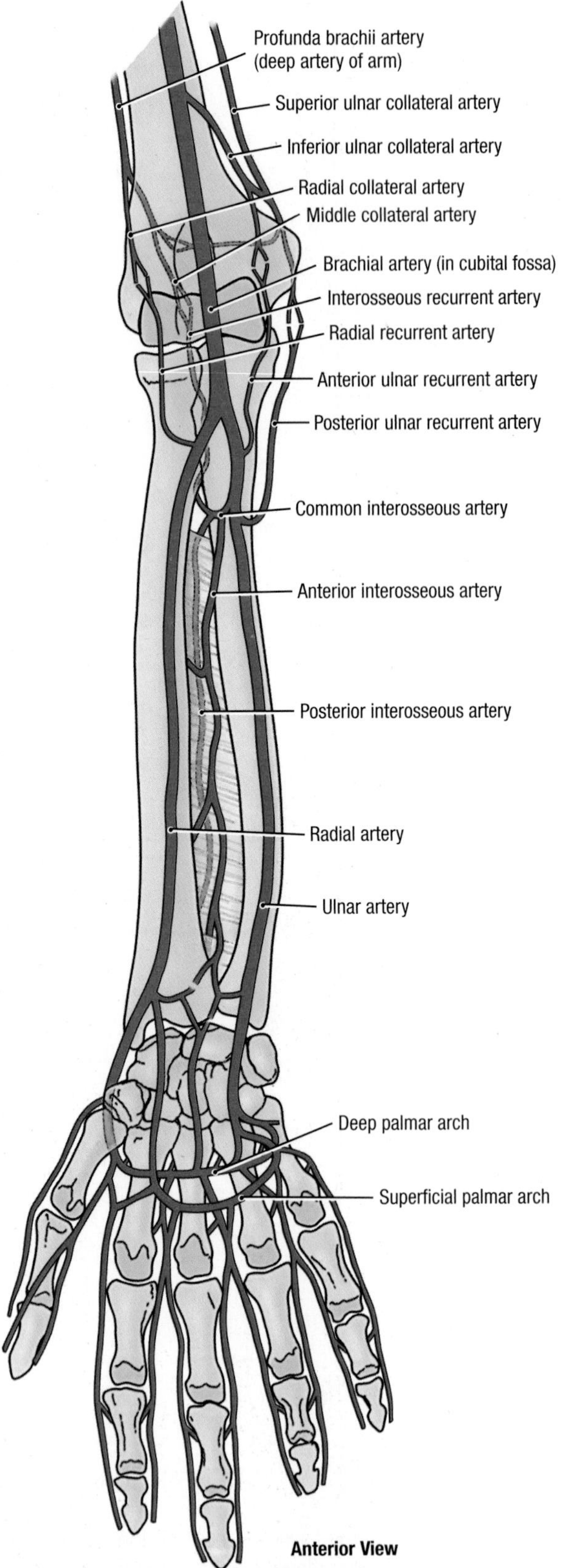
Profunda brachii artery
(deep artery of arm)
Superior ulnar collateral artery
Inferior ulnar collateral artery
Radial collateral artery
Middle collateral artery
Brachial artery (in cubital fossa)
Interosseous recurrent artery
Radial recurrent artery
Anterior ulnar recurrent artery
Posterior ulnar recurrent artery
Common interosseous artery
Anterior interosseous artery
Posterior interosseous artery
Radial artery
Ulnar artery
Deep palmar arch
Superficial palmar arch
Anterior View

6.59 ARTERIES OF FOREARM

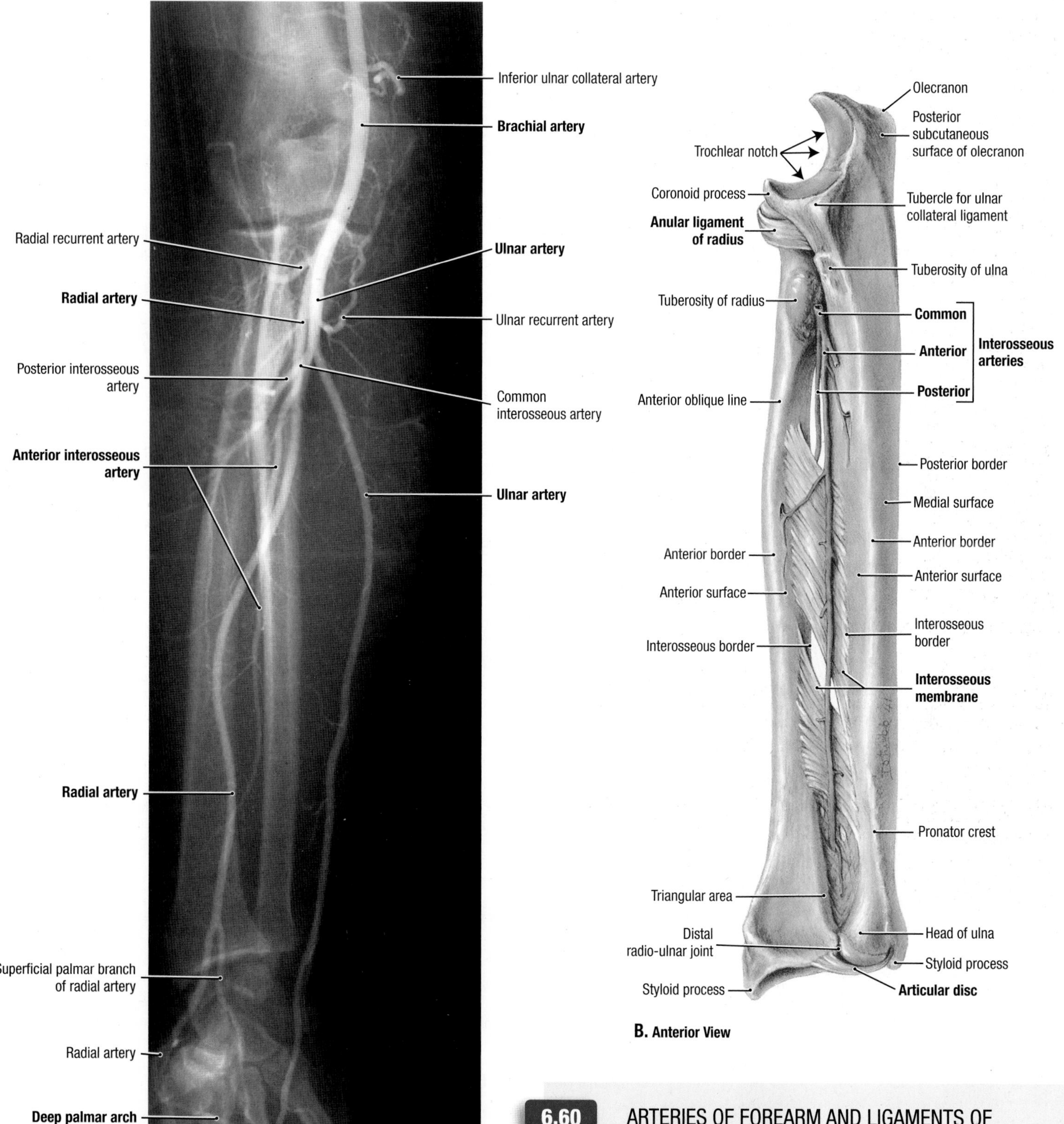
Inferior ulnar collateral artery
Brachial artery
Radial recurrent artery
Ulnar artery
Radial artery
Ulnar recurrent artery
Posterior interosseous artery
Common interosseous artery
Anterior interosseous artery
Ulnar artery
Radial artery
Superficial palmar branch of radial artery
Radial artery
Deep palmar arch
Superficial palmar arch
Olecranon
Posterior subcutaneous surface of olecranon
Trochlear notch
Coronoid process
Tubercle for ulnar collateral ligament
Anular ligament of radius
Tuberosity of ulna
Tuberosity of radius
Common
Anterior
Posterior
Interosseous arteries
Anterior oblique line
Posterior border
Medial surface
Anterior border
Anterior border
Anterior surface
Anterior surface
Interosseous border
Interosseous border
Interosseous membrane
Pronator crest
Triangular area
Head of ulna
Distal radio-ulnar joint
Styloid process
Styloid process
Articular disc

A. Anteroposterior View

B. Anterior View

6.60 ARTERIES OF FOREARM AND LIGAMENTS OF RADIO-ULNAR JOINTS

A. Brachial arteriogram. **B.** Radio-ulnar ligaments and interosseous arteries. The ligament maintaining the proximal radio-ulnar joint is the anular ligament, that for the distal joint is the articular disc, and that for the middle joint is the interosseous membrane. The interosseous membrane is attached to the interosseous borders of the radius and ulna, but it also spreads onto their surfaces.

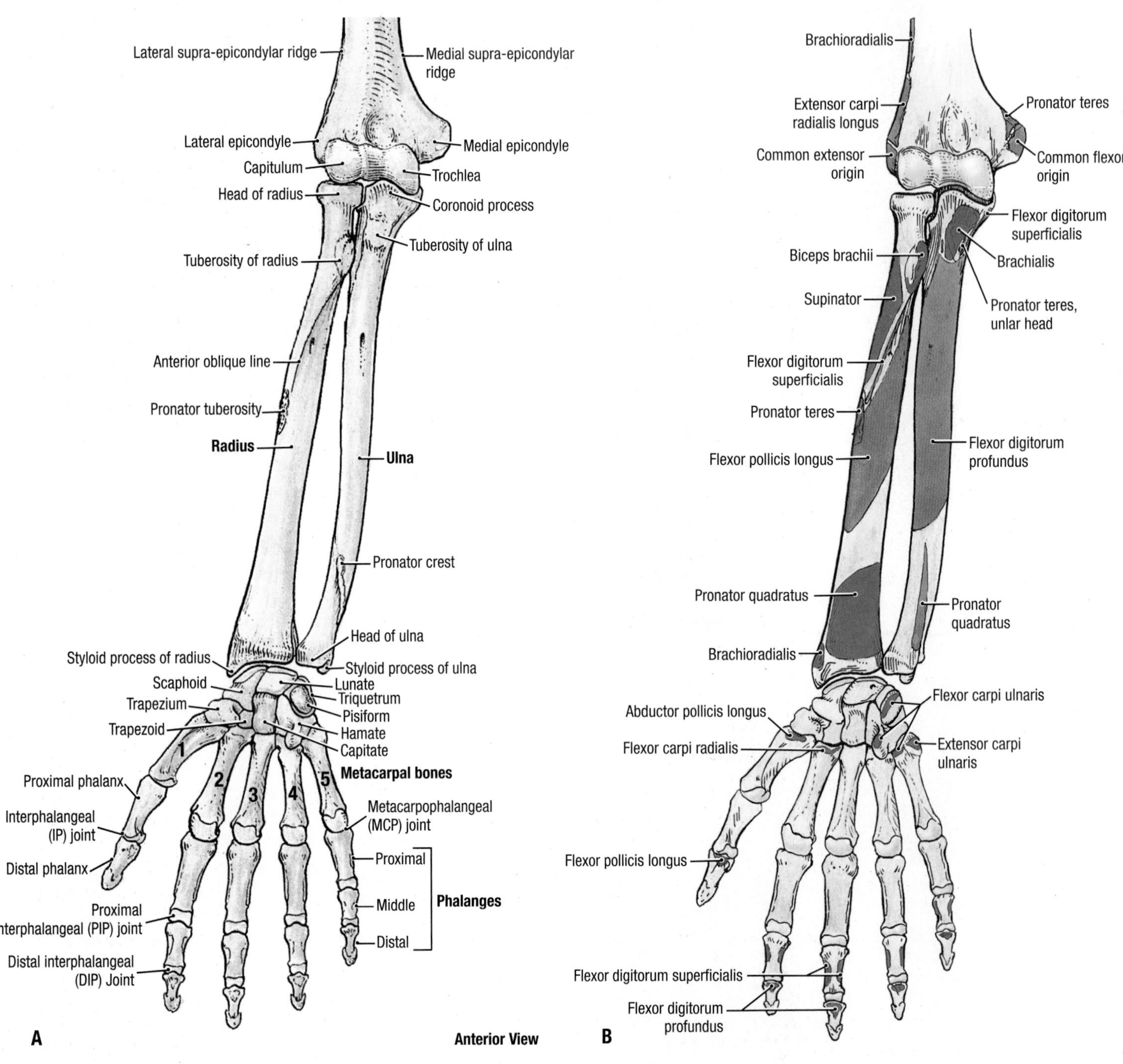
Lateral supra-epicondylar ridge
Medial supra-epicondylar ridge
Lateral epicondyle
Medial epicondyle
Capitulum
Trochlea
Head of radius
Coronoid process
Tuberosity of ulna
Tuberosity of radius
Anterior oblique line
Pronator tuberosity
Radius
Ulna
Pronator crest
Head of ulna
Styloid process of radius
Styloid process of ulna
Scaphoid
Lunate
Trapezium
Triquetrum
Pisiform
Trapezoid
Hamate
Capitate
1
2
3
4
5
Metacarpal bones
Proximal phalanx
Interphalangeal (IP) joint
Metacarpophalangeal (MCP) joint
Distal phalanx
Proximal
Middle
Distal
Phalanges
Proximal interphalangeal (PIP) joint
Distal interphalangeal (DIP) Joint
A
Anterior View
Brachioradialis
Extensor carpi radialis longus
Pronator teres
Common extensor origin
Common flexor origin
Flexor digitorum superficialis
Biceps brachii
Brachialis
Supinator
Pronator teres, unlar head
Flexor digitorum superficialis
Pronator teres
Flexor pollicis longus
Flexor digitorum profundus
Pronator quadratus
Pronator quadratus
Brachioradialis
Abductor pollicis longus
Flexor carpi ulnaris
Flexor carpi radialis
Extensor carpi ulnaris
Flexor pollicis longus
Flexor digitorum superficialis
Flexor digitorum profundus
B

6.61 BONES OF FOREARM AND HAND AND ATTACHMENTS OF FOREARM MUSCLES

A. Bony features. **B.** Sites of muscle attachments.

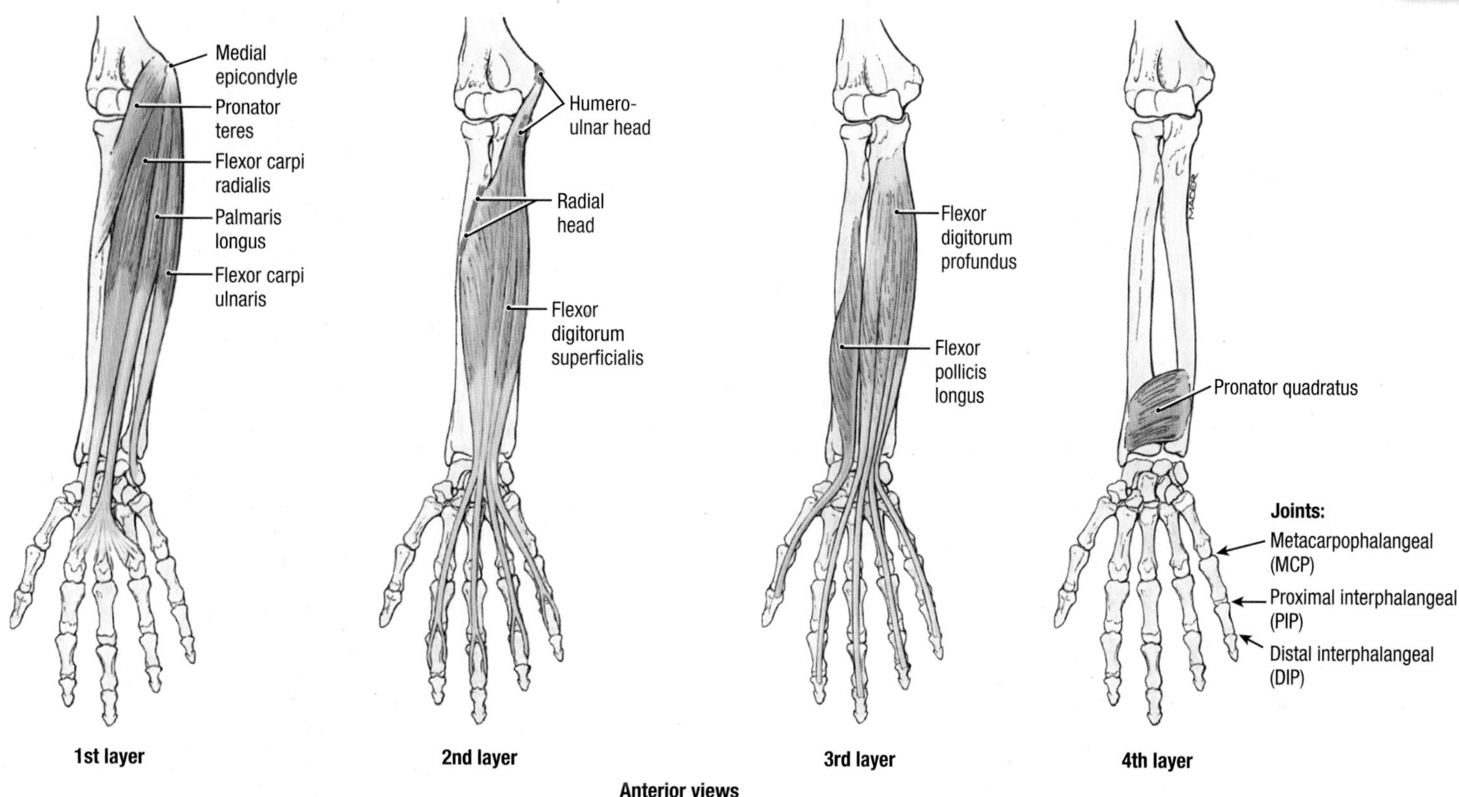
Medial epicondyle
Pronator teres
Flexor carpi radialis
Palmaris longus
Flexor carpi ulnaris
Humero-ulnar head
Radial head
Flexor digitorum superficialis
Flexor digitorum profundus
Flexor pollicis longus
Pronator quadratus
Joints:
Metacarpophalangeal (MCP)
Proximal interphalangeal (PIP)
Distal interphalangeal (DIP)
1st layer
2nd layer
3rd layer
4th layer
Anterior views

6.62 MUSCLES OF ANTERIOR ASPECT OF FOREARM

TABLE 6.12 MUSCLES OF ANTERIOR ASPECT OF FOREARM

Muscle	Proximal Attachment	Distal Attachment	Innervation	Main Actions
Pronator teres	Medial epicondyle of humerus and coronoid process of ulna	Middle of lateral surface of radius (pronator tuberosity)	Median nerve (C6–**C7**)	Pronates forearm and flexes elbow joint
Flexor carpi radialis	Medial epicondyle of humerus	Base of 2nd and 3rd metacarpals		Flexes and abducts wrist joint
Palmaris longus		Distal half of flexor retinaculum and palmar aponeurosis	Median nerve (C7–**C8**)	Flexes wrist joint and tightens palmar aponeurosis
Flexor carpi ulnaris	*Humeral head:* medial epicondyle of humerus; *Ulnar head:* olecranon and posterior border of ulna	Pisiform, hook of hamate, and 5th metacarpal	Ulnar nerve (C7–**C8**)	Flexes and adducts wrist joint
Flexor digitorum superficialis	*Humero-ulnar head:* medial epicondyle of humerus, ulnar collateral ligament, and coronoid process of ulna *Radial head:* superior half of anterior border of radius	Bodies of middle phalanges of medial four digits	Median nerve (C7, **C8**, and T1)	Flexes PIPs of medial four digits; acting more strongly, it flexes MCPs and wrist joint
Flexor digitorum profundus	Proximal three quarters of medial and anterior surfaces of ulna and interosseous membrane	Bases of distal phalanges of medial four digits	*Medial part:* ulnar nerve (**C8**–T1) *Lateral part:* median nerve (**C8**–T1)	Flexes DIPs of medial four digits; assists with flexion of wrist joint
Flexor pollicis longus	Anterior surface of radius and adjacent interosseous membrane	Base of distal phalanx of thumb	Anterior interosseous nerve from median (**C8**–T1)	Flexes IP joints of 1st digit (thumb) and assists flexion of wrist joint
Pronator quadratus	Distal fourth of anterior surface of ulna	Distal fourth of anterior surface of radius		Pronates forearm; deep fibers bind radius and ulna together

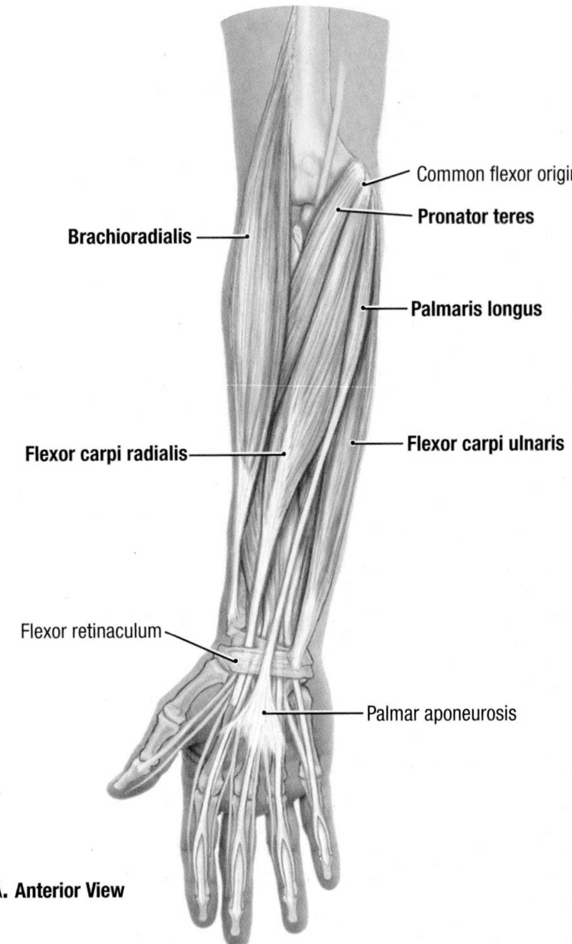
Common flexor origin
Pronator teres
Brachioradialis
Palmaris longus
Flexor carpi radialis
Flexor carpi ulnaris
Flexor retinaculum
Palmar aponeurosis

A. Anterior View

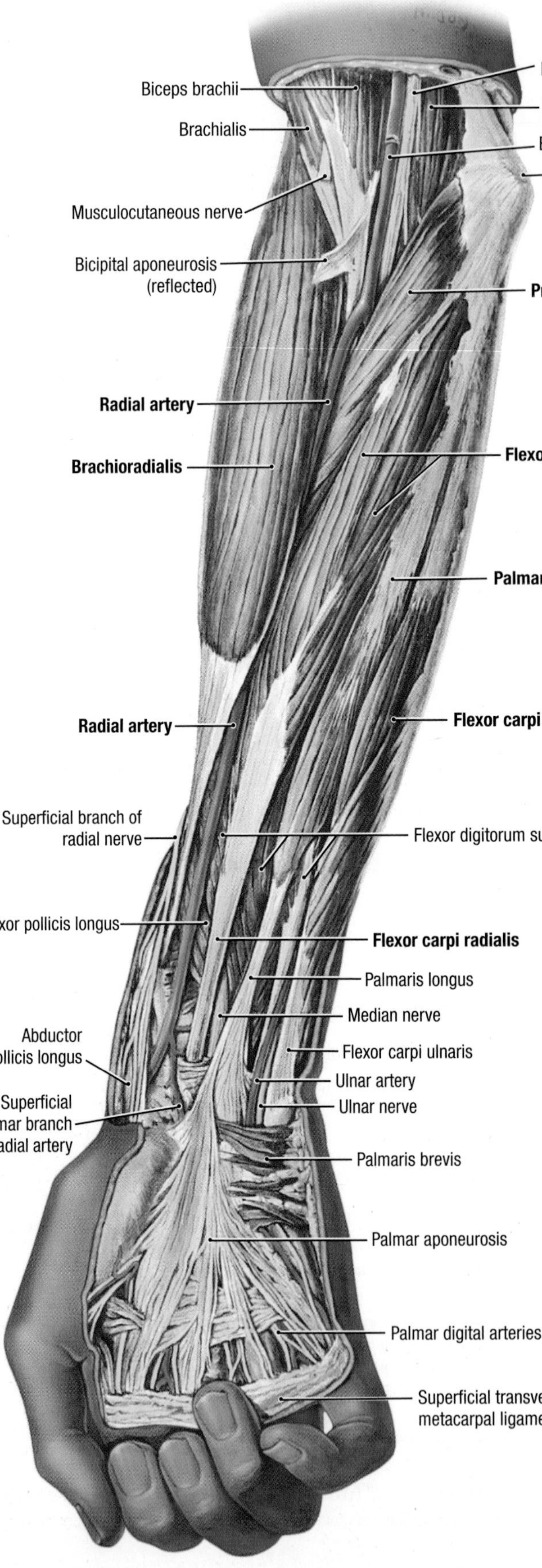

Biceps brachii
Median nerve
Brachialis
Brachialis
Brachial artery
Medial epicondyle of humerus (common flexor origin)
Musculocutaneous nerve
Bicipital aponeurosis (reflected)
Pronator teres
Radial artery
Flexor carpi radialis
Brachioradialis
Palmaris longus
Radial artery
Flexor carpi ulnaris
Superficial branch of radial nerve
Flexor digitorum superficialis
Flexor pollicis longus
Flexor carpi radialis
Palmaris longus
Median nerve
Abductor pollicis longus
Flexor carpi ulnaris
Ulnar artery
Superficial palmar branch of radial artery
Ulnar nerve
Palmaris brevis
Palmar aponeurosis
Palmar digital arteries and nerves
Superficial transverse metacarpal ligament

B. Anterior View

6.63 SUPERFICIAL MUSCLES OF FOREARM AND PALMAR APONEUROSIS

- At the elbow, the brachial artery lies between the biceps tendon and median nerve. It then bifurcates into the radial and ulnar arteries.
- At the wrist, the radial artery is lateral to the flexor carpi radialis tendon, and the ulnar artery is lateral to flexor carpi ulnaris tendon.
- In the forearm, the radial artery lies between the flexor and extensor compartments. The muscles lateral to the artery are supplied by the radial nerve, and those medial to it by the median and ulnar nerves; thus, no motor nerve crosses the radial artery.
- The brachioradialis muscle slightly overlaps the radial artery, which is otherwise superficial.
- The four superficial muscles all attach proximally to the medial epicondyle of the humerus (common flexor origin).
- The palmaris longus muscle, in this specimen, has an anomalous distal belly; this muscle usually has a small belly at the common flexor origin and a long tendon that is continued into the palm as the palmar aponeurosis. The palmaris longus is absent unilaterally or bilaterally in approximately 14% of limbs.

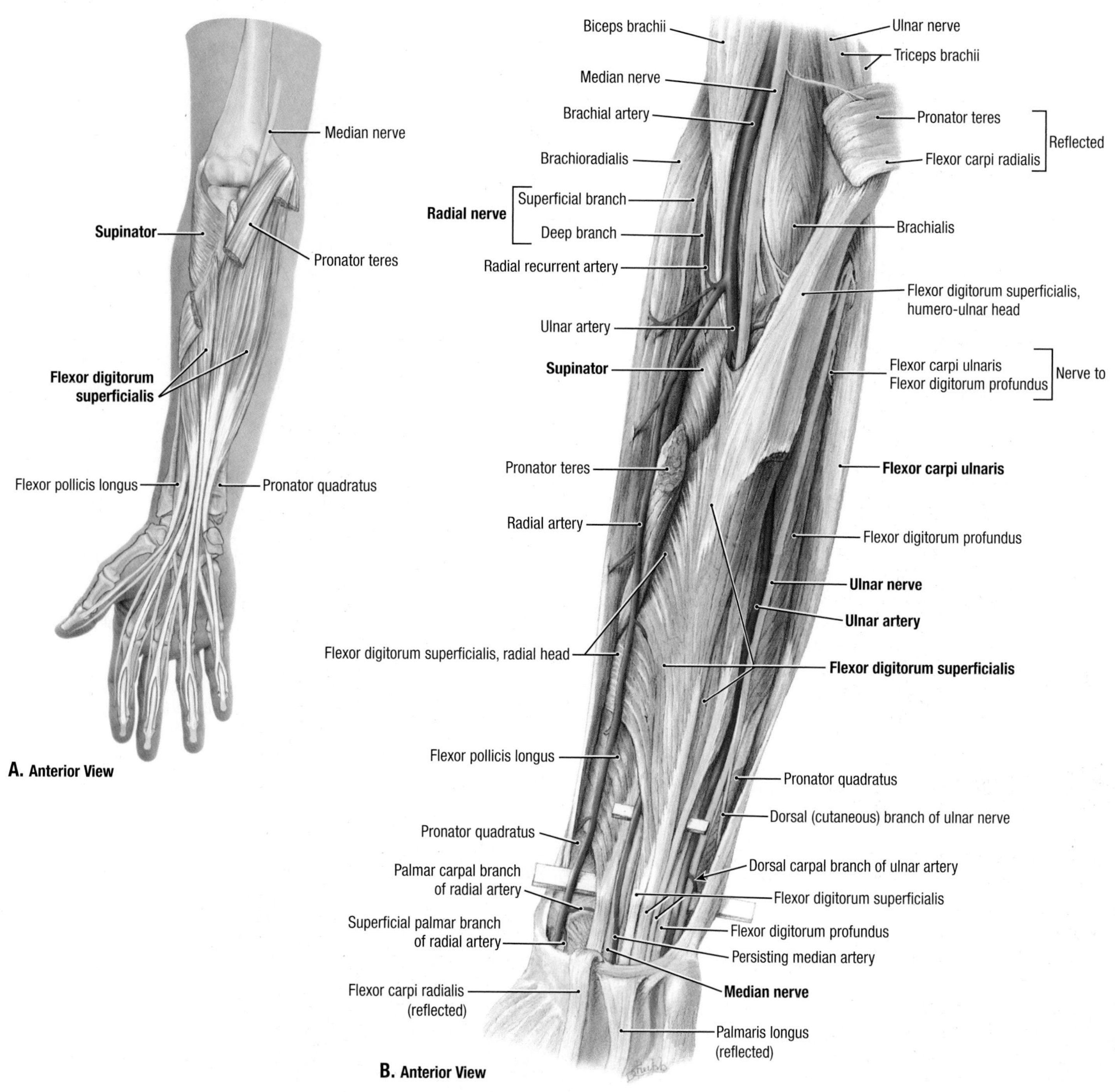
Median nerve
Supinator
Pronator teres
Flexor digitorum superficialis
Flexor pollicis longus
Pronator quadratus
A. Anterior View
Biceps brachii
Ulnar nerve
Triceps brachii
Median nerve
Brachial artery
Pronator teres
Reflected
Brachioradialis
Flexor carpi radialis
Radial nerve
Superficial branch
Deep branch
Brachialis
Radial recurrent artery
Flexor digitorum superficialis, humero-ulnar head
Ulnar artery
Supinator
Flexor carpi ulnaris
Flexor digitorum profundus
Nerve to
Pronator teres
Flexor carpi ulnaris
Radial artery
Flexor digitorum profundus
Ulnar nerve
Ulnar artery
Flexor digitorum superficialis, radial head
Flexor digitorum superficialis
Flexor pollicis longus
Pronator quadratus
Dorsal (cutaneous) branch of ulnar nerve
Pronator quadratus
Palmar carpal branch of radial artery
Dorsal carpal branch of ulnar artery
Flexor digitorum superficialis
Superficial palmar branch of radial artery
Flexor digitorum profundus
Persisting median artery
Flexor carpi radialis (reflected)
Median nerve
Palmaris longus (reflected)
B. Anterior View

6.64 FLEXOR DIGITORUM SUPERFICIALIS AND RELATED STRUCTURES

- The flexor digitorum superficialis muscle is attached proximally to the humerus, ulna, and radius.
- The ulnar artery passes obliquely posterior to the flexor digitorum superficialis; at the medial border of the muscle, the ulnar artery joins the ulnar nerve.
- The ulnar nerve lies between the flexor digitorum profundus and flexor carpi ulnaris.
- The median nerve descends vertically posterior to the flexor digitorum superficialis and appears distally at its lateral border.
- The median artery of this specimen is a variation resulting from persistence of an embryologic vessel that usually disappears.

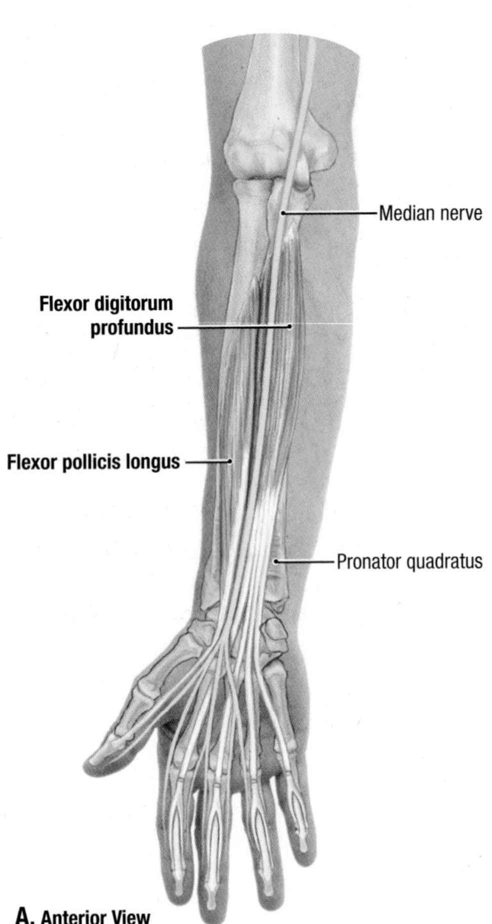
Median nerve
Flexor digitorum profundus
Flexor pollicis longus
Pronator quadratus

A. Anterior View

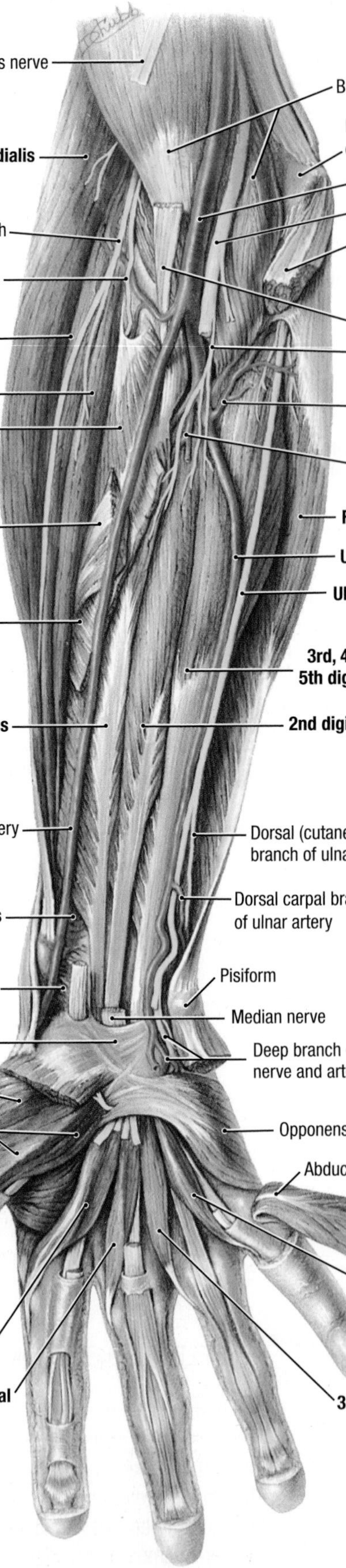

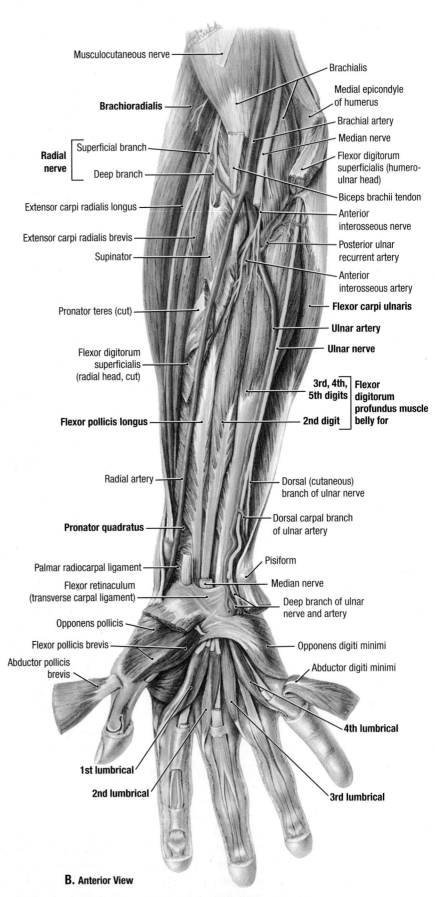

Musculocutaneous nerve
Brachialis
Medial epicondyle of humerus
Brachioradialis
Brachial artery
Median nerve
Radial nerve: Superficial branch; Deep branch
Flexor digitorum superficialis (humero-ulnar head)
Biceps brachii tendon
Extensor carpi radialis longus
Anterior interosseous nerve
Extensor carpi radialis brevis
Posterior ulnar recurrent artery
Supinator
Anterior interosseous artery
Flexor carpi ulnaris
Pronator teres (cut)
Ulnar artery
Ulnar nerve
Flexor digitorum superficialis (radial head, cut)
Flexor digitorum profundus muscle belly for: 3rd, 4th, 5th digits; 2nd digit
Flexor pollicis longus
Radial artery
Dorsal (cutaneous) branch of ulnar nerve
Dorsal carpal branch of ulnar artery
Pronator quadratus
Pisiform
Palmar radiocarpal ligament
Median nerve
Flexor retinaculum (transverse carpal ligament)
Deep branch of ulnar nerve and artery
Opponens pollicis
Flexor pollicis brevis
Opponens digiti minimi
Abductor pollicis brevis
Abductor digiti minimi
4th lumbrical
1st lumbrical
2nd lumbrical
3rd lumbrical

B. Anterior View

6.65 DEEP FLEXORS OF DIGITS AND RELATED STRUCTURES

- The ulnar nerve enters the forearm posterior to the medial epicondyle, then descends between the flexor digitorum profundus and flexor carpi ulnaris and is joined by the ulnar artery. At the wrist the ulnar nerve and artery pass anterior to the flexor retinaculum and lateral to the pisiform to enter the palm.
- At the elbow, the ulnar nerve supplies the flexor carpi ulnaris and the medial half of the flexor digitorum profundus muscles; proximal to the wrist, it gives off the dorsal (cutaneous) branch.
- The four lumbricals arise from the flexor digitorum profundus tendons.

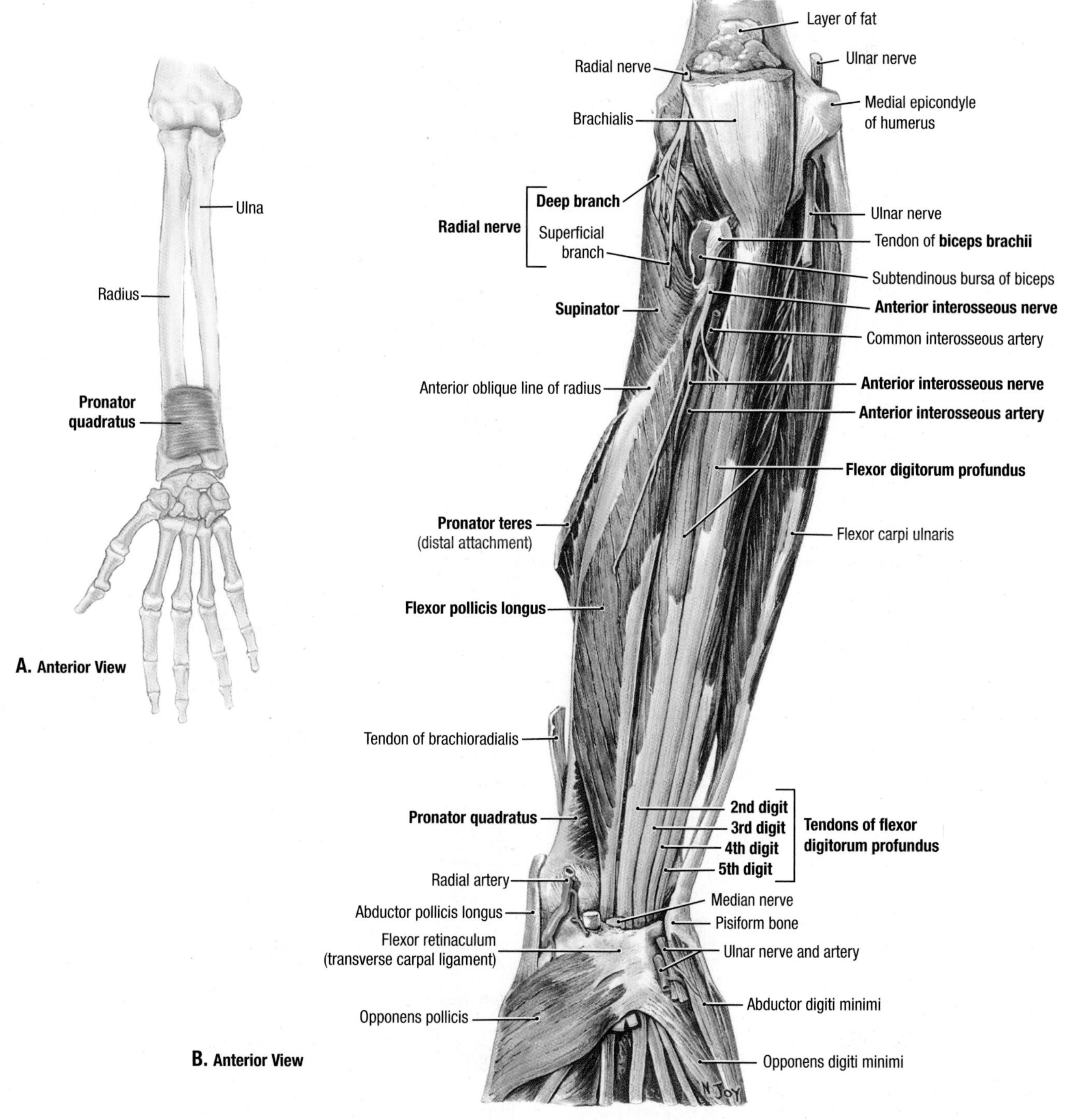
Ulna
Radius
Pronator quadratus
A. Anterior View
Layer of fat
Radial nerve
Ulnar nerve
Medial epicondyle of humerus
Brachialis
Radial nerve
Deep branch
Superficial branch
Ulnar nerve
Tendon of biceps brachii
Subtendinous bursa of biceps
Supinator
Anterior interosseous nerve
Common interosseous artery
Anterior oblique line of radius
Anterior interosseous nerve
Anterior interosseous artery
Flexor digitorum profundus
Pronator teres (distal attachment)
Flexor carpi ulnaris
Flexor pollicis longus
Tendon of brachioradialis
Pronator quadratus
2nd digit
3rd digit
4th digit
5th digit
Tendons of flexor digitorum profundus
Radial artery
Median nerve
Abductor pollicis longus
Pisiform bone
Flexor retinaculum (transverse carpal ligament)
Ulnar nerve and artery
Abductor digiti minimi
Opponens pollicis
Opponens digiti minimi
B. Anterior View

6.66 DEEP FLEXORS OF DIGITS AND SUPINATOR

- The five tendons of the deep digital flexors (flexor pollicis longus and flexor digitorum profundus) lie side by side as they enter the carpal tunnel.
- The deep branch of the radial nerve pierces and innervates the supinator muscle.
- The anterior interosseous nerve and artery pass deeply between the flexor pollicis longus and flexor digitorum profundus muscles to lie on the interosseous membrane.

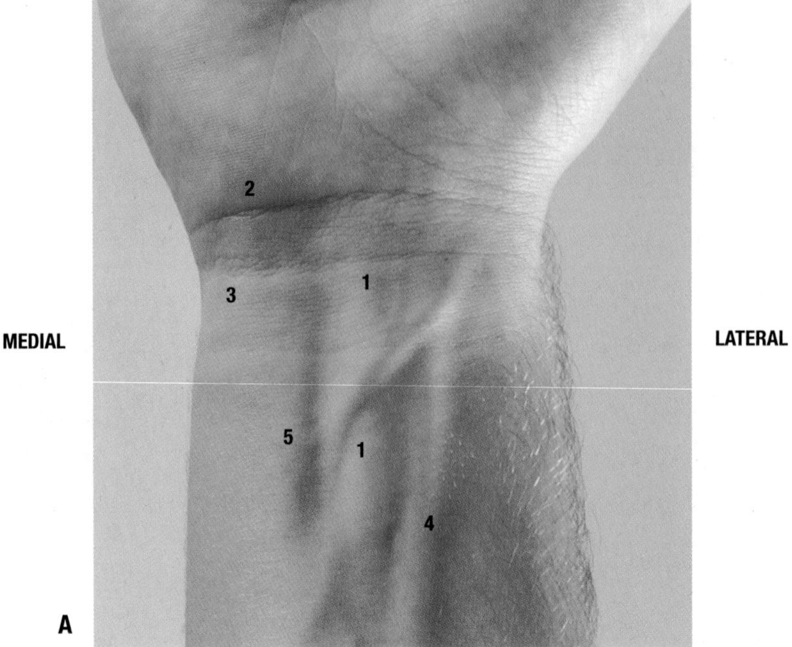

MEDIAL
LATERAL
2
3
1
5
1
4
A

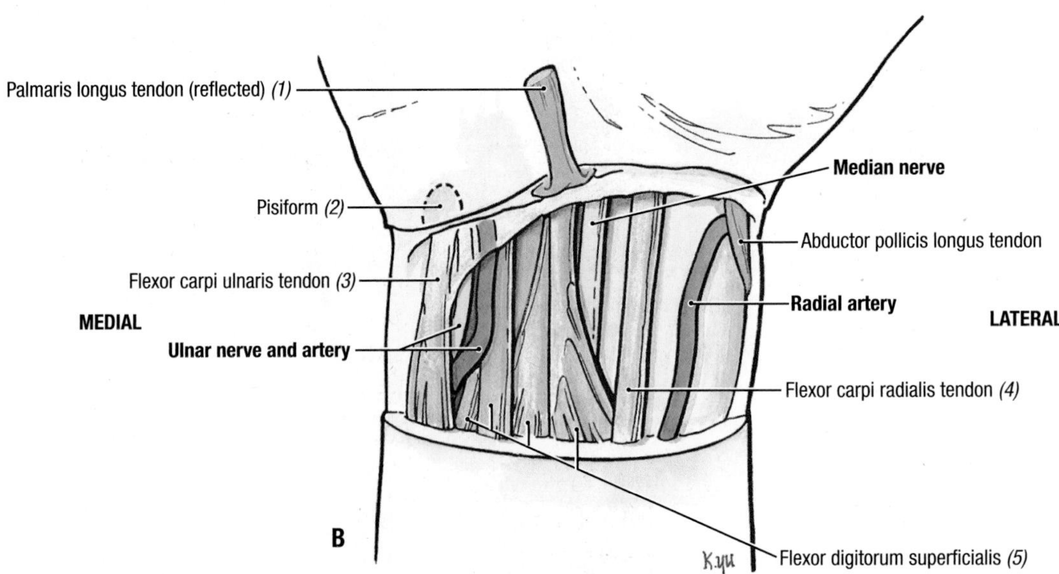

Palmaris longus tendon (reflected) (1)
Pisiform (2)
Flexor carpi ulnaris tendon (3)
MEDIAL
Ulnar nerve and artery
Median nerve
Abductor pollicis longus tendon
Radial artery
LATERAL
Flexor carpi radialis tendon (4)
Flexor digitorum superficialis (5)
B

Anterior Views of Right Hand and Wrist

6.67 STRUCTURES OF ANTERIOR ASPECT OF WRIST

A. Surface anatomy. **B.** Schematic illustration. **C.** Dissection.

- The distal skin incision follows the transverse skin crease at the wrist. The incision crosses the pisiform, to which the flexor carpi ulnaris muscle attaches, and the tubercle of the scaphoid, to which the tendon of flexor carpi radialis muscle is a guide.
- The palmaris longus tendon bisects the transverse skin crease; deep to the lateral margin of the tendon is the median nerve.
- The radial artery passes deep to the tendon of the abductor pollicis longus muscle.
- The flexor digitorum superficialis tendons to the 3rd and 4th digits become anterior to those of the 2nd and 5th digits.
- The recurrent branch of the median nerve to the thenar muscles lies within a circle whose center is 2.5 to 4 cm distal to the tubercle of the scaphoid.

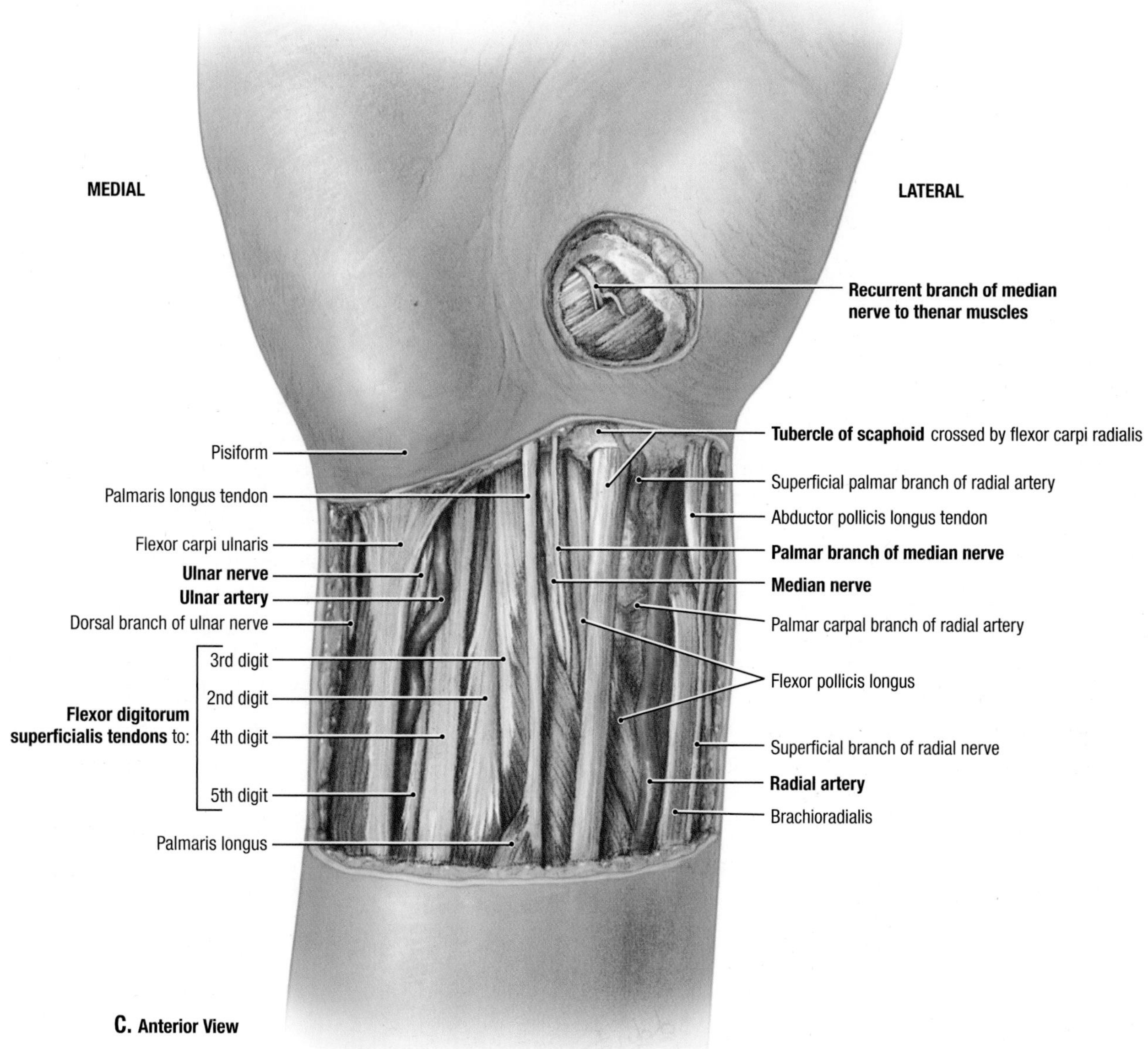
MEDIAL
LATERAL
Recurrent branch of median nerve to thenar muscles
Pisiform
Palmaris longus tendon
Flexor carpi ulnaris
Ulnar nerve
Ulnar artery
Dorsal branch of ulnar nerve
3rd digit
2nd digit
Flexor digitorum superficialis tendons to:
4th digit
5th digit
Palmaris longus
Tubercle of scaphoid crossed by flexor carpi radialis
Superficial palmar branch of radial artery
Abductor pollicis longus tendon
Palmar branch of median nerve
Median nerve
Palmar carpal branch of radial artery
Flexor pollicis longus
Superficial branch of radial nerve
Radial artery
Brachioradialis

C. **Anterior View**

6.67 STRUCTURES OF ANTERIOR ASPECT OF WRIST *(CONTINUED)*

Lesions of the median nerve usually occur in two places: the forearm and wrist. The most common site is where the nerve passes though the carpal tunnel. Lacerations of the wrist often cause median nerve injury because this nerve is relatively close to the surface. This results in paralysis of the thenar muscles and the first two lumbricals. Hence opposition of the thumb is not possible and fine control movements of the 2nd and 3rd digits are impaired. Sensation is also lost over the thumb and adjacent two and a half digits.

Median nerve injury resulting from a perforating wound in the elbow region results in loss of flexion of the proximal and distal interphalangeal joints of the 2nd and 3rd digits. The ability to flex the metacarpophalangeal joints of these digits is also affected because digital branches of the median nerve supply the 1st and 2nd lumbricals. The palmar cutaneous branch of the median nerve does not traverse the carpal tunnel. It supplies the skin of the central palm, which remains sensitive in carpal tunnel syndrome.

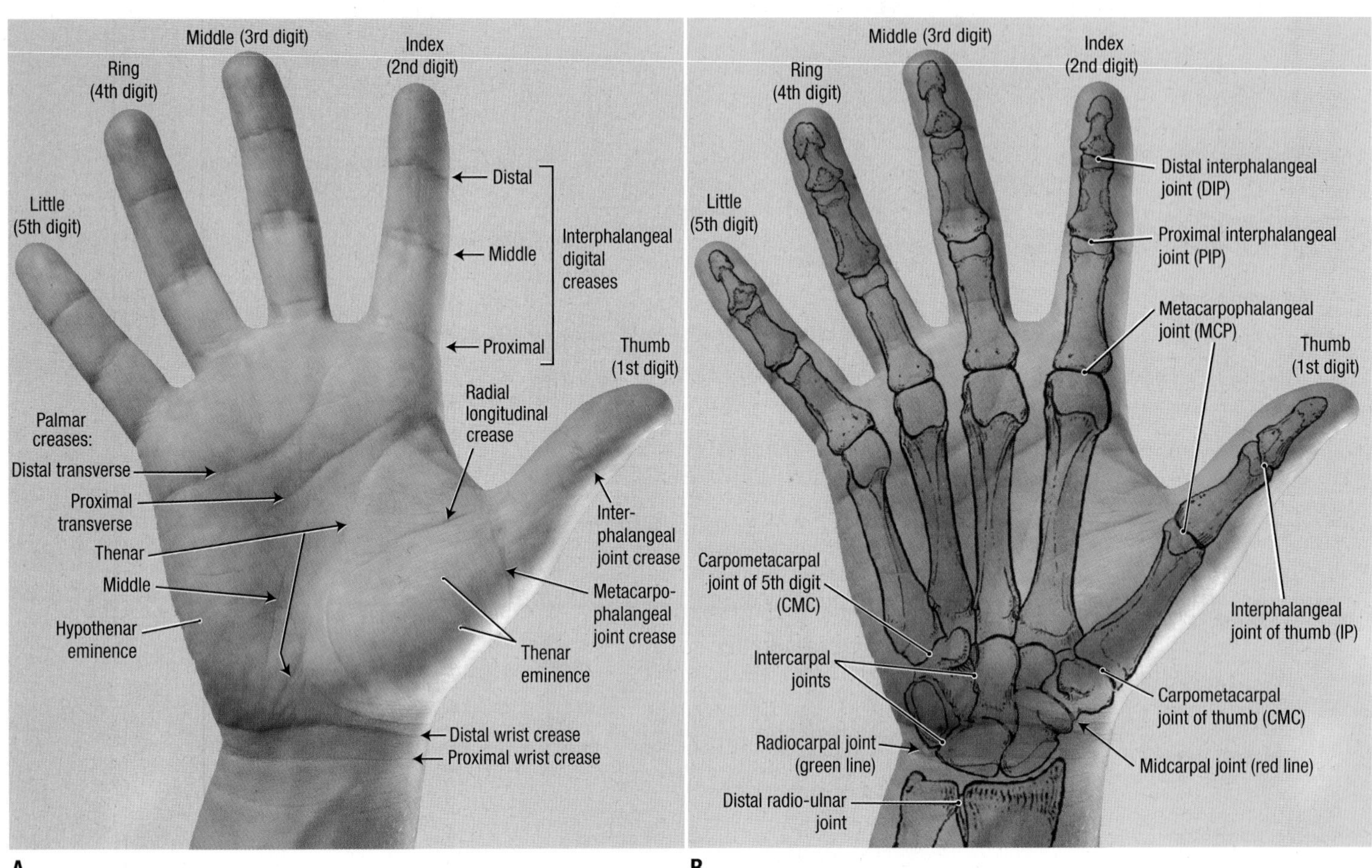

Middle (3rd digit)
Ring (4th digit)
Index (2nd digit)
Little (5th digit)
Distal
Middle
Proximal
Interphalangeal digital creases
Thumb (1st digit)
Radial longitudinal crease
Palmar creases:
Distal transverse
Proximal transverse
Thenar
Middle
Hypothenar eminence
Inter-phalangeal joint crease
Metacarpo-phalangeal joint crease
Thenar eminence
Distal wrist crease
Proximal wrist crease
A
Middle (3rd digit)
Ring (4th digit)
Index (2nd digit)
Little (5th digit)
Distal interphalangeal joint (DIP)
Proximal interphalangeal joint (PIP)
Metacarpophalangeal joint (MCP)
Thumb (1st digit)
Carpometacarpal joint of 5th digit (CMC)
Interphalangeal joint of thumb (IP)
Intercarpal joints
Carpometacarpal joint of thumb (CMC)
Radiocarpal joint (green line)
Midcarpal joint (red line)
Distal radio-ulnar joint
B

Anterior Views

6.68 SURFACE ANATOMY OF SKELETON OF HAND AND WRIST

A. Skin creases of wrist and hand. **B.** Surface projection of joints of wrist and hand. Note relationship of bones and joints to features of the hand.

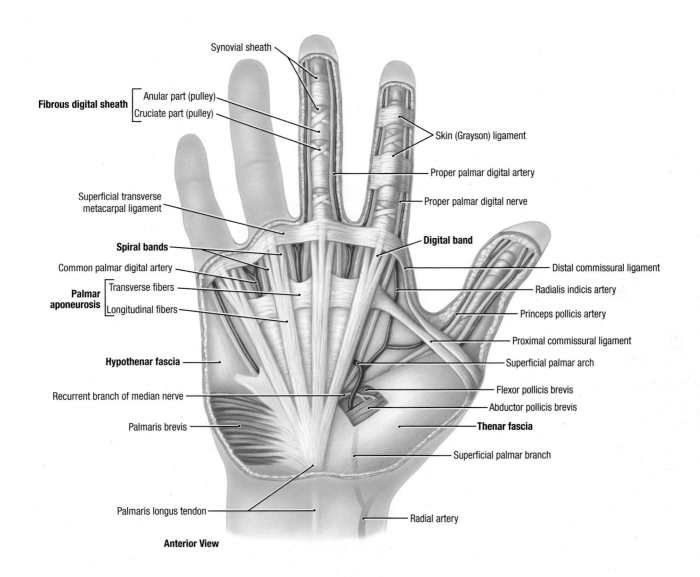

Synovial sheath
Fibrous digital sheath
Anular part (pulley)
Cruciate part (pulley)
Skin (Grayson) ligament
Proper palmar digital artery
Superficial transverse metacarpal ligament
Proper palmar digital nerve
Digital band
Spiral bands
Common palmar digital artery
Distal commissural ligament
Palmar aponeurosis
Transverse fibers
Longitudinal fibers
Radialis indicis artery
Princeps pollicis artery
Proximal commissural ligament
Hypothenar fascia
Superficial palmar arch
Recurrent branch of median nerve
Flexor pollicis brevis
Abductor pollicis brevis
Palmaris brevis
Thenar fascia
Superficial palmar branch
Palmaris longus tendon
Radial artery
Anterior View

6.69 PALMAR (DEEP) FASCIA: PALMAR APONEUROSIS, THENAR AND HYPOTHENAR FASCIA

A. Anterior view.

- The palmar fascia is thin over the thenar and hypothenar eminences, but thick centrally, where it forms the palmar aponeurosis, and in the digits, where it forms the fibrous digital sheaths.
- At the distal end (base) of the palmar aponeurosis, four bundles of digital and spiral bands continue to the bases and fibrous digital sheaths of digits 2 to 5.

B. Dupuytren contracture is a disease of the palmar fascia resulting in progressive shortening, thickening, and fibrosis of the palmar fascia and palmar aponeurosis. The fibrous degeneration of the longitudinal digital bands of the aponeurosis on the medial side of the hand pulls the 4th and 5th fingers into partial flexion at the metacarpophalangeal and proximal interphalangeal joints. The contracture is frequently bilateral. Treatment of Dupuytren contracture usually involves surgical excision of all fibrotic parts of the palmar fascia to free the fingers.

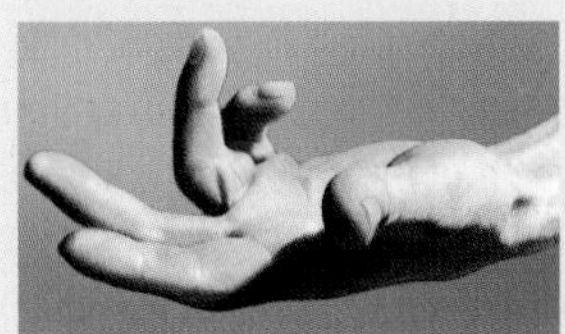

B. Dupuytren contracture

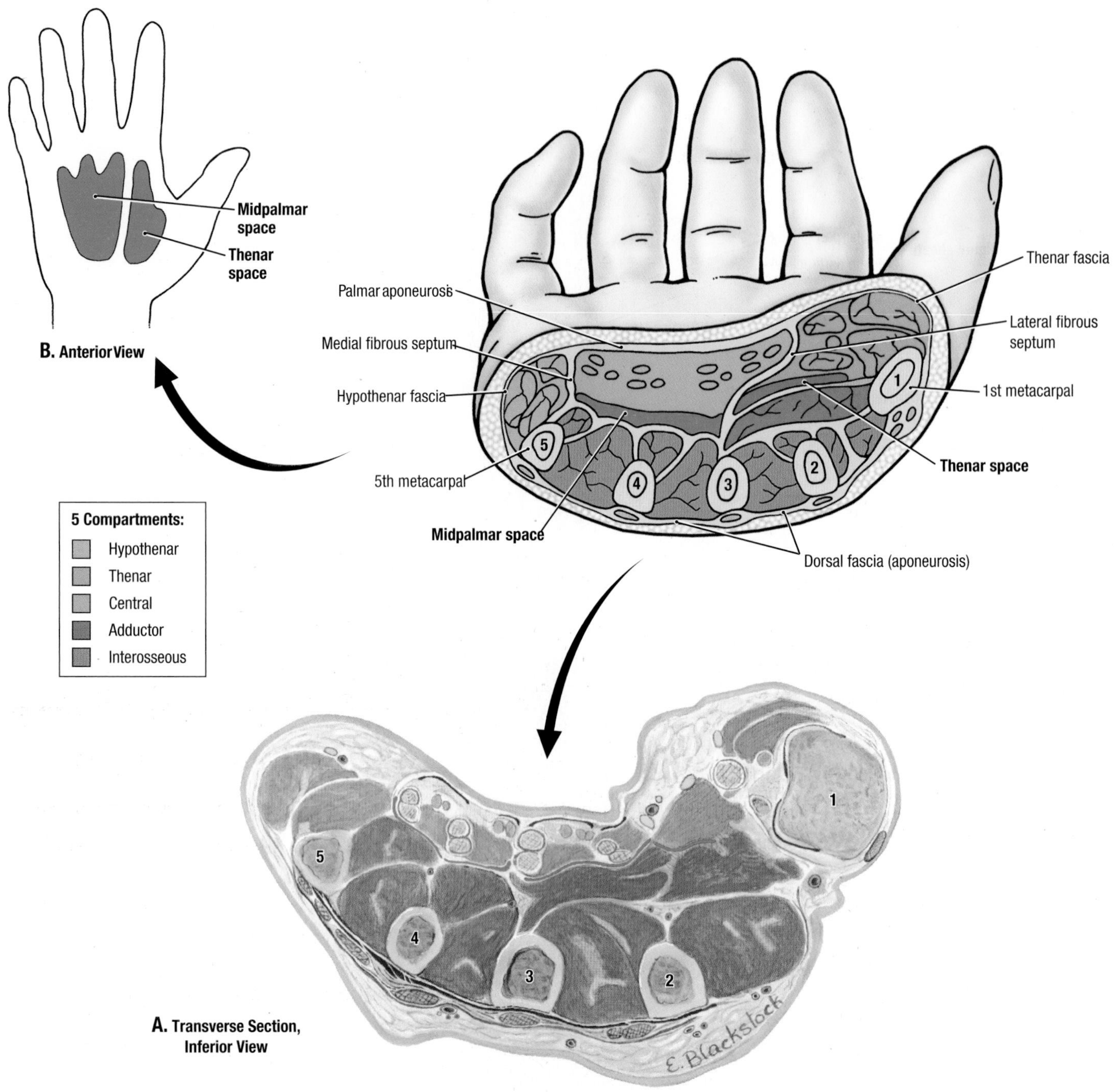

Midpalmar space
Thenar space
B. Anterior View
Palmar aponeurosis
Medial fibrous septum
Hypothenar fascia
5th metacarpal
Midpalmar space
Thenar fascia
Lateral fibrous septum
1st metacarpal
Thenar space
Dorsal fascia (aponeurosis)
5 Compartments:
Hypothenar
Thenar
Central
Adductor
Interosseous
1
2
3
4
5
A. Transverse Section, Inferior View
E. Blackstock

6.70 SYNOVIAL CAPSULE OF ELBOW JOINT AND ANULAR LIGAMENT

A. Transverse section through the middle of the palm showing the fascial compartments for the musculotendinous structures of the hand. **B.** Potential fascial spaces of palm.

- The potential midpalmar space lies posterior to the central compartment, is bounded medially by the hypothenar compartment, and is related distally to the synovial sheath of the 3rd, 4th, and 5th digits.
- The potential thenar space lies posterior to the thenar compartment and is related distally to the synovial sheath of the index finger.
- The potential midpalmar and thenar spaces are separated by a septum that passes from the palmar aponeurosis to the third metacarpal.

Because the palmar fascia is thick and strong, **swellings resulting from hand infections** usually appear on the dorsum of the hand where the fascia is thinner. The potential fascial spaces of the palm are important because they may become infected. The fascial spaces determine the extent and direction of the spread of pus formed in the infected areas. Depending on the site of infection, pus will accumulate in the thenar, hypothenar, or adductor compartments. Antibiotic therapy has made infections that spread beyond one of these fascial compartments rare, but an untreated infection can spread proximally through the carpal tunnel into the forearm anterior to the pronator quadratus and its fascia.

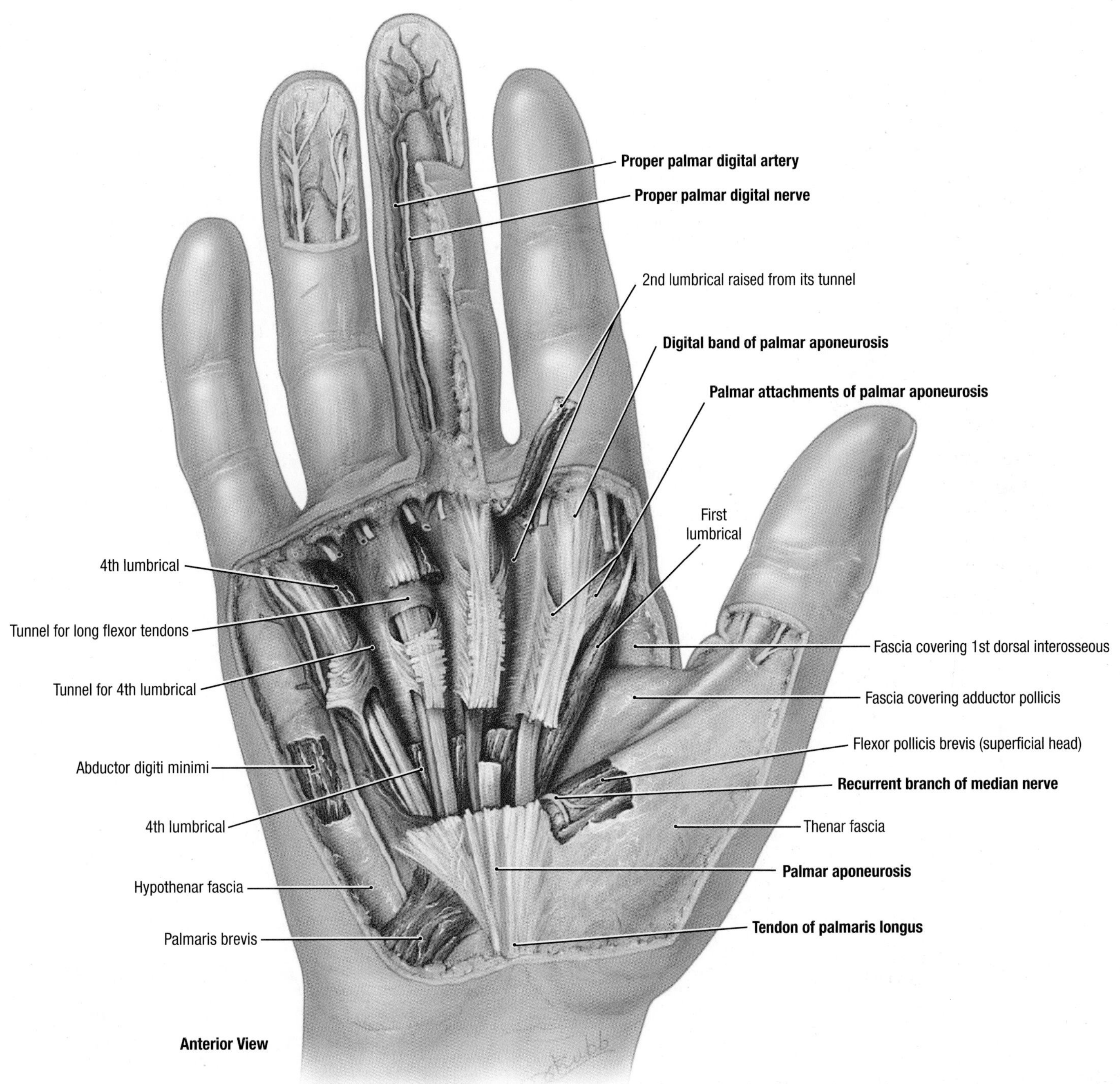
Proper palmar digital artery
Proper palmar digital nerve
2nd lumbrical raised from its tunnel
Digital band of palmar aponeurosis
Palmar attachments of palmar aponeurosis
First lumbrical
4th lumbrical
Tunnel for long flexor tendons
Tunnel for 4th lumbrical
Fascia covering 1st dorsal interosseous
Fascia covering adductor pollicis
Flexor pollicis brevis (superficial head)
Abductor digiti minimi
Recurrent branch of median nerve
4th lumbrical
Thenar fascia
Hypothenar fascia
Palmar aponeurosis
Palmaris brevis
Tendon of palmaris longus
Anterior View

6.71 PALMAR APONEUROSIS

- From the palmar aponeurosis, four longitudinal digital bands enter the fingers; the other fibers form extensive fibro-areolar septa that pass posteriorly to the palmar ligaments (see Fig. 6.78) and, more proximally, to the fascia covering the interossei. Thus, two sets of tunnels exist in the distal half of the palm: (1) tunnels for long flexor tendons and (2) tunnels for lumbricals, digital vessels, and digital nerves.
- In the dissected middle finger, note the absence of fat deep to the skin creases of the fingers.

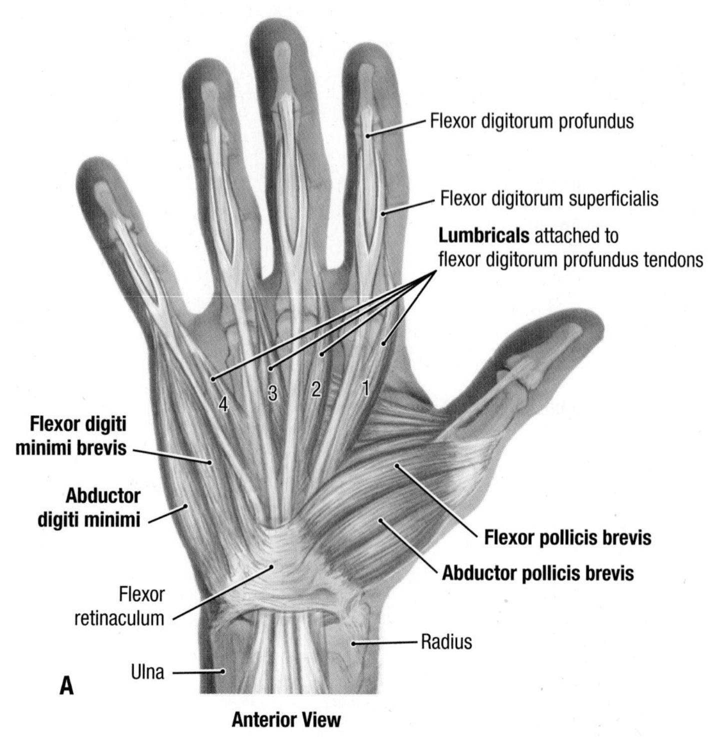
Flexor digitorum profundus
Flexor digitorum superficialis
Lumbricals attached to flexor digitorum profundus tendons
4
3
2
1
Flexor digiti minimi brevis
Abductor digiti minimi
Flexor pollicis brevis
Abductor pollicis brevis
Flexor retinaculum
Radius
Ulna
A
Anterior View

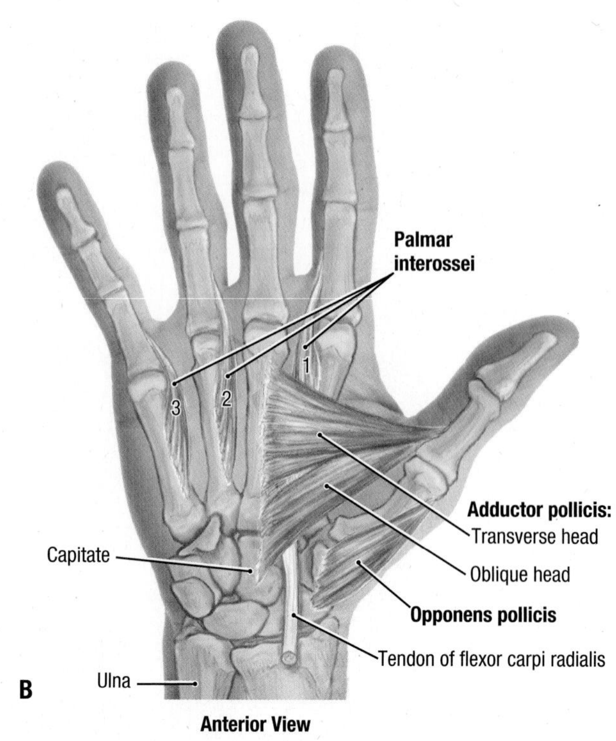
Palmar interossei
3
2
1
Adductor pollicis:
Transverse head
Oblique head
Capitate
Opponens pollicis
Tendon of flexor carpi radialis
Ulna
B
Anterior View

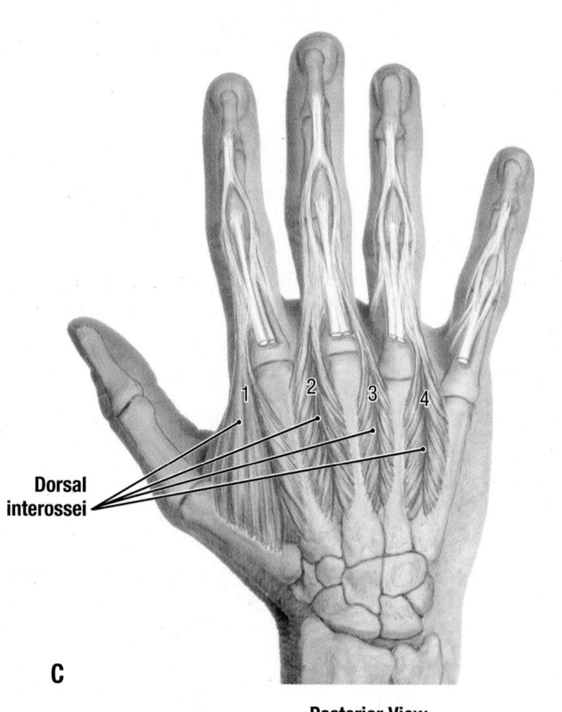
1
2
3
4
Dorsal interossei
C
Posterior View

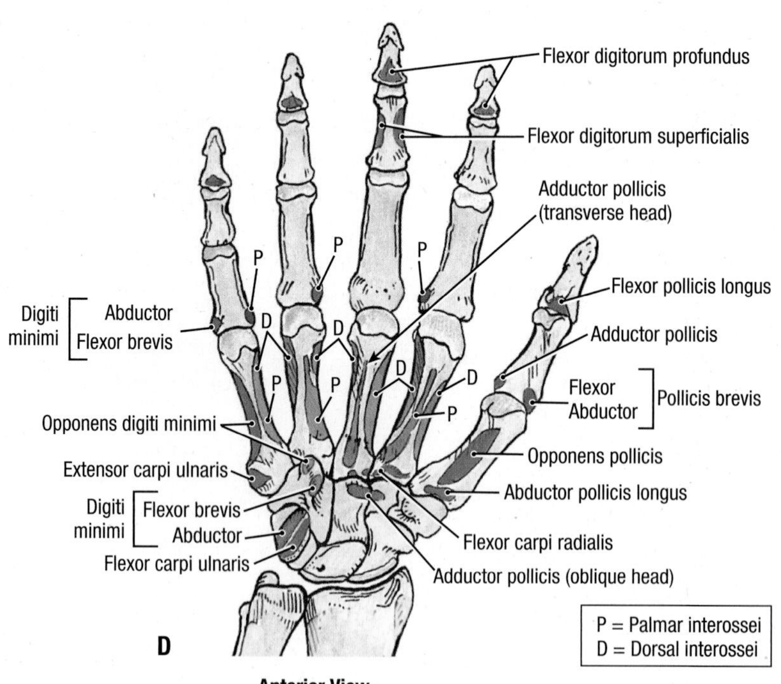
Flexor digitorum profundus
Flexor digitorum superficialis
Adductor pollicis (transverse head)
Flexor pollicis longus
Adductor pollicis
Digiti minimi
Abductor
Flexor brevis
Flexor
Abductor
Pollicis brevis
Opponens digiti minimi
Opponens pollicis
Extensor carpi ulnaris
Abductor pollicis longus
Digiti minimi
Flexor brevis
Abductor
Flexor carpi radialis
Flexor carpi ulnaris
Adductor pollicis (oblique head)
P = Palmar interossei
D = Dorsal interossei
D
Anterior View

6.72 MUSCULAR LAYERS OF PALM

A. Lumbricals. **B.** Adductor pollicis. **C.** Dorsal (*D*) and palmar (*P*) interossei. **D.** Bony attachments.

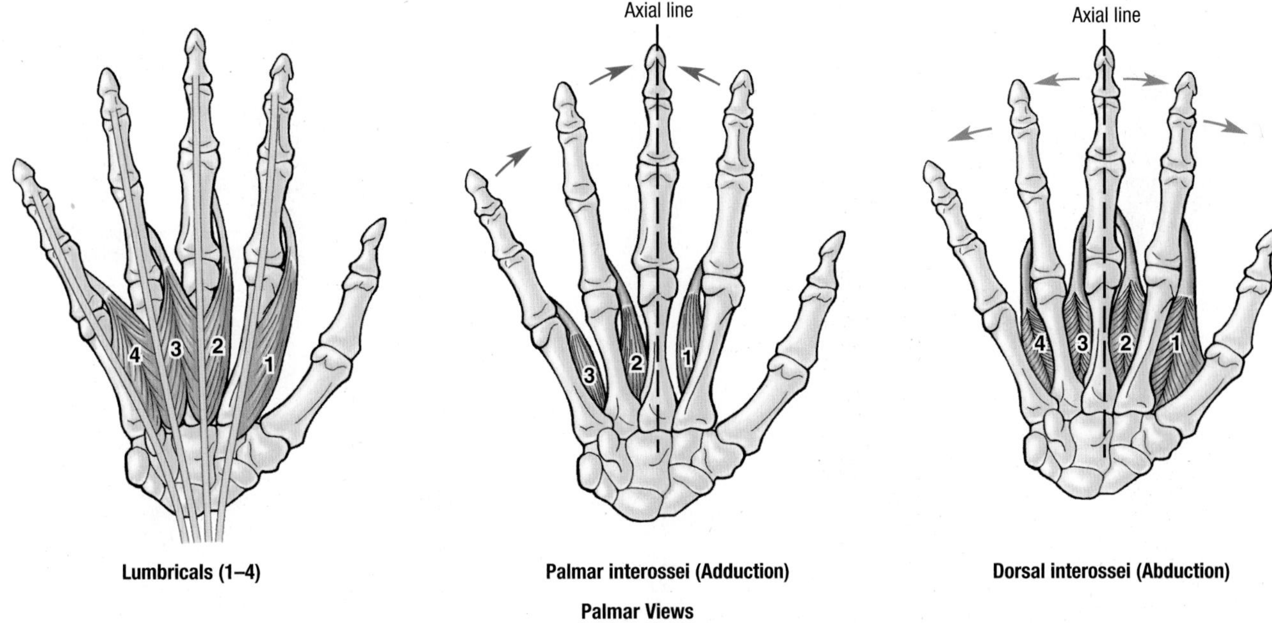
Axial line
Axial line
4
3
2
1
3
2
1
4
3
2
1
Lumbricals (1–4)
Palmar interossei (Adduction)
Dorsal interossei (Abduction)
Palmar Views

6.73 LUMBRICALS AND INTEROSSEI

TABLE 6.13 MUSCLES OF HAND

Muscle	Proximal Attachment	Distal Attachment	Innervation	Main Actions
Abductor pollicis brevis	Flexor retinaculum and tubercles of scaphoid and trapezium	Lateral side of base of proximal phalanx of thumb	Recurrent branch of median nerve (**C8** and T1)	Abducts thumb and helps oppose it
Flexor pollicis brevis	Flexor retinaculum (transverse carpal ligament) and tubercle of trapezium			Flexes thumb
Opponens pollicis		Lateral side of first metacarpal		Opposes thumb toward center of palm and rotates it medially
Adductor pollicis	*Oblique head:* bases of second and third metacarpals, capitate, and adjacent carpal bones *Transverse head:* anterior surface of shaft of third metacarpal	Medial side of base of proximal phalanx of thumb	Deep branch of ulnar nerve (C8 and **T1**)	Adducts thumb toward lateral border of palm
Abductor digiti minimi	Pisiform	Medial side of base of proximal phalanx of digit 5	Deep branch of ulnar nerve (C8 and T1)	Abducts digit 5, assists in flexion of its PIP joint
Flexor digiti minimi brevis	Hook of hamate and flexor retinaculum (transverse carpal ligament)	Medial border of fifth metacarpal		Flexes PIP joint of digit 5
Opponens digiti minimi				Draws fifth metacarpal anteriorly and rotates it, bringing digit 5 into opposition with thumb
Lumbricals 1 and 2	Lateral two tendons of flexor digitorum profundus	Lateral sides of extensor expansions of digits 2–5	Median nerve (C8 and **T1**)	Flex MCP joints and extend IP joints of digits 2–5
Lumbricals 3 and 4	Medial three tendons of flexor digitorum profundus		Deep branch of ulnar nerve (C8 and **T1**)	
Dorsal interossei 1–4	Adjacent sides of two metacarpals	Extensor expansions and bases of proximal phalanges of digits 2–4		Abduct 2–4 MCP joints; act with lumbricals to flex MCP and extend IP joints
Palmar interossei 1–3	Palmar surfaces of second, fourth, and fifth metacarpals	Extensor expansions of digits and bases of proximal phalanges of digits 2, 4, and 5		Adduct 2, 4, and 5 MCP joints; act with lumbricals to flex MCP and extend IP joints

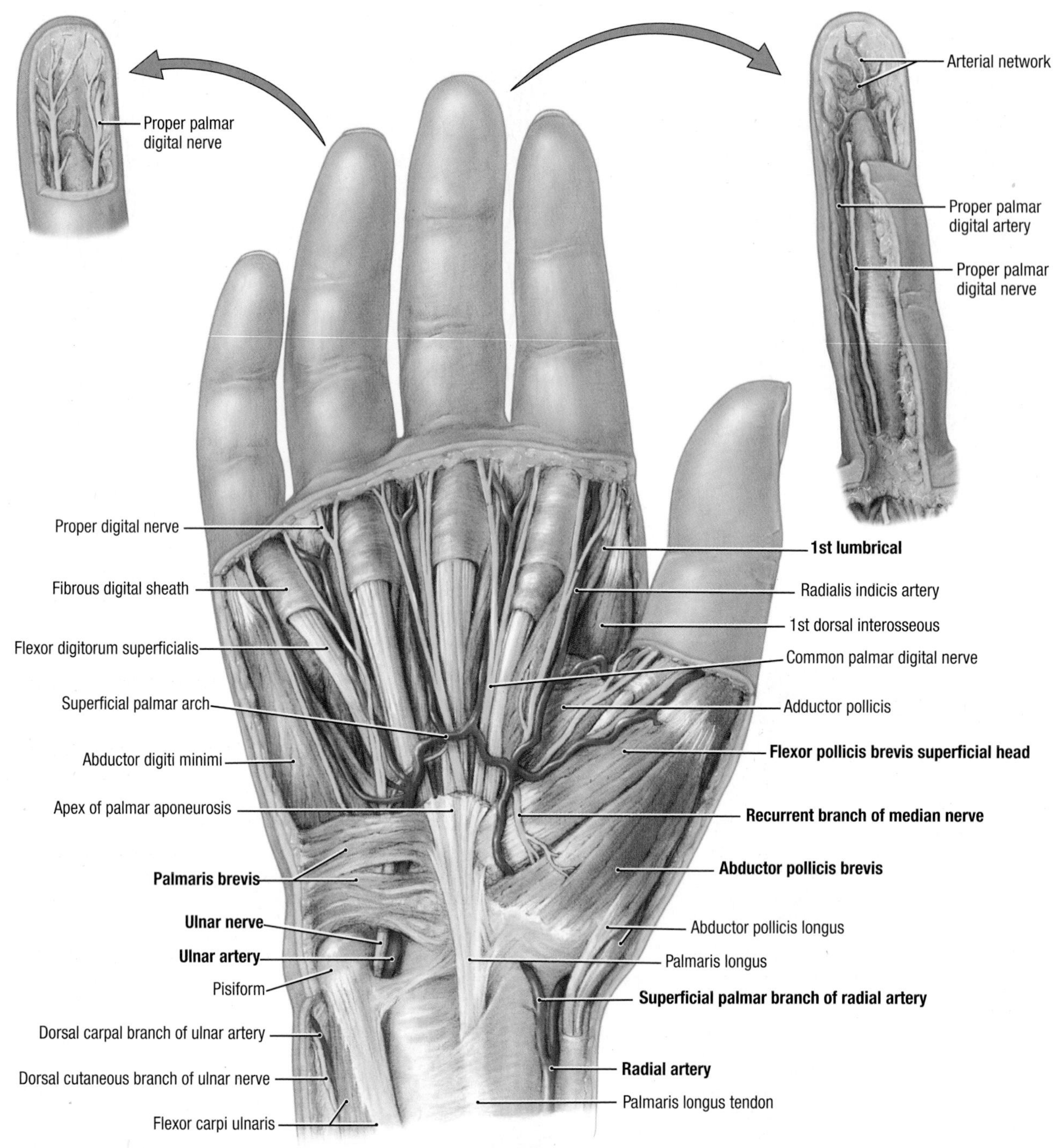

Proper palmar digital nerve
Arterial network
Proper palmar digital artery
Proper palmar digital nerve
Proper digital nerve
Fibrous digital sheath
Flexor digitorum superficialis
Superficial palmar arch
Abductor digiti minimi
Apex of palmar aponeurosis
Palmaris brevis
Ulnar nerve
Ulnar artery
Pisiform
Dorsal carpal branch of ulnar artery
Dorsal cutaneous branch of ulnar nerve
Flexor carpi ulnaris
1st lumbrical
Radialis indicis artery
1st dorsal interosseous
Common palmar digital nerve
Adductor pollicis
Flexor pollicis brevis superficial head
Recurrent branch of median nerve
Abductor pollicis brevis
Abductor pollicis longus
Palmaris longus
Superficial palmar branch of radial artery
Radial artery
Palmaris longus tendon

A. Anterior View

6.74 SUPERFICIAL DISSECTION OF PALM, ULNAR, AND MEDIAN NERVES

A. Superficial palmar arch and digital nerves and vessels.

- The skin, superficial fascia, palmar aponeurosis, and thenar and hypothenar fasciae have been removed.
- The superficial palmar arch is formed by the ulnar artery and completed by the superficial palmar branch of the radial artery.
- The four lumbricals lie posterior to the digital vessels and nerves. The lumbricals arise from the lateral sides of the flexor digitorum profundus tendons and are inserted into the lateral sides of the dorsal expansions of the corresponding digits. The medial two lumbricals are bipennate and also arise from the medial sides of adjacent flexor digitorum profundus tendons.
- In the digits, a proper palmar digital artery and nerve lie on each side of the fibrous digital sheath.
- Note the canal (Guyon) through which the ulnar vessels and nerve pass medial to the pisiform.

Laceration of palmar (arterial) arches. Bleeding is usually profuse when the palmar (arterial) arches are lacerated. It may not be sufficient to ligate (tie off) only one forearm artery when the arches are lacerated, because these vessels usually have numerous communications in the forearm and hand and thus bleed from both ends.

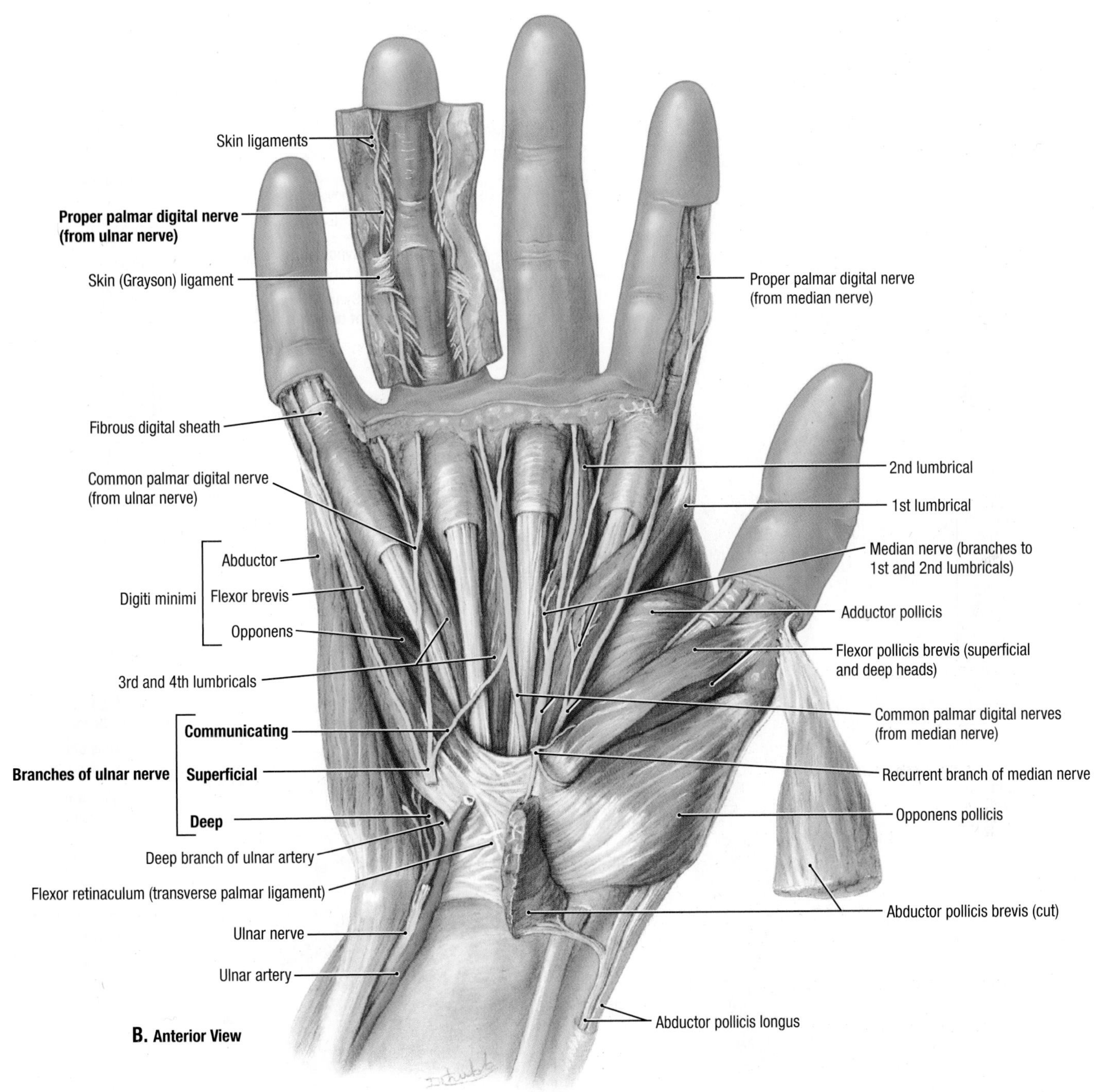
Skin ligaments
Proper palmar digital nerve (from ulnar nerve)
Skin (Grayson) ligament
Proper palmar digital nerve (from median nerve)
Fibrous digital sheath
Common palmar digital nerve (from ulnar nerve)
2nd lumbrical
1st lumbrical
Digiti minimi
Abductor
Flexor brevis
Opponens
Median nerve (branches to 1st and 2nd lumbricals)
Adductor pollicis
Flexor pollicis brevis (superficial and deep heads)
3rd and 4th lumbricals
Common palmar digital nerves (from median nerve)
Branches of ulnar nerve
Communicating
Superficial
Deep
Recurrent branch of median nerve
Opponens pollicis
Deep branch of ulnar artery
Flexor retinaculum (transverse palmar ligament)
Abductor pollicis brevis (cut)
Ulnar nerve
Ulnar artery
Abductor pollicis longus

B. Anterior View

6.74 SUPERFICIAL DISSECTION OF PALM, ULNAR, AND MEDIAN NERVES *(CONTINUED)*

B. Ulnar and median nerves.

Carpal tunnel syndrome results from any lesion that significantly reduces the size of the carpal tunnel or, more commonly, increases the size of some of the structures (or their coverings) that pass though it (e.g., inflammation of the synovial sheaths). The median nerve is the most sensitive structure in the carpal tunnel. The median nerve has two terminal sensory branches that supply the skin of the hand; hence paresthesia (tingling), hypothesia (diminished sensation), or anesthesia (absence of tactile sensation) may occur in the lateral three and a half digits. Recall, however, that the palmar cutaneous branch of the median nerve arises proximal to and does not pass through the carpal tunnel; thus sensation in the central palm remains unaffected. This nerve also has one terminal motor branch, the recurrent branch, which innervates the three thenar muscles. Wasting of the thenar eminence and progressive loss of coordination and strength in the thumb may occur. To relieve the compression and resulting symptoms, partial or complete surgical division of the flexor retinaculum, a procedure called **carpal tunnel release,** may be necessary. The incision for carpal tunnel release is made toward the medial side of the wrist and flexor retinaculum to avoid possible injury to the recurrent branch of the median nerve.

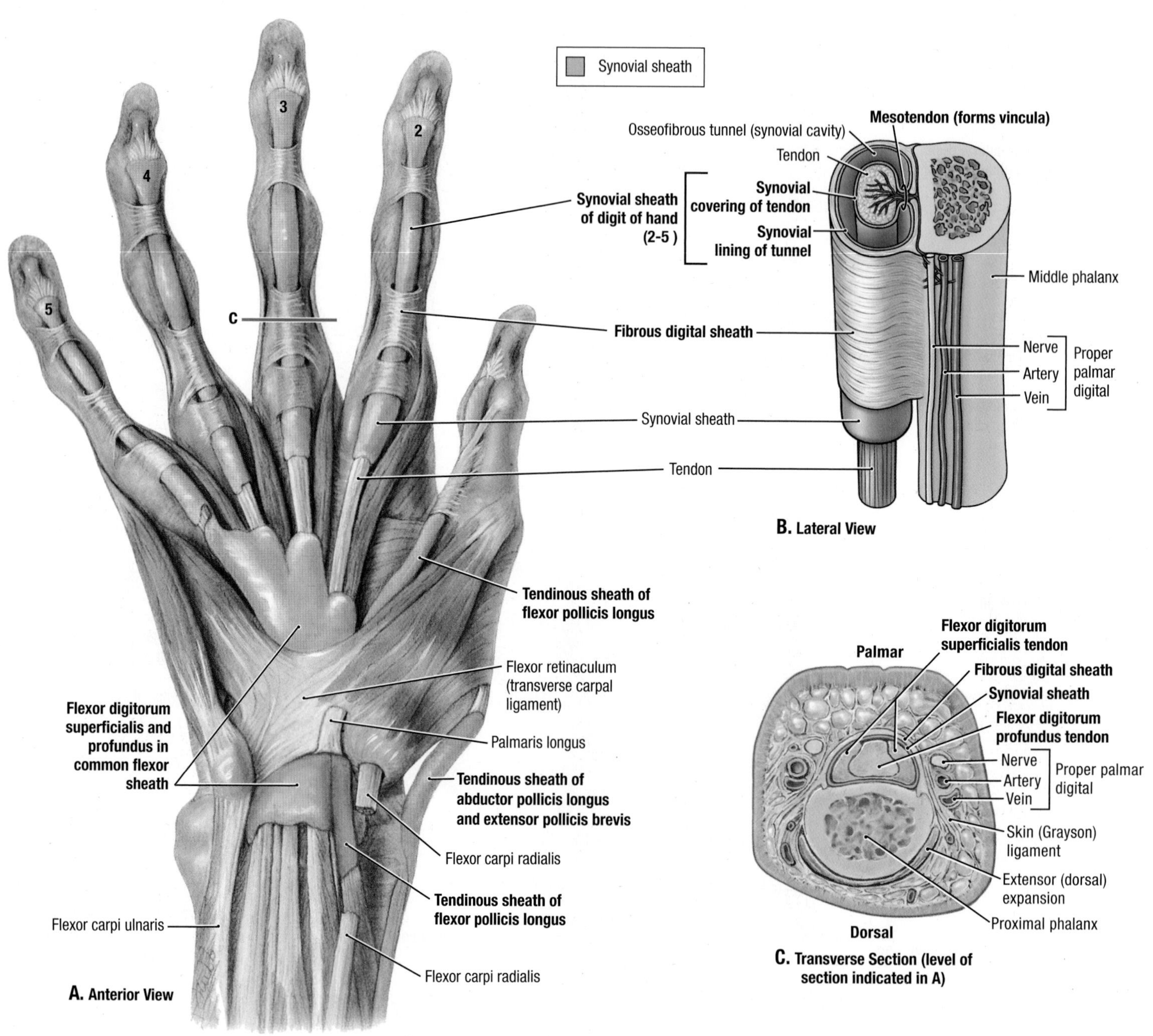
Synovial sheath
3
2
4
5
C
Synovial sheath of digit of hand (2-5)
Fibrous digital sheath
Synovial sheath
Tendon
Tendinous sheath of flexor pollicis longus
Flexor retinaculum (transverse carpal ligament)
Palmaris longus
Flexor digitorum superficialis and profundus in common flexor sheath
Tendinous sheath of abductor pollicis longus and extensor pollicis brevis
Flexor carpi radialis
Tendinous sheath of flexor pollicis longus
Flexor carpi ulnaris
Flexor carpi radialis
A. Anterior View
Osseofibrous tunnel (synovial cavity)
Mesotendon (forms vincula)
Tendon
Synovial covering of tendon
Synovial lining of tunnel
Middle phalanx
Nerve
Artery
Vein
Proper palmar digital
B. Lateral View
Palmar
Flexor digitorum superficialis tendon
Fibrous digital sheath
Synovial sheath
Flexor digitorum profundus tendon
Nerve
Artery
Vein
Proper palmar digital
Skin (Grayson) ligament
Extensor (dorsal) expansion
Proximal phalanx
Dorsal
C. Transverse Section (level of section indicated in A)

6.75 SYNOVIAL SHEATHS OF PALM OF HAND

A. Tendinous (synovial) sheaths of long flexor tendons of the digits. **B.** Osseofibrous tunnel and tendinous (synovial) sheath. **C.** Transverse section through the proximal phalanx.

Injuries such as puncture of a finger by a rusty nail can cause **infection of the digital synovial sheaths.** When inflammation of the tendon and synovial sheath **(tenosynovitis)** occurs, the digit swells and movement becomes painful. Because the tendons of the 2nd to 4th digits nearly always have separate synovial sheaths, the infection usually is confined to the infected digits. If the infection is untreated, however, the proximal ends of these sheaths may rupture, allowing the infection to spread to the midpalmar space. Because the synovial sheath of the little finger is usually continuous with the common flexor sheath, tenosynovitis in this finger may spread to the common flexor sheath and thus through the palm and carpal tunnel to the anterior forearm. Likewise, tenosynovitis in the thumb may spread through the continuous tendinous sheath of flexor pollicis longus.

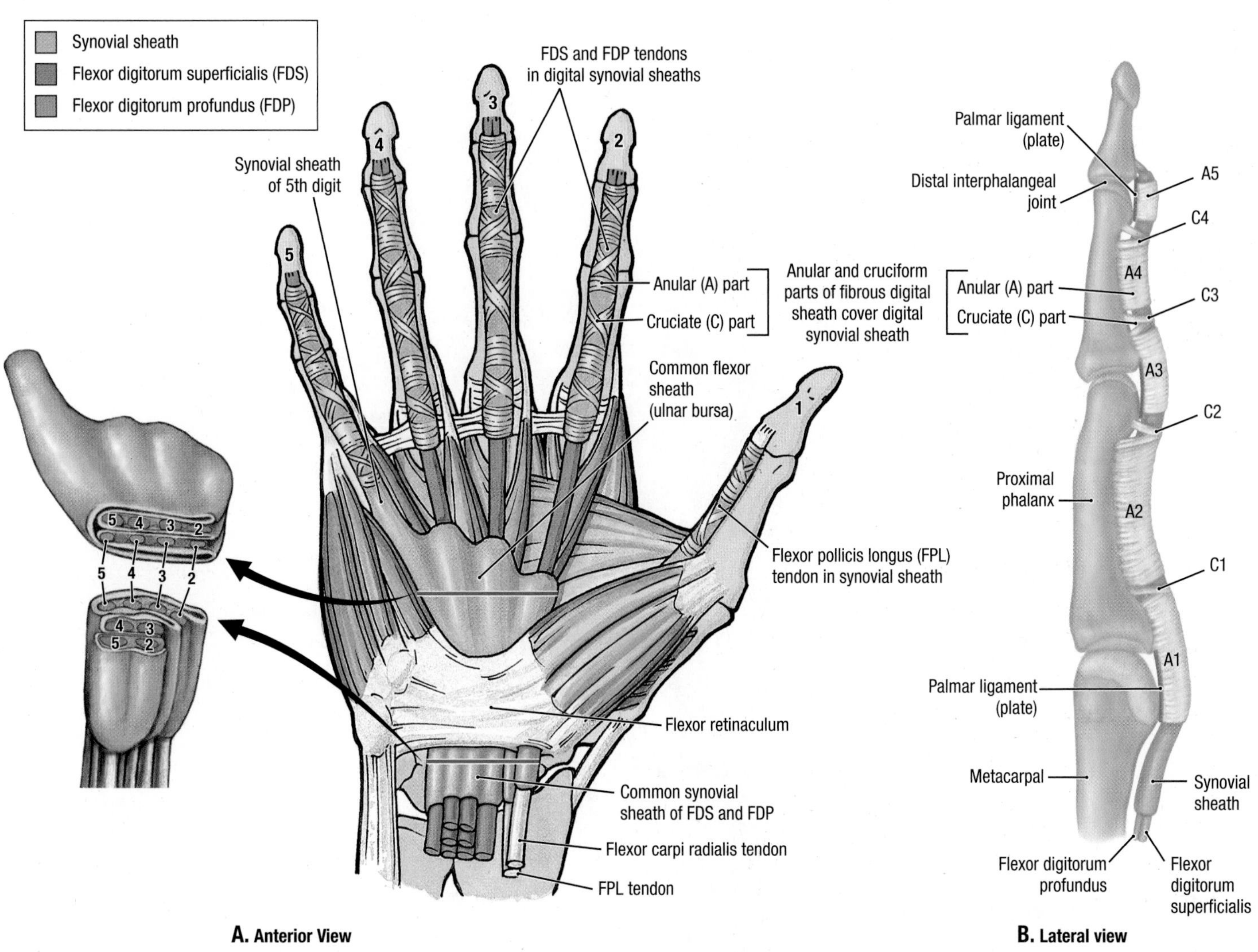
Synovial sheath
Flexor digitorum superficialis (FDS)
Flexor digitorum profundus (FDP)
FDS and FDP tendons in digital synovial sheaths
Synovial sheath of 5th digit
Anular (A) part
Cruciate (C) part
Anular and cruciform parts of fibrous digital sheath cover digital synovial sheath
Common flexor sheath (ulnar bursa)
Flexor pollicis longus (FPL) tendon in synovial sheath
Flexor retinaculum
Common synovial sheath of FDS and FDP
Flexor carpi radialis tendon
FPL tendon
A. Anterior View
Palmar ligament (plate)
Distal interphalangeal joint
A5
C4
A4
C3
A3
C2
Proximal phalanx
A2
C1
A1
Palmar ligament (plate)
Metacarpal
Synovial sheath
Flexor digitorum profundus
Flexor digitorum superficialis
B. Lateral view

6.76 FIBROUS DIGITAL SHEATHS

A. Fibrous digital and synovial sheaths. **B.** Anular and cruciate parts (pulleys) of the fibrous digital sheath.

Fibrous digital sheaths are the strong ligamentous tunnels containing the flexor tendons and their synovial sheaths. The sheaths extend from the heads of the metacarpals to the bases of the distal phalanges. These sheaths prevent the tendons from pulling away from the digits (bowstringing). The fibrous digital sheaths combine with the bones to form osseofibrous tunnels through which the tendons pass to reach the digits. The anular and cruciform (cruciate) parts, often referred to clinically as "pulleys," are thickened reinforcements of the fibrous digital sheaths.

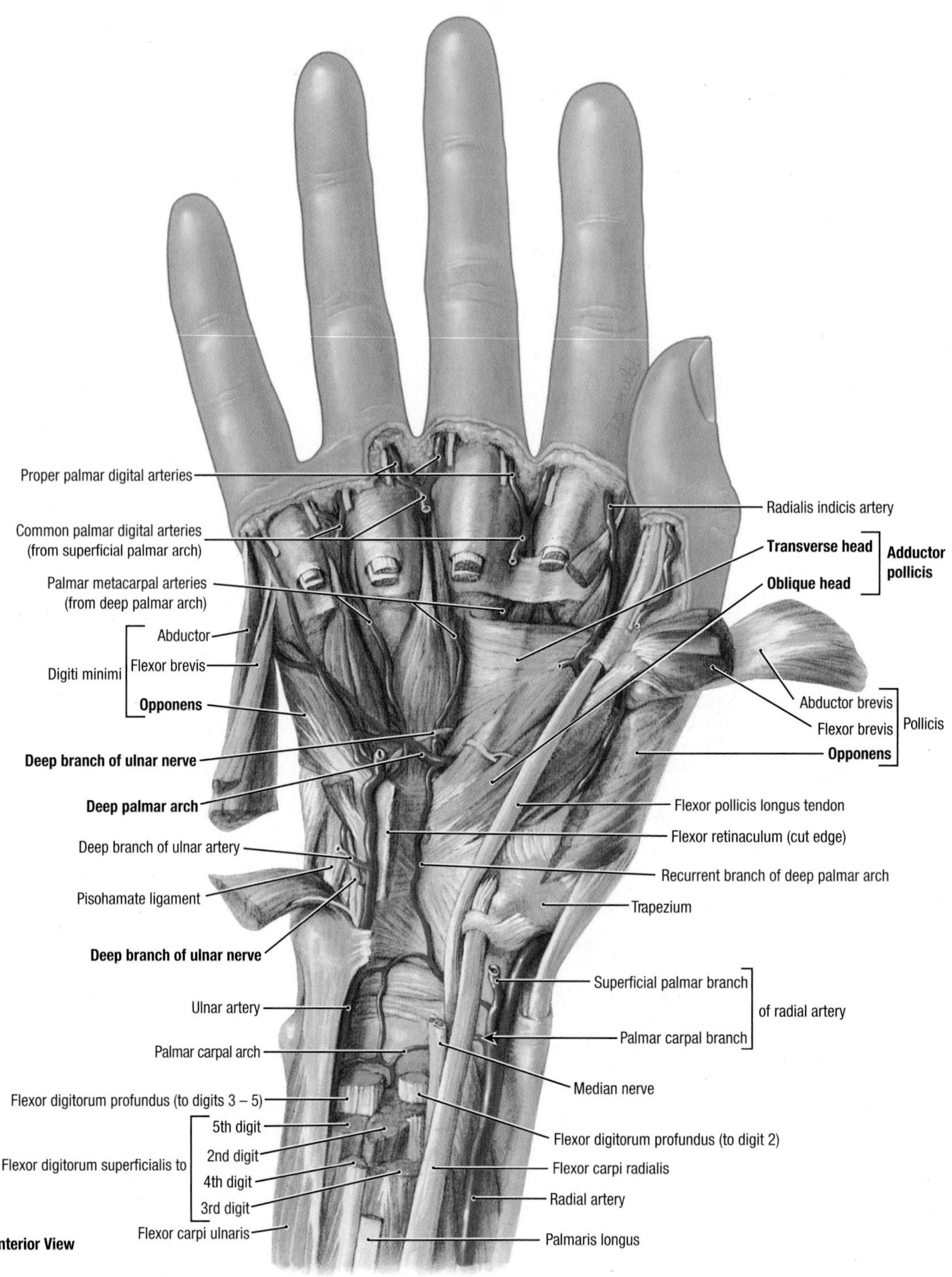
Proper palmar digital arteries
Common palmar digital arteries (from superficial palmar arch)
Palmar metacarpal arteries (from deep palmar arch)
Digiti minimi
Abductor
Flexor brevis
Opponens
Deep branch of ulnar nerve
Deep palmar arch
Deep branch of ulnar artery
Pisohamate ligament
Deep branch of ulnar nerve
Ulnar artery
Palmar carpal arch
Flexor digitorum profundus (to digits 3 – 5)
Flexor digitorum superficialis to
5th digit
2nd digit
4th digit
3rd digit
Flexor carpi ulnaris
Anterior View
Radialis indicis artery
Transverse head
Oblique head
Adductor pollicis
Abductor brevis
Flexor brevis
Opponens
Pollicis
Flexor pollicis longus tendon
Flexor retinaculum (cut edge)
Recurrent branch of deep palmar arch
Trapezium
Superficial palmar branch
Palmar carpal branch
of radial artery
Median nerve
Flexor digitorum profundus (to digit 2)
Flexor carpi radialis
Radial artery
Palmaris longus

6.77 DEEP DISSECTION OF PALM

- The deep branch of the ulnar artery joins the radial artery to form the deep palmar arch.
- The pisohamate ligament is often considered a continuation of the tendon of flexor carpi ulnaris; thus making the pisiform a sesamoid bone.

Compression of the ulnar nerve may occur at the wrist where it passes between the pisiform and the hook of hamate. The depression between these bones is converted by the pisohamate ligament into an osseofibrous ulnar canal. **Ulnar canal syndrome** is manifest by hypoesthesia in the medial one and one half digits and weakness of the intrinsic hand muscles. Clawing of the 4th and 5th digits may occur, but in contrast to proximal nerve injury, their ability to flex is unaffected and there is no radial deviation of the wrist joint.

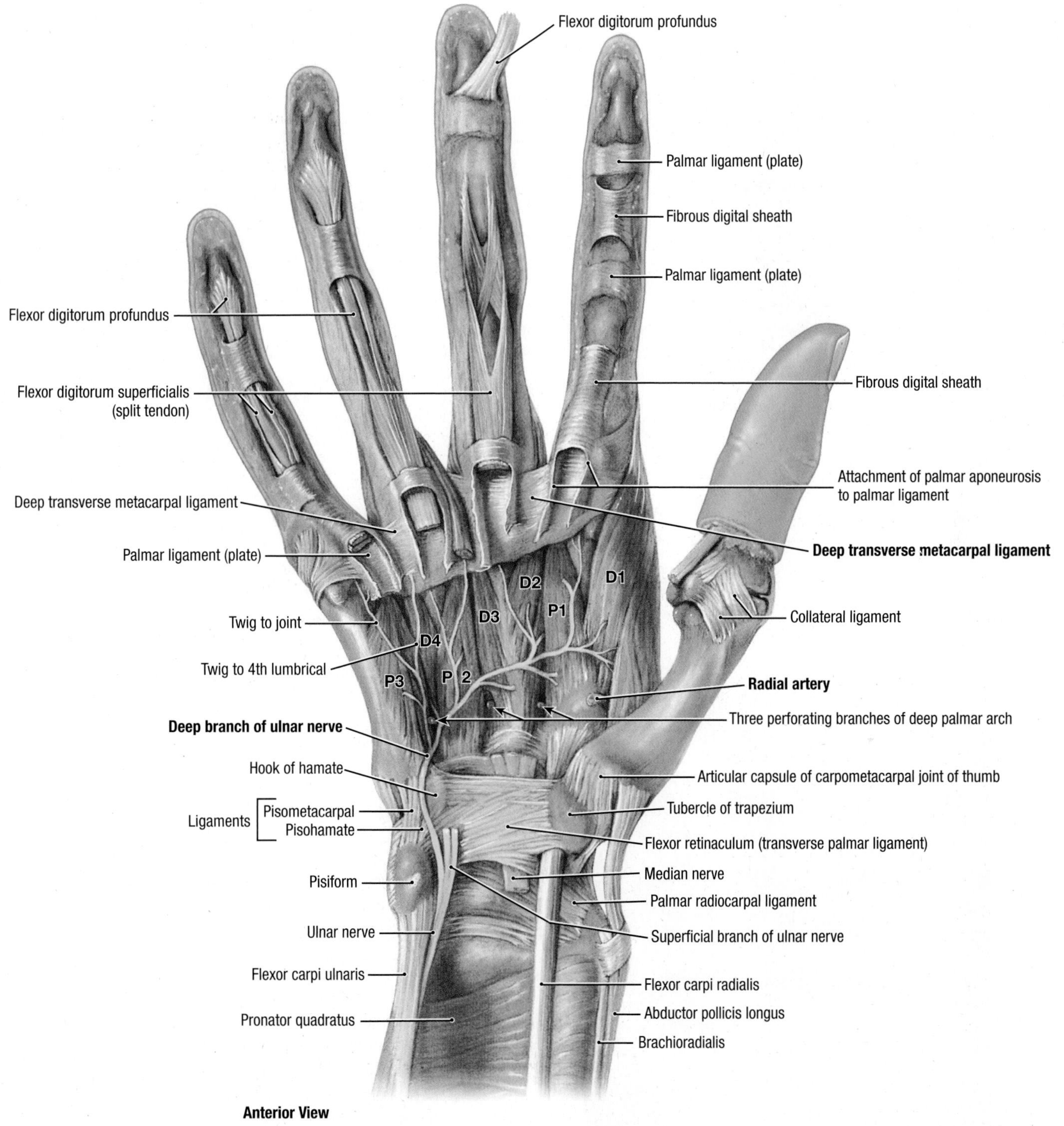
Flexor digitorum profundus
Palmar ligament (plate)
Fibrous digital sheath
Palmar ligament (plate)
Flexor digitorum profundus
Fibrous digital sheath
Flexor digitorum superficialis (split tendon)
Attachment of palmar aponeurosis to palmar ligament
Deep transverse metacarpal ligament
Deep transverse metacarpal ligament
Palmar ligament (plate)
D2
D1
Collateral ligament
D3
P1
Twig to joint
D4
Twig to 4th lumbrical
P3
P 2
Radial artery
Three perforating branches of deep palmar arch
Deep branch of ulnar nerve
Hook of hamate
Articular capsule of carpometacarpal joint of thumb
Tubercle of trapezium
Ligaments
Pisometacarpal
Pisohamate
Flexor retinaculum (transverse palmar ligament)
Median nerve
Pisiform
Palmar radiocarpal ligament
Ulnar nerve
Superficial branch of ulnar nerve
Flexor carpi ulnaris
Flexor carpi radialis
Abductor pollicis longus
Pronator quadratus
Brachioradialis
Anterior View

6.78 DEEP DISSECTION OF PALM AND DIGITS WITH DEEP BRANCH OF ULNAR NERVE

- Three unipennate palmar *(P1–P3)* and four bipennate dorsal *(D1–D4)* interosseous muscles are illustrated; the palmar interossei adduct the fingers, and the dorsal interossei abduct the fingers in relation to the axial line, an imaginary line drawn through the long axis of the 3rd digit (see Table 6.13).
- The deep transverse metacarpal ligaments unite the palmar ligaments; the lumbricals pass anterior to the deep transverse metacarpal ligament, and the interossei pass posterior to the ligament.
- Note the ulnar (Guyon) canal through which the ulnar vessels and nerve pass medial to the pisiform.
- The pisohamate and pisometacarpal ligaments form the distal attachment of flexor carpi ulnaris.

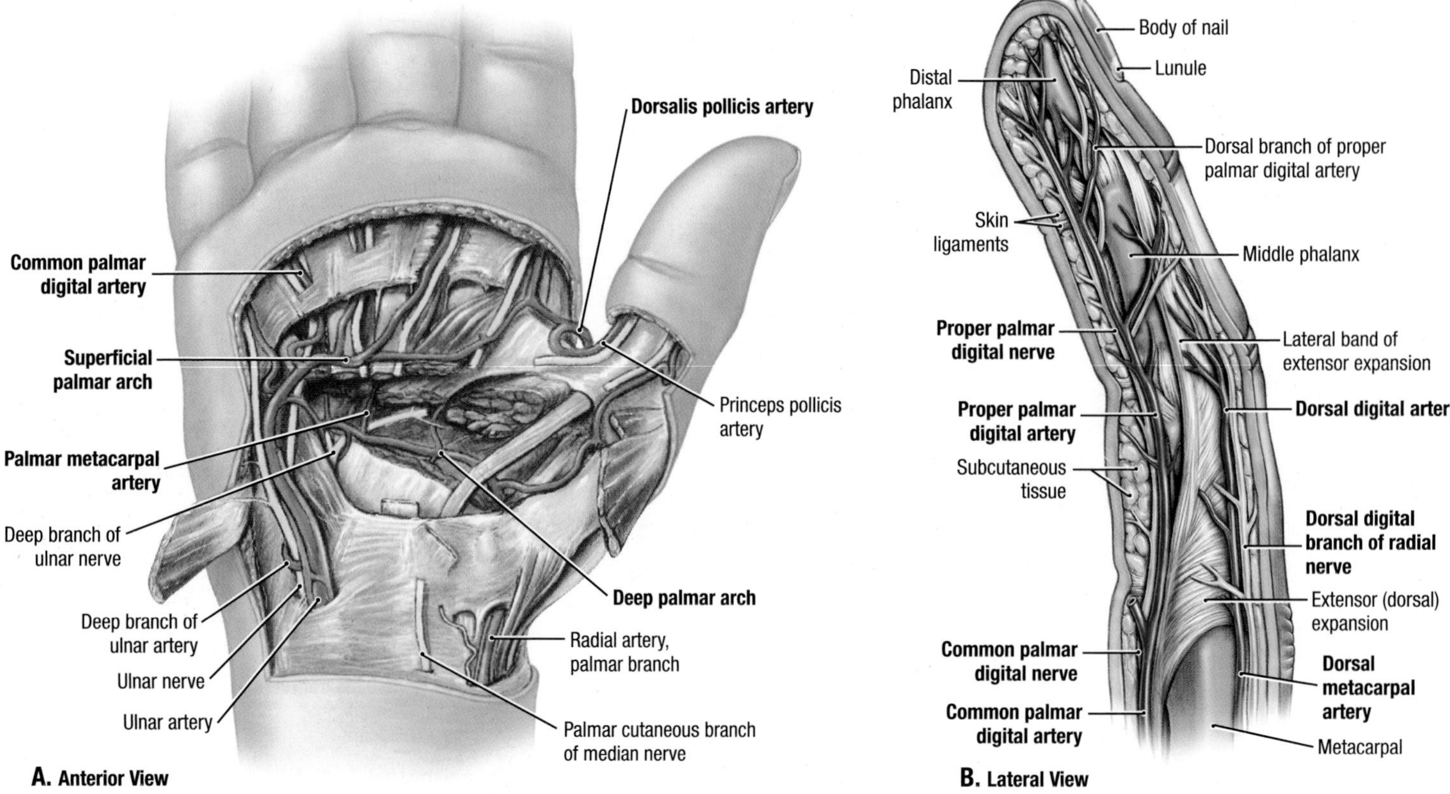
Dorsalis pollicis artery
Common palmar digital artery
Superficial palmar arch
Princeps pollicis artery
Palmar metacarpal artery
Deep branch of ulnar nerve
Deep palmar arch
Deep branch of ulnar artery
Radial artery, palmar branch
Ulnar nerve
Ulnar artery
Palmar cutaneous branch of median nerve
A. Anterior View
Body of nail
Lunule
Distal phalanx
Dorsal branch of proper palmar digital artery
Skin ligaments
Middle phalanx
Proper palmar digital nerve
Lateral band of extensor expansion
Proper palmar digital artery
Dorsal digital artery
Subcutaneous tissue
Dorsal digital branch of radial nerve
Extensor (dorsal) expansion
Common palmar digital nerve
Dorsal metacarpal artery
Common palmar digital artery
Metacarpal
B. Lateral View

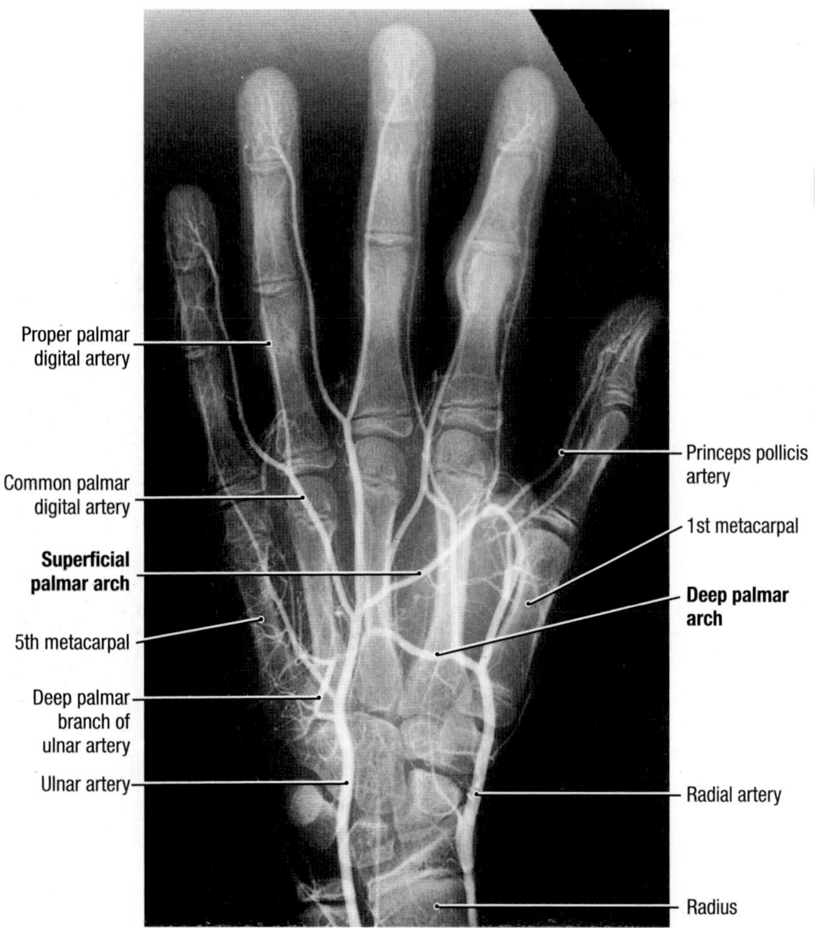
Proper palmar digital artery
Princeps pollicis artery
Common palmar digital artery
1st metacarpal
Superficial palmar arch
Deep palmar arch
5th metacarpal
Deep palmar branch of ulnar artery
Ulnar artery
Radial artery
Radius
C. Anteroposterior View

6.79 ARTERIAL SUPPLY OF HAND

A. Dissection of palmar arterial arches. **B.** Digital vessels and nerves. **C.** Arteriogram of the hand.

- The superficial palmar arch is usually completed by the superficial palmar branch of the radial artery, but in this specimen the dorsalis pollicis artery completes the arch.

The **superficial and deep palmar (arterial) arches** are not palpable, but their surface markings are visible. The superficial palmar arch occurs at the level of the distal border of the fully extended thumb. The deep palmar arch lies approximately 1 cm proximal to the superficial palmar arch. The location of these arches should be borne in mind in wounds of the palm and when palmar incisions are made.

Intermittent bilateral attacks of **ischemia of the digits,** marked by cyanosis and often accompanied by paresthesia and pain, are characteristically brought on by cold and emotional stimuli. The condition may result from an anatomical abnormality or an underlying disease. When the cause of the condition is idiopathic (unknown) or primary, it is called **Raynaud syndrome** (disease). Since arteries receive innervation from postsynaptic fibers from the sympathetic ganglia, it may be necessary to perform a cervicodorsal presynaptic sympathectomy to dilate the digital arteries.

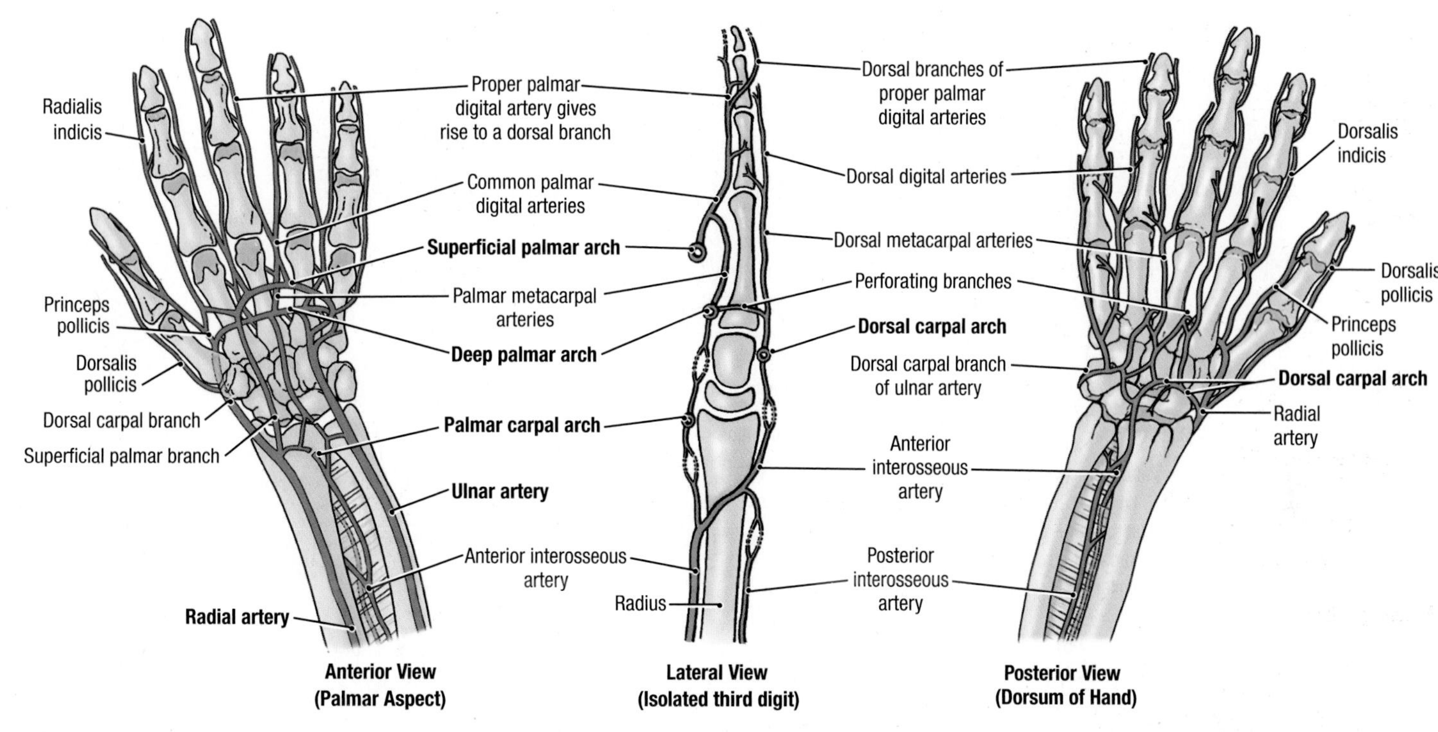
Radialis indicis
Proper palmar digital artery gives rise to a dorsal branch
Common palmar digital arteries
Superficial palmar arch
Palmar metacarpal arteries
Deep palmar arch
Princeps pollicis
Dorsalis pollicis
Dorsal carpal branch
Superficial palmar branch
Palmar carpal arch
Ulnar artery
Anterior interosseous artery
Radial artery
Radius
Dorsal branches of proper palmar digital arteries
Dorsal digital arteries
Dorsal metacarpal arteries
Perforating branches
Dorsal carpal arch
Dorsal carpal branch of ulnar artery
Anterior interosseous artery
Posterior interosseous artery
Dorsalis indicis
Dorsalis pollicis
Princeps pollicis
Dorsal carpal arch
Radial artery
Anterior View (Palmar Aspect)
Lateral View (Isolated third digit)
Posterior View (Dorsum of Hand)

6.80 ARTERIES OF HAND

TABLE 6.14 ARTERIES OF HAND

Artery	Origin	Course
Superficial palmar arch	Direct continuation of ulnar artery; arch is completed on lateral side by superficial branch of radial artery or another of its branches	Curves laterally deep to palmar aponeurosis and superficial to long flexor tendons; curve of arch lies across palm at level of distal border of extended thumb
Deep palmar arch	Direct continuation of radial artery; arch is completed on medial side by deep branch of ulnar artery	Curves medially, deep to long flexor tendons and is in contact with bases of metacarpals
Common palmar digital	Superficial palmar arch	Pass directly on lumbricals to webbings of digits
Proper palmar digital	Common palmar digital arteries	Run along sides of digits 2–5
Princeps pollicis	Radial artery as it turns into palm	Descends on palmar aspect of first metacarpal and divides at the base of proximal phalanx into two branches that run along sides of thumb
Radialis indicis	Radial artery, but may arise from princeps pollicis artery	Passes along lateral side of index finger to its distal end
Dorsal carpal arch	Radial and ulnar arteries	Arches within fascia on dorsum of hand

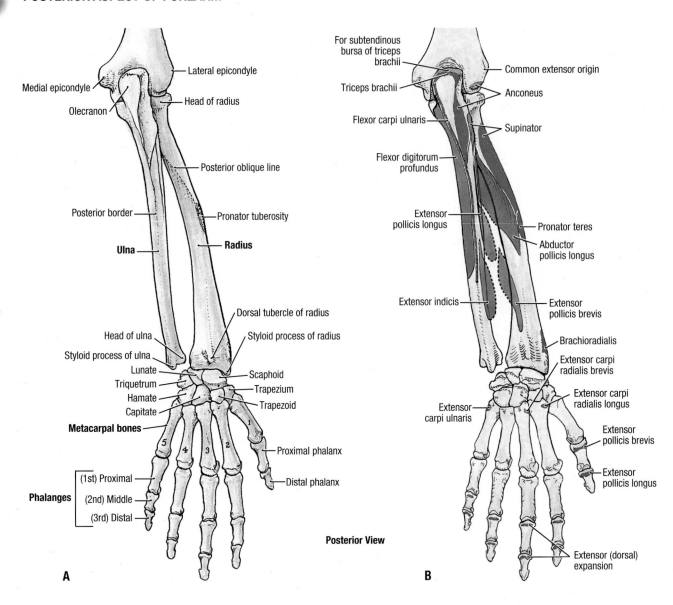

Lateral epicondyle
Medial epicondyle
Head of radius
Olecranon
Posterior oblique line
Posterior border
Pronator tuberosity
Ulna
Radius
Dorsal tubercle of radius
Head of ulna
Styloid process of radius
Styloid process of ulna
Lunate
Scaphoid
Triquetrum
Trapezium
Hamate
Trapezoid
Capitate
Metacarpal bones
Proximal phalanx
(1st) Proximal
Distal phalanx
Phalanges
(2nd) Middle
(3rd) Distal
A

For subtendinous bursa of triceps brachii
Common extensor origin
Triceps brachii
Anconeus
Flexor carpi ulnaris
Supinator
Flexor digitorum profundus
Extensor pollicis longus
Pronator teres
Abductor pollicis longus
Extensor indicis
Extensor pollicis brevis
Brachioradialis
Extensor carpi radialis brevis
Extensor carpi radialis longus
Extensor carpi ulnaris
Extensor pollicis brevis
Extensor pollicis longus
Extensor (dorsal) expansion
B

Posterior View

6.81 BONES AND MUSCLE ATTACHMENTS ON POSTERIOR ASPECT OF FOREARM AND HAND

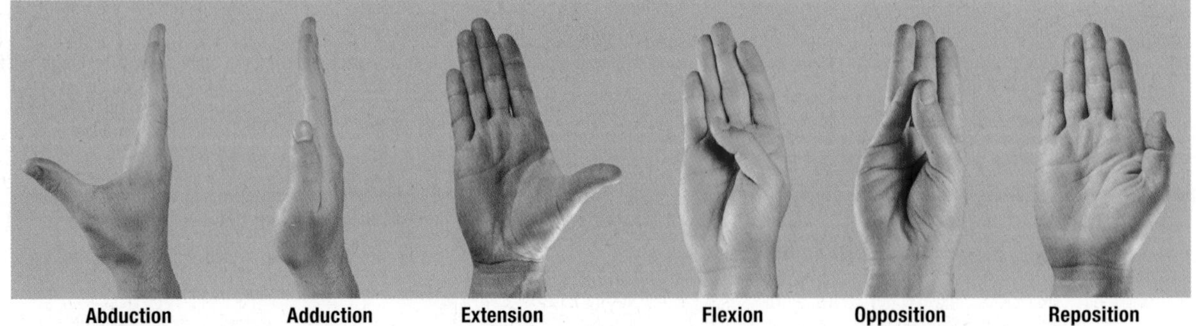

Abduction **Adduction** **Extension** **Flexion** **Opposition** **Reposition**

6.82 MOVEMENTS OF THUMB

The thumb is rotated 90° compared to the other digits. Abduction and adduction at the MCP joint occur in a sagittal plane; flexion and extension at the MCP and IP joints occur in frontal planes, opposite to these movements at other joints.

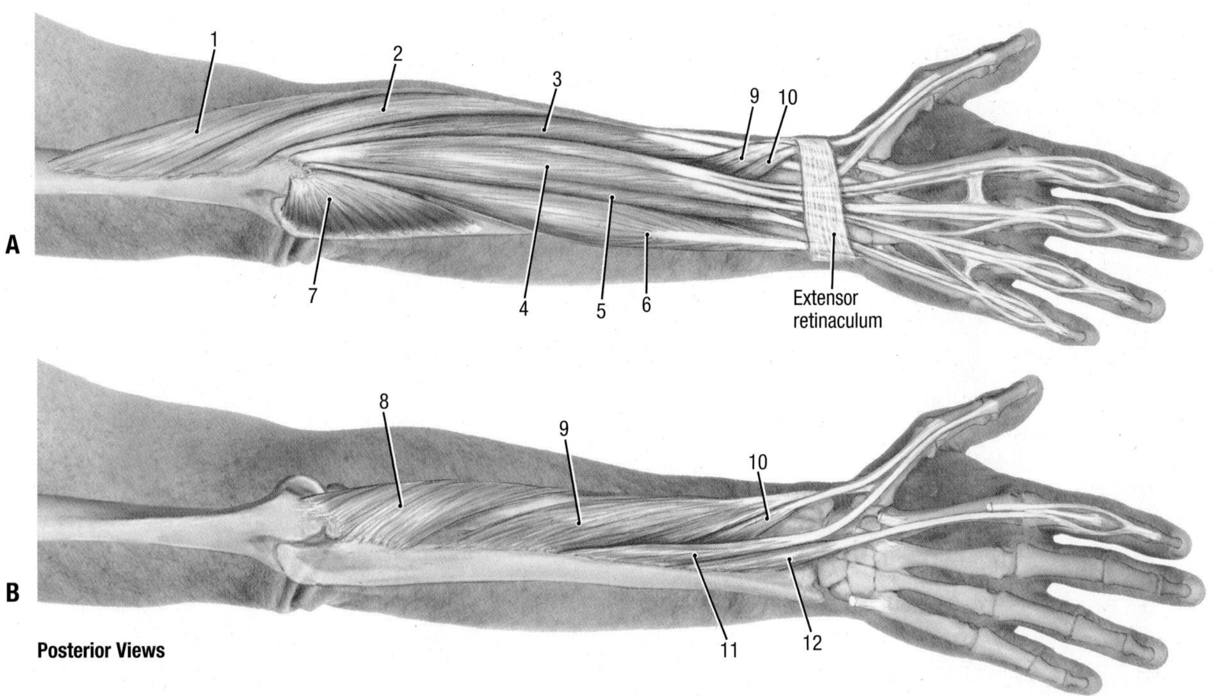
1
2
3
9 10
A
7
4
5
6
Extensor retinaculum
8
9
10
B
11
12
Posterior Views

6.83 MUSCLES ON POSTERIOR ASPECT OF FOREARM

A. Superficial. **B.** Deep

TABLE 6.15 MUSCLES OF POSTERIOR SURFACE OF FOREARM

Muscle	Proximal Attachment	Distal Attachment	Innervation	Main Actions
Brachioradialis (1)	Proximal two thirds of lateral supra-epicondylar ridge of humerus	Lateral surface of distal end of radius	Radial nerve (C5, **C6**, and C7)	Flexes elbow joint
Extensor carpi radialis longus (2)	Lateral supra-epicondylar ridge of humerus	Base of second metacarpal bone	Radial nerve (C6 and C7)	Extend and abduct wrist joint
Extensor carpi radialis brevis (3)	Lateral epicondyle of humerus	Base of third metacarpal bone	Deep branch of radial nerve (**C7** and C8)	
Extensor digitorum (4)		Extensor expansions of medial four digits	Posterior interosseous nerve (C7 and C8), a branch of the radial nerve	Extends medial four metacarpophalangeal joints; extends wrist joint
Extensor digiti minimi (5)		Extensor expansion of fifth digit		Extends metacarpophalangeal and interphalangeal joints of 5th digit
Extensor carpi ulnaris (6)	Lateral epicondyle of humerus and posterior border of ulna	Base of fifth metacarpal bone		Extends and adducts wrist joint
Anconeus (7)	Lateral epicondyle of humerus	Lateral surface of olecranon and superior part of posterior surface of ulna	Radial nerve (C7, C8, and T1)	Assists triceps brachii in extending elbow joint; stabilizes elbow joint; abducts ulna during pronation
Supinator (8)	Lateral epicondyle of humerus, radial collateral and anular ligaments, supinator fossa, and crest of ulna	Lateral, posterior, and anterior surfaces of proximal third of radius	Deep branch of radial nerve (C5 and **C6**)	Supinates forearm
Abductor pollicis longus (9)	Posterior surface of ulna, radius, and interosseous membrane	Base of first metacarpal bone	Posterior interosseous nerve (C7 and **C8**)	Abducts and extends carpometacarpal joint of thumb
Extensor pollicis brevis (10)	Posterior surface of radius and interosseous membrane	Base of proximal phalanx of thumb		Extends metacarpophalangeal joint of thumb
Extensor pollicis longus (11)	Posterior surface of middle third of ulna and interosseous membrane	Base of distal phalanx of thumb		Extends metacarpophalangeal and interphalangeal joints of thumb
Extensor indicis (12)	Posterior surface of ulna and interosseous membrane	Extensor expansion of second digit		Extends MCP and IP joints of 2nd digit and helps to extend wrist joint

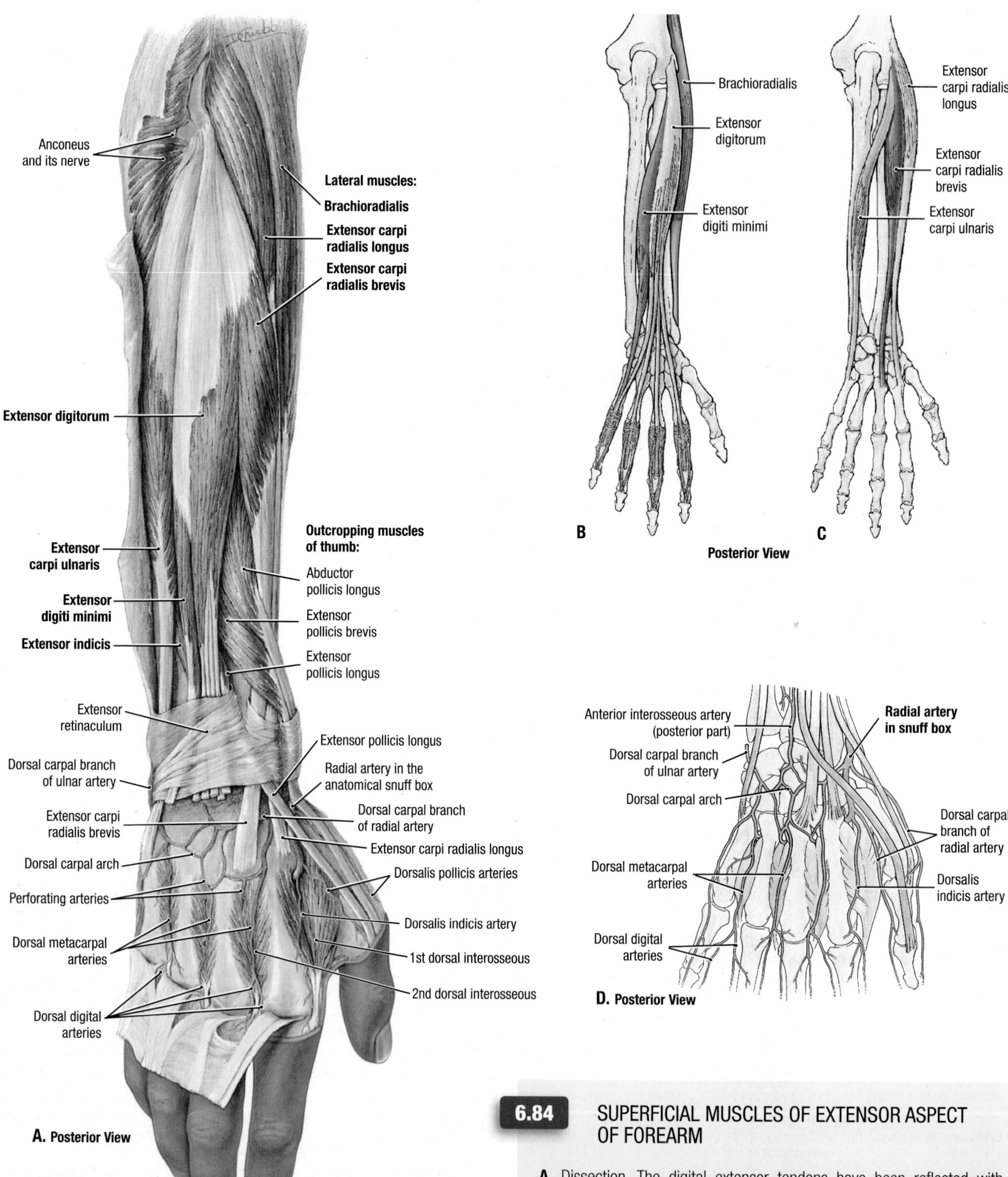

Anconeus and its nerve
Lateral muscles:
Brachioradialis
Extensor carpi radialis longus
Extensor carpi radialis brevis
Extensor digitorum
Outcropping muscles of thumb:
Abductor pollicis longus
Extensor pollicis brevis
Extensor pollicis longus
Extensor carpi ulnaris
Extensor digiti minimi
Extensor indicis
Extensor retinaculum
Extensor pollicis longus
Dorsal carpal branch of ulnar artery
Radial artery in the anatomical snuff box
Extensor carpi radialis brevis
Dorsal carpal branch of radial artery
Extensor carpi radialis longus
Dorsal carpal arch
Dorsalis pollicis arteries
Perforating arteries
Dorsalis indicis artery
Dorsal metacarpal arteries
1st dorsal interosseous
2nd dorsal interosseous
Dorsal digital arteries
A. Posterior View
Brachioradialis
Extensor digitorum
Extensor digiti minimi
Extensor carpi radialis longus
Extensor carpi radialis brevis
Extensor carpi ulnaris
B
C
Posterior View
Anterior interosseous artery (posterior part)
Radial artery in snuff box
Dorsal carpal branch of ulnar artery
Dorsal carpal arch
Dorsal carpal branch of radial artery
Dorsal metacarpal arteries
Dorsalis indicis artery
Dorsal digital arteries
D. Posterior View

6.84 SUPERFICIAL MUSCLES OF EXTENSOR ASPECT OF FOREARM

A. Dissection. The digital extensor tendons have been reflected without disturbing the arteries because they lie on the skeletal plane. **B.** and **C.** Schematic illustrations of superficial extensor muscles. **D.** Arteries on dorsum of hand.

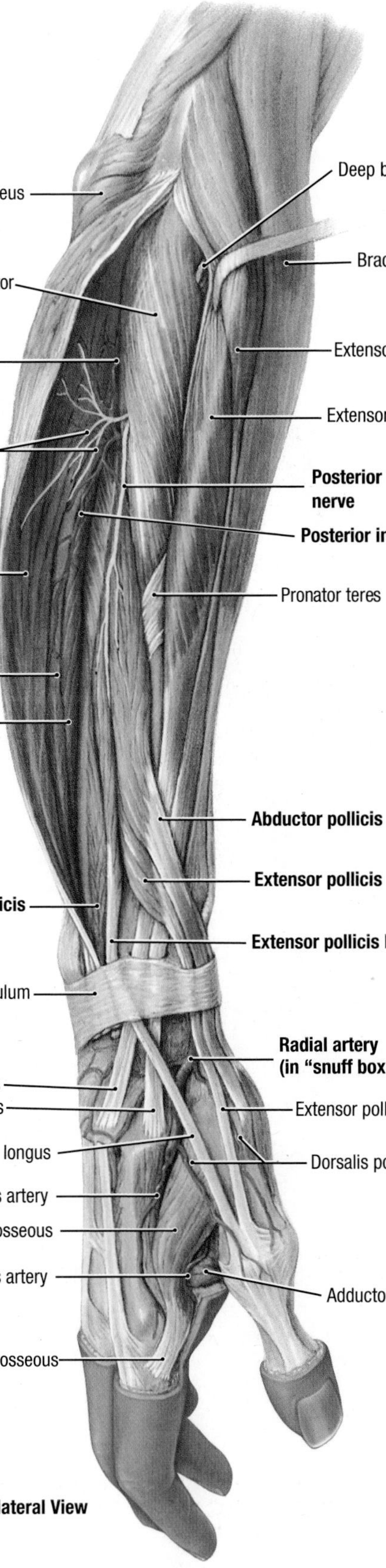

Anconeus
Supinator
Posterior interosseous recurrent artery
Branches of posterior interosseous nerve
Extensor digitorum
Extensor digiti minimi
Extensor carpi ulnaris
Extensor indicis
Extensor retinaculum
Extensor carpi radialis Brevis
Extensor carpi radialis Longus
Extensor pollicis longus
Dorsalis indicis artery
1st dorsal interosseous
Radialis indicis artery
1st dorsal interosseous
Deep branch of radial nerve
Brachioradialis
Extensor carpi radialis longus
Extensor carpi radialis brevis
Posterior interosseous nerve
Posterior interosseous artery
Pronator teres
Abductor pollicis longus
Extensor pollicis brevis
Extensor pollicis longus
Radial artery (in "snuff box")
Extensor pollicis brevis
Dorsalis pollicis arteries
Adductor pollicis

A. Posterolateral View

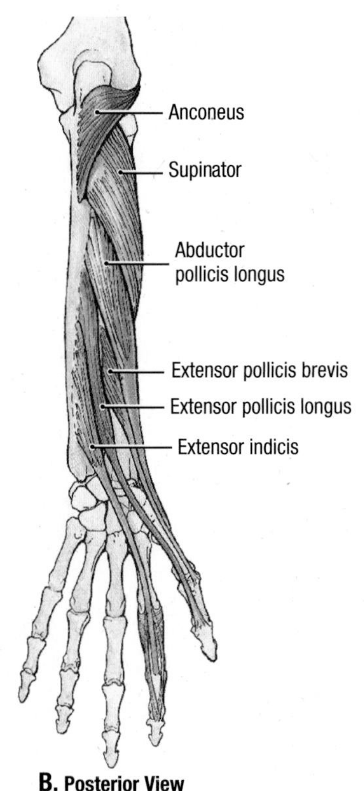
Anconeus
Supinator
Abductor pollicis longus
Extensor pollicis brevis
Extensor pollicis longus
Extensor indicis

B. Posterior View

6.85 DEEP STRUCTURES ON EXTENSOR ASPECT OF FOREARM

A. Dissection. **B.** Schematic illustration of deep extensor muscles.

- Three "outcropping" muscles of the thumb (abductor pollicis longus, extensor pollicis brevis, and extensor pollicis longus) emerge between the extensor carpi radialis brevis and the extensor digitorum.
- The laterally retracted brachioradialis and extensor carpi radialis longus and brevis muscles and supinator muscle are innervated by the deep branch of the radial nerve; the other extensor muscles are supplied by the posterior interosseous nerve, which is a continuation of the deep branch of the radial nerve that pierced the supinator.

Severance of the deep branch of the radial nerve results in an inability to extend the thumb and the metacarpophalangeal joints of the other digits. Loss of sensation does not occur because the deep branch is entirely muscular and articular in distribution.

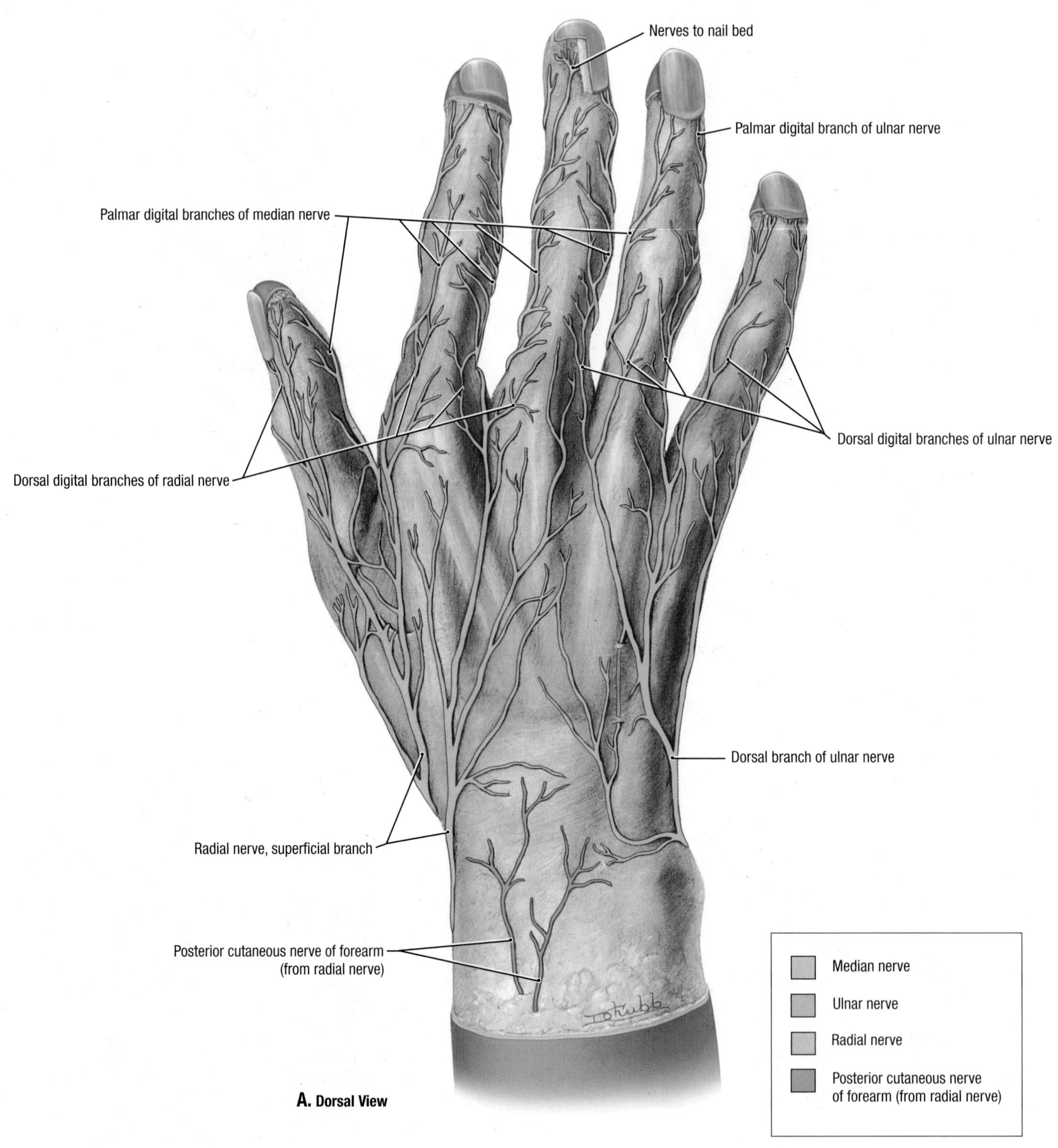
Nerves to nail bed
Palmar digital branch of ulnar nerve
Palmar digital branches of median nerve
Dorsal digital branches of ulnar nerve
Dorsal digital branches of radial nerve
Dorsal branch of ulnar nerve
Radial nerve, superficial branch
Posterior cutaneous nerve of forearm (from radial nerve)
Median nerve
Ulnar nerve
Radial nerve
Posterior cutaneous nerve of forearm (from radial nerve)

A. **Dorsal View**

6.86 CUTANEOUS INNERVATION OF HAND

A. Dissection of nerves of dorsum of hand.

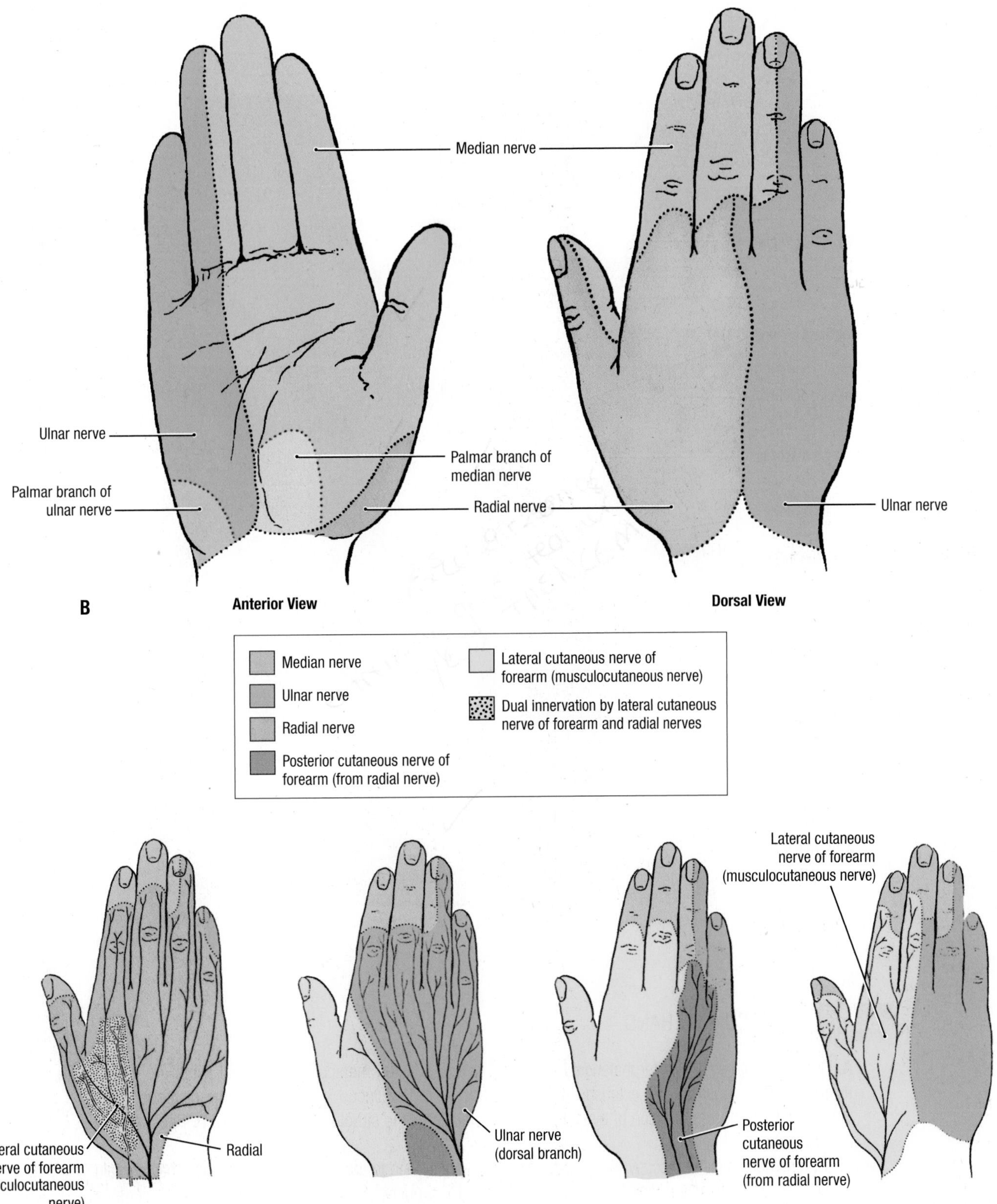
Median nerve
Ulnar nerve
Palmar branch of median nerve
Palmar branch of ulnar nerve
Radial nerve
Ulnar nerve
B
Anterior View
Dorsal View
Median nerve
Ulnar nerve
Radial nerve
Posterior cutaneous nerve of forearm (from radial nerve)
Lateral cutaneous nerve of forearm (musculocutaneous nerve)
Dual innervation by lateral cutaneous nerve of forearm and radial nerves
Lateral cutaneous nerve of forearm (musculocutaneous nerve)
Radial
Ulnar nerve (dorsal branch)
Posterior cutaneous nerve of forearm (from radial nerve)
Lateral cutaneous nerve of forearm (musculocutaneous nerve)
C. Dorsal Views

6.86 CUTANEOUS INNERVATION OF HAND *(CONTINUED)*

B. Distribution of the cutaneous nerves to the palm and dorsum of the hand, schematic illustration. **C.** Variations in pattern of cutaneous nerves in dorsum of hand.

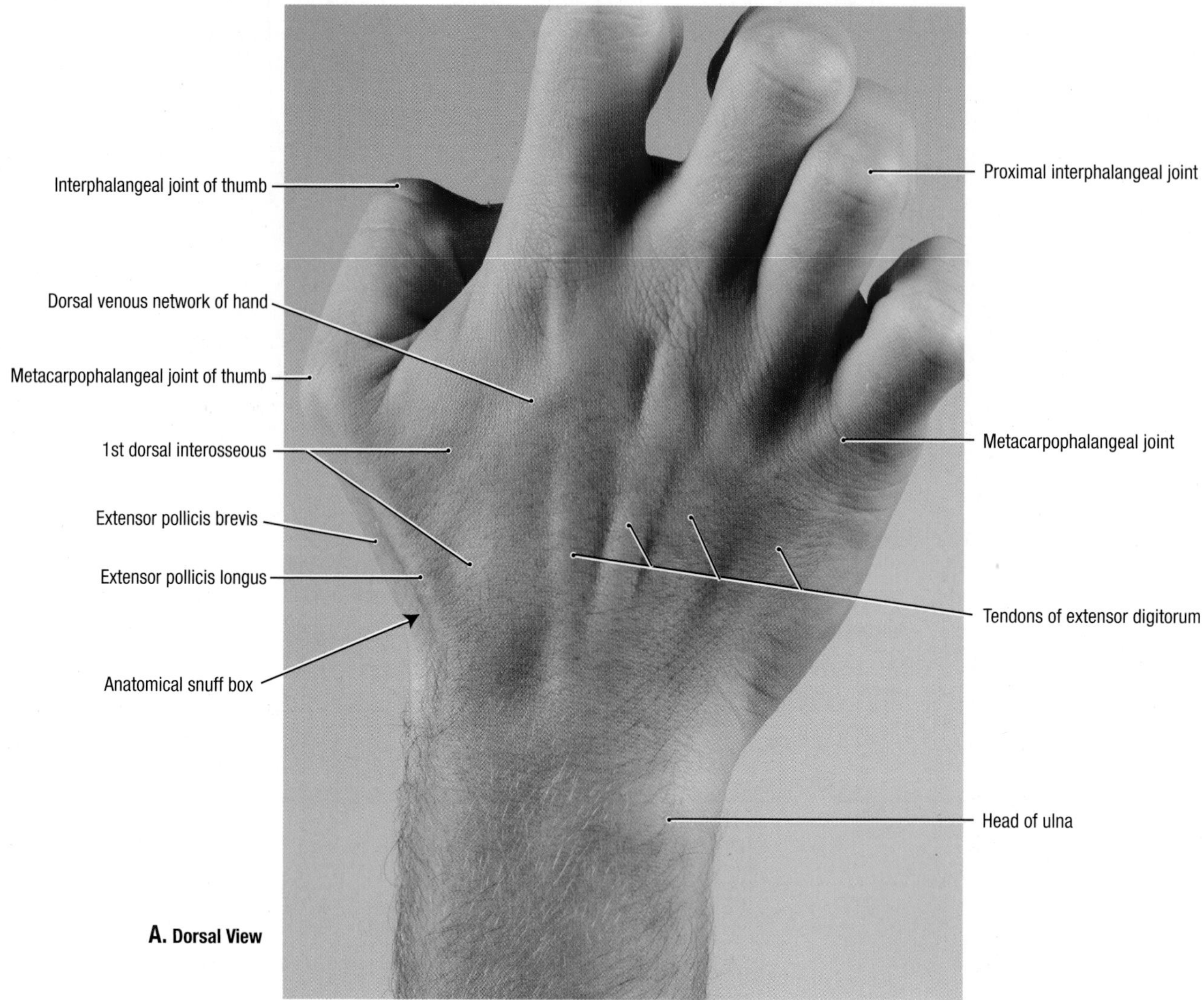
Interphalangeal joint of thumb
Dorsal venous network of hand
Metacarpophalangeal joint of thumb
1st dorsal interosseous
Extensor pollicis brevis
Extensor pollicis longus
Anatomical snuff box
Proximal interphalangeal joint
Metacarpophalangeal joint
Tendons of extensor digitorum
Head of ulna

A. Dorsal View

6.87 DORSUM OF HAND

A. Surface anatomy. The interphalangeal joints are flexed, and the metacarpophalangeal joints are hyperextended to demonstrate the extensor digitorum tendons. **B.** Tendinous (synovial) sheaths distended with blue fluid. **C.** Transverse section of distal forearm (*numbers* refer to structures labeled in B). **D.** Sites of bony attachments.

- Six tendinous sheaths occupy the six osseofibrous tunnels deep to the extensor retinaculum. They contain nine tendons: tendons for the thumb in sheaths 1 and 3, tendons for the extensors of the wrist in sheaths 2 and 6, and tendons for the extensors of the wrist and fingers in sheaths 4 and 5.
- The tendon of the extensor pollicis longus hooks around the dorsal tubercle of radius to pass obliquely across the tendons of the extensor carpi radialis longus and brevis to the thumb.

The tendons of the abductor pollicis longus and extensor pollicis brevis are in the same tendinous sheath on the dorsum of the wrist. Excessive friction of these tendons results in fibrous thickening of the sheath and stenosis of the osseofibrous tunnel, **Quervain tenovaginitis stenosans.** This condition causes pain in the wrist that radiates proximally to the forearm and distally to the thumb.

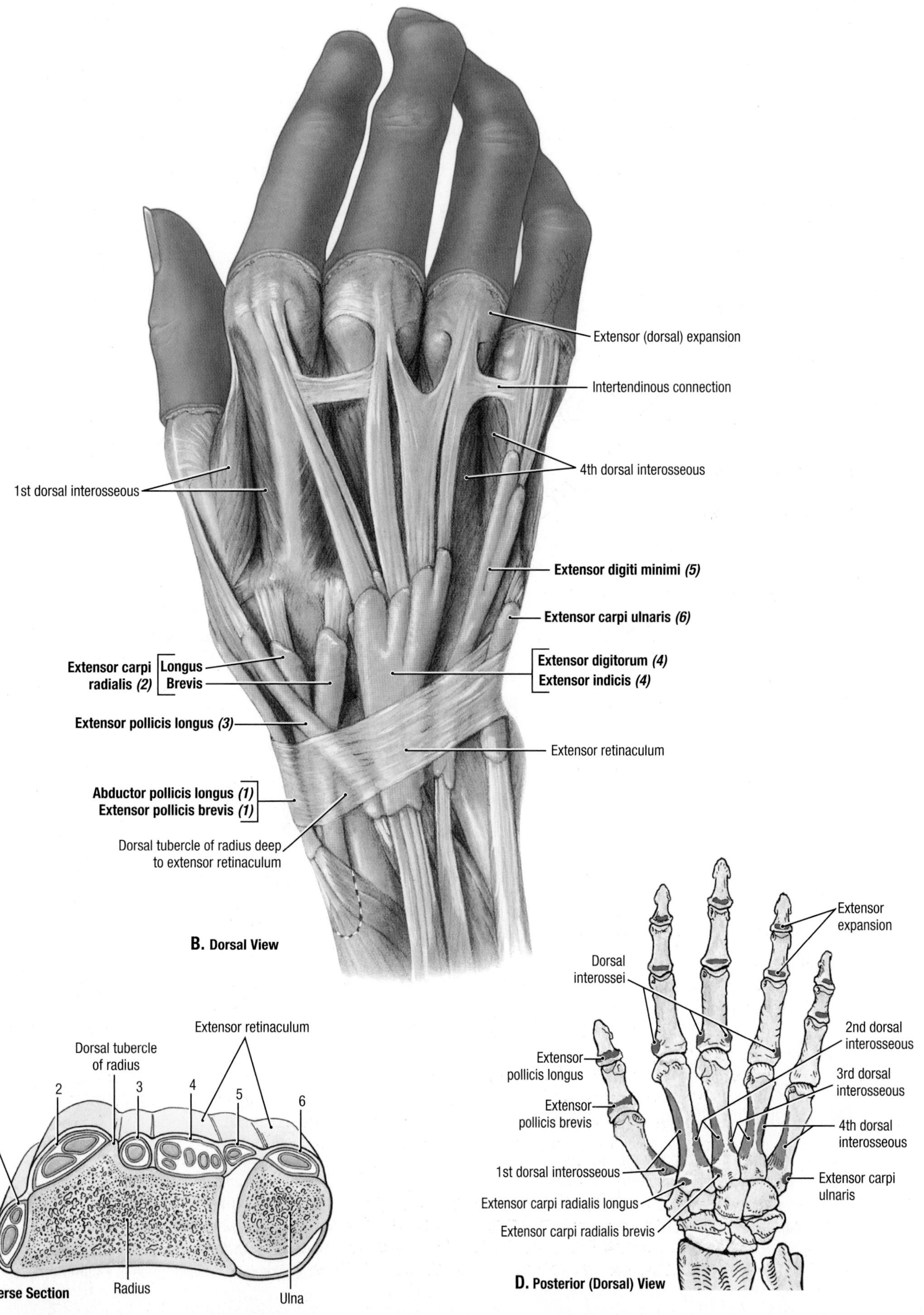
Extensor (dorsal) expansion
Intertendinous connection
4th dorsal interosseous
1st dorsal interosseous
Extensor digiti minimi (5)
Extensor carpi ulnaris (6)
Extensor carpi radialis (2)
Longus
Brevis
Extensor digitorum (4)
Extensor indicis (4)
Extensor pollicis longus (3)
Extensor retinaculum
Abductor pollicis longus (1)
Extensor pollicis brevis (1)
Dorsal tubercle of radius deep to extensor retinaculum
Extensor retinaculum
Dorsal tubercle of radius
1
2
3
4
5
6
Radius
Ulna
Extensor expansion
Dorsal interossei
Extensor pollicis longus
Extensor pollicis brevis
2nd dorsal interosseous
3rd dorsal interosseous
4th dorsal interosseous
1st dorsal interosseous
Extensor carpi ulnaris
Extensor carpi radialis longus
Extensor carpi radialis brevis

B. Dorsal View

C. Transverse Section

D. Posterior (Dorsal) View

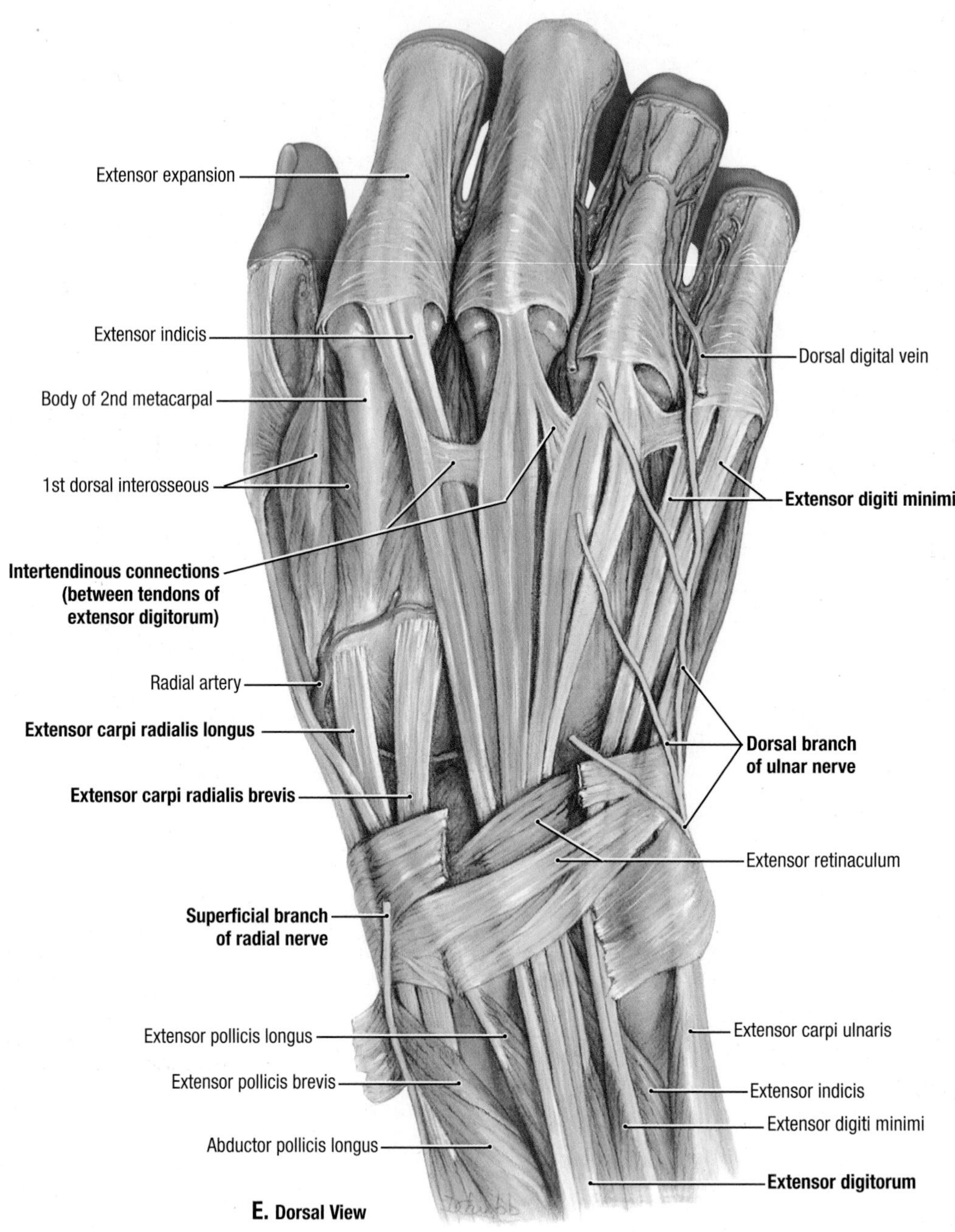

Extensor expansion
Extensor indicis
Body of 2nd metacarpal
1st dorsal interosseous
Intertendinous connections (between tendons of extensor digitorum)
Radial artery
Extensor carpi radialis longus
Extensor carpi radialis brevis
Superficial branch of radial nerve
Extensor pollicis longus
Extensor pollicis brevis
Abductor pollicis longus
Dorsal digital vein
Extensor digiti minimi
Dorsal branch of ulnar nerve
Extensor retinaculum
Extensor carpi ulnaris
Extensor indicis
Extensor digiti minimi
Extensor digitorum

E. Dorsal View

6.87 DORSUM OF HAND *(CONTINUED)*

E. Tendons on dorsum of hand and extensor retinaculum.

- The deep fascia is thickened to form the extensor retinaculum.
- Proximal to the knuckles, intertendinous connections extend between the tendons of the digital extensors and, thereby, restrict the independent action of the fingers.

"Ganglion" cyst. Sometimes a nontender cystic swelling appears on the hand, most commonly on the dorsum of the wrist. The thin-walled cyst contains clear mucinous fluid. Clinically, this type of swelling is called a "ganglion" (G. swelling or knot). These synovial cysts are close to and often communicate with the synovial sheaths. The distal attachment of the extensor carpi radialis brevis tendon is a common site for such a cyst.

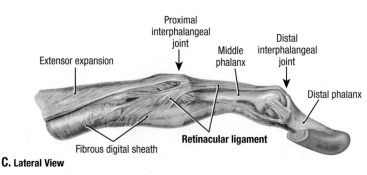

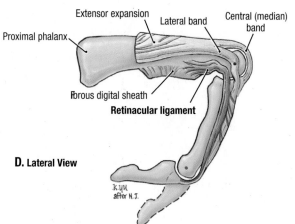

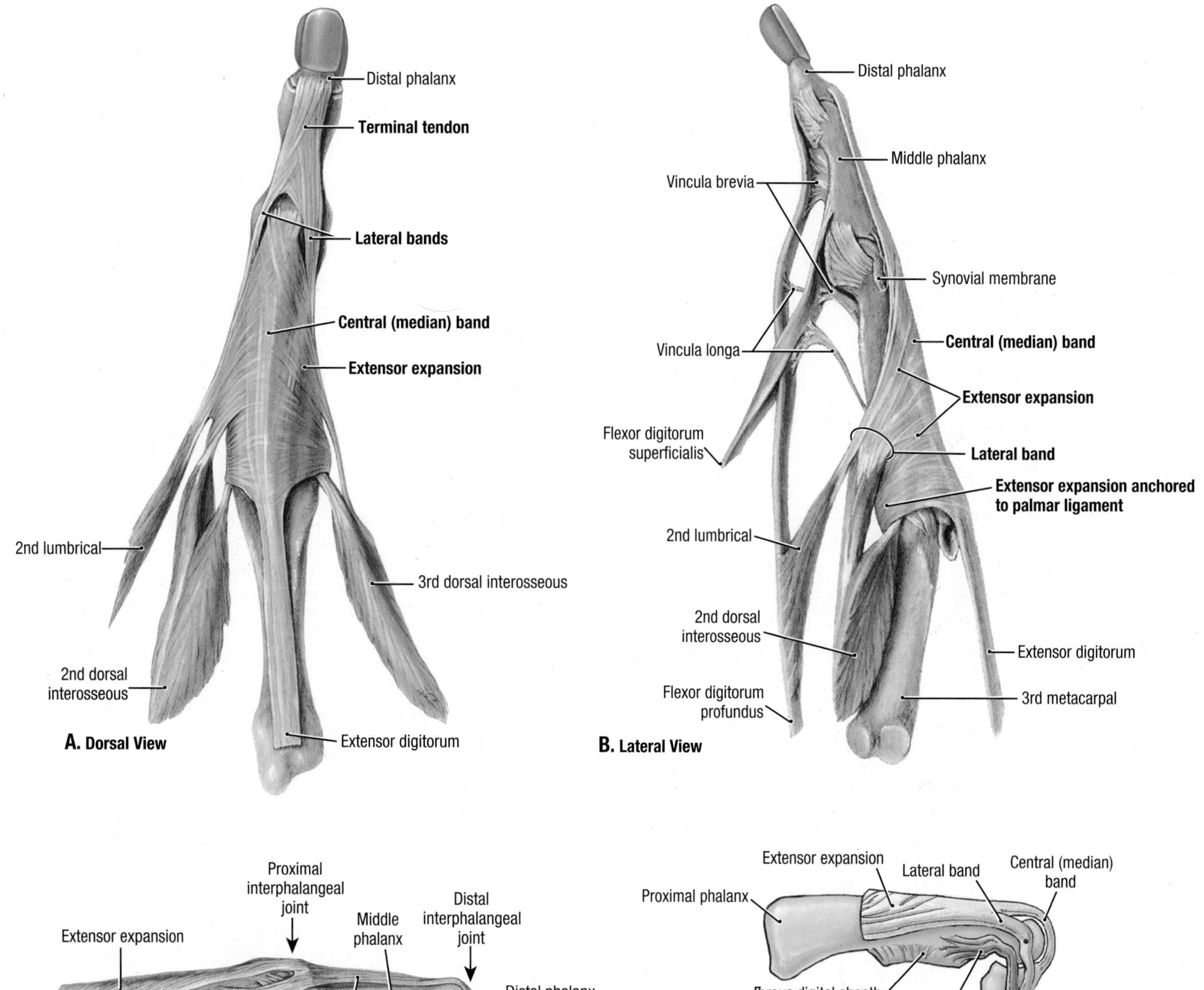
Distal phalanx
Terminal tendon
Lateral bands
Central (median) band
Extensor expansion
2nd lumbrical
3rd dorsal interosseous
2nd dorsal interosseous
Extensor digitorum
A. Dorsal View
Distal phalanx
Middle phalanx
Vincula brevia
Synovial membrane
Vincula longa
Central (median) band
Extensor expansion
Flexor digitorum superficialis
Lateral band
Extensor expansion anchored to palmar ligament
2nd lumbrical
2nd dorsal interosseous
Extensor digitorum
Flexor digitorum profundus
3rd metacarpal
B. Lateral View
Proximal interphalangeal joint
Distal interphalangeal joint
Middle phalanx
Extensor expansion
Distal phalanx
Fibrous digital sheath
Retinacular ligament
C. Lateral View
Extensor expansion
Lateral band
Central (median) band
Proximal phalanx
Fibrous digital sheath
Retinacular ligament
D. Lateral View
K.Yu after N.J.

6.88 EXTENSOR (DORSAL) EXPANSION OF THIRD DIGIT

A. Dorsal aspect. **B.** Lateral aspect. **C.** Retinacular ligaments of extended digit. **D.** Retinacular ligaments of flexed digit.

- The hood covering the head of the metacarpal is attached to the palmar ligament.
- Contraction of the muscles attaching to the lateral band will produce flexion of the metacarpophalangeal joint and extension of the interphalangeal joints.
- The retinacular ligament is a fibrous band that runs from the proximal phalanx and fibrous digital sheath obliquely across the middle phalanx and two interphalangeal joints to join the extensor (dorsal) expansion, and then to the distal phalanx.
- On flexion of the distal interphalangeal joint, the retinacular ligament becomes taut and pulls the proximal joint into flexion; on extension of the proximal joint, the distal joint is pulled by the ligament into nearly complete extension.

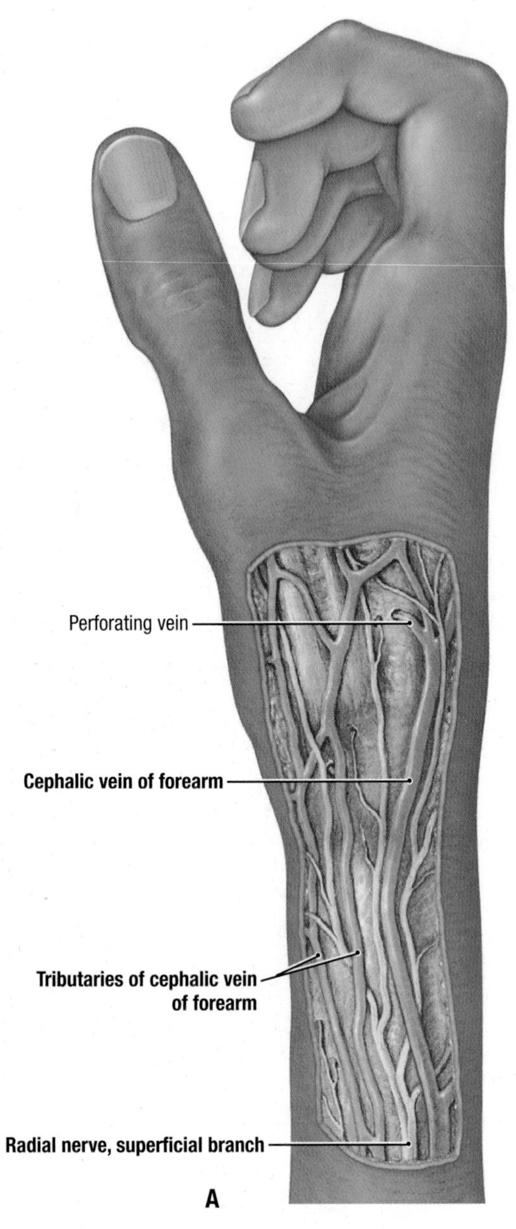
Perforating vein
Cephalic vein of forearm
Tributaries of cephalic vein of forearm
Radial nerve, superficial branch
A

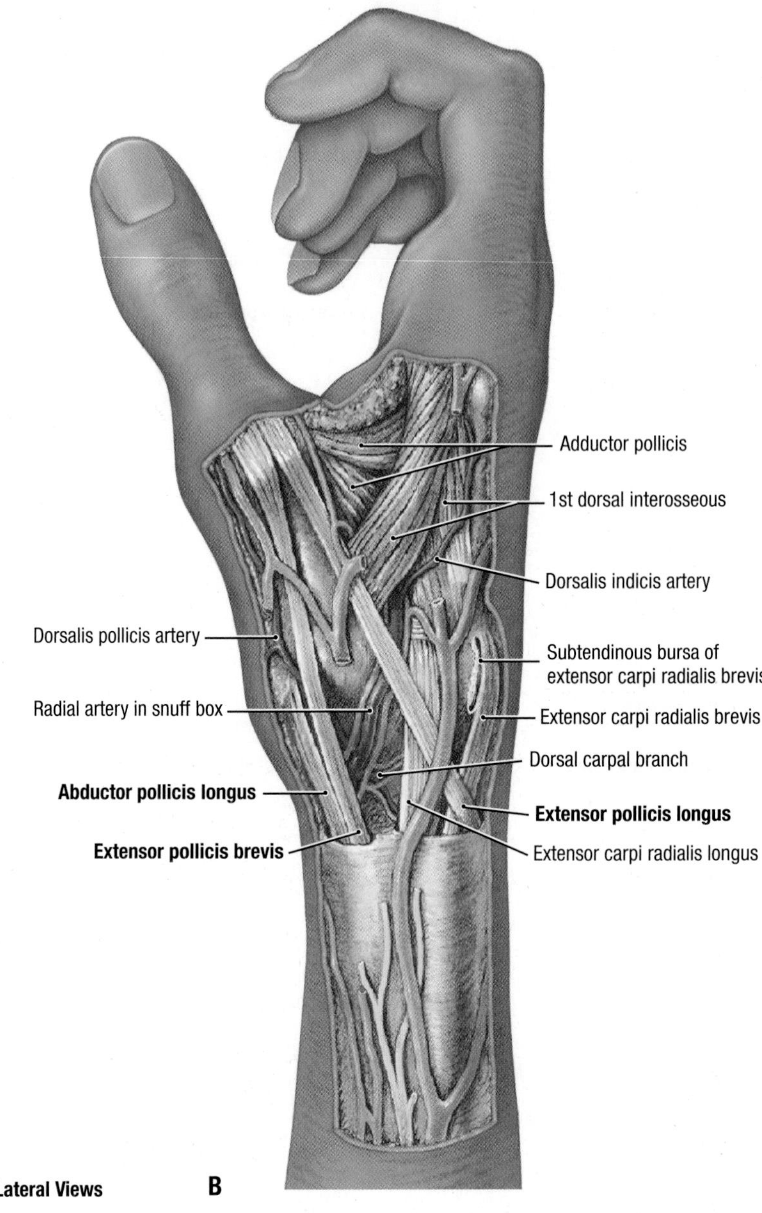
Adductor pollicis
1st dorsal interosseous
Dorsalis indicis artery
Dorsalis pollicis artery
Subtendinous bursa of extensor carpi radialis brevis
Radial artery in snuff box
Extensor carpi radialis brevis
Dorsal carpal branch
Abductor pollicis longus
Extensor pollicis longus
Extensor pollicis brevis
Extensor carpi radialis longus
Lateral Views
B

6.89 LATERAL ASPECT OF WRIST AND HAND

A. Anatomical snuff box—I. **B.** Anatomical snuff box—II.

In **A**:

- The depression at the base of the thumb, the "anatomical snuff box," retains its name from an archaic habit.
- Note the superficial veins, including the cephalic vein of forearm and/or its tributaries, and cutaneous nerves crossing the snuff box.

In **B**:

- Three long tendons of the thumb form the boundaries of the snuff box; the extensor pollicis longus forms the medial boundary and the abductor pollicis longus and extensor pollicis brevis the lateral boundary.
- The radial artery crosses the floor of the snuff box and travels between the two heads of the 1st dorsal interosseous.
- The adductor pollicis and 1st dorsal interosseous are supplied by the ulnar nerve.

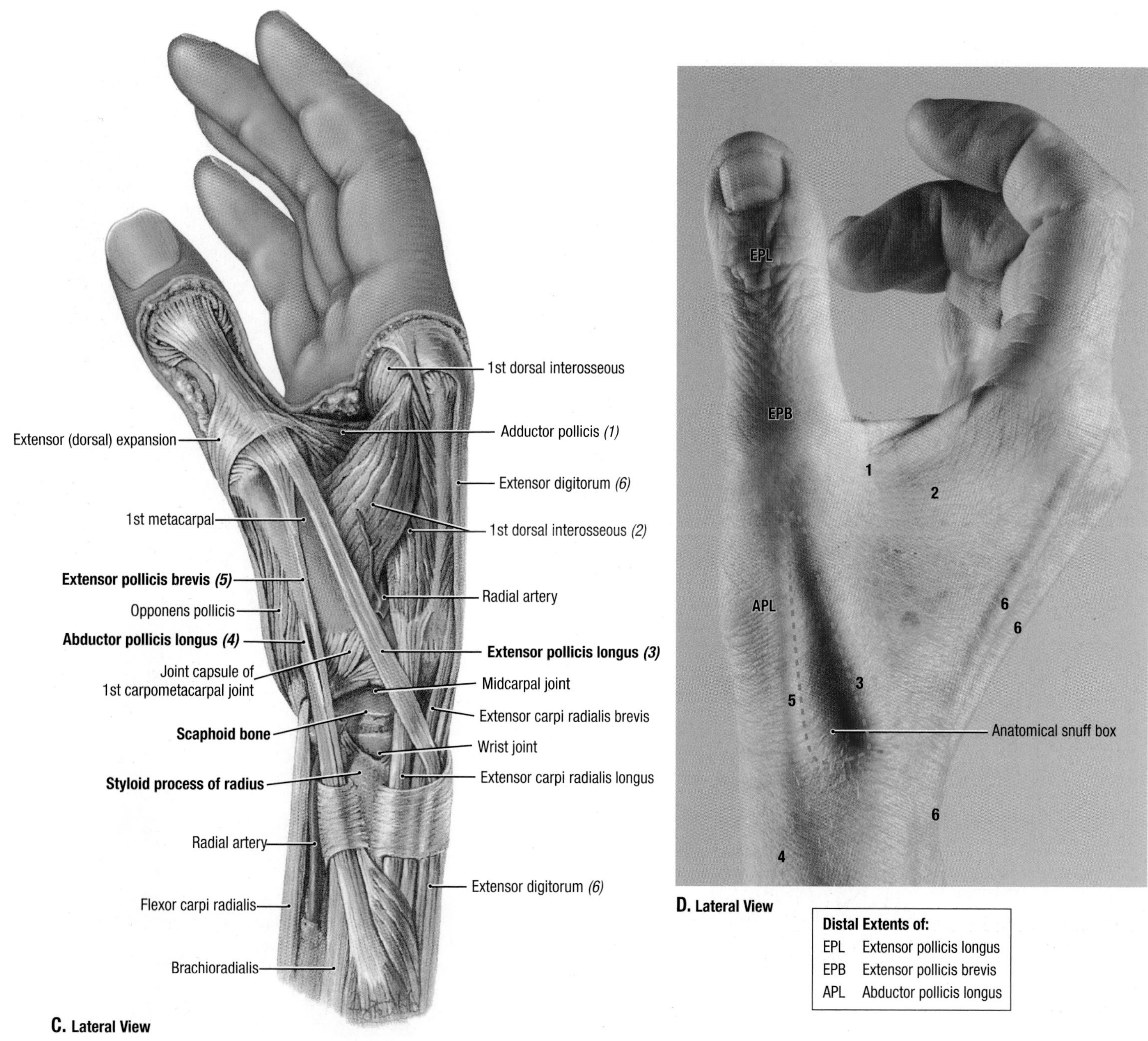
1st dorsal interosseous
Extensor (dorsal) expansion
Adductor pollicis (1)
Extensor digitorum (6)
1st metacarpal
1st dorsal interosseous (2)
Extensor pollicis brevis (5)
Radial artery
Opponens pollicis
Abductor pollicis longus (4)
Extensor pollicis longus (3)
Joint capsule of 1st carpometacarpal joint
Midcarpal joint
Extensor carpi radialis brevis
Scaphoid bone
Wrist joint
Styloid process of radius
Extensor carpi radialis longus
Radial artery
Extensor digitorum (6)
Flexor carpi radialis
Brachioradialis
EPL
EPB
1
2
APL
6
6
3
5
Anatomical snuff box
6
4
Distal Extents of:
EPL Extensor pollicis longus
EPB Extensor pollicis brevis
APL Abductor pollicis longus

C. Lateral View

D. Lateral View

6.89 LATERAL ASPECT OF WRIST AND HAND *(CONTINUED)*

C. Anatomical snuff box—III. **D.** Surface anatomy.

In **C**: Note the scaphoid bone, the wrist joint proximal to the scaphoid, and the midcarpal joint distal to it.

Fracture of the scaphoid often results from a fall on the palm with the hand abducted. The fracture occurs across the narrow part ("waist") of the scaphoid. Pain occurs primarily on the lateral side of the wrist, especially during dorsiflexion and abduction of the hand. Initial radiographs of the wrist may not reveal a fracture, but radiographs taken 10 to 14 days later reveal a fracture because bone resorption has occurred. Owing to the poor blood supply to the proximal part of the scaphoid, union of the fractured parts may take several months. **Avascular necrosis of the proximal fragment of the scaphoid** (pathological death of bone resulting from poor blood supply) may occur and produce degenerative joint disease of the wrist.

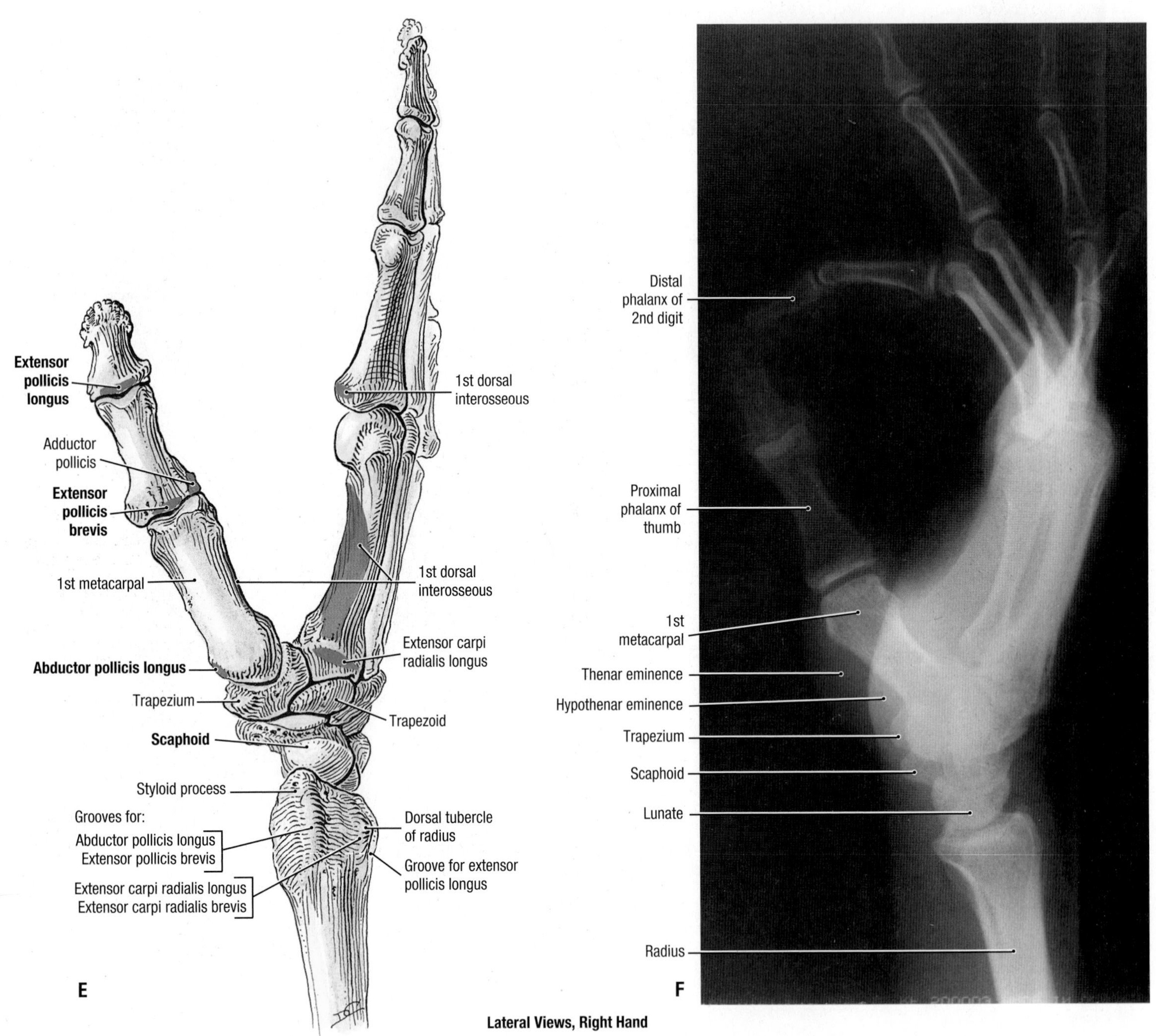
Extensor pollicis longus
Adductor pollicis
Extensor pollicis brevis
1st metacarpal
Abductor pollicis longus
Trapezium
Scaphoid
Styloid process
Grooves for:
Abductor pollicis longus
Extensor pollicis brevis
Extensor carpi radialis longus
Extensor carpi radialis brevis
1st dorsal interosseous
1st dorsal interosseous
Extensor carpi radialis longus
Trapezoid
Dorsal tubercle of radius
Groove for extensor pollicis longus
E
Distal phalanx of 2nd digit
Proximal phalanx of thumb
1st metacarpal
Thenar eminence
Hypothenar eminence
Trapezium
Scaphoid
Lunate
Radius
F

Lateral Views, Right Hand

6.89 LATERAL ASPECT OF WRIST AND HAND *(CONTINUED)*

E. Bony hand showing muscle attachments. **F.** Radiograph.

- The anatomical snuff box is limited proximally by the styloid process of the radius and distally by the base of the 1st metacarpal; aspects of the two lateral bones of the carpus (scaphoid and trapezium) form the floor of the snuff box.

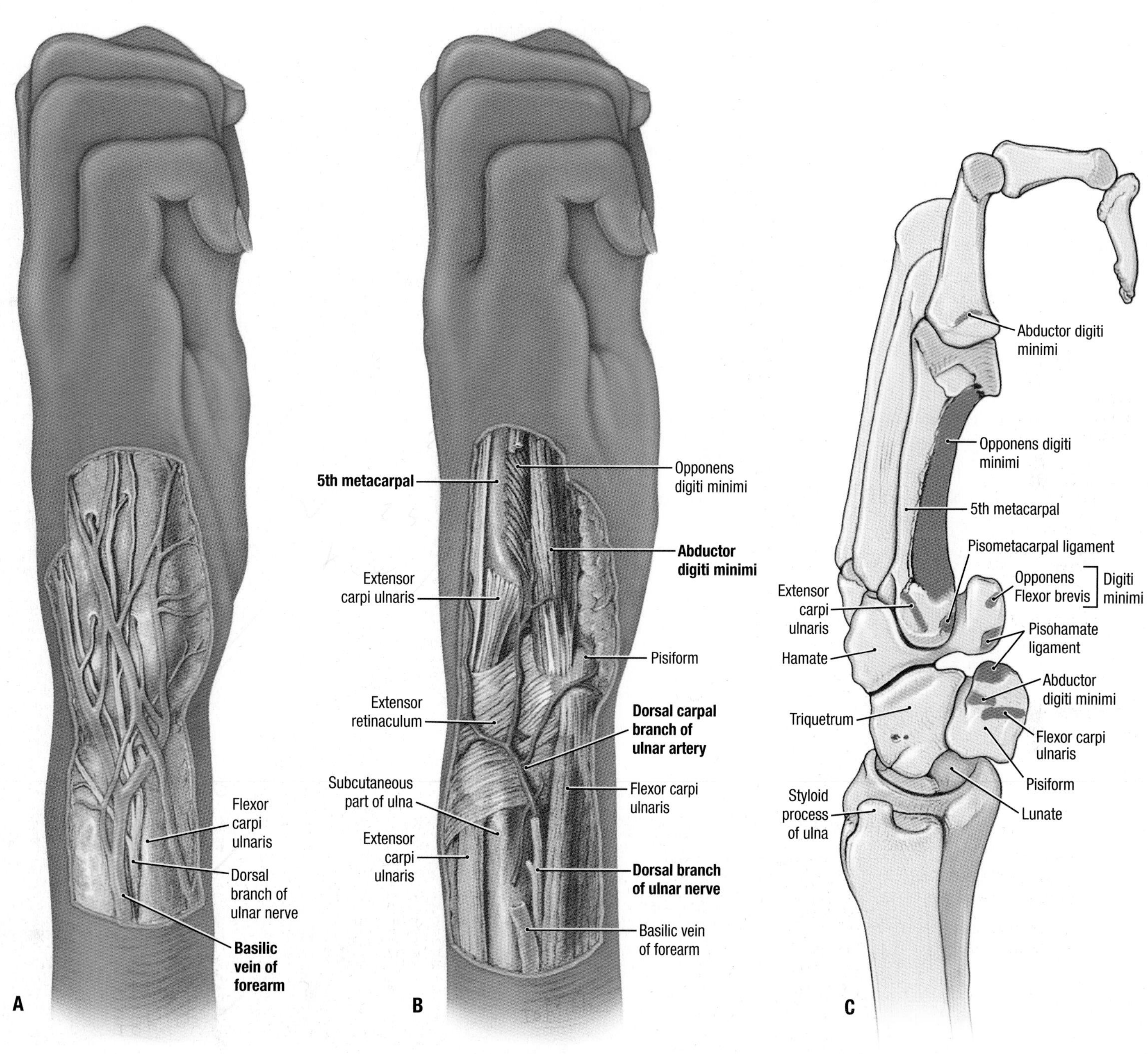
Flexor carpi ulnaris
Dorsal branch of ulnar nerve
Basilic vein of forearm
A
5th metacarpal
Extensor carpi ulnaris
Extensor retinaculum
Subcutaneous part of ulna
Extensor carpi ulnaris
Opponens digiti minimi
Abductor digiti minimi
Pisiform
Dorsal carpal branch of ulnar artery
Flexor carpi ulnaris
Dorsal branch of ulnar nerve
Basilic vein of forearm
B
Abductor digiti minimi
Opponens digiti minimi
5th metacarpal
Pisometacarpal ligament
Opponens
Flexor brevis
Digiti minimi
Extensor carpi ulnaris
Hamate
Pisohamate ligament
Abductor digiti minimi
Triquetrum
Flexor carpi ulnaris
Pisiform
Styloid process of ulna
Lunate
C
Medial Views

6.90 MEDIAL ASPECT OF WRIST AND HAND

A. Superficial dissection. **B.** Deep dissection. **C.** Bony hand showing sites of muscular and ligamentous attachments. The extensor carpi ulnaris is inserted directly into the base of the fifth metacarpal, but the flexor carpi ulnaris inserts indirectly to the base of the fifth metacarpal via the pisiform and pisohamate and pisometacarpal ligaments. These ligaments are often considered to be a part of the distal attachment of flexor carpi ulnaris.

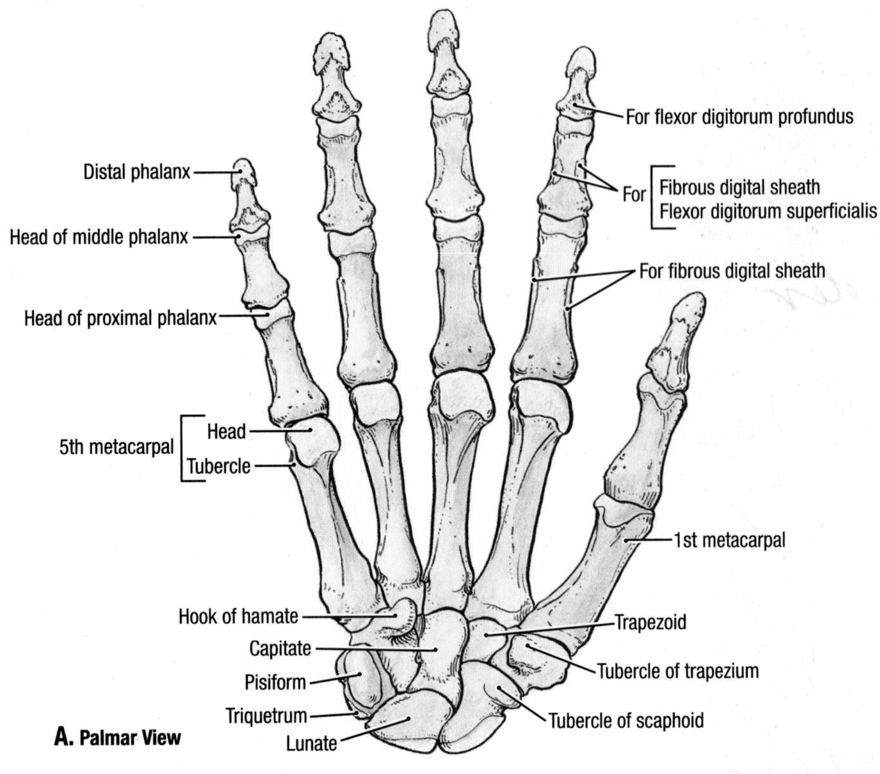
For flexor digitorum profundus
Distal phalanx
For
Fibrous digital sheath
Flexor digitorum superficialis
Head of middle phalanx
For fibrous digital sheath
Head of proximal phalanx
5th metacarpal
Head
Tubercle
1st metacarpal
Hook of hamate
Trapezoid
Capitate
Tubercle of trapezium
Pisiform
Triquetrum
Tubercle of scaphoid
Lunate

A. Palmar View

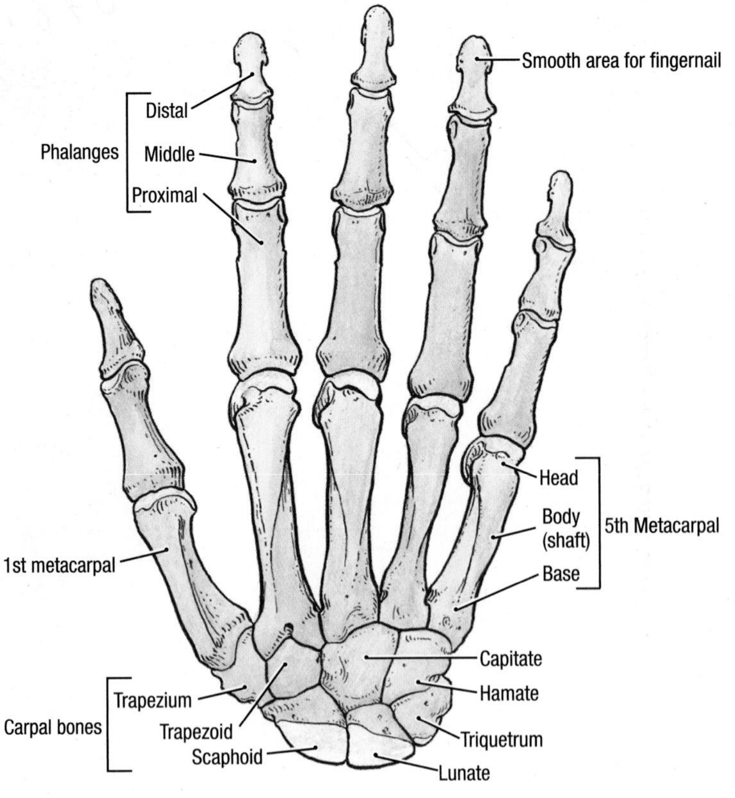
Smooth area for fingernail
Phalanges
Distal
Middle
Proximal
Head
Body (shaft)
5th Metacarpal
Base
1st metacarpal
Capitate
Hamate
Carpal bones
Trapezium
Trapezoid
Scaphoid
Triquetrum
Lunate

B. Dorsal View

6.91 BONES OF HAND

A. Palmar view. **B.** Dorsal view.

The eight carpal bones form two rows: in the distal row, the hamate, capitate, trapezoid, and trapezium, the trapezium forming a saddle-shaped joint with the 1st metacarpal, and in the proximal row, the scaphoid, lunate, and pisiform, the pisiform being superimposed on the triquetrum.

Severe **crushing injuries of the hand** may produce multiple metacarpal fractures, resulting in instability of the hand. Similar injuries of the distal phalanges are common (e.g., when a finger is caught in a car door).

A **fracture of a distal phalanx** is usually comminuted, and a painful **hematoma** (collection of blood) develops. **Fractures of the proximal and middle phalanges** are usually the result of crushing or hypertension injuries.

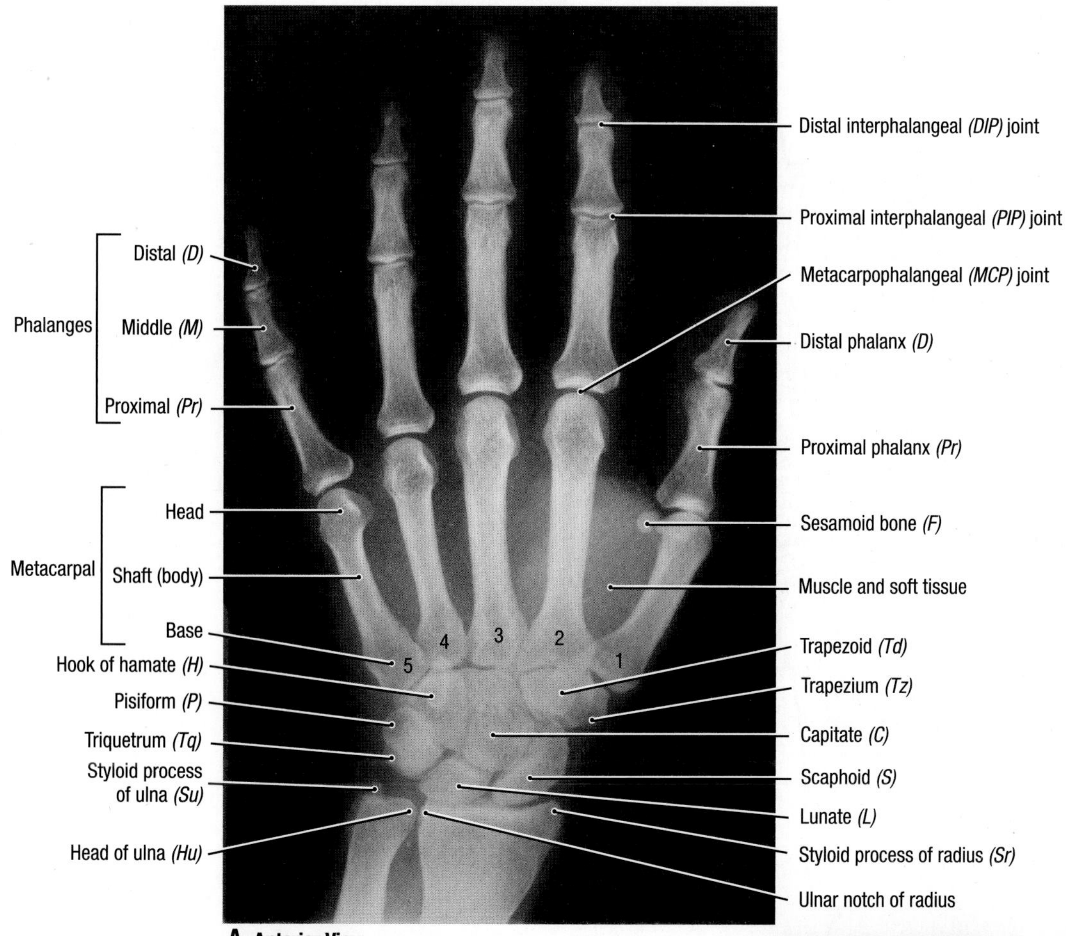
Distal interphalangeal (DIP) joint
Proximal interphalangeal (PIP) joint
Metacarpophalangeal (MCP) joint
Distal phalanx (D)
Proximal phalanx (Pr)
Sesamoid bone (F)
Muscle and soft tissue
Trapezoid (Td)
Trapezium (Tz)
Capitate (C)
Scaphoid (S)
Lunate (L)
Styloid process of radius (Sr)
Ulnar notch of radius
Phalanges
Distal (D)
Middle (M)
Proximal (Pr)
Metacarpal
Head
Shaft (body)
Base
Hook of hamate (H)
Pisiform (P)
Triquetrum (Tq)
Styloid process of ulna (Su)
Head of ulna (Hu)
1
2
3
4
5

A. Anterior View

DIP
PIP
MCP
D
M
Pr
D
Pr
F
F
1
2
3
4
5
H
C
Td
Tz
Su
P
T
L
S
Sr
Hu

B. Anterior View

6.92 IMAGING OF BONES OF WRIST AND HAND

A. Radiograph. **B.** Three-dimensional computer-generated image of wrist and hand (letters correspond to structures labeled in **A**).

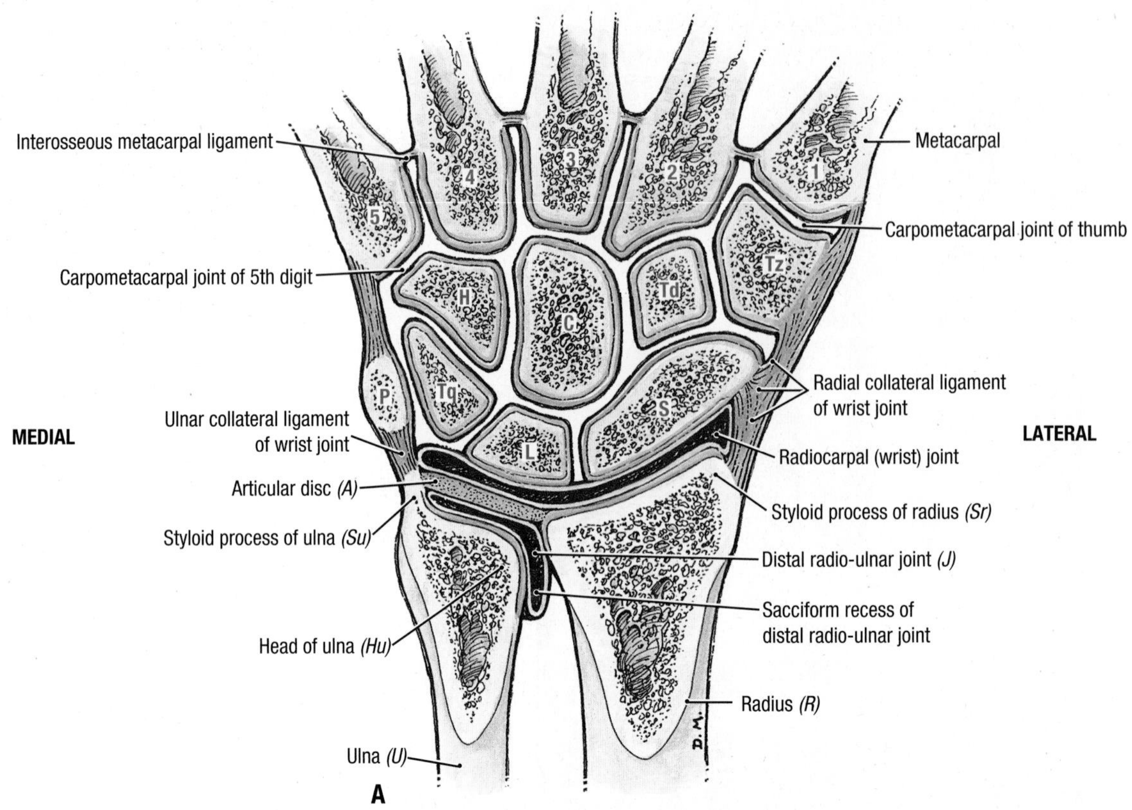
Interosseous metacarpal ligament
Metacarpal
Carpometacarpal joint of thumb
Carpometacarpal joint of 5th digit
Radial collateral ligament of wrist joint
MEDIAL
Ulnar collateral ligament of wrist joint
Radiocarpal (wrist) joint
LATERAL
Articular disc (A)
Styloid process of radius (Sr)
Styloid process of ulna (Su)
Distal radio-ulnar joint (J)
Sacciform recess of distal radio-ulnar joint
Head of ulna (Hu)
Radius (R)
Ulna (U)
1
2
3
4
5
H
C
Td
Tz
P
Tq
S
L
D.M.
A

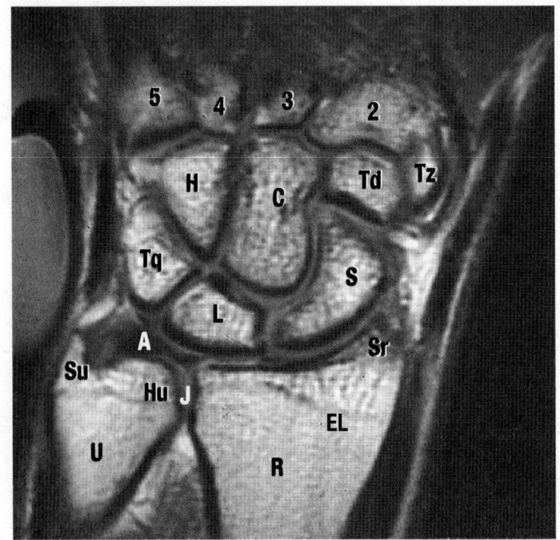
5
4
3
2
H
C
Td
Tz
Tq
S
L
A
Sr
Su
Hu
J
EL
U
R
B

6.93 CORONAL SECTION OF WRIST

A. Schematic illustration. **B.** Coronal MRI. *EL*, epiphysial line; letters correspond to structures labeled in **A**.

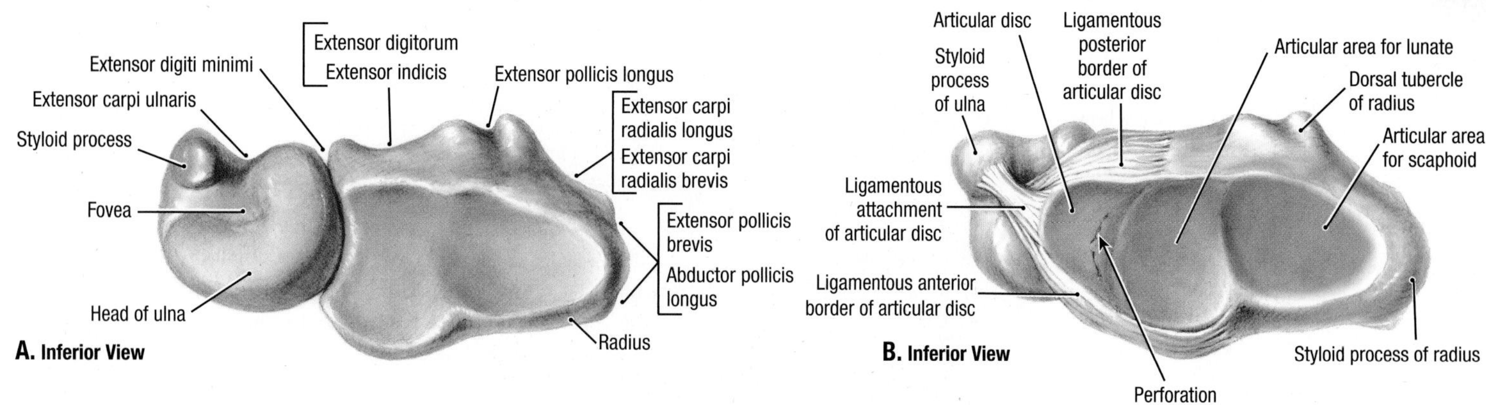
Extensor digitorum
Extensor indicis
Extensor digiti minimi
Extensor pollicis longus
Extensor carpi ulnaris
Extensor carpi radialis longus
Extensor carpi radialis brevis
Styloid process
Fovea
Extensor pollicis brevis
Abductor pollicis longus
Head of ulna
Radius
A. Inferior View
Articular disc
Ligamentous posterior border of articular disc
Styloid process of ulna
Articular area for lunate
Dorsal tubercle of radius
Articular area for scaphoid
Ligamentous attachment of articular disc
Ligamentous anterior border of articular disc
B. Inferior View
Styloid process of radius
Perforation

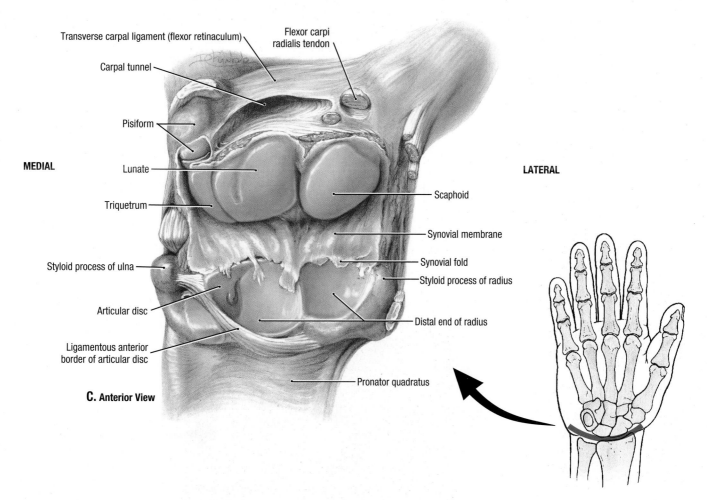

Transverse carpal ligament (flexor retinaculum)
Flexor carpi radialis tendon
Carpal tunnel
Pisiform
MEDIAL
Lunate
LATERAL
Scaphoid
Triquetrum
Synovial membrane
Synovial fold
Styloid process of ulna
Styloid process of radius
Articular disc
Distal end of radius
Ligamentous anterior border of articular disc
Pronator quadratus
C. Anterior View

6.94 RADIOCARPAL (WRIST) JOINT

A. Distal ends of radius and ulna showing grooves for tendons on the posterior aspects. **B.** Articular disc. The articular disc unites the distal ends of the radius and ulna; it is fibrocartilaginous at the triangular area between the head of the ulna and the lunate bone, but ligamentous and pliable elsewhere. The cartilaginous part of the articular disc commonly has a fissure or perforation, as shown here, associated with a roughened surface of the lunate. **C.** Articular surface of the radiocarpal joint, which is opened anteriorly. The lunate articulates with the radius and articular disc; only during adduction of the wrist does the triquetrum come into articulation with the disc.

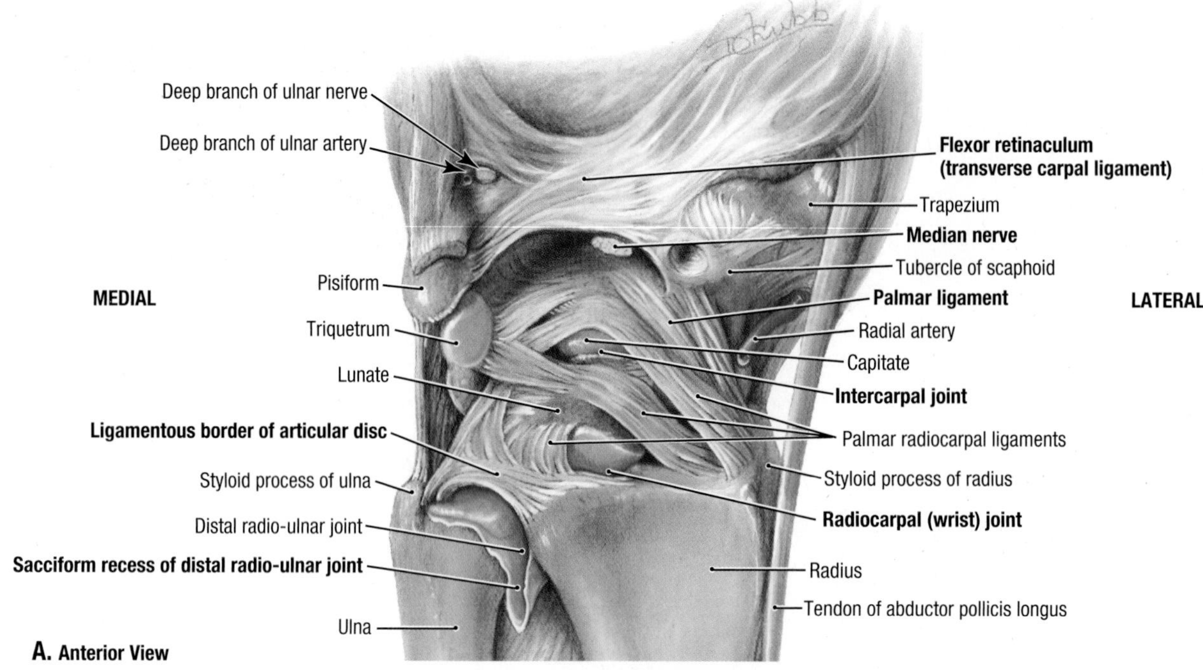
Deep branch of ulnar nerve
Deep branch of ulnar artery
Flexor retinaculum (transverse carpal ligament)
Trapezium
Median nerve
Tubercle of scaphoid
MEDIAL
Pisiform
Palmar ligament
LATERAL
Triquetrum
Radial artery
Capitate
Lunate
Intercarpal joint
Ligamentous border of articular disc
Palmar radiocarpal ligaments
Styloid process of ulna
Styloid process of radius
Distal radio-ulnar joint
Radiocarpal (wrist) joint
Sacciform recess of distal radio-ulnar joint
Radius
Tendon of abductor pollicis longus
Ulna

A. Anterior View

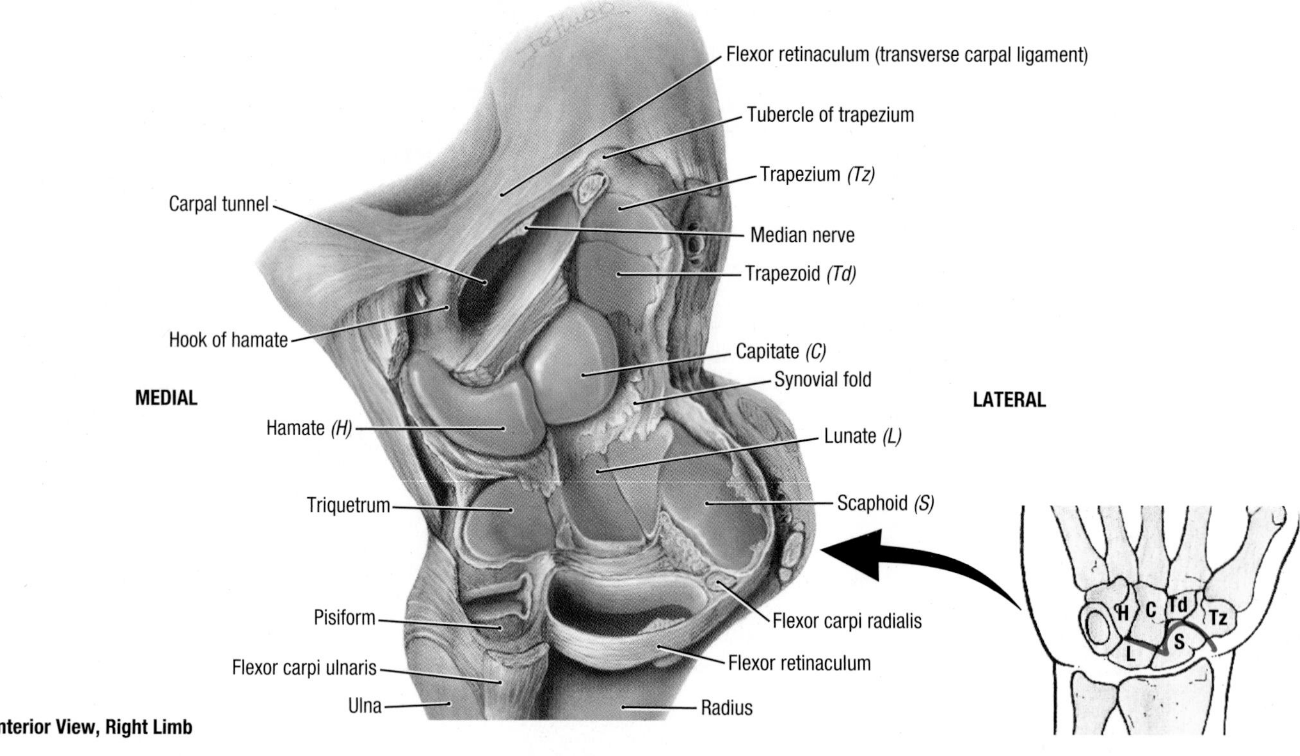
Flexor retinaculum (transverse carpal ligament)
Tubercle of trapezium
Trapezium (Tz)
Carpal tunnel
Median nerve
Trapezoid (Td)
Hook of hamate
Capitate (C)
Synovial fold
MEDIAL
LATERAL
Hamate (H)
Lunate (L)
Triquetrum
Scaphoid (S)
Pisiform
Flexor carpi radialis
Flexor carpi ulnaris
Flexor retinaculum
Ulna
Radius
H
C
Td
Tz
L
S

B. Anterior View, Right Limb

6.95 RADIOCARPAL (WRIST) AND MIDCARPAL (TRANSVERSE CARPAL) JOINT

A. Ligaments. The hand is forcibly extended. The palmar radiocarpal ligaments pass from the radius to the two rows of carpal bones; they are strong and directed so that the hand moves with the radius during supination.
B. Articular surfaces of midcarpal (transverse carpal) joint, opened anteriorly.

- The flexor retinaculum (transverse carpal ligament) is cut; the proximal part of the ligament, which spans from the pisiform to the scaphoid, is relatively weak; the distal part, which passes from the hook of the hamate to the tubercle of the trapezium, is strong.
- The opposed bones have sinuous surfaces: the trapezium and trapezoid together form a concave, oval surface for the scaphoid, and the capitate and hamate together form a convex surface for the scaphoid, lunate, and triquetrum.

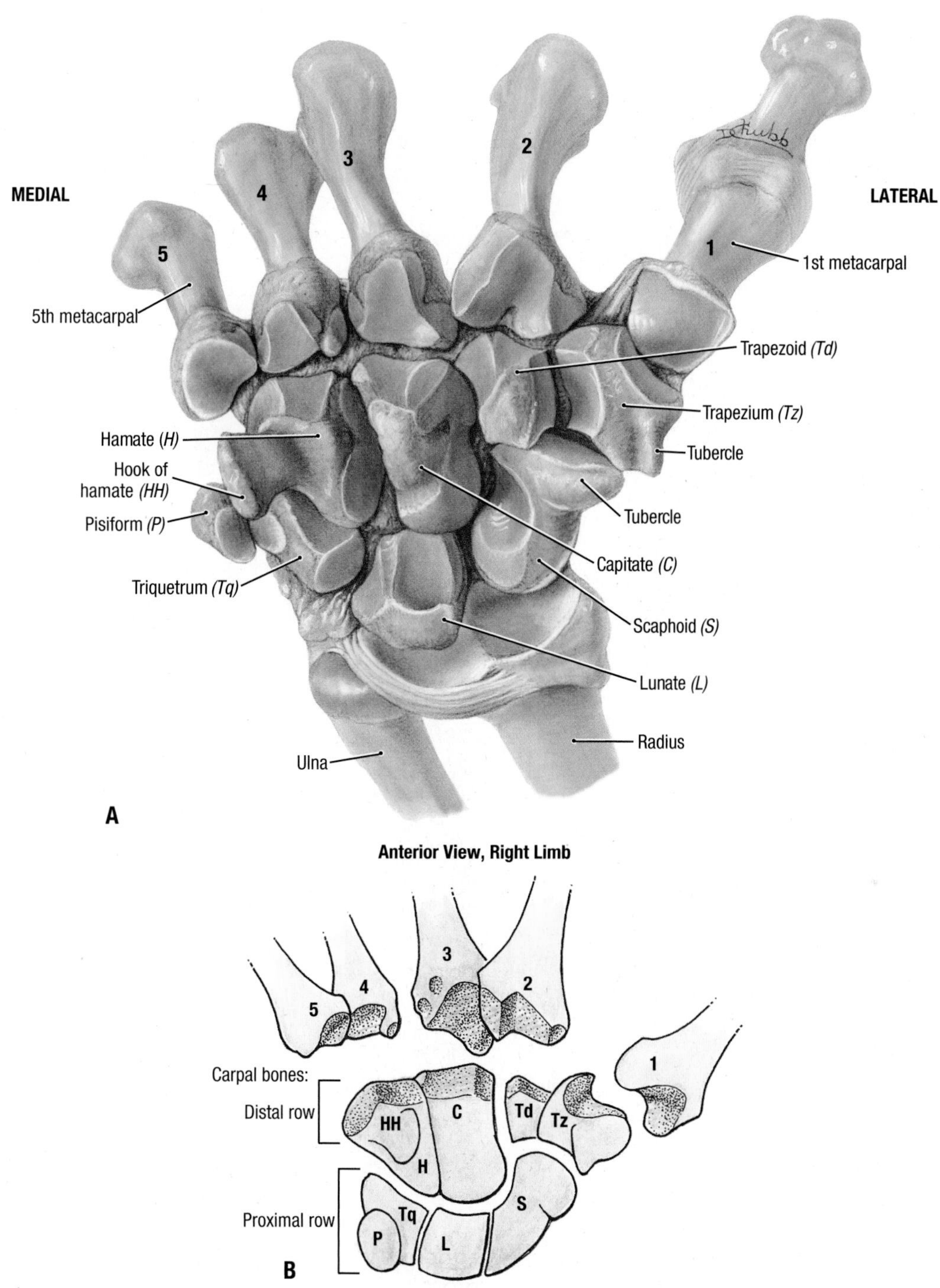
MEDIAL
LATERAL
5
4
3
2
1
1st metacarpal
5th metacarpal
Trapezoid (Td)
Trapezium (Tz)
Tubercle
Hamate (H)
Hook of hamate (HH)
Pisiform (P)
Tubercle
Capitate (C)
Triquetrum (Tq)
Scaphoid (S)
Lunate (L)
Radius
Ulna
A
Anterior View, Right Limb
Carpal bones:
Distal row
Proximal row
HH
H
C
Td
Tz
Tq
P
L
S
B

6.96 CARPAL BONES AND BASES OF METACARPALS

A. Open intercarpal and carpometacarpal (CMC) joints. The dorsal ligaments remain intact, and all the joints have been hyperextended, permitting study of articular facets. **B.** Diagram of the articular surfaces of the CMC joints (*letters* refer to structures labeled in **A**).

- The capitate articulates with three metacarpals (2nd, 3rd, and 4th).
- The 2nd metacarpal articulates with three carpals (trapezium, trapezoid, and capitate).
- The 1st CMC joint is saddle-shaped and especially mobile, allowing opposition of the thumb; the 2nd and 3rd CMC joints have interlocking surfaces and are practically immobile; and the 4th and 5th are hinge-shaped synovial joints with limited movement.

Anterior dislocation of the lunate is a serious injury that usually results from a fall on the extended wrist. The lunate is pushed to the palmar surface of the wrist and may compress the median nerve and lead to carpal tunnel syndrome. Because of poor blood supply, **avascular necrosis of the lunate** may occur.

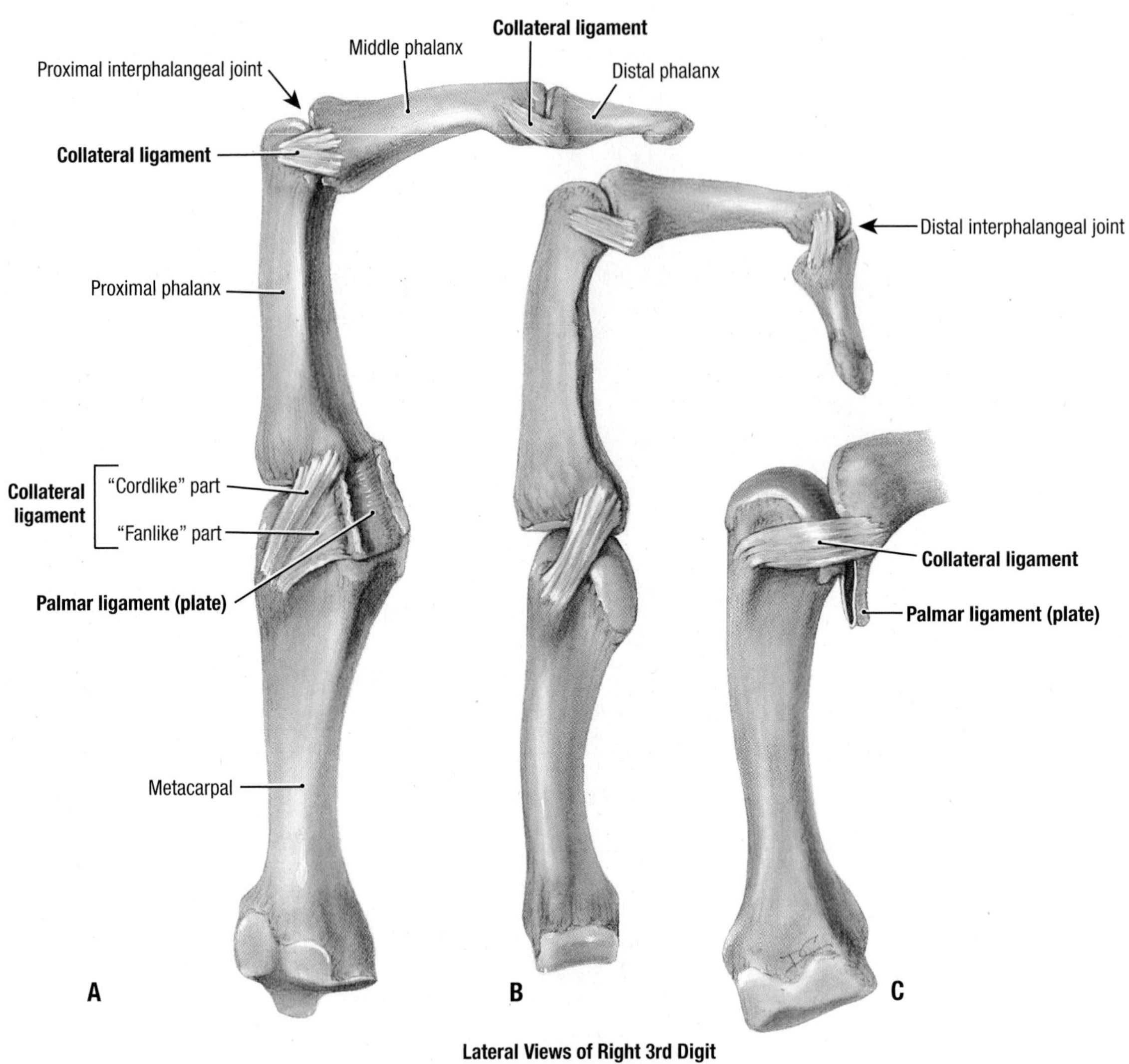
Collateral ligament
Middle phalanx
Proximal interphalangeal joint
Distal phalanx
Collateral ligament
Distal interphalangeal joint
Proximal phalanx
Collateral ligament
"Cordlike" part
"Fanlike" part
Palmar ligament (plate)
Collateral ligament
Palmar ligament (plate)
Metacarpal
A
B
C

Lateral Views of Right 3rd Digit

6.97 COLLATERAL LIGAMENTS OF METACARPOPHALANGEAL AND INTERPHALANGEAL JOINTS OF THIRD DIGIT

A. Extended metacarpophalangeal (MCP) and distal interphalangeal (IP) joints. **B.** Flexed interphalangeal joints. **C.** Flexed MCP joint.

- A fibrocartilaginous plate, the palmar ligament, hangs from the base of the proximal phalanx; is fixed to the head of the metacarpal by the weaker, fanlike part of the collateral ligament (**A**); and moves like a visor across the metacarpal head (**C**). The IP joints have similar palmar ligaments.
- The extremely strong, cordlike parts of the collateral ligaments of this joint (**A** and **B**) are eccentrically attached to the metacarpal heads; they are slack during extension and taut during flexion (**C**), so the fingers cannot be spread (abducted) unless the hand is open; the IP joints have similar collateral ligaments.

Skier's thumb refers to the rupture or chronic laxity of the collateral ligament of the 1st metacarpophalangeal joint. The injury results from hyperextension of the joint, which occurs when the thumb is held by the ski pole while the rest of the hand hits the ground or enters the snow.

TABLE 6.16 LESIONS OF NERVES OF UPPER LIMB

Nerve Injury	Injury Description	Impairments	Clinical Aspect
Long thoracic nerve	Stab wound Mastectomy	Abduction of shoulder joint and protraction of the scapula is compromised	Test: Pushing against a wall causes winging of scapula
Axillary nerve	Surgical neck fracture of humerus Anterior dislocation of shoulder joint	Abduction of shoulder joint to horizontal is compromised; sensory loss on lateral side of upper arm	Test: Abduct shoulder joint to horizontal and ask patient to hold position against a downward pull
Radial nerve	Midshaft fracture of humerus Badly fitted crutch Arm draped over a chair	Extension at wrist and joints of digits is lost; supination of forearm is compromised; sensory loss on posterior arm and forearm, and lateral aspect of dorsum of hand	Wrist drop
Median nerve at elbow	Supra-epicondylar fracture of humerus	Flexion of wrist joint is weakened; hand will deviate to ulnar side during flexion of wrist joint; flexion of DIP, PIP and MP joints of index and middle digits is lost; abduction, opposition and flexion of thumb joints are lost; sensory loss on palmar and dorsal aspects of index, middle, and lateral half of ring fingers and palmar aspect of thumb	Absence of thumb opposition Hand of benediction
Median nerve at wrist	Slashing of wrist Carpal tunnel syndrome	Weakened flexion of MP joints of index and middle fingers; opposition and abduction of CMC and MP joint of thumb lost; sensory loss same as for median nerve injury at elbow	Test: Make an "O" with thumb and index finger
Ulnar nerve at elbow	Fracture of medial epicondyle of humerus	Hand will deviate to radial side during flexion of wrist joint; flexion of DIP joints of ring and little finger lost; flexion at MP joint and extension at PIP and DIP joints of little and ring finger are lost; adduction and abduction of MP joints of digits 2–5 lost; adduction of thumb lost; sensory loss on palmar and dorsal aspects of little and medial half of ring fingers	Claw hand
Ulnar nerve at wrist	Slashing of wrist	Flexion at MP joint and extension at PIP and DIP joints of little and ring fingers lost; adduction and abduction of MP joints of digits 2–5 lost; adduction of thumb lost; sensory loss same as for ulnar nerve injury at elbow	Test: Hold paper between middle and ring fingers

CMC, carpometacarpal joint; MP, metacarpophalangeal joint; PIP, proximal interphalangeal joint; DIP, distal interphalangeal joint.

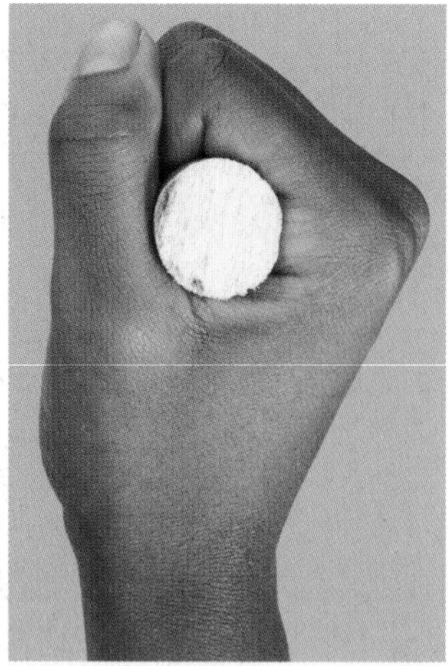

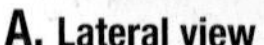

A. Lateral view

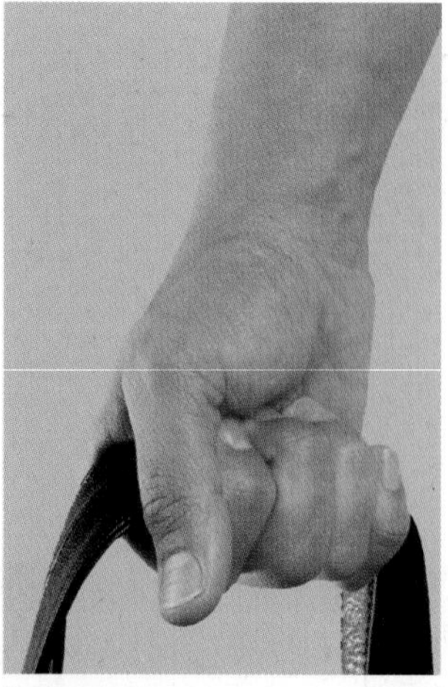

B. Anterior view

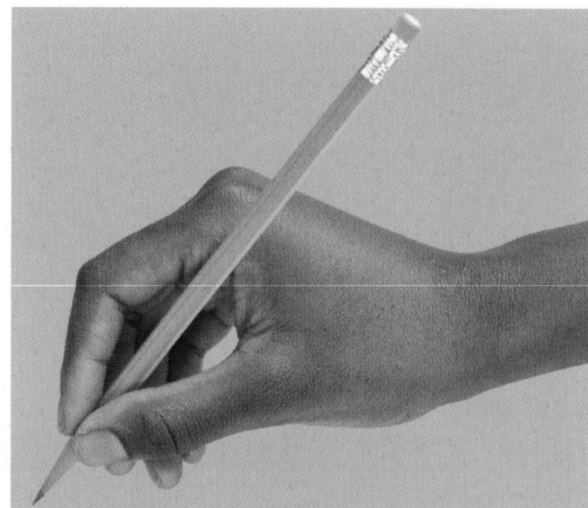

C. Medial view

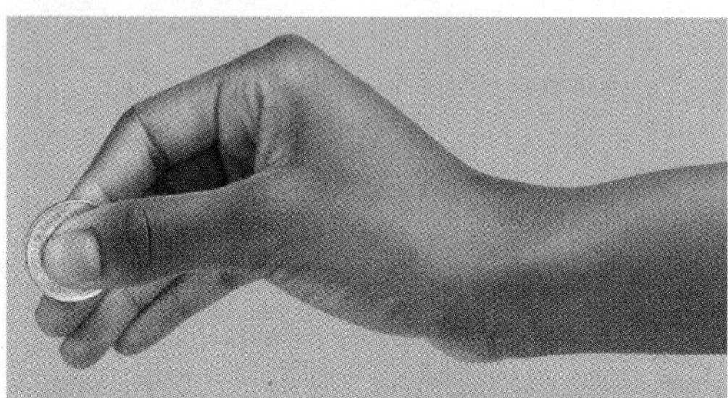

D. Medial view

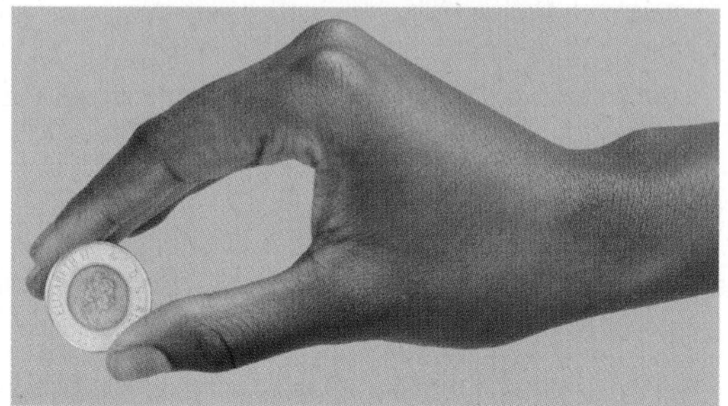

E. Medial view

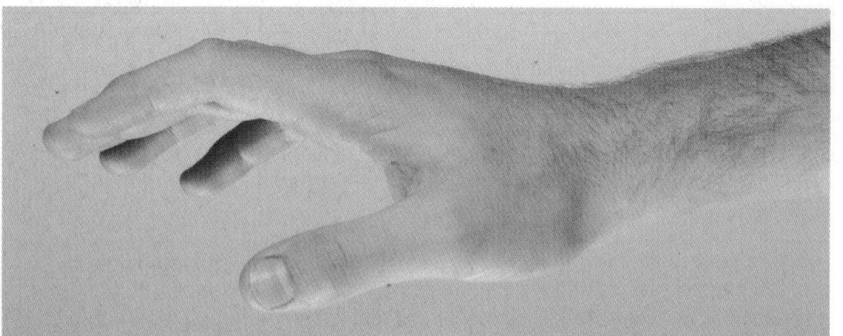

F. Medial view

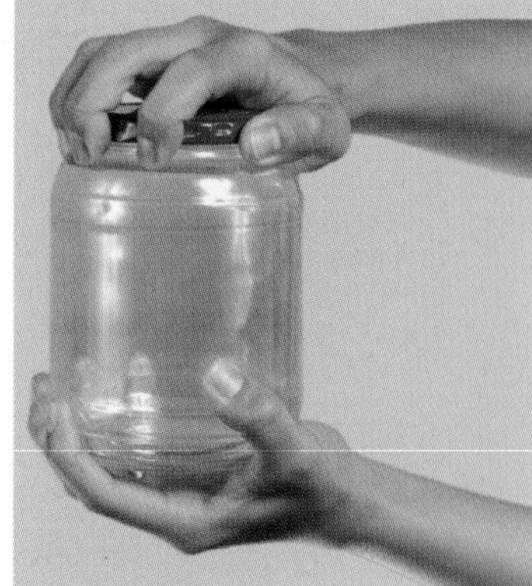

I. Lateral view

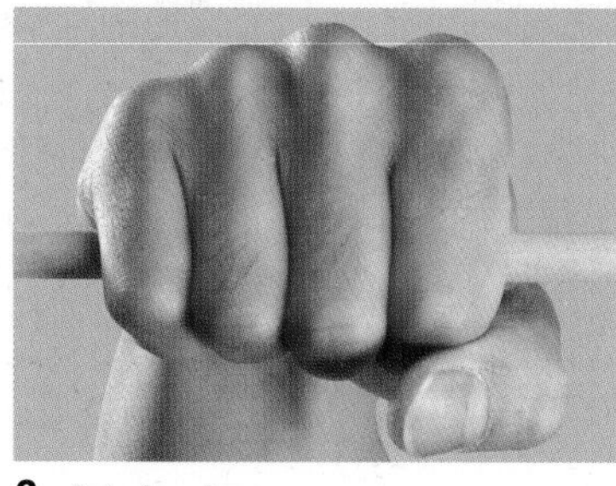

G. Anterior view

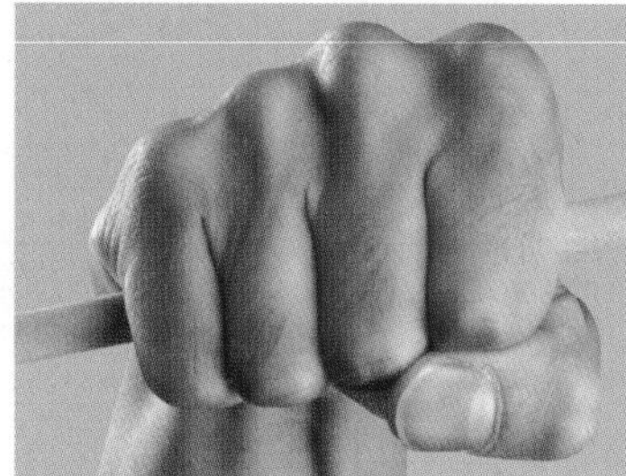

H. Anterior view

6.98 FUNCTIONAL POSITIONS OF HAND

A. Cylindrical (power) grasp. When grasping an object, the metacarpophalangeal and interphalangeal joints are flexed, but the radiocarpal joints are extended. Without wrist extension the grip is weak and insecure. **B.** Hook grasp. This grasp involves primarily the long flexors of the fingers, which are flexed to a varying degree depending on the size of the object. **C.** Tripod (three-jaw chuck) pinch. **D. and E.** Fingertip pinch. **F.** Rest position of hand. Casts for fractures are applied most often with the hand in this position. **G.** Loose cylindrical grasp. **H.** Firm cylindrical (power) grasp. **I.** Disc (power) grasp.

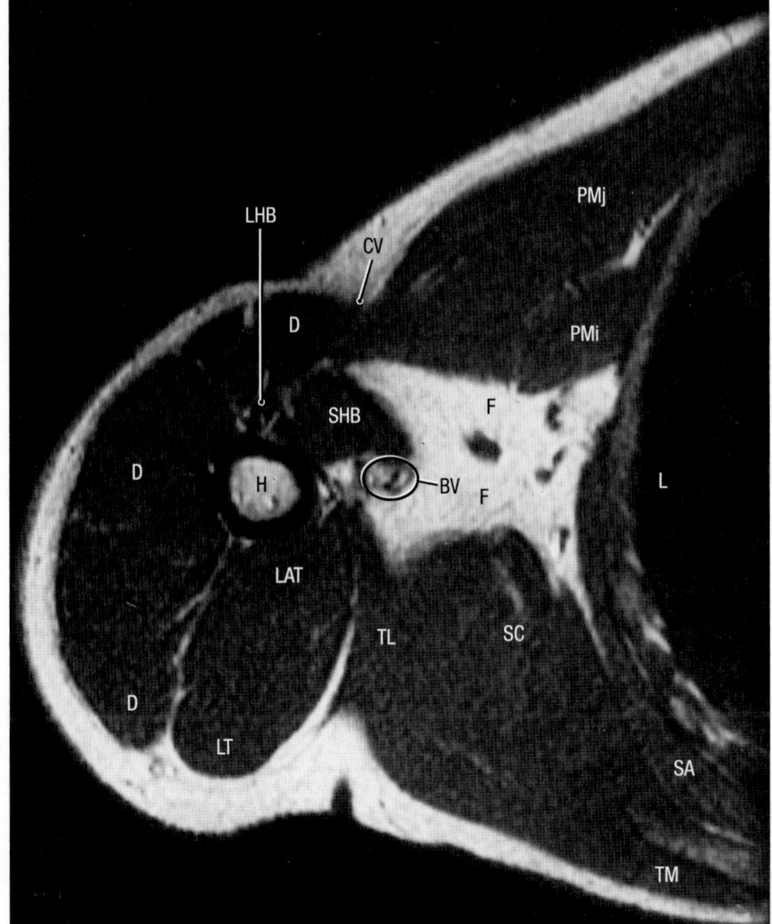
ANTERIOR
LHB
CV
PMj
D
PMi
SHB
F
D
H
BV
F
L
LAT
TL
SC
D
LT
SA
TM
A
POSTERIOR

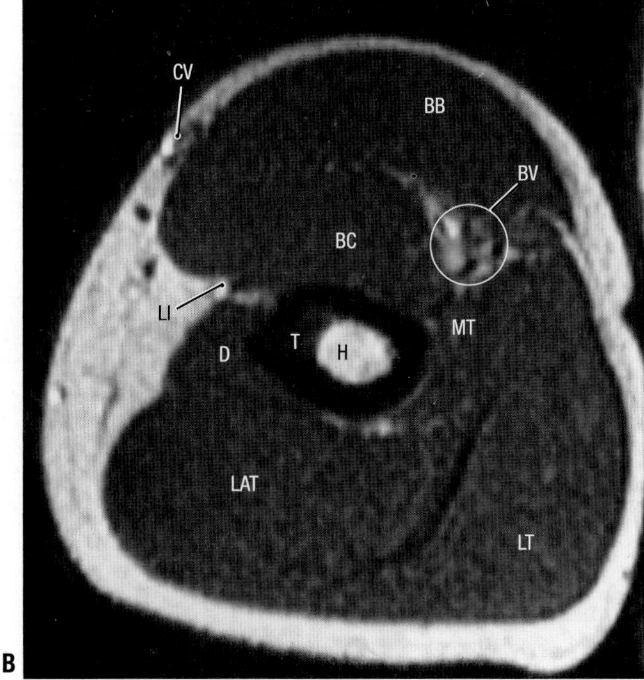
ANTERIOR
CV
BB
BV
BC
LI
T
H
MT
D
LAT
LT
B
POSTERIOR

ANTERIOR

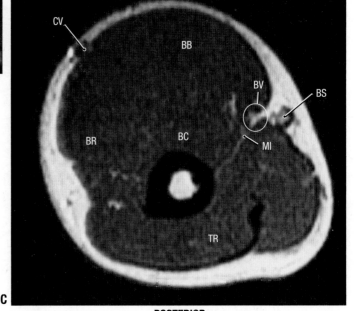

CV
BB
BV
BS
BR
BC
MI
TR
C

POSTERIOR

A
B
C

Key for A, B, and C:

BB	Biceps brachii
BC	Brachialis
BR	Brachioradialis
BS	Basilic Vein
BV	Brachial vessels and nerves
CV	Cephalic vein
D	Deltoid
F	Fat in axilla
H	Humerus
L	Lung
LAT	Lateral head of triceps brachii
LHB	Long head of biceps brachii
LI	Lateral intermuscular septum
LT	Long head of triceps brachii
MI	Medial intermuscular septum
MT	Medial head of triceps brachii
PMi	Pectoralis minor
PMj	Pectoralis major
SA	Serratus anterior
SC	Subscapularis
SHB	Short head of biceps brachii
T	Deltoid tuberosity
TL	Teres major and latissimus dorsi
TM	Teres minor
TR	Triceps brachii

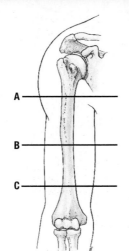

6.99 TRANSVERSE (AXIAL) MRIs OF ARM

A. Transverse MRI through the proximal arm. **B.** Transverse MRI though the middle of the arm. **C.** Transverse MRI through the distal arm.

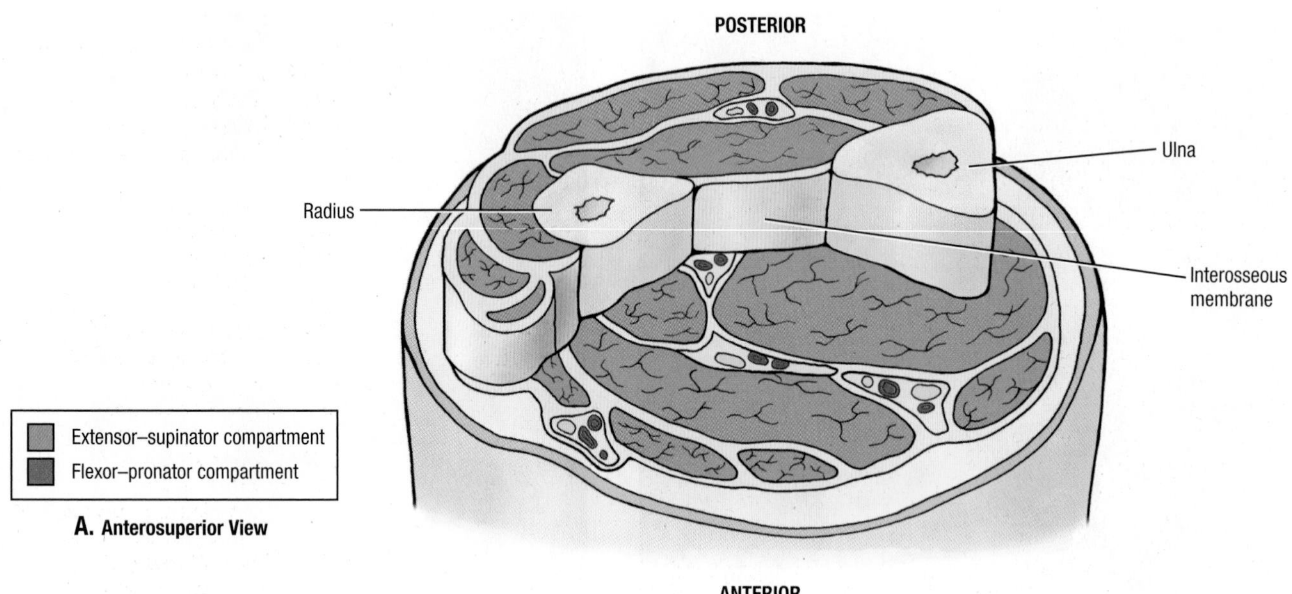
POSTERIOR
Ulna
Radius
Interosseous membrane
Extensor–supinator compartment
Flexor–pronator compartment
ANTERIOR

A. Anterosuperior View

Flexors:

1 Pronator teres
2 Flexor carpi radialis
3 Palmaris longus
4 Flexor carpi ulnaris
5 Flexor digitorum superficialis
6 Flexor digitorum profundus
7 Flexor pollicis longus

Extensors:

8 Brachioradialis
9 Extensor carpi radialis longus
10 Extensor carpi radialis brevis
11 Extensor digitorum
12 Extensor digiti minimi
13 Extensor carpi ulnaris
14 Abductor pollicis longus
15 Extensor pollicis brevis
16 Extensor pollicis longus and extensor indicis

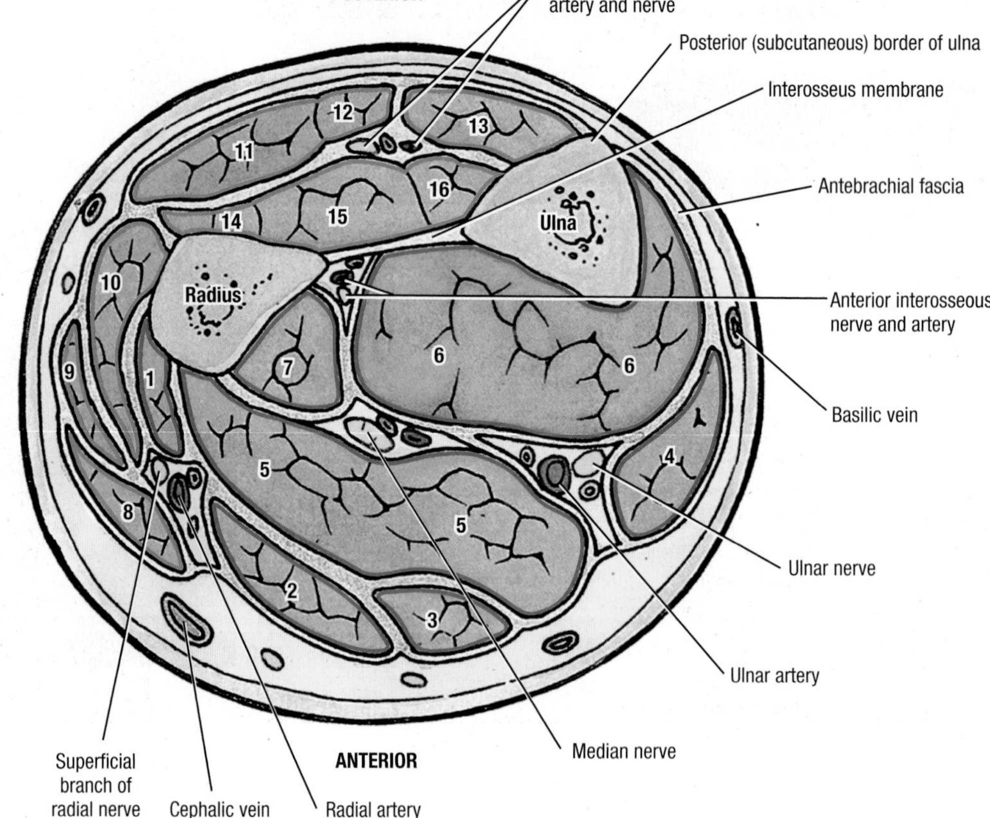
POSTERIOR
Posterior interosseous artery and nerve
Posterior (subcutaneous) border of ulna
Interosseus membrane
Antebrachial fascia
Ulna
Radius
Anterior interosseous nerve and artery
Basilic vein
Ulnar nerve
Ulnar artery
Median nerve
ANTERIOR
Superficial branch of radial nerve
Cephalic vein
Radial artery
1
2
3
4
5
6
7
8
9
10
11
12
13
14
15
16

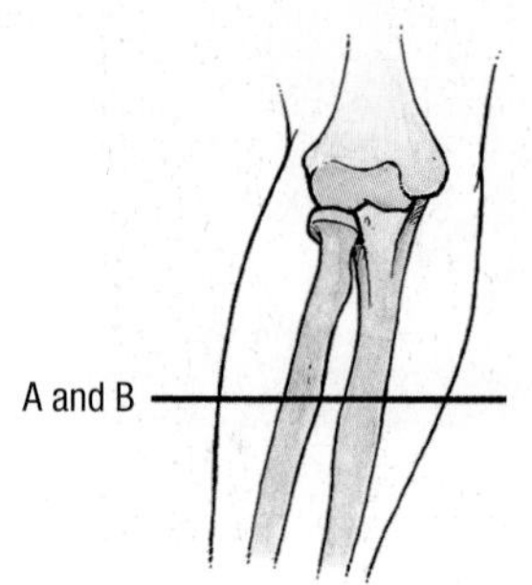
A and B

B. Transverse Section

6.100 TRANSVERSE SECTIONS AND TRANSVERSE (AXIAL) MRIs OF FOREARM

A. Stepped transverse sections of the anterior and posterior compartments. **B.** Contents of the anterior and posterior compartments.

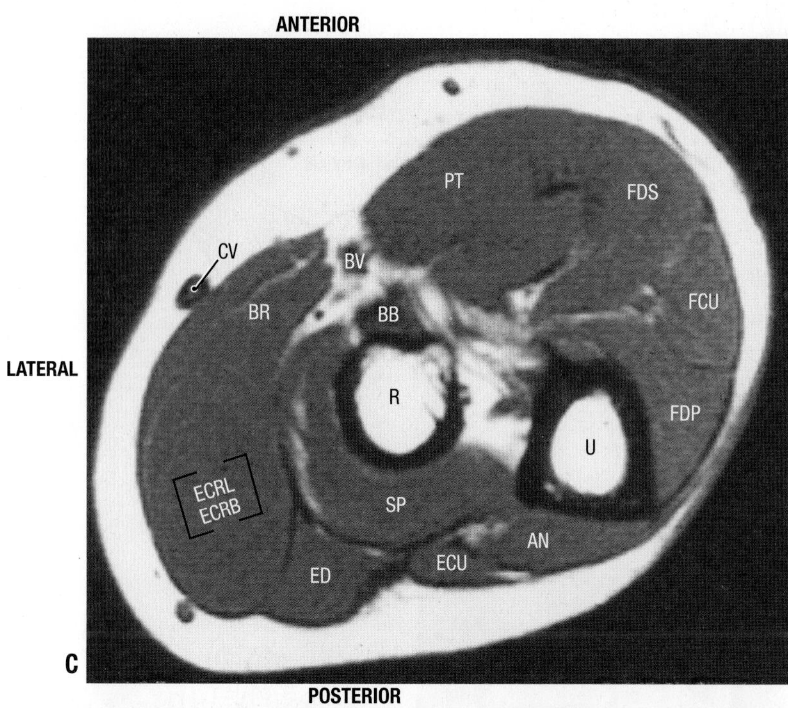
ANTERIOR
LATERAL
MEDIAL
POSTERIOR
C
PT
FDS
CV
BV
BR
BB
FCU
R
U
FDP
ECRL
ECRB
SP
AN
ED
ECU

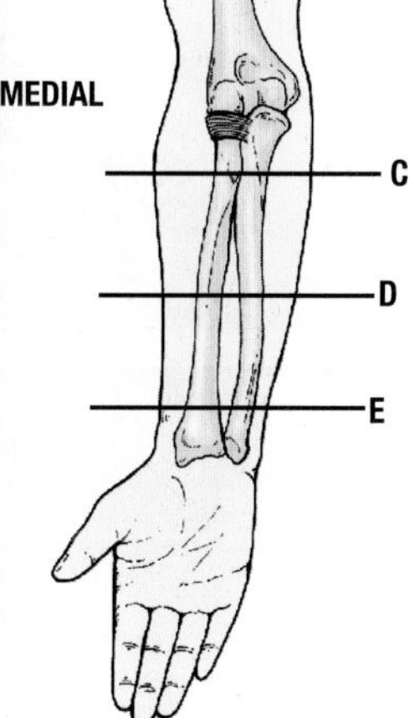
C
D
E

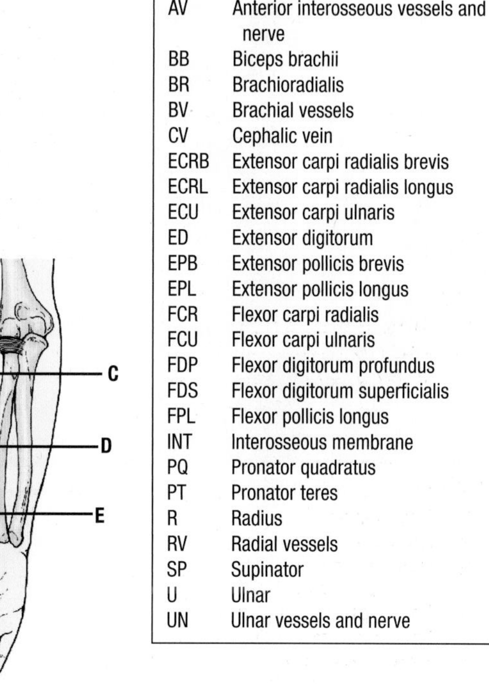

Key for C, D, and E:

AN	Anconeus
APL	Abductor pollicis longus
AV	Anterior interosseous vessels and nerve
BB	Biceps brachii
BR	Brachioradialis
BV	Brachial vessels
CV	Cephalic vein
ECRB	Extensor carpi radialis brevis
ECRL	Extensor carpi radialis longus
ECU	Extensor carpi ulnaris
ED	Extensor digitorum
EPB	Extensor pollicis brevis
EPL	Extensor pollicis longus
FCR	Flexor carpi radialis
FCU	Flexor carpi ulnaris
FDP	Flexor digitorum profundus
FDS	Flexor digitorum superficialis
FPL	Flexor pollicis longus
INT	Interosseous membrane
PQ	Pronator quadratus
PT	Pronator teres
R	Radius
RV	Radial vessels
SP	Supinator
U	Ulnar
UN	Ulnar vessels and nerve

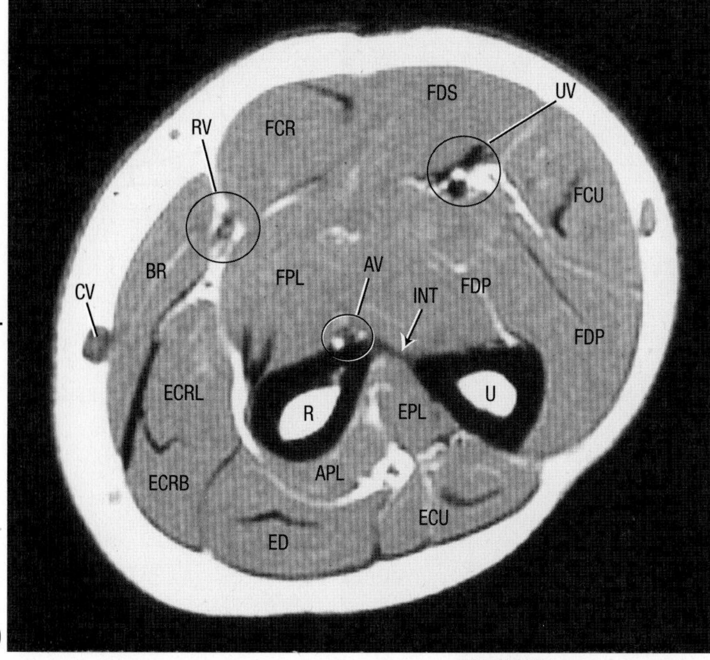
ANTERIOR
LATERAL
MEDIAL
POSTERIOR
D
FDS
UV
RV
FCR
FCU
BR
FPL
AV
INT
FDP
CV
FDP
ECRL
R
EPL
U
ECRB
APL
ECU
ED
ANTERIOR
LATERAL
MEDIAL
POSTERIOR
E
FCR
UV
FDS
FCU
FDP
PQ
U
FPL
EPL
R
EPB
ECU
ED
APL

6.100 TRANSVERSE SECTIONS AND TRANSVERSE (AXIAL) MRIs OF FOREARM *(CONTINUED)*

C. Transverse MRI through the proximal forearm. **D.** Transverse MRI through the middle forearm. **E.** Transverse MRI through the distal forearm.

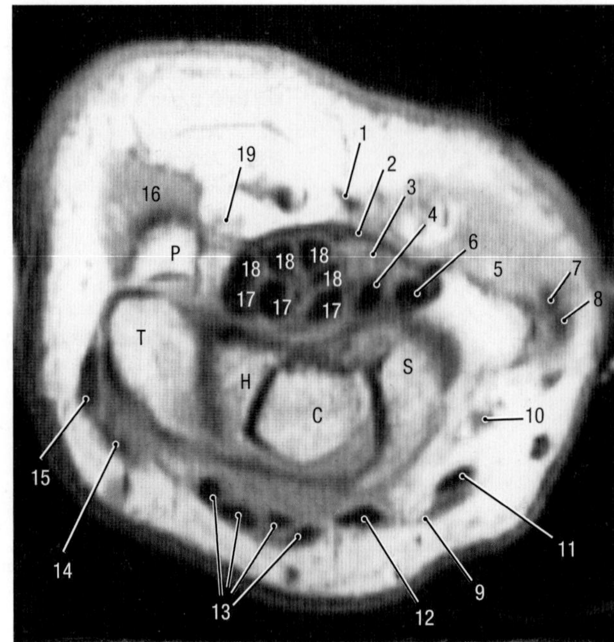
1
2
3
4
5
6
7
8
9
10
11
12
13
14
15
16
17
18
19
P
T
H
C
S

A. Transverse MRI

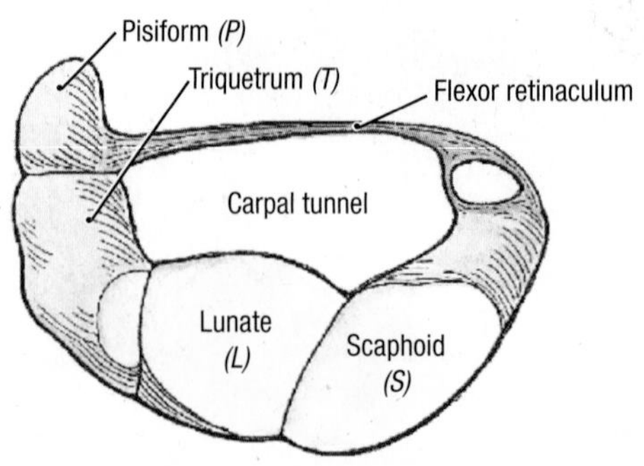
Pisiform (P)
Triquetrum (T)
Flexor retinaculum
Carpal tunnel
Lunate (L)
Scaphoid (S)

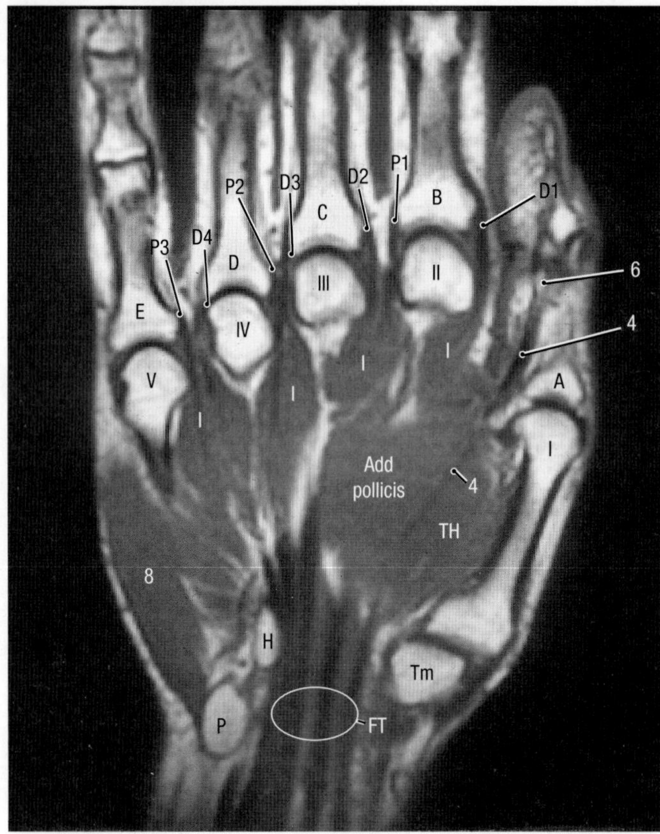
P1
P2
P3
D1
D2
D3
D4
A
B
C
D
E
I
II
III
IV
V
Add pollicis
TH
Tm
H
P
FT
4
6
8

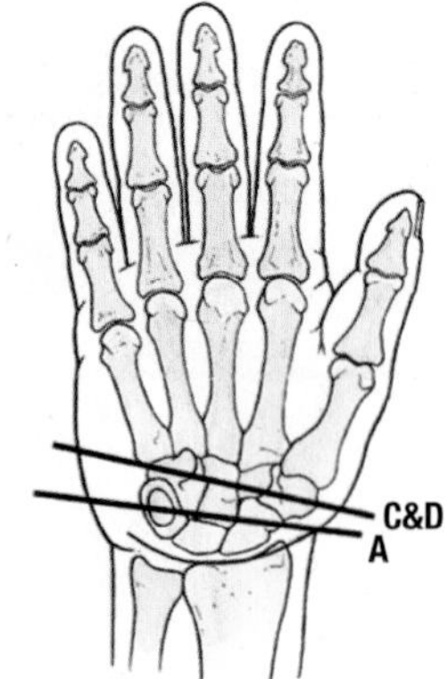
C&D
A

B. Coronal MRI

6.101 TRANSVERSE (AXIAL) SECTION AND MRIs THROUGH CARPAL TUNNEL

A. Transverse MRI through the proximal carpal tunnel (*numbers* and *letters* in MRIs refer to structures in **D**). **B.** Coronal MRI of wrist and hand showing the course of the long flexor tendons in the carpal tunnel (*numbers* and *letters* in MRIs refer to structures in **D**). *FT*, long flexor tendons in carpal tunnel; *TH*, thenar muscles; *P*, pisiform; *H*, hook of hamate; *Tm,* trapezium; *I*, interossei, *A–E,* proximal phalanges.

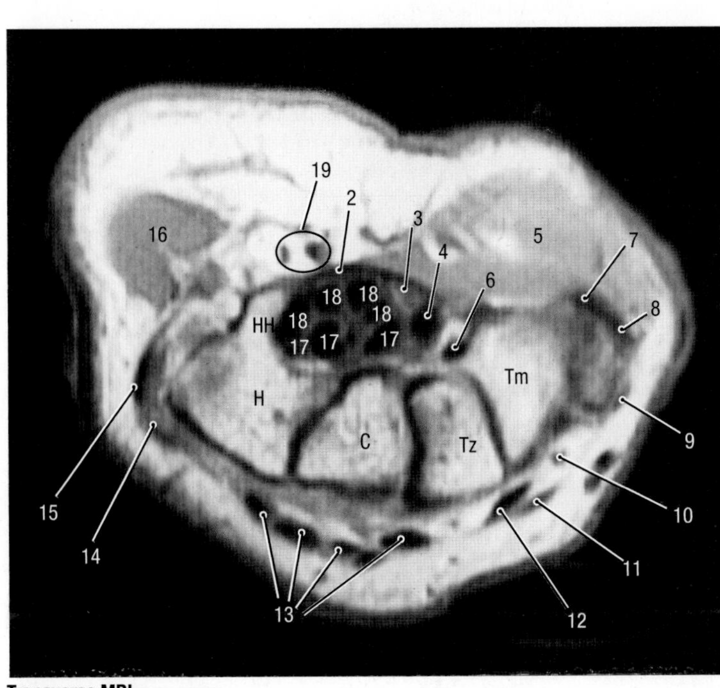
19
2
3
4
5
6
7
8
16
18 18
HH 18 18
17 17 17
H
Tm
C
Tz
9
10
11
12
13
14
15
C. Transverse MRI

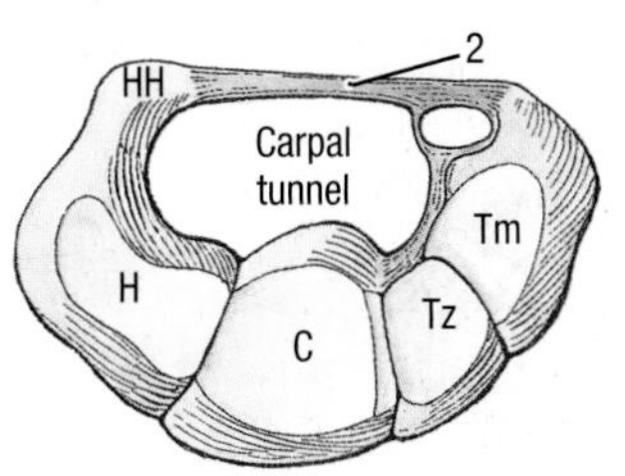
HH
2
Carpal tunnel
Tm
H
C
Tz

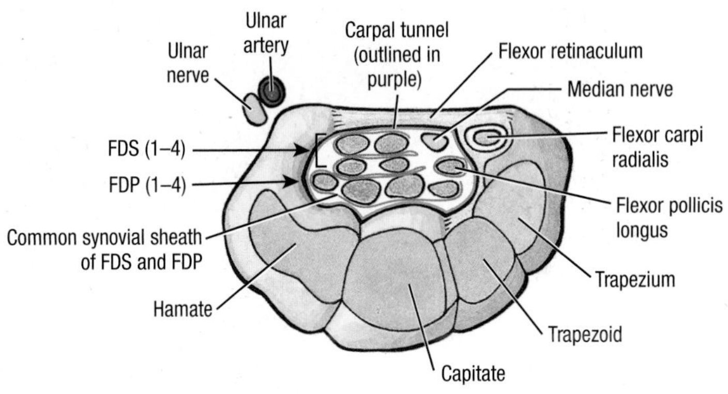
Ulnar nerve
Ulnar artery
Carpal tunnel (outlined in purple)
Flexor retinaculum
Median nerve
FDS (1–4)
FDP (1–4)
Flexor carpi radialis
Flexor pollicis longus
Common synovial sheath of FDS and FDP
Trapezium
Hamate
Trapezoid
Capitate

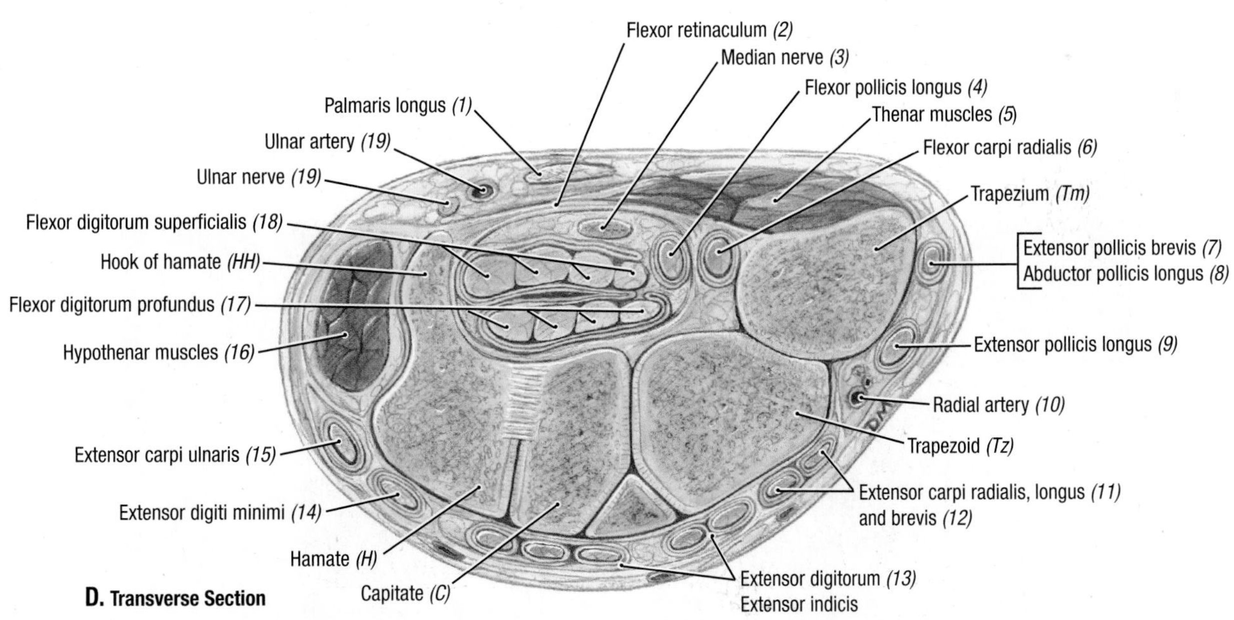
Flexor retinaculum (2)
Median nerve (3)
Flexor pollicis longus (4)
Palmaris longus (1)
Thenar muscles (5)
Ulnar artery (19)
Flexor carpi radialis (6)
Ulnar nerve (19)
Trapezium (Tm)
Flexor digitorum superficialis (18)
Extensor pollicis brevis (7)
Abductor pollicis longus (8)
Hook of hamate (HH)
Flexor digitorum profundus (17)
Extensor pollicis longus (9)
Hypothenar muscles (16)
Radial artery (10)
Trapezoid (Tz)
Extensor carpi ulnaris (15)
Extensor carpi radialis, longus (11) and brevis (12)
Extensor digiti minimi (14)
Hamate (H)
Extensor digitorum (13)
Extensor indicis
Capitate (C)
D. Transverse Section

6.101 TRANSVERSE (AXIAL) SECTION AND MRIs THROUGH CARPAL TUNNEL *(CONTINUED)*

C. Transverse MRI through the distal carpal tunnel (*numbers* and *letters* in MRIs refer to structures in **D**).
D. Transverse section of carpal tunnel through the distal row of carpal bones.

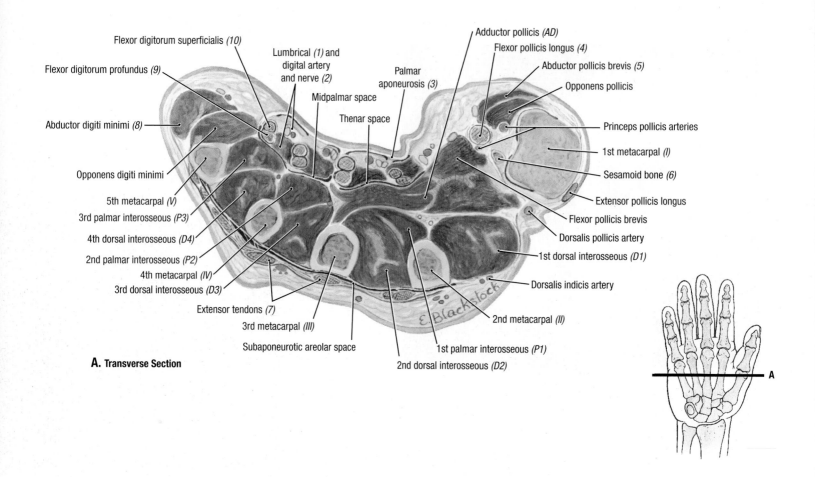

Flexor digitorum superficialis *(10)*
Flexor digitorum profundus *(9)*
Lumbrical *(1)* and digital artery and nerve *(2)*
Palmar aponeurosis *(3)*
Midpalmar space
Thenar space
Adductor pollicis *(AD)*
Flexor pollicis longus *(4)*
Abductor pollicis brevis *(5)*
Opponens pollicis
Princeps pollicis arteries
1st metacarpal *(I)*
Sesamoid bone *(6)*
Extensor pollicis longus
Flexor pollicis brevis
Dorsalis pollicis artery
1st dorsal interosseous *(D1)*
Dorsalis indicis artery
2nd metacarpal *(II)*
1st palmar interosseous *(P1)*
2nd dorsal interosseous *(D2)*
Subaponeurotic areolar space
3rd metacarpal *(III)*
Extensor tendons *(7)*
3rd dorsal interosseous *(D3)*
4th metacarpal *(IV)*
2nd palmar interosseous *(P2)*
4th dorsal interosseous *(D4)*
3rd palmar interosseous *(P3)*
5th metacarpal *(V)*
Opponens digiti minimi
Abductor digiti minimi *(8)*
E Blackstock
A

A. Transverse Section

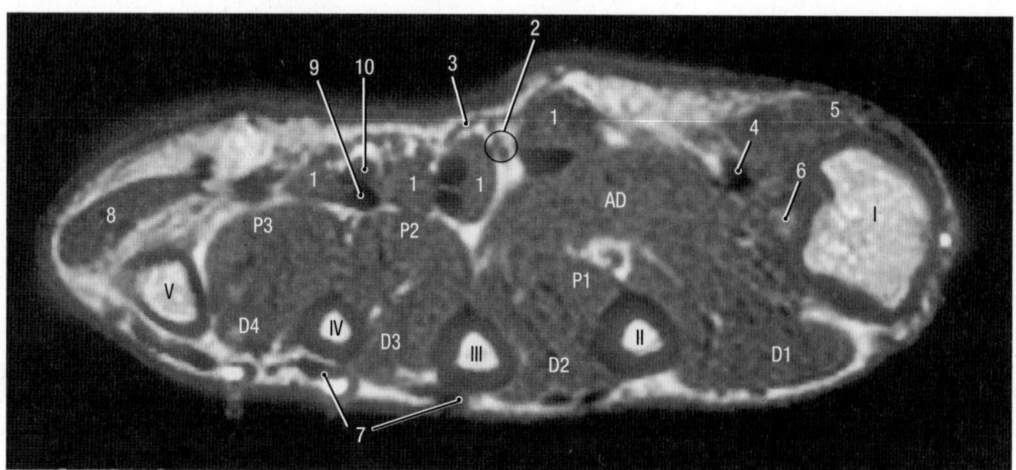

2
9
10
3
1
5
4
6
1
1
1
AD
8
P3
P2
I
P1
V
D4
IV
D3
III
II
D2
D1
7

B. Transverse MRI

6.102 TRANSVERSE SECTION AND MRI THROUGH PALM (METACARPALS) AT LEVEL OF ADDUCTOR POLLICIS

CHAPTER 7

Head

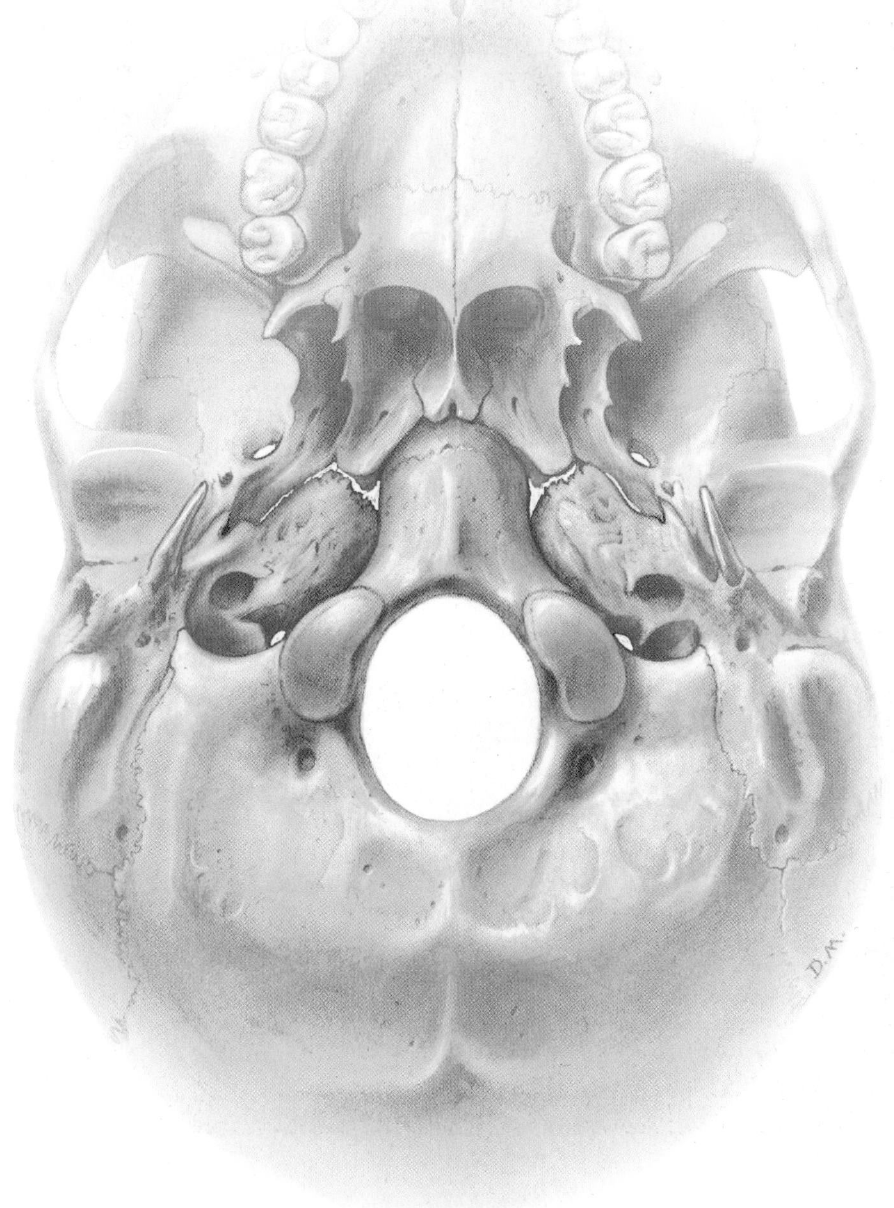

Cranium	612
Face and Scalp	632
Meninges and Meningeal Spaces	641
Cranial Base and Cranial Nerves	646
Blood Supply of Brain	652
Orbit and Eyeball	656
Parotid Region	668
Temporal Region and Infratemporal Fossa	670
Temporomandibular Joint	678
Tongue	682
Palate	688
Teeth	691
Nose, Paranasal Sinuses, and Pterygopalatine Fossa	696
Ear	709
Lymphatic Drainage of Head	722
Autonomic Innervation of Head	723
Imaging of Head	724
Neuroanatomy: Overview and Ventricular System	728
Telencephalon (Cerebrum) and Diencephalon	731
Brainstem and Cerebellum	740
Imaging of Brain	746

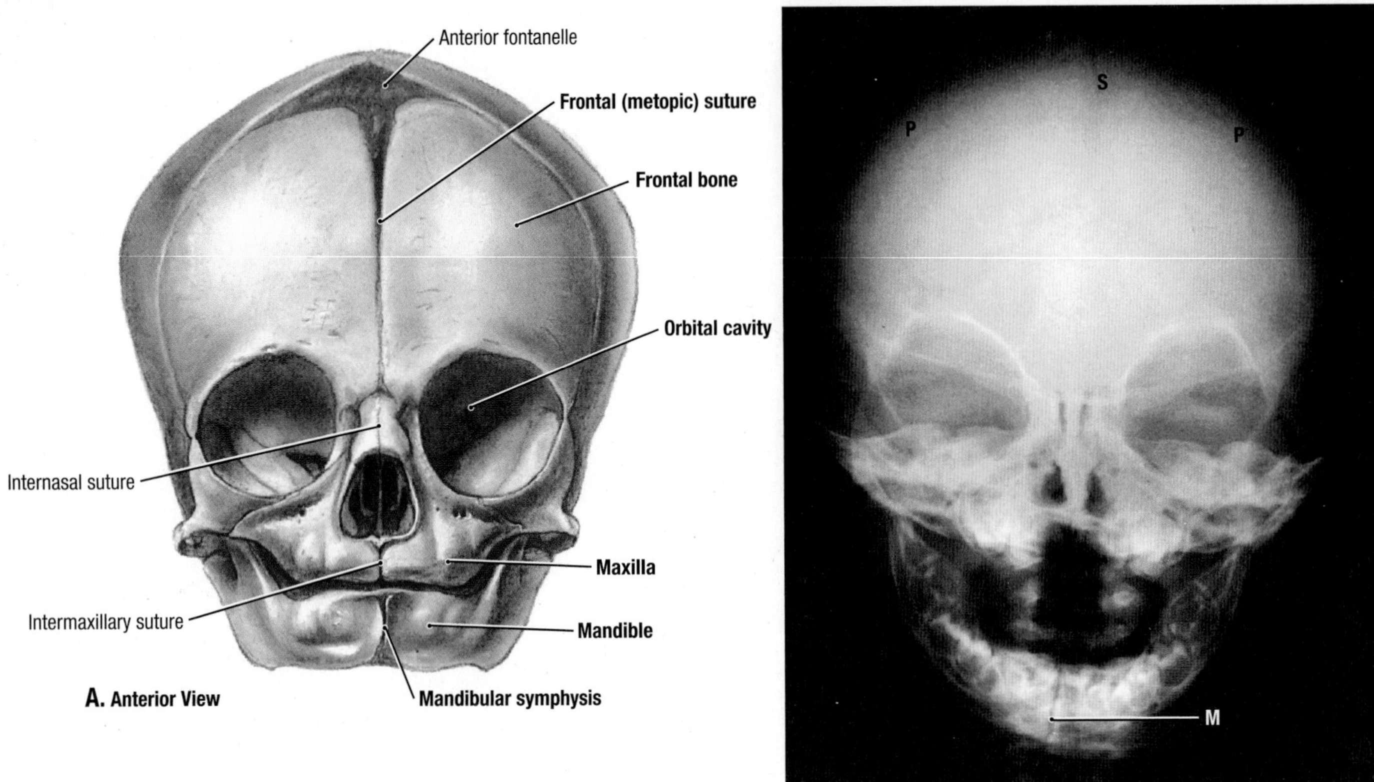

Anterior fontanelle
Frontal (metopic) suture
Frontal bone
Orbital cavity
Internasal suture
Maxilla
Intermaxillary suture
Mandible
Mandibular symphysis
A. Anterior View
S
P
P
M

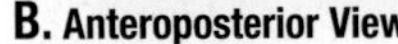

B. Anteroposterior View

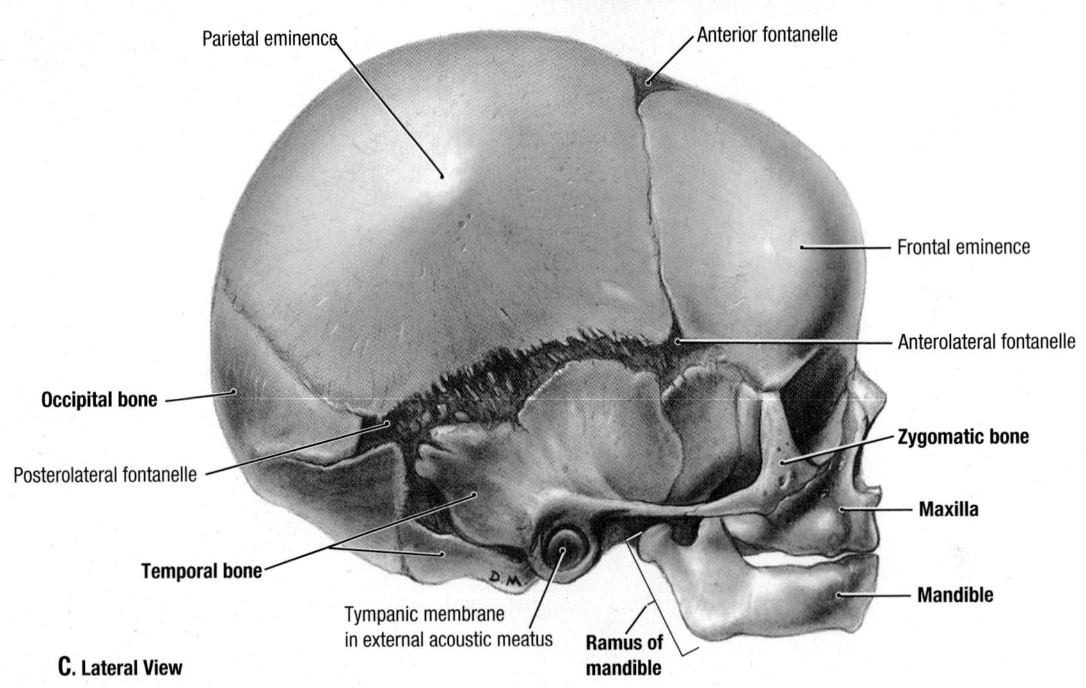

Parietal eminence
Anterior fontanelle
Frontal eminence
Anterolateral fontanelle
Occipital bone
Zygomatic bone
Posterolateral fontanelle
Maxilla
Temporal bone
Mandible
Tympanic membrane in external acoustic meatus
Ramus of mandible

C. Lateral View

7.1 CRANIUM AT BIRTH AND IN EARLY CHILDHOOD

A. Cranium at birth, anterior aspect. **B.** Radiograph of $6^1/_2$-month-old child. **C.** Cranium at birth, lateral aspect.

Compared with the adult skull (Figs. 7.2–7.4):

- The maxilla and mandible are proportionately small.
- The mandibular symphysis, which closes during the second year, and the frontal suture, which closes during the sixth year, are still open (unfused).
- The orbital cavities are proportionately large, but the face is small; the facial skeleton forming only one eighth of the whole cranium, while in the adult, it forms one third.

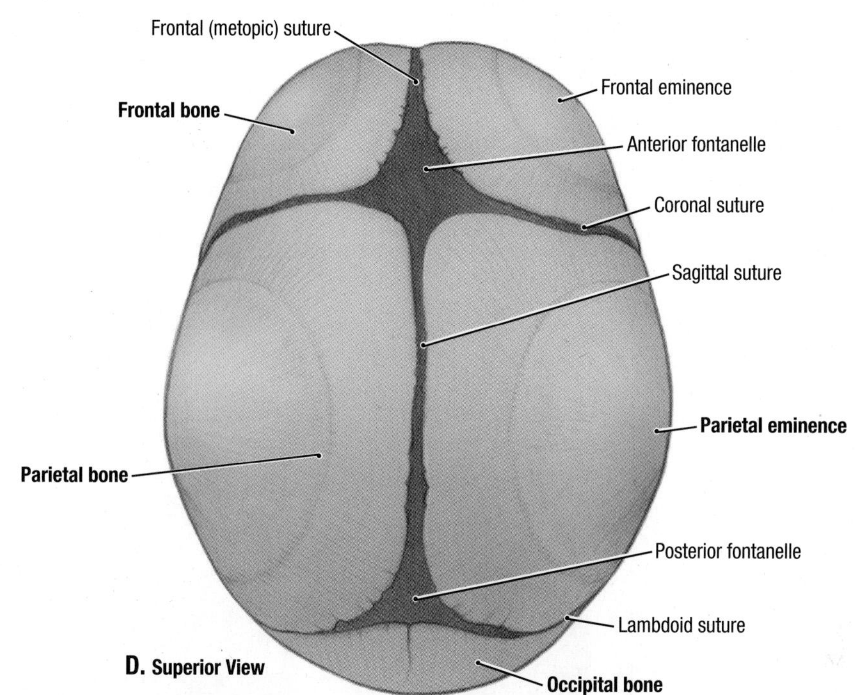
Frontal (metopic) suture
Frontal bone
Frontal eminence
Anterior fontanelle
Coronal suture
Sagittal suture
Parietal eminence
Parietal bone
Posterior fontanelle
Lambdoid suture
Occipital bone
D. Superior View

Key for B, E and F

A	Angle of mandible
B	Body of mandible
C	Coronal suture
F	Frontal bone
L	Lambdoid suture
M	Mandibular symphysis
O	Occipital bone
P	Parietal eminence
S	Sagittal suture
SP	Sphenoid
T	Temporal bone
X	Maxilla
Y	Mastoid process
Z	Zygomatic bone

Arrowheads = Membranous outline of parietal bone

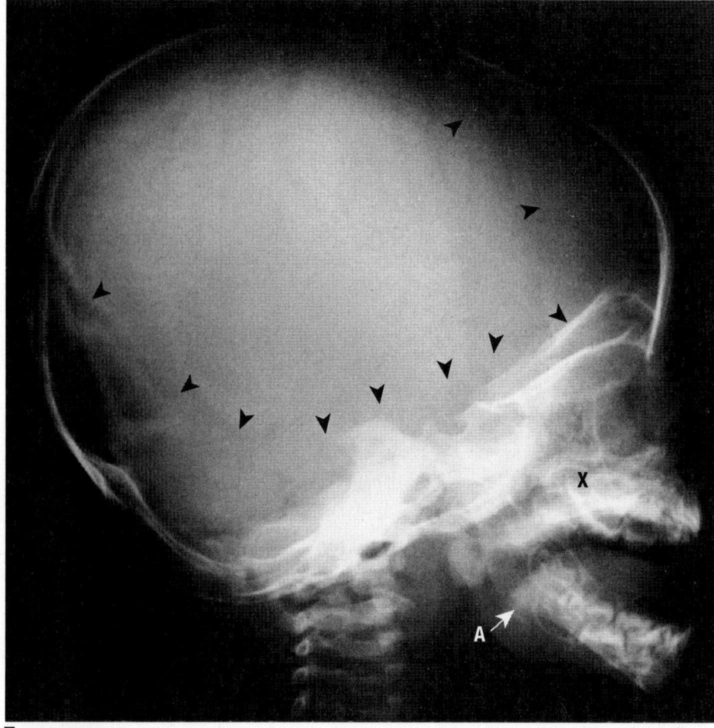
X
A
E. Lateral View

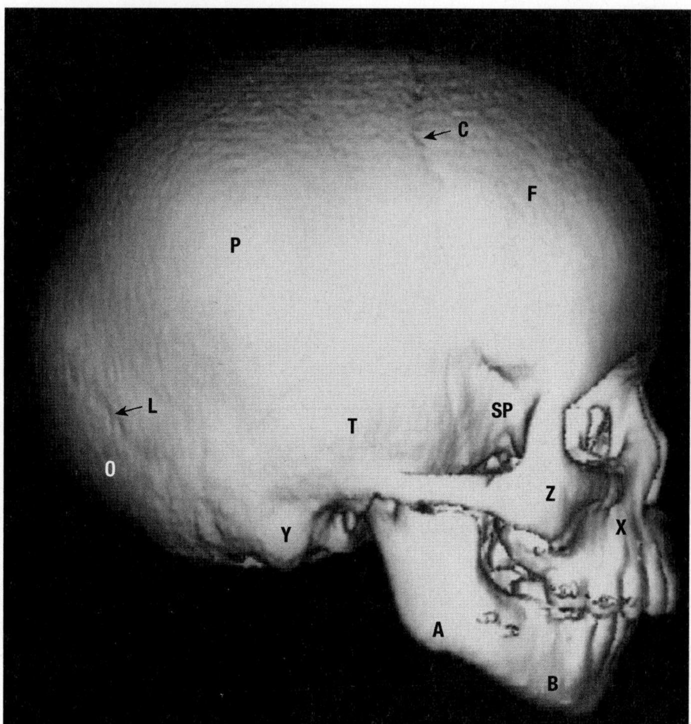
C
F
P
L
T
SP
O
Z
Y
X
A
B
F. Lateral View

7.1 CRANIUM AT BIRTH AND IN EARLY CHILDHOOD *(CONTINUED)*

D. Cranium at birth, superior aspect. **E.** Radiograph of $6^1/_2$-month-old child. **F.** Three-dimensional computer-generated images of 3-year-old child's cranium.

- The parietal eminence is a shallow, rounded cone. Ossification, which starts at the eminences, has not yet reached the ultimate four angles of the parietal bone; accordingly, these regions are membranous, and the membrane is blended with the pericranium externally and the dura mater internally to form the fontanelles. The fontanelles are usually closed by the second year. There is no mastoid process until the second year.

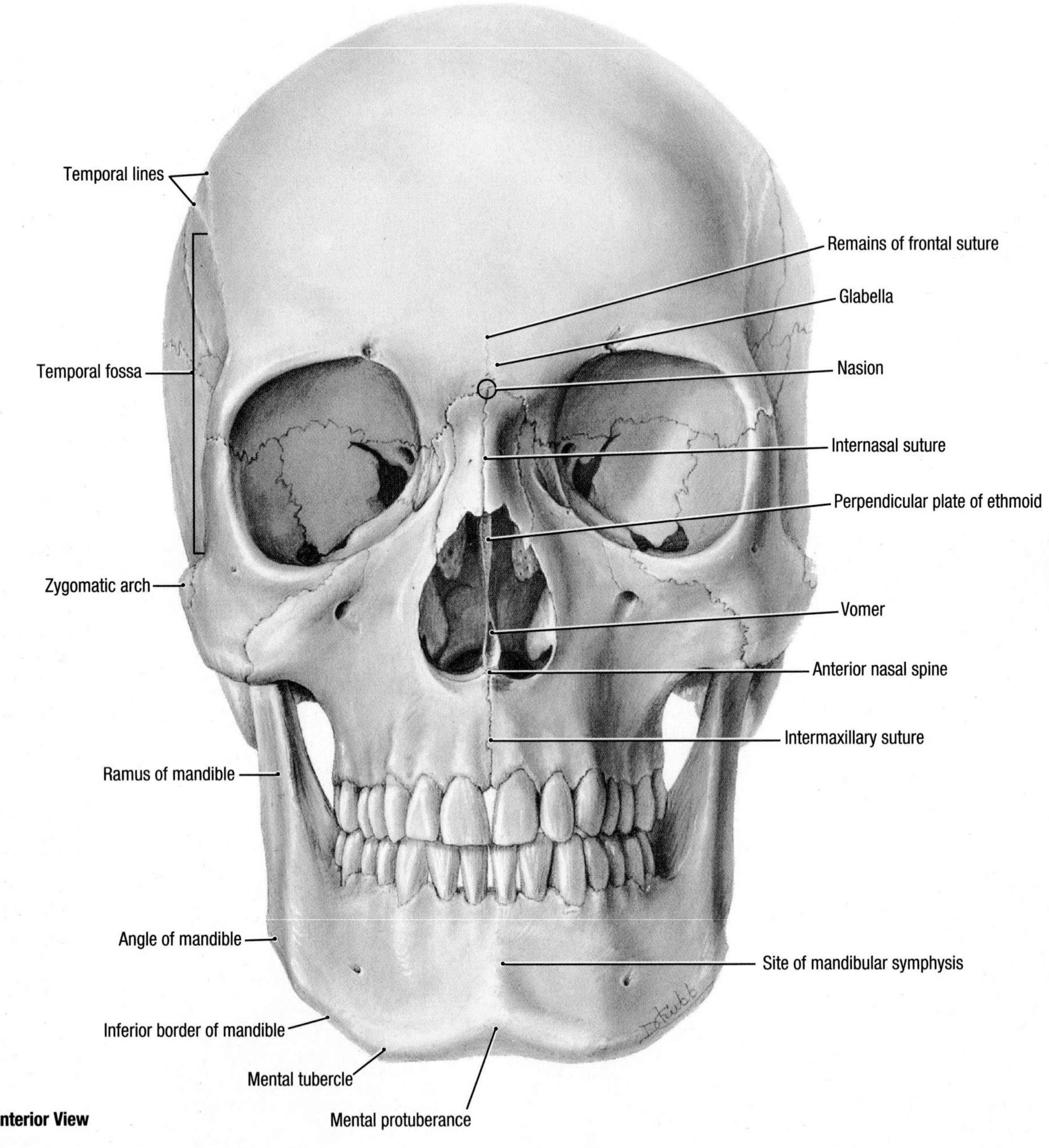

Temporal lines
Temporal fossa
Zygomatic arch
Ramus of mandible
Angle of mandible
Inferior border of mandible
Mental tubercle
Mental protuberance
Remains of frontal suture
Glabella
Nasion
Internasal suture
Perpendicular plate of ethmoid
Vomer
Anterior nasal spine
Intermaxillary suture
Site of mandibular symphysis

A. Anterior View

7.2 CRANIUM, FACIAL (FRONTAL) ASPECT

A. Formations of the bony cranium. **B.** Bones of cranium and their features. The individual bones forming the cranium are color coded. For the orbital cavity, see also Figure 7.36A.

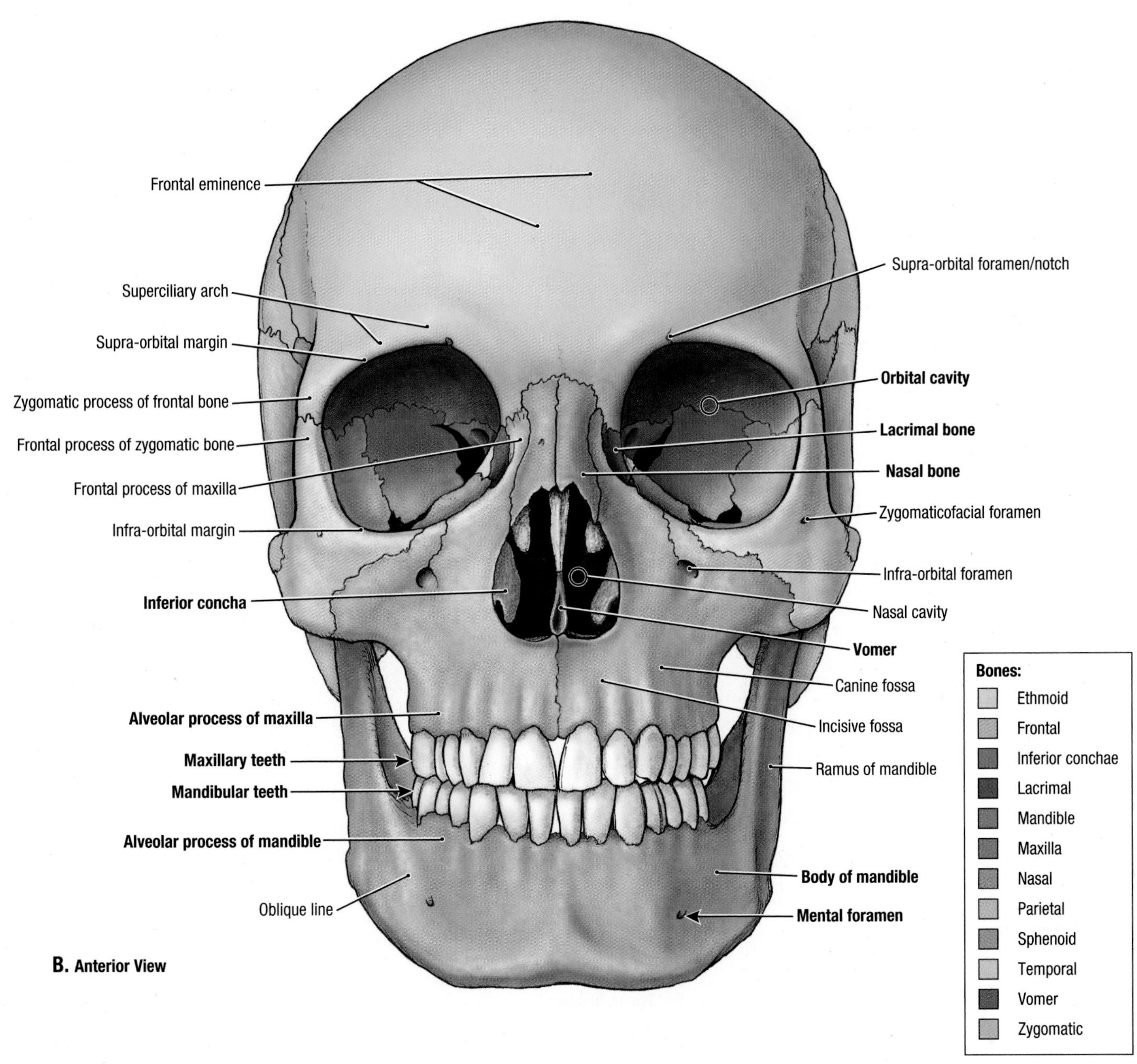
Frontal eminence
Superciliary arch
Supra-orbital margin
Zygomatic process of frontal bone
Frontal process of zygomatic bone
Frontal process of maxilla
Infra-orbital margin
Inferior concha
Alveolar process of maxilla
Maxillary teeth
Mandibular teeth
Alveolar process of mandible
Oblique line
Supra-orbital foramen/notch
Orbital cavity
Lacrimal bone
Nasal bone
Zygomaticofacial foramen
Infra-orbital foramen
Nasal cavity
Vomer
Canine fossa
Incisive fossa
Ramus of mandible
Body of mandible
Mental foramen
Bones:
Ethmoid
Frontal
Inferior conchae
Lacrimal
Mandible
Maxilla
Nasal
Parietal
Sphenoid
Temporal
Vomer
Zygomatic

B. Anterior View

7.2 CRANIUM, FACIAL (FRONTAL) ASPECT *(CONTINUED)*

Extraction of teeth causes the alveolar bone to resorb in the affected regions(s). Following complete loss or extraction of maxillary teeth, the sockets begin to fill in with bone, and the alveolar process begins to resorb. Similarly, extraction of mandibular teeth causes the bone of the alveolar process to resorb. The mental foramen may eventually lie near the superior border of the body of the mandible. In some cases, the mental foramina disappear, exposing the mental nerves to injury.

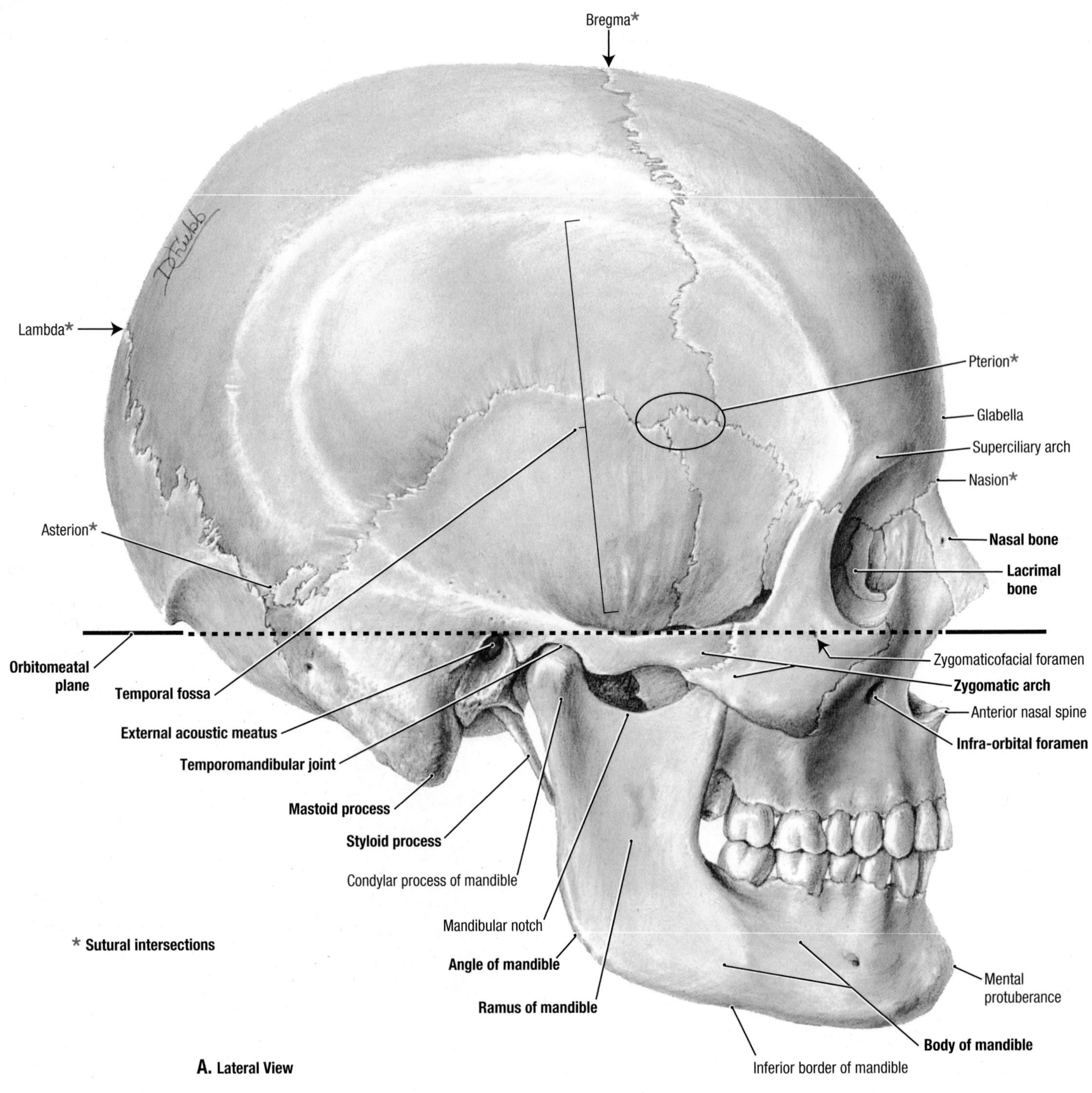
Bregma*
Lambda*
Pterion*
Glabella
Superciliary arch
Nasion*
Nasal bone
Lacrimal bone
Asterion*
Orbitomeatal plane
Temporal fossa
Zygomaticofacial foramen
Zygomatic arch
Anterior nasal spine
Infra-orbital foramen
External acoustic meatus
Temporomandibular joint
Mastoid process
Styloid process
Condylar process of mandible
Mandibular notch
* Sutural intersections
Angle of mandible
Ramus of mandible
Mental protuberance
Body of mandible
Inferior border of mandible

A. Lateral View

7.3 CRANIUM, LATERAL ASPECT

A. Bony cranium. **B.** Cranium with bones color coded. The cranium is in the anatomical position when the orbitomeatal plane is horizontal. **C.** Buttresses of cranium. The buttresses are thicker portions of cranial bones that transfer forces around the weaker regions of the orbits and nasal cavity.

The convexity of the neurocranium (braincase) distributes and thereby minimizes the effects of a blow to it. However, hard blows to the head in thin areas of the cranium (e.g., in the temporal fossa) are likely to produce **depressed fractures**, in which a fragment of bone is depressed inward, compressing and/or injuring the brain. In **comminuted fractures**, the bone is broken into several pieces. **Linear fractures**, the most frequent type, usually occur at the point of impact, but fracture lines often radiate away from it in two or more directions.

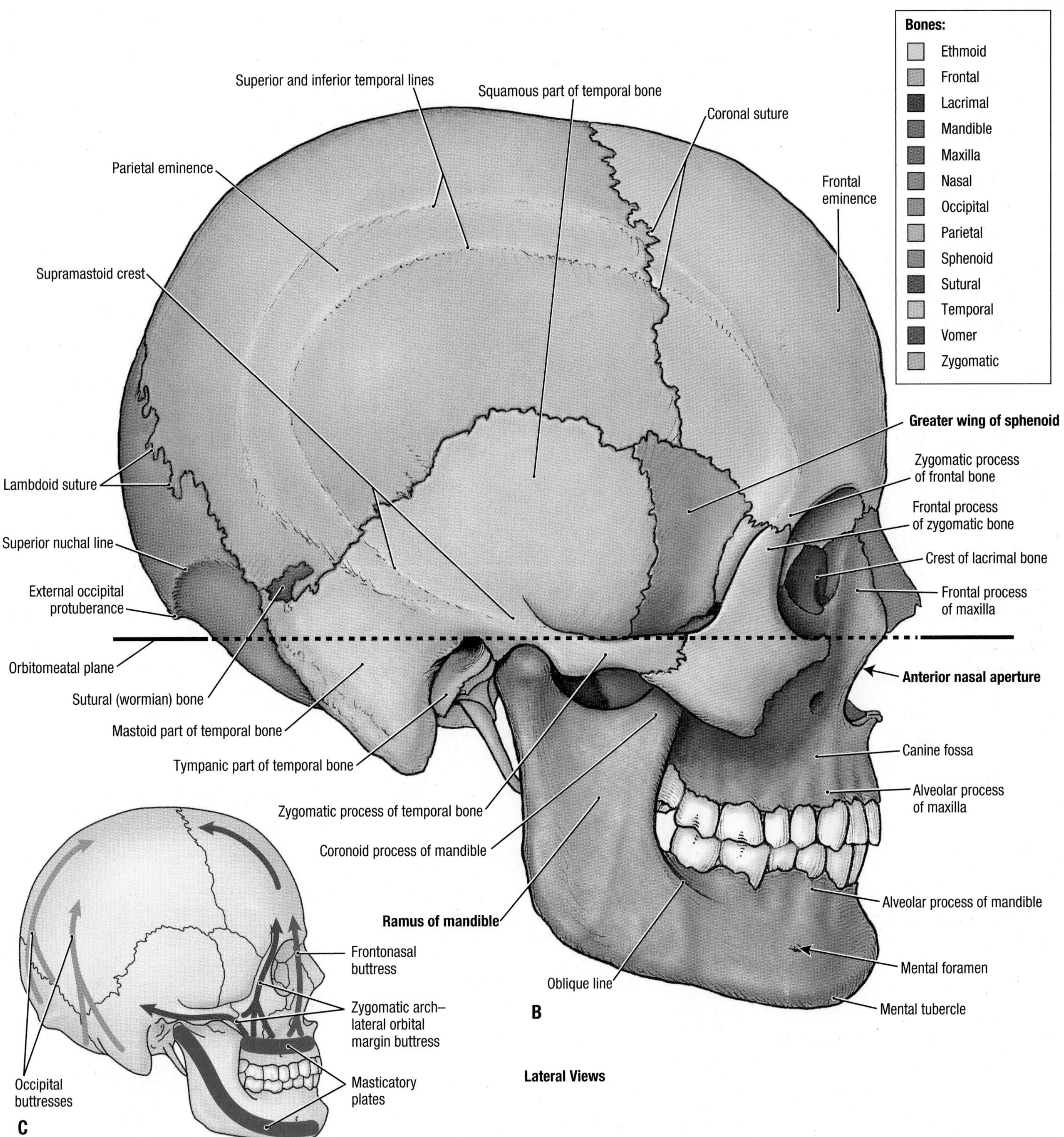
Bones:
Ethmoid
Frontal
Lacrimal
Mandible
Maxilla
Nasal
Occipital
Parietal
Sphenoid
Sutural
Temporal
Vomer
Zygomatic
Superior and inferior temporal lines
Squamous part of temporal bone
Coronal suture
Parietal eminence
Frontal eminence
Supramastoid crest
Greater wing of sphenoid
Zygomatic process of frontal bone
Lambdoid suture
Frontal process of zygomatic bone
Superior nuchal line
Crest of lacrimal bone
External occipital protuberance
Frontal process of maxilla
Orbitomeatal plane
Anterior nasal aperture
Sutural (wormian) bone
Mastoid part of temporal bone
Canine fossa
Tympanic part of temporal bone
Alveolar process of maxilla
Zygomatic process of temporal bone
Coronoid process of mandible
Alveolar process of mandible
Ramus of mandible
Frontonasal buttress
Mental foramen
Oblique line
Zygomatic arch–lateral orbital margin buttress
B
Mental tubercle
Masticatory plates
Occipital buttresses
C

Lateral Views

7.3 CRANIUM, LATERAL ASPECT *(CONTINUED)*

If the area of the neurocranium is thick at the site of impact, the bone usually bends inward without fracturing; however, a fracture may occur some distance from the site of direct trauma where the calvaria is thinner. In a **contrecoup (counterblow) fracture**, the fracture occurs on the opposite side of the cranium rather than at the point of impact. One or more sutural (accessory) bones may be located at the lambda or near the mastoid process.

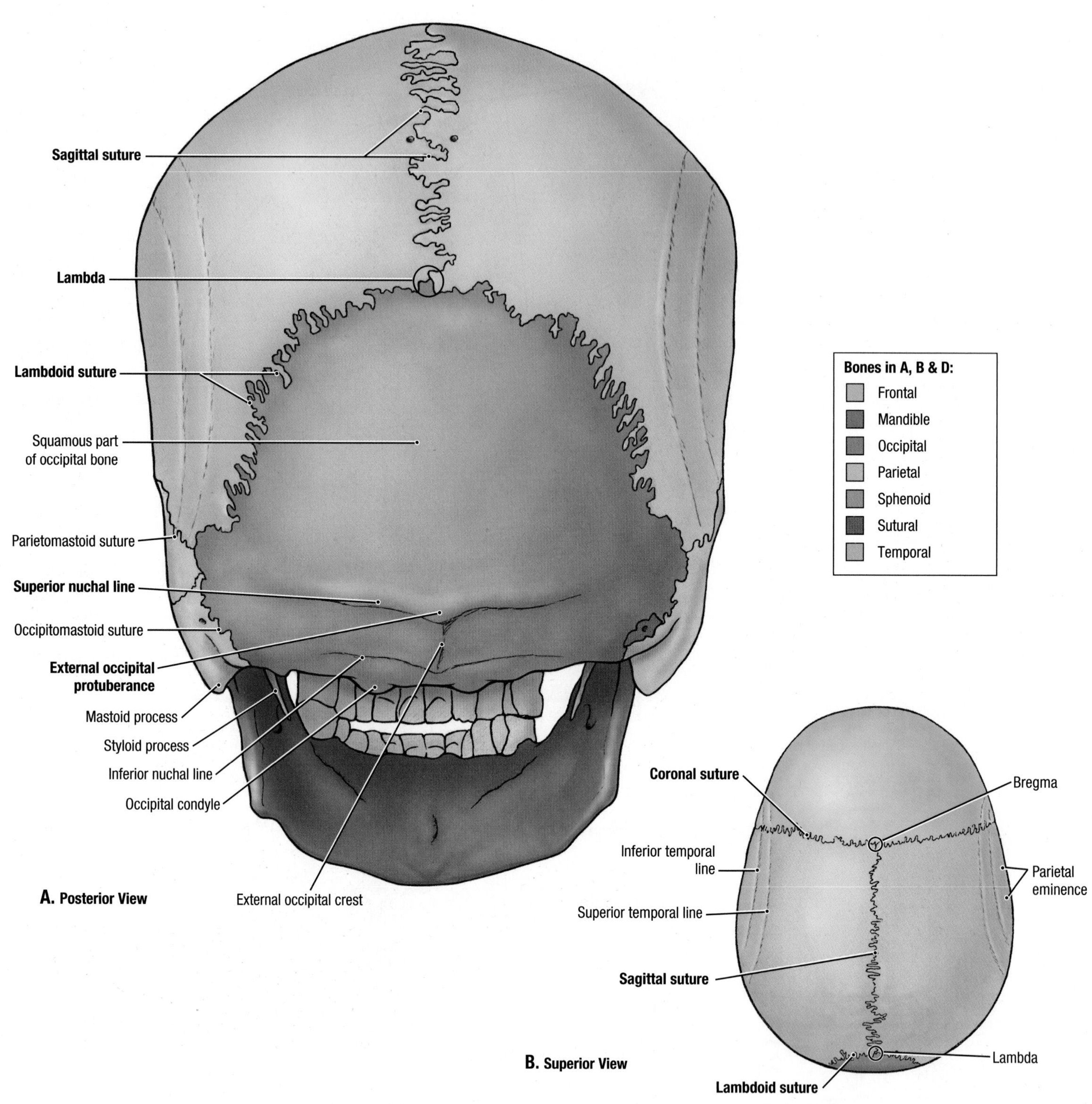
Sagittal suture
Lambda
Lambdoid suture
Squamous part of occipital bone
Parietomastoid suture
Superior nuchal line
Occipitomastoid suture
External occipital protuberance
Mastoid process
Styloid process
Inferior nuchal line
Occipital condyle
External occipital crest
A. Posterior View
Bones in A, B & D:
Frontal
Mandible
Occipital
Parietal
Sphenoid
Sutural
Temporal
Coronal suture
Bregma
Inferior temporal line
Parietal eminence
Superior temporal line
Sagittal suture
Lambda
Lambdoid suture
B. Superior View

7.4 CRANIUM, OCCIPITAL ASPECT, CALVARIA, AND ANTERIOR PART OF POSTERIOR CRANIAL FOSSA

A. The lambda, near the center of this convex surface, is located at the junction of the sagittal and lambdoid sutures. **B.** The roof of the neurocranium, or calvaria (skullcap), is formed primarily by the paired parietal bones, the frontal bone, and the occipital bone.

Premature closure of the coronal suture results in a high, tower-like cranium, called **oxycephaly** or **turricephaly**. Premature closure of sutures usually does not affect brain development. When premature closure occurs on one side only, the cranium is asymmetrical, a condition known as **plagiocephaly**.

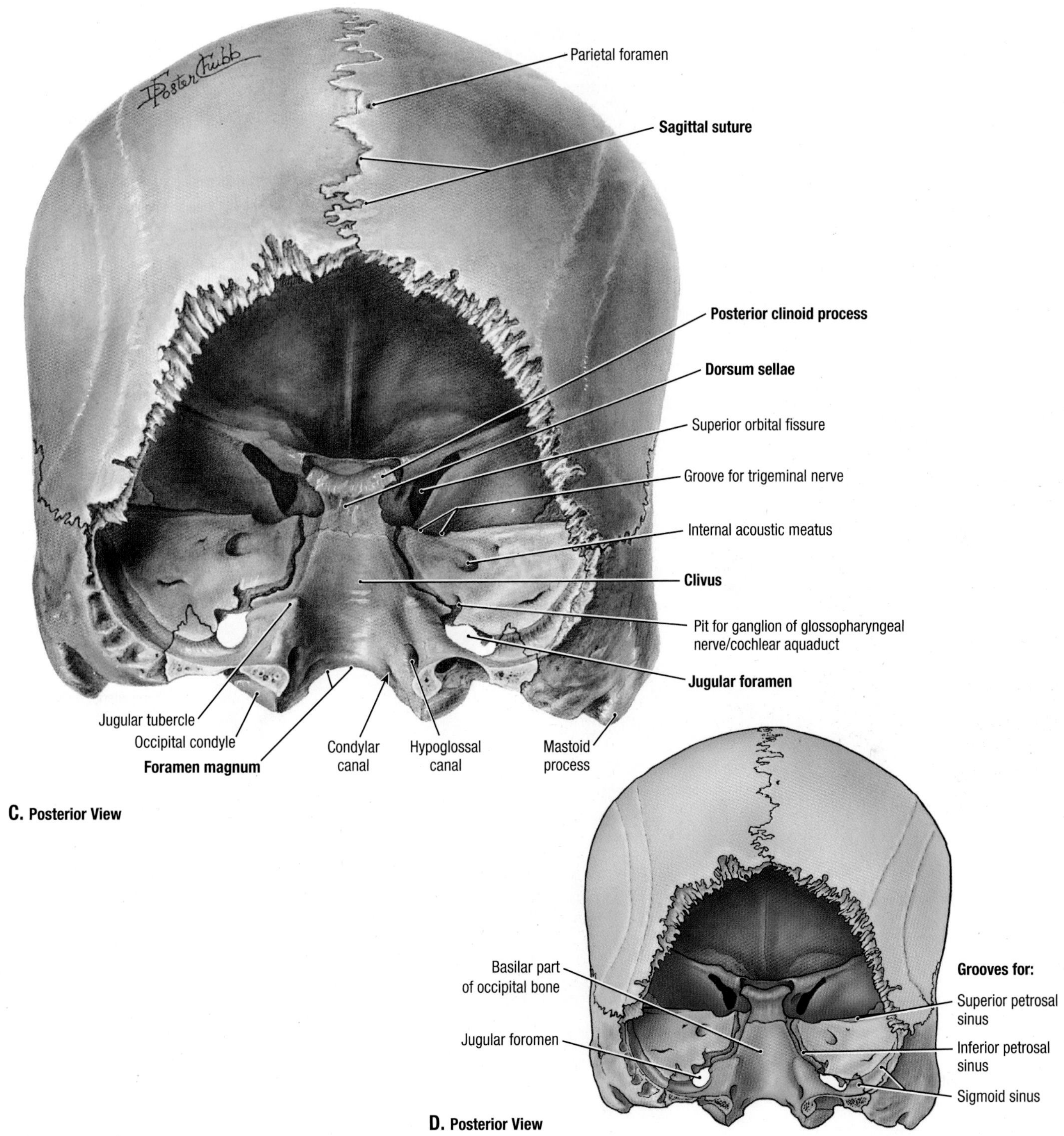
Parietal foramen
Sagittal suture
Posterior clinoid process
Dorsum sellae
Superior orbital fissure
Groove for trigeminal nerve
Internal acoustic meatus
Clivus
Pit for ganglion of glossopharyngeal nerve/cochlear aquaduct
Jugular foramen
Jugular tubercle
Occipital condyle
Foramen magnum
Condylar canal
Hypoglossal canal
Mastoid process
Basilar part of occipital bone
Jugular foromen
Grooves for:
Superior petrosal sinus
Inferior petrosal sinus
Sigmoid sinus

C. Posterior View

D. Posterior View

7.4 CRANIUM, OCCIPITAL ASPECT, CALVARIA, AND ANTERIOR PART OF POSTERIOR CRANIAL FOSSA *(CONTINUED)*

C. and D. Cranium after removal of squamous part of occipital bone.

- The dorsum sellae projects from the body of the sphenoid; the posterior clinoid processes form its superolateral corners.
- The clivus is the slope descending from the dorsum sellae to the foramen magnum.
- The grooves for the sigmoid sinus and inferior petrosal sinus lead inferiorly to the jugular foramen.

Premature closure of the sagittal suture, in which the anterior fontanelle is small or absent, results in a long, narrow, wedge-shaped cranium, a condition called **scaphocephaly**.

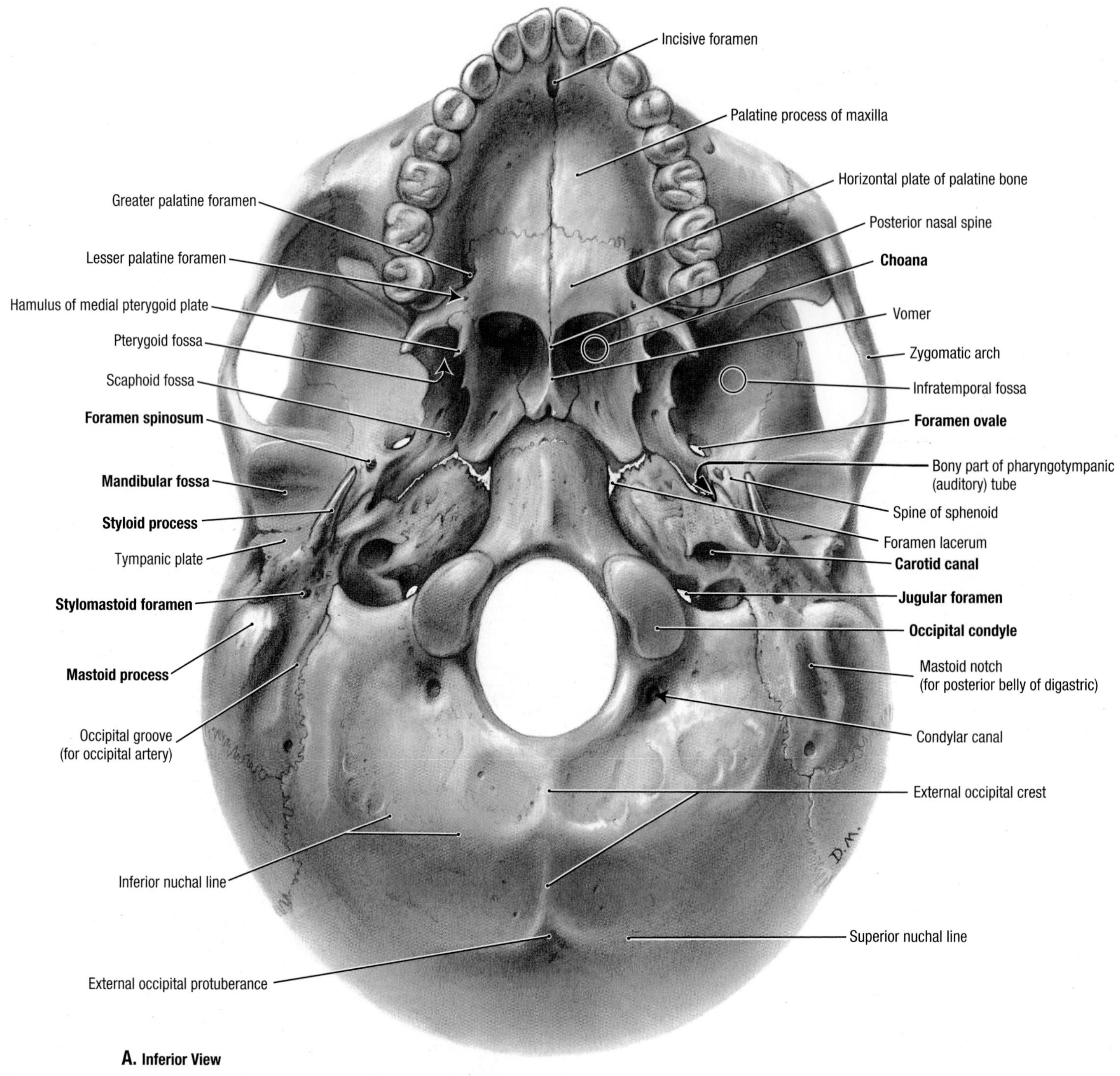
Incisive foramen
Palatine process of maxilla
Horizontal plate of palatine bone
Posterior nasal spine
Choana
Vomer
Zygomatic arch
Infratemporal fossa
Foramen ovale
Bony part of pharyngotympanic (auditory) tube
Spine of sphenoid
Foramen lacerum
Carotid canal
Jugular foramen
Occipital condyle
Mastoid notch (for posterior belly of digastric)
Condylar canal
External occipital crest
Superior nuchal line
Greater palatine foramen
Lesser palatine foramen
Hamulus of medial pterygoid plate
Pterygoid fossa
Scaphoid fossa
Foramen spinosum
Mandibular fossa
Styloid process
Tympanic plate
Stylomastoid foramen
Mastoid process
Occipital groove (for occipital artery)
Inferior nuchal line
External occipital protuberance
D.M.

A. **Inferior View**

7.5 CRANIUM, INFERIOR ASPECT

A. Bony cranium. **B.** Diagram of cranium with bones color coded.

TABLE 7.1 FORAMINA AND OTHER APERTURES OF CRANIAL FOSSAE, AND CONTENTS (SEE FIGS. 7.2–7.6)

Foramen cecum: Nasal emissary vein (1% of population)	Optic canals: Optic nerve (CN II) and ophthalmic arteries
Cribriform plate: Olfactory nerves (CN I)	Superior orbital fissure: Ophthalmic veins; ophthalmic nerve (CN V_1); CN III, IV and VI; and sympathetic fibers
Anterior and posterior ethmoidal foramina: Vessels and nerves with same names	Foramen rotundum: Maxillary nerve (CN V_2)

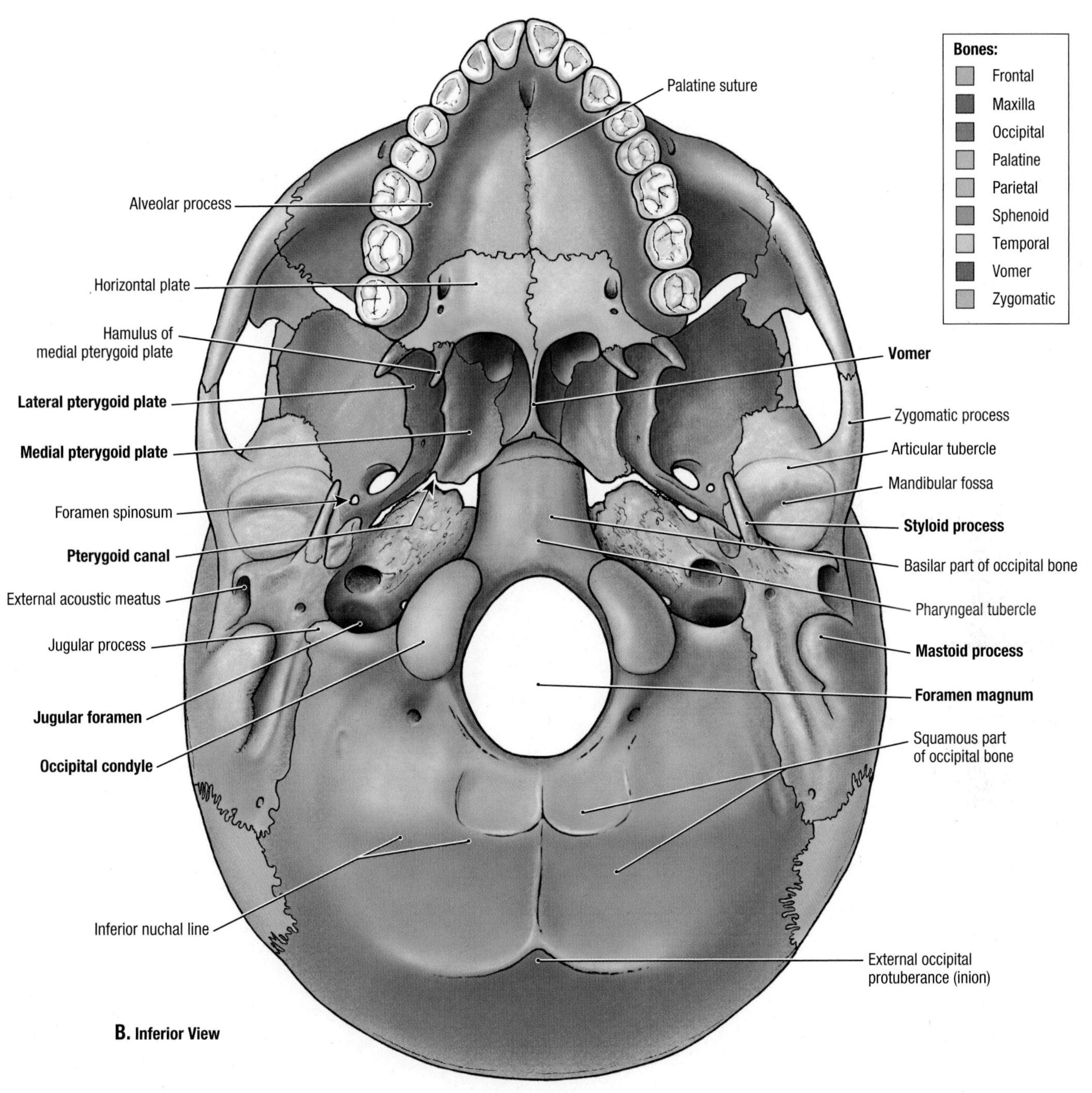
Bones:
Frontal
Maxilla
Occipital
Palatine
Parietal
Sphenoid
Temporal
Vomer
Zygomatic
Palatine suture
Alveolar process
Horizontal plate
Hamulus of medial pterygoid plate
Lateral pterygoid plate
Medial pterygoid plate
Foramen spinosum
Pterygoid canal
External acoustic meatus
Jugular process
Jugular foramen
Occipital condyle
Inferior nuchal line
Vomer
Zygomatic process
Articular tubercle
Mandibular fossa
Styloid process
Basilar part of occipital bone
Pharyngeal tubercle
Mastoid process
Foramen magnum
Squamous part of occipital bone
External occipital protuberance (inion)

B. **Inferior View**

7.5 CRANIUM, INFERIOR ASPECT *(CONTINUED)*

TABLE 7.1 FORAMINA AND OTHER APERTURES OF CRANIAL FOSSAE, AND CONTENTS (SEE FIGS. 7.2–7.6) (CONTINUED)

Foramen ovale: Mandibular nerve (CN V_3) and accessory meningeal artery	Jugular foramen: CN IX, X, and XI; superior bulb of internal jugular vein; inferior petrosal and sigmoid sinuses; meningeal branches of ascending pharyngeal and occipital arteries.
Foramen spinosum: Middle meningeal artery/vein and meningeal branch of CN V_3	Hypoglossal canal: Hypoglossal nerve (CN XII)
Foramen lacerum[a]: Deep petrosal nerve, some meningeal arterial branches and small veins.	Foramen magnum: Spinal cord; spinal accessory nerve (CN XI); vertebral arteries; internal vertebral venous plexus.
Groove of greater petrosal nerve: Greater petrosal nerve and petrosal branch of middle meningeal artery	Condylar canal: Condyloid emissary vein (passes from sigmoid sinus to vertebral veins in neck)
Carotid canal: Internal carotid artery and accompanying sympathetic and venous plexuses	Stylomastoid foramen: Facial nerve (CN VII)
Internal acoustic meatus: Facial nerve/ intermediate nerve (CN VII); vestibulocochlear nerve (CN VIII); labyrinthine artery	Mastoid foramina: Mastoid emissary vein from sigmoid sinus and meningeal branch of occipital artery

[a]The internal carotid artery and its accompanying sympathetic and venous plexuses actually pass horizontally across (rather than vertically through) the area of the foramen lacerum, an artifact of dry crania, which is closed by cartilage in life.

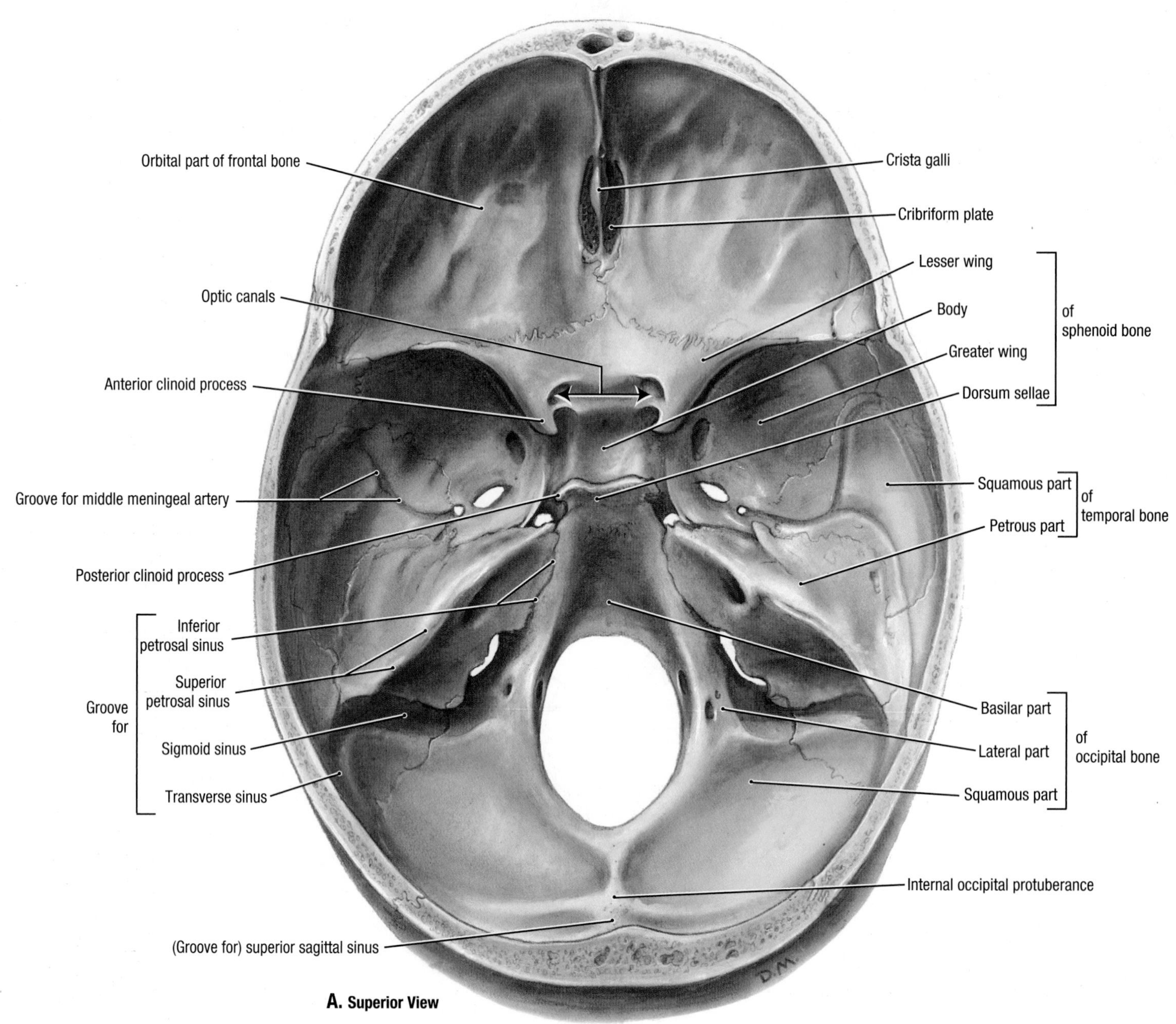

Orbital part of frontal bone
Crista galli
Cribriform plate
Lesser wing
Body
Greater wing
Dorsum sellae
of sphenoid bone
Optic canals
Anterior clinoid process
Groove for middle meningeal artery
Squamous part
Petrous part
of temporal bone
Posterior clinoid process
Groove for
Inferior petrosal sinus
Superior petrosal sinus
Sigmoid sinus
Transverse sinus
Basilar part
Lateral part
Squamous part
of occipital bone
Internal occipital protuberance
(Groove for) superior sagittal sinus

A. **Superior View**

7.6 INTERIOR OF THE CRANIAL BASE

A. Bony cranial base. **B.** Diagrammatic cranial base with bones color coded.

In **A:**

- Three bones contribute to the anterior cranial fossa: the orbital part of the frontal bone, the cribriform plate of the ethmoid, and the lesser wing of the sphenoid.
- The four parts of the occipital bone are the basilar, right and left lateral, and squamous.
- **Fractures in the floor of the anterior cranial fossa** may involve the cribriform plate of the ethmoid, resulting in leakage of CSF through the nose (CSF rhinorrhea). **CSF rhinorrhea** may be a primary indication of a cranial base fracture which increases the risk of meningitis, because an infection could spread to the meninges from the ear or nose.

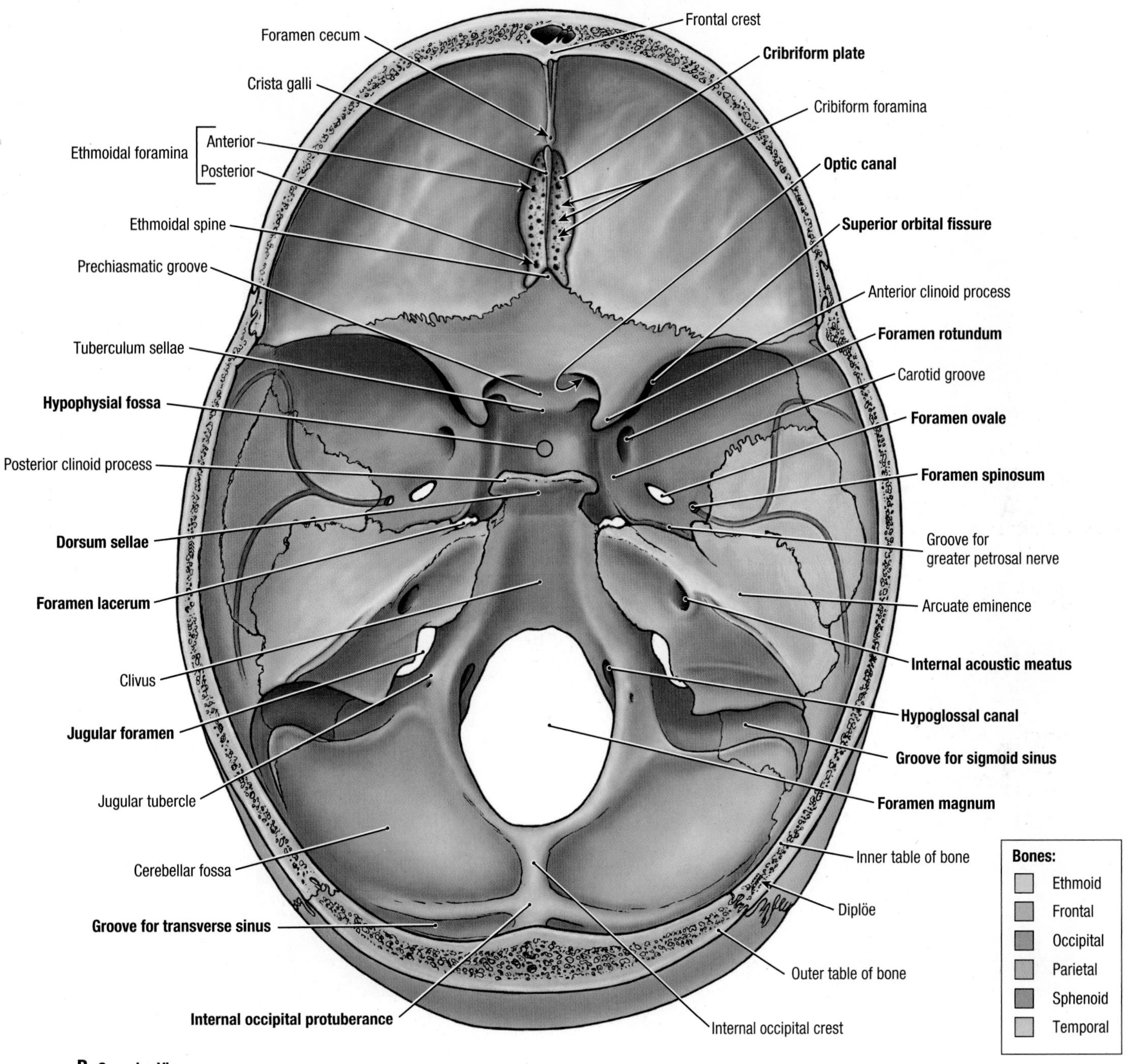
Frontal crest
Foramen cecum
Cribriform plate
Crista galli
Cribiform foramina
Ethmoidal foramina
Anterior
Posterior
Optic canal
Ethmoidal spine
Superior orbital fissure
Prechiasmatic groove
Anterior clinoid process
Foramen rotundum
Tuberculum sellae
Carotid groove
Hypophysial fossa
Foramen ovale
Posterior clinoid process
Foramen spinosum
Dorsum sellae
Groove for greater petrosal nerve
Foramen lacerum
Arcuate eminence
Internal acoustic meatus
Clivus
Hypoglossal canal
Jugular foramen
Groove for sigmoid sinus
Jugular tubercle
Foramen magnum
Inner table of bone
Cerebellar fossa
Diplöe
Groove for transverse sinus
Outer table of bone
Internal occipital protuberance
Internal occipital crest
Bones:
Ethmoid
Frontal
Occipital
Parietal
Sphenoid
Temporal

B. Superior View

7.6 INTERIOR OF THE CRANIAL BASE *(CONTINUED)*

In **B,** note the following midline features:

- In the anterior cranial fossa, the frontal crest and crista galli for anterior attachment of the falx cerebri have between them the foramen cecum, which, during development, transmits a vein connecting the superior sagittal sinus with the veins of the frontal sinus and root of the nose.
- In the middle cranial fossa, the tuberculum sellae, hypophysial fossa, dorsum sellae, and posterior clinoid processes constitute the sella turcica (L. Turkish saddle).
- In the posterior cranial fossa, note the clivus, foramen magnum, internal occipital crest for attachment of the falx cerebelli, and the internal occipital protuberance, from which the grooves for the transverse sinuses course laterally.

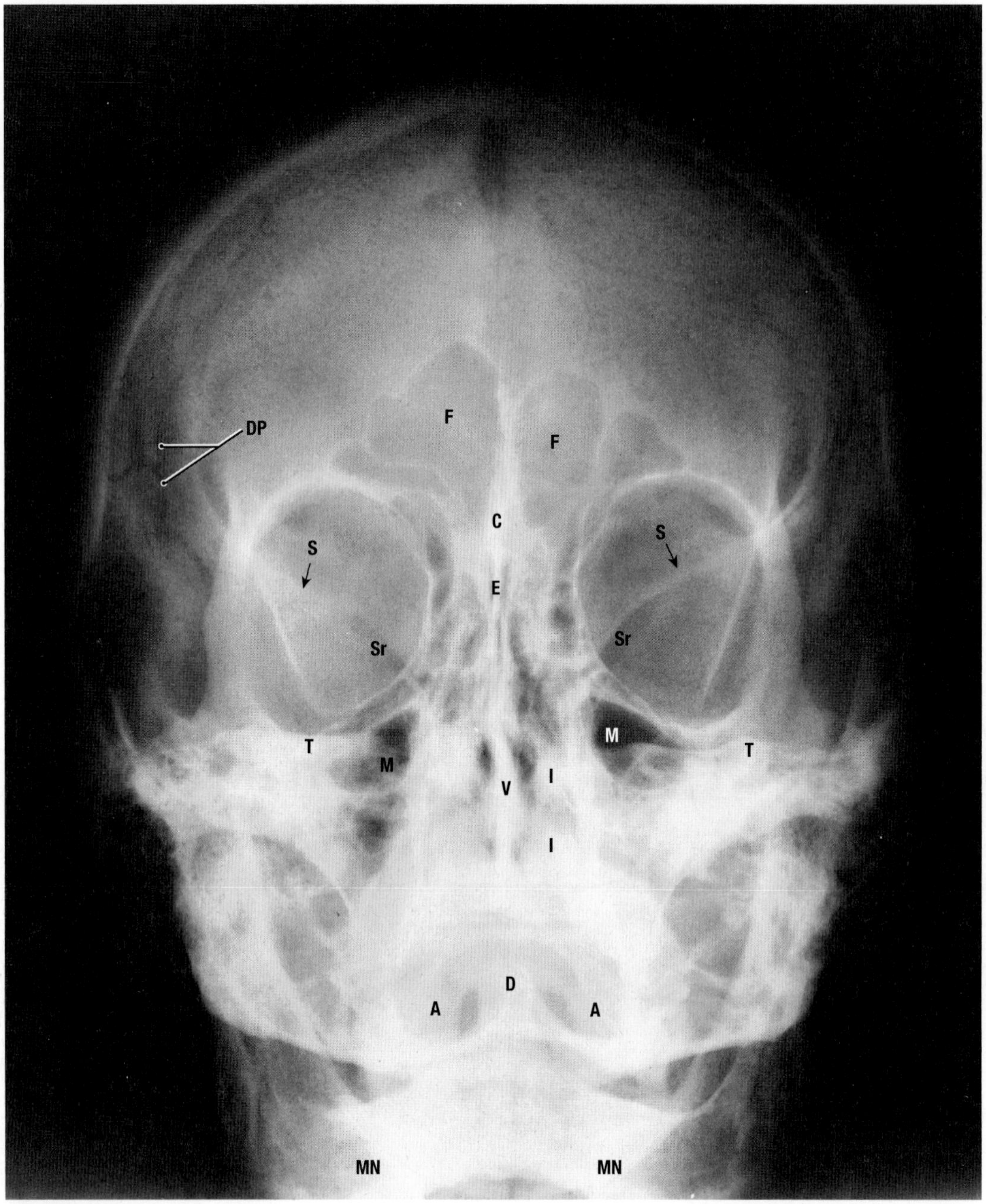

A. **Anteroposterior View**

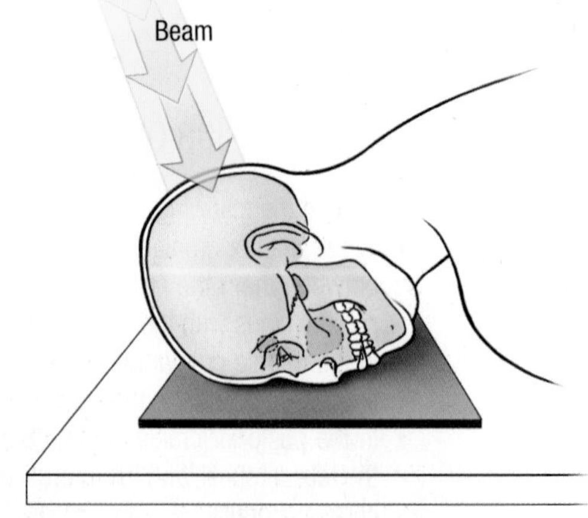
Beam

7.7 RADIOGRAPHS OF THE CRANIUM

A. Postero-anterior (*Caldwell*) radiograph. This view places the orbits centrally in the head and is used to examine the orbits and paranasal sinuses. Observe in **A:**

- The labeled features include the superior orbital fissure *(Sr)*, lesser wing of the sphenoid *(S)*, superior surface of the petrous part of the temporal bone *(T)*, crista galli *(C)*, frontal sinus *(F)*, mandible *(MN)*, maxillary sinus *(M)*, and diploic veins *(DP)*.
- The nasal septum is formed by the perpendicular plate of the ethmoid (*E*) and the vomer (*V*); note the inferior and middle conchae (*I*) of the lateral wall of the nose.
- Superimposed on the facial skeleton are the dens (*D*) and lateral masses of the atlas (*A*).

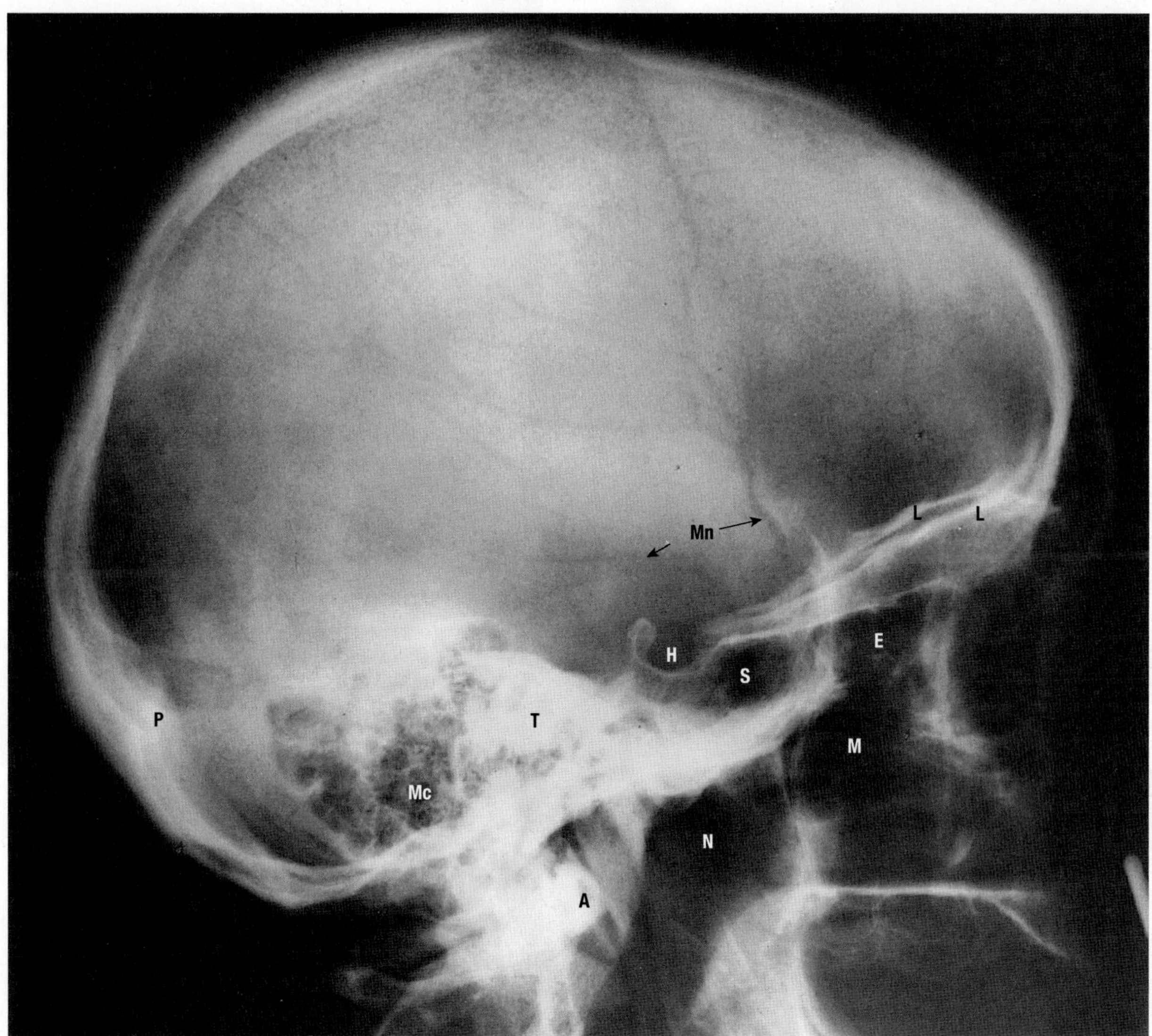
Mn
L
L
E
H
S
P
T
M
Mc
N
A

B. Lateral View

7.7 RADIOGRAPHS OF THE CRANIUM *(CONTINUED)*

B. Lateral radiograph of the cranium. Most of the relatively thin bone of the facial skeleton (viscerocranium) is radiolucent (appears *black*).

- The labeled features include the ethmoidal cells (*E*), sphenoidal (*S*) and maxillary (*M*) sinuses, the hypophysial fossa (*H*) for the pituitary gland, the petrous part of the temporal bone (*T*), mastoid cells (*Mc*), grooves for the branches of the middle meningeal vessels (*Mn*), anterior arch of the atlas (*A*), internal occipital protuberance (*P*), and the nasopharynx (*N*).
- The right and left orbital plates of the frontal bone are not superimposed; thus, the floor of the anterior cranial fossa appears as two lines (*L*).

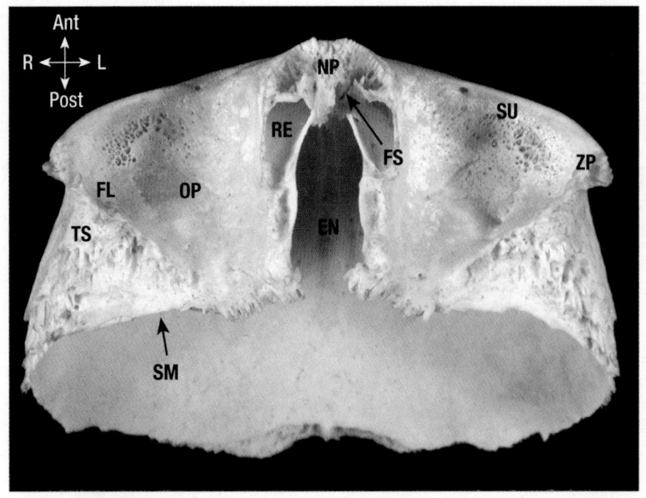
Ant
R
L
Post
NP
SU
RE
FS
ZP
FL
OP
EN
TS
SM

A. **Inferior View**

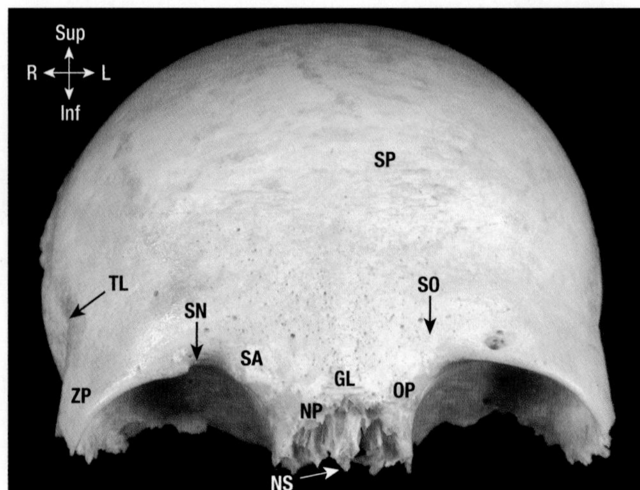
Sup
R
L
Inf
SP
TL
SN
SO
SA
GL
OP
ZP
NP
NS

B. **Anterior View**

Key for A and B: Frontal Bone

EN	Ethmoidal notch	NP	Nasal part	SA	Superciliary arch	SU	Supra-orbital margin
FL	Fossa for lacrimal gland	NS	Nasal spine	SM	Sphenoidal margin	TL	Temporal line
FS	Opening of frontal sinus	OP	Orbital part	SN	Supra-orbital notch	TS	Temporal surface
GL	Glabella	RE	Root of ethmoid cells	SO	Supra-orbital foramen	ZP	Zygomatic process
				SP	Squamous part		

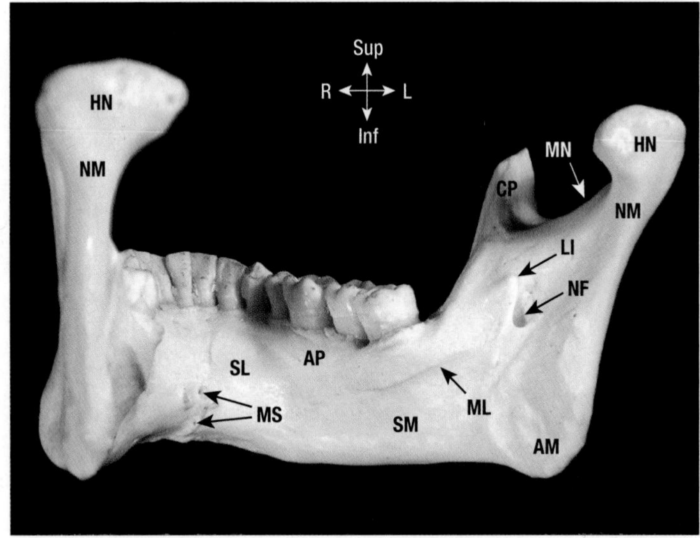
Sup
R
L
Inf
HN
NM
MN
HN
CP
NM
LI
NF
SL
AP
MS
SM
ML
AM

C. **Posteromedial View**

D. **Lateral View**

Key for C and D: Mandible

AM	Angle of mandible	ML	Mylohyoid groove	NM	Neck of mandible
AP	Alveolar part	MN	Mandibular notch	PF	Pterygoid fovea
CP	Coronoid process	MS	Mental (genial) spines	RM	Ramus of mandible
HM	Head of mandible	MT	Mental foramen	SL	Sublingual fossa
LI	Lingula	NF	Mandibular foramen	SM	Submandibular fossa

7.8 MANDIBLE, MAXILLA, FRONTAL, ETHMOID, AND LACRIMAL BONES

A. and B. Frontal bone. **C. and D.** Mandible.

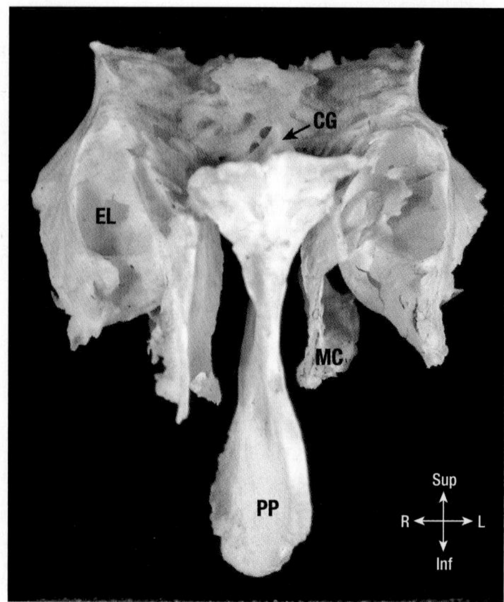
CG
EL
MC
PP
Sup
R
L
Inf

E. Anterior View

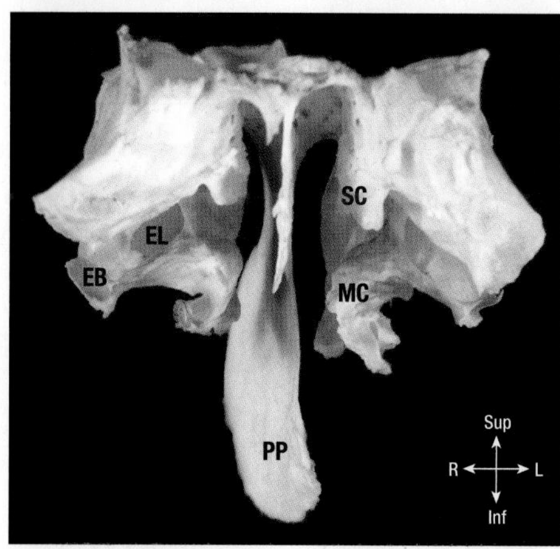
SC
EL
EB
MC
PP
Sup
R
L
Inf

F. Posterior View

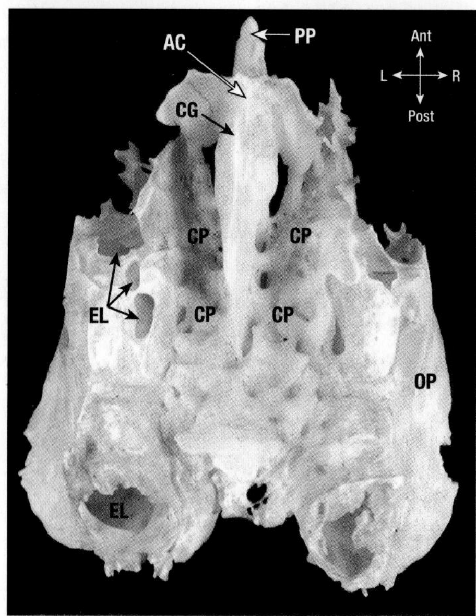
AC
PP
Ant
L
R
Post
CG
CP
CP
EL
CP
CP
OP
EL

G. Superior View

Key for E-G: Ethmoid Bone

AC	Ala of crista galli	EB	Ethmoidal bulla	OP	Orbital plate
CG	Crista galli	EL	Ethmoidal labyrinth (cells)	PP	Perpendicular plate
CP	Cribriform plate	MC	Middle nasal concha	SC	Superior nasal concha

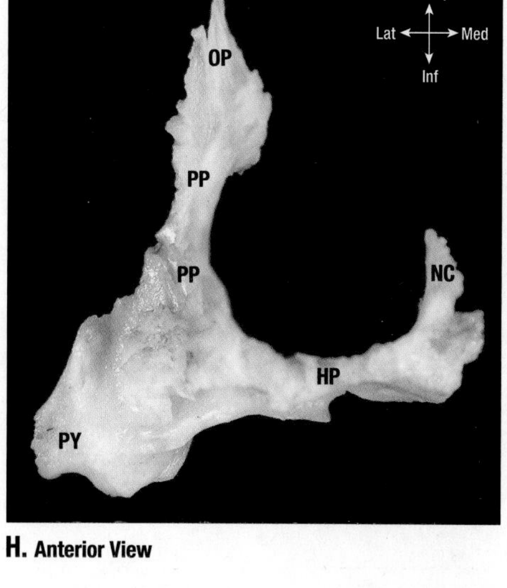
Sup
Lat
Med
Inf
OP
PP
PP
NC
HP
PY

H. Anterior View

Key for H: Palatine Bone

HP	Horizontal plate	PP	Perpendicular plate
NC	Nasal crest	PY	Pyramidal process
OP	Orbital process		

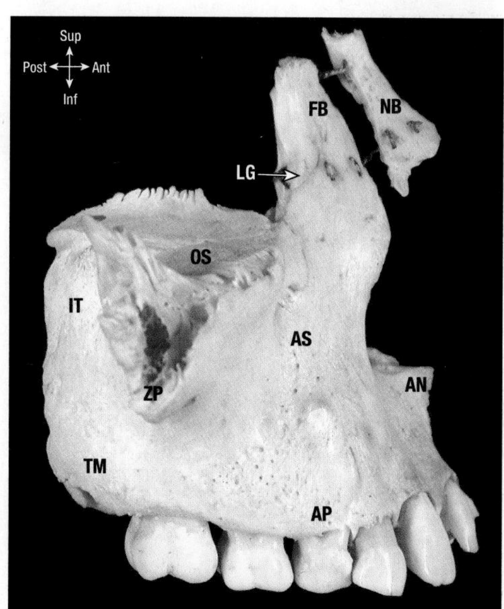
Sup
Post
Ant
Inf
FB
NB
LG
OS
IT
AS
AN
ZP
TM
AP

I. Lateral View

Key for I: Maxilla and Nasal Bone

AN	Anterior nasal spine	LG	Lacrimal groove
AP	Alveolar part	NB	Nasal bone
AS	Anterior surface	OS	Orbital surface
FP	Frontal process	TM	Tuberosity
IT	Infratemporal surface	ZP	Zygomatic process

7.8 MANDIBLE, MAXILLA, FRONTAL, ETHMOID, AND LACRIMAL BONES *(CONTINUED)*

E.–G. Ethmoid bone. **H.** Lacrimal bone. **I.** Maxilla

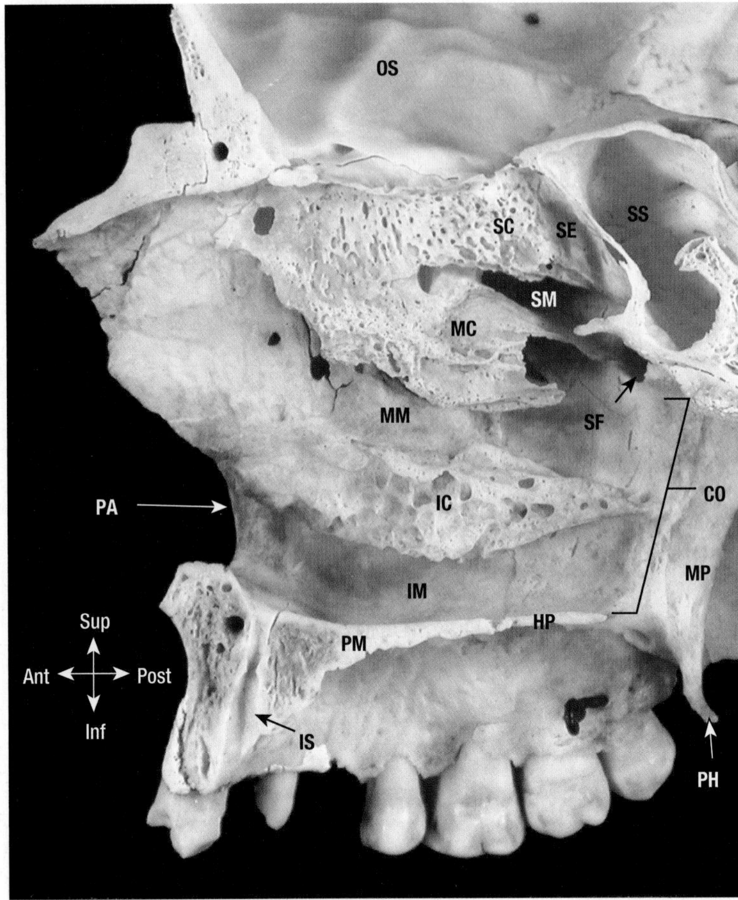
OS
SC
SE
SS
SM
MC
MM
SF
PA
IC
CO
MP
IM
HP
PM
Sup
Ant
Post
Inf
IS
PH

A. Lateral Wall of Nose, Medial View

Key for A: Lateral Wall of Nose

CO	Choana (posterior nasal aperture)
HP	Horizontal plate of palatine bone
IC	Inferior nasal concha
IS	Incisive canal
IM	Inferior nasal meatus
MC	Middle nasal concha
MM	Middle nasal meatus
PH	Pterygoid hamulus
PM	Palatine process of maxilla
OS	Orbital surface of frontal bone
PA	Piriform aperture
PM	Palatine process of maxilla
SC	Superior nasal concha
SE	Spheno-ethmoidal recess
SF	Sphenopalatine foramen
SM	Superior nasal meatus
SS	Sphenoidal sinus

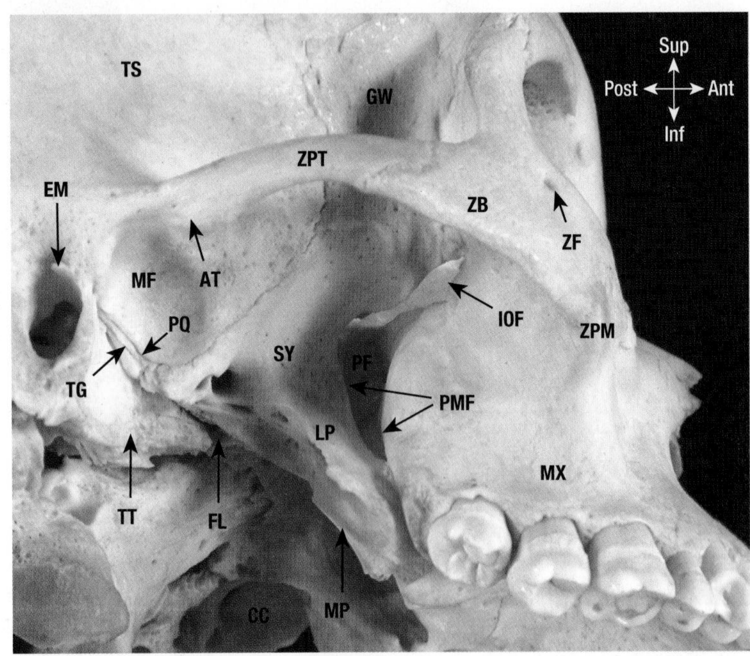
TS
GW
Sup
Post
Ant
Inf
ZPT
EM
ZB
ZF
MF
AT
IOF
PQ
ZPM
SY
PF
TG
PMF
LP
MX
TT
FL
CC
MP

B. Infratemporal Region, Inferolateral View

Key for B: Infratemporal Region

PF	Pterygopalatine fossa
MF	Mandibular fossa
AT	Articular tubercle
ZPT	Zygomatic process of temporal bone
CC	Carotid canal
FL	Foramen lacerum
ZF	Zygomaticofacial foramen
PQ	Petrosquamous fissure
TG	Tegmen tympani
TT	Temporal bone (tympanic part)
ZB	Zygomatic bone
MX	Maxilla
IOF	Inferior orbital fissure
PMF	Pterygomaxillary fissure
ZPM	Zygomatic process of maxilla
EM	External acoustic meatus
GW	Greater wing of sphenoid
LP	Lateral pterygoid plate
MP	Medial pterygoid plate
SY	Stylomastoid foramen

7.9 LATERAL WALL OF NOSE AND INFRATEMPORAL REGION

A. Lateral wall of nose. **B.** Infratemporal region.

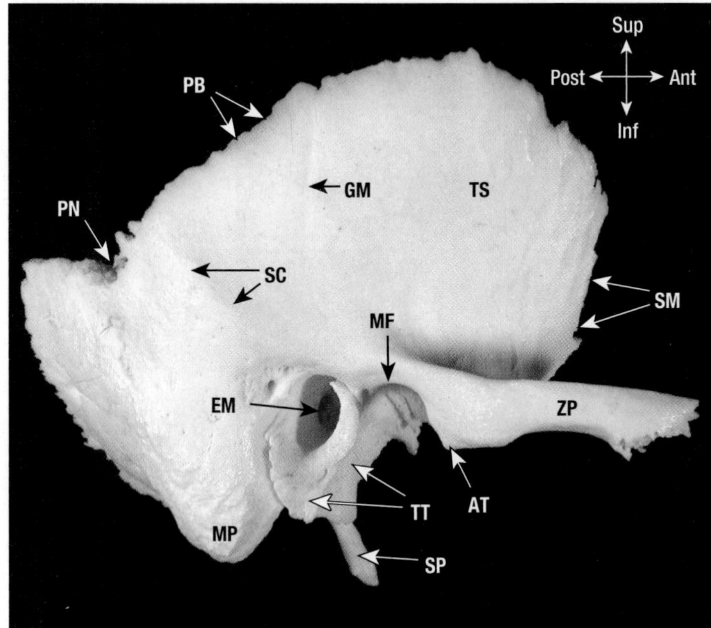
Sup
Post
Ant
Inf
PB
PN
GM
TS
SC
SM
MF
EM
ZP
TT
AT
MP
SP

A. Lateral View

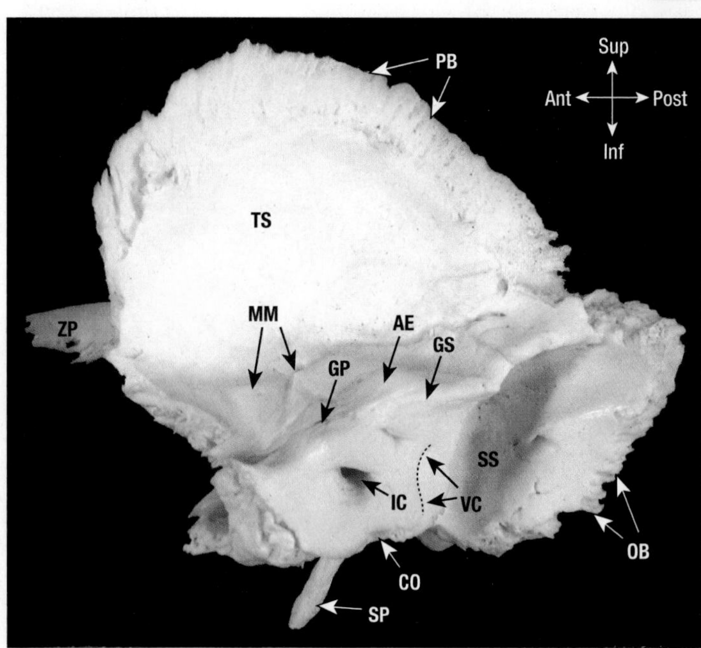
PB
Sup
Ant
Post
Inf
TS
ZP
MM
AE
GS
GP
SS
IC
VC
OB
CO
SP

B. Medial View

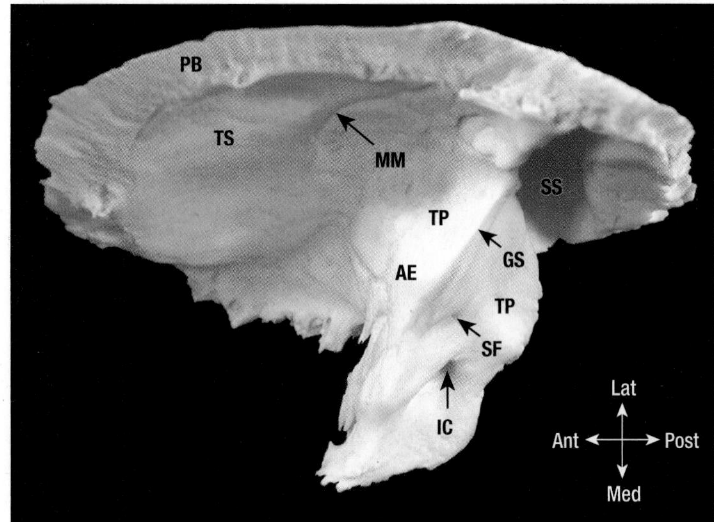
PB
TS
MM
SS
TP
GS
AE
TP
SF
IC
Lat
Ant
Post
Med

C. Superior View

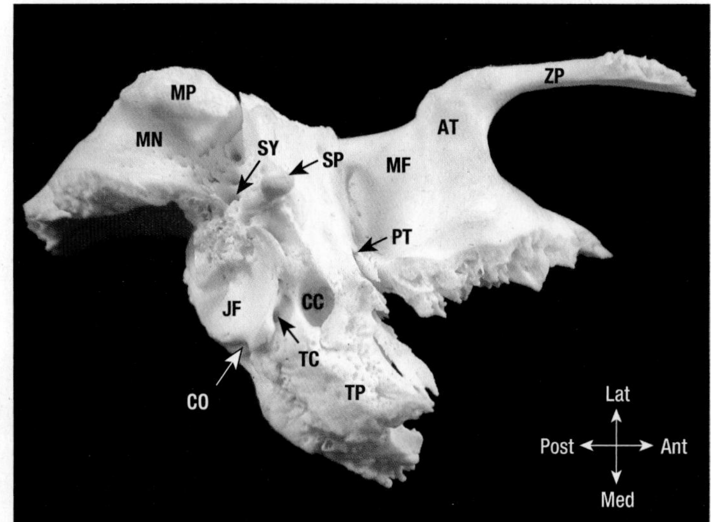
ZP
MP
AT
MN
SY
SP
MF
PT
JF
CC
TC
CO
TP
Lat
Post
Ant
Med

D. Inferior View

Key for A-D: Temporal Bone

AE	Arcuate eminence	MF	Mandibular fossa	SM	Sphenoid margin
AT	Articular tubercle	MM	Groove for middle meningeal artery	SP	Styloid process
CC	Carotid canal	MN	Mastoid notch	SS	Groove for sigmoid sinus
CO	Cochlear canaliculus	MP	Mastoid process	SY	Stylomastoid foramen
EM	External acoustic meatus	OB	Occipital border	TC	Tympanic canaliculus
GM	Groove for middle temporal artery	PB	Parietal border	TP	Temporal bone (petrous part)
GP	Hiatus for greater petrosal nerve	PN	Parietal notch	TS	Temporal bone (squamous part)
GS	Groove for superior petrosal sinus	PT	Petrotympanic fissure	TT	Temporal bone (tympanic part)
IC	Internal acoustic meatus	SC	Supramastoid crest	VC	Vestibular canaliculus
JF	Jugular fossa	SF	Subarcuate fossa	ZP	Zygomatic process

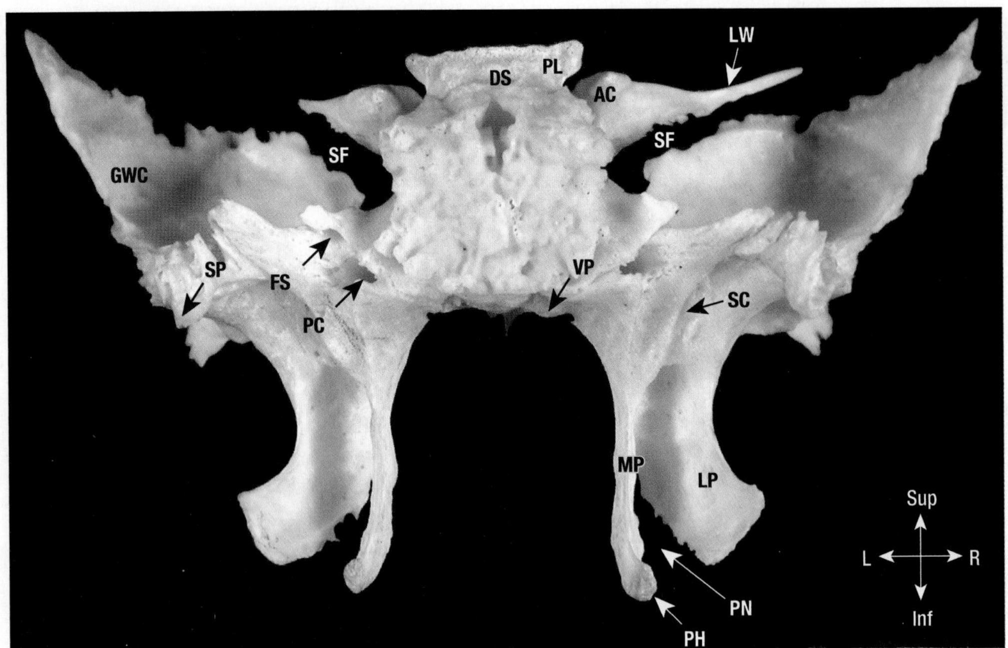
LW
DS
PL
AC
SF
SF
GWC
SP
FS
PC
VP
SC
MP
LP
PN
PH
Sup
L
R
Inf

A. **Posterior View**

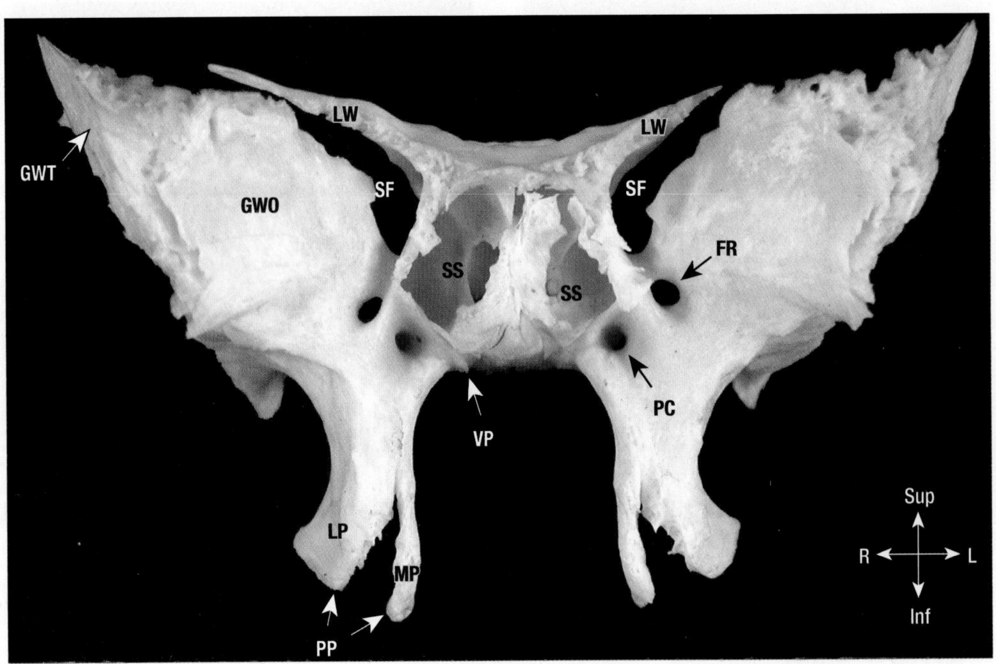
LW
LW
GWT
SF
SF
GWO
FR
SS
SS
VP
PC
LP
MP
PP
Sup
R
L
Inf

B. **Anterior View**

Key for A-D: Sphenoid Bone

AC	Anterior clinoid process	FO	Foramen ovale	GWO	Greater wing (orbital surface)
CG	Carotid sulcus	FR	Foramen rotundum	GWT	Greater wing (temporal surface)
CS	Prechiasmatic sulcus	FS	Foramen spinosum	H	Hypophysial fossa
DS	Dorsum sellae	GWC	Greater wing (cerebral surface)	LP	Lateral pterygoid plate
ES	Ethmoidal spine	GWI	Greater wing (infratemporal surface)	LW	Lesser wing

7.11 SPHENOID BONE

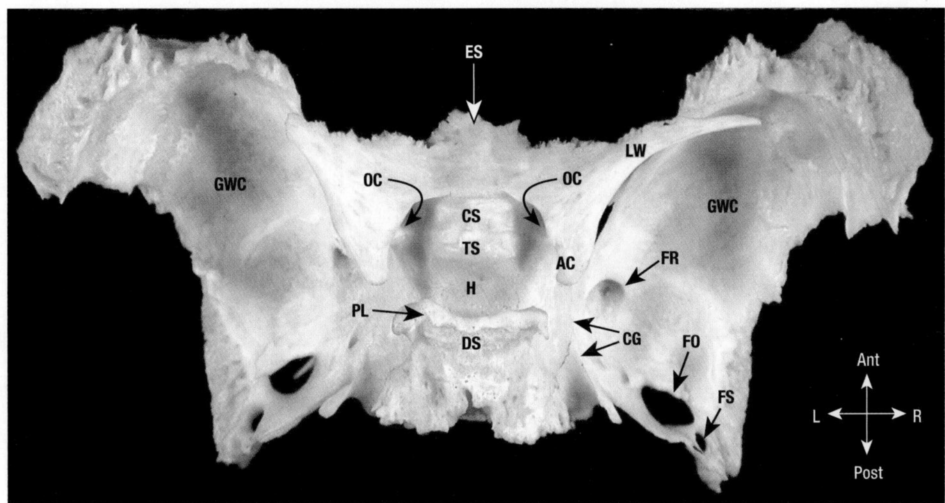
ES
LW
GWC
OC
OC
GWC
CS
TS
AC
FR
H
PL
DS
CG
FO
FS
Ant
L
R
Post

C. Superior View

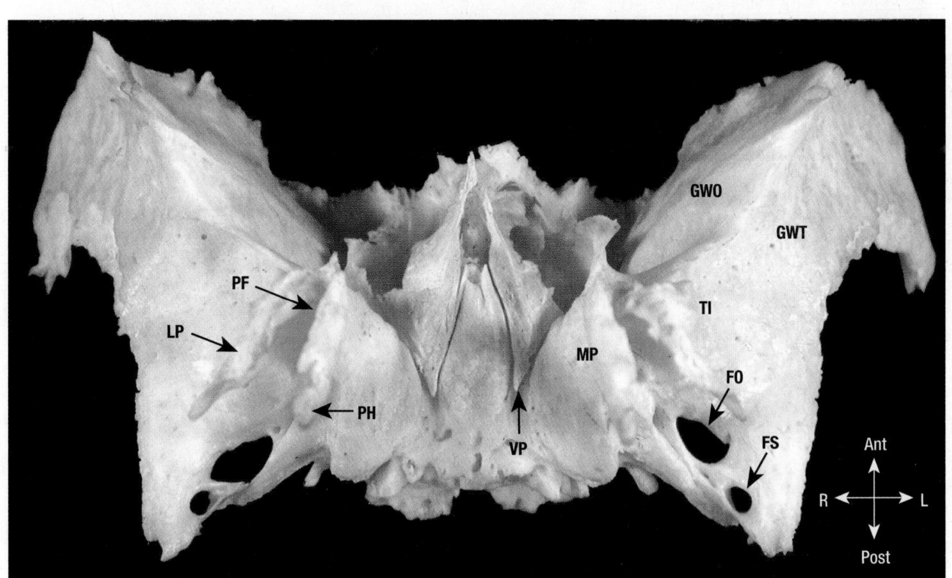
GWO
GWT
PF
TI
LP
MP
FO
PH
VP
FS
Ant
R
L
Post

D. Inferior View

Key for A-D: Sphenoid Bone (Continued)

MP	Medial pterygoid plate	PL	Posterior clinoid process	SP	Spine of sphenoid bone
OC	Optic canal	PN	Pterygoid notch	SS	Sphenoidal sinus (in body of sphenoid)
PC	Pterygoid canal	PP	Pterygoid process	TS	Tuberculum sellae
PF	Pterygoid fossa	SC	Scaphoid fossa	VP	Vaginal process
PH	Pterygoid hamulus	SF	Superior orbital fissure		

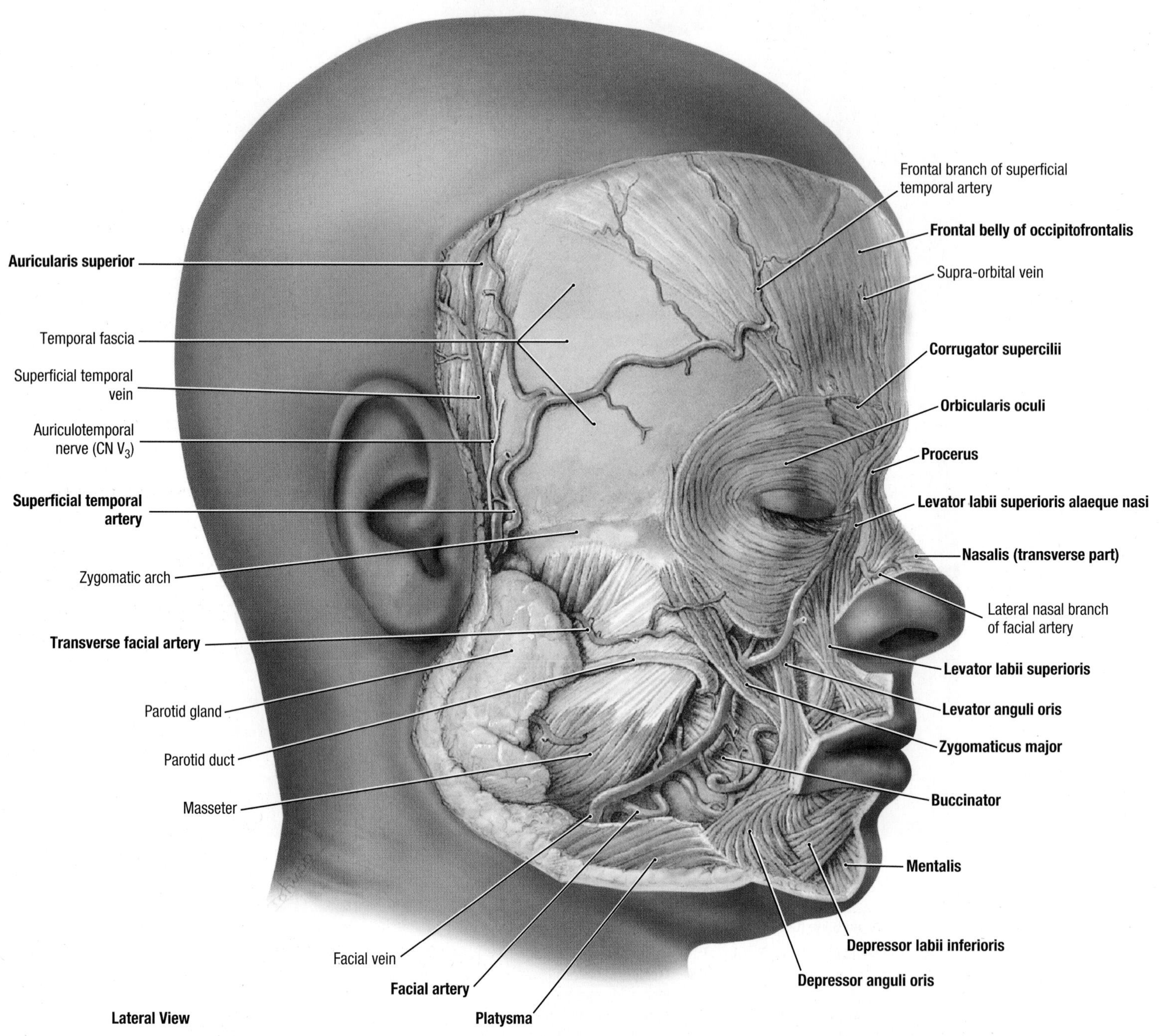
Frontal branch of superficial temporal artery
Frontal belly of occipitofrontalis
Supra-orbital vein
Auricularis superior
Temporal fascia
Superficial temporal vein
Auriculotemporal nerve (CN V_3)
Corrugator supercilii
Orbicularis oculi
Procerus
Superficial temporal artery
Levator labii superioris alaeque nasi
Nasalis (transverse part)
Zygomatic arch
Lateral nasal branch of facial artery
Transverse facial artery
Levator labii superioris
Parotid gland
Levator anguli oris
Parotid duct
Zygomaticus major
Masseter
Buccinator
Mentalis
Depressor labii inferioris
Facial vein
Depressor anguli oris
Facial artery
Lateral View
Platysma

7.12 MUSCLES OF FACIAL EXPRESSION AND ARTERIES OF THE FACE

- The muscles of facial expression are the superficial sphincters and dilators of the openings of the head; all are supplied by the facial nerve (CN VII). The masseter and temporalis (the latter covered here by temporal fascia) are muscles of mastication that are innervated by the trigeminal nerve (CN V).
- **Superficial temporal and facial artery pulses.** Anesthesiologists, usually stationed at the head of the operating table, take these pulses. The superficial temporal pulse is palpated anterior to the auricle as the artery crosses the zygomatic arch. The facial pulse is palpated where the facial artery crosses the inferior border of the mandible immediately anterior to the masseter.

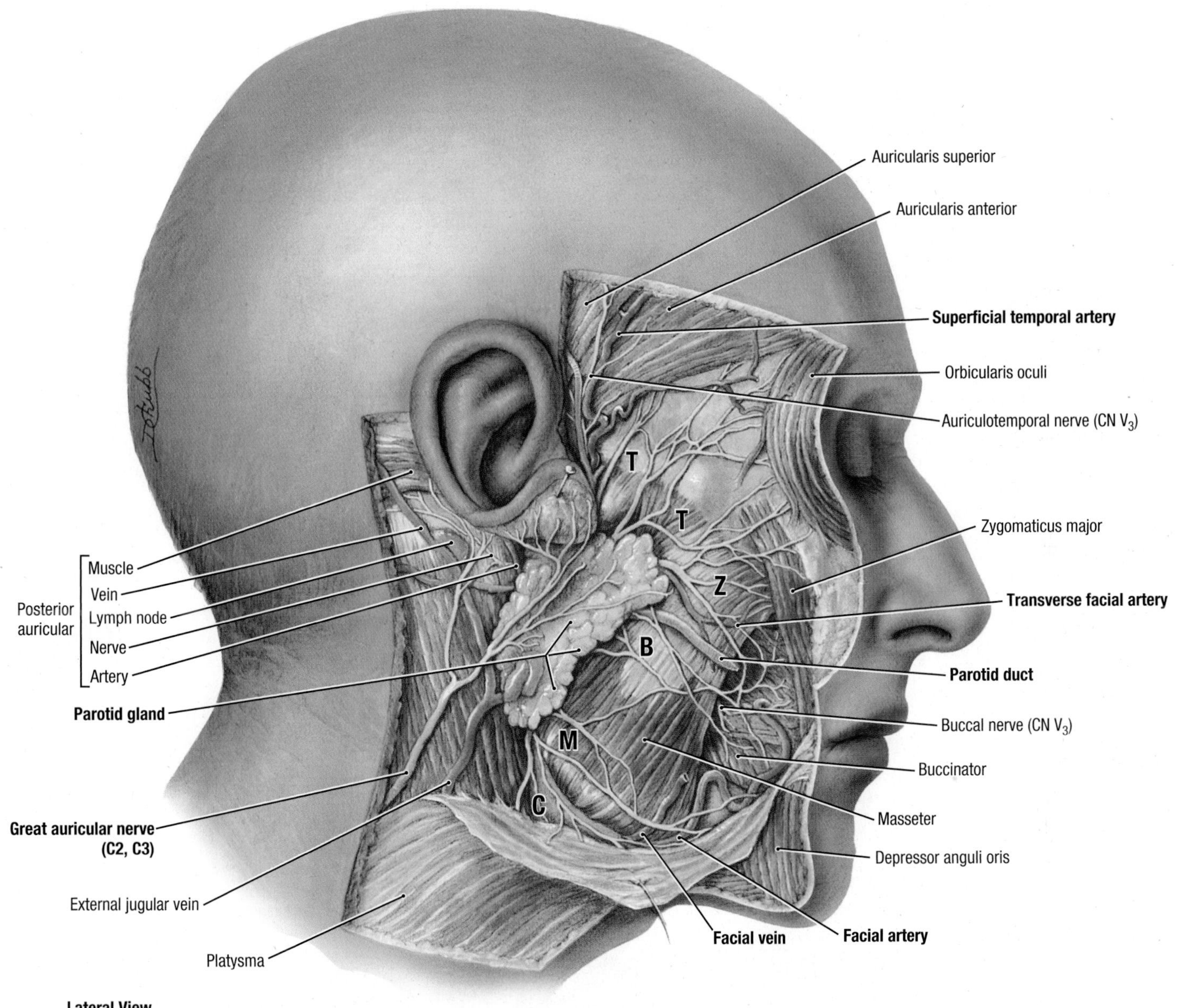
Auricularis superior
Auricularis anterior
Superficial temporal artery
Orbicularis oculi
Auriculotemporal nerve (CN V_3)
T
T
Z
Zygomaticus major
Transverse facial artery
B
Parotid duct
Posterior auricular
Muscle
Vein
Lymph node
Nerve
Artery
Parotid gland
M
Buccal nerve (CN V_3)
Buccinator
C
Masseter
Great auricular nerve (C2, C3)
Depressor anguli oris
External jugular vein
Facial vein
Facial artery
Platysma
Lateral View

7.13 RELATIONSHIPS OF BRANCHES OF FACIAL NERVE AND VESSELS TO THE PAROTID GLAND AND DUCT

- The parotid duct extends across the masseter muscle just inferior to the zygomatic arch; the duct turns medially to pierce the buccinator and opens into the oral vestibule.
- The facial nerve (CN VII) innervates the muscles of facial expression. After emerging from the stylomastoid foramen, the main stem of the facial nerve has posterior auricular, digastric, and stylohyoid branches; the parotid plexus gives rise to temporal (T), zygomatic (Z), buccal (B), marginal mandibular (M), cervical (C), and posterior auricular branches. These branches form a plexus within the parotid gland, the branches of which radiate over the face, anastomosing with each other and the branches of the trigeminal nerve.
- During **parotidectomy** (surgical excision of the parotid gland), identification, dissection, and preservation of the branches of the facial nerve are critical.
- The parotid gland may become infected by infectious agents that pass through the bloodstream, as occurs in mumps, an acute communicable viral disease. Infection of the gland causes inflammation, **parotiditis**, and swelling of the gland. Severe pain occurs because the parotid sheath, innervated by the great auricular nerve, is distended by swelling.

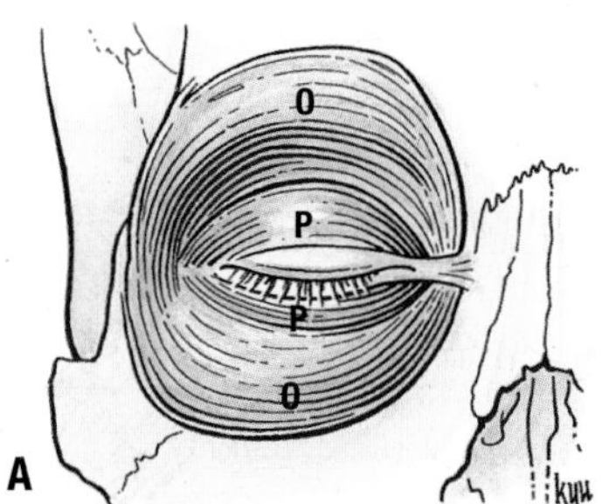
O
P
P
O
A

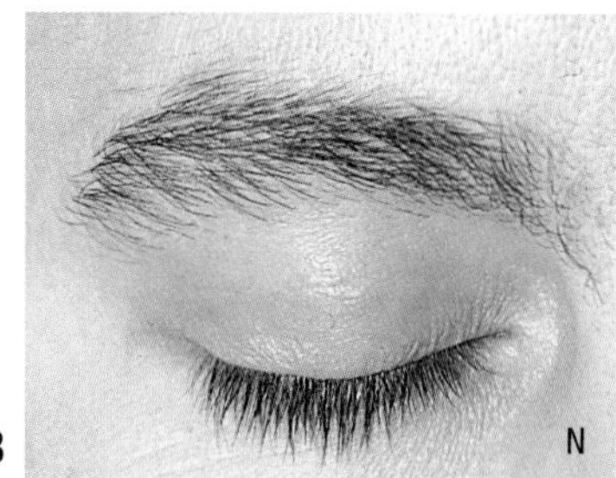
N
B

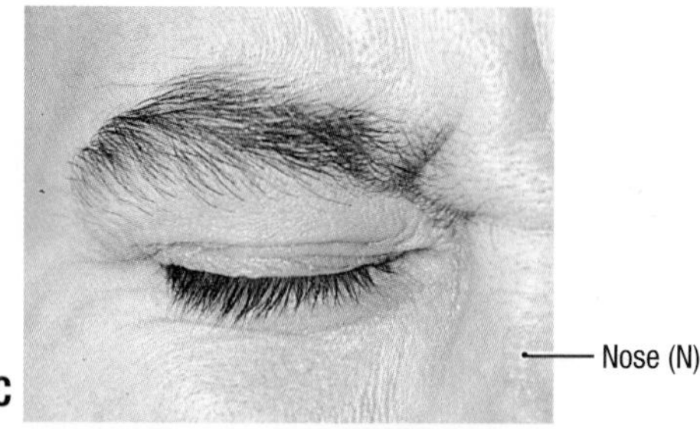
Nose (N)
C

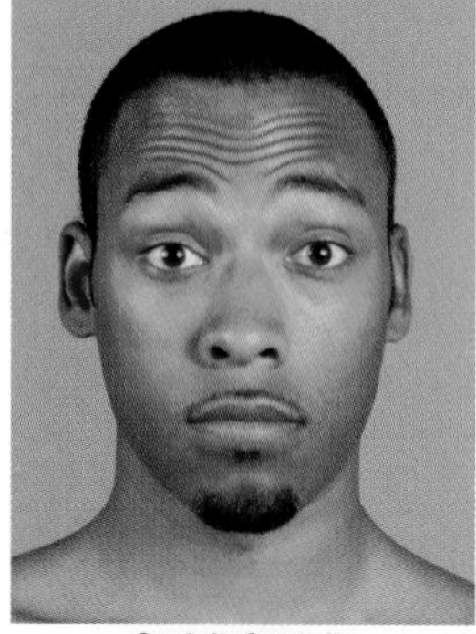
Occipitofrontalis

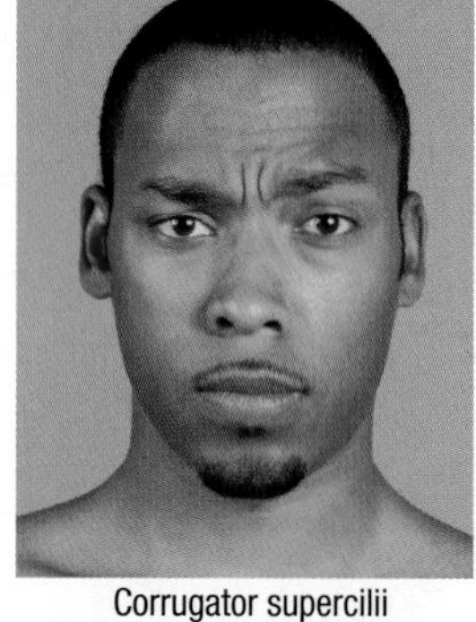
Corrugator supercilii

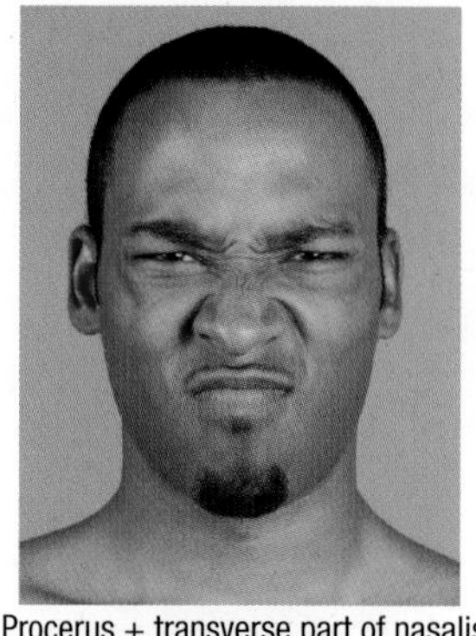
Procerus + transverse part of nasalis

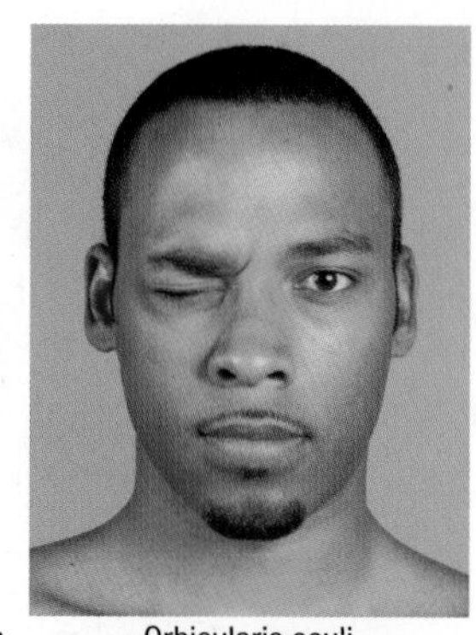
Orbicularis oculi

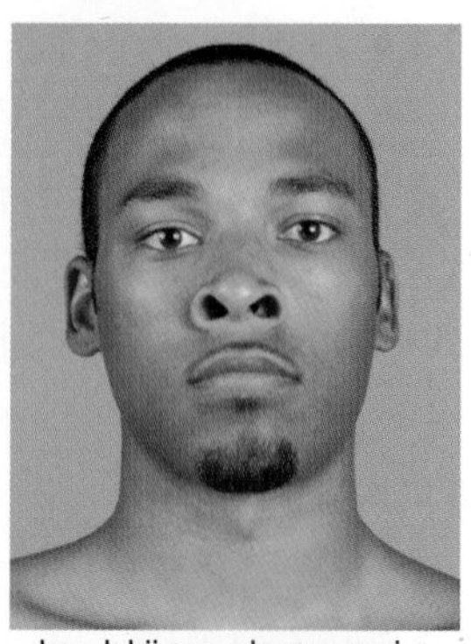
Lev. labii sup. alaeque nasi + alar part of nasalis

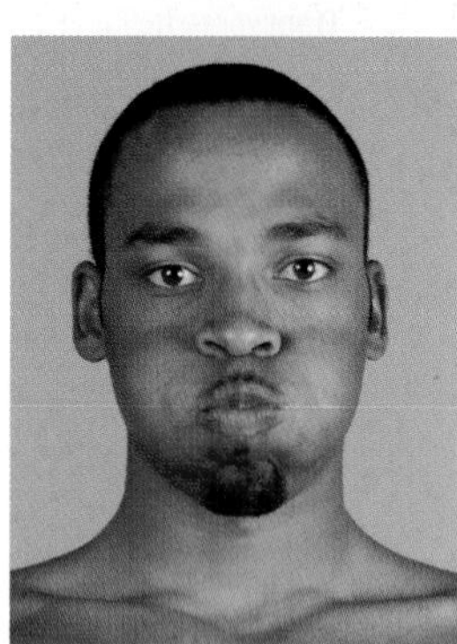
Buccinator + orbicularis oris

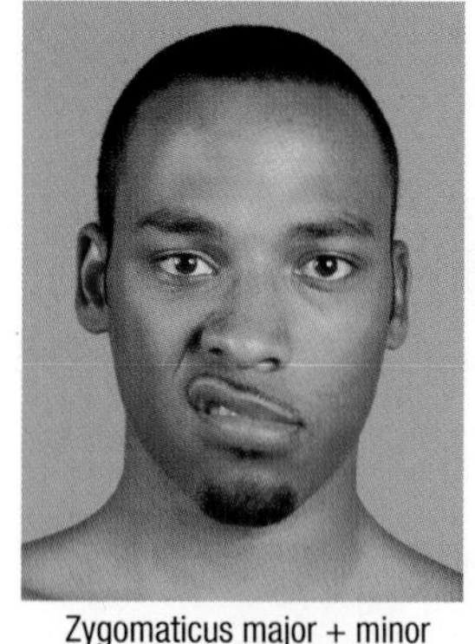
Zygomaticus major + minor

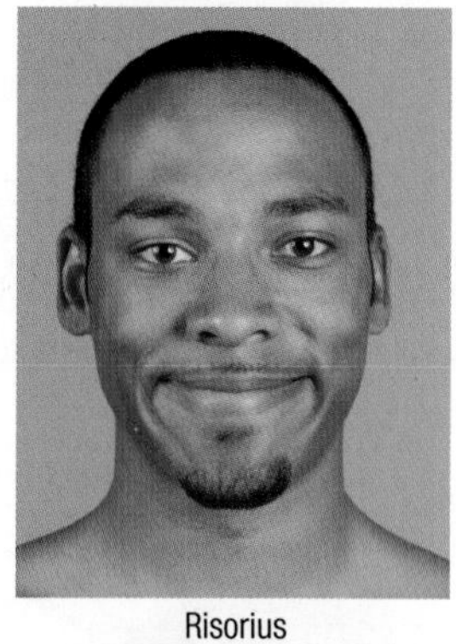
Risorius

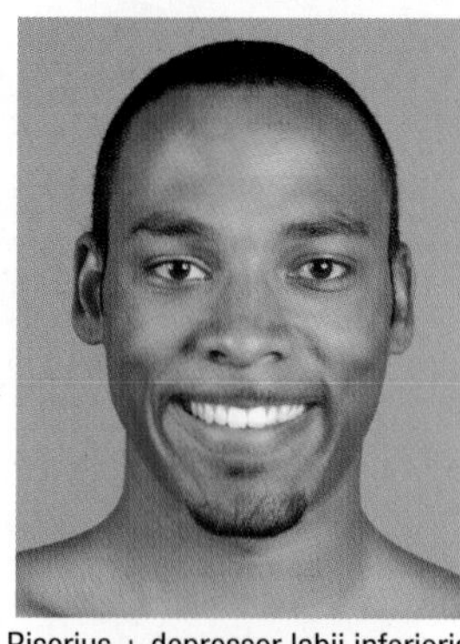
Risorius + depressor labii inferioris

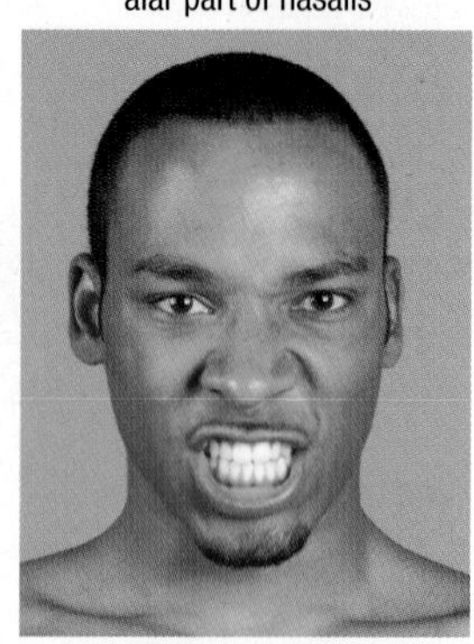
Levator labii sup. + depressor labii

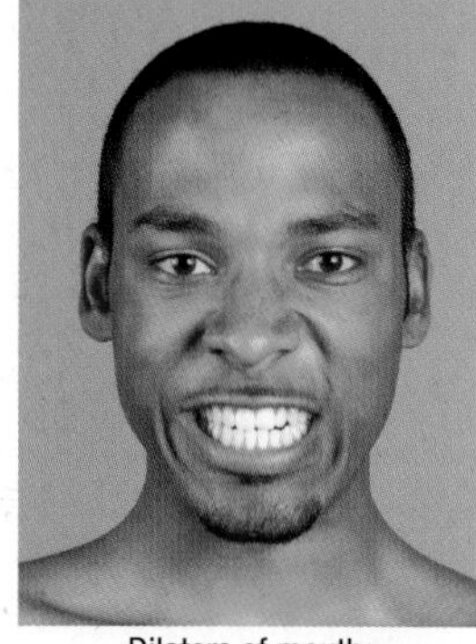
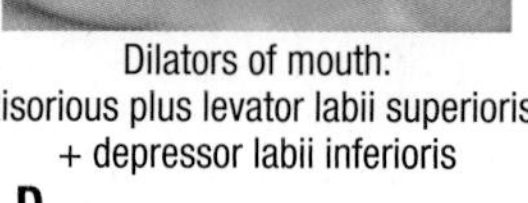
Dilators of mouth: Risorious plus levator labii superioris + depressor labii inferioris

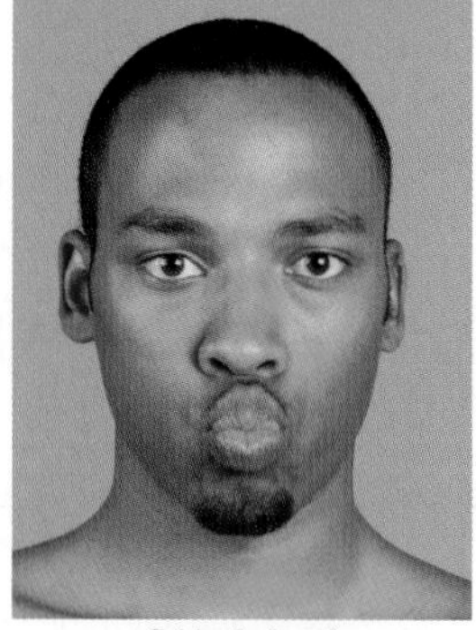
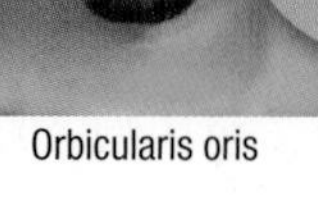
Orbicularis oris

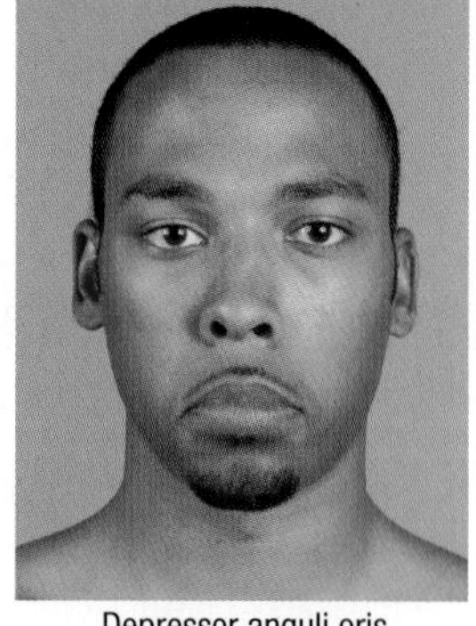
Depressor anguli oris

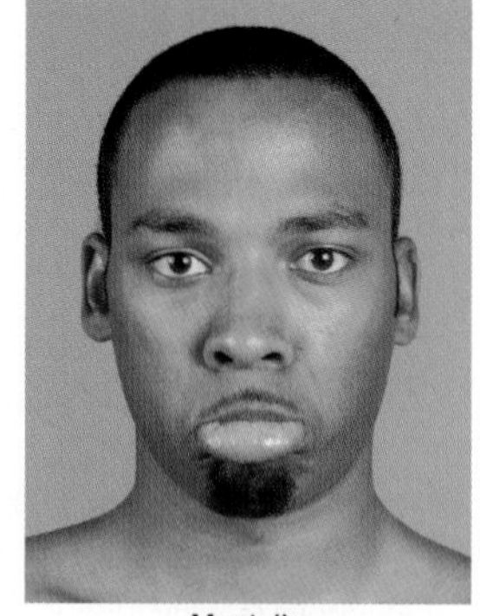
Mentalis

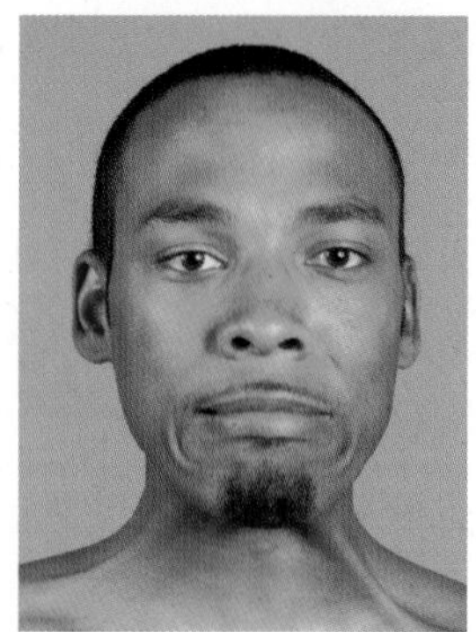
Platysma

D

Anterior Views

7.14 MUSCLES OF FACIAL EXPRESSION

A. Orbicularis oculi: palpebral (P) and orbital (O) parts. Eyelids close lateral to medial washing lacrimal fluid across the cornea. **B.** Gentle closure of eyelid—palpebral part. **C.** Tight closure of eyelid—orbital part. **D.** Actions of selected muscles of facial expression.

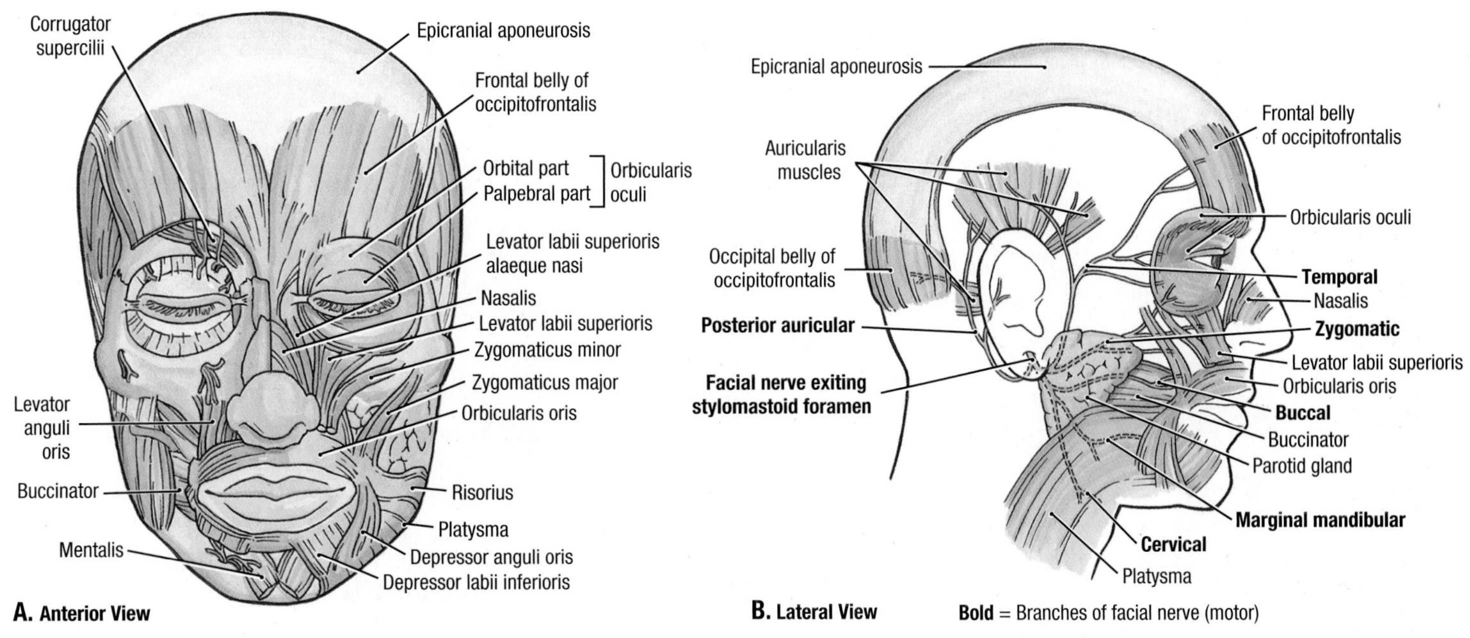
Corrugator supercilii
Epicranial aponeurosis
Frontal belly of occipitofrontalis
Orbital part
Palpebral part
Orbicularis oculi
Levator labii superioris alaeque nasi
Nasalis
Levator labii superioris
Zygomaticus minor
Zygomaticus major
Orbicularis oris
Levator anguli oris
Buccinator
Risorius
Platysma
Mentalis
Depressor anguli oris
Depressor labii inferioris
A. Anterior View
Epicranial aponeurosis
Frontal belly of occipitofrontalis
Auricularis muscles
Orbicularis oculi
Occipital belly of occipitofrontalis
Temporal
Nasalis
Posterior auricular
Zygomatic
Levator labii superioris
Facial nerve exiting stylomastoid foramen
Orbicularis oris
Buccal
Buccinator
Parotid gland
Marginal mandibular
Cervical
Platysma
B. Lateral View
Bold = Branches of facial nerve (motor)

7.15 BRANCHES OF FACIAL NERVE AND MUSCLES OF FACIAL EXPRESSION

A. Muscles. **B.** Branches of facial nerve.

TABLE 7.2 MAIN MUSCLES OF FACIAL EXPRESSION [a]

Muscle[a]	Origin	Insertion	Action
Occipitofrontalis, frontal belly	Epicranial aponeurosis	Skin of and subcutaneous tissue of eyebrows and forehead	Elevates eyebrows and wrinkles skin of forehead; protracts scalp (indicating surprise or curiosity)
Occipitofrontalis, occipital belly	Lateral two-thirds of superior nuchal line	Epicranial aponeurosis	Retracts scalp; increasing effectiveness of frontal belly
Orbicularis oculi	Medial orbital margin, medial palpebral ligament; lacrimal bone	Skin around margin of orbit; superior and inferior tarsal plates	Closes eyelids; palpebral part does so gently; orbital part tightly (winking)
Orbicularis oris	Medial maxilla and mandible; deep surface of perioral skin; angle of mouth (modiolus)	Mucous membrane of lips	Tonus closes oral fissure; phasic contraction compresses and protrudes lips (kissing) or resists distension (when blowing)
Levator labii superioris	Infra-orbital margin (maxilla)	Skin of upper lip	Part of dilators of mouth; retract (elevate) and/or evert upper lip; deepen nasolabial sulcus (showing sadness)
Zygomaticus minor	Anterior aspect, zygomatic bone		
Buccinator	Mandible, alveolar processes of maxilla and mandible; pterygomandibular raphe	Angle of mouth (modiolus); orbicularis oris	Presses cheek against molar teeth; works with tongue to keep food between occlusal surfaces and out of oral vestibule; resists distension (when blowing)
Zygomaticus major	Lateral aspect of zygomatic bone	Angle of mouth (modiolus)	Part of dilators of mouth; elevate labial commissure—bilaterally to smile (happiness); unilaterally to sneer (disdain)
Rizorius	Parotid fascia and buccal skin (highly variable)		Part of dilators of mouth; widens oral fissure
Platysma	Subcutaneous tissue of infraclavicular and supraclavicular regions	Base of mandible; skin of cheek and lower lip; angle of mouth (modiolus); orbicularis oris	Depresses mandible (against resistance); tenses skin of inferior face and neck (conveying tension and stress)

[a]All of these muscles are supplied by the facial nerve (CN VII).

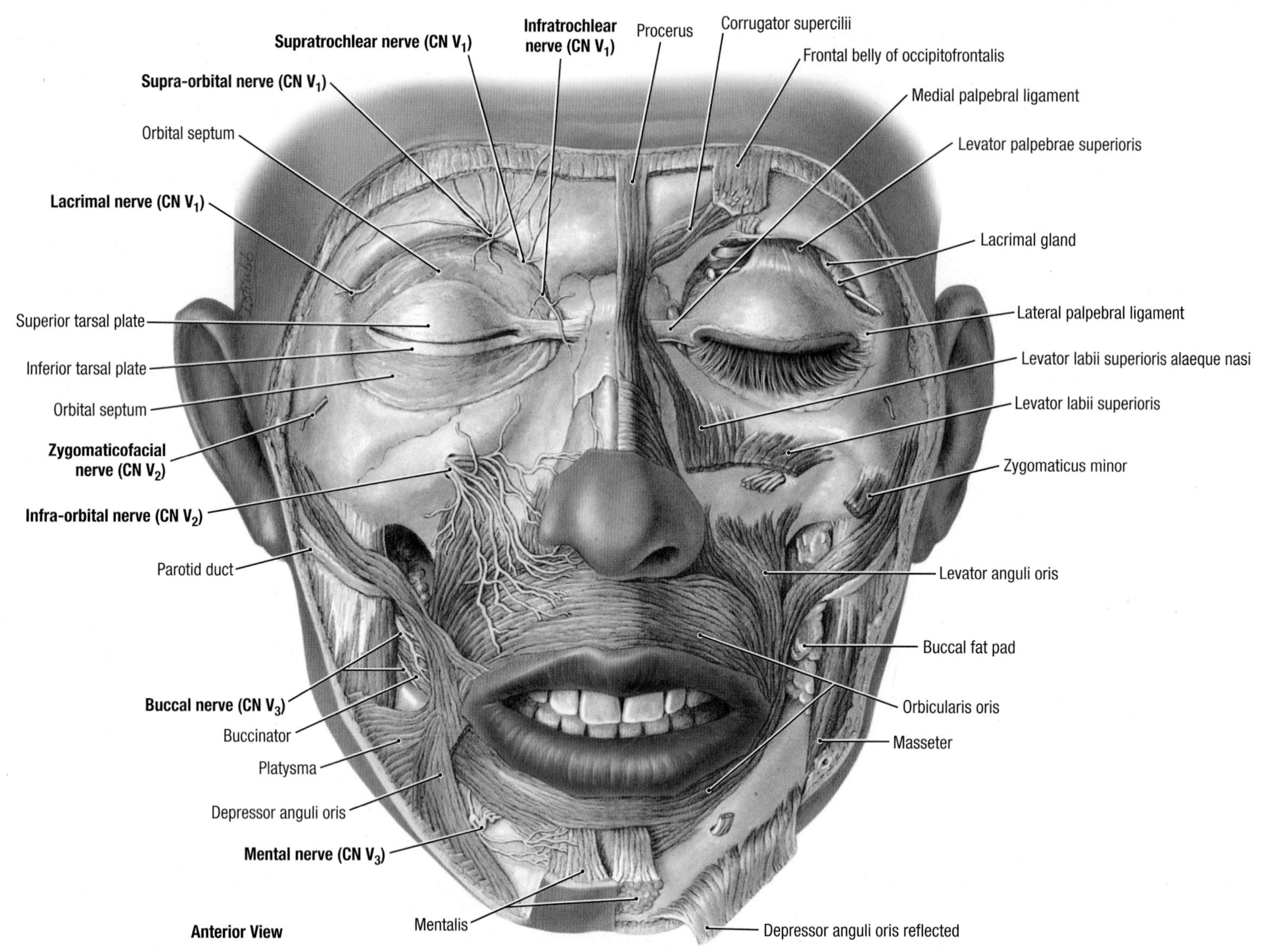

Supratrochlear nerve (CN V_1)
Infratrochlear nerve (CN V_1)
Procerus
Corrugator supercilii
Frontal belly of occipitofrontalis
Supra-orbital nerve (CN V_1)
Medial palpebral ligament
Orbital septum
Levator palpebrae superioris
Lacrimal nerve (CN V_1)
Lacrimal gland
Lateral palpebral ligament
Superior tarsal plate
Inferior tarsal plate
Levator labii superioris alaeque nasi
Orbital septum
Levator labii superioris
Zygomaticofacial nerve (CN V_2)
Zygomaticus minor
Infra-orbital nerve (CN V_2)
Parotid duct
Levator anguli oris
Buccal fat pad
Buccal nerve (CN V_3)
Orbicularis oris
Buccinator
Masseter
Platysma
Depressor anguli oris
Mental nerve (CN V_3)
Anterior View
Mentalis
Depressor anguli oris reflected

7.16 CUTANEOUS BRANCHES OF TRIGEMINAL NERVE, MUSCLES OF FACIAL EXPRESSION, AND EYELID

Injury to the facial nerve (CN VII) or its branches produces paralysis of some or all of the facial muscles on the affected side (Bell palsy). The affected area sags, and facial expression is distorted. The loss of tonus of the orbicularis oculi causes the inferior lid to evert (fall away from the surface of the eyeball). As a result, the lacrimal fluid is not spread over the cornea, preventing adequate lubrication, hydration, and flushing of the cornea. This makes the cornea vulnerable to ulceration. If the injury weakens or paralyzes the buccinator and orbicularis oris, food will accumulate in the oral vestibule during chewing, usually requiring continual removal with a finger. When the sphincters or dilators of the mouth are affected, displacement of the mouth (drooping of the corner) is produced by gravity and contraction of unopposed contralateral facial muscles, resulting in food and saliva dribbling out of the side of the mouth. Weakened lip muscles affect speech. Affected people cannot whistle or blow a wind instrument effectively. They frequently dab their eyes and mouth with a handkerchief to wipe the fluid (tears and saliva) that runs from the drooping lid and mouth.

Because the face does not have a distinct layer of deep fascia and the subcutaneous tissue is loose between the attachments of facial muscles, **facial lacerations** tend to gap (part widely). Consequently, the skin must be sutured carefully to prevent scarring. The looseness of the subcutaneous tissue also enables fluid and blood to accumulate in the loose connective tissue after **bruising of the face**.

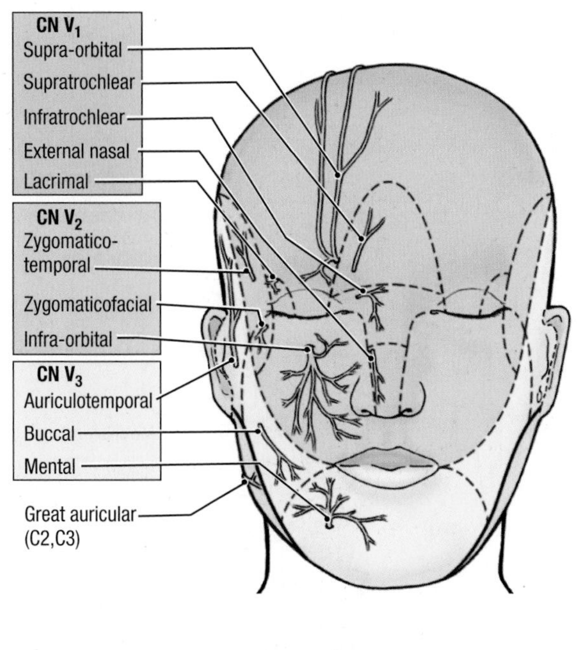
CN V_1
Supra-orbital
Supratrochlear
Infratrochlear
External nasal
Lacrimal
CN V_2
Zygomatico-
temporal
Zygomaticofacial
Infra-orbital
CN V_3
Auriculotemporal
Buccal
Mental
Great auricular
(C2,C3)

A. Anterior view

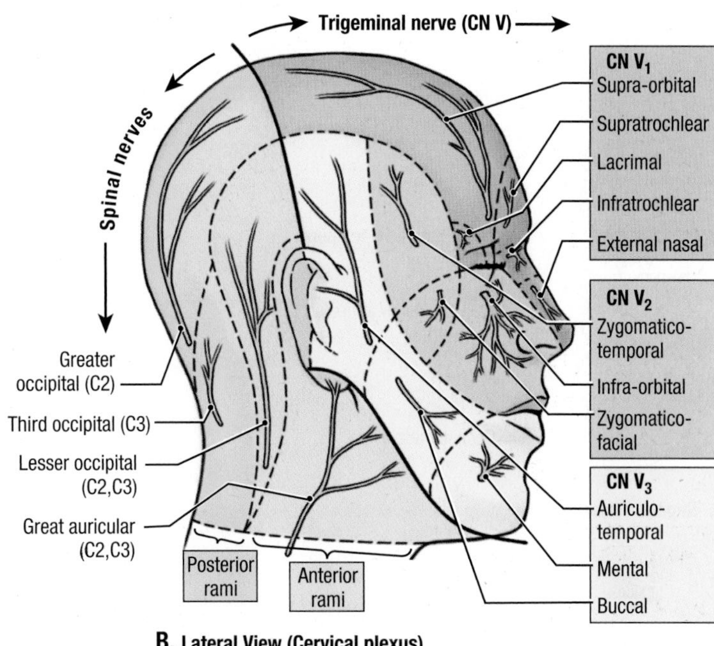
Trigeminal nerve (CN V)
Spinal nerves
CN V_1
Supra-orbital
Supratrochlear
Lacrimal
Infratrochlear
External nasal
CN V_2
Zygomatico-
temporal
Infra-orbital
Zygomatico-
facial
CN V_3
Auriculo-
temporal
Mental
Buccal
Greater
occipital (C2)
Third occipital (C3)
Lesser occipital
(C2,C3)
Great auricular
(C2,C3)
Posterior
rami
Anterior
rami

B. Lateral View (Cervical plexus)

7.17 NERVES OF FACE AND SCALP

TABLE 7.3 NERVES OF FACE AND SCALP

Nerve	Origin	Course	Distribution
Frontal	Ophthalmic nerve (CN V_1)	Crosses orbit on superior aspect of levator palpebrae superioris; divides into supra-orbital and supratrochlear branches	Skin of forehead, scalp, superior eyelid, and nose; conjunctiva of superior lid and mucosa of frontal sinus
Supra-orbital	Continuation of frontal nerve (CN V_1)	Emerges through supra-orbital notch, or foramen, and breaks up into small branches	Mucous membrane of frontal sinus and conjunctiva (lining) of superior eyelid; skin of forehead as far as vertex
Supratrochlear	Frontal nerve (CN V_1)	Continues anteromedially along roof of orbit, passing lateral to trochlea	Skin in middle of forehead to hairline
Infratrochlear	Nasociliary nerve (CN V_1)	Follows medial wall of orbit passing inferior to trochlea to superior eyelid	Skin and conjunctiva (lining) of superior eye lid
Lacrimal	Ophthalmic nerve (CN V_1)	Passes through palpebral fascia of superior eyelid near lateral angle (canthus) of eye	Lacrimal gland and small area of skin and conjunctiva of lateral part of superior eyelid
External nasal	Anterior ethmoidal nerve (CN V_1)	Runs in nasal cavity and emerges on face between nasal bone and lateral nasal cartilage	Skin on dorsum of nose, including tip of nose
Zygomatic	Maxillary nerve (CN V_2)	Arises in floor of orbit, divides into zygomaticofacial and zygomaticotemporal nerves, which traverse foramina of same name	Skin over zygomatic arch and anterior temporal region
Infra-orbital	Terminal branch of maxillary nerve (CN V_2)	Runs in floor of orbit and emerges at infra-orbital foramen	Skin of cheek, inferior lid, lateral side of nose and inferior septum and superior lip, upper premolar incisors and canine teeth; mucosa of maxillary sinus and superior lip
Auriculotemporal	Mandibular nerve (CN V_3)	From posterior division of CN V_3, it passes between neck of mandible and external acoustic meatus to accompany superficial temporal artery	Skin anterior to ear and posterior temporal region, tragus and part of helix of auricle, and roof of external acoustic meatus and upper tympanic membrane
Buccal	Mandibular nerve (CN V_3)	From the anterior division of CN V_3 in infratemporal fossa, it passes anteriorly to reach cheek	Skin and mucosa of cheek, buccal gingiva adjacent to 2nd and 3rd molar teeth
Mental	Terminal branch of inferior alveolar nerve (CN V_3)	Emerges from mandibular canal at mental foramen	Skin of chin and inferior lip and mucosa of lower lip

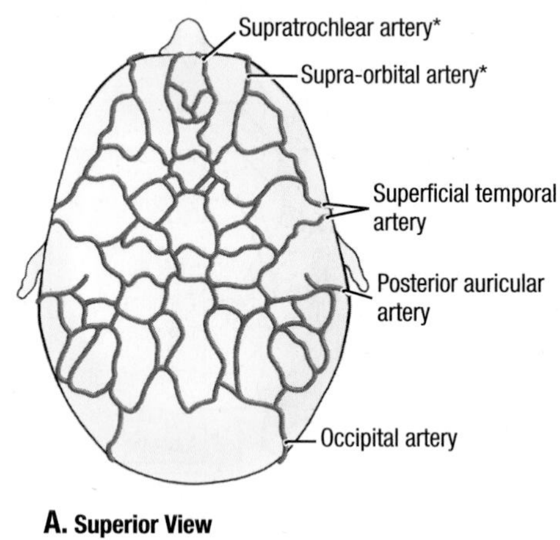
Supratrochlear artery*
Supra-orbital artery*
Superficial temporal artery
Posterior auricular artery
Occipital artery

A. Superior View

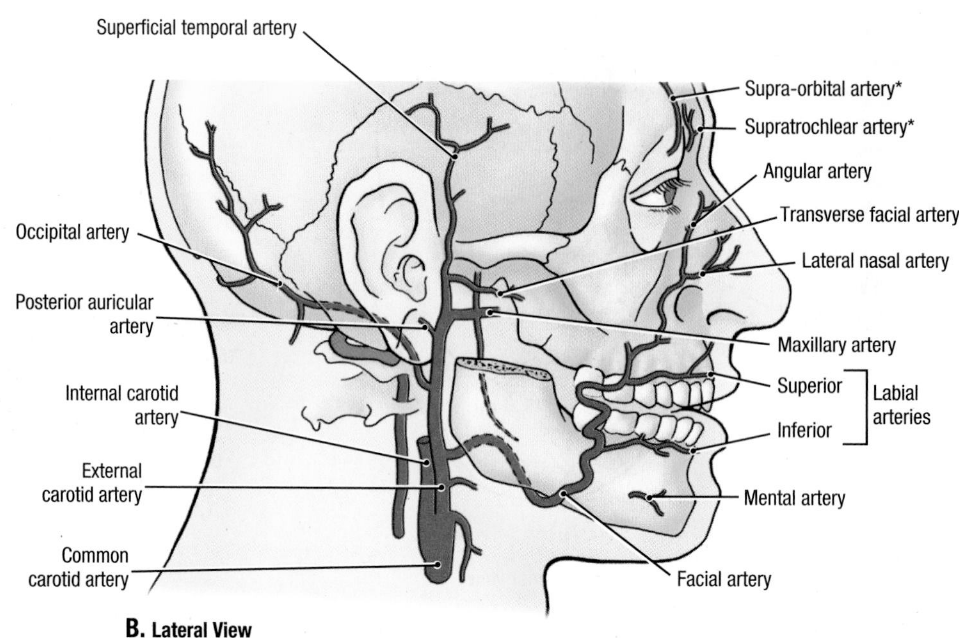
Superficial temporal artery
Supra-orbital artery*
Supratrochlear artery*
Angular artery
Transverse facial artery
Lateral nasal artery
Occipital artery
Posterior auricular artery
Maxillary artery
Superior
Labial arteries
Inferior
Internal carotid artery
External carotid artery
Mental artery
Common carotid artery
Facial artery

B. Lateral View

*Source= internal carotid artery (ophthalmic artery); all other labeled arteries are from external carotid

7.18 ARTERIES OF FACE AND SCALP

TABLE 7.4 ARTERIES OF SUPERFICIAL FACE AND SCALP

Artery	Origin	Course	Distribution
Facial	External carotid artery	Ascends deep to submandibular gland, winds around inferior border of mandible and enters face	Muscles of facial expression and face
Inferior labial	Facial artery near angle of mouth	Runs medially in lower lip	Lower lip and chin
Superior labial		Runs medially in upper lip	Upper lip and ala (side) and septum of nose
Lateral nasal	Facial artery as it ascends alongside nose	Passes to ala of nose	Skin on ala and dorsum of nose
Angular	Terminal branch of facial artery	Passes to medial angle (canthus) of eye	Superior part of cheek and lower eyelid
Occipital	External carotid artery	Passes medial to posterior belly of digastric and mastoid process; accompanies occipital nerve in occipital region	Scalp of back of head, as far as vertex
Posterior auricular		Passes posteriorly, deep to parotid, along styloid process between mastoid and ear	Scalp posterior to auricle and auricle
Superficial temporal	Smaller terminal branch of external carotid artery	Ascends anterior to ear to temporal region and ends in scalp	Facial muscles and skin of frontal and temporal regions
Transverse facial	Superficial temporal artery within parotid gland	Crosses face superficial to masseter and inferior to zygomatic arch	Parotid gland and duct, muscles and skin of face
Mental	Terminal branch of inferior alveolar artery	Emerges from mental foramen and passes to chin	Facial muscles and skin of chin
***Supra-orbital**	Terminal branch of ophthalmic artery, a branch of internal carotid	Passes superiorly from supra-orbital foramen	Muscles and skin of forehead and scalp
***Supratrochlear**		Passes superiorly from supratrochlear notch	Muscles and skin of scalp

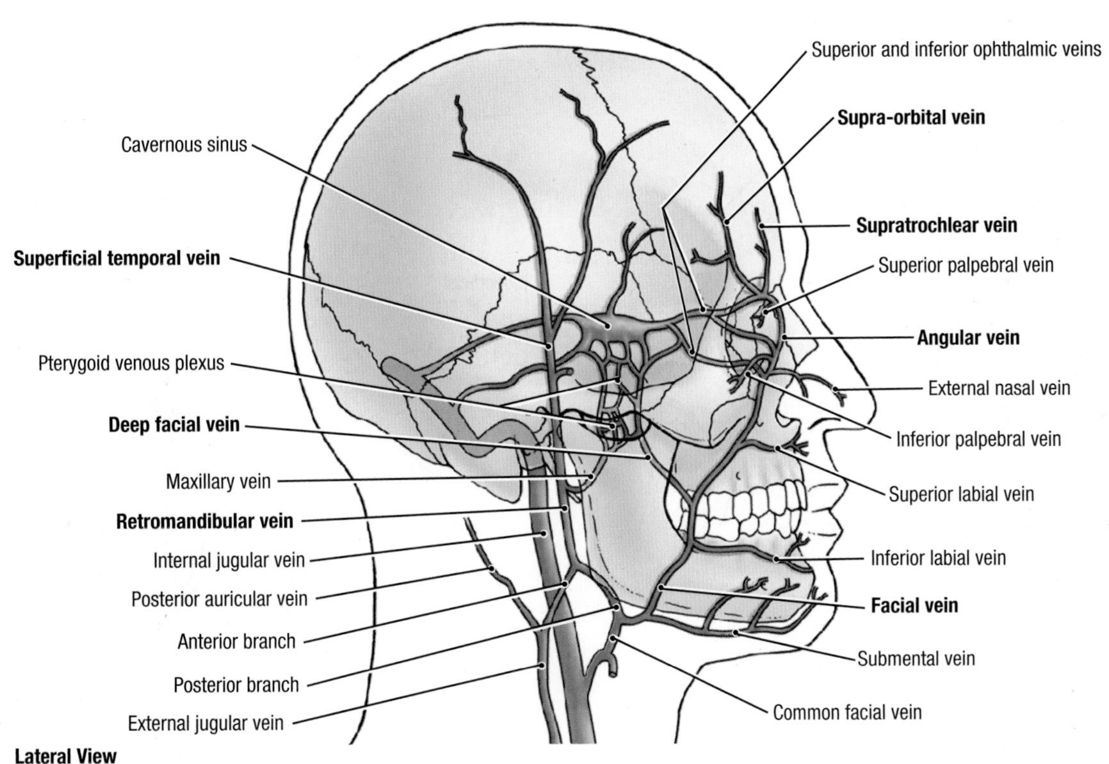
Superior and inferior ophthalmic veins
Supra-orbital vein
Cavernous sinus
Supratrochlear vein
Superficial temporal vein
Superior palpebral vein
Angular vein
Pterygoid venous plexus
External nasal vein
Deep facial vein
Inferior palpebral vein
Maxillary vein
Superior labial vein
Retromandibular vein
Internal jugular vein
Inferior labial vein
Posterior auricular vein
Facial vein
Anterior branch
Submental vein
Posterior branch
External jugular vein
Common facial vein
Lateral View

7.19 VEINS OF FACE

TABLE 7.5 VEINS OF FACE

Vein	Origin	Course	Termination	Area Drained
Supratrochlear	Begins from a venous plexus on the forehead and scalp, through which it communicates with the frontal branch of the superficial temporal vein, its contralateral partner, and the supra-orbital vein	Descends near the midline of the forehead to the root of the nose where it joins the supra-orbital vein	Angular vein at the root of the nose	Anterior part of scalp and forehead
Supra-orbital	Begins in the forehead by anastomosing with a frontal tributary of the superficial temporal vein	Passes medially superior to the orbit and joins the supratrochlear vein; a branch passes through the supra-orbital notch and joins with the superior ophthalmic vein		
Angular	Begins at root of nose by union of supratrochlear and supra-orbital veins	Descends obliquely along the root and side of the nose to the inferior margin of the orbit	Becomes the facial vein at the inferior margin of the orbit	In addition to above, drains upper and lower lids and conjunctiva; may receive drainage from cavernous sinus
Facial	Continuation of angular vein past inferior margin of orbit	Descends along lateral border of the nose, receiving external nasal and inferior palpebral veins, then obliquely across face to mandible; receives anterior division of retromandibular vein, after which it is sometimes called the common facial vein	Internal jugular vein at or inferior to the level of the hyoid bone	Anterior scalp and forehead, eyelids, external nose, and anterior cheek, lips, chin, and submandibular gland
Deep facial	Pterygoid venous plexus	Runs anteriorly on maxilla above buccinator and deep to masseter, emerging medial to anterior border of masseter onto face	Enters posterior aspect of facial vein	Infratemporal fossa (most areas supplied by maxillary artery)
Superficial temporal	Begins from a widespread plexus of veins on the side of the scalp and along the zygomatic arch	Its frontal and parietal tributaries unite anterior to the auricle; it crosses the temporal root of the zygomatic arch to pass from the temporal region and enters the substance of the parotid gland	Joins the maxillary vein posterior to the neck of the mandible to form the retromandibular vein	Side of the scalp, superficial aspect of the temporal muscle, and external ear
Retromandibular	Formed anterior to the ear by the union of the superficial temporal and maxillary veins	Runs posterior and deep to the ramus of the mandible through the substance of the parotid gland; communicates at its inferior end with the facial vein	*Anterior branch* unites with facial vein to form common facial vein; *posterior branch* unites with the posterior auricular vein to form the external jugular vein	Parotid gland and masseter muscle

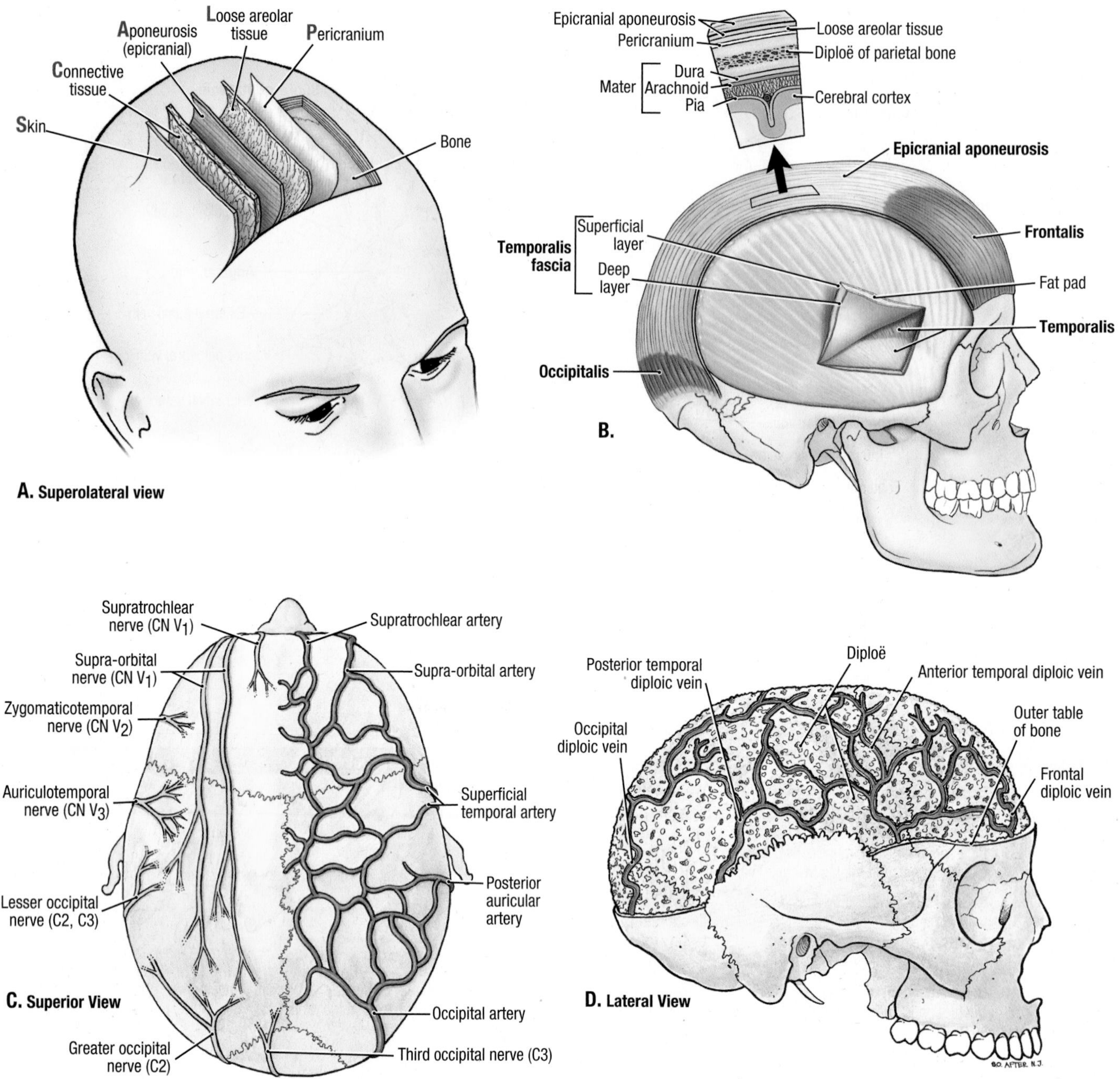

Loose areolar tissue
Aponeurosis (epicranial)
Pericranium
Connective tissue
Skin
Bone
A. Superolateral view
Epicranial aponeurosis
Pericranium
Mater
Dura
Arachnoid
Pia
Loose areolar tissue
Diploë of parietal bone
Cerebral cortex
Epicranial aponeurosis
Temporalis fascia
Superficial layer
Deep layer
Frontalis
Fat pad
Temporalis
Occipitalis
B.
Supratrochlear nerve (CN V1)
Supra-orbital nerve (CN V1)
Zygomaticotemporal nerve (CN V2)
Auriculotemporal nerve (CN V3)
Lesser occipital nerve (C2, C3)
C. Superior View
Greater occipital nerve (C2)
Supratrochlear artery
Supra-orbital artery
Superficial temporal artery
Posterior auricular artery
Occipital artery
Third occipital nerve (C3)
Posterior temporal diploic vein
Diploë
Anterior temporal diploic vein
Occipital diploic vein
Outer table of bone
Frontal diploic vein
D. Lateral View

7.20 BRANCHES OF FACIAL NERVE, MUSCLES OF FACIAL EXPRESSION, AND SCALP

A. Layers of scalp. **B.** Occipitofrontalis and temporal muscles and fascia. **C.** Sensory nerves and arteries of the scalp. **D.** Diploic veins. The outer layer of the compact bone of the cranium has been filed away, exposing the channels for the diploic veins in the cancellous bone that composes the diploë (see Fig. 7.7).

Scalp injuries and infections. The loose areolar tissue layer is the danger area of the scalp because pus or blood spreads easily in it. Infection in this layer can pass into the cranial cavity through emissary veins, which pass through parietal foramina in the calvaria and reach intracranial structures such as the meninges. An infection cannot pass into the neck because the occipital belly of the occipitofrontalis attaches to the occipital bone and mastoid parts of the temporal bones. Neither can a scalp infection spread laterally beyond the zygomatic arches because the epicranial aponeurosis is continuous with the temporalis fascia that attaches to these arches. An infection or fluid (e.g., pus or blood) can enter the eyelids and the root of the nose because the frontal belly of the occipitofrontalis inserts into the skin and dense subcutaneous tissue and does not attach to the bone. **Ecchymoses**, or purple patches, develop as a result of extravasation of blood into the subcutaneous tissue and skin of the eyelids and surrounding regions.

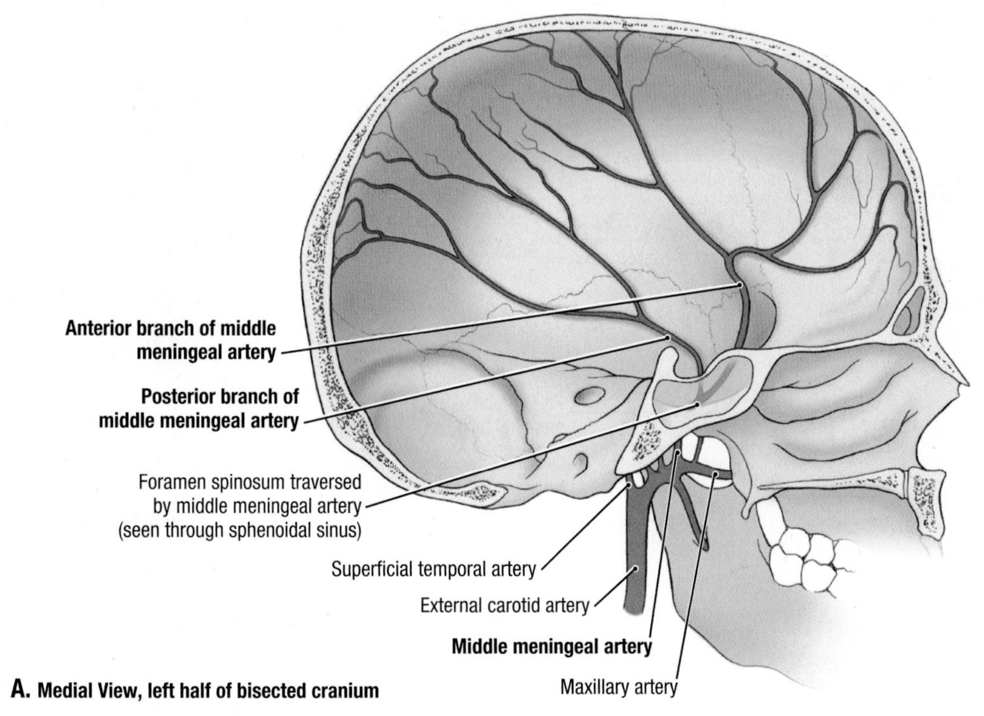
Anterior branch of middle meningeal artery
Posterior branch of middle meningeal artery
Foramen spinosum traversed by middle meningeal artery (seen through sphenoidal sinus)
Superficial temporal artery
External carotid artery
Middle meningeal artery
Maxillary artery

A. Medial View, left half of bisected cranium

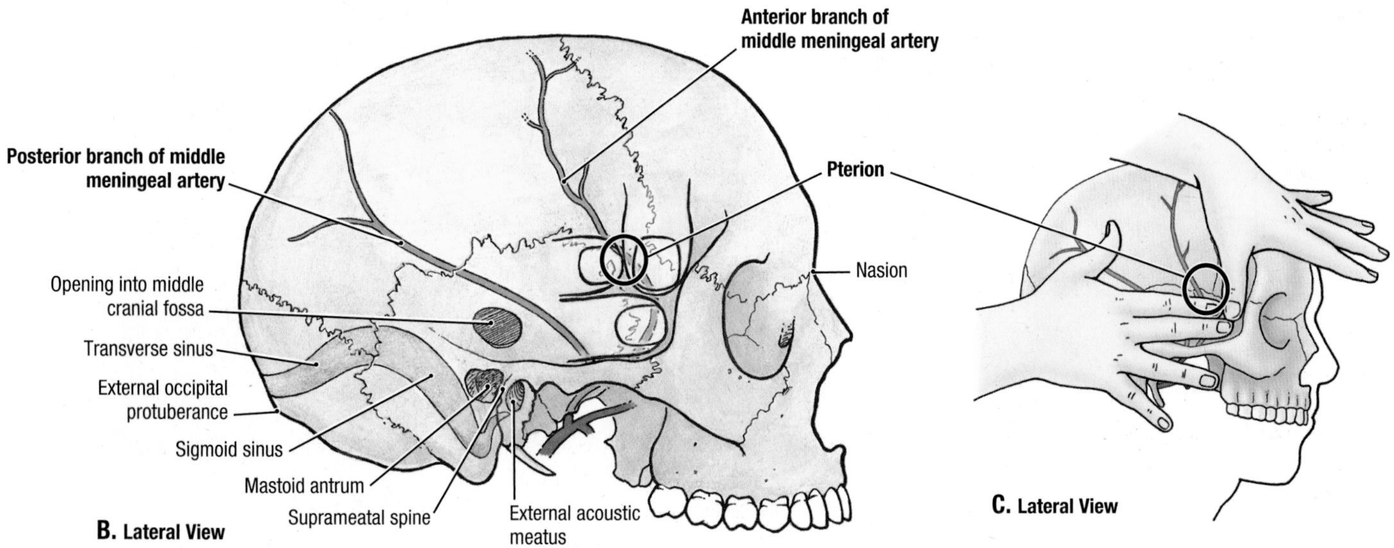
Anterior branch of middle meningeal artery
Posterior branch of middle meningeal artery
Pterion
Nasion
Opening into middle cranial fossa
Transverse sinus
External occipital protuberance
Sigmoid sinus
Mastoid antrum
Suprameatal spine
External acoustic meatus

B. Lateral View

C. Lateral View

7.21 MIDDLE MENINGEAL ARTERY AND PTERION

A. Course of the middle meningeal artery in the cranium. **B.** Surface projections of internal features of the neurocranium. **C.** Locating the pterion. The pterion is located two fingers breadth superior to the zygomatic arch and one thumb breadth posterior to the frontal process of the zygomatic bone (approximately 4 cm superior to the midpoint of the zygomatic arch); the anterior branch of the middle meningeal artery crosses the pterion.

A hard blow to the side of the head may fracture the thin bones forming the pterion, rupturing the anterior branch of the middle meningeal artery crossing the pterion. The resulting **extradural (epidural) hematoma** exerts pressure on the underlying cerebral cortex. Untreated middle meningeal artery hemorrhage may cause death in a few hours.

Superior sagittal sinus
Scalp
Skin
Connective tissue
Aponeurosis (epicranial)
Loose areolar tissue
Pericranium
Diploë of parietal bone
Mater
Dura
Arachnoid
Pia
Arachnoid granulations
Cerebral cortex
Falx cerebri (cerebral falx)
Cerebral artery in subarachnoid space
Inferior sagittal sinus

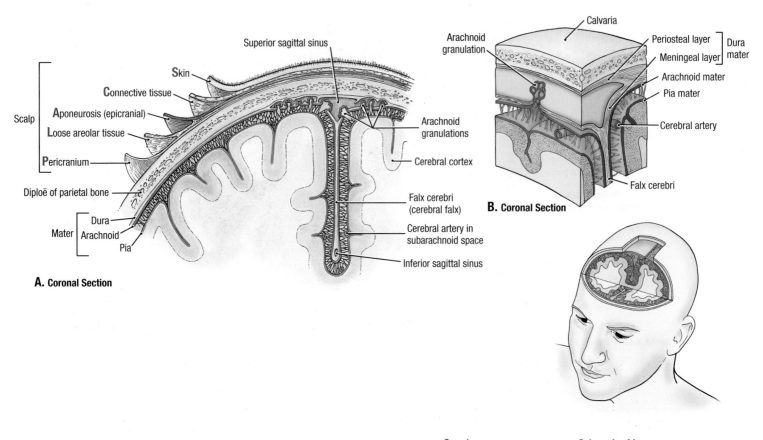

A. Coronal Section

Calvaria
Arachnoid granulation
Periosteal layer
Meningeal layer
Dura mater
Arachnoid mater
Pia mater
Cerebral artery
Falx cerebri

B. Coronal Section

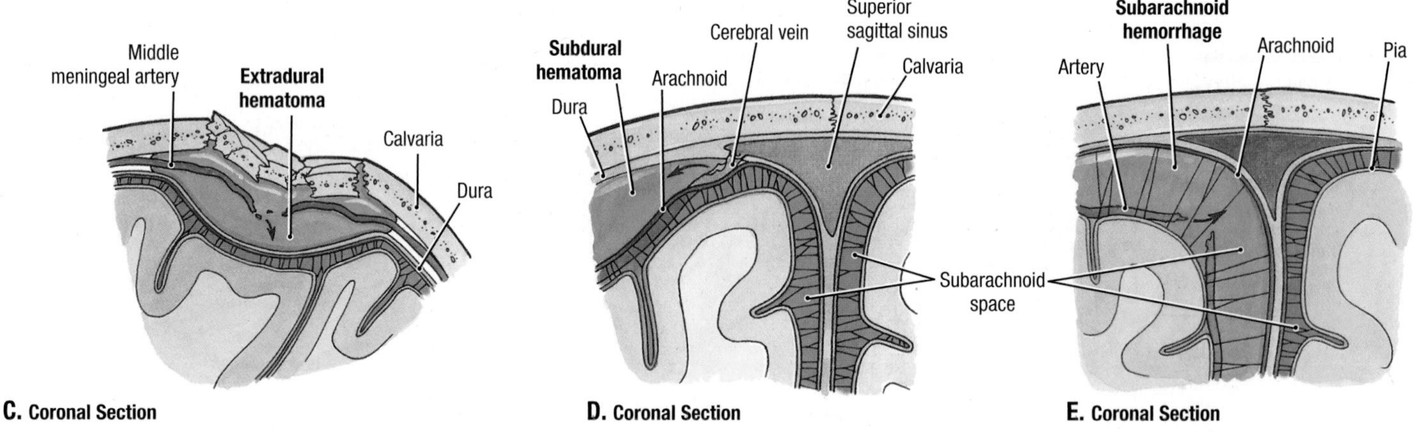
Middle meningeal artery
Extradural hematoma
Calvaria
Dura
Subdural hematoma
Dura
Arachnoid
Cerebral vein
Superior sagittal sinus
Calvaria
Subarachnoid space
Subarachnoid hemorrhage
Artery
Arachnoid
Pia

C. Coronal Section

D. Coronal Section

E. Coronal Section

7.22 LAYERS OF THE SCALP AND MENINGES

A. Scalp, cranium, and meninges. **B.** Meninges and their relationship to the calvaria. The three meningeal spaces include the extradural (epidural) space between the cranial bones and dura, which is a potential space normally (it becomes a real space pathologically if blood accumulates in it); the similarly potential subdural space between the dura and arachnoid; and the subarachnoid space, the normal realized space between the arachnoid and pia, which contains cerebrospinal fluid (CSF). **C. Extradural (epidural) hematomas** result from bleeding from a torn middle meningeal artery. **D. Subdural hematomas** commonly result from tearing of a cerebral vein as it enters the superior sagittal sinus. **E. Subarachnoid hemorrhage** results from bleeding within the subarachnoid space, e.g., from rupture of an aneurysm.

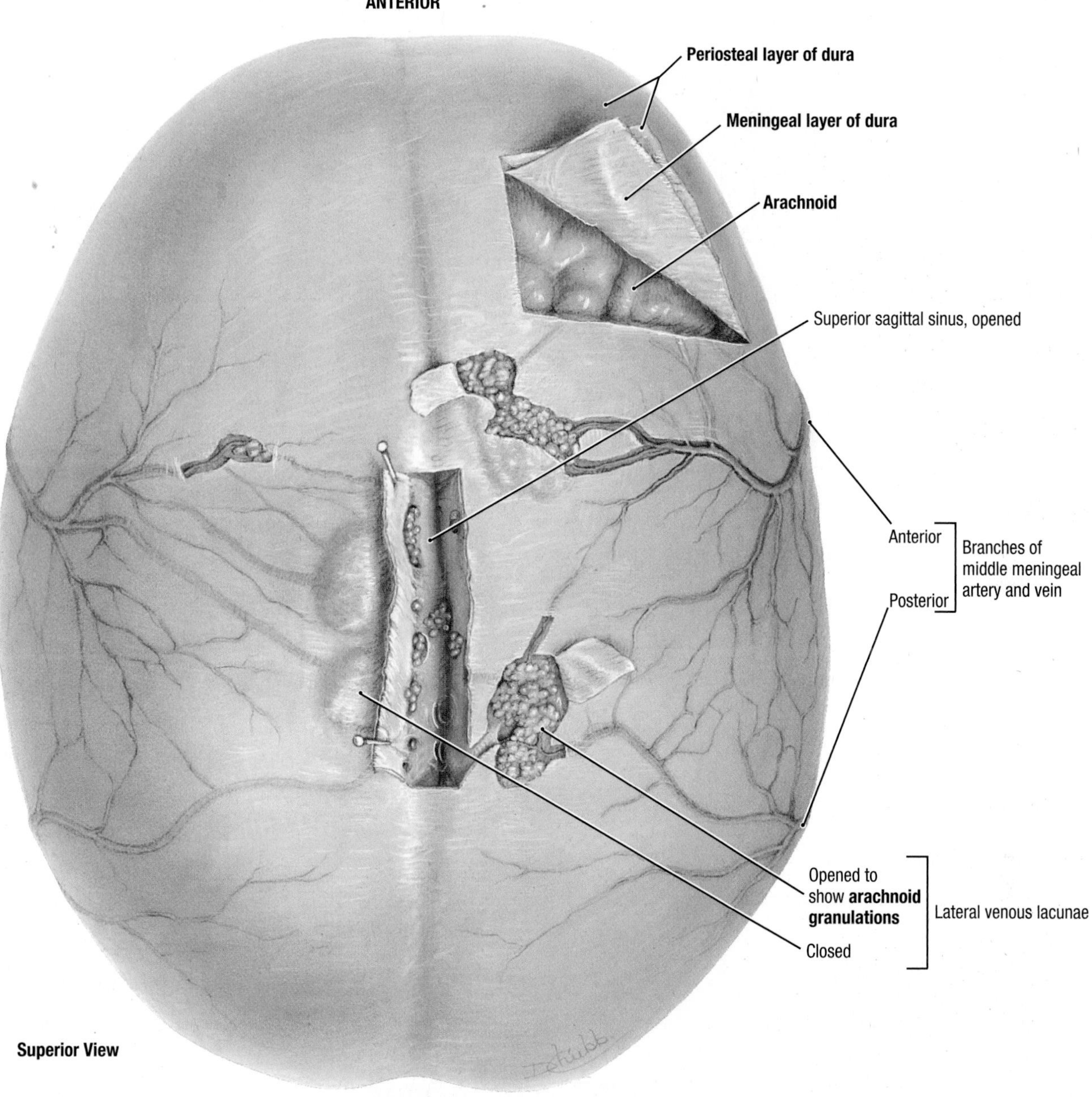
ANTERIOR
Periosteal layer of dura
Meningeal layer of dura
Arachnoid
Superior sagittal sinus, opened
Anterior
Posterior
Branches of middle meningeal artery and vein
Opened to show arachnoid granulations
Closed
Lateral venous lacunae
Superior View
POSTERIOR

7.23 DURA MATER AND ARACHNOID GRANULATIONS

- The calvaria is removed. In the median plane, the thick roof of the superior sagittal sinus is partly pinned aside, and laterally, the thin roofs of two lateral lacunae are reflected.
- The middle meningeal artery lies in a venous channel (middle meningeal vein), which enlarges superiorly into a lateral lacunae. Other channels drain the lateral lacunae into the superior sagittal sinus.
- Arachnoid granulations in the lacunae are responsible for absorption of CSF from the subarachnoid space into the venous system.
- The dura is sensitive to pain, especially where it is related to the dural venous sinuses and meningeal arteries. Although the causes of **headache** are numerous, distention of the scalp or meningeal vessels (or both) is believed to be one cause of headache. Many headaches appear to be dural in origin, such as the headache occurring after a lumbar spinal puncture for removal of CSF. These headaches are thought to result from stimulation of sensory nerve endings in the dura.

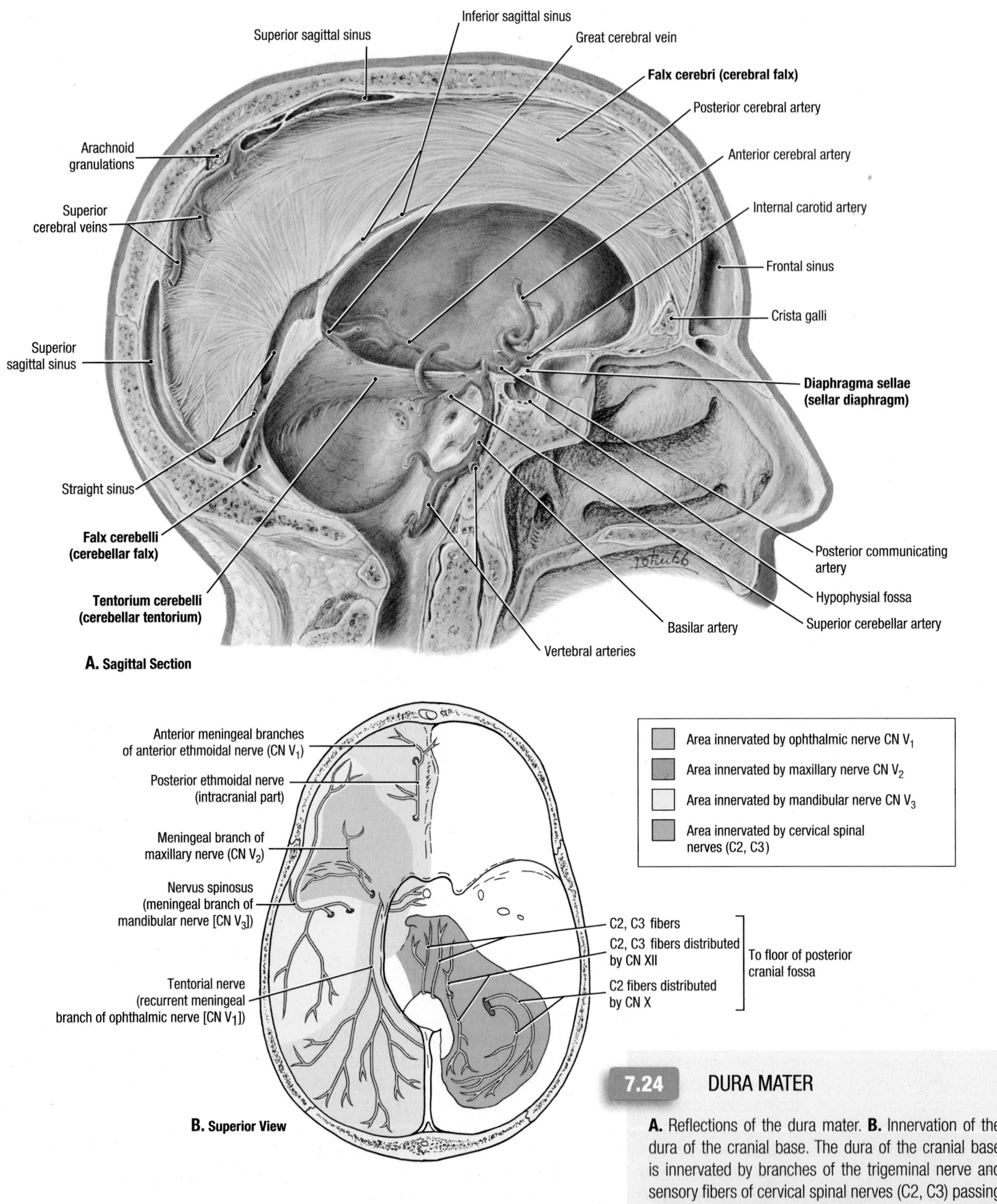

Inferior sagittal sinus
Superior sagittal sinus
Great cerebral vein
Falx cerebri (cerebral falx)
Posterior cerebral artery
Arachnoid granulations
Anterior cerebral artery
Internal carotid artery
Superior cerebral veins
Frontal sinus
Crista galli
Superior sagittal sinus
Diaphragma sellae (sellar diaphragm)
Straight sinus
Falx cerebelli (cerebellar falx)
Posterior communicating artery
Hypophysial fossa
Tentorium cerebelli (cerebellar tentorium)
Basilar artery
Superior cerebellar artery
Vertebral arteries
A. Sagittal Section
Anterior meningeal branches of anterior ethmoidal nerve (CN V1)
Posterior ethmoidal nerve (intracranial part)
Meningeal branch of maxillary nerve (CN V2)
Nervus spinosus (meningeal branch of mandibular nerve [CN V3])
Tentorial nerve (recurrent meningeal branch of ophthalmic nerve [CN V1])
Area innervated by ophthalmic nerve CN V1
Area innervated by maxillary nerve CN V2
Area innervated by mandibular nerve CN V3
Area innervated by cervical spinal nerves (C2, C3)
C2, C3 fibers
C2, C3 fibers distributed by CN XII
C2 fibers distributed by CN X
To floor of posterior cranial fossa
B. Superior View

7.24 DURA MATER

A. Reflections of the dura mater. **B.** Innervation of the dura of the cranial base. The dura of the cranial base is innervated by branches of the trigeminal nerve and sensory fibers of cervical spinal nerves (C2, C3) passing directly from those nerves or via meningeal branches of the vagus (CN X) and hypoglossal (CN XII) nerves.

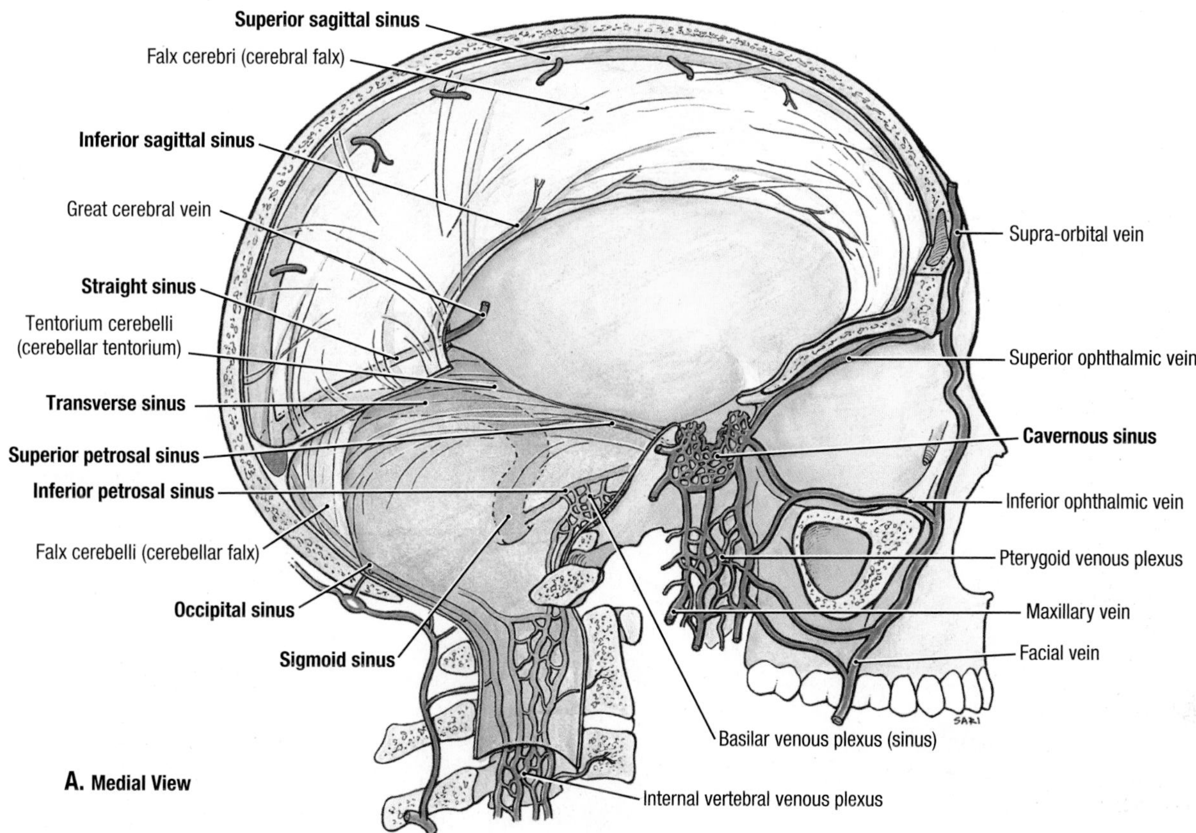
Superior sagittal sinus
Falx cerebri (cerebral falx)
Inferior sagittal sinus
Great cerebral vein
Straight sinus
Tentorium cerebelli (cerebellar tentorium)
Transverse sinus
Superior petrosal sinus
Inferior petrosal sinus
Falx cerebelli (cerebellar falx)
Occipital sinus
Sigmoid sinus
Supra-orbital vein
Superior ophthalmic vein
Cavernous sinus
Inferior ophthalmic vein
Pterygoid venous plexus
Maxillary vein
Facial vein
Basilar venous plexus (sinus)
Internal vertebral venous plexus
A. Medial View

7.25 VENOUS SINUSES OF DURA MATER

A. Schematic of left half of cranial cavity and right facial skeleton. **B.** Venous sinuses of the cranial base.

- The superior sagittal sinus is at the superior border of the falx cerebri, and the inferior sagittal sinus is in its free border. The great cerebral vein joins the inferior sagittal sinus to form the straight sinus.
- The superior sagittal sinus usually becomes the right transverse sinus, which drains into the right sigmoid sinus, and next into the right internal jugular vein; the straight sinus similarly drains through the left transverse sinus, left sigmoid sinus, and left internal jugular vein.
- The cavernous sinus communicates with the veins of the face through the ophthalmic veins and pterygoid plexus of veins and with the sigmoid sinus through the superior and inferior petrosal sinuses.
- **Metastasis of tumor cells to dural sinuses.** The basilar and occipital sinuses communicate through the foramen magnum with the internal vertebral venous plexuses. Because these venous channels are valveless, increased intra-abdominopelvic or intrathoracic pressure, as occurs during heavy coughing and straining, may force venous blood from these regions into the internal vertebral venous system and from it into the dural venous sinuses. As a result, pus in abscesses and tumor cells in these regions may spread to the vertebrae and brain.

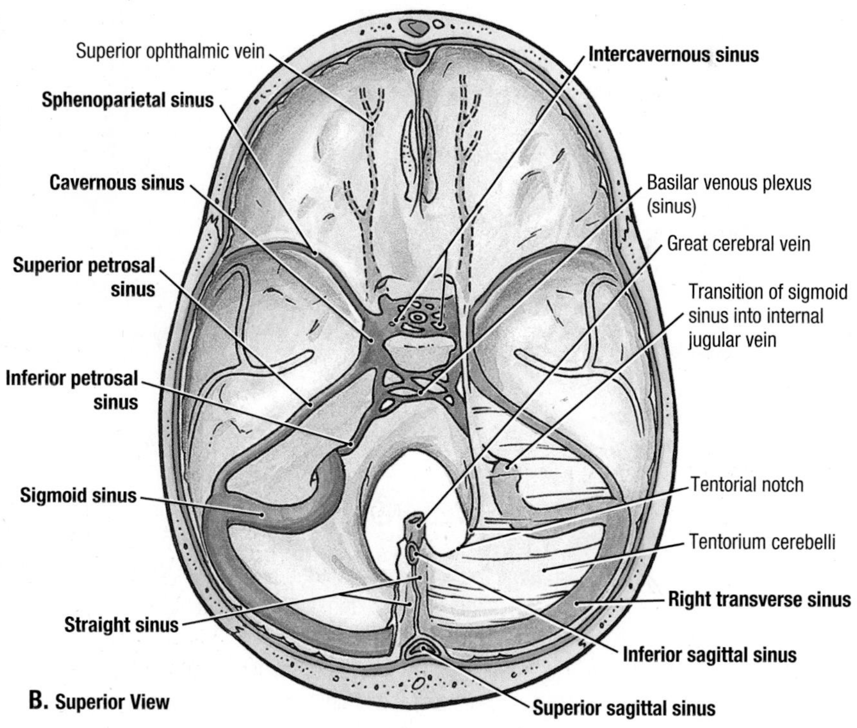
Superior ophthalmic vein
Intercavernous sinus
Sphenoparietal sinus
Cavernous sinus
Basilar venous plexus (sinus)
Great cerebral vein
Superior petrosal sinus
Transition of sigmoid sinus into internal jugular vein
Inferior petrosal sinus
Sigmoid sinus
Tentorial notch
Tentorium cerebelli
Right transverse sinus
Straight sinus
Inferior sagittal sinus
Superior sagittal sinus
B. Superior View

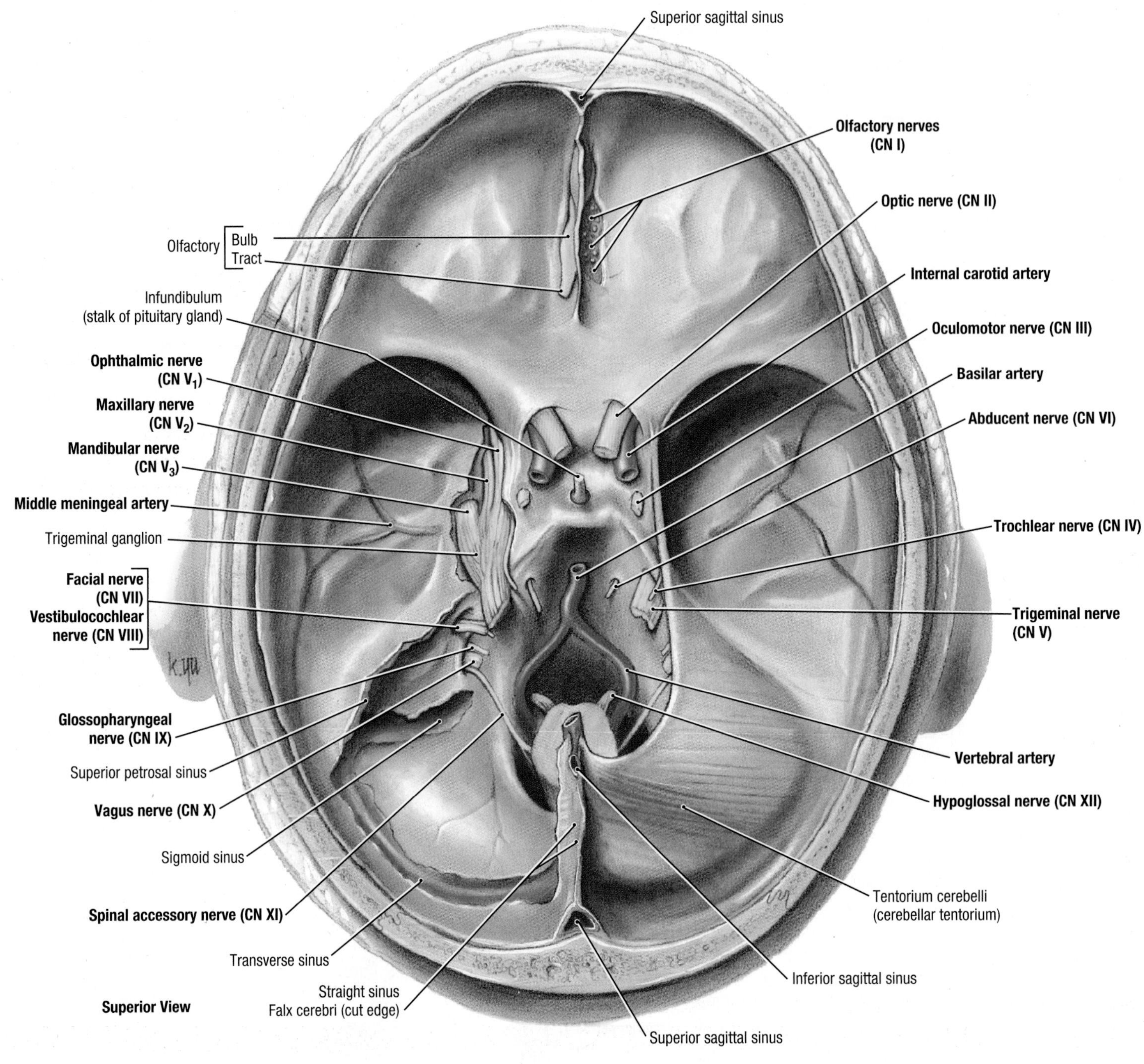

Superior sagittal sinus
Olfactory nerves (CN I)
Optic nerve (CN II)
Olfactory
Bulb
Tract
Internal carotid artery
Infundibulum (stalk of pituitary gland)
Oculomotor nerve (CN III)
Ophthalmic nerve (CN V_1)
Basilar artery
Maxillary nerve (CN V_2)
Abducent nerve (CN VI)
Mandibular nerve (CN V_3)
Middle meningeal artery
Trigeminal ganglion
Trochlear nerve (CN IV)
Facial nerve (CN VII)
Vestibulocochlear nerve (CN VIII)
Trigeminal nerve (CN V)
Glossopharyngeal nerve (CN IX)
Vertebral artery
Superior petrosal sinus
Hypoglossal nerve (CN XII)
Vagus nerve (CN X)
Sigmoid sinus
Tentorium cerebelli (cerebellar tentorium)
Spinal accessory nerve (CN XI)
Transverse sinus
Inferior sagittal sinus
Superior View
Straight sinus
Falx cerebri (cut edge)
Superior sagittal sinus

7.26 NERVES AND VESSELS OF THE INTERIOR OF THE BASE OF CRANIUM

- On the left of the specimen, the dura mater forming the roof of the trigeminal cave is cut away to expose the trigeminal ganglion and its three branches. The tentorium cerebelli is removed to reveal the transverse and superior petrosal sinuses.
- The frontal lobes of the cerebrum are located in the anterior cranial fossa, the temporal lobes in the middle cranial fossa, and the brainstem and cerebellum in the posterior cranial fossa; the occipital lobes rest on the tentorium cerebelli.
- The sites where the 12 cranial nerves and the internal carotid, vertebral, basilar, and middle meningeal arteries penetrate the dura mater are shown.

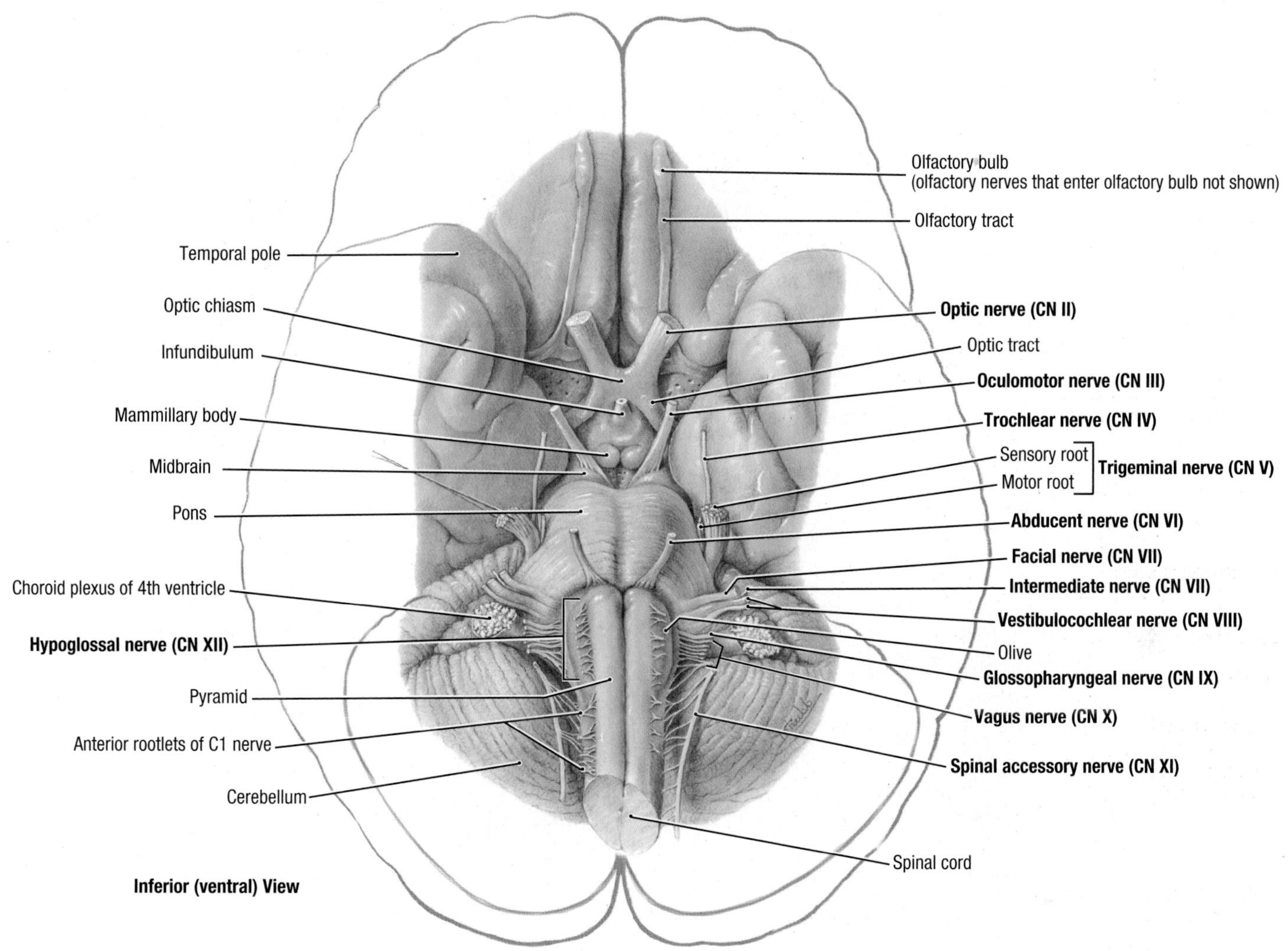
Olfactory bulb
(olfactory nerves that enter olfactory bulb not shown)
Olfactory tract
Temporal pole
Optic chiasm
Optic nerve (CN II)
Infundibulum
Optic tract
Oculomotor nerve (CN III)
Mammillary body
Trochlear nerve (CN IV)
Sensory root
Motor root
Trigeminal nerve (CN V)
Midbrain
Pons
Abducent nerve (CN VI)
Facial nerve (CN VII)
Choroid plexus of 4th ventricle
Intermediate nerve (CN VII)
Vestibulocochlear nerve (CN VIII)
Hypoglossal nerve (CN XII)
Olive
Glossopharyngeal nerve (CN IX)
Pyramid
Vagus nerve (CN X)
Anterior rootlets of C1 nerve
Spinal accessory nerve (CN XI)
Cerebellum
Spinal cord
Inferior (ventral) View

7.27 BASE OF BRAIN AND SUPERFICIAL ORIGINS OF CRANIAL NERVES

Foramina of skull and their associated cranial nerve(s) are listed below.

TABLE 7.6 OPENINGS BY WHICH CRANIAL NERVES EXIT CRANIAL CAVITY

Foramina/Apertures	Cranial nerve
Anterior cranial fossa	
Cribriform foramina in cribriform plate	Axons of olfactory cells in olfactory epithelium form olfactory nerves (CN I)
Middle cranial fossa	
Optic canal	Optic nerve (CN II)
Superior orbital fissure	Ophthalmic nerve (CN V_1), oculomotor nerve (CN III), trochlear nerve (CN IV), abducent nerve (CN VI) and branches of ophthalmic nerve (CN V_1)
Foramen rotundum	Maxillary nerve (CN V_2)
Foramen ovale	Mandibular nerve (CN V_3)
Posterior cranial fossa	
Foramen magnum	Spinal accessory nerve (CN XI)
Jugular foramen	Glossopharyngeal nerve (CN IX), vagus nerve (CN X), and spinal accessory nerve (CN XI)
Hypoglossal canal	Hypoglossal nerve (CN XII)

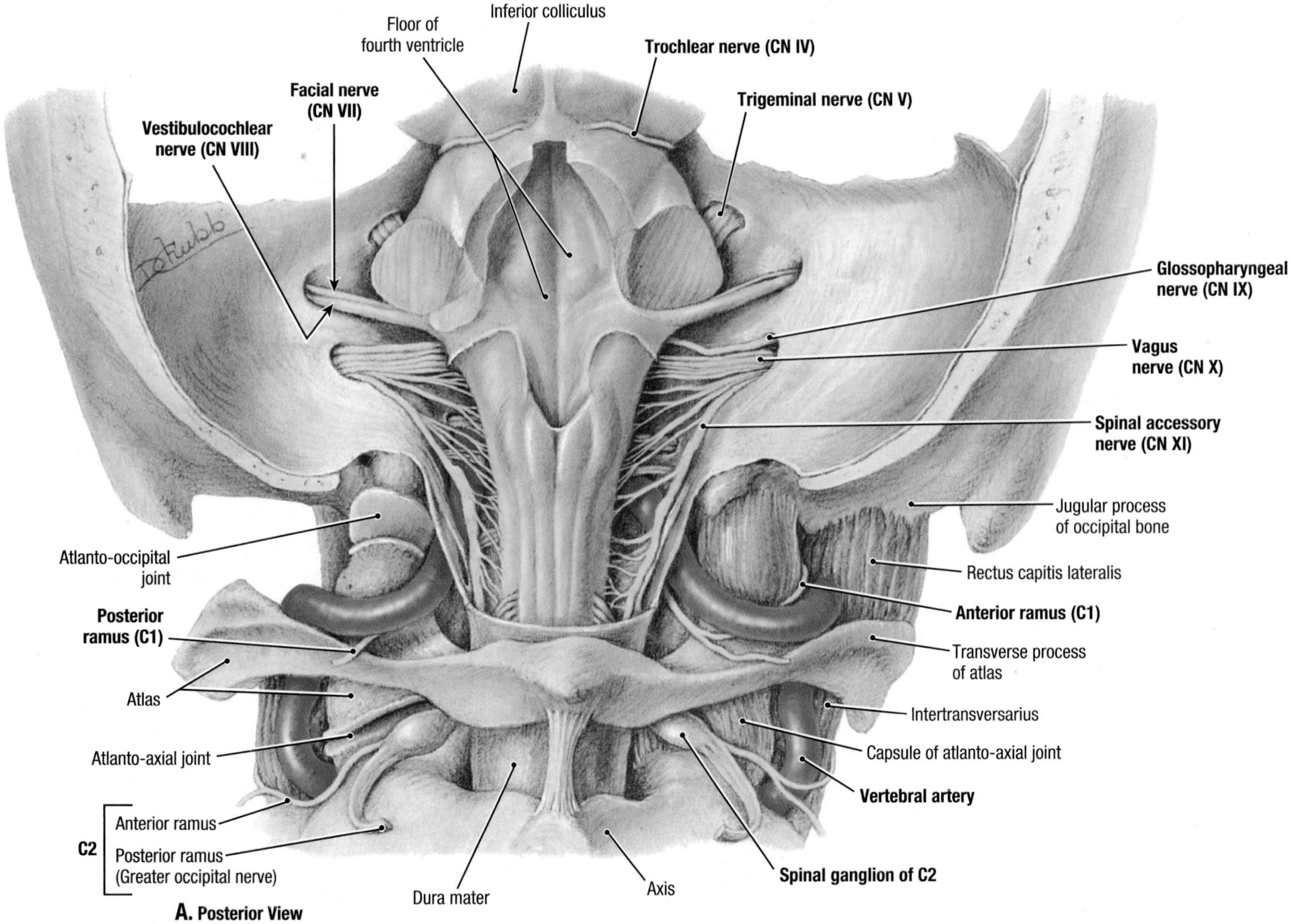

Inferior colliculus
Floor of fourth ventricle
Trochlear nerve (CN IV)
Facial nerve (CN VII)
Trigeminal nerve (CN V)
Vestibulocochlear nerve (CN VIII)
Glossopharyngeal nerve (CN IX)
Vagus nerve (CN X)
Spinal accessory nerve (CN XI)
Jugular process of occipital bone
Atlanto-occipital joint
Rectus capitis lateralis
Posterior ramus (C1)
Anterior ramus (C1)
Transverse process of atlas
Atlas
Intertransversarius
Atlanto-axial joint
Capsule of atlanto-axial joint
Vertebral artery
C2 Anterior ramus
Posterior ramus (Greater occipital nerve)
Dura mater
Axis
Spinal ganglion of C2

A. Posterior View

7.28 POSTERIOR EXPOSURES OF CRANIAL NERVES

A. and B. Squamous part of occipital bone has been removed posterior to foramen magnum to reveal posterior cranial fossa. **A.** Brainstem in situ. **B.** Right side, with brainstem removed. The trochlear nerves (CN IV) arise from the dorsal aspect of the midbrain, just inferior to the inferior colliculi.

- The sensory and motor roots of the trigeminal nerves (CN V) pass anterolaterally to enter the mouth of the trigeminal cave.
- The facial (CN VII) and vestibulocochlear (CN VIII) nerves course laterally to enter the internal acoustic meatus.
- The glossopharyngeal nerve (CN IX) pierces the dura mater separately but passes with the vagus (CN X) and spinal accessory (CN XI) nerves through the jugular foramen.
- An **acoustic neuroma** (neurofibroma) is a slow-growing benign tumor of the neurolemma (Schwann) cells. The tumor begins in the vestibulocochlear nerve (CN VIII) while it is in the internal acoustic meatus. The early symptom of an acoustic neuroma is usually loss of hearing. Dysequilibrium and tinnitus also may occur.

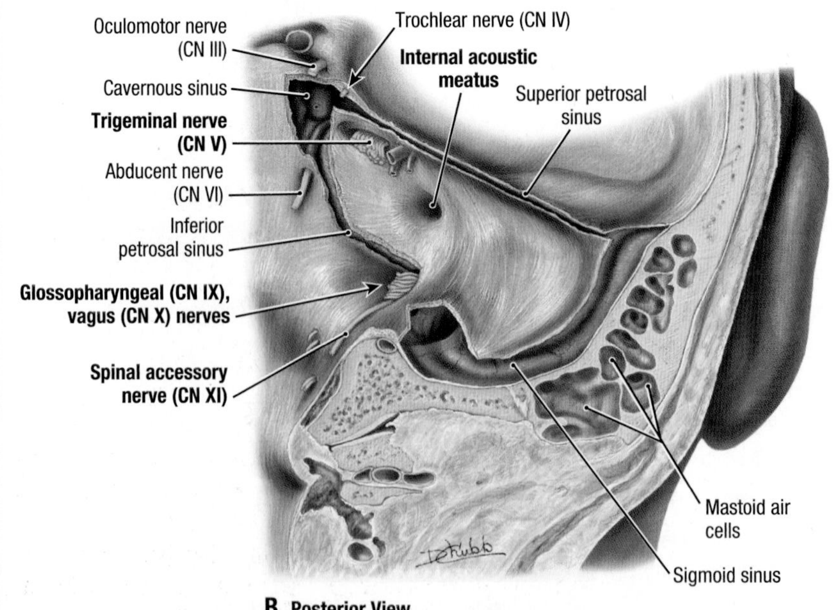
Oculomotor nerve (CN III)
Trochlear nerve (CN IV)
Internal acoustic meatus
Cavernous sinus
Superior petrosal sinus
Trigeminal nerve (CN V)
Abducent nerve (CN VI)
Inferior petrosal sinus
Glossopharyngeal (CN IX), vagus (CN X) nerves
Spinal accessory nerve (CN XI)
Mastoid air cells
Sigmoid sinus

B. Posterior View

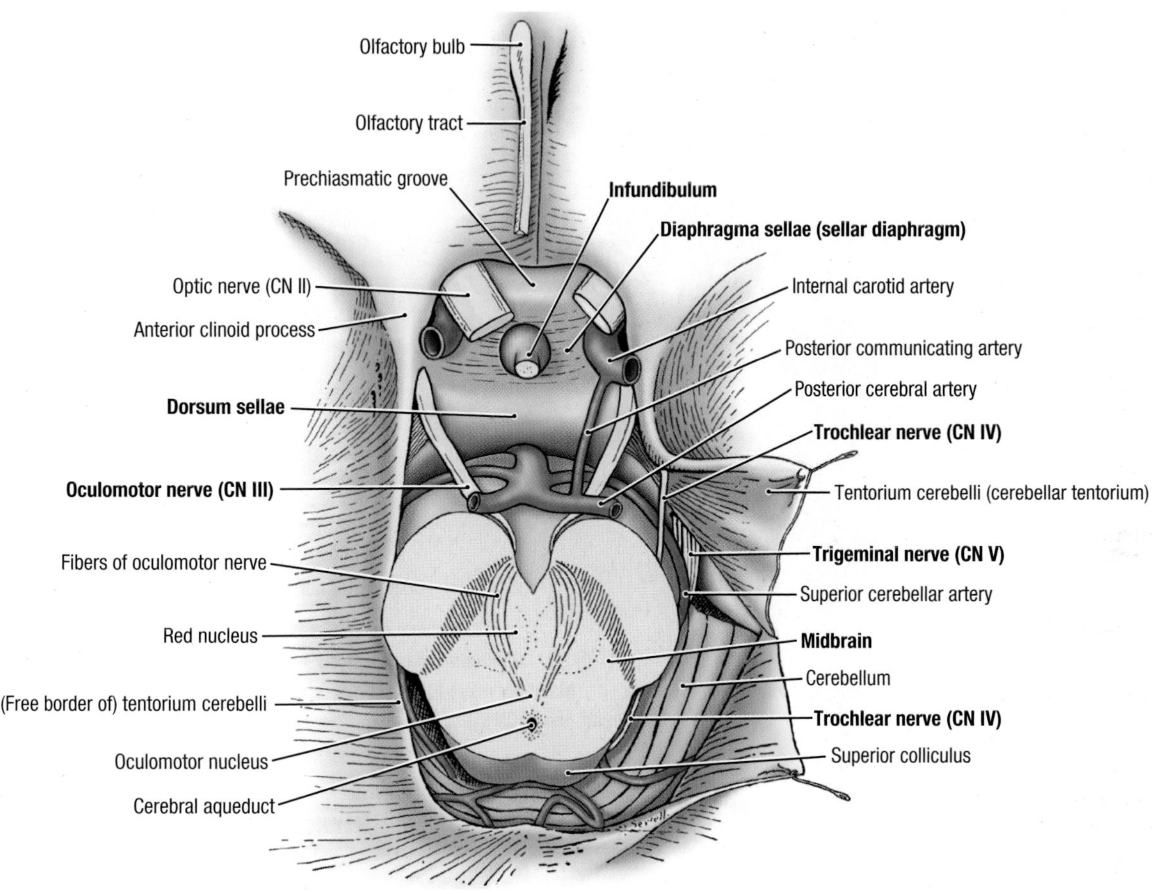
Olfactory bulb
Olfactory tract
Prechiasmatic groove
Infundibulum
Diaphragma sellae (sellar diaphragm)
Optic nerve (CN II)
Internal carotid artery
Anterior clinoid process
Posterior communicating artery
Posterior cerebral artery
Dorsum sellae
Trochlear nerve (CN IV)
Oculomotor nerve (CN III)
Tentorium cerebelli (cerebellar tentorium)
Trigeminal nerve (CN V)
Fibers of oculomotor nerve
Superior cerebellar artery
Red nucleus
Midbrain
Cerebellum
(Free border of) tentorium cerebelli
Trochlear nerve (CN IV)
Oculomotor nucleus
Superior colliculus
Cerebral aqueduct

Superior View

7.29 TENTORIAL NOTCH

- The brain has been removed by cutting through the midbrain, revealing the tentorial notch through which the brainstem extends from the posterior into the middle cranial fossa.
- On the right side of the specimen, the tentorium cerebelli is divided and reflected. The trochlear nerve (CN IV) passes around the midbrain under the free edge of the tentorium cerebelli; the roots of the trigeminal nerve (CN V) enter the mouth of the trigeminal cave.
- There is a circular opening in the diaphragma sellae for the infundibulum, the stalk of the pituitary gland.
- The oculomotor nerve (CN III) passes between the posterior cerebral and superior cerebellar arteries and then laterally around the posterior clinoid process.
- The tentorial notch is the opening in the tentorium cerebelli for the brainstem, which is slightly larger than is necessary to accommodate the midbrain. Hence, space-occupying lesions, such as tumors in the supratentorial compartment, produce increased intracranial pressure that may cause part of the adjacent temporal lobe of the brain to herniate through the tentorial notch. During **tentorial herniation**, the temporal lobe may be lacerated by the tough tentorium cerebelli, and the oculomotor nerve (CN III) may be stretched, compressed, or both. Oculomotor lesions may produce paralysis of the extrinsic eye muscles supplied by CN III.

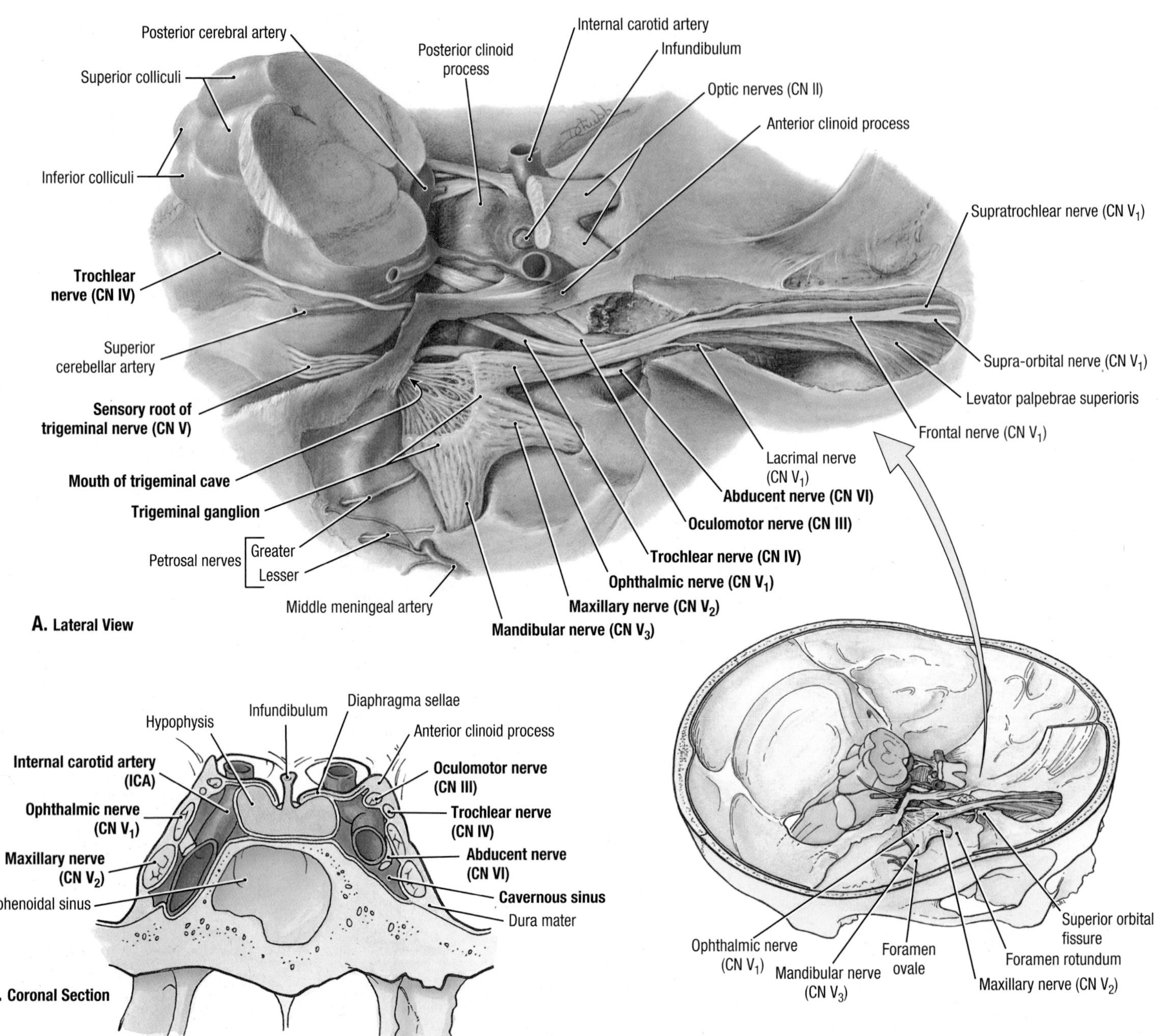
Posterior cerebral artery
Superior colliculi
Inferior colliculi
Posterior clinoid process
Internal carotid artery
Infundibulum
Optic nerves (CN II)
Anterior clinoid process
Supratrochlear nerve (CN V1)
Trochlear nerve (CN IV)
Superior cerebellar artery
Sensory root of trigeminal nerve (CN V)
Mouth of trigeminal cave
Trigeminal ganglion
Petrosal nerves
Greater
Lesser
Middle meningeal artery
Supra-orbital nerve (CN V1)
Levator palpebrae superioris
Frontal nerve (CN V1)
Lacrimal nerve (CN V1)
Abducent nerve (CN VI)
Oculomotor nerve (CN III)
Trochlear nerve (CN IV)
Ophthalmic nerve (CN V1)
Maxillary nerve (CN V2)
Mandibular nerve (CN V3)
A. Lateral View
Hypophysis
Infundibulum
Diaphragma sellae
Anterior clinoid process
Internal carotid artery (ICA)
Ophthalmic nerve (CN V1)
Maxillary nerve (CN V2)
Sphenoidal sinus
Oculomotor nerve (CN III)
Trochlear nerve (CN IV)
Abducent nerve (CN VI)
Cavernous sinus
Dura mater
B. Coronal Section
Ophthalmic nerve (CN V1)
Mandibular nerve (CN V3)
Foramen ovale
Superior orbital fissure
Foramen rotundum
Maxillary nerve (CN V2)

7.30 NERVES AND VESSELS OF MIDDLE CRANIAL FOSSA I

A. Superficial dissection. The tentorium cerebelli is cut away. The dura mater is largely removed from the middle cranial fossa. The roof of the orbit is partly removed. **B.** Coronal section through the cavernous sinus.

In **fractures of the cranial base**, the internal carotid artery may be torn, producing an arteriovenous fistula within the cavernous sinus. Arterial blood rushes into the sinus, enlarging it and forcing retrograde blood flow into its venous tributaries, especially the ophthalmic veins. As a result, the eyeball protrudes (**exophthalmos**) and the conjunctiva becomes engorged (**chemosis**). Because CN III, CN IV, CN VI, CN V_1, and CN V_2 lie in or close to the lateral wall of the cavernous sinus, these nerves may also be affected.

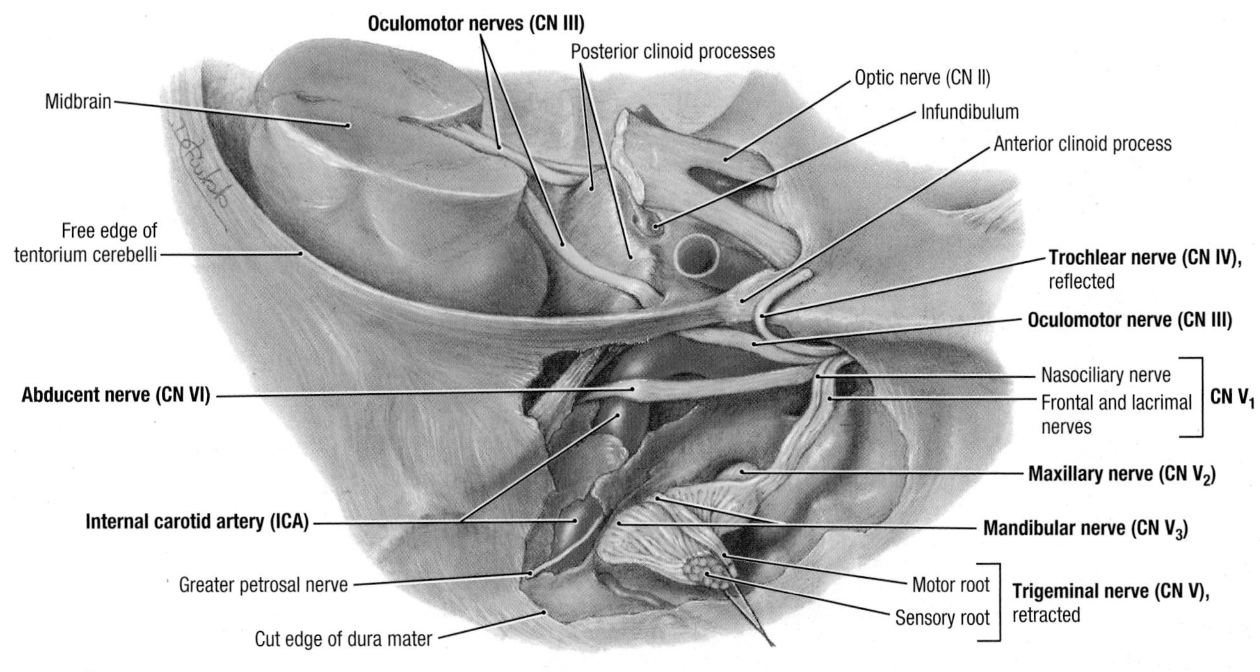
Oculomotor nerves (CN III)
Posterior clinoid processes
Optic nerve (CN II)
Midbrain
Infundibulum
Anterior clinoid process
Free edge of tentorium cerebelli
Trochlear nerve (CN IV), reflected
Oculomotor nerve (CN III)
Nasociliary nerve
Frontal and lacrimal nerves
CN V_1
Abducent nerve (CN VI)
Maxillary nerve (CN V_2)
Internal carotid artery (ICA)
Mandibular nerve (CN V_3)
Motor root
Greater petrosal nerve
Trigeminal nerve (CN V), retracted
Sensory root
Cut edge of dura mater

A. **Lateral View**

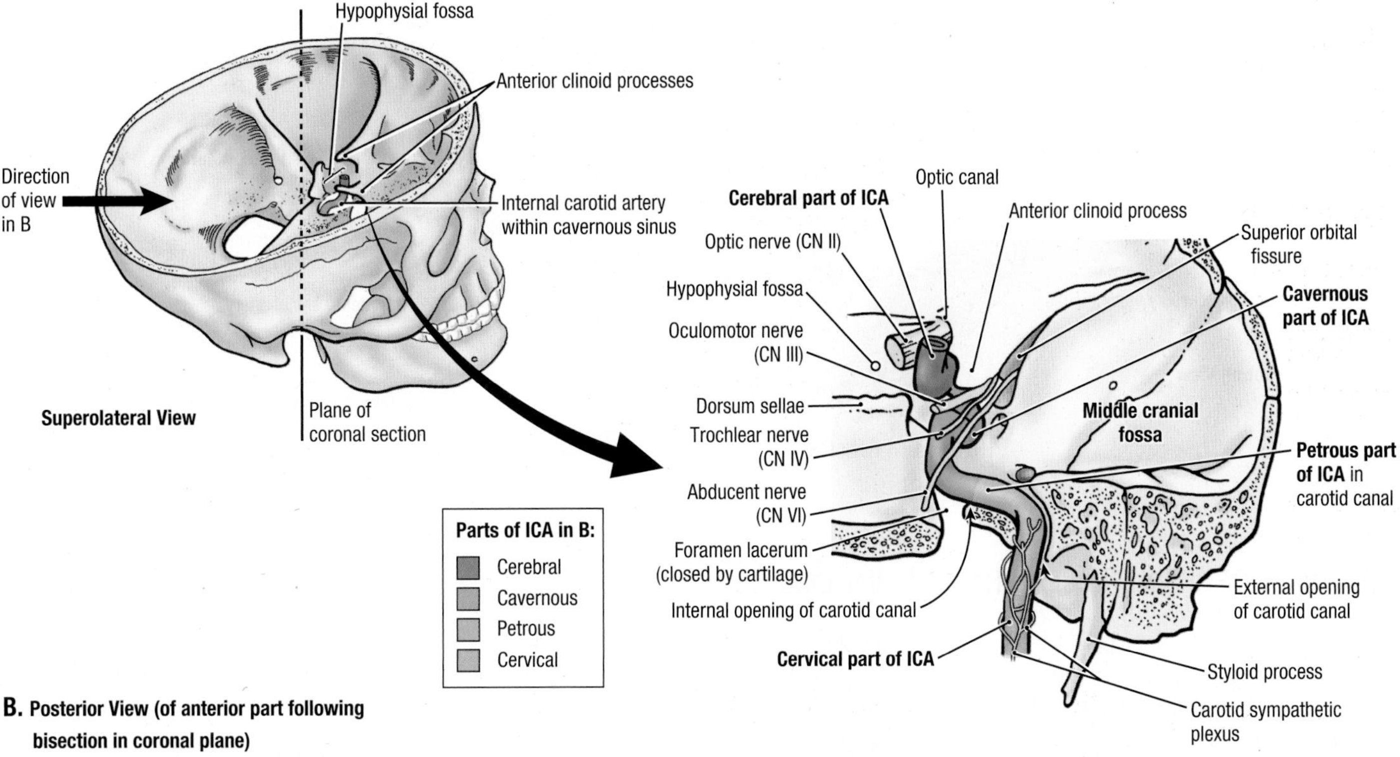
Hypophysial fossa
Anterior clinoid processes
Direction of view in B
Internal carotid artery within cavernous sinus
Superolateral View
Plane of coronal section
Optic canal
Cerebral part of ICA
Anterior clinoid process
Optic nerve (CN II)
Superior orbital fissure
Hypophysial fossa
Cavernous part of ICA
Oculomotor nerve (CN III)
Dorsum sellae
Middle cranial fossa
Trochlear nerve (CN IV)
Petrous part of ICA in carotid canal
Abducent nerve (CN VI)
Parts of ICA in B:
Cerebral
Cavernous
Petrous
Cervical
Foramen lacerum (closed by cartilage)
Internal opening of carotid canal
External opening of carotid canal
Cervical part of ICA
Styloid process
Carotid sympathetic plexus

B. **Posterior View (of anterior part following bisection in coronal plane)**

7.31 NERVES AND VESSELS OF MIDDLE CRANIAL FOSSA II

A. Deep dissection. The roots of the trigeminal nerve are divided, withdrawn from the mouth of the trigeminal cave, and turned anteriorly. The trochlear nerve is reflected anteriorly. **B.** Course of the internal carotid artery.

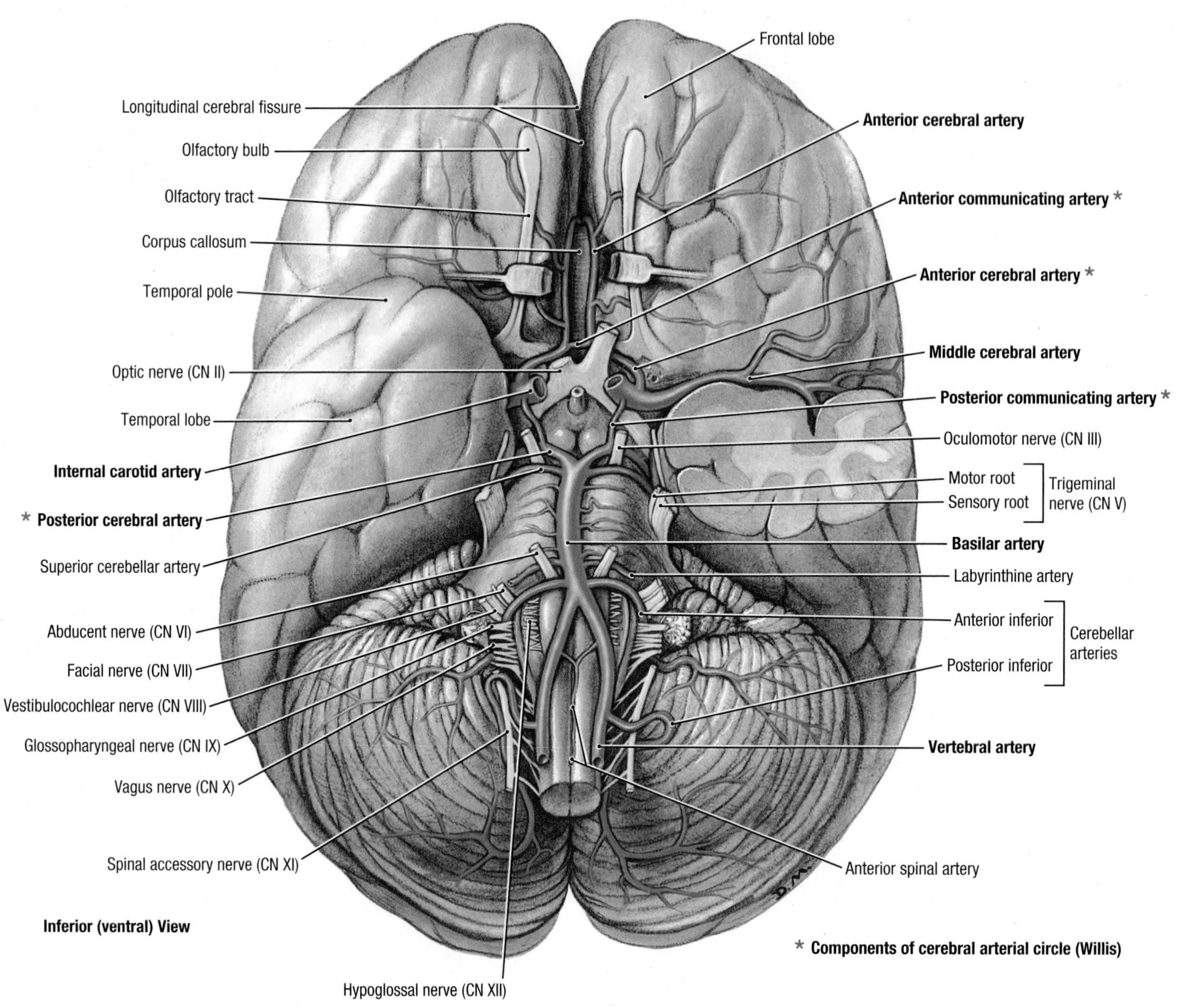
Frontal lobe
Longitudinal cerebral fissure
Anterior cerebral artery
Olfactory bulb
Olfactory tract
Anterior communicating artery *
Corpus callosum
Anterior cerebral artery *
Temporal pole
Middle cerebral artery
Optic nerve (CN II)
Posterior communicating artery *
Temporal lobe
Oculomotor nerve (CN III)
Internal carotid artery
Motor root
Sensory root
Trigeminal nerve (CN V)
* Posterior cerebral artery
Basilar artery
Superior cerebellar artery
Labyrinthine artery
Anterior inferior
Abducent nerve (CN VI)
Cerebellar arteries
Facial nerve (CN VII)
Posterior inferior
Vestibulocochlear nerve (CN VIII)
Glossopharyngeal nerve (CN IX)
Vertebral artery
Vagus nerve (CN X)
Spinal accessory nerve (CN XI)
Anterior spinal artery
Inferior (ventral) View
* Components of cerebral arterial circle (Willis)
Hypoglossal nerve (CN XII)

7.32 BASE OF BRAIN AND CEREBRAL ARTERIAL CIRCLE

The anterior part of the left temporal lobe is removed to enable visualization of the middle cerebral artery in the lateral fissure. The frontal lobes are separated to expose the anterior cerebral arteries and corpus callosum.

An **ischemic stroke** denotes the sudden development of neurological deficits that are consequences of impaired cerebral blood flow. The most common causes of strokes are spontaneous cerebrovascular accidents such as cerebral embolism, cerebral thrombosis, cerebral hemorrhage, and subarachnoid hemorrhage (Rowland, 2000). The cerebral arterial circle is an important means of collateral circulation in the event of gradual obstruction of one of the major arteries forming the circle. Sudden occlusion, even if only partial, results in neurological deficits. In elderly persons, the anastomoses are often inadequate when a large artery (e.g., internal carotid) is occluded, even if the occlusion is gradual. In such cases function is impaired at least to some degree.

Hemorrhagic stroke follows the rupture of an artery or a saccular aneurysm, a saclike dilation on a weak part of the arterial wall. The most common type of saccular aneurysm is a berry aneurysm, occurring in the vessels of or near the cerebral arterial circle. In time, especially in people with hypertension (high blood pressure), the weak part of the arterial wall expands and may rupture, allowing blood to enter the subarachnoid space.

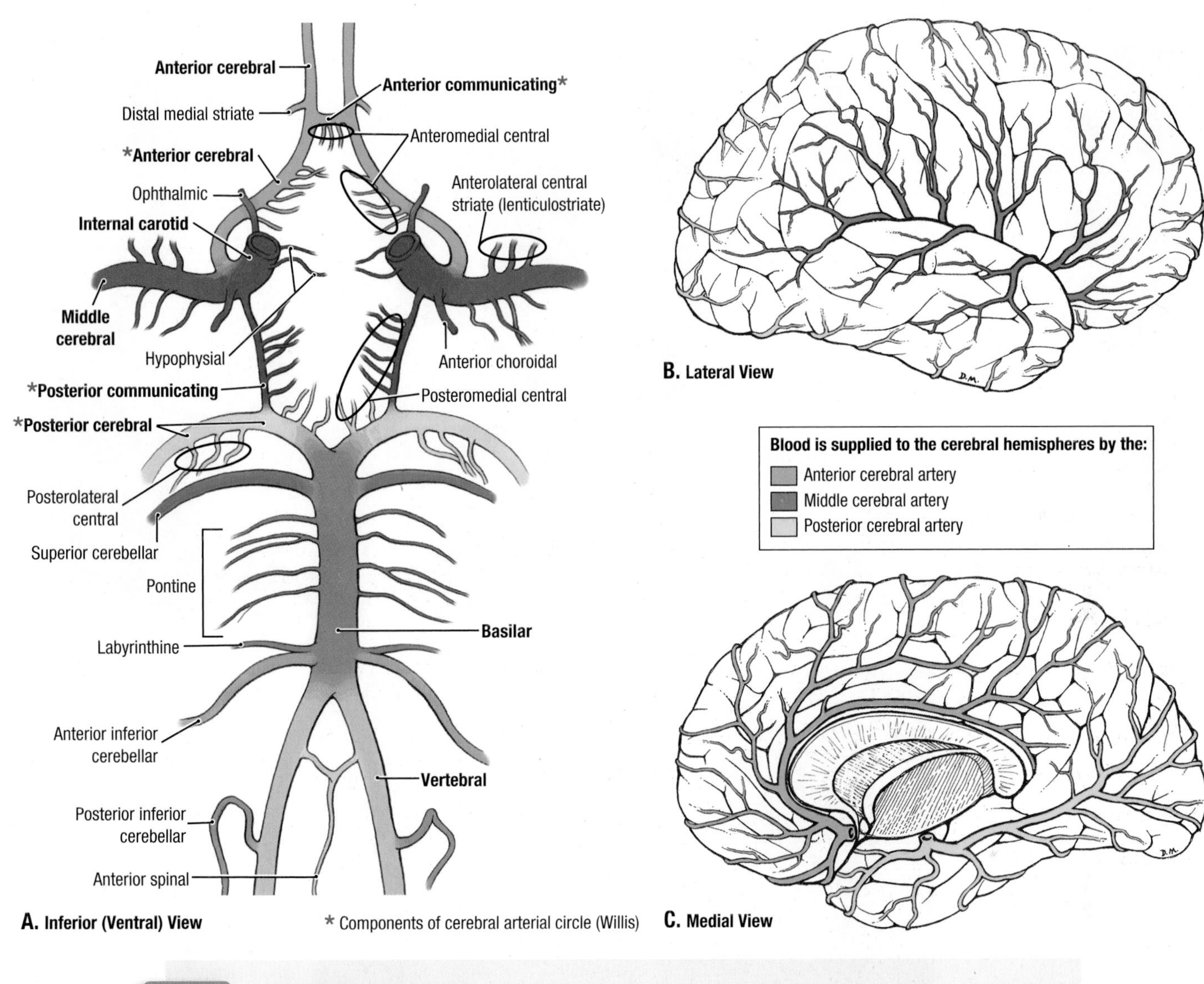
Anterior cerebral
Anterior communicating*
Distal medial striate
Anteromedial central
*Anterior cerebral
Anterolateral central striate (lenticulostriate)
Ophthalmic
Internal carotid
Middle cerebral
Hypophysial
Anterior choroidal
*Posterior communicating
Posteromedial central
*Posterior cerebral
Posterolateral central
Superior cerebellar
Pontine
Basilar
Labyrinthine
Anterior inferior cerebellar
Vertebral
Posterior inferior cerebellar
Anterior spinal
A. Inferior (Ventral) View
* Components of cerebral arterial circle (Willis)
B. Lateral View
Blood is supplied to the cerebral hemispheres by the:
Anterior cerebral artery
Middle cerebral artery
Posterior cerebral artery
C. Medial View

7.33 ARTERIES OF BRAIN

A. Schematic overview. **B and C.** Distribution of cerebral arteries.

TABLE 7.7 ARTERIAL SUPPLY TO BRAIN

Artery	Origin	Distribution
Vertebral	Subclavian artery	Cranial meninges and cerebellum
Posterior inferior cerebellar	Vertebral artery	Postero-inferior aspect of cerebellum
Basilar	Formed by junction of vertebral arteries	Brainstem, cerebellum, and cerebrum
Pontine	Basilar artery	Numerous branches to brainstem
Anterior inferior cerebellar		Inferior aspect of cerebellum
Superior cerebellar		Superior aspect of cerebellum
Internal carotid	Common carotid artery at superior border of thyroid cartilage	Gives branches in cavernous sinus and provides supply to brain
Anterior cerebral	Internal carotid artery	Cerebral hemispheres, except for occipital lobes
Middle cerebral	Continuation of the internal carotid artery distal to anterior cerebral artery	Most of lateral surface of cerebral hemispheres
Posterior cerebral	Terminal branch of basilar artery	Inferior aspect of cerebral hemisphere and occipital lobe
Anterior communicating	Anterior cerebral artery	Cerebral arterial circle
Posterior communicating	Internal carotid artery	

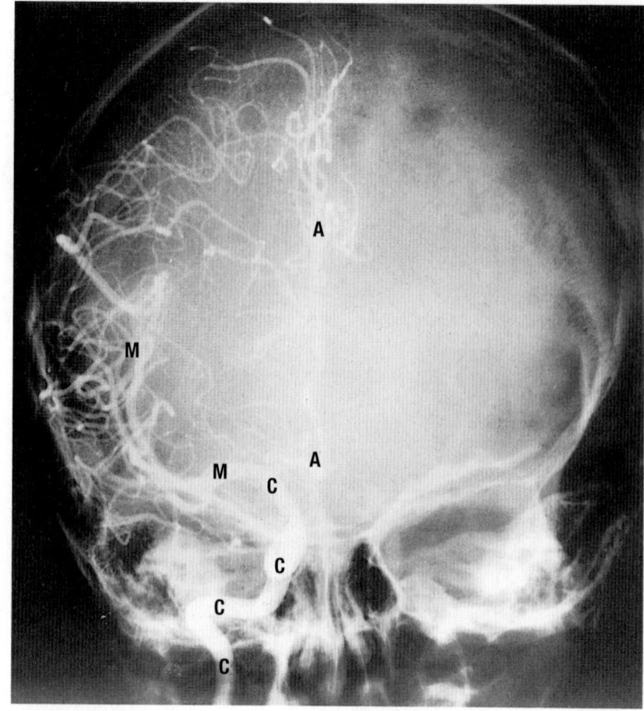
A
M
M
C
A
C
C
C

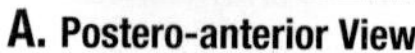
A. Postero-anterior View

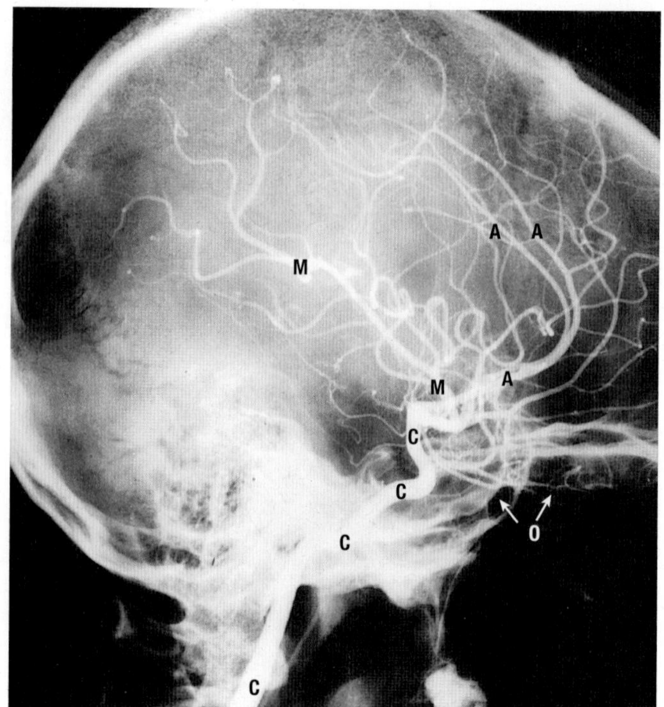
M
A A
M
A
C
C
C
O
C

B. Lateral View

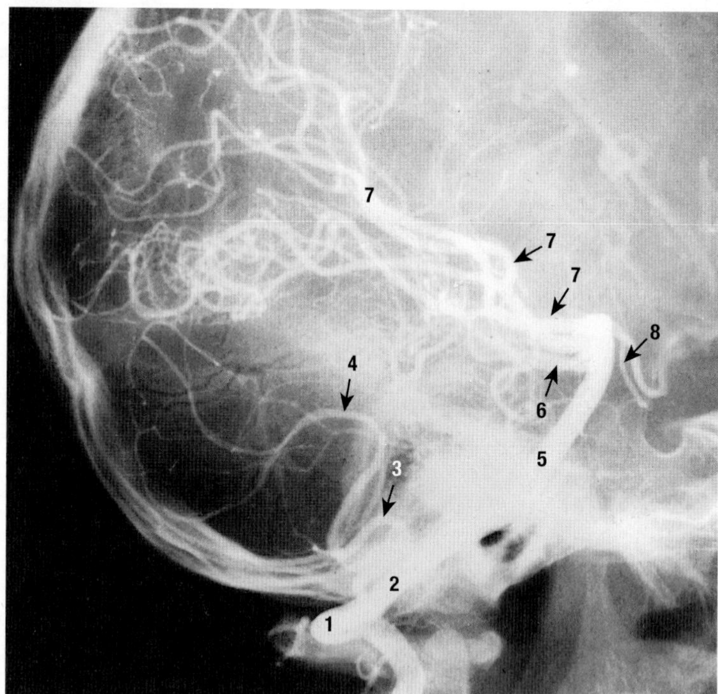
7
7
7
8
4
6
5
3
2
1

C. Lateral View

Key for A, B and C:

- A Anterior cerebral artery
- M Middle cerebral artery
- C Internal carotid artery
- O Ophthalmic artery
- 1 Vertebral artery on posterior arch of atlas
- 2 Vertebral artery entering skull through foramen magnum
- 3 Posterior inferior cerebellar artery
- 4 Anterior inferior cerebellar artery
- 5 Basilar artery
- 6 Superior cerebellar artery
- 7 Posterior cerebellar artery
- 8 Posterior communicating artery

7.34 ARTERIOGRAMS

A. and B. Carotid arteriogram. The four *C*s indicate the parts of the internal carotid artery: cervical, before entering the cranium; petrous, within the temporal bone; cavernous, within the sinus; and cerebral, within the cranial subarachnoid space. **C.** Vertebral arteriogram. **Transient ischemic attacks (TIAs)** refer to neurological symptoms resulting from ischemia (deficient blood supply) of the brain. The symptoms of a TIA may be ambiguous: staggering, dizziness, light-headedness, fainting, and paresthesias (e.g., tingling in a limb). Most TIAs last a few minutes, but some persist longer. Individuals with TIAs are at increased risk for myocardial infarction and *ischemic stroke* (Brust, 2000).

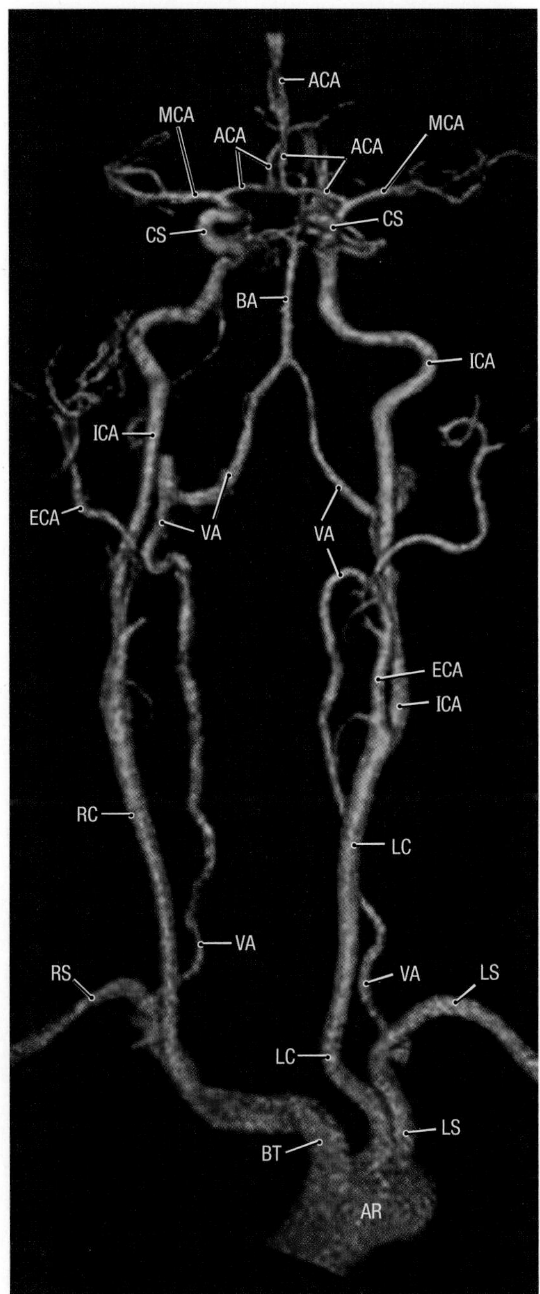
ACA
MCA
ACA
ACA
MCA
CS
CS
BA
ICA
ICA
ECA
VA
VA
ECA
ICA
RC
LC
VA
RS
VA
LS
LC
LS
BT
AR
A. Anterior View

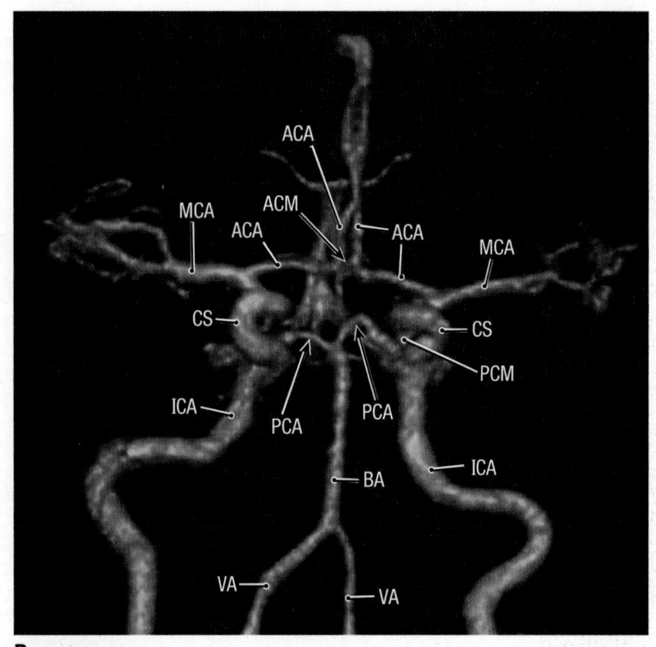
ACA
MCA
ACM
ACA
ACA
MCA
CS
CS
PCM
ICA
PCA
PCA
ICA
BA
VA
VA
B. Anterior View

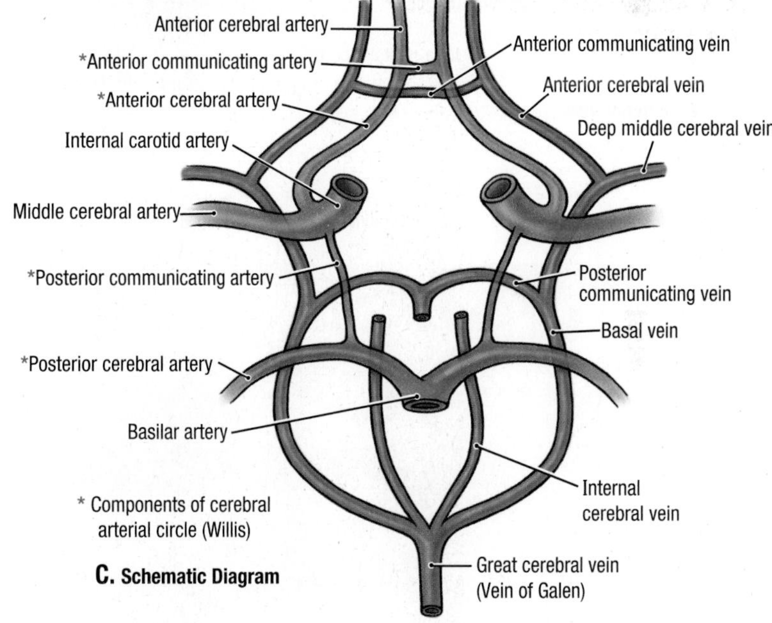
Anterior cerebral artery
*Anterior communicating artery
*Anterior cerebral artery
Internal carotid artery
Middle cerebral artery
*Posterior communicating artery
*Posterior cerebral artery
Basilar artery
* Components of cerebral arterial circle (Willis)
Anterior communicating vein
Anterior cerebral vein
Deep middle cerebral vein
Posterior communicating vein
Basal vein
Internal cerebral vein
Great cerebral vein (Vein of Galen)
C. Schematic Diagram

Key for A and B:

ACM	Anterior communicating artery	BT	Brachiocephalic trunk	LC	Left common carotid artery	PCM	Posterior communicating artery
ACA	Anterior cerebral artery	CS	Carotid siphon	LS	Left subclavian artery	RC	Right common carotid artery
AR	Arch of aorta	ECA	External carotid artery	MCA	Middle cerebral artery	RS	Right subclavian artery
BA	Basilar artery	ICA	Internal carotid artery	PCA	Posterior cerebral artery	VA	Vertebral artery

7.35 BLOOD SUPPLY OF HEAD AND NECK

A. CT angiogram of arteries of head and neck. **B.** CT angiogram of cerebral arterial circle (circle of Willis). **C.** Schematic diagram of cerebral arterial circle and veins of cerebral base.

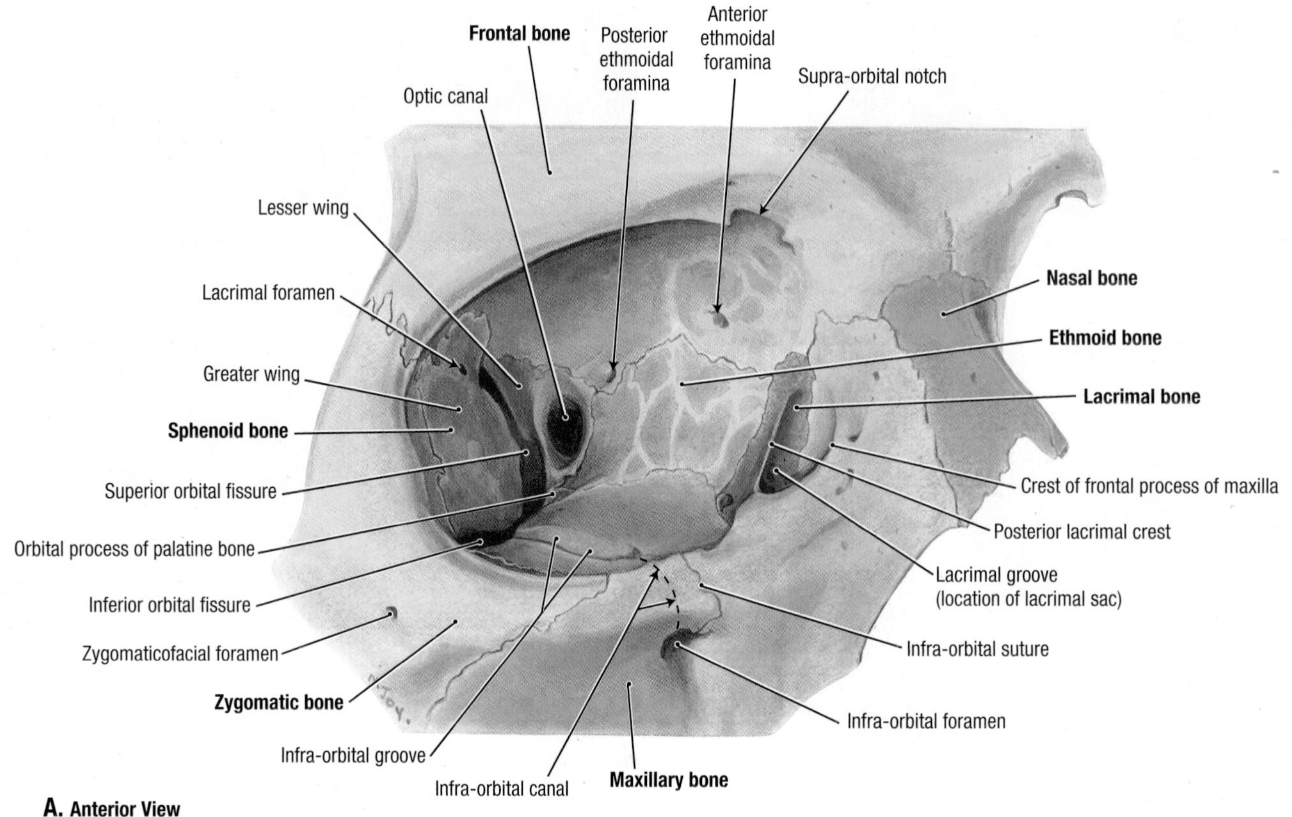
Frontal bone
Posterior ethmoidal foramina
Anterior ethmoidal foramina
Supra-orbital notch
Optic canal
Lesser wing
Lacrimal foramen
Greater wing
Sphenoid bone
Superior orbital fissure
Orbital process of palatine bone
Inferior orbital fissure
Zygomaticofacial foramen
Zygomatic bone
Infra-orbital groove
Infra-orbital canal
Maxillary bone
Nasal bone
Ethmoid bone
Lacrimal bone
Crest of frontal process of maxilla
Posterior lacrimal crest
Lacrimal groove (location of lacrimal sac)
Infra-orbital suture
Infra-orbital foramen

A. Anterior View

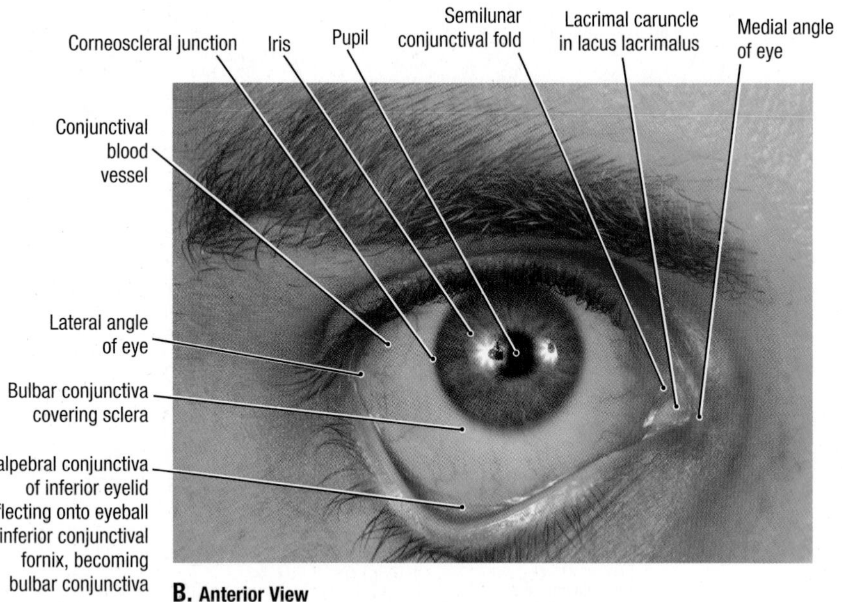
Corneoscleral junction
Iris
Pupil
Semilunar conjunctival fold
Lacrimal caruncle in lacus lacrimalus
Medial angle of eye
Conjunctival blood vessel
Lateral angle of eye
Bulbar conjunctiva covering sclera
Palpebral conjunctiva of inferior eyelid reflecting onto eyeball at inferior conjunctival fornix, becoming bulbar conjunctiva

B. Anterior View

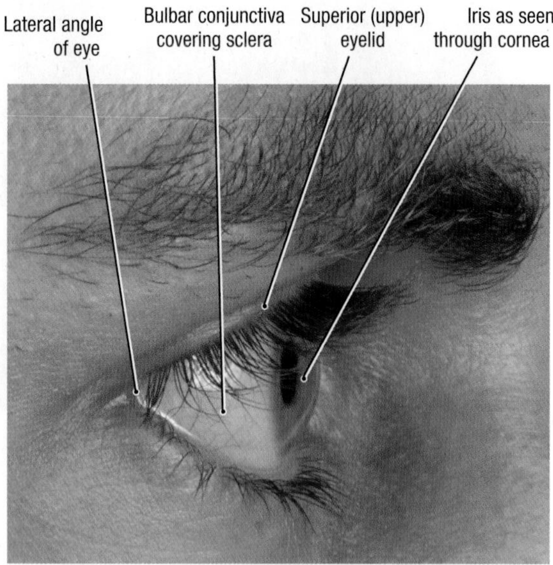
Lateral angle of eye
Bulbar conjunctiva covering sclera
Superior (upper) eyelid
Iris as seen through cornea

C. Lateral View

7.36 ORBITAL CAVITY AND SURFACE ANATOMY OF THE EYE

A. Bones and features of the orbital cavity. **B. and C.** Surface anatomy of the eye. In **B,** the inferior eyelid is everted to demonstrate the palpebral conjunctiva. When powerful blows impact directly on the bony rim of the orbit, the resulting **orbital fractures** usually occur at the sutures between the bones forming the orbital margin. Fractures of the medial wall may involve the ethmoidal and sphenoidal sinuses, whereas fractures in the inferior wall may involve the maxillary sinus. Although the superior wall is stronger than the medial and inferior walls, it is thin enough to be translucent and may be readily penetrated. Thus, a sharp object may pass through it into the frontal lobe of the brain. Orbital fractures often result in intraorbital bleeding, which exerts pressure on the eyeball, causing **exophthalmos** (protrusion of the eyeball).

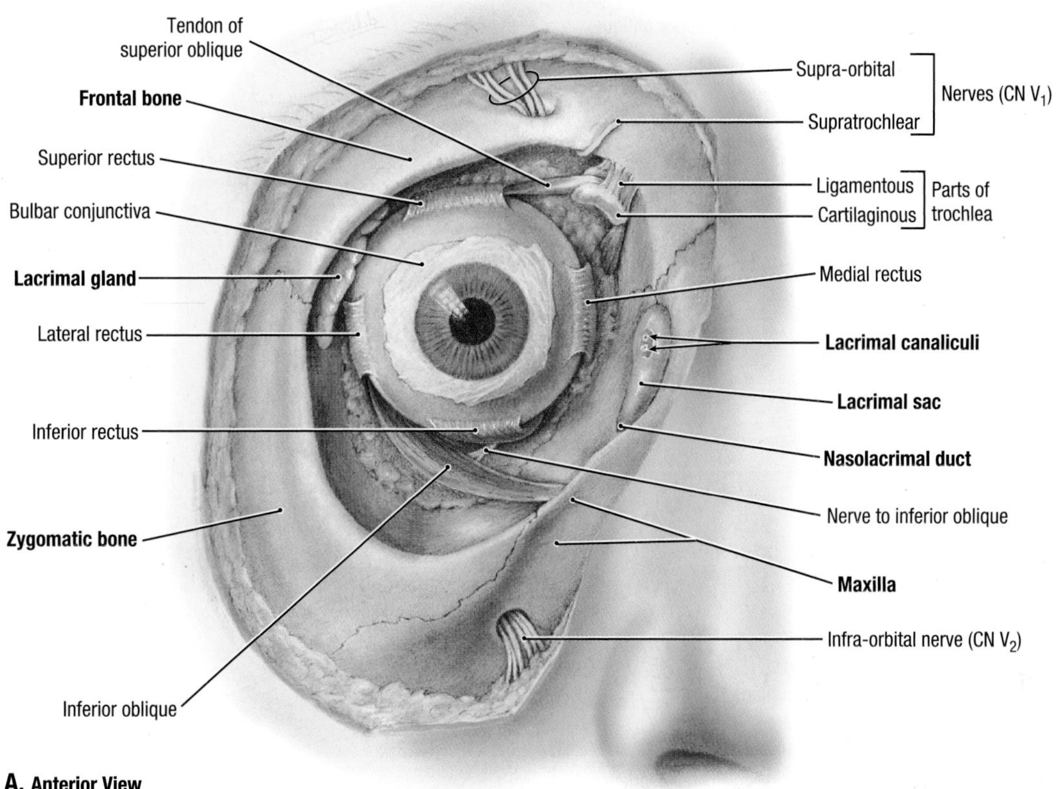
Tendon of superior oblique
Frontal bone
Superior rectus
Bulbar conjunctiva
Lacrimal gland
Lateral rectus
Inferior rectus
Zygomatic bone
Inferior oblique
Supra-orbital
Supratrochlear
Nerves (CN V_1)
Ligamentous
Cartilaginous
Parts of trochlea
Medial rectus
Lacrimal canaliculi
Lacrimal sac
Nasolacrimal duct
Nerve to inferior oblique
Maxilla
Infra-orbital nerve (CN V_2)

A. Anterior View

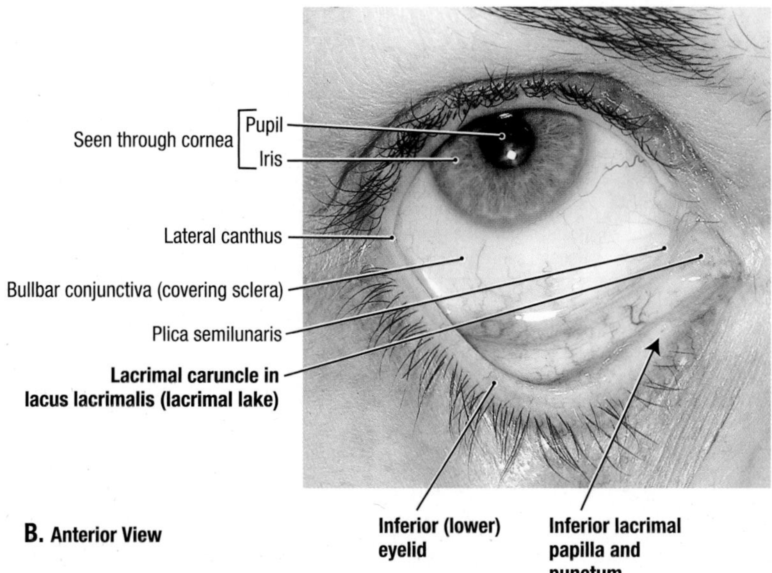
Seen through cornea
Pupil
Iris
Lateral canthus
Bullbar conjunctiva (covering sclera)
Plica semilunaris
Lacrimal caruncle in lacus lacrimalis (lacrimal lake)
Inferior (lower) eyelid
Inferior lacrimal papilla and punctum

B. Anterior View

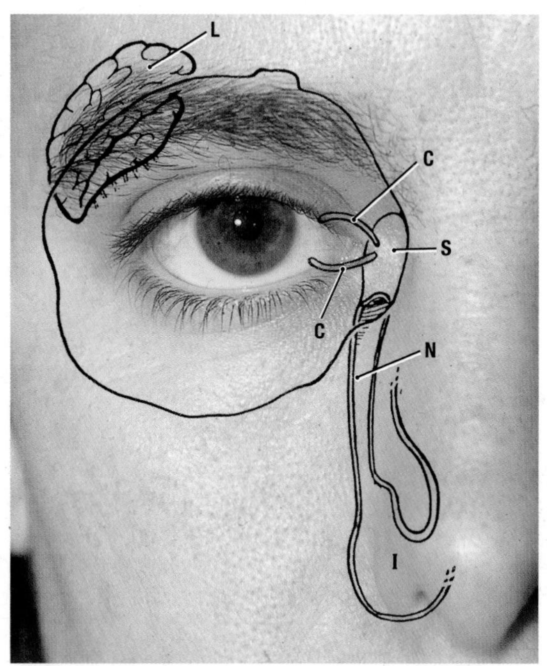
L
C
S
C
N
I

C. Anterior View

7.37 EYE AND LACRIMAL APPARATUS

A. Anterior dissection of orbital cavity. The eyelids, orbital septum, levator palpebrae superioris, and some fat are removed. **B.** Surface features, with the inferior eyelid everted. **C.** Surface projection of lacrimal apparatus. Tears, secreted by the lacrimal gland *(L)* in the superolateral angle of the bony orbit, pass across the eyeball and enter the lacus lacrimalis (lacrimal lake) at the medial angle of the eye; from here they drain through the lacrimal puncta and lacrimal canaliculi *(C)* to the lacrimal sac *(S)*. The lacrimal sac drains into the nasolacrimal duct *(N)*, which empties into the inferior meatus *(I)* of the nose.

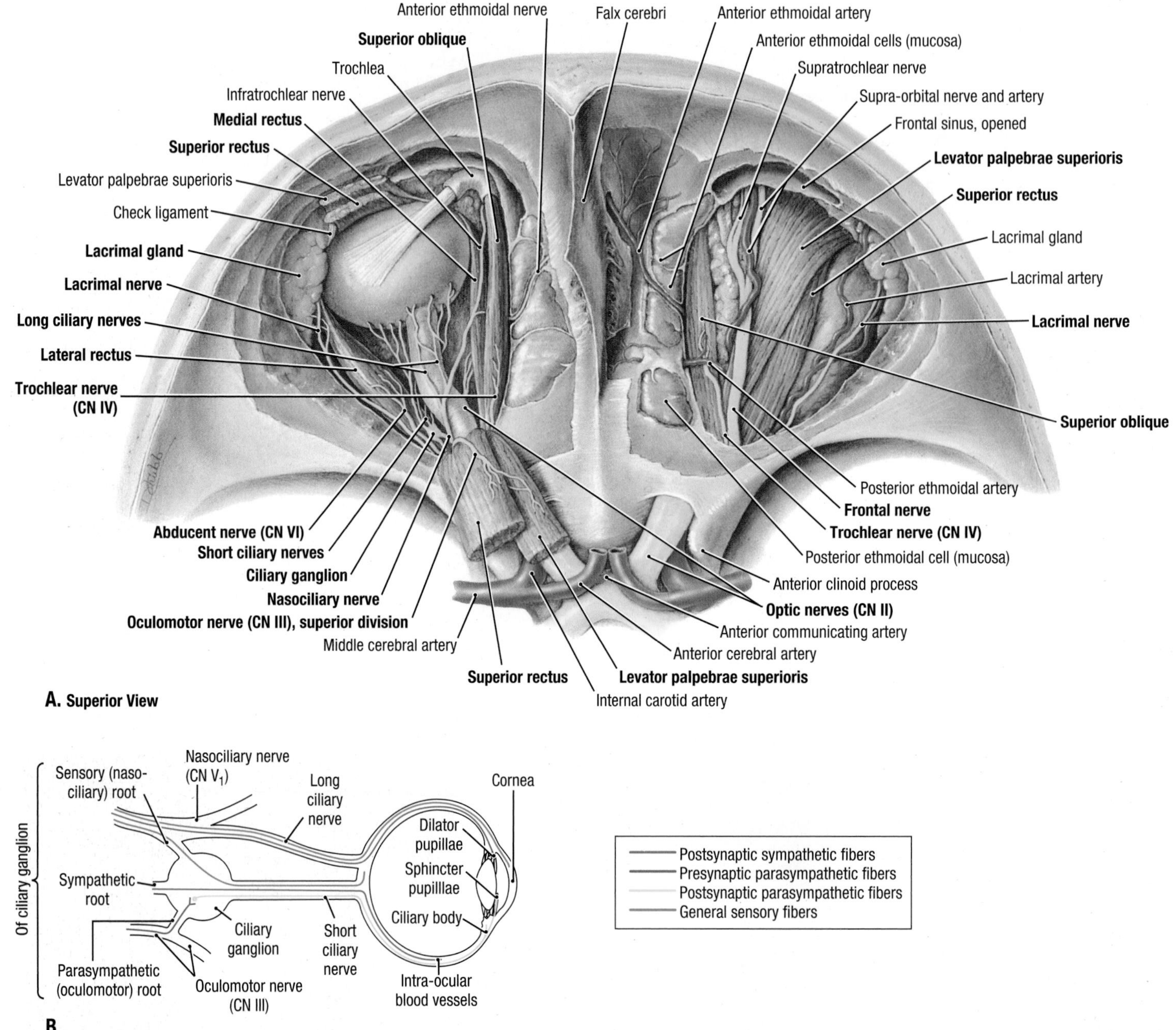

Anterior ethmoidal nerve
Falx cerebri
Anterior ethmoidal artery
Superior oblique
Anterior ethmoidal cells (mucosa)
Trochlea
Supratrochlear nerve
Infratrochlear nerve
Supra-orbital nerve and artery
Medial rectus
Frontal sinus, opened
Superior rectus
Levator palpebrae superioris
Levator palpebrae superioris
Superior rectus
Check ligament
Lacrimal gland
Lacrimal gland
Lacrimal artery
Lacrimal nerve
Lacrimal nerve
Long ciliary nerves
Lateral rectus
Trochlear nerve (CN IV)
Superior oblique
Posterior ethmoidal artery
Frontal nerve
Abducent nerve (CN VI)
Trochlear nerve (CN IV)
Short ciliary nerves
Posterior ethmoidal cell (mucosa)
Ciliary ganglion
Anterior clinoid process
Nasociliary nerve
Optic nerves (CN II)
Oculomotor nerve (CN III), superior division
Anterior communicating artery
Middle cerebral artery
Anterior cerebral artery
Superior rectus
Levator palpebrae superioris
Internal carotid artery
A. Superior View
Of ciliary ganglion
Sensory (naso-ciliary) root
Nasociliary nerve (CN V1)
Long ciliary nerve
Cornea
Dilator pupillae
Sphincter pupilllae
Ciliary body
Sympathetic root
Ciliary ganglion
Short ciliary nerve
Parasympathetic (oculomotor) root
Oculomotor nerve (CN III)
Intra-ocular blood vessels
B
Postsynaptic sympathetic fibers
Presynaptic parasympathetic fibers
Postsynaptic parasympathetic fibers
General sensory fibers

7.38 ORBITAL CAVITY, SUPERIOR APPROACH

A. Superficial dissection. On the right side of figure **A,** the orbital plate of the frontal bone is removed. On the left side of figure **A,** the levator palpebrae and superior rectus muscles are reflected.

- The trochlear nerve (CN IV) lies on the medial side of the superior oblique muscle, and the abducent nerve (CN VI) on the medial side of the lateral rectus muscle.
- The lacrimal nerve runs superior to the lateral rectus muscle supplying sensory fibers to the conjunctiva and skin of the superior eyelid; it receives a communicating branch of the zygomaticotemporal nerve carrying secretory motor fibers from the pterygopalatine ganglion to the lacrimal gland.
- The parasympathetic ciliary ganglion, placed between the lateral rectus muscle and the optic nerve (CN II), gives rise to many short ciliary nerves; the nasociliary nerve gives rise to two long ciliary nerves that anastomose with each other and the short ciliary nerves.

B. Distribution of nerve fibers to ciliary ganglion and eyeball.

Horner syndrome results from interruption of a cervical sympathetic trunk and is manifest by the absence of sympathetically stimulated functions on the ipsilateral side of the head. The syndrome includes the following signs: constriction of the pupil *(miosis),* drooping of the superior eyelid (**ptosis**), redness and increased temperature of the skin (**vasodilatation**), and absence of sweating (**anhydrosis**).

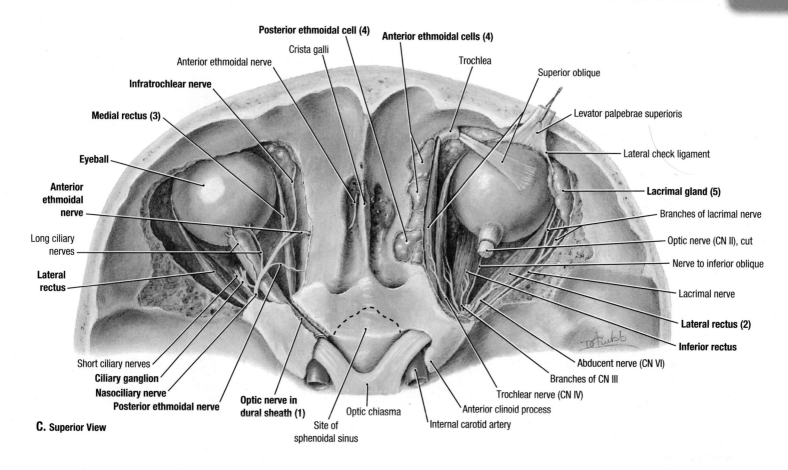

Posterior ethmoidal cell (4)
Anterior ethmoidal cells (4)
Crista galli
Anterior ethmoidal nerve
Trochlea
Superior oblique
Infratrochlear nerve
Levator palpebrae superioris
Medial rectus (3)
Lateral check ligament
Eyeball
Lacrimal gland (5)
Anterior ethmoidal nerve
Branches of lacrimal nerve
Long ciliary nerves
Optic nerve (CN II), cut
Nerve to inferior oblique
Lateral rectus
Lacrimal nerve
Lateral rectus (2)
Inferior rectus
Short ciliary nerves
Abducent nerve (CN VI)
Ciliary ganglion
Branches of CN III
Nasociliary nerve
Trochlear nerve (CN IV)
Posterior ethmoidal nerve
Optic nerve in dural sheath (1)
Optic chiasma
Anterior clinoid process
Site of sphenoidal sinus
Internal carotid artery

C. Superior View

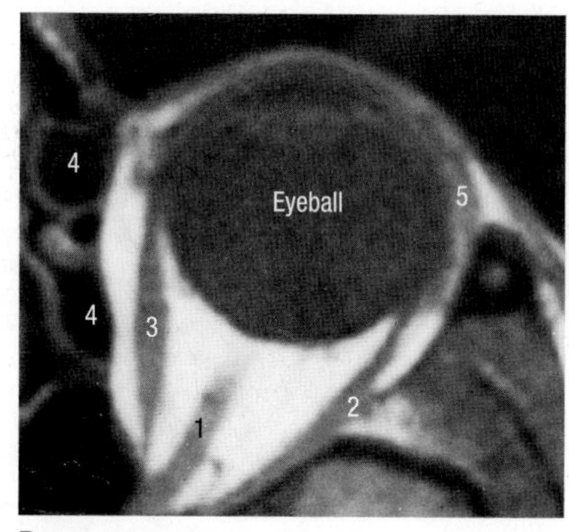
4
Eyeball
5
4
3
2
1

D. Axial MRI

7.38 ORBITAL CAVITY, SUPERIOR APPROACH *(CONTINUED)*

C. Deep dissection before *(left side of specimen)* and after *(right side of specimen)* section of the optic nerve (CN II). **D.** Transverse (axial) MRI of orbital cavity. (The *numbers* refer to structures labeled in **C**).

Observe on the right side of figure **C:**

- The eyeball occupies the anterior half of the orbital cavity.

Observe on the left of figure **C:**

- The parasympathetic ciliary ganglion lies posteriorly between the lateral rectus muscle and the sheath of the optic nerve.
- The nasociliary nerve (CN V_1) sends a branch to the ciliary ganglion and crosses the optic nerve (CN II), where it gives off two long ciliary nerves (sensory to the eyeball and cornea) and the posterior ethmoidal nerve (to the sphenoidal sinus and posterior ethmoidal cells). The nasociliary nerve then divides into the anterior ethmoidal and infratrochlear nerves.
- The ciliary ganglion receives sensory fibers from the nasociliary branches of CN VI, postsynaptic sympathetic fibers from the continuation of the internal carotid plexus extending along the ophthalmic artery, and presynaptic parasympathetic fibers from the inferior branch of the oculomotor nerve; only the latter synapse in the ganglion.
- Complete **oculomotor nerve palsy** affects most of the ocular muscles, the levator palpebrae superioris, and the sphincter pupillae. The superior eyelid droops (**ptosis**) and cannot be raised voluntarily because of the unopposed activity of the orbicularis oculi (supplied by the facial nerve). The pupil is also fully dilated and nonreactive because of the unopposed dilator pupillae. The pupil is fully abducted and depressed ("down and out") because of the unopposed activity of the lateral rectus and superior oblique, respectively.
- A **lesion of the abducent nerve** results in loss of lateral gaze to the ipsilateral side because of paralysis of the lateral rectus muscle. On forward gaze, the eye is diverted medially because of the lack of normal resting tone in the lateral rectus, resulting in diplopia (double vision).

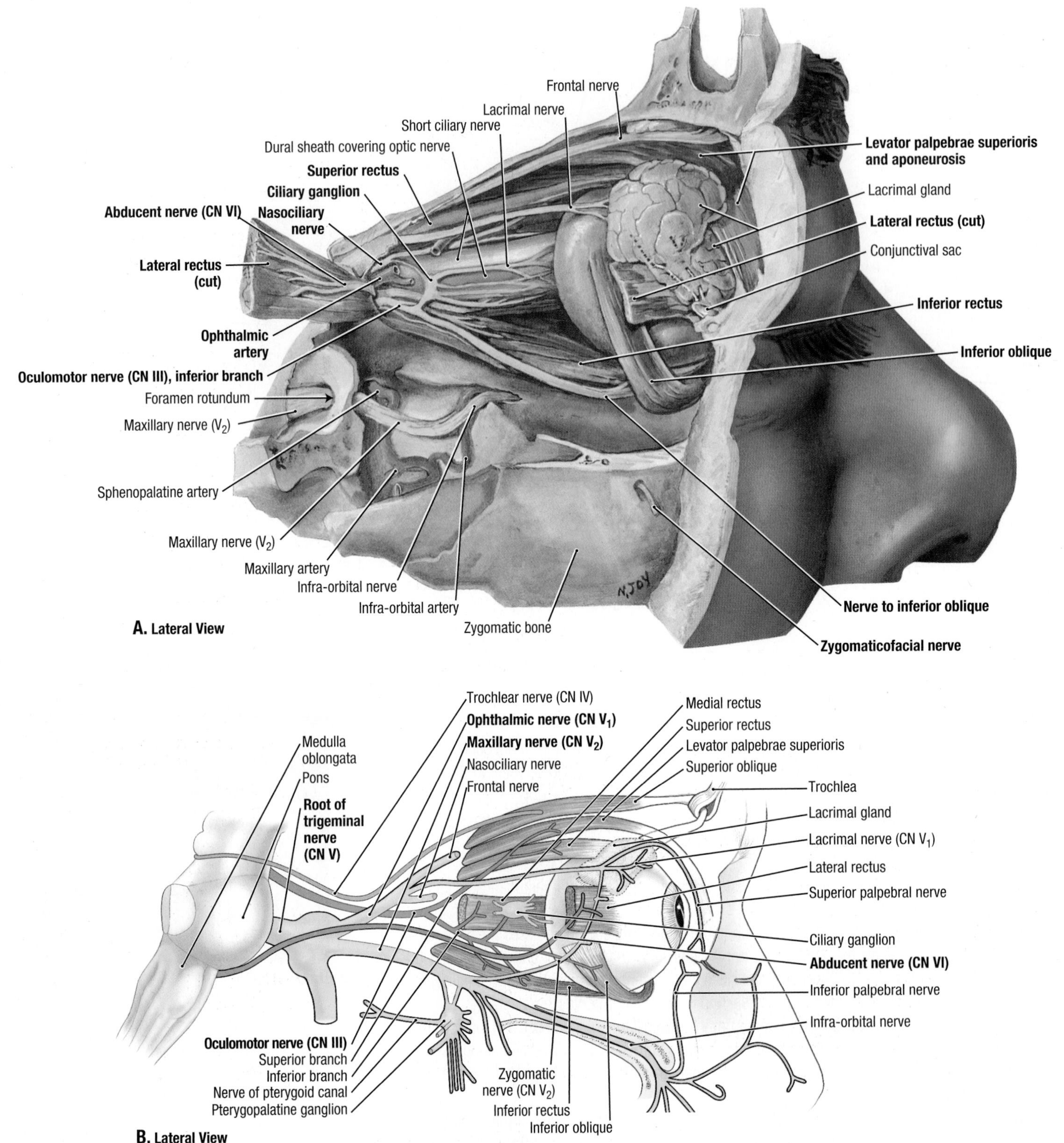

Frontal nerve
Lacrimal nerve
Short ciliary nerve
Dural sheath covering optic nerve
Superior rectus
Ciliary ganglion
Abducent nerve (CN VI)
Nasociliary nerve
Lateral rectus (cut)
Ophthalmic artery
Oculomotor nerve (CN III), inferior branch
Foramen rotundum
Maxillary nerve (V_2)
Sphenopalatine artery
Maxillary nerve (V_2)
Maxillary artery
Infra-orbital nerve
Infra-orbital artery
Zygomatic bone
Levator palpebrae superioris and aponeurosis
Lacrimal gland
Lateral rectus (cut)
Conjunctival sac
Inferior rectus
Inferior oblique
Nerve to inferior oblique
Zygomaticofacial nerve
A. Lateral View
Trochlear nerve (CN IV)
Ophthalmic nerve (CN V_1)
Maxillary nerve (CN V_2)
Nasociliary nerve
Frontal nerve
Medulla oblongata
Pons
Root of trigeminal nerve (CN V)
Medial rectus
Superior rectus
Levator palpebrae superioris
Superior oblique
Trochlea
Lacrimal gland
Lacrimal nerve (CN V_1)
Lateral rectus
Superior palpebral nerve
Ciliary ganglion
Abducent nerve (CN VI)
Inferior palpebral nerve
Infra-orbital nerve
Oculomotor nerve (CN III)
Superior branch
Inferior branch
Nerve of pterygoid canal
Pterygopalatine ganglion
Zygomatic nerve (CN V_2)
Inferior rectus
Inferior oblique
B. Lateral View

7.39 LATERAL ASPECT OF THE ORBIT AND STRUCTURE OF THE EYELID

A. Dissection. **B.** Nerves. **C.** Sagittal and cross section through optic nerve. The subarachnoid space around the optic nerve is continuous with the subarachnoid space around the brain. **D.** Sagittal MRI. The *numbers* refer to structures labeled in *C; S,* superior ophthalmic vein; *M,* maxillary sinus; *circled,* optic foramen. **E.** Structure of eyelid.

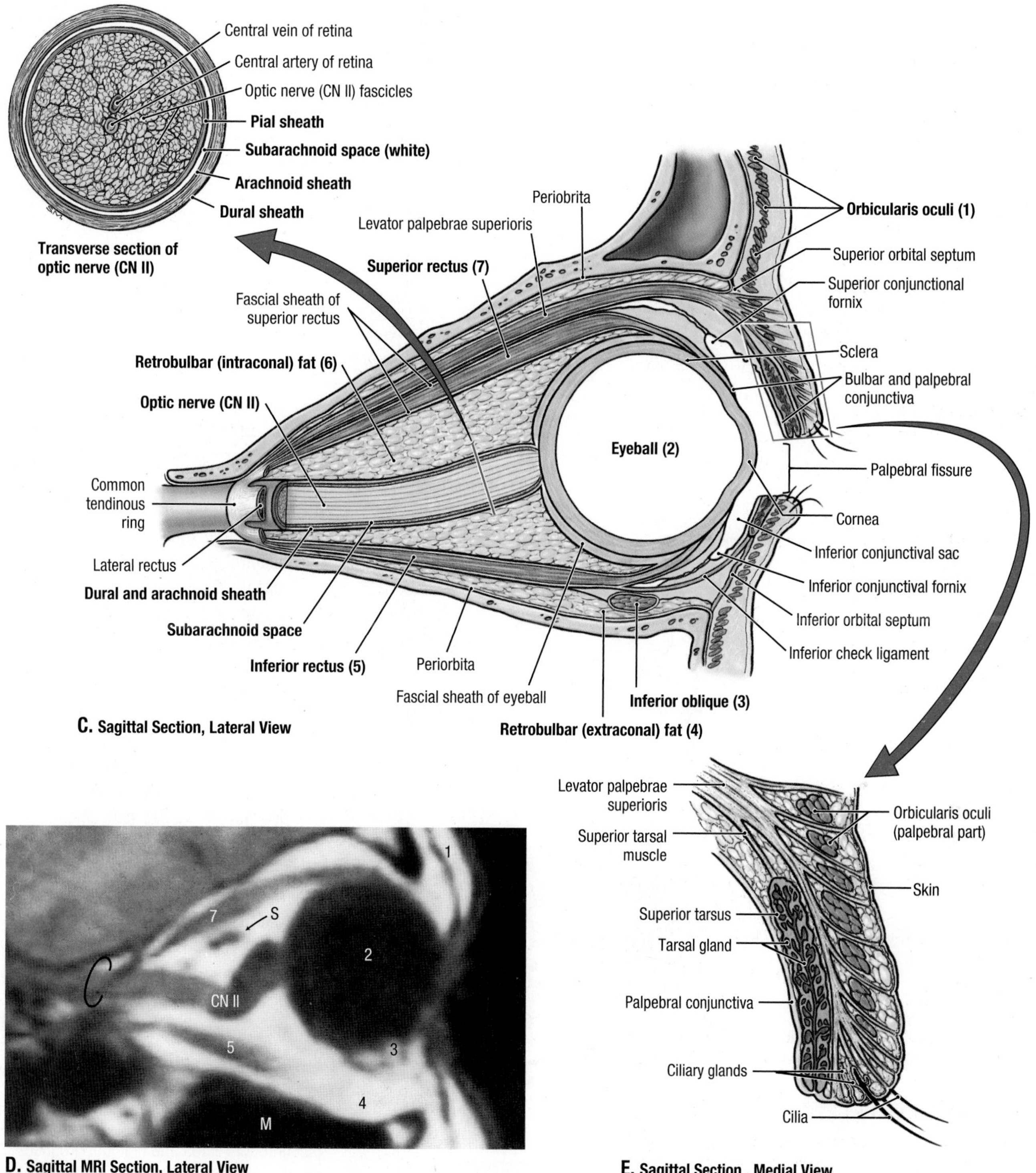
Central vein of retina
Central artery of retina
Optic nerve (CN II) fascicles
Pial sheath
Subarachnoid space (white)
Arachnoid sheath
Dural sheath
Transverse section of optic nerve (CN II)
Periobrita
Levator palpebrae superioris
Orbicularis oculi (1)
Superior orbital septum
Superior rectus (7)
Superior conjunctional fornix
Fascial sheath of superior rectus
Sclera
Retrobulbar (intraconal) fat (6)
Bulbar and palpebral conjunctiva
Optic nerve (CN II)
Eyeball (2)
Palpebral fissure
Common tendinous ring
Cornea
Inferior conjunctival sac
Lateral rectus
Inferior conjunctival fornix
Dural and arachnoid sheath
Inferior orbital septum
Subarachnoid space
Inferior check ligament
Inferior rectus (5)
Periorbita
Fascial sheath of eyeball
Inferior oblique (3)
Retrobulbar (extraconal) fat (4)
Levator palpebrae superioris
Orbicularis oculi (palpebral part)
Superior tarsal muscle
Skin
Superior tarsus
Tarsal gland
Palpebral conjunctiva
Ciliary glands
Cilia
1
7
S
2
C
CN II
5
3
4
M

C. Sagittal Section, Lateral View

D. Sagittal MRI Section, Lateral View

E. Sagittal Section , Medial View

7.39 LATERAL ASPECT OF THE ORBIT AND STRUCTURE OF THE EYELID *(CONTINUED)*

- Foreign objects, such as sand or metal filings, produce **corneal abrasions** that cause sudden, stabbing eye pain and tears. Opening and closing the eyelids is also painful. **Corneal lacerations** are caused by sharp objects such as fingernails or the corner of a page of a book.
- Any of the glands in the eyelid may become inflamed and swollen from infection or obstruction of their ducts. If the ducts of the ciliary glands are obstructed, a painful red suppurative (pus-producing) swelling, a sty (hordeolum), develops on the eyelid. **Obstruction of a tarsal gland** produces inflammation, a tarsal chalazion, that protrudes toward the eyeball and rubs against it as the eyelids blink.

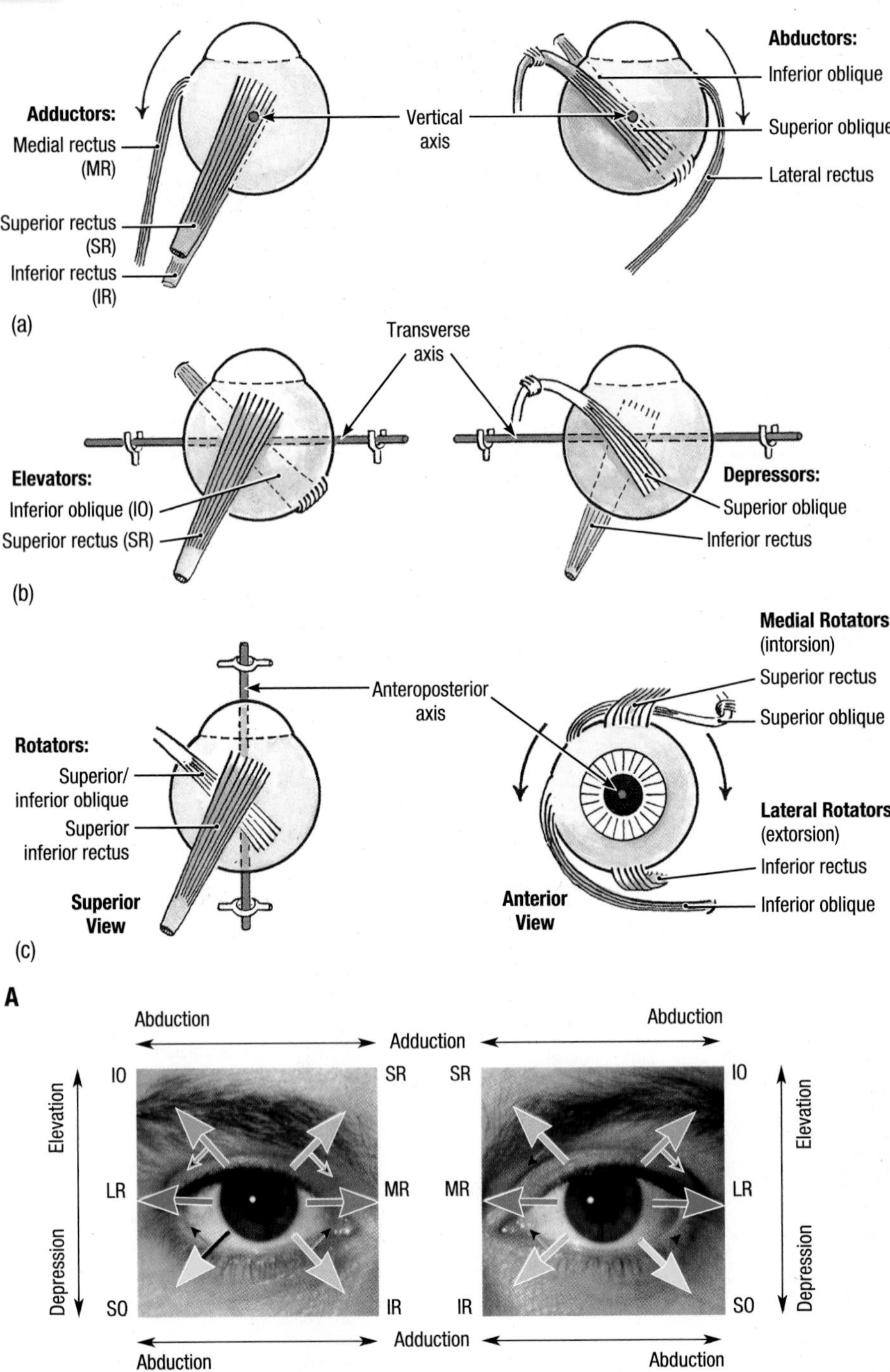
Adductors:
Medial rectus (MR)
Superior rectus (SR)
Inferior rectus (IR)
Vertical axis
Abductors:
Inferior oblique
Superior oblique
Lateral rectus
(a)
Transverse axis
Elevators:
Inferior oblique (IO)
Superior rectus (SR)
Depressors:
Superior oblique
Inferior rectus
(b)
Anteroposterior axis
Rotators:
Superior/ inferior oblique
Superior inferior rectus
Superior View
Medial Rotators: (intorsion)
Superior rectus
Superior oblique
Lateral Rotators (extorsion)
Inferior rectus
Inferior oblique
Anterior View
(c)
A
Abduction
Adduction
Abduction
Elevation
Depression
IO
SR
SR
IO
LR
MR
MR
LR
SO
IR
IR
SO
Adduction
Abduction
Abduction

B. **Anterior View of Right and Left Eyes**

7.40 EXTRA-OCULAR MUSCLES AND THEIR MOVEMENTS

A. The line of pull of the muscles relative to the eyeball and the axes around which movements occur. The orientation of the orbit is important in understanding the actions of the extra-ocular muscles. The common tendinous ring (origin of the recti), the origin of the inferior oblique, and the trochlea of the superior oblique all lie medial to the eyeball and to the A-P and vertical axes **(a)** The medial and lateral recti are the primary adductors and abductors of the eyeball. However, when movements begin from the primary position (gaze directed anteriorly along the A-P axis): (1) the line of pull of the superior and inferior rectus muscles passes medial and anterior to the vertical axis, resulting in secondary actions of a<u>d</u>duction; and (2) the line of pull of the superior and inferior oblique muscles passes medial and posterior to the vertical axis, resulting in secondary actions of a<u>b</u>duction. **(b)** Pulling in opposite directions relative to the transverse axis, the superior rectus and inferior oblique muscles are synergistic elevators, and the inferior rectus and superior oblique are synergistic depressors. **(c)** Medial pull produced by the muscles attaching to the superior eyeball (superior rectus and oblique) produces secondary actions of medial rotation (intorsion), and that produced by muscles attaching to the inferior eyeball (inferior rectus and oblique) produces lateral rotation (extorsion). **B.** Movements produced by isolated contraction of the four rectus and two oblique muscles, starting from the primary position. Large arrows indicate prime movers for the six cardinal movements. Movements in directions between large arrows (e.g., vertical elevation or depression) require synergistic actions of adjacent muscles. Contralaterally-paired muscles that work synergistically to direct parallel binocular gaze are called yoke muscles. For example, the right LR and left MR act as yoke muscles in directing gaze to the right.

TABLE 7.8 ACTIONS OF MUSCLES OF ORBIT STARTING FROM PRIMARY POSITION[a]

Muscle	Main Action		
	Vertical Axis (A)	**Horizontal Axis (B)**	**Anteroposterior Axis (C)**
Superior rectus (SR)	Elevates	Adducts	Rotates medially (intorsion)
Inferior rectus (IR)	Depresses	Adducts	Rotates laterally (extorsion)
Superior oblique (SO)	Depresses	Abducts	Rotates medially (intorsion)
Inferior oblique (IO)	Elevates	Abducts	Rotates laterally (extorsion)
Medial rectus (MR)	N/A	Adducts	N/A
Lateral rectus (LR)	N/A	Abducts	N/A

[a]Primary position, gaze directed anteriorly.

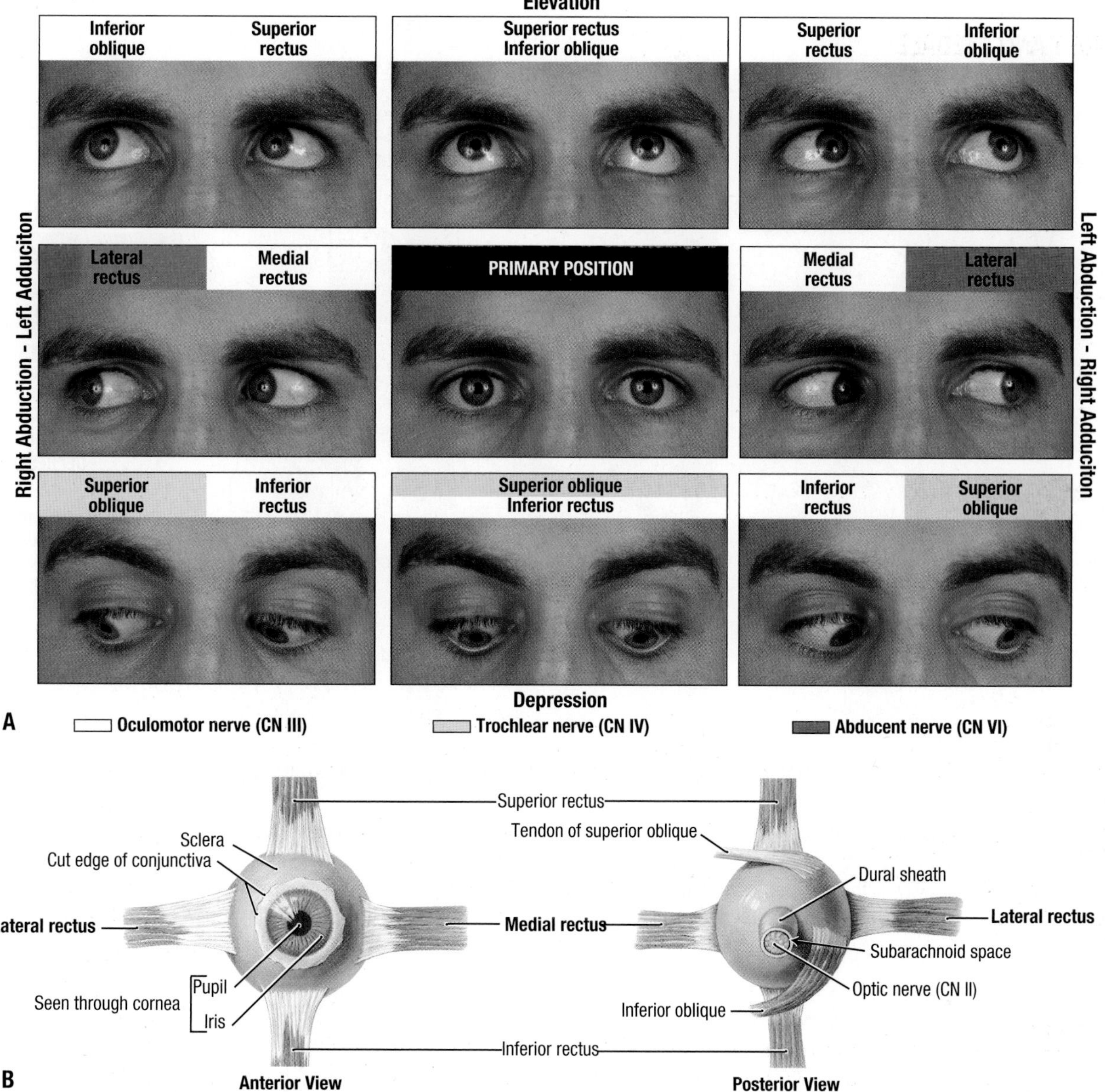

Elevation
Inferior oblique
Superior rectus
Superior rectus
Inferior oblique
Superior rectus
Inferior oblique
Right Abduction - Left Adduciton
Lateral rectus
Medial rectus
PRIMARY POSITION
Medial rectus
Lateral rectus
Left Abduction - Right Adduciton
Superior oblique
Inferior rectus
Superior oblique
Inferior rectus
Inferior rectus
Superior oblique
Depression
A
Oculomotor nerve (CN III)
Trochlear nerve (CN IV)
Abducent nerve (CN VI)
Superior rectus
Tendon of superior oblique
Sclera
Cut edge of conjunctiva
Dural sheath
Lateral rectus
Medial rectus
Lateral rectus
Subarachnoid space
Seen through cornea
Pupil
Iris
Optic nerve (CN II)
Inferior oblique
Inferior rectus
B
Anterior View
Posterior View

7.41 EXTRA-OCULAR MUSCLES AND THEIR MOVEMENTS *(CONTINUED)*

A. Binocular movements of eyeball from primary position, and muscles and nerves producing them. **B.** Muscles of eyeball.

TABLE 7.9 MUSCLES OF ORBIT

Muscle	Origin	Insertion	Innervation	Main Action(s)[a]
Levator palpebrae superioris	Lesser wing of sphenoid bone, superior and anterior to optic canal	Superior tarsus and skin of superior eyelid	Oculomotor nerve; deep layer (superior tarsal muscle) supplied by sympathetic fibers	Elevates superior eyelid
Superior oblique (SO)	Body of sphenoid bone	Tendon passes through trochlea to insert into sclera, deep to SR	Trochlear nerve (CN IV)	Abducts, depresses, and rotates eyeball medially (intorsion)
Inferior oblique (IO)	Anterior part of floor of orbit	Sclera deep to lateral rectus muscle	Oculomotor nerve (CN III)	Abducts, elevates, and rotates eyeball laterally (extorsion)
Superior rectus (SR)	Common tendinous ring	Sclera just posterior to corneoscleral junction		Elevates, adducts, and (SR) rotates eyeball medially (intorsion)
Inferior rectus (IR)				Depresses, adducts, and rotates eyeball laterally (extorsion)
Medial rectus (MR)				Adducts eyeball
Lateral rectus (LR)			Abducent nerve (CN VI)	Abducts eyeball

[a]It is essential to appreciate that all muscles are continuously involved in eyeball movements; thus the individual actions are not usually tested clinically.

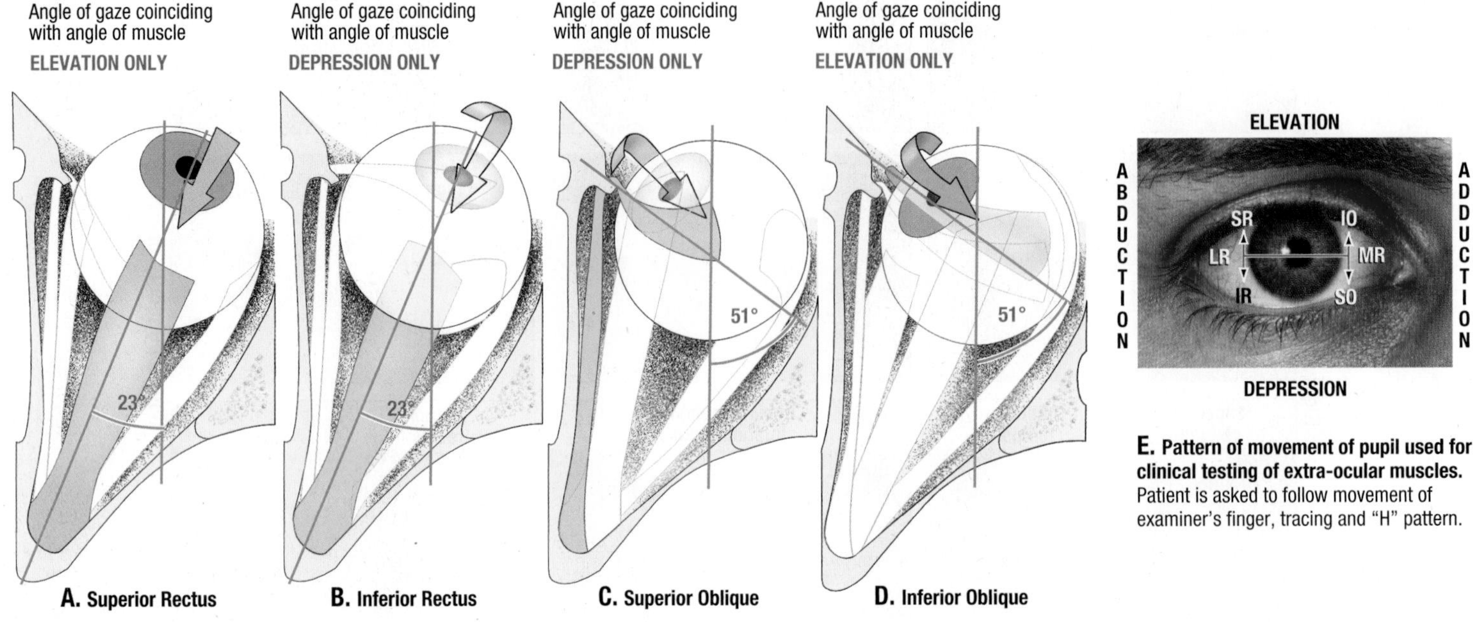
Angle of gaze coinciding with angle of muscle
ELEVATION ONLY
Angle of gaze coinciding with angle of muscle
DEPRESSION ONLY
Angle of gaze coinciding with angle of muscle
DEPRESSION ONLY
Angle of gaze coinciding with angle of muscle
ELEVATION ONLY
23°
23°
51°
51°
ELEVATION
ABDUCTION
ADDUCTION
SR
IO
LR
MR
IR
SO
DEPRESSION

A. **Superior Rectus** **B.** **Inferior Rectus** **C.** **Superior Oblique** **D.** **Inferior Oblique**

E. Pattern of movement of pupil used for clinical testing of extra-ocular muscles. Patient is asked to follow movement of examiner's finger, tracing and "H" pattern.

7.42 CLINICAL TESTING OF EXTRA-OCULAR MUSCLES AND MOTOR NERVES (CN III, IV, AND VI)

Most movements from the primary position involve synergists. When testing muscles (usually to determine the integrity of the involved motor nerve), it is desirable to isolate muscle activity. If the pupil is first adducted (MR—CN III) so that the direction of gaze coincides with the line of pull of the oblique muscles, only the SO (CN IV) can depress and only the IO (CN III) can elevate the pupil. If the pupil is first abducted (LR—CN VI) so that the direction of gaze coincides with the line of pull of the superior and inferior recti, only these muscles can elevate and depress the pupil (superior and inferior divisions of CN III)

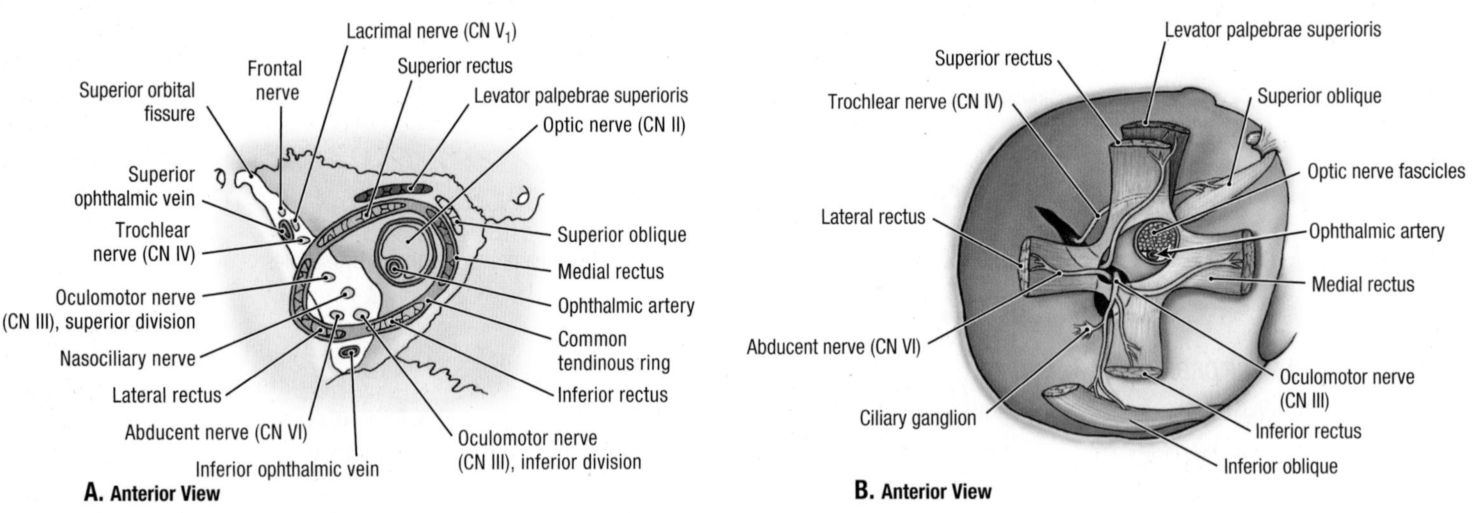
Lacrimal nerve (CN V_1)
Frontal nerve
Superior rectus
Superior orbital fissure
Levator palpebrae superioris
Optic nerve (CN II)
Superior ophthalmic vein
Trochlear nerve (CN IV)
Superior oblique
Medial rectus
Oculomotor nerve (CN III), superior division
Ophthalmic artery
Common tendinous ring
Nasociliary nerve
Lateral rectus
Inferior rectus
Abducent nerve (CN VI)
Oculomotor nerve (CN III), inferior division
Inferior ophthalmic vein
Levator palpebrae superioris
Superior rectus
Trochlear nerve (CN IV)
Superior oblique
Optic nerve fascicles
Lateral rectus
Ophthalmic artery
Medial rectus
Abducent nerve (CN VI)
Oculomotor nerve (CN III)
Ciliary ganglion
Inferior rectus
Inferior oblique

A. Anterior View **B. Anterior View**

7.43 NERVES OF ORBIT

A. Overview. **B.** Relationships at apex of orbit. **C.** Common tendinous ring, structural relationships.

Orbital tumors. Because of the closeness of the optic nerve to the sphenoidal and posterior ethmoidal sinuses, a malignant tumor in these sinuses may erode the thin bony walls of the orbit and compress the optic nerve and orbital contents. Tumors in the orbit produce **exophthalmos** (protrusion of eyeball). Tumors in the middle cranial fossa enter the orbital cavity through the superior orbital fissure. Tumors in the temporal or infratemporal fossae enter the orbit through the inferior orbital fissure.

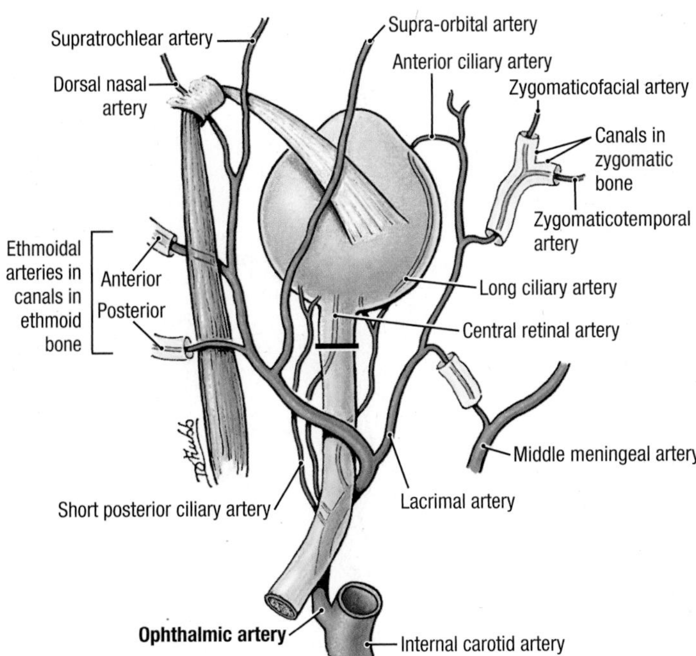
Supratrochlear artery
Supra-orbital artery
Anterior ciliary artery
Zygomaticofacial artery
Dorsal nasal artery
Canals in zygomatic bone
Zygomaticotemporal artery
Ethmoidal arteries in canals in ethmoid bone
Anterior
Posterior
Long ciliary artery
Central retinal artery
Middle meningeal artery
Short posterior ciliary artery
Lacrimal artery
Ophthalmic artery
Internal carotid artery

A. **Superior View**

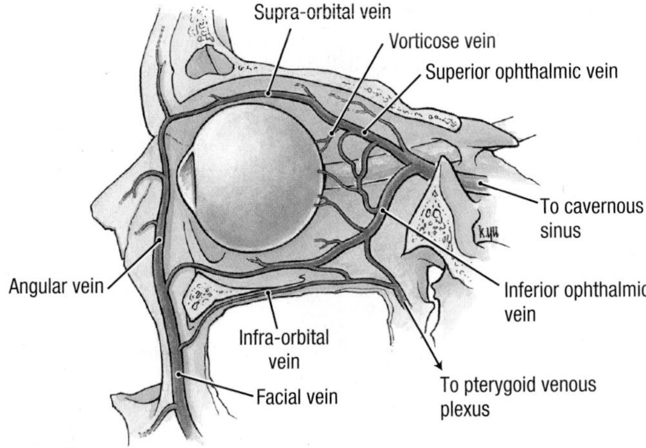
Supra-orbital vein
Vorticose vein
Superior ophthalmic vein
To cavernous sinus
Angular vein
Inferior ophthalmic vein
Infra-orbital vein
To pterygoid venous plexus
Facial vein

B. **Lateral View**

7.44 ARTERIES AND VEINS OF ORBIT

A. Arteries.

Blockage of central retinal artery. The terminal branches of the central retinal artery are end arteries. Obstruction of the artery by an embolus results in instant and total blindness. Blockage of the artery is usually unilateral and occurs in older people. **B.** Veins. The superior and inferior ophthalmic veins receive the vorticose veins from the eyeball and drain into the cavernous sinus posteriorly and the pterygoid plexus inferiorly. They communicate with the facial and supra-orbital veins anteriorly.

- The facial veins make clinically important connections with the cavernous sinus through the superior ophthalmic veins. **Cavernous sinus thrombosis** usually results from infections in the orbit, nasal sinuses, and superior part of the face (the danger triangle). In persons with thrombophlebitis of the facial vein, pieces of an infected thrombus may extend into the cavernous sinus, producing **thrombophlebitis of the cavernous sinus.** The infection usually involves only one sinus initially but may spread to the opposite side through the intercavernous sinuses.
- **Blockade of central retinal vein.** The central retinal vein enters the cavernous sinus. Thrombophlebitis of this sinus may result in passage of a thrombus to the central retinal vein and produce a blockage in one of the small retinal veins. Occlusion of a branch of the central vein of the retina usually results in slow, painless loss of vision.

TABLE 7.10 ARTERIES OF ORBIT

Artery	Origin	Course and Distribution
Ophthalmic	Internal carotid artery	Traverses optic foramen to reach orbital cavity
Central retinal	Ophthalmic artery	Runs in dural sheath of optic nerve, entering nerve near eyeball; appears at center of optic disc; supplies optic retina (except cones and rods)
Supra-orbital		Passes superiorly and posteriorly from supra-orbital foramen to supply forehead and scalp
Supratrochlear		Passes from supra-orbital margin to forehead and scalp
Lacrimal		Passes along superior border of lateral rectus muscle to supply lacrimal gland, conjunctiva, and eyelids
Dorsal nasal		Courses along dorsal aspect of nose and supplies its surface
Short posterior ciliary		Pierces sclera at periphery of optic nerve to supply choroid, which, in turn, supplies cones and rods of optic retina
Long posterior ciliary		Pierces sclera to supply ciliary body and iris
Posterior ethmoidal		Passes through posterior ethmoidal foramen to posterior ethmoidal cells
Anterior ethmoidal		Passes through anterior ethmoidal foramen to anterior cranial fossa; supplies anterior and middle ethmoidal cells, frontal sinus, nasal cavity, and skin on dorsum of nose
Anterior ciliary	Muscular rami of the opthalmic and infra-orbital arteries	Pierces sclera at attachments of rectus muscles and forms network in iris and ciliary body
Infra-orbital	Third part of maxillary artery	Passes along infra-orbital groove and exits through infra-orbital foramen to face

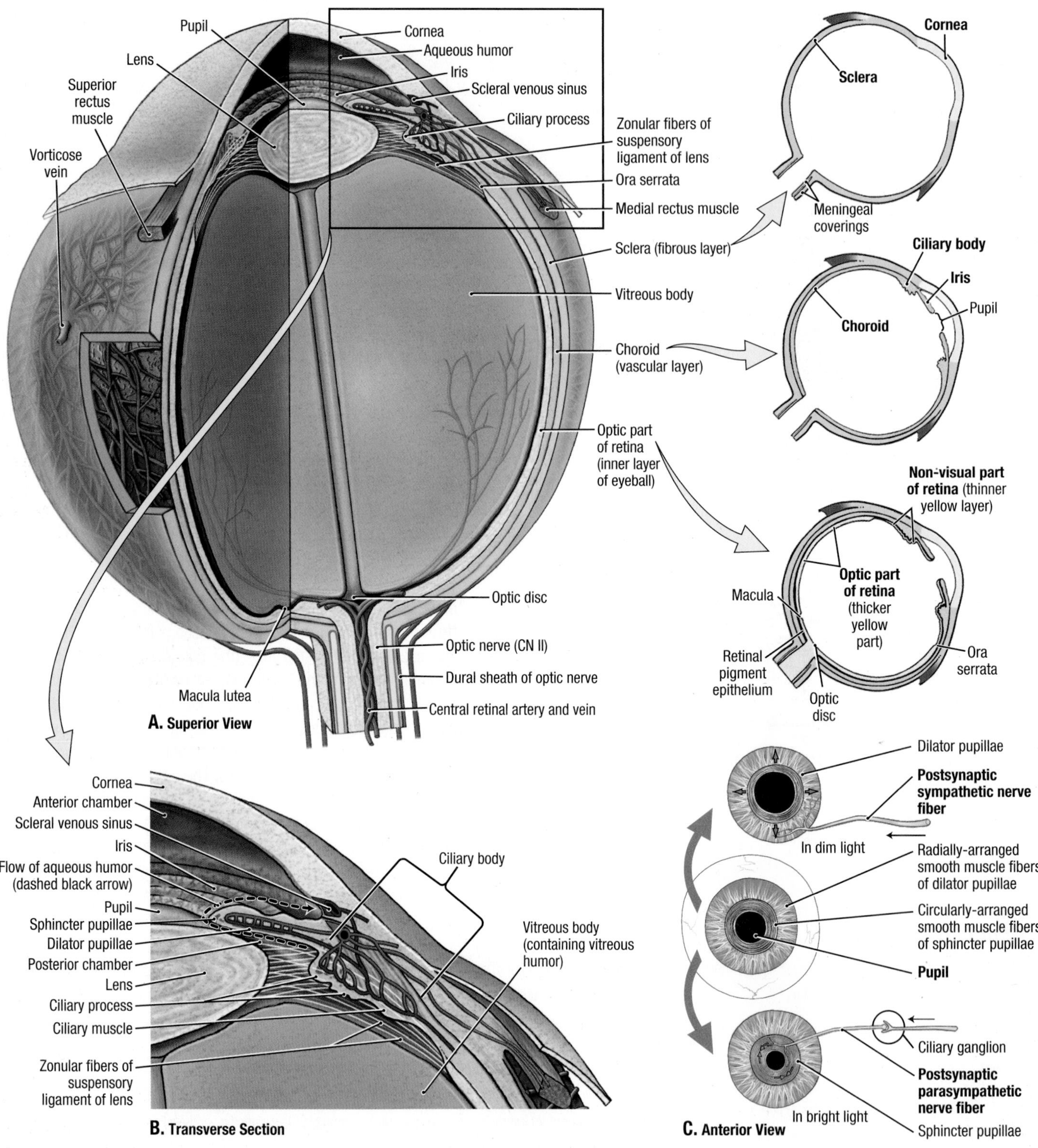

Pupil
Lens
Superior rectus muscle
Vorticose vein
Cornea
Aqueous humor
Iris
Scleral venous sinus
Ciliary process
Zonular fibers of suspensory ligament of lens
Ora serrata
Medial rectus muscle
Sclera (fibrous layer)
Vitreous body
Choroid (vascular layer)
Optic part of retina (inner layer of eyeball)
Optic disc
Optic nerve (CN II)
Dural sheath of optic nerve
Central retinal artery and vein
Macula lutea
A. Superior View
Cornea
Sclera
Meningeal coverings
Ciliary body
Iris
Pupil
Choroid
Non-visual part of retina (thinner yellow layer)
Optic part of retina (thicker yellow part)
Macula
Retinal pigment epithelium
Optic disc
Ora serrata
Cornea
Anterior chamber
Scleral venous sinus
Iris
Flow of aqueous humor (dashed black arrow)
Pupil
Sphincter pupillae
Dilator pupillae
Posterior chamber
Lens
Ciliary process
Ciliary muscle
Zonular fibers of suspensory ligament of lens
Ciliary body
Vitreous body (containing vitreous humor)
B. Transverse Section
Dilator pupillae
Postsynaptic sympathetic nerve fiber
In dim light
Radially-arranged smooth muscle fibers of dilator pupillae
Circularly-arranged smooth muscle fibers of sphincter pupillae
Pupil
Ciliary ganglion
Postsynaptic parasympathetic nerve fiber
In bright light
Sphincter pupillae
C. Anterior View

7.45 ILLUSTRATION OF A DISSECTED EYEBALL

A. Parts of the eyeball. **B.** Ciliary region. **C.** Structure and function of iris. The aqueous humor is produced by the ciliary processes and provides nutrients for the avascular cornea and lens; the aqueous humor drains into the scleral venous sinus (also called the sinus venosus sclerae or canal of Schlemm). **Glaucoma.** If drainage of the aqueous humor is reduced significantly, pressure builds up in the chambers of the eye (glaucoma). Blindness can result from compression of the inner layer of the retina and retinal arteries if aqueous humor production is not reduced to maintain normal intraocular pressure.

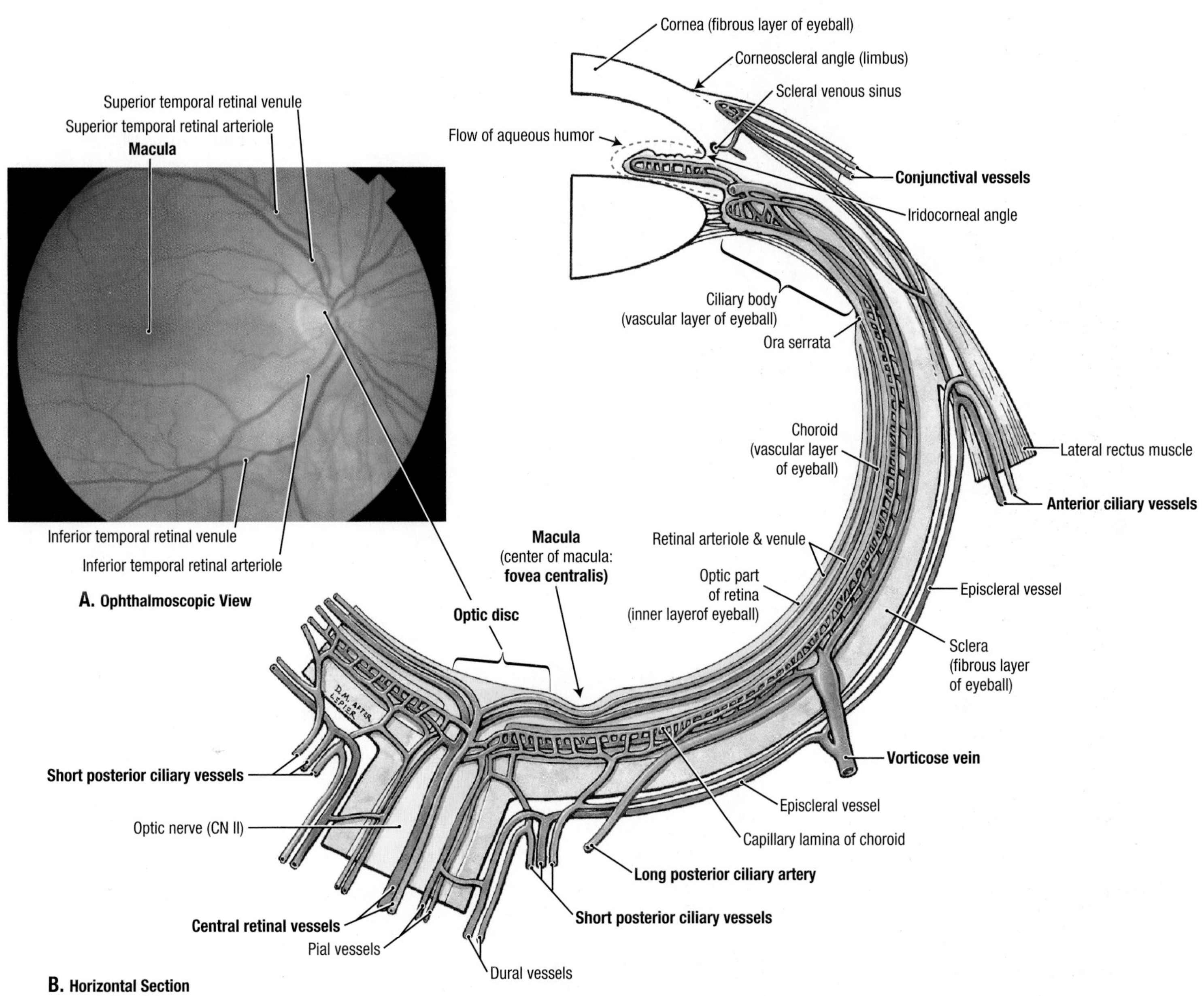
Superior temporal retinal venule
Superior temporal retinal arteriole
Macula
Inferior temporal retinal venule
Inferior temporal retinal arteriole
A. Ophthalmoscopic View
Cornea (fibrous layer of eyeball)
Corneoscleral angle (limbus)
Scleral venous sinus
Flow of aqueous humor
Conjunctival vessels
Iridocorneal angle
Ciliary body (vascular layer of eyeball)
Ora serrata
Choroid (vascular layer of eyeball)
Lateral rectus muscle
Anterior ciliary vessels
Macula (center of macula: fovea centralis)
Retinal arteriole & venule
Optic part of retina (inner layerof eyeball)
Optic disc
Episcleral vessel
Sclera (fibrous layer of eyeball)
Vorticose vein
Short posterior ciliary vessels
Optic nerve (CN II)
Episcleral vessel
Capillary lamina of choroid
Long posterior ciliary artery
Short posterior ciliary vessels
Central retinal vessels
Pial vessels
Dural vessels
B. Horizontal Section

7.46 OCULAR FUNDUS AND BLOOD SUPPLY TO THE EYEBALL

A. Right ocular fundus, ophthalmoscopic view. Retinal venules (wider) and retinal arterioles (narrower) radiate from the center of the oval optic disc, formed in relation to the entry of the optic nerve into the eyeball. The round, dark area lateral to the disc is the macula; branches of vessels extend to this area, but do not reach its center, the fovea centralis, a depressed spot that is the area of most acute vision. It is avascular but, like the rest of the outermost (cones and rods) layer of the retina, is nourished by the adjacent choriocapillaris. Increased intracranial pressure is transmitted through the CSF in the subarachnoid space surrounding the optic nerve, causing the optic disc to protrude. The protrusion, called **papilledema,** is apparent during ophthalmoscopy. **B.** Blood supply to eyeball. The eyeball has three layers: (1) the external, fibrous layer is the sclera and cornea; (2) the middle, vascular layer is the choroid, ciliary body, and iris; and (3) the internal, neural layer or retina consists of a pigment cell layer and a neural layer. The central artery of the retina, a branch of the ophthalmic artery, is an end artery. Of the eight posterior ciliary arteries, six are short posterior ciliary arteries and supply the choroid, which in turn nourishes the outer, nonvascular layer of the retina. Two long posterior ciliary arteries, one on each side of the eyeball, run between the sclera and choroid to anastomose with the anterior ciliary arteries, which are derived from muscular branches. The choroid is drained by posterior ciliary veins, and four to five vorticose veins drain into the ophthalmic veins.

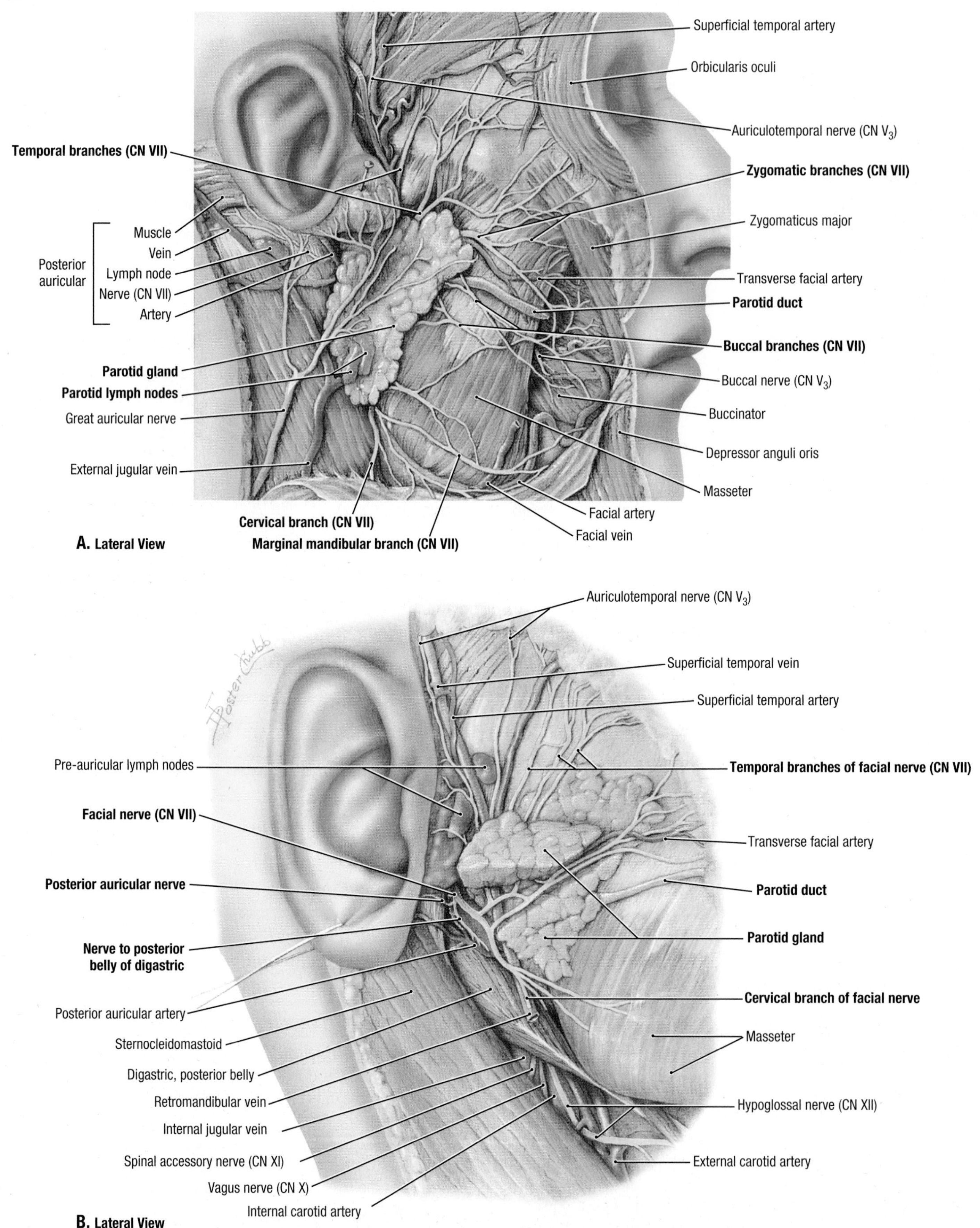
Superficial temporal artery
Orbicularis oculi
Auriculotemporal nerve (CN V_3)
Temporal branches (CN VII)
Zygomatic branches (CN VII)
Zygomaticus major
Posterior auricular
Muscle
Vein
Lymph node
Nerve (CN VII)
Artery
Transverse facial artery
Parotid duct
Buccal branches (CN VII)
Parotid gland
Parotid lymph nodes
Buccal nerve (CN V_3)
Great auricular nerve
Buccinator
Depressor anguli oris
External jugular vein
Masseter
Facial artery
Facial vein
Cervical branch (CN VII)
Marginal mandibular branch (CN VII)
Auriculotemporal nerve (CN V_3)
Superficial temporal vein
Superficial temporal artery
Pre-auricular lymph nodes
Temporal branches of facial nerve (CN VII)
Facial nerve (CN VII)
Transverse facial artery
Posterior auricular nerve
Parotid duct
Parotid gland
Nerve to posterior belly of digastric
Cervical branch of facial nerve
Posterior auricular artery
Sternocleidomastoid
Masseter
Digastric, posterior belly
Retromandibular vein
Hypoglossal nerve (CN XII)
Internal jugular vein
Spinal accessory nerve (CN XI)
External carotid artery
Vagus nerve (CN X)
Internal carotid artery

A. **Lateral View**

B. **Lateral View**

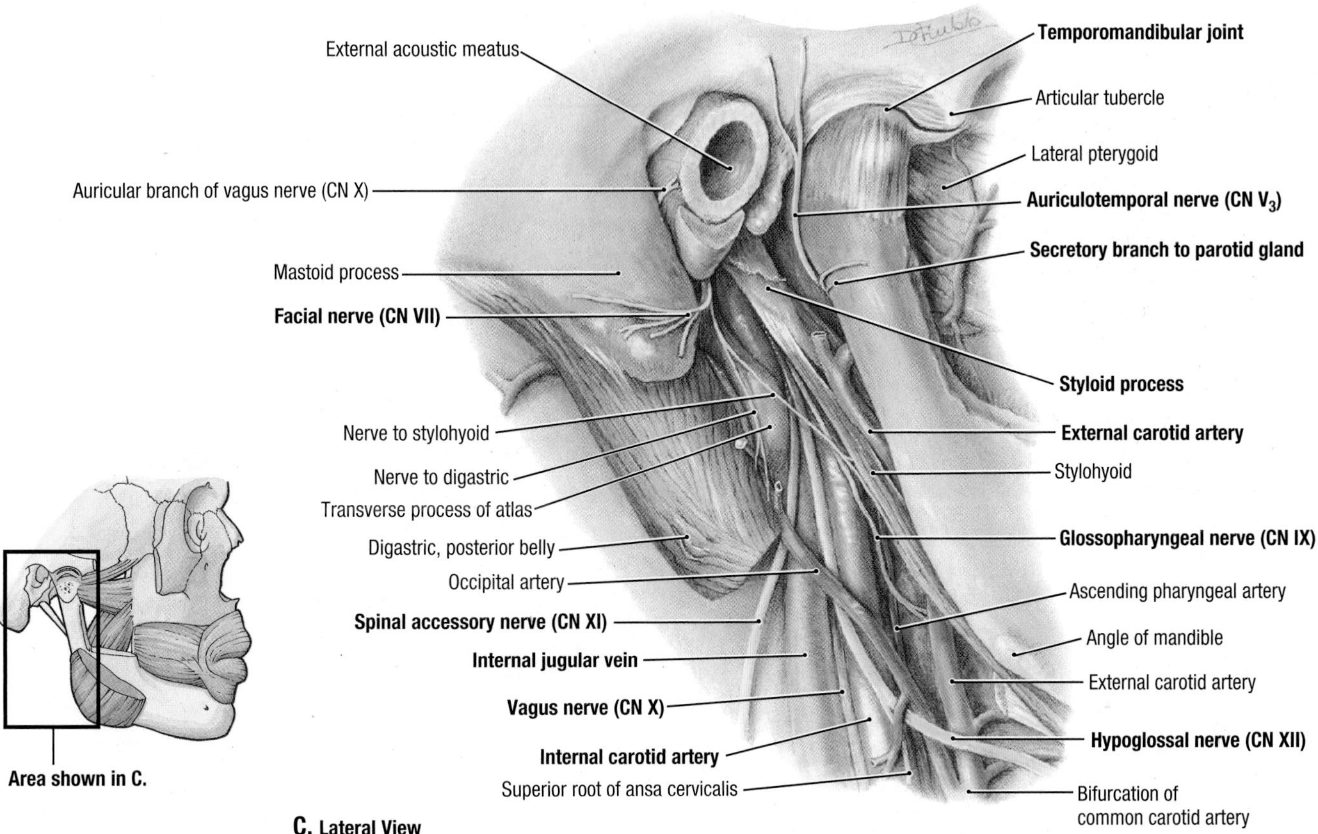
External acoustic meatus
Temporomandibular joint
Articular tubercle
Lateral pterygoid
Auricular branch of vagus nerve (CN X)
Auriculotemporal nerve (CN V_3)
Secretory branch to parotid gland
Mastoid process
Facial nerve (CN VII)
Styloid process
Nerve to stylohyoid
External carotid artery
Stylohyoid
Nerve to digastric
Transverse process of atlas
Digastric, posterior belly
Glossopharyngeal nerve (CN IX)
Occipital artery
Ascending pharyngeal artery
Spinal accessory nerve (CN XI)
Angle of mandible
Internal jugular vein
External carotid artery
Vagus nerve (CN X)
Hypoglossal nerve (CN XII)
Internal carotid artery
Superior root of ansa cervicalis
Bifurcation of common carotid artery
Area shown in C.

C. Lateral View

7.47 PAROTID REGION

A. Superficial dissection. **B.** Deep dissection with part of the gland removed. During **parotidectomy** (surgical excision of the parotid gland), identification, dissection, and preservation of the facial nerve are critical. The parotid gland has superficial and deep parts. In parotidectomy the superficial part is removed, then the plexus may be retracted to remove the deep part. **C.** Deep dissection following removal of the parotid gland. The facial nerve, posterior belly of the digastric muscle, and its nerve are retracted; the external carotid artery, stylohyoid muscle, and the nerve to the stylohyoid remain in situ. The internal jugular vein, internal carotid artery, and glossopharyngeal (CN IX), vagus (CN X), accessory (CN XI), and hypoglossal (CN XII) nerves cross anterior to the transverse process of the atlas and deep to the styloid process.

Trauma, such as a **fractured mandible,** may injure the hypoglossal nerve (CN XII), resulting in paralysis and eventual atrophy of one side of the tongue. The tongue deviates to the paralyzed side during protrusion.

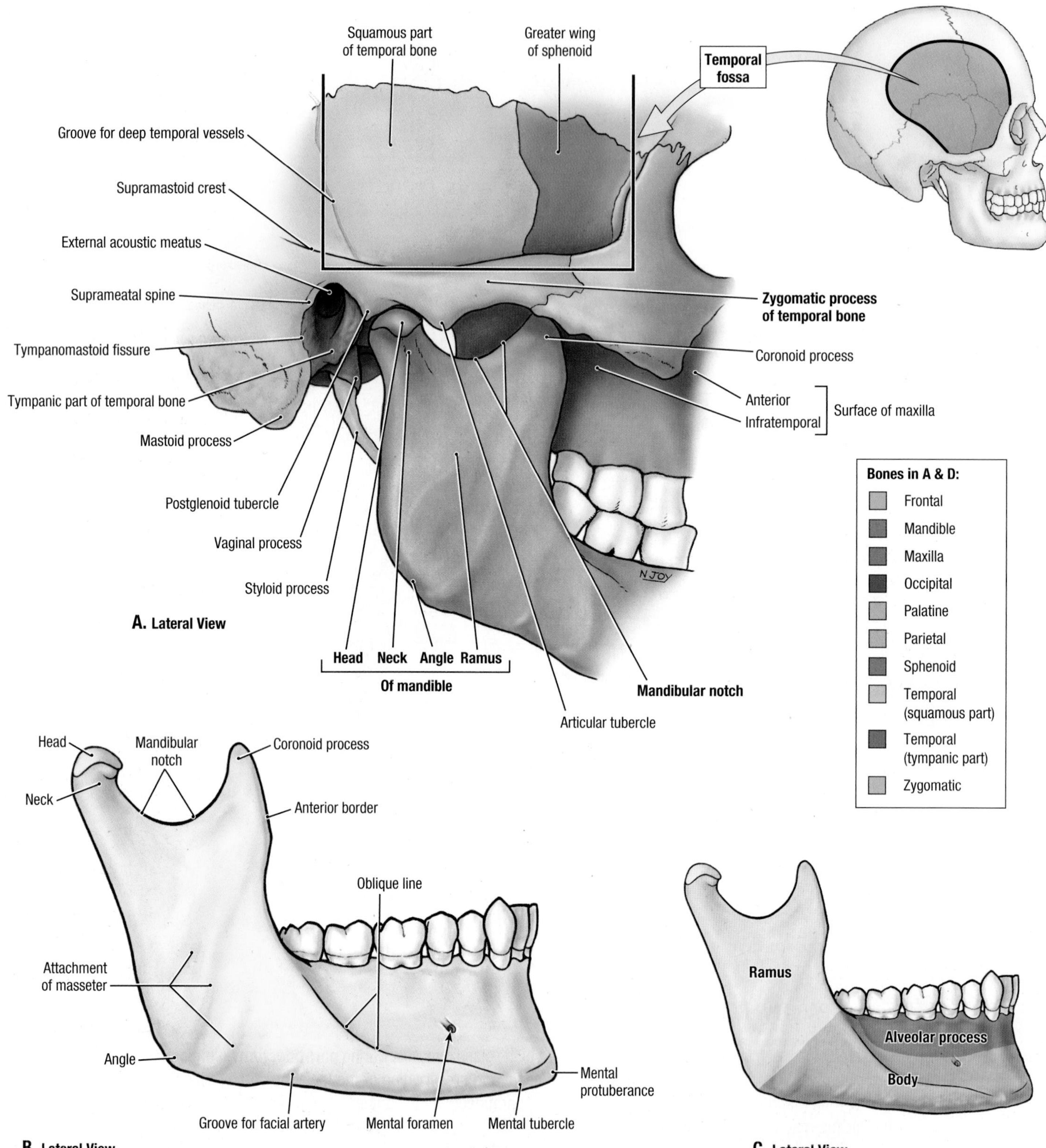
Squamous part of temporal bone
Greater wing of sphenoid
Temporal fossa
Groove for deep temporal vessels
Supramastoid crest
External acoustic meatus
Suprameatal spine
Tympanomastoid fissure
Tympanic part of temporal bone
Mastoid process
Postglenoid tubercle
Vaginal process
Styloid process
Zygomatic process of temporal bone
Coronoid process
Anterior
Infratemporal
Surface of maxilla
Bones in A & D:
Frontal
Mandible
Maxilla
Occipital
Palatine
Parietal
Sphenoid
Temporal (squamous part)
Temporal (tympanic part)
Zygomatic
A. Lateral View
Head Neck Angle Ramus
Of mandible
Mandibular notch
Articular tubercle
Head
Mandibular notch
Coronoid process
Neck
Anterior border
Oblique line
Attachment of masseter
Angle
Mental protuberance
Groove for facial artery
Mental foramen
Mental tubercle
B. Lateral View
Ramus
Alveolar process
Body
C. Lateral View

7.48 TEMPORAL AND INFRATEMPORAL FOSSAE AND MANDIBLE

A. Bones and bony features. Note that superficially the zygomatic process of the temporal bone is the boundary between the temporal fossa superiorly and the infratemporal fossa inferiorly. **B.** External surface of the mandible. **C.** Parts of mandible.

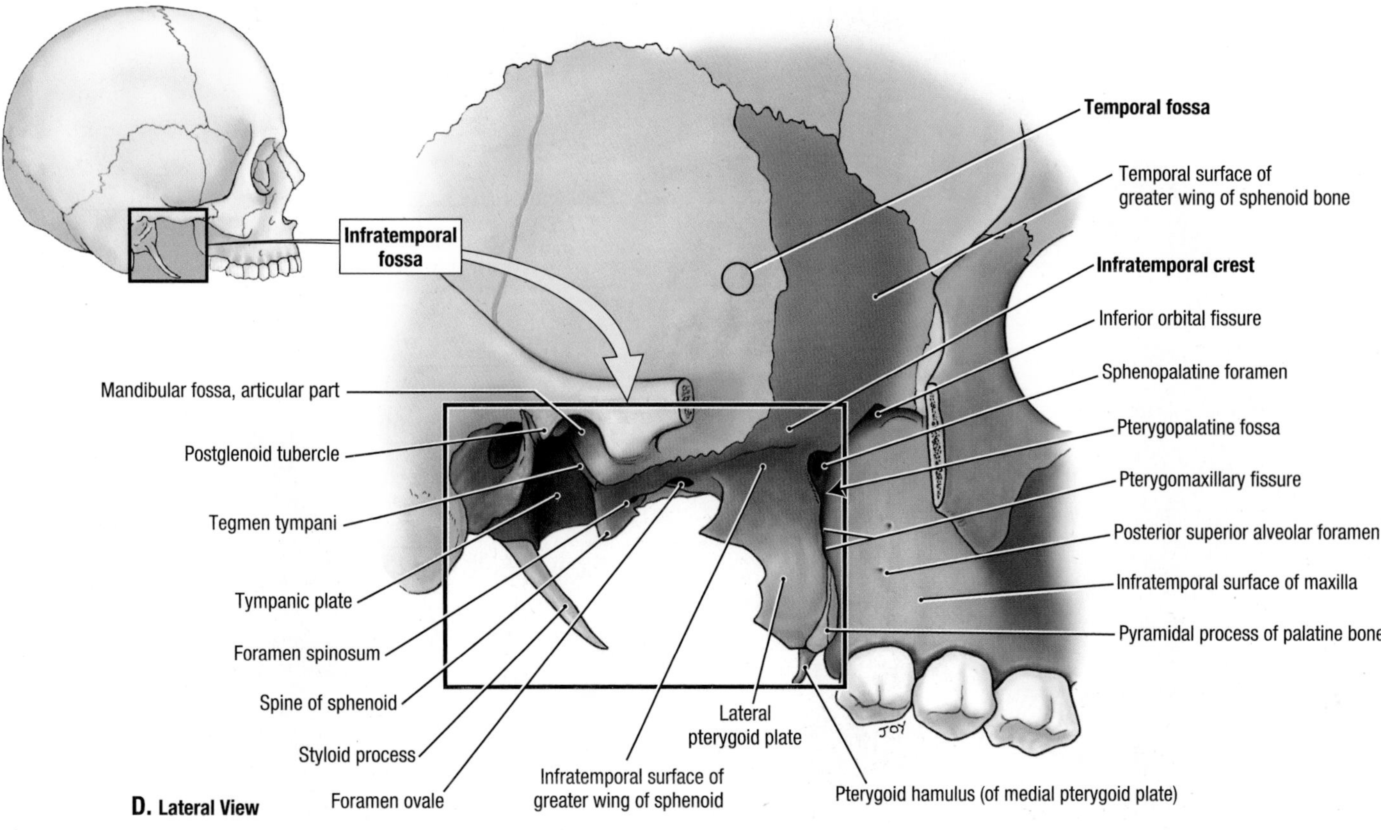
Infratemporal fossa
Temporal fossa
Temporal surface of greater wing of sphenoid bone
Infratemporal crest
Inferior orbital fissure
Sphenopalatine foramen
Pterygopalatine fossa
Pterygomaxillary fissure
Posterior superior alveolar foramen
Infratemporal surface of maxilla
Pyramidal process of palatine bone
Mandibular fossa, articular part
Postglenoid tubercle
Tegmen tympani
Tympanic plate
Foramen spinosum
Spine of sphenoid
Styloid process
Foramen ovale
Lateral pterygoid plate
Infratemporal surface of greater wing of sphenoid
Pterygoid hamulus (of medial pterygoid plate)

D. Lateral View

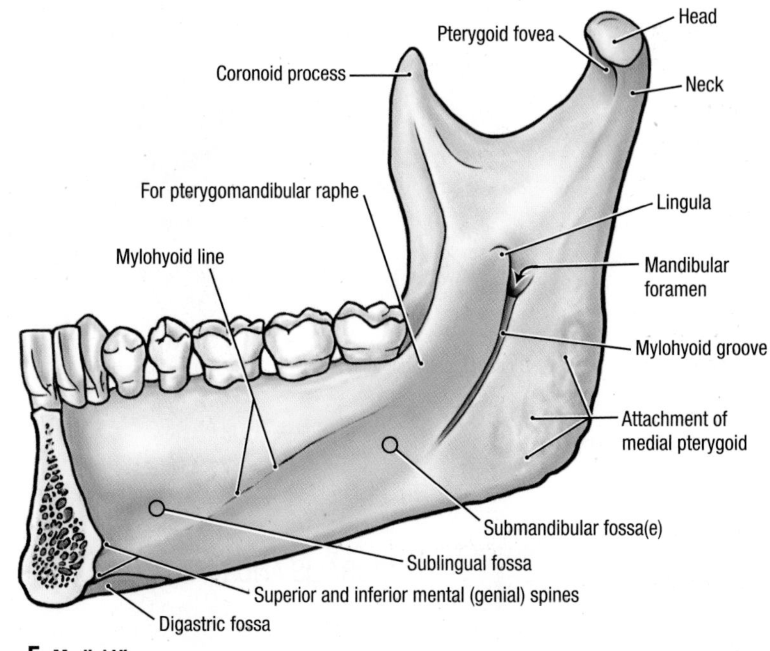
Head
Pterygoid fovea
Coronoid process
Neck
For pterygomandibular raphe
Lingula
Mylohyoid line
Mandibular foramen
Mylohyoid groove
Attachment of medial pterygoid
Submandibular fossa(e)
Sublingual fossa
Superior and inferior mental (genial) spines
Digastric fossa

E. Medial View

7.48 TEMPORAL AND INFRATEMPORAL FOSSAE AND MANDIBLE *(CONTINUED)*

D. Bones and bony features of the infratemporal fossa. The mandible and part of the zygomatic arch have been removed. Deeply, the infratemporal crest separates the temporal and infratemporal fossae. **E.** Internal surface of the mandible.

- The temporal region is the region of the head that includes the lateral area of the scalp and the deeper soft tissues overlying the temporal fossa of the cranium, superior to the zygomatic arch. The temporal fossa, occupied primarily by the upper portion of the temporalis muscle, is bounded by the inferior temporal lines (see Fig. 7.3B).
- The infratemporal fossa is an irregularly shaped space deep and inferior to the zygomatic arch, deep to the ramus of the mandible and posterior to the maxilla. It communicates with the temporal fossa through the interval between the zygomatic arch and the cranial bones.

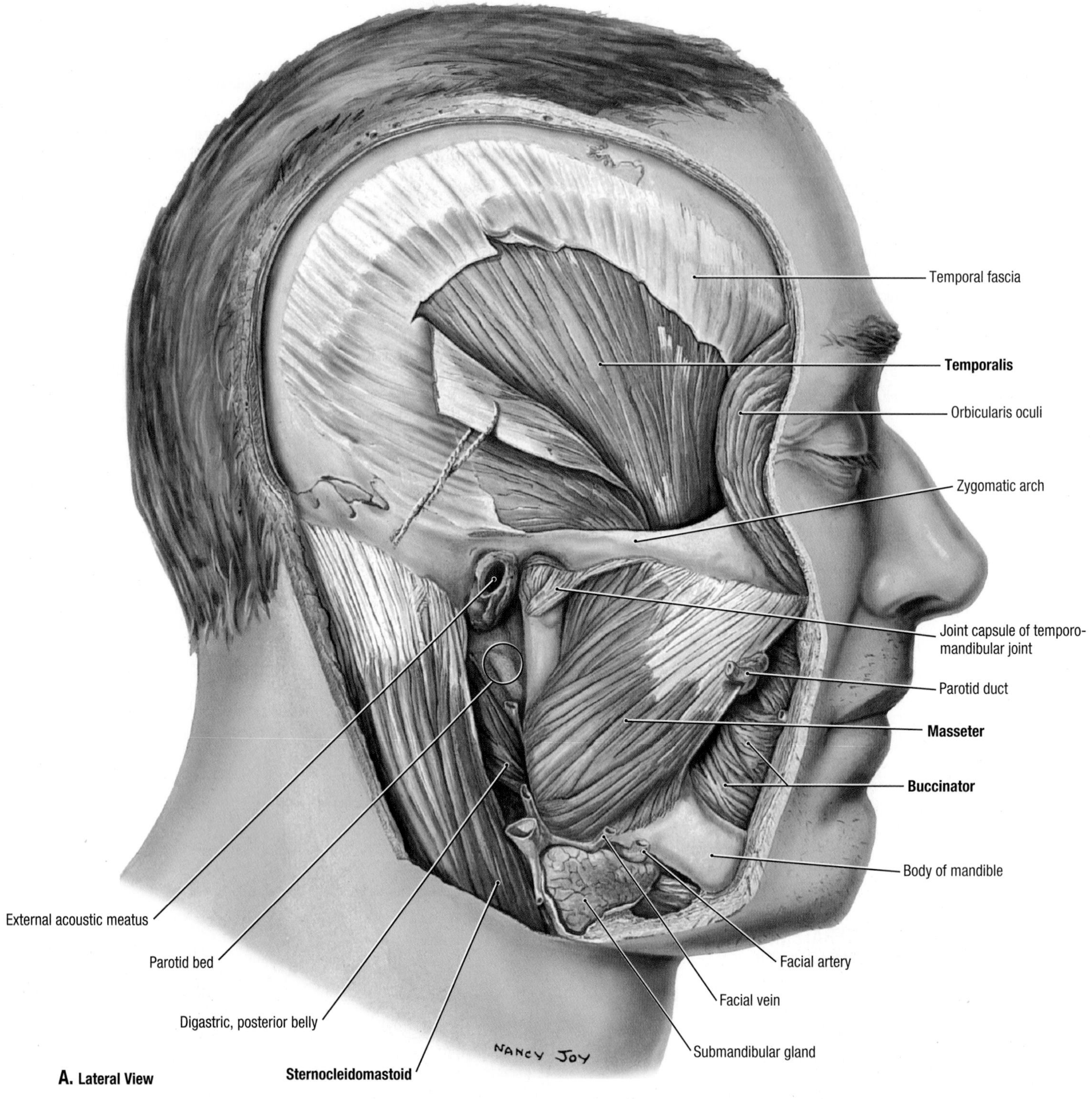
Temporal fascia
Temporalis
Orbicularis oculi
Zygomatic arch
Joint capsule of temporo-mandibular joint
Parotid duct
Masseter
Buccinator
Body of mandible
External acoustic meatus
Parotid bed
Digastric, posterior belly
Sternocleidomastoid
Facial artery
Facial vein
Submandibular gland
NANCY JOY

A. Lateral View

7.49 TEMPORALIS AND MASSETER

A. Superficial dissection.

- The temporalis and masseter muscles are supplied by the trigeminal nerve (CN V), and both elevate the mandible. The buccinator muscle, supplied by the facial nerve (CN VII), functions during chewing to keep food between the teeth but does not act on the mandible.
- The sternocleidomastoid muscle, supplied by the spinal accessory nerve (CN XI), is the chief flexor of the head and neck; it forms the lateral part of the posterior boundary of the parotid region/parotid bed.

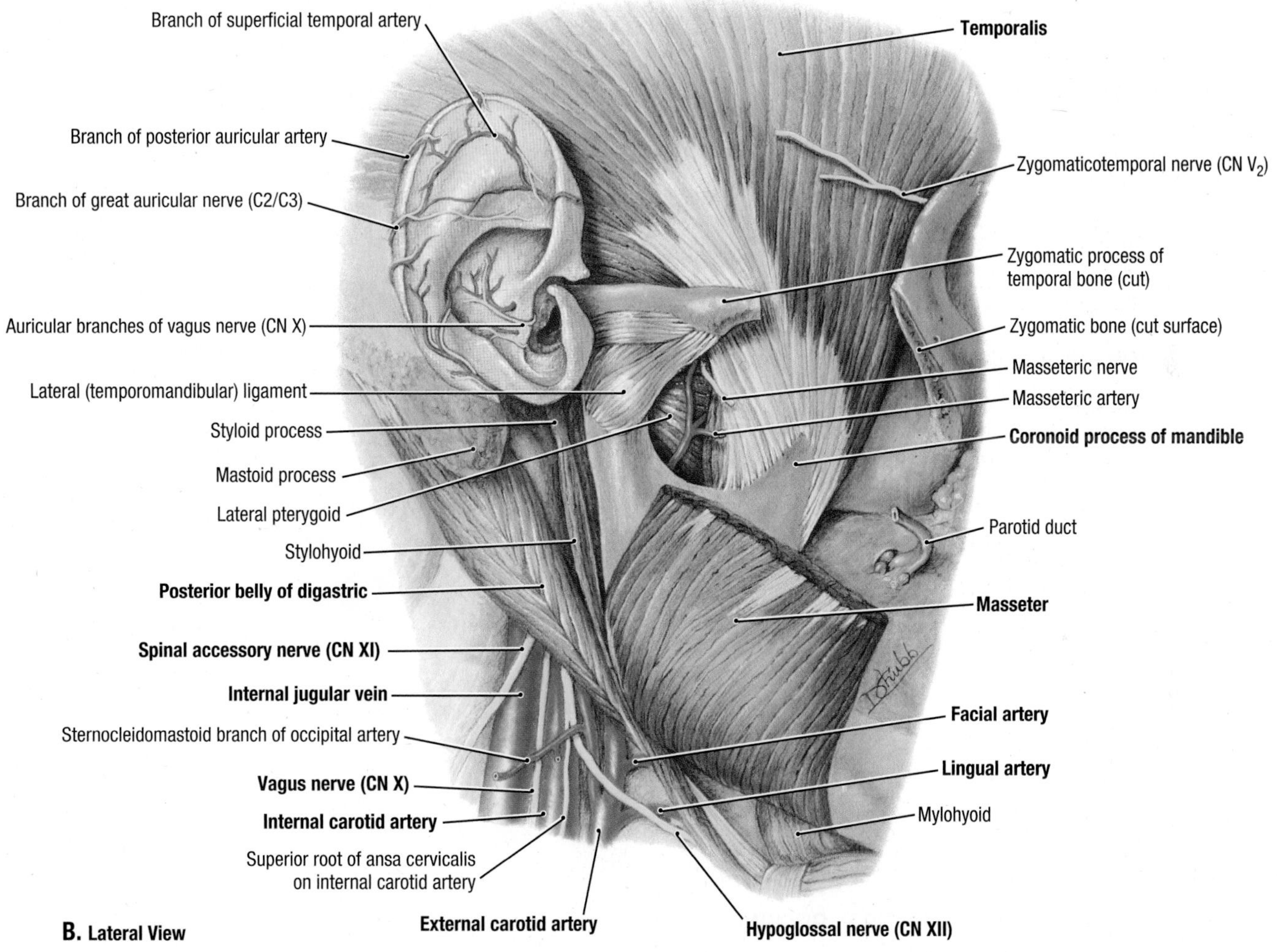
Branch of superficial temporal artery
Temporalis
Branch of posterior auricular artery
Zygomaticotemporal nerve (CN V_2)
Branch of great auricular nerve (C2/C3)
Zygomatic process of temporal bone (cut)
Auricular branches of vagus nerve (CN X)
Zygomatic bone (cut surface)
Masseteric nerve
Lateral (temporomandibular) ligament
Masseteric artery
Styloid process
Coronoid process of mandible
Mastoid process
Lateral pterygoid
Parotid duct
Stylohyoid
Posterior belly of digastric
Masseter
Spinal accessory nerve (CN XI)
Internal jugular vein
Facial artery
Sternocleidomastoid branch of occipital artery
Lingual artery
Vagus nerve (CN X)
Internal carotid artery
Mylohyoid
Superior root of ansa cervicalis on internal carotid artery
External carotid artery
Hypoglossal nerve (CN XII)

B. Lateral View

7.49 TEMPORALIS AND MASSETER *(CONTINUED)*

B. Deep dissection.

- Parts of the zygomatic arch and the attached masseter muscle have been removed to expose the attachment of the temporalis muscle to the coronoid process of the mandible.
- The carotid sheath surrounding the internal jugular vein, internal carotid artery, and the vagus nerve (CN X) has been removed. The external carotid artery and its lingual, facial, and occipital branches, and the spinal accessory (CN XI) and hypoglossal (CN XII) nerves pass deep to the posterior belly of the digastric muscle.

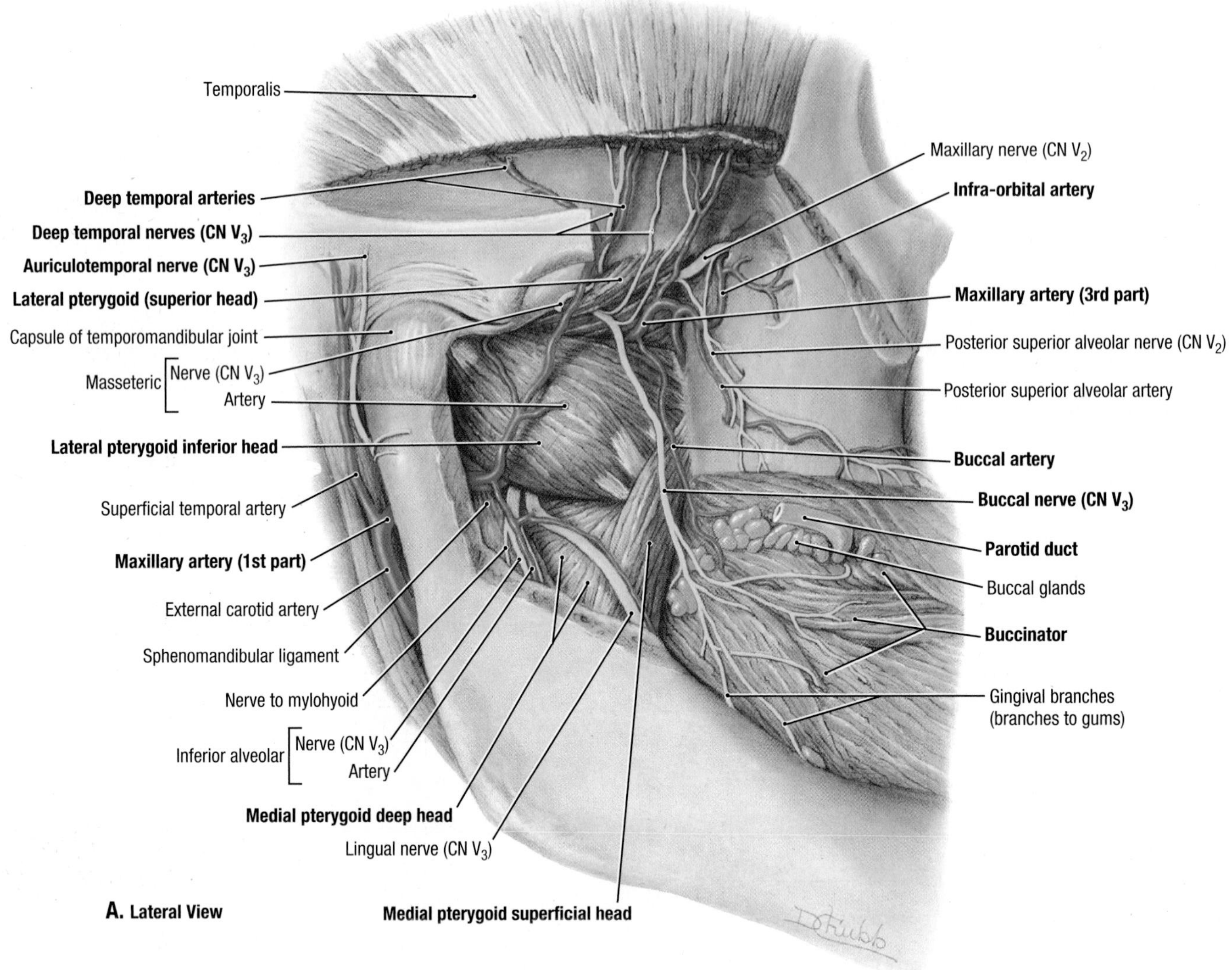

Temporalis
Deep temporal arteries
Deep temporal nerves (CN V_3)
Auriculotemporal nerve (CN V_3)
Lateral pterygoid (superior head)
Capsule of temporomandibular joint
Masseteric
Nerve (CN V_3)
Artery
Lateral pterygoid inferior head
Superficial temporal artery
Maxillary artery (1st part)
External carotid artery
Sphenomandibular ligament
Nerve to mylohyoid
Inferior alveolar
Nerve (CN V_3)
Artery
Medial pterygoid deep head
Lingual nerve (CN V_3)
Medial pterygoid superficial head
Maxillary nerve (CN V_2)
Infra-orbital artery
Maxillary artery (3rd part)
Posterior superior alveolar nerve (CN V_2)
Posterior superior alveolar artery
Buccal artery
Buccal nerve (CN V_3)
Parotid duct
Buccal glands
Buccinator
Gingival branches
(branches to gums)

A. Lateral View

7.50 INFRATEMPORAL REGION

A. Superficial dissection.

- The maxillary artery, the larger of two terminal branches of the external carotid, is divided into three parts relative to the lateral pterygoid muscle.
- The buccinator is pierced by the parotid duct, the ducts of the buccal glands, and sensory branches of the buccal nerve.
- The lateral pterygoid muscle arises by two heads (parts), one head from the roof, and the other head from the medial wall of the infratemporal fossa; both heads insert in relation to the temporomandibular joint—the superior head attaching primarily to the articular disc of the joint and the inferior head primarily to the anterior aspect of the neck of the mandible (pterygoid fovea).
- Because of the close relationship of the facial and auriculotemporal nerves to the temporomandibular joint (TMJ), care must be taken during **surgical procedures on the temporomandibular joint** to preserve both the branches of the facial nerve overlying it and the articular branches of the auriculotemporal nerve that enter the posterior part of the joint. Injury to articular branches of the auriculotemporal nerve supplying the TMJ—associated with traumatic dislocation and rupture of the joint capsule and lateral ligament—leads to laxity and instability of the TMJ.

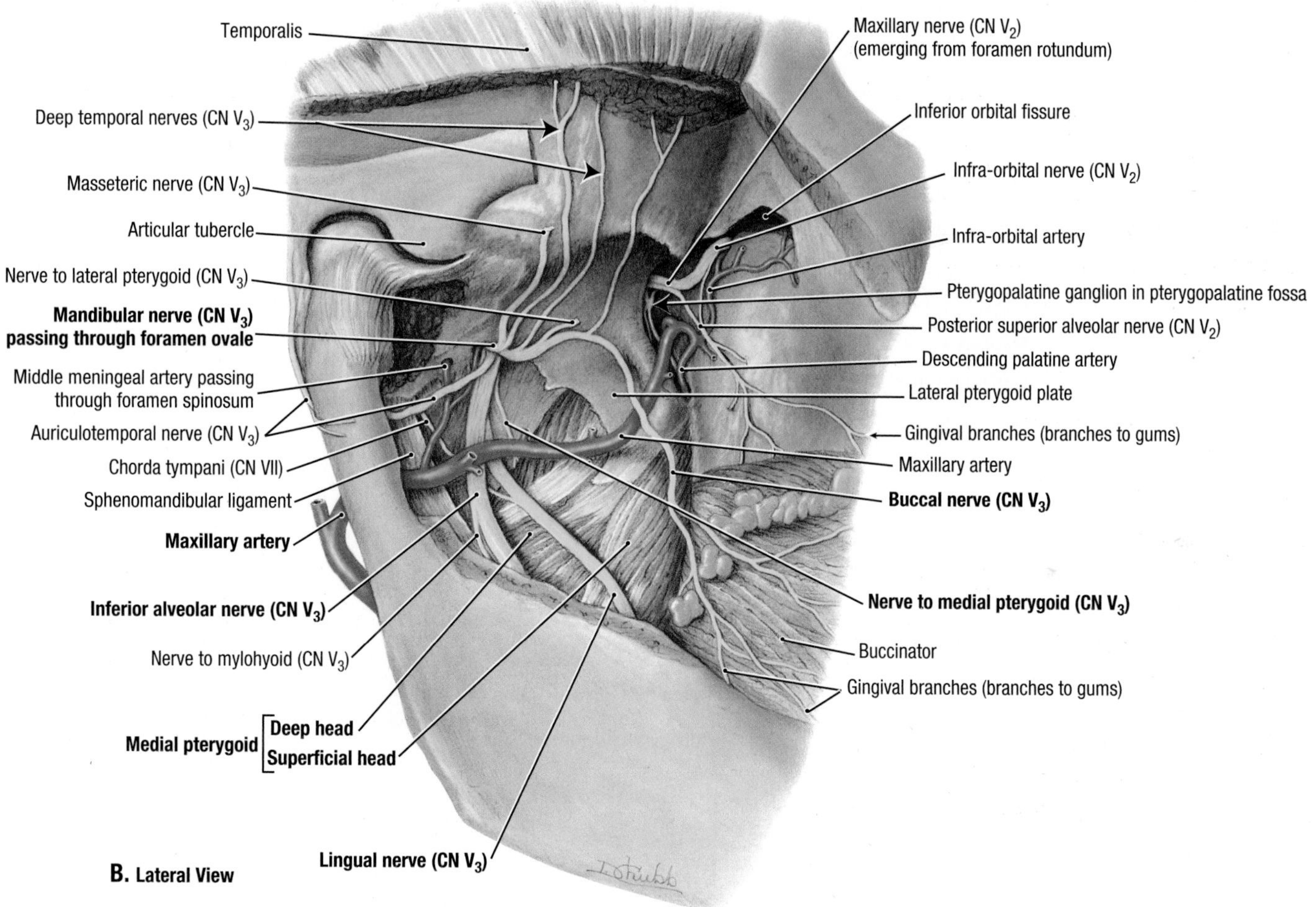
Temporalis
Deep temporal nerves (CN V_3)
Masseteric nerve (CN V_3)
Articular tubercle
Nerve to lateral pterygoid (CN V_3)
Mandibular nerve (CN V_3) passing through foramen ovale
Middle meningeal artery passing through foramen spinosum
Auriculotemporal nerve (CN V_3)
Chorda tympani (CN VII)
Sphenomandibular ligament
Maxillary artery
Inferior alveolar nerve (CN V_3)
Nerve to mylohyoid (CN V_3)
Medial pterygoid
Deep head
Superficial head
Lingual nerve (CN V_3)
Maxillary nerve (CN V_2) (emerging from foramen rotundum)
Inferior orbital fissure
Infra-orbital nerve (CN V_2)
Infra-orbital artery
Pterygopalatine ganglion in pterygopalatine fossa
Posterior superior alveolar nerve (CN V_2)
Descending palatine artery
Lateral pterygoid plate
Gingival branches (branches to gums)
Maxillary artery
Buccal nerve (CN V_3)
Nerve to medial pterygoid (CN V_3)
Buccinator
Gingival branches (branches to gums)

B. Lateral View

7.50 INFRATEMPORAL REGION *(CONTINUED)*

B. Deeper dissection.

- The lateral pterygoid muscle and most of the branches of the maxillary artery have been removed to expose the mandibular nerve (CN V_3) entering the infratemporal fossa through the foramen ovale and the middle meningeal artery passing through the foramen spinosum.
- The deep head of the medial pterygoid muscle arises from the medial surface of the lateral pterygoid plate and the pyramidal process of the palatine bone. It has a small, superficial head that arises from the tuberosity of the maxilla.
- The inferior alveolar and lingual nerves descend on the medial pterygoid muscle. The inferior alveolar nerve gives off the nerve to mylohyoid and nerve to anterior belly of the digastric muscle, and the lingual nerve receives the chorda tympani, which carries secretory parasympathetic fibers and fibers of taste.
- Motor nerves arising from CN V_3 supply the four muscles of mastication: the masseter, temporalis, and lateral and medial pterygoids. The buccal nerve from the mandibular nerve is sensory; the buccal branch of the facial nerve is the motor supply to the buccinator muscle.
- To perform a **mandibular nerve block,** an anesthetic agent is injected near the mandibular nerve where it enters the infratemporal fossa. This block usually anesthetizes the auriculotemporal, inferior alveolar, lingual, and buccal branches of the mandibular nerve.

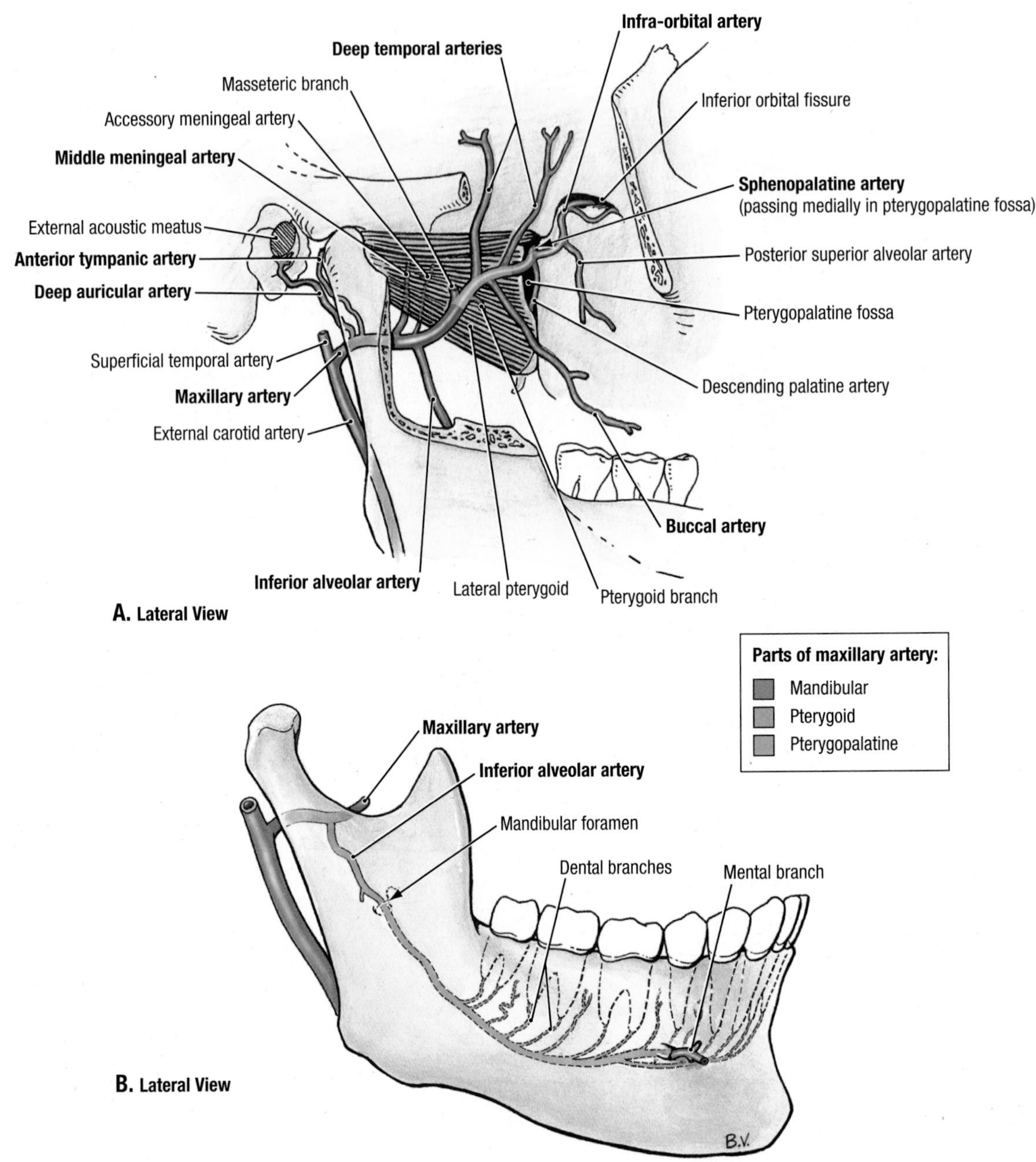
Infra-orbital artery
Deep temporal arteries
Masseteric branch
Accessory meningeal artery
Middle meningeal artery
Inferior orbital fissure
Sphenopalatine artery
(passing medially in pterygopalatine fossa)
External acoustic meatus
Anterior tympanic artery
Deep auricular artery
Posterior superior alveolar artery
Pterygopalatine fossa
Superficial temporal artery
Maxillary artery
External carotid artery
Descending palatine artery
Buccal artery
Inferior alveolar artery
Lateral pterygoid
Pterygoid branch
A. Lateral View
Parts of maxillary artery:
Mandibular
Pterygoid
Pterygopalatine
Maxillary artery
Inferior alveolar artery
Mandibular foramen
Dental branches
Mental branch
B. Lateral View
B.V.

7.51 BRANCHES OF MAXILLARY ARTERY

A. Infratemporal region. **B.** Mandible.

- The maxillary artery arises at the neck of the mandible and is divided into three parts (mandibular, pterygoid, and pterygopalatine) by the lateral pterygoid; it can pass medial or lateral to the lateral pterygoid.
- The branches of the *first (mandibular) part* pass through foramina or canals: the deep auricular to the external acoustic meatus, the anterior tympanic to the tympanic cavity, the middle and accessory meningeal to the cranial cavity, and the inferior alveolar to the mandible and teeth.
- The branches of the *second (pterygoid) part*, directly related to the lateral pterygoid, supply muscles via the masseteric, deep temporal, pterygoid, and buccal branches.
- The branches of the *third (pterygopalatine) part* (posterior superior alveolar, infra-orbital, descending palatine, and sphenopalatine arteries) arise immediately proximal to and within the pterygopalatine fossa.

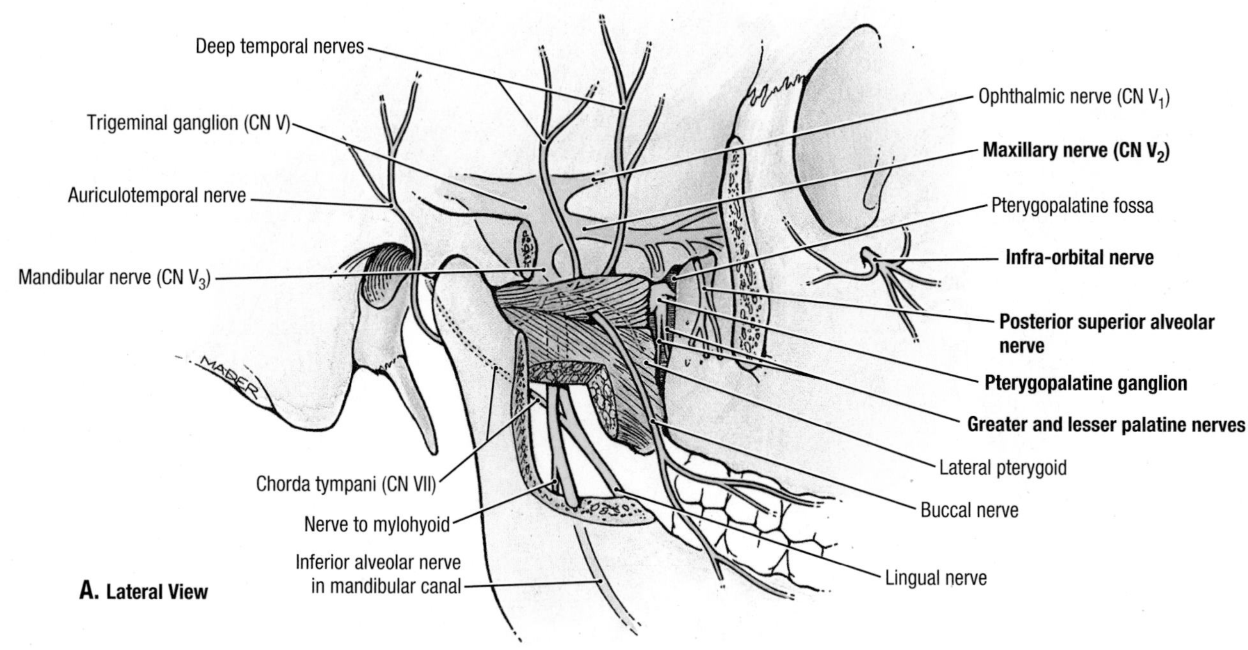
Deep temporal nerves
Trigeminal ganglion (CN V)
Auriculotemporal nerve
Mandibular nerve (CN V3)
Ophthalmic nerve (CN V1)
Maxillary nerve (CN V2)
Pterygopalatine fossa
Infra-orbital nerve
Posterior superior alveolar nerve
Pterygopalatine ganglion
Greater and lesser palatine nerves
Lateral pterygoid
Buccal nerve
Lingual nerve
Chorda tympani (CN VII)
Nerve to mylohyoid
Inferior alveolar nerve in mandibular canal
A. Lateral View

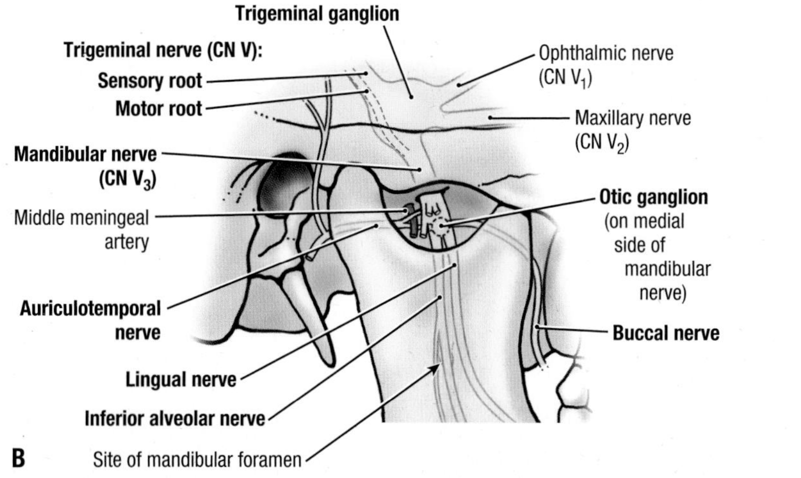
Trigeminal ganglion
Trigeminal nerve (CN V):
Sensory root
Motor root
Mandibular nerve (CN V3)
Middle meningeal artery
Auriculotemporal nerve
Lingual nerve
Inferior alveolar nerve
Site of mandibular foramen
Ophthalmic nerve (CN V1)
Maxillary nerve (CN V2)
Otic ganglion (on medial side of mandibular nerve)
Buccal nerve
B

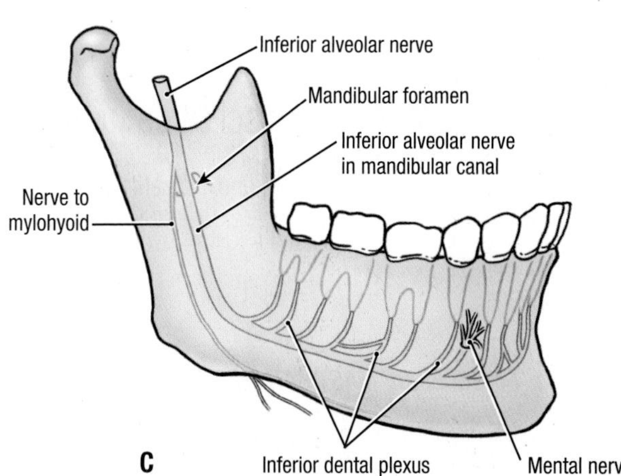
Inferior alveolar nerve
Mandibular foramen
Inferior alveolar nerve in mandibular canal
Nerve to mylohyoid
C
Inferior dental plexus
Mental nerve

7.52 BRANCHES OF MAXILLARY AND MANDIBULAR NERVES

A. Infratemporal region and pterygopalatine fossa. Branches of the maxillary (CN V_2) and mandibular (CN V_3) nerves accompany branches from the three parts of the maxillary artery. **B.** Nerves of infratemporal fossa and otic ganglion. **C.** Mandible and inferior alveolar nerve.

An **alveolar nerve block**—commonly used by dentists when repairing mandibular teeth—anesthetizes the inferior alveolar nerve, a branch of CN V_3. The anesthetic agent is injected around the mandibular foramen, the opening into the mandibular canal on the medial aspect of the ramus of the mandible. This canal gives passage to the inferior alveolar nerve, artery, and vein. When this nerve block is successful, all mandibular teeth are anesthetized to the median plane. The skin and mucous membrane of the lower lip, the labial alveolar mucosa and gingiva, and the skin of the chin are also anesthetized because they are supplied by the mental branch of this nerve.

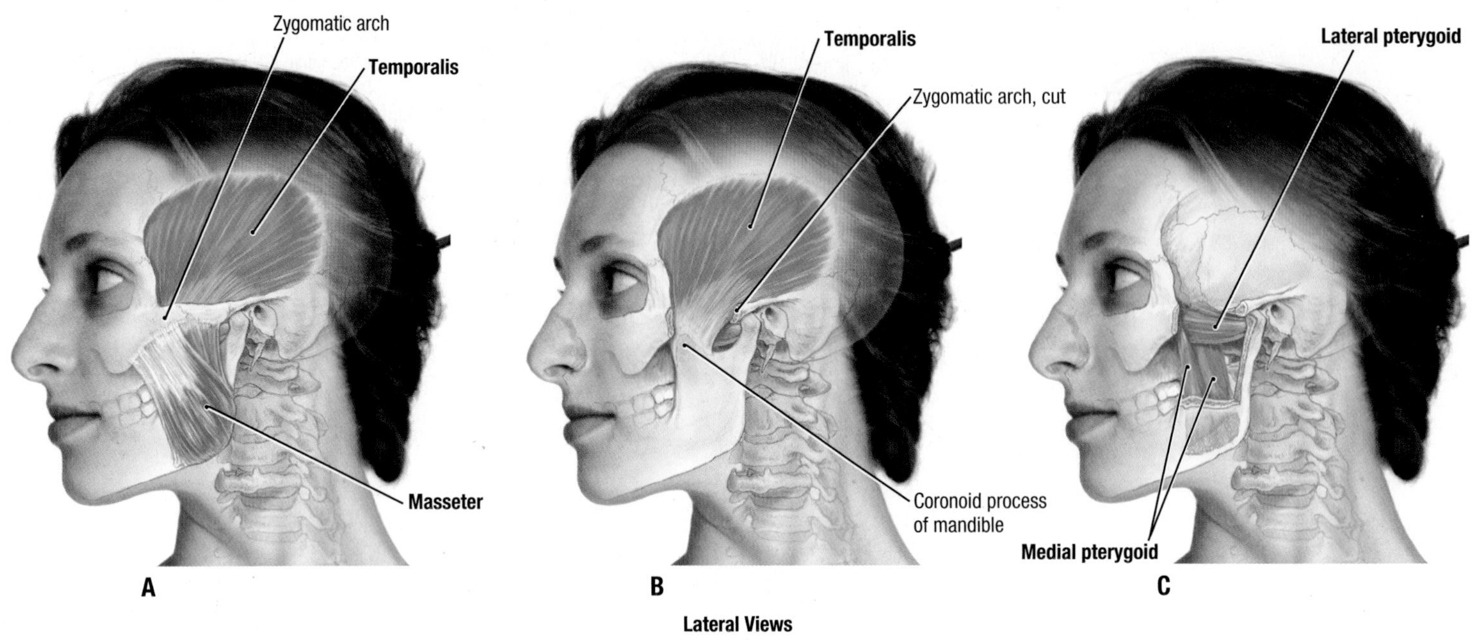

Zygomatic arch
Temporalis
Masseter
A
Temporalis
Zygomatic arch, cut
Coronoid process of mandible
B
Lateral pterygoid
Medial pterygoid
C
Lateral Views

7.53 MUSCLES OF MASTICATION

A. Temporalis and masseter. **B.** Temporalis. Zygomatic arch has been removed. **C.** Medial and lateral pterygoid.

TABLE 7.11 MUSCLES OF MASTICATION (ACTING ON TEMPOROMANDIBULAR JOINT)

Muscle	Origin	Insertion	Innervation	Main Action
Temporalis	Floor of temporal fossa and deep surface of temporal fascia	Tip and medial surface of coronoid process and anterior border of ramus of mandible	Deep temporal branches of mandibular nerve (CN V_3)	Elevates mandible, closing jaws; posterior fibers retrude mandible after protrusion
Masseter	Inferior border and medial surface of zygomatic arch	Lateral surface of ramus of mandible and coronoid process	Mandibular nerve (CN V_3) through masseteric nerve that enters deep surface of the muscle	Elevates and protrudes mandible, thus closing jaws; deep fibers retrude it
Lateral pterygoid	*Superior head:* infratemporal surface and infratemporal crest of greater wing of sphenoid bone *Inferior head:* lateral surface of lateral pterygoid plate	Neck of mandible, articular disc, and capsule of temporomandibular joint	Mandibular nerve (CN V_3) through lateral pterygoid nerve which enters its deep surface	*Acting bilaterally,* protrude mandible and depress chin; *Acting unilaterally* alternately, they produce side-to-side movements of mandible
Medial pterygoid	*Deep head:* medial surface of lateral pterygoid plate and pyramidal process of palatine bone *Superficial head:* tuberosity of maxilla	Medial surface of ramus of mandible, inferior to mandibular foramen	Mandibular nerve (CN V_3) through medial pterygoid nerve	Helps elevate mandible, closing jaws; *acting bilaterally* protrude mandible; *acting unilaterally,* protrudes side of jaw; acting alternately, they produce a grinding motion

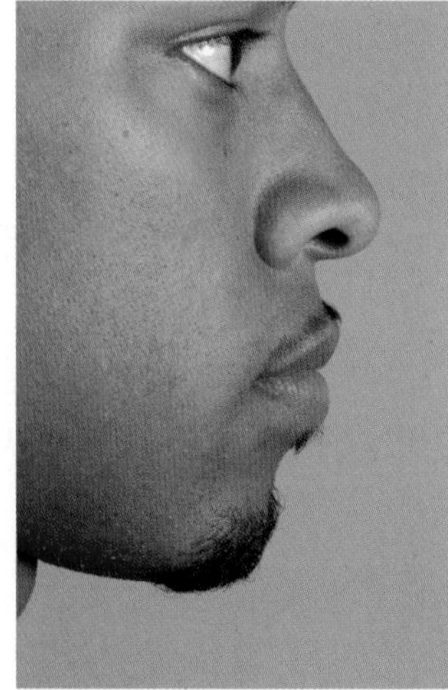

A. Elevation of mandible

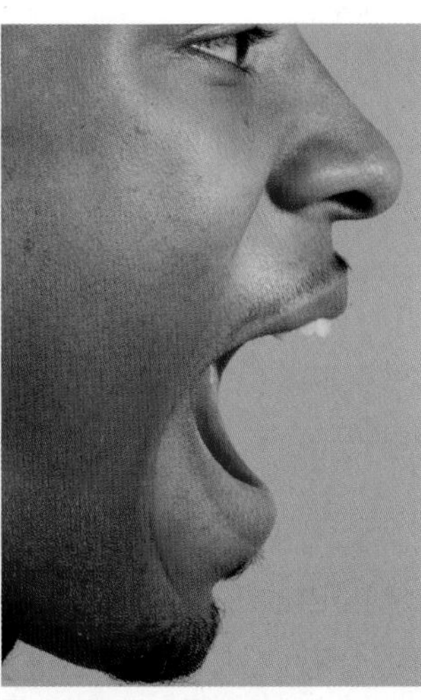

B. Depression of mandible

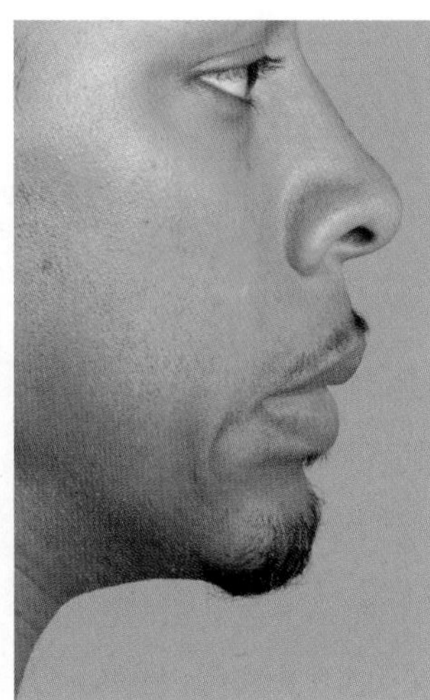

C. Retrusion

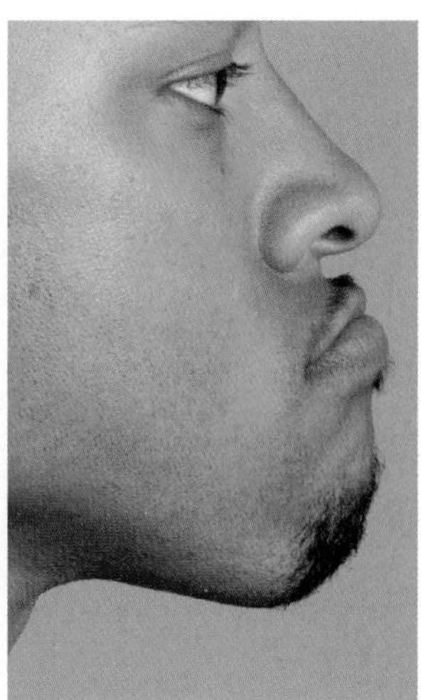

D. Protrusion

Lateral Views

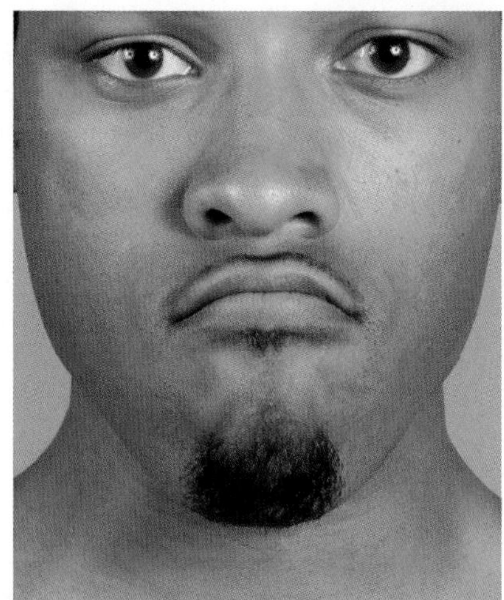

E. Protrusion

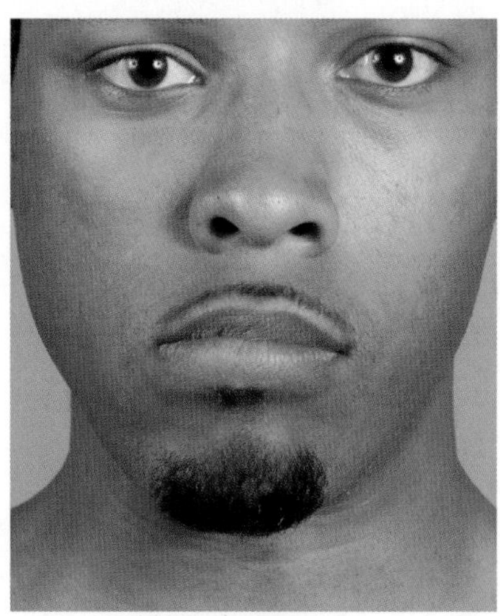

F. Lateral movement to right side

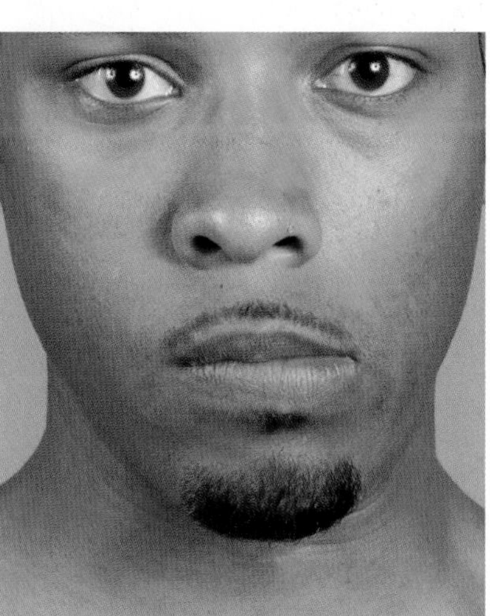

G. Lateral movement to left side

Anterior Views

7.54 MOVEMENTS OF TEMPOROMANDIBULAR JOINT

TABLE 7.12 MOVEMENTS OF TEMPOROMANDIBULAR JOINT

Movements	Muscles
Elevation (close mouth) (A)	Temporalis, masseter, and medial pterygoid
Depression (open mouth) (B)	Lateral pterygoid; suprahyoid and infrahyoid muscles; gravity
Retrusion (retrude chin) (C)	Temporalis (posterior oblique and near horizontal fibers) and masseter
Protrusion (protrude chin) (D and E)	Lateral pterygoid, masseter, and medial pterygoid
Lateral movements (grinding and chewing) (F and G)	Temporalis of same side, pterygoids of opposite side, and masseter

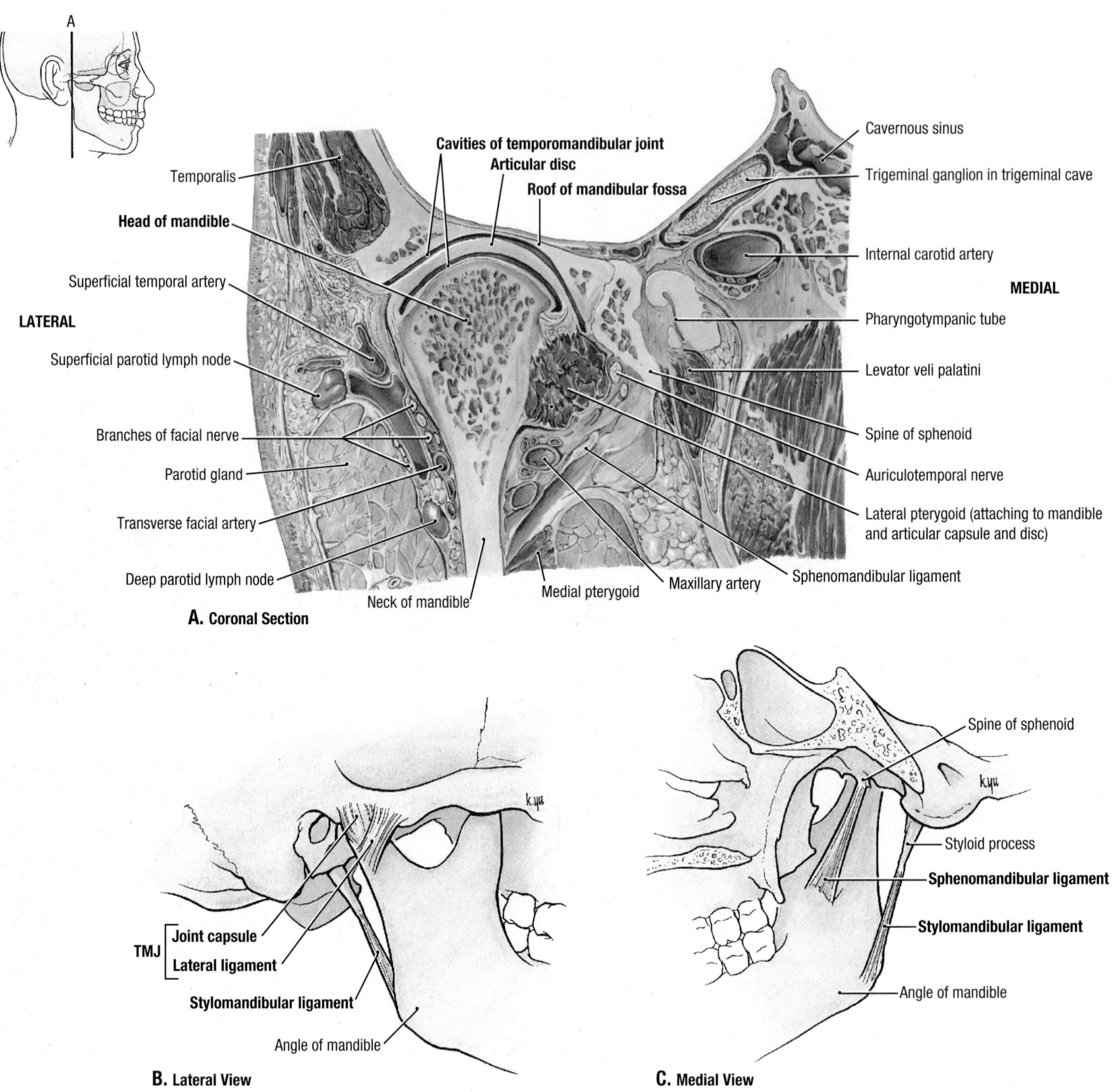
A
Cavities of temporomandibular joint
Articular disc
Roof of mandibular fossa
Temporalis
Head of mandible
Superficial temporal artery
LATERAL
Superficial parotid lymph node
Branches of facial nerve
Parotid gland
Transverse facial artery
Deep parotid lymph node
Neck of mandible
Medial pterygoid
Maxillary artery
Sphenomandibular ligament
Cavernous sinus
Trigeminal ganglion in trigeminal cave
Internal carotid artery
MEDIAL
Pharyngotympanic tube
Levator veli palatini
Spine of sphenoid
Auriculotemporal nerve
Lateral pterygoid (attaching to mandible and articular capsule and disc)
A. Coronal Section
TMJ
Joint capsule
Lateral ligament
Stylomandibular ligament
Angle of mandible
B. Lateral View
Spine of sphenoid
Styloid process
Sphenomandibular ligament
Stylomandibular ligament
Angle of mandible
C. Medial View

7.55 TEMPOROMANDIBULAR JOINT

A. Coronal section. **B.** Temporomandibular joint and stylomandibular ligament. The joint capsule of the temporomandibular joint attaches to the margins of the mandibular fossa and articular tubercle of the temporal bone and around the neck of the mandible; the lateral (temporomandibular) ligament strengthens the lateral aspect of the joint. **C.** Stylomandibular and sphenomandibular ligaments. The strong sphenomandibular ligament descends from near the spine of the sphenoid to the lingula of the mandible and is the "swinging hinge" by which the mandible is suspended; the weaker stylomandibular ligament is a thickened part of the parotid sheath that joins the styloid process to the angle of the mandible.

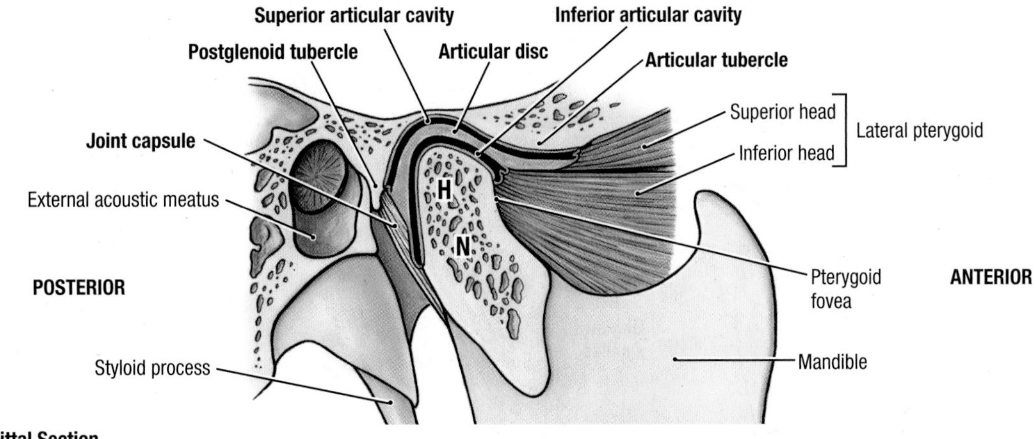
Superior articular cavity
Inferior articular cavity
Postglenoid tubercle
Articular disc
Articular tubercle
Superior head
Inferior head
Lateral pterygoid
Joint capsule
External acoustic meatus
H
N
POSTERIOR
Pterygoid fovea
ANTERIOR
Styloid process
Mandible

A. Sagittal Section

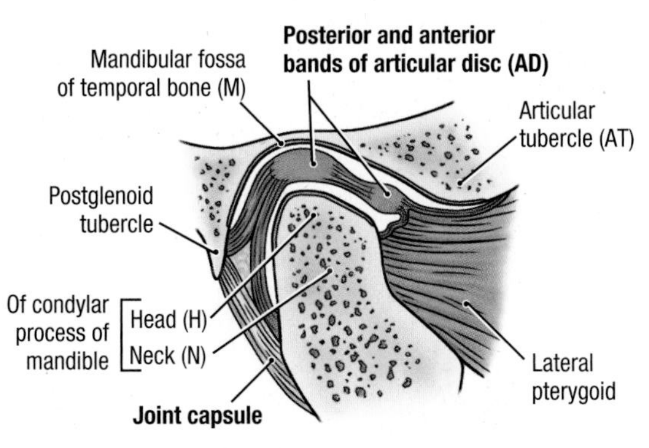
Mandibular fossa of temporal bone (M)
Posterior and anterior bands of articular disc (AD)
Articular tubercle (AT)
Postglenoid tubercle
Of condylar process of mandible
Head (H)
Neck (N)
Joint capsule
Lateral pterygoid

B. Closed Mouth, Sagittal Section

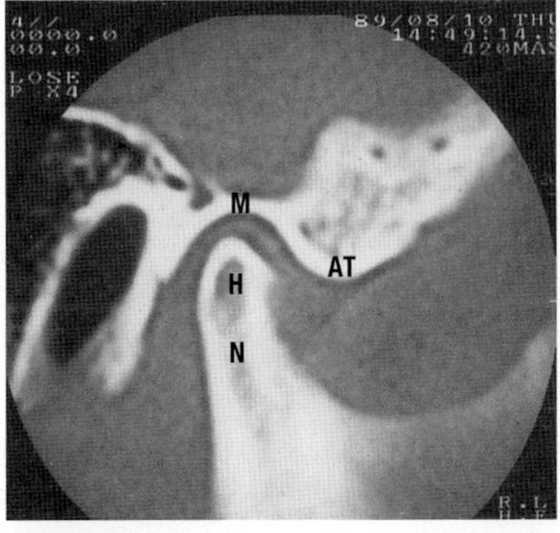
M
AT
H
N

Sagittal CT

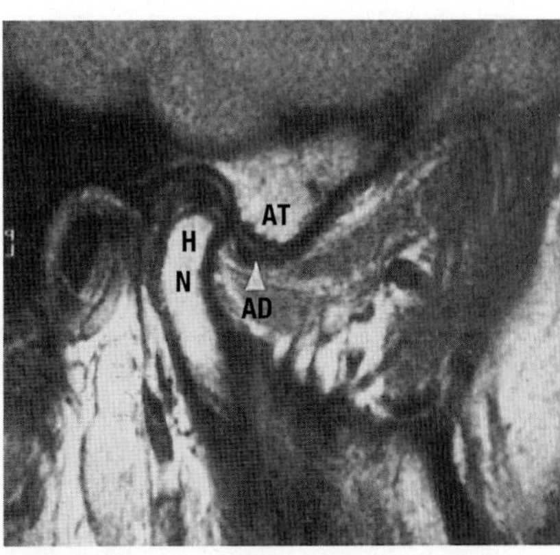
AT
H
N
AD

Sagittal MRI

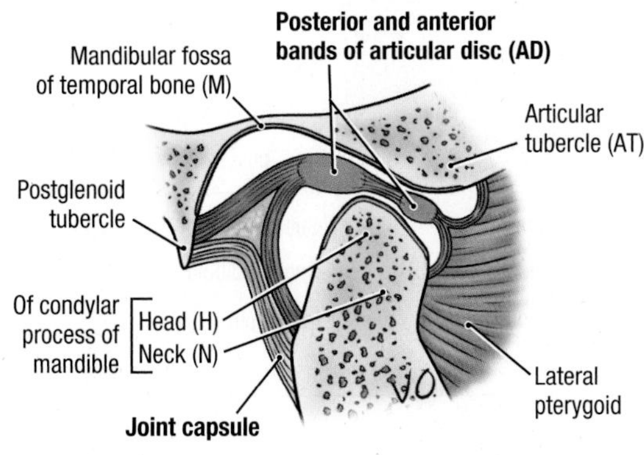
Mandibular fossa of temporal bone (M)
Posterior and anterior bands of articular disc (AD)
Articular tubercle (AT)
Postglenoid tubercle
Of condylar process of mandible
Head (H)
Neck (N)
Joint capsule
Lateral pterygoid

C. Open Mouth, Sagittal Section

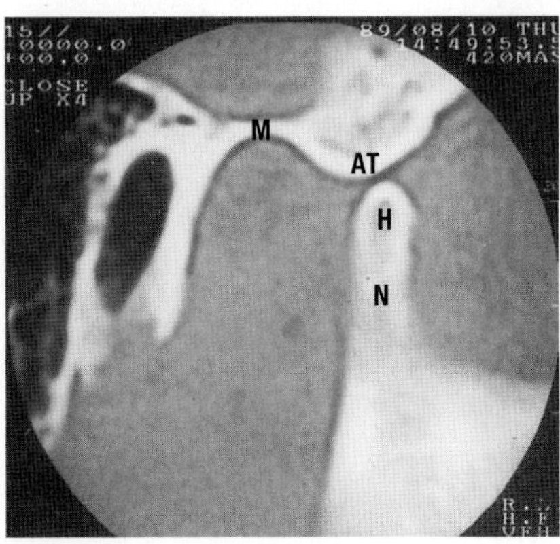
M
AT
H
N

Sagittal CT

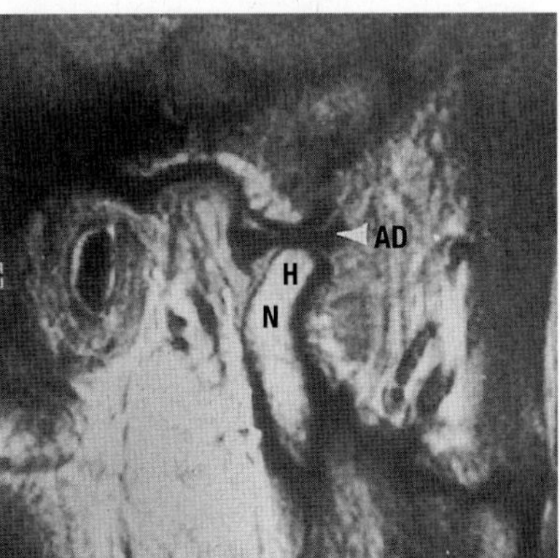
AD
H
N

Sagittal MRI

7.56 SECTIONAL ANATOMY OF TEMPOROMANDIBULAR JOINT

A. TMJ and related structures, sagittal section. **B.** Sagittal orientation figure, CT, and MRI—mouth closed. **C.** Sagittal orientation figure, CT, and MRI—mouth opened widely. The articular disc divides the articular cavity into superior and inferior compartments, each lined by a separate synovial membrane.

Dislocation of mandible. During yawning or taking large bites, excessive contraction of the lateral pterygoids can cause the head of the mandible to dislocate (pass anterior to the articular tubercle). In this position, the mouth remains wide open, and the person cannot close it without manual distraction.

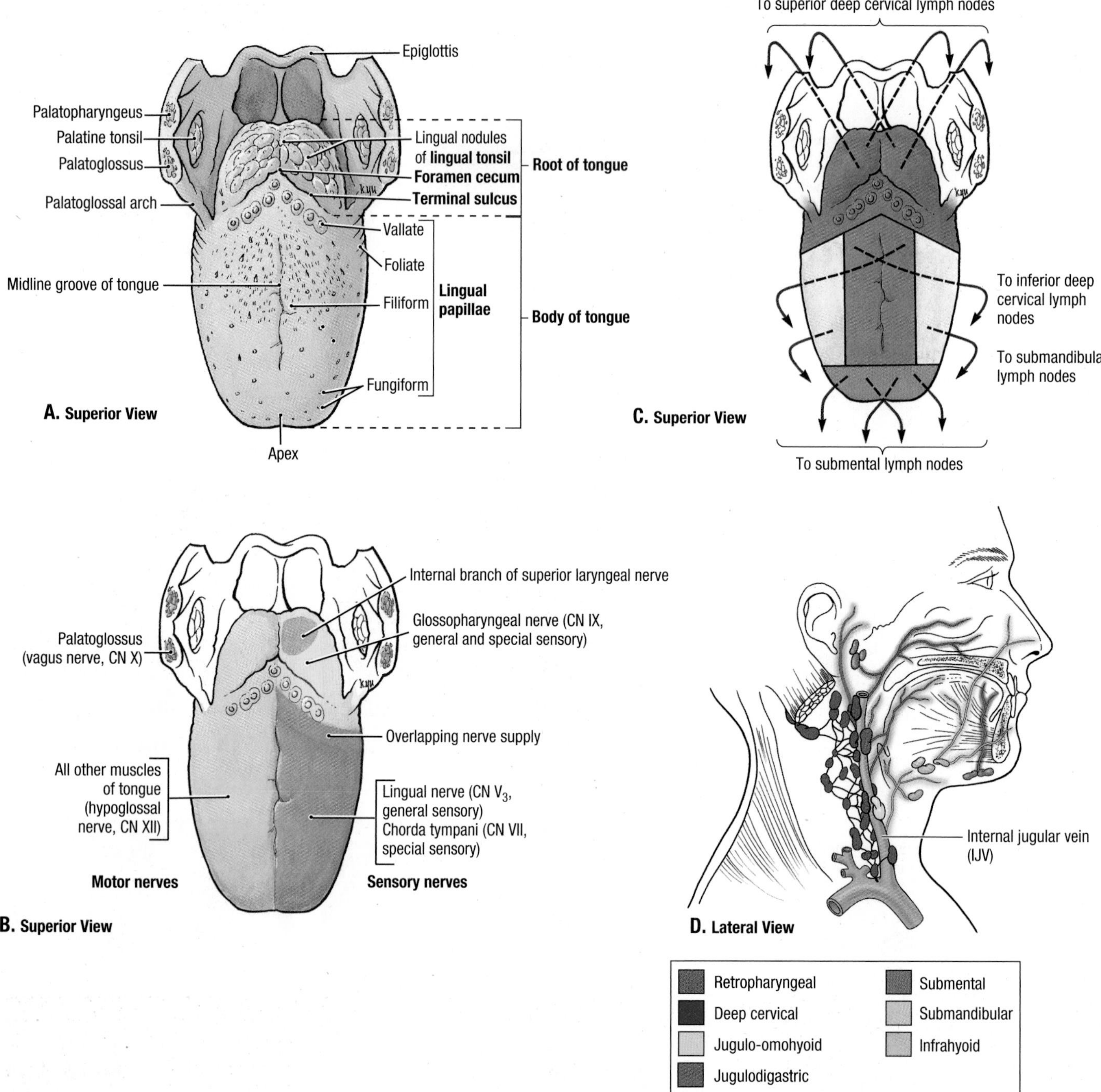
Epiglottis
Palatopharyngeus
Palatine tonsil
Palatoglossus
Palatoglossal arch
Lingual nodules of lingual tonsil
Foramen cecum
Terminal sulcus
Root of tongue
Vallate
Foliate
Midline groove of tongue
Filiform
Lingual papillae
Body of tongue
Fungiform
Apex
A. Superior View
To superior deep cervical lymph nodes
To inferior deep cervical lymph nodes
To submandibular lymph nodes
To submental lymph nodes
C. Superior View
Internal branch of superior laryngeal nerve
Glossopharyngeal nerve (CN IX, general and special sensory)
Palatoglossus (vagus nerve, CN X)
Overlapping nerve supply
All other muscles of tongue (hypoglossal nerve, CN XII)
Lingual nerve (CN V_3, general sensory)
Chorda tympani (CN VII, special sensory)
Motor nerves
Sensory nerves
B. Superior View
Internal jugular vein (IJV)
D. Lateral View
Retropharyngeal
Deep cervical
Jugulo-omohyoid
Jugulodigastric
Submental
Submandibular
Infrahyoid

7.57 TONGUE

A. Features of dorsum of the tongue. The foramen cecum is the upper end of the primitive thyroglossal duct; the arms of the V-shaped terminal sulcus diverge from the foramen, demarcating the posterior third of the tongue from the anterior two thirds. **B.** General sensory, special sensory (taste), and motor innervation of tongue. **C.** Lymphatic drainage of dorsum of tongue. **D.** Lymphatic drainage of tongue, mouth, nasal cavity, and nose.

Carcinoma of tongue. Malignant tumors in the posterior part of the tongue metastasize to the superior deep cervical lymph nodes on both sides. In contrast, tumors in the apex and anterolateral parts usually do not metastasize to the inferior deep cervical nodes until late in the disease. Because the deep nodes are closely related to the internal jugular vein, metastases from the carcinoma may spread to the submental and submandibular regions and along the IJV into the neck.

Gag reflex. One may touch the anterior part of the tongue without feeling discomfort; however, when the posterior part is touched, one usually gags. CN IX and CN X are responsible for the muscular contraction of each side of the pharynx. Glossopharyngeal branches (CN IX) provide the afferent limb of the gag reflex.

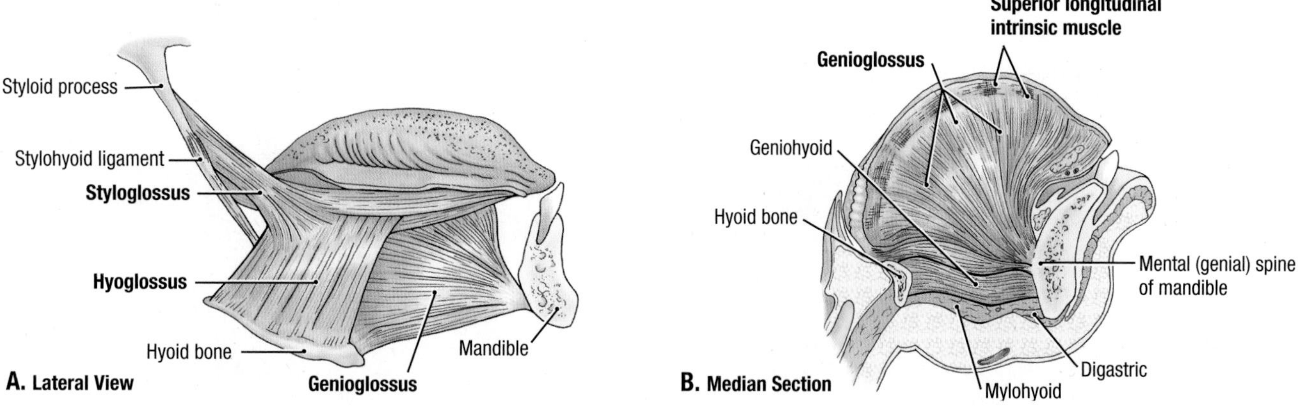
Styloid process
Stylohyoid ligament
Styloglossus
Hyoglossus
Hyoid bone
Genioglossus
Mandible
A. Lateral View
Superior longitudinal intrinsic muscle
Genioglossus
Geniohyoid
Hyoid bone
Mental (genial) spine of mandible
Digastric
Mylohyoid
B. Median Section

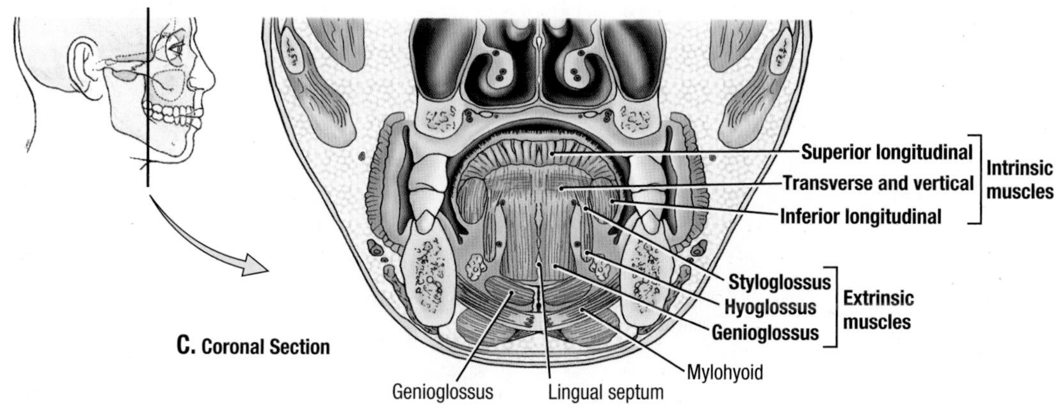
Superior longitudinal
Transverse and vertical
Inferior longitudinal
Intrinsic muscles
Styloglossus
Hyoglossus
Genioglossus
Extrinsic muscles
Mylohyoid
Genioglossus
Lingual septum
C. Coronal Section

7.58 MUSCLES OF TONGUE

The extrinsic muscles of the tongue originate outside the tongue and attach to it, whereas the intrinsic muscles have their attachments entirely within the tongue and are not attached to bone.

TABLE 7.13 MUSCLES OF TONGUE

Extrinsic Muscles				
Muscle	**Origin**	**Insertion**	**Innervation**	**Main Action**
Genioglossus	Superior part of mental spine of mandible	Dorsum of tongue and body of hyoid bone	Hypoglossal nerve (CN XII)	Depresses tongue; its posterior part pulls tonguew anteriorly for protrusion[a]
Hyoglossus	Body and greater horn of hyoid bone	Side and inferior aspect of tongue		Depresses and retracts tongue
Styloglossus	Styloid process of temporal bone and stylohyoid ligament	Side and inferior aspect of tongue		Retracts tongue and draws it up to create a trough for swallowing
Palatoglossus	Palatine aponeurosis of soft palate	Side of tongue	CN X and pharyngeal plexus	Elevates posterior part of tongue plexus
Intrinsic Muscles				
Muscle	**Origin**	**Insertion**	**Innervation**	**Main Action**
Superior longitudinal	Submucous fibrous layer and lingual septum	Margins and mucous membrane of tongue	Hypoglossal nerve (CN XII)	Curls tip and sides of tongue superiorly and shortens tongue
Inferior longitudinal	Root of tongue and body of hyoid bone	Apex of tongue		Curls tip of tongue inferiorly and shortens tongue
Transverse	Lingual septum	Fibrous tissue at margins of tongue		Narrows and elongates the tongue[a]
Vertical	Superior surface of borders of tongue	Inferior surface of borders of tongue		Flattens and broadens the tongue[a]

[a]Acts simultaneously to protrude tongue.

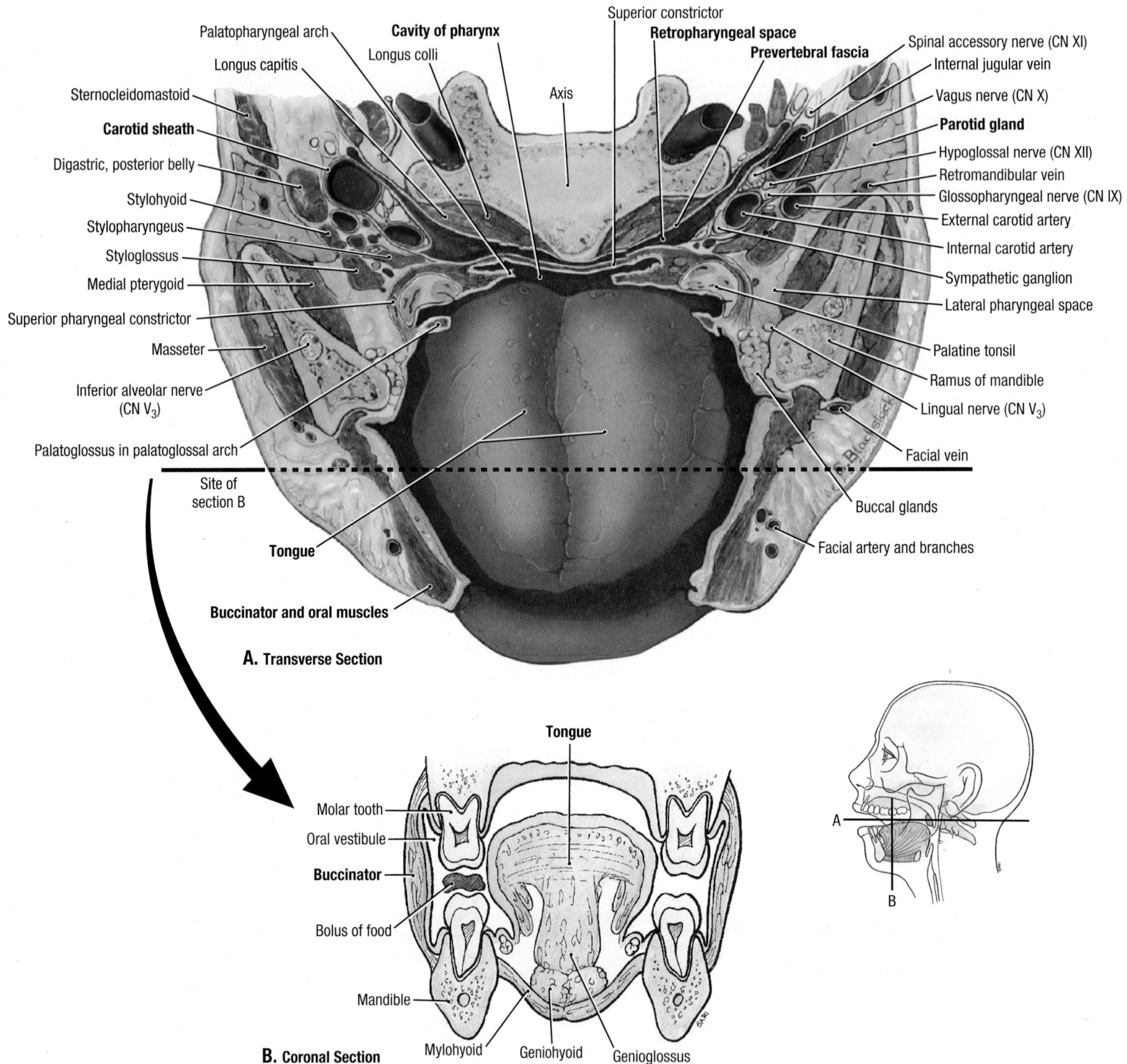

Superior constrictor
Palatopharyngeal arch
Cavity of pharynx
Retropharyngeal space
Spinal accessory nerve (CN XI)
Longus colli
Prevertebral fascia
Longus capitis
Internal jugular vein
Axis
Sternocleidomastoid
Vagus nerve (CN X)
Carotid sheath
Parotid gland
Digastric, posterior belly
Hypoglossal nerve (CN XII)
Retromandibular vein
Stylohyoid
Glossopharyngeal nerve (CN IX)
Stylopharyngeus
External carotid artery
Internal carotid artery
Styloglossus
Sympathetic ganglion
Medial pterygoid
Lateral pharyngeal space
Superior pharyngeal constrictor
Masseter
Palatine tonsil
Ramus of mandible
Inferior alveolar nerve (CN V_3)
Lingual nerve (CN V_3)
Palatoglossus in palatoglossal arch
Facial vein
Site of section B
Buccal glands
Tongue
Facial artery and branches
Buccinator and oral muscles
A. Transverse Section
Tongue
Molar tooth
Oral vestibule
Buccinator
Bolus of food
Mandible
B. Coronal Section
Mylohyoid
Geniohyoid
Genioglossus
A
B

7.59 SECTIONS THROUGH MOUTH

A. The viscerocranium has been sectioned at the C1 vertebral level, the plane of section passing through the oral fissure anteriorly. The retropharyngeal space (opened up in this specimen) allows the pharynx to contract and relax during swallowing; the retropharyngeal space is closed laterally at the carotid sheath and limited posteriorly by the prevertebral fascia. The beds of the parotid glands are also demonstrated. **B.** Schematic coronal section demonstrating how the tongue and buccinator (or, anteriorly, the orbicularis oris) work together to retain food between the teeth when chewing. The buccinator and superior part of the orbicularis oris are innervated by the buccal branch of the facial nerve (CN VII).

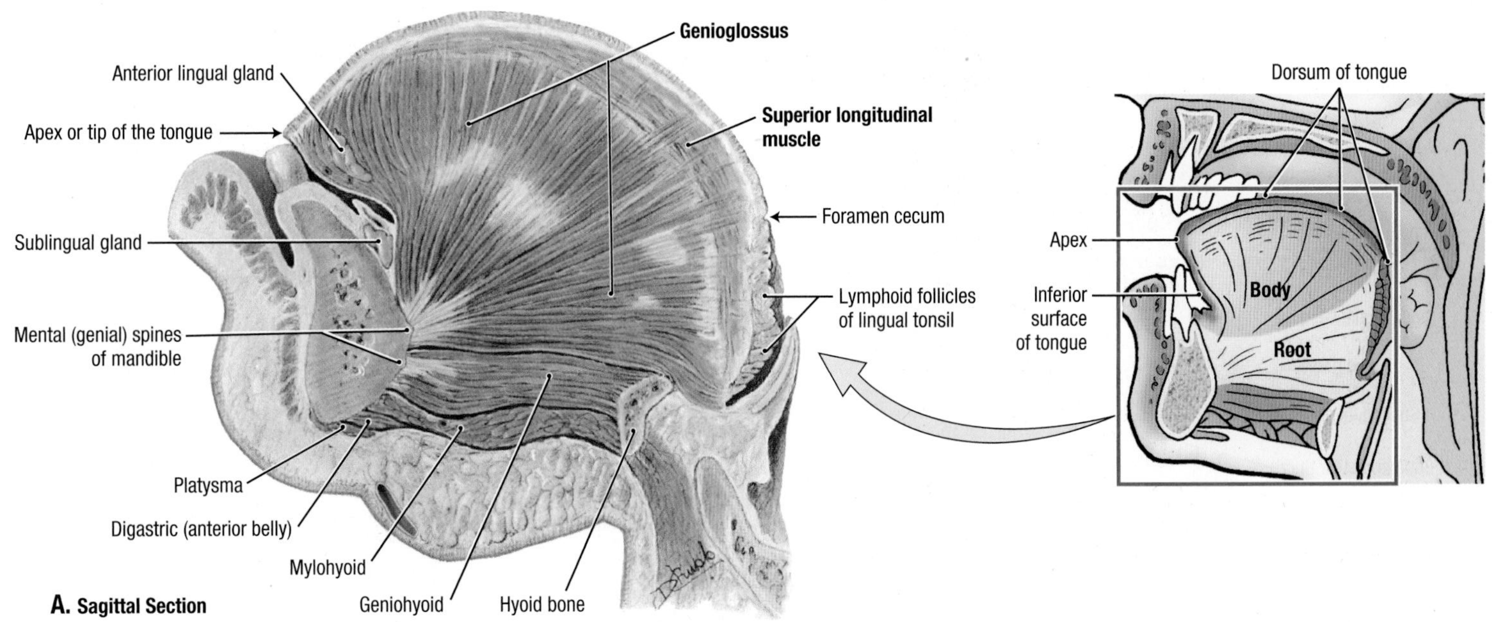
Anterior lingual gland
Apex or tip of the tongue
Sublingual gland
Mental (genial) spines of mandible
Platysma
Digastric (anterior belly)
Mylohyoid
Geniohyoid
Hyoid bone
Genioglossus
Superior longitudinal muscle
Foramen cecum
Lymphoid follicles of lingual tonsil
Dorsum of tongue
Apex
Inferior surface of tongue
Body
Root
A. Sagittal Section

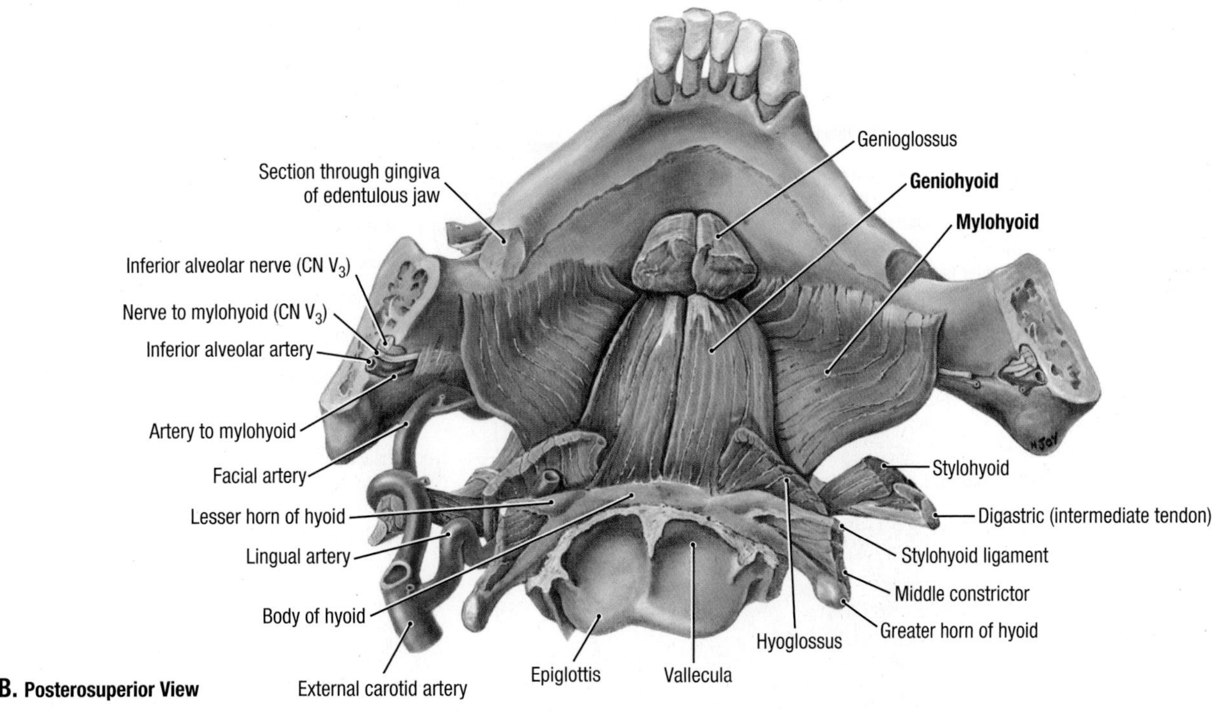
Section through gingiva of edentulous jaw
Inferior alveolar nerve (CN V_3)
Nerve to mylohyoid (CN V_3)
Inferior alveolar artery
Artery to mylohyoid
Facial artery
Lesser horn of hyoid
Lingual artery
Body of hyoid
External carotid artery
Epiglottis
Vallecula
Hyoglossus
Genioglossus
Geniohyoid
Mylohyoid
Stylohyoid
Digastric (intermediate tendon)
Stylohyoid ligament
Middle constrictor
Greater horn of hyoid
B. Posterosuperior View

7.60 TONGUE AND FLOOR OF MOUTH

A. Median section though the tongue and lower jaw. The tongue is composed mainly of muscle; extrinsic muscles alter the position of the tongue, and intrinsic muscles alter its shape. The genioglossus is the extrinsic muscle apparent in this plane, and the superior longitudinal muscle is the intrinsic muscle. **B.** Muscles of the floor of the mouth viewed posterosuperiorly. The mylohyoid muscle extends between the two mylohyoid lines of the mandible. It has a thick, free posterior border and becomes thinner anteriorly.

Genioglossus paralysis. When the genioglossus is paralyzed, the tongue mass has a tendency to shift posteriorly, obstructing the airway and presenting the risk of suffocation. Total relaxation of the genioglossus muscles occurs during general anesthesia; therefore, the tongue of an anesthetized patient must be prevented from relapsing by inserting an airway.

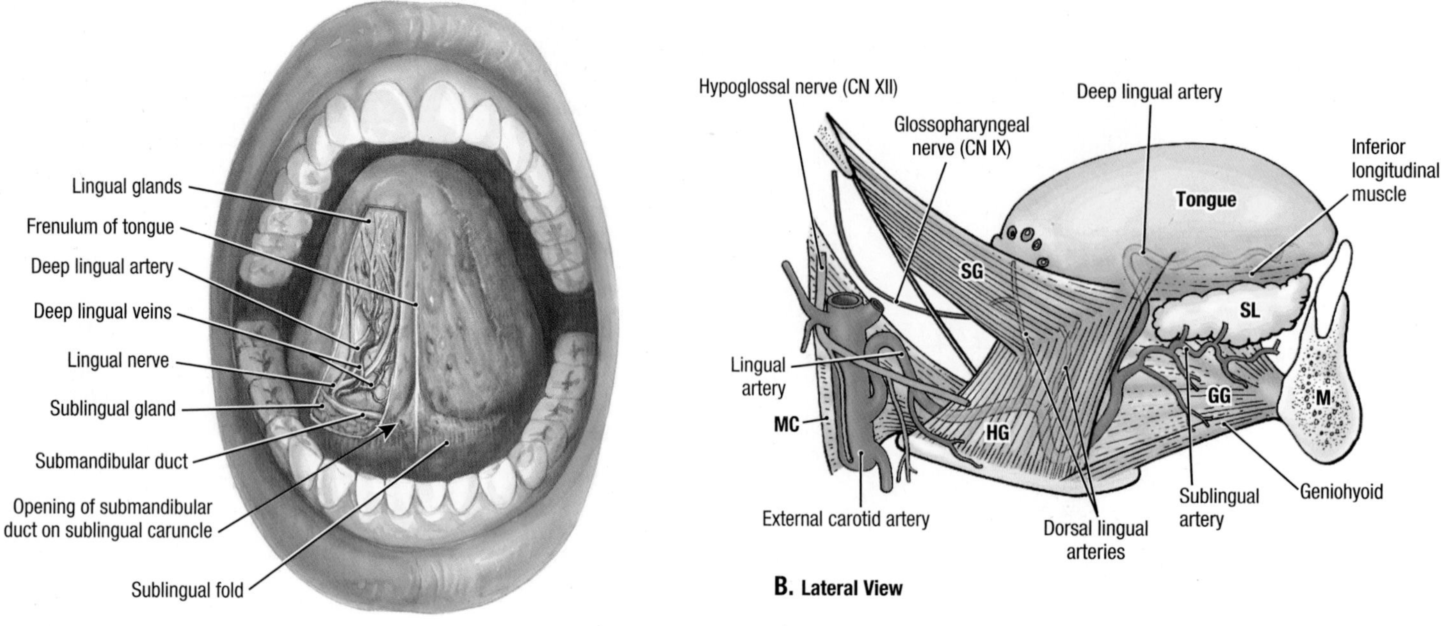
Lingual glands
Frenulum of tongue
Deep lingual artery
Deep lingual veins
Lingual nerve
Sublingual gland
Submandibular duct
Opening of submandibular duct on sublingual caruncle
Sublingual fold
A. Anterior View
Hypoglossal nerve (CN XII)
Glossopharyngeal nerve (CN IX)
Deep lingual artery
Inferior longitudinal muscle
Tongue
SG
SL
Lingual artery
MC
HG
GG
M
External carotid artery
Dorsal lingual arteries
Sublingual artery
Geniohyoid
B. Lateral View

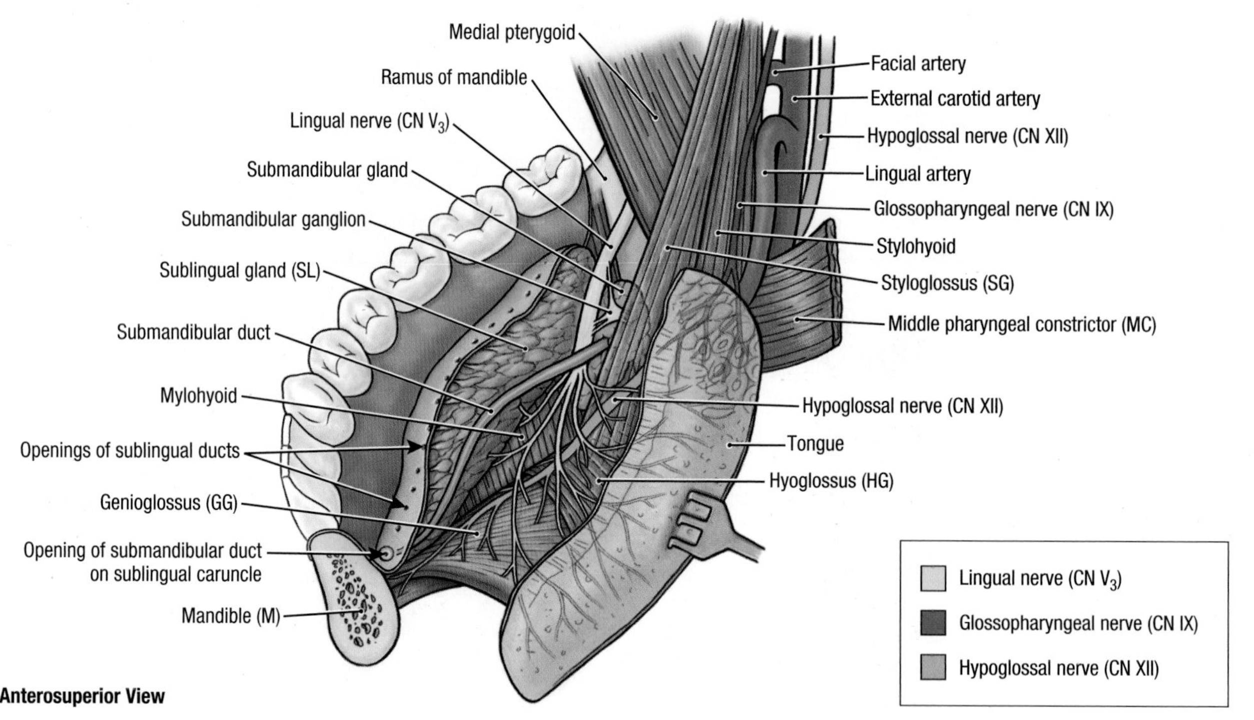
Medial pterygoid
Ramus of mandible
Lingual nerve (CN V3)
Submandibular gland
Submandibular ganglion
Sublingual gland (SL)
Submandibular duct
Mylohyoid
Openings of sublingual ducts
Genioglossus (GG)
Opening of submandibular duct on sublingual caruncle
Mandible (M)
Facial artery
External carotid artery
Hypoglossal nerve (CN XII)
Lingual artery
Glossopharyngeal nerve (CN IX)
Stylohyoid
Styloglossus (SG)
Middle pharyngeal constrictor (MC)
Hypoglossal nerve (CN XII)
Tongue
Hyoglossus (HG)
Lingual nerve (CN V3)
Glossopharyngeal nerve (CN IX)
Hypoglossal nerve (CN XII)
C. Anterosuperior View

7.61 ARTERIES AND NERVES OF THE TONGUE

A. Inferior surface of the tongue and floor of the mouth. The thin sublingual mucosa has been removed on the left side. **B.** Course and distribution of the lingual artery. **C.** Dissection of right side of floor of mouth. Letters in parentheses refer to **B**.

Sialography. The parotid and submandibular salivary glands may be examined radiographically after the injection of a contrast medium into their ducts. This special type of radiograph (sialogram) demonstrates the salivary ducts and some secretory units. Because of the small size and number of sublingual ducts of the sublingual glands, one cannot usually inject contrast medium into them.

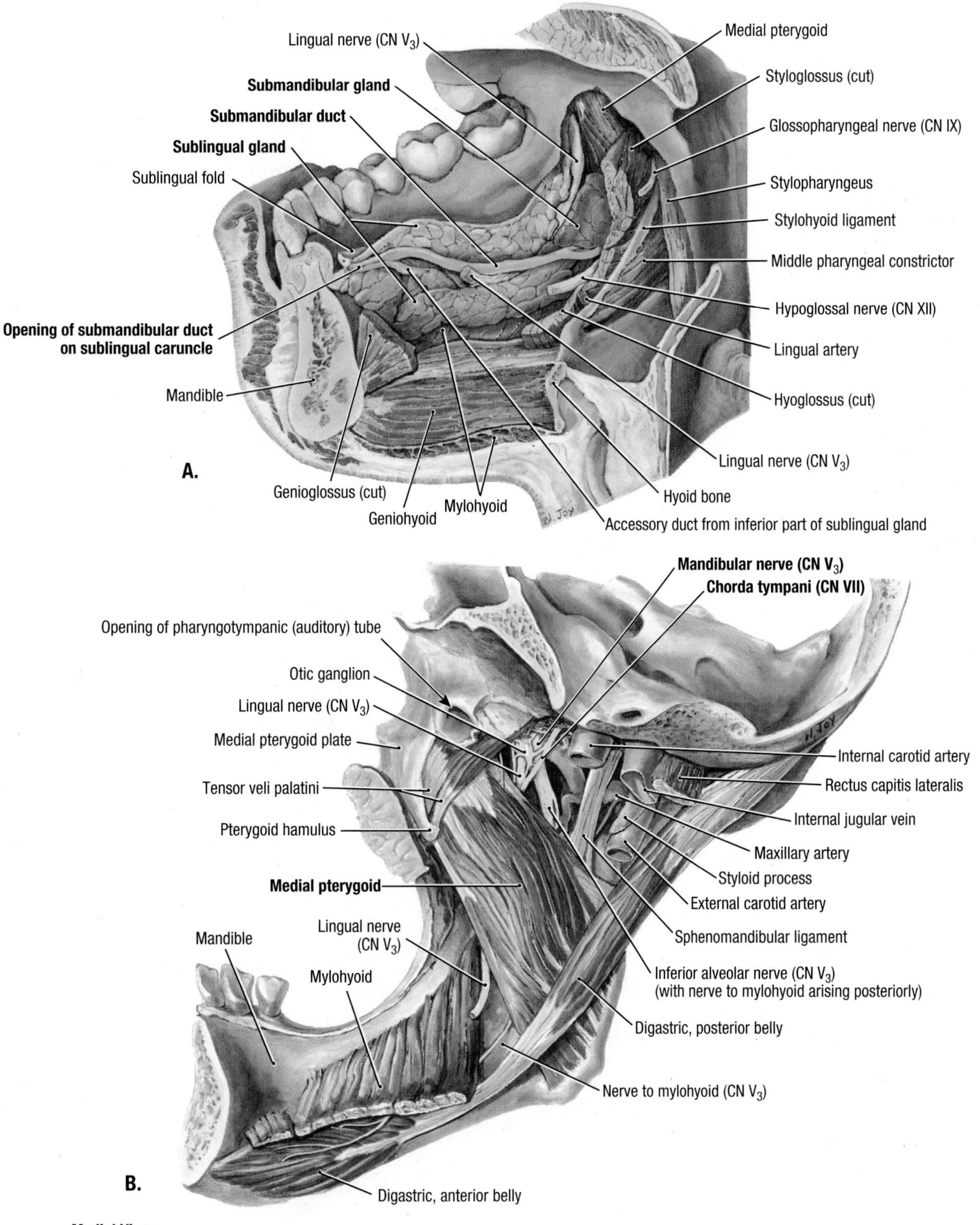
Lingual nerve (CN V_3)
Submandibular gland
Submandibular duct
Sublingual gland
Sublingual fold
Opening of submandibular duct on sublingual caruncle
Mandible
A.
Genioglossus (cut)
Geniohyoid
Mylohyoid
Medial pterygoid
Styloglossus (cut)
Glossopharyngeal nerve (CN IX)
Stylopharyngeus
Stylohyoid ligament
Middle pharyngeal constrictor
Hypoglossal nerve (CN XII)
Lingual artery
Hyoglossus (cut)
Lingual nerve (CN V_3)
Hyoid bone
Accessory duct from inferior part of sublingual gland
Mandibular nerve (CN V_3)
Chorda tympani (CN VII)
Opening of pharyngotympanic (auditory) tube
Otic ganglion
Lingual nerve (CN V_3)
Medial pterygoid plate
Tensor veli palatini
Pterygoid hamulus
Medial pterygoid
Mandible
Lingual nerve (CN V_3)
Mylohyoid
Internal carotid artery
Rectus capitis lateralis
Internal jugular vein
Maxillary artery
Styloid process
External carotid artery
Sphenomandibular ligament
Inferior alveolar nerve (CN V_3) (with nerve to mylohyoid arising posteriorly)
Digastric, posterior belly
Nerve to mylohyoid (CN V_3)
B.
Digastric, anterior belly

Medial Views

7.62 MUSCLES, GLANDS, AND VESSELS OF FLOOR OF MOUTH AND MEDIAL ASPECT OF MANDIBLE

A. Sublingual and submandibular glands. The tongue has been excised. **B.** Structures related to the medial surface of the mandible. The otic ganglion lies medial to the mandibular nerve (CN V_3) and between the foramen ovale superiorly and the medial pterygoid muscle inferiorly.

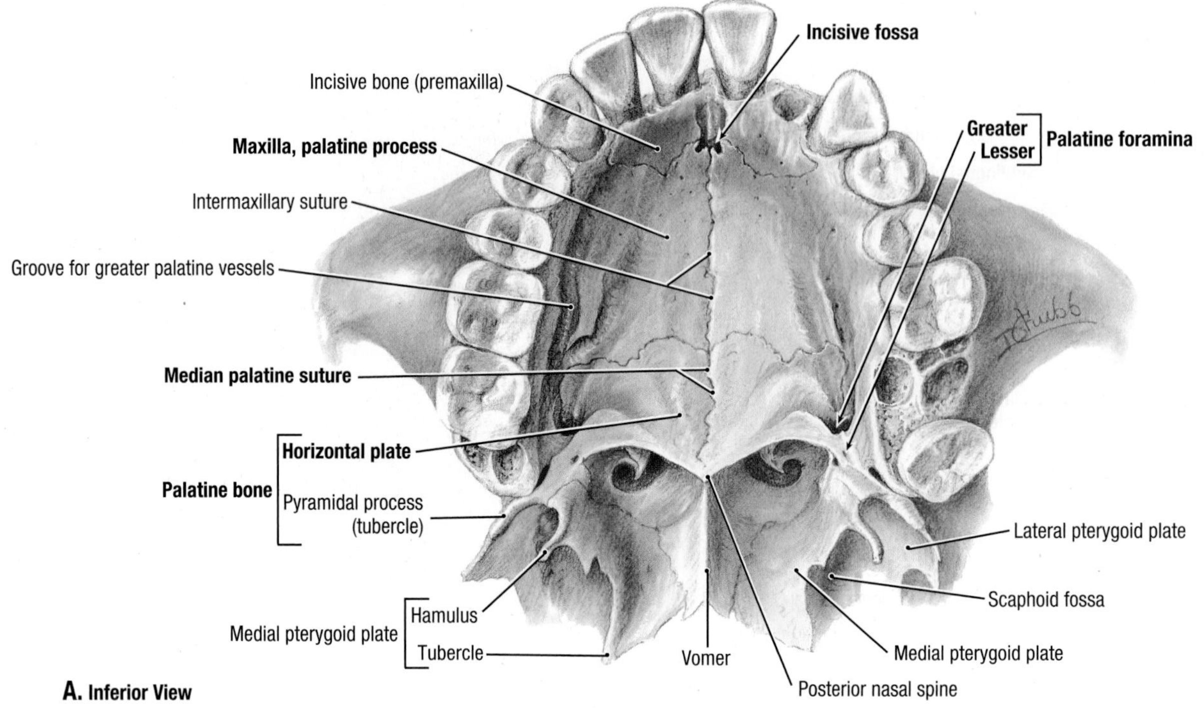
Incisive fossa
Incisive bone (premaxilla)
Maxilla, palatine process
Intermaxillary suture
Groove for greater palatine vessels
Greater
Lesser
Palatine foramina
Median palatine suture
Horizontal plate
Palatine bone
Pyramidal process (tubercle)
Lateral pterygoid plate
Scaphoid fossa
Medial pterygoid plate
Hamulus
Tubercle
Medial pterygoid plate
Vomer
Posterior nasal spine

A. **Inferior View**

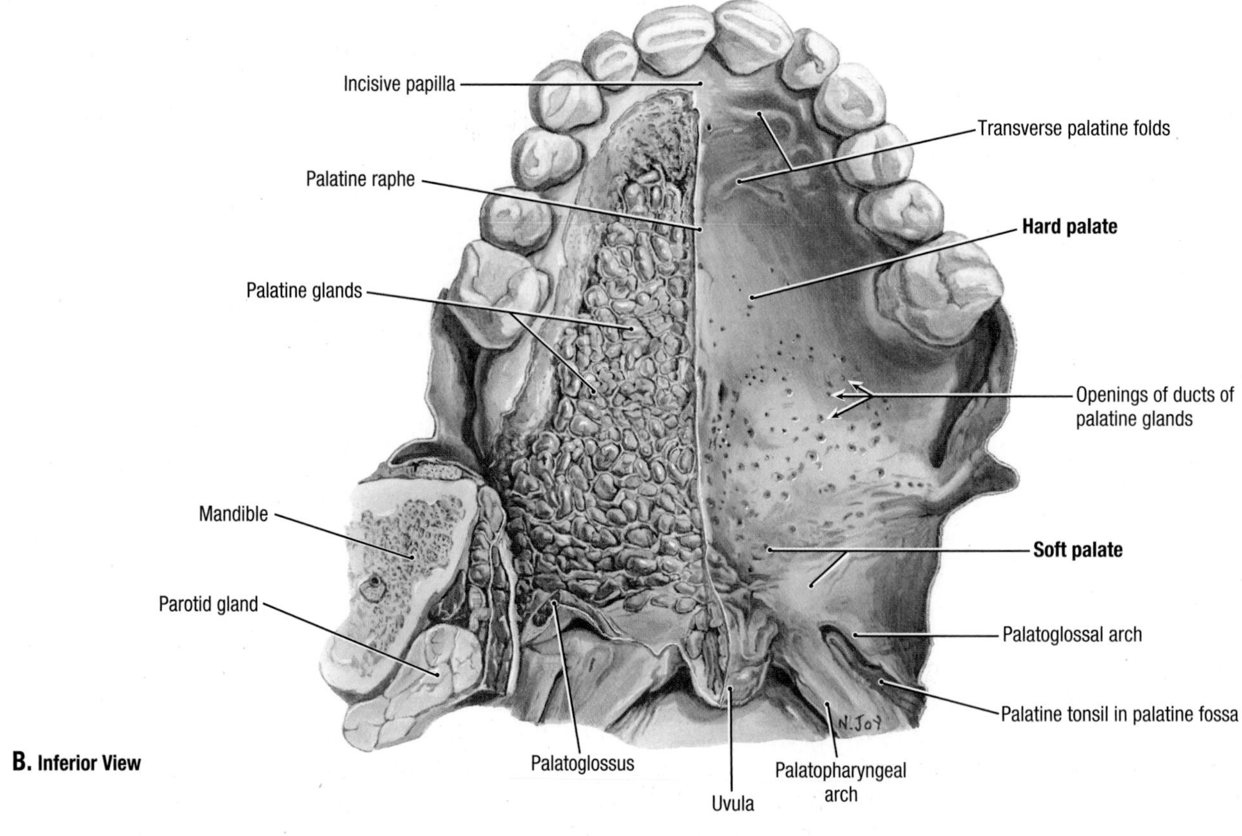
Incisive papilla
Transverse palatine folds
Palatine raphe
Hard palate
Palatine glands
Openings of ducts of palatine glands
Mandible
Soft palate
Parotid gland
Palatoglossal arch
Palatine tonsil in palatine fossa
Palatoglossus
Uvula
Palatopharyngeal arch
N. JOY

B. **Inferior View**

7.63 PALATE

A. Bones of the hard palate. The palatine aponeurosis, which forms the fibrous "skeleton" of the soft palate, stretches between the hamuli of the medial pterygoid plates. **B.** Mucous membrane and glands of palate.

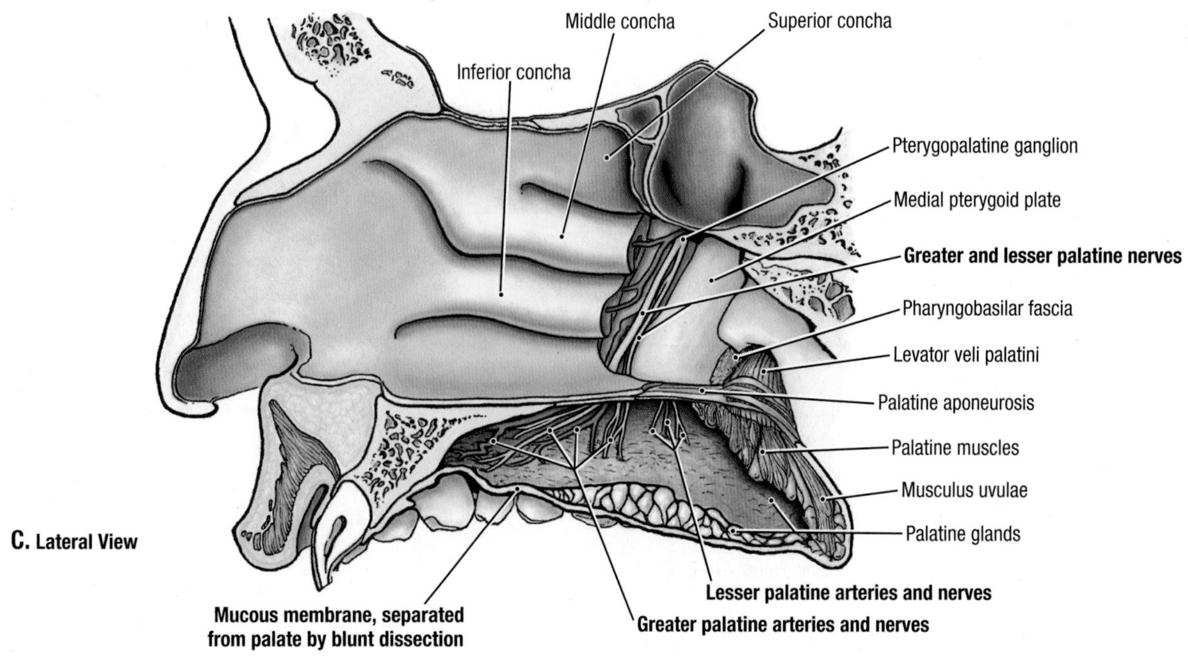
Middle concha
Superior concha
Inferior concha
Pterygopalatine ganglion
Medial pterygoid plate
Greater and lesser palatine nerves
Pharyngobasilar fascia
Levator veli palatini
Palatine aponeurosis
Palatine muscles
Musculus uvulae
Palatine glands
Lesser palatine arteries and nerves
Greater palatine arteries and nerves
Mucous membrane, separated from palate by blunt dissection

C. **Lateral View**

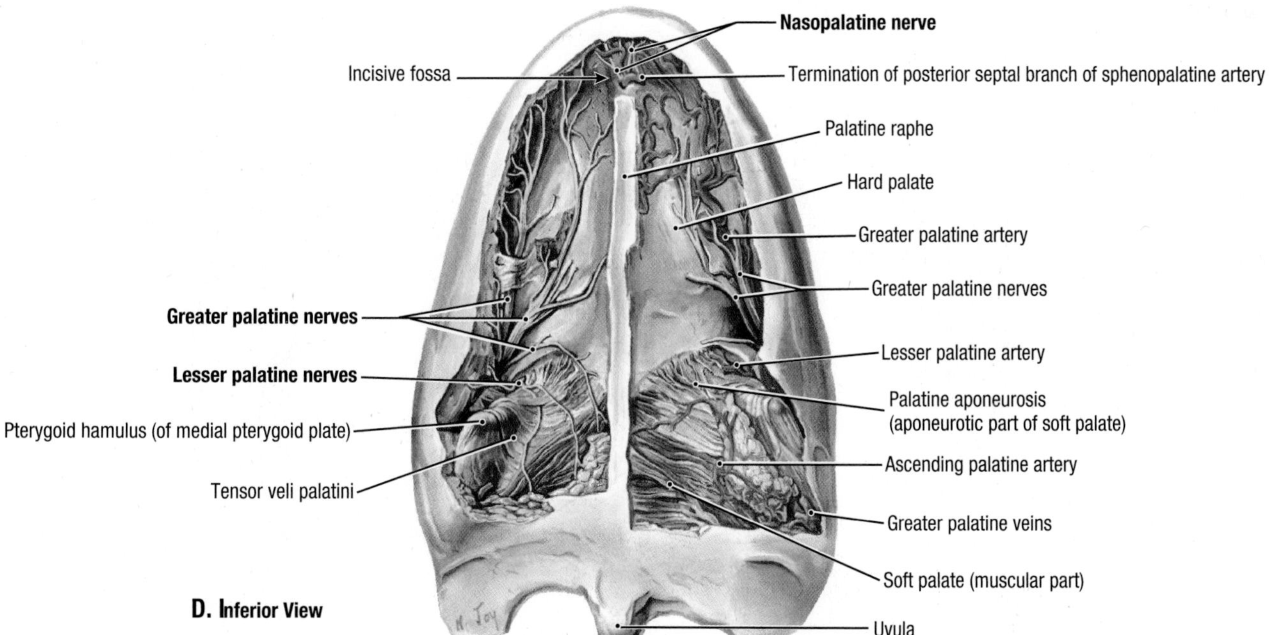
Nasopalatine nerve
Incisive fossa
Termination of posterior septal branch of sphenopalatine artery
Palatine raphe
Hard palate
Greater palatine artery
Greater palatine nerves
Greater palatine nerves
Lesser palatine nerves
Lesser palatine artery
Palatine aponeurosis (aponeurotic part of soft palate)
Pterygoid hamulus (of medial pterygoid plate)
Ascending palatine artery
Tensor veli palatini
Greater palatine veins
Soft palate (muscular part)
Uvula

D. **Inferior View**

7.63 PALATE *(CONTINUED)*

C. Nerves and vessels of palatine canal. The lateral wall of the nasal cavity is shown. The posterior ends of the middle and inferior conchae are excised along with the mucoperiosteum; the thin, perpendicular plate of the palatine bone is removed to expose the palatine nerves and arteries. **D.** Dissection of an edentulous palate. The greater palatine nerve supplies the gingivae and hard palate, the nasopalatine nerve the incisive region, and the lesser palatine nerves the soft palate. **Anesthesia of palatine nerves.** The nasopalatine nerves can be anesthetized by injecting anesthetic into the mouth of the incisive fossa in the hard palate. The anesthetized tissues are the palatal mucosa, the lingual gingivae, the six anterior maxillary teeth, and associated alveolar bone. The greater palatine nerve can be anesthetized by injecting anesthetic into the greater palatine foramen. The nerve emerges between the second and third maxillary molar teeth. This nerve block anesthetizes the palatal mucosa and lingual gingivae posterior to the maxillary canine teeth, and the underlying bone of the palate.

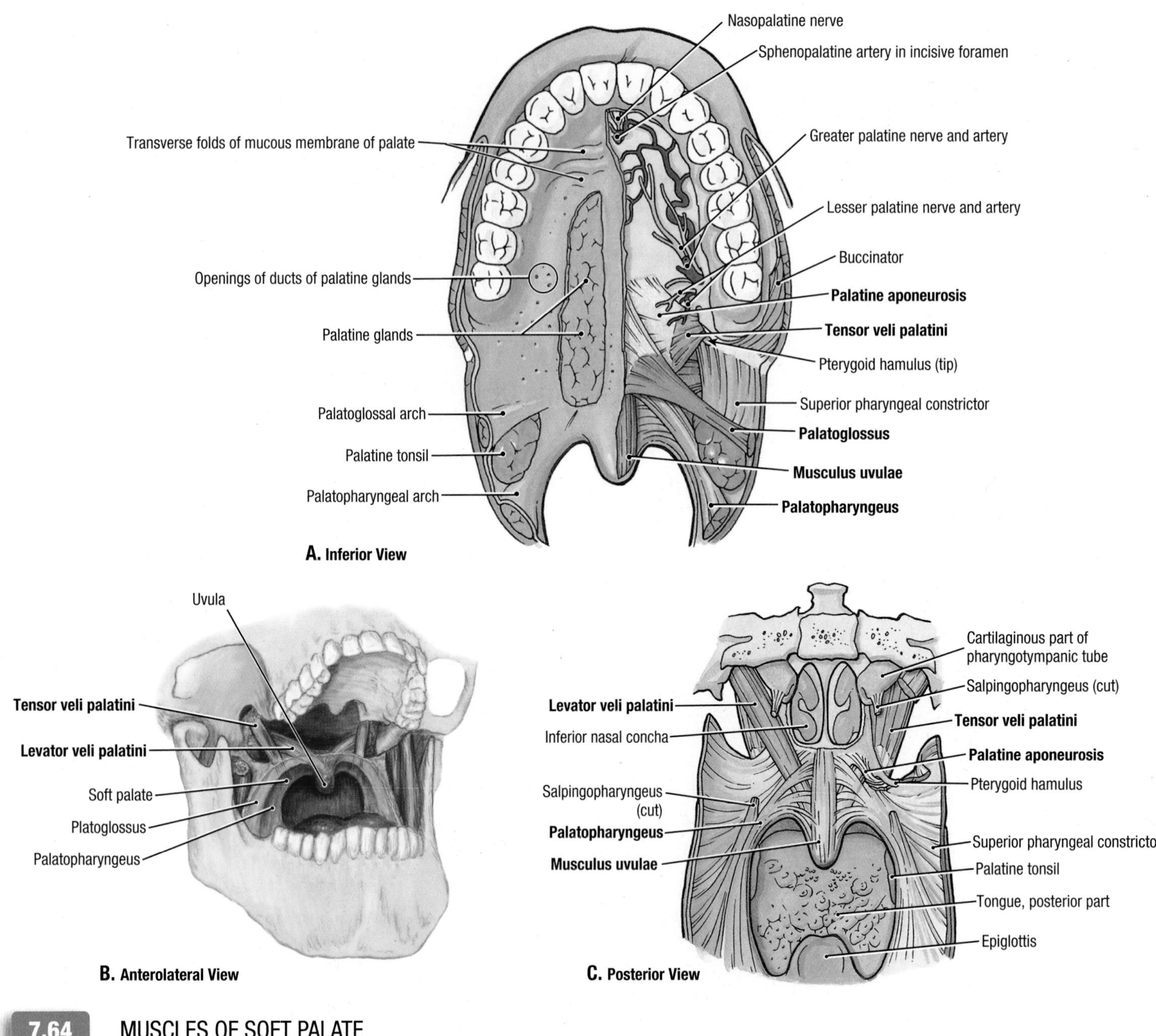
Nasopalatine nerve
Sphenopalatine artery in incisive foramen
Transverse folds of mucous membrane of palate
Greater palatine nerve and artery
Lesser palatine nerve and artery
Buccinator
Openings of ducts of palatine glands
Palatine aponeurosis
Palatine glands
Tensor veli palatini
Pterygoid hamulus (tip)
Superior pharyngeal constrictor
Palatoglossal arch
Palatoglossus
Palatine tonsil
Musculus uvulae
Palatopharyngeal arch
Palatopharyngeus
A. Inferior View
Uvula
Tensor veli palatini
Levator veli palatini
Soft palate
Platoglossus
Palatopharyngeus
B. Anterolateral View
Cartilaginous part of pharyngotympanic tube
Salpingopharyngeus (cut)
Levator veli palatini
Tensor veli palatini
Inferior nasal concha
Palatine aponeurosis
Pterygoid hamulus
Salpingopharyngeus (cut)
Palatopharyngeus
Superior pharyngeal constrictor
Musculus uvulae
Palatine tonsil
Tongue, posterior part
Epiglottis
C. Posterior View

7.64 MUSCLES OF SOFT PALATE

TABLE 7.14 MUSCLES OF SOFT PALATE

Muscle	Superior Attachment	Inferior Attachment	Innervation	Main Action(s)
Levator veli palatini	Cartilage of pharyngotympanic tube and petrous part of temporal bone	Palatine aponeurosis	Pharyngeal branch of vagus nerve through pharyngeal plexus	Elevates soft palate during swallowing and yawning
Tensor veli palatini	Scaphoid fossa of medial pterygoid plate, spine of sphenoid bone, and cartilage of pharyngotympanic tube		Medial pterygoid nerve (CN V_3) through otic ganglion	Tenses soft palate and opens mouth of pharyngotympanic tube during swallowing and yawning
Palatoglossus	Palatine aponeurosis	Side of tongue	Pharyngeal branch of vagus nerve (CN X) via pharyngeal plexus	Elevates posterior part of tongue and draws soft palate onto tongue
Palatopharyngeus	Hard palate and palatine aponeurosis	Lateral wall of pharynx		Tenses soft palate and pulls walls of pharynx superiorly, anteriorly, and medially during swallowing
Musculus uvulae	Posterior nasal spine and palatine aponeurosis	Mucosa of uvula		Shortens uvula and pulls it superiorly

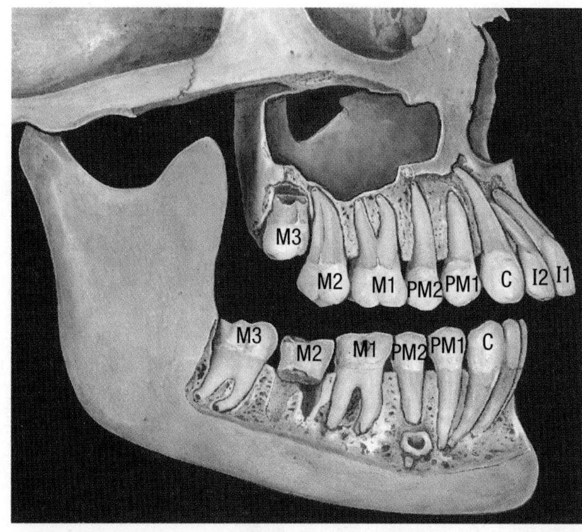
M3
M2
M1
PM2
PM1
C
I2
I1
M3
M2
M1
PM2
PM1
C

A. **Lateral View**

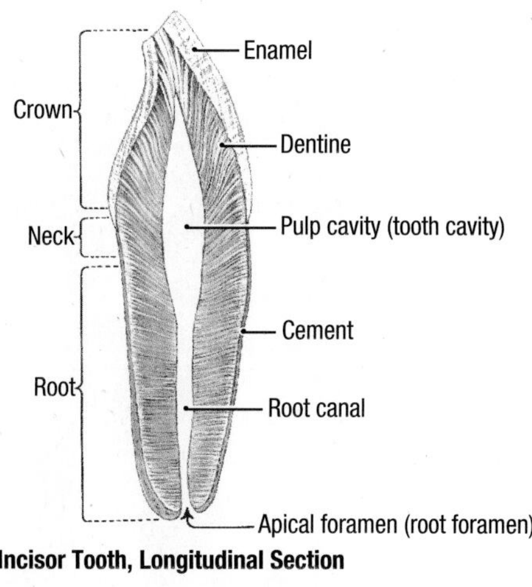
Enamel
Crown
Dentine
Pulp cavity (tooth cavity)
Neck
Cement
Root
Root canal
Apical foramen (root foramen)

Incisor Tooth, Longitudinal Section

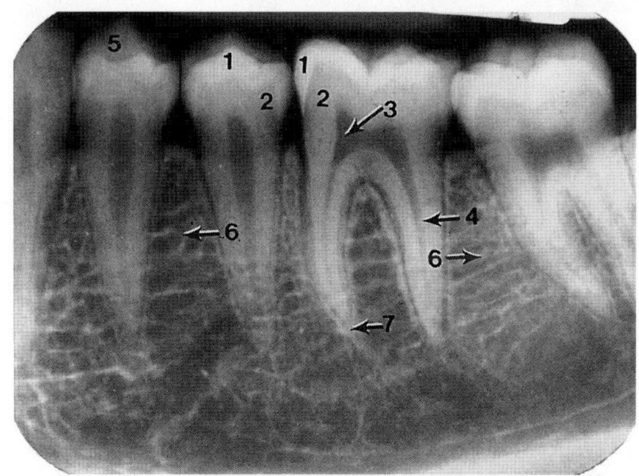
5
1
1
2
2
3
4
6
6
7

B. **Lateral Radiograph**

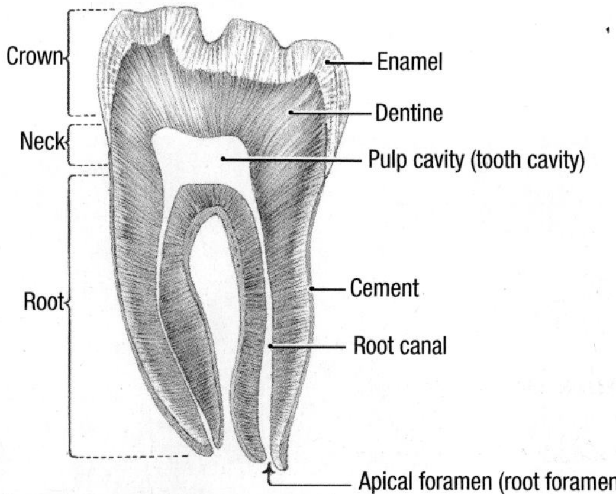
Crown
Enamel
Dentine
Neck
Pulp cavity (tooth cavity)
Root
Cement
Root canal
Apical foramen (root foramen)

C. **Molar Tooth, Longitudinal Section**

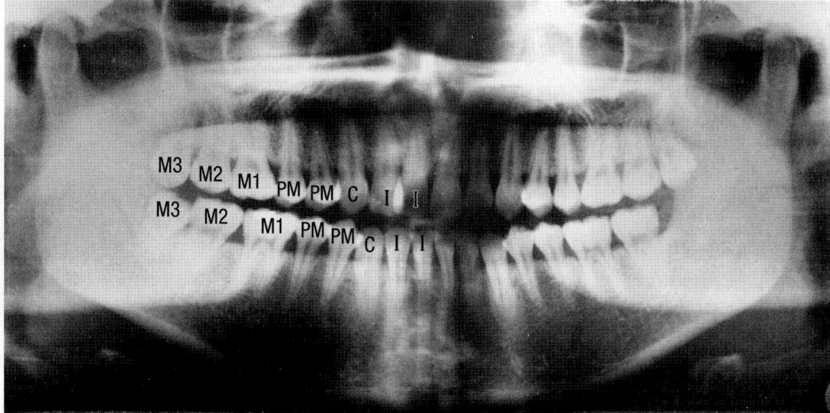
M3
M2
M1
PM
PM
C
I
I
M3
M2
M1
PM
PM
C
I
I

D. **Pantomographic Radiograph**

7.65 PERMANENT TEETH I

A. Teeth in situ with roots exposed. Incisors *(I1, I2)*, canine *(C1)*, premolars *(PM1, PM2)*, and molars *(M1, M2, M3)*. The roots of the 2nd lower molar have been removed. **B.** Lateral radiograph. *(1)* enamel, *(2)* dentin, *(3)* pulp chamber, *(4)* pulp canal, *(5)* buccal cusp, (*6*) alveolar bone, and *(7)* root apex. **C.** Longitudinal sections of an incisor and a molar tooth. **D.** Pantomographic radiograph of mandible and maxilla. The left lower third molar is not present.

Decay of the hard tissues of a tooth results in the formation of **dental caries** (cavities). Invasion of the pulp of the tooth by a carious lesion (cavity) results in infection and irritation of the tissues in the pulp cavity. This condition causes an inflammatory process (pulpitis). Because the pulp cavity is a rigid space, the swollen pulpal tissues cause pain (toothache).

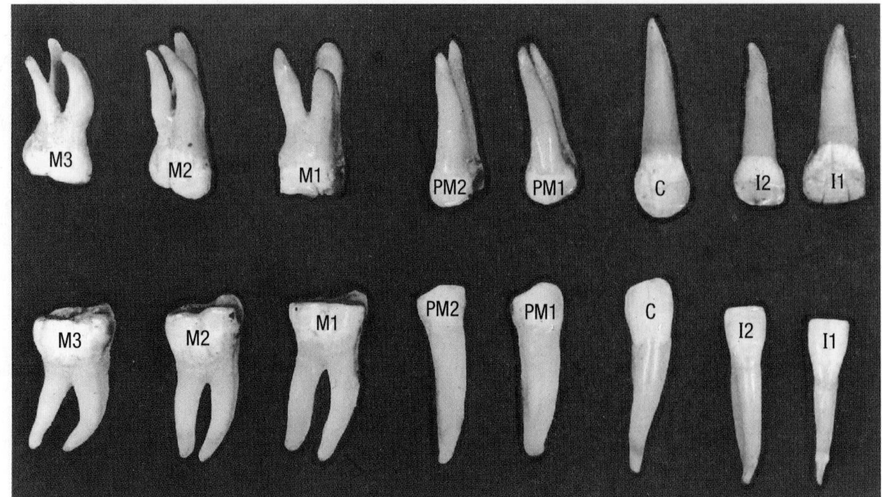
M3
M2
M1
PM2
PM1
C
I2
I1
Maxillary Teeth
M3
M2
M1
PM2
PM1
C
I2
I1
Mandibular Teeth

A. Vestibular View

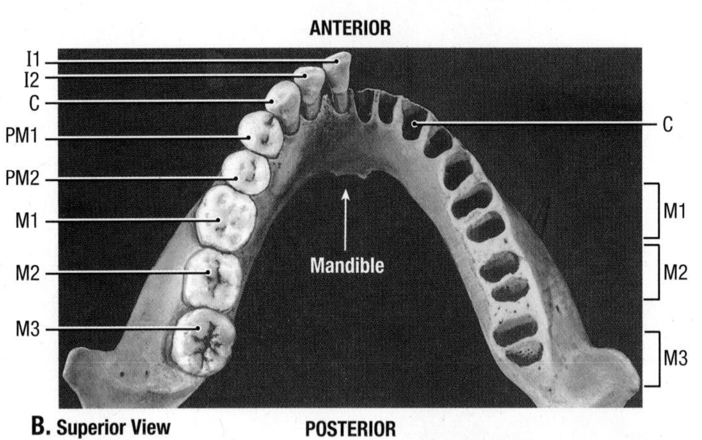
ANTERIOR
I1
I2
C
PM1
PM2
M1
M2
M3
C
Mandible
M1
M2
M3
POSTERIOR

B. Superior View

ANTERIOR
I1
I2
C
PM1
PM2
M1
M2
M3
C
M1
M2
M3
Hard palate
POSTERIOR

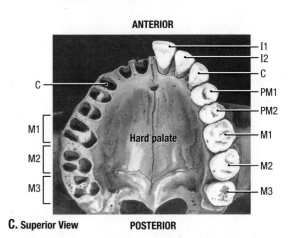

C. Superior View

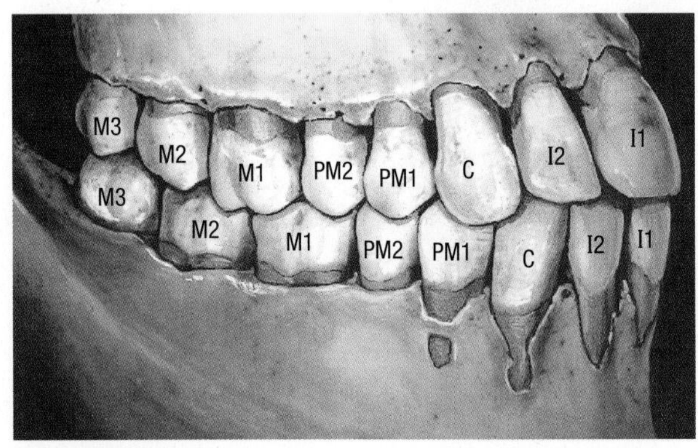
M3
M2
M1
PM2
PM1
C
I2
I1
M3
M2
M1
PM2
PM1
C
I2
I1

D. Anterolateral View

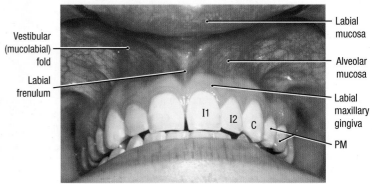

Labial mucosa
Vestibular (mucolabial) fold
Alveolar mucosa
Labial frenulum
Labial maxillary gingiva
I1
I2
C
PM

E. Anterior View

7.66 PERMANENT TEETH II

A. Removed teeth, displaying roots. There are 32 permanent teeth; 8 are on each side of each dental arch on the top (maxillary teeth) and bottom (mandibular teeth): 2 incisors *(I1–2)*, 1 canine *(C)*, 2 premolars *(PM1–2)*, and 3 molars *(M1–3)*. **B.** Permanent mandibular teeth and their sockets. **C.** Permanent maxillary teeth and their sockets. **D.** Teeth in occlusion. **E.** Vestibule and gingivae of the maxilla

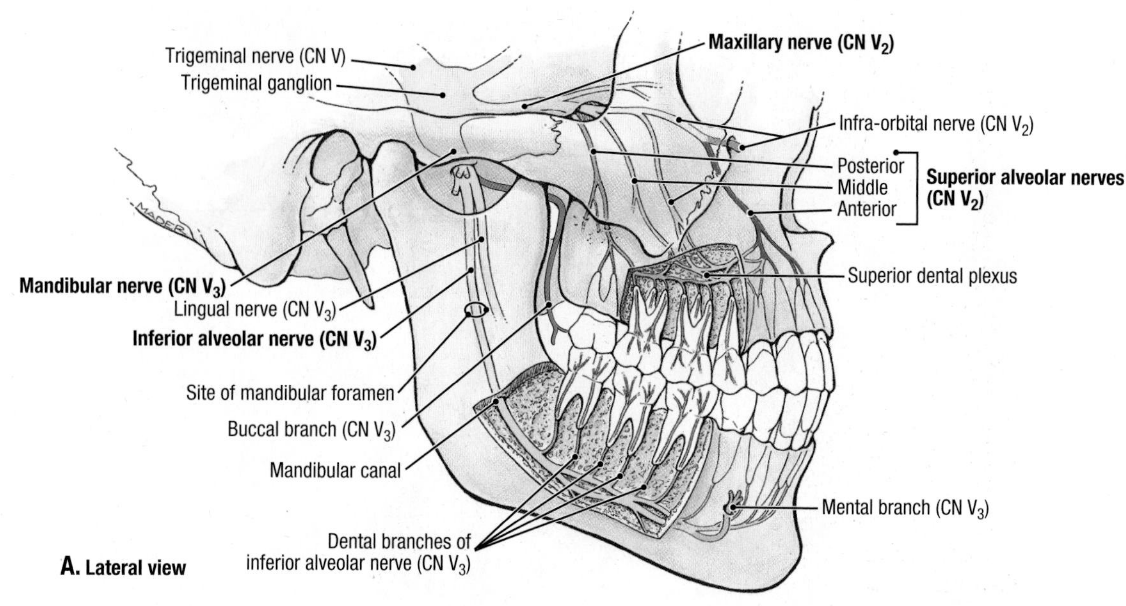
Trigeminal nerve (CN V)
Trigeminal ganglion
Maxillary nerve (CN V_2)
Infra-orbital nerve (CN V_2)
Posterior
Middle
Anterior
Superior alveolar nerves (CN V_2)
Superior dental plexus
Mandibular nerve (CN V_3)
Lingual nerve (CN V_3)
Inferior alveolar nerve (CN V_3)
Site of mandibular foramen
Buccal branch (CN V_3)
Mandibular canal
Mental branch (CN V_3)
Dental branches of inferior alveolar nerve (CN V_3)
A. Lateral view

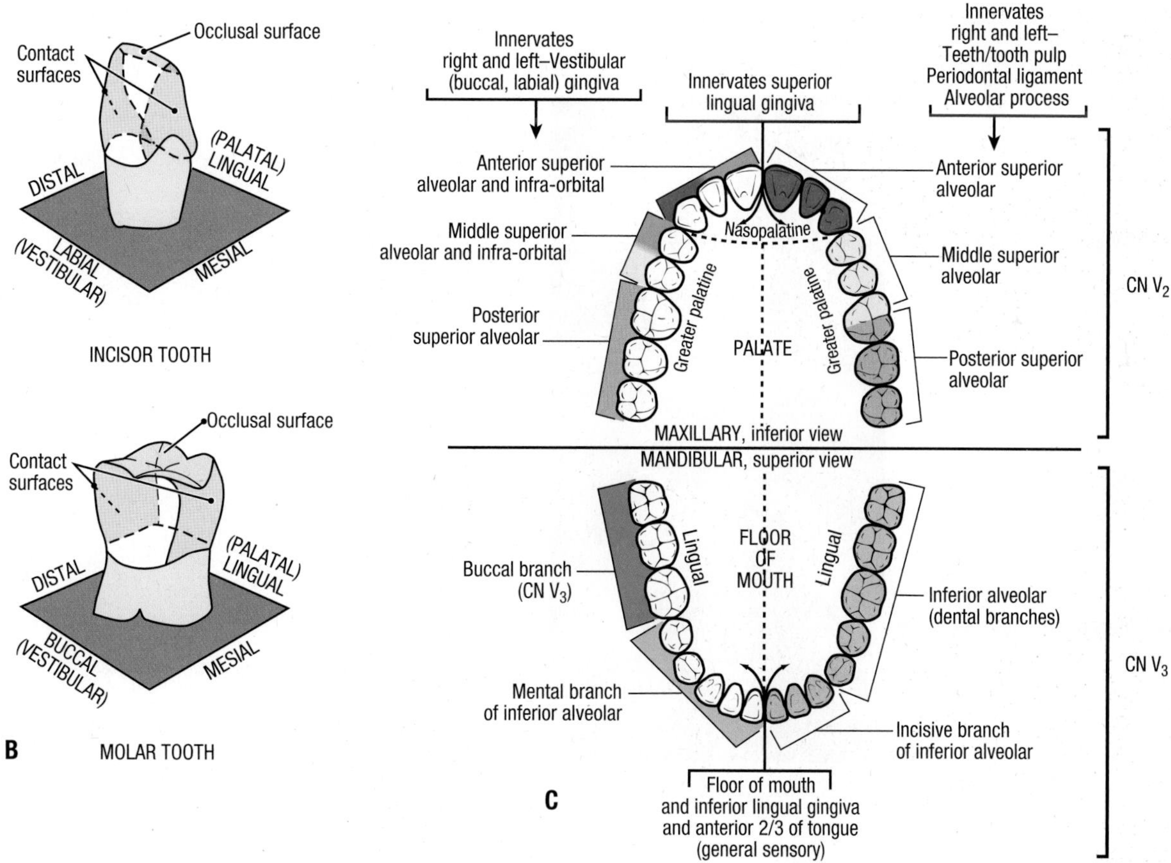
Contact surfaces
Occlusal surface
(PALATAL) LINGUAL
DISTAL
LABIAL (VESTIBULAR)
MESIAL
INCISOR TOOTH
Contact surfaces
Occlusal surface
(PALATAL) LINGUAL
DISTAL
BUCCAL (VESTIBULAR)
MESIAL
B
MOLAR TOOTH
Innervates right and left–Vestibular (buccal, labial) gingiva
Innervates superior lingual gingiva
Innervates right and left– Teeth/tooth pulp Periodontal ligament Alveolar process
Anterior superior alveolar and infra-orbital
Middle superior alveolar and infra-orbital
Posterior superior alveolar
Nasopalatine
Greater palatine
PALATE
Greater palatine
Anterior superior alveolar
Middle superior alveolar
Posterior superior alveolar
CN V_2
MAXILLARY, inferior view
MANDIBULAR, superior view
Buccal branch (CN V_3)
Lingual
FLOOR OF MOUTH
Lingual
Inferior alveolar (dental branches)
Mental branch of inferior alveolar
Incisive branch of inferior alveolar
CN V_3
Floor of mouth and inferior lingual gingiva and anterior 2/3 of tongue (general sensory)
C

7.67 INNERVATION OF TEETH

A. Superior and inferior alveolar nerves. **B.** Surfaces of an incisor and molar tooth. **C.** Innervation of the mouth and teeth.

Improper oral hygiene results in food deposits in tooth and gingival crevices, which may cause inflammation of the gingivae, **gingivitis**. If untreated, the disease spreads to other supporting structures (including the alveolar bone), producing **periodontitis**. Periodontitis results in inflammation of the gingivae and may result in absorption of alveolar bone and gingival recession. Gingival recession exposes the sensitive cement of the teeth.

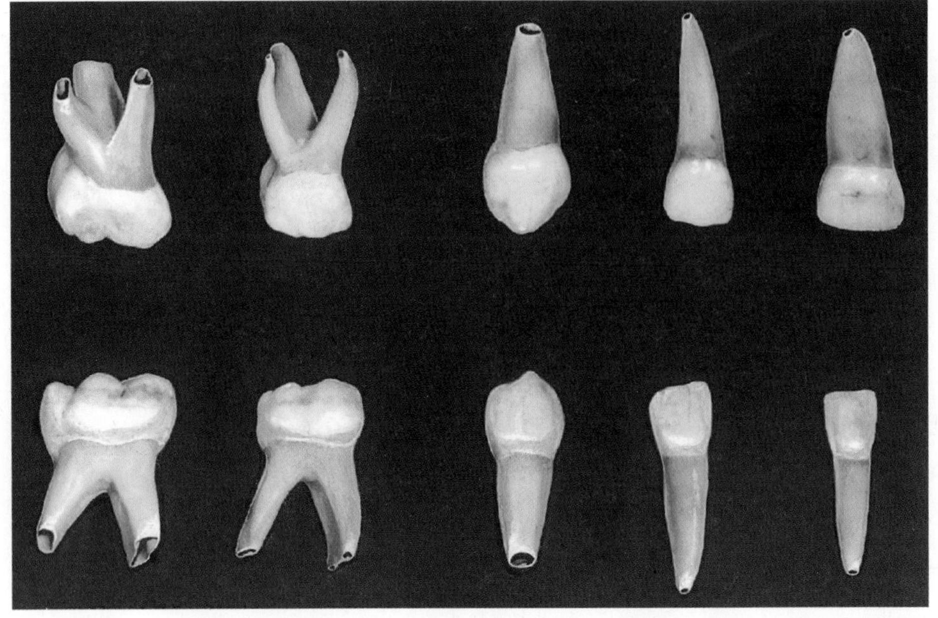
MAXILLARY TEETH
MANDIBULAR TEETH
2nd molar
1st molar
Canine
Lateral incisor
Central incisor

A. Vestibular View

INFERIOR VIEW OF MAXILLARY TEETH

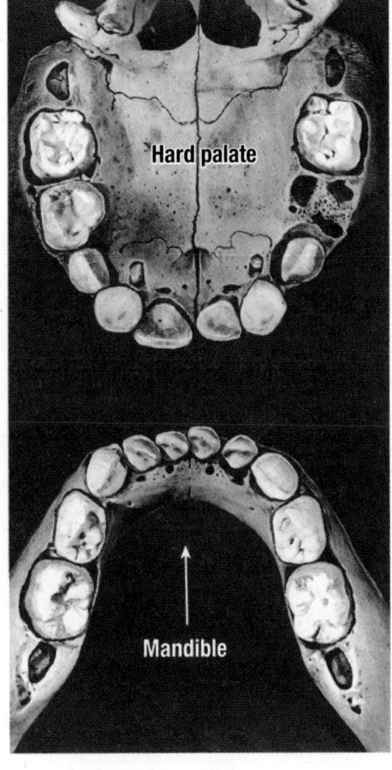
Hard palate
Mandible

M1
M2
Socket for M1
Canine
Alveolus for permanent incisor
Central and lateral incisors

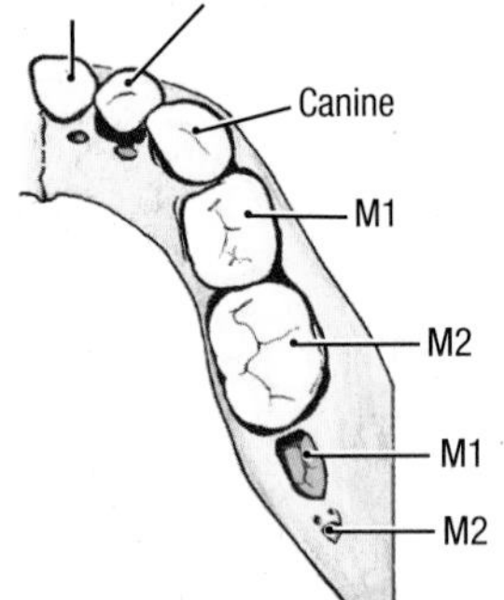
Canine
M1
M2
M1
M2

SUPERIOR VIEW OF MANDIBULAR TEETH

B

7.68 PRIMARY TEETH

A. Removed teeth. There are 20 primary (deciduous) teeth, 5 in each half of the mandible and 5 in each maxilla. They are named central incisor, lateral incisor, canine, 1st molar *(M1)*, and 2nd molar *(M2)*. Primary teeth differ from permanent teeth in that the primary teeth are smaller and whiter; the molars also have more bulbous crowns and more divergent roots. **B.** Teeth in situ, younger than 2 years of age. Permanent teeth are colored orange; the crowns of the unerupted first and second permanent molars are partly visible.

TABLE 7.15 PRIMARY AND SECONDARY DENTITION

Deciduous Teeth	Central Incisor	Lateral Incisor	Canine	First Molar	Second Molar
Eruption (months)[a]	6–8	8–10	16–20	12–16	20–24
Shedding (years)	6–7	7–8	10–12	9–11	10–12

[a]In some normal infants, the first teeth (medial incisors) may not erupt until 12 to 13 months of age

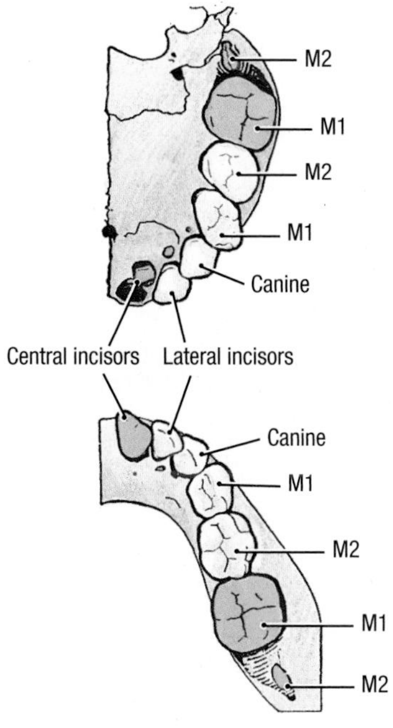
M2
M1
M2
M1
Canine
Central incisors
Lateral incisors
Canine
M1
M2
M1
M2

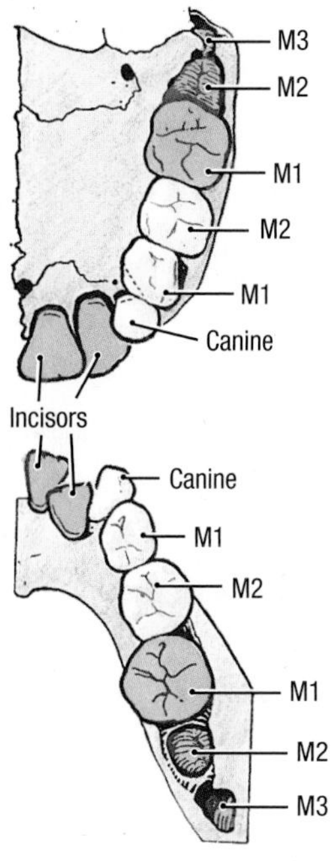
M3
M2
M1
M2
M1
Canine
Incisors
Canine
M1
M2
M1
M2
M3

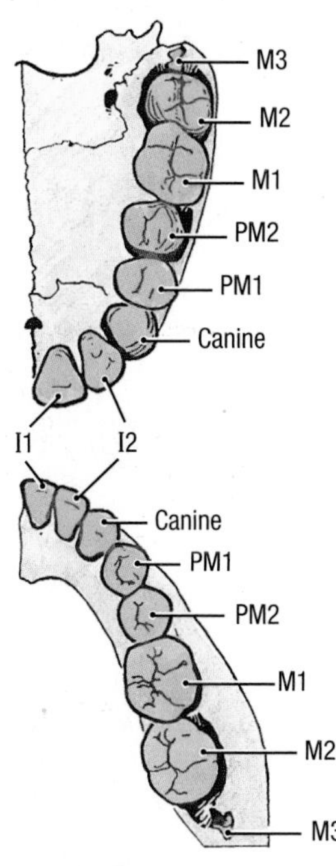
M3
M2
M1
PM2
PM1
Canine
I1
I2
Canine
PM1
PM2
M1
M2
M3

Age: 6–7 years

The 1st molars (6-year molars) have fully erupted, the primary central incisor has been shed, the lower central incisor is almost fully erupted, and the upper central incisor is descending into the vacated socket.

Age: 8 years

All of the permanent incisors have erupted; however, the lower lateral incisor is only partially erupted.

Age: 12 years

The primary teeth have been replaced by 20 permanent teeth, and the 1st and 2nd molars (12-year molars) have erupted; the canines, 2nd premolars, and 2nd molars (especially those in the upper jaw) have not erupted fully, nor have their bony sockets closed around them. By age 12, 28 permanent teeth are in evidence; the last 4 teeth, the 3rd molars, may erupt any time after this, or never.

Permanent Teeth	Central Incisor	Lateral Incisor	Canine	First Premolar	Second Premolar	First Molar	Second Molar	Third Molar
Eruption (years)	7–8	8–9	10–12	10–11	11–12	6–7	12	13–25

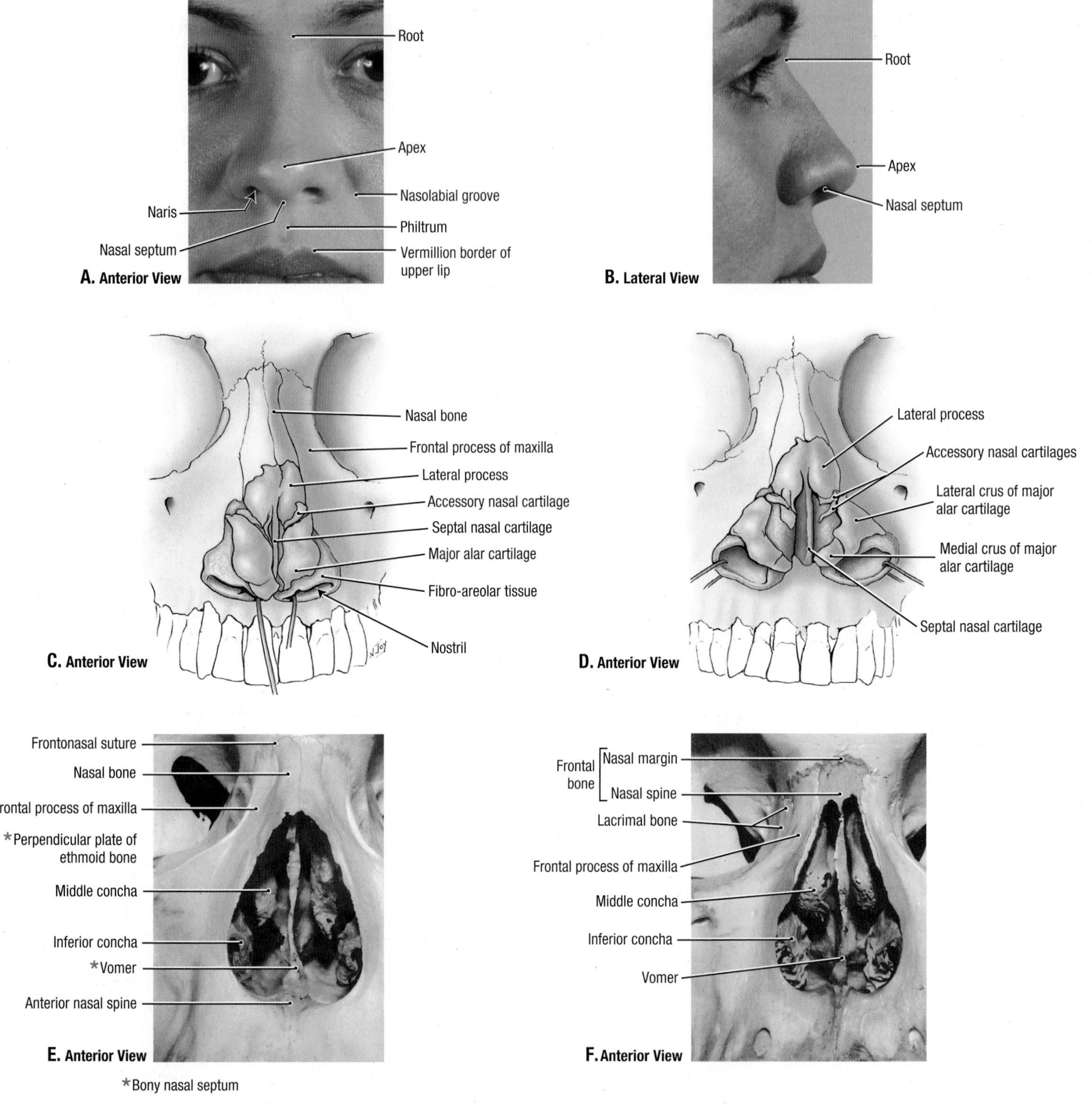
Root
Apex
Nasolabial groove
Naris
Philtrum
Nasal septum
Vermillion border of upper lip
A. Anterior View
Root
Apex
Nasal septum
B. Lateral View
Nasal bone
Frontal process of maxilla
Lateral process
Accessory nasal cartilage
Septal nasal cartilage
Major alar cartilage
Fibro-areolar tissue
Nostril
C. Anterior View
Lateral process
Accessory nasal cartilages
Lateral crus of major alar cartilage
Medial crus of major alar cartilage
Septal nasal cartilage
D. Anterior View
Frontonasal suture
Nasal bone
Frontal process of maxilla
*Perpendicular plate of ethmoid bone
Middle concha
Inferior concha
*Vomer
Anterior nasal spine
E. Anterior View
*Bony nasal septum
Frontal bone
Nasal margin
Nasal spine
Lacrimal bone
Frontal process of maxilla
Middle concha
Inferior concha
Vomer
F. Anterior View

7.69 SURFACE ANATOMY, CARTILAGES, AND BONES OF NOSE

A. Surface features of anterior aspect of nose. **B.** Surface features of lateral aspect of nose. **C.** Nasal cartilages, with the septum pulled inferiorly. **D.** Nasal cartilages, separated and retracted laterally. **E.** Lower conchae and bony septum seen through the piriform aperture. The margin of the piriform aperture is sharp and formed by the maxillae and nasal bones. **F.** Nasal bones removed. The areas of the frontal processes of the maxillae *(yellow)* and of the frontal bone *(blue)* that articulate with the nasal bones can be seen.

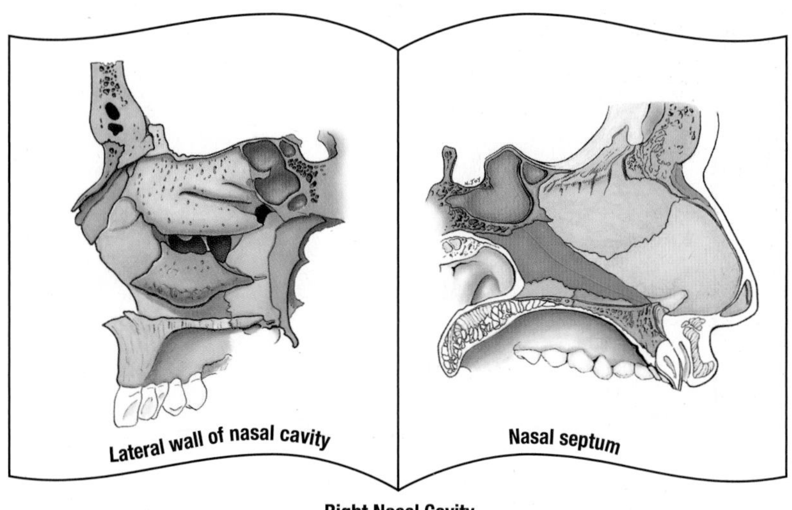
Lateral wall of nasal cavity
Nasal septum

Right Nasal Cavity

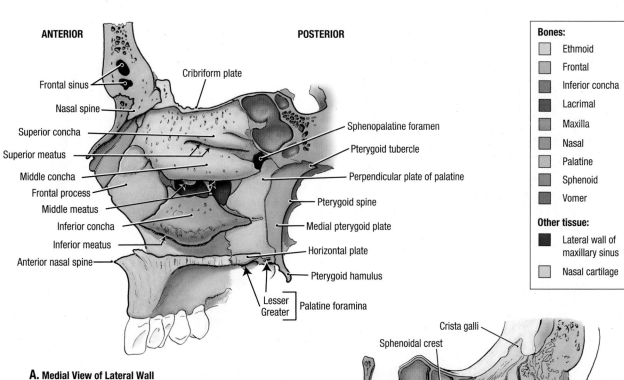

ANTERIOR
POSTERIOR
Frontal sinus
Cribriform plate
Nasal spine
Superior concha
Sphenopalatine foramen
Superior meatus
Pterygoid tubercle
Middle concha
Perpendicular plate of palatine
Frontal process
Pterygoid spine
Middle meatus
Inferior concha
Medial pterygoid plate
Inferior meatus
Horizontal plate
Anterior nasal spine
Pterygoid hamulus
Lesser
Greater
Palatine foramina

Bones:
Ethmoid
Frontal
Inferior concha
Lacrimal
Maxilla
Nasal
Palatine
Sphenoid
Vomer

Other tissue:
Lateral wall of maxillary sinus
Nasal cartilage

A. Medial View of Lateral Wall

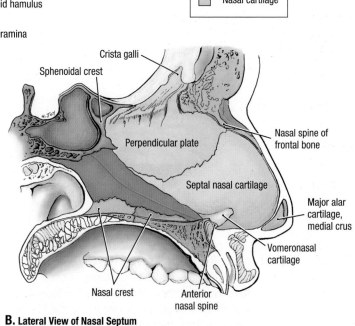

Crista galli
Sphenoidal crest
Nasal spine of frontal bone
Perpendicular plate
Septal nasal cartilage
Major alar cartilage, medial crus
Vomeronasal cartilage
Nasal crest
Anterior nasal spine

B. Lateral View of Nasal Septum

7.70 BONES OF THE NASAL WALL AND SEPTUM

A. Lateral wall of nose. The superior and middle conchae are parts of the ethmoid bone, whereas the inferior concha is itself a bone. **B.** Nasal septum.

Deformity of the external nose usually is present with a fracture, particularly when a lateral force is applied by someone's elbow, for example. When the injury results from a direct blow (e.g., from a hockey stick), the cribriform plate of the ethmoid bone may fracture, resulting in CSF rhinorrhea.

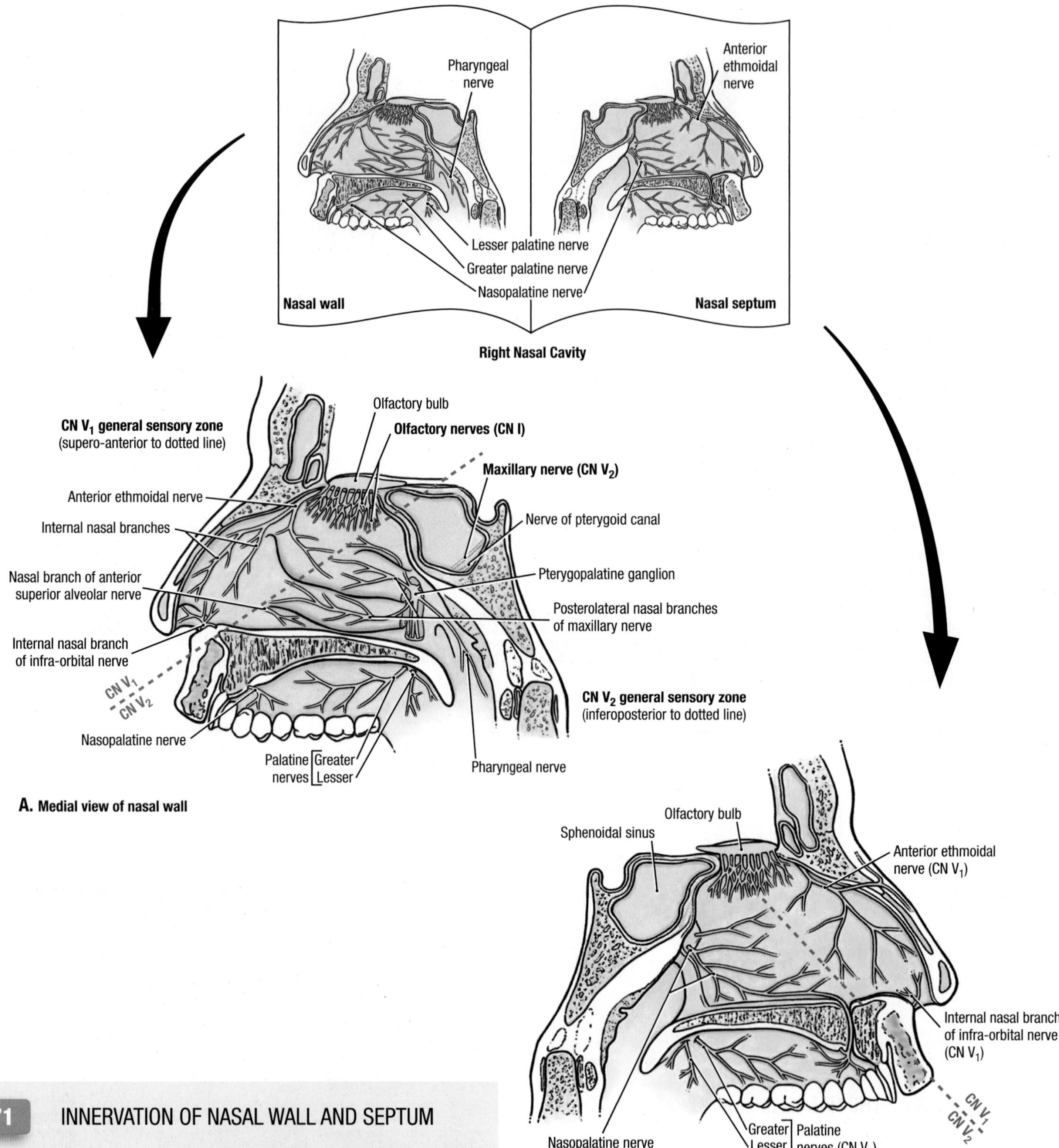
Pharyngeal nerve
Anterior ethmoidal nerve
Lesser palatine nerve
Greater palatine nerve
Nasopalatine nerve
Nasal wall
Nasal septum
Right Nasal Cavity
CN V_1 general sensory zone
(supero-anterior to dotted line)
Olfactory bulb
Olfactory nerves (CN I)
Maxillary nerve (CN V_2)
Anterior ethmoidal nerve
Internal nasal branches
Nerve of pterygoid canal
Pterygopalatine ganglion
Nasal branch of anterior superior alveolar nerve
Posterolateral nasal branches of maxillary nerve
Internal nasal branch of infra-orbital nerve
CN V_1
CN V_2
CN V_2 general sensory zone
(inferoposterior to dotted line)
Nasopalatine nerve
Palatine nerves Greater Lesser
Pharyngeal nerve
A. Medial view of nasal wall
Olfactory bulb
Sphenoidal sinus
Anterior ethmoidal nerve (CN V_1)
Internal nasal branch of infra-orbital nerve (CN V_1)
CN V_1
CN V_2
Nasopalatine nerve (CN V_2)
Greater Lesser Palatine nerves (CN V_2)
B. Lateral view of nasal septum

7.71 INNERVATION OF NASAL WALL AND SEPTUM

A. Lateral wall of nose. *Dashed diagonal lines* demarcate CN V_1 and CN V_2 general sensory zones. The olfactory neuroepithelium is in the superior part of the lateral and septal walls of the nasal cavity. The central processes of the olfactory neurosensory cells of each side form approximately 20 bundles that together form an olfactory nerve (CN I). **B.** Nasal septum. The nasopalatine nerve from the pterygopalatine ganglion supplies the posteroinferior septum, and the anterior ethmoidal nerve (branch of V_1) supplies the anterosuperior septum.

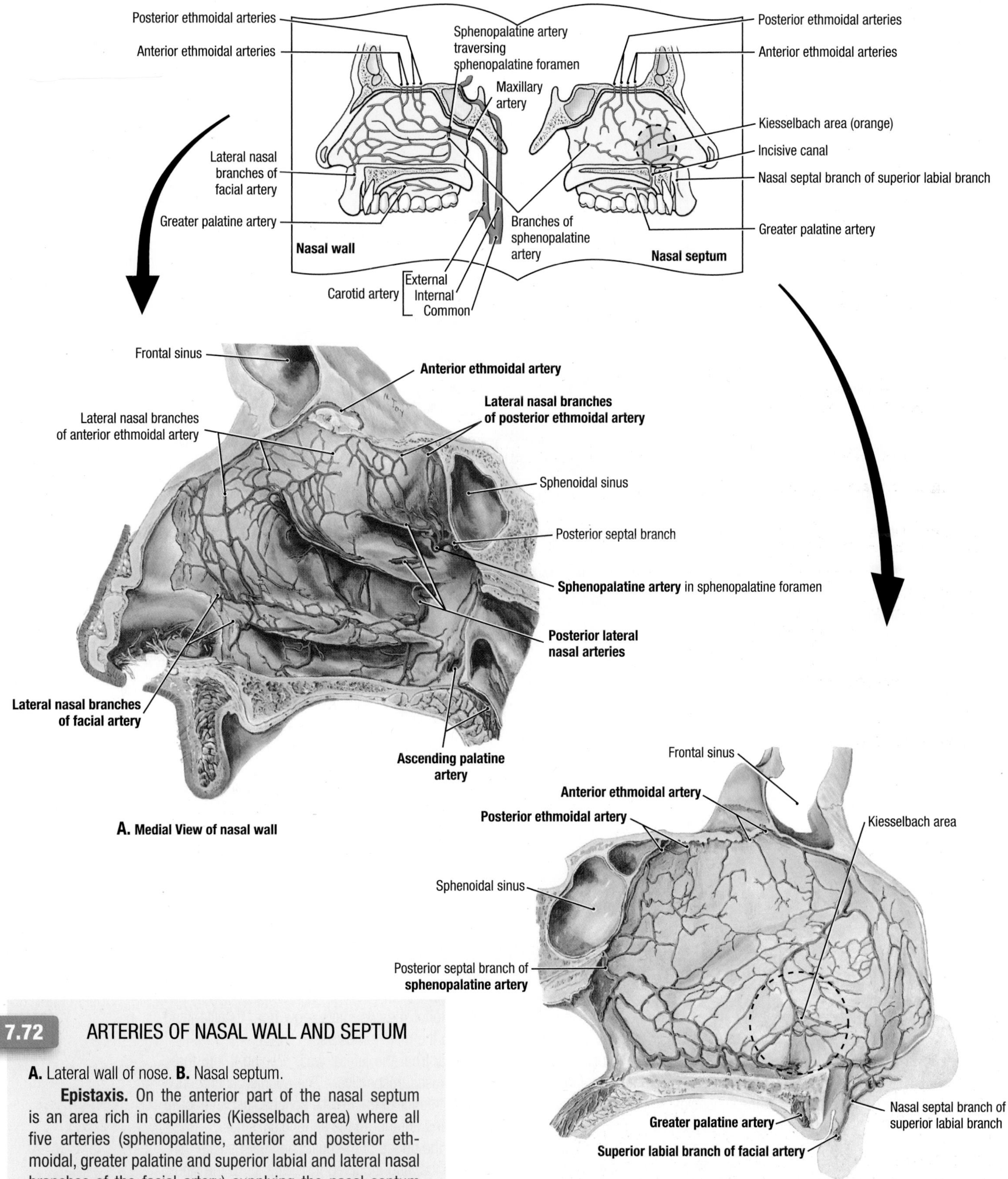
Posterior ethmoidal arteries
Anterior ethmoidal arteries
Sphenopalatine artery traversing sphenopalatine foramen
Maxillary artery
Lateral nasal branches of facial artery
Greater palatine artery
Nasal wall
Branches of sphenopalatine artery
Carotid artery
External
Internal
Common
Posterior ethmoidal arteries
Anterior ethmoidal arteries
Kiesselbach area (orange)
Incisive canal
Nasal septal branch of superior labial branch
Greater palatine artery
Nasal septum
Frontal sinus
Anterior ethmoidal artery
Lateral nasal branches of anterior ethmoidal artery
Lateral nasal branches of posterior ethmoidal artery
Sphenoidal sinus
Posterior septal branch
Sphenopalatine artery in sphenopalatine foramen
Posterior lateral nasal arteries
Lateral nasal branches of facial artery
Ascending palatine artery
Frontal sinus
Anterior ethmoidal artery
Posterior ethmoidal artery
Kiesselbach area
Sphenoidal sinus
Posterior septal branch of sphenopalatine artery
Greater palatine artery
Nasal septal branch of superior labial branch
Superior labial branch of facial artery

A. Medial View of nasal wall

B. Lateral View of Nasal Septum

7.72 ARTERIES OF NASAL WALL AND SEPTUM

A. Lateral wall of nose. **B.** Nasal septum.

Epistaxis. On the anterior part of the nasal septum is an area rich in capillaries (Kiesselbach area) where all five arteries (sphenopalatine, anterior and posterior ethmoidal, greater palatine and superior labial and lateral nasal branches of the facial artery) supplying the nasal septum anastomose. This area is often where profuse bleeding from the nose (epistaxis) occurs.

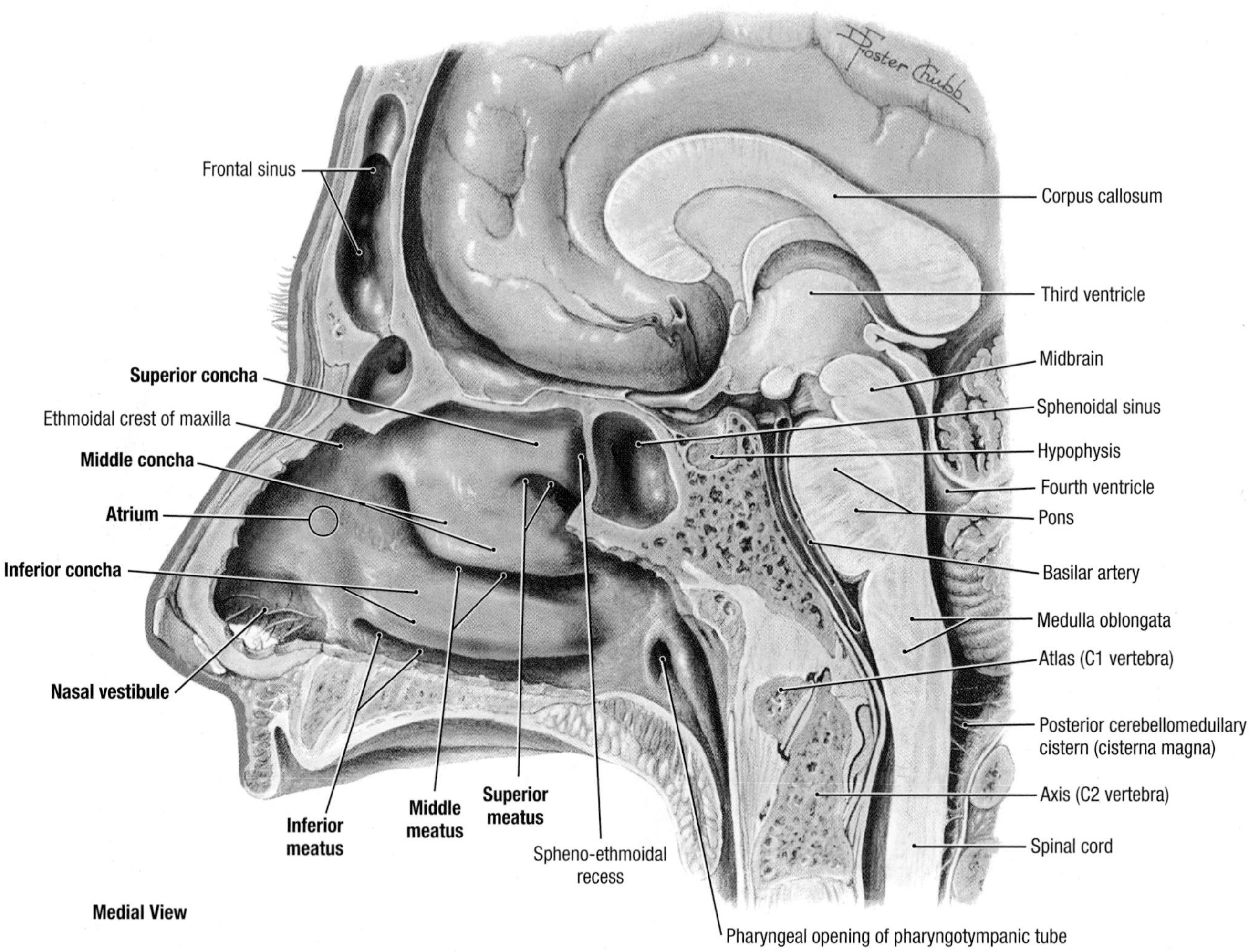
Frontal sinus
Corpus callosum
Third ventricle
Midbrain
Superior concha
Sphenoidal sinus
Ethmoidal crest of maxilla
Hypophysis
Middle concha
Fourth ventricle
Atrium
Pons
Inferior concha
Basilar artery
Medulla oblongata
Atlas (C1 vertebra)
Nasal vestibule
Posterior cerebellomedullary cistern (cisterna magna)
Axis (C2 vertebra)
Superior meatus
Middle meatus
Inferior meatus
Spinal cord
Spheno-ethmoidal recess
Medial View
Pharyngeal opening of pharyngotympanic tube

7.73 RIGHT HALF OF HEMISECTED HEAD DEMONSTRATING UPPER RESPIRATORY TRACT

- The vestibule is superior to the nostril and anterior to the inferior meatus; hairs grow from its skin-lined surface. The atrium is superior to the vestibule and anterior to the middle meatus.
- The inferior and middle conchae curve inferiorly and medially from the lateral wall, dividing it into three nearly equal parts and covering the inferior and middle meatuses, respectively. The middle concha ends inferior to the sphenoidal sinus, and the inferior concha ends inferior to the middle concha, just anterior to the orifice of the auditory tube. The superior concha is small and anterior to the sphenoidal sinus.
- The roof comprises an anterior sloping part corresponding to the bridge of the nose; an intermediate horizontal part; a perpendicular part anterior to the sphenoidal sinus; and a curved part, inferior to the sinus, that is continuous with the roof of the nasopharynx.

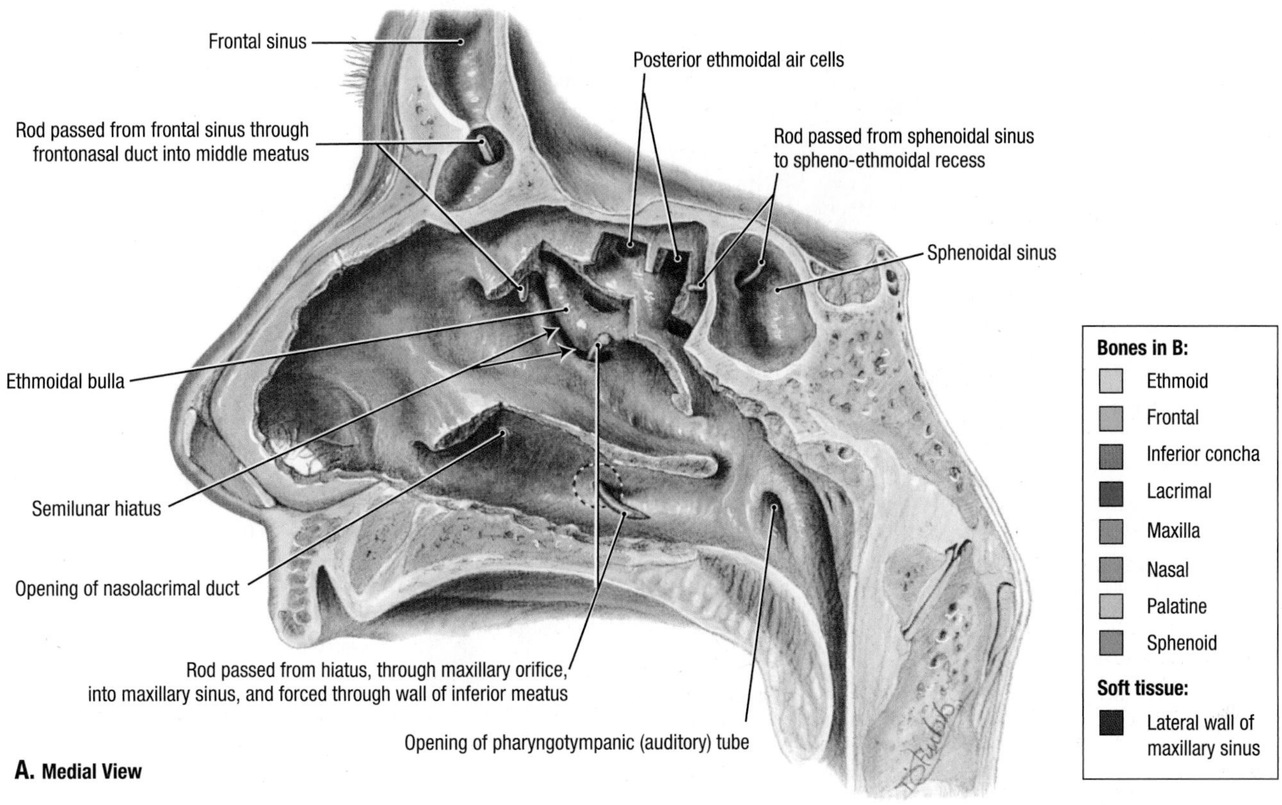
Frontal sinus
Posterior ethmoidal air cells
Rod passed from frontal sinus through frontonasal duct into middle meatus
Rod passed from sphenoidal sinus to spheno-ethmoidal recess
Sphenoidal sinus
Ethmoidal bulla
Semilunar hiatus
Opening of nasolacrimal duct
Rod passed from hiatus, through maxillary orifice, into maxillary sinus, and forced through wall of inferior meatus
Opening of pharyngotympanic (auditory) tube
Bones in B:
Ethmoid
Frontal
Inferior concha
Lacrimal
Maxilla
Nasal
Palatine
Sphenoid
Soft tissue:
Lateral wall of maxillary sinus

A. Medial View

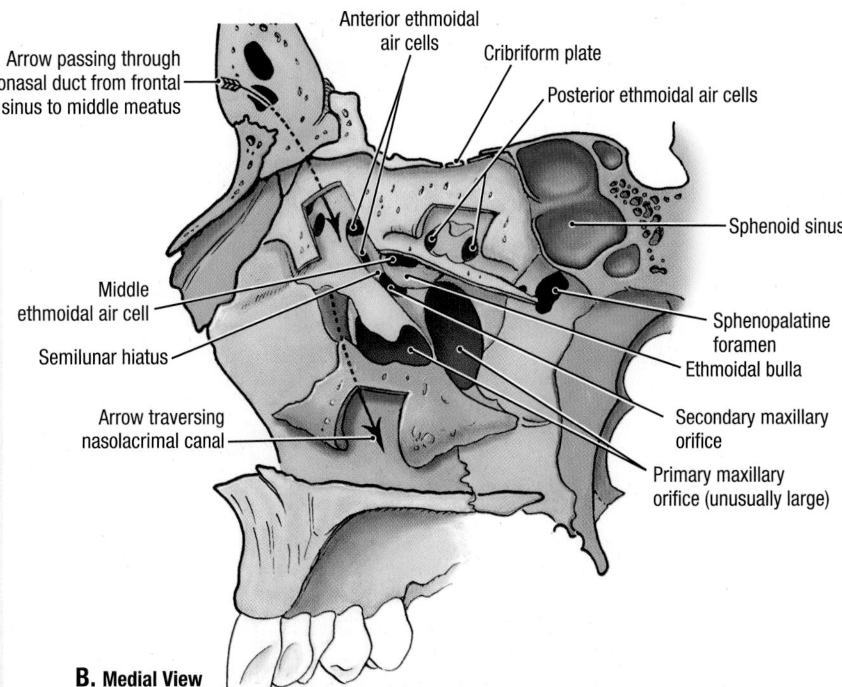
Anterior ethmoidal air cells
Cribriform plate
Arrow passing through frontonasal duct from frontal sinus to middle meatus
Posterior ethmoidal air cells
Sphenoid sinus
Middle ethmoidal air cell
Sphenopalatine foramen
Semilunar hiatus
Ethmoidal bulla
Secondary maxillary orifice
Arrow traversing nasolacrimal canal
Primary maxillary orifice (unusually large)

B. Medial View

7.74 COMMUNICATIONS THROUGH NASAL WALL

A. Dissection. Parts of the superior, middle, and inferior conchae are cut away to reveal the openings of the air sinuses. **B.** Diagrams of the bones and openings of the lateral wall of nasal cavity following dissection. Note one *arrow* passing from the frontal sinus through the frontonasal duct into the middle meatus and another *arrow* coming from the anteromedial orbit via the nasolacrimal canal.

Rhinits. The nasal mucosa becomes swollen and inflamed (rhinitis) during upper respiratory infections and allergic reactions (e.g., hay fever). Swelling of this mucous membrane occurs readily because of its vascularity and abundant mucosal glands. Infections of the nasal cavities may spread to the anterior cranial fossa through the cribriform plate, nasopharynx and retropharyngeal soft tissues, middle ear through the pharyngotympanic (auditory) tube, paranasal sinuses, lacrimal apparatus, and conjunctiva.

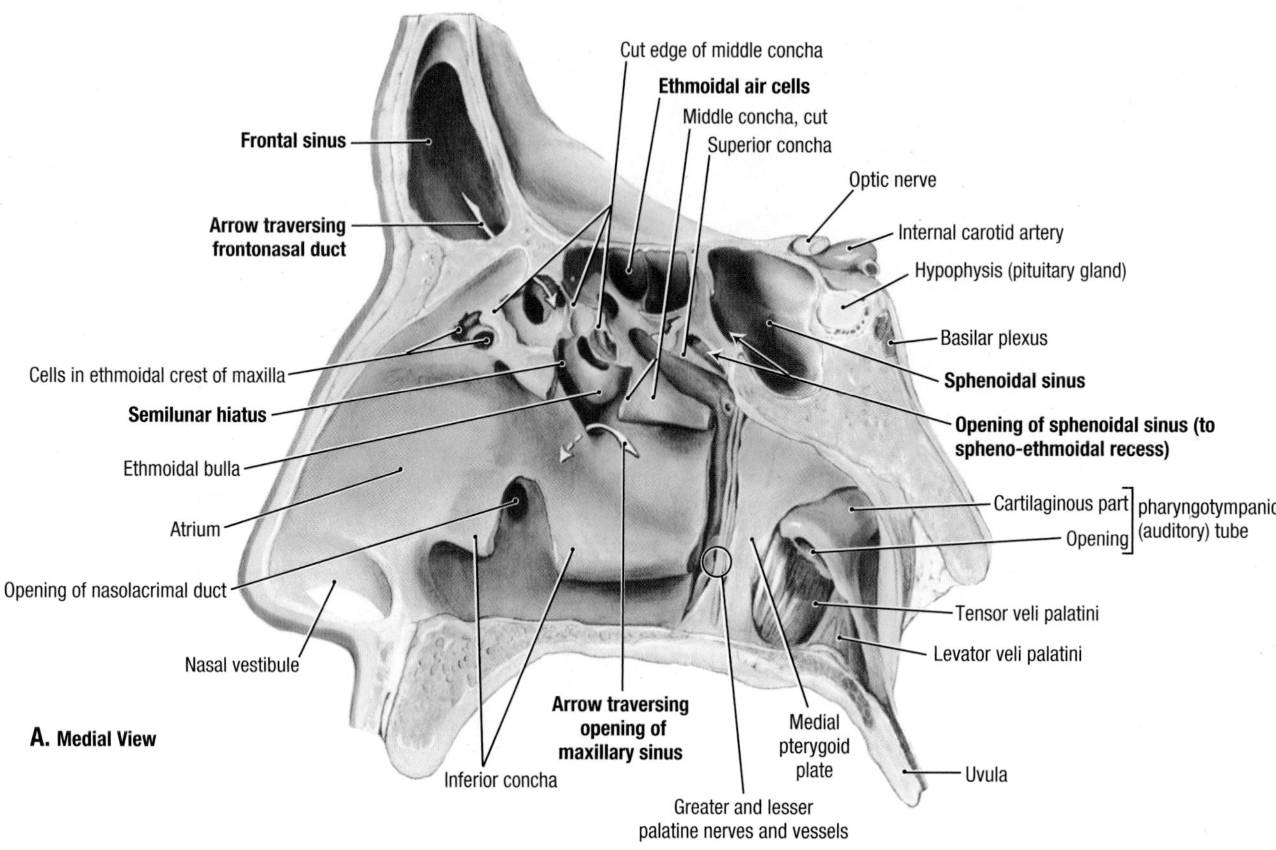
Cut edge of middle concha
Ethmoidal air cells
Middle concha, cut
Superior concha
Frontal sinus
Optic nerve
Internal carotid artery
Arrow traversing frontonasal duct
Hypophysis (pituitary gland)
Basilar plexus
Sphenoidal sinus
Cells in ethmoidal crest of maxilla
Semilunar hiatus
Opening of sphenoidal sinus (to spheno-ethmoidal recess)
Ethmoidal bulla
Atrium
Cartilaginous part
Opening
pharyngotympanic (auditory) tube
Opening of nasolacrimal duct
Tensor veli palatini
Levator veli palatini
Nasal vestibule
Arrow traversing opening of maxillary sinus
Medial pterygoid plate
Uvula
Inferior concha
Greater and lesser palatine nerves and vessels

A. Medial View

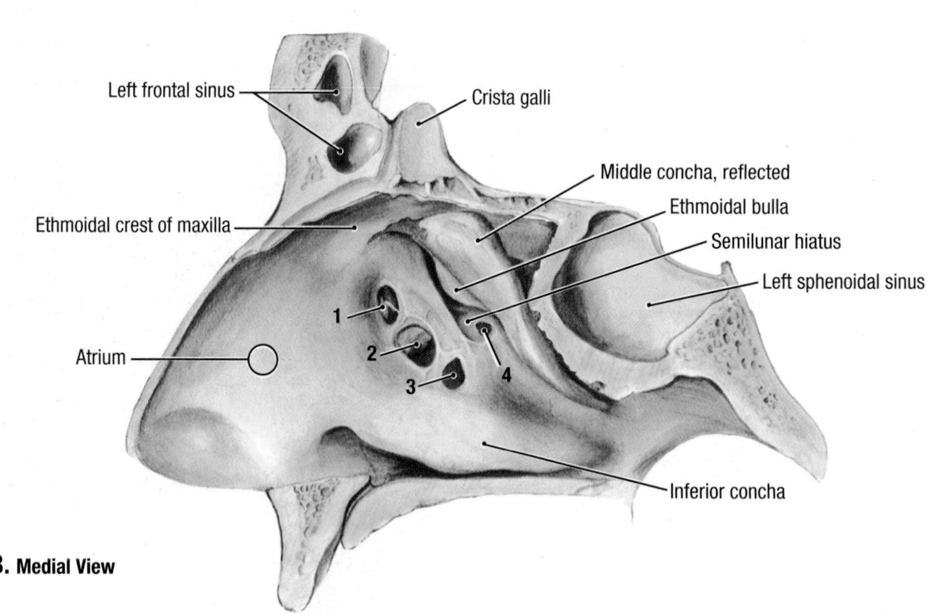
Left frontal sinus
Crista galli
Middle concha, reflected
Ethmoidal bulla
Ethmoidal crest of maxilla
Semilunar hiatus
Left sphenoidal sinus
1
2
3
4
Atrium
Inferior concha

B. Medial View

7.75 PARANASAL SINUSES, OPENINGS, AND PALATINE MUSCLES IN NASAL WALL

A. Dissection. Parts of the middle and inferior conchae and lateral wall of the nasal cavity are cut away to expose the nerves and vessels in the palatine canal and the extrinsic palatine muscles. **B.** Accessory maxillary orifices. In addition to the primary, or normal, ostium (not shown), there are four secondary, or acquired, ostia (numbered 1 to 4).

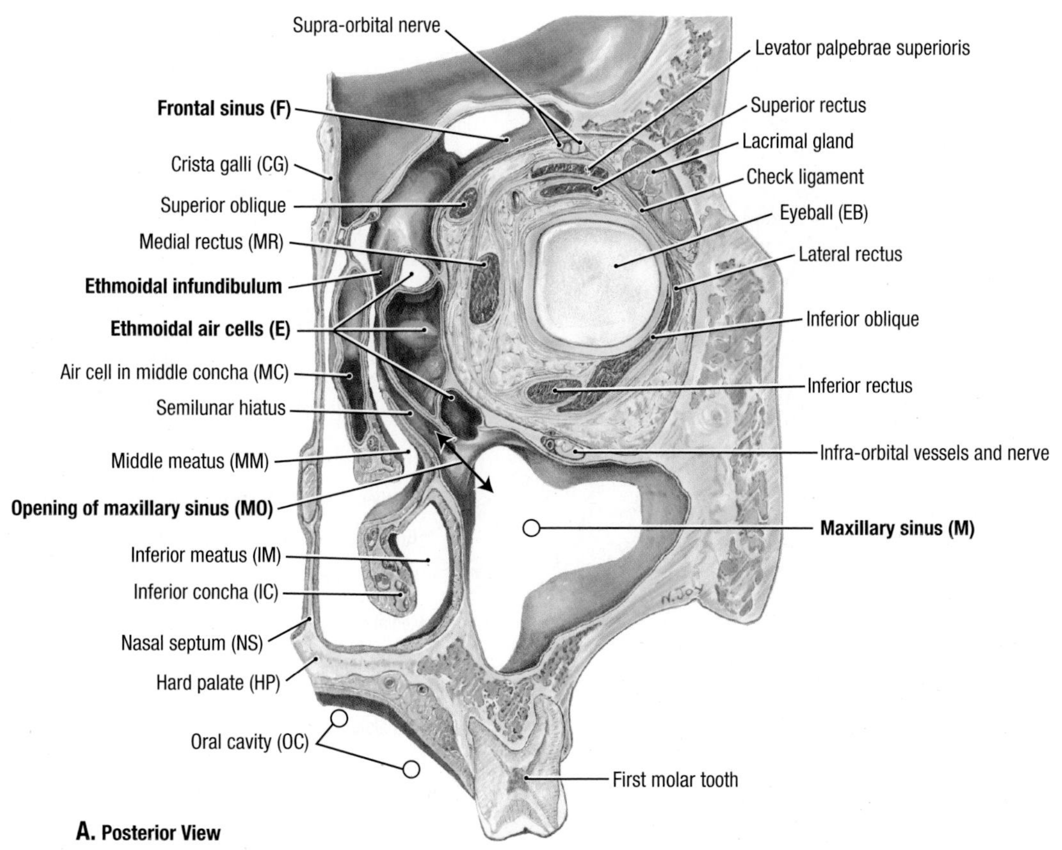
Supra-orbital nerve
Levator palpebrae superioris
Frontal sinus (F)
Superior rectus
Lacrimal gland
Crista galli (CG)
Check ligament
Superior oblique
Eyeball (EB)
Medial rectus (MR)
Lateral rectus
Ethmoidal infundibulum
Ethmoidal air cells (E)
Inferior oblique
Air cell in middle concha (MC)
Inferior rectus
Semilunar hiatus
Middle meatus (MM)
Infra-orbital vessels and nerve
Opening of maxillary sinus (MO)
Maxillary sinus (M)
Inferior meatus (IM)
Inferior concha (IC)
Nasal septum (NS)
Hard palate (HP)
Oral cavity (OC)
First molar tooth

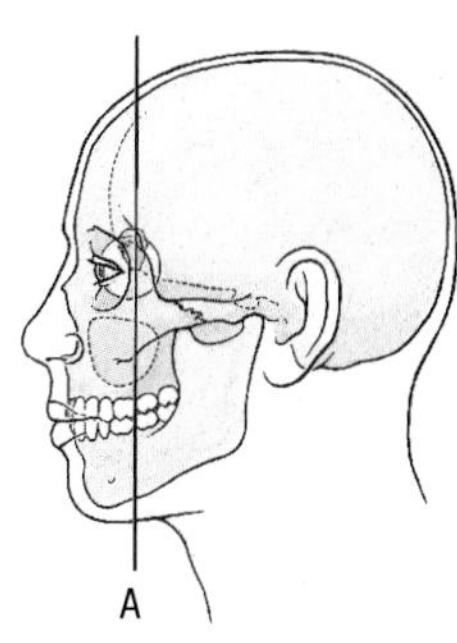
A

A. Posterior View

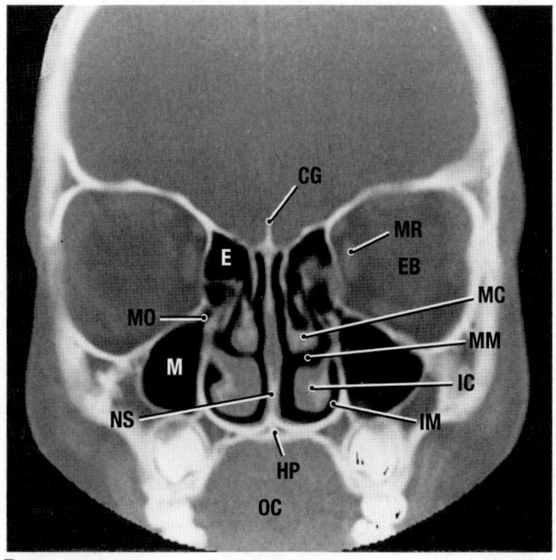
CG
MR
E
EB
MC
MO
MM
M
IC
NS
IM
HP
OC

B. Posterior View

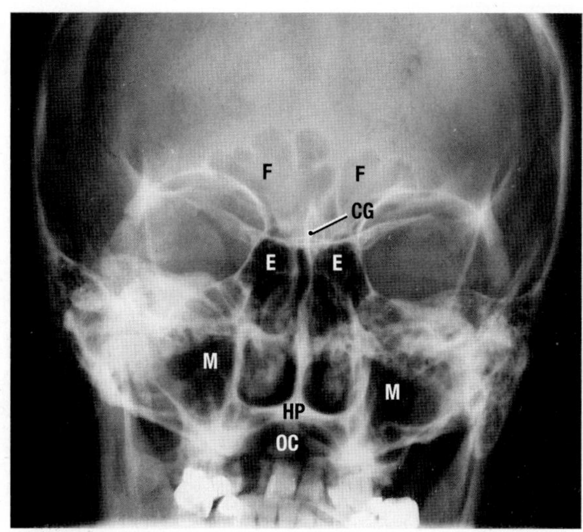
F
F
CG
E
E
M
M
HP
OC

C. Anteroposterior View

7.76 PARANASAL SINUSES AND NASAL CAVITY

A. Coronal section of right side of the head. **B.** CT scan. **C.** Radiograph of cranium. Letters in **B** and **C** refer to structures labeled in **A**.

If nasal drainage is blocked, **infections of the ethmoidal cells** of the ethmoidal sinuses may break through the fragile medial wall of the orbit. Severe infections from this source may cause blindness but could also affect the dural sheath of the optic nerve, causing **optic neuritis**.

During **removal of a maxillary molar tooth,** a fracture of a root may occur. If proper retrieval methods are not used, a piece of the root may be driven superiorly into the maxillary sinus.

Radiographs/CT scans of the frontal sinuses may be used for forensic identification of unknown individuals. The frontal sinuses are unique to each person, much like fingerprints.

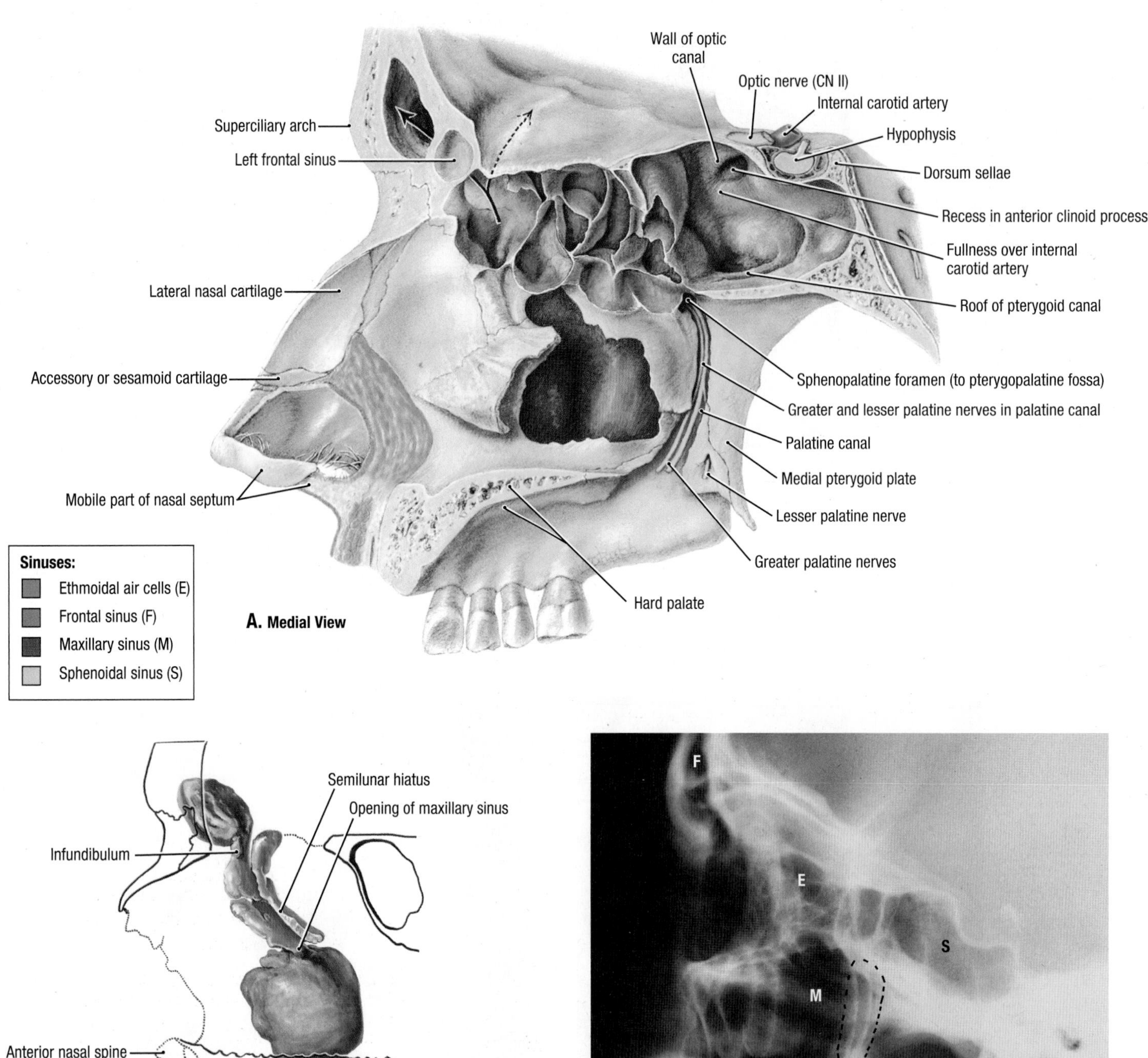

Wall of optic canal
Optic nerve (CN II)
Internal carotid artery
Hypophysis
Dorsum sellae
Recess in anterior clinoid process
Fullness over internal carotid artery
Roof of pterygoid canal
Superciliary arch
Left frontal sinus
Lateral nasal cartilage
Accessory or sesamoid cartilage
Sphenopalatine foramen (to pterygopalatine fossa)
Greater and lesser palatine nerves in palatine canal
Palatine canal
Medial pterygoid plate
Mobile part of nasal septum
Lesser palatine nerve
Greater palatine nerves
Hard palate
Sinuses:
Ethmoidal air cells (E)
Frontal sinus (F)
Maxillary sinus (M)
Sphenoidal sinus (S)
A. Medial View
Semilunar hiatus
Opening of maxillary sinus
Infundibulum
Anterior nasal spine
Hard palate (HP)
B. Medial View
F
E
S
M
HP
P
C. Lateral View

7.77 PARANASAL SINUSES

A. Opened sinuses, color coded. **B.** Cast of frontal and maxillary sinuses. **C.** Radiograph of cranium. *P*, pharynx; *dotted lines*, pterygopalatine fossa. Letters refer to structures labeled in **B. Maxillary sinusitis.** The maxillary sinuses are the most commonly infected, probably because their ostia are small and located high on their superomedial walls, a poor location for natural drainage of the sinus. When the mucous membrane of the sinus is congested, the maxillary ostia often are obstructed. The maxillary sinus can be cannulated and drained by passing a canula from the nares through the maxillary ostium into the sinus.

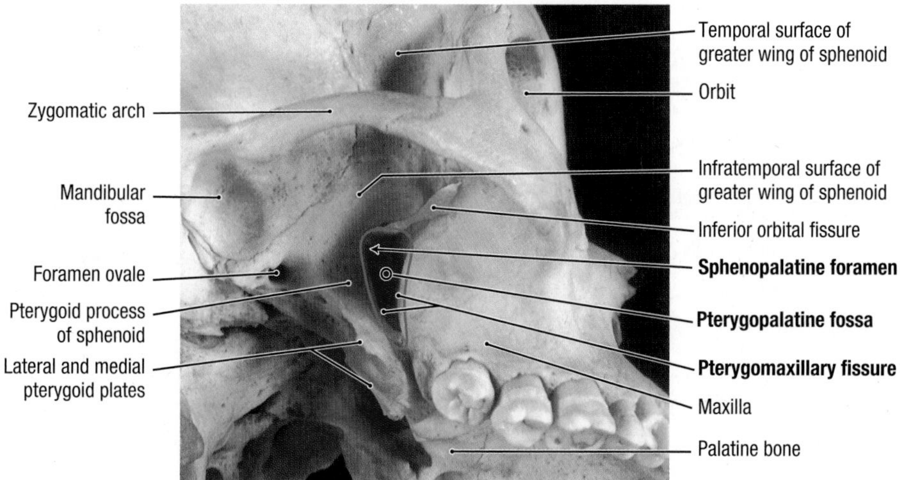
Temporal surface of greater wing of sphenoid
Orbit
Zygomatic arch
Infratemporal surface of greater wing of sphenoid
Mandibular fossa
Inferior orbital fissure
Sphenopalatine foramen
Foramen ovale
Pterygopalatine fossa
Pterygoid process of sphenoid
Pterygomaxillary fissure
Lateral and medial pterygoid plates
Maxilla
Palatine bone

A. **Inferolateral and slightly posterior view, looking into infratemporal and pterygopalatine fossae**

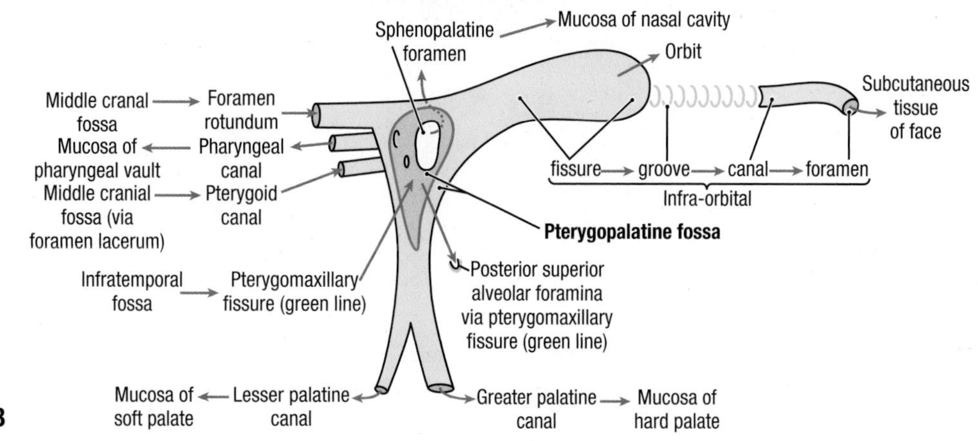
Sphenopalatine foramen
Mucosa of nasal cavity
Orbit
Subcutaneous tissue of face
Middle cranial fossa
Foramen rotundum
Mucosa of pharyngeal vault
Pharyngeal canal
Middle cranial fossa (via foramen lacerum)
Pterygoid canal
fissure
groove
canal
foramen
Infra-orbital
Pterygopalatine fossa
Infratemporal fossa
Pterygomaxillary fissure (green line)
Posterior superior alveolar foramina via pterygomaxillary fissure (green line)
Mucosa of soft palate
Lesser palatine canal
Greater palatine canal
Mucosa of hard palate

B

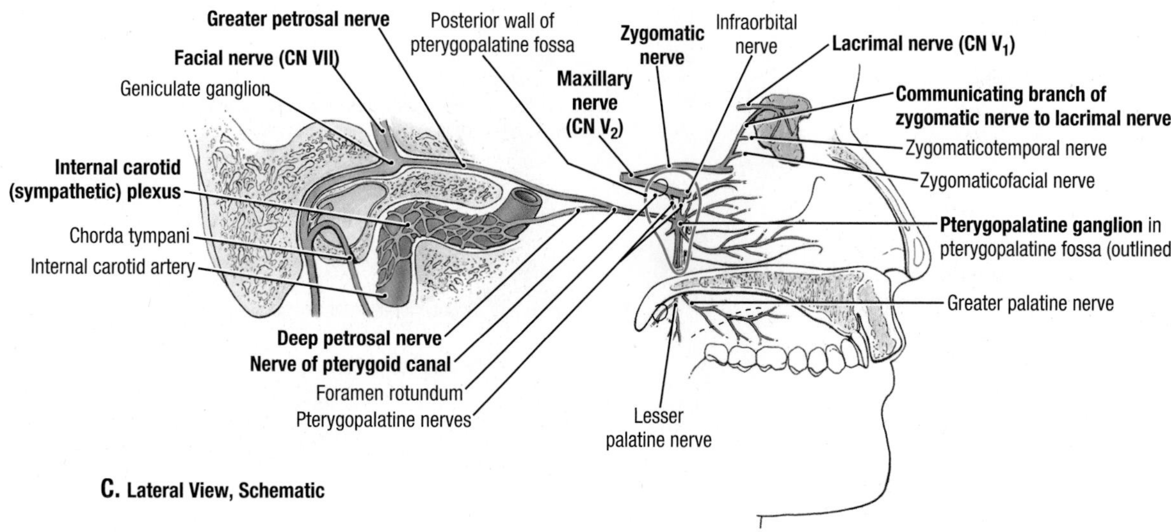
Greater petrosal nerve
Posterior wall of pterygopalatine fossa
Zygomatic nerve
Infraorbital nerve
Lacrimal nerve (CN V1)
Facial nerve (CN VII)
Geniculate ganglion
Maxillary nerve (CN V2)
Communicating branch of zygomatic nerve to lacrimal nerve
Zygomaticotemporal nerve
Internal carotid (sympathetic) plexus
Zygomaticofacial nerve
Chorda tympani
Pterygopalatine ganglion in pterygopalatine fossa (outlined)
Internal carotid artery
Greater palatine nerve
Deep petrosal nerve
Nerve of pterygoid canal
Foramen rotundum
Pterygopalatine nerves
Lesser palatine nerve

C. **Lateral View, Schematic**

7.78 PTERYGOPALATINE FOSSA

A. Bony relationships. The pterygopalatine fossa is a small pyramidal space inferior to the apex of the orbit. It lies between the pterygoid process of the sphenoid and the posterior aspect of the maxilla anteriorly. **B.** Communications. **C.** Pterygopalatine ganglion and related nerves.

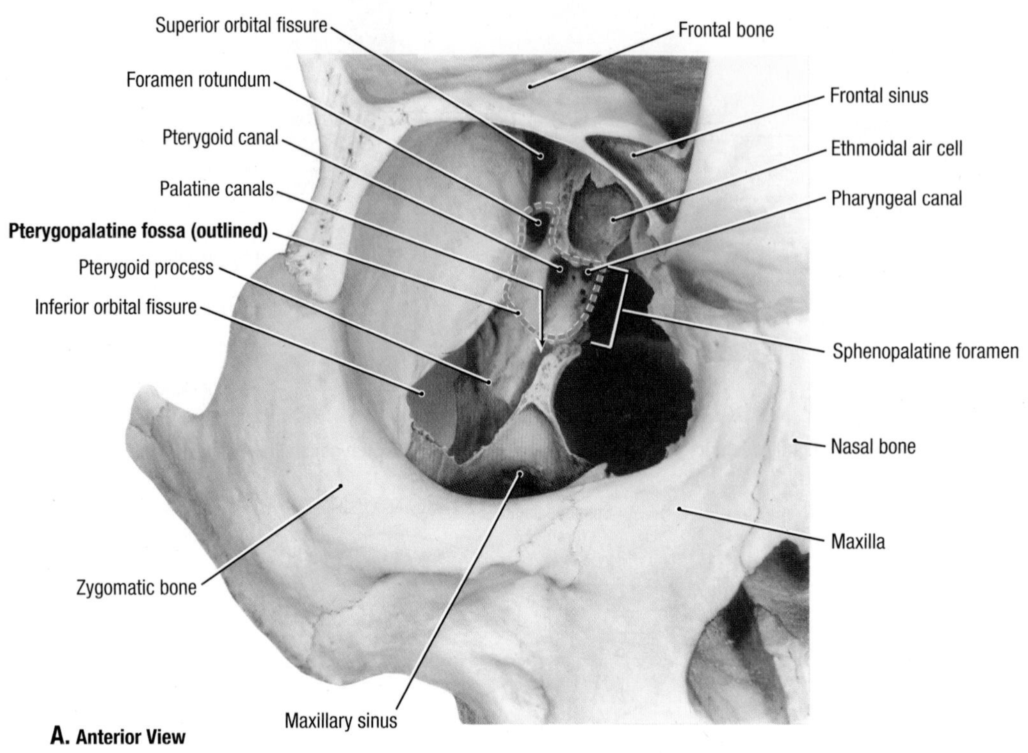
Superior orbital fissure
Foramen rotundum
Pterygoid canal
Palatine canals
Pterygopalatine fossa (outlined)
Pterygoid process
Inferior orbital fissure
Zygomatic bone
Maxillary sinus
Frontal bone
Frontal sinus
Ethmoidal air cell
Pharyngeal canal
Sphenopalatine foramen
Nasal bone
Maxilla

A. Anterior View

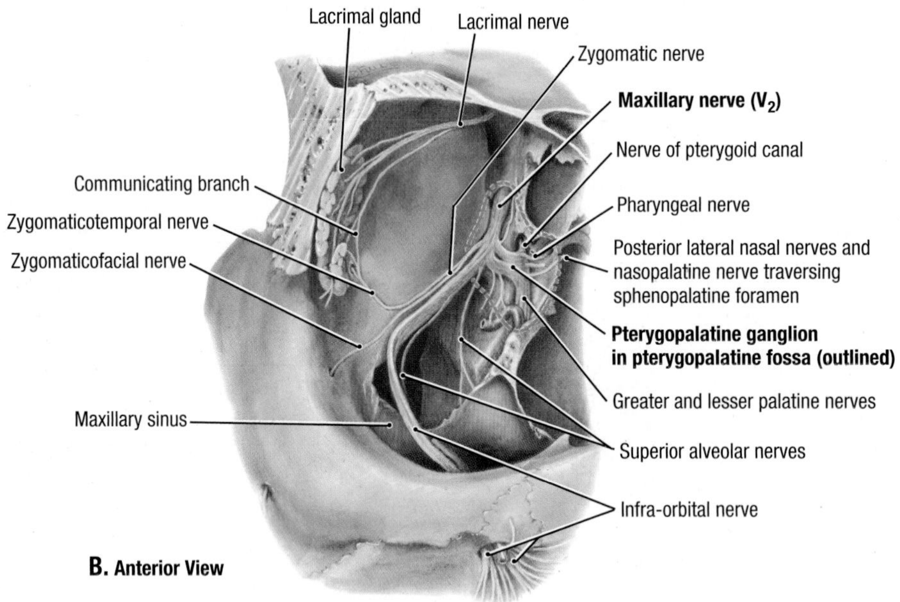
Lacrimal gland
Lacrimal nerve
Zygomatic nerve
Maxillary nerve (V_2)
Nerve of pterygoid canal
Pharyngeal nerve
Posterior lateral nasal nerves and nasopalatine nerve traversing sphenopalatine foramen
Pterygopalatine ganglion in pterygopalatine fossa (outlined)
Greater and lesser palatine nerves
Superior alveolar nerves
Infra-orbital nerve
Communicating branch
Zygomaticotemporal nerve
Zygomaticofacial nerve
Maxillary sinus

B. Anterior View

7.79 NERVES OF THE PTERYGOPALATINE FOSSA

A. Bones and foramina, orbital approach. **B.** Vessels and nerves, orbital approach. In **A** and **B,** the pterygopalatine fossa has been exposed through the floor of the orbit and maxillary sinus.

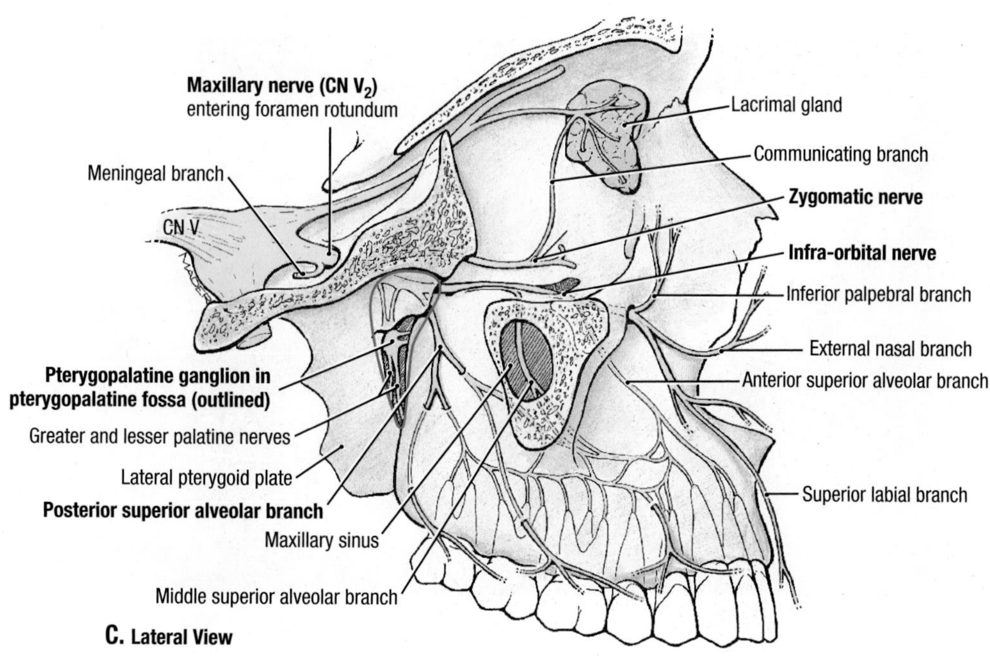
Maxillary nerve (CN V_2) entering foramen rotundum
Meningeal branch
CN V
Lacrimal gland
Communicating branch
Zygomatic nerve
Infra-orbital nerve
Inferior palpebral branch
External nasal branch
Anterior superior alveolar branch
Pterygopalatine ganglion in pterygopalatine fossa (outlined)
Greater and lesser palatine nerves
Lateral pterygoid plate
Posterior superior alveolar branch
Maxillary sinus
Middle superior alveolar branch
Superior labial branch

C. Lateral View

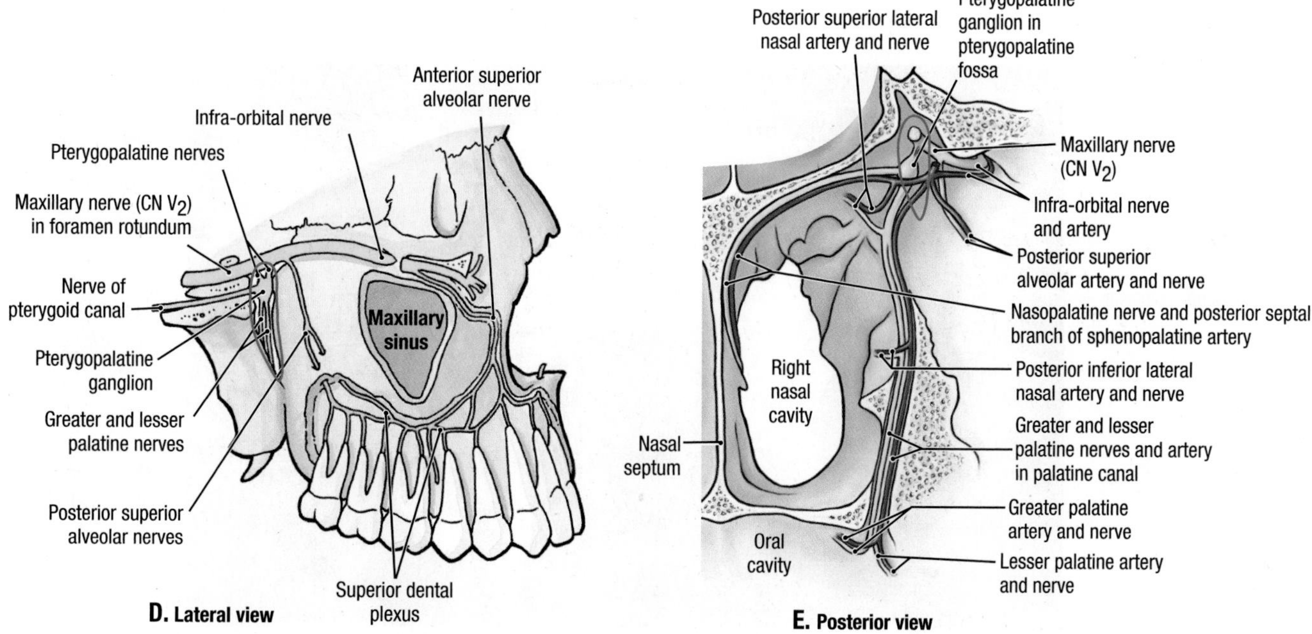
Anterior superior alveolar nerve
Infra-orbital nerve
Pterygopalatine nerves
Maxillary nerve (CN V_2) in foramen rotundum
Nerve of pterygoid canal
Pterygopalatine ganglion
Greater and lesser palatine nerves
Posterior superior alveolar nerves
Maxillary sinus
Superior dental plexus
Posterior superior lateral nasal artery and nerve
Pterygopalatine ganglion in pterygopalatine fossa
Maxillary nerve (CN V_2)
Infra-orbital nerve and artery
Posterior superior alveolar artery and nerve
Nasopalatine nerve and posterior septal branch of sphenopalatine artery
Posterior inferior lateral nasal artery and nerve
Greater and lesser palatine nerves and artery in palatine canal
Greater palatine artery and nerve
Lesser palatine artery and nerve
Right nasal cavity
Nasal septum
Oral cavity

D. Lateral view

E. Posterior view

7.79 NERVES OF THE PTERYGOPALATINE FOSSA *(CONTINUED)*

C. Maxillary nerve (CN V_2) and branches. **D.** The fossa is viewed laterally. Part of the wall of the maxillary sinus has been removed. **E.** Nasopalatine and greater and lesser palatine nerves.

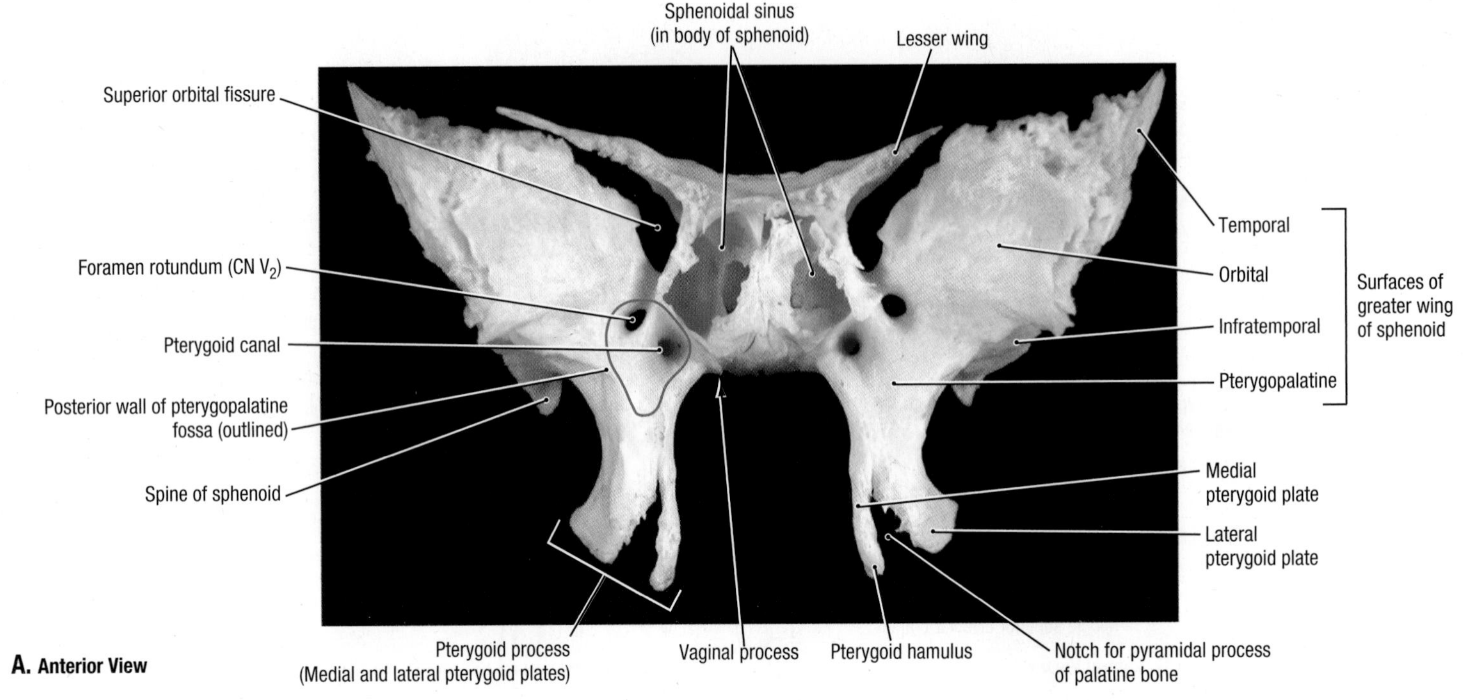
Sphenoidal sinus (in body of sphenoid)
Lesser wing
Superior orbital fissure
Foramen rotundum (CN V_2)
Pterygoid canal
Posterior wall of pterygopalatine fossa (outlined)
Spine of sphenoid
Temporal
Orbital
Infratemporal
Pterygopalatine
Surfaces of greater wing of sphenoid
Medial pterygoid plate
Lateral pterygoid plate
Pterygoid process (Medial and lateral pterygoid plates)
Vaginal process
Pterygoid hamulus
Notch for pyramidal process of palatine bone

A. Anterior View

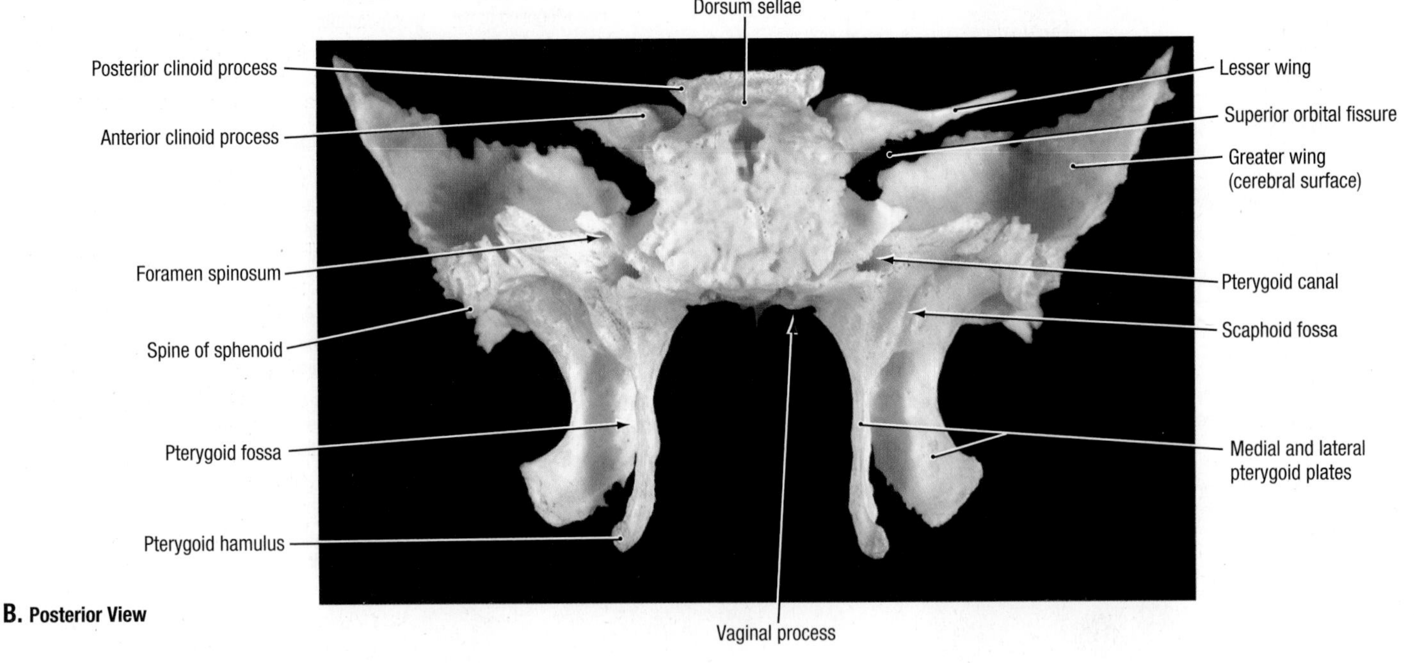
Dorsum sellae
Posterior clinoid process
Anterior clinoid process
Foramen spinosum
Spine of sphenoid
Pterygoid fossa
Pterygoid hamulus
Lesser wing
Superior orbital fissure
Greater wing (cerebral surface)
Pterygoid canal
Scaphoid fossa
Medial and lateral pterygoid plates
Vaginal process

B. Posterior View

7.80 SPHENOID BONE: FEATURES AND RELATIONSHIP TO PTERYGOPALATINE FOSSA

A. The pterygopalatine fossa communicates posterosuperiorly with the middle cranial fossa through the foramen rotundum and pterygoid canal. **B.** Bony features and tensor veli palatini.

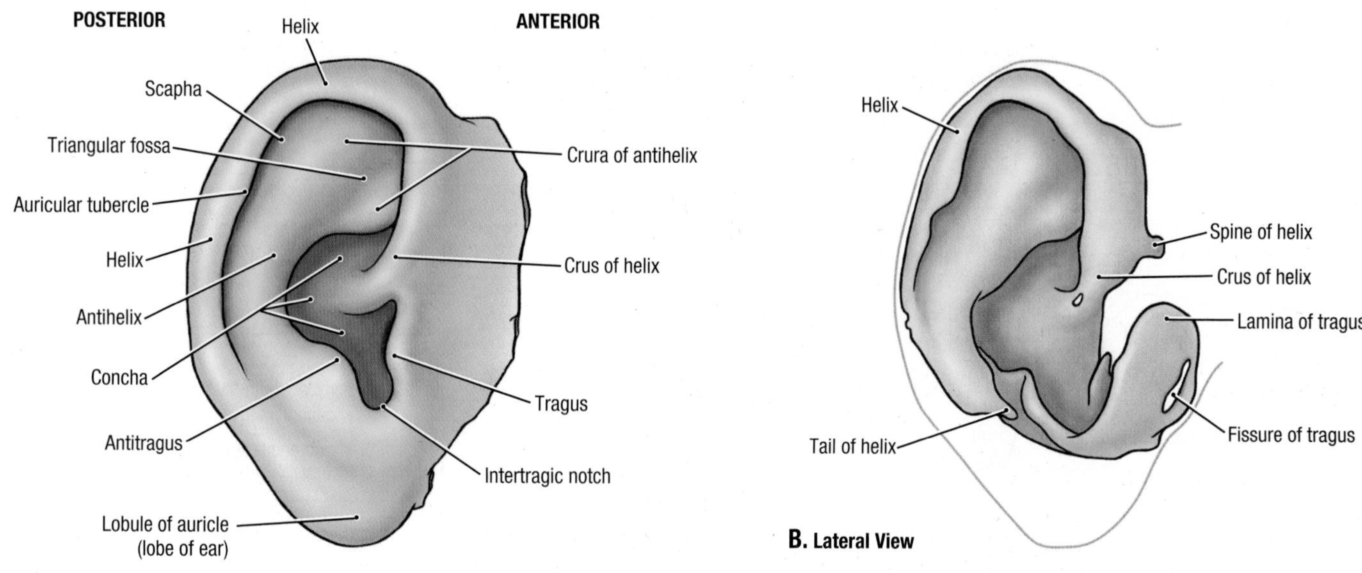
POSTERIOR
Helix
ANTERIOR
Scapha
Triangular fossa
Crura of antihelix
Auricular tubercle
Helix
Crus of helix
Antihelix
Concha
Tragus
Antitragus
Intertragic notch
Lobule of auricle
(lobe of ear)
Helix
Spine of helix
Crus of helix
Lamina of tragus
Fissure of tragus
Tail of helix

A. Lateral View

B. Lateral View

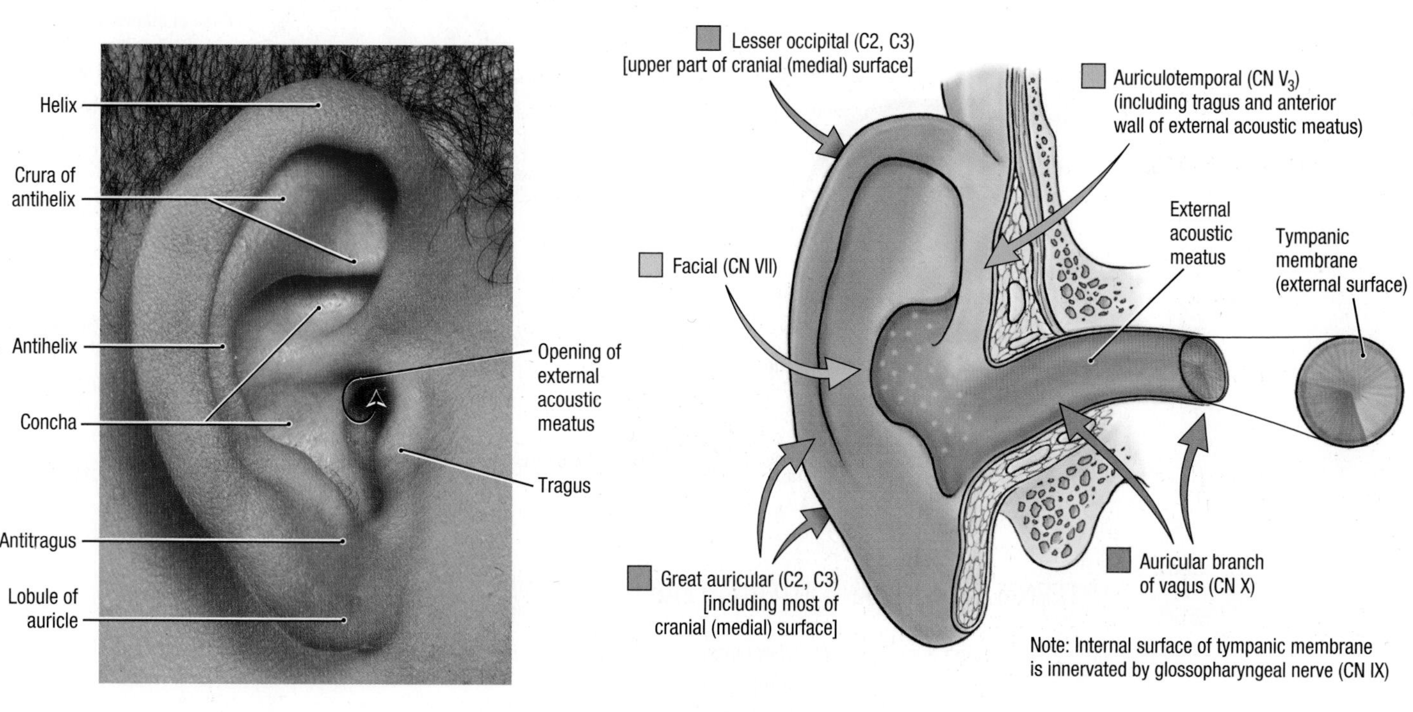
Helix
Crura of antihelix
Antihelix
Concha
Antitragus
Lobule of auricle
Opening of external acoustic meatus
Tragus
Lesser occipital (C2, C3) [upper part of cranial (medial) surface]
Auriculotemporal (CN V_3) (including tragus and anterior wall of external acoustic meatus)
Facial (CN VII)
External acoustic meatus
Tympanic membrane (external surface)
Great auricular (C2, C3) [including most of cranial (medial) surface]
Auricular branch of vagus (CN X)
Note: Internal surface of tympanic membrane is innervated by glossopharyngeal nerve (CN IX)

C. Lateral View

D. Schematic Section

7.81 AURICLE

A. Features of auricle. **B.** Cartilage of auricle. **C.** Surface anatomy of auricle. **D.** Sensory innervation.

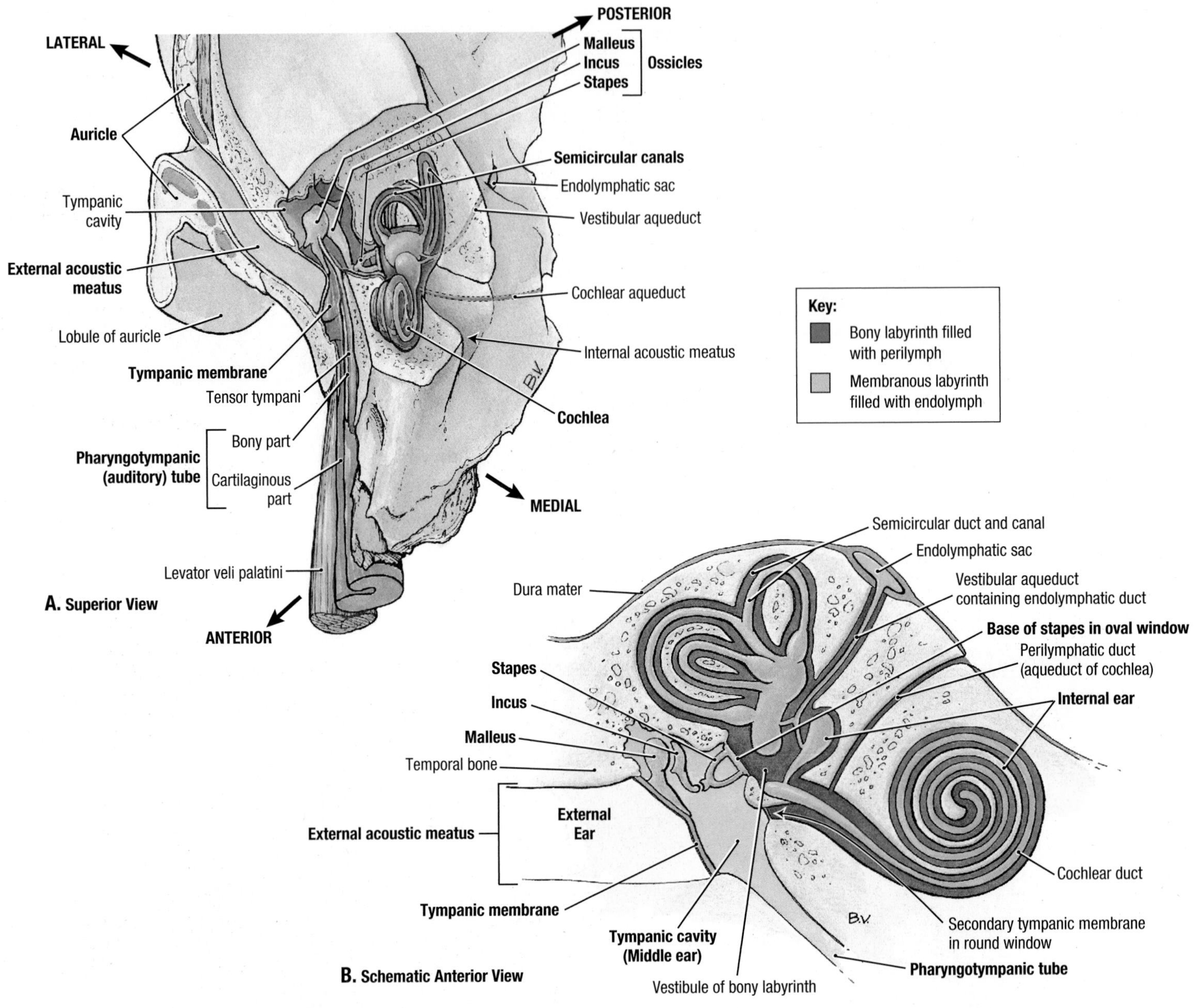
POSTERIOR
LATERAL
Malleus
Incus
Stapes
Ossicles
Auricle
Semicircular canals
Endolymphatic sac
Tympanic cavity
Vestibular aqueduct
External acoustic meatus
Cochlear aqueduct
Lobule of auricle
Internal acoustic meatus
Tympanic membrane
Tensor tympani
Cochlea
Pharyngotympanic (auditory) tube
Bony part
Cartilaginous part
MEDIAL
Levator veli palatini
A. Superior View
ANTERIOR
Key:
Bony labyrinth filled with perilymph
Membranous labyrinth filled with endolymph
Semicircular duct and canal
Endolymphatic sac
Dura mater
Vestibular aqueduct containing endolymphatic duct
Base of stapes in oval window
Perilymphatic duct (aqueduct of cochlea)
Stapes
Incus
Internal ear
Malleus
Temporal bone
External Ear
External acoustic meatus
Cochlear duct
Tympanic membrane
Secondary tympanic membrane in round window
Tympanic cavity (Middle ear)
Pharyngotympanic tube
B. Schematic Anterior View
Vestibule of bony labyrinth

7.82 EXTERNAL, MIDDLE, AND INTERNAL EAR I: OVERVIEWS

A. Right temporal bone and auricle, sectioned in planes of (1) externa acoustic meatus and (2) pharyngotympanic tube. **B.** Schematic section of petrous temporal bone.

- The external ear comprises the auricle and external acoustic (auditory) meatus.
- The middle ear (tympanum) lies between the tympanic membrane and internal ear. Three ossicles extend from the lateral to the medial walls of the tympanum. Of these, the malleus is attached to the tympanic membrane. The stapes is attached by the anular ligament to the oval window, and the incus connects to the malleus and stapes. The pharyngotympanic tube, extending from the nasopharynx, opens into the anterior wall of the tympanic cavity.
- The membranous labyrinth comprises a closed system of membranous tubes and bulbs filled with fluid, endolymph (*orange* in **A** and **B**) and bathed in surrounding fluid, called perilymph (*purple* in **A** and **B**); both membranous labyrinth and perilymph are contained within the bony labyrinth.

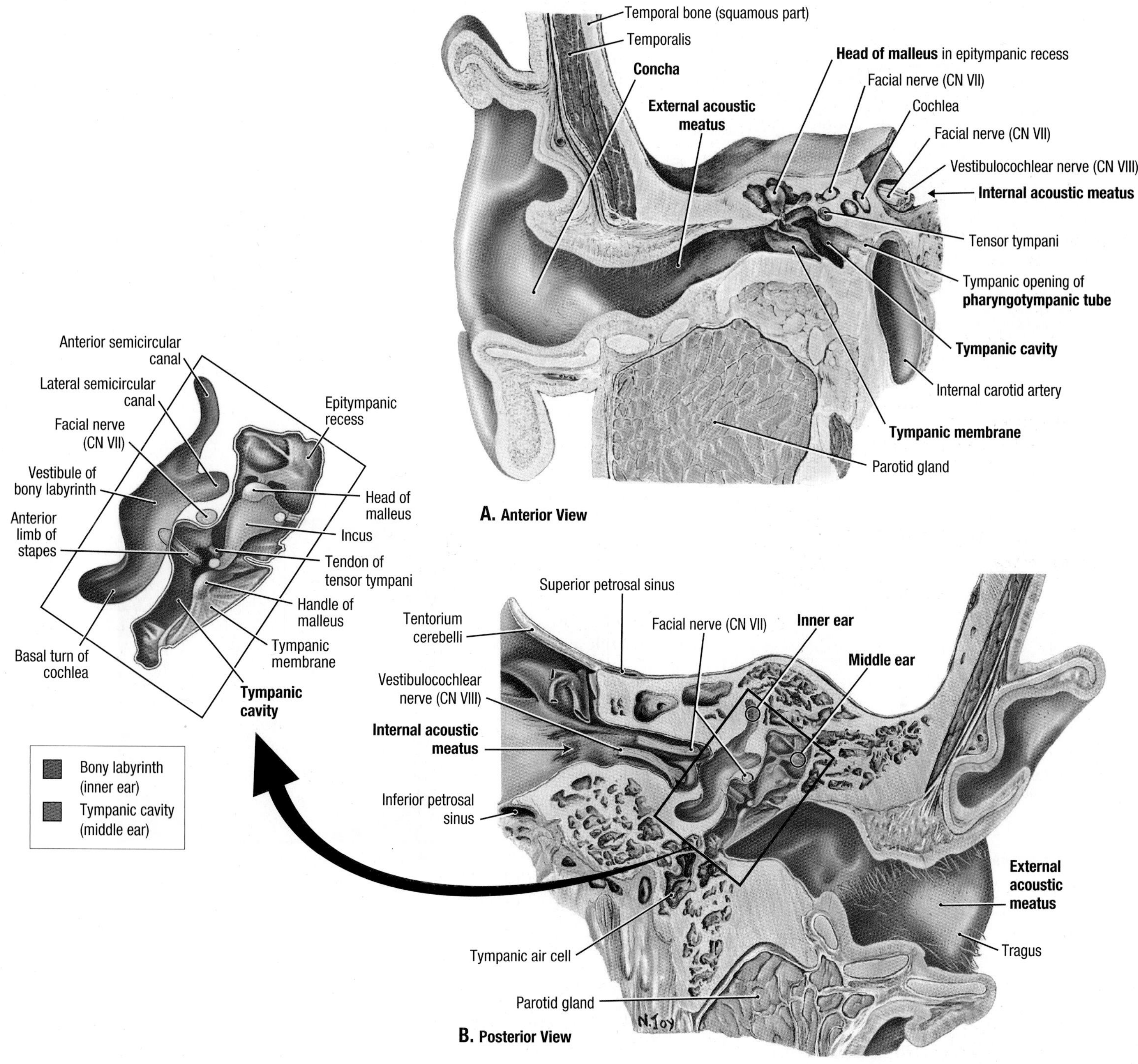
Temporal bone (squamous part)
Temporalis
Concha
External acoustic meatus
Head of malleus in epitympanic recess
Facial nerve (CN VII)
Cochlea
Facial nerve (CN VII)
Vestibulocochlear nerve (CN VIII)
Internal acoustic meatus
Tensor tympani
Tympanic opening of pharyngotympanic tube
Tympanic cavity
Internal carotid artery
Tympanic membrane
Parotid gland
A. Anterior View
Anterior semicircular canal
Lateral semicircular canal
Facial nerve (CN VII)
Vestibule of bony labyrinth
Anterior limb of stapes
Basal turn of cochlea
Epitympanic recess
Head of malleus
Incus
Tendon of tensor tympani
Handle of malleus
Tympanic membrane
Tympanic cavity
Bony labyrinth (inner ear)
Tympanic cavity (middle ear)
Superior petrosal sinus
Tentorium cerebelli
Facial nerve (CN VII)
Inner ear
Middle ear
Vestibulocochlear nerve (CN VIII)
Internal acoustic meatus
Inferior petrosal sinus
External acoustic meatus
Tragus
Tympanic air cell
Parotid gland
B. Posterior View

7.83 EXTERNAL, MIDDLE, AND INTERNAL EAR II: CORONALLY SECTIONED

A. Anterior portion. **B.** Posterior portion. The inset *(outlined by the box)* is an enlargement of the structures of the middle and internal ear as they appear in **B.**

- The external acoustic meatus is about 3 cm long; half is cartilaginous and half is bony. It is narrowest at the isthmus, near the junction of the cartilaginous and bony parts.
- The external acoustic meatus is innervated by the auriculotemporal branch of the mandibular nerve (CN V_3) and the auricular branches of the vagus nerve (CN X); the middle ear is innervated by the glossopharyngeal nerve (CN IX).
- The cartilaginous part of the external acoustic meatus is lined with thick skin; the bony part is lined with thin skin that adheres to the periosteum and forms the outermost layer of the tympanic membrane.

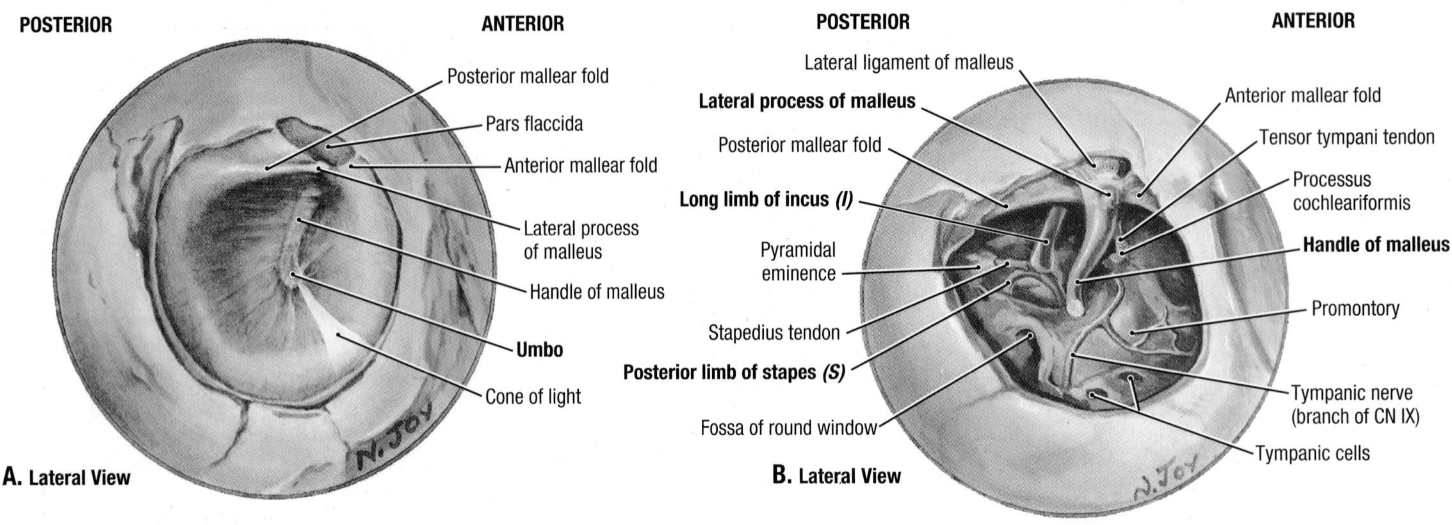
POSTERIOR
ANTERIOR
Posterior mallear fold
Pars flaccida
Anterior mallear fold
Lateral process of malleus
Handle of malleus
Umbo
Cone of light
A. Lateral View
POSTERIOR
ANTERIOR
Lateral ligament of malleus
Lateral process of malleus
Posterior mallear fold
Long limb of incus (I)
Pyramidal eminence
Stapedius tendon
Posterior limb of stapes (S)
Fossa of round window
Anterior mallear fold
Tensor tympani tendon
Processus cochleariformis
Handle of malleus
Promontory
Tympanic nerve (branch of CN IX)
Tympanic cells
B. Lateral View

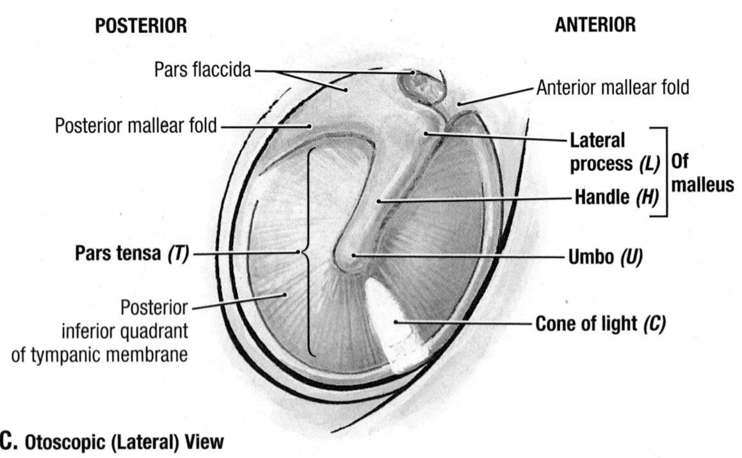
POSTERIOR
ANTERIOR
Pars flaccida
Posterior mallear fold
Pars tensa (T)
Posterior inferior quadrant of tympanic membrane
Anterior mallear fold
Lateral process (L)
Handle (H)
Of malleus
Umbo (U)
Cone of light (C)
C. Otoscopic (Lateral) View

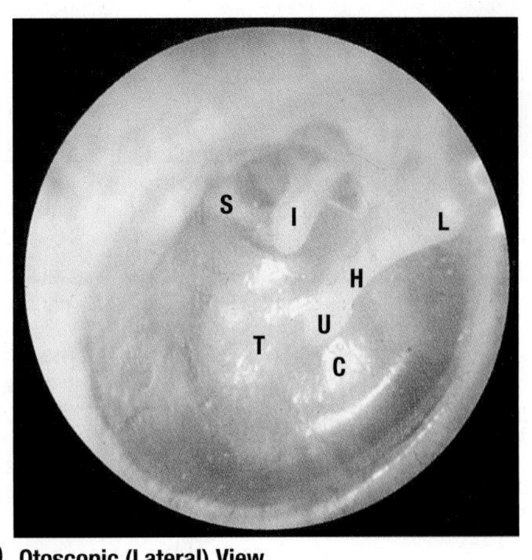
S
I
L
H
U
T
C
D. Otoscopic (Lateral) View

7.84 TYMPANIC MEMBRANE

A. External (lateral) surface of tympanic membrane. **B.** Tympanic membrane removed, demonstrating structures that lie medially. **C.** Diagram of otoscopic view of tympanic membrane. **D.** Otoscopic view of tympanic membrane. Letter labels are identified in **C**.

- The oval tympanic membrane is a shallow cone deepest at the central apex, the umbo, where the membrane is attached to the tip of the handle of the malleus. The handle of the malleus is attached to the membrane along its entire length as it extends anterosuperiorly toward the periphery of the membrane.
- Superior to the lateral process of the malleus, the membrane is thin (pars flaccida); the flaccid part lacks the radial and circular fibers present in the remainder of the membrane (pars tensa). The junction between the two parts is marked by anterior and posterior mallear folds.
- The lateral surface of the tympanic membrane is innervated by the auricular branch of the auriculotemporal nerve (CN V_3) and the auricular branch of the vagus nerve (CN X); the medial surface is innervated by tympanic branches of CN IX.

Examination of the external acoustic meatus and tympanic membrane begins by straightening the meatus. In adults, the helix is grasped and pulled posterosuperiorly (up, out, and back). These movements reduce the curvature of the external acoustic meatus, facilitating insertion of the otoscope. The external acoustic meatus is relatively short in infants; therefore, extra care must be taken to prevent damage to the tympanic membrane.

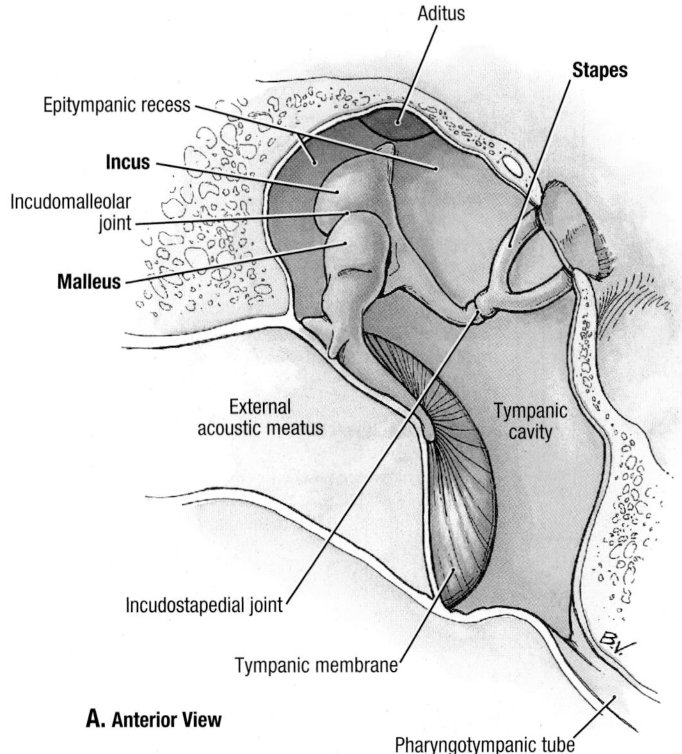
Aditus
Stapes
Epitympanic recess
Incus
Incudomalleolar joint
Malleus
External acoustic meatus
Tympanic cavity
Incudostapedial joint
Tympanic membrane
Pharyngotympanic tube
A. Anterior View

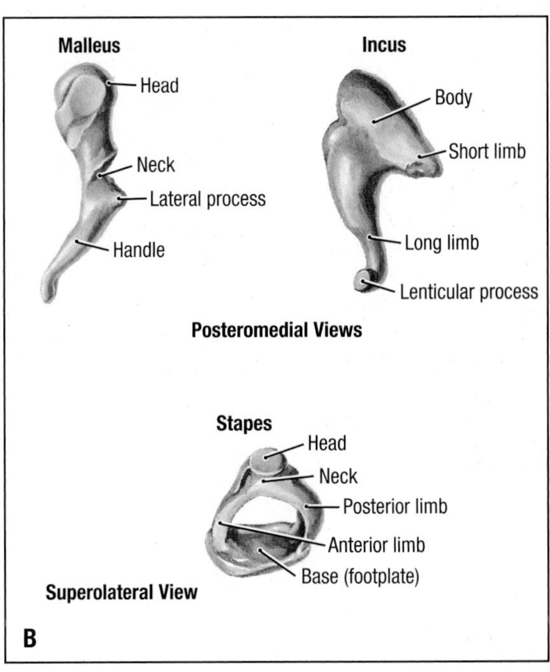
Malleus
Head
Neck
Lateral process
Handle
Incus
Body
Short limb
Long limb
Lenticular process
Posteromedial Views
Stapes
Head
Neck
Posterior limb
Anterior limb
Base (footplate)
Superolateral View
B

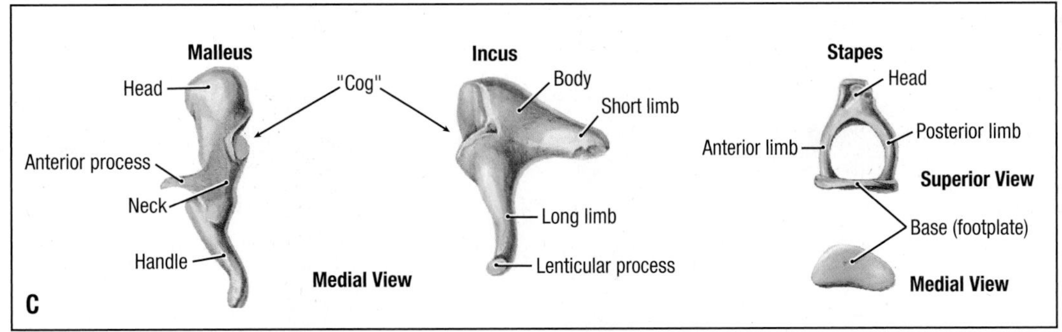
Malleus
Head
Anterior process
Neck
Handle
"Cog"
Medial View
Incus
Body
Short limb
Long limb
Lenticular process
Stapes
Head
Posterior limb
Anterior limb
Superior View
Base (footplate)
Medial View
C

7.85 OSSICLES OF THE MIDDLE EAR

A. Ossicles in situ, as revealed by a coronal section of the temporal bone. **B. and C.** Isolated ossicles.

- The head of the malleus and body and short process of the incus lie in the epitympanic recess, and the handle of the malleus is embedded in the tympanic membrane.
- The saddle-shaped articular surface of the head of the malleus and the reciprocally shaped articular surface of the body of the incus form the incudomalleolar synovial joint.
- A convex articular facet at the end of the long process of the incus articulates with the head of the stapes to compose the incudostapedial synovial joint.
- An earache and bulging red tympanic membrane may indicate pus or fluid in the middle ear, a sign of **otitis media.** Infection of the middle ear often is secondary to upper respiratory infections. Inflammation and swelling of the mucous membrane lining the tympanic cavity may cause partial or complete blockage of the pharyngotympanic tube. The tympanic membrane becomes red and bulges, and the person may complain of "ear popping." If untreated, otitis media may produce impaired hearing as the result of scarring of the auditory ossicles, limiting the ability of these bones to move in response to sound.

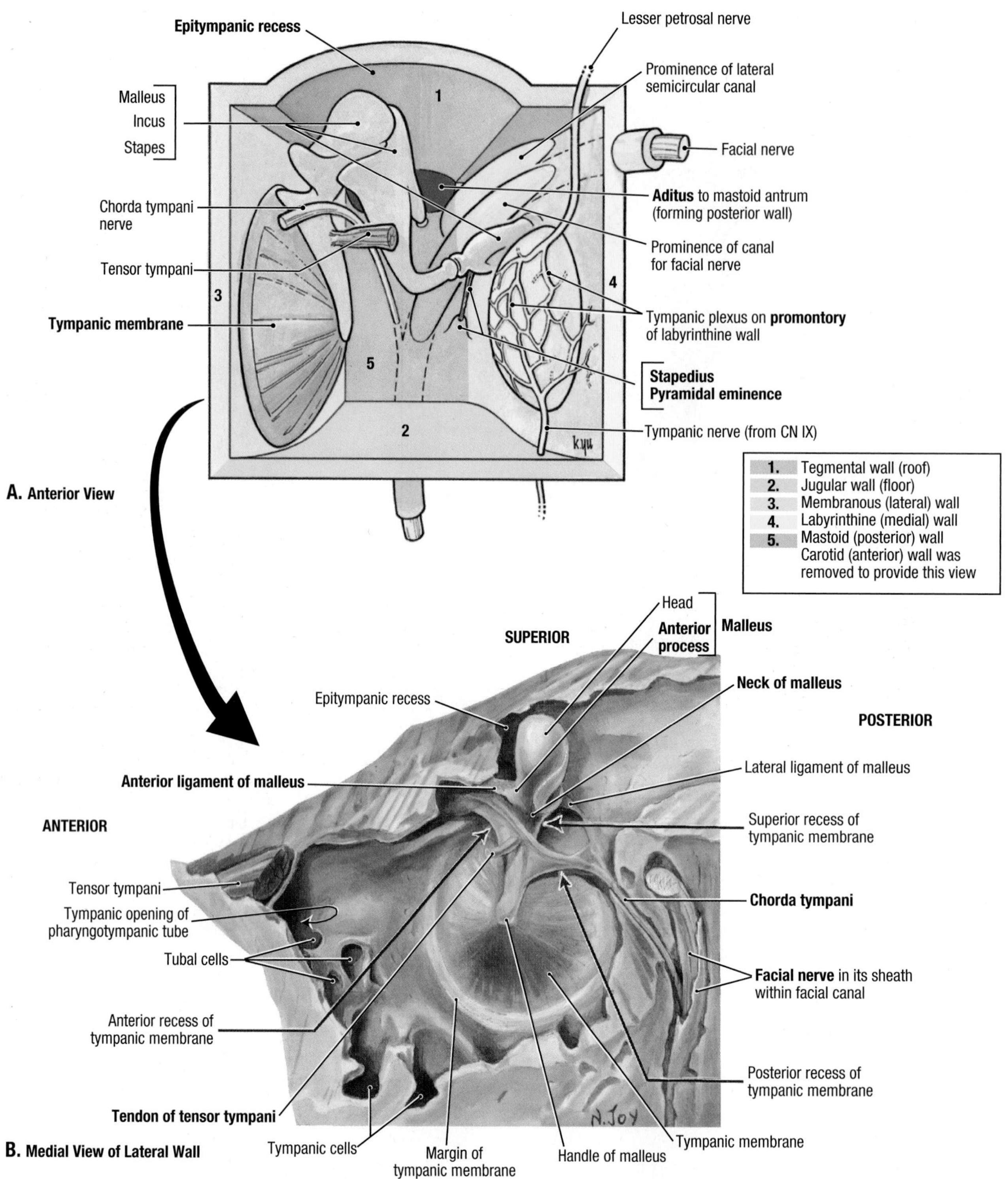
Epitympanic recess
Lesser petrosal nerve
Prominence of lateral semicircular canal
Malleus
Incus
Stapes
1
Facial nerve
Aditus to mastoid antrum (forming posterior wall)
Chorda tympani nerve
Prominence of canal for facial nerve
Tensor tympani
4
3
Tympanic plexus on promontory of labyrinthine wall
Tympanic membrane
5
Stapedius
Pyramidal eminence
2
Tympanic nerve (from CN IX)
A. Anterior View
1. Tegmental wall (roof)
2. Jugular wall (floor)
3. Membranous (lateral) wall
4. Labyrinthine (medial) wall
5. Mastoid (posterior) wall
Carotid (anterior) wall was removed to provide this view
Head
Anterior process
Malleus
SUPERIOR
Neck of malleus
Epitympanic recess
POSTERIOR
Lateral ligament of malleus
Anterior ligament of malleus
ANTERIOR
Superior recess of tympanic membrane
Tensor tympani
Chorda tympani
Tympanic opening of pharyngotympanic tube
Tubal cells
Facial nerve in its sheath within facial canal
Anterior recess of tympanic membrane
Posterior recess of tympanic membrane
Tendon of tensor tympani
B. Medial View of Lateral Wall
Tympanic cells
Margin of tympanic membrane
Handle of malleus
Tympanic membrane

7.86 TRUCTURES OF THE TYMPANIC CAVITY

A. Schematic illustration of the tympanic cavity with the anterior wall removed. **B.** Lateral wall of the tympanic cavity. The facial nerve lies within the facial canal surrounded by a tough periosteal tube; the chorda tympani leaves the facial nerve and lies within two crescentic folds of mucous membrane, crossing the neck of the malleus superior to the tendon of tensor tympani.

Perforation of the tympanic membrane (ruptured eardrum) may result from otitis media. Perforation may also result from foreign bodies in the external acoustic meatus, trauma, or excessive pressure. Because the superior half of the tympanic membrane is much more vascular than the inferior half, incisions are made posteroinferiorly through the membrane. This incision also avoids injury to the chorda tympani nerve and auditory ossicles.

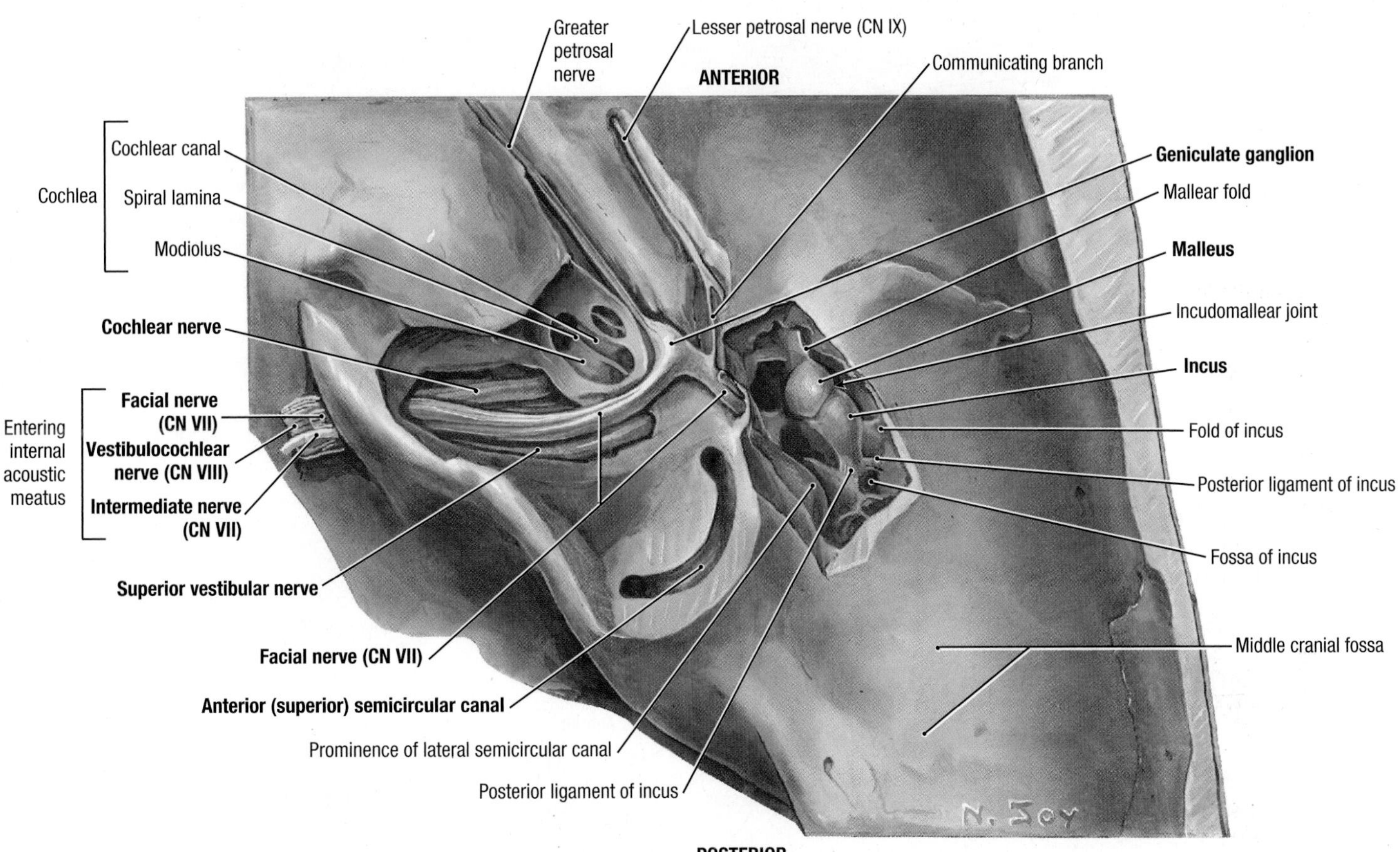
Greater petrosal nerve
Lesser petrosal nerve (CN IX)
ANTERIOR
Communicating branch
Cochlea
Cochlear canal
Spiral lamina
Modiolus
Cochlear nerve
Entering internal acoustic meatus
Facial nerve (CN VII)
Vestibulocochlear nerve (CN VIII)
Intermediate nerve (CN VII)
Superior vestibular nerve
Facial nerve (CN VII)
Anterior (superior) semicircular canal
Prominence of lateral semicircular canal
Posterior ligament of incus
POSTERIOR
Geniculate ganglion
Mallear fold
Malleus
Incudomallear joint
Incus
Fold of incus
Posterior ligament of incus
Fossa of incus
Middle cranial fossa

7.87 MIDDLE AND INNER EAR IN SITU

The tegmen tympani has been removed to expose the middle ear, the arcuate eminence has been removed to expose the anterior semicircular canal, and the course of the facial and vestibulocochlear nerves through the internal acoustic meatus and internal ear is demonstrated. At the geniculate ganglion, the facial nerve executes a sharp bend, called the genu, and then curves posteroinferiorly within the bony facial canal; the thin lateral wall of the facial canal separates the facial nerve from the tympanic cavity of the middle ear.

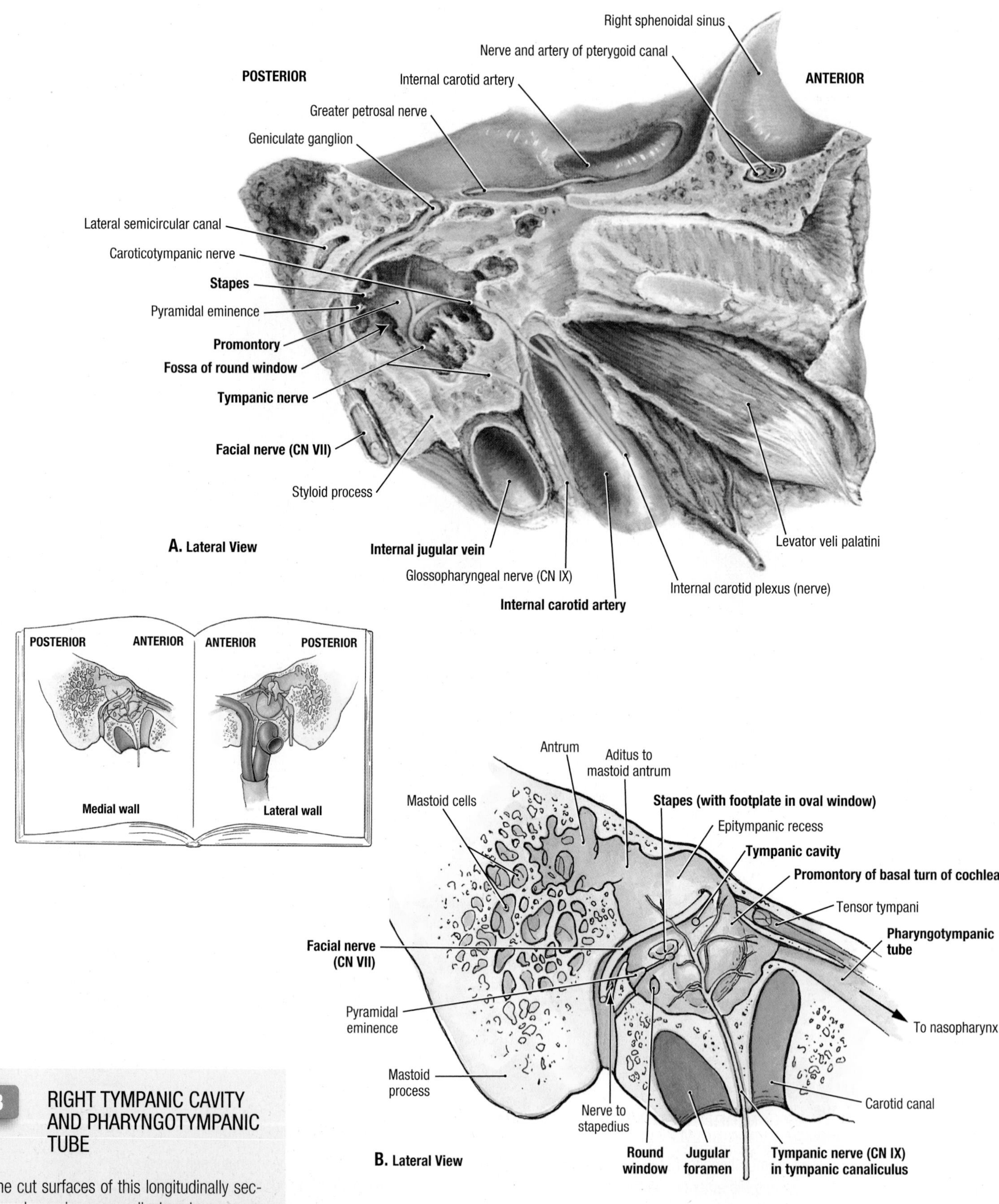
POSTERIOR
ANTERIOR
Right sphenoidal sinus
Nerve and artery of pterygoid canal
Internal carotid artery
Greater petrosal nerve
Geniculate ganglion
Lateral semicircular canal
Caroticotympanic nerve
Stapes
Pyramidal eminence
Promontory
Fossa of round window
Tympanic nerve
Facial nerve (CN VII)
Styloid process
Internal jugular vein
Glossopharyngeal nerve (CN IX)
Internal carotid artery
Internal carotid plexus (nerve)
Levator veli palatini
A. Lateral View
POSTERIOR
ANTERIOR
ANTERIOR
POSTERIOR
Medial wall
Lateral wall
Antrum
Aditus to mastoid antrum
Mastoid cells
Stapes (with footplate in oval window)
Epitympanic recess
Tympanic cavity
Promontory of basal turn of cochlea
Tensor tympani
Pharyngotympanic tube
Facial nerve (CN VII)
Pyramidal eminence
To nasopharynx
Mastoid process
Carotid canal
Nerve to stapedius
Round window
Jugular foramen
Tympanic nerve (CN IX) in tympanic canaliculus
B. Lateral View

7.88 RIGHT TYMPANIC CAVITY AND PHARYNGOTYMPANIC TUBE

The cut surfaces of this longitudinally sectioned specimen are displayed as pages in a book. **A.** Dissection of medial wall. **B.** Schematic illustration of medial wall.

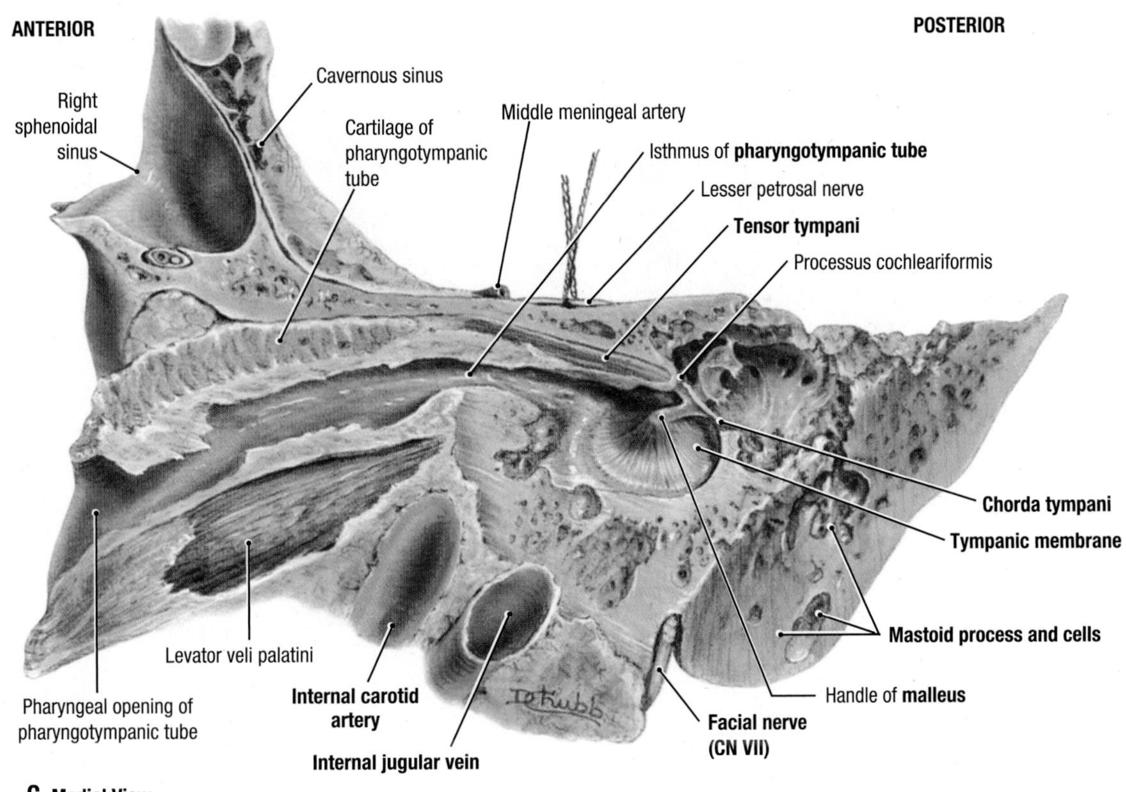
ANTERIOR
POSTERIOR
Cavernous sinus
Right sphenoidal sinus
Cartilage of pharyngotympanic tube
Middle meningeal artery
Isthmus of pharyngotympanic tube
Lesser petrosal nerve
Tensor tympani
Processus cochleariformis
Chorda tympani
Tympanic membrane
Mastoid process and cells
Handle of malleus
Facial nerve (CN VII)
Internal jugular vein
Internal carotid artery
Levator veli palatini
Pharyngeal opening of pharyngotympanic tube

C. Medial View

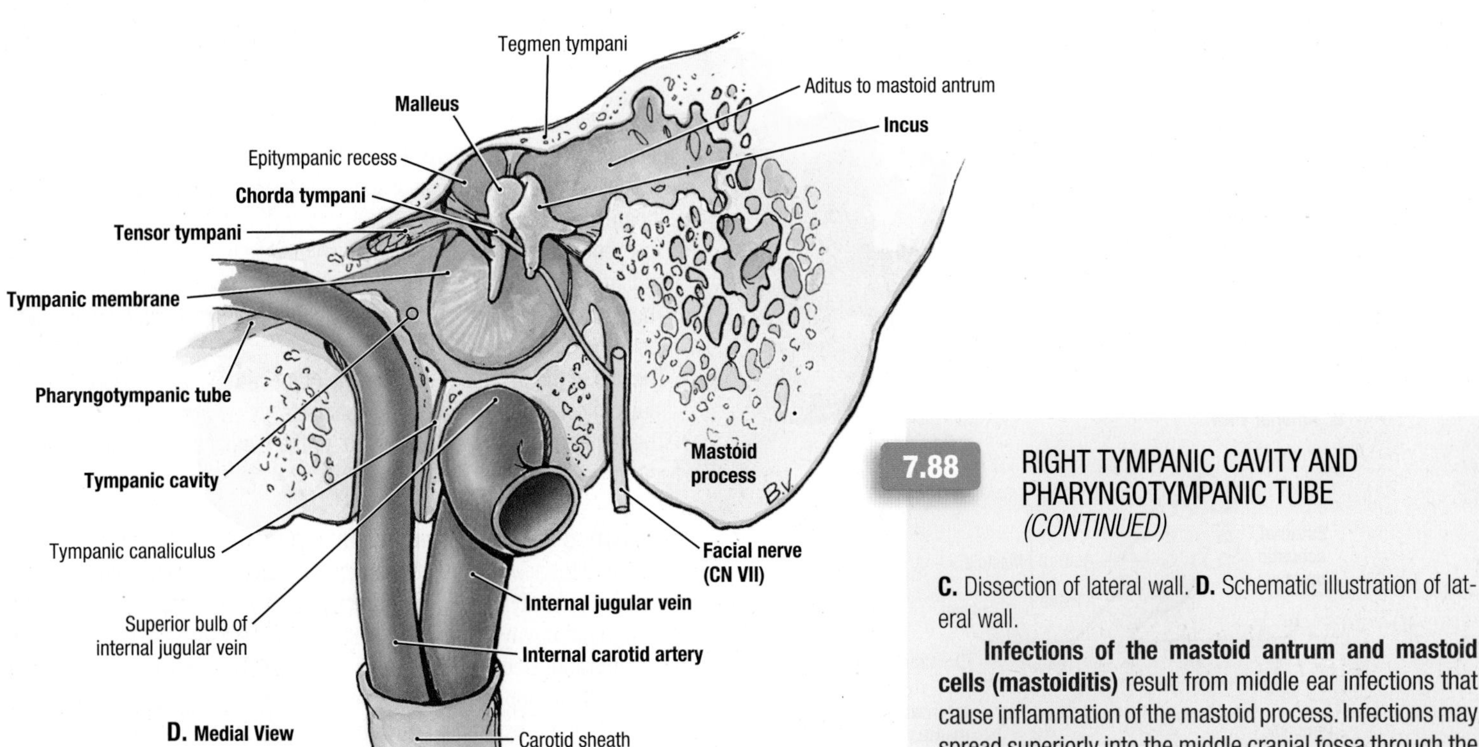
Tegmen tympani
Aditus to mastoid antrum
Malleus
Incus
Epitympanic recess
Chorda tympani
Tensor tympani
Tympanic membrane
Pharyngotympanic tube
Tympanic cavity
Tympanic canaliculus
Superior bulb of internal jugular vein
Mastoid process
Facial nerve (CN VII)
Internal jugular vein
Internal carotid artery
Carotid sheath

D. Medial View

7.88 RIGHT TYMPANIC CAVITY AND PHARYNGOTYMPANIC TUBE *(CONTINUED)*

C. Dissection of lateral wall. **D.** Schematic illustration of lateral wall.

Infections of the mastoid antrum and mastoid cells (mastoiditis) result from middle ear infections that cause inflammation of the mastoid process. Infections may spread superiorly into the middle cranial fossa through the petrosquamous fissure in children or may cause osteomyelitis (bone infection) of the tegmen tympani. Since the advent of antibiotics, mastoiditis is uncommon.

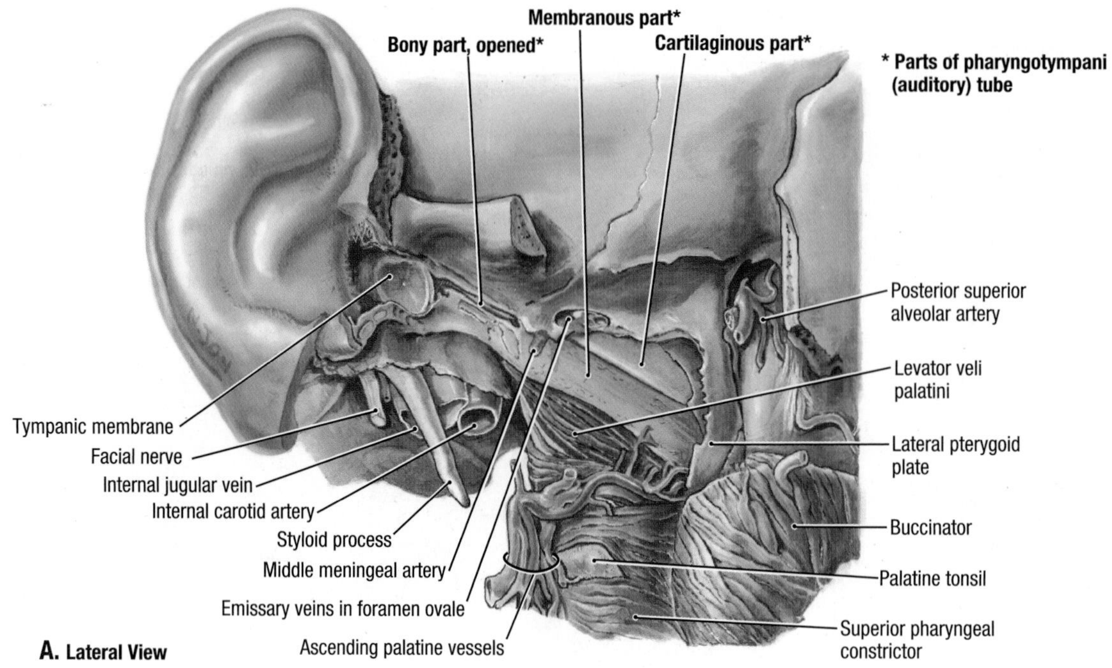
Membranous part*
Bony part, opened*
Cartilaginous part*
* Parts of pharyngotympani (auditory) tube
Posterior superior alveolar artery
Levator veli palatini
Lateral pterygoid plate
Buccinator
Palatine tonsil
Superior pharyngeal constrictor
Tympanic membrane
Facial nerve
Internal jugular vein
Internal carotid artery
Styloid process
Middle meningeal artery
Emissary veins in foramen ovale
Ascending palatine vessels

A. Lateral View

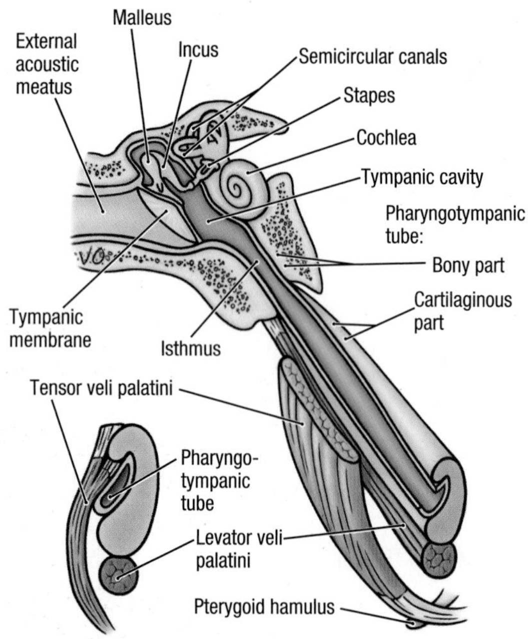
Malleus
External acoustic meatus
Incus
Semicircular canals
Stapes
Cochlea
Tympanic cavity
Pharyngotympanic tube:
Bony part
Cartilaginous part
Tympanic membrane
Isthmus
Tensor veli palatini
Pharyngo-tympanic tube
Levator veli palatini
Pterygoid hamulus

B. Anterior view

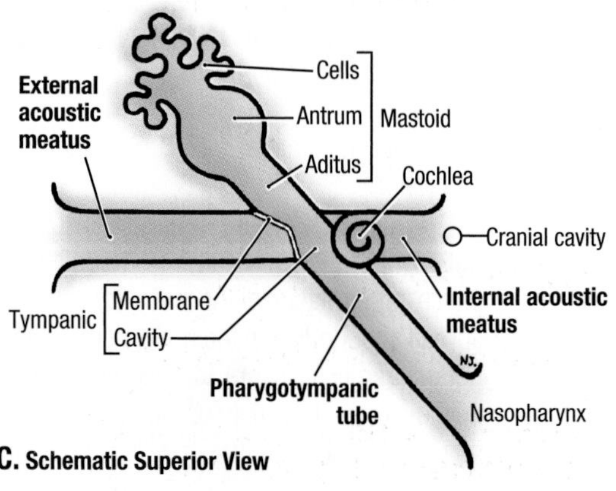
External acoustic meatus
Cells
Antrum
Aditus
Mastoid
Cochlea
Cranial cavity
Tympanic
Membrane
Cavity
Internal acoustic meatus
Pharygotympanic tube
Nasopharynx

C. Schematic Superior View

7.89 RIGHT TYMPANIC CAVITY AND PHARYNGOTYMPANIC TUBE

A. Dissection demonstrating lateral aspect of pharyngotympanic tube and structures located medially. **B.** Right pharyngotympanic tube. **C.** Schematic illustration demonstrating relationship between internal and external acoustic meatuses.

- The general direction of the pharyngotympanic tube is superior, posterior, and lateral from the nasopharynx to the tympanic cavity.
- The cartilaginous part of the tube rests throughout its length on the levator veli palatini muscle.
- The line of the meatuses and the line of the airway, from nasopharynx to mastoid cells, intersect at the tympanic cavity.
- The tegmen tympani forms the roof of the tympanic cavity and mastoid antrum.

The **function of the pharyngotympanic tube** is to equalize pressure in the middle ear with the atmospheric pressure, thereby allowing free movement of the tympanic membrane. By allowing air to enter and leave the tympanic cavity, this tube balances the pressure on both sides of the membrane. Because the walls of the cartilaginous part of the tube are normally in apposition, the tube must be actively opened. The tube is opened by the expanding girth of the belly of the levator veli palatini as it contracts longitudinally, pushing against one wall while the tensor veli palatini pulls on the other. Because these are muscles of the soft palate, equalizing pressure (popping the eardrums) is commonly associated with activities such as yawning and swallowing.

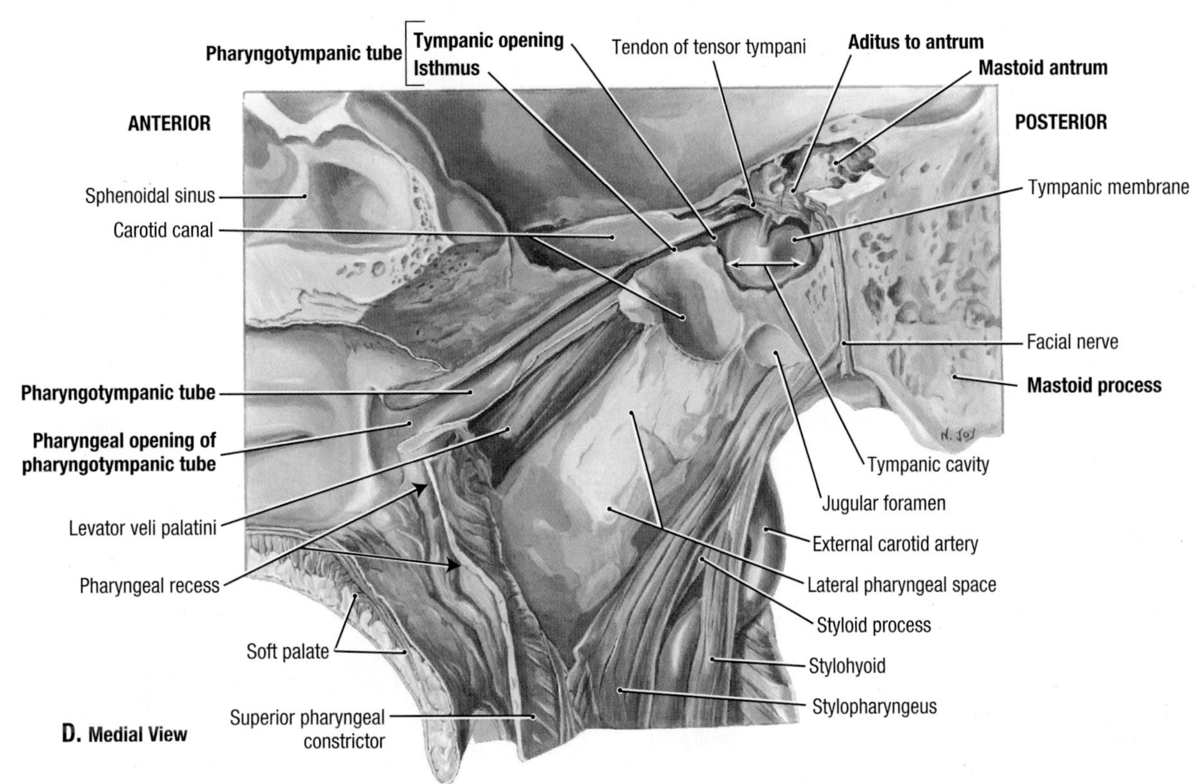
Pharyngotympanic tube
Tympanic opening
Isthmus
Tendon of tensor tympani
Aditus to antrum
Mastoid antrum
ANTERIOR
POSTERIOR
Sphenoidal sinus
Carotid canal
Tympanic membrane
Facial nerve
Mastoid process
Pharyngotympanic tube
Pharyngeal opening of pharyngotympanic tube
Levator veli palatini
Pharyngeal recess
Soft palate
Superior pharyngeal constrictor
Tympanic cavity
Jugular foramen
External carotid artery
Lateral pharyngeal space
Styloid process
Stylohyoid
Stylopharyngeus

D. Medial View

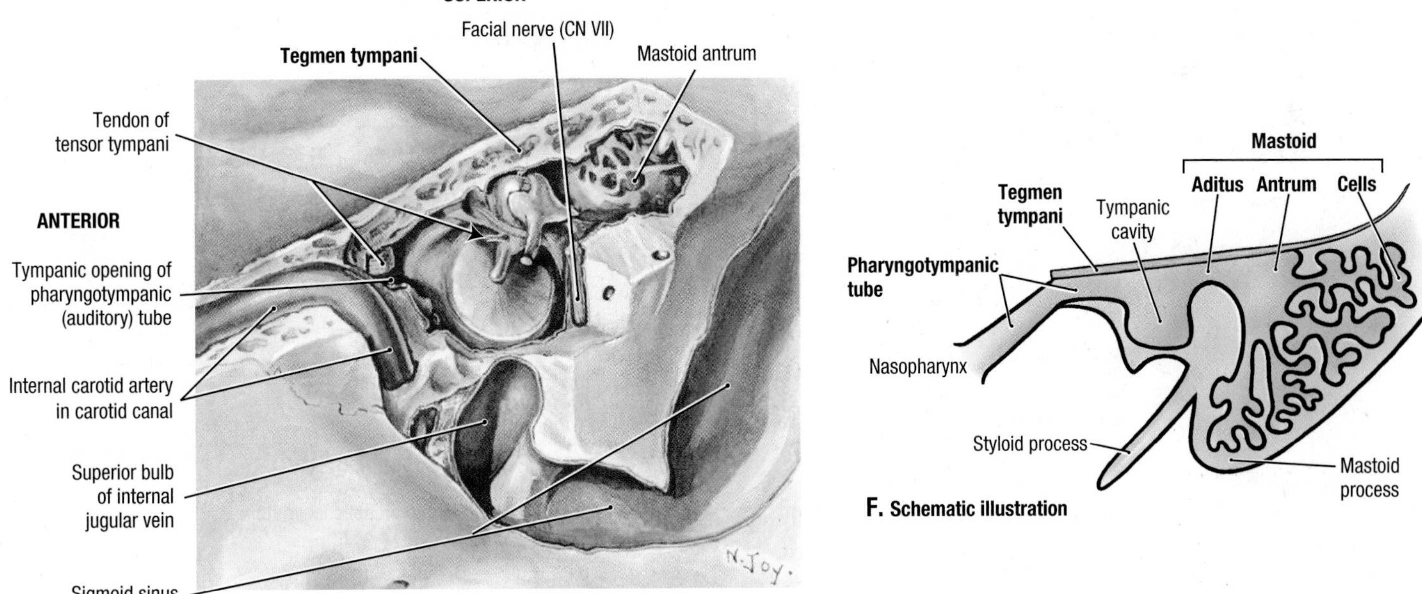
SUPERIOR
Facial nerve (CN VII)
Tegmen tympani
Mastoid antrum
Tendon of tensor tympani
ANTERIOR
Tympanic opening of pharyngotympanic (auditory) tube
Internal carotid artery in carotid canal
Superior bulb of internal jugular vein
Sigmoid sinus
Mastoid
Aditus
Antrum
Cells
Tegmen tympani
Tympanic cavity
Pharyngotympanic tube
Nasopharynx
Styloid process
Mastoid process

E. Medial View

F. Schematic illustration

7.89 RIGHT TYMPANIC CAVITY AND PHARYNGOTYMPANIC TUBE *(CONTINUED)*

D. Spaces of tympanic bone. **E.** Relationship of tympanic cavity to internal carotid artery, sigmoid sinus, and middle cranial fossa. **F.** Diagram of tegmen tympani.

- The internal carotid artery is the primary relationship of the anterior wall, the internal jugular vein is the primary relationship of the floor, and the facial nerve is the primary relationship of the posterior wall.

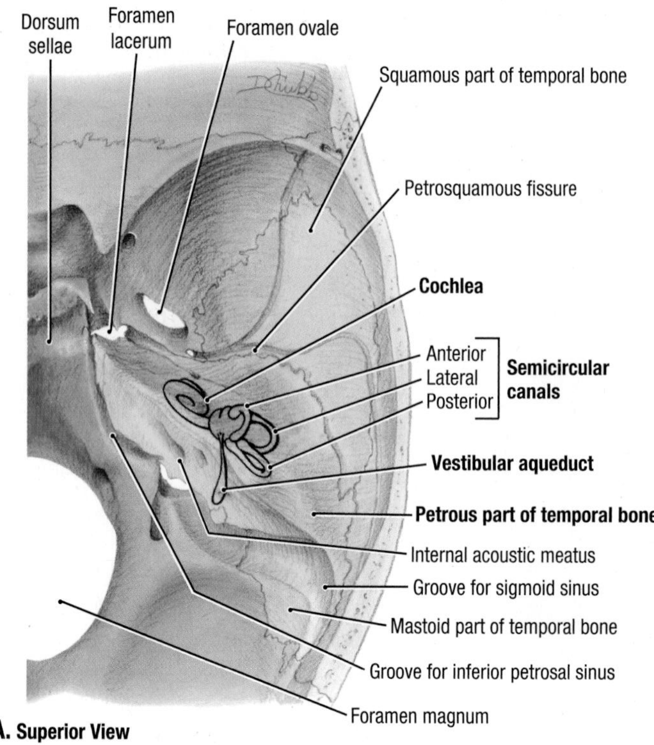

Dorsum sellae
Foramen lacerum
Foramen ovale
Squamous part of temporal bone
Petrosquamous fissure
Cochlea
Anterior
Lateral
Posterior
Semicircular canals
Vestibular aqueduct
Petrous part of temporal bone
Internal acoustic meatus
Groove for sigmoid sinus
Mastoid part of temporal bone
Groove for inferior petrosal sinus
Foramen magnum

A. Superior View

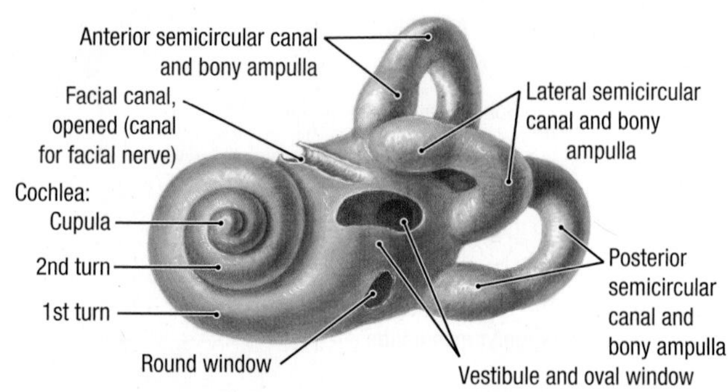

Anterior semicircular canal and bony ampulla
Facial canal, opened (canal for facial nerve)
Cochlea:
Cupula
2nd turn
1st turn
Round window
Lateral semicircular canal and bony ampulla
Posterior semicircular canal and bony ampulla
Vestibule and oval window

C. Anterolateral view of left otic capsule

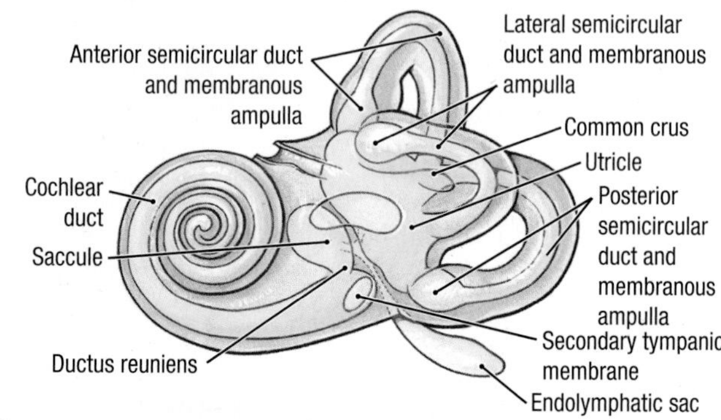

Anterior semicircular duct and membranous ampulla
Lateral semicircular duct and membranous ampulla
Common crus
Utricle
Cochlear duct
Saccule
Posterior semicircular duct and membranous ampulla
Secondary tympanic membrane
Ductus reuniens
Endolymphatic sac

C. Anterolateral view of left membranous labyrinth (through transparent otic capsule)

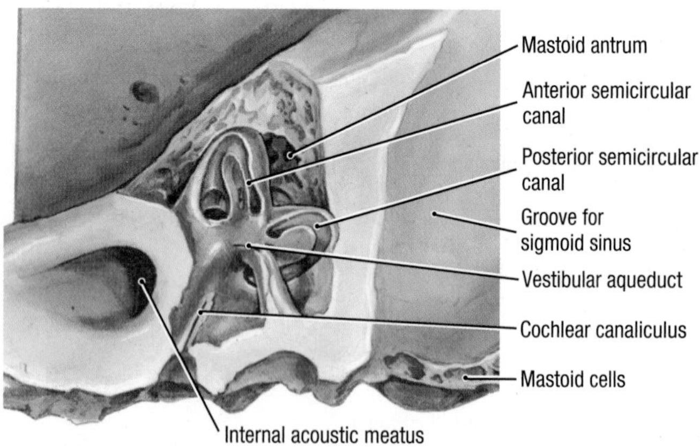

Mastoid antrum
Anterior semicircular canal
Posterior semicircular canal
Groove for sigmoid sinus
Vestibular aqueduct
Cochlear canaliculus
Mastoid cells
Internal acoustic meatus

B. Posterosuperior View

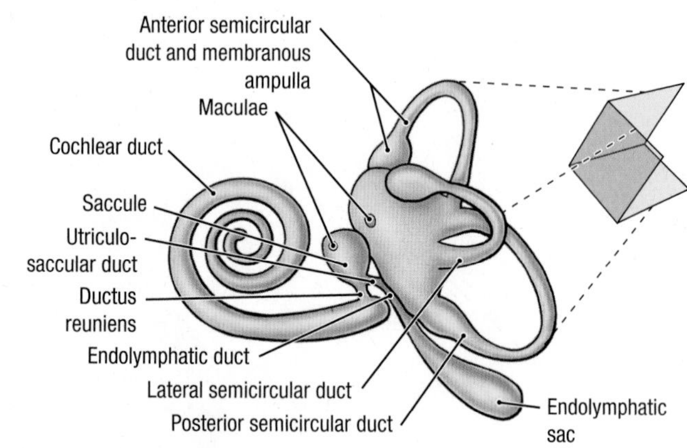

Anterior semicircular duct and membranous ampulla
Maculae
Cochlear duct
Saccule
Utriculo-saccular duct
Ductus reuniens
Endolymphatic duct
Lateral semicircular duct
Posterior semicircular duct
Endolymphatic sac

D. Anterolateral view of left membranous labyrinth

7.90 BONY AND MEMBRANOUS LABYRINTHS

A. Location and orientation of bony labyrinth within petrous temporal bone. **B.** Semicircular canals and aqueducts *in situ*. The tegmen tympani has been excised, and the softer bone surrounding the harder bone of the otic capsule has been drilled away. **C.** Walls of left bony labyrinth (otic capsule). The bony labyrinth is the fluid-filled space contained within this formation. **D.** Membranous labyrinth as it lies within the surrounding bony labyrinth. **E.** Isolated left membranous labyrinth.

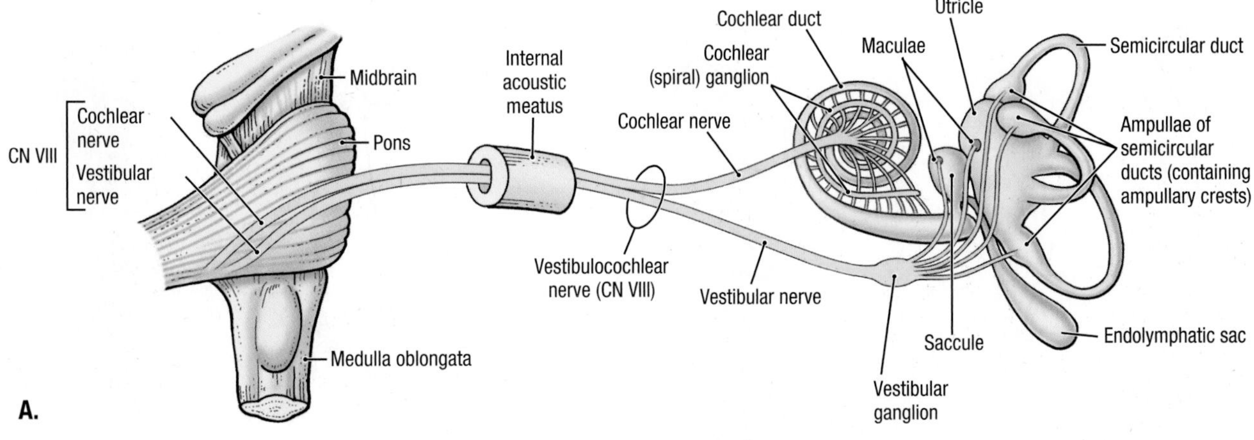
CN VIII
Cochlear nerve
Vestibular nerve
Midbrain
Pons
Medulla oblongata
Internal acoustic meatus
Vestibulocochlear nerve (CN VIII)
Cochlear nerve
Vestibular nerve
Cochlear duct
Cochlear (spiral) ganglion
Maculae
Utricle
Semicircular duct
Ampullae of semicircular ducts (containing ampullary crests)
Endolymphatic sac
Saccule
Vestibular ganglion
A.

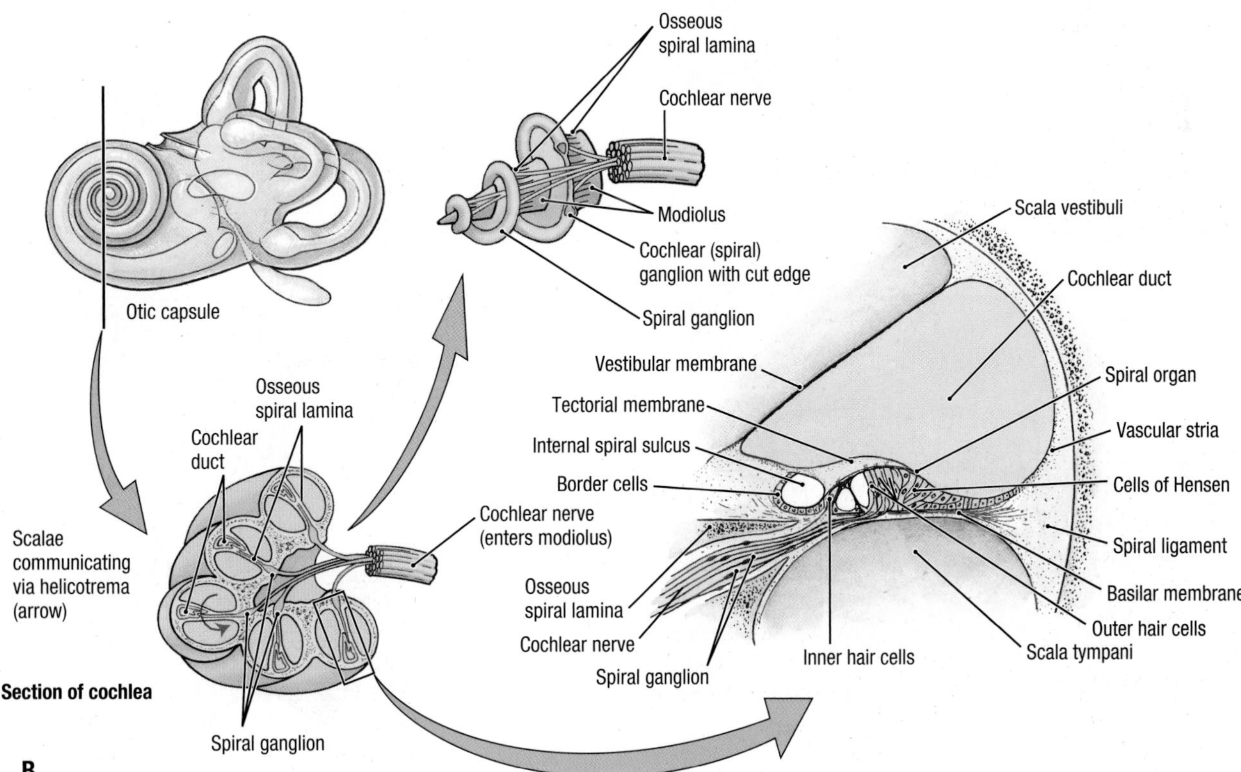
Otic capsule
Osseous spiral lamina
Cochlear nerve
Modiolus
Cochlear (spiral) ganglion with cut edge
Spiral ganglion
Osseous spiral lamina
Cochlear duct
Scalae communicating via helicotrema (arrow)
Cochlear nerve (enters modiolus)
Section of cochlea
Spiral ganglion
Scala vestibuli
Cochlear duct
Vestibular membrane
Tectorial membrane
Internal spiral sulcus
Border cells
Osseous spiral lamina
Cochlear nerve
Spiral ganglion
Inner hair cells
Spiral organ
Vascular stria
Cells of Hensen
Spiral ligament
Basilar membrane
Outer hair cells
Scala tympani
B.

7.91 VESTIBULOCOCHLEAR NERVE (CN VIII) AND STRUCTURE OF COCHLEA

A. Distribution of vestibulocochlear nerve (schematic). **B.** Structure of cochlea. The cochlea has been sectioned along the bony core of the cochlea (modiolus), the axis about which the cochlea winds. An isolated modiolus is shown after the turns of the cochlea are removed, leaving only the spiral lamina winding around it. The *large drawing* shows the details of the *area enclosed in the rectangle,* including a cross section of the cochlear duct of the membranous labyrinth.

- The maculae of the membranous labyrinth are primarily static organs, which have small dense particles (otoliths) embedded among the hair cells. Under the influence of gravity, the otoliths cause bending of the hair cells, which stimulate the vestibular nerve and provide awareness of the position of the head in space; the hairs also respond to quick tilting movements and to linear acceleration and deceleration. **Motion sickness** results mainly from discordance between vestibular and visual stimuli.
- Persistent exposure to excessively loud sound causes degenerative changes in the spiral organ, resulting in **high-tone deafness.** This type of hearing loss commonly occurs in workers who are exposed to loud noises and do not wear protective earmuffs.

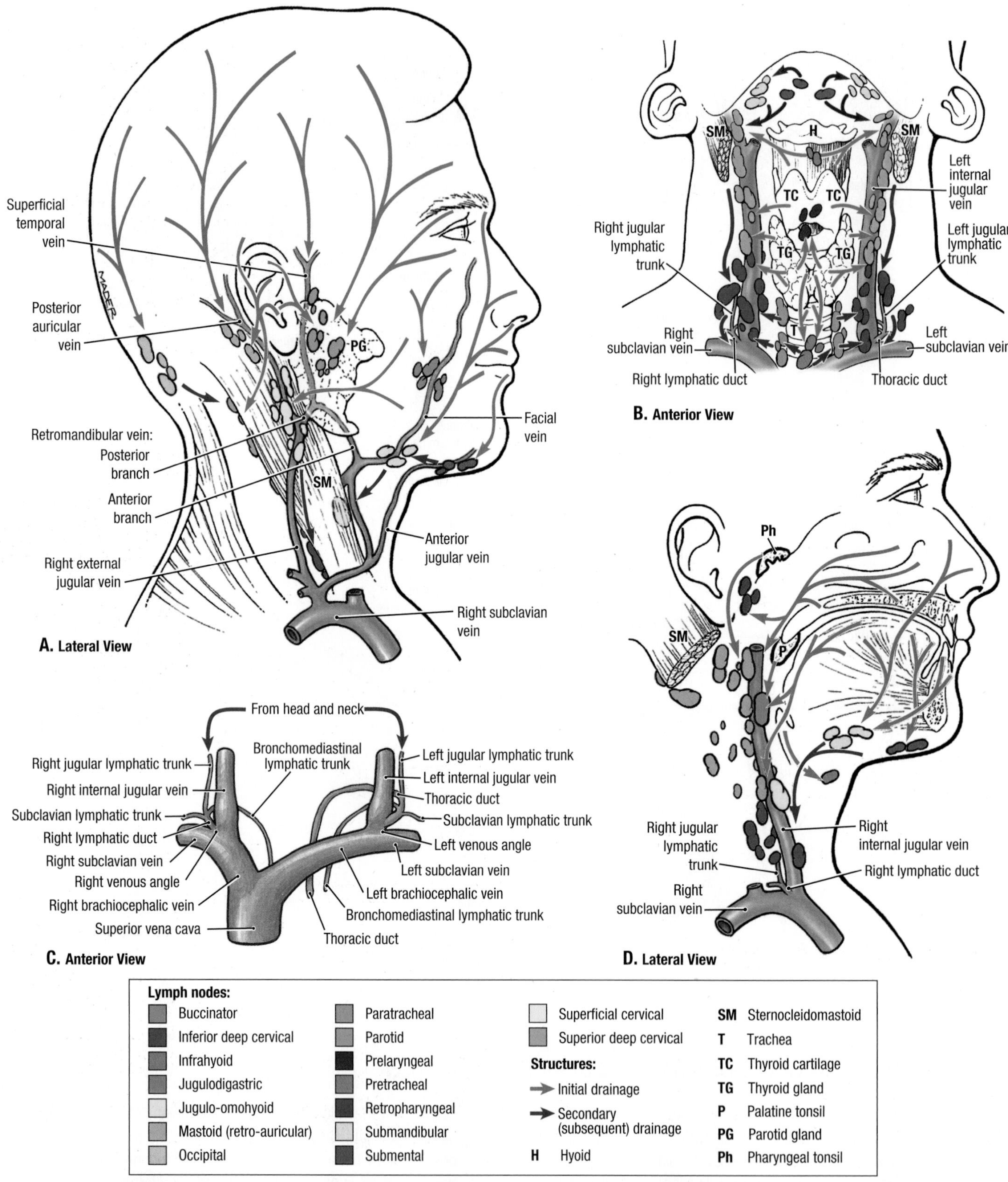

Superficial temporal vein
Posterior auricular vein
MADER
PG
Retromandibular vein:
Posterior branch
Anterior branch
SM
Facial vein
Anterior jugular vein
Right external jugular vein
Right subclavian vein
A. Lateral View
SM
H
SM
Left internal jugular vein
TC
TC
TG
TG
Right jugular lymphatic trunk
Left jugular lymphatic trunk
T
Right subclavian vein
Left subclavian vein
Right lymphatic duct
Thoracic duct
B. Anterior View
Ph
SM
P
Right jugular lymphatic trunk
Right internal jugular vein
Right lymphatic duct
Right subclavian vein
D. Lateral View
From head and neck
Bronchomediastinal lymphatic trunk
Right jugular lymphatic trunk
Right internal jugular vein
Subclavian lymphatic trunk
Right lymphatic duct
Right subclavian vein
Right venous angle
Right brachiocephalic vein
Superior vena cava
Left jugular lymphatic trunk
Left internal jugular vein
Thoracic duct
Subclavian lymphatic trunk
Left venous angle
Left subclavian vein
Left brachiocephalic vein
Bronchomediastinal lymphatic trunk
Thoracic duct
C. Anterior View

Lymph nodes:

- Buccinator
- Inferior deep cervical
- Infrahyoid
- Jugulodigastric
- Jugulo-omohyoid
- Mastoid (retro-auricular)
- Occipital
- Paratracheal
- Parotid
- Prelaryngeal
- Pretracheal
- Retropharyngeal
- Submandibular
- Submental
- Superficial cervical
- Superior deep cervical

Structures:

- Initial drainage
- Secondary (subsequent) drainage

H Hyoid

SM Sternocleidomastoid
T Trachea
TC Thyroid cartilage
TG Thyroid gland
P Palatine tonsil
PG Parotid gland
Ph Pharyngeal tonsil

7.92 LYMPHATIC AND VENOUS DRAINAGE OF HEAD AND NECK

A. Superficial drainage. **B.** Drainage of the trachea, thyroid gland, larynx, and floor of mouth. **C.** Termination of right and left jugular lymphatic trunks. **D.** Deep drainage.

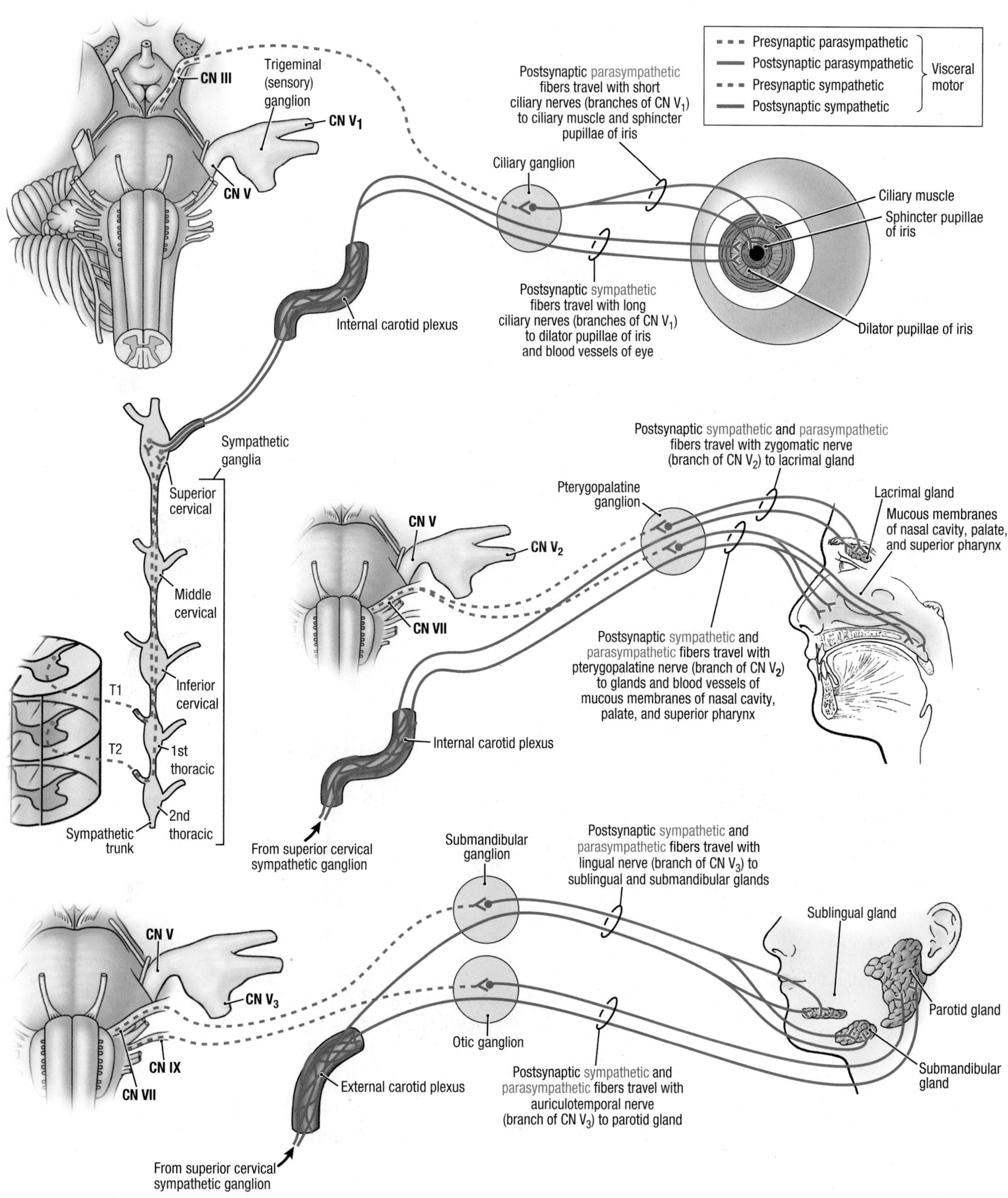
Presynaptic parasympathetic
Postsynaptic parasympathetic
Presynaptic sympathetic
Postsynaptic sympathetic
Visceral motor
CN III
Trigeminal (sensory) ganglion
CN V_1
CN V
Postsynaptic parasympathetic fibers travel with short ciliary nerves (branches of CN V_1) to ciliary muscle and sphincter pupillae of iris
Ciliary ganglion
Ciliary muscle
Sphincter pupillae of iris
Internal carotid plexus
Postsynaptic sympathetic fibers travel with long ciliary nerves (branches of CN V_1) to dilator pupillae of iris and blood vessels of eye
Dilator pupillae of iris
Sympathetic ganglia
Superior cervical
Middle cervical
Inferior cervical
T1
T2
1st thoracic
2nd thoracic
Sympathetic trunk
Postsynaptic sympathetic and parasympathetic fibers travel with zygomatic nerve (branch of CN V_2) to lacrimal gland
Pterygopalatine ganglion
CN V
CN V_2
CN VII
Lacrimal gland
Mucous membranes of nasal cavity, palate, and superior pharynx
Postsynaptic sympathetic and parasympathetic fibers travel with pterygopalatine nerve (branch of CN V_2) to glands and blood vessels of mucous membranes of nasal cavity, palate, and superior pharynx
Internal carotid plexus
From superior cervical sympathetic ganglion
Submandibular ganglion
Postsynaptic sympathetic and parasympathetic fibers travel with lingual nerve (branch of CN V_3) to sublingual and submandibular glands
Sublingual gland
CN V
CN V_3
Parotid gland
CN IX
CN VII
Otic ganglion
External carotid plexus
Postsynaptic sympathetic and parasympathetic fibers travel with auriculotemporal nerve (branch of CN V_3) to parotid gland
Submandibular gland
From superior cervical sympathetic ganglion

7.93 AUTONOMIC INNERVATION OF HEAD

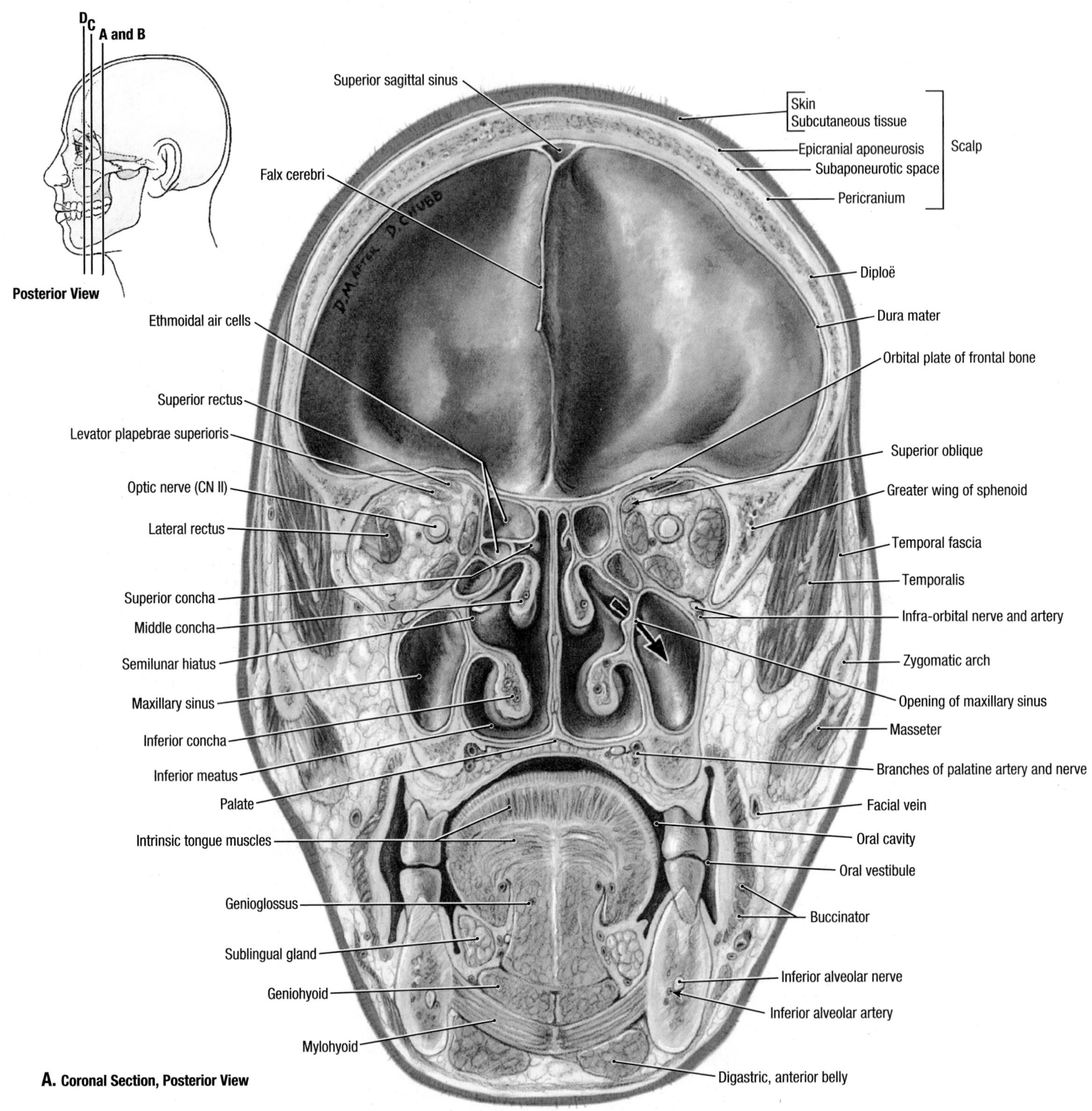
D
C
A and B
Posterior View
Superior sagittal sinus
Skin
Subcutaneous tissue
Epicranial aponeurosis
Subaponeurotic space
Pericranium
Scalp
Falx cerebri
Diploë
Dura mater
Ethmoidal air cells
Orbital plate of frontal bone
Superior rectus
Levator plapebrae superioris
Superior oblique
Optic nerve (CN II)
Greater wing of sphenoid
Lateral rectus
Temporal fascia
Temporalis
Superior concha
Middle concha
Infra-orbital nerve and artery
Semilunar hiatus
Zygomatic arch
Maxillary sinus
Opening of maxillary sinus
Inferior concha
Masseter
Inferior meatus
Branches of palatine artery and nerve
Palate
Facial vein
Intrinsic tongue muscles
Oral cavity
Oral vestibule
Genioglossus
Buccinator
Sublingual gland
Inferior alveolar nerve
Geniohyoid
Inferior alveolar artery
Mylohyoid
Digastric, anterior belly

A. **Coronal Section, Posterior View**

7.94 CORONAL SECTION AND MRI IMAGING OF NASOPHARYNX AND ORAL CAVITY

A. Coronal section. **B.–D.** Coronal MRIs.

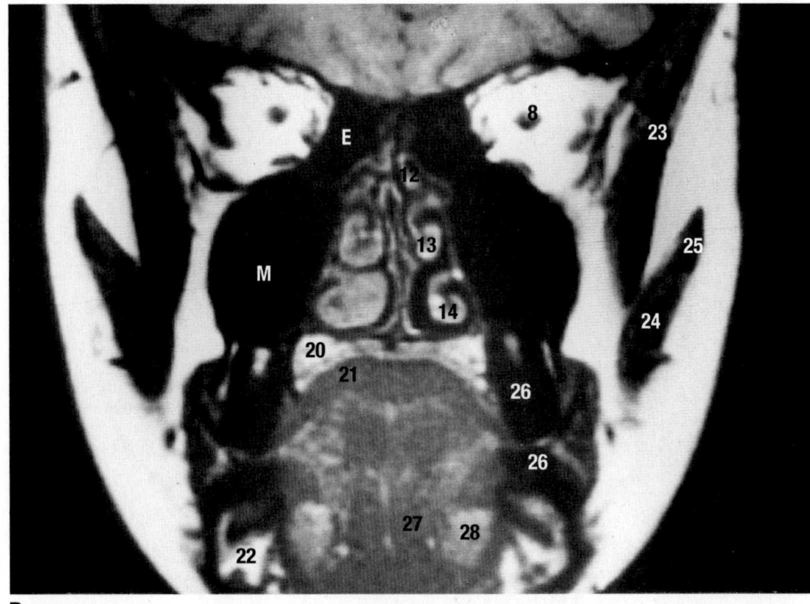
E
8
23
12
13
25
M
14
24
20
21
26
26
27
28
22

B

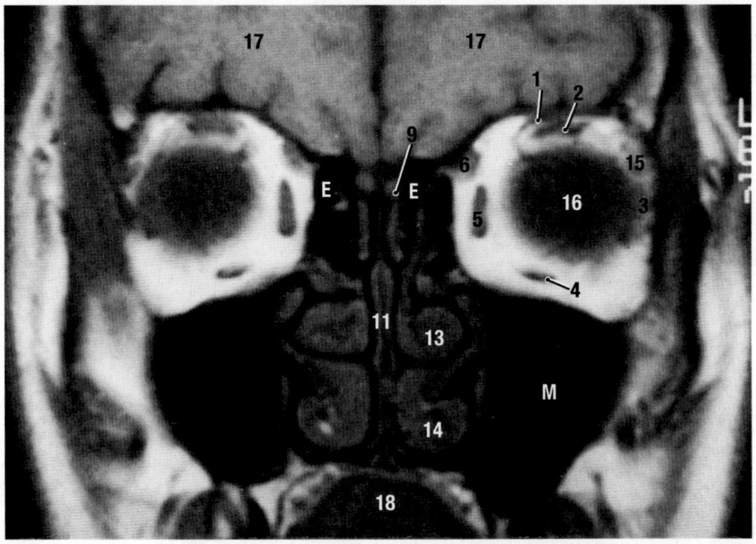

C

1	Levator palpebrae superioris
2	Superior rectus
3	Lateral rectus
4	Inferior rectus
5	Medial rectus
6	Superior oblique
7	Inferior oblique
8	Optic nerve
9	Olfactory bulb
10	Crista galli
11	Nasal septum
12	Superior concha
13	Middle concha
14	Inferior concha
15	Lacrimal gland
16	Eyeball
17	Frontal lobe
18	Tongue
19	Infra-orbital vessels and nerve
20	Hard palate
21	Intrinsic muscles of tongue
22	Mandible
23	Temporalis
24	Masseter
25	Zygomatic arch
26	Molar teeth
27	Genioglossus
28	Sublingual gland
M	Maxillary sinus
E	Ethmoidal air cell

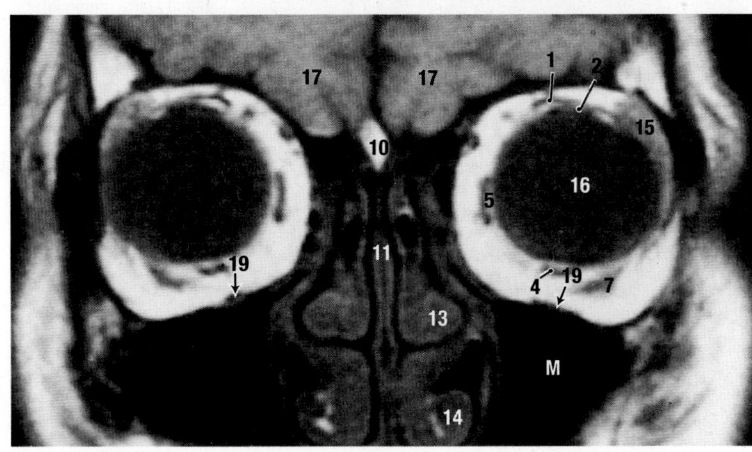
17
17
1
2
15
10
16
5
11
19
4
19
7
13
M
14

Posterior Views

D

7.94 CORONAL SECTION AND MRI IMAGING OF NASOPHARYNX AND ORAL CAVITY *(CONTINUED)*

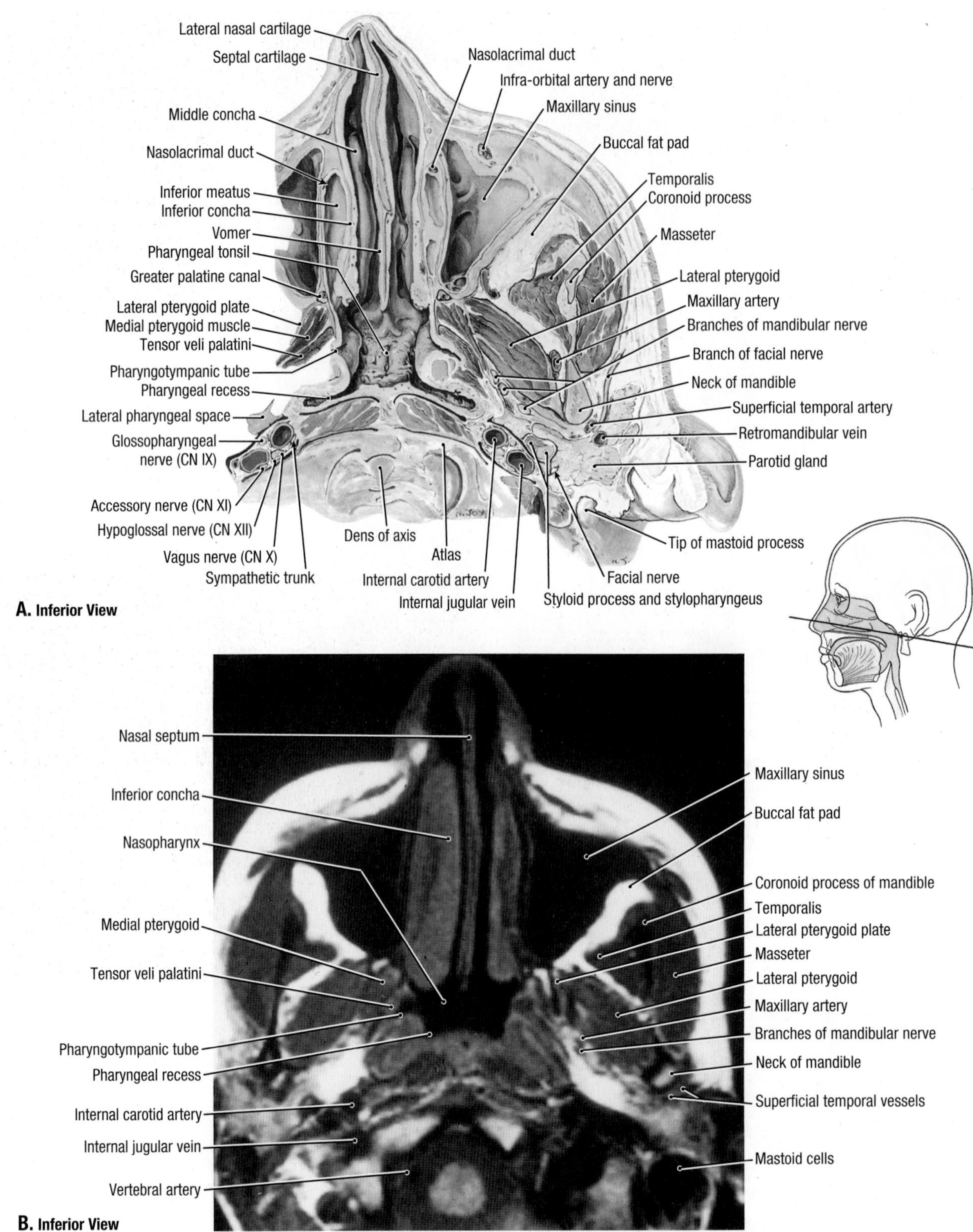
Lateral nasal cartilage
Septal cartilage
Middle concha
Nasolacrimal duct
Inferior meatus
Inferior concha
Vomer
Pharyngeal tonsil
Greater palatine canal
Lateral pterygoid plate
Medial pterygoid muscle
Tensor veli palatini
Pharyngotympanic tube
Pharyngeal recess
Lateral pharyngeal space
Glossopharyngeal nerve (CN IX)
Accessory nerve (CN XI)
Hypoglossal nerve (CN XII)
Vagus nerve (CN X)
Sympathetic trunk
Dens of axis
Atlas
Internal carotid artery
Internal jugular vein
Styloid process and stylopharyngeus
Facial nerve
Tip of mastoid process
Parotid gland
Retromandibular vein
Superficial temporal artery
Neck of mandible
Branch of facial nerve
Branches of mandibular nerve
Maxillary artery
Lateral pterygoid
Masseter
Coronoid process
Temporalis
Buccal fat pad
Maxillary sinus
Infra-orbital artery and nerve
Nasolacrimal duct
A. Inferior View
Nasal septum
Inferior concha
Nasopharynx
Medial pterygoid
Tensor veli palatini
Pharyngotympanic tube
Pharyngeal recess
Internal carotid artery
Internal jugular vein
Vertebral artery
Maxillary sinus
Buccal fat pad
Coronoid process of mandible
Temporalis
Lateral pterygoid plate
Masseter
Lateral pterygoid
Maxillary artery
Branches of mandibular nerve
Neck of mandible
Superficial temporal vessels
Mastoid cells
B. Inferior View

7.95 TRANSVERSE SECTION AND MRI IMAGE OF NASAL CAVITY AND NASOPHARYNX

A. Transverse section of left side of head. **B.** Transverse (axial) MRI scan.

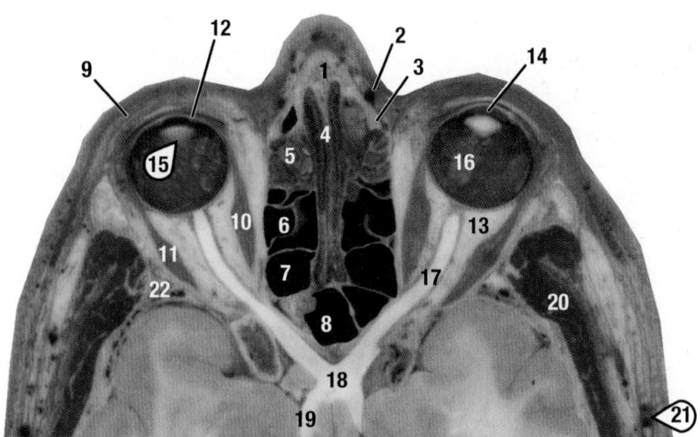
12
2
9
3
14
1
4
5
15
16
10
6
13
11
7
17
22
20
8
18
19
21

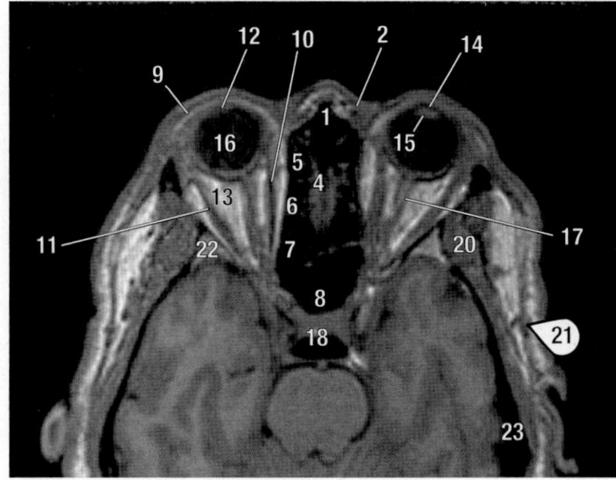
12
10
2
14
9
1
16
15
5
4
13
6
11
22
7
20
17
8
18
21
23

A. Transverse Section and Transverse (axial) MRI Scan

Key

1	Nasal bones	7	Posterior ethmoidal air cell	13	Retrobulbar fat	19	Optic tract
2	Angular artery	8	Sphenoid sinus	14	Anterior chamber	20	Temporalis muscle
3	Frontal process of maxilla	9	Orbicularis oculi muscle	15	Lens	21	Superficial temporal vessels
4	Nasal septum	10	Medial rectus muscle	16	Vitreous body	22	Greater wing of sphenoid
5	Anterior ethmoidal cell	11	Lateral rectus muscle	17	Optic nerve	23	Squamous part of temporal bone
6	Middle ethmoidal cell	12	Cornea	18	Optic chiasm		

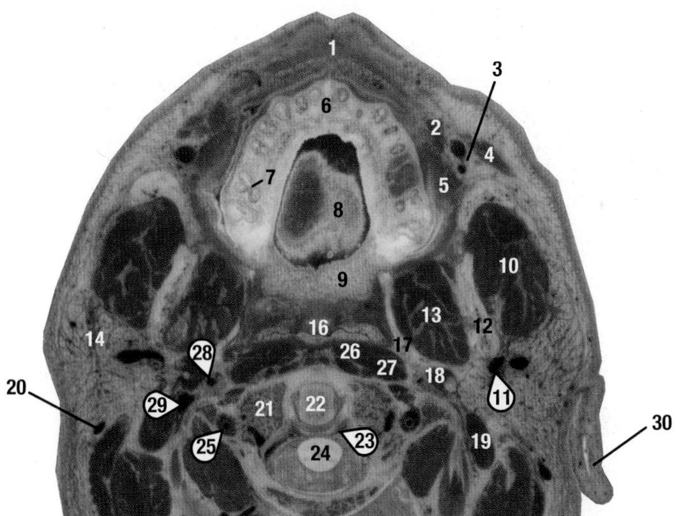
1
3
6
2
4
7
5
8
9
10
16
13
12
14
28
26
17
27
18
20
29
21
22
11
25
23
24
19
30

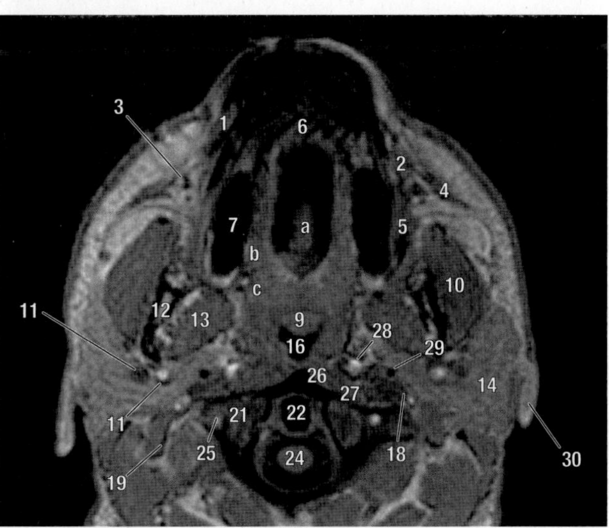
3
1
6
2
4
7
a
5
b
c
10
11
12
13
9
28
29
16
26
14
27
11
21
22
25
24
18
30
19

B. Transverse Section and Transverse (axial) MRI Scan

Key

1	Orbicularis oris muscle	12	Ramus of mandible	23	Transverse ligament of atlas
2	Levator anguli oris muscle	13	Lateral pterygoid muscle	24	Spinal cord
3	Facial artery and vein	14	Parotid gland	25	Vertebral artery in foramina transversaria
4	Zygomaticus major muscle	15	Superficial temporal vessels	26	Longus colli muscle
5	Buccinator muscle	16	Region of pharyngeal tubercle	27	Longus capitis muscle
6	Maxilla	17	Sphenoid bone	28	Internal carotid artery
7	Alveolar process of maxilla	18	Stylohyoid ligament and muscle	29	Internal jugular vein
8	Dorsum of tongue	19	Posterior belly of digastric muscle	30	Inferior portion of helix of auricle
9	Soft palate (uvula apparent in image)	20	Occipital artery	a	Hard palate
10	Masseter muscle	21	First cervical vertebrae (atlas)	b	Palatoglossus muscle
11	Retromandibular vein	22	Dens (axis)	c	Palatopharyngeus muscle

7.96 IMAGING OF ORBIT AND ORAL CAVITY/MAXILLARY REGION

A. Transverse section and MRI through in plane of optic nerve. **B.** Transverse section and MRI at level of atlas/dens.

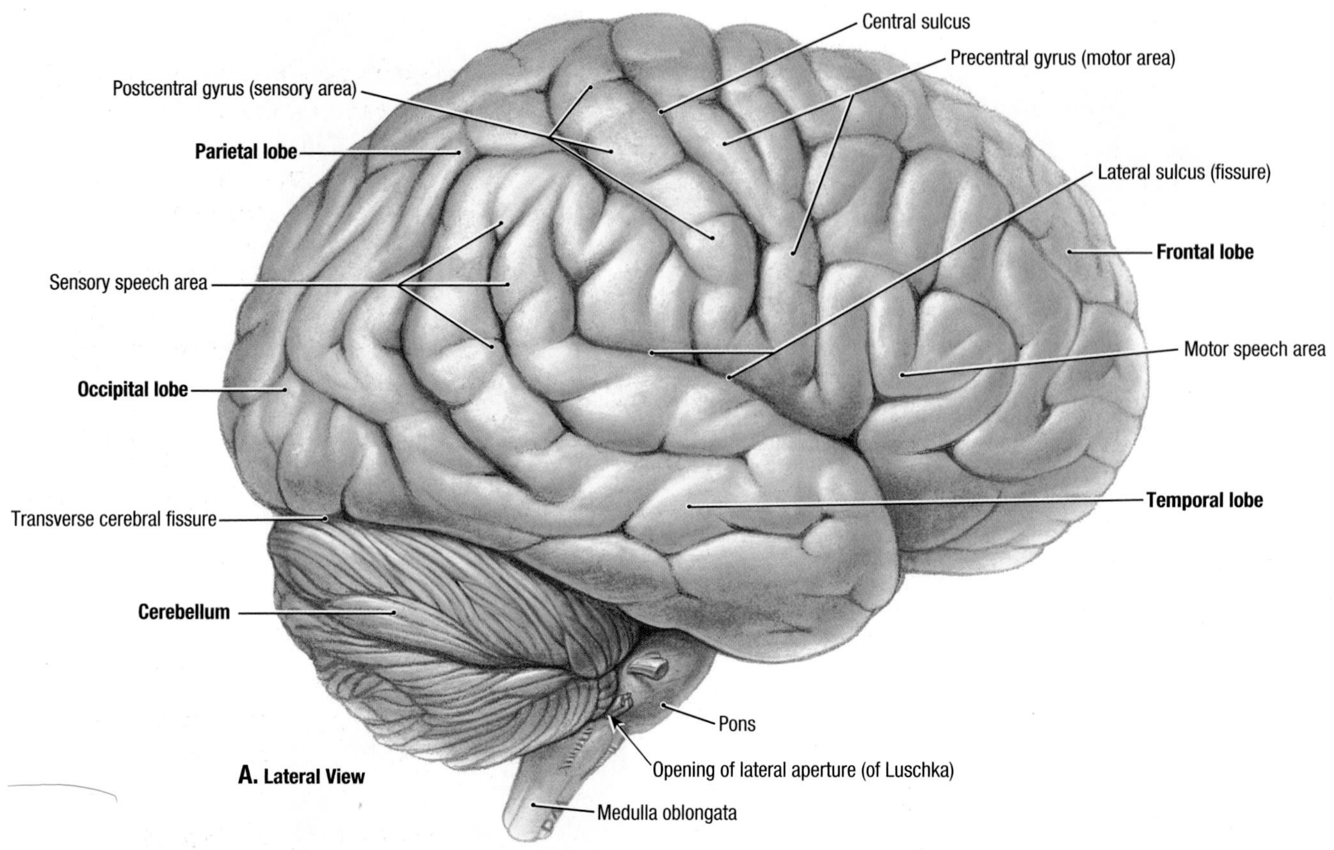
Central sulcus
Precentral gyrus (motor area)
Postcentral gyrus (sensory area)
Parietal lobe
Lateral sulcus (fissure)
Frontal lobe
Sensory speech area
Motor speech area
Occipital lobe
Temporal lobe
Transverse cerebral fissure
Cerebellum
Pons
Opening of lateral aperture (of Luschka)
Medulla oblongata

A. Lateral View

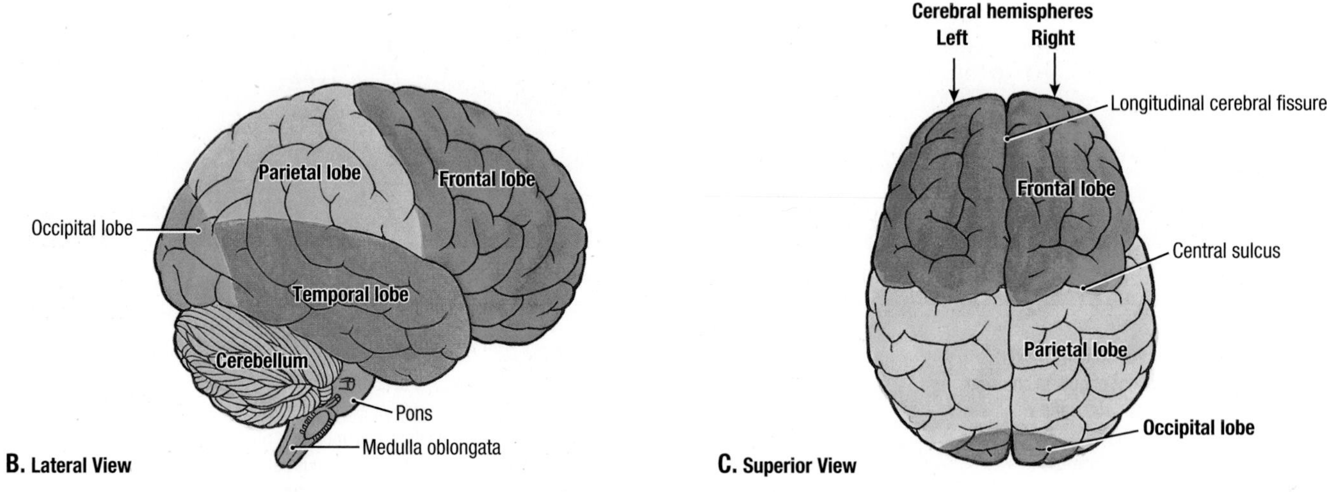
Parietal lobe
Frontal lobe
Occipital lobe
Temporal lobe
Cerebellum
Pons
Medulla oblongata
Cerebral hemispheres
Left
Right
Longitudinal cerebral fissure
Frontal lobe
Central sulcus
Parietal lobe
Occipital lobe

B. Lateral View

C. Superior View

7.97 BRAIN

A. Cerebrum, cerebellum, and brainstem, lateral aspect. **B.** Lobes of the cerebral hemispheres, lateral aspect. **C.** Lobes of the cerebral hemispheres, superior aspect.

Cerebral contusion (bruising) results from brain trauma in which the pia is stripped from the injured surface of the brain and may be torn, allowing blood to enter the subarachnoid space. The bruising results from the sudden impact of the moving brain against the stationary cranium or from the suddenly moving cranium against the stationary brain. Cerebral contusion may result in an extended loss of consciousness.

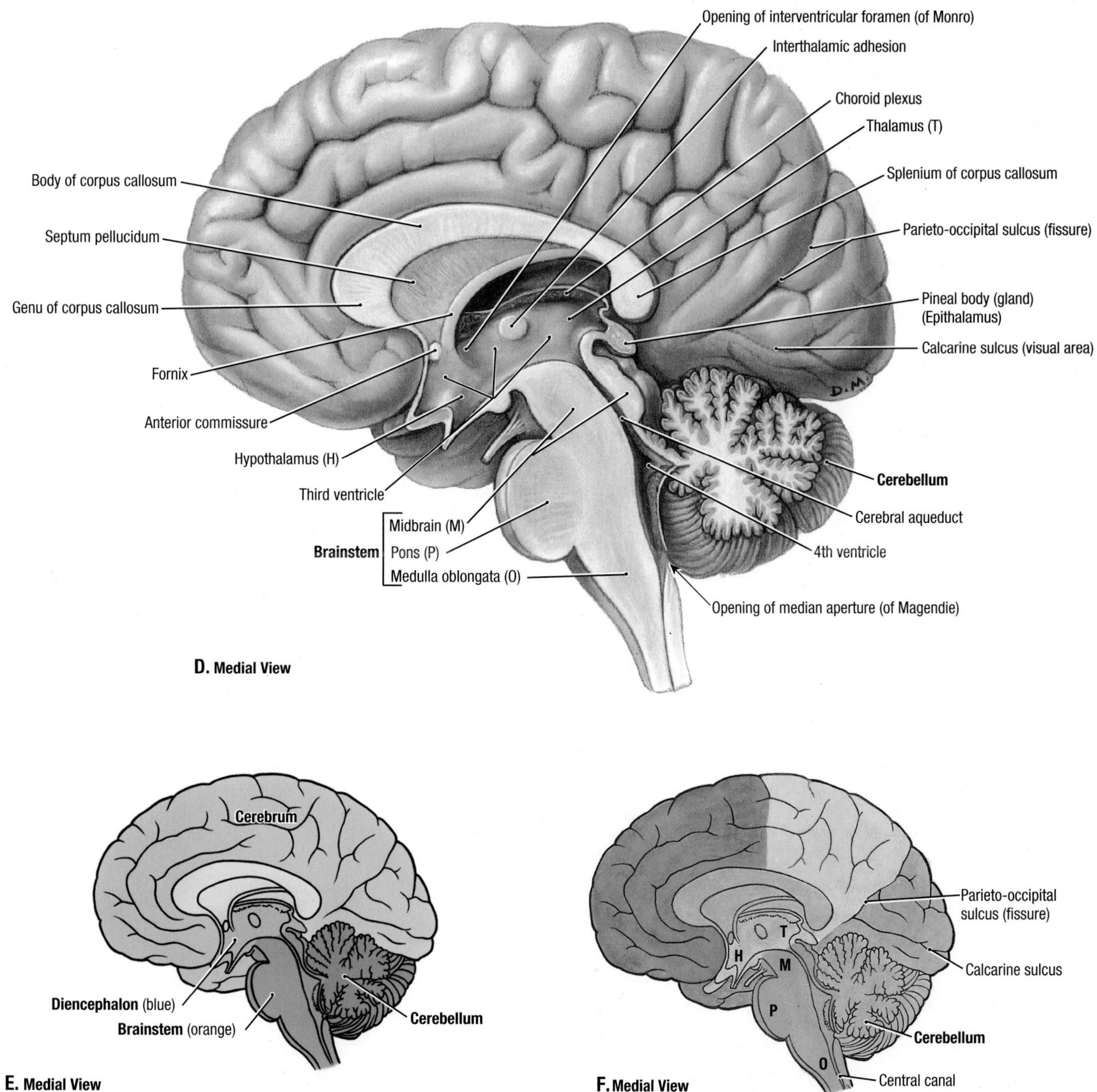
Opening of interventricular foramen (of Monro)
Interthalamic adhesion
Choroid plexus
Thalamus (T)
Splenium of corpus callosum
Parieto-occipital sulcus (fissure)
Pineal body (gland) (Epithalamus)
Calcarine sulcus (visual area)
Body of corpus callosum
Septum pellucidum
Genu of corpus callosum
Fornix
Anterior commissure
Hypothalamus (H)
Third ventricle
Cerebellum
Cerebral aqueduct
4th ventricle
Brainstem
Midbrain (M)
Pons (P)
Medulla oblongata (O)
Opening of median aperture (of Magendie)
D. Medial View
Cerebrum
Diencephalon (blue)
Brainstem (orange)
Cerebellum
E. Medial View
T
H
M
P
O
Parieto-occipital sulcus (fissure)
Calcarine sulcus
Cerebellum
Central canal
F. Medial View

7.97 BRAIN *(CONTINUED)*

D. Cerebrum, cerebellum, and brainstem, median section. **E.** Parts of the brain, median section. **F.** Lobes of the cerebral hemisphere, median section. See **D** for labeling key.

Cerebral compression may be produced by intracranial collections of blood, obstruction of CSF circulation or absorption, intracranial tumors or abscesses, and brain swelling caused by brain edema, an increase in brain volume resulting from an increase in water and sodium content.

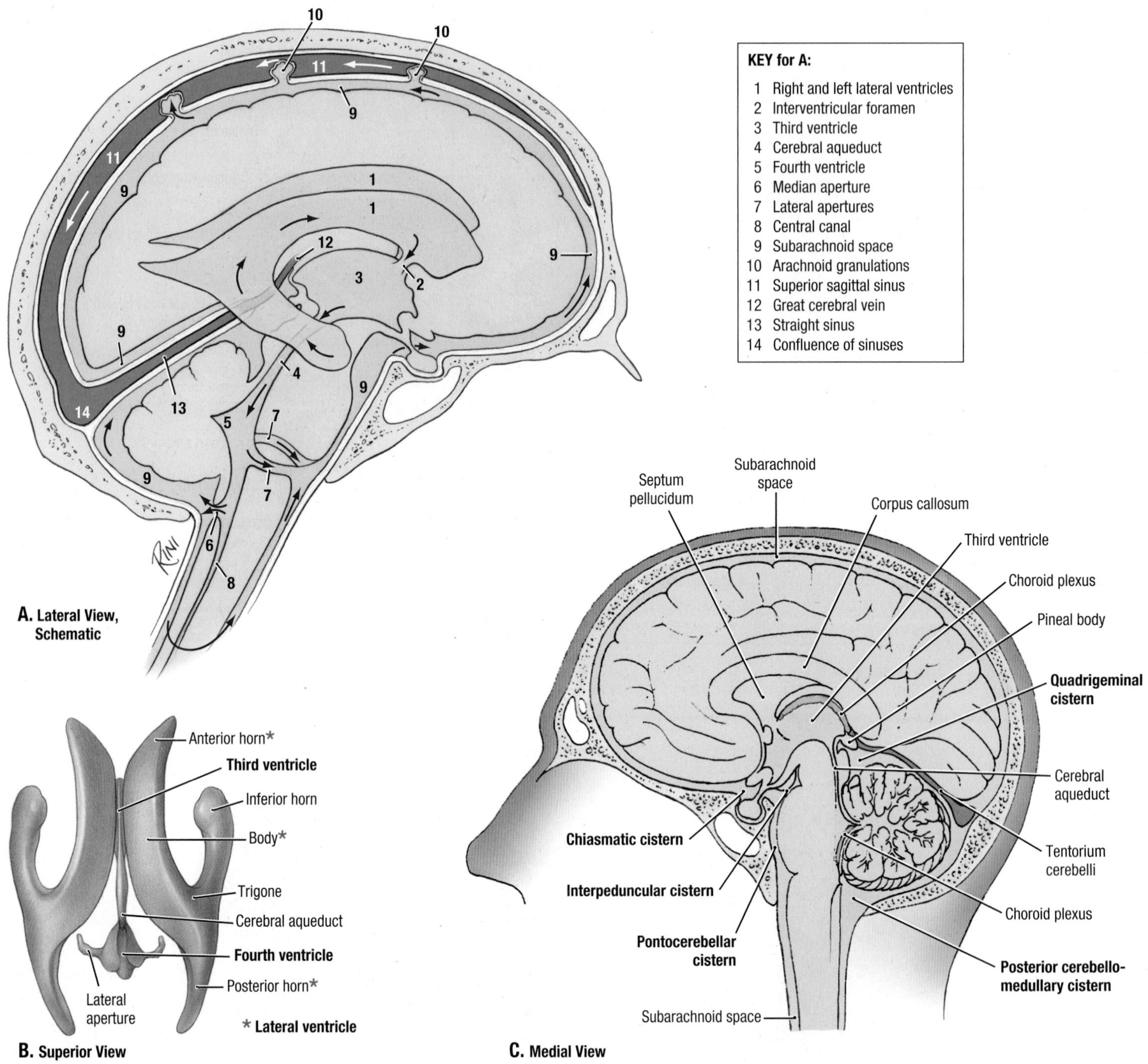
KEY for A:
1 Right and left lateral ventricles
2 Interventricular foramen
3 Third ventricle
4 Cerebral aqueduct
5 Fourth ventricle
6 Median aperture
7 Lateral apertures
8 Central canal
9 Subarachnoid space
10 Arachnoid granulations
11 Superior sagittal sinus
12 Great cerebral vein
13 Straight sinus
14 Confluence of sinuses
A. Lateral View, Schematic
Anterior horn*
Third ventricle
Inferior horn
Body*
Trigone
Cerebral aqueduct
Fourth ventricle
Posterior horn*
Lateral aperture
* Lateral ventricle
B. Superior View
Septum pellucidum
Subarachnoid space
Corpus callosum
Third ventricle
Choroid plexus
Pineal body
Quadrigeminal cistern
Cerebral aqueduct
Tentorium cerebelli
Choroid plexus
Chiasmatic cistern
Interpeduncular cistern
Pontocerebellar cistern
Posterior cerebello-medullary cistern
Subarachnoid space
C. Medial View

7.98 VENTRICULAR SYSTEM

A. Circulation of cerebrospinal fluid (CSF). **B.** Ventricles: lateral, third, and fourth.

- The ventricular system consists of two lateral ventricles located in the cerebral hemispheres, a third ventricle located between the right and left halves of the diencephalon, and a fourth ventricle located in the posterior parts of the pons and medulla.
- CSF secreted by choroid plexus in the ventricles drains via the interventricular foramen from the lateral to the third ventricle, via the cerebral aqueduct from the third to the fourth ventricle, and via median and lateral apertures into the subarachnoid space. CSF is absorbed by arachnoid granulations into the venous sinuses (especially the superior sagittal sinus).
- **Hydrocephalus.** Overproduction of CSF, obstruction of its flow, or interference with its absorption results in an excess of CSF in the ventricles and enlargement of the head, a condition known as hydrocephalus. Excess CSF dilates the ventricles; thins the brain; and, in infants, separates the bones of the calvaria because the sutures and fontanelles are still open.

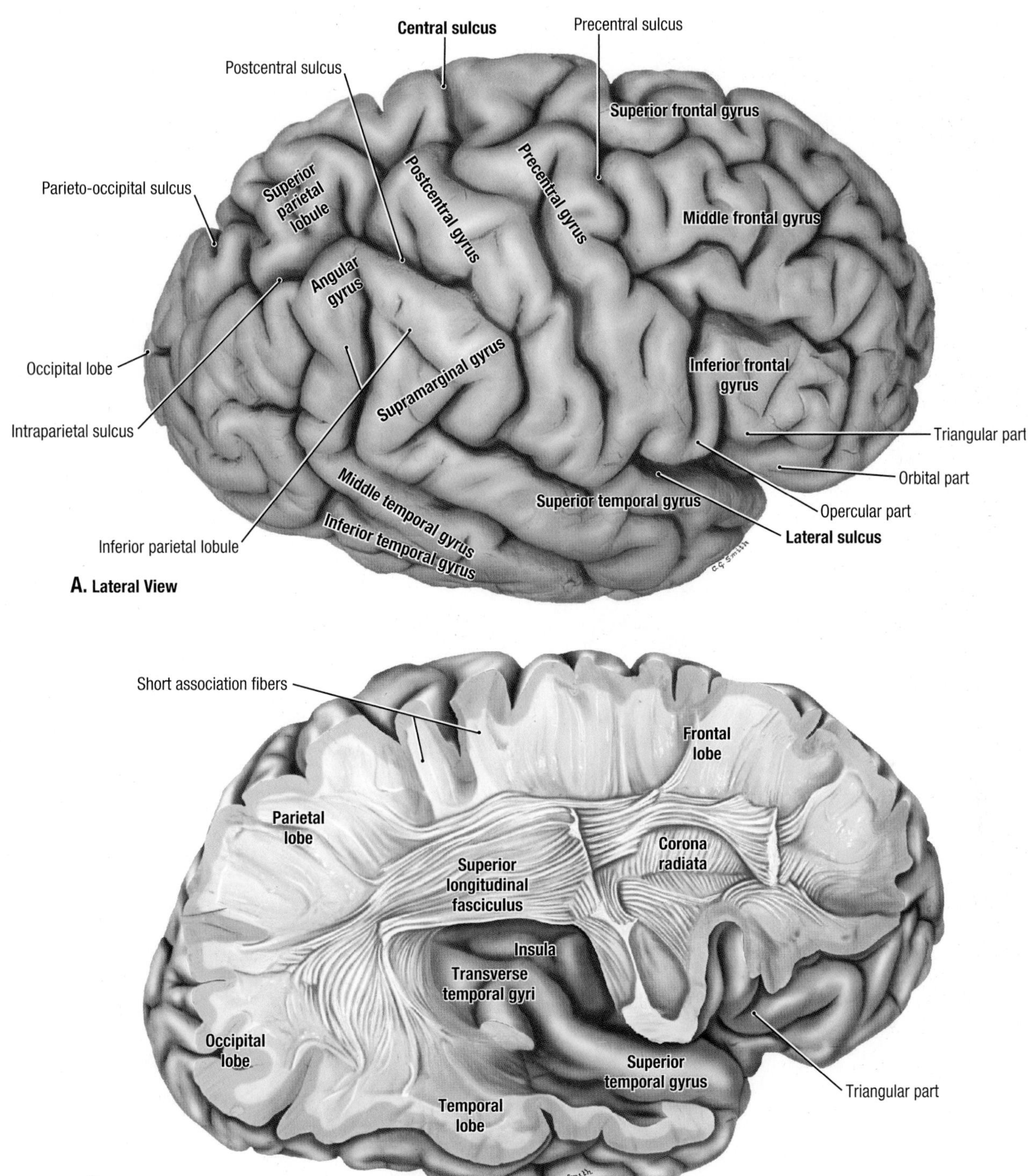
Central sulcus
Precentral sulcus
Postcentral sulcus
Superior frontal gyrus
Parieto-occipital sulcus
Superior parietal lobule
Postcentral gyrus
Precentral gyrus
Middle frontal gyrus
Angular gyrus
Occipital lobe
Inferior frontal gyrus
Supramarginal gyrus
Intraparietal sulcus
Triangular part
Orbital part
Middle temporal gyrus
Superior temporal gyrus
Opercular part
Inferior temporal gyrus
Lateral sulcus
Inferior parietal lobule
A. Lateral View
Short association fibers
Frontal lobe
Parietal lobe
Corona radiata
Superior longitudinal fasciculus
Insula
Transverse temporal gyri
Occipital lobe
Superior temporal gyrus
Triangular part
Temporal lobe
B. Lateral View

7.99 SERIAL DISSECTIONS OF LATERAL ASPECT OF CEREBRAL HEMISPHERE

The dissections begin from the lateral surface of the cerebral hemisphere **(A)** and proceed sequentially medially **(B.–F)**.

A. Sulci and gyri of the lateral surface of one cerebral hemisphere. Each gyrus is a fold of cerebral cortex with a core of white matter. The furrows are called *sulci*. The pattern of sulci and gyri, formed shortly before birth, is recognizable in some adult brains, as shown in this specimen. Usually the expanding cortex acquires secondary foldings, which make identification of this basic pattern more difficult. **B.** Superior longitudinal fasciculus, transverse temporal gyri, and insula. The cortex and short association fiber bundles around the lateral fissure have been removed.

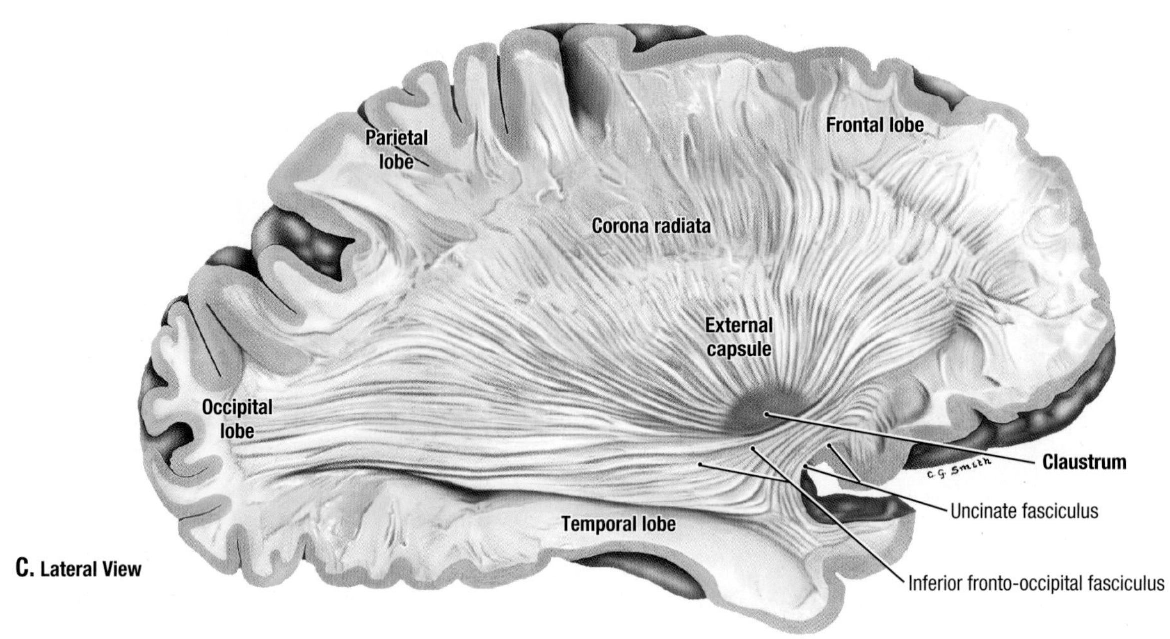
Parietal lobe
Frontal lobe
Corona radiata
External capsule
Occipital lobe
Claustrum
Uncinate fasciculus
Temporal lobe
Inferior fronto-occipital fasciculus
C. G. Smith

C. Lateral View

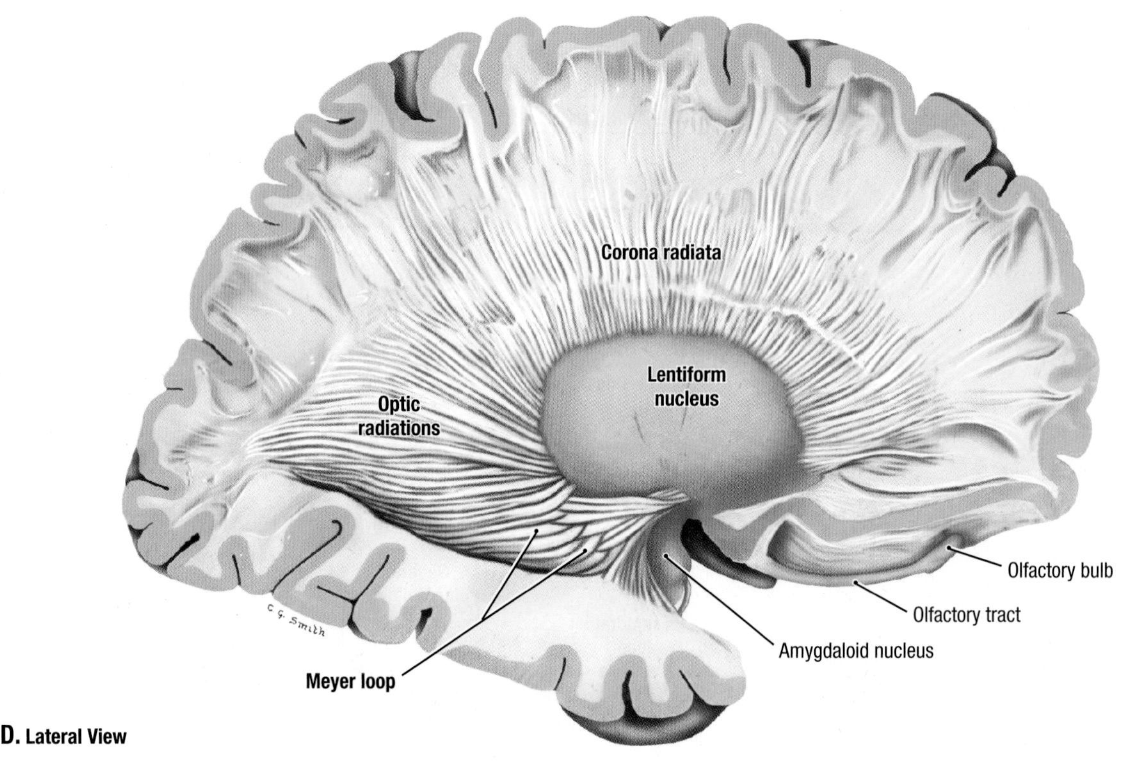
Corona radiata
Lentiform nucleus
Optic radiations
Olfactory bulb
Olfactory tract
Amygdaloid nucleus
Meyer loop
C. G. Smith

D. Lateral View

7.99 SERIAL DISSECTIONS OF LATERAL ASPECT OF CEREBRAL HEMISPHERE *(CONTINUED)*

C. Uncinate and inferior fronto-occipital fasciculi and external capsule. The external capsule consists of projection fibers that pass between the claustrum laterally and the lentiform nucleus medially. **D.** Lentiform nucleus and corona radiata. The inferior longitudinal and uncinate fasciculi, claustrum, and external capsule have been removed. The fibers of the optic radiations convey impulses from the right half of the retina of each eye; the fibers extending closest to the temporal pole (Meyer's loop) carry impulses from the lower portion of each retina.

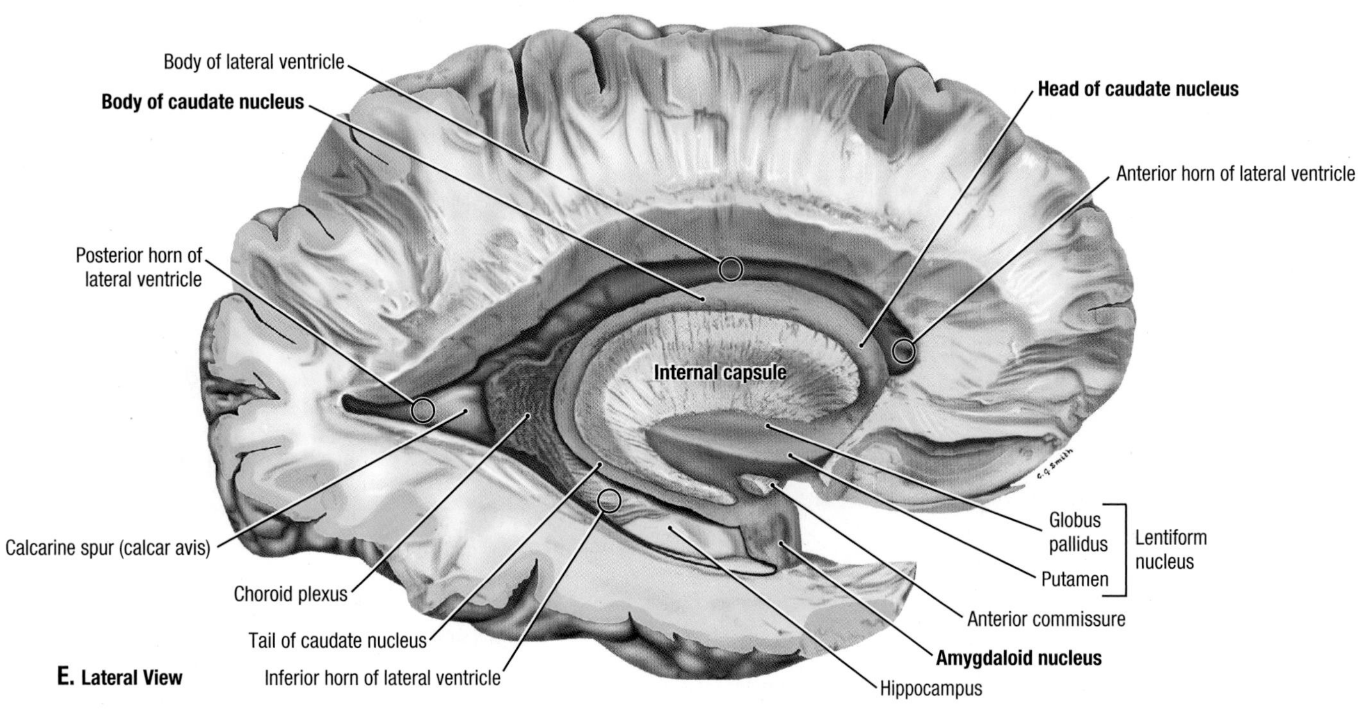
Body of lateral ventricle
Body of caudate nucleus
Head of caudate nucleus
Anterior horn of lateral ventricle
Posterior horn of lateral ventricle
Internal capsule
Calcarine spur (calcar avis)
Choroid plexus
Tail of caudate nucleus
Inferior horn of lateral ventricle
Globus pallidus
Putamen
Lentiform nucleus
Anterior commissure
Amygdaloid nucleus
Hippocampus

E. Lateral View

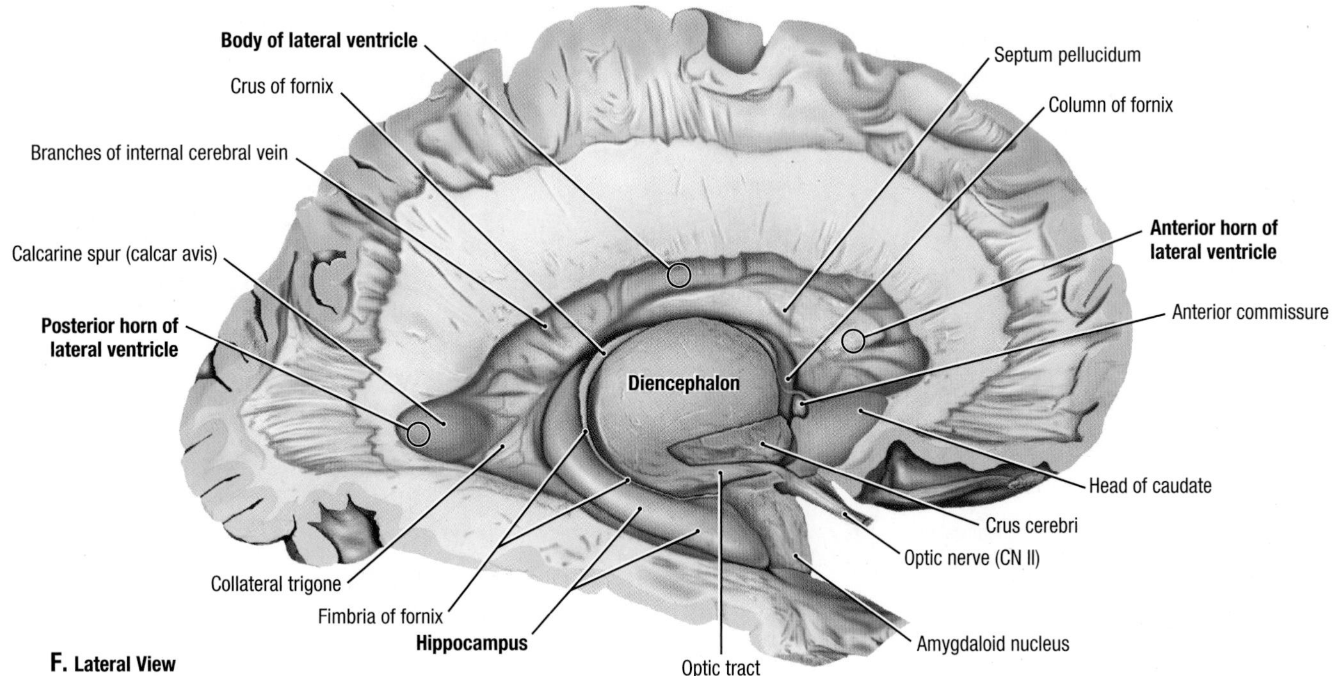
Body of lateral ventricle
Crus of fornix
Branches of internal cerebral vein
Calcarine spur (calcar avis)
Posterior horn of lateral ventricle
Septum pellucidum
Column of fornix
Anterior horn of lateral ventricle
Anterior commissure
Diencephalon
Head of caudate
Crus cerebri
Optic nerve (CN II)
Collateral trigone
Fimbria of fornix
Hippocampus
Optic tract
Amygdaloid nucleus

F. Lateral View

7.99 SERIAL DISSECTIONS OF LATERAL ASPECT OF CEREBRAL HEMISPHERE *(CONTINUED)*

E. Caudate and amygdaloid nuclei and internal capsule. The lateral wall of the lateral ventricle, the marginal part of the internal capsule, the anterior commissure, and the superior part of the lentiform nucleus have been removed. **F.** Lateral ventricle, hippocampus, and diencephalon. The inferior parts of the lentiform nucleus, internal capsule, and caudate nucleus have been removed.

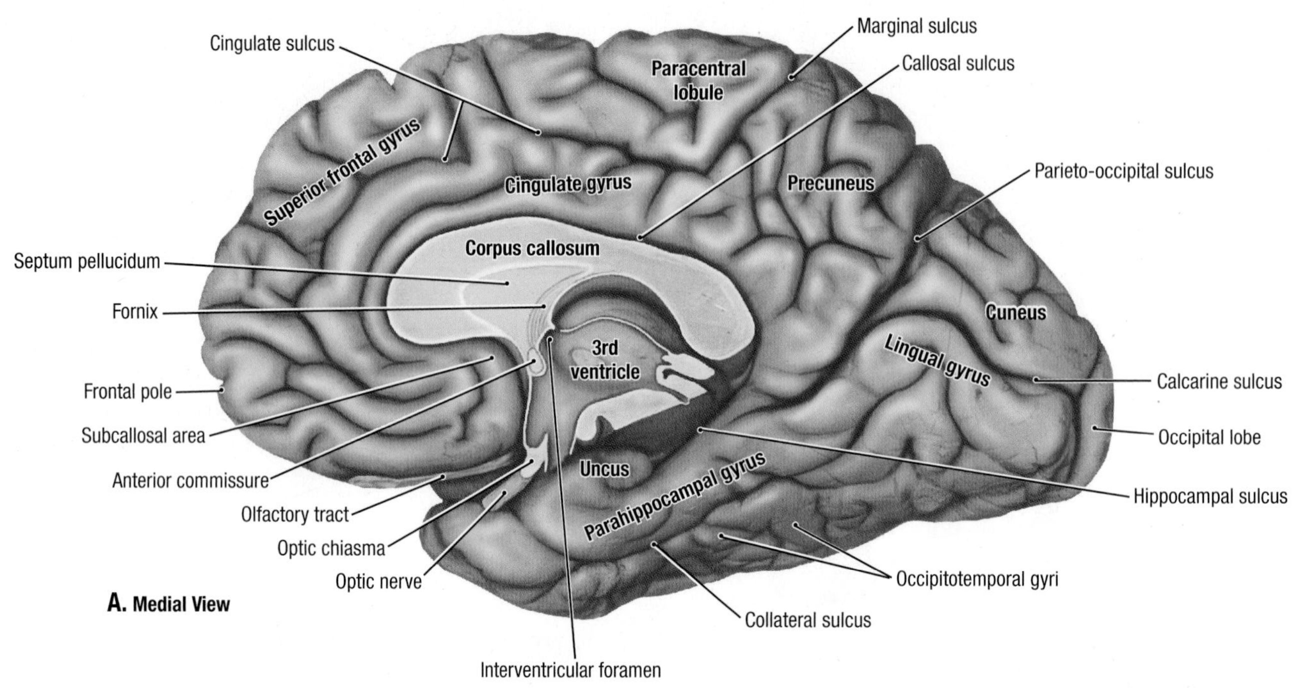
Cingulate sulcus
Marginal sulcus
Callosal sulcus
Paracentral lobule
Superior frontal gyrus
Cingulate gyrus
Precuneus
Parieto-occipital sulcus
Corpus callosum
Septum pellucidum
Fornix
Cuneus
3rd ventricle
Lingual gyrus
Frontal pole
Calcarine sulcus
Subcallosal area
Occipital lobe
Anterior commissure
Uncus
Hippocampal sulcus
Parahippocampal gyrus
Olfactory tract
Optic chiasma
Optic nerve
Occipitotemporal gyri
Collateral sulcus
Interventricular foramen

A. Medial View

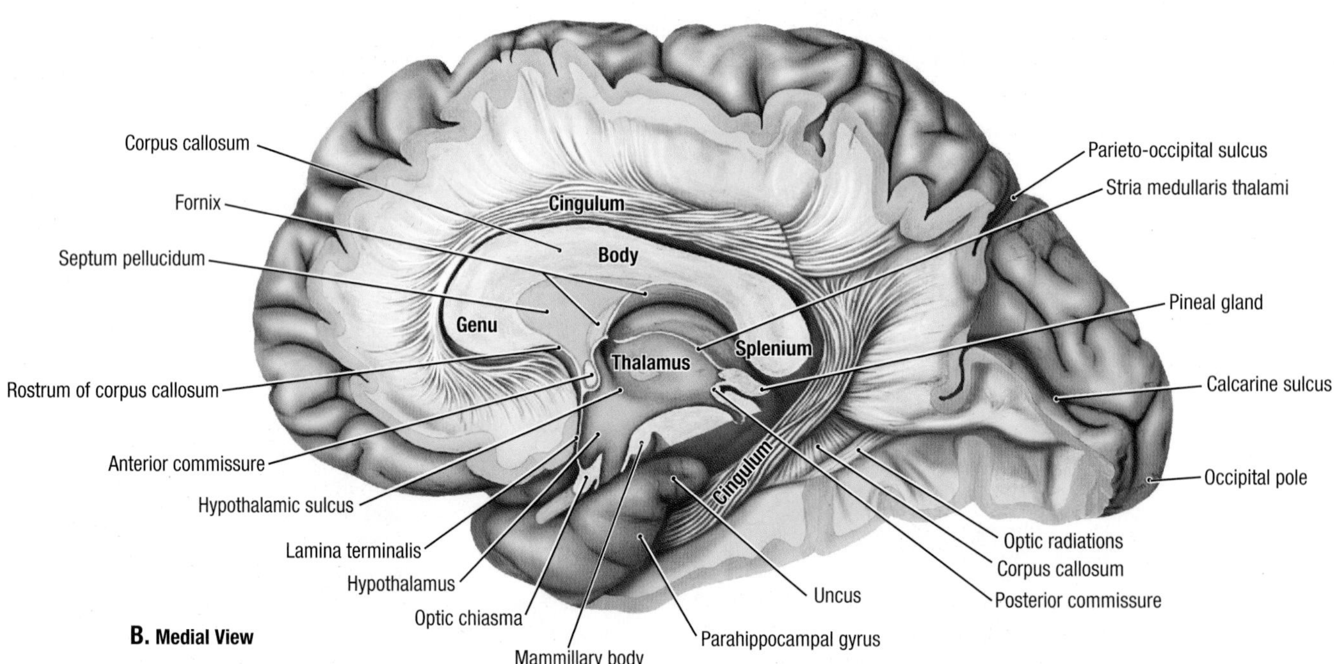
Corpus callosum
Parieto-occipital sulcus
Stria medullaris thalami
Fornix
Cingulum
Body
Septum pellucidum
Pineal gland
Genu
Splenium
Thalamus
Rostrum of corpus callosum
Calcarine sulcus
Anterior commissure
Cingulum
Occipital pole
Hypothalamic sulcus
Lamina terminalis
Optic radiations
Corpus callosum
Hypothalamus
Uncus
Posterior commissure
Optic chiasma
Parahippocampal gyrus
Mammillary body

B. Medial View

7.100 SERIAL DISSECTIONS OF MEDIAL ASPECT OF CEREBRAL HEMISPHERE

The dissections begin from the medial surface of the cerebral hemisphere **(A)** and proceed sequentially laterally **(B.–D)**.

A. Sulci and gyri of medial surface of cerebral hemisphere. The corpus callosum consists of the rostrum, genu, body, and splenium; the cingulate and parahippocampal gyri from the limbic lobe. **B.** Cingulum. The cortex and short association fibers were removed from the medial aspect of the hemisphere. The cingulum is a long association fiber bundle that lies in the core of the cingulate and parahippocampal gyri.

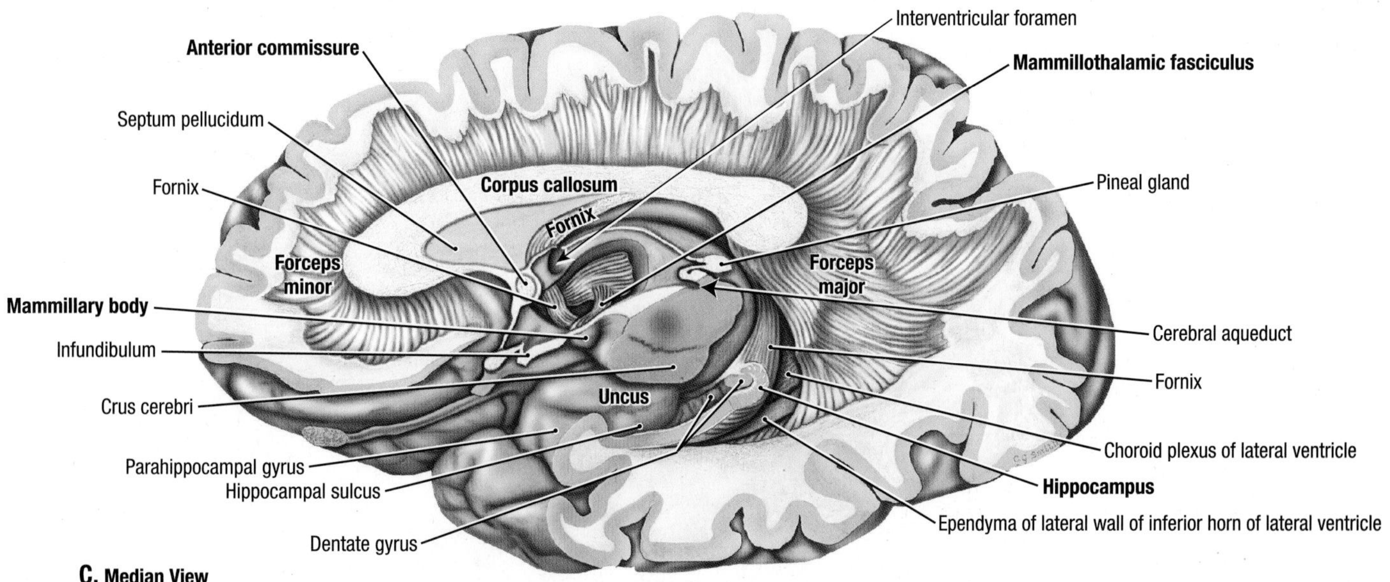
Interventricular foramen
Anterior commissure
Mammillothalamic fasciculus
Septum pellucidum
Pineal gland
Fornix
Corpus callosum
Fornix
Forceps minor
Forceps major
Mammillary body
Cerebral aqueduct
Infundibulum
Fornix
Crus cerebri
Uncus
Choroid plexus of lateral ventricle
Parahippocampal gyrus
Hippocampal sulcus
Hippocampus
Ependyma of lateral wall of inferior horn of lateral ventricle
Dentate gyrus

C. Median View

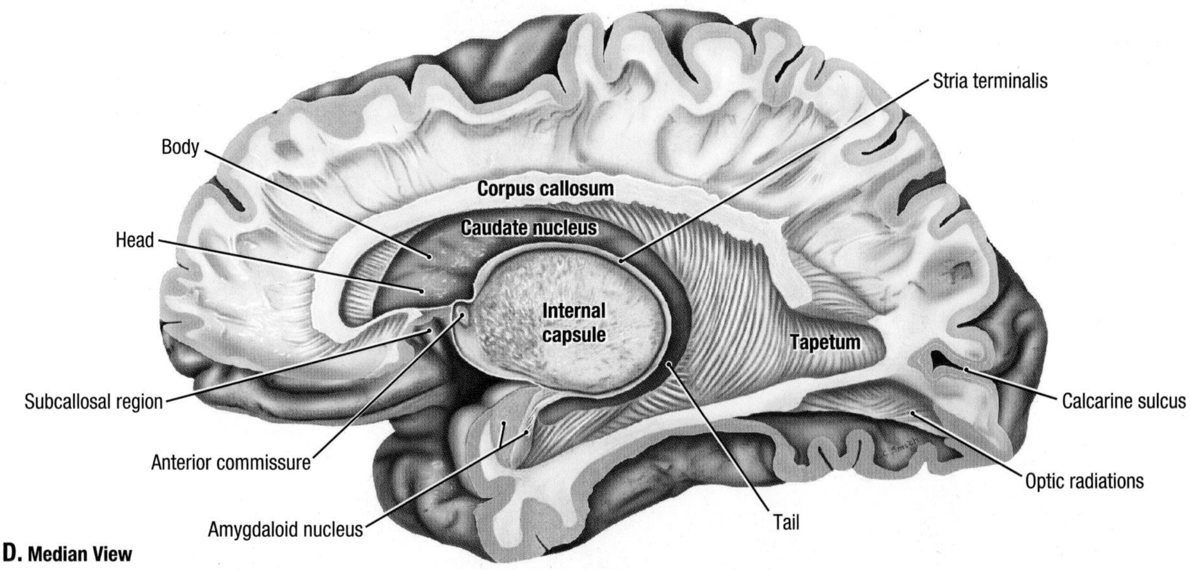
Stria terminalis
Body
Corpus callosum
Head
Caudate nucleus
Internal capsule
Tapetum
Subcallosal region
Calcarine sulcus
Anterior commissure
Optic radiations
Amygdaloid nucleus
Tail

D. Median View

7.100 SERIAL DISSECTIONS OF THE MEDIAL ASPECT OF CEREBRAL HEMISPHERE *(CONTINUED)*

C. Fornix, mammillothalamic fasciculus, and forceps major and minor. The cingulum and a portion of the wall of the third ventricle have been removed. The fornix begins at the hippocampus and terminates in the mammillary body by passing anterior to the interventricular foramen and posterior to the anterior commissure. The mammillothalamic fasciculus emerges from the mammillary body and terminates in the anterior nucleus of the thalamus. **D.** Caudate nucleus and internal capsule. The diencephalon was removed, along with the ependyma of the lateral ventricle, except where it covers the caudate and amygdaloid nuclei. **E.** Corpus callosum. The body of the corpus callosum connects the two cerebral hemispheres; the minor (frontal) forceps (at the genu of corpus callosum) connects the frontal lobes, and the major (occipital) forceps (at splenium) connects the occipital lobes.

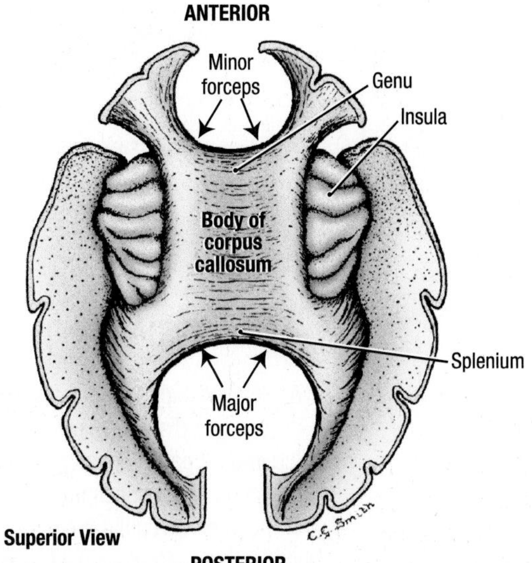
ANTERIOR
Minor forceps
Genu
Insula
Body of corpus callosum
Splenium
Major forceps
POSTERIOR

E. Superior View

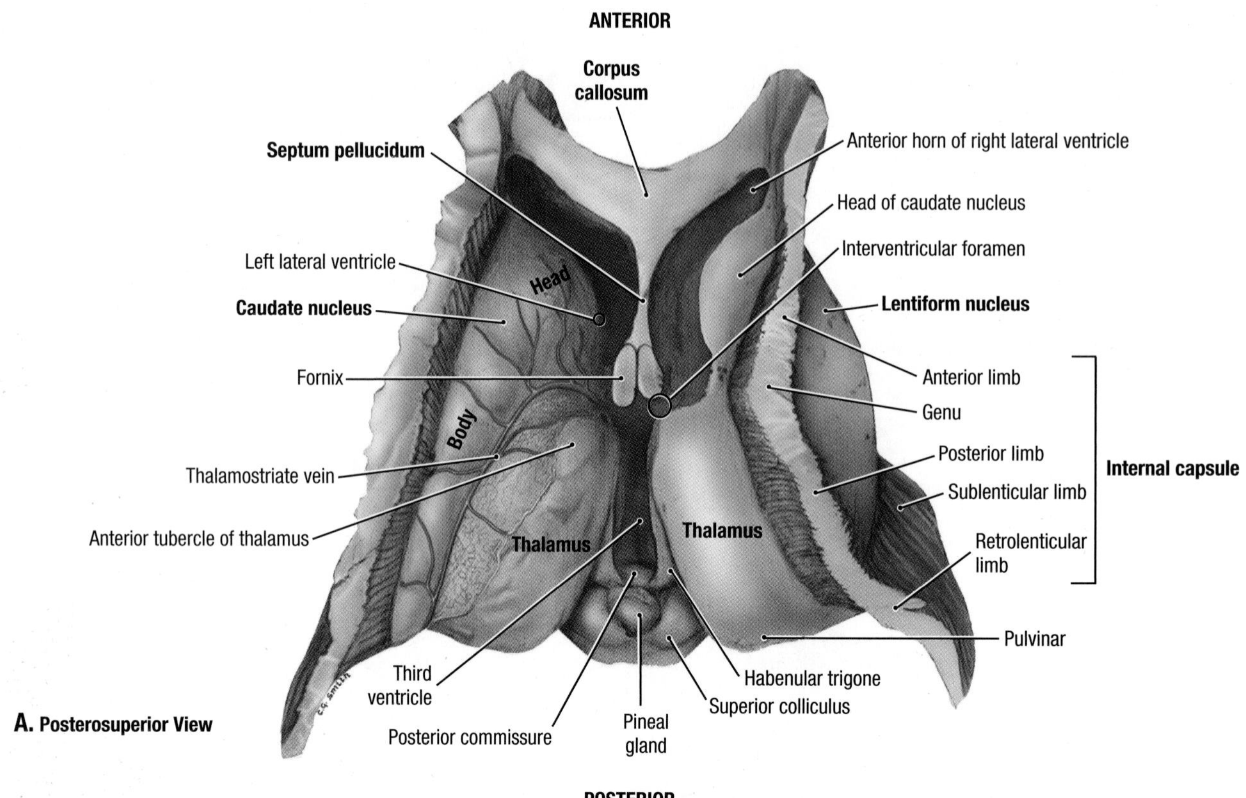
ANTERIOR
Corpus callosum
Septum pellucidum
Anterior horn of right lateral ventricle
Head of caudate nucleus
Interventricular foramen
Left lateral ventricle
Head
Caudate nucleus
Lentiform nucleus
Fornix
Anterior limb
Genu
Body
Posterior limb
Internal capsule
Thalamostriate vein
Sublenticular limb
Anterior tubercle of thalamus
Thalamus
Thalamus
Retrolenticular limb
Pulvinar
Third ventricle
Habenular trigone
Superior colliculus
Posterior commissure
Pineal gland
POSTERIOR

A. **Posterosuperior View**

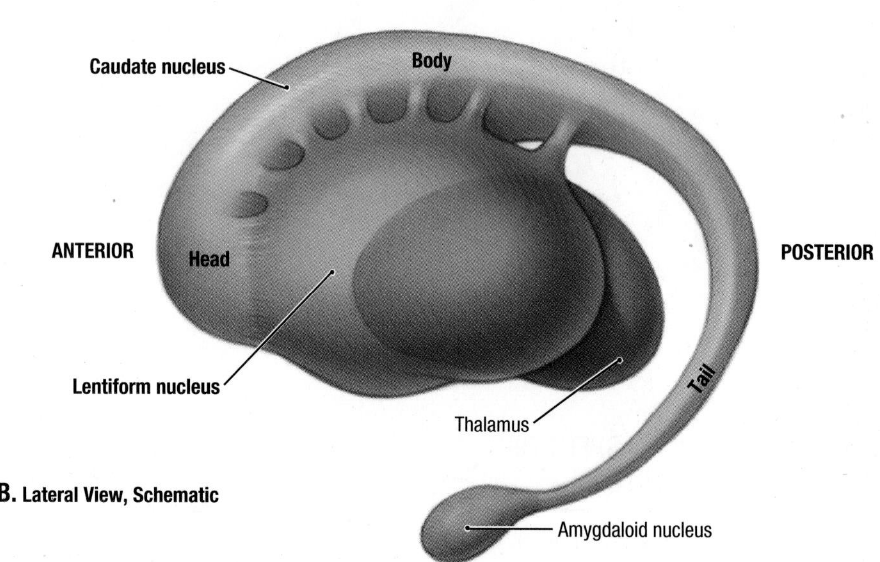
Caudate nucleus
Body
ANTERIOR
Head
POSTERIOR
Lentiform nucleus
Tail
Thalamus
Amygdaloid nucleus

B. **Lateral View, Schematic**

7.101 CAUDATE AND LENTIFORM NUCLEI

A. Relationship to the lateral ventricles and internal capsule. The dorsal surface of the diencephalon has been exposed by dissecting away the two cerebral hemispheres, except the anterior part of the corpus callosum, the inferior part of the septum pellucidum, the internal capsule, and the caudate and lentiform nuclei. On the right side of the specimen, the thalamus, caudate, and lentiform nuclei have been cut horizontally at the level of the interventricular foramen. The parts of the internal capsule include the anterior, posterior, retrolenticular sublenticular limbs, and genu. **B.** Schematic illustration of nuclei.

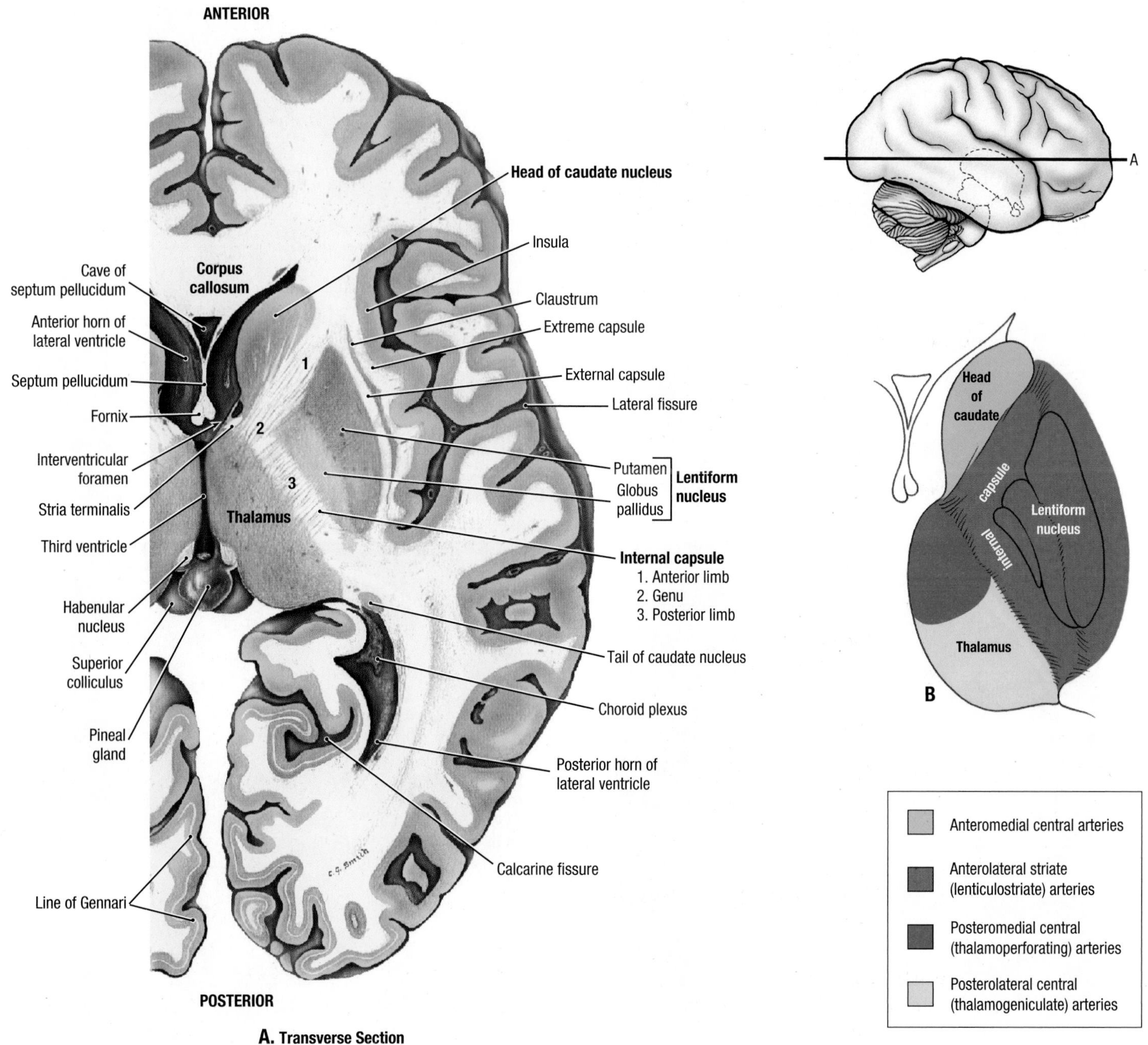
ANTERIOR
Head of caudate nucleus
Insula
Cave of septum pellucidum
Corpus callosum
Claustrum
Anterior horn of lateral ventricle
Extreme capsule
1
Septum pellucidum
External capsule
Lateral fissure
Fornix
2
Interventricular foramen
Putamen
Globus pallidus
Lentiform nucleus
3
Stria terminalis
Thalamus
Third ventricle
Internal capsule
1. Anterior limb
2. Genu
3. Posterior limb
Habenular nucleus
Superior colliculus
Tail of caudate nucleus
Choroid plexus
Pineal gland
Posterior horn of lateral ventricle
Calcarine fissure
Line of Gennari
POSTERIOR
A
Head of caudate
capsule
internal
Lentiform nucleus
Thalamus
B
Anteromedial central arteries
Anterolateral striate (lenticulostriate) arteries
Posteromedial central (thalamoperforating) arteries
Posterolateral central (thalamogeniculate) arteries

A. Transverse Section

7.102 AXIAL SECTIONS THROUGH THALAMUS, CAUDATE NUCLEUS, AND LENTIFORM NUCLEUS

A. Relationships of the internal capsule. **B.** Blood supply of region.

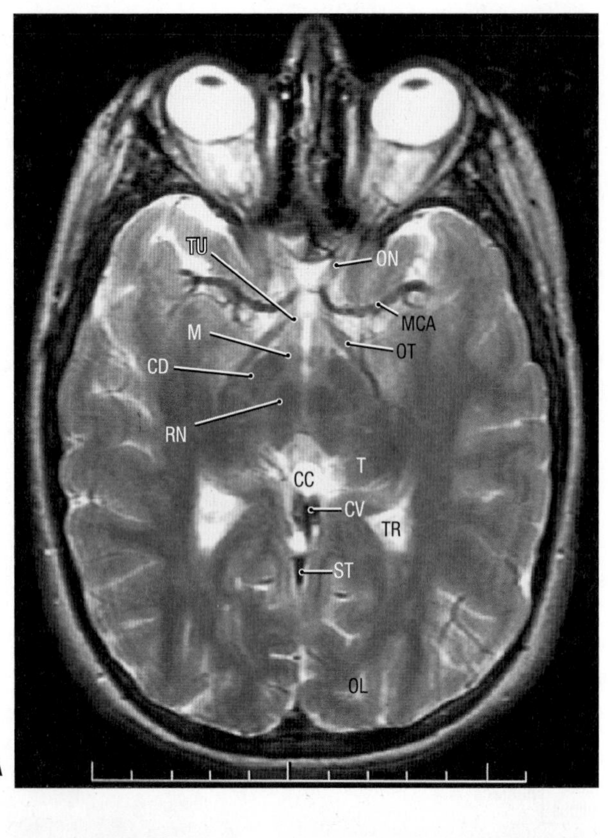

TU
ON
MCA
M
OT
CD
RN
T
CC
CV
TR
ST
OL
A

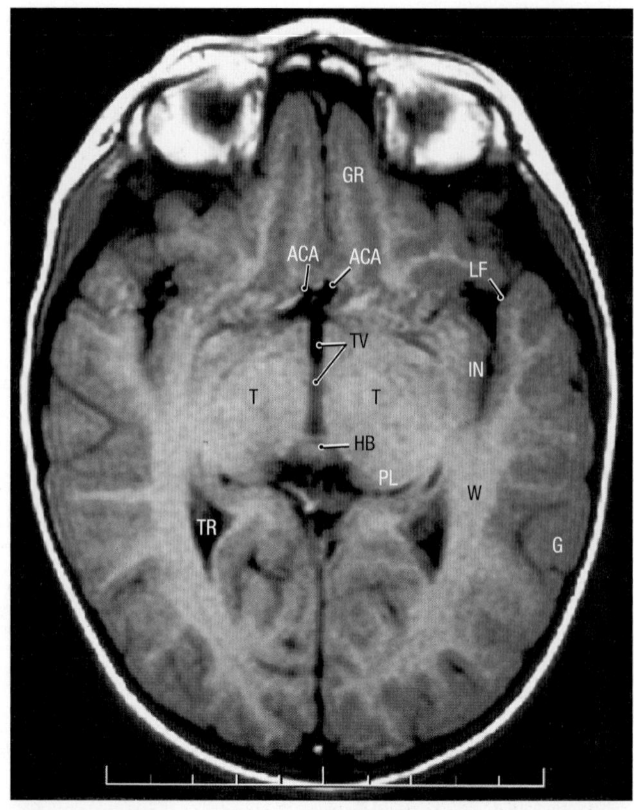

GR
ACA
ACA
LF
TV
IN
T
T
HB
PL
W
TR
G
B

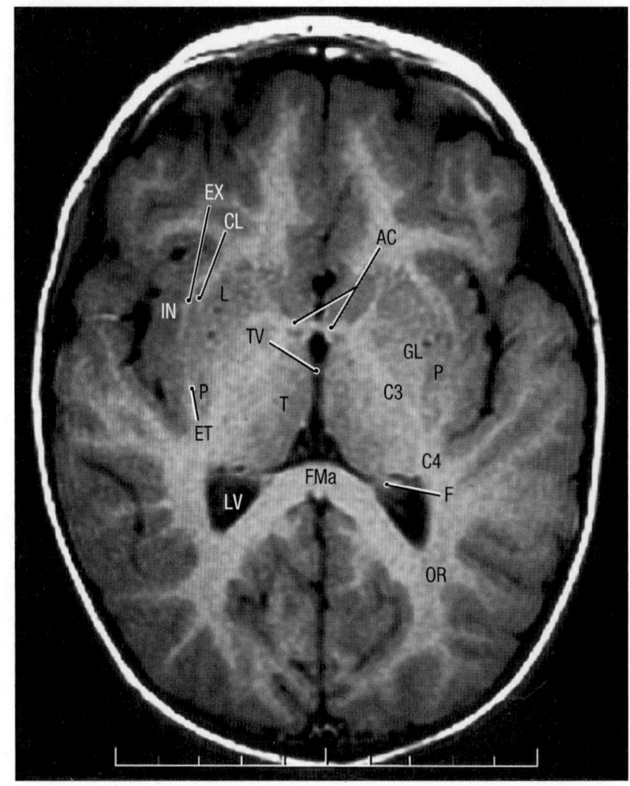

EX
CL
AC
L
IN
TV
GL
P
P
T
C3
ET
C4
FMa
F
LV
OR
C

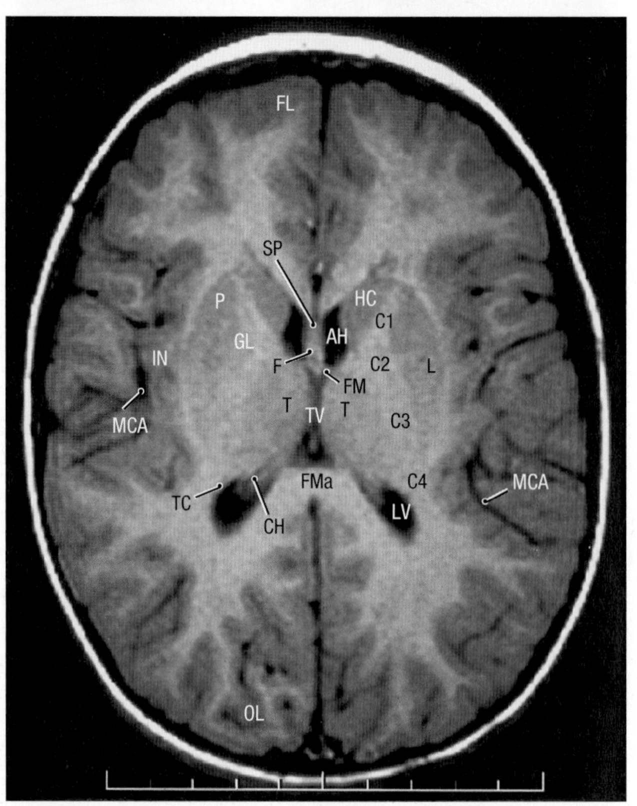

FL
SP
HC
P
C1
GL
AH
F
C2
L
IN
FM
T
TV
T
C3
MCA
FMa
C4
MCA
TC
CH
LV
OL
D

7.103 AXIAL (TRANSVERSE) MRIs THROUGH CEREBRAL HEMISPHERES

See orientation drawing for sites of scans **A.–F. A** is T2 weighted, and **B.–F.** are T1 weighted.

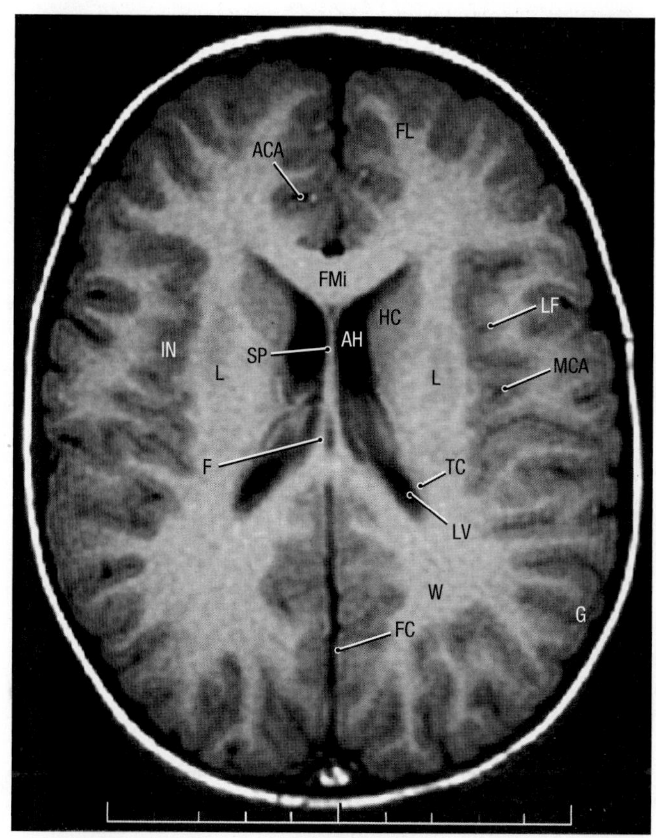
ACA
FL
FMi
HC
LF
AH
IN
SP
L
L
MCA
F
TC
LV
W
G
FC
E

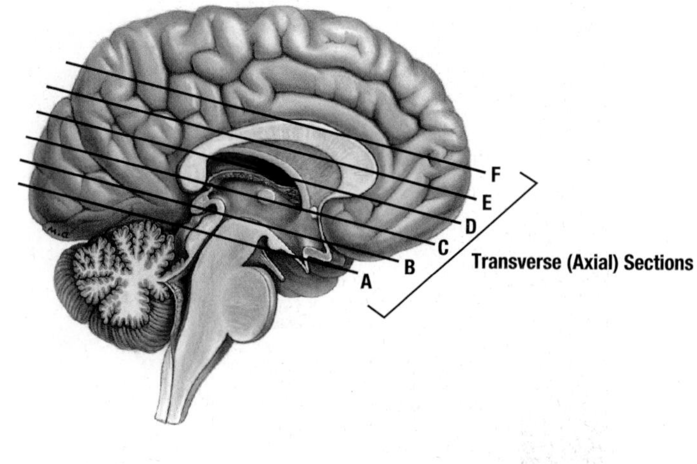
F
E
D
C
B
A
Transverse (Axial) Sections

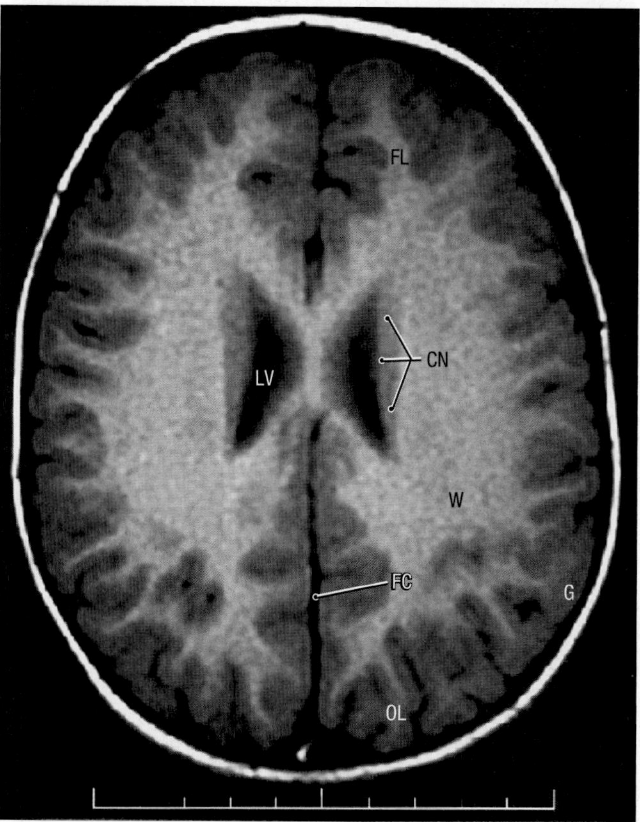
FL
LV
CN
W
FC
G
OL
F

AC	Anterior commissure	GL	Globus pallidus
ACA	Anterior cerebral artery	GR	Gyrus rectus
AH	Anterior horn of lateral ventricle	HB	Habenular commissure
C1	Anterior limb of internal capsule	HC	Head of caudate nucleus
C2	Genu of internal capsule	IN	Insular cortex
C3	Posterior limb of internal capsule	L	Lentiform nucleus
C4	Retrolenticular limb of internal capsule	LF	Lateral fissure
CC	Collicular cistern	LV	Lateral ventricle
CD	Cerebral peduncle	M	Mammillary body
CH	Choroid plexus	MCA	Middle cerebral artery
CL	Claustrum	OL	Occipital lobe
CN	Caudate nucleus	ON	Optic nerve
CV	Great cerebral vein	OR	Optic radiations
ET	External capsule	OT	Optic tract
EX	Extreme capsule	P	Putamen
F	Fornix	PL	Pulvinar
FC	Falx cerebri	RN	Red nucleus
FL	Frontal lobe	SP	Septum pellucidum
FM	Interventricular foramen	ST	Straight sinus
FMa	Forceps major	T	Thalamus
FMi	Forceps minor	TC	Tail of caudate nucleus
G	Gray matter	TR	Trigone of lateral ventricle
		TU	Tuber cinereum
		TV	Third ventricle
		W	White matter

7.103 AXIAL (TRANSVERSE) MRIs THROUGH CEREBRAL HEMISPHERES *(CONTINUED)*

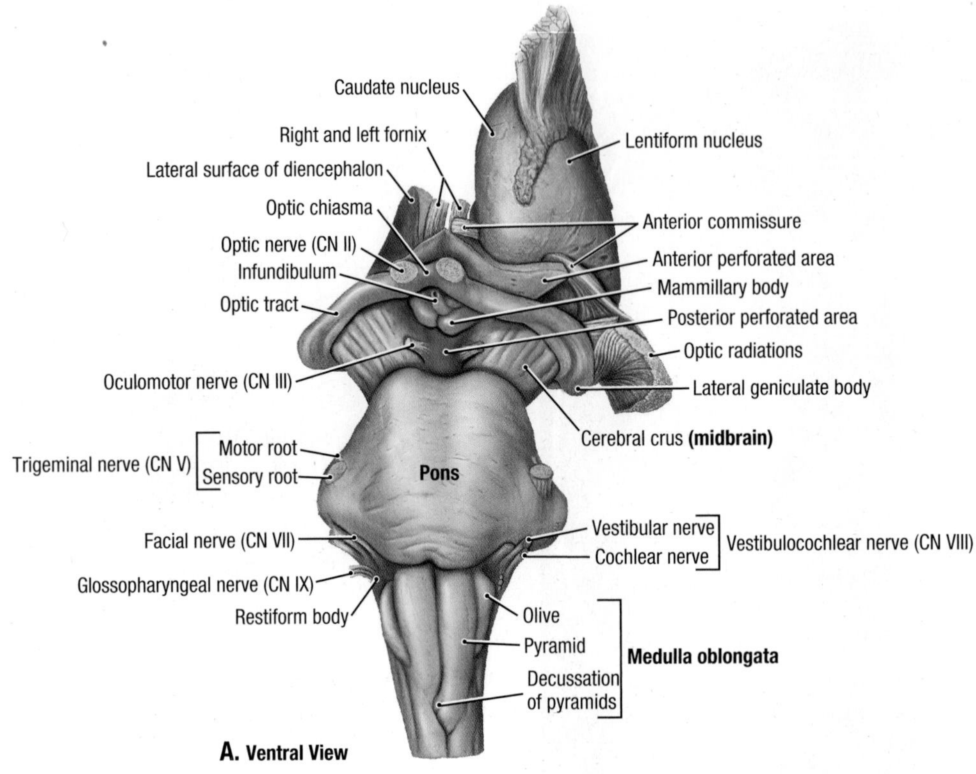
Caudate nucleus
Right and left fornix
Lateral surface of diencephalon
Optic chiasma
Optic nerve (CN II)
Infundibulum
Optic tract
Oculomotor nerve (CN III)
Trigeminal nerve (CN V)
Motor root
Sensory root
Pons
Facial nerve (CN VII)
Glossopharyngeal nerve (CN IX)
Restiform body
Lentiform nucleus
Anterior commissure
Anterior perforated area
Mammillary body
Posterior perforated area
Optic radiations
Lateral geniculate body
Cerebral crus (midbrain)
Vestibular nerve
Cochlear nerve
Vestibulocochlear nerve (CN VIII)
Olive
Pyramid
Decussation of pyramids
Medulla oblongata

A. Ventral View

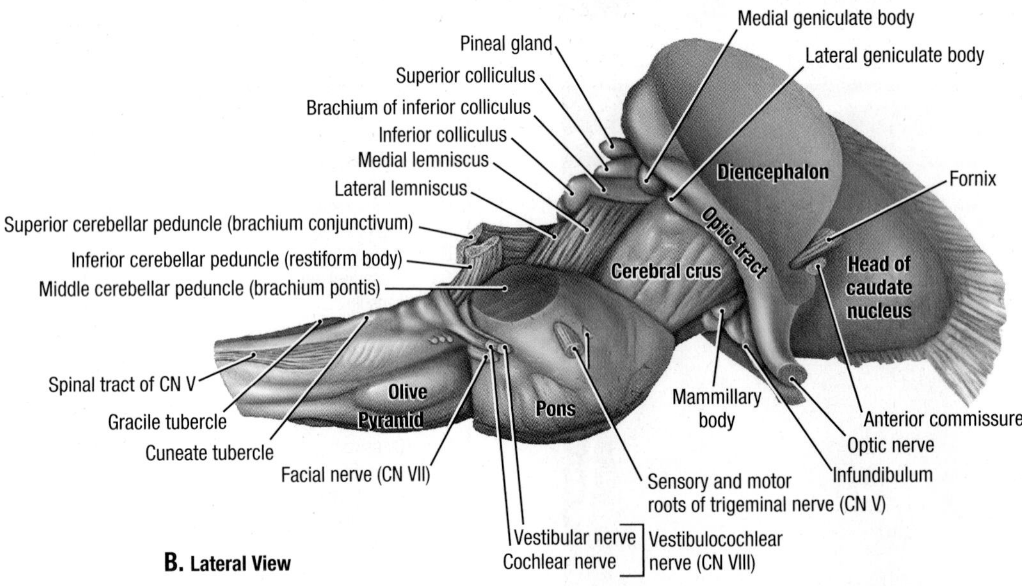
Medial geniculate body
Pineal gland
Lateral geniculate body
Superior colliculus
Brachium of inferior colliculus
Inferior colliculus
Medial lemniscus
Lateral lemniscus
Diencephalon
Fornix
Optic tract
Superior cerebellar peduncle (brachium conjunctivum)
Inferior cerebellar peduncle (restiform body)
Middle cerebellar peduncle (brachium pontis)
Cerebral crus
Head of caudate nucleus
Spinal tract of CN V
Olive
Pyramid
Gracile tubercle
Cuneate tubercle
Facial nerve (CN VII)
Pons
Mammillary body
Anterior commissure
Optic nerve
Infundibulum
Sensory and motor roots of trigeminal nerve (CN V)
Vestibular nerve
Cochlear nerve
Vestibulocochlear nerve (CN VIII)

B. Lateral View

7.104 BRAINSTEM

The brainstem has been exposed by removing the cerebellum, all of the right cerebral hemisphere, and the major portion of the left hemisphere. **A.** Ventral aspect.

- The brainstem consists of the medulla oblongata, pons, and midbrain.
- The pyramid is on the ventral surface of the medulla; the decussation of the pyramids is formed by the decussating (crossing) lateral corticospinal tract.
- The trigeminal nerve (CN V) emerges as sensory and motor roots.
- The crus cerebri are part of the midbrain.
- The oculomotor nerve emerges from the interpeduncular fossa.

B. Lateral aspect.

- The vestibulocochlear nerve (CN VIII) consists of two nerves, the vestibular and cochlear nerves.
- The spinal tract of the trigeminal nerve is exposed where it comes to the surface of the medulla to form the tuber cinereum.
- The three are cerebellar peduncles: superior, middle, and inferior.
- The medial and lateral lemnisci on the lateral aspect of the midbrain

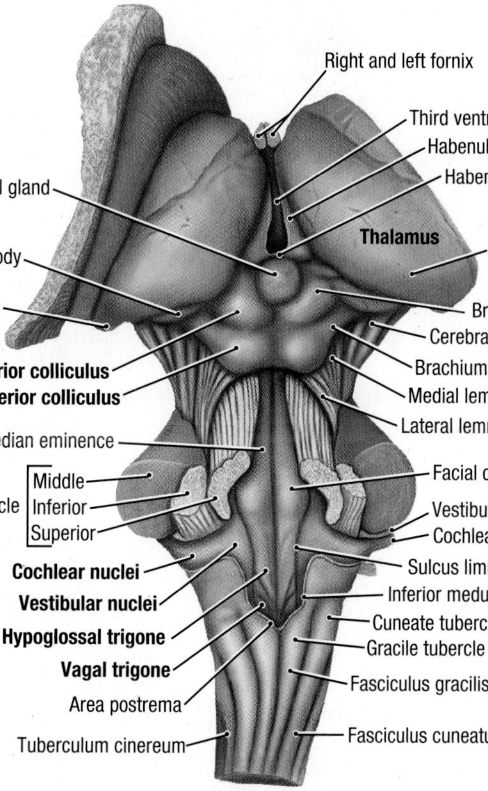

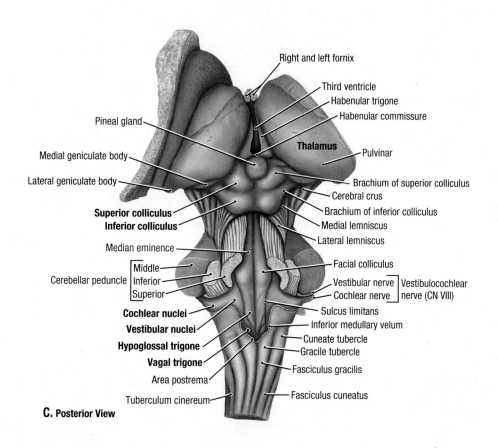

Right and left fornix
Third ventricle
Habenular trigone
Habenular commissure
Pineal gland
Thalamus
Pulvinar
Medial geniculate body
Lateral geniculate body
Brachium of superior colliculus
Cerebral crus
Superior colliculus
Inferior colliculus
Brachium of inferior colliculus
Medial lemniscus
Lateral lemniscus
Median eminence
Facial colliculus
Cerebellar peduncle: Middle, Inferior, Superior
Vestibular nerve, Cochlear nerve — Vestibulocochlear nerve (CN VIII)
Cochlear nuclei
Sulcus limitans
Vestibular nuclei
Inferior medullary velum
Cuneate tubercle
Hypoglossal trigone
Gracile tubercle
Vagal trigone
Fasciculus gracilis
Area postrema
Tuberculum cinereum
Fasciculus cuneatus

C. Posterior View

7.104 BRAINSTEM *(CONTINUED)*

C. Dorsal aspect.

- Ridges are formed by the fasciculus gracilis and cuneatus.
- The gracile and cuneate tubercles are the sites of the nucleus gracilis and nucleus cuneatus.
- The diamond-shaped floor of the fourth ventricle; lateral to the sulcus limitans are the vestibular and cochlear nuclei and medially are the hypoglossal and vagal trigones and the facial colliculus.
- The superior and inferior colliculi form the dorsal surface of the midbrain.

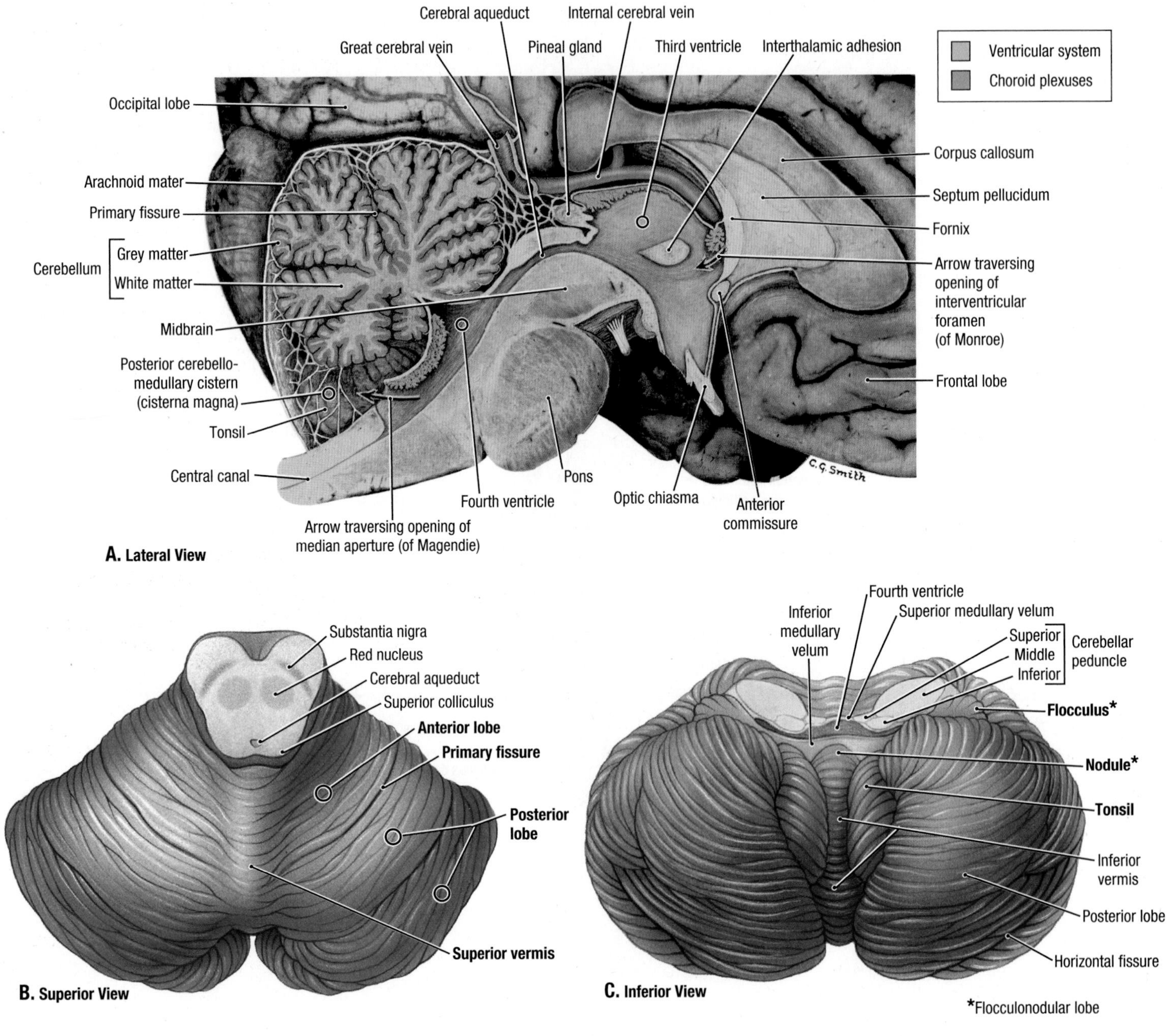

Cerebral aqueduct
Internal cerebral vein
Great cerebral vein
Pineal gland
Third ventricle
Interthalamic adhesion
Ventricular system
Choroid plexuses
Occipital lobe
Arachnoid mater
Primary fissure
Cerebellum
Grey matter
White matter
Midbrain
Posterior cerebello-medullary cistern (cisterna magna)
Tonsil
Central canal
Corpus callosum
Septum pellucidum
Fornix
Arrow traversing opening of interventricular foramen (of Monroe)
Frontal lobe
Pons
Fourth ventricle
Optic chiasma
Anterior commissure
Arrow traversing opening of median aperture (of Magendie)
C.G. Smith

A. Lateral View

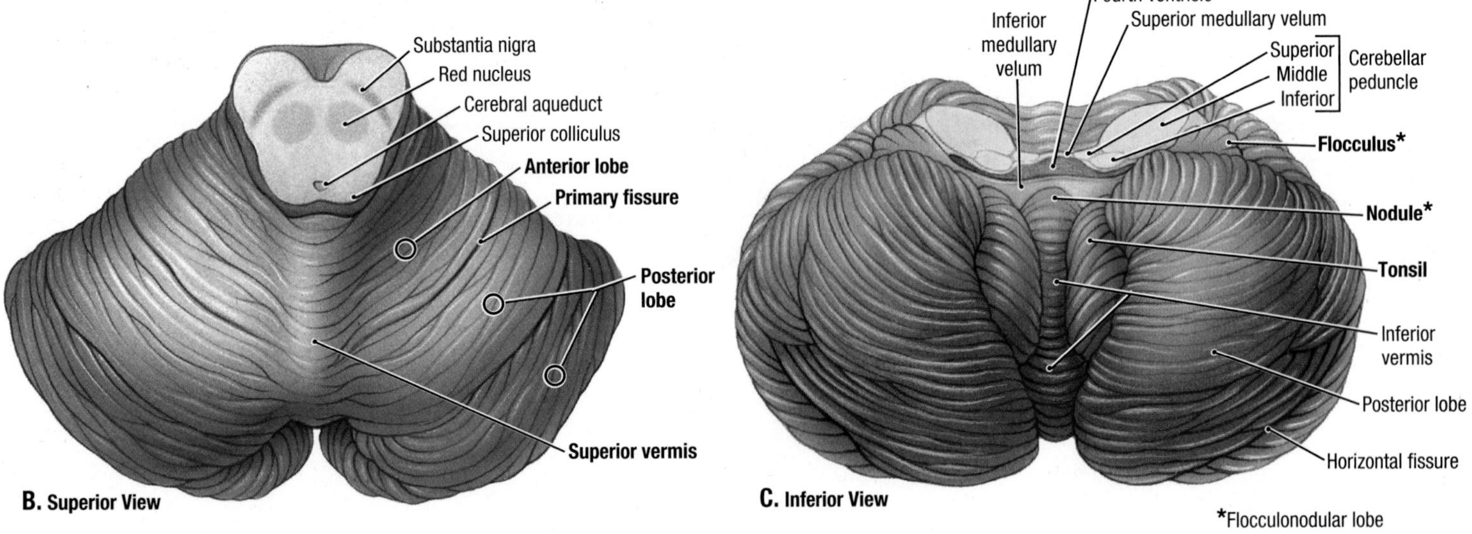

Substantia nigra
Red nucleus
Cerebral aqueduct
Superior colliculus
Anterior lobe
Primary fissure
Posterior lobe
Superior vermis
Fourth ventricle
Superior medullary velum
Inferior medullary velum
Superior
Middle
Inferior
Cerebellar peduncle
Flocculus*
Nodule*
Tonsil
Inferior vermis
Posterior lobe
Horizontal fissure

B. Superior View

C. Inferior View

*Flocculonodular lobe

7.105 CEREBELLUM

A. Median section. The arachnoid mater was removed except where it covered the cerebellum and the occipital lobe. **Cisternal puncture.** CSF may be obtained, for diagnostic purposes, from the posterior cerebellomedullary cistern, using a procedure known as cisternal puncture. The subarachnoid space or the ventricular system may also be entered for measuring or monitoring CSF pressure, injecting antibiotics, or administering contrast media for radiography. **B.** Superior view of the cerebellum. The right and left cerebellar hemispheres are united by the superior vermis; the anterior and posterior lobes are separated by the primary fissure. **C.** Inferior view of cerebellum. The flocculonodular lobe, the oldest part of the cerebellum, consists of the flocculus and nodule; the cerebellar tonsils typically extend into the foramen magnum.

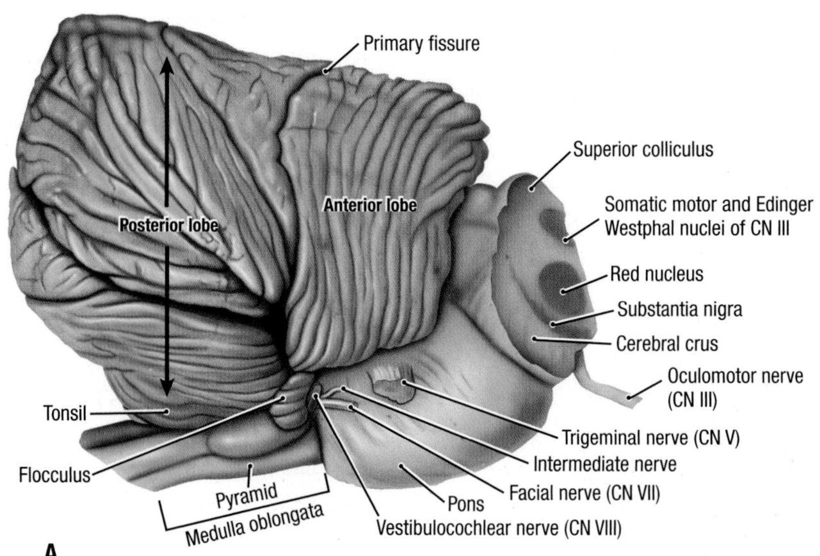
Primary fissure
Superior colliculus
Somatic motor and Edinger Westphal nuclei of CN III
Posterior lobe
Anterior lobe
Red nucleus
Substantia nigra
Cerebral crus
Oculomotor nerve (CN III)
Tonsil
Trigeminal nerve (CN V)
Intermediate nerve
Flocculus
Facial nerve (CN VII)
Pyramid
Pons
Medulla oblongata
Vestibulocochlear nerve (CN VIII)
A

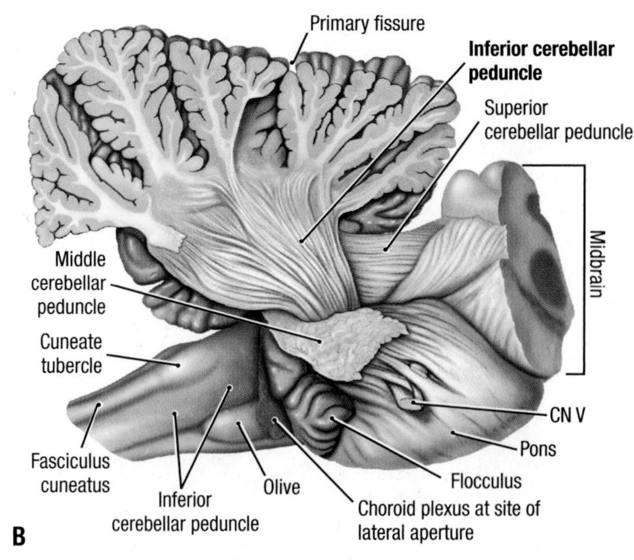
Primary fissure
Inferior cerebellar peduncle
Superior cerebellar peduncle
Midbrain
Middle cerebellar peduncle
Cuneate tubercle
CN V
Pons
Fasciculus cuneatus
Flocculus
Olive
Inferior cerebellar peduncle
Choroid plexus at site of lateral aperture
B

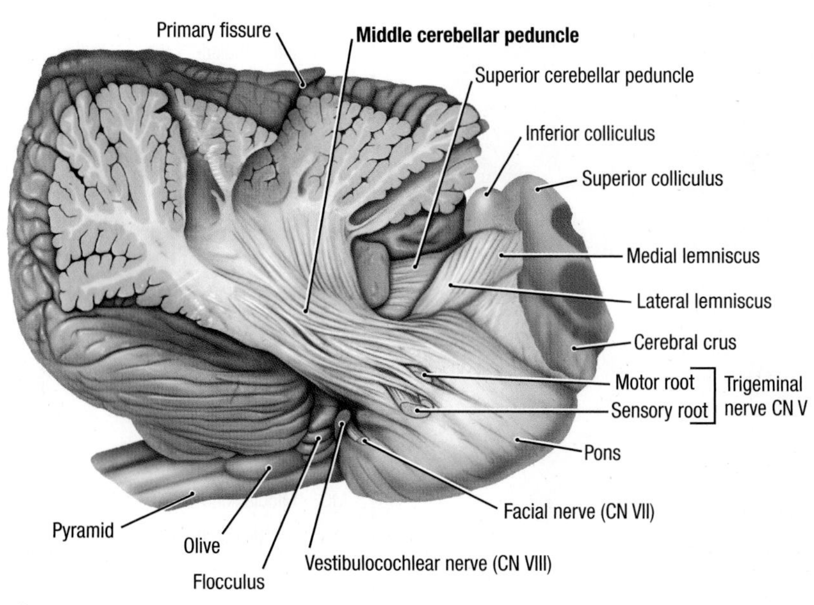
Primary fissure
Middle cerebellar peduncle
Superior cerebellar peduncle
Inferior colliculus
Superior colliculus
Medial lemniscus
Lateral lemniscus
Cerebral crus
Motor root
Sensory root
Trigeminal nerve CN V
Pons
Facial nerve (CN VII)
Pyramid
Olive
Flocculus
Vestibulocochlear nerve (CN VIII)
C

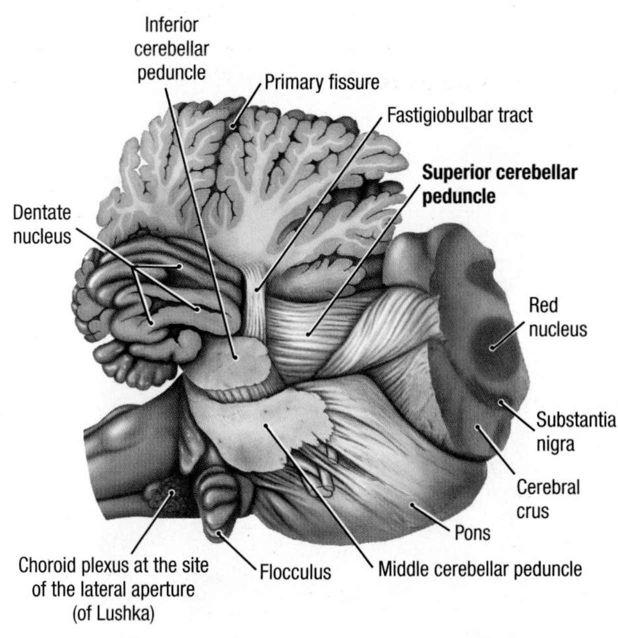
Inferior cerebellar peduncle
Primary fissure
Fastigiobulbar tract
Superior cerebellar peduncle
Dentate nucleus
Red nucleus
Substantia nigra
Cerebral crus
Pons
Choroid plexus at the site of the lateral aperture (of Lushka)
Flocculus
Middle cerebellar peduncle
D

Lateral Views

7.106 SERIAL DISSECTIONS OF THE CEREBELLUM

The series begins with the lateral surface of the cerebellar hemispheres **(A)** and proceeds medially in sequence **(B–D)**.

A. Cerebellum and brainstem. **B.** Inferior cerebellar peduncle. The fibers of the middle cerebellar peduncle were cut dorsal to the trigeminal nerve and peeled away to expose the fibers of the inferior cerebellar peduncle. **C.** Middle cerebellar peduncle. The fibers of the middle cerebellar peduncle were exposed by peeling away the lateral portion of the lobules of the cerebellar hemisphere. **D.** Superior cerebellar peduncle and dentate nucleus. The fibers of the inferior cerebellar peduncle were cut just dorsal to the previously sectioned middle cerebellar peduncle and peeled away until the gray matter of the dentate nucleus could be seen.

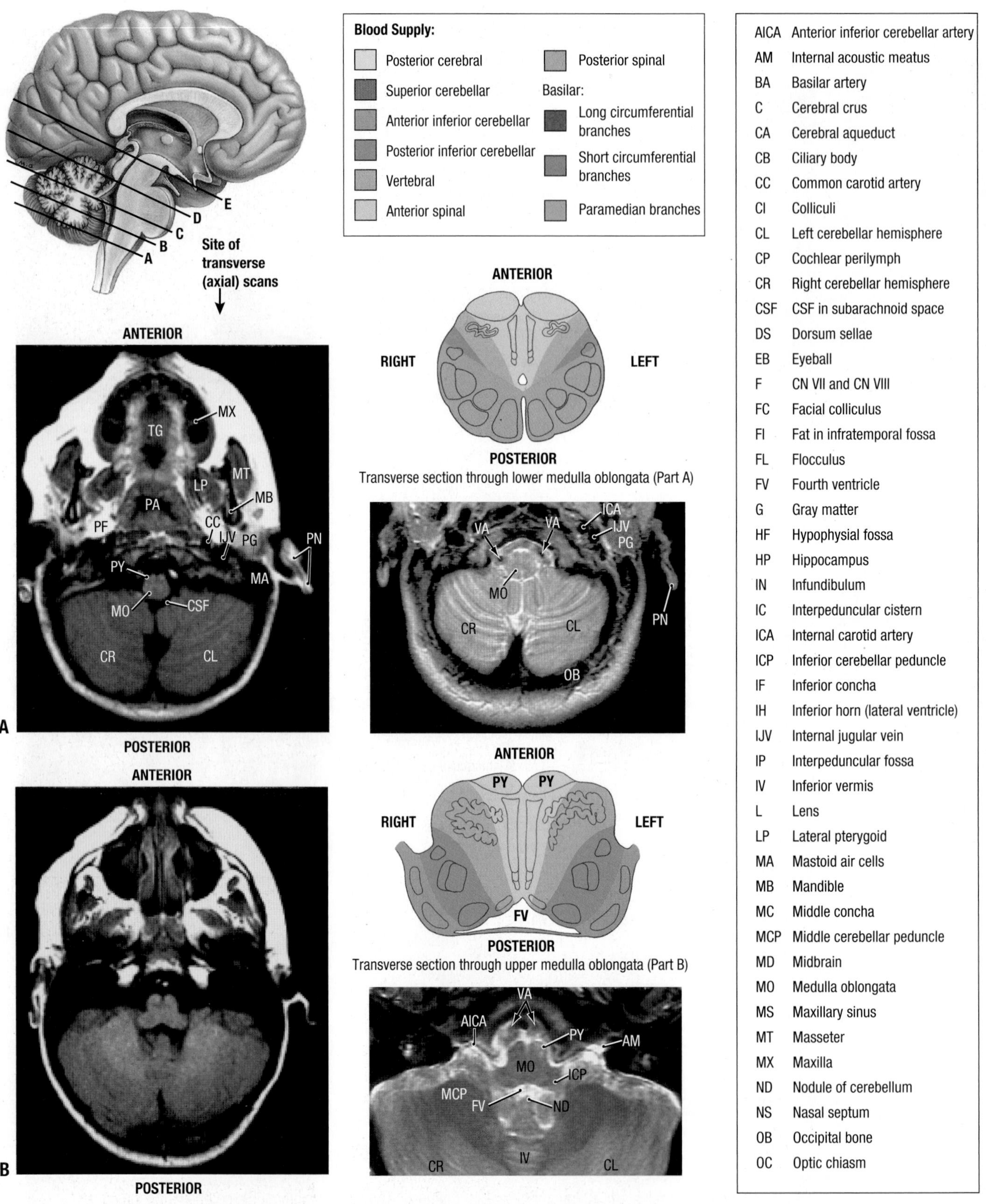
E
D
C
B
A
Site of transverse (axial) scans
Blood Supply:
Posterior cerebral
Superior cerebellar
Anterior inferior cerebellar
Posterior inferior cerebellar
Vertebral
Anterior spinal
Posterior spinal
Basilar:
Long circumferential branches
Short circumferential branches
Paramedian branches
AICA Anterior inferior cerebellar artery
AM Internal acoustic meatus
BA Basilar artery
C Cerebral crus
CA Cerebral aqueduct
CB Ciliary body
CC Common carotid artery
CI Colliculi
CL Left cerebellar hemisphere
CP Cochlear perilymph
CR Right cerebellar hemisphere
CSF CSF in subarachnoid space
DS Dorsum sellae
EB Eyeball
F CN VII and CN VIII
FC Facial colliculus
FI Fat in infratemporal fossa
FL Flocculus
FV Fourth ventricle
G Gray matter
HF Hypophysial fossa
HP Hippocampus
IN Infundibulum
IC Interpeduncular cistern
ICA Internal carotid artery
ICP Inferior cerebellar peduncle
IF Inferior concha
IH Inferior horn (lateral ventricle)
IJV Internal jugular vein
IP Interpeduncular fossa
IV Inferior vermis
L Lens
LP Lateral pterygoid
MA Mastoid air cells
MB Mandible
MC Middle concha
MCP Middle cerebellar peduncle
MD Midbrain
MO Medulla oblongata
MS Maxillary sinus
MT Masseter
MX Maxilla
ND Nodule of cerebellum
NS Nasal septum
OB Occipital bone
OC Optic chiasm
ANTERIOR
MX
TG
MT
LP
MB
PA
PF
CC
IJV
PG
PN
PY
MA
MO
CSF
CR
CL
A
POSTERIOR
ANTERIOR
RIGHT
LEFT
POSTERIOR
Transverse section through lower medulla oblongata (Part A)
ICA
VA
VA
IJV
PG
MO
CR
CL
PN
OB
ANTERIOR
B
POSTERIOR
ANTERIOR
PY
PY
RIGHT
LEFT
FV
POSTERIOR
Transverse section through upper medulla oblongata (Part B)
VA
AICA
PY
AM
MO
ICP
MCP
FV
ND
IV
CR
CL

7.107 AXIAL (TRANSVERSE) MRIs THROUGH BRAINSTEM, INFERIOR VIEWS

Images on left side of the page are T1 weighted, and images on the right side are T2 weighted.

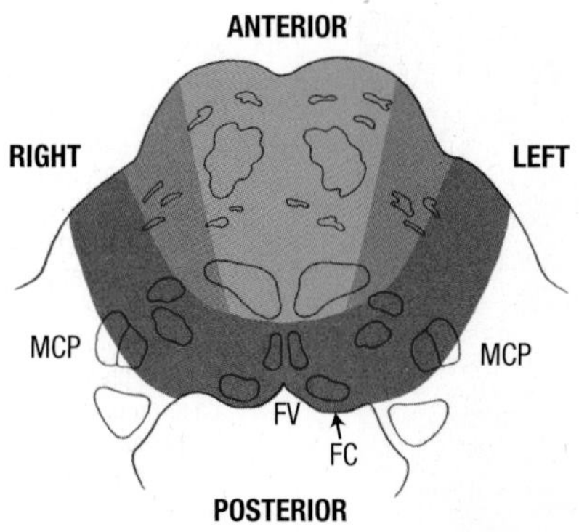
ANTERIOR
RIGHT
LEFT
MCP
MCP
FV
FC
POSTERIOR

Transverse section through pons (Parts C & D)

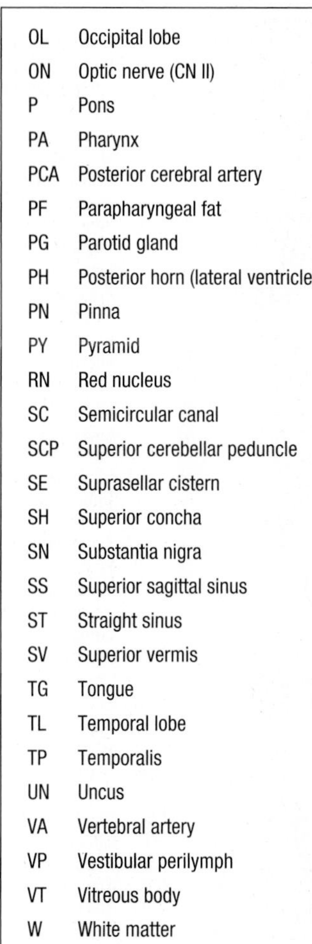

OL	Occipital lobe
ON	Optic nerve (CN II)
P	Pons
PA	Pharynx
PCA	Posterior cerebral artery
PF	Parapharyngeal fat
PG	Parotid gland
PH	Posterior horn (lateral ventricle)
PN	Pinna
PY	Pyramid
RN	Red nucleus
SC	Semicircular canal
SCP	Superior cerebellar peduncle
SE	Suprasellar cistern
SH	Superior concha
SN	Substantia nigra
SS	Superior sagittal sinus
ST	Straight sinus
SV	Superior vermis
TG	Tongue
TL	Temporal lobe
TP	Temporalis
UN	Uncus
VA	Vertebral artery
VP	Vestibular perilymph
VT	Vitreous body
W	White matter

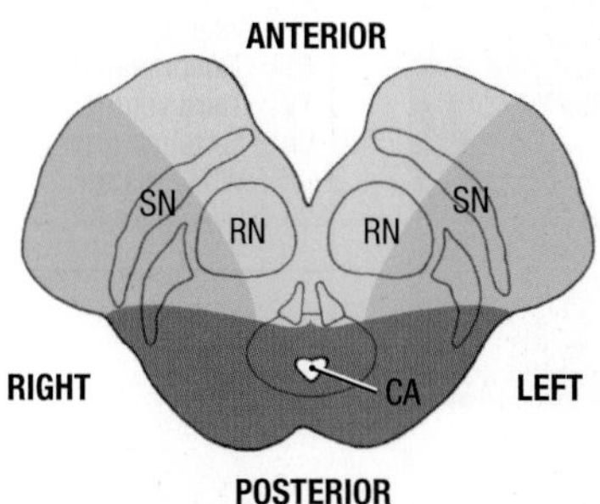
ANTERIOR
SN
RN
RN
SN
RIGHT
CA
LEFT
POSTERIOR

Transverse section through midbrain (Part E)

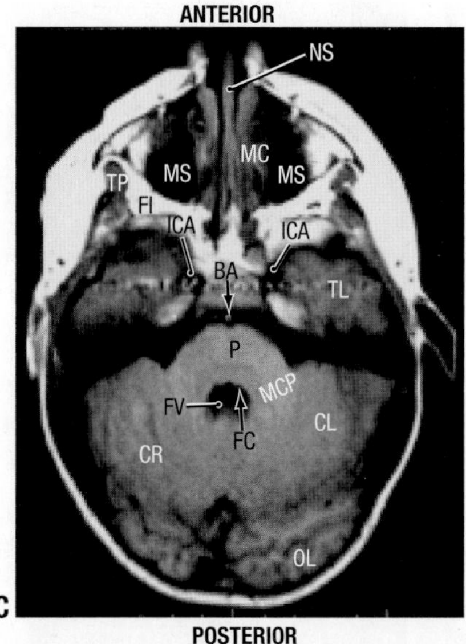
ANTERIOR
NS
MC
MS
MS
TP
FI
ICA
ICA
BA
TL
P
FV
MCP
FC
CL
CR
OL
C
POSTERIOR

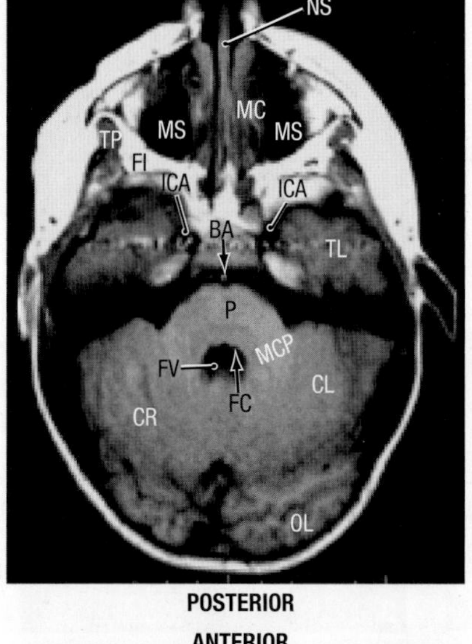

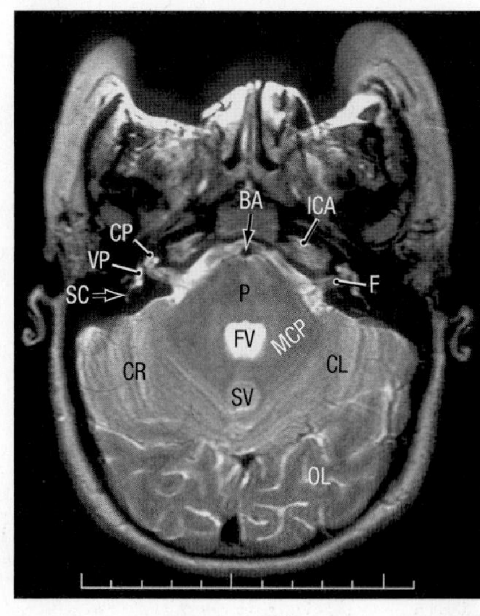
BA
ICA
CP
VP
SC
F
P
FV
MCP
CR
CL
SV
OL

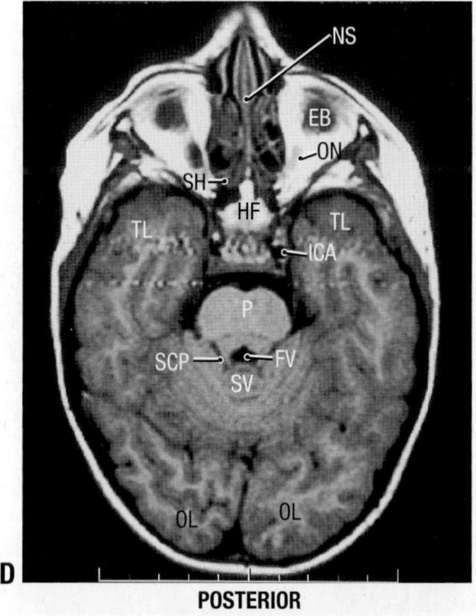
ANTERIOR
NS
EB
ON
SH
HF
TL
TL
ICA
P
SCP
FV
SV
OL
OL
D
POSTERIOR

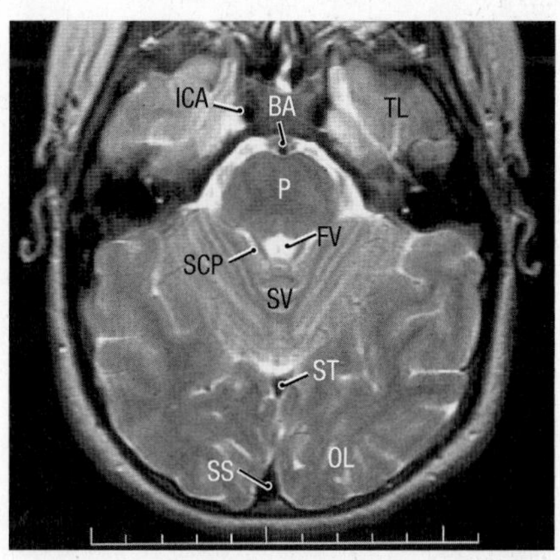
ICA
BA
TL
P
SCP
FV
SV
ST
SS
OL

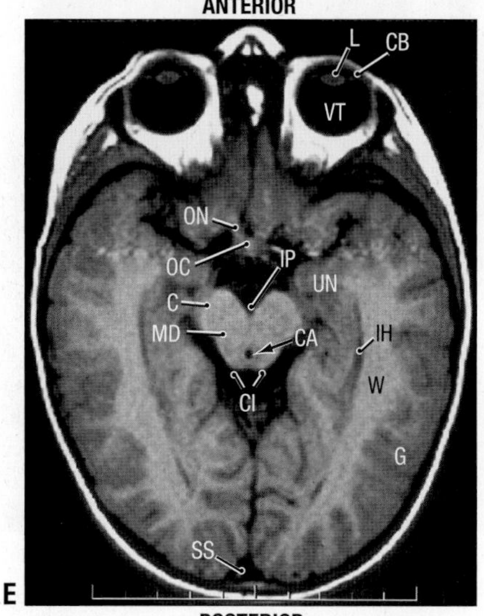
ANTERIOR
L
CB
VT
ON
OC
IP
UN
C
MD
CA
IH
CI
W
G
SS
E
POSTERIOR

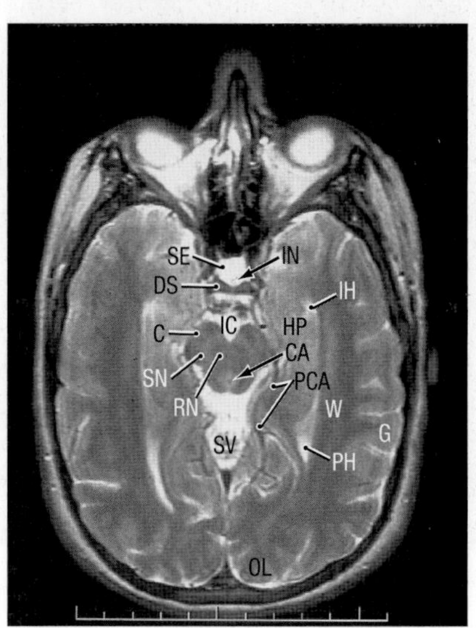
SE
IN
DS
IH
C
IC
HP
CA
SN
RN
PCA
W
G
SV
PH
OL

7.107 AXIAL (TRANSVERSE) MRIs THROUGH BRAINSTEM, INFERIOR VIEWS *(CONTINUED)*

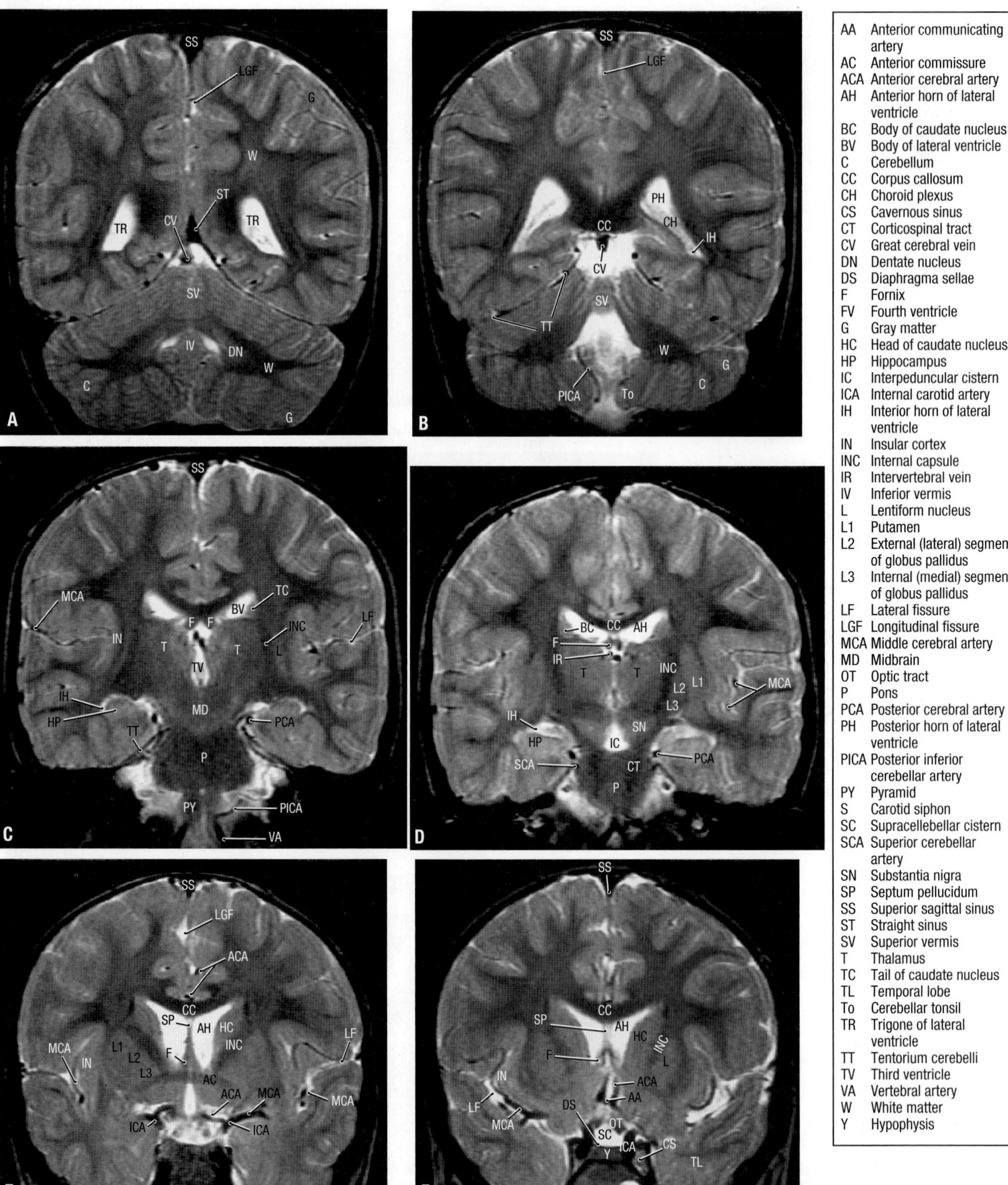
AA Anterior communicating artery
AC Anterior commissure
ACA Anterior cerebral artery
AH Anterior horn of lateral ventricle
BC Body of caudate nucleus
BV Body of lateral ventricle
C Cerebellum
CC Corpus callosum
CH Choroid plexus
CS Cavernous sinus
CT Corticospinal tract
CV Great cerebral vein
DN Dentate nucleus
DS Diaphragma sellae
F Fornix
FV Fourth ventricle
G Gray matter
HC Head of caudate nucleus
HP Hippocampus
IC Interpeduncular cistern
ICA Internal carotid artery
IH Interior horn of lateral ventricle
IN Insular cortex
INC Internal capsule
IR Intervertebral vein
IV Inferior vermis
L Lentiform nucleus
L1 Putamen
L2 External (lateral) segment of globus pallidus
L3 Internal (medial) segment of globus pallidus
LF Lateral fissure
LGF Longitudinal fissure
MCA Middle cerebral artery
MD Midbrain
OT Optic tract
P Pons
PCA Posterior cerebral artery
PH Posterior horn of lateral ventricle
PICA Posterior inferior cerebellar artery
PY Pyramid
S Carotid siphon
SC Supracellebellar cistern
SCA Superior cerebellar artery
SN Substantia nigra
SP Septum pellucidum
SS Superior sagittal sinus
ST Straight sinus
SV Superior vermis
T Thalamus
TC Tail of caudate nucleus
TL Temporal lobe
To Cerebellar tonsil
TR Trigone of lateral ventricle
TT Tentorium cerebelli
TV Third ventricle
VA Vertebral artery
W White matter
Y Hypophysis

7.108 CORONAL MRIs (T2 WEIGHTED) AND SECTIONS OF BRAIN

A.–F. Coronal MRIs. **G.–H.** Coronal sections, posterior views.

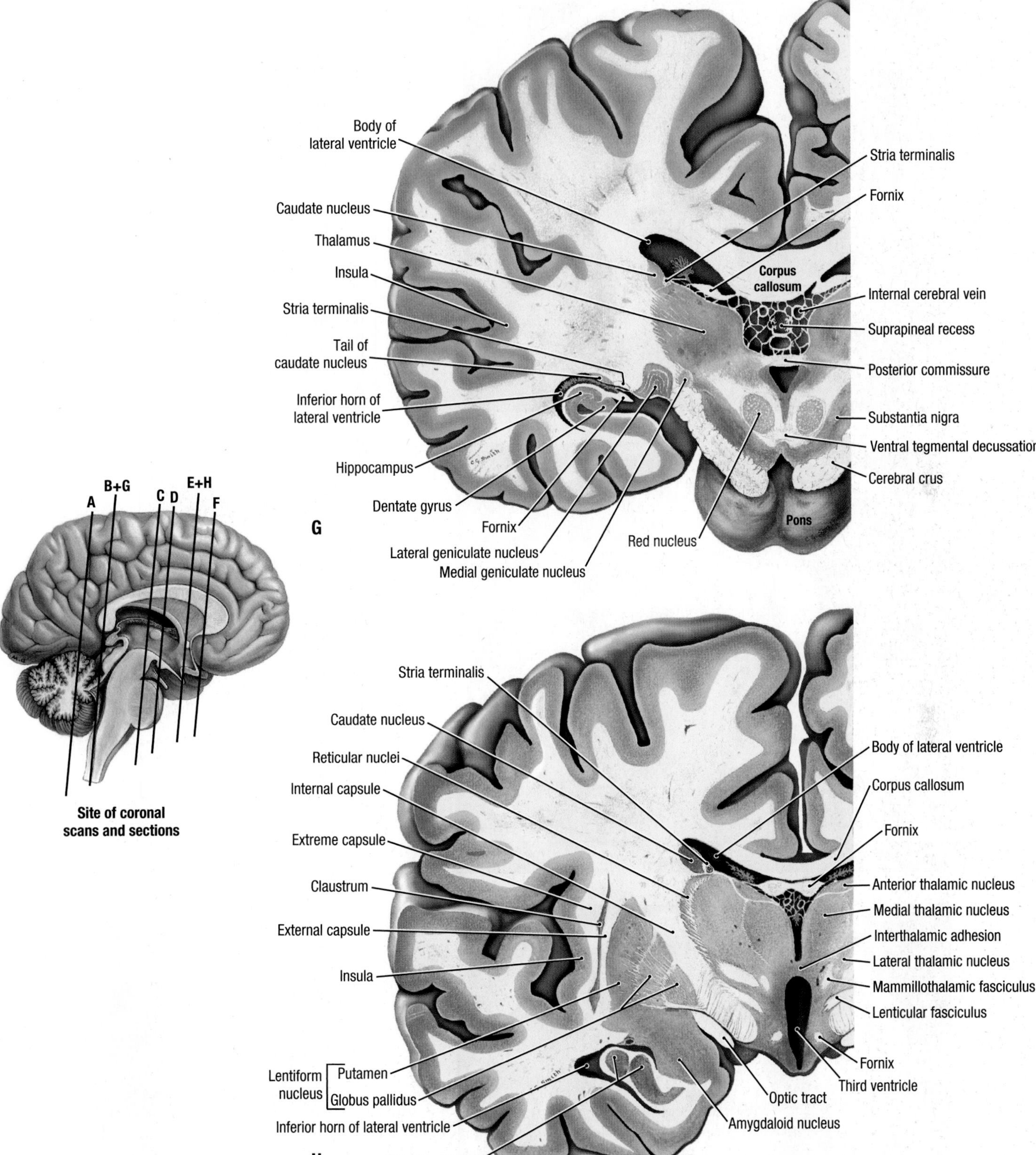
Body of lateral ventricle
Caudate nucleus
Thalamus
Insula
Stria terminalis
Tail of caudate nucleus
Inferior horn of lateral ventricle
Hippocampus
Dentate gyrus
G
Fornix
Lateral geniculate nucleus
Medial geniculate nucleus
Red nucleus
Pons
Stria terminalis
Fornix
Corpus callosum
Internal cerebral vein
Suprapineal recess
Posterior commissure
Substantia nigra
Ventral tegmental decussation
Cerebral crus
A
B+G
C
D
E+H
F
Site of coronal scans and sections
Stria terminalis
Caudate nucleus
Reticular nuclei
Internal capsule
Extreme capsule
Claustrum
External capsule
Insula
Lentiform nucleus
Putamen
Globus pallidus
Inferior horn of lateral ventricle
H
Pes hippocampi
Body of lateral ventricle
Corpus callosum
Fornix
Anterior thalamic nucleus
Medial thalamic nucleus
Interthalamic adhesion
Lateral thalamic nucleus
Mammillothalamic fasciculus
Lenticular fasciculus
Fornix
Third ventricle
Optic tract
Amygdaloid nucleus

7.108 CORONAL MRIs (T2 WEIGHTED) AND SECTIONS OF BRAIN *(CONTINUED)*

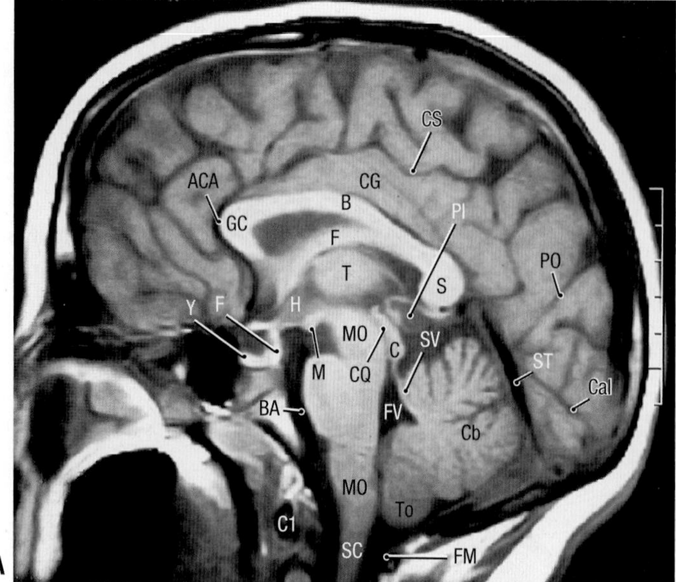
CS
ACA
CG
GC
B
PI
F
T
S
PO
Y
F
H
MO
SV
C
M
CQ
ST
Cal
BA
FV
Cb
MO
To
C1
SC
FM
A

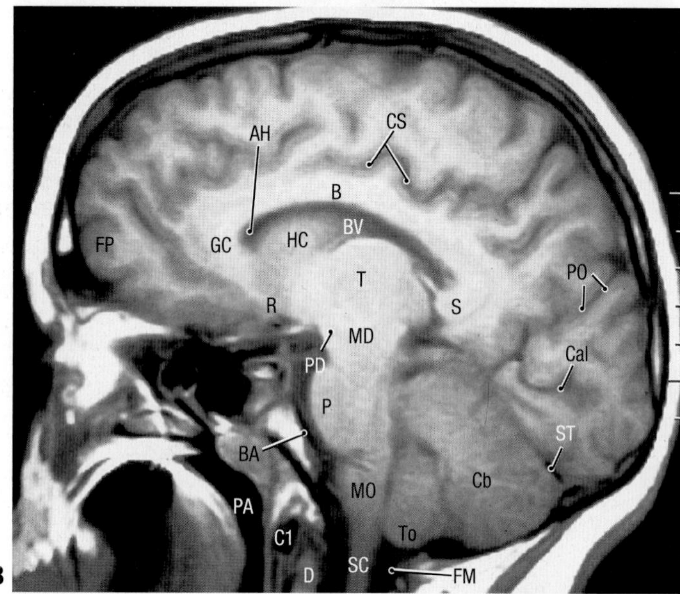
CS
AH
B
BV
FP
GC
HC
T
PO
R
S
MD
PD
Cal
P
ST
BA
Cb
MO
PA
C1
To
D
SC
FM
B

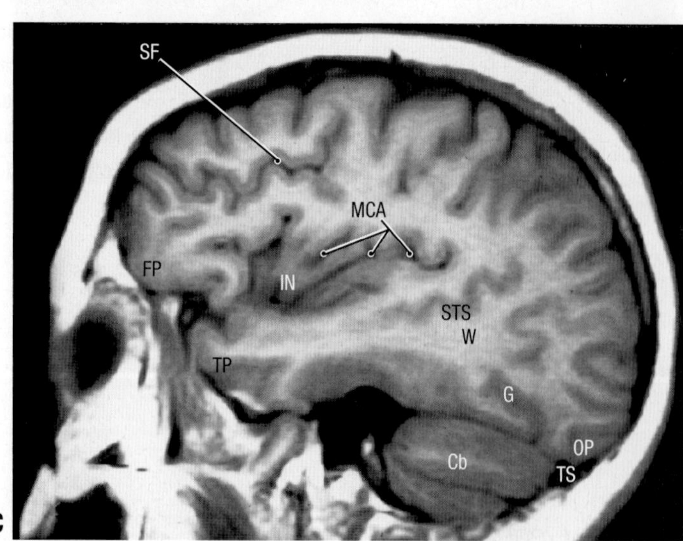
SF
MCA
FP
IN
STS
W
TP
G
Cb
OP
TS
C

ACA	Anterior cerebral artery
AH	Anterior horn of lateral ventricle
B	Body of corpus callosum
BA	Basilar artery
BV	Body of lateral ventricle
C	Colliculi
C1	Anterior tubercle of atlas
Cal	Calcarine sulcus
Cb	Cerebellum
CG	Cingulate nucleus
CQ	Cerebral aqueduct
CS	Cingulate sulcus
D	Dens (odontoid process)
F	Fornix
FM	Foramen magnum
FP	Frontal pole
FV	Fourth ventricle
G	Cerebral cortex (gray matter)
GC	Genus of corpus callosum
H	Hypothalamus
HC	Head of caudate nucleus
I	Infundibulum
IN	Insular cortex
M	Mammillary body
MCA	Middle cerebral artery
MD	Midbrain
OP	Occipital pole
P	Pons
PA	Pharynx
PD	Cerebral peduncle
PI	Pineal
PO	Parieto-occipital fissure
R	Rostrum of corpus callosum
S	Splenium of corpus callosum
SC	Spinal cord
SF	Superior frontal sulcus
ST	Straight sinus
STS	Superior temporal sulcus
SV	Superior medullary vellum
T	Thalamus
To	Cerebellar tonsil
TP	Temporal pole
TS	Transverse sinus
W	White matter
Y	Hypophysis

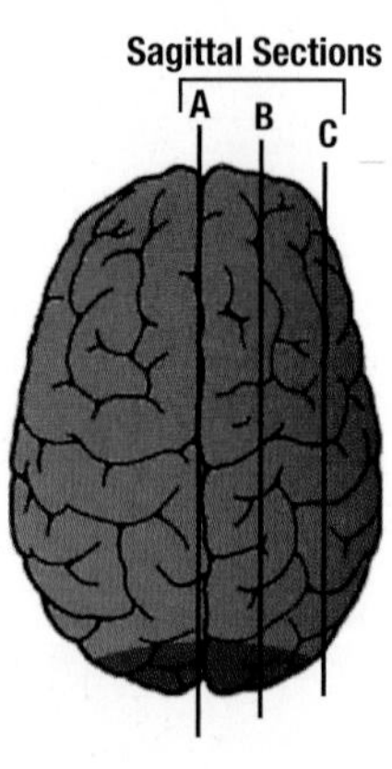
Sagittal Sections
A
B
C

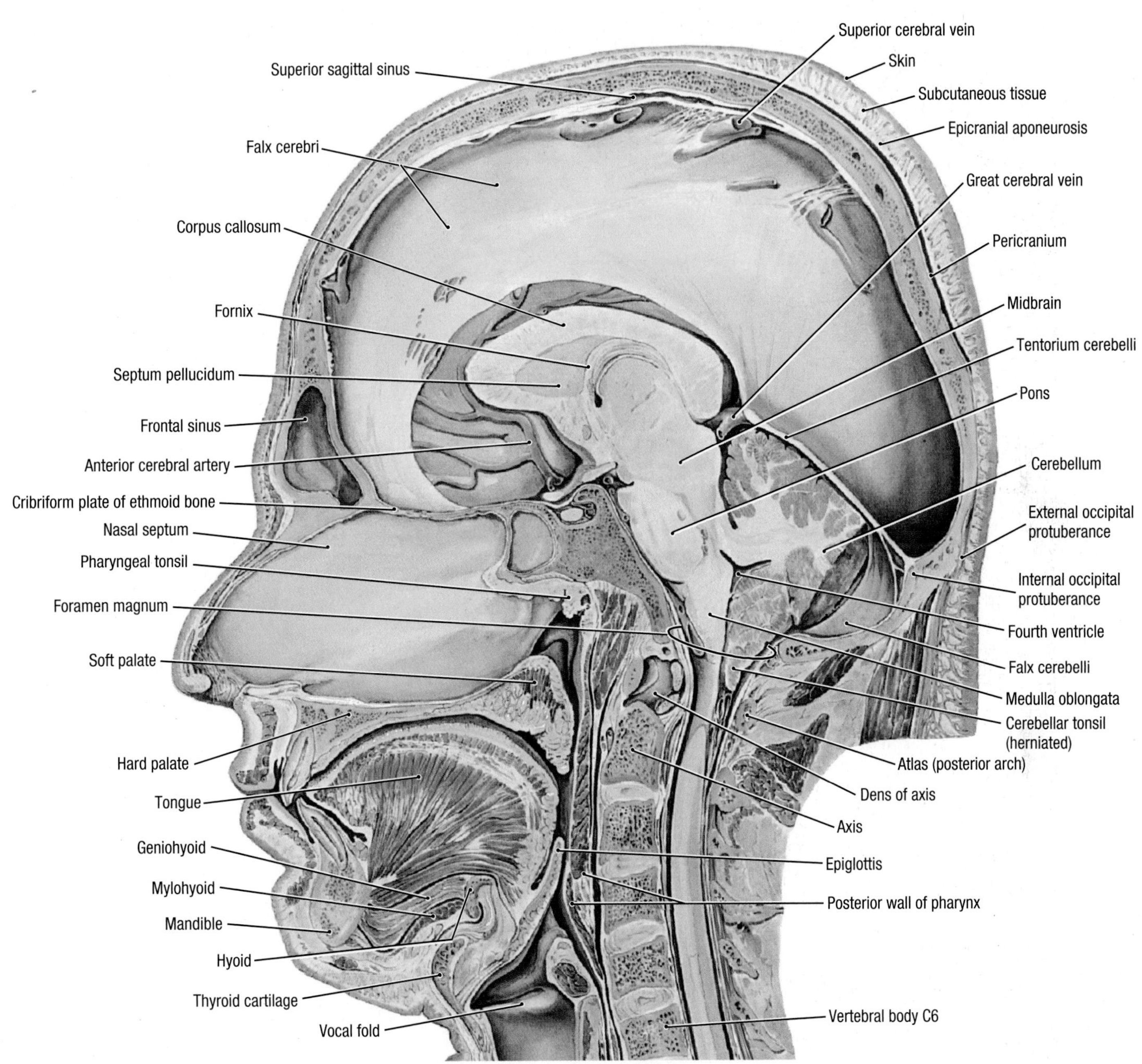
Superior cerebral vein
Skin
Subcutaneous tissue
Epicranial aponeurosis
Great cerebral vein
Pericranium
Midbrain
Tentorium cerebelli
Pons
Cerebellum
External occipital protuberance
Internal occipital protuberance
Fourth ventricle
Falx cerebelli
Medulla oblongata
Cerebellar tonsil (herniated)
Atlas (posterior arch)
Dens of axis
Axis
Epiglottis
Posterior wall of pharynx
Vertebral body C6
Superior sagittal sinus
Falx cerebri
Corpus callosum
Fornix
Septum pellucidum
Frontal sinus
Anterior cerebral artery
Cribriform plate of ethmoid bone
Nasal septum
Pharyngeal tonsil
Foramen magnum
Soft palate
Hard palate
Tongue
Geniohyoid
Mylohyoid
Mandible
Hyoid
Thyroid cartilage
Vocal fold

D. **Median Section**

7.109 SAGITTAL MRIs (T1 WEIGHTED) AND MEDIAN SECTION OF BRAIN

See orientation drawing for sites of scans **A.–C.**

Increased intracranial pressure (e.g., due to a tumor) may cause displacement of the cerebellar tonsils through the foramen magnum, resulting in a foraminal (tonsillar) herniation. Compression of the brainstem, if severe, may result in respiratory and cardiac arrest.

CHAPTER 8

Neck

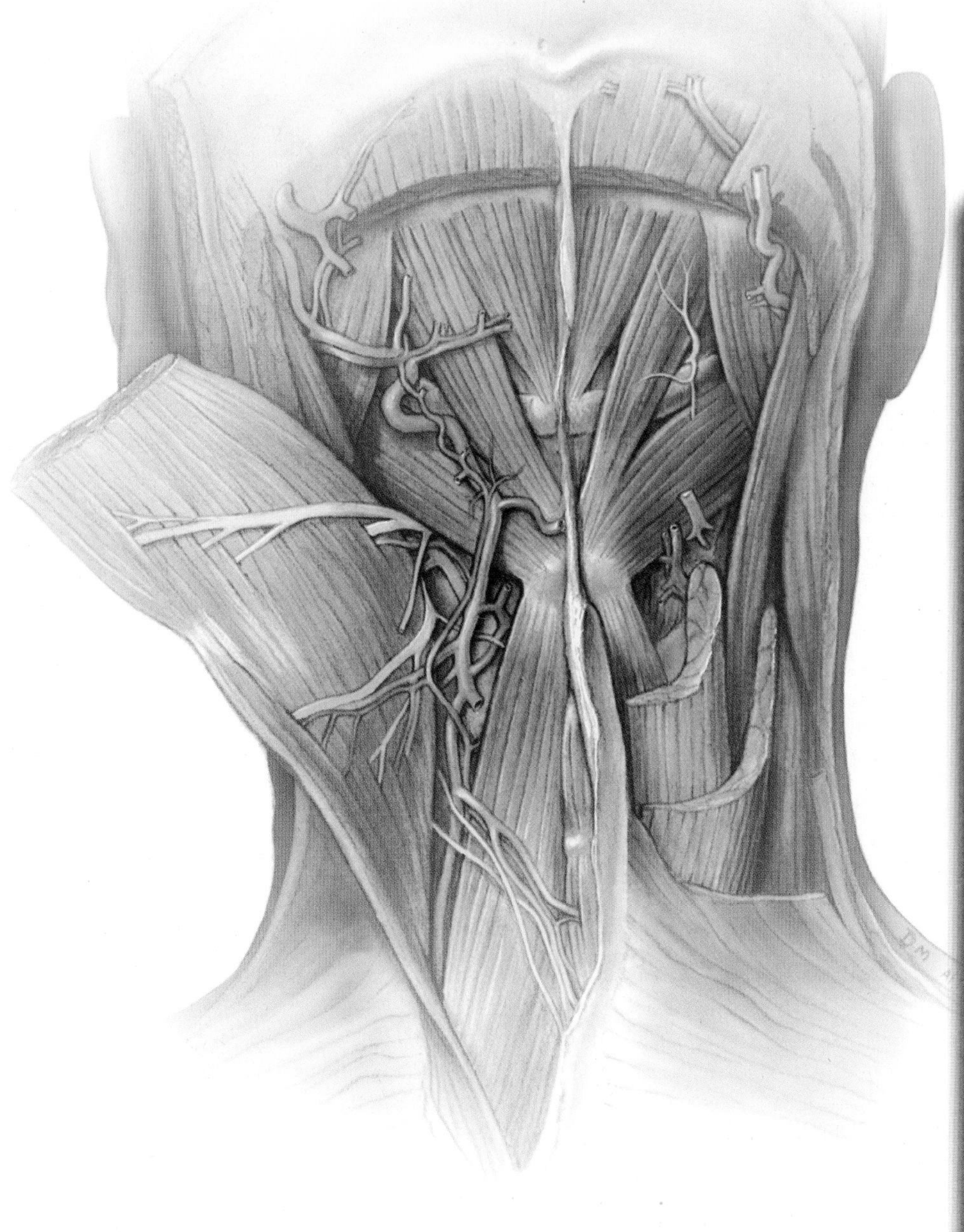

Subcutaneous Structures and Cervical Fascia	752
Skeleton of Neck	756
Regions of Neck	758
Lateral Region (Posterior Triangle) of Neck	760
Anterior Region (Anterior Triangle) of Neck	764
Neurovascular Structures of Neck	768
Visceral Compartment of Neck	774
Root and Prevertebral Region of Neck	778
Submandibular Region and Floor of Mouth	784
Posterior Cervical Region	789
Pharynx	792
Isthmus of Fauces	798
Larynx	804
Sectional Anatomy and Imaging of Neck	812

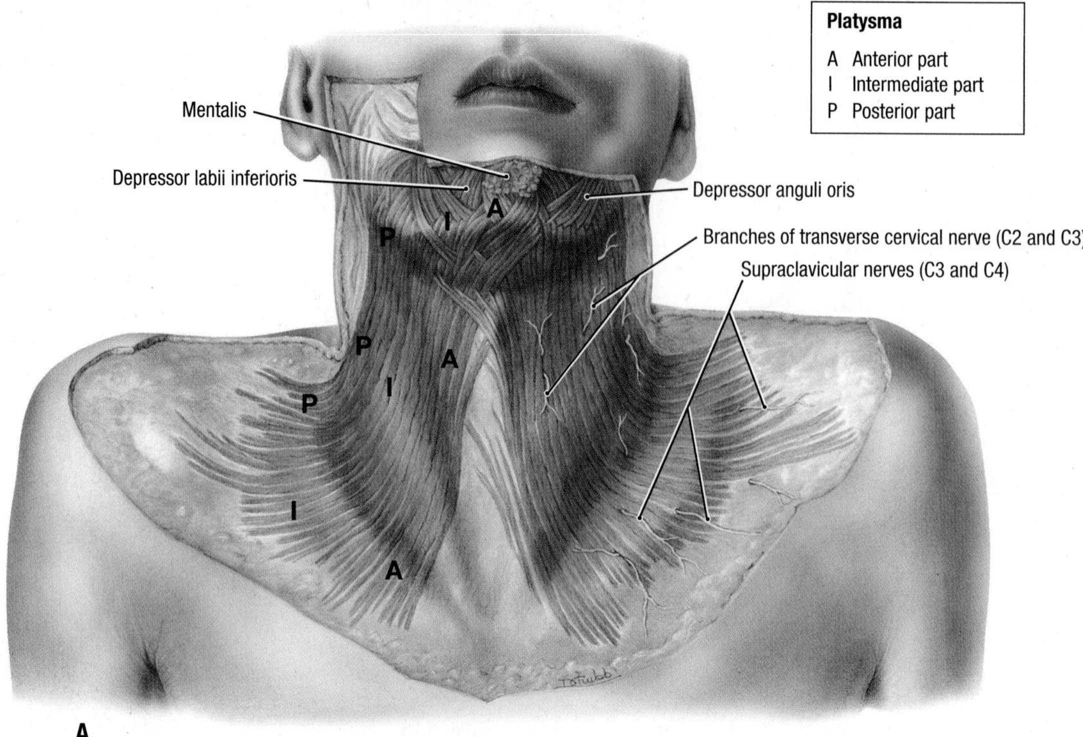
Platysma
A Anterior part
I Intermediate part
P Posterior part
Mentalis
Depressor labii inferioris
Depressor anguli oris
Branches of transverse cervical nerve (C2 and C3)
Supraclavicular nerves (C3 and C4)
A
I
P
A.

Anterior Views

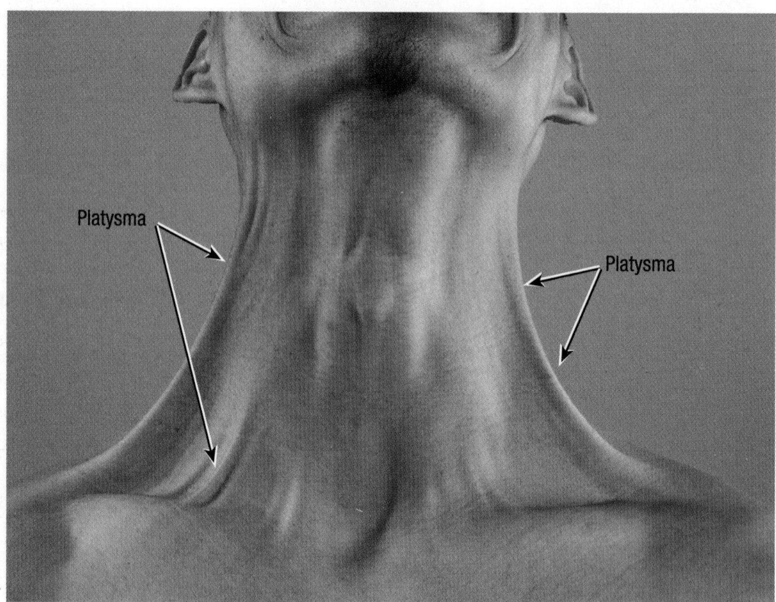
Platysma
Platysma
B.

8.1 PLATYSMA

A. Parts of platysma. **B.** Surface anatomy.

TABLE 8.1 PLATYSMA

Muscle	Superior Attachment	Inferior Attachment	Innervation	Main Action
Platysma	*Anterior part:* Fibers interlace with contralateral muscle *Intermediate part:* Fibers pass deep to depressors anguli oris and labii inferioris to attach to inferior border of mandible *Posterior part:* Skin/subcutaneous tissue of lower face lateral to mouth	Subcutaneous tissue overlying superior parts of pectoralis major and sometimes deltoid muscles	Cervical branch of facial nerve (CN VII)	Draws corner of mouth inferiorly and widens it as in expressions of sadness and fright; draws the skin of the neck superiorly, forming tense vertical and oblique ridges over the anterior neck

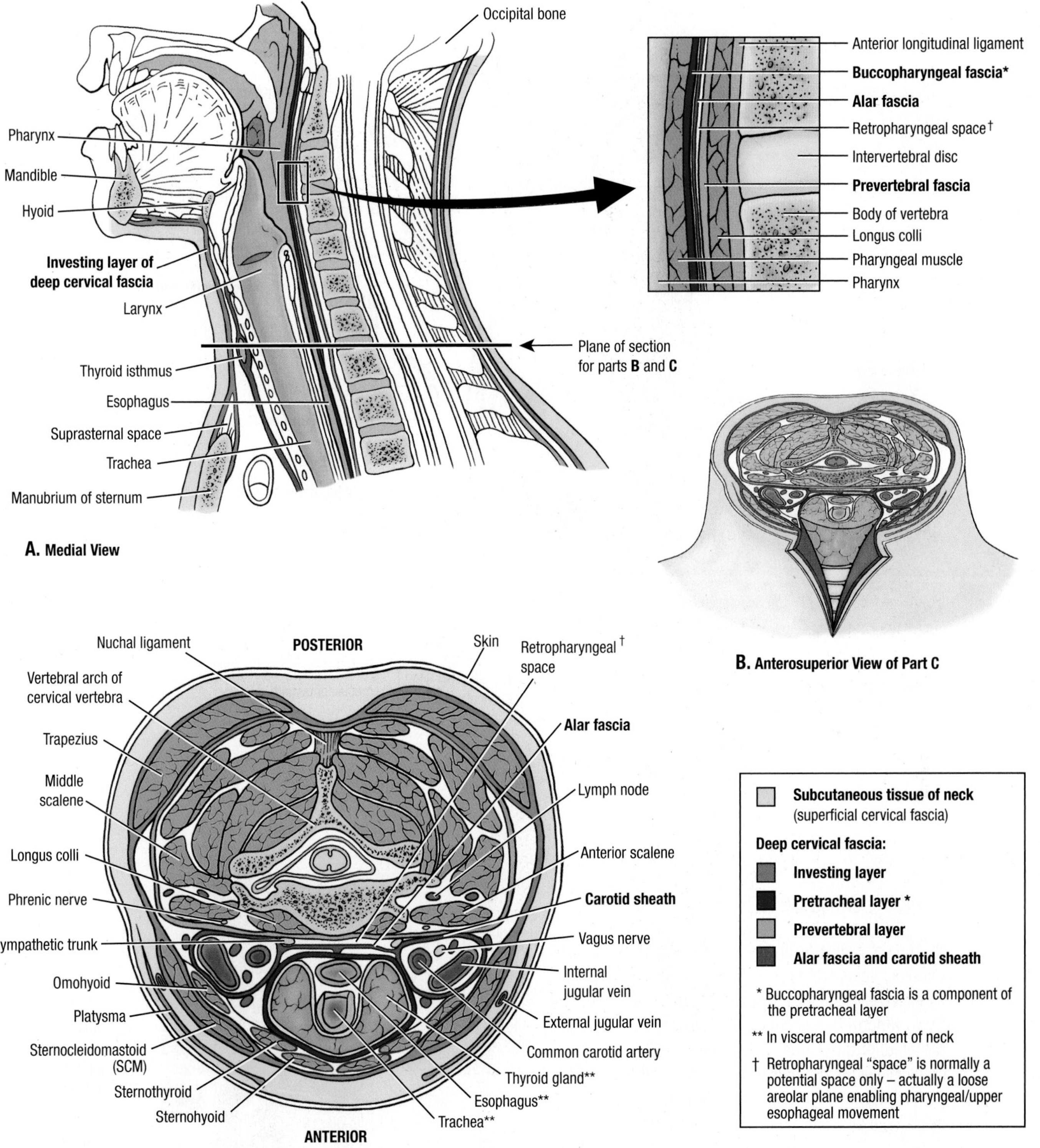
Occipital bone
Pharynx
Mandible
Hyoid
Investing layer of deep cervical fascia
Larynx
Thyroid isthmus
Esophagus
Suprasternal space
Trachea
Manubrium of sternum
Plane of section for parts B and C
Anterior longitudinal ligament
Buccopharyngeal fascia*
Alar fascia
Retropharyngeal space†
Intervertebral disc
Prevertebral fascia
Body of vertebra
Longus colli
Pharyngeal muscle
Pharynx
A. Medial View
B. Anterosuperior View of Part C
POSTERIOR
Nuchal ligament
Skin
Retropharyngeal† space
Vertebral arch of cervical vertebra
Trapezius
Alar fascia
Middle scalene
Lymph node
Longus colli
Anterior scalene
Phrenic nerve
Carotid sheath
Sympathetic trunk
Vagus nerve
Omohyoid
Internal jugular vein
Platysma
External jugular vein
Sternocleidomastoid (SCM)
Common carotid artery
Sternothyroid
Thyroid gland**
Sternohyoid
Esophagus**
Trachea**
ANTERIOR
Subcutaneous tissue of neck (superficial cervical fascia)
Deep cervical fascia:
Investing layer
Pretracheal layer *
Prevertebral layer
Alar fascia and carotid sheath
* Buccopharyngeal fascia is a component of the pretracheal layer
** In visceral compartment of neck
† Retropharyngeal "space" is normally a potential space only – actually a loose areolar plane enabling pharyngeal/upper esophageal movement

C. Superior View of Transverse Section (at level of C7 vertebra)

8.2 SUBCUTANEOUS TISSUE AND DEEP FASCIA OF NECK

Sectional demonstrations of the fasciae of the neck. **A.** Fasciae of the neck are continuous inferiorly and superiorly with thoracic and cranial fasciae. The *inset* illustrates the fascia of the retropharyngeal region. **B.** Relationship of the main layers of deep cervical fascia and the carotid sheath. Midline access to the cervical viscera is possible with minimal disruption of tissues. **C.** The concentric layers of fascia are apparent in this transverse section of neck at the level indicated in **A.**

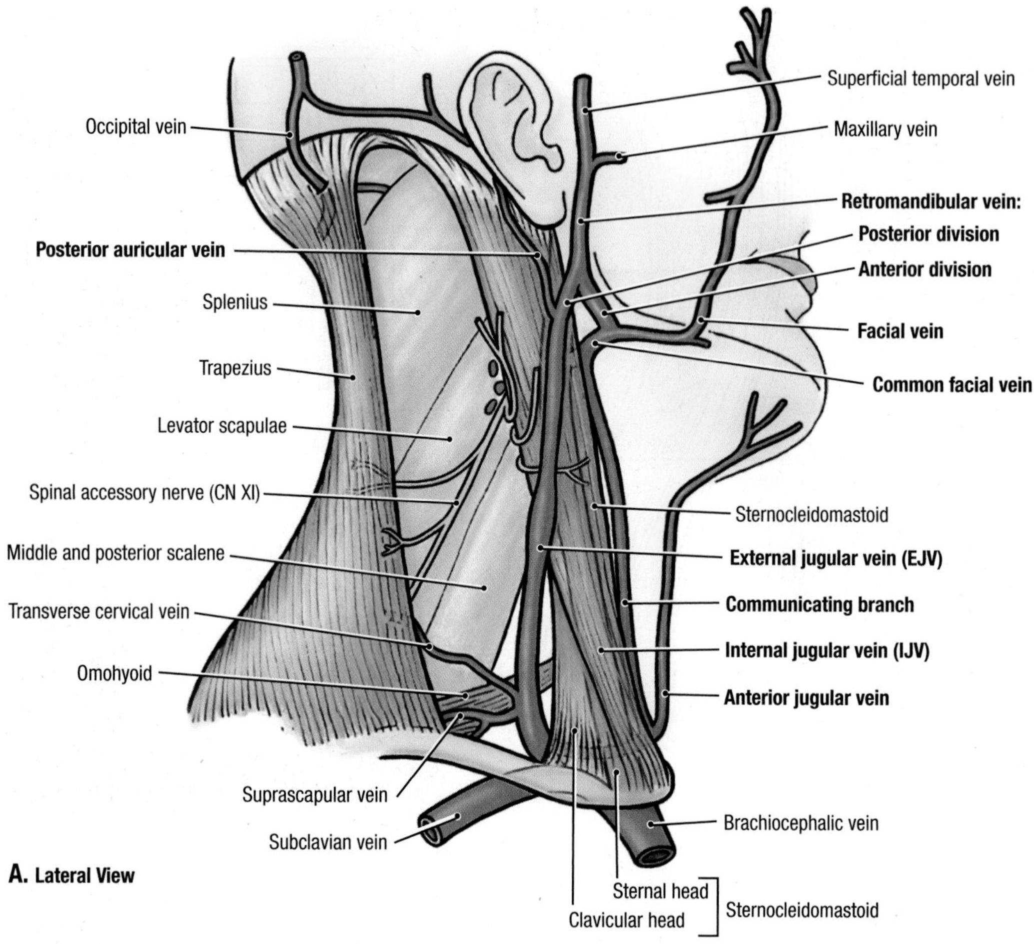
Superficial temporal vein
Occipital vein
Maxillary vein
Retromandibular vein:
Posterior division
Anterior division
Posterior auricular vein
Splenius
Facial vein
Trapezius
Common facial vein
Levator scapulae
Spinal accessory nerve (CN XI)
Sternocleidomastoid
Middle and posterior scalene
External jugular vein (EJV)
Communicating branch
Transverse cervical vein
Internal jugular vein (IJV)
Omohyoid
Anterior jugular vein
Suprascapular vein
Brachiocephalic vein
Subclavian vein
Sternal head
Clavicular head
Sternocleidomastoid

A. **Lateral View**

8.3 SUPERFICIAL VEINS OF NECK

A. Schematic illustration of superficial veins of the neck. The superficial temporal and maxillary veins merge to form the retromandibular vein. The posterior division of the retromandibular vein unites with the posterior auricular vein to form the external jugular vein (EJV). The facial vein receives the anterior division of the retromandibular vein, forming the common facial vein that empties into the internal jugular vein. Variations are common. **B.** Surface anatomy of the external jugular vein and the muscles bounding the lateral cervical region (posterior triangle) of the neck.

External jugular vein (EJV). The EJV may serve as an "internal barometer." When venous pressure is in the normal range, the EJV is usually visible superior to the clavicle for only a short distance. However, when venous pressure rises (e.g., as in heart failure) the vein is prominent throughout its course along the side of the neck. Consequently, routine observation for distention of the EJVs during physical examinations may reveal diagnostic signs of heart failure, obstruction of the superior vena cava, enlarged supraclavicular lymph nodes, or increased intrathoracic pressure.

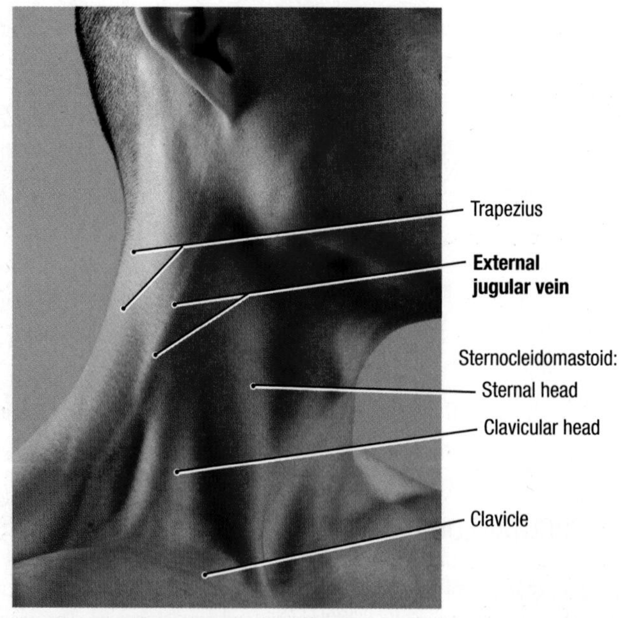
Trapezius
External jugular vein
Sternocleidomastoid:
Sternal head
Clavicular head
Clavicle

B. **Right Anterolateral View**

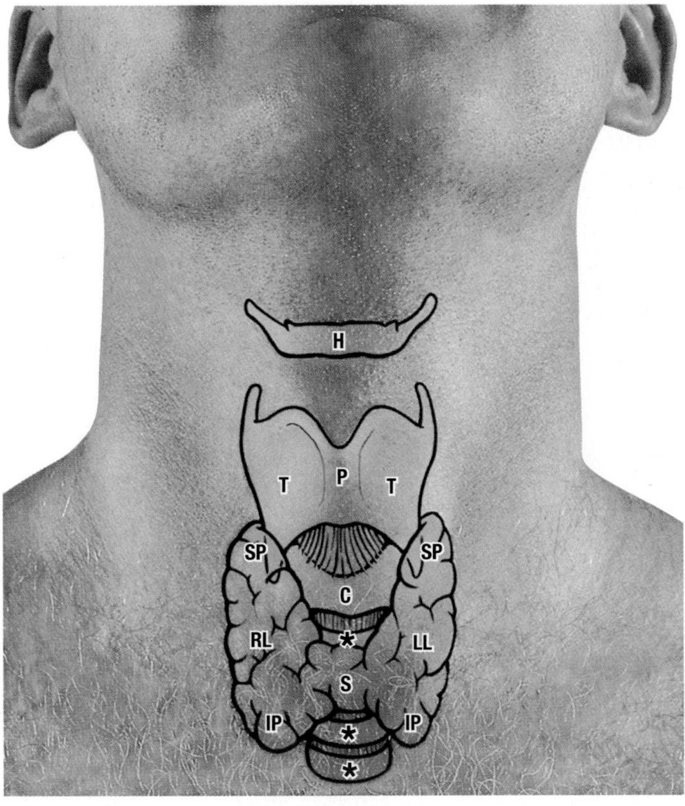
H
T
P
T
SP
SP
C
RL
LL
S
IP
IP
*
*
*

C	Cricoid cartilage
H	Hyoid bone
IP	Inferior pole of thyroid gland
LL	Left lobe of thyroid gland
P	Laryngeal prominence
RL	Right lobe of thyroid gland
S	Isthmus
SP	Superior pole of thyroid gland
T	Thyroid cartilage
*	Tracheal rings

A. Anterior View

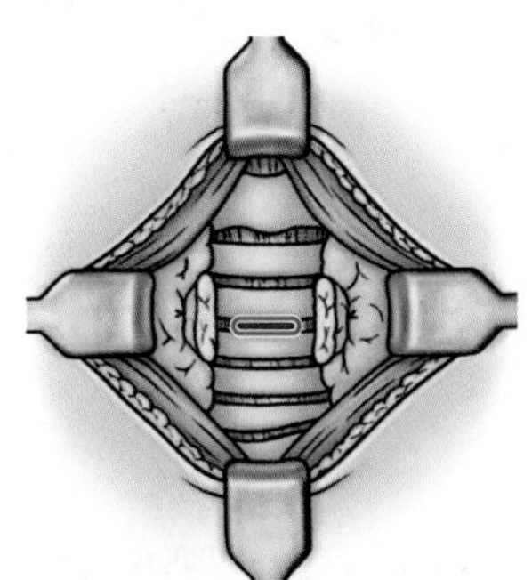

Incision in trachea after retracting infrahyoid muscles and incising isthmus of thyroid gland

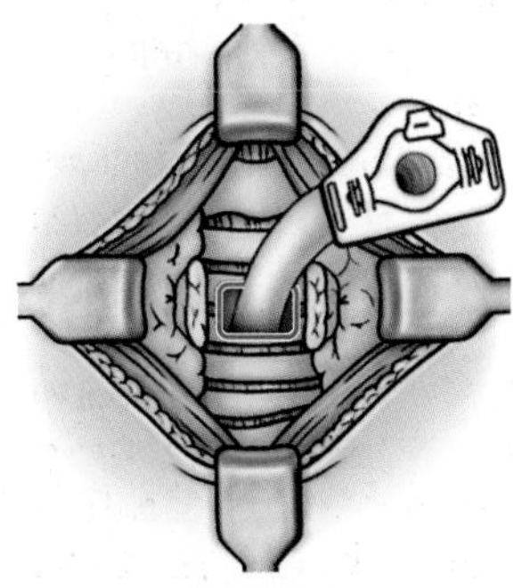

Tracheostomy tube inserted in tracheal opening

B. Tracheostomy

8.4 SURFACE ANATOMY OF HYOID AND CARTILAGES OF ANTERIOR NECK

A. Surface anatomy. **B.** Tracheostomy. The U-shaped hyoid bone lies superior to the thyroid cartilage at the level of the C4 and C5 vertebrae. The laryngeal prominence is produced by the fused laminae of the thyroid cartilage, which meet in the median plane. The cricoid cartilage can be felt inferior to the laryngeal prominence. It lies at the level of the C6 vertebra. The cartilaginous tracheal rings are palpable in the inferior part of the neck. The 2nd to 4th rings cannot be felt because the isthmus of the thyroid, connecting its right and left lobes, covers them. The first tracheal ring is just superior to the isthmus.

Tracheostomy. A transverse incision through the skin of the neck and anterior wall of the trachea (*tracheostomy*) establishes an airway in patients with upper airway obstruction or respiratory failure. The infrahyoid muscles are retracted laterally, and the isthmus of the thyroid gland is either divided or retracted superiorly. An opening is made in the trachea between the 1st and 2nd tracheal rings or through the 2nd through 4th rings. A *tracheostomy tube* is then inserted into the trachea and secured. To avoid complications during a tracheostomy, the following anatomical relationships are important:

- The inferior thyroid veins arise from a venous plexus on the thyroid gland and descend anterior to the trachea (see Fig. 8.10).
- A small thyroid ima artery is present in approximately 10% of people; it ascends from the brachiocephalic trunk or the arch of the aorta to the isthmus of the thyroid gland (see Fig. 8.21).
- The left brachiocephalic vein, jugular venous arch, and pleurae may be encountered, particularly in infants and children.
- The thymus covers the inferior part of the trachea in infants and children.
- The trachea is small, mobile, and soft in infants, making it easy to cut through its posterior wall and damage the esophagus.

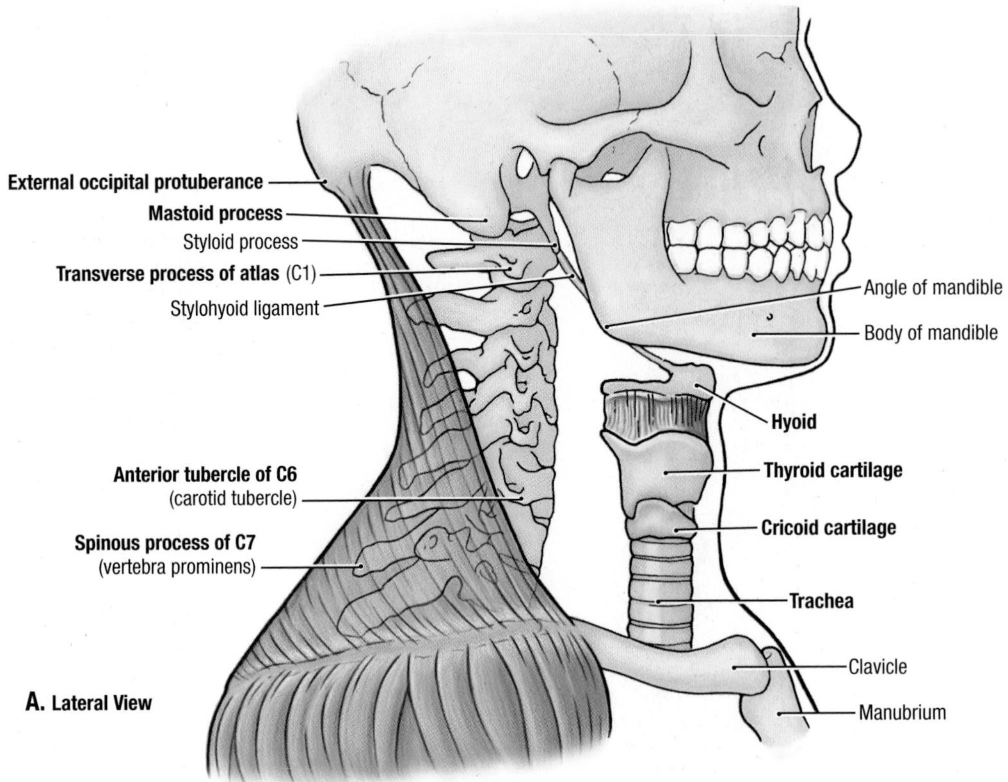
External occipital protuberance
Mastoid process
Styloid process
Transverse process of atlas (C1)
Stylohyoid ligament
Angle of mandible
Body of mandible
Hyoid
Thyroid cartilage
Cricoid cartilage
Trachea
Clavicle
Manubrium
Anterior tubercle of C6
(carotid tubercle)
Spinous process of C7
(vertebra prominens)
A. Lateral View

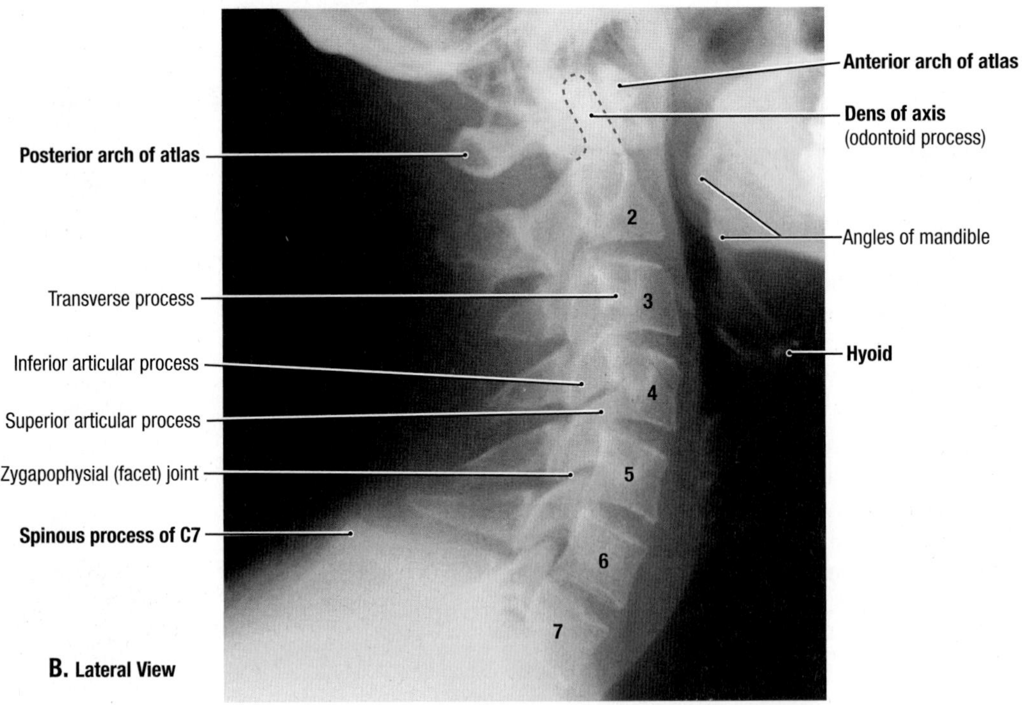
Anterior arch of atlas
Dens of axis
(odontoid process)
Posterior arch of atlas
Angles of mandible
Transverse process
Hyoid
Inferior articular process
Superior articular process
Zygapophysial (facet) joint
Spinous process of C7
2
3
4
5
6
7
B. Lateral View

8.5 BONES AND CARTILAGES OF NECK

A. Bony and cartilaginous landmarks of the neck. **B.** Radiograph of hyoid bone and cervical vertebrae. Because the upper cervical vertebrae lie posterior to the upper and lower jaws and teeth, they are best seen radiographically in lateral views.

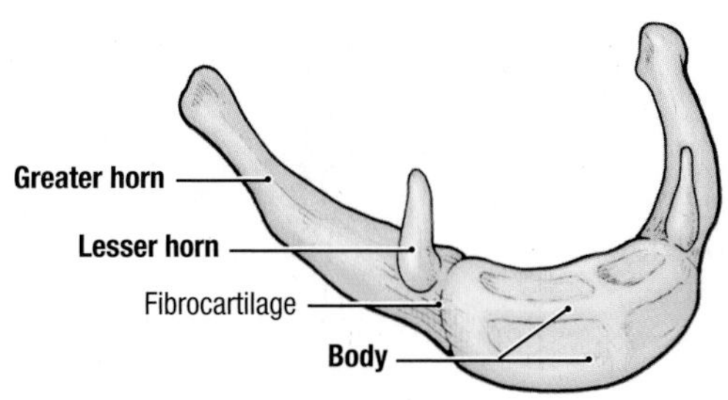
Greater horn
Lesser horn
Fibrocartilage
Body

C. Right Anterolateral View of Hyoid

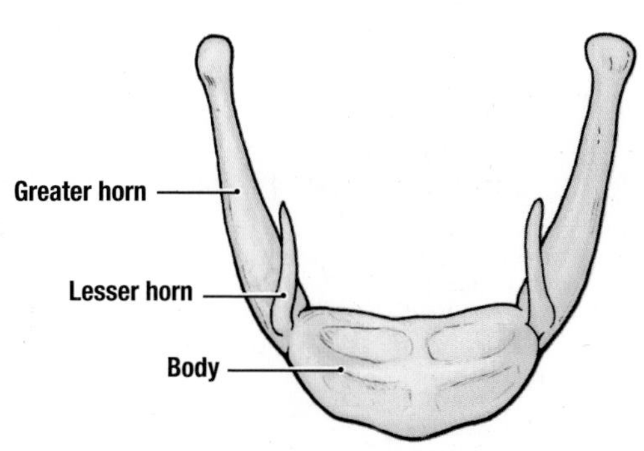
Greater horn
Lesser horn
Body

D. Anterosuperior View of Hyoid

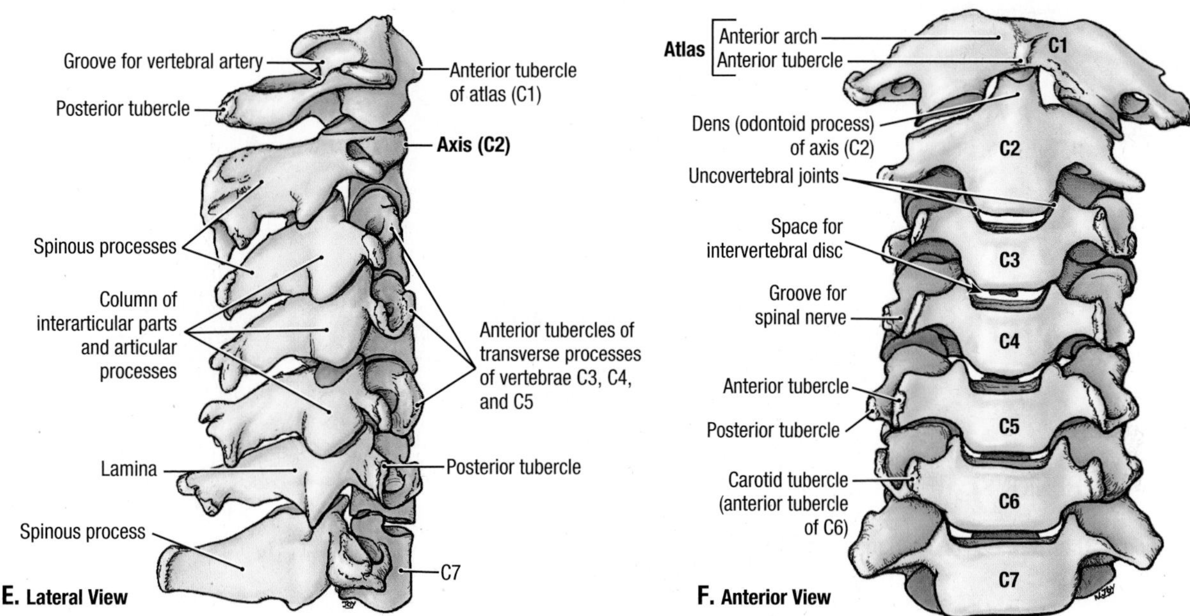
Groove for vertebral artery
Posterior tubercle
Anterior tubercle of atlas (C1)
Axis (C2)
Spinous processes
Column of interarticular parts and articular processes
Anterior tubercles of transverse processes of vertebrae C3, C4, and C5
Lamina
Posterior tubercle
Spinous process
C7
Atlas
Anterior arch
Anterior tubercle
C1
Dens (odontoid process) of axis (C2)
C2
Uncovertebral joints
Space for intervertebral disc
C3
Groove for spinal nerve
C4
Anterior tubercle
Posterior tubercle
C5
Carotid tubercle (anterior tubercle of C6)
C6
C7

E. Lateral View

F. Anterior View

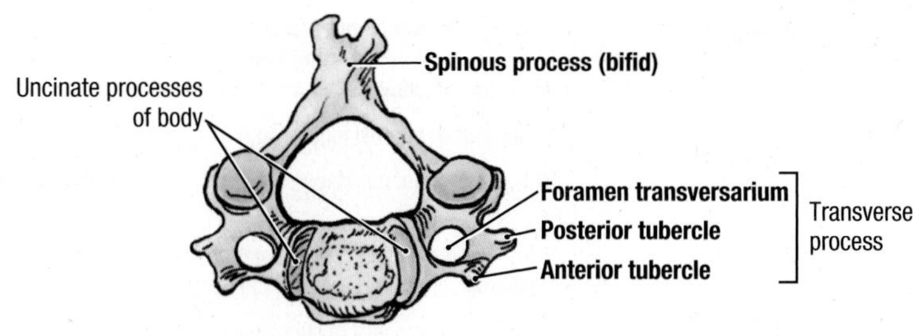
Spinous process (bifid)
Uncinate processes of body
Foramen transversarium
Posterior tubercle
Anterior tubercle
Transverse process

G. Superior View of Typical Cervical Vertebra (e.g., C4)

8.5 BONES AND CARTILAGES OF NECK *(CONTINUED)*

C. and D. Features of hyoid bone. **E. and F.** Articulated cervical vertebrae. **G.** Features of typical cervical vertebrae.

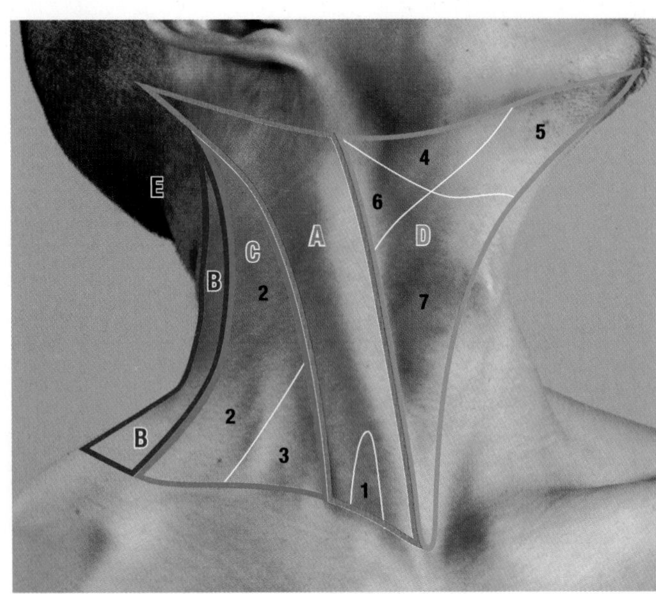
E
B
C
A
D
B
1
2
2
3
4
5
6
7
A. Anterolateral view

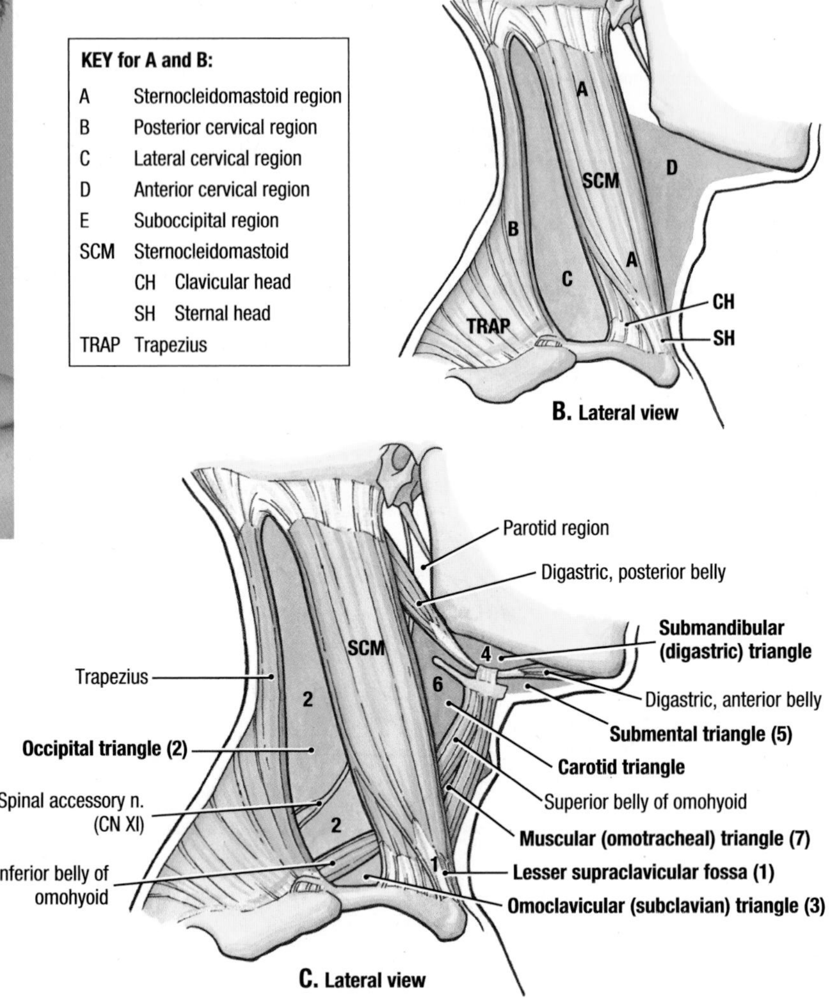
KEY for A and B:
A Sternocleidomastoid region
B Posterior cervical region
C Lateral cervical region
D Anterior cervical region
E Suboccipital region
SCM Sternocleidomastoid
CH Clavicular head
SH Sternal head
TRAP Trapezius
A
SCM
D
B
C
A
TRAP
CH
SH
Parotid region
Digastric, posterior belly
Submandibular (digastric) triangle
Digastric, anterior belly
Submental triangle (5)
Carotid triangle
Superior belly of omohyoid
Muscular (omotracheal) triangle (7)
Lesser supraclavicular fossa (1)
Omoclavicular (subclavian) triangle (3)
Trapezius
Occipital triangle (2)
Spinal accessory n. (CN XI)
Inferior belly of omohyoid
SCM
2
2
4
6
1
B. Lateral view

C. Lateral view

8.6 CERVICAL REGIONS

A. Surface anatomy. **B. and C.** Regions and triangles of neck.

TABLE 8.2 CERVICAL REGIONS AND CONTENTS[a]

Region	Main Contents and Underlying Structures
Sternocleidomastoid region *(A)*	Sternocleidomastoid (SCM) muscle; superior part of the external jugular vein; greater auricular nerve; transverse cervical nerve
Lesser supraclavicular fossa *(1)*	Inferior part of internal jugular vein
Posterior cervical region *(B)*	Trapezius muscle; cutaneous branches of posterior rami of cervical spinal nerves; suboccipital region (E) lies deep to superior part of this region
Lateral cervical region (posterior triangle) *(C)* Occipital triangle *(2)*	Part of external jugular vein; posterior branches of cervical plexus of nerves; spinal accessory nerve; trunks of brachial plexus; transverse cervical artery; cervical lymph nodes
Omoclavicular triangle *(3)*	Subclavian artery; part of subclavian vein (variable); suprascapular artery; supraclavicular lymph nodes
Anterior cervical region (anterior triangle) *(D)* Submandibular (digastric) triangle *(4)*	Submandibular gland almost fills triangle; submandibular lymph nodes; hypoglossal nerve; mylohyoid nerve; parts of facial artery and vein
Submental triangle *(5)*	Submental lymph nodes and small veins that unite to form anterior jugular vein
Carotid triangle *(6)*	Common carotid artery and its branches; internal jugular vein and its tributaries; vagus nerve; external carotid artery and some of its branches; hypoglossal nerve and superior root of ansa cervicalis; spinal accessory nerve; thyroid gland, larynx, and pharynx; deep cervical lymph nodes; branches of cervical plexus
Muscular (omotracheal) triangle (7)	Sternothyroid and sternohyoid muscles; thyroid and parathyroid glands

[a]Letters and numbers in parentheses refer to Figures A, B and C.

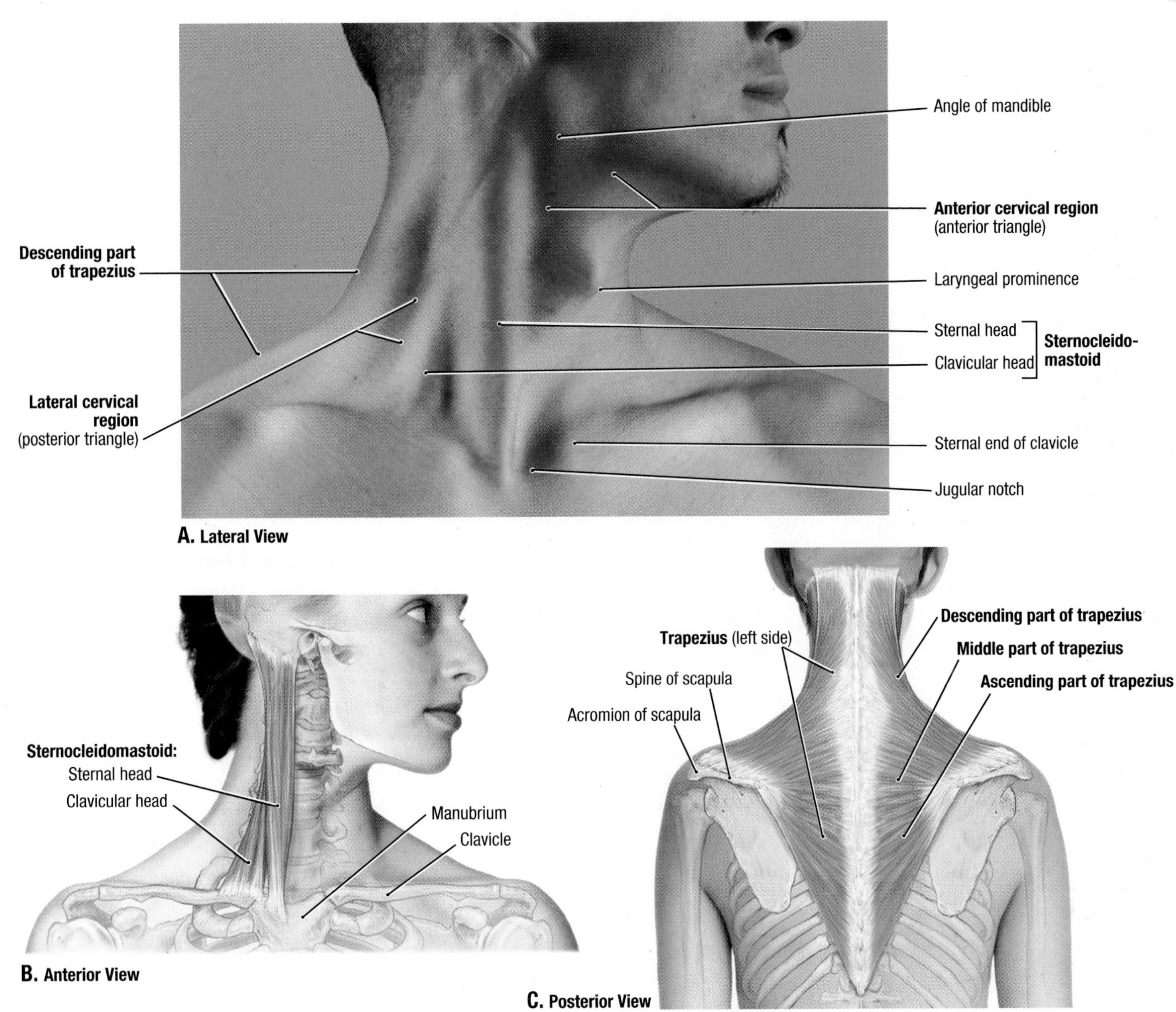
Angle of mandible
Anterior cervical region (anterior triangle)
Descending part of trapezius
Laryngeal prominence
Sternal head
Clavicular head
Sternocleido-mastoid
Lateral cervical region (posterior triangle)
Sternal end of clavicle
Jugular notch
A. Lateral View
Sternocleidomastoid:
Sternal head
Clavicular head
Manubrium
Clavicle
B. Anterior View
Trapezius (left side)
Spine of scapula
Acromion of scapula
Descending part of trapezius
Middle part of trapezius
Ascending part of trapezius
C. Posterior View

8.7 STERNOCLEIDOMASTOID AND TRAPEZIUS.

A. Surface anatomy. **B.** Sternocleidomastoid. **C.** Trapezius.

TABLE 8.3 STERNOCLEIDOMASTOID AND TRAPEZIUS

Muscle	Superior Attachment	Inferior Attachment	Innervation	Main Action
Sternocleidomastoid	Lateral surface of mastoid process of temporal bone; lateral half of superior nuchal line	*Sternal head:* anterior surface of manubrium of sternum *Clavicular head:* superior surface of medial third of clavicle	Spinal accessory nerve (CN XI) [motor] and C2 and C3 nerves (pain and proprioception)	*Unilateral contraction:* laterally flexes neck; rotates neck so face is turned superiorly toward opposite side; *Bilateral contraction:* (1) extends neck at atlanto-occipital joints, (2) flexes cervical vertebrae so that chin approaches manubrium, or (3) extends superior cervical vertebrae while flexing inferior vertebrae, so chin is thrust forward with head kept level; with cervical vertebrae fixed, may elevate manubrium and medial end of clavicles, assisting deep respiration.
Trapezius	Medial third of superior nuchal line, external occipital protuberance, nuchal ligament, spinous processes of C7–T12 vertebrae, lumbar and sacral spinous processes	Lateral third of clavicle, acromion, spine of scapula	Spinal accessory nerve (CN XI) [motor] and C2 and C3 nerves (pain and proprioception)	*Descending fibers* elevate pectoral girdle, maintain level of shoulders against gravity or resistance; *middle fibers* retract scapula; and *ascending fibers* depress shoulders; *superior* and *inferior fibers* work together to rotate scapula upward; *when shoulders are fixed,* bilateral contraction extends neck; unilateral contraction produces lateral flexion to same side

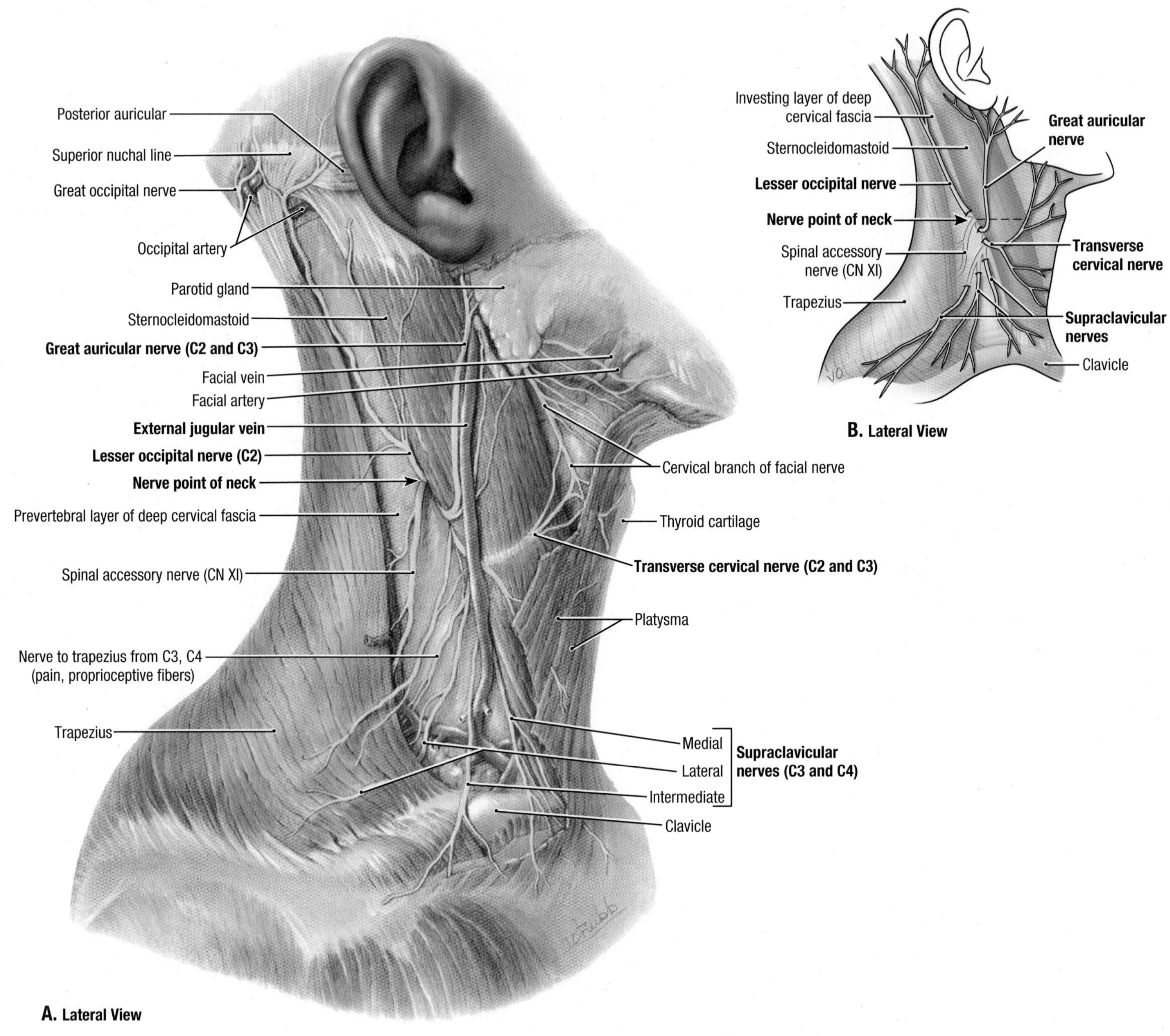

Posterior auricular
Superior nuchal line
Great occipital nerve
Occipital artery
Parotid gland
Sternocleidomastoid
Great auricular nerve (C2 and C3)
Facial vein
Facial artery
External jugular vein
Lesser occipital nerve (C2)
Nerve point of neck
Prevertebral layer of deep cervical fascia
Spinal accessory nerve (CN XI)
Nerve to trapezius from C3, C4 (pain, proprioceptive fibers)
Trapezius
Cervical branch of facial nerve
Thyroid cartilage
Transverse cervical nerve (C2 and C3)
Platysma
Medial
Lateral
Intermediate
Supraclavicular nerves (C3 and C4)
Clavicle
A. Lateral View
Investing layer of deep cervical fascia
Sternocleidomastoid
Lesser occipital nerve
Nerve point of neck
Spinal accessory nerve (CN XI)
Trapezius
Great auricular nerve
Transverse cervical nerve
Supraclavicular nerves
Clavicle
B. Lateral View

8.8 SERIAL DISSECTIONS OF LATERAL CERVICAL REGION (POSTERIOR TRIANGLE OF NECK)

A. External jugular vein and cutaneous branches of cervical plexus. Subcutaneous fat, the part of the plasma overlying the inferior part of the lateral cervical region, and the investing layer of deep cervical fascia have all been removed. The external jugular vein descends vertically across the sternocleidomastoid and pierces the prevertebral layer of deep cervical fascia superior to the clavicle.

B. and C. Branches of the cervical plexus.

- Branches arising from the nerve loop between the anterior rami of C2 and C3 are the lesser occipital, great auricular, and transverse cervical nerves.
- Branches arising from the loop formed between the anterior rami of C3 and C4 are the supraclavicular nerves, which emerge as a common trunk under cover of the SCM.

Regional anesthesia is often used for surgical procedures in the neck region or upper limb. In a **cervical plexus block,** an anesthetic agent is injected at several points along the posterior border of the SCM, mainly at its midpoint, the nerve point of the neck.

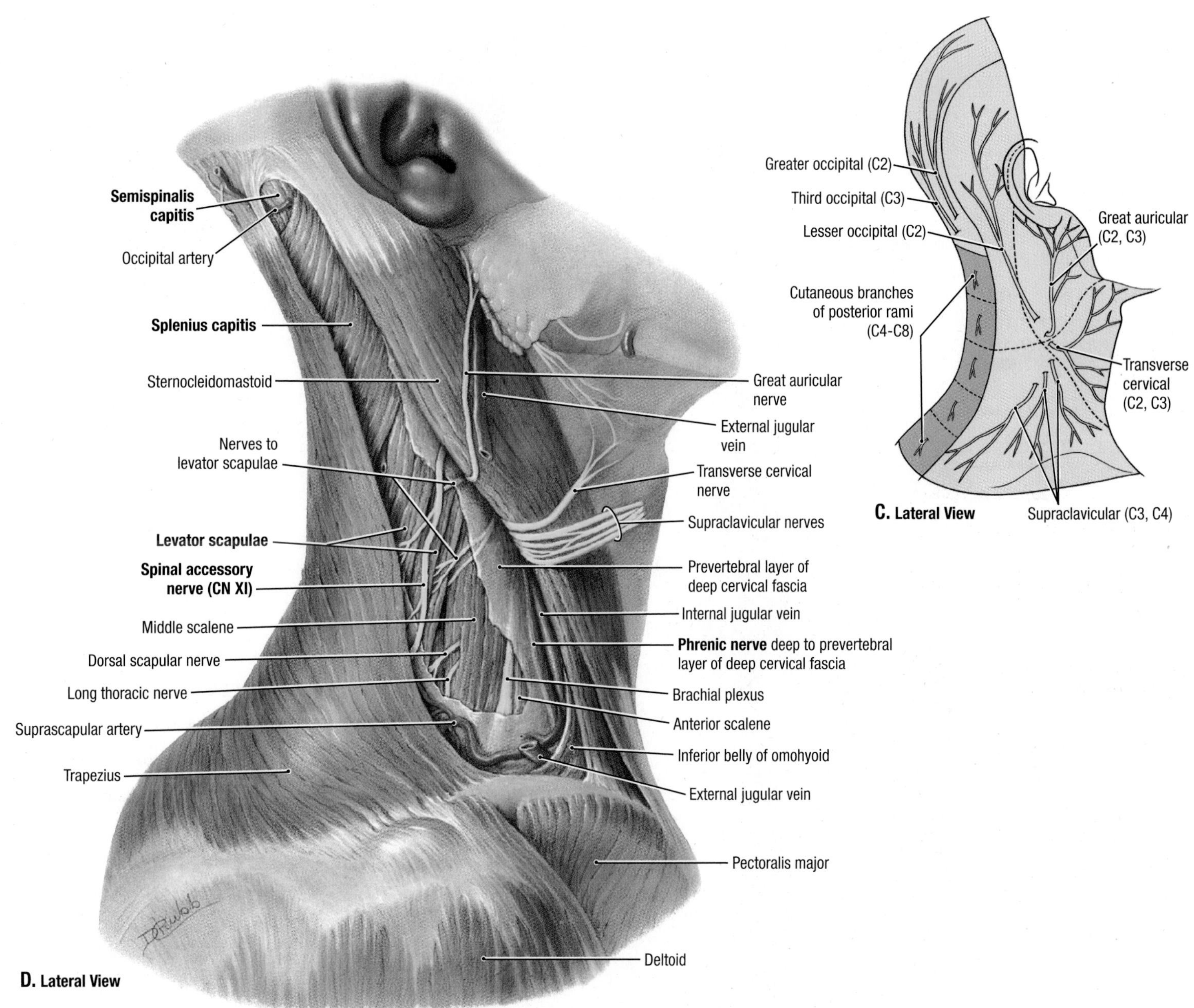
Greater occipital (C2)
Third occipital (C3)
Lesser occipital (C2)
Great auricular (C2, C3)
Cutaneous branches of posterior rami (C4-C8)
Transverse cervical (C2, C3)
Supraclavicular (C3, C4)
Semispinalis capitis
Occipital artery
Splenius capitis
Sternocleidomastoid
Nerves to levator scapulae
Levator scapulae
Spinal accessory nerve (CN XI)
Middle scalene
Dorsal scapular nerve
Long thoracic nerve
Suprascapular artery
Trapezius
Great auricular nerve
External jugular vein
Transverse cervical nerve
Supraclavicular nerves
Prevertebral layer of deep cervical fascia
Internal jugular vein
Phrenic nerve deep to prevertebral layer of deep cervical fascia
Brachial plexus
Anterior scalene
Inferior belly of omohyoid
External jugular vein
Pectoralis major
Deltoid

C. **Lateral View**

D. **Lateral View**

8.8 SERIAL DISSECTIONS OF LATERAL CERVICAL REGION *(CONTINUED)*

D. Muscles forming the floor of the lateral cervical region. The prevertebral layer of deep cervical fascia has been partially removed, and the motor nerves and most of the floor of the region are exposed.

- The spinal accessory nerve (CN XI) supplies the SCM and trapezius muscles; between them, it courses along the levator scapulae muscle but is separated from it by the prevertebral layer of deep cervical fascia.
- The phrenic nerve (C3, C4, C5) supplies the diaphragm and is located deep to the prevertebral layer of deep cervical fascia on the anterior surface of the anterior scalene muscle.

Severance of a phrenic nerve results in an ipsilateral paralysis of the diaphragm. A phrenic nerve block produces a short period of paralysis of the diaphragm on one side (e.g., for a lung operation). The anesthetic agent is injected around the nerve where it lies on the anterior surface of the anterior scalene muscle.

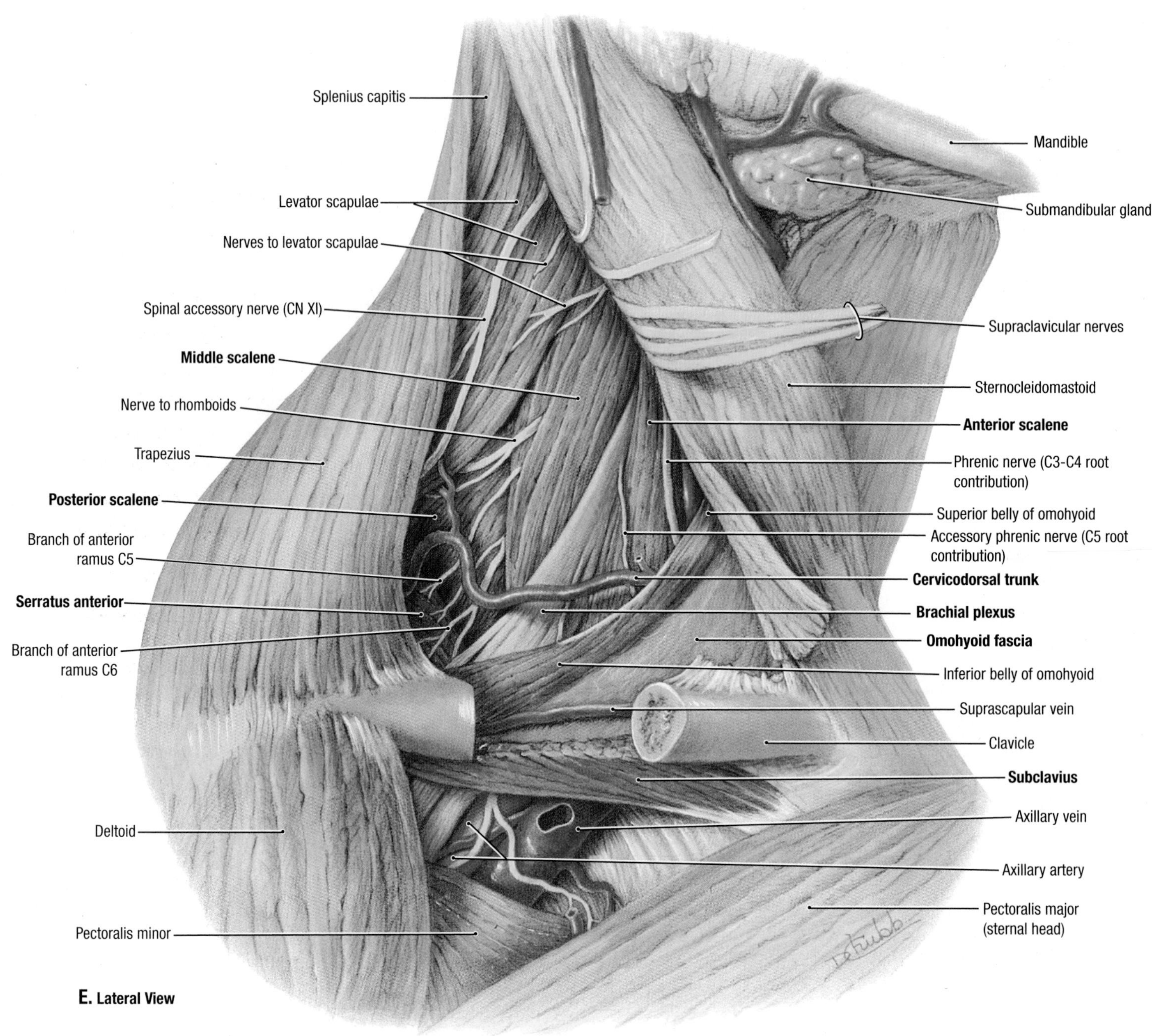
Splenius capitis
Mandible
Submandibular gland
Levator scapulae
Nerves to levator scapulae
Spinal accessory nerve (CN XI)
Supraclavicular nerves
Middle scalene
Sternocleidomastoid
Nerve to rhomboids
Anterior scalene
Trapezius
Phrenic nerve (C3-C4 root contribution)
Posterior scalene
Superior belly of omohyoid
Branch of anterior ramus C5
Accessory phrenic nerve (C5 root contribution)
Cervicodorsal trunk
Serratus anterior
Brachial plexus
Branch of anterior ramus C6
Omohyoid fascia
Inferior belly of omohyoid
Suprascapular vein
Clavicle
Subclavius
Deltoid
Axillary vein
Axillary artery
Pectoralis major (sternal head)
Pectoralis minor

E. Lateral View

8.8 SERIAL DISSECTIONS OF LATERAL CERVICAL REGION *(CONTINUED)*

E. Vessels and motor nerves of the lateral cervical region. The clavicular head of the pectoralis major muscle and part of the clavicle have been removed.

The muscles that form the floor of the region are the semispinalis capitis, splenius capitis and levator scapulae superiorly and the anterior, middle and posterior scalenes and serratus anterior inferiorly.

- The brachial plexus emerges between the anterior and middle scalene muscles.

A **supraclavicular brachial plexus block** may be utilized for anesthesia of the upper limb. The anesthetic agent is injected around the supraclavicular part of the brachial plexus. The main injection site is superior to the midpoint of the clavicle.

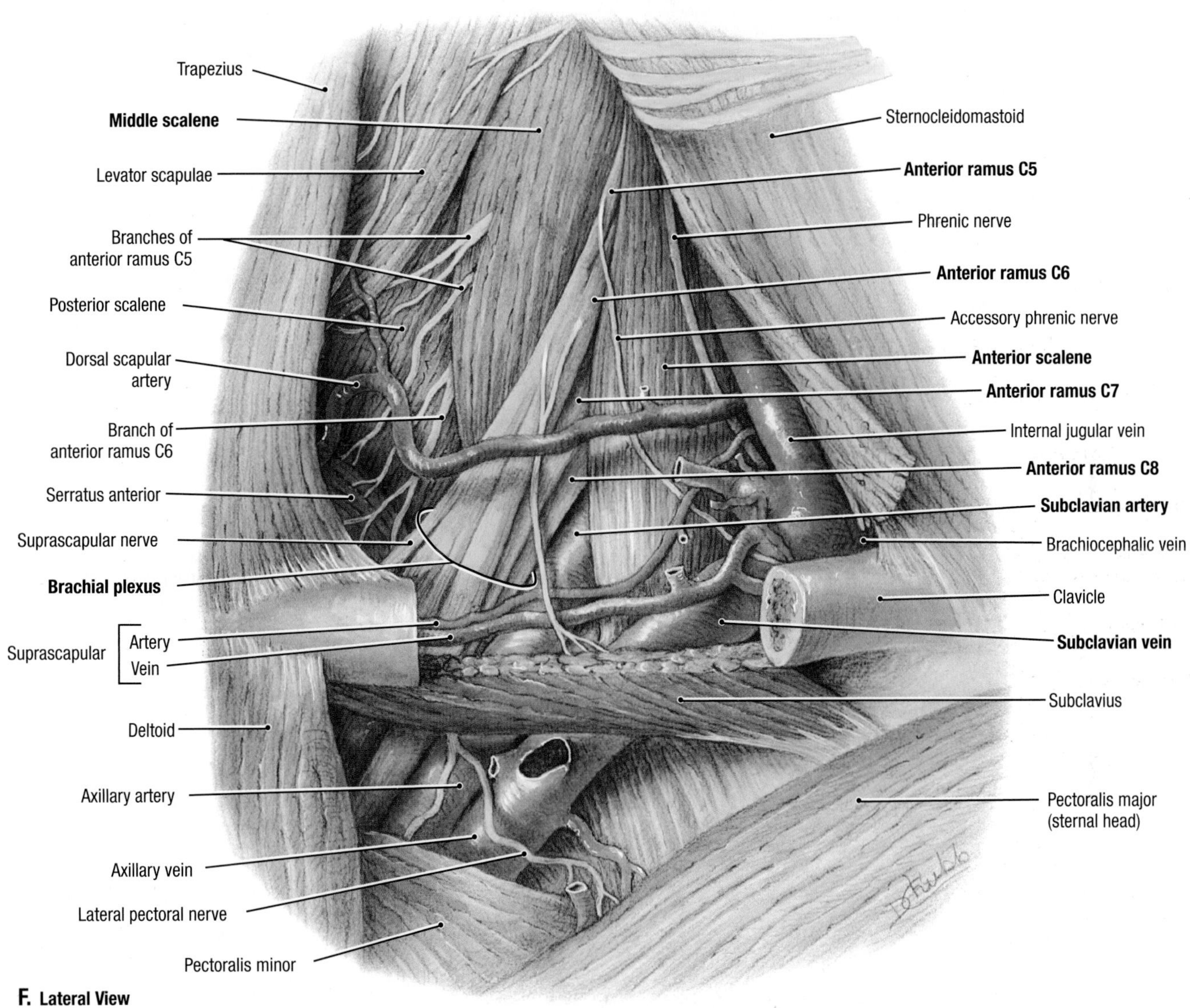
Trapezius
Middle scalene
Levator scapulae
Branches of anterior ramus C5
Posterior scalene
Dorsal scapular artery
Branch of anterior ramus C6
Serratus anterior
Suprascapular nerve
Brachial plexus
Suprascapular Artery
Vein
Deltoid
Axillary artery
Axillary vein
Lateral pectoral nerve
Pectoralis minor
Sternocleidomastoid
Anterior ramus C5
Phrenic nerve
Anterior ramus C6
Accessory phrenic nerve
Anterior scalene
Anterior ramus C7
Internal jugular vein
Anterior ramus C8
Subclavian artery
Brachiocephalic vein
Clavicle
Subclavian vein
Subclavius
Pectoralis major (sternal head)

F. Lateral View

8.8 SERIAL DISSECTIONS OF LATERAL CERVICAL REGION *(CONTINUED)*

F. Structures of the omoclavicular (subclavian) triangle. The omohyoid muscle and fascia have been removed, exposing the brachial plexus and subclavian vessels.

- The anterior rami of C5–T1 form the brachial plexus; the anterior ramus of T1 lies posterior to the subclavian artery.
- The brachial plexus and subclavian artery emerge between the middle and anterior scalene muscles.
- The anterior scalene muscle lies between the subclavian artery and vein.

The right or left subclavian vein is often the site of **placement for a central venous catheter**, used to insert intravenous tubes ("central venous lines") for the administration of parenteral nutritional fluids or medications, for testing blood chemistry or central venous pressure, or inserting electrode wires for heart pacemaker devices. The relationships of the subclavian vein to the sternocleidomastoid muscle, clavicle, sternoclavicular joint and 1st rib are of clinical importance in line placement, and there is danger of puncture of the pleura or subclavian artery if the procedure is not performed correctly.

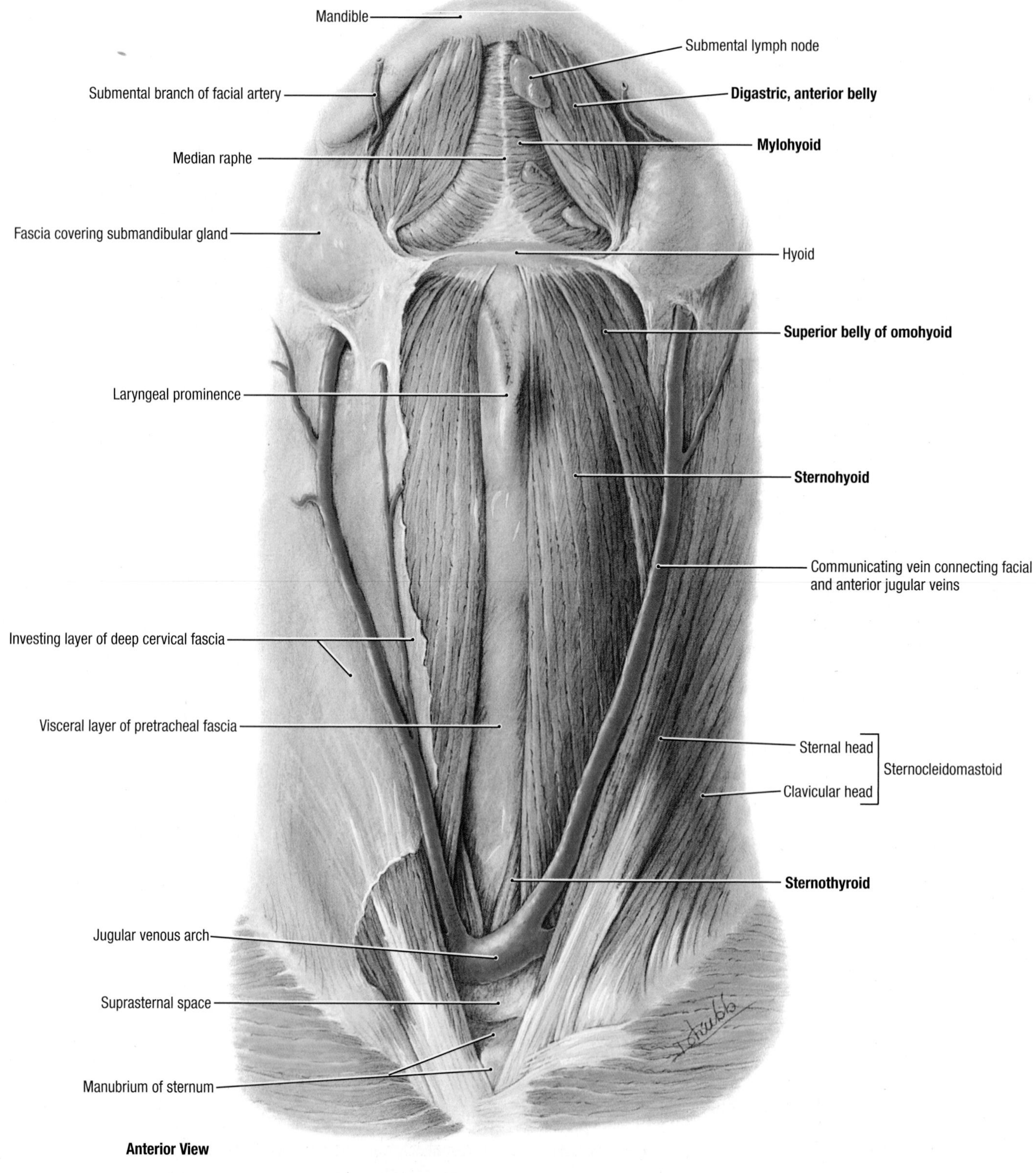
Mandible
Submental lymph node
Submental branch of facial artery
Digastric, anterior belly
Median raphe
Mylohyoid
Fascia covering submandibular gland
Hyoid
Superior belly of omohyoid
Laryngeal prominence
Sternohyoid
Communicating vein connecting facial and anterior jugular veins
Investing layer of deep cervical fascia
Visceral layer of pretracheal fascia
Sternal head
Sternocleidomastoid
Clavicular head
Sternothyroid
Jugular venous arch
Suprasternal space
Manubrium of sternum

Anterior View

8.9 SUPRAHYOID AND INFRAHYOID MUSCLES

Much of the investing layer of deep cervical fascia has been removed.

- The anterior bellies of the digastric muscles form the sides of the suprahyoid part of the anterior cervical region, or submental triangle (floor of mouth). The hyoid bone forms the triangle's base, and the mylohyoid muscles are its floor.
- The infrahyoid part of the anterior cervical region is shaped like an elongated diamond bounded by the sternohyoid muscle superiorly and sternothyroid muscle inferiorly.

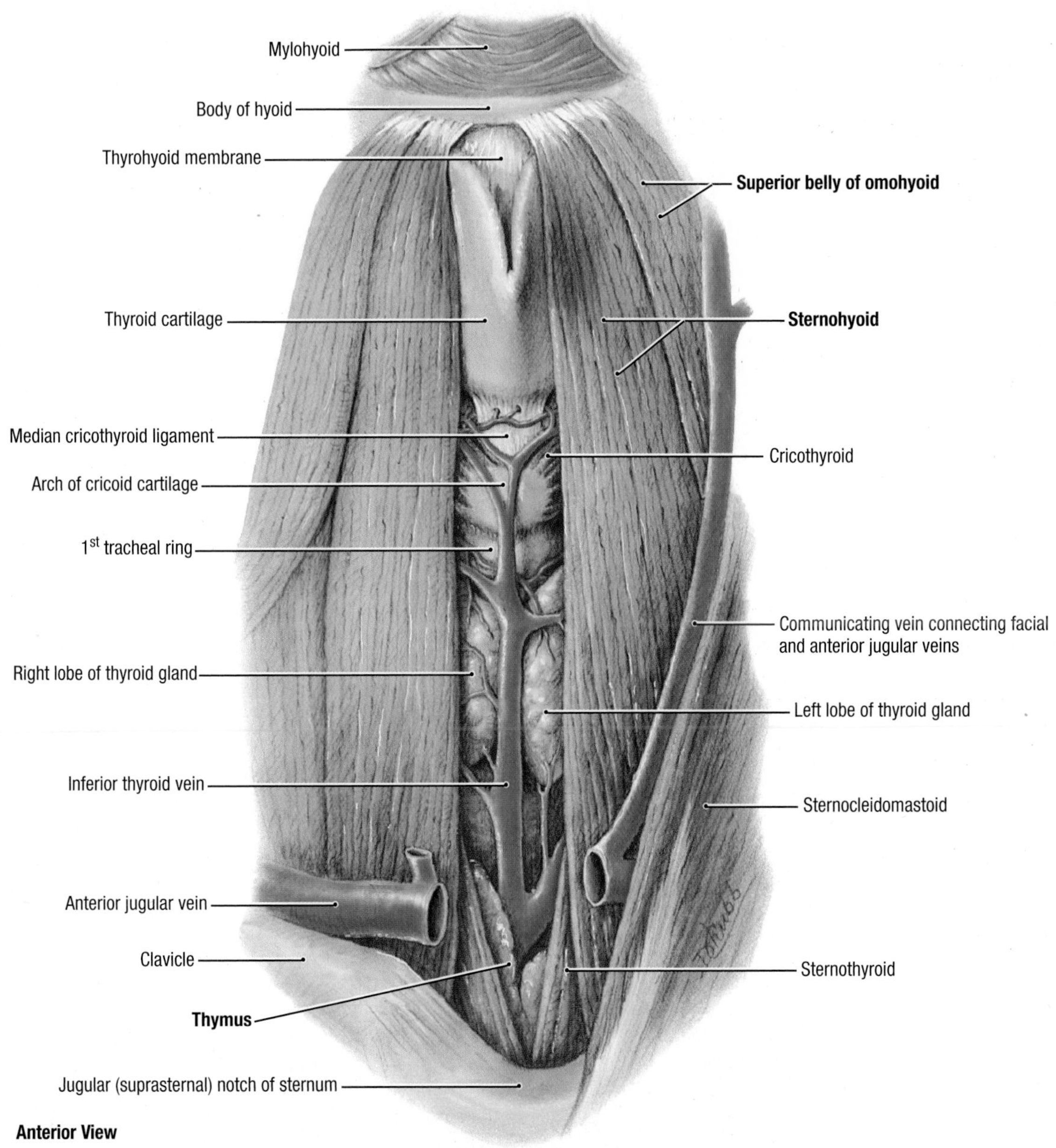
Mylohyoid
Body of hyoid
Thyrohyoid membrane
Superior belly of omohyoid
Thyroid cartilage
Sternohyoid
Median cricothyroid ligament
Cricothyroid
Arch of cricoid cartilage
1st tracheal ring
Communicating vein connecting facial and anterior jugular veins
Right lobe of thyroid gland
Left lobe of thyroid gland
Inferior thyroid vein
Sternocleidomastoid
Anterior jugular vein
Clavicle
Sternothyroid
Thymus
Jugular (suprasternal) notch of sternum
Anterior View

8.10 INFRAHYOID REGION, SUPERFICIAL MUSCULAR LAYER

A. Muscular attachments onto the hyoid bone. **B.** The pretracheal fascia, right anterior jugular vein, and jugular venous arch have been removed.

- A persistent thymus projects superiorly from the thorax.
- The two superficial depressors of the larynx ("strap muscles") are the omohyoid (only the superior belly of which is seen here) and sternohyoid.

Fracture of the hyoid. This results in depression of the body of the hyoid onto the thyroid cartilage. Inability to elevate the hyoid and move it anteriorly beneath the tongue makes swallowing and maintenance of the separation of the alimentary and respiratory tracts difficult and may result in **aspiration pneumonia.**

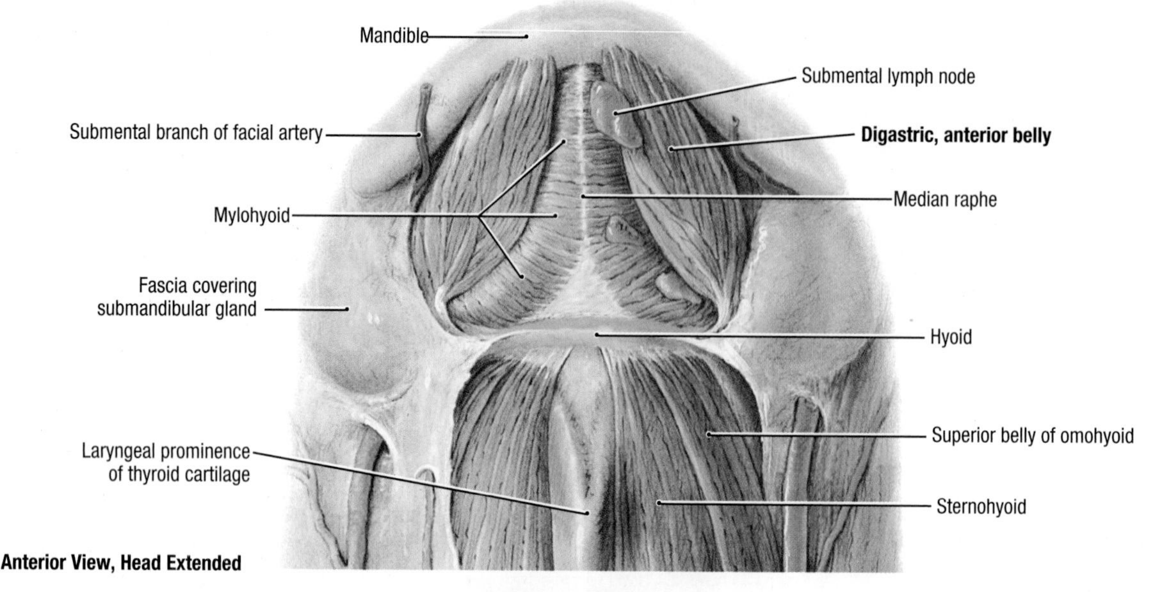
Mandible
Submental lymph node
Submental branch of facial artery
Digastric, anterior belly
Median raphe
Mylohyoid
Fascia covering submandibular gland
Hyoid
Superior belly of omohyoid
Laryngeal prominence of thyroid cartilage
Sternohyoid

A. Anterior View, Head Extended

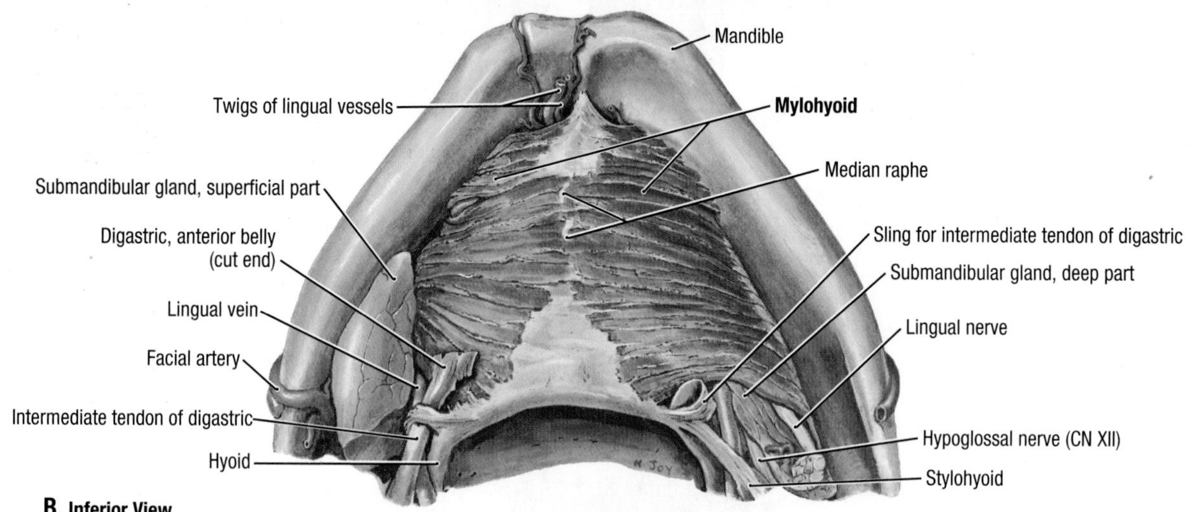
Mandible
Twigs of lingual vessels
Mylohyoid
Median raphe
Submandibular gland, superficial part
Digastric, anterior belly (cut end)
Sling for intermediate tendon of digastric
Submandibular gland, deep part
Lingual vein
Lingual nerve
Facial artery
Intermediate tendon of digastric
Hypoglossal nerve (CN XII)
Hyoid
Stylohyoid

B. Inferior View

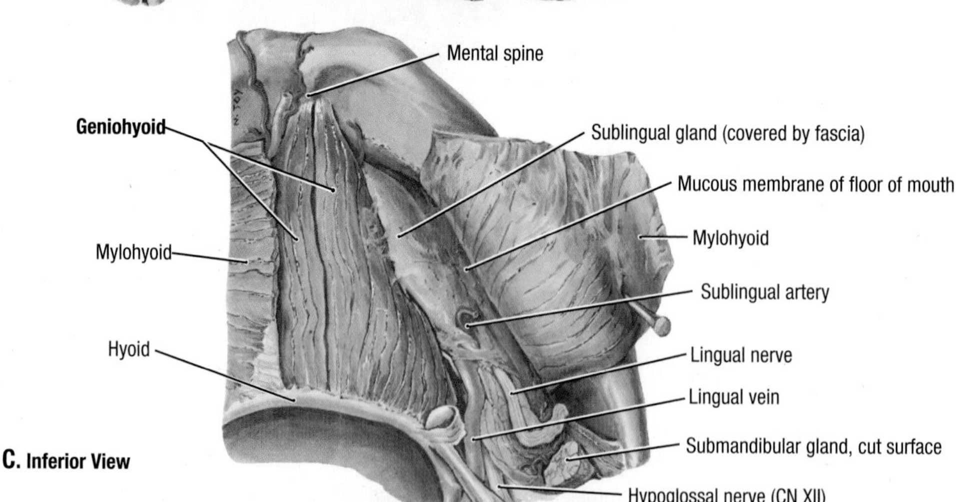
Mental spine
Geniohyoid
Sublingual gland (covered by fascia)
Mucous membrane of floor of mouth
Mylohyoid
Mylohyoid
Sublingual artery
Hyoid
Lingual nerve
Lingual vein
Submandibular gland, cut surface
Hypoglossal nerve (CN XII)

C. Inferior View

8.11 SUPRAHYOID REGION (SUBMENTAL TRIANGLE)

A. Superficial layer—anterior belly of digastric. **B.** Intermediate layer—mylohyoid muscles. **C.** Deep layer—geniohyoid muscles.

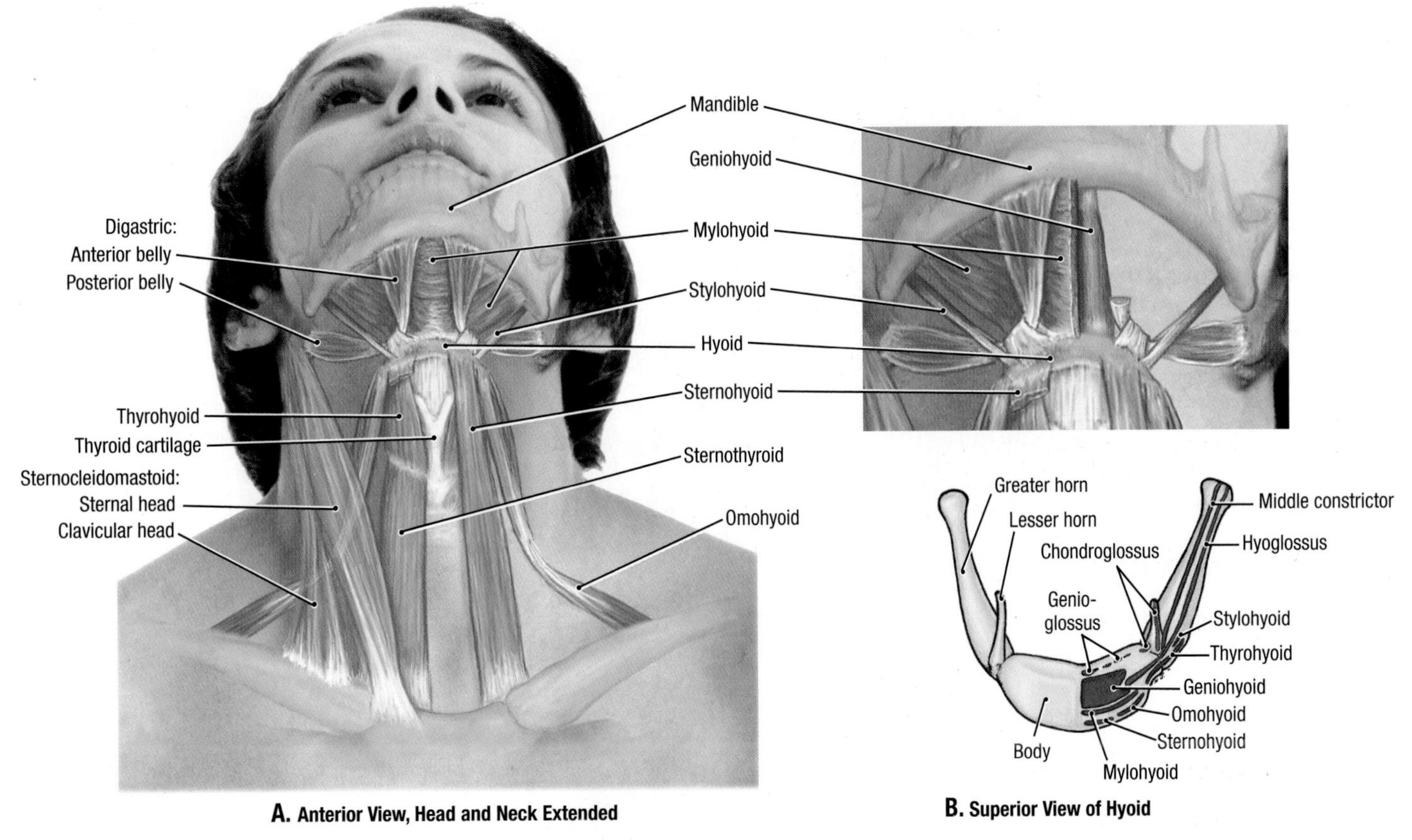
Mandible
Geniohyoid
Digastric:
Anterior belly
Posterior belly
Mylohyoid
Stylohyoid
Hyoid
Sternohyoid
Thyrohyoid
Thyroid cartilage
Sternothyroid
Sternocleidomastoid:
Sternal head
Clavicular head
Omohyoid
Greater horn
Lesser horn
Chondroglossus
Genio-
glossus
Body
Mylohyoid
Middle constrictor
Hyoglossus
Stylohyoid
Thyrohyoid
Geniohyoid
Omohyoid
Sternohyoid

A. Anterior View, Head and Neck Extended

B. Superior View of Hyoid

8.12 SUPRAHYOID AND INFRAHYOID MUSCLES

A. Overview. **B.** Muscular attachments onto the hyoid bone.

TABLE 8.4 SUPRAHYOID AND INFRAHYOID MUSCLES

Muscle	Superior Attachment	Inferior Attachment	Innervation	Main Action
Suprahyoid muscles				
Mylohyoid	Mylohyoid line of mandible	Raphe and body of hyoid bone	Nerve to mylohyoid, a branch of inferior alveolar nerve (CN V^3)	Elevates hyoid bone, floor of mouth and tongue during swallowing and speaking
Digastric	*Anterior belly:* digastric fossa of mandible *Posterior belly:* mastoid notch of temporal bone	Intermediate tendon to body and greater horn of hyoid bone	*Anterior belly:* nerve to mylohyoid, a branch of inferior alveolar nerve (CN V^3) *Posterior belly:* facial nerve (CN VII)	Elevates hyoid bone and steadies it during swallowing and speaking; depresses mandible against resistance
Geniohyoid	Inferior mental spine of mandible	Body of hyoid bone	C1 via the hypoglossal nerve (CN XII)	Pulls hyoid bone anterosuperiorly, shortens floor of mouth, and widens pharynx
Stylohyoid	Styloid process of temporal bone		Cervical branch of facial nerve (CN VII)	Elevates and retracts hyoid bone, thereby elongating floor of mouth
Infrahyoid muscles				
Sternohyoid	Body of hyoid bone	Manubrium of sternum and medial end of clavicle	C1–C3 by a branch of ansa cervicalis	Depresses hyoid bone after it has been elevated during swallowing
Omohyoid	Inferior border of hyoid bone	Superior border of scapula near suprascapular notch		Depresses, retracts, and steadies hyoid bone
Sternothyroid	Oblique line of thyroid cartilage	Posterior surface of manubrium of sternum	C2 and C3 by a branch of ansa cervicalis	Depresses hyoid bone and larynx
Thyrohyoid	Inferior border of body and greater horn of hyoid bone	Oblique line of thyroid cartilage	C1 via hypoglossal nerve(CN XII)	Depresses hyoid bone and elevates larynx

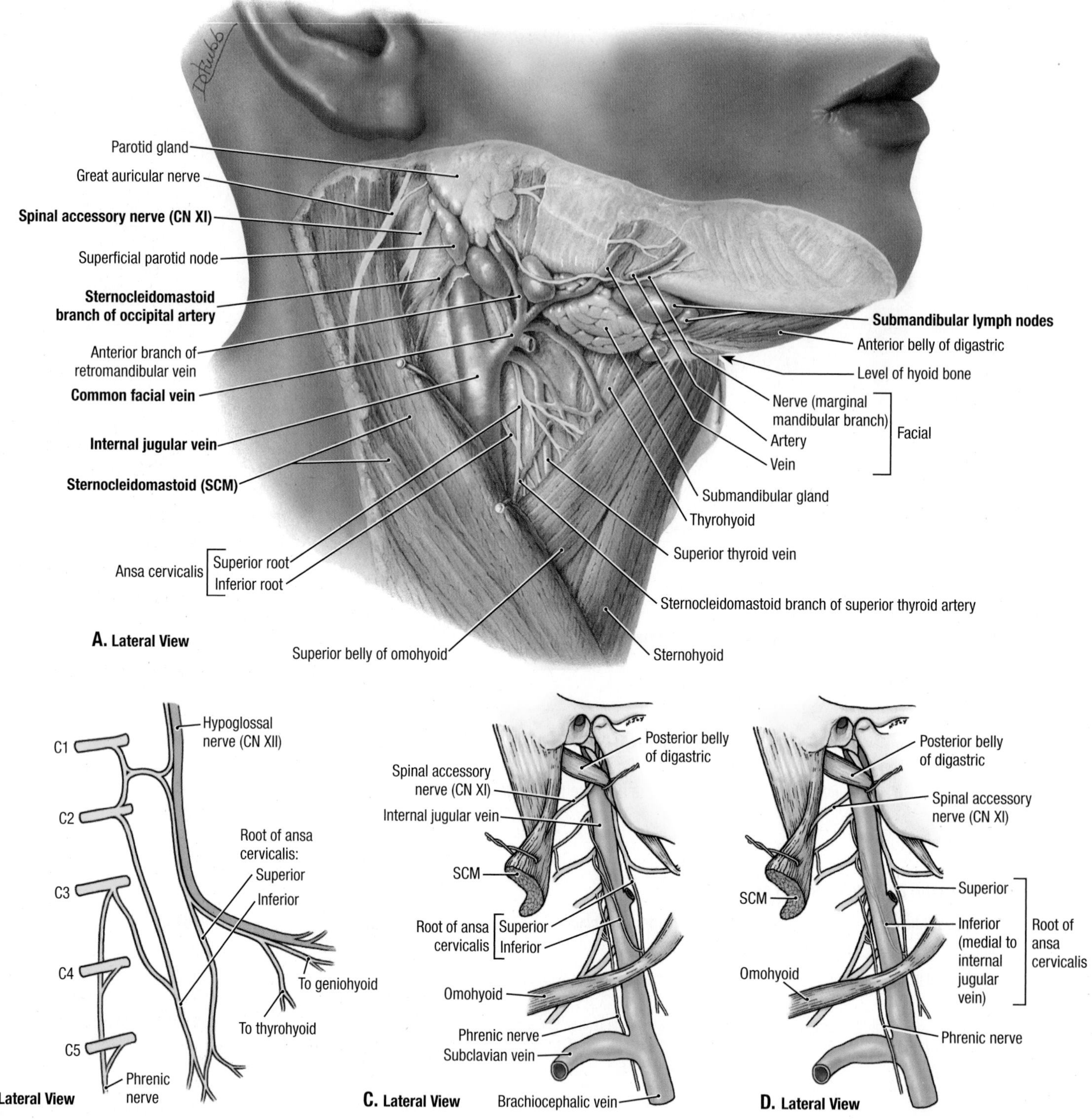
Parotid gland
Great auricular nerve
Spinal accessory nerve (CN XI)
Superficial parotid node
Sternocleidomastoid branch of occipital artery
Anterior branch of retromandibular vein
Common facial vein
Internal jugular vein
Sternocleidomastoid (SCM)
Ansa cervicalis
Superior root
Inferior root
Submandibular lymph nodes
Anterior belly of digastric
Level of hyoid bone
Nerve (marginal mandibular branch)
Artery
Vein
Facial
Submandibular gland
Thyrohyoid
Superior thyroid vein
Sternocleidomastoid branch of superior thyroid artery
Superior belly of omohyoid
Sternohyoid
A. Lateral View
C1
C2
C3
C4
C5
Hypoglossal nerve (CN XII)
Root of ansa cervicalis:
Superior
Inferior
To geniohyoid
To thyrohyoid
Phrenic nerve
B. Lateral View
Posterior belly of digastric
Spinal accessory nerve (CN XI)
Internal jugular vein
SCM
Root of ansa cervicalis
Superior
Inferior
Omohyoid
Phrenic nerve
Subclavian vein
Brachiocephalic vein
C. Lateral View
Posterior belly of digastric
Spinal accessory nerve (CN XI)
SCM
Superior
Inferior (medial to internal jugular vein)
Root of ansa cervicalis
Omohyoid
Phrenic nerve
D. Lateral View

8.13 SUPERFICIAL DISSECTION OF CAROTID TRIANGLE

A. The skin, subcutaneous tissue (with platysma), and the investing layer of deep cervical fascia, including the sheaths of the parotid and submandibular glands, have been removed.

- The spinal accessory nerve (CN XI) enters the deep surface of the sternocleidomastoid muscle and is joined along its anterior border by the sternocleidomastoid branch of the occipital artery.
- The (common) facial vein joins the internal jugular vein near the level of the hyoid bone; here, the facial vein is joined by several other veins.
- The submandibular lymph nodes lie deep to the investing layer of deep cervical fascia in the submandibular triangle; some of the nodes lie deep in the submandibular gland.

B. Diagram of the motor branches of cervical plexus. **C.** Typical relationships of ansa cervicalis, spinal accessory nerve (CN XI), and phrenic nerve to the internal jugular and subclavian veins. **D.** Atypical relationships.

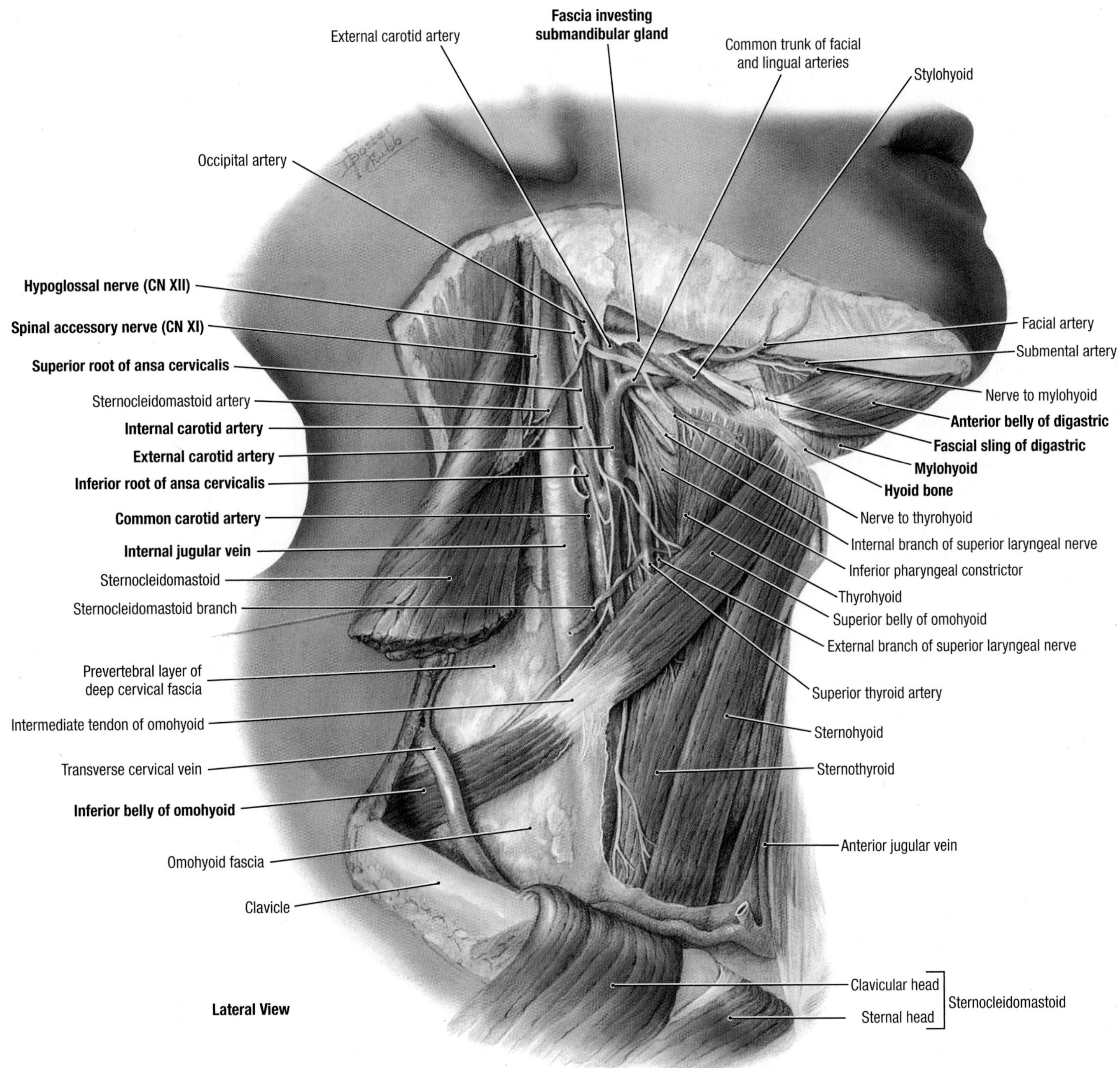
External carotid artery
Fascia investing submandibular gland
Common trunk of facial and lingual arteries
Stylohyoid
Occipital artery
Hypoglossal nerve (CN XII)
Spinal accessory nerve (CN XI)
Superior root of ansa cervicalis
Sternocleidomastoid artery
Internal carotid artery
External carotid artery
Inferior root of ansa cervicalis
Common carotid artery
Internal jugular vein
Sternocleidomastoid
Sternocleidomastoid branch
Prevertebral layer of deep cervical fascia
Intermediate tendon of omohyoid
Transverse cervical vein
Inferior belly of omohyoid
Omohyoid fascia
Clavicle
Lateral View
Facial artery
Submental artery
Nerve to mylohyoid
Anterior belly of digastric
Fascial sling of digastric
Mylohyoid
Hyoid bone
Nerve to thyrohyoid
Internal branch of superior laryngeal nerve
Inferior pharyngeal constrictor
Thyrohyoid
Superior belly of omohyoid
External branch of superior laryngeal nerve
Superior thyroid artery
Sternohyoid
Sternothyroid
Anterior jugular vein
Clavicular head
Sternal head
Sternocleidomastoid

8.14 DEEP DISSECTION OF CAROTID TRIANGLE

The sternocleidomastoid muscle has been severed; the inferior portion reflected inferiorly and superior portion posteriorly.

- The tendon of the digastric muscle is connected to the hyoid bone by a fascial sling derived from the muscular part of the pretracheal layer of deep cervical fascia; the tendon of the omohyoid muscle is similarly tethered to the clavicle.
- In this specimen, the facial and lingual arteries arise from a common trunk and pass deep to the stylohyoid and digastric muscles.
- The hypoglossal nerve (CN XII) crosses the internal and external carotid arteries and gives off two branches, the superior root of the ansa cervicalis and the nerve to the thyrohyoid, before passing anteriorly deep to the mylohyoid muscle. In this specimen, the inferior root of the ansa cervicalis lies deep to the internal jugular vein and emerges at its medial aspect.

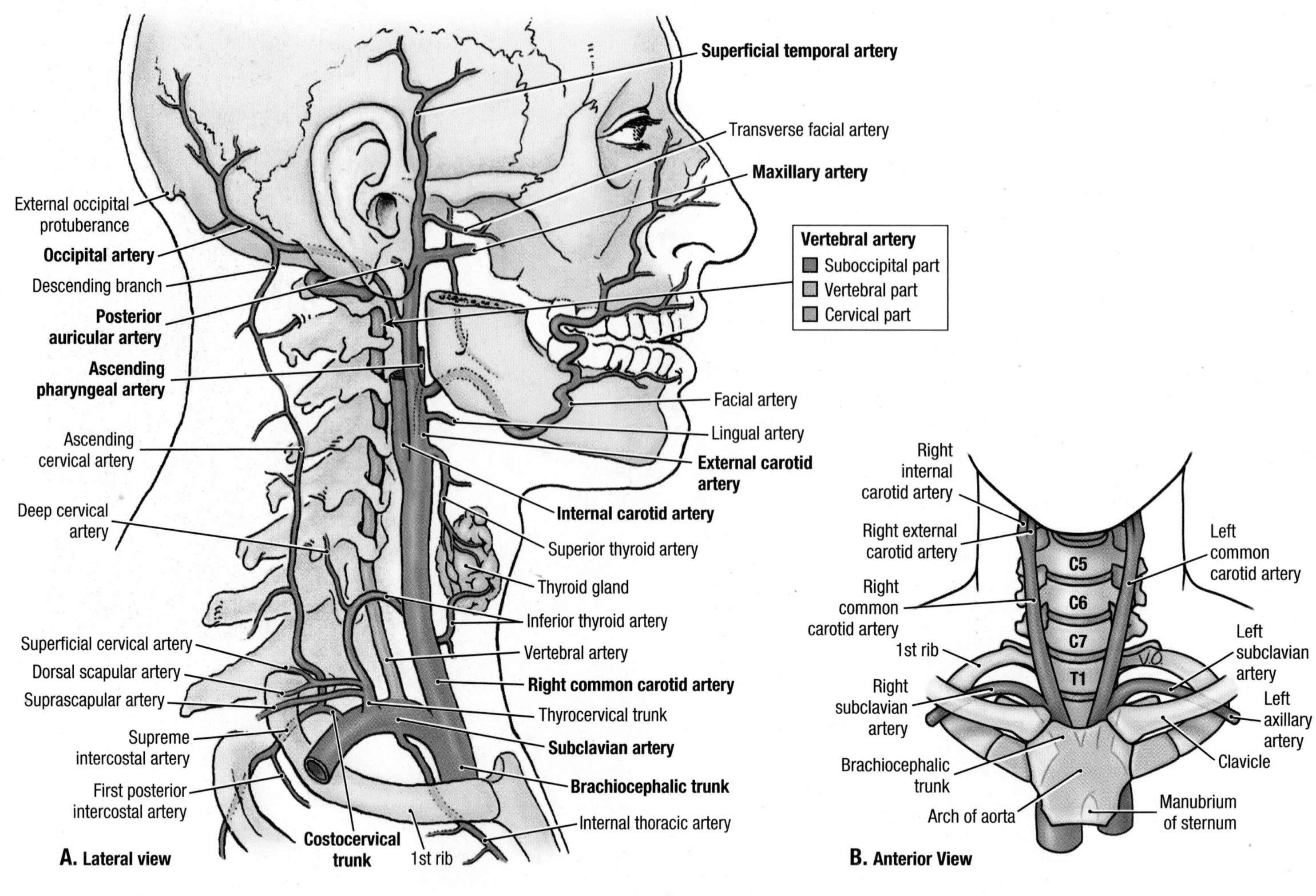
Superficial temporal artery
Transverse facial artery
Maxillary artery
External occipital protuberance
Occipital artery
Descending branch
Posterior auricular artery
Ascending pharyngeal artery
Ascending cervical artery
Deep cervical artery
Vertebral artery
Suboccipital part
Vertebral part
Cervical part
Facial artery
Lingual artery
External carotid artery
Internal carotid artery
Superior thyroid artery
Thyroid gland
Inferior thyroid artery
Vertebral artery
Right common carotid artery
Thyrocervical trunk
Subclavian artery
Brachiocephalic trunk
Internal thoracic artery
Superficial cervical artery
Dorsal scapular artery
Suprascapular artery
Supreme intercostal artery
First posterior intercostal artery
Costocervical trunk
1st rib
A. Lateral view
Right internal carotid artery
Right external carotid artery
Right common carotid artery
1st rib
Right subclavian artery
Brachiocephalic trunk
Arch of aorta
C5
C6
C7
T1
Left common carotid artery
Left subclavian artery
Left axillary artery
Clavicle
Manubrium of sternum
B. Anterior View

8.15 ARTERIES OF NECK

A. Overview. **B.** Common carotid and subclavian arteries.

TABLE 8.5 ARTERIES OF NECK

Artery	Origin	Course and Distribution
Right common carotid	Bifurcation of brachiocephalic trunk	Ascends in neck within carotid sheath with the internal jugular vein and vagus nerve (CN X). Terminates at superior border of thyroid cartilage (C4 vertebral level) by dividing into internal and external carotid arteries
Left common carotid	Arch of aorta	
Right and left internal carotid	Right and left common carotid	No branches in the neck. Enters cranium via carotid canal to supply brain and orbits. Proximal part location of carotid sinus, a baroreceptor that reacts to change in arterial blood pressure. The carotid body, a chemoreceptor that monitors oxygen level in blood, is located in bifurcation of common carotid
Right and left external carotid		Supplies most structures external to cranium; the orbit, part of forehead, and scalp are major exceptions (supplied by ophthalmic artery from intra-cranial internal carotid artery)
Ascending pharyngeal	External carotid	Ascends on pharynx to supply pharynx, prevertebral muscles, middle ear, and cranial meninges
Occipital		Passes posteriorly, medial and parallel to the posterior belly of digastric, ending in the posterior scalp
Posterior auricular		Ascends posteriorly between external acoustic meatus and mastoid process to supply adjacent muscles, parotid gland, facial nerve, auricle, and scalp

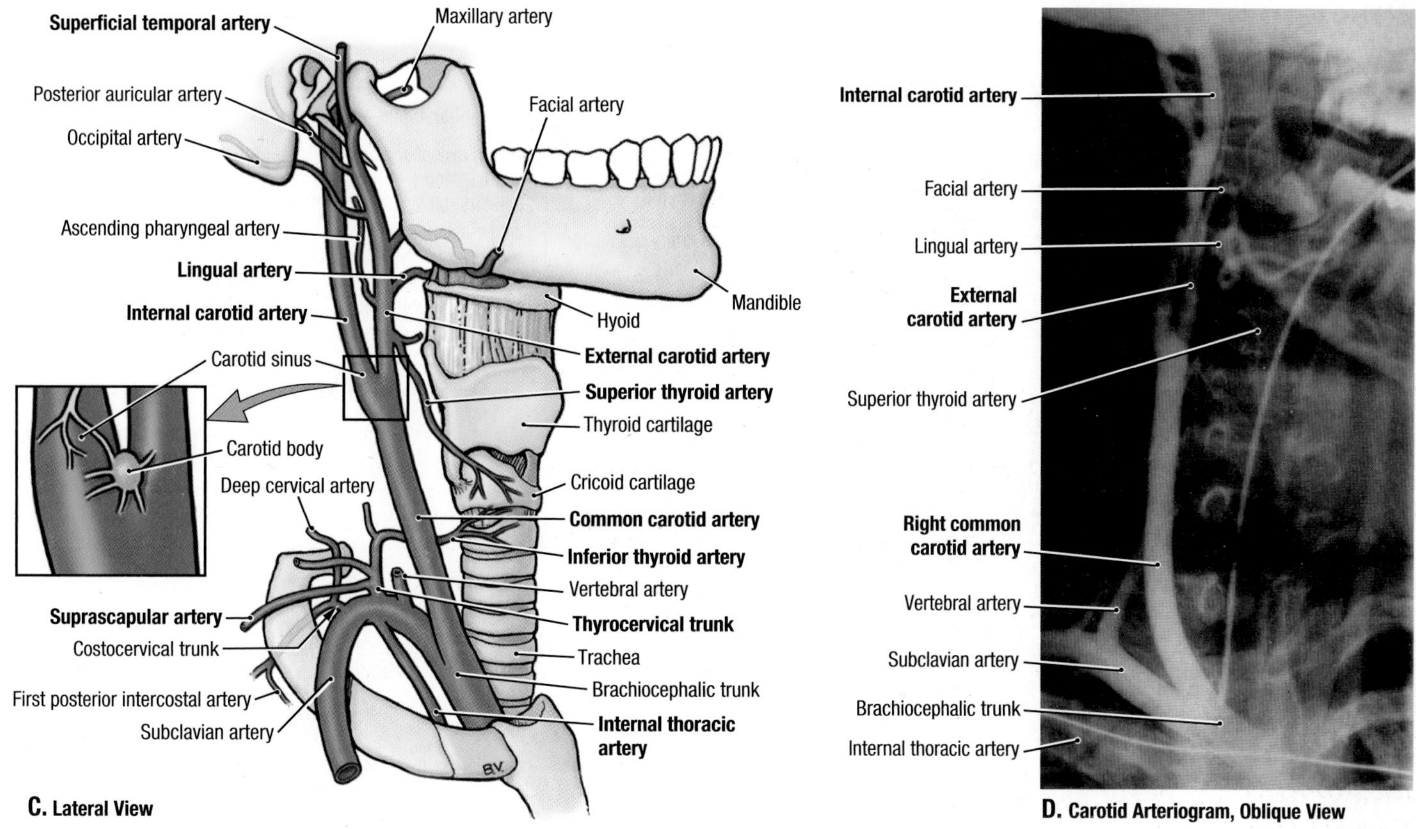
Superficial temporal artery
Maxillary artery
Posterior auricular artery
Facial artery
Occipital artery
Ascending pharyngeal artery
Lingual artery
Internal carotid artery
Mandible
Hyoid
Carotid sinus
External carotid artery
Superior thyroid artery
Thyroid cartilage
Carotid body
Deep cervical artery
Cricoid cartilage
Common carotid artery
Inferior thyroid artery
Vertebral artery
Suprascapular artery
Thyrocervical trunk
Costocervical trunk
Trachea
Brachiocephalic trunk
First posterior intercostal artery
Subclavian artery
Internal thoracic artery
Internal carotid artery
Facial artery
Lingual artery
External carotid artery
Superior thyroid artery
Right common carotid artery
Vertebral artery
Subclavian artery
Brachiocephalic trunk
Internal thoracic artery

C. Lateral View

D. Carotid Arteriogram, Oblique View

8.15 ARTERIES OF NECK *(CONTINUED)*

C. Branches of external carotid and subclavian arteries. The carotid sinus is a baroreceptor that reacts to changes in arterial blood pressure and is located in the dilatation of the proximal part of the internal carotid artery. The carotid body is an ovoid mass of tissue that lies at the bifurcation of the common carotid artery. It is a chemoreceptor that monitors the level of oxygen in the blood.

TABLE 8.5 ARTERIES OF NECK (CONTINUED)

Artery	Origin	Course and Distribution
Superior thyroid	External carotid	Runs antero-inferiorly deep to infrahyoid muscles to reach thyroid gland. Supplies thyroid gland, infrahyoid muscles, SCM, and larynx via *superior laryngeal artery*
Lingual		Lies on middle constrictor muscle of pharynx; arches supero-anteriorly and passes deep to CN XII, stylohyoid muscle, and posterior belly of digastric then passes deep to hyoglossus, giving branches to the posterior tongue and bifurcating into *deep lingual* and *sublingual arteries*
Facial		After giving rise to *ascending palatine artery* and a tonsillar branch, it passes superiorly under cover of the angle of the mandible. It then loops anteriorly to supply the submandibular gland and give rise to the *submental artery* to the floor of the mouth before entering the face
Maxillary	Terminal branches of external carotid	Passes posterior to neck of mandible, enters infratemporal fossa then pterygopalatine fossa to supply teeth, nose, ear, and face
Superficial temporal		Ascends anterior to auricle to temporal region and ends in scalp
Vertebral	Subclavian	Passes through the foramina transversaria of the transverse processes of vertebrae C1–C6, runs in a groove on the posterior arch of the atlas, and enters the cranial cavity through the foramen magnum
Internal thoracic		No branches in neck; enters thorax
Thyrocervical trunk		Has two branches: the *inferior thyroid artery*, the main visceral artery of the neck; the cervicodorsal trunk sending branches to the lateral cervical region, trapezius, and medial scapular arteries
Costocervical trunk		Trunk passes posterosuperiorly and divides into *superior intercostal* and *deep cervical arteries* to supply the 1st and 2nd intercostal spaces and posterior deep cervical muscles, respectively

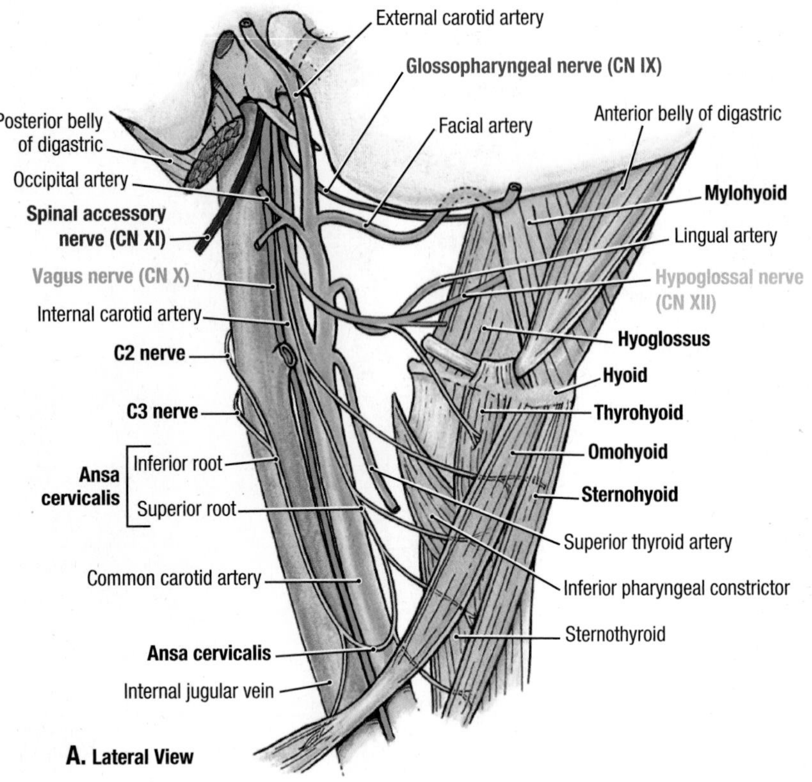
External carotid artery
Glossopharyngeal nerve (CN IX)
Posterior belly of digastric
Facial artery
Anterior belly of digastric
Occipital artery
Spinal accessory nerve (CN XI)
Mylohyoid
Lingual artery
Vagus nerve (CN X)
Hypoglossal nerve (CN XII)
Internal carotid artery
C2 nerve
Hyoglossus
Hyoid
C3 nerve
Thyrohyoid
Ansa cervicalis
Inferior root
Superior root
Omohyoid
Sternohyoid
Superior thyroid artery
Common carotid artery
Inferior pharyngeal constrictor
Sternothyroid
Ansa cervicalis
Internal jugular vein
A. Lateral View

Glossopharyngeal—CN IX	Vagus—CN X
Motor: stylopharyngeus, parotid gland **Sensory:** taste: posterior third of tongue; general sensation: pharynx, tonsillar sinus, pharyngotympanic tube, middle ear cavity	**Motor:** palate, pharynx, larynx, trachea, bronchial tree, heart, GI tract to left colic flexure **Sensory:** pharynx, larynx; reflex sensory from tracheo-bronchial tree, lungs, heart, GI tract to left colic flexure
Spinal accessory—CN XI	**Hypoglossal—CN XII**
Motor: sternocleidomastoid and trapezius	**Motor:** all intrinsic and extrinsic muscles of tongue (excluding palatoglossus—a palatine muscle)

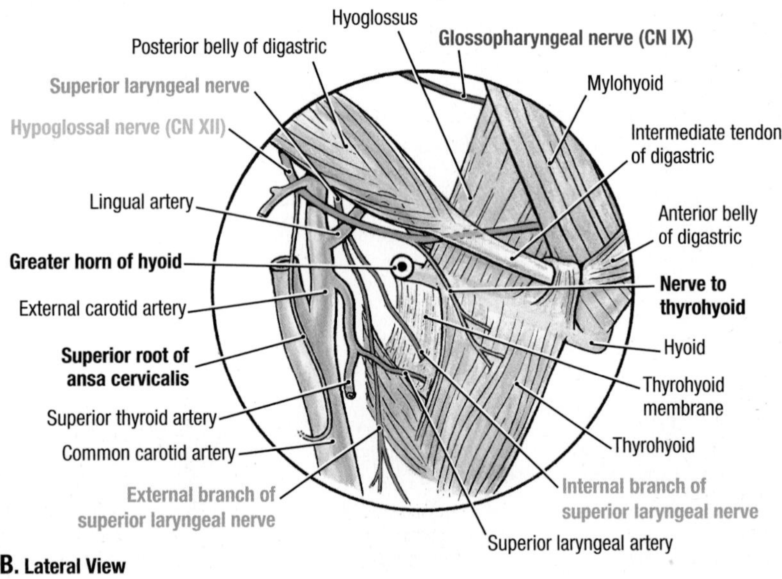
Hyoglossus
Posterior belly of digastric
Glossopharyngeal nerve (CN IX)
Superior laryngeal nerve
Mylohyoid
Hypoglossal nerve (CN XII)
Intermediate tendon of digastric
Lingual artery
Anterior belly of digastric
Greater horn of hyoid
Nerve to thyrohyoid
External carotid artery
Hyoid
Superior root of ansa cervicalis
Thyrohyoid membrane
Superior thyroid artery
Thyrohyoid
Common carotid artery
External branch of superior laryngeal nerve
Internal branch of superior laryngeal nerve
Superior laryngeal artery
B. Lateral View

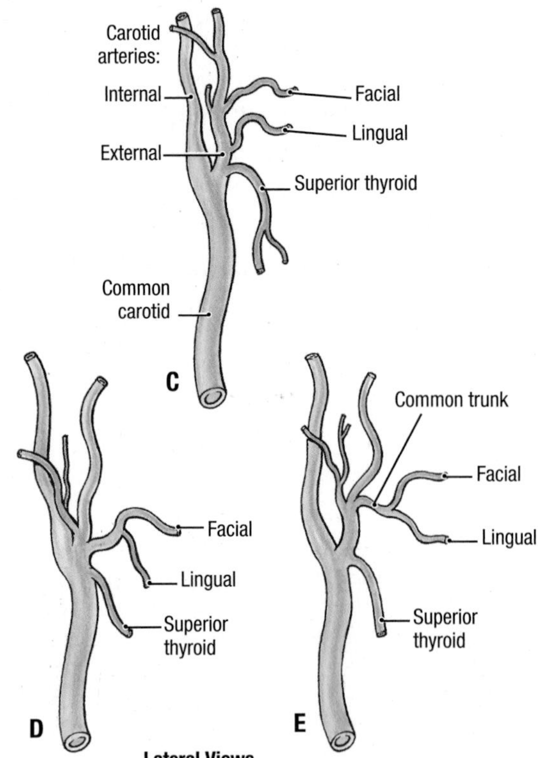
Carotid arteries:
Internal
External
Facial
Lingual
Superior thyroid
Common carotid
C
Facial
Lingual
Superior thyroid
D
Common trunk
Facial
Lingual
Superior thyroid
E
Lateral Views

8.16 RELATIONSHIPS OF NERVES AND VESSELS IN CAROTID TRIANGLE OF NECK

A. Ansa cervicalis and the strap muscles. **B.** Hypoglossal nerve (CN XII) and internal and external branches of superior laryngeal nerve (CN X). The tip of the greater hyoid bone, indicated with a *circle* is the reference point for many structures. **C.–E.** Variation in the origin of the lingual artery as studied by Dr. Grant in 211 specimens. In 80%, the superior thyroid, lingual, and facial arteries arose separately **(C)**; in 20%, the lingual and facial arteries arose from a common stem inferiorly **(D)** or high on the external carotid artery **(E)**. In one specimen, the superior thyroid and lingual arteries arose from a common stem.

Carotid occlusion, causing stenosis (narrowing), can be relieved by opening the artery at its origin and stripping off the atherosclerotic plaque with the artery's lining (intima). This procedure is called carotid endarterectomy. Because of the relationships of the internal carotid artery, there is a risk of cranial nerve injury during the procedure involving one or more of the following nerves: CN IX, CN X (or its branch, the superior laryngeal nerve), CN XI, or CN XII.

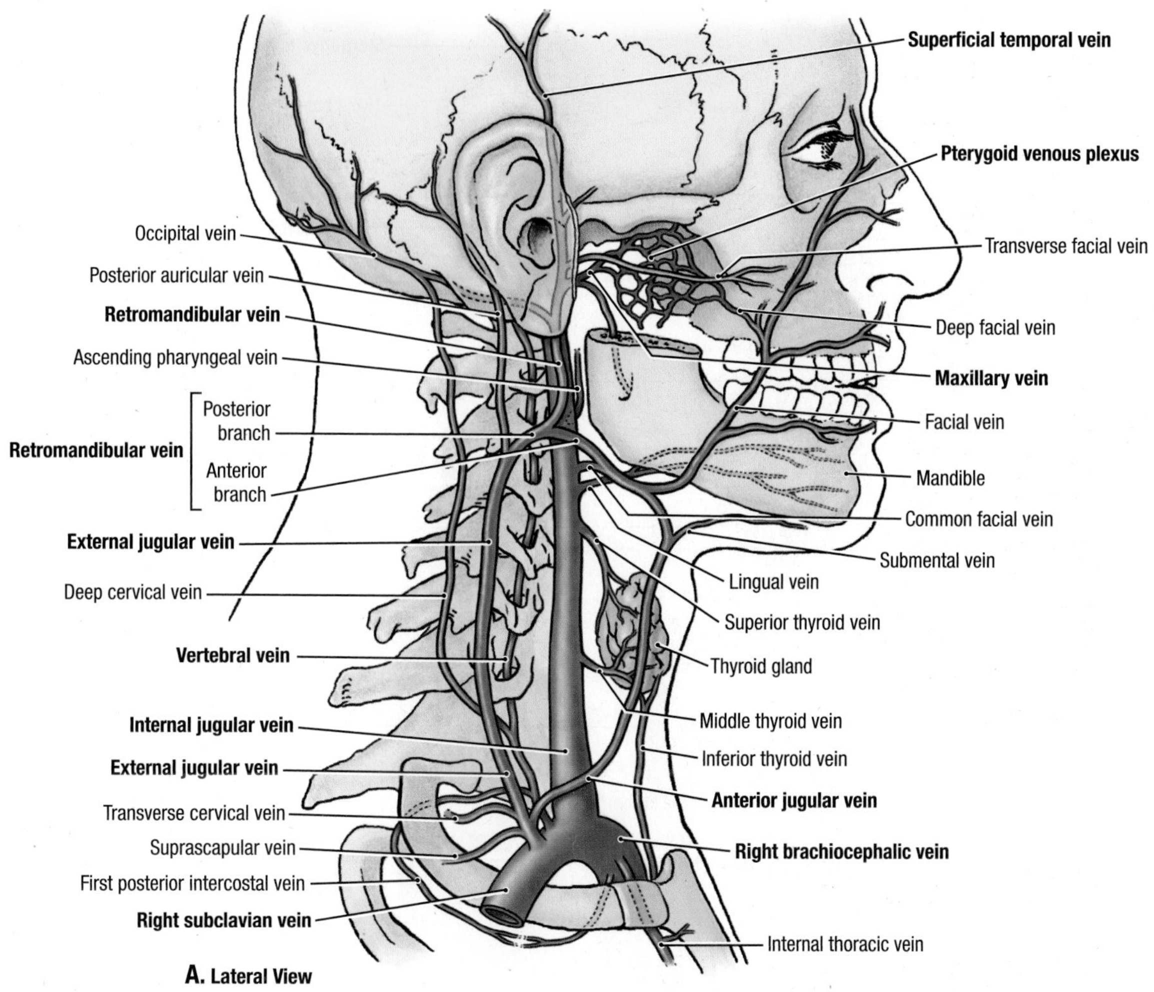
Superficial temporal vein
Pterygoid venous plexus
Transverse facial vein
Occipital vein
Posterior auricular vein
Retromandibular vein
Ascending pharyngeal vein
Deep facial vein
Maxillary vein
Posterior branch
Retromandibular vein
Anterior branch
Facial vein
Mandible
Common facial vein
External jugular vein
Submental vein
Deep cervical vein
Lingual vein
Superior thyroid vein
Vertebral vein
Thyroid gland
Internal jugular vein
Middle thyroid vein
External jugular vein
Inferior thyroid vein
Anterior jugular vein
Transverse cervical vein
Suprascapular vein
Right brachiocephalic vein
First posterior intercostal vein
Right subclavian vein
Internal thoracic vein

A. **Lateral View**

8.17 DEEP VEINS OF NECK

A. Overview. The IJV begins at the jugular foramen as the continuation of the sigmoid sinus. From a dilated origin, the superior bulb of the IJV, the vein runs inferiorly through the neck in the carotid sheath. Posterior to the sternal end of the clavicle the vein merges perpendicularly with the subclavian vein, forming the "venous angle" that marks the origin of the brachiocephalic vein. The inferior end of the IJV dilates superior to its terminal valve, forming the inferior bulb of the IJV. The valve permits blood to flow toward the heart while preventing backflow into the IJV. The external jugular vein drains blood from the occipital region and posterior neck to the subclavian vein, and the anterior jugular vein the anterior aspect of the neck. **B. Internal jugular vein puncture**. A needle and catheter may be inserted into the IJV, using ultrasonic guidance, for diagnostic or therapeutic purposes. The right internal jugular vein is preferable to the left because it is usually larger and straighter. During this procedure, the clinician palpates the common carotid artery and inserts the needle into the IJV just lateral to it at a 30° angle, aiming at the apex of the triangle between the sternal and clavicular heads of the SCM. The needle is then directed inferolaterally toward the ipsilateral nipple.

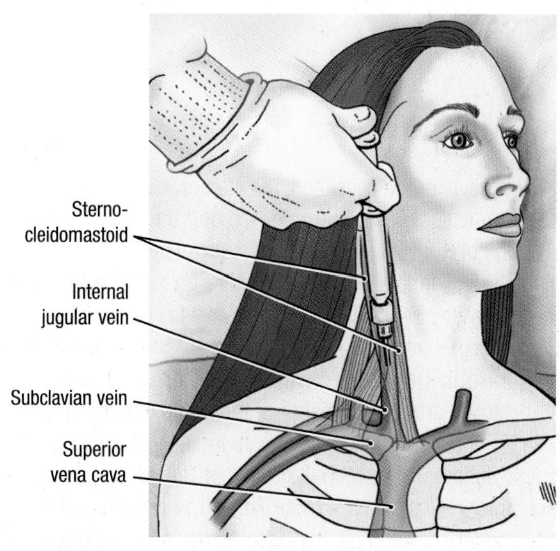
Sterno-
cleidomastoid
Internal
jugular vein
Subclavian vein
Superior
vena cava

B. **Internal jugular vein puncture**

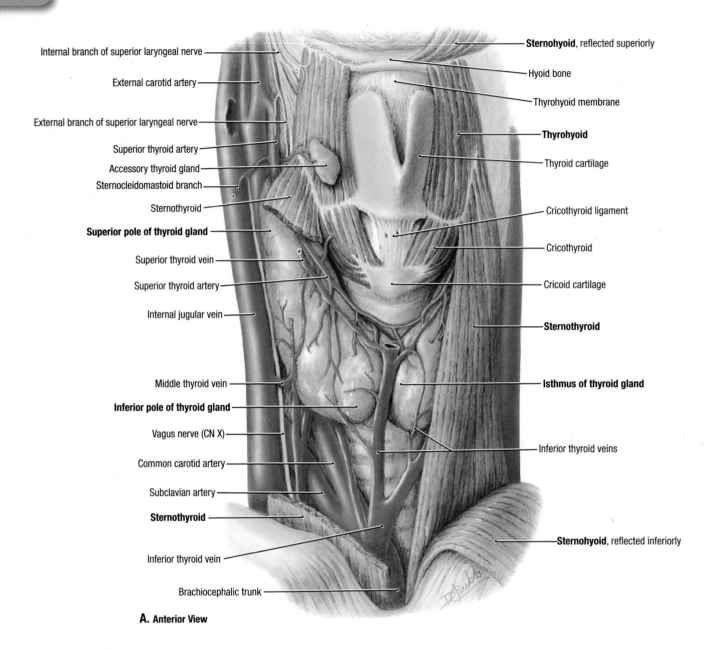

Internal branch of superior laryngeal nerve
External carotid artery
External branch of superior laryngeal nerve
Superior thyroid artery
Accessory thyroid gland
Sternocleidomastoid branch
Sternothyroid
Superior pole of thyroid gland
Superior thyroid vein
Superior thyroid artery
Internal jugular vein
Middle thyroid vein
Inferior pole of thyroid gland
Vagus nerve (CN X)
Common carotid artery
Subclavian artery
Sternothyroid
Inferior thyroid vein
Brachiocephalic trunk
Sternohyoid, reflected superiorly
Hyoid bone
Thyrohyoid membrane
Thyrohyoid
Thyroid cartilage
Cricothyroid ligament
Cricothyroid
Cricoid cartilage
Sternothyroid
Isthmus of thyroid gland
Inferior thyroid veins
Sternohyoid, reflected inferiorly

A. Anterior View

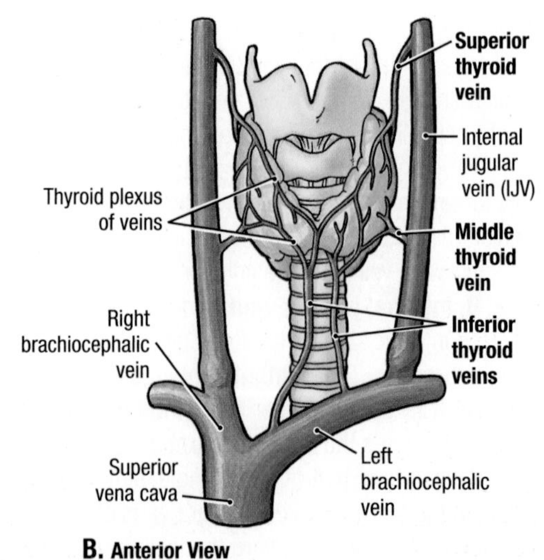
Superior thyroid vein
Internal jugular vein (IJV)
Thyroid plexus of veins
Middle thyroid vein
Right brachiocephalic vein
Inferior thyroid veins
Superior vena cava
Left brachiocephalic vein

B. Anterior View

8.18 ENDOCRINE LAYER OF VISCERAL COMPARTMENT I

A. On the left side of the specimen, the sternohyoid and omohyoid muscles are reflected, exposing the sternothyroid and the thyrohyoid muscles; on the right side of the specimen, the sternothyroid muscle is largely excised. **B.** Schematic illustration of the venous drainage of the thyroid gland. Except for the superior thyroid veins, the thyroid veins are not paired with arteries of corresponding names.

The **carotid pulse (neck pulse)** is easily felt by palpating the common carotid artery in the side of the neck, where it lies in a groove between the trachea and the infrahyoid muscles. It is usually easily palpated just deep to the anterior border of the SCM at the level of the superior border of the thyroid cartilage. It is routinely checked during cardiopulmonary resuscitation (CPR). Absence of a carotid pulse indicates cardiac arrest.

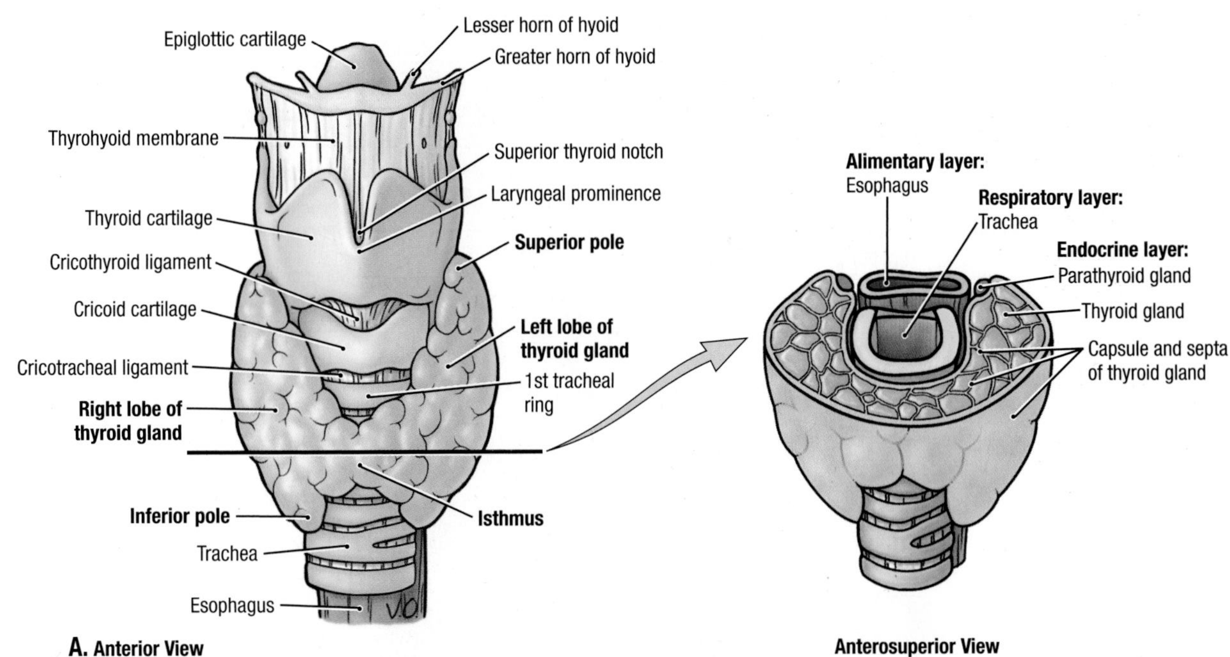
Epiglottic cartilage
Lesser horn of hyoid
Greater horn of hyoid
Thyrohyoid membrane
Superior thyroid notch
Laryngeal prominence
Thyroid cartilage
Superior pole
Cricothyroid ligament
Cricoid cartilage
Left lobe of thyroid gland
Cricotracheal ligament
1st tracheal ring
Right lobe of thyroid gland
Inferior pole
Isthmus
Trachea
Esophagus
A. Anterior View
Alimentary layer:
Esophagus
Respiratory layer:
Trachea
Endocrine layer:
Parathyroid gland
Thyroid gland
Capsule and septa of thyroid gland
Anterosuperior View

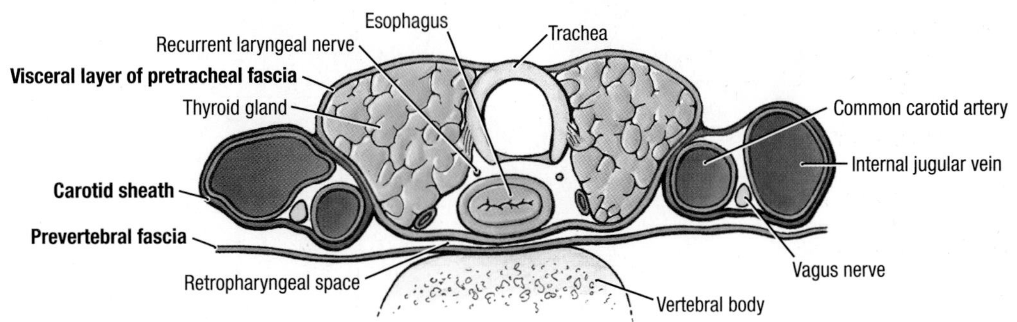
Esophagus
Trachea
Recurrent laryngeal nerve
Visceral layer of pretracheal fascia
Thyroid gland
Common carotid artery
Internal jugular vein
Carotid sheath
Prevertebral fascia
Vagus nerve
Retropharyngeal space
Vertebral body
B. Transverse Section, Inferior View

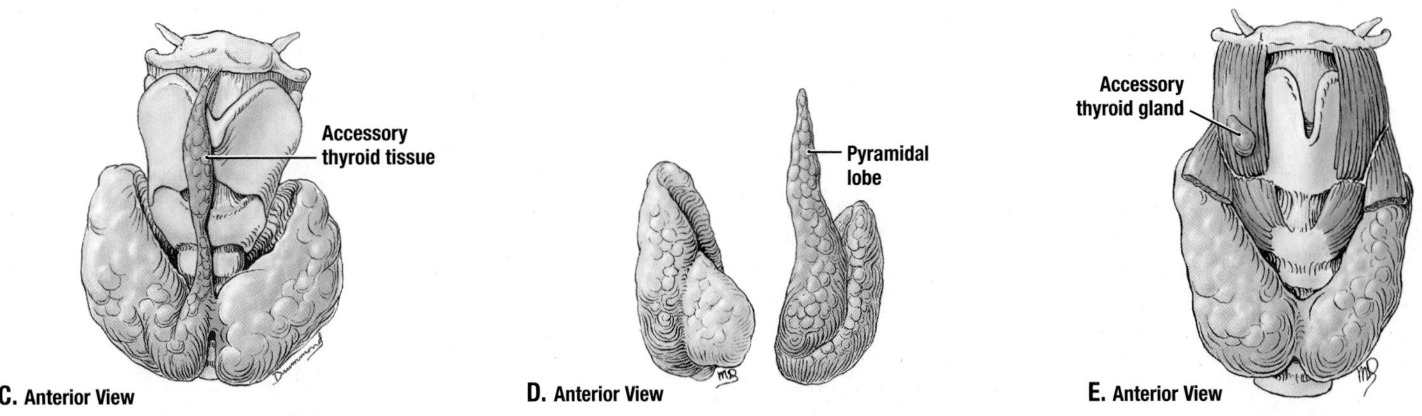
Accessory thyroid tissue
Pyramidal lobe
Accessory thyroid gland
C. Anterior View
D. Anterior View
E. Anterior View

8.19 ENDOCRINE LAYER OF VISCERAL COMPARTMENT II

A. Relations of thyroid gland with transverse section showing alimentary, respiratory, and endocrine layers of visceral compartment. **B.** Fascia. **C.** Accessory thyroid tissue along the course of the thyroglossal duct, which was the path of migration of thyroid tissue from its embryonic site of development. **D.** Approximately 50% of glands have a pyramidal lobe that extends from near the isthmus to or toward the hyoid bone; the isthmus is occasionally absent, in which case the gland is in two parts. **E.** An accessory thyroid gland can occur between the suprahyoid region and arch of the aorta (see Fig. 8.18A).

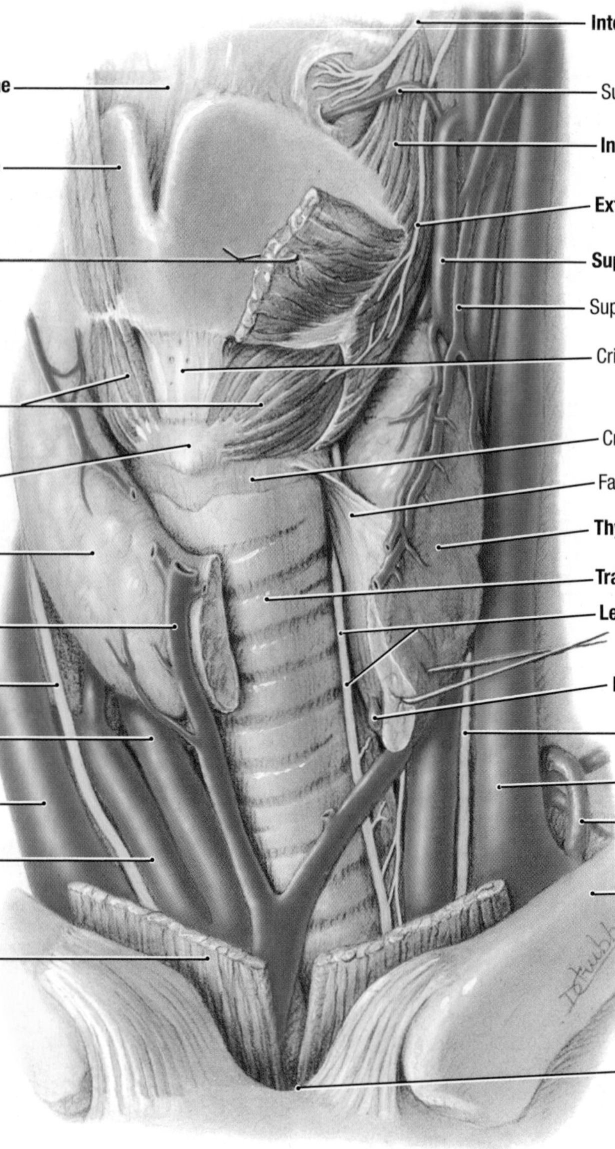

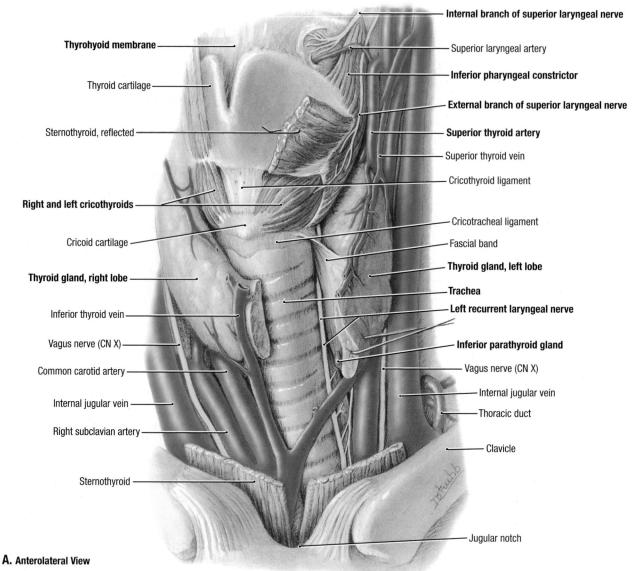

Internal branch of superior laryngeal nerve
Thyrohyoid membrane
Superior laryngeal artery
Inferior pharyngeal constrictor
Thyroid cartilage
External branch of superior laryngeal nerve
Sternothyroid, reflected
Superior thyroid artery
Superior thyroid vein
Cricothyroid ligament
Right and left cricothyroids
Cricotracheal ligament
Cricoid cartilage
Fascial band
Thyroid gland, left lobe
Thyroid gland, right lobe
Trachea
Left recurrent laryngeal nerve
Inferior thyroid vein
Vagus nerve (CN X)
Inferior parathyroid gland
Common carotid artery
Vagus nerve (CN X)
Internal jugular vein
Internal jugular vein
Thoracic duct
Right subclavian artery
Clavicle
Sternothyroid
Jugular notch

A. Anterolateral View

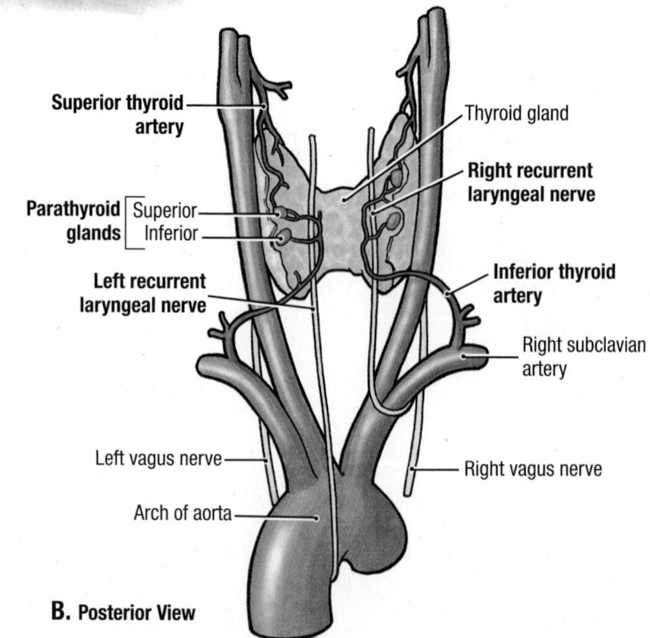

Superior thyroid artery
Thyroid gland
Right recurrent laryngeal nerve
Parathyroid glands
Superior
Inferior
Left recurrent laryngeal nerve
Inferior thyroid artery
Right subclavian artery
Left vagus nerve
Right vagus nerve
Arch of aorta

B. Posterior View

8.20 RESPIRATORY LAYER OF VISCERAL COMPARTMENT

A. The isthmus of the thyroid gland is divided, and the left lobe is retracted. The left recurrent laryngeal nerve ascends on the lateral aspect of the trachea between the trachea and esophagus. The internal branch of the superior laryngeal nerve runs along the superior border of the inferior pharyngeal constrictor muscle and pierces the thyrohyoid membrane. The external branch of the superior laryngeal nerve lies adjacent to the inferior pharyngeal constrictor muscle and supplies its lower portion; it continues to run along the anterior border of the superior thyroid artery, passing deep to the superior attachment of the sternothyroid muscle, and then supplies the cricothyroid muscle. **B.** Blood supply of the parathyroid glands and courses of the left and right recurrent laryngeal nerves.

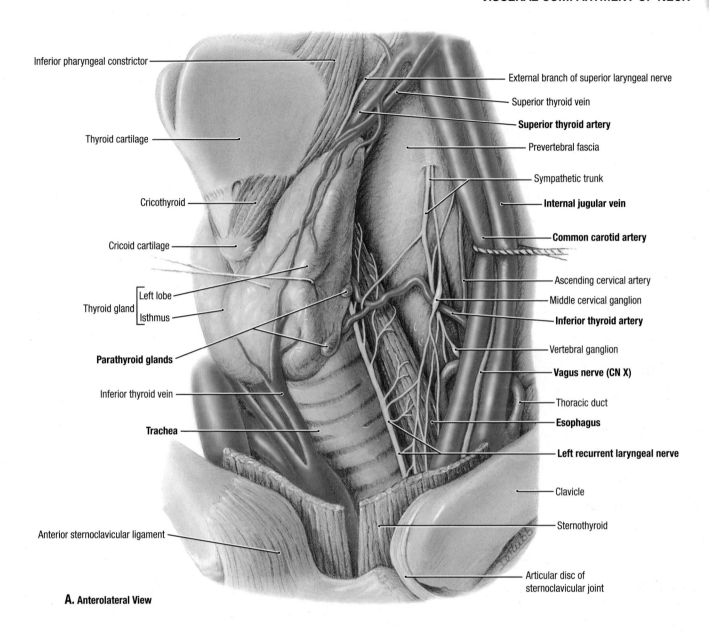

Inferior pharyngeal constrictor
External branch of superior laryngeal nerve
Superior thyroid vein
Superior thyroid artery
Thyroid cartilage
Prevertebral fascia
Sympathetic trunk
Cricothyroid
Internal jugular vein
Common carotid artery
Cricoid cartilage
Ascending cervical artery
Thyroid gland: Left lobe, Isthmus
Middle cervical ganglion
Inferior thyroid artery
Parathyroid glands
Vertebral ganglion
Vagus nerve (CN X)
Inferior thyroid vein
Thoracic duct
Trachea
Esophagus
Left recurrent laryngeal nerve
Clavicle
Sternothyroid
Anterior sternoclavicular ligament
Articular disc of sternoclavicular joint

A. Anterolateral View

8.21 ALIMENTARY LAYER OF VISCERAL COMPARTMENT

A. Dissection of the left side of the root of the neck. The three structures contained in the carotid sheath (internal jugular vein, common carotid artery, and vagus nerve) are retracted. The left recurrent laryngeal nerve ascends on the lateral aspect of the trachea, just anterior to the recess between the trachea and esophagus. **B.** Arterial supply of thyroid gland. The thyroid ima artery is infrequent (10%) and variable in its origin.

During a **total thyroidectomy** (e.g., excision of a malignant thyroid gland), the parathyroid glands are in danger of being inadvertently damaged or removed. These glands are safe during **subtotal thyroidectomy** because the most posterior part of the thyroid gland usually is preserved. Variability in the position of the parathyroid glands, especially the inferior ones, puts them in danger of being removed during surgery on the thyroid gland. If the parathyroid glands are inadvertently removed during surgery, the patient suffers from **tetany,** a severe convulsive disorder. The generalized convulsive muscle spasms result from a fall in blood calcium levels.

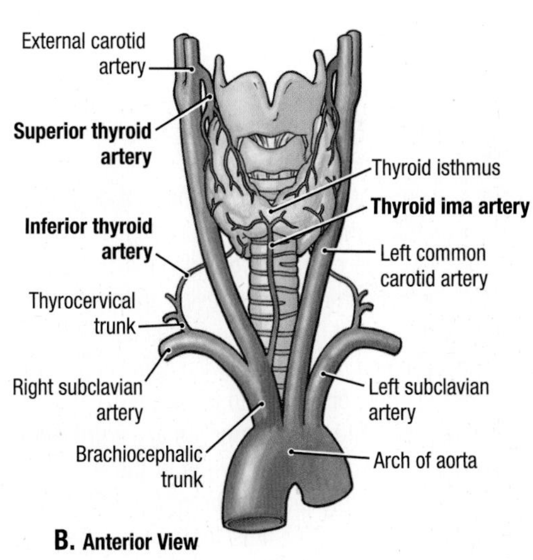
External carotid artery
Superior thyroid artery
Thyroid isthmus
Thyroid ima artery
Inferior thyroid artery
Left common carotid artery
Thyrocervical trunk
Right subclavian artery
Left subclavian artery
Brachiocephalic trunk
Arch of aorta

B. Anterior View

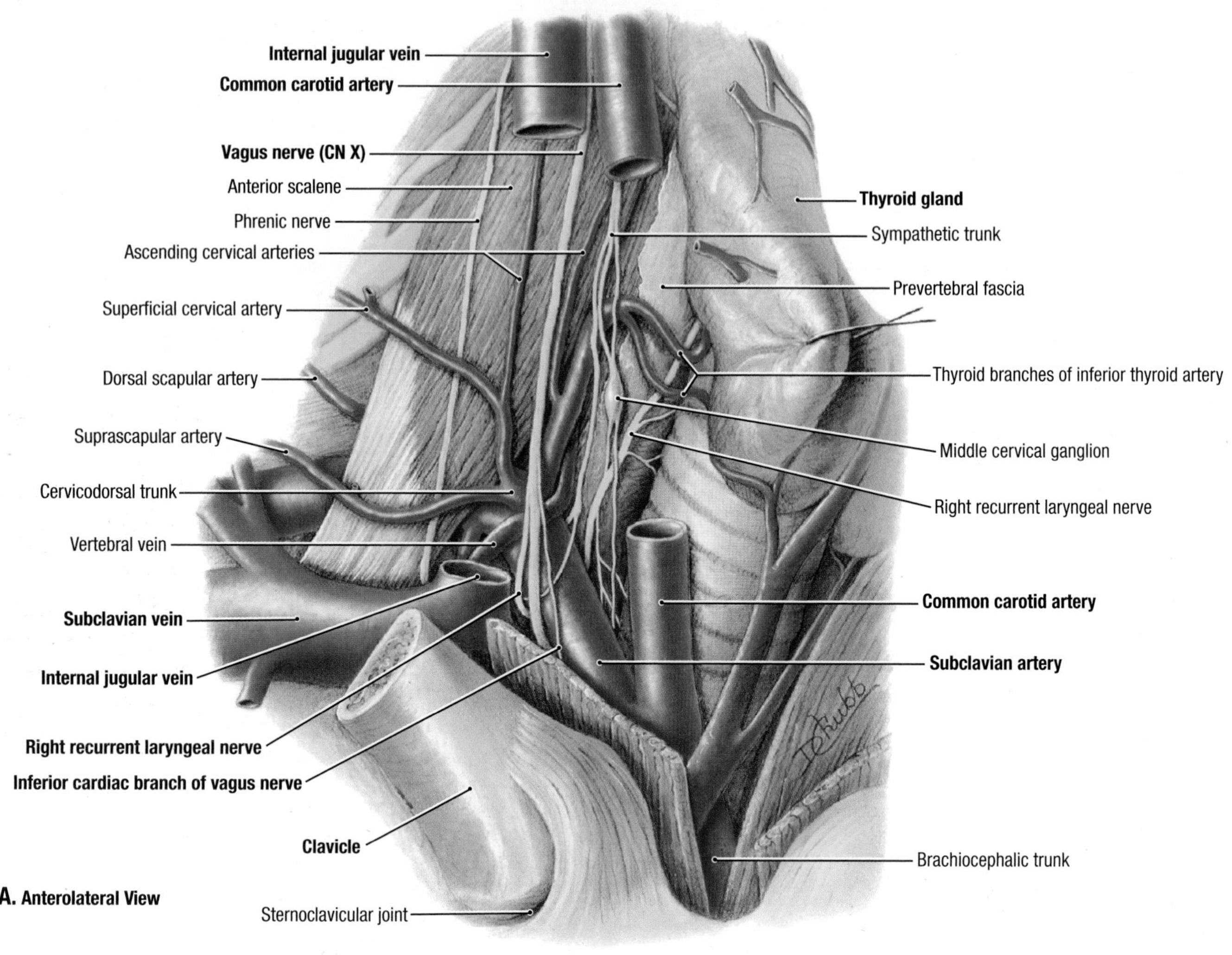

Internal jugular vein
Common carotid artery
Vagus nerve (CN X)
Anterior scalene
Phrenic nerve
Ascending cervical arteries
Superficial cervical artery
Dorsal scapular artery
Suprascapular artery
Cervicodorsal trunk
Vertebral vein
Subclavian vein
Internal jugular vein
Right recurrent laryngeal nerve
Inferior cardiac branch of vagus nerve
Clavicle
Sternoclavicular joint
Thyroid gland
Sympathetic trunk
Prevertebral fascia
Thyroid branches of inferior thyroid artery
Middle cervical ganglion
Right recurrent laryngeal nerve
Common carotid artery
Subclavian artery
Brachiocephalic trunk

A. **Anterolateral View**

8.22 ROOT OF NECK

A. Dissection of the right side of the root of the neck. The clavicle is cut, sections of the common carotid artery and internal jugular vein are removed, and the right lobe of the thyroid gland is retracted. The right vagus nerve crosses the first part of the subclavian artery and gives off an inferior cardiac branch and the right recurrent laryngeal nerve. The right recurrent laryngeal nerve loops inferior to the subclavian artery and passes posterior to the common carotid artery on its way to the posterolateral aspect of the trachea.

- The **recurrent laryngeal nerves are vulnerable to injury** during thyroidectomy and other surgeries in the anterior cervical region of the neck. Because the terminal branch of this nerve, the inferior laryngeal nerve, innervates the muscles moving the vocal folds, injury to the nerve results in **paralysis of the vocal folds.**
- A non-neoplastic and noninflammatory enlargement of the thyroid gland, other than the variable enlargement that may occur during menstruation and pregnancy, is called a goiter. A **goiter** results from a lack of iodine. It is common in certain parts of the world where the soil and water are deficient in iodine and iodized salt is unavailable. The enlarged gland causes a swelling in the neck that may compress the trachea, esophagus, and recurrent laryngeal nerves. When the gland enlarges, it may do so anteriorly, posteriorly, inferiorly, or laterally. It cannot move superiorly because of the superior attachments of the sternothyroid and sternohyoid muscles. Substernal extension of a goiter is also common.

Esophagus
Sympathetic trunk
Ascending cervical artery
Carotid tubercle (C6 vertebra)
Anterior ramus C5
Vertebral artery
Anterior ramus C6
Inferior thyroid artery
Dorsal scapular artery
Anterior scalene
Anterior ramus C8
Phrenic nerve
Right subclavian artery
Suprascapular artery
Right vagus nerve (CN X)
Right common carotid artery
1st rib
Cervical parietal pleura
Right brachiocephalic vein
Brachiocephalic trunk
Inferior thyroid vein
Thymic branch of inferior thyroid artery
Thyroid gland
Longus colli
Longus capitis
Phrenic nerve
Anterior vertebral vein
Middle scalene
Anterior scalene
Trachea
Dorsal scapular artery
Inferior thyroid artery
Thyrocervical trunk
Vertebral vein
Thoracic duct
Subclavian artery
Subclavian vein
Left subclavian artery
Left vagus nerve
Left common carotid artery
Internal jugular vein
Internal thoracic artery
Phrenic nerve
Internal thoracic vein
Left brachiocephalic vein

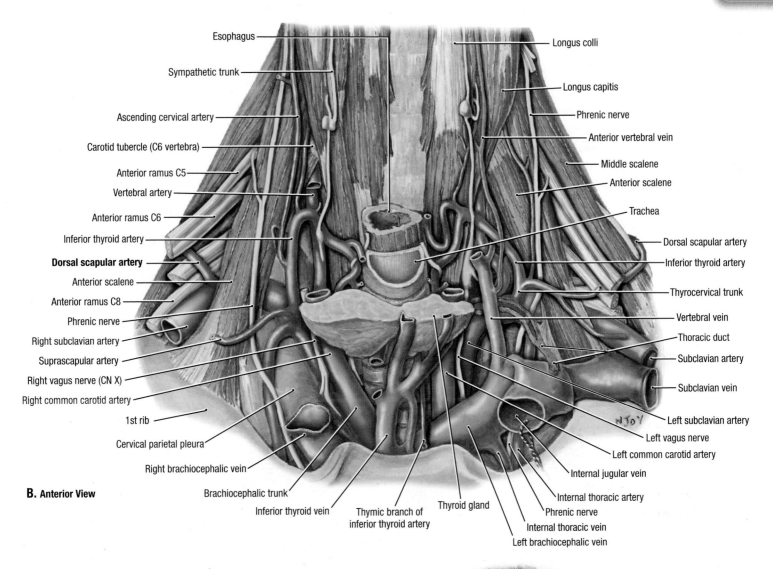

B. Anterior View

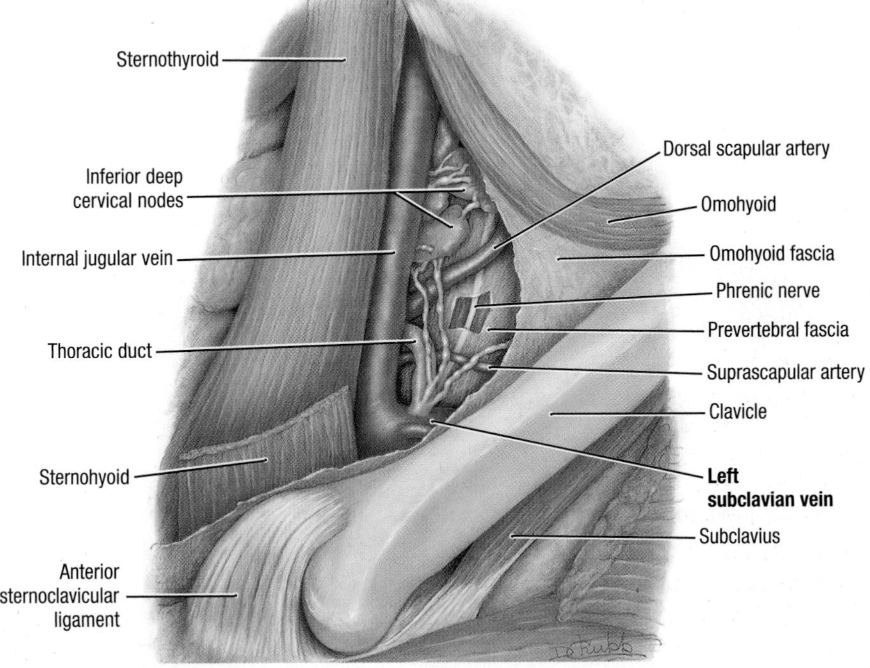
Sternothyroid
Inferior deep cervical nodes
Internal jugular vein
Thoracic duct
Sternohyoid
Anterior sternoclavicular ligament
Dorsal scapular artery
Omohyoid
Omohyoid fascia
Phrenic nerve
Prevertebral fascia
Suprascapular artery
Clavicle
Left subclavian vein
Subclavius

C. Anterolateral View

8.22 ROOT OF NECK *(CONTINUED)*

B. Deep anterior dissection. Note that the right dorsal scapular artery arises directly from the subclavian artery, a common variation. **C.** Dissection of termination of the thoracic duct. The sternocleidomastoid muscle is removed, the sternohyoid muscle is resected, and the omohyoid portion of the pretracheal fascia is partially removed. The thoracic duct arches laterally in the neck, passing posterior to the carotid sheath and anterior to the vertebral artery, thyrocervical trunk, and subclavian arteries; it enters the angle formed by the junction of the left subclavian and internal jugular veins to form the left brachiocephalic vein (the left venous angle).

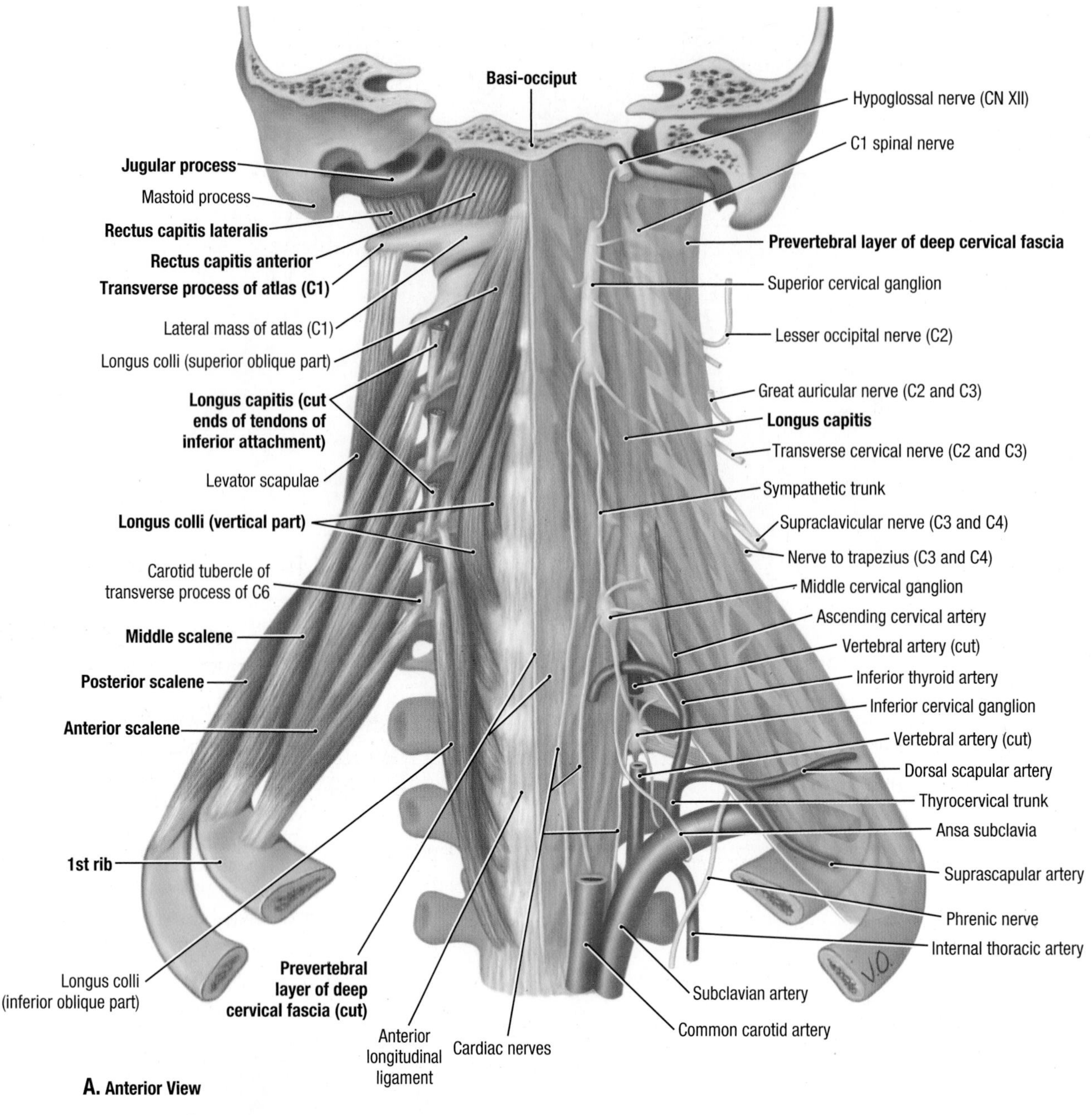
Basi-occiput
Hypoglossal nerve (CN XII)
C1 spinal nerve
Jugular process
Mastoid process
Rectus capitis lateralis
Prevertebral layer of deep cervical fascia
Rectus capitis anterior
Transverse process of atlas (C1)
Superior cervical ganglion
Lateral mass of atlas (C1)
Lesser occipital nerve (C2)
Longus colli (superior oblique part)
Great auricular nerve (C2 and C3)
Longus capitis (cut ends of tendons of inferior attachment)
Longus capitis
Transverse cervical nerve (C2 and C3)
Levator scapulae
Sympathetic trunk
Longus colli (vertical part)
Supraclavicular nerve (C3 and C4)
Nerve to trapezius (C3 and C4)
Carotid tubercle of transverse process of C6
Middle cervical ganglion
Ascending cervical artery
Middle scalene
Vertebral artery (cut)
Inferior thyroid artery
Posterior scalene
Inferior cervical ganglion
Anterior scalene
Vertebral artery (cut)
Dorsal scapular artery
Thyrocervical trunk
Ansa subclavia
1st rib
Suprascapular artery
Phrenic nerve
Internal thoracic artery
Longus colli (inferior oblique part)
Prevertebral layer of deep cervical fascia (cut)
Subclavian artery
Common carotid artery
Anterior longitudinal ligament
Cardiac nerves
A. Anterior View

8.23 PREVERTEBRAL REGION

A. and B. Overview of muscles, nerves and vessels.

TABLE 8.6 PREVERTEBRAL AND SCALENE MUSCLES

Muscle	Superior Attachment	Inferior Attachment	Innervation	Main Action
Longus colli				
Superior oblique part	Anterior tubercle of atlas (C1)	Anterior tubercles of TVP C3–C5	Anterior rami of C2–C6 spinal nerves (cervical plexus)	Rotation of cervical spine to opposite side (acting unilaterally)
Vertical part	Vertebral bodies of C2–C4	Vertebral bodies C5–T3		
Inferior oblique part	Anterior tubercles of TVP C5–C6	Vertebral bodies T1–T3		Flexion of cervical spine (acting bilaterally)
Longus capitis	Basilar part of occipital bone	Anterior tubercles of TVP C3–C6	Anterior rami of C1–C3 spinal nerves (cervical plexus)	Flexion of head (atlanto-occipital joints)

TVP, transverse process

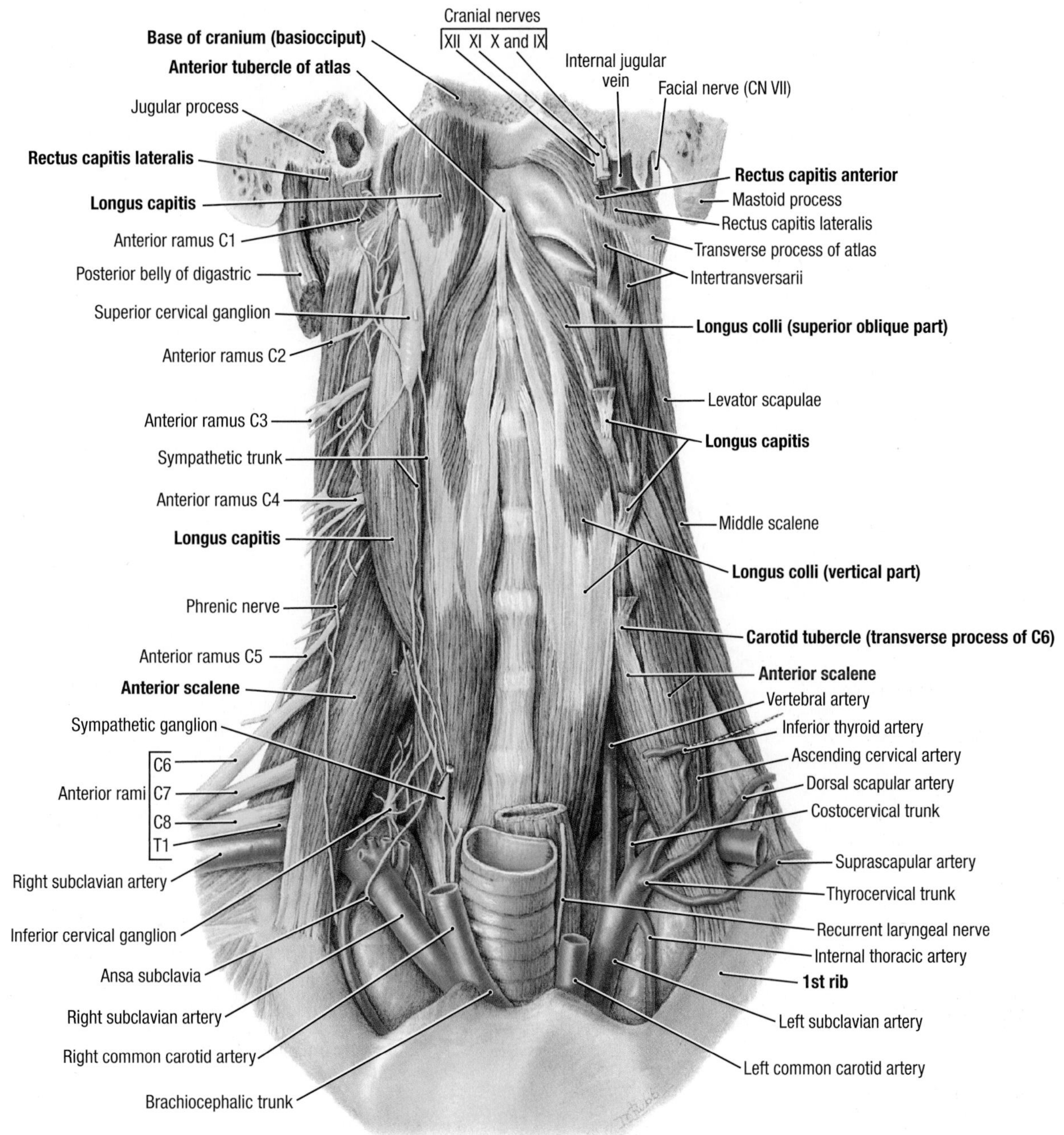
Cranial nerves
XII XI X and IX
Base of cranium (basiocciput)
Anterior tubercle of atlas
Internal jugular vein
Facial nerve (CN VII)
Jugular process
Rectus capitis lateralis
Rectus capitis anterior
Longus capitis
Mastoid process
Rectus capitis lateralis
Anterior ramus C1
Transverse process of atlas
Posterior belly of digastric
Intertransversarii
Superior cervical ganglion
Longus colli (superior oblique part)
Anterior ramus C2
Levator scapulae
Anterior ramus C3
Longus capitis
Sympathetic trunk
Anterior ramus C4
Middle scalene
Longus capitis
Longus colli (vertical part)
Phrenic nerve
Carotid tubercle (transverse process of C6)
Anterior ramus C5
Anterior scalene
Anterior scalene
Vertebral artery
Sympathetic ganglion
Inferior thyroid artery
Ascending cervical artery
C6
Dorsal scapular artery
Anterior rami C7
Costocervical trunk
C8
T1
Suprascapular artery
Right subclavian artery
Thyrocervical trunk
Recurrent laryngeal nerve
Inferior cervical ganglion
Internal thoracic artery
1st rib
Ansa subclavia
Left subclavian artery
Right subclavian artery
Right common carotid artery
Left common carotid artery
Brachiocephalic trunk

B. Anterior View

8.23 PREVERTEBRAL REGION *(CONTINUED)*

TABLE 8.6 PREVERTEBRAL AND SCALENE MUSCLES

Muscle	Superior Attachment	Inferior Attachment	Innervation	Main Action
Rectus capitis anterior	Base of cranium, just anterior to occipital condyle	Anterior surface of lateral mass of atlas (C1)	Branches from loop between C1 and C2 spinal nerves	Lateral flexion at atlanto-occipital joints (acting unilaterally)
Rectus capitis lateralis	Base of cranium just lateral to occipital condyle	Transverse process of atlas (C1)		Flexion at atlanto-occipital joints (acting bilaterally)
Anterior scalene	Anterior tubercles of TVP C3–C6	Scalene tubercle of 1st rib	Anterior rami of C3–C8 (cervical and brachial plexus)	Forced inspiration (ribs mobile): elevate superior ribs
Middle scalene	TVP C1–C2	Superior surface of 1st rib; posterior to groove for subclavian artery		
	Posterior tubercles of TVP C3–C7			Ribs fixed: lateral flexion of cervical spine (acting unilaterally) Flexes neck (acting bilaterally)
Posterior scalene	Posterior tubercles of TVP C5–C7	External border of 2nd rib		

TVP, Transverse process.

Sympathetic trunk
Cervical cardiac branch
Middle scalene
Rami communicantes
Vertebral artery
Transverse process, C7
Cervicothoracic (stellate) ganglion:
Inferior cervical ganglion
1st thoracic ganglion
1st rib
2nd rib
Trunks of **brachial plexus**
Dorsal scapular artery
Subclavian artery
Anterior scalene
Cervical parietal pleura
Pericardiacophrenic artery
Vagus nerve (CN X)
Longus cervicis
Vertebral body C5
C5
C6
C7
C8
T1
Anterior rami (roots of brachial plexus)
Trachea
Right common carotid artery
Ansa subclavia
Right recurrent laryngeal nerve
N'Joy

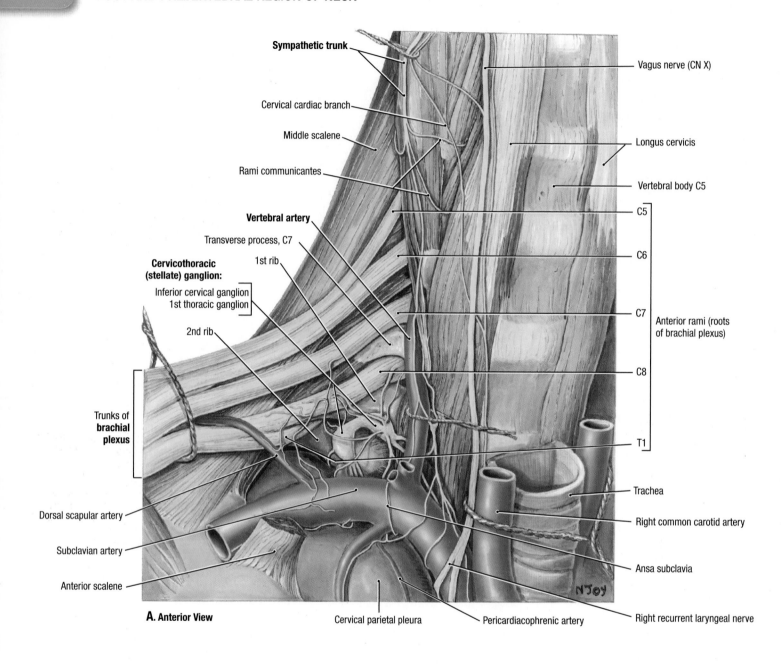

A. Anterior View

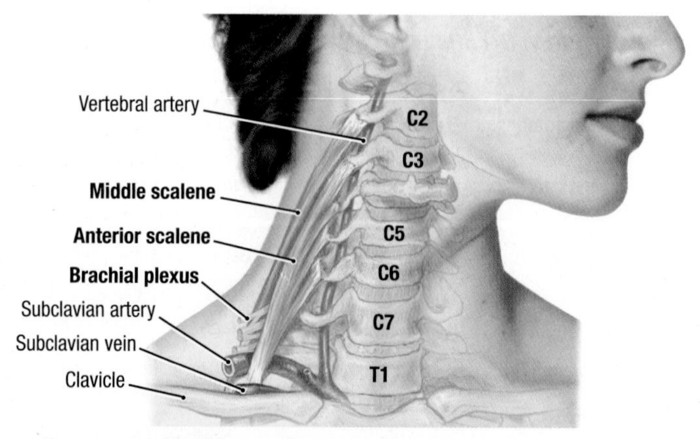
Vertebral artery
Middle scalene
Anterior scalene
Brachial plexus
Subclavian artery
Subclavian vein
Clavicle
C2
C3
C5
C6
C7
T1

B. Anterolateral View

8.24 BRACHIAL PLEXUS AND SYMPATHETIC TRUNK IN ROOT OF NECK

A. Dissection of right side of specimen. The pleura has been depressed, the vertebral artery retracted medially, and the brachial plexus retracted superiorly to reveal the cervicothoracic (stellate) ganglion (the combined inferior cervical and 1st thoracic ganglia). Anesthetic injected around the cervicothoracic (stellate) ganglion blocks transmission of stimuli through the cervical and superior thoracic ganglia. This **stellate ganglion block** may relieve vascular spasms involving the brain and upper limb. It is also useful when deciding if surgical resection of the ganglion would be beneficial to a person with excess vasoconstriction of the ipsilateral limb. **B.** Relation of brachial plexus and subclavian artery to anterior and middle scalene muscles.

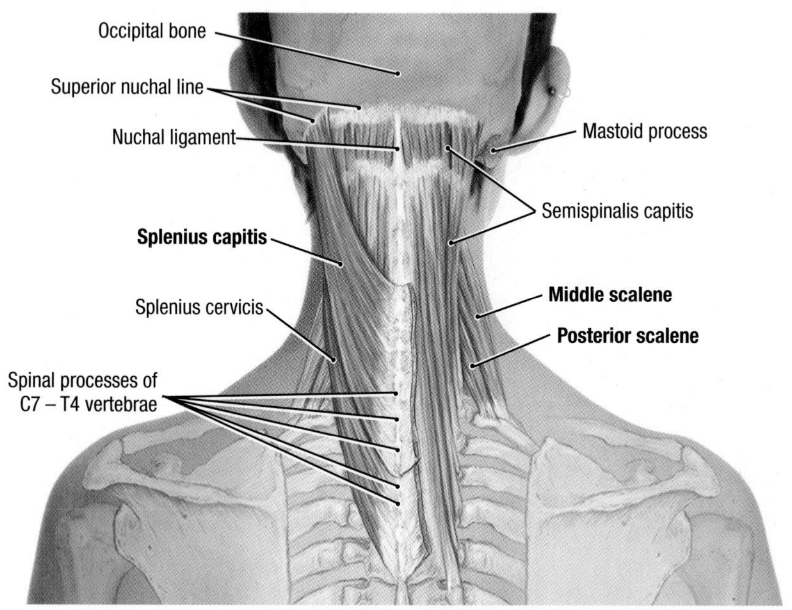
Occipital bone
Superior nuchal line
Nuchal ligament
Mastoid process
Semispinalis capitis
Splenius capitis
Splenius cervicis
Middle scalene
Posterior scalene
Spinal processes of C7 – T4 vertebrae

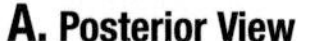

A. Posterior View

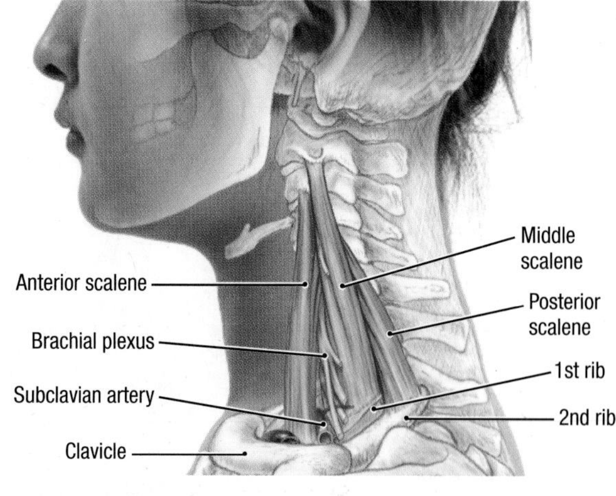
Anterior scalene
Middle scalene
Posterior scalene
Brachial plexus
1st rib
Subclavian artery
2nd rib
Clavicle

B. Lateral View

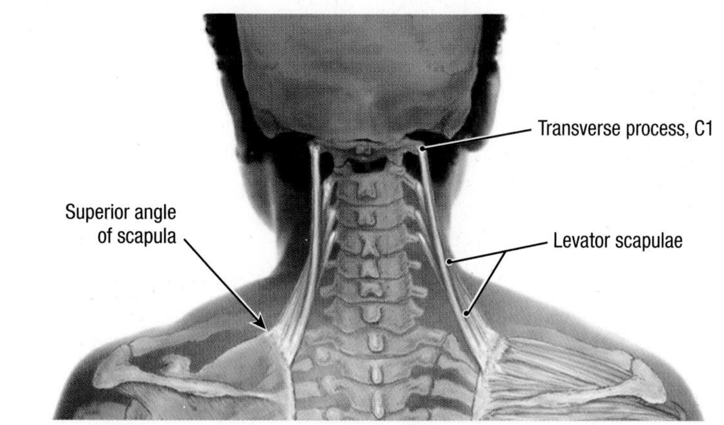
Transverse process, C1
Superior angle of scapula
Levator scapulae

C. Posterior View

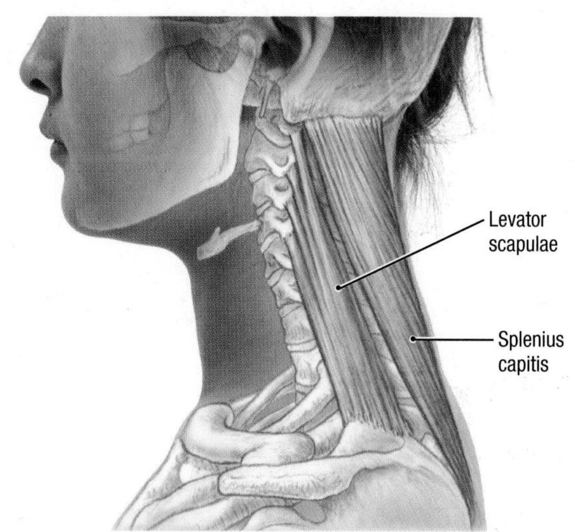
Levator scapulae
Splenius capitis

D. Lateral View

8.25 LATERAL VERTEBRAL MUSCLES

A. Overview. **B.** Scalene muscles. **C.** Levator scapulae. **D.** Levator scapulae and splenius capitis.

TABLE 8.7 LATERAL VERTEBRAL MUSCLES

Muscle	Superior Attachment	Inferior Attachment	Innervation	Main Action
Splenius capitis	Inferior half of nuchal ligament and spinous processes of C7 and superior 3–4 thoracic vertebrae	Lateral aspect of mastoid process and lateral third of superior nuchal line	Posterior rami of middle cervical spinal nerves	Laterally flexes and rotates head and neck to same side; acting bilaterally, extends head and neck[a]
Levator scapulae	Posterior tubercles of transverse processes of C1–C4 vertebrae	Superior part of medial border of scapula	Dorsal scapular nerve (C5) and cervical spinal nerves C3 and C4	Elevates scapula and tilts glenoid cavity inferiorly by rotating scapula
Middle scalene	See Table 8.6.			
Posterior scalene				

[a]Rotation of head occurs at atlanto-axial joints.

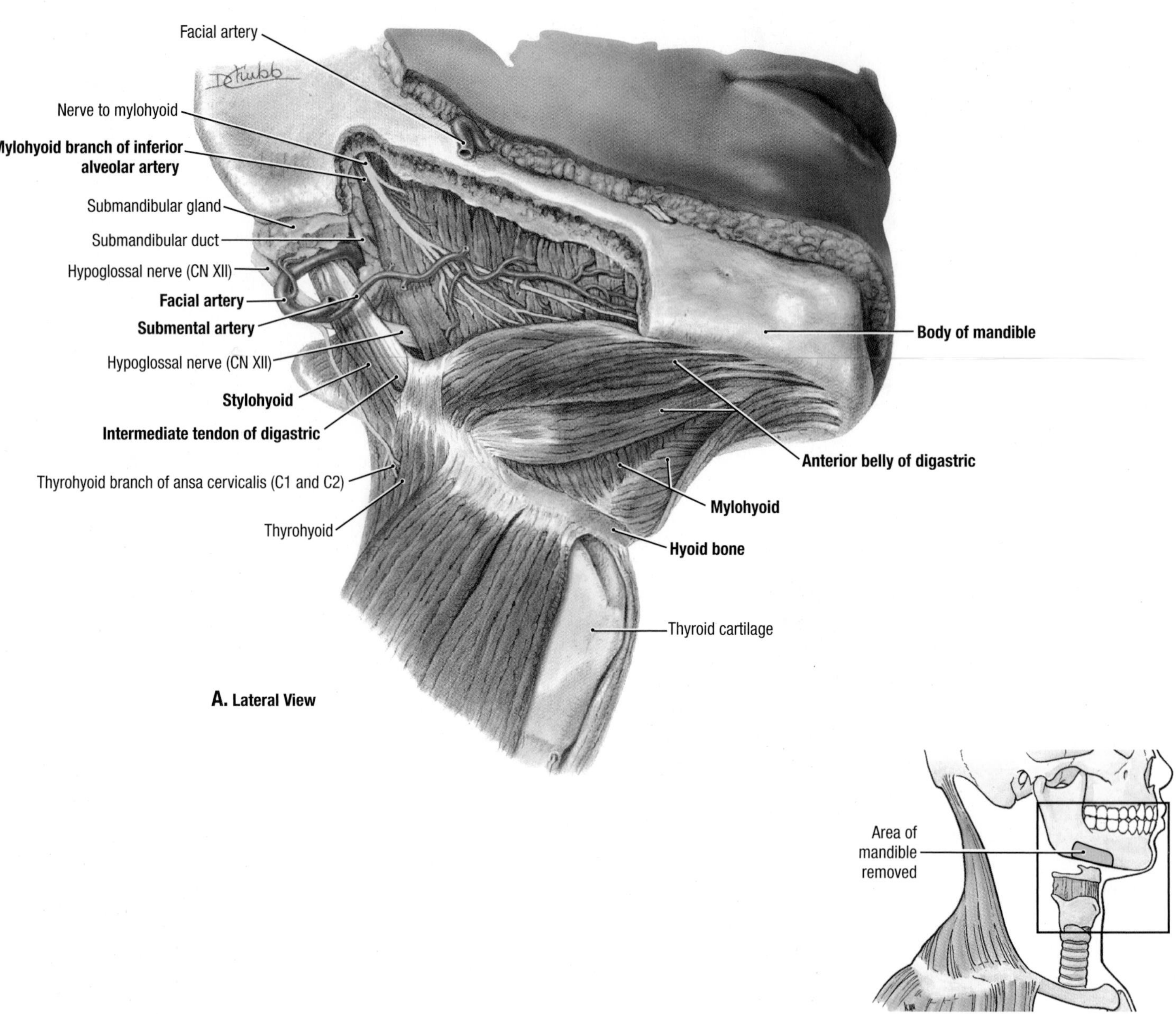
Facial artery
Nerve to mylohyoid
Mylohyoid branch of inferior alveolar artery
Submandibular gland
Submandibular duct
Hypoglossal nerve (CN XII)
Facial artery
Submental artery
Hypoglossal nerve (CN XII)
Stylohyoid
Intermediate tendon of digastric
Thyrohyoid branch of ansa cervicalis (C1 and C2)
Thyrohyoid
Body of mandible
Anterior belly of digastric
Mylohyoid
Hyoid bone
Thyroid cartilage
Area of mandible removed

A. **Lateral View**

8.26 SERIAL DISSECTION OF SUBMANDIBULAR REGION AND FLOOR OF MOUTH I

Mylohyoid and digastric muscles. **A.** Structures overlying the mandible and a portion of the body of the mandible have been removed.

- The stylohyoid and posterior belly and intermediate tendon of the digastric muscle form the posterior border of the submandibular triangle; the facial artery passes superficial to these muscles.
- The anterior belly of the digastric muscle forms the anterior border of the submandibular triangle. In this specimen, the anterior belly has an additional origin from the hyoid bone; the mylohyoid muscle forms the medial wall of the triangle and has a thick, free posterior border.
- The nerve to mylohyoid, which supplies the mylohyoid muscle and anterior belly of the digastric muscle, is accompanied by the mylohyoid branch of the inferior alveolar artery posteriorly and the submental artery from the facial artery anteriorly.

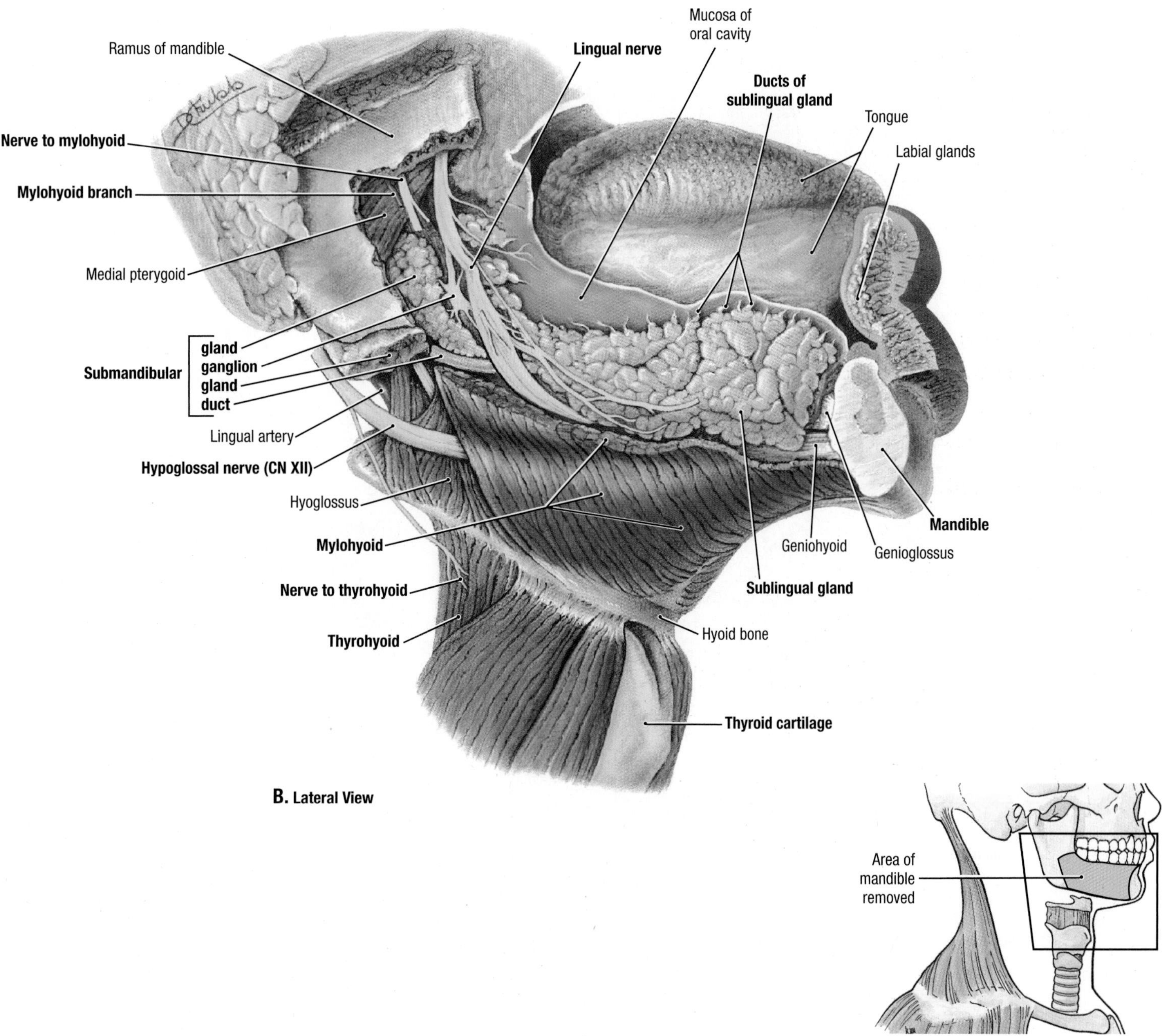
Ramus of mandible
Nerve to mylohyoid
Mylohyoid branch
Medial pterygoid
Submandibular
gland
ganglion
gland
duct
Lingual artery
Hypoglossal nerve (CN XII)
Hyoglossus
Mylohyoid
Nerve to thyrohyoid
Thyrohyoid
Lingual nerve
Mucosa of
oral cavity
Ducts of
sublingual gland
Tongue
Labial glands
Mandible
Geniohyoid
Genioglossus
Sublingual gland
Hyoid bone
Thyroid cartilage
Area of
mandible
removed

B. Lateral View

8.26 SERIAL DISSECTION OF SUBMANDIBULAR REGION AND FLOOR OF MOUTH II

B. Sublingual and submandibular glands. The body and adjacent portion of the ramus of the mandible have been removed.

- The sublingual salivary gland lies posterior to the mandible and is in contact with the deep part of the submandibular gland posteriorly.
- Numerous fine ducts pass from the superior border of the sublingual gland to open on the sublingual fold of the overlying mucosa.
- The lingual nerve lies between the sublingual gland and the deep part of the submandibular gland; the submandibular ganglion is suspended from this nerve.
- Spinal nerve C1 fibers, conveyed by the hypoglossal nerve (CN XII), pass to the thyrohyoid muscle before the hypoglossal nerve passes deep to the mylohyoid muscle.

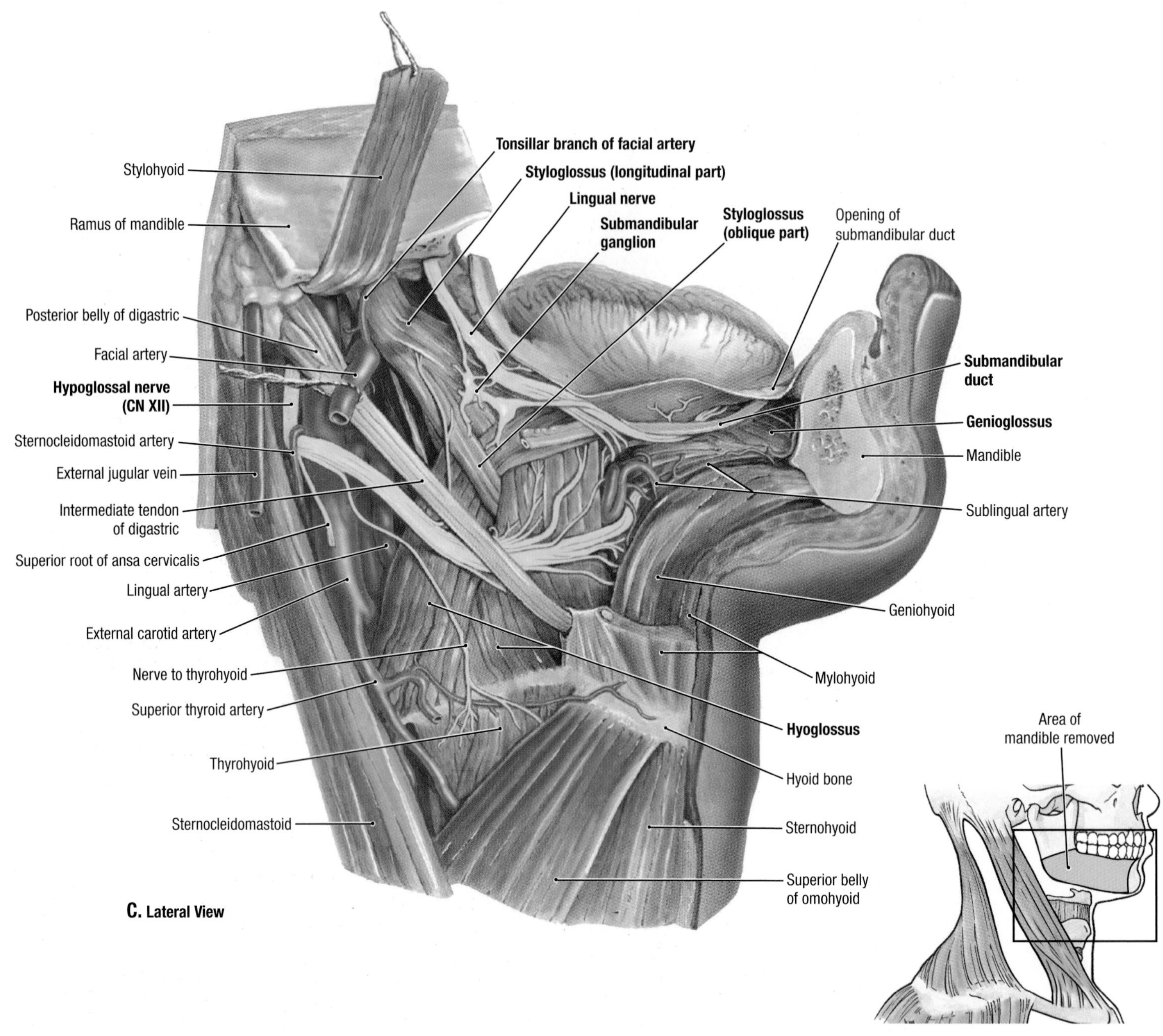
Tonsillar branch of facial artery
Styloglossus (longitudinal part)
Lingual nerve
Submandibular ganglion
Styloglossus (oblique part)
Opening of submandibular duct
Stylohyoid
Ramus of mandible
Posterior belly of digastric
Facial artery
Hypoglossal nerve (CN XII)
Sternocleidomastoid artery
External jugular vein
Intermediate tendon of digastric
Superior root of ansa cervicalis
Lingual artery
External carotid artery
Nerve to thyrohyoid
Superior thyroid artery
Thyrohyoid
Sternocleidomastoid
Submandibular duct
Genioglossus
Mandible
Sublingual artery
Geniohyoid
Mylohyoid
Hyoglossus
Hyoid bone
Sternohyoid
Superior belly of omohyoid
Area of mandible removed

C. Lateral View

8.26 SERIAL DISSECTION OF SUBMANDIBULAR REGION AND FLOOR OF MOUTH III

C. Hyoglossus muscle, lingual (CN V_3) and hypoglossal nerves (CN XII). All of the right half of the mandible, except the superior part of the ramus, has been removed. The stylohyoid muscle is reflected superiorly, and the posterior belly of the digastric muscle is left in situ.

- The hyoglossus muscle ascends from the greater horn and body of the hyoid bone to the side of the tongue.
- The styloglossus muscle is crossed by the tonsillar branch of the facial artery posterosuperiorly, and its oblique part interdigitates with bundles of the hyoglossus muscle inferiorly.
- The hypoglossal nerve (CN XII) supplies all of the muscles of the tongue, both extrinsic and intrinsic, except the palatoglossus (a palatine muscle, innervated by CN X).
- The submandibular duct runs anteriorly in contact with the hyoglossus and genioglossus muscles to its opening on the side of the frenulum of the tongue.
- The lingual nerve is in contact with the mandible posteriorly, looping inferior to the submandibular duct and ending in the tongue. The submandibular ganglion is suspended from the lingual nerve; twigs leave the nerve to supply the mucous membrane.

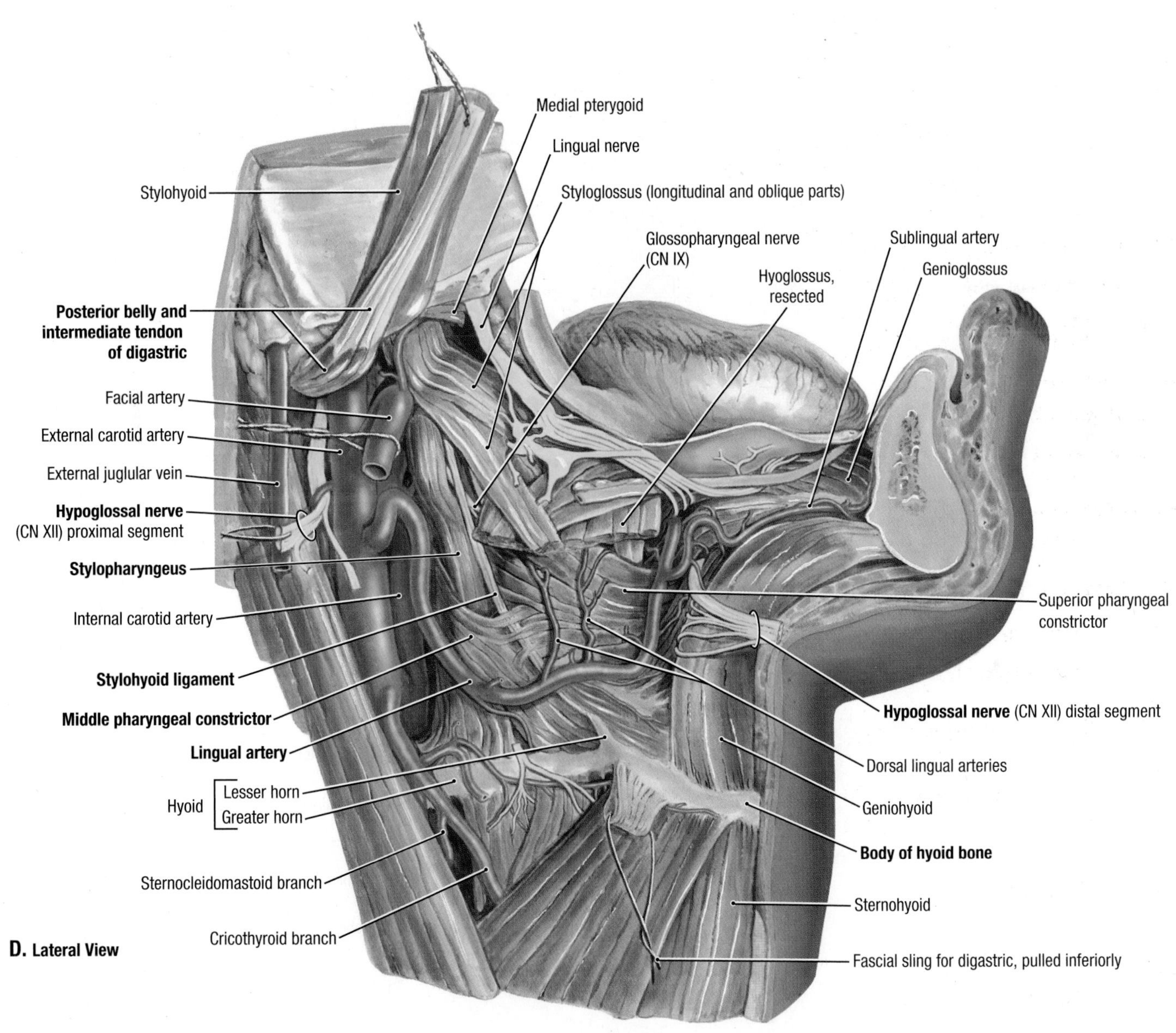
Medial pterygoid
Lingual nerve
Stylohyoid
Styloglossus (longitudinal and oblique parts)
Glossopharyngeal nerve (CN IX)
Sublingual artery
Hyoglossus, resected
Genioglossus
Posterior belly and intermediate tendon of digastric
Facial artery
External carotid artery
External juglular vein
Hypoglossal nerve (CN XII) proximal segment
Stylopharyngeus
Superior pharyngeal constrictor
Internal carotid artery
Stylohyoid ligament
Hypoglossal nerve (CN XII) distal segment
Middle pharyngeal constrictor
Lingual artery
Dorsal lingual arteries
Hyoid
Lesser horn
Greater horn
Geniohyoid
Body of hyoid bone
Sternocleidomastoid branch
Sternohyoid
Cricothyroid branch
Fascial sling for digastric, pulled inferiorly

D. Lateral View

8.26 SERIAL DISSECTION OF SUBMANDIBULAR REGION AND FLOOR OF MOUTH IV

D. Genioglossus and geniohyoid muscles. The stylohyoid, posterior belly and intermediate tendon of the digastric muscle are reflected superiorly, the hypoglossal nerve (CN XII) is divided, and the hyoglossus muscle is mostly removed.

- The lingual artery passes deep to the hyoglossus muscle (resected here), close to the greater horn of the hyoid, and then passes lateral to the middle pharyngeal constrictor muscle, stylohyoid ligament, and genioglossus muscle and turns into the tongue as the deep lingual arteries.

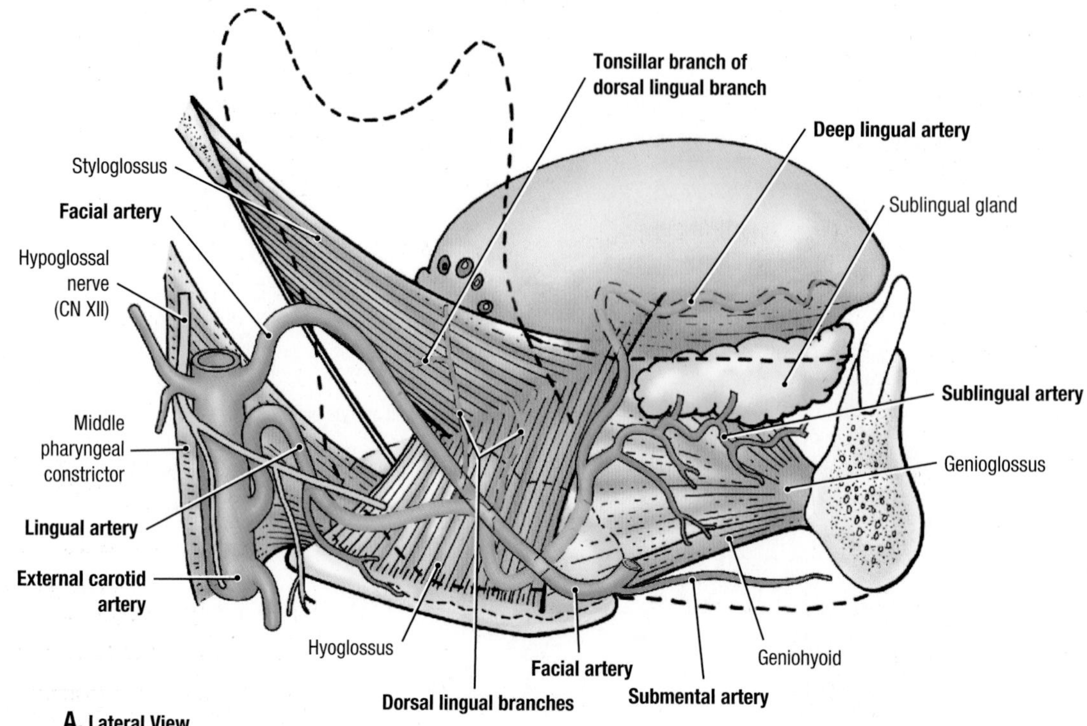
Tonsillar branch of
dorsal lingual branch
Deep lingual artery
Sublingual gland
Styloglossus
Facial artery
Hypoglossal
nerve
(CN XII)
Sublingual artery
Genioglossus
Middle
pharyngeal
constrictor
Lingual artery
External carotid
artery
Hyoglossus
Facial artery
Geniohyoid
Dorsal lingual branches
Submental artery

A. Lateral View

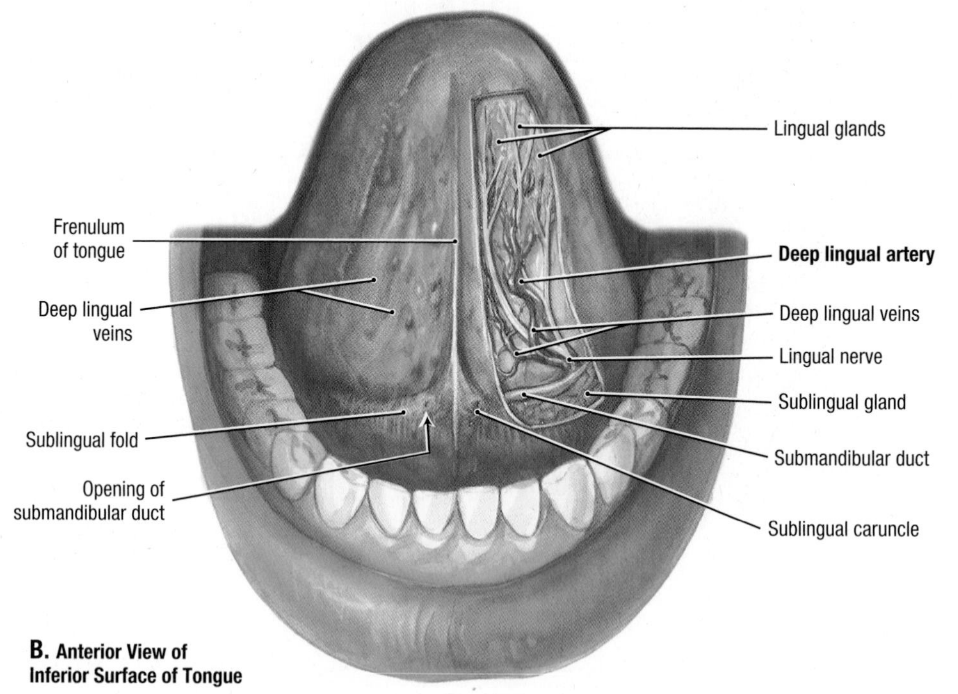
Lingual glands
Frenulum
of tongue
Deep lingual artery
Deep lingual
veins
Deep lingual veins
Lingual nerve
Sublingual gland
Sublingual fold
Submandibular duct
Opening of
submandibular duct
Sublingual caruncle

B. Anterior View of Inferior Surface of Tongue

8.27 LINGUAL AND FACIAL ARTERIES IN SUBMANDIBULAR REGION AND FLOOR OF MOUTH

A. Course of the lingual artery. **B.** Inferior surface of the tongue and floor of the mouth.

In **A**: The lingual artery arises from the anterior aspect of the external carotid artery, where it lies on the middle pharyngeal constrictor. Then it arches supero-anteriorly, passes deep to CN XII and disappears deep to the hyoglossus muscle, giving branches to the posterior tongue (dorsal lingual branches). It then turns superiorly at the anterior border of hyoglossus, bifurcating into the deep lingual and sublingual arteries.

In **B**: The inferior (sublingual) surface of the tongue is covered by mucous membrane through which the underlying deep lingual veins can be seen.

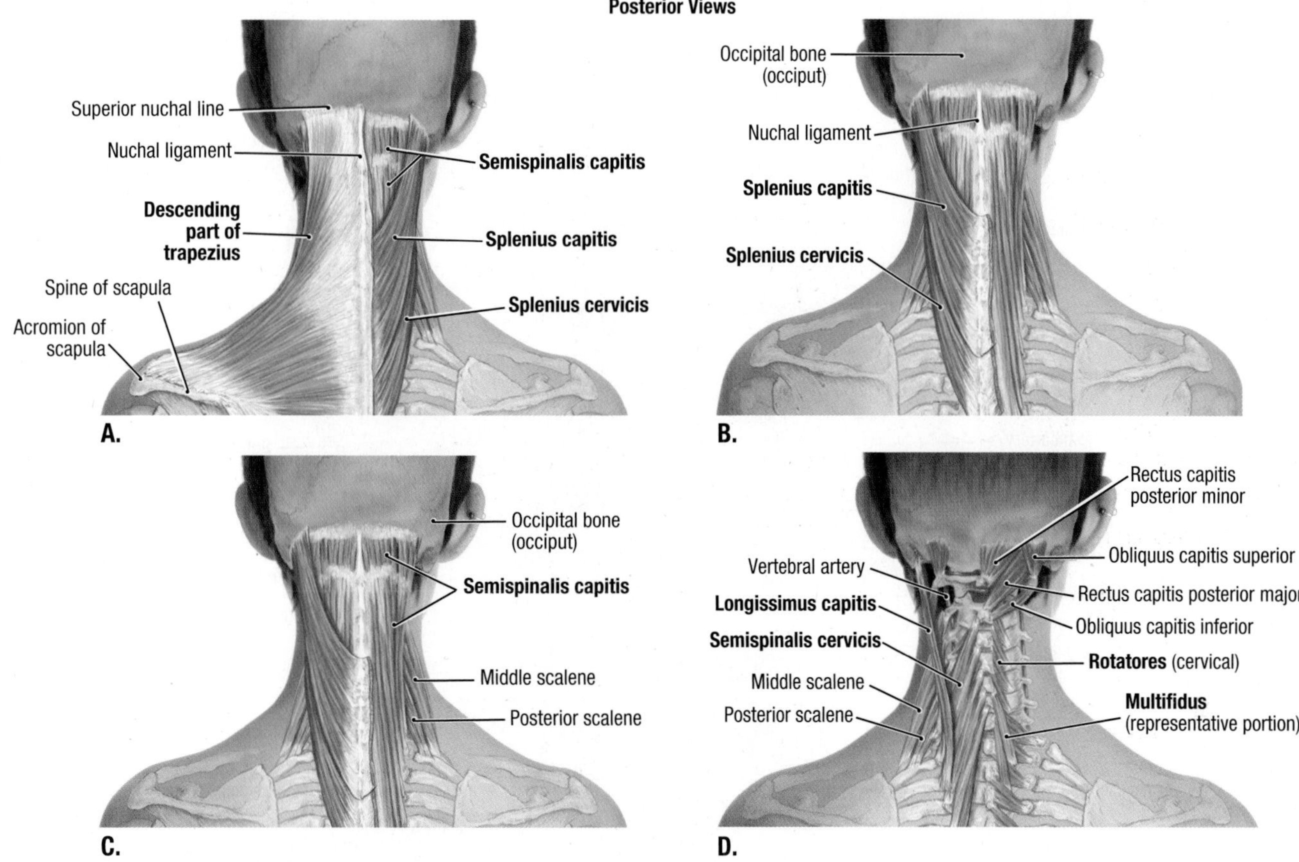
Posterior Views
Superior nuchal line
Nuchal ligament
Semispinalis capitis
Descending part of trapezius
Splenius capitis
Spine of scapula
Splenius cervicis
Acromion of scapula
A.
Occipital bone (occiput)
Nuchal ligament
Splenius capitis
Splenius cervicis
B.
Occipital bone (occiput)
Semispinalis capitis
Middle scalene
Posterior scalene
C.
Rectus capitis posterior minor
Vertebral artery
Obliquus capitis superior
Longissimus capitis
Rectus capitis posterior major
Obliquus capitis inferior
Semispinalis cervicis
Rotatores (cervical)
Middle scalene
Multifidus (representative portion)
Posterior scalene
D.

8.28 MUSCLES OF POSTERIOR CERVICAL REGION

A. Trapezius. **B.** Splenius. **C.** Semispinalis. **D.** Deep muscles.

TABLE 8.8 MUSCLES OF POSTERIOR CERVICAL REGION

Muscle	Superior Attachment	Inferior Attachment	Innervation	Main Action
Extrinsic muscle of back (superior axioappendicular muscle)				
Descending part of trapezius	Medial third of superior nuchal line; external occipital protuberance; nuchal ligament	Lateral third of clavicle and lateral aspect of acromion of scapula	Spinal accessory nerve (CN XI)	Elevates scapulae and works with other parts of muscle to retract scapulae; with shoulder fixed, contributes to extension of head, side bending (lateral flexion) of neck
Intrinsic muscles of back—superficial layer				
Splenius	Nuchal ligament and spinous processes of C7 toT3–T4 vertebrae	*Splenius capitis:* fibers run superolaterally to mastoid process of temporal bone and lateral third of superior nuchal line of occipital bone *Splenius cervicis:* Tubercles of transverse processes of C1–C4 vertebrae	Posterior rami of spinal nerves	*Acting unilaterally:* laterally flex and rotate head to side of active muscle *Acting bilaterally:* extend head and neck
Intrinsic muscles of back—intermediate layer				
Longissimus	Transverse processes of T1–T5 vertebrae	*Longissimus capitis:* posterior mastoid process *Longissimus cervicis:* transverse processes of C2–C6	Posterior rami of spinal nerves	Extends vertebral column; longissimus capitis turns face ipsilaterally
Intrinsic muscles of back—deep layer				
Semispinalis	Transverse processes of C4–T5 vertebrae	*Semispinalis capitis:* Superior nuchal line of occipital bone *Semispinalis cervicis:* Spinous processes of cervical vertebrae	Posterior rami of spinal nerves	*Acting unilaterally:* contribute to contralateral rotation; *Acting bilaterally:* extend head and neck
Multifidus of cervical region	Transverse processes of T1–T3 Articular processes of C4–C7 vertebrae	Spinous processes 2–4 segments inferior to attachment		Stabilizes vertebrae during local movements of vertebral column
Rotatores	Transverse processes	Junction of lamina and transverse process, or spinous process of vertebra immediately (brevis) or two segments (longus) superior to origin		Stabilize, assist with local extension and rotatory movements; may function as proprioceptive organs

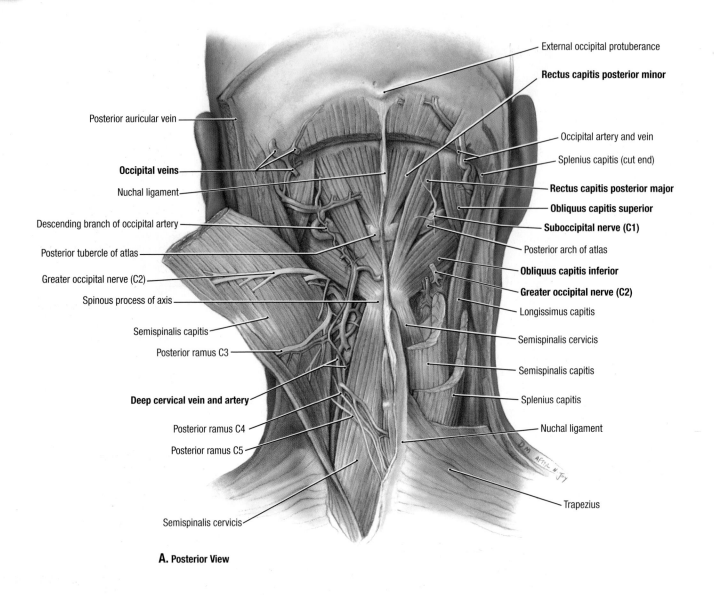

External occipital protuberance
Rectus capitis posterior minor
Posterior auricular vein
Occipital artery and vein
Splenius capitis (cut end)
Occipital veins
Nuchal ligament
Rectus capitis posterior major
Obliquus capitis superior
Descending branch of occipital artery
Suboccipital nerve (C1)
Posterior arch of atlas
Posterior tubercle of atlas
Obliquus capitis inferior
Greater occipital nerve (C2)
Greater occipital nerve (C2)
Spinous process of axis
Longissimus capitis
Semispinalis capitis
Semispinalis cervicis
Posterior ramus C3
Semispinalis capitis
Deep cervical vein and artery
Splenius capitis
Posterior ramus C4
Nuchal ligament
Posterior ramus C5
Trapezius
Semispinalis cervicis

A. Posterior View

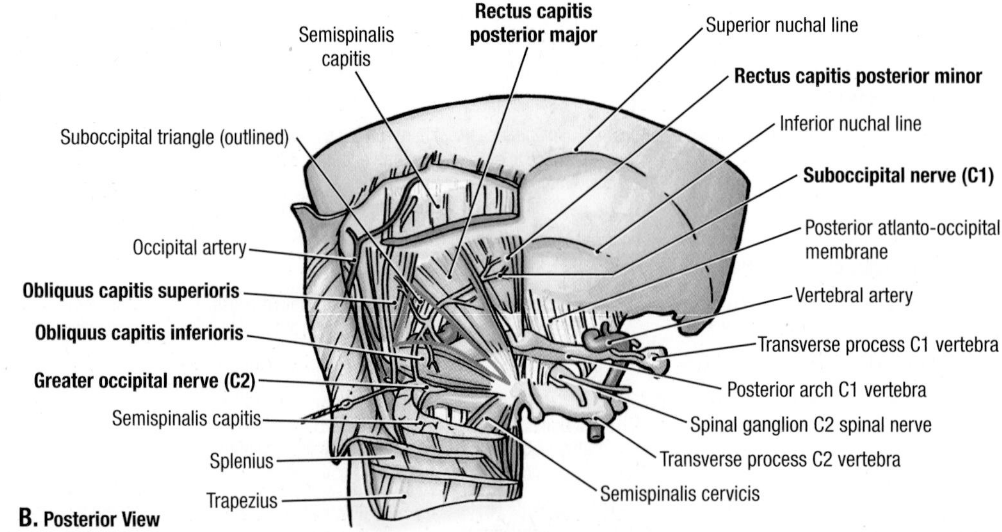
Semispinalis capitis
Rectus capitis posterior major
Superior nuchal line
Rectus capitis posterior minor
Inferior nuchal line
Suboccipital triangle (outlined)
Suboccipital nerve (C1)
Occipital artery
Posterior atlanto-occipital membrane
Obliquus capitis superioris
Vertebral artery
Obliquus capitis inferioris
Transverse process C1 vertebra
Greater occipital nerve (C2)
Posterior arch C1 vertebra
Semispinalis capitis
Spinal ganglion C2 spinal nerve
Splenius
Transverse process C2 vertebra
Trapezius
Semispinalis cervicis

B. Posterior View

8.29 SUBOCCIPITAL REGION

A. Dissection. **B.** Schematic illustration.

- The suboccipital triangle is bounded by three muscles: obliquus capitis inferior and superior, and rectus capitis posterior major.
- The suboccipital nerve (posterior ramus of C1 spinal nerve) emerges through the suboccipital triangle to innervate the muscles forming the triangle.

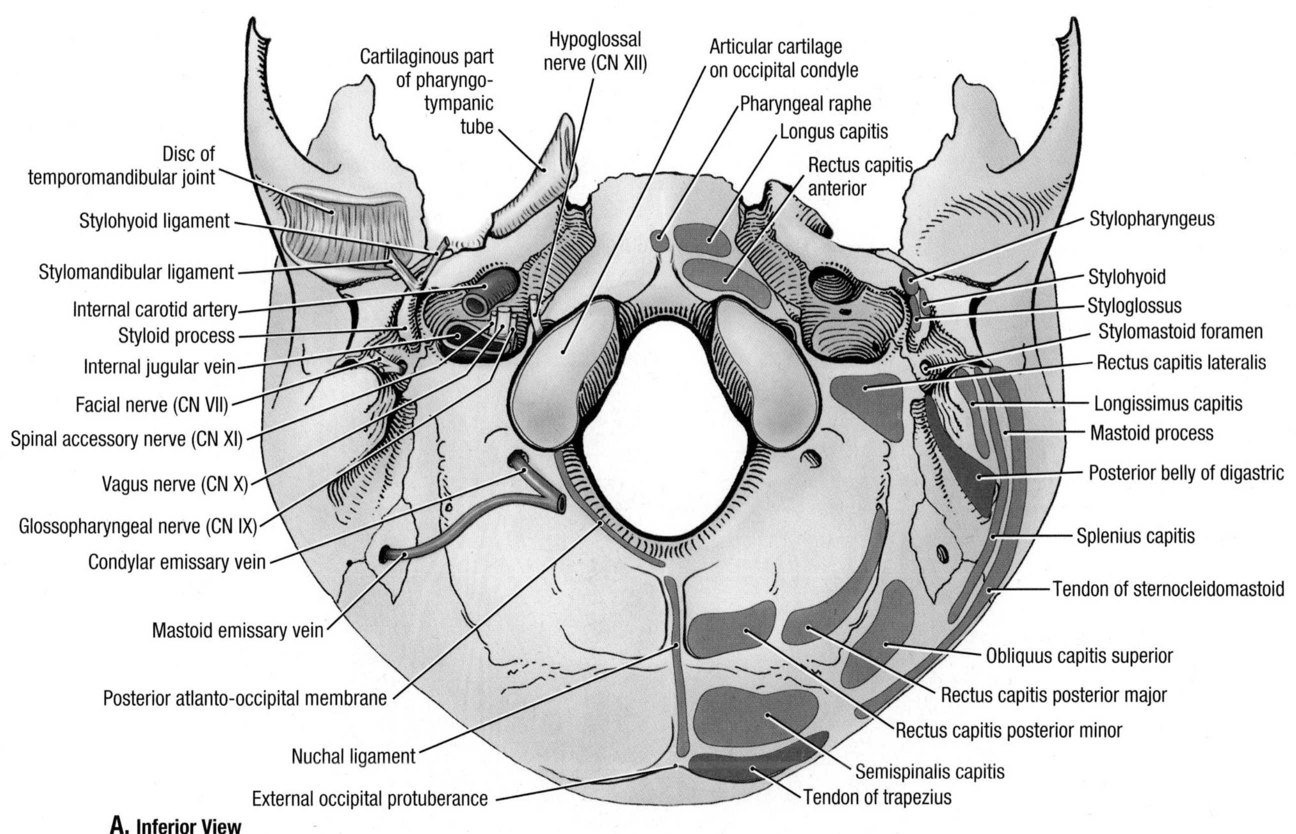
Cartilaginous part of pharyngo-tympanic tube
Hypoglossal nerve (CN XII)
Articular cartilage on occipital condyle
Pharyngeal raphe
Longus capitis
Rectus capitis anterior
Disc of temporomandibular joint
Stylohyoid ligament
Stylomandibular ligament
Internal carotid artery
Styloid process
Internal jugular vein
Facial nerve (CN VII)
Spinal accessory nerve (CN XI)
Vagus nerve (CN X)
Glossopharyngeal nerve (CN IX)
Condylar emissary vein
Mastoid emissary vein
Posterior atlanto-occipital membrane
Nuchal ligament
External occipital protuberance
Stylopharyngeus
Stylohyoid
Styloglossus
Stylomastoid foramen
Rectus capitis lateralis
Longissimus capitis
Mastoid process
Posterior belly of digastric
Splenius capitis
Tendon of sternocleidomastoid
Obliquus capitis superior
Rectus capitis posterior major
Rectus capitis posterior minor
Semispinalis capitis
Tendon of trapezius
A. Inferior View

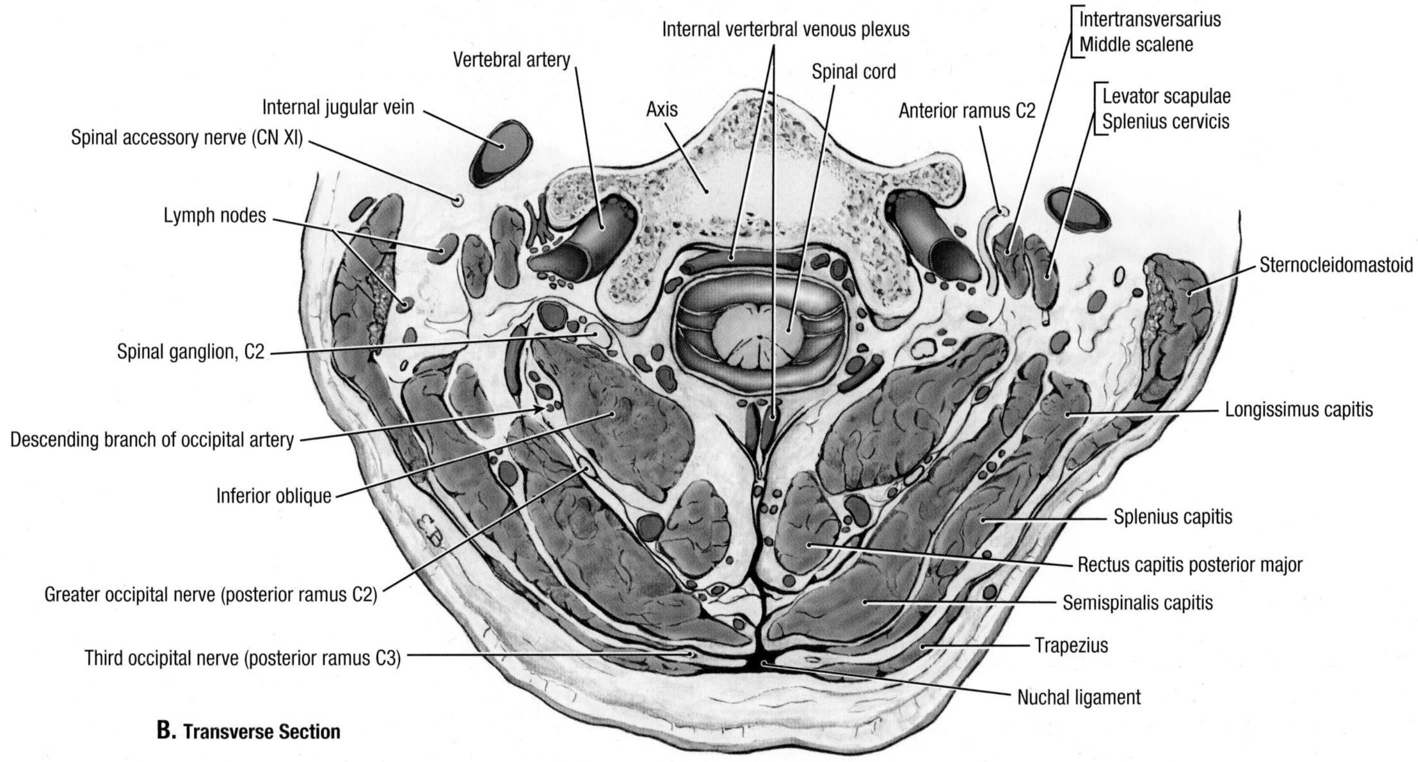
Internal verterbral venous plexus
Vertebral artery
Spinal cord
Axis
Anterior ramus C2
Intertransversarius
Middle scalene
Levator scapulae
Splenius cervicis
Internal jugular vein
Spinal accessory nerve (CN XI)
Lymph nodes
Spinal ganglion, C2
Descending branch of occipital artery
Inferior oblique
Greater occipital nerve (posterior ramus C2)
Third occipital nerve (posterior ramus C3)
Sternocleidomastoid
Longissimus capitis
Splenius capitis
Rectus capitis posterior major
Semispinalis capitis
Trapezius
Nuchal ligament
B. Transverse Section

8.30 POSTERIOR CERVICAL REGION—BASE OF SKULL AND TRANSVERSE SECTION

A. Muscular attachments to and neurovascular relationships at the base of the skull. **B.** Transverse section through the axis (C2 vertebra).

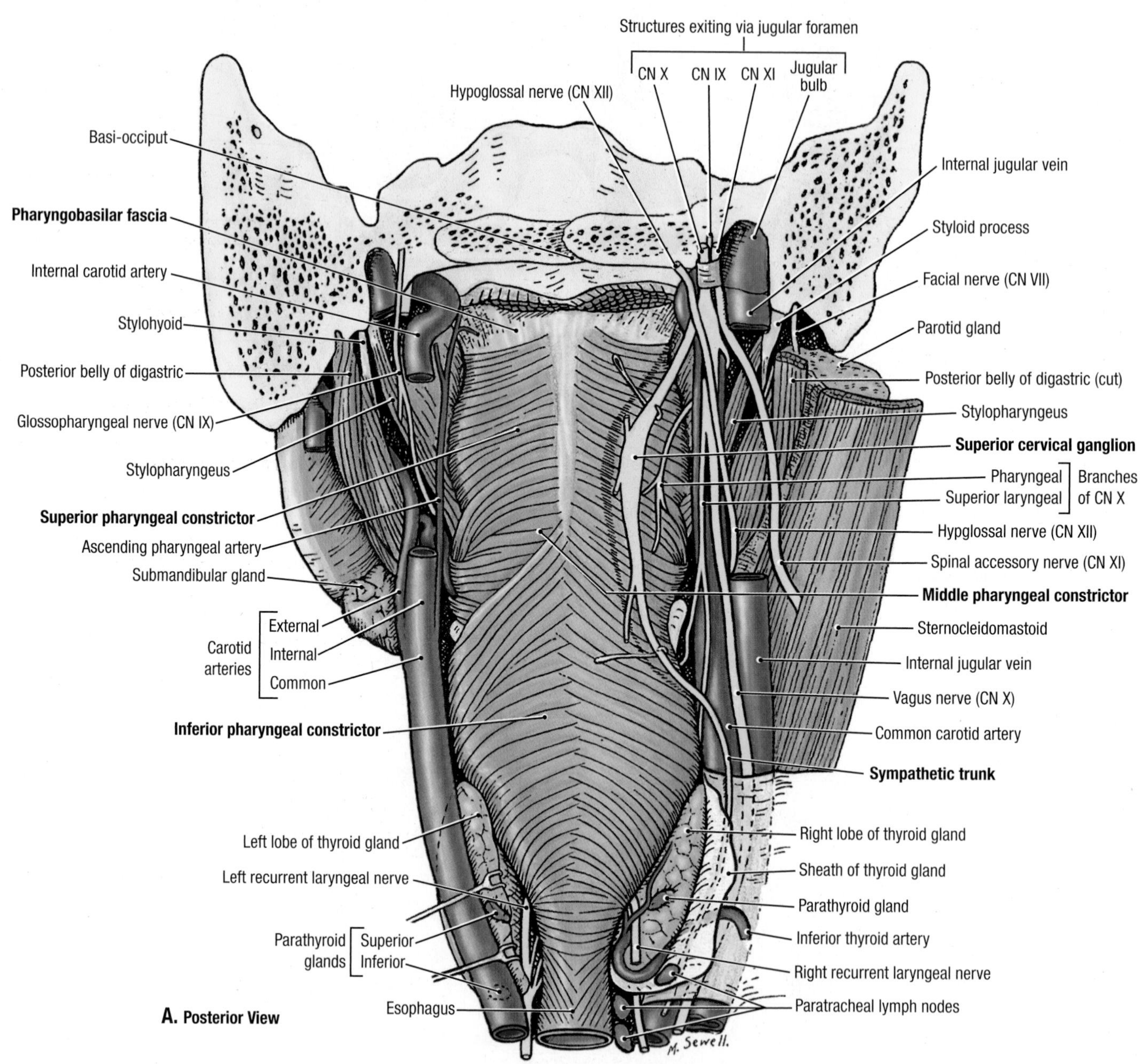
Structures exiting via jugular foramen
CN X
CN IX
CN XI
Jugular bulb
Hypoglossal nerve (CN XII)
Basi-occiput
Pharyngobasilar fascia
Internal carotid artery
Stylohyoid
Posterior belly of digastric
Glossopharyngeal nerve (CN IX)
Stylopharyngeus
Superior pharyngeal constrictor
Ascending pharyngeal artery
Submandibular gland
Carotid arteries
External
Internal
Common
Inferior pharyngeal constrictor
Left lobe of thyroid gland
Left recurrent laryngeal nerve
Parathyroid glands
Superior
Inferior
Esophagus
Internal jugular vein
Styloid process
Facial nerve (CN VII)
Parotid gland
Posterior belly of digastric (cut)
Stylopharyngeus
Superior cervical ganglion
Pharyngeal
Superior laryngeal
Branches of CN X
Hypglossal nerve (CN XII)
Spinal accessory nerve (CN XI)
Middle pharyngeal constrictor
Sternocleidomastoid
Internal jugular vein
Vagus nerve (CN X)
Common carotid artery
Sympathetic trunk
Right lobe of thyroid gland
Sheath of thyroid gland
Parathyroid gland
Inferior thyroid artery
Right recurrent laryngeal nerve
Paratracheal lymph nodes
M. Sewell.

A. Posterior View

8.31 EXTERNAL PHARYNX—POSTERIOR VIEWS

A. Illustration of a dissection similar to **B.** The sympathetic trunk (including the superior cervical ganglion), which normally lies posterior to the internal carotid artery, has been retracted medially.

- The pharyngobasilar fascia, between the superior pharyngeal constrictor muscle and the base of the skull, attaches the pharynx to the occipital bone and forms the wall of the noncollapsible pharyngeal recesses.
- As they exit the jugular foramen, CN IX lies anterior to CN X, and CN XI; CN XII, exiting the hypoglossal canal, lies medially.

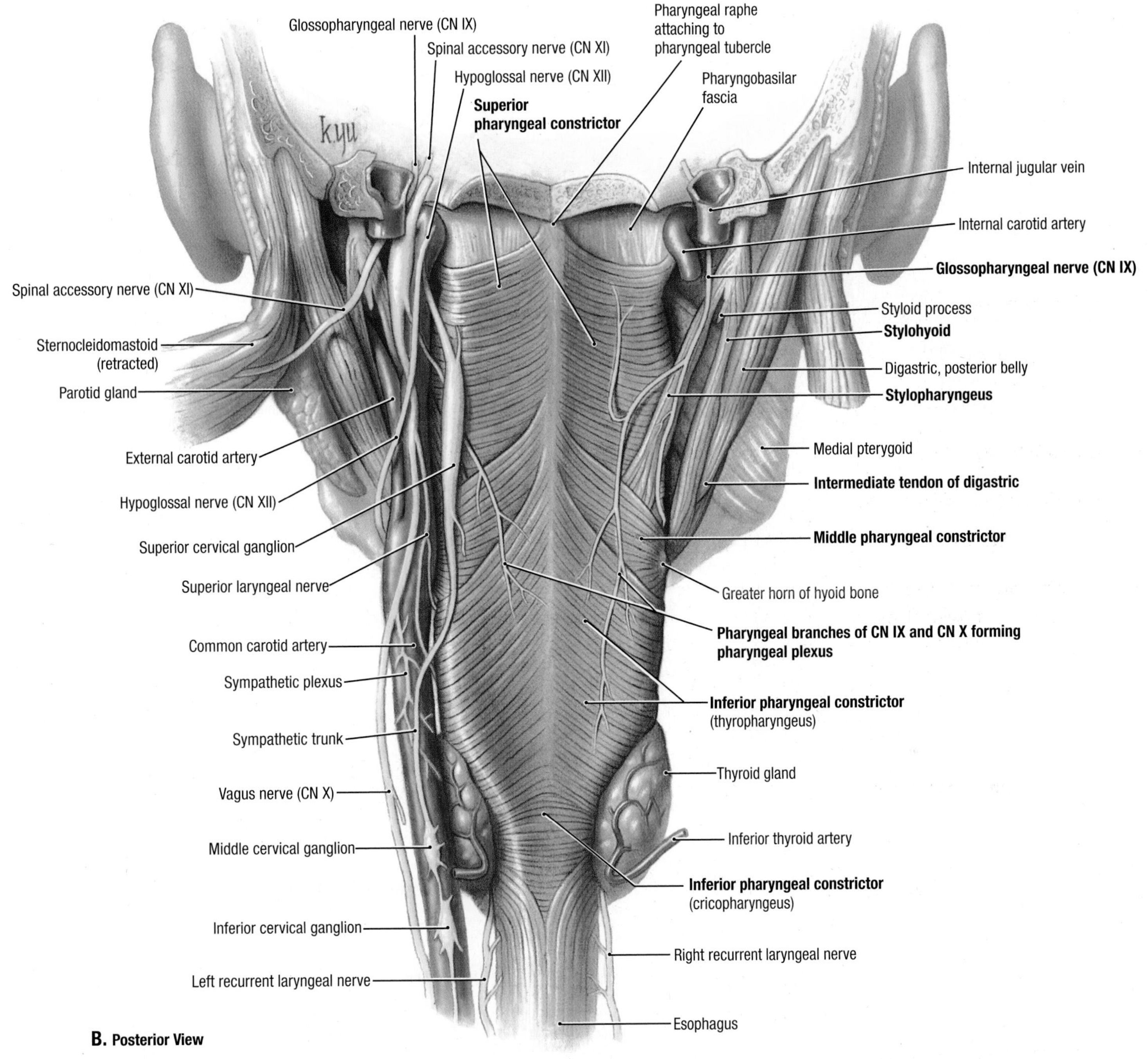
Glossopharyngeal nerve (CN IX)
Spinal accessory nerve (CN XI)
Hypoglossal nerve (CN XII)
Superior pharyngeal constrictor
Pharyngeal raphe attaching to pharyngeal tubercle
Pharyngobasilar fascia
kyu
Internal jugular vein
Internal carotid artery
Glossopharyngeal nerve (CN IX)
Styloid process
Stylohyoid
Digastric, posterior belly
Stylopharyngeus
Medial pterygoid
Intermediate tendon of digastric
Middle pharyngeal constrictor
Greater horn of hyoid bone
Pharyngeal branches of CN IX and CN X forming pharyngeal plexus
Inferior pharyngeal constrictor (thyropharyngeus)
Thyroid gland
Inferior thyroid artery
Inferior pharyngeal constrictor (cricopharyngeus)
Right recurrent laryngeal nerve
Esophagus
Spinal accessory nerve (CN XI)
Sternocleidomastoid (retracted)
Parotid gland
External carotid artery
Hypoglossal nerve (CN XII)
Superior cervical ganglion
Superior laryngeal nerve
Common carotid artery
Sympathetic plexus
Sympathetic trunk
Vagus nerve (CN X)
Middle cervical ganglion
Inferior cervical ganglion
Left recurrent laryngeal nerve

B. Posterior View

8.31 EXTERNAL PHARYNX—POSTERIOR VIEWS *(CONTINUED)*

B. Dissection. A large wedge of occipital bone (including the foramen magnum) and the articulated cervical vertebrae have been separated from the remainder (anterior portion) of the head and cervical viscera at the retropharyngeal space and removed.

- The pharynx is a unique portion of the alimentary tract, having a circular layer of muscle externally and a longitudinal layer internally.
- The circular layer of the pharynx consists of the three pharyngeal constrictor muscles (superior, middle, and inferior), which overlap one another.
- On the right side of the specimen, the stylopharyngeus muscle and glossopharyngeal nerve (IX) pass from the medial side of the styloid process anteromedially through the interval between the superior and middle pharyngeal constrictor muscles to become part of the internal longitudinal layer. The stylohyoid muscle passes from the lateral side of the styloid process anterolaterally and splits on its way to the hyoid bone to accommodate passage of the intermediate tendon of the digastric.
- Pharyngeal branches of the glossopharyngeal nerve (CN IX) and the vagus nerve (CN X) form the pharyngeal plexus, which provides most of the pharyngeal innervation. The glossopharyngeal nerve supplies the sensory component, while the vagus supplies motor innervation.

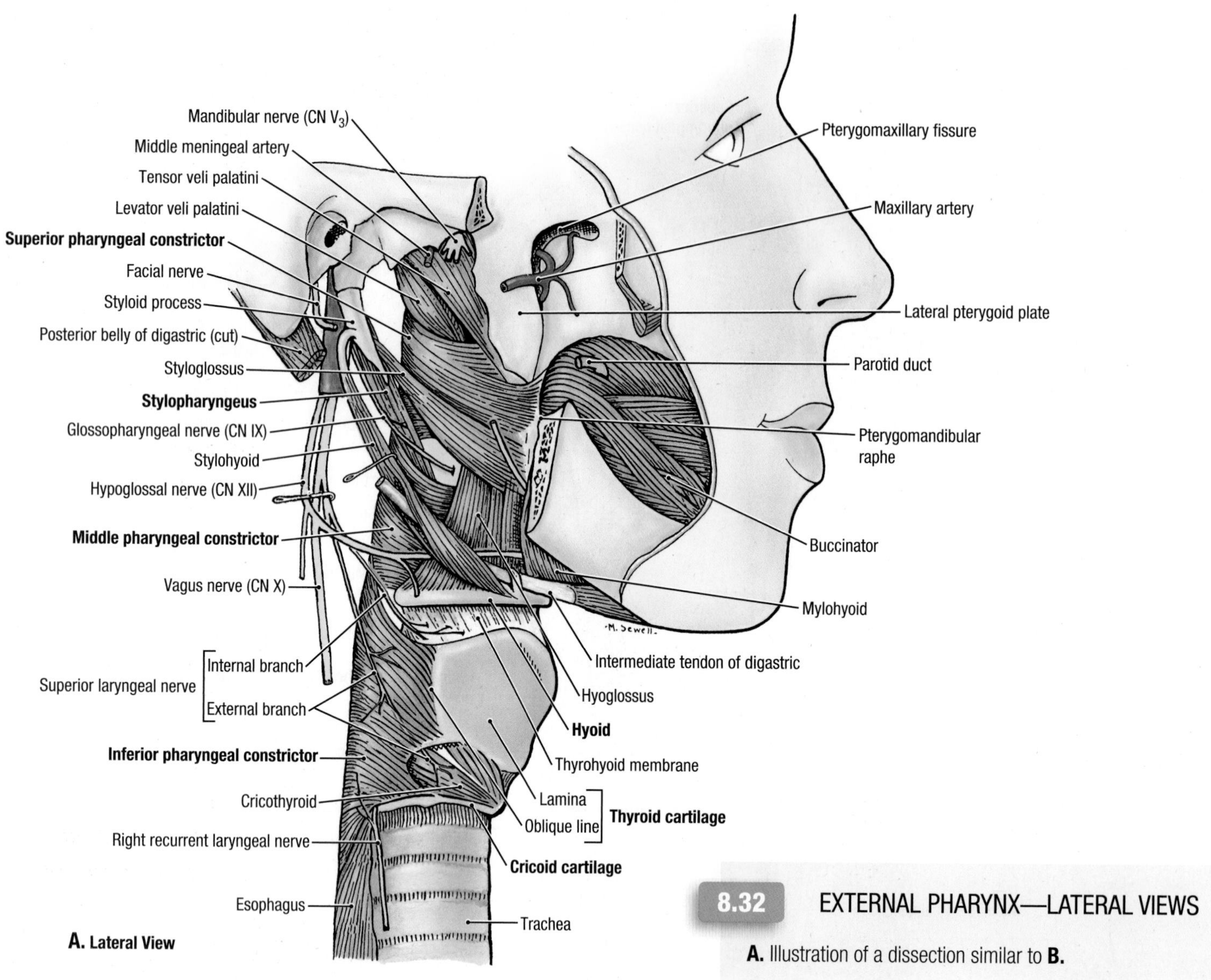

Mandibular nerve (CN V_3)
Middle meningeal artery
Tensor veli palatini
Levator veli palatini
Superior pharyngeal constrictor
Facial nerve
Styloid process
Posterior belly of digastric (cut)
Styloglossus
Stylopharyngeus
Glossopharyngeal nerve (CN IX)
Stylohyoid
Hypoglossal nerve (CN XII)
Middle pharyngeal constrictor
Vagus nerve (CN X)
Superior laryngeal nerve
Internal branch
External branch
Inferior pharyngeal constrictor
Cricothyroid
Right recurrent laryngeal nerve
Esophagus
Pterygomaxillary fissure
Maxillary artery
Lateral pterygoid plate
Parotid duct
Pterygomandibular raphe
Buccinator
Mylohyoid
M. Sewell
Intermediate tendon of digastric
Hyoglossus
Hyoid
Thyrohyoid membrane
Lamina
Oblique line
Thyroid cartilage
Cricoid cartilage
Trachea

A. Lateral View

8.32 EXTERNAL PHARYNX—LATERAL VIEWS

A. Illustration of a dissection similar to **B.**

TABLE 8.9 MUSCLES OF PHARYNX

Muscle	Origin	Insertion	Innervation	Main Action(s)
Superior pharyngeal constrictor	Pterygoid hamulus, pterygo-mandibular raphe, posterior end of mylohyoid line of mandible, and side of tongue			
Middle pharyngeal constrictor	Stylohyoid ligament and superior (greater) and inferior (lesser) horns of hyoid bone	Pharyngeal raphe	Pharyngeal and superior laryngeal branches of vagus (CN X) through pharyngeal plexus	Constrict wall of pharynx during swallowing
Inferior pharyngeal constrictor	Oblique line of thyroid cartilage			
Thyropharyngeus				
Cricopharyngeus (see Fig. 8.20B)	Side of cricoid cartilage	Contralateral side of cricoid cartilage	Pharyngeal and superior laryngeal branches of vagus (CN X) through pharyngeal plexus + external laryngeal plexus	Serves as superior esophageal sphincter
Palatopharyngeus (see Fig. 8.31B)	Hard palate and palatine aponeurosis	Posterior border of lamina of thyroid cartilage and side of pharynx and esophagus	Pharyngeal and superior laryngeal branches of vagus (CN X) through pharyngeal plexus	
Salpingopharyngeus (see Fig. 8.33B)	Cartilaginous part of pharyngotympanic tube	Blends with palatopharyngeus		Elevate pharynx and larynx during swallowing and speaking
Stylopharyngeus	Styloid process of temporal bone	Posterior and superior borders of thyroid cartilage with palatopharyngeus	Glossopharyngeal nerve (CN IX)	

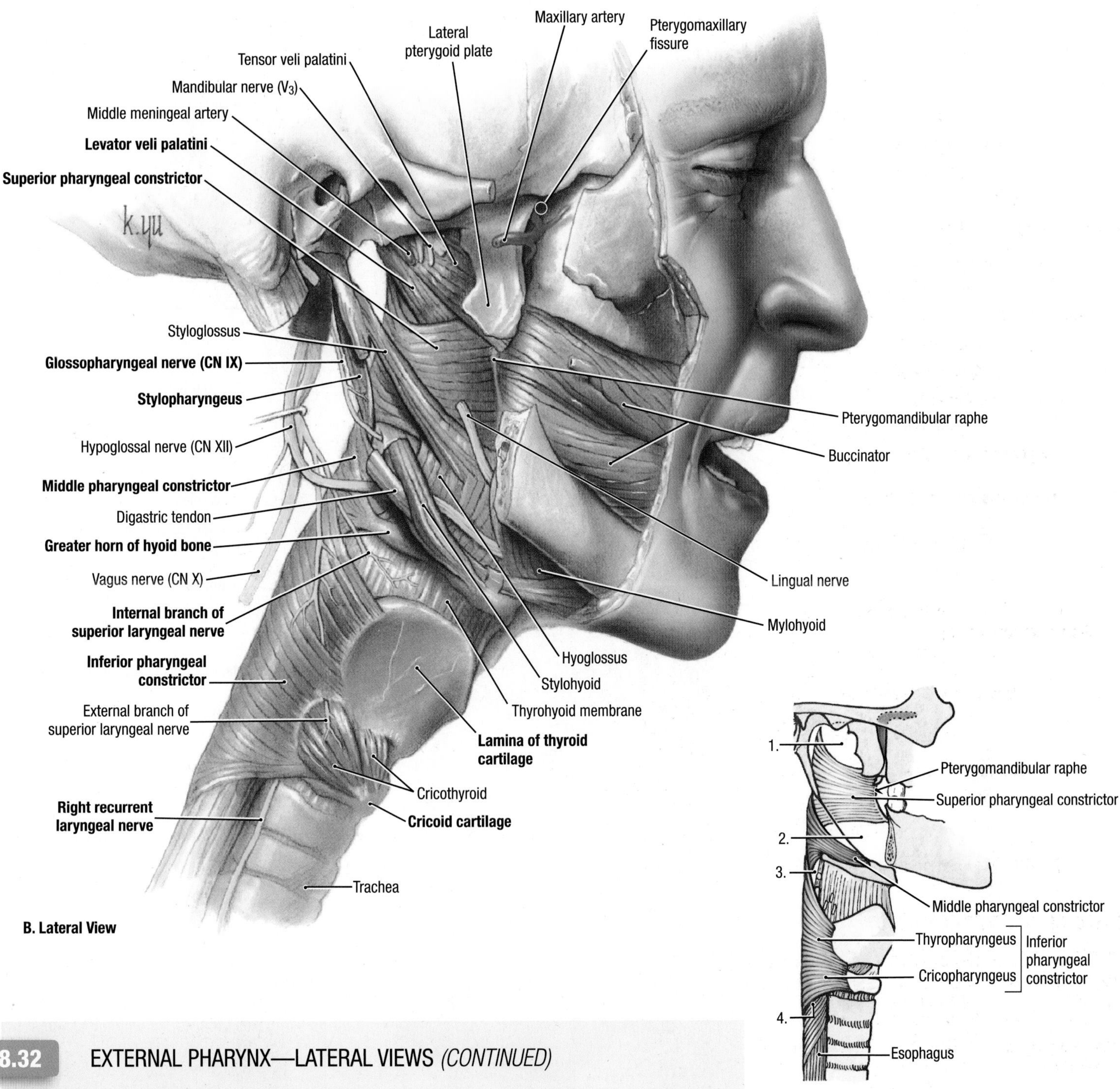
Maxillary artery
Pterygomaxillary fissure
Lateral pterygoid plate
Tensor veli palatini
Mandibular nerve (V_3)
Middle meningeal artery
Levator veli palatini
Superior pharyngeal constrictor
Styloglossus
Glossopharyngeal nerve (CN IX)
Stylopharyngeus
Hypoglossal nerve (CN XII)
Middle pharyngeal constrictor
Digastric tendon
Greater horn of hyoid bone
Vagus nerve (CN X)
Internal branch of superior laryngeal nerve
Inferior pharyngeal constrictor
External branch of superior laryngeal nerve
Right recurrent laryngeal nerve
Trachea
Cricoid cartilage
Cricothyroid
Lamina of thyroid cartilage
Thyrohyoid membrane
Stylohyoid
Hyoglossus
Mylohyoid
Lingual nerve
Buccinator
Pterygomandibular raphe
1.
2.
3.
4.
Pterygomandibular raphe
Superior pharyngeal constrictor
Middle pharyngeal constrictor
Thyropharyngeus
Cricopharyngeus
Inferior pharyngeal constrictor
Esophagus

B. Lateral View

C. Lateral View

8.32 EXTERNAL PHARYNX—LATERAL VIEWS *(CONTINUED)*

B. Dissection. **C. and D.** Observe that there are gaps in the pharyngeal musculature (1-4 in **D**) allowing the entry of structures:

1. Superior to the superior constrictor muscle: levator veli palatini muscle and pharyngotympanic (auditory) tube (see Fig. 8.33B)
2. Between the superior and middle constrictors: stylopharyngeus muscle, CN IX, and stylohyoid ligament
3. Between the middle and inferior constrictors: internal branch of superior laryngeal nerve and superior laryngeal artery and nerve (not shown)
4. Inferior to the inferior constrictor muscle: recurrent laryngeal nerve

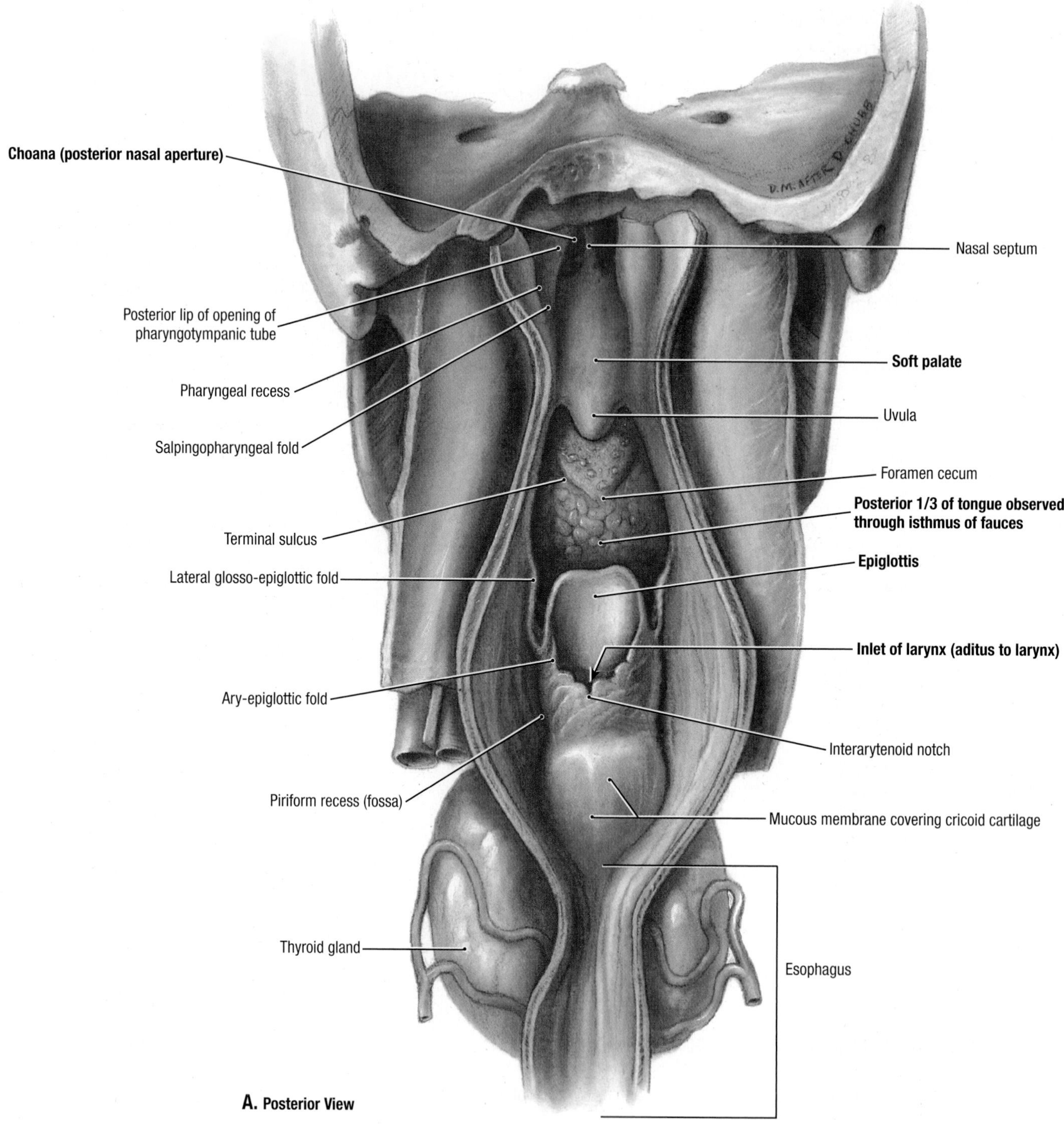

Choana (posterior nasal aperture)
Nasal septum
Posterior lip of opening of pharyngotympanic tube
Pharyngeal recess
Salpingopharyngeal fold
Soft palate
Uvula
Foramen cecum
Posterior 1/3 of tongue observed through isthmus of fauces
Terminal sulcus
Lateral glosso-epiglottic fold
Epiglottis
Inlet of larynx (aditus to larynx)
Ary-epiglottic fold
Interarytenoid notch
Piriform recess (fossa)
Mucous membrane covering cricoid cartilage
Thyroid gland
Esophagus

A. Posterior View

8.33 INTERNAL PHARYNX I

A. Dissection. The posterior wall of the pharynx has been split in the midline and the halves retracted laterally to reveal the internal aspect of the anterior wall of the pharynx, occupied by communications that define three parts of the pharynx: (1) the nasal part (nasopharynx), superior to the level of the soft palate, communicates anteriorly through the choanae with the nasal cavities; (2) the oral part (oropharynx), between the soft palate and the epiglottis, communicates anteriorly through the isthmus of the fauces with the oral cavity; and (3) the laryngeal part (laryngopharynx), posterior to the larynx, communicates with the vestibule of the larynx through the inlet of (aditus to) the larynx. The pharynx extends from the cranial base to the inferior border of the cricoid cartilage. Inferiorly, it is narrowed by the encircling cricopharyngeus.

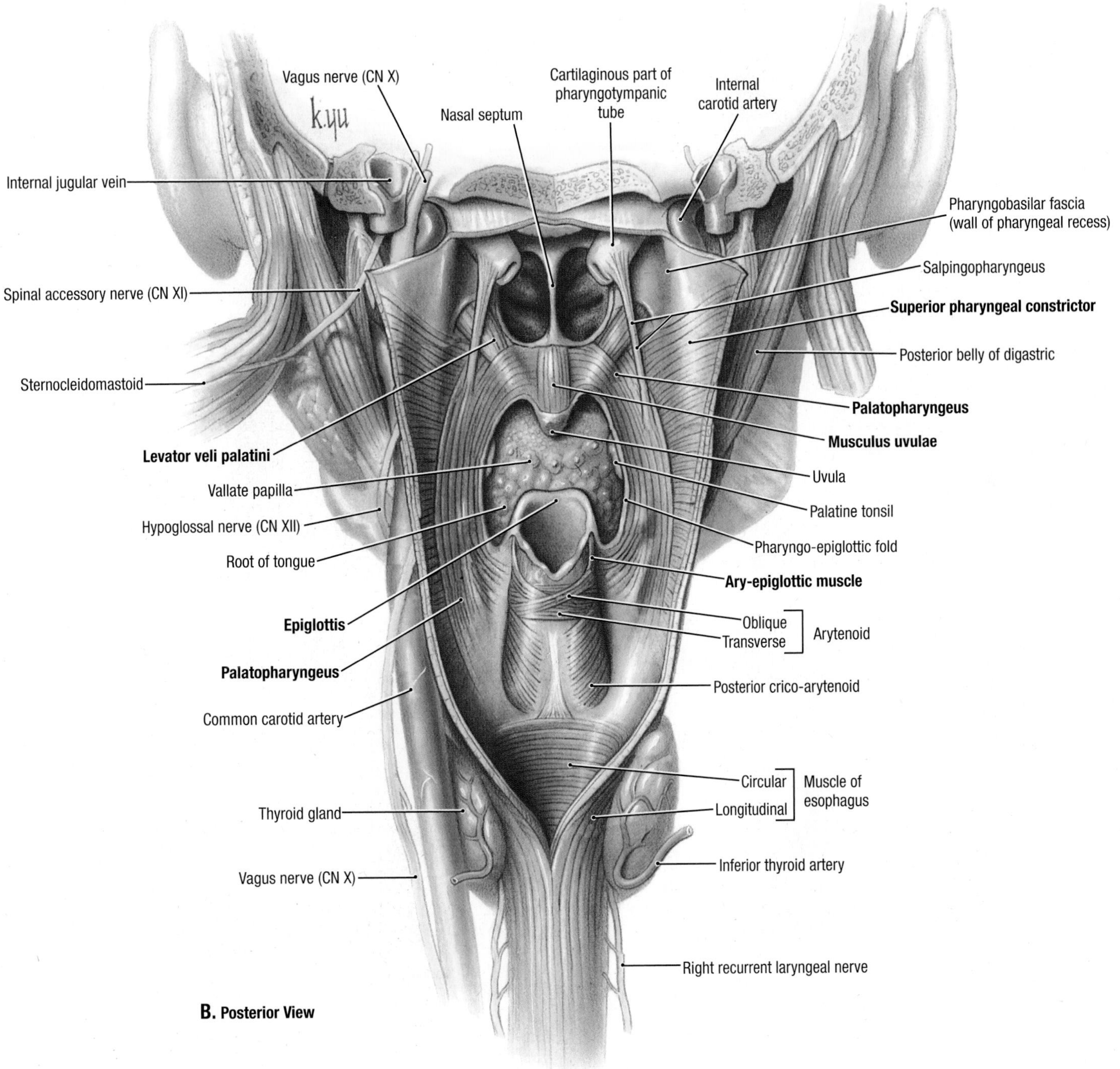

Vagus nerve (CN X)
k.yu
Nasal septum
Cartilaginous part of pharyngotympanic tube
Internal carotid artery
Internal jugular vein
Pharyngobasilar fascia (wall of pharyngeal recess)
Salpingopharyngeus
Spinal accessory nerve (CN XI)
Superior pharyngeal constrictor
Posterior belly of digastric
Sternocleidomastoid
Palatopharyngeus
Musculus uvulae
Levator veli palatini
Uvula
Vallate papilla
Palatine tonsil
Hypoglossal nerve (CN XII)
Pharyngo-epiglottic fold
Root of tongue
Ary-epiglottic muscle
Epiglottis
Oblique
Transverse
Arytenoid
Palatopharyngeus
Posterior crico-arytenoid
Common carotid artery
Circular
Longitudinal
Muscle of esophagus
Thyroid gland
Inferior thyroid artery
Vagus nerve (CN X)
Right recurrent laryngeal nerve

B. **Posterior View**

8.33 INTERNAL PHARYNX II

B. Illustration. The posterior wall of the pharynx has been split in the midline and reflected laterally as in **A;** then, the mucous membrane was removed to expose the underlying musculature. The muscles of the soft palate, pharynx, and larynx work together during swallowing, elevating the soft palate, narrowing the pharyngeal isthmus (passageway between the nasal and oral parts of the pharynx) and laryngeal inlet, retracting the epiglottis, and closing the glottis, to keep food and drink out of the nasopharynx and larynx as they pass from oral cavity to esophagus. At other times, as when blowing one's nose, the palatopharyngeus muscles, partially encircling the opening to the oral cavity, constrict this opening and depress the soft palate, working with placement and expansion of the posterior tongue to direct expired air through the nasal cavity.

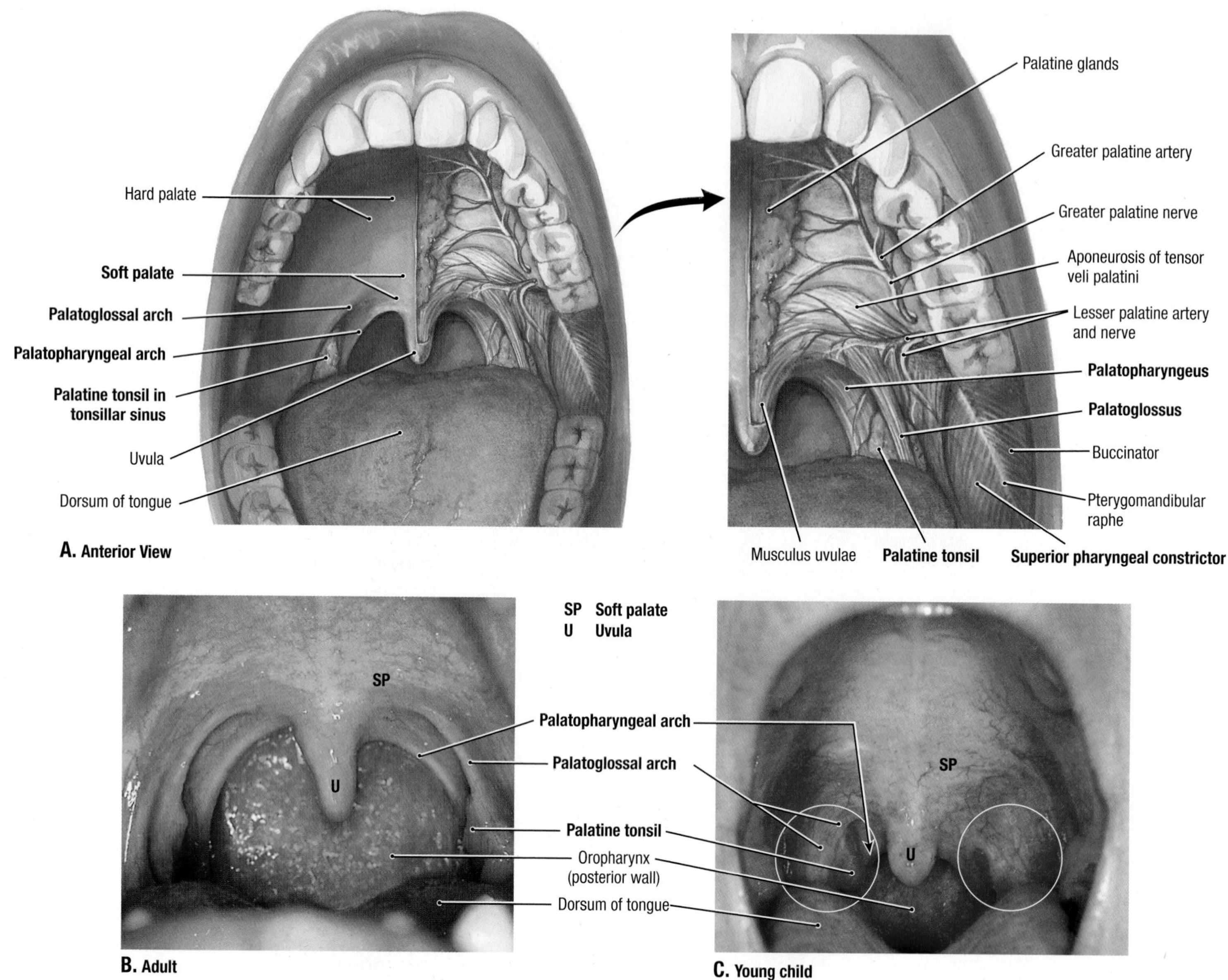

Hard palate
Soft palate
Palatoglossal arch
Palatopharyngeal arch
Palatine tonsil in tonsillar sinus
Uvula
Dorsum of tongue
A. Anterior View
Palatine glands
Greater palatine artery
Greater palatine nerve
Aponeurosis of tensor veli palatini
Lesser palatine artery and nerve
Palatopharyngeus
Palatoglossus
Buccinator
Pterygomandibular raphe
Musculus uvulae
Palatine tonsil
Superior pharyngeal constrictor
SP Soft palate
U Uvula
SP
U
Palatopharyngeal arch
Palatoglossal arch
Palatine tonsil
Oropharynx (posterior wall)
Dorsum of tongue
B. Adult
C. Young child

8.34 SURFACE ANATOMY OF ISTHMUS OF THE FAUCES (OROPHARYNGEAL ISTHMUS)

A. Oral cavity and isthmus demonstrating the sinus (bed) of the tonsils. **B. and C.** Tonsillar sinuses with palatine tonsils in situ, and oropharynx in adult **(B)** and young child (**C**).

- The fauces (throat), the passage from the mouth to the pharynx, is bounded superiorly by the soft palate, inferiorly by the root (base) of the tongue, and laterally by the palatoglossal and palatopharyngeal arches.
- The palatine tonsils are located between the palatoglossal and palatopharyngeal arches, formed by mucosa overlying the similarly named muscles; the arches form the boundaries, and the superior pharyngeal constrictor the floor, of the tonsillar sinuses.
- **Normal palatine tonsils.** In the adult the palatine tonsils are normally involuted, with little glandular tissue in the tonsillar sinuses (B). In contrast in young children the palatine tonsils are large relative to the adult, since most of the development of the lymphoid system occurs prior to puberty. Despite their large size, as long as the tonsils are not inflamed and not interfering with swallowing/breathing they are considered normal.

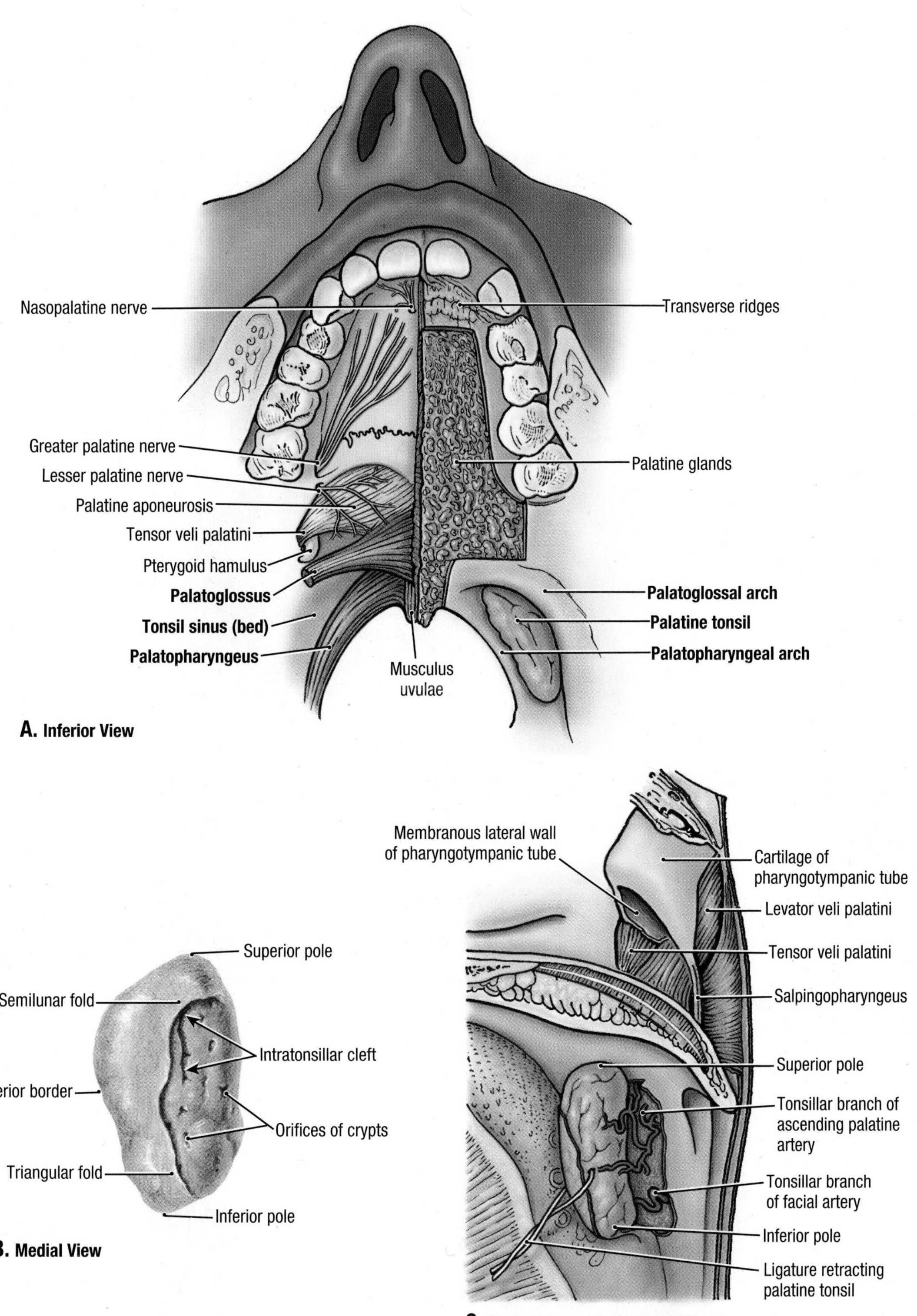
Nasopalatine nerve
Transverse ridges
Greater palatine nerve
Lesser palatine nerve
Palatine aponeurosis
Tensor veli palatini
Pterygoid hamulus
Palatoglossus
Tonsil sinus (bed)
Palatopharyngeus
Palatine glands
Palatoglossal arch
Palatine tonsil
Palatopharyngeal arch
Musculus uvulae
A. Inferior View
Superior pole
Semilunar fold
Intratonsillar cleft
Anterior border
Orifices of crypts
Triangular fold
Inferior pole
B. Medial View
Membranous lateral wall of pharyngotympanic tube
Cartilage of pharyngotympanic tube
Levator veli palatini
Tensor veli palatini
Salpingopharyngeus
Superior pole
Tonsillar branch of ascending palatine artery
Tonsillar branch of facial artery
Inferior pole
Ligature retracting palatine tonsil
C. Medial View of Right Half of Head

8.35 PALATINE TONSIL

A. Left side: Palatine tonsil in situ and glands of palatine mucosa. Right side: Palatine mucosa and tonsils removed demonstrating palatine nerves and muscles. **B.** Isolated palatine tonsil. **C. Tonsillectomy.** The procedure involves removal of the tonsil and the fascial sheet covering the tonsillar sinus. Because of the rich blood supply of the tonsil, bleeding commonly arises from the large external palatine vein or less commonly from the tonsillar artery or other arterial twigs. The glossopharyngeal nerve accompanies the tonsillar artery on the lateral wall of the pharynx and is vulnerable to injury because this wall is thin. The internal carotid artery is especially vulnerable when it is tortuous, as it lies directly lateral to the tonsil.

Middle nasal concha
Inferior nasal concha
Opening of pharyngotympanic tube
Palatine bone (bony palate)
Palatine glands
Palatoglossal arch
Tonsillar fossa
Dorsum of tongue
Pharyngeal tonsil
Torus tubarius
Torus levatorius (ridge of levator veli palatini)
Pharyngeal recess
Salpingopharyngeal fold
Soft palate
Uvula
Palatopharyngeal arch
Vallate papillae
Lingual follicles
Epiglottis

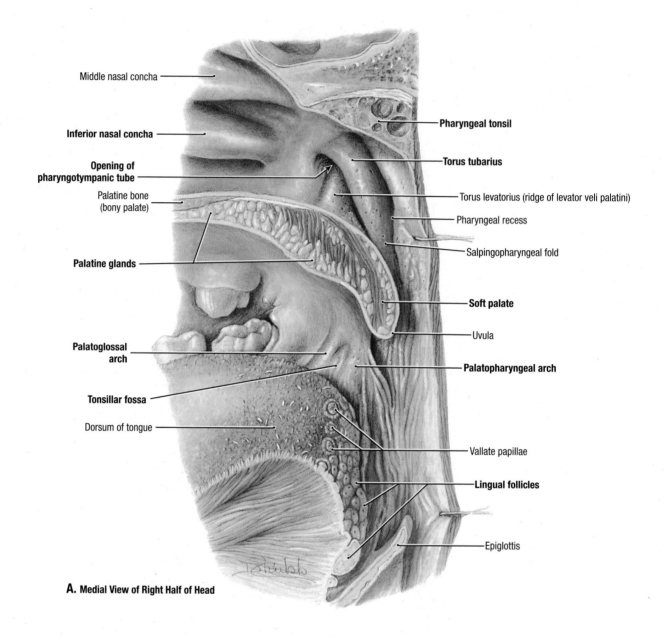

A. Medial View of Right Half of Head

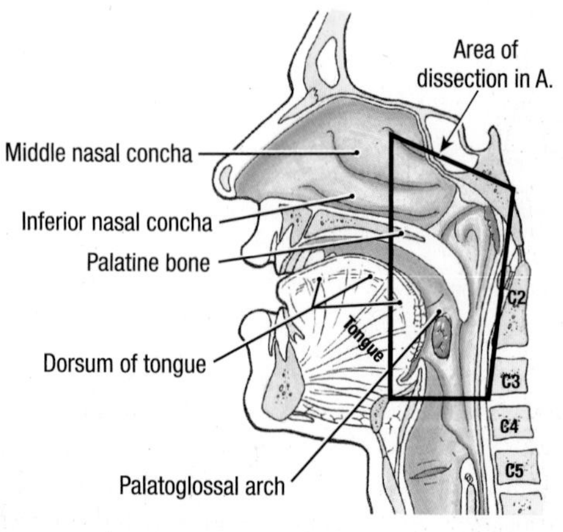
Area of dissection in A.
Middle nasal concha
Inferior nasal concha
Palatine bone
Dorsum of tongue
Palatoglossal arch
Tongue
C2
C3
C4
C5

8.36 SERIAL DISSECTION OF ISTHMUS OF FAUCES AND LATERAL WALL OF NASOPHARYNX I

- The pharyngeal opening of the pharyngotympanic tube is located approximately 1 cm posterior to the inferior concha.
- The numerous pinpoint orifices of the ducts of the mucous glands can be seen in the mucosa of the torus.
- The pharyngeal tonsil lies in the mucous membrane of the roof and posterior wall of the nasopharynx.
- The palatine glands lie in the soft palate.
- The palatine tonsil lies in the tonsillar sinus between the palatoglossal and palatopharyngeal arches.
- Each lingual follicle has the duct of a mucous gland opening onto its surface; collectively, the follicles are known as the lingual tonsil.

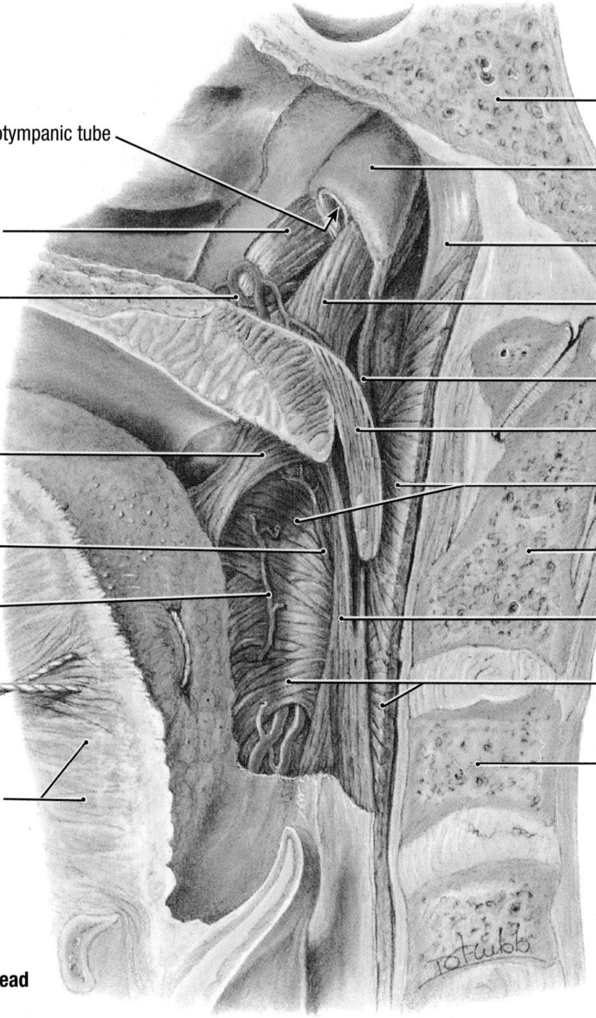

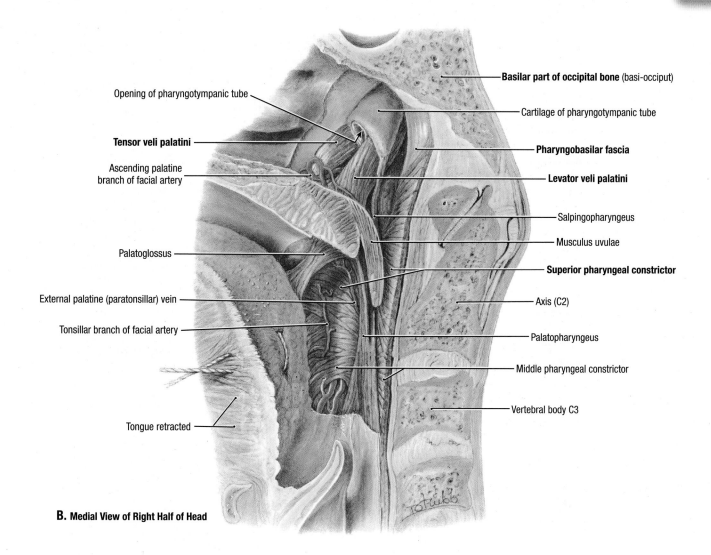

Basilar part of occipital bone (basi-occiput)
Opening of pharyngotympanic tube
Cartilage of pharyngotympanic tube
Tensor veli palatini
Pharyngobasilar fascia
Ascending palatine branch of facial artery
Levator veli palatini
Salpingopharyngeus
Musculus uvulae
Palatoglossus
Superior pharyngeal constrictor
External palatine (paratonsillar) vein
Axis (C2)
Tonsillar branch of facial artery
Palatopharyngeus
Middle pharyngeal constrictor
Vertebral body C3
Tongue retracted

B. Medial View of Right Half of Head

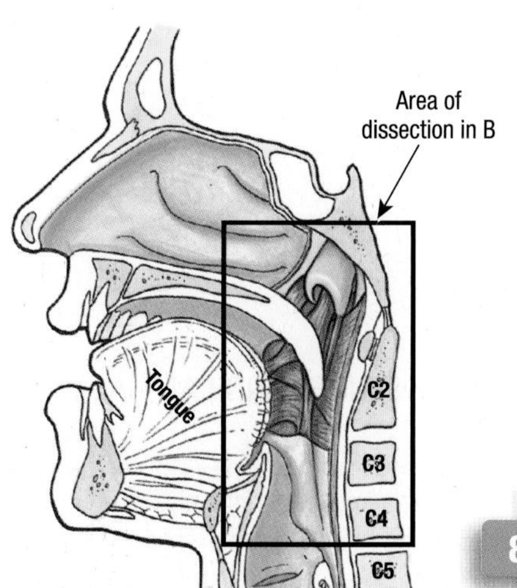
Area of dissection in B
Tongue
C2
C3
C4
C5

8.36 SERIAL DISSECTION OF ISTHMUS OF FAUCES AND LATERAL WALL OF NASOPHARYNX II

Muscles underlying tonsillar sinus and wall of nasopharynx. The palatine and pharyngeal tonsils and mucous membrane have been removed. The pharyngobasilar fascia, which attaches the pharynx to the basilar part of the occipital bone was also removed, except at the superior, arched border of the superior pharyngeal constrictor.

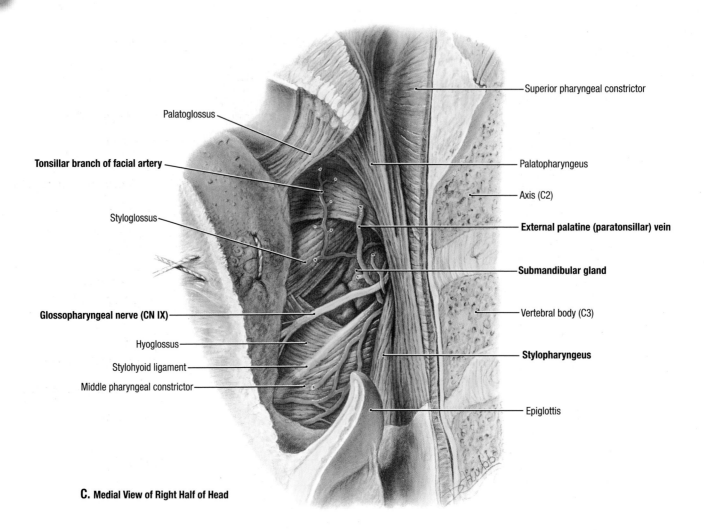

Superior pharyngeal constrictor
Palatoglossus
Tonsillar branch of facial artery
Palatopharyngeus
Axis (C2)
Styloglossus
External palatine (paratonsillar) vein
Submandibular gland
Glossopharyngeal nerve (CN IX)
Vertebral body (C3)
Hyoglossus
Stylopharyngeus
Stylohyoid ligament
Middle pharyngeal constrictor
Epiglottis

C. Medial View of Right Half of Head

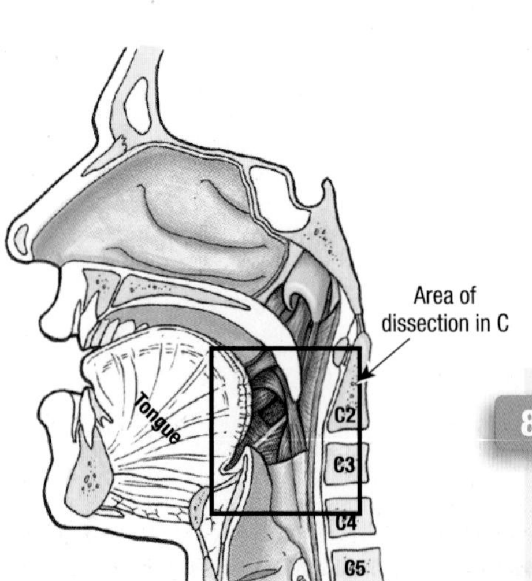
Area of dissection in C
Tongue
C2
C3
C4
C5

8.36 SERIAL DISSECTION OF ISTHMUS OF FAUCES AND LATERAL WALL OF NASOPHARYNX III

Neurovascular structures of tonsillar sinus and longitudinal muscles of the pharynx.

- In this deeper dissection, the tongue was pulled anteriorly, and the inferior part of the origin of the superior pharyngeal constrictor muscle was cut away.
- The glossopharyngeal nerve passes to the posterior one third of the tongue and lies anterior to the stylopharyngeus muscle.
- The tonsillar branch of the facial artery sends a branch (cut short here) to accompany the glossopharyngeal nerve to the tongue; the submandibular gland is seen lateral to the artery and external palatine (paratonsillar) vein.

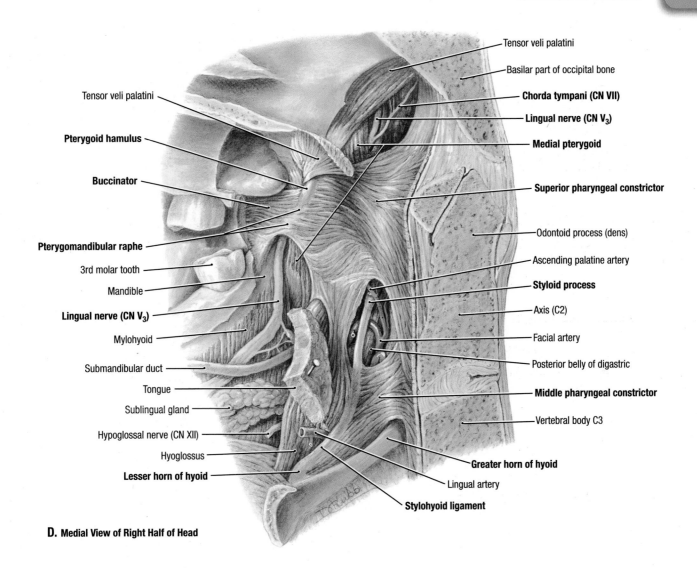

Tensor veli palatini
Basilar part of occipital bone
Tensor veli palatini
Chorda tympani (CN VII)
Pterygoid hamulus
Lingual nerve (CN V_3)
Medial pterygoid
Buccinator
Superior pharyngeal constrictor
Odontoid process (dens)
Pterygomandibular raphe
Ascending palatine artery
3rd molar tooth
Styloid process
Mandible
Axis (C2)
Lingual nerve (CN V_3)
Mylohyoid
Facial artery
Submandibular duct
Posterior belly of digastric
Tongue
Middle pharyngeal constrictor
Sublingual gland
Vertebral body C3
Hypoglossal nerve (CN XII)
Hyoglossus
Greater horn of hyoid
Lesser horn of hyoid
Lingual artery
Stylohyoid ligament

D. Medial View of Right Half of Head

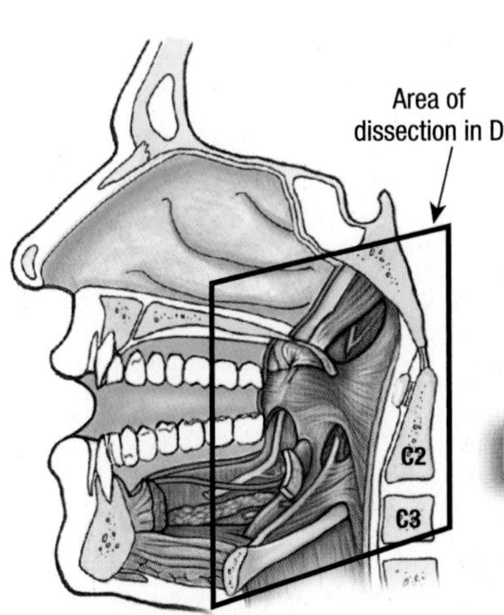
Area of dissection in D
C2
C3

8.36 SERIAL DISSECTION OF ISTHMUS OF FAUCES AND LATERAL WALL OF NASOPHARYNX IV

- The superior pharyngeal constrictor muscle arises from (1) the pterygomandibular raphe, which unites it to the buccinator muscle; (2) the bones at each end of the raphe, the hamulus of the medial pterygoid plate superiorly and the mandible inferiorly; and (3) the root (posterior part) of the tongue.
- The middle pharyngeal constrictor muscle arises from the angle formed by the greater and lesser horns of the hyoid bone and from the stylohyoid ligament; in this specimen, the styloid process is long and, therefore, a lateral relation of the tonsil.
- The lingual nerve is joined by the chorda tympani, disappears at the posterior border of the medial pterygoid muscle, and reappears at the anterior border to follow the mandible.

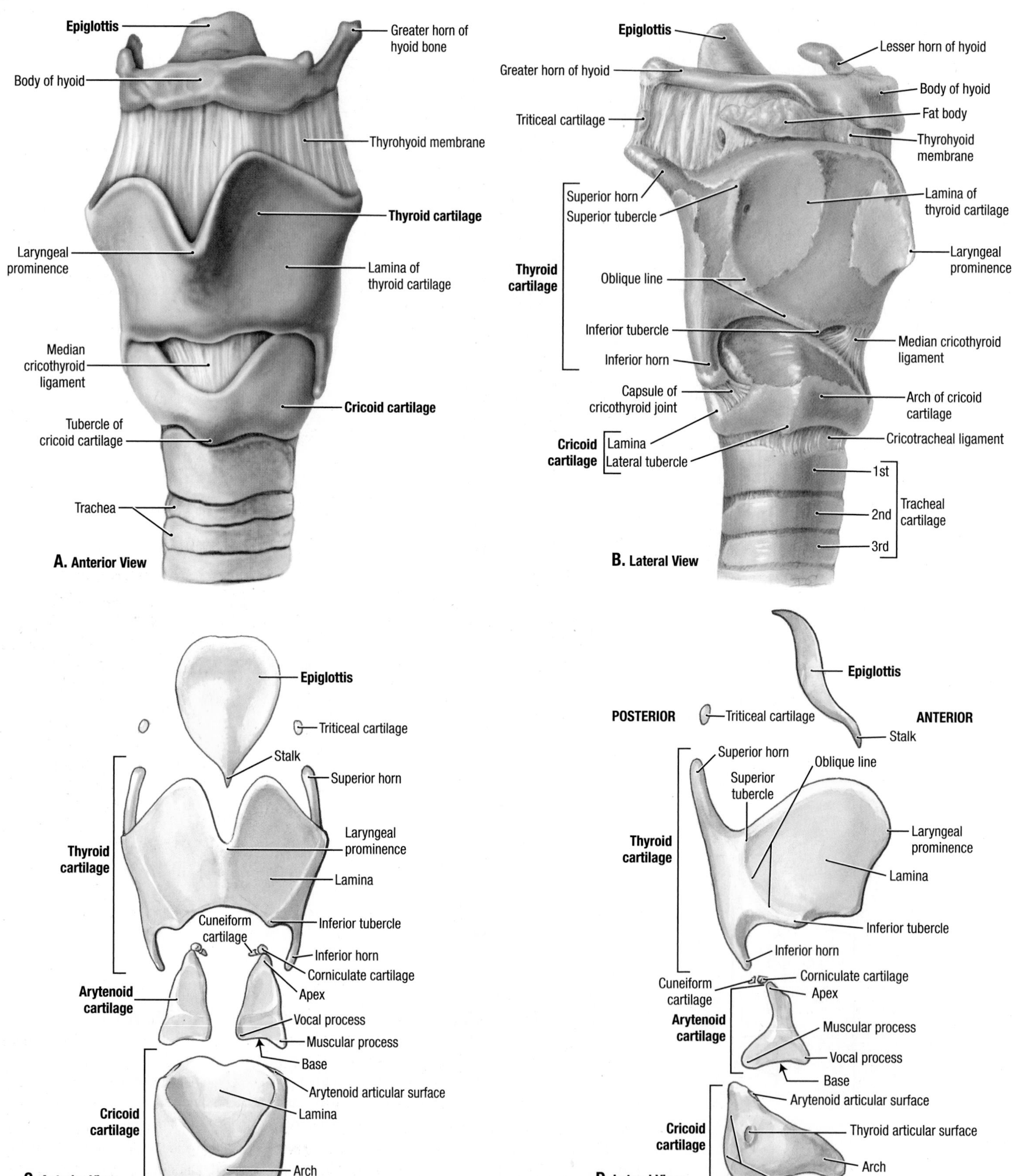
Epiglottis
Greater horn of hyoid bone
Body of hyoid
Thyrohyoid membrane
Thyroid cartilage
Laryngeal prominence
Lamina of thyroid cartilage
Median cricothyroid ligament
Cricoid cartilage
Tubercle of cricoid cartilage
Trachea
A. Anterior View
Epiglottis
Lesser horn of hyoid
Greater horn of hyoid
Body of hyoid
Fat body
Triticeal cartilage
Thyrohyoid membrane
Superior horn
Superior tubercle
Lamina of thyroid cartilage
Thyroid cartilage
Laryngeal prominence
Oblique line
Inferior tubercle
Median cricothyroid ligament
Inferior horn
Capsule of cricothyroid joint
Arch of cricoid cartilage
Cricoid cartilage
Lamina
Lateral tubercle
Cricotracheal ligament
1st
2nd
3rd
Tracheal cartilage
B. Lateral View
Epiglottis
Triticeal cartilage
Stalk
Superior horn
Laryngeal prominence
Thyroid cartilage
Lamina
Inferior tubercle
Cuneiform cartilage
Inferior horn
Corniculate cartilage
Apex
Arytenoid cartilage
Vocal process
Muscular process
Base
Arytenoid articular surface
Cricoid cartilage
Lamina
Arch
C. Anterior View
Epiglottis
POSTERIOR
Triticeal cartilage
ANTERIOR
Stalk
Superior horn
Oblique line
Superior tubercle
Laryngeal prominence
Thyroid cartilage
Lamina
Inferior tubercle
Inferior horn
Cuneiform cartilage
Corniculate cartilage
Apex
Arytenoid cartilage
Muscular process
Vocal process
Base
Arytenoid articular surface
Cricoid cartilage
Thyroid articular surface
Arch
Lamina
D. Lateral View

8.37 CARTILAGES OF LARYNGEAL SKELETON

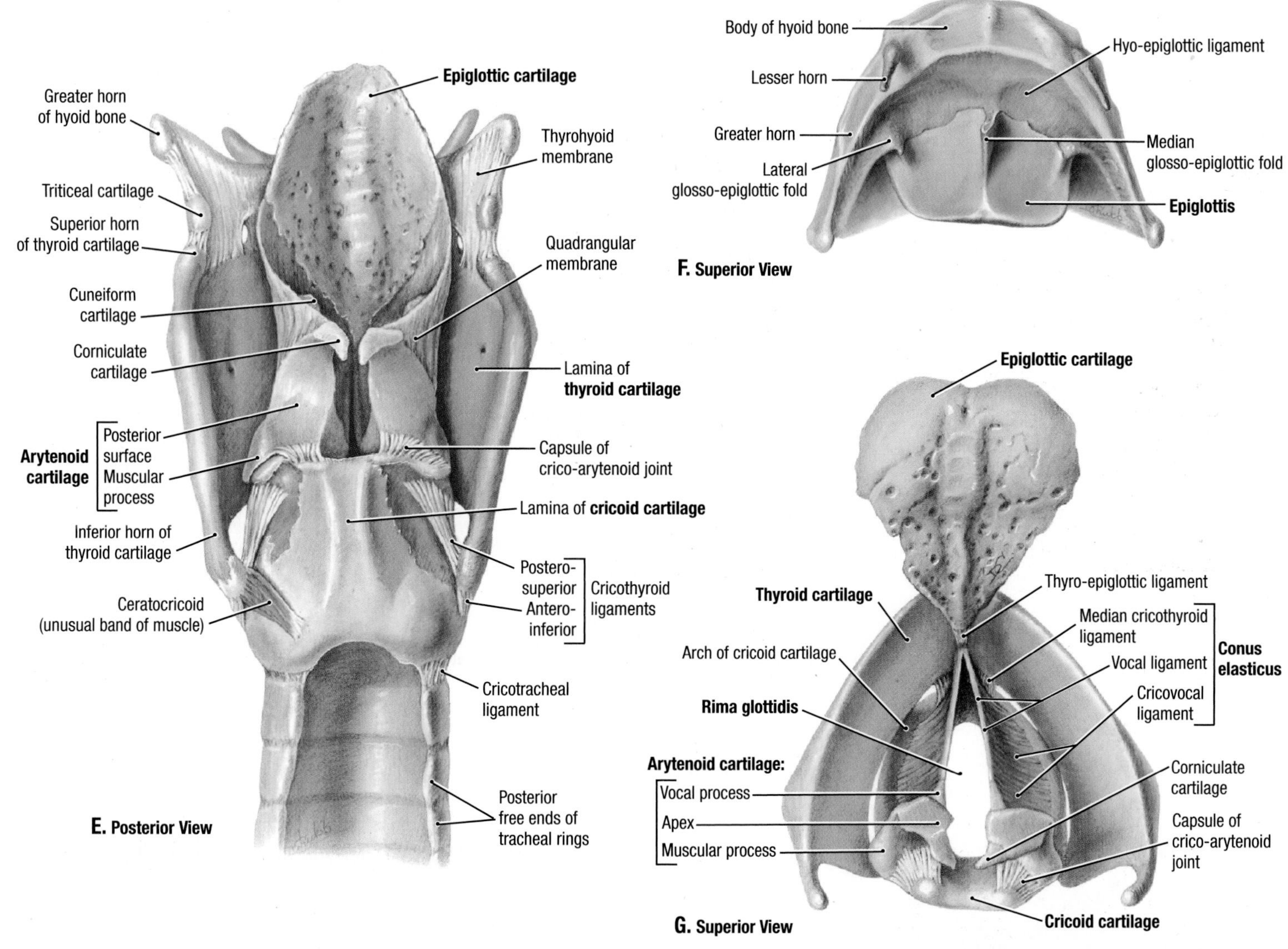
Epiglottic cartilage
Greater horn of hyoid bone
Thyrohyoid membrane
Triticeal cartilage
Superior horn of thyroid cartilage
Quadrangular membrane
Cuneiform cartilage
Corniculate cartilage
Lamina of thyroid cartilage
Arytenoid cartilage
Posterior surface
Muscular process
Capsule of crico-arytenoid joint
Lamina of cricoid cartilage
Inferior horn of thyroid cartilage
Postero-superior
Antero-inferior
Cricothyroid ligaments
Ceratocricoid (unusual band of muscle)
Cricotracheal ligament
Posterior free ends of tracheal rings
E. Posterior View
Body of hyoid bone
Hyo-epiglottic ligament
Lesser horn
Greater horn
Median glosso-epiglottic fold
Lateral glosso-epiglottic fold
Epiglottis
F. Superior View
Epiglottic cartilage
Thyroid cartilage
Thyro-epiglottic ligament
Median cricothyroid ligament
Arch of cricoid cartilage
Vocal ligament
Conus elasticus
Cricovocal ligament
Rima glottidis
Arytenoid cartilage:
Vocal process
Apex
Muscular process
Corniculate cartilage
Capsule of crico-arytenoid joint
Cricoid cartilage
G. Superior View

8.37 CARTILAGES OF THE LARYNGEAL SKELETON *(CONTINUED)*

A., B. and E. Articulated laryngeal skeleton. **C. and D.** Cartilages disarticulated and separated. **F.** Epiglottis and hyo-epiglottic ligament. **G.** Conus elasticus and rima glottidis.

- The larynx extends vertically from the tip of the epiglottis to the inferior border of the cricoid cartilage. The hyoid bone is generally not regarded as part of the larynx.
- The cricoid cartilage is the only cartilage that totally encircles the airway.
- The rima glottidis is the aperture between the vocal folds. During normal respiration, it is narrow and wedge shaped; during forced respiration, it is wide. Variations in the tension and length of the vocal folds, in the width of the rima glottidis, and in the intensity of the expiratory effort produce changes in the pitch of the voice.
- **Laryngeal fractures** may result from blows received in sports such as kickboxing and hockey or from compression by a shoulder strap during an automobile accident. Laryngeal fractures produce submucous hemorrhage and edema, respiratory obstruction, hoarseness, and sometimes a temporary inability to speak. The thyroid, cricoid, and most of the arytenoid cartilages often ossify as age advances, commencing at approximately 25 years of age in the thyroid cartilage.

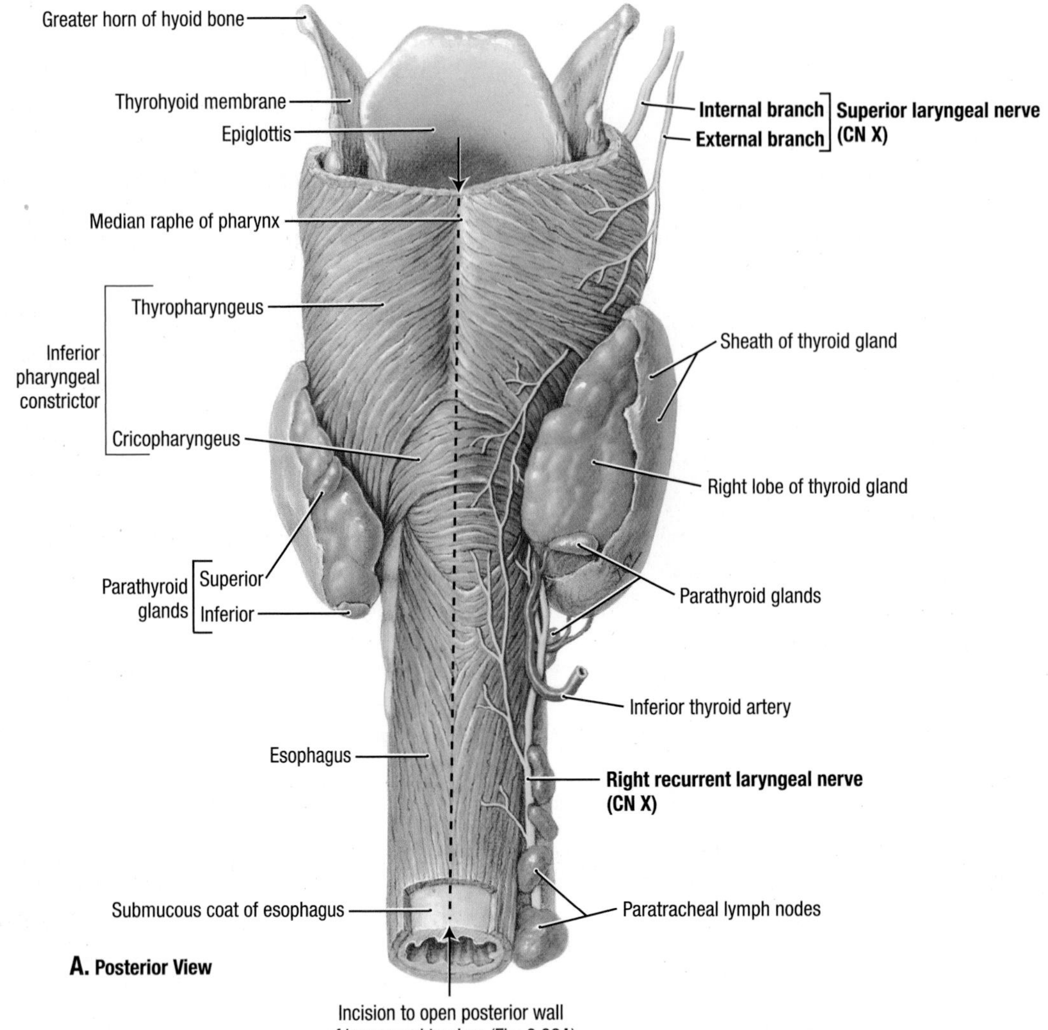
Greater horn of hyoid bone
Thyrohyoid membrane
Epiglottis
Internal branch
External branch
Superior laryngeal nerve (CN X)
Median raphe of pharynx
Thyropharyngeus
Inferior pharyngeal constrictor
Cricopharyngeus
Sheath of thyroid gland
Right lobe of thyroid gland
Parathyroid glands
Superior
Inferior
Parathyroid glands
Inferior thyroid artery
Esophagus
Right recurrent laryngeal nerve (CN X)
Submucous coat of esophagus
Paratracheal lymph nodes
Incision to open posterior wall of larynx and trachea (Fig. 8.39A)

A. Posterior View

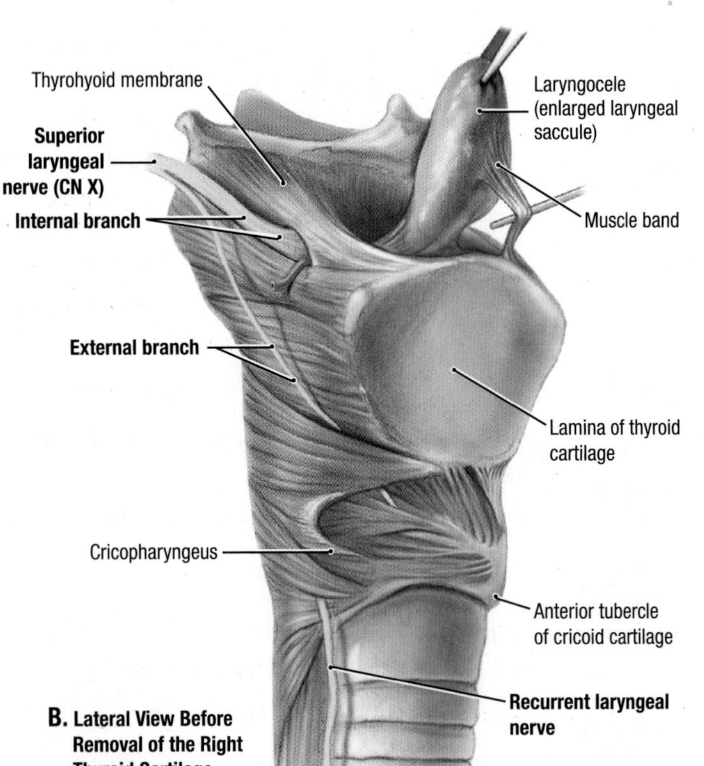
Thyrohyoid membrane
Superior laryngeal nerve (CN X)
Internal branch
Laryngocele (enlarged laryngeal saccule)
Muscle band
External branch
Lamina of thyroid cartilage
Cricopharyngeus
Anterior tubercle of cricoid cartilage
Recurrent laryngeal nerve

B. Lateral View Before Removal of the Right Thyroid Cartilage

8.38 EXTERNAL LARYNX AND LARYNGEAL NERVES

A. Posterior aspect.

- The internal branch of the superior laryngeal nerve innervates the mucous membrane superior to the vocal folds, and the external laryngeal branch supplies the inferior pharyngeal constrictor and cricothyroid muscles.
- The recurrent laryngeal nerve supplies the esophagus, trachea, and inferior pharyngeal constrictor muscle. It supplies sensory innervation inferior to the vocal folds and motor innervation to the intrinsic muscles of the larynx, except the cricothyroid.

B. Laryngocele. A laryngocele (enlarged laryngeal saccule) projects through the thyrohyoid membrane and communicates with the larynx through the ventricle. This air sac can form a bulge in the neck, especially on coughing. The inferior laryngeal nerves are vulnerable to injury during operations in the anterior triangles of the neck. **Injury of the inferior laryngeal nerve** results in paralysis of the vocal fold. The voice is initially poor because the paralyzed fold cannot adduct to meet the normal vocal fold. In a bilateral paralysis, the voice is almost absent. **Injury to the external branch of the superior laryngeal nerve** results in a voice that is monotonous in character because the cricothyroid muscle is unable to vary the tension of the vocal fold. Hoarseness is the most common symptom of serious disorders of the larynx.

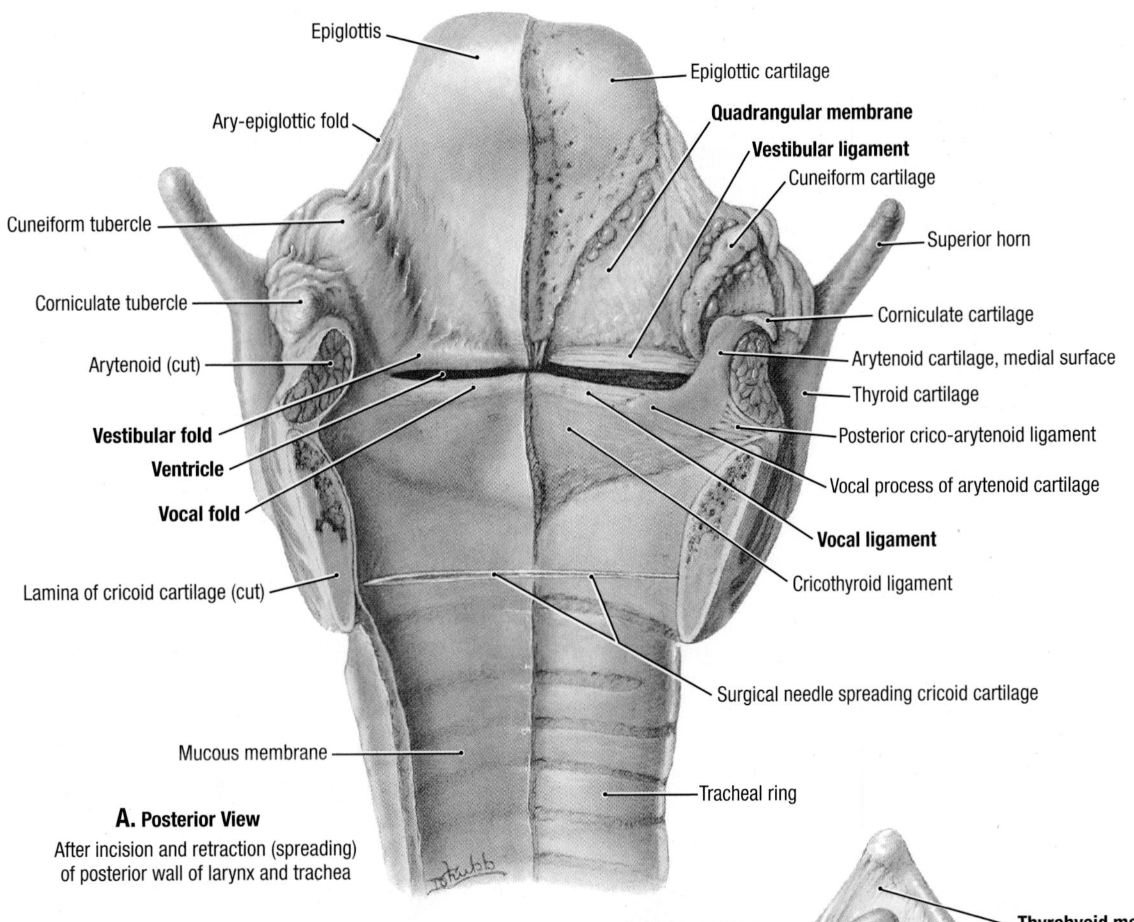
Epiglottis
Epiglottic cartilage
Ary-epiglottic fold
Quadrangular membrane
Vestibular ligament
Cuneiform cartilage
Cuneiform tubercle
Superior horn
Corniculate tubercle
Corniculate cartilage
Arytenoid (cut)
Arytenoid cartilage, medial surface
Thyroid cartilage
Vestibular fold
Posterior crico-arytenoid ligament
Ventricle
Vocal process of arytenoid cartilage
Vocal fold
Vocal ligament
Lamina of cricoid cartilage (cut)
Cricothyroid ligament
Surgical needle spreading cricoid cartilage
Mucous membrane
Tracheal ring

A. Posterior View
After incision and retraction (spreading) of posterior wall of larynx and trachea

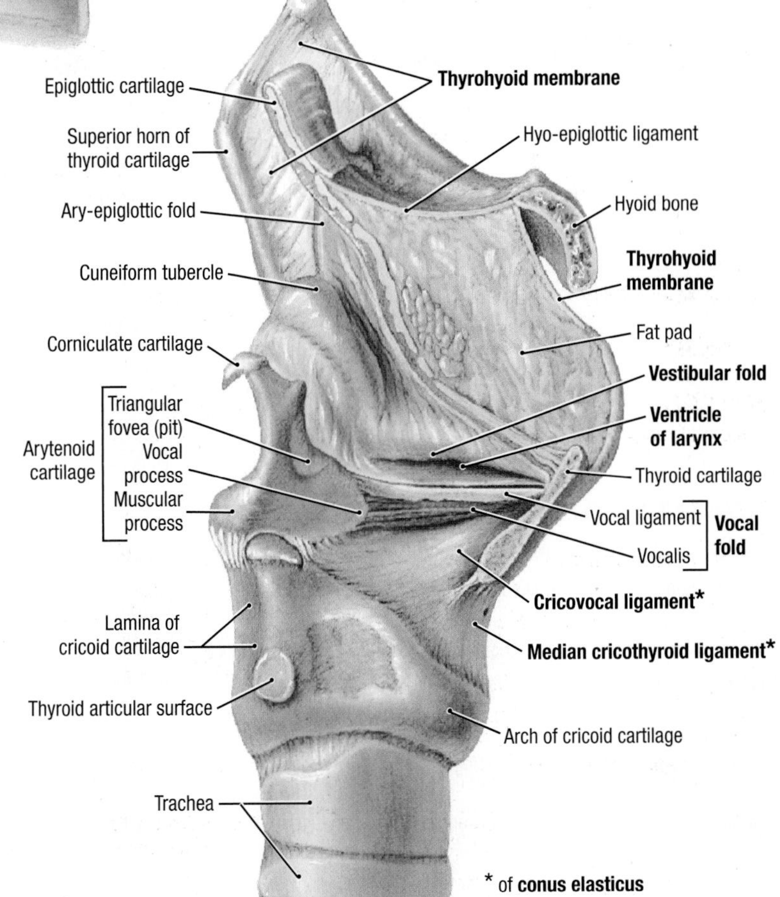
Epiglottic cartilage
Thyrohyoid membrane
Superior horn of thyroid cartilage
Hyo-epiglottic ligament
Ary-epiglottic fold
Hyoid bone
Cuneiform tubercle
Thyrohyoid membrane
Fat pad
Corniculate cartilage
Vestibular fold
Arytenoid cartilage
Triangular fovea (pit)
Vocal process
Muscular process
Ventricle of larynx
Thyroid cartilage
Vocal ligament
Vocalis
Vocal fold
Cricovocal ligament*
Lamina of cricoid cartilage
Median cricothyroid ligament*
Thyroid articular surface
Arch of cricoid cartilage
Trachea
* of conus elasticus

B. Lateral View After Removal of the Right Thyroid Cartilage

8.39 INTERNAL LARYNX

A. The posterior wall of the larynx is split in the median plane (see Fig. 8.29A), and the two sides held apart. On the left side of the specimen, the mucous membrane, which is the innermost coat of the larynx, is intact; on the right side of the specimen, the mucous and submucous coats are peeled off, and the next coat, consisting of cartilages, ligaments, and fibro-elastic membrane, is uncovered.
B. Interior of the larynx superior to the vocal folds. The larynx is sectioned near the median plane to reveal the interior of its left side. Inferior to this level, the right side of the intact larynx is dissected.

- The three compartments of the larynx are (1) the superior compartment of the vestibule, superior to the level of the vestibular folds (false cords); (2) the middle, between the levels of the vestibular and vocal folds; and (3) the inferior, or infraglottic, cavity, inferior to the level of the vocal folds.
- The quadrangular membrane underlies the ary-epiglottic fold superiorly and is thickened inferiorly to form the vestibular ligament. The cricothyroid ligament (conus elasticus) begins inferiorly as the strong median cricothyroid ligament and is thickened superiorly as the vocal ligament. The lateral recess between the vocal and vestibular ligaments, lined with mucous membrane, is the ventricle.

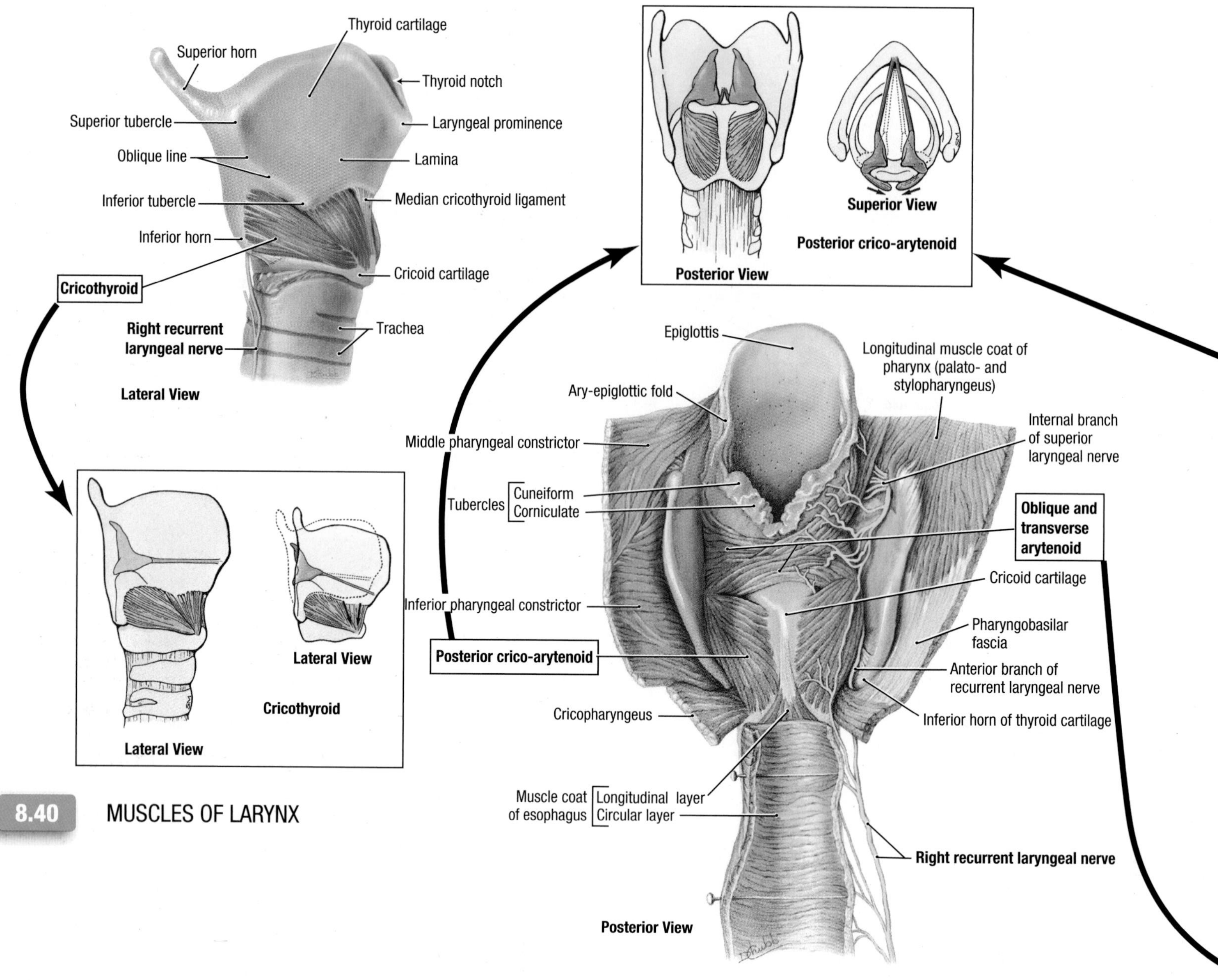
Thyroid cartilage
Superior horn
Thyroid notch
Superior tubercle
Laryngeal prominence
Oblique line
Lamina
Inferior tubercle
Median cricothyroid ligament
Inferior horn
Cricothyroid
Cricoid cartilage
Right recurrent laryngeal nerve
Trachea
Lateral View
Lateral View
Cricothyroid
Lateral View
Superior View
Posterior crico-arytenoid
Posterior View
Epiglottis
Longitudinal muscle coat of pharynx (palato- and stylopharyngeus)
Ary-epiglottic fold
Internal branch of superior laryngeal nerve
Middle pharyngeal constrictor
Tubercles
Cuneiform
Corniculate
Oblique and transverse arytenoid
Cricoid cartilage
Inferior pharyngeal constrictor
Pharyngobasilar fascia
Posterior crico-arytenoid
Anterior branch of recurrent laryngeal nerve
Cricopharyngeus
Inferior horn of thyroid cartilage
Muscle coat of esophagus
Longitudinal layer
Circular layer
Right recurrent laryngeal nerve
Posterior View

8.40 MUSCLES OF LARYNX

TABLE 8.10 MUSCLES OF LARYNX

Muscle	Origin	Insertion	Innervation	Main Action(s)
Cricothyroid	Anterolateral part of cricoid cartilage	Inferior margin and inferior horn of thyroid cartilage	External branch of superior laryngeal nerve (CN X)	Tenses vocal fold
Posterior cricoarytenoid	Posterior surface of laminae of cricoid cartilage	Muscular process of arytenoid cartilage	Recurrent laryngeal nerve (CN X)	Abducts vocal fold
Lateral cricoarytenoid	Arch of cricoid cartilage			Adducts vocal fold
Thyroarytenoid[a]	Posterior surface of thyroid cartilage			Relaxes vocal fold
Transverse and oblique arytenoids[b]	One arytenoid cartilage	Opposite arytenoid cartilage		Close inlet of larynx by approximating arytenoid cartilages
Vocalis[c]	Angle between laminae of thyroid cartilage	Vocal ligament, between origin and vocal process of arytenoid cartilage		Alters vocal fold during phonation

[a]Superior fibers of the thyroarytenoid muscle pass into the aryepiglottic fold, and some of them reach the epiglottic cartilage. These fibers constitute the thyroepiglottic muscle, which widens the inlet of the larynx.
[b]Some fibers of the oblique arytenoid muscle continue as the aryepiglottic muscle.
[c]This slender muscular slip is derived from inferior deeper fibers of the thyroarytenoid muscle.

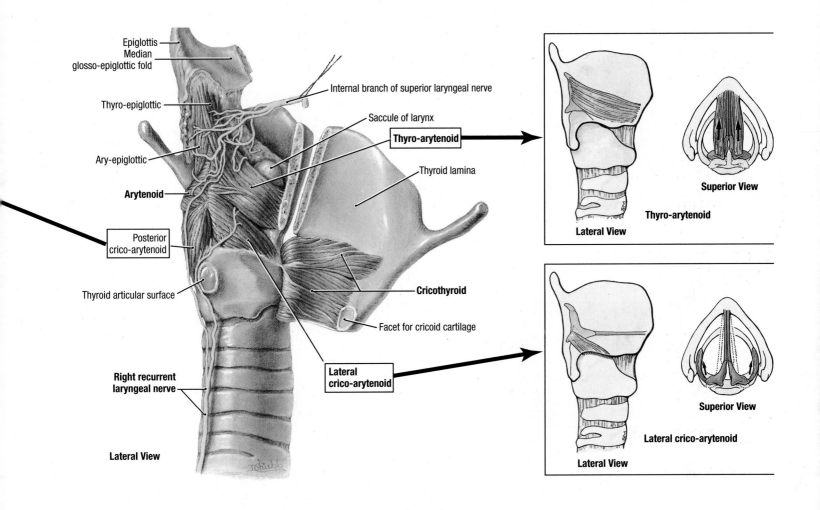

Epiglottis
Median glosso-epiglottic fold
Internal branch of superior laryngeal nerve
Thyro-epiglottic
Saccule of larynx
Thyro-arytenoid
Ary-epiglottic
Thyroid lamina
Arytenoid
Posterior crico-arytenoid
Thyroid articular surface
Cricothyroid
Facet for cricoid cartilage
Lateral crico-arytenoid
Right recurrent laryngeal nerve

Lateral View

Superior View
Thyro-arytenoid
Lateral View

Superior View
Lateral crico-arytenoid
Lateral View

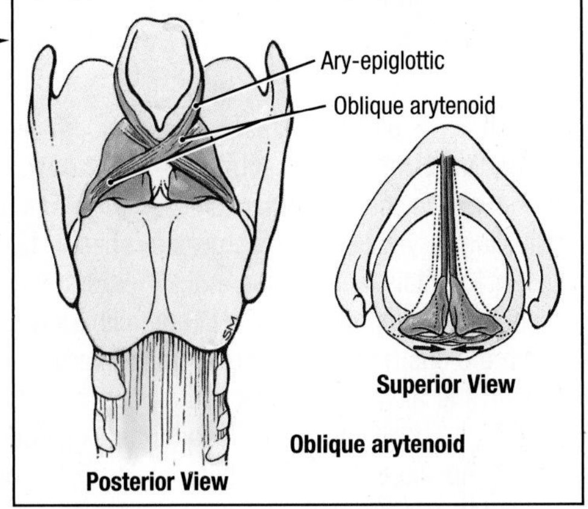
Ary-epiglottic
Oblique arytenoid
Superior View
Oblique arytenoid
Posterior View

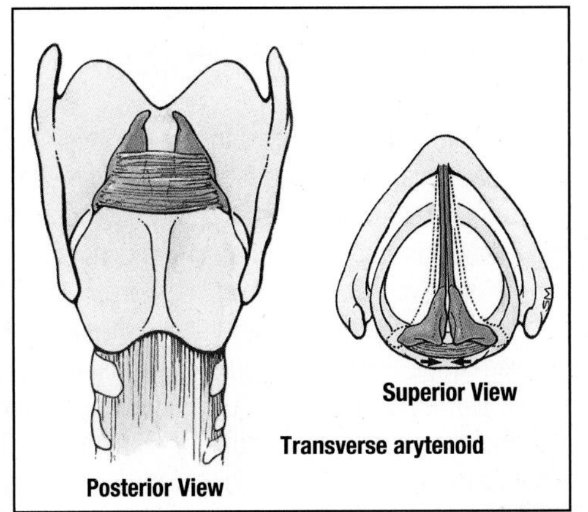
Superior View
Transverse arytenoid
Posterior View

8.40 MUSCLES OF LARYNX *(CONTINUED)*

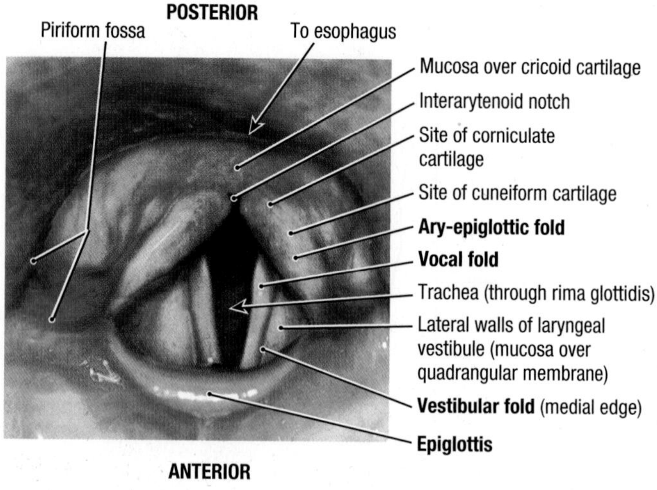
POSTERIOR
Piriform fossa
To esophagus
Mucosa over cricoid cartilage
Interarytenoid notch
Site of corniculate cartilage
Site of cuneiform cartilage
Ary-epiglottic fold
Vocal fold
Trachea (through rima glottidis)
Lateral walls of laryngeal vestibule (mucosa over quadrangular membrane)
Vestibular fold (medial edge)
Epiglottis
ANTERIOR

A. Laryngoscopic Examination

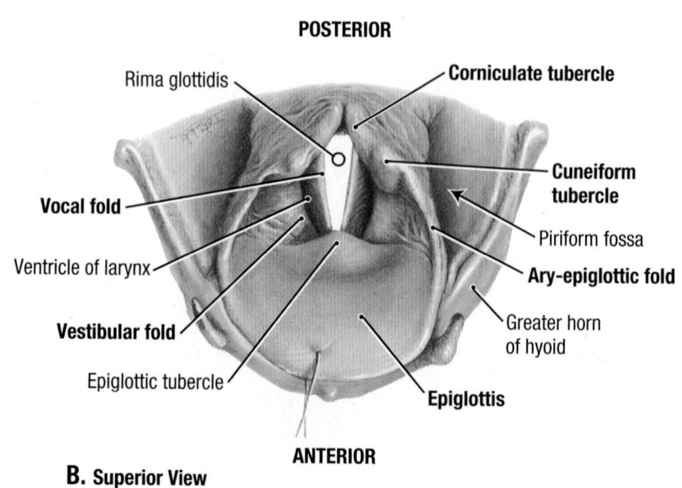
POSTERIOR
Rima glottidis
Corniculate tubercle
Cuneiform tubercle
Vocal fold
Piriform fossa
Ventricle of larynx
Ary-epiglottic fold
Vestibular fold
Greater horn of hyoid
Epiglottic tubercle
Epiglottis
ANTERIOR

B. Superior View

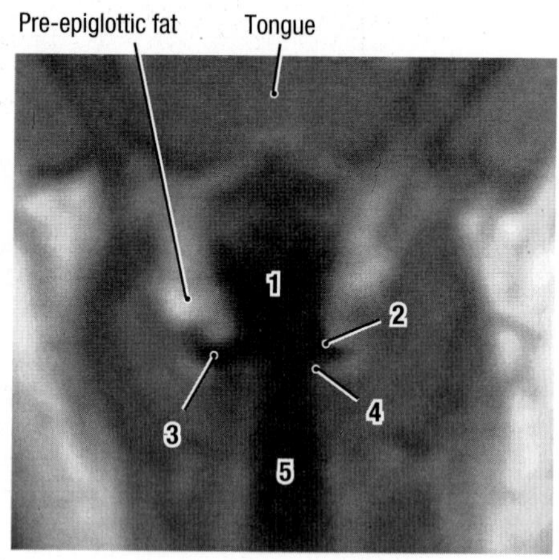
Pre-epiglottic fat
Tongue
1
2
3
4
5

C. Coronal MRI

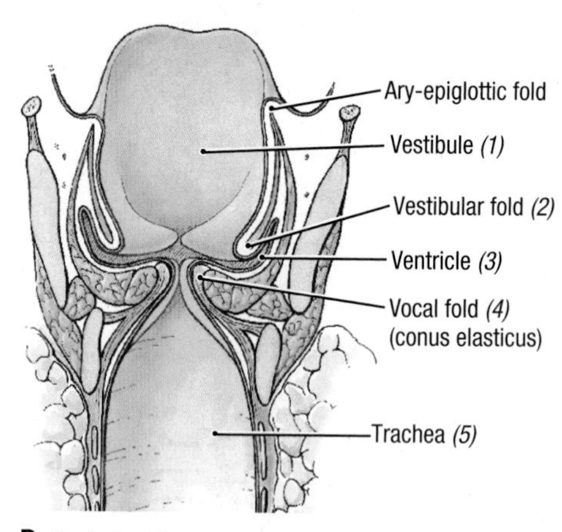
Ary-epiglottic fold
Vestibule (1)
Vestibular fold (2)
Ventricle (3)
Vocal fold (4)
(conus elasticus)
Trachea (5)

D. Posterior View

8.41 LARYNGOSCOPIC EXAMINATION AND MRI IMAGING OF LARYNX

A. Laryngoscopic examination. Laryngoscopy is the procedure used to examine the interior of the larynx. The larynx may be examined visually by indirect laryngoscopy using a laryngeal mirror or it may be viewed by direct laryngoscopy using a tubular and endoscopic instrument, a laryngoscope. The vestibular and vocal folds can be observed. **B.** Vocal folds and rima glottidis. The inlet, or aditus, to the larynx is bounded anteriorly by the epiglottis; posteriorly by the arytenoid cartilages, the corniculate cartilages that cap them, and the interarytenoid fold that unites them; and on each side by the ary-epiglottic fold, which contains the superior end of the cuneiform cartilage. The vocal apparatus of the larynx, the glottis, includes the vocal folds, vocal processes of the arytenoid cartilages and the rima glottidis, the aperture between the vocal folds. **C.** Coronal MRI. **D.** Coronal section. Numbers in parentheses on diagram refer to numbered structures on MRI.

A foreign object, such as a piece of steak, may accidentally aspirate through the laryngeal inlet into the vestibule of the larynx, where it becomes trapped superior to the vestibular folds. When a foreign object enters the vestibule, the laryngeal muscles go into spasm, tensing the vocal folds. The rima glottidis closes and no air enters the trachea. **Asphyxiation** occurs, and the person will die in approximately 5 minutes from lack of oxygen if the obstruction is not removed. Emergency therapy must be given to open the airway. The procedure used depends on the condition of the patient, the facilities available, and the experience of the person giving first aid. Because the lungs still contain air, sudden compression of the abdomen **(Heimlich maneuver)** causes the diaphragm to elevate and compress the lungs, expelling air from the trachea into the larynx. This maneuver may dislodge the food or other material from the larynx.

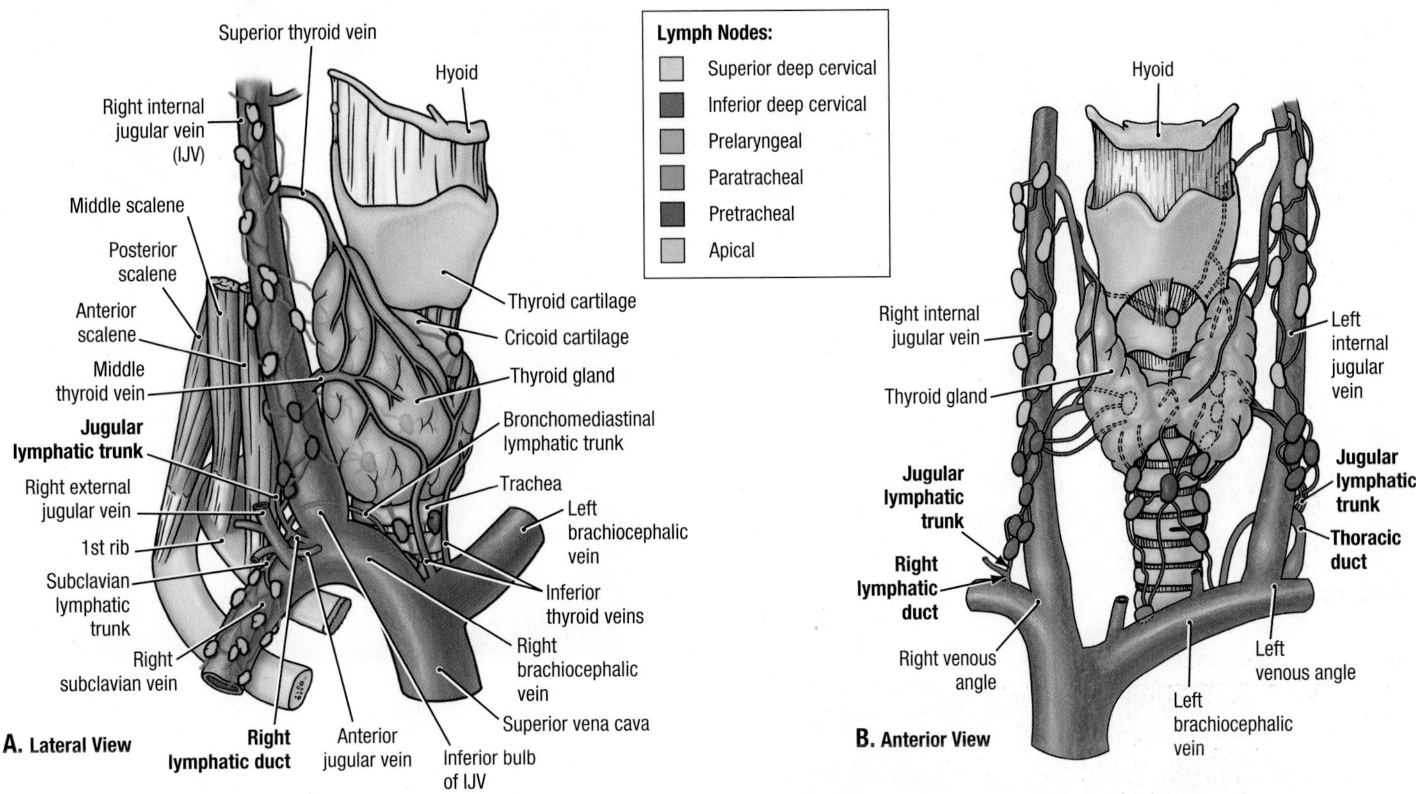
Superior thyroid vein
Hyoid
Right internal jugular vein (IJV)
Middle scalene
Posterior scalene
Anterior scalene
Middle thyroid vein
Jugular lymphatic trunk
Right external jugular vein
1st rib
Subclavian lymphatic trunk
Right subclavian vein
Thyroid cartilage
Cricoid cartilage
Thyroid gland
Bronchomediastinal lymphatic trunk
Trachea
Left brachiocephalic vein
Inferior thyroid veins
Right brachiocephalic vein
Superior vena cava
Inferior bulb of IJV
Anterior jugular vein
Right lymphatic duct
A. Lateral View
Lymph Nodes:
Superior deep cervical
Inferior deep cervical
Prelaryngeal
Paratracheal
Pretracheal
Apical
Hyoid
Right internal jugular vein
Thyroid gland
Jugular lymphatic trunk
Right lymphatic duct
Right venous angle
Left internal jugular vein
Jugular lymphatic trunk
Thoracic duct
Left venous angle
Left brachiocephalic vein
B. Anterior View

8.42 LYMPHATIC DRAINAGE OF THYROID GLAND, LARYNX, AND TRACHEA

Radical neck dissections are performed when cancer invades the lymphatics. During the procedure, the deep cervical lymph nodes and the tissues around them are removed as completely as possible. Although major arteries, the brachial plexus, CN X, and the phrenic nerve are preserved, most cutaneous branches of the cervical plexus are removed. The aim of the dissection is to remove all tissue that contains lymph nodes in one piece.

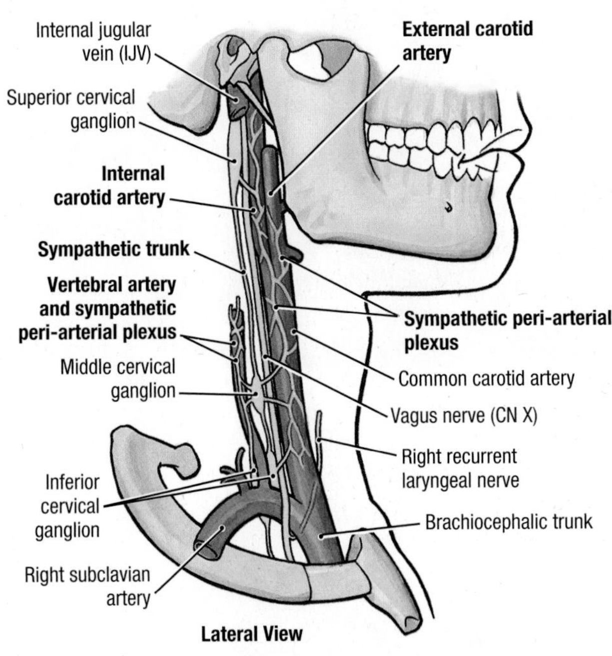
Internal jugular vein (IJV)
Superior cervical ganglion
Internal carotid artery
Sympathetic trunk
Vertebral artery and sympathetic peri-arterial plexus
Middle cervical ganglion
Inferior cervical ganglion
Right subclavian artery
External carotid artery
Sympathetic peri-arterial plexus
Common carotid artery
Vagus nerve (CN X)
Right recurrent laryngeal nerve
Brachiocephalic trunk
Lateral View

8.43 SYMPATHETIC TRUNK AND SYMPATHETIC PERIARTERIAL PLEXUS

A **lesion of a sympathetic trunk** in the neck results in a sympathetic disturbance called **Horner syndrome,** which is characterized by the following:

- Pupillary constriction resulting from paralysis of the dilator pupillae muscle.
- Ptosis (drooping of the superior eyelid), resulting from paralysis of the smooth (tarsal) muscle intermingled with striated muscle of the levator palpebrae superioris.
- Sinking in of the eyeball (enophthalmos), possibly caused by paralysis of smooth (orbitalis) muscle in the floor of the orbit.
- Vasodilation and absence of sweating on the face and neck (anhydrosis), caused by a lack of sympathetic (vasoconstrictive) nerve supply to the blood vessels and sweat glands.

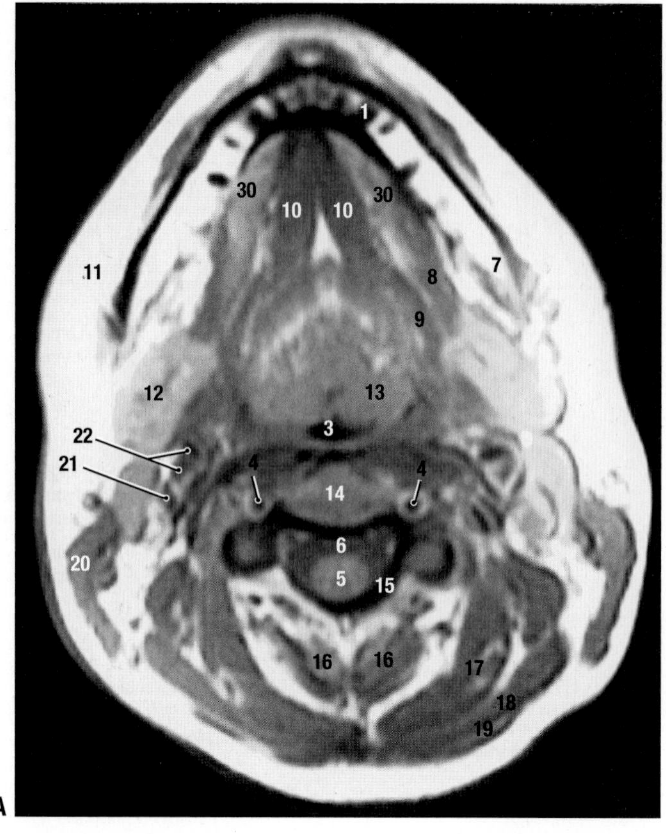
A

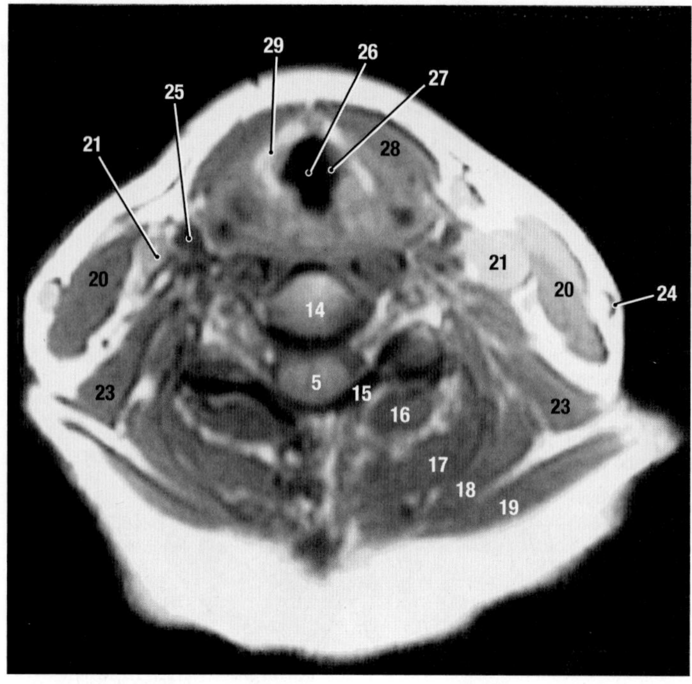
B

Tongue
C2
C3 A
C4
C5 B
C6 C
C7

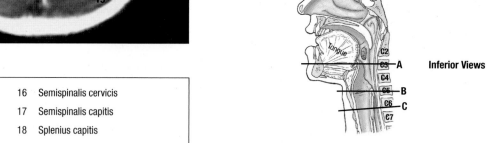

Inferior Views

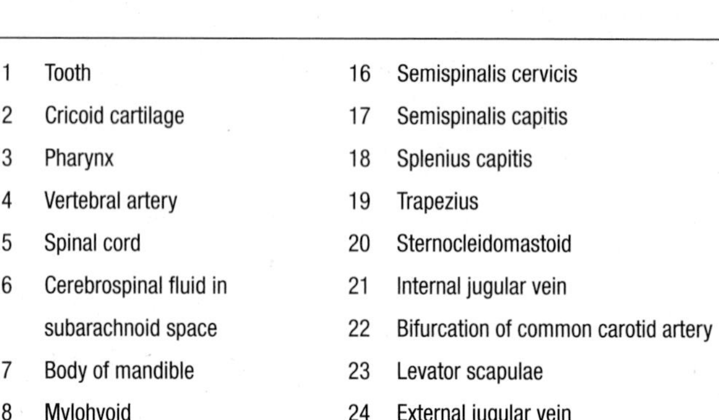

1	Tooth	16	Semispinalis cervicis
2	Cricoid cartilage	17	Semispinalis capitis
3	Pharynx	18	Splenius capitis
4	Vertebral artery	19	Trapezius
5	Spinal cord	20	Sternocleidomastoid
6	Cerebrospinal fluid in subarachnoid space	21	Internal jugular vein
		22	Bifurcation of common carotid artery
7	Body of mandible	23	Levator scapulae
8	Mylohyoid	24	External jugular vein
9	Hyoglossus	25	Common carotid artery
10	Genioglossus	26	Rima glottidis
11	Buccal fat pad	27	Vocal fold
12	Submandibular gland	28	Strap muscles
13	Intrinsic muscles of tongue	29	Thyroid cartilage
14	Vertebral body	30	Sublingual gland
15	Lamina of vertebra	31	Inferior pharyngeal constrictor

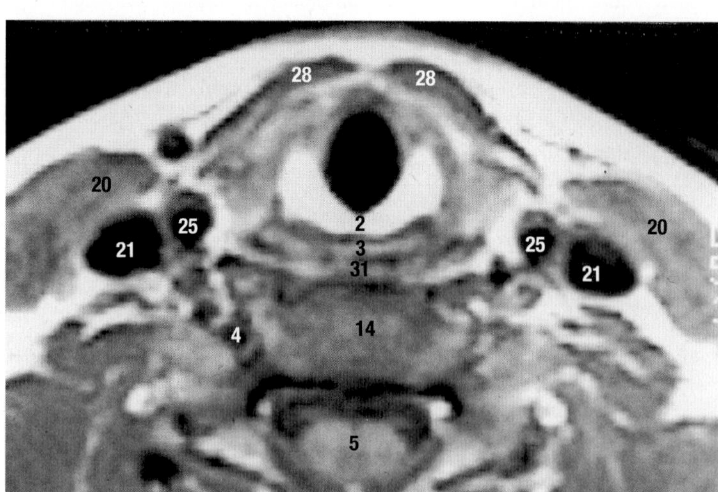
C

8.44 TRANSVERSE MRIs OF NECK

The orientation figure indicates the vertebral level of the MRI sections.

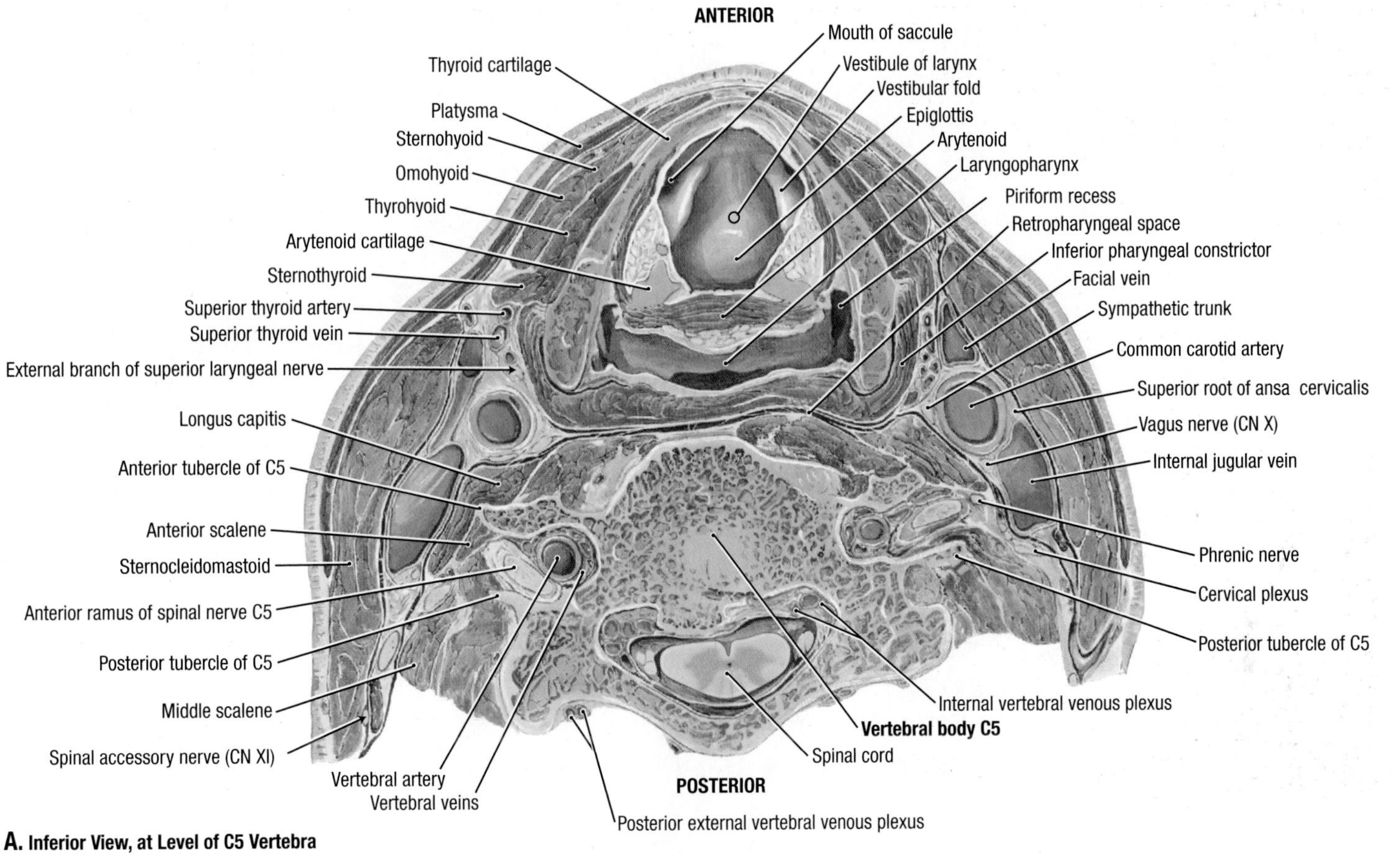

ANTERIOR
Mouth of saccule
Thyroid cartilage
Vestibule of larynx
Vestibular fold
Platysma
Sternohyoid
Epiglottis
Arytenoid
Omohyoid
Laryngopharynx
Thyrohyoid
Piriform recess
Retropharyngeal space
Arytenoid cartilage
Inferior pharyngeal constrictor
Facial vein
Sternothyroid
Sympathetic trunk
Superior thyroid artery
Superior thyroid vein
Common carotid artery
External branch of superior laryngeal nerve
Superior root of ansa cervicalis
Longus capitis
Vagus nerve (CN X)
Internal jugular vein
Anterior tubercle of C5
Anterior scalene
Phrenic nerve
Sternocleidomastoid
Cervical plexus
Anterior ramus of spinal nerve C5
Posterior tubercle of C5
Posterior tubercle of C5
Internal vertebral venous plexus
Middle scalene
Vertebral body C5
Spinal accessory nerve (CN XI)
Spinal cord
Vertebral artery
Vertebral veins
POSTERIOR
Posterior external vertebral venous plexus

A. Inferior View, at Level of C5 Vertebra

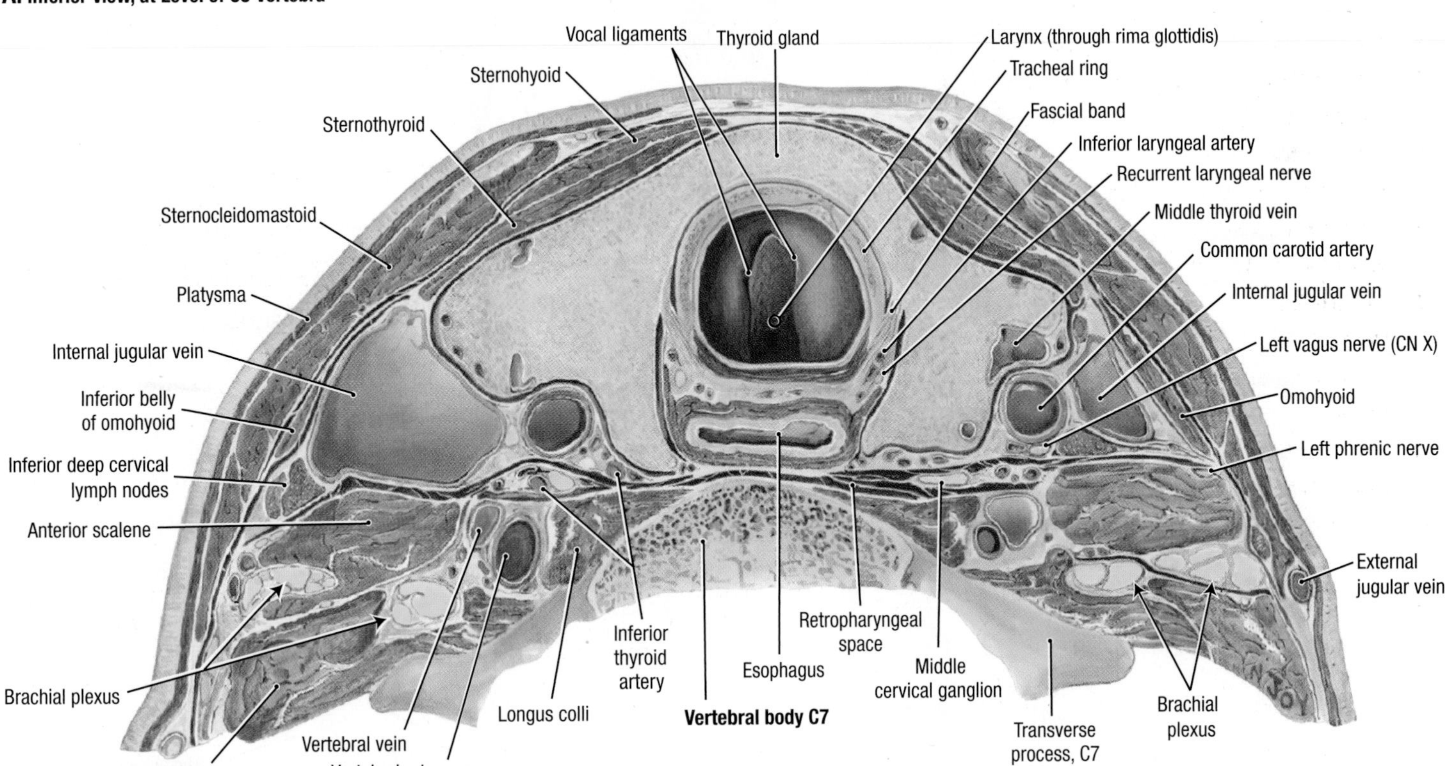
Vocal ligaments
Thyroid gland
Larynx (through rima glottidis)
Tracheal ring
Sternohyoid
Fascial band
Sternothyroid
Inferior laryngeal artery
Recurrent laryngeal nerve
Sternocleidomastoid
Middle thyroid vein
Common carotid artery
Platysma
Internal jugular vein
Internal jugular vein
Left vagus nerve (CN X)
Inferior belly of omohyoid
Omohyoid
Inferior deep cervical lymph nodes
Left phrenic nerve
Anterior scalene
External jugular vein
Inferior thyroid artery
Retropharyngeal space
Esophagus
Middle cervical ganglion
Brachial plexus
Brachial plexus
Longus colli
Vertebral body C7
Transverse process, C7
Vertebral vein
Middle scalene
Vertebral artery

B. Inferior View, at Level of C7 Vertebra

8.45 TRANSVERSE ANATOMICAL SECTIONS OF NECK

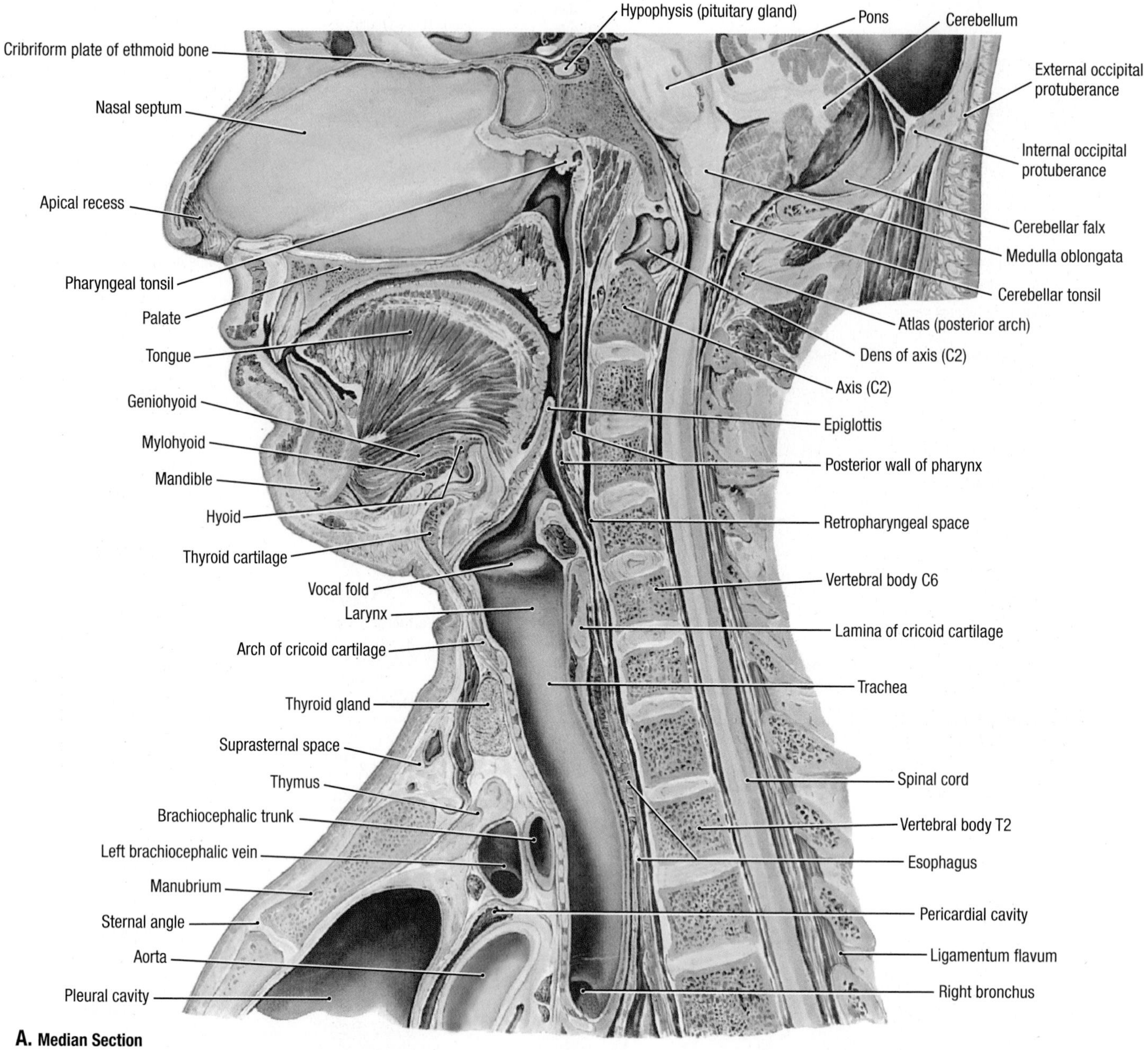

Hypophysis (pituitary gland)
Pons
Cerebellum
Cribriform plate of ethmoid bone
External occipital protuberance
Nasal septum
Internal occipital protuberance
Apical recess
Cerebellar falx
Medulla oblongata
Pharyngeal tonsil
Cerebellar tonsil
Palate
Atlas (posterior arch)
Tongue
Dens of axis (C2)
Axis (C2)
Geniohyoid
Epiglottis
Mylohyoid
Posterior wall of pharynx
Mandible
Hyoid
Retropharyngeal space
Thyroid cartilage
Vocal fold
Vertebral body C6
Larynx
Lamina of cricoid cartilage
Arch of cricoid cartilage
Trachea
Thyroid gland
Suprasternal space
Spinal cord
Thymus
Brachiocephalic trunk
Vertebral body T2
Left brachiocephalic vein
Esophagus
Manubrium
Sternal angle
Pericardial cavity
Aorta
Ligamentum flavum
Pleural cavity
Right bronchus

A. Median Section

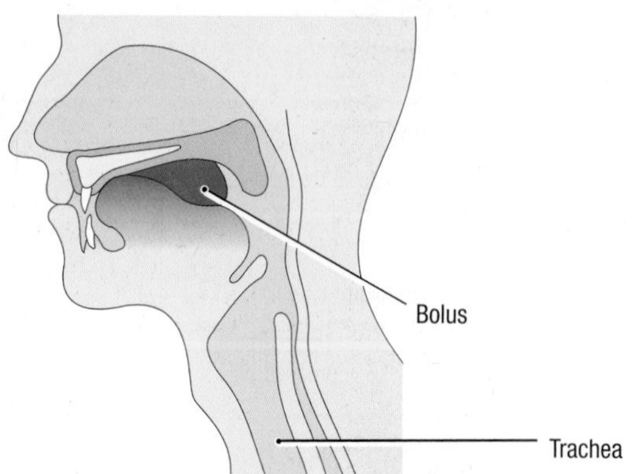
Bolus
Trachea

(1) The bolus of food is squeezed to the back of the mouth by pushing the tongue against the palate.

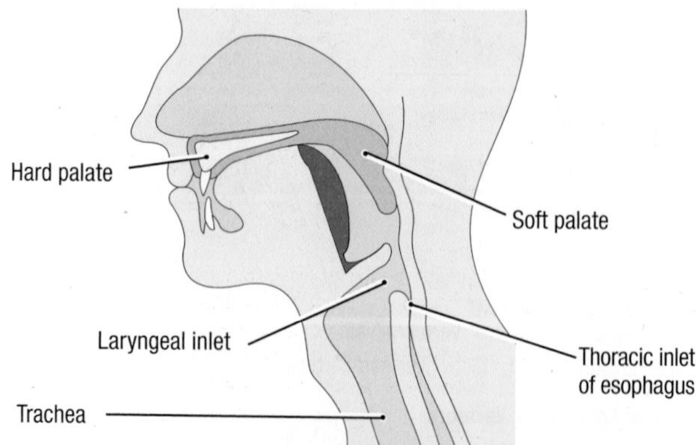
Hard palate
Soft palate
Laryngeal inlet
Thoracic inlet of esophagus
Trachea

(2) The nasopharynx is sealed off, and the larynx is elevated, enlarging the pharynx to receive food.

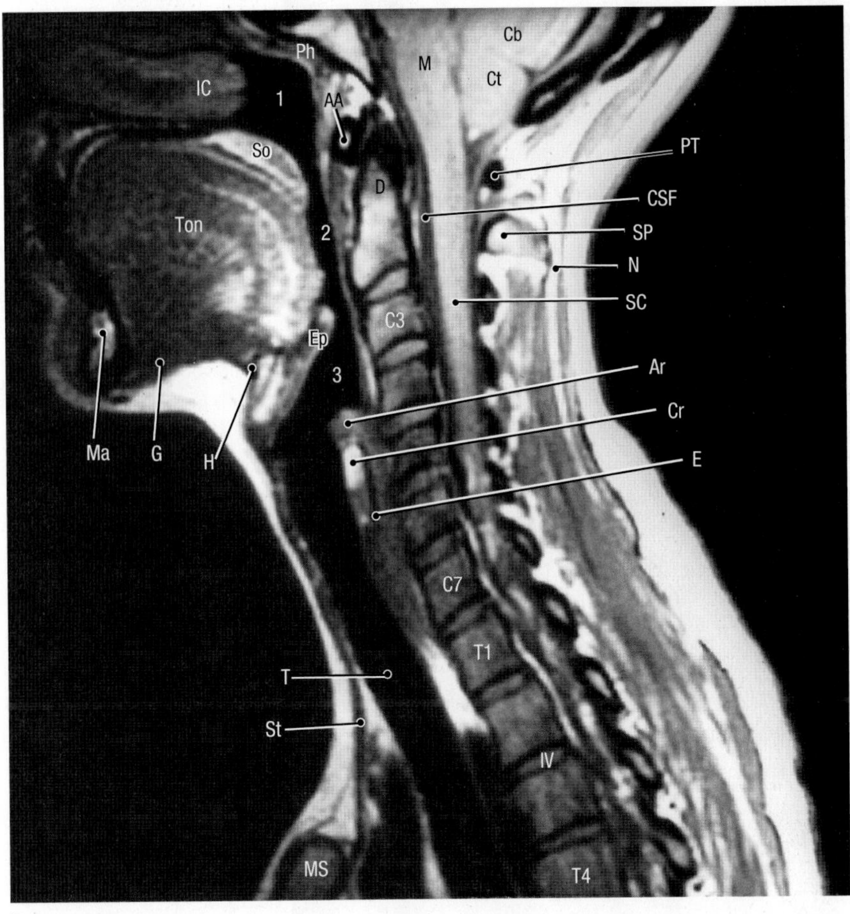
Ph
Cb
M
Ct
IC
1
AA
So
PT
D
CSF
Ton
2
SP
N
SC
C3
Ep
3
Ar
Cr
Ma
G
H
E
C7
T1
T
St
IV
MS
T4

B. Median MRI Scan

AA	Anterior arch of C1
Ar	Arytenoid cartilage
C3-T4	Vertebral bodies
Cb	Cerebellum
Cr	Cricoid cartilage
CSF	Cerebrospinal fluid in subarachnoid space
Ct	Tonsil of cerebellum
D	Dens
E	Esophagus
Ep	Epiglottis
G	Genioglossus
H	Hyoid
IC	Inferior concha
IV	Intervertebral disc
M	Medulla oblongata
Ma	Mandible
MS	Manubrium of sternum
N	Nuchal ligament
Ph	Pharyngeal tonsil (adenoid)
PT	Posterior tubercle of C1
SC	Spinal cord
So	Soft palate
SP	Spinous process
St	Strap muscles
T	Trachea
Ton	Tongue
1	Nasopharynx
2	Oropharynx
3	Laryngopharynx

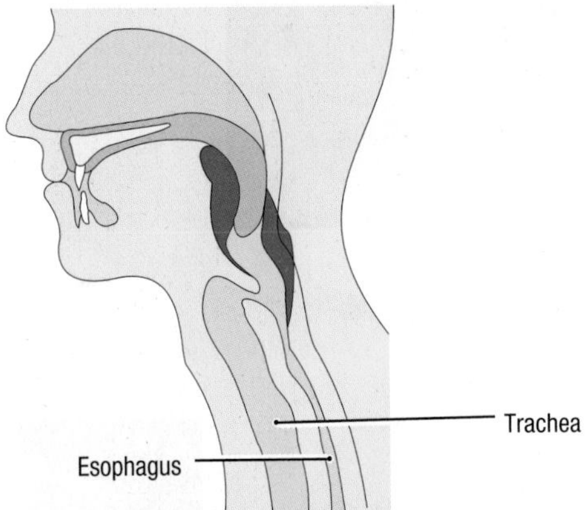
Trachea
Esophagus

(3) The pharyngeal sphincters contract sequentially, squeezing food into the esophagus. The epiglottis deflects the bolus from but does not close the inlet to the larynx and trachia.

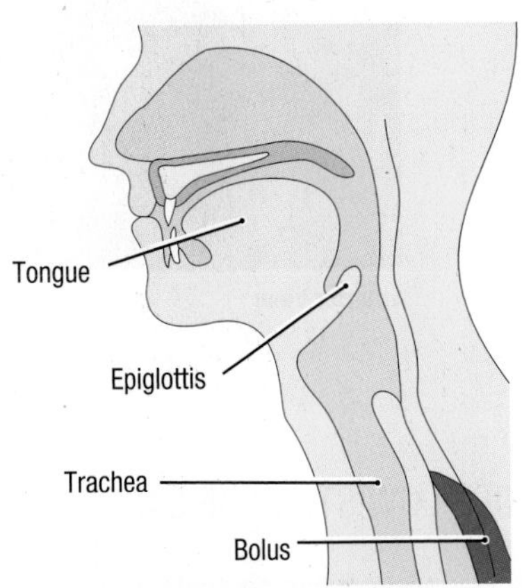
Tongue
Epiglottis
Trachea
Bolus

(4) The bolus of food moves down the esophagus by peristaltic contractions.

8.46 MEDIAN SECTION AND MRI SCAN OF HEAD AND NECK

A. Median anatomical section. **B.** Median MRI scan. **C.** Swallowing.

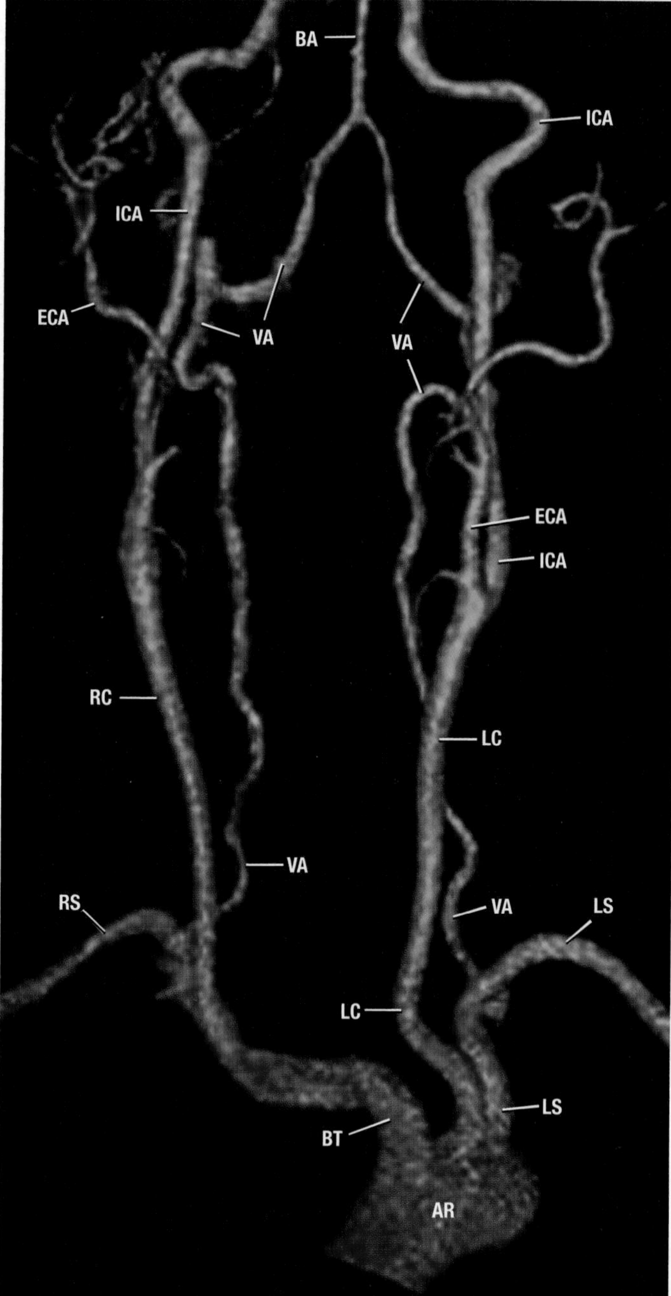
BA
ICA
ICA
ECA
VA
VA
ECA
ICA
RC
LC
VA
RS
VA
LS
LC
LS
BT
AR

Anterior View

Key	
AR	Arch of aorta
BA	Basilar artery
BT	Brachiocephalic trunk
ECA	External carotid artery
ICA	Internal carotid artery
LC	Left common carotid artery
LS	Left subclavian artery
RC	Right common carotid artery
RS	Right subclavian artery
VA	Vertebral artery

8.47 DOPPLER US COLOR FLOW STUDY OF CAROTID ARTERY

Ultrasonography is a useful diagnostic imaging technique for studying soft tissues of the neck. Ultrasound provides images of many abnormal conditions noninvasively, at relatively low cost, and with minimal discomfort. Ultrasound is useful for distinguishing solid from cystic masses, for example, which may be difficult to determine during physical examination. Vascular imaging of arteries and veins of the neck is possible using intravascular ultrasonography. The images are produced by placing the transducer over the blood vessel. Doppler ultrasound techniques help evaluate blood flow through a vessel (e.g., for detecting stenosis [narrowing] of a carotid artery).

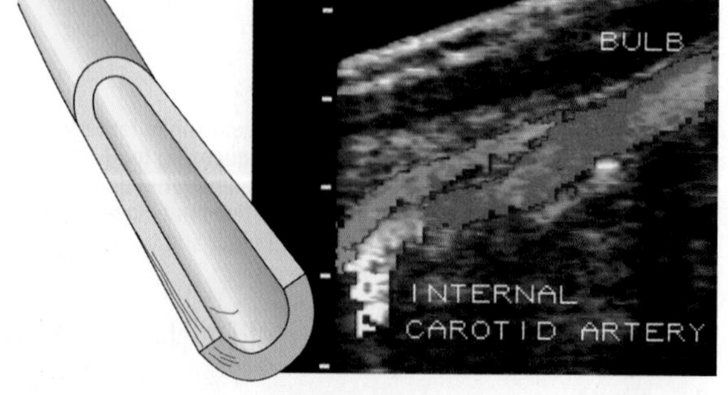
BULB
INTERNAL
CAROTID ARTERY

CHAPTER 9

Cranial Nerves

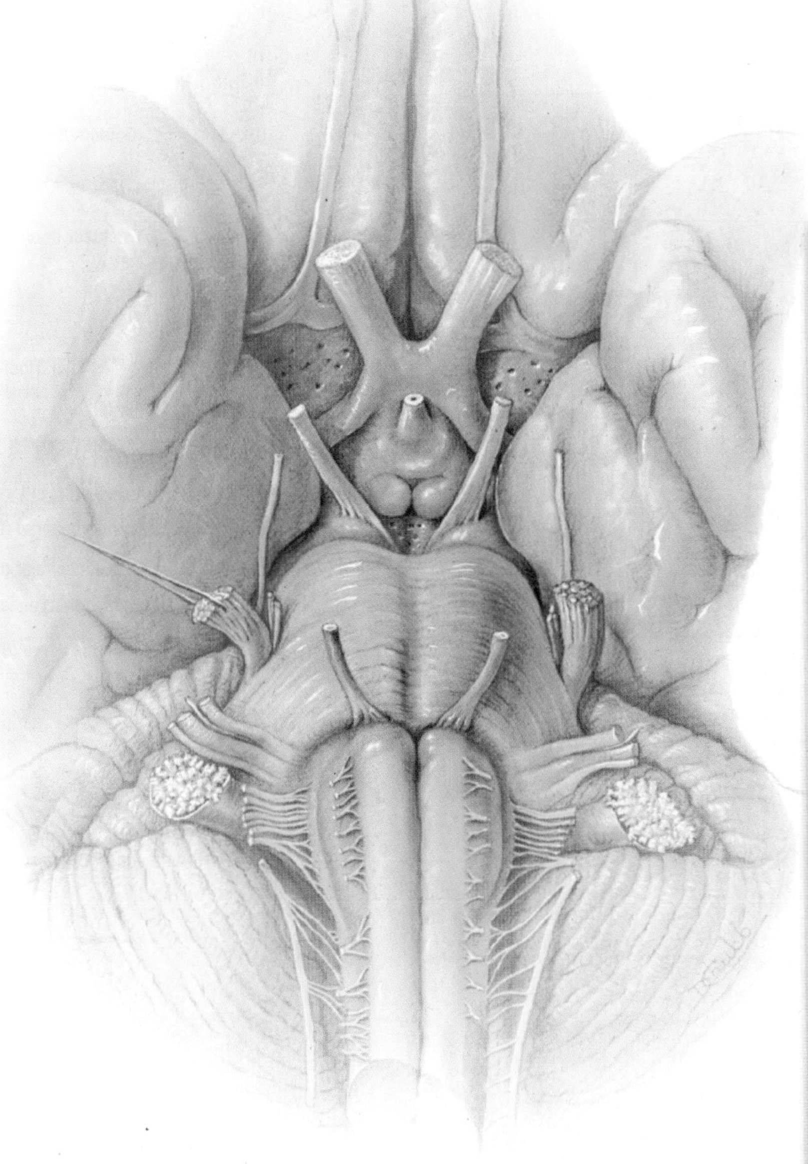

Overview of Cranial Nerves	818
Cranial Nerve Nuclei	822
Cranial Nerve I: Olfactory	824
Cranial Nerve II: Optic	825
Cranial Nerves III, IV, and VI: Oculomotor, Trochlear, and Abducent	827
Cranial Nerve V: Trigeminal	830
Cranial Nerve VII: Facial	837
Cranial Nerve VIII: Vestibulocochlear	838
Cranial Nerve IX: Glossopharyngeal	840
Cranial Nerve X: Vagus	843
Cranial Nerve XI: Spinal Accessory	844
Cranial Nerve XII: Hypoglossal	845
Summary of Autonomic Ganglia of Head	846
Summary of Cranial Nerve Lesions	847
Sectional Imaging of Cranial Nerves	848

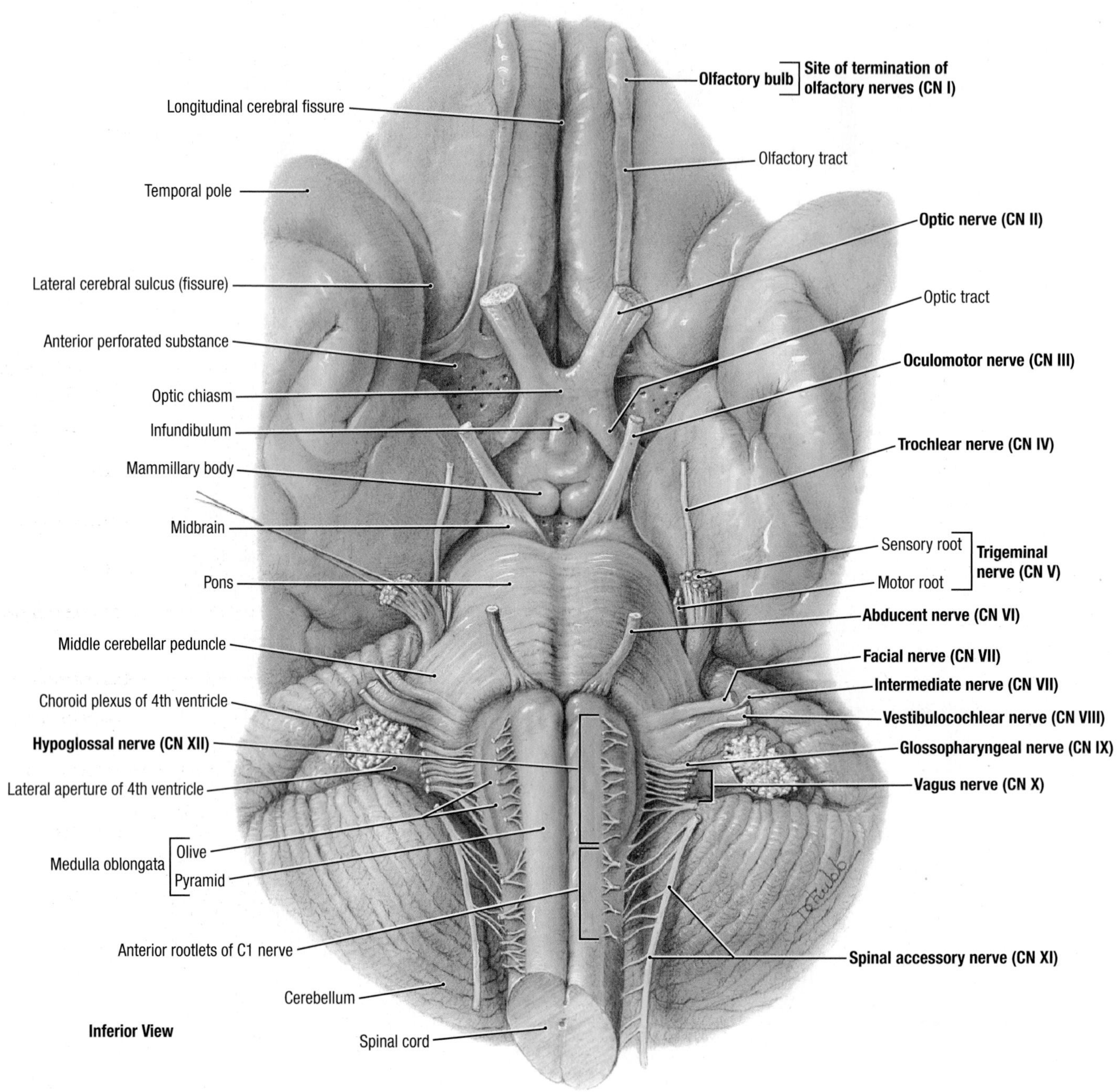
Olfactory bulb
Site of termination of olfactory nerves (CN I)
Longitudinal cerebral fissure
Olfactory tract
Temporal pole
Optic nerve (CN II)
Lateral cerebral sulcus (fissure)
Optic tract
Anterior perforated substance
Oculomotor nerve (CN III)
Optic chiasm
Infundibulum
Trochlear nerve (CN IV)
Mammillary body
Midbrain
Sensory root
Trigeminal nerve (CN V)
Pons
Motor root
Abducent nerve (CN VI)
Middle cerebellar peduncle
Facial nerve (CN VII)
Intermediate nerve (CN VII)
Choroid plexus of 4th ventricle
Vestibulocochlear nerve (CN VIII)
Hypoglossal nerve (CN XII)
Glossopharyngeal nerve (CN IX)
Lateral aperture of 4th ventricle
Vagus nerve (CN X)
Medulla oblongata
Olive
Pyramid
Anterior rootlets of C1 nerve
Spinal accessory nerve (CN XI)
Cerebellum
Inferior View
Spinal cord

9.1 CRANIAL NERVES IN RELATION TO THE BASE OF THE BRAIN

Cranial nerves are nerves that exit from the cranial cavity through openings in the cranium. There are 12 pairs of cranial nerves that are named and numbered in rostrocaudal sequence of their superficial origins from the brain, brainstem, and superior spinal cord. The olfactory nerves (CN I, not shown) end in the olfactory bulb. The entire origin of the spinal accessory nerve (CN XI) from the spinal cord is not included here; it extends inferiorly as far as the C6 spinal cord segment.

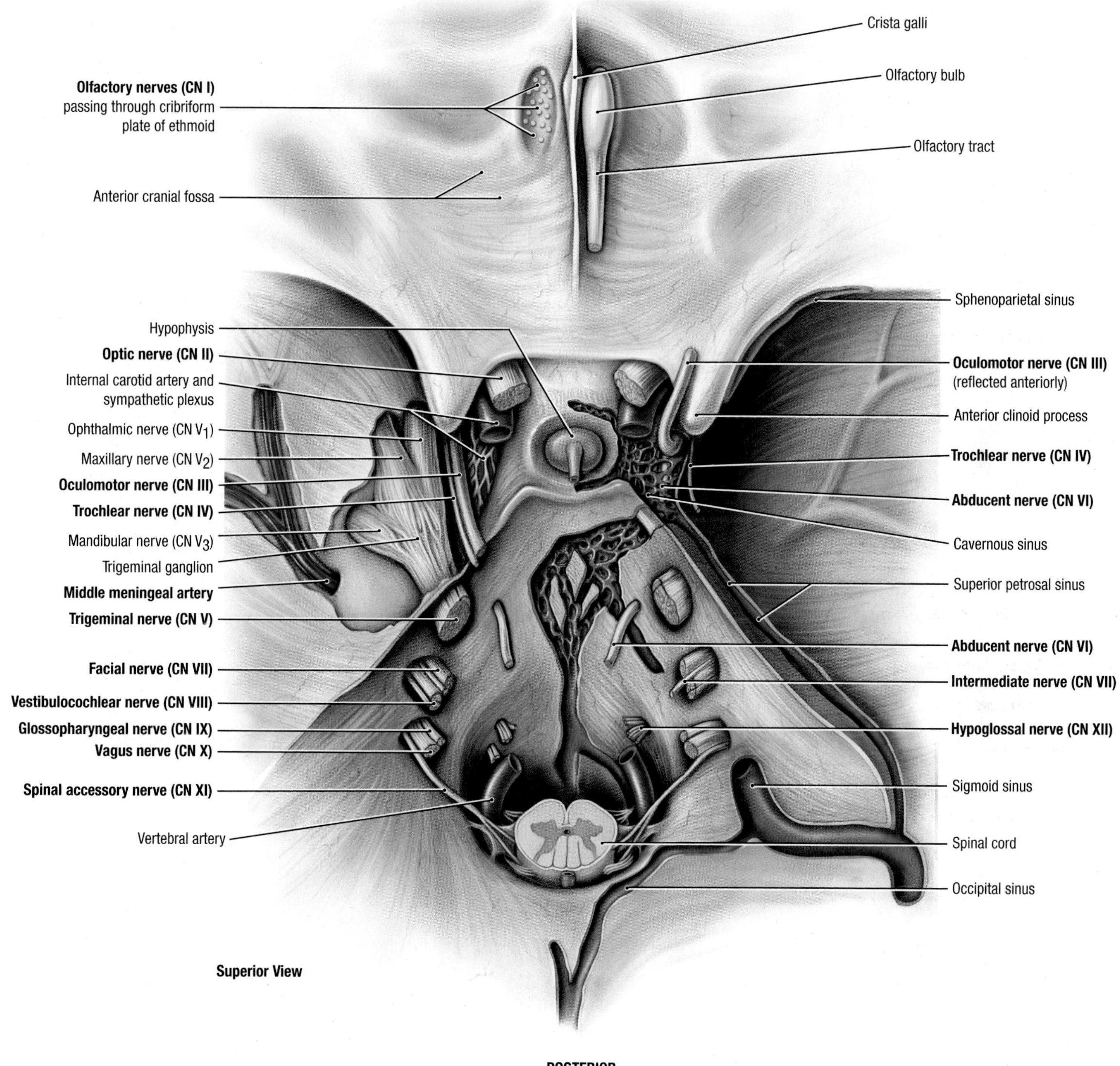
ANTERIOR
Crista galli
Olfactory nerves (CN I) passing through cribriform plate of ethmoid
Olfactory bulb
Olfactory tract
Anterior cranial fossa
Sphenoparietal sinus
Hypophysis
Optic nerve (CN II)
Internal carotid artery and sympathetic plexus
Oculomotor nerve (CN III) (reflected anteriorly)
Anterior clinoid process
Ophthalmic nerve (CN V1)
Maxillary nerve (CN V2)
Trochlear nerve (CN IV)
Oculomotor nerve (CN III)
Trochlear nerve (CN IV)
Abducent nerve (CN VI)
Mandibular nerve (CN V3)
Cavernous sinus
Trigeminal ganglion
Middle meningeal artery
Superior petrosal sinus
Trigeminal nerve (CN V)
Abducent nerve (CN VI)
Facial nerve (CN VII)
Intermediate nerve (CN VII)
Vestibulocochlear nerve (CN VIII)
Glossopharyngeal nerve (CN IX)
Hypoglossal nerve (CN XII)
Vagus nerve (CN X)
Spinal accessory nerve (CN XI)
Sigmoid sinus
Vertebral artery
Spinal cord
Occipital sinus
Superior View
POSTERIOR

9.2 CRANIAL NERVES IN RELATION TO THE INTERNAL ASPECT OF THE CRANIAL BASE

The venous sinuses have been opened on the right side. The ophthalmic division of the trigeminal nerve (CN V_1) and the trochlear (CN IV) and oculomotor (CN III) nerves have been dissected from the lateral wall of the cavernous sinus. Although there are no sympathetic fibers in cranial nerves as they leave the brain, postsynaptic sympathetic nerve fibers "hitch-hike" onto branches of cranial nerves having traveled to the region via major blood vessels.

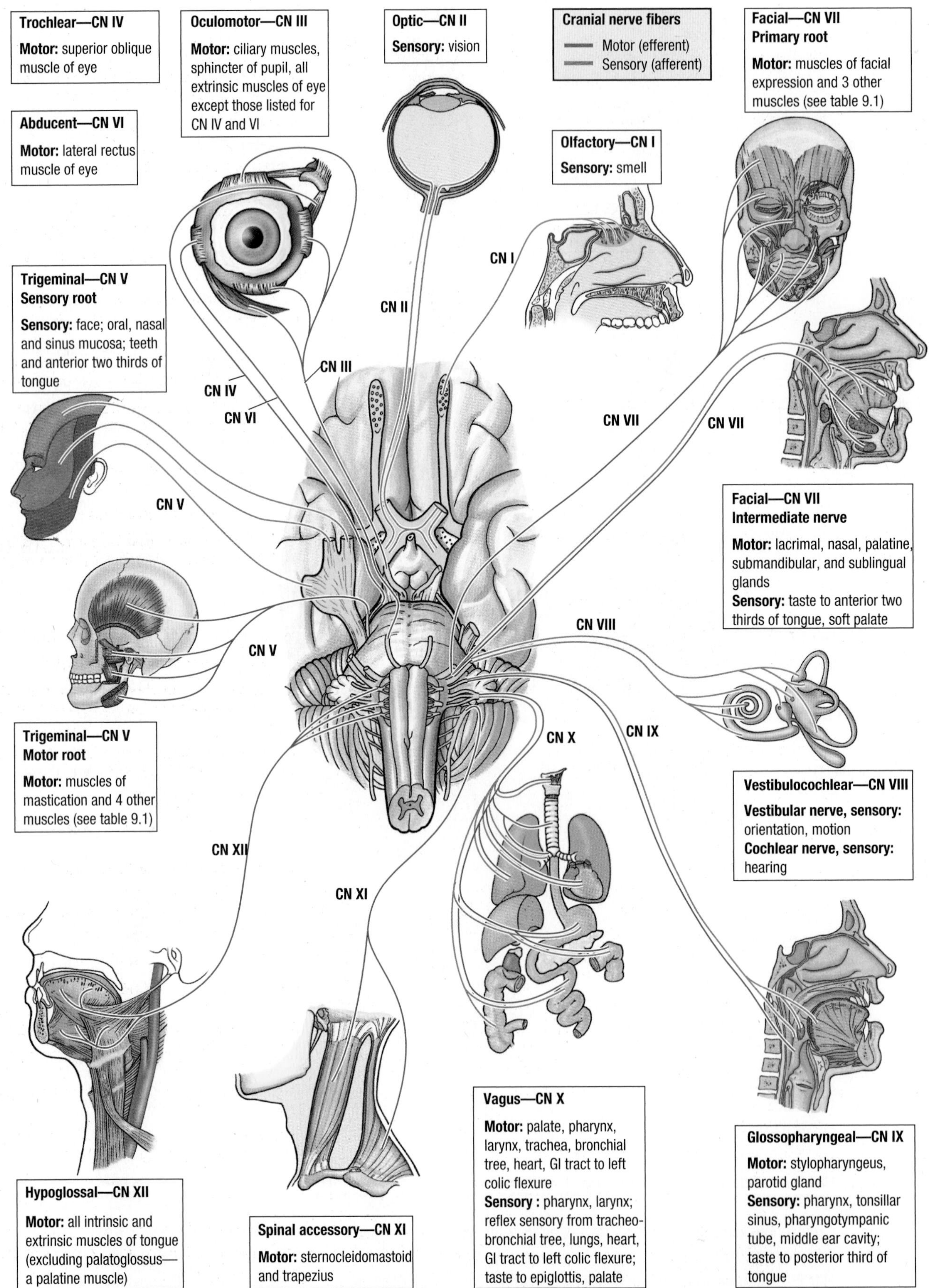
Trochlear—CN IV
Motor: superior oblique muscle of eye
Oculomotor—CN III
Motor: ciliary muscles, sphincter of pupil, all extrinsic muscles of eye except those listed for CN IV and VI
Optic—CN II
Sensory: vision
Cranial nerve fibers
Motor (efferent)
Sensory (afferent)
Facial—CN VII
Primary root
Motor: muscles of facial expression and 3 other muscles (see table 9.1)
Abducent—CN VI
Motor: lateral rectus muscle of eye
Olfactory—CN I
Sensory: smell
Trigeminal—CN V
Sensory root
Sensory: face; oral, nasal and sinus mucosa; teeth and anterior two thirds of tongue
CN I
CN II
CN III
CN IV
CN VI
CN VII
CN VII
CN V
Facial—CN VII
Intermediate nerve
Motor: lacrimal, nasal, palatine, submandibular, and sublingual glands
Sensory: taste to anterior two thirds of tongue, soft palate
CN VIII
CN V
CN X
CN IX
Trigeminal—CN V
Motor root
Motor: muscles of mastication and 4 other muscles (see table 9.1)
Vestibulocochlear—CN VIII
Vestibular nerve, sensory: orientation, motion
Cochlear nerve, sensory: hearing
CN XII
CN XI
Vagus—CN X
Motor: palate, pharynx, larynx, trachea, bronchial tree, heart, GI tract to left colic flexure
Sensory : pharynx, larynx; reflex sensory from tracheobronchial tree, lungs, heart, GI tract to left colic flexure; taste to epiglottis, palate
Glossopharyngeal—CN IX
Motor: stylopharyngeus, parotid gland
Sensory: pharynx, tonsillar sinus, pharyngotympanic tube, middle ear cavity; taste to posterior third of tongue
Hypoglossal—CN XII
Motor: all intrinsic and extrinsic muscles of tongue (excluding palatoglossus—a palatine muscle)
Spinal accessory—CN XI
Motor: sternocleidomastoid and trapezius

TABLE 9.1 SUMMARY OF CRANIAL NERVES

Nerve	Components	Location of Nerve Cell Bodies	Cranial Exit	Function
Olfactory (CN I)	Special sensory	Olfactory epithelium (olfactory cells)	Foramina in cribriform plate of ethmoid bone	Smell from nasal mucosa of roof of each nasal cavity, superior sides of nasal septum and superior concha
Optic (CN II)	Special sensory	Retina (ganglion cells)	Optic canal	Vision from retina
Oculomotor (CN III)	Somatic motor	Midbrain (nucleus of CN III)	Superior orbital fissure	Motor to superior, inferior, and medial rectus, inferior oblique, and levator palpebrae superioris that raise upper eyelid and direct gaze superiorly, inferiorly, and medially
	Visceral motor	Presynaptic: midbrain (Edinger-Westphal nucleus); Postsynaptic: ciliary ganglion		Parasympathetic innervation to sphincter pupillae and ciliary muscles that constrict pupil and accommodate lens of eye
Trochlear (CN IV)	Somatic motor	Midbrain (nucleus of CN IV)		Motor to superior oblique that assists in directing gaze inferolaterally
Trigeminal (CN V) Ophthalmic division (CN V^1)	Somatic (general) sensory	Trigeminal ganglion Synapse: sensory nucleus of CN V		Sensation from cornea, skin of forehead, scalp, eyelids, nose, and mucosa of nasal cavity and paranasal sinuses
Maxillary division (CN V^2)			Foramen rotundum	Sensation from skin of face over maxilla including upper lip, maxillary teeth, mucosa of nose, maxillary sinuses, and palate
Mandibular division (CN V^3)	Somatic (branchial) motor	Pons (motor nucleus of CN V)	Foramen ovale	Sensation from the skin over mandible, including lower lip and side of head, mandibular teeth, temporomandibular joint, and mucosa of mouth and anterior two thirds of tongue
				Motor to muscles of mastication, mylohyoid, anterior belly of digastric, tensor veli palatini, and tensor tympani
Abducent (CN VI)	Somatic motor	Pons (nucleus of CN VI)	Superior orbital fissure	Motor to lateral rectus to direct gaze laterally
Facial (CN VII)	Somatic (branchial) motor	Pons (motor nucleus of CN VII)	Internal acoustic meatus, facial canal, and stylomastoid foramen	Motor to muscles of facial expression and scalp; also supplies stapedius of middle ear, stylohyoid, and posterior belly of digastric
	Special sensory	Geniculate ganglion Synapse: nuclei of solitary tract		Taste from anterior two thirds of tongue, and palate
	General sensory	Geniculate ganglion Synapse: sensory nucleus of CN V		Sensation from skin of external acoustic meatus
	Visceral motor	Presynaptic: pons (superior salivatory nucleus); Postsynaptic: pterygopalatine ganglion and submandibular ganglion		Parasympathetic innervation to submandibular and sublingual salivary glands, lacrimal gland, and glands of nose and palate
Vestibulocochlear (CN VIII) Vestibular	Special sensory	Vestibular ganglion Synapse: vestibular nuclei	Internal acoustic meatus	Vestibular sensation from semicircular ducts, utricle, and saccule related to position and movement of head
Cochlear	Special sensory	Spiral ganglion Synapse: cochlear nuclei		Hearing from spiral organ
Glossopharyngeal (CN IX)	Somatic (branchial) motor	Medulla (nucleus ambiguus)	Jugular foramen	Motor to stylopharyngeus that assists with swallowing
	Visceral motor	Presynaptic: medulla (inferior salivatory nucleus); Postsynaptic: otic ganglion		Parasympathetic innervation to parotid gland
	Visceral sensory	Inferior ganglion		Visceral sensation from parotid gland, carotid body and sinus, pharynx, and middle ear
	Special sensory	Inferior ganglion Synapse: nuclei of solitary tract		Taste from posterior third of tongue
	General sensory	Superior ganglion Synapse: sensory nucleus of CN V		Cutaneous sensation from external ear
Vagus (CN X)	Somatic (branchial) motor	Medulla (nucleus ambiguus)		Motor to constrictor muscles of pharynx, intrinsic muscles of larynx, muscles of palate (except tensor veli palatini), and striated muscle in superior two thirds of esophagus
	Visceral motor	Presynaptic: medulla; Postsynaptic: neurons in, on, or near viscera		Smooth muscle of trachea, bronchi, and digestive tract, cardiac muscle
	Visceral sensory	Inferior ganglion Synapse: nuclei of solitary tract		Visceral sensation from base of tongue, pharynx, larynx, trachea, bronchi, heart, esophagus, stomach, and intestine
	Special sensory	Inferior ganglion Synapse: nuclei of solitary tract		Taste from epiglottis and palate
	Somatic (general) sensory	Superior ganglion Synapse: sensory nucleus of trigeminal nerve		Sensation from auricle, external acoustic meatus, and dura mater of posterior cranial fossa
Spinal accessory nerve (CN XI)	Somatic motor	Cervical spinal cord		Motor to sternocleidomastoid and trapezius
Hypoglossal (CN XII)	Somatic motor	Medulla (Nucleus of CN XII)	Hypoglossal canal	Motor to muscles of tongue (except palatoglossus)

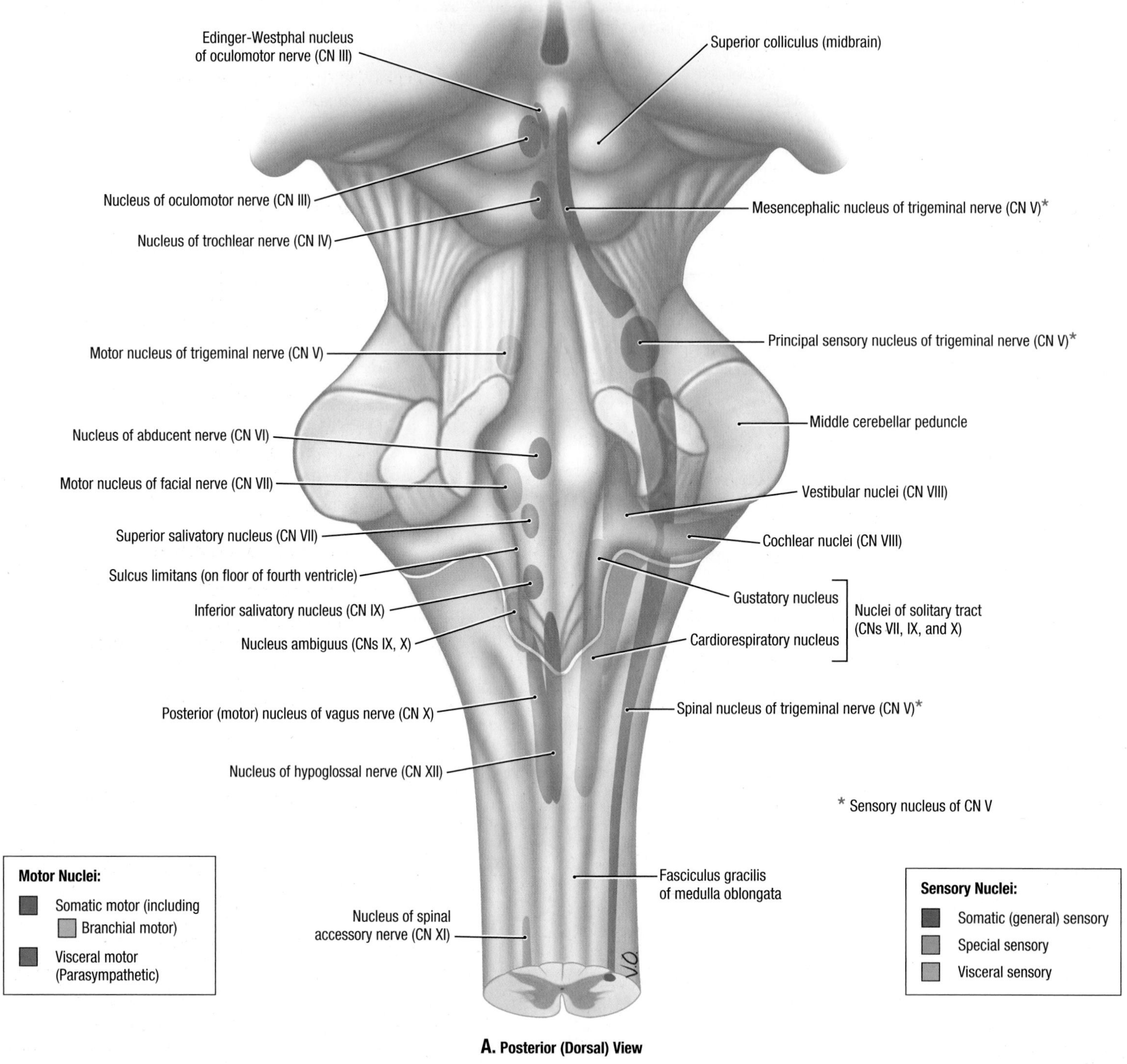
Edinger-Westphal nucleus of oculomotor nerve (CN III)
Superior colliculus (midbrain)
Nucleus of oculomotor nerve (CN III)
Mesencephalic nucleus of trigeminal nerve (CN V)*
Nucleus of trochlear nerve (CN IV)
Motor nucleus of trigeminal nerve (CN V)
Principal sensory nucleus of trigeminal nerve (CN V)*
Middle cerebellar peduncle
Nucleus of abducent nerve (CN VI)
Motor nucleus of facial nerve (CN VII)
Vestibular nuclei (CN VIII)
Superior salivatory nucleus (CN VII)
Cochlear nuclei (CN VIII)
Sulcus limitans (on floor of fourth ventricle)
Gustatory nucleus
Nuclei of solitary tract (CNs VII, IX, and X)
Inferior salivatory nucleus (CN IX)
Nucleus ambiguus (CNs IX, X)
Cardiorespiratory nucleus
Posterior (motor) nucleus of vagus nerve (CN X)
Spinal nucleus of trigeminal nerve (CN V)*
Nucleus of hypoglossal nerve (CN XII)
* Sensory nucleus of CN V
Motor Nuclei:
Somatic motor (including
Branchial motor)
Visceral motor (Parasympathetic)
Fasciculus gracilis of medulla oblongata
Nucleus of spinal accessory nerve (CN XI)
Sensory Nuclei:
Somatic (general) sensory
Special sensory
Visceral sensory

A. Posterior (Dorsal) View

9.4 CRANIAL NERVE NUCLEI

The fibers of the cranial nerves are connected to nuclei (groups of nerve cell bodies in the central nervous system), in which afferent (sensory) fibers terminate and from which efferent (motor) fibers originate. Nuclei of common functional types (motor, sensory, parasympathetic, and special sensory nuclei) have a generally columnar placement within the brainstem, with the sulcus limitans demarcating motor and sensory columns.

Somatic motor: motor fibers innervating voluntary (striated muscle). For the muscles derived from the embryonic pharyngeal arches, their somatic motor innervation can be referred to more specifically as *branchial motor.*

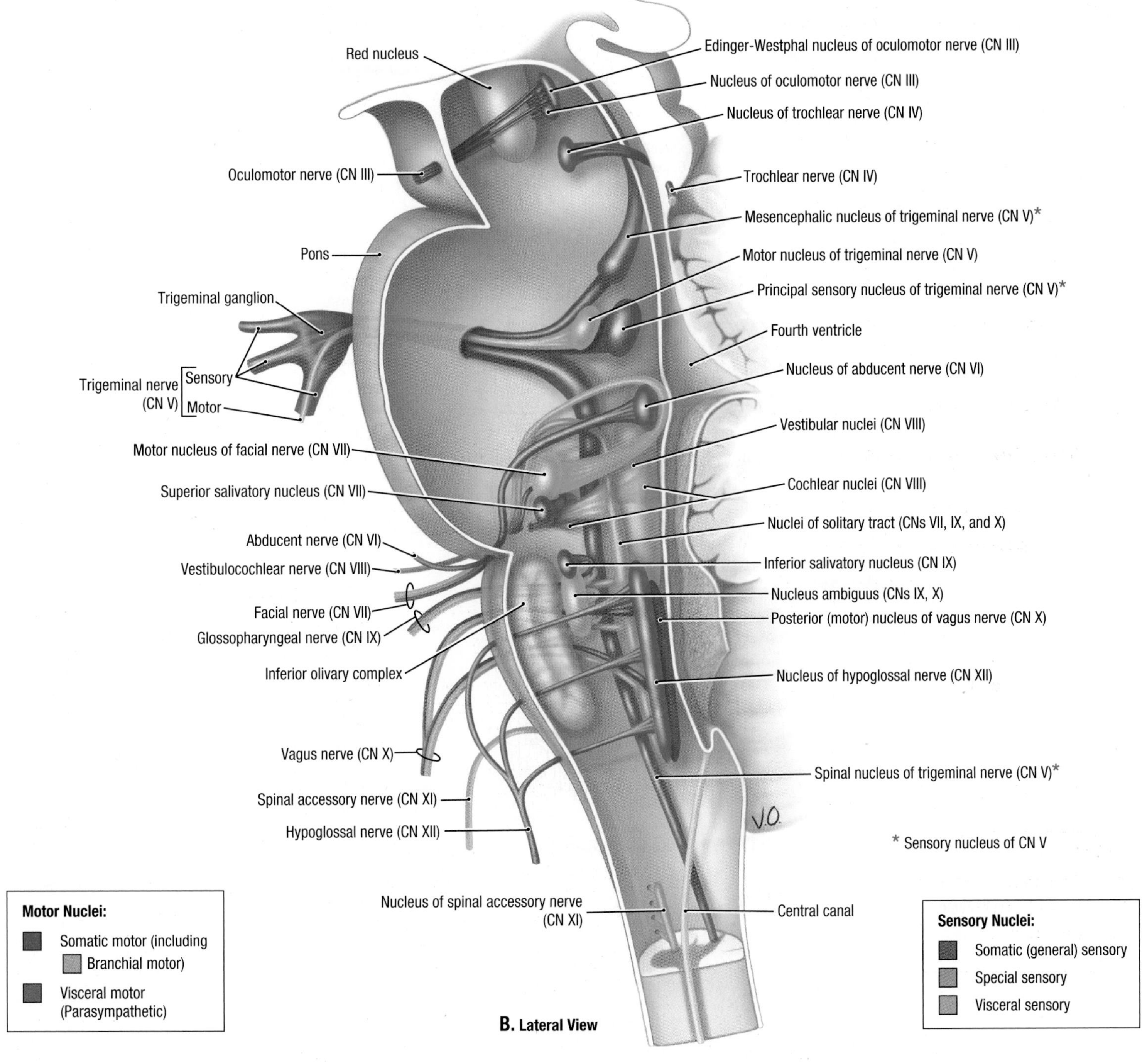
Red nucleus
Edinger-Westphal nucleus of oculomotor nerve (CN III)
Nucleus of oculomotor nerve (CN III)
Nucleus of trochlear nerve (CN IV)
Oculomotor nerve (CN III)
Trochlear nerve (CN IV)
Mesencephalic nucleus of trigeminal nerve (CN V)*
Pons
Motor nucleus of trigeminal nerve (CN V)
Trigeminal ganglion
Principal sensory nucleus of trigeminal nerve (CN V)*
Fourth ventricle
Trigeminal nerve (CN V)
Sensory
Motor
Nucleus of abducent nerve (CN VI)
Vestibular nuclei (CN VIII)
Motor nucleus of facial nerve (CN VII)
Cochlear nuclei (CN VIII)
Superior salivatory nucleus (CN VII)
Nuclei of solitary tract (CNs VII, IX, and X)
Abducent nerve (CN VI)
Inferior salivatory nucleus (CN IX)
Vestibulocochlear nerve (CN VIII)
Nucleus ambiguus (CNs IX, X)
Facial nerve (CN VII)
Posterior (motor) nucleus of vagus nerve (CN X)
Glossopharyngeal nerve (CN IX)
Inferior olivary complex
Nucleus of hypoglossal nerve (CN XII)
Vagus nerve (CN X)
Spinal nucleus of trigeminal nerve (CN V)*
Spinal accessory nerve (CN XI)
V.O.
Hypoglossal nerve (CN XII)
* Sensory nucleus of CN V
Nucleus of spinal accessory nerve (CN XI)
Central canal
Motor Nuclei:
Somatic motor (including
Branchial motor)
Visceral motor (Parasympathetic)
Sensory Nuclei:
Somatic (general) sensory
Special sensory
Visceral sensory

B. Lateral View

9.4 CRANIAL NERVE NUCLEI *(CONTINUED)*

Visceral motor: Parasympathetic innervation to glands and involuntary (smooth) muscle.

Somatic (general) sensory: Fibers transmitting general sensation from skin and membranes (e.g., touch, pressure, heat, cold).

Visceral sensory: Fibers conveying sensation from viscera (organs) and mucous membranes.

Special sensory: Taste, smell, vision, hearing, and balance.

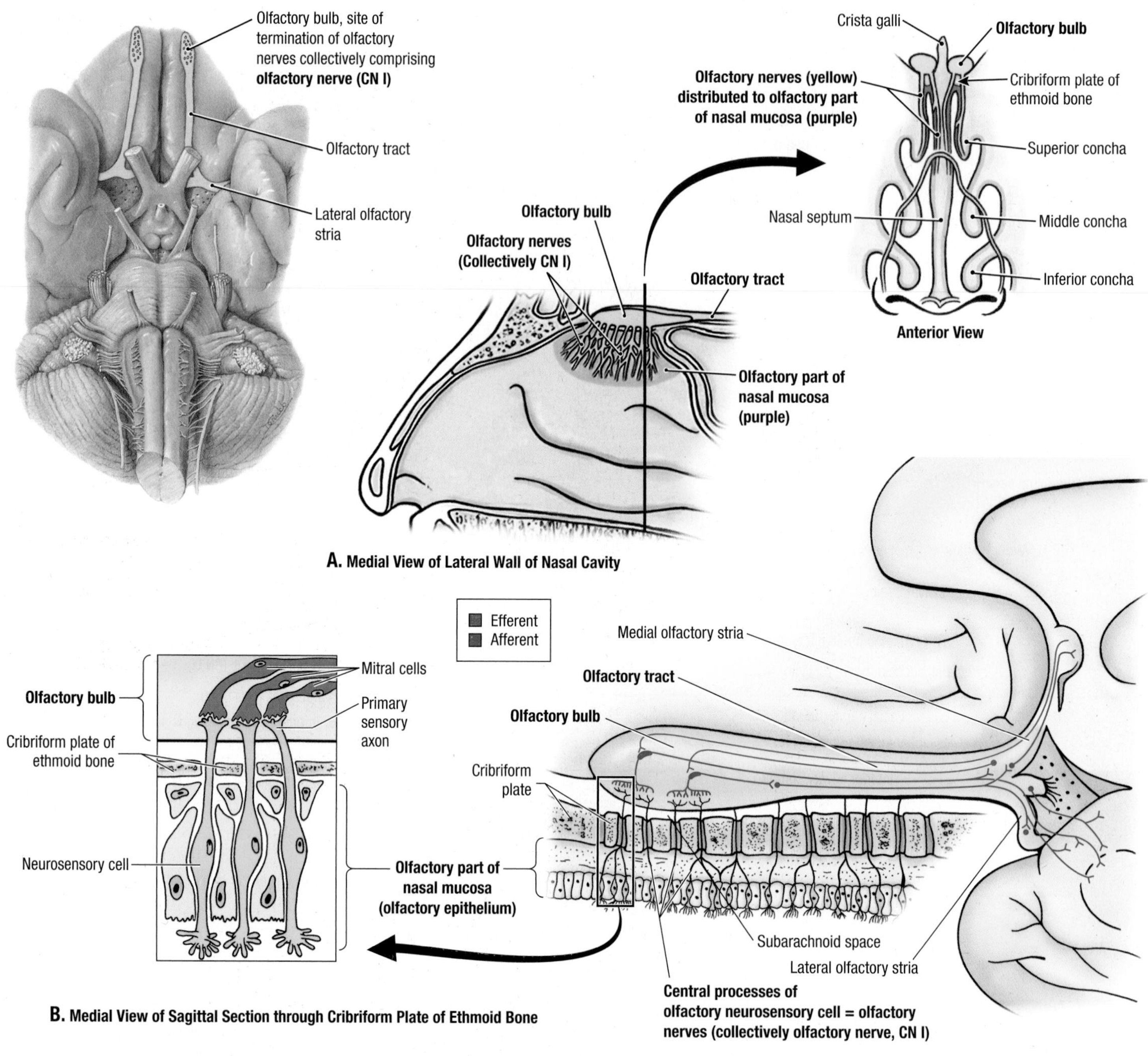
Olfactory bulb, site of termination of olfactory nerves collectively comprising **olfactory nerve (CN I)**
Olfactory tract
Lateral olfactory stria
Crista galli
Olfactory bulb
Olfactory nerves (yellow) distributed to olfactory part of nasal mucosa (purple)
Cribriform plate of ethmoid bone
Superior concha
Nasal septum
Middle concha
Inferior concha
Anterior View
Olfactory bulb
Olfactory nerves (Collectively CN I)
Olfactory tract
Olfactory part of nasal mucosa (purple)
A. Medial View of Lateral Wall of Nasal Cavity
Efferent
Afferent
Olfactory bulb
Mitral cells
Primary sensory axon
Cribriform plate of ethmoid bone
Neurosensory cell
Olfactory part of nasal mucosa (olfactory epithelium)
Medial olfactory stria
Olfactory tract
Olfactory bulb
Cribriform plate
Subarachnoid space
Lateral olfactory stria
Central processes of olfactory neurosensory cell = olfactory nerves (collectively olfactory nerve, CN I)
B. Medial View of Sagittal Section through Cribriform Plate of Ethmoid Bone

9.5 OLFACTORY NERVE (CN I)

A. Relationship of olfactory mucosa to olfactory bulb. **B.** Olfactory epithelium.

TABLE 9.2 OLFACTORY NERVE (CN I)

Nerve	Functional Components	Cells of Origin/Termination	Cranial Exit	Distribution and Functions
Olfactory	Special sensory	Olfactory epithelium (olfactory cells/olfactory bulb)	Foramina in cribriform plate of ethmoid bone	Smell from nasal mucosa of roof and superior sides of nasal septum and superior concha of each nasal cavity

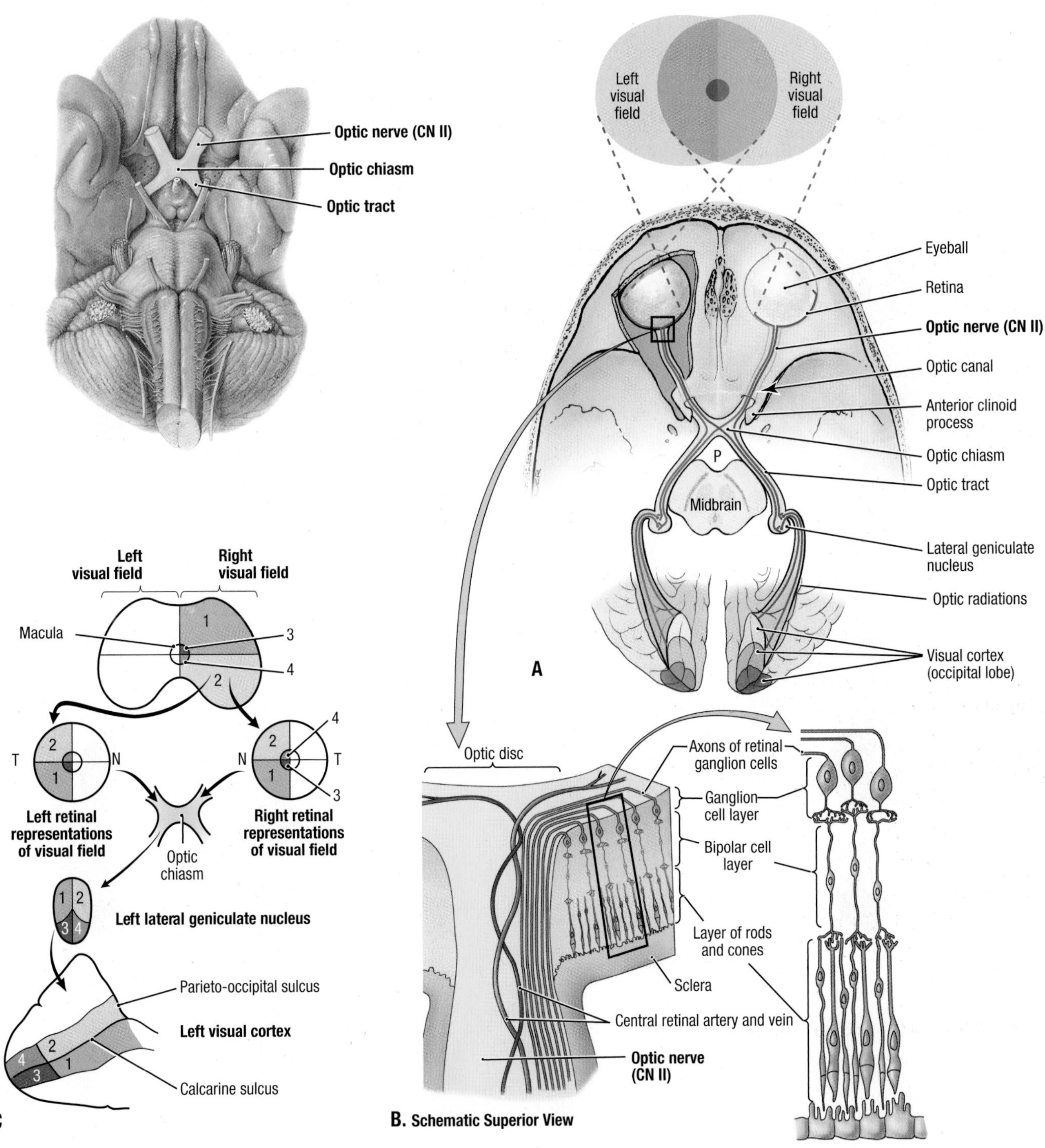
Optic nerve (CN II)
Optic chiasm
Optic tract
Left visual field
Right visual field
Eyeball
Retina
Optic nerve (CN II)
Optic canal
Anterior clinoid process
Optic chiasm
P
Optic tract
Midbrain
Lateral geniculate nucleus
Optic radiations
Visual cortex (occipital lobe)
A
Left visual field
Right visual field
Macula
1
2
3
4
T
N
Left retinal representations of visual field
Optic chiasm
Right retinal representations of visual field
Left lateral geniculate nucleus
Parieto-occipital sulcus
Left visual cortex
Calcarine sulcus
C
Optic disc
Axons of retinal ganglion cells
Ganglion cell layer
Bipolar cell layer
Layer of rods and cones
Sclera
Central retinal artery and vein
Optic nerve (CN II)
B. Schematic Superior View

9.6 OPTIC NERVE (CN II)

A. Origin and course of visual pathway. **B.** Rods and cones in retina. **C.** Right visual field representation on retinae, left lateral geniculate nucleus, and left visual cortex.

TABLE 9.3 OPTIC NERVE (CN II)

Nerve	Functional Components	Cells of Origin/Termination	Cranial Exit	Distribution and Functions
Optic	Special sensory	Retina (ganglion cells)/lateral geniculate body (nucleus)	Optic canal	Vision from retina

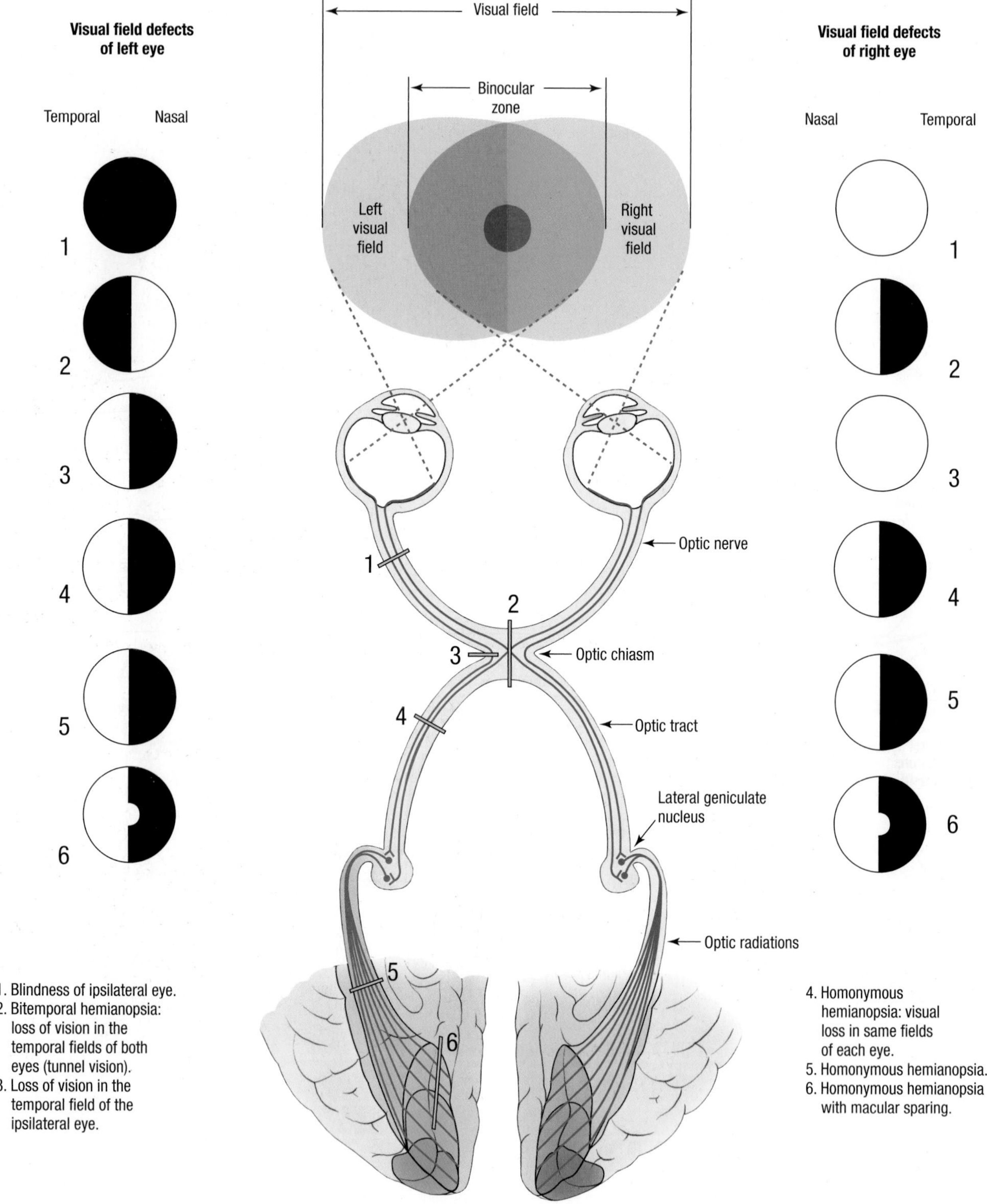
Visual field defects of left eye
Temporal
Nasal
1
2
3
4
5
6
Visual field
Binocular zone
Left visual field
Right visual field
Visual field defects of right eye
Nasal
Temporal
1
2
3
4
5
6
Optic nerve
Optic chiasm
Optic tract
Lateral geniculate nucleus
Optic radiations
1. Blindness of ipsilateral eye.
2. Bitemporal hemianopsia: loss of vision in the temporal fields of both eyes (tunnel vision).
3. Loss of vision in the temporal field of the ipsilateral eye.
4. Homonymous hemianopsia: visual loss in same fields of each eye.
5. Homonymous hemianopsia.
6. Homonymous hemianopsia with macular sparing.

9.7 VISUAL FIELD DEFECTS (CN II)

Visual field defects may result from a large number of neurologic diseases. It is clinically important to be able to link the defects to a likely location of the lesion.

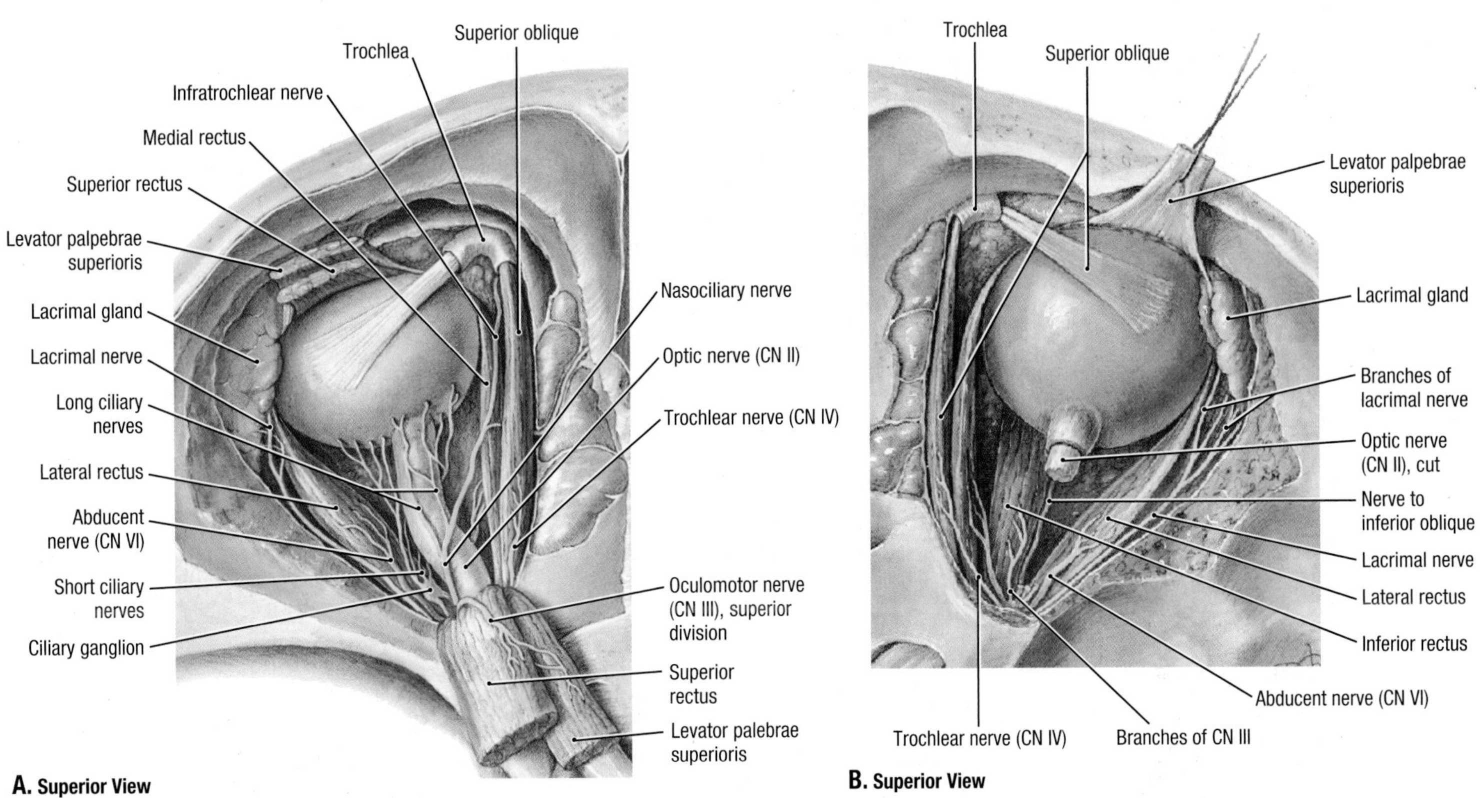
Trochlea
Superior oblique
Infratrochlear nerve
Medial rectus
Superior rectus
Levator palpebrae superioris
Lacrimal gland
Lacrimal nerve
Long ciliary nerves
Lateral rectus
Abducent nerve (CN VI)
Short ciliary nerves
Ciliary ganglion
Nasociliary nerve
Optic nerve (CN II)
Trochlear nerve (CN IV)
Oculomotor nerve (CN III), superior division
Superior rectus
Levator palebrae superioris
Trochlea
Superior oblique
Levator palpebrae superioris
Lacrimal gland
Branches of lacrimal nerve
Optic nerve (CN II), cut
Nerve to inferior oblique
Lacrimal nerve
Lateral rectus
Inferior rectus
Abducent nerve (CN VI)
Trochlear nerve (CN IV)
Branches of CN III

A. **Superior View**

B. **Superior View**

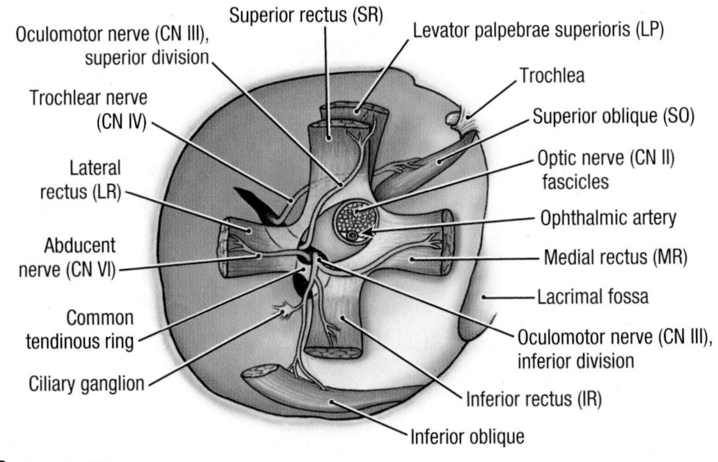
Superior rectus (SR)
Oculomotor nerve (CN III), superior division
Levator palpebrae superioris (LP)
Trochlea
Trochlear nerve (CN IV)
Superior oblique (SO)
Optic nerve (CN II) fascicles
Lateral rectus (LR)
Ophthalmic artery
Abducent nerve (CN VI)
Medial rectus (MR)
Lacrimal fossa
Common tendinous ring
Oculomotor nerve (CN III), inferior division
Ciliary ganglion
Inferior rectus (IR)
Inferior oblique

C. **Anterior View**

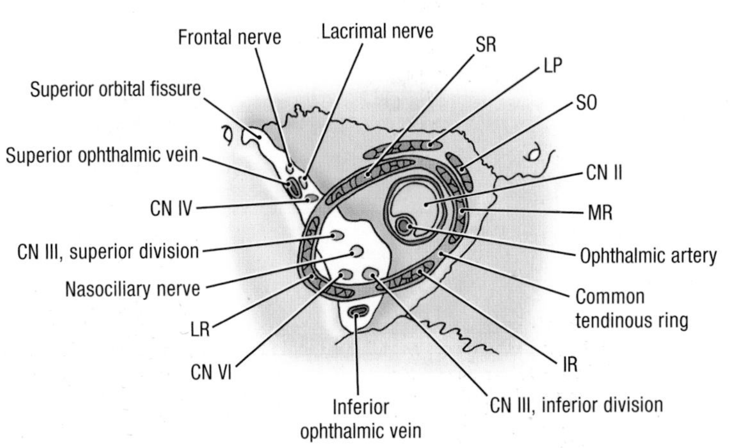
Frontal nerve
Lacrimal nerve
SR
LP
Superior orbital fissure
SO
Superior ophthalmic vein
CN II
CN IV
MR
CN III, superior division
Ophthalmic artery
Nasociliary nerve
Common tendinous ring
LR
IR
CN VI
Inferior ophthalmic vein
CN III, inferior division

D. **Anterior View**

9.8 OVERVIEW OF MUSCLES AND NERVES OF ORBIT

A. and B. Orbital cavities, dissected from a superior approach. The optic nerve is intact in **A** and cut away in **B.**, **C. and D.** Relationship of muscle attachments and nerves at apex of orbit.

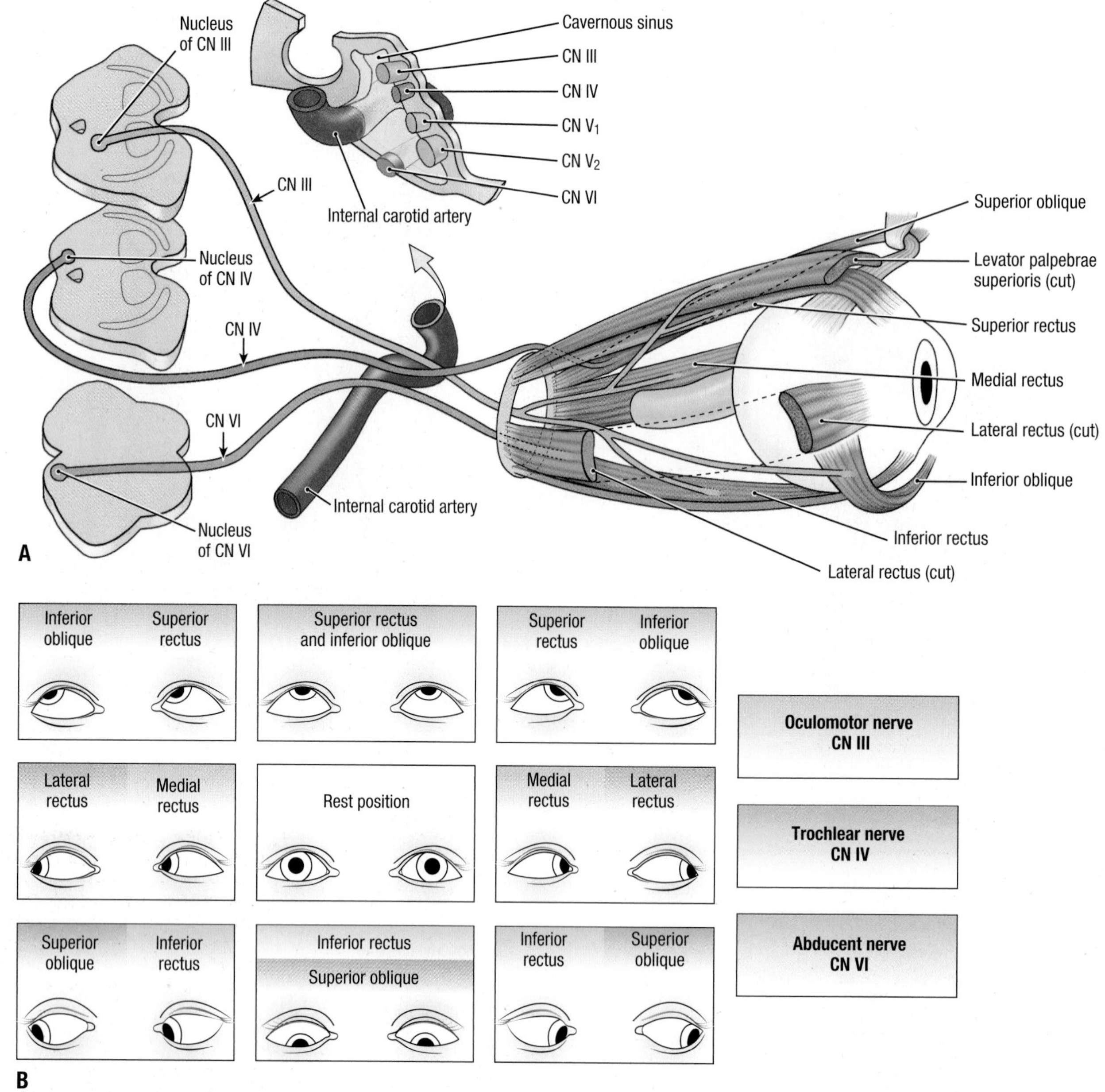

Nucleus of CN III
Cavernous sinus
CN III
CN IV
CN V_1
CN V_2
CN VI
CN III
Internal carotid artery
Superior oblique
Levator palpebrae superioris (cut)
Nucleus of CN IV
Superior rectus
CN IV
Medial rectus
CN VI
Lateral rectus (cut)
Inferior oblique
Internal carotid artery
Nucleus of CN VI
Inferior rectus
A
Lateral rectus (cut)
Inferior oblique
Superior rectus
Superior rectus and inferior oblique
Superior rectus
Inferior oblique
Oculomotor nerve CN III
Lateral rectus
Medial rectus
Rest position
Medial rectus
Lateral rectus
Trochlear nerve CN IV
Superior oblique
Inferior rectus
Inferior rectus
Superior oblique
Inferior rectus
Superior oblique
Abducent nerve CN VI
B

9.9 OCULOMOTOR (CN III), TROCHLEAR (CN IV), AND ABDUCENT (CN VI) NERVES

A. Schematic overview. **B.** Binocular movements and muscles producing them. All movements start from the rest (primary) position.

TABLE 9.4 OCULOMOTOR (CN III), TROCHLEAR (CN IV), AND ABDUCENT (CN VI) NERVES[a]

Nerve	Functional Components	Cells of Origin/Termination	Cranial Exit	Distribution and Functions
Oculomotor	Somatic motor	Nucleus of CN III	Superior orbital fissure	Motor to superior, inferior, and medial recti, inferior oblique, and levator palpebrae superioris muscles; raises upper eyelid, directing gaze superiorly, inferiorly, and medially
	Visceral motor (parasympathetic)	Presynaptic: midbrain (Edinger-Westphal nucleus); Postsynaptic: ciliary ganglion		Motor to sphincter pupillae and ciliary muscle that constrict pupil and accommodate lens of eyeball
Trochlear	Somatic motor	Nucleus of CN IV		Motor to superior oblique that assists in directing gaze inferolaterally
Abducent	Somatic motor	Nucleus of CN VI		Motor to lateral rectus that directs gaze laterally

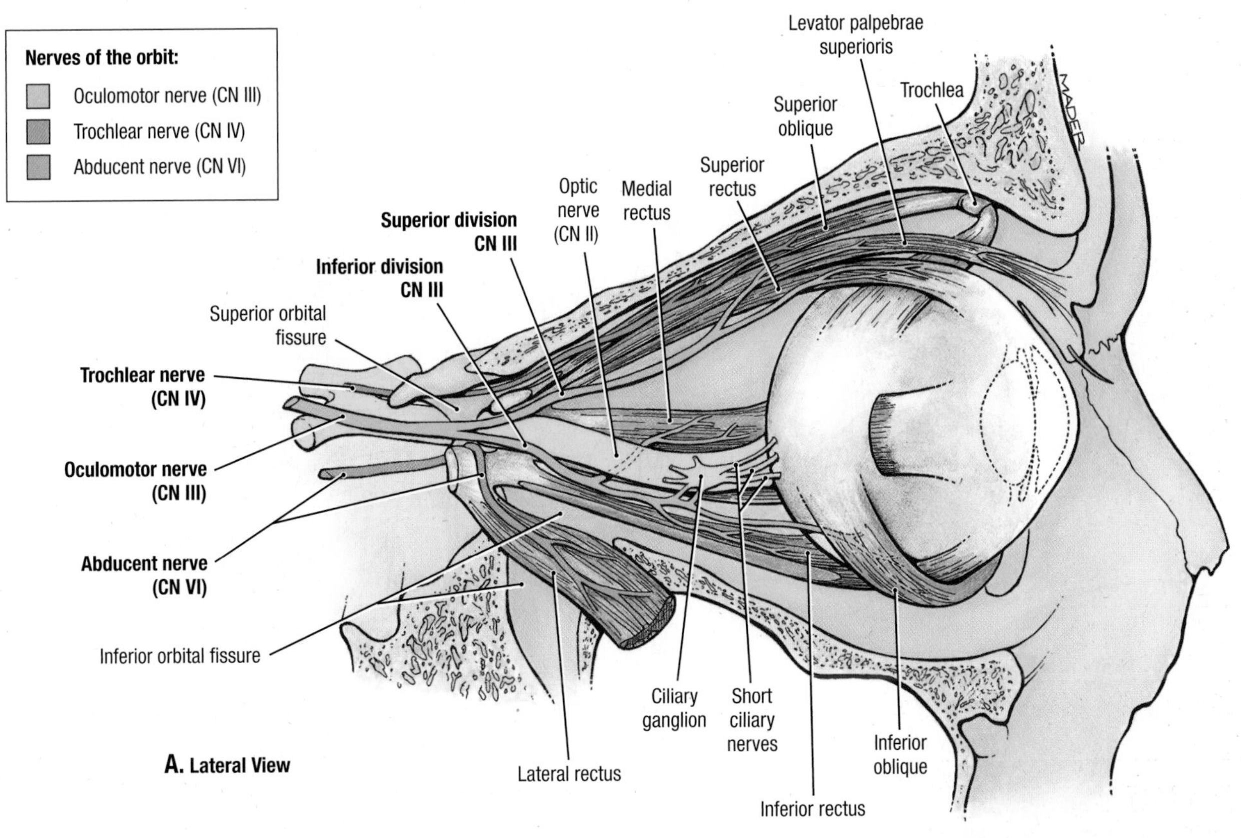
Nerves of the orbit:
Oculomotor nerve (CN III)
Trochlear nerve (CN IV)
Abducent nerve (CN VI)
Levator palpebrae superioris
Trochlea
Superior oblique
Superior rectus
Optic nerve (CN II)
Medial rectus
Superior division CN III
Inferior division CN III
Superior orbital fissure
Trochlear nerve (CN IV)
Oculomotor nerve (CN III)
Abducent nerve (CN VI)
Inferior orbital fissure
Ciliary ganglion
Short ciliary nerves
Inferior oblique
Lateral rectus
Inferior rectus
A. Lateral View

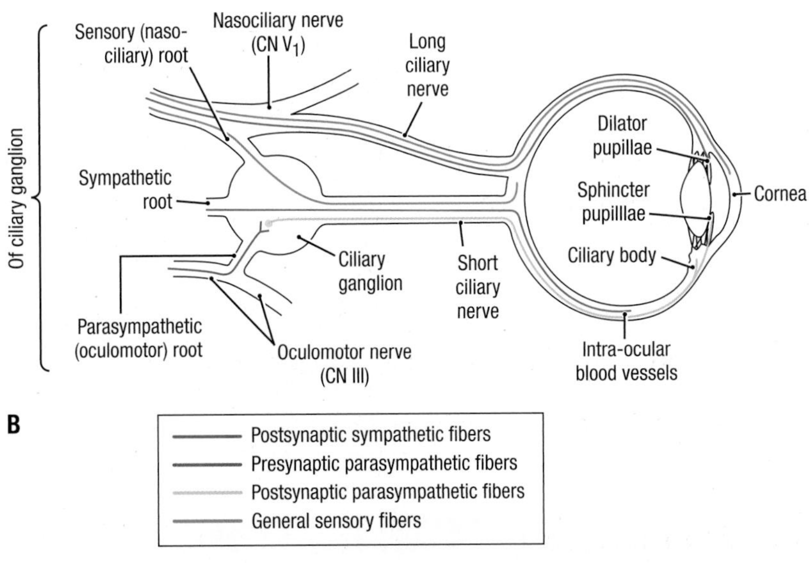
Sensory (naso-ciliary) root
Nasociliary nerve (CN V_1)
Long ciliary nerve
Dilator pupillae
Sympathetic root
Sphincter pupilllae
Cornea
Of ciliary ganglion
Ciliary body
Ciliary ganglion
Short ciliary nerve
Parasympathetic (oculomotor) root
Oculomotor nerve (CN III)
Intra-ocular blood vessels
B
Postsynaptic sympathetic fibers
Presynaptic parasympathetic fibers
Postsynaptic parasympathetic fibers
General sensory fibers

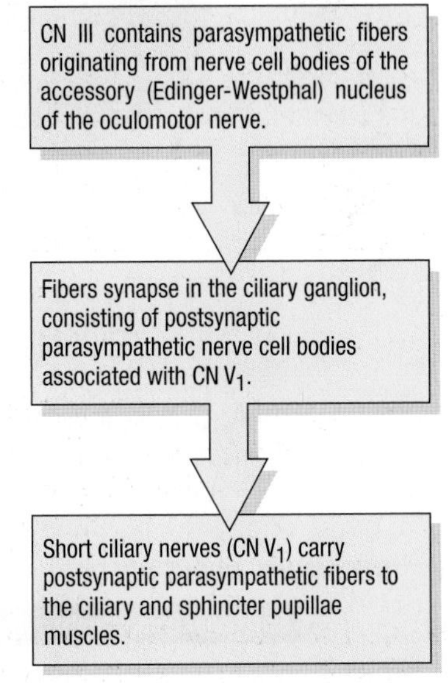
Visceral (parasympathetic) motor innervation of ciliary and sphincter pupillae muscles
CN III contains parasympathetic fibers originating from nerve cell bodies of the accessory (Edinger-Westphal) nucleus of the oculomotor nerve.
Fibers synapse in the ciliary ganglion, consisting of postsynaptic parasympathetic nerve cell bodies associated with CN V_1.
Short ciliary nerves (CN V_1) carry postsynaptic parasympathetic fibers to the ciliary and sphincter pupillae muscles.

9.10 INNERVATION OF EYEBALL

A. Nerves of orbit. **B.** Somatic and autonomic innervation of eyeball.

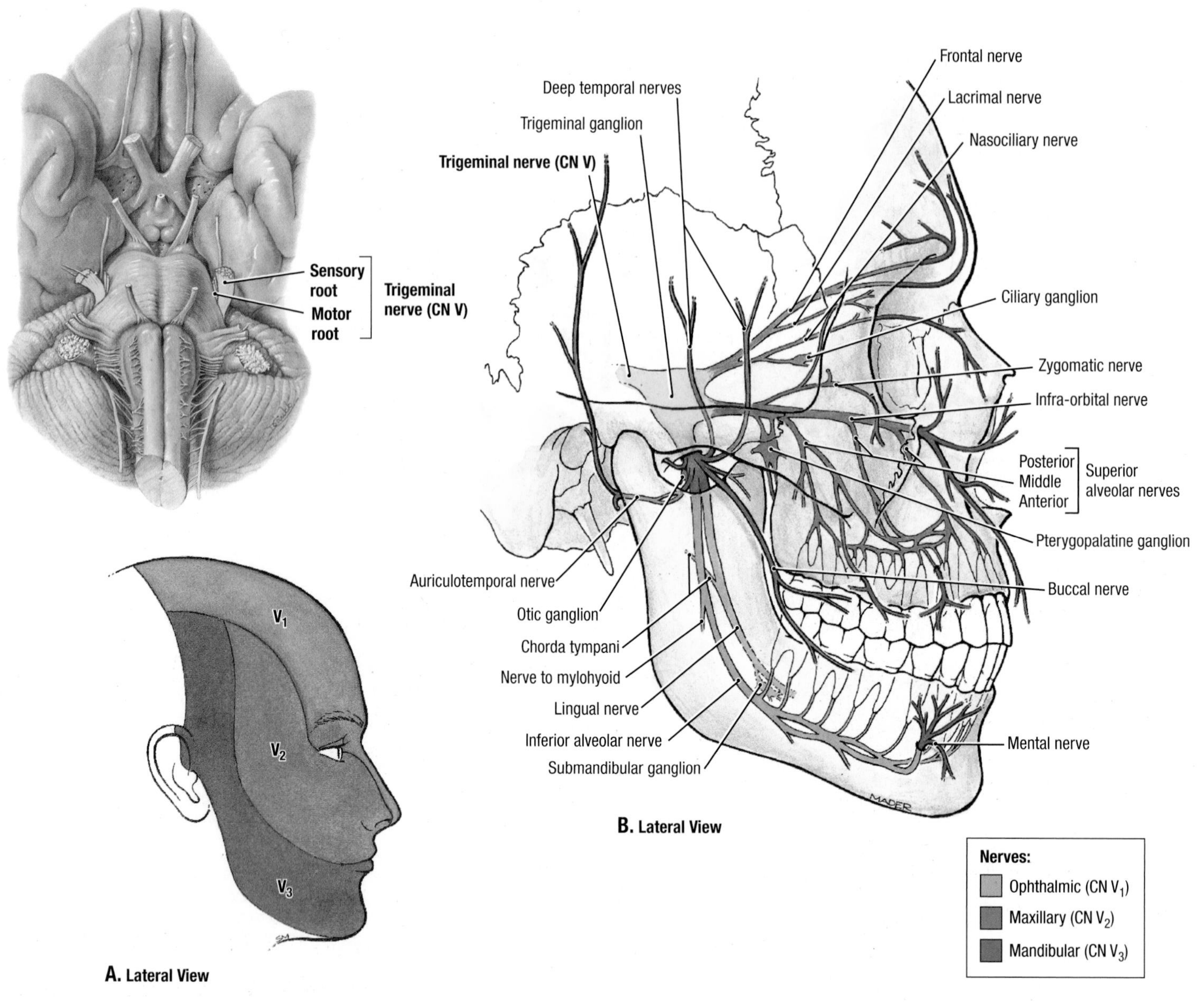

Sensory root
Motor root
Trigeminal nerve (CN V)
V1
V2
V3
A. Lateral View
Frontal nerve
Deep temporal nerves
Lacrimal nerve
Trigeminal ganglion
Nasociliary nerve
Trigeminal nerve (CN V)
Ciliary ganglion
Zygomatic nerve
Infra-orbital nerve
Posterior
Middle
Anterior
Superior alveolar nerves
Pterygopalatine ganglion
Auriculotemporal nerve
Buccal nerve
Otic ganglion
Chorda tympani
Nerve to mylohyoid
Lingual nerve
Inferior alveolar nerve
Mental nerve
Submandibular ganglion
B. Lateral View
Nerves:
Ophthalmic (CN V1)
Maxillary (CN V2)
Mandibular (CN V3)

9.11 TRIGEMINAL NERVE (CN V)

A. Cutaneous (somatic sensory) distribution. **B.** Branches of ophthalmic (CN V_1), maxillary (CN V_2), and mandibular (CN V_3) divisions.

TABLE 9.5 TRIGEMINAL NERVE (CN V)

Nerve	Functional Components	Cells of Origin/Termination	Cranial Exit	Distribution and Functions
Ophthalmic division (CN V_1)	Somatic (general sensory)	Trigeminal ganglion/spinal, principal and mesencephalic nucleus of CN V	Superior orbital fissure	Sensation from cornea, skin of forehead, scalp, eyelids, nose, and mucosa of nasal cavity and paranasal sinuses
Maxillary division (CN V_2)			Foramen rotundum	Sensation from skin of face over maxilla including upper lip, maxillary teeth, mucosa of nose, maxillary sinuses, and palate
Mandibular division (CN V_3)			Foramen ovale	Sensation from the skin over mandible, including lower lip and side of head, mandibular teeth, temporomandibular joint, and mucosa of mouth and anterior two thirds of tongue
	Somatic (branchial) motor	Motor nucleus of CN V		Motor to muscles of mastication, mylohyoid, anterior belly of digastric, tensor veli palatini, and tensor tympani

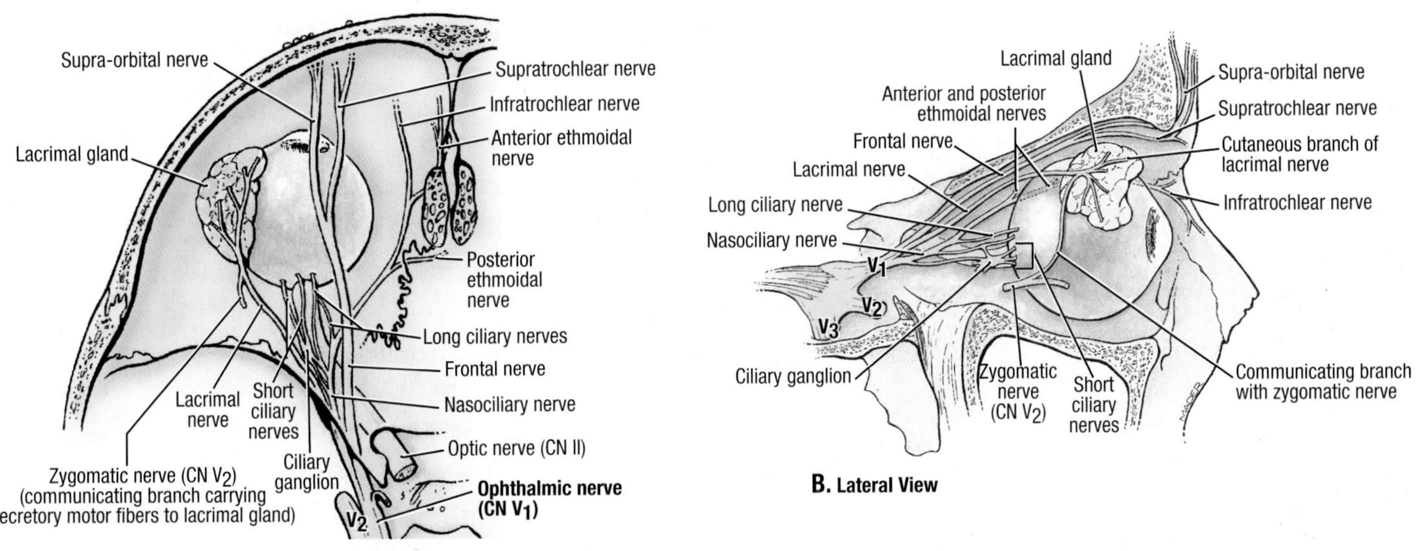
Supra-orbital nerve
Supratrochlear nerve
Infratrochlear nerve
Anterior ethmoidal nerve
Lacrimal gland
Posterior ethmoidal nerve
Long ciliary nerves
Frontal nerve
Nasociliary nerve
Lacrimal nerve
Short ciliary nerves
Optic nerve (CN II)
Ciliary ganglion
Zygomatic nerve (CN V_2) (communicating branch carrying secretory motor fibers to lacrimal gland)
Ophthalmic nerve (CN V_1)
V_2
Lacrimal gland
Anterior and posterior ethmoidal nerves
Frontal nerve
Lacrimal nerve
Long ciliary nerve
Nasociliary nerve
V_1
V_2
V_3
Supra-orbital nerve
Supratrochlear nerve
Cutaneous branch of lacrimal nerve
Infratrochlear nerve
Ciliary ganglion
Zygomatic nerve (CN V_2)
Short ciliary nerves
Communicating branch with zygomatic nerve

A. Superior View

B. Lateral View

Internal carotid artery
Posterior clinoid process
Infundibulum
Optic nerves (CN II)
Anterior clinoid process
Midbrain
Supratrochlear nerve (CN V_1)
Trochlear nerve (CN IV)
Supra-orbital nerve (CN V_1)
Levator palpebrae superioris
Sensory root of trigeminal nerve (CN V)
Frontal nerve (CN V_1)
Lacrimal nerve (CN V_1)
Mouth of trigeminal cave
Abducent nerve (CN VI)
Oculomotor nerve (CN III)
Trigeminal ganglion
Trochlear nerve (CN IV)
Petrosal nerves Greater Lesser
Ophthalmic nerve (CN V_1)
Maxillary nerve (CN V_2)
Mandibular nerve (CN V_3)

C. Lateral View

9.12 OPHTHALMIC NERVE (CN V_1)

A. and B. Overview. **C.** Course through cavernous sinus.

TABLE 9.6 BRANCHES OF OPHTHALMIC NERVE (CN V_1)

Function	Branches
Ophthalmic nerve (CN V_1) Somatic sensory only at origin from trigeminal ganglion Visceral motor: extracranially, conveys (1) postsynaptic parasympathetic fibers from ciliary ganglion to ciliary body and sphincter of pupillae; (2) postsynaptic parasympathetic fibers from communicating branch of zygomatic nerve (CN V_2) to lacrimal gland; and (3) postsynaptic sympathetic fibers from internal carotid plexus to dilator pupillae and intra-ocular blood vessels. Passes through superior orbital fissure to enter orbit Supplies general sensory innervation to cornea, superior bulbar and palpebral conjunctiva, mucosa of anterosuperior nasal cavity, frontal, ethmoidal, and sphenoidal sinuses, anterior and supratentorial dura mater, skin of dorsum of external nose, superior eyelid, forehead and anterior scalp. Somatic sensory CN V_1	*Somatic sensory branches:* Tentorial nerve (an intracranial meningeal branch) Lacrimal nerve [terminal portion also receives postsynaptic parasympathetic fibers from zygomatic nerve (CN V_2) and conveys them to lacrimal gland] Frontal nerve Supra-orbital nerve Supratrochlear nerve Nasociliary nerve Sensory root of ciliary ganglion Long and short ciliary nerves [also convey postsynaptic sympathetic fibers (from internal carotid plexus to eyeball additionally, short ciliary nerves convey postsynaptic parasympathetic fibers from ciliary ganglion to eyeball] Anterior and posterior ethmoidal nerves Anterior meningeal nerves Internal and external nasal branches Infratrochlear nerve

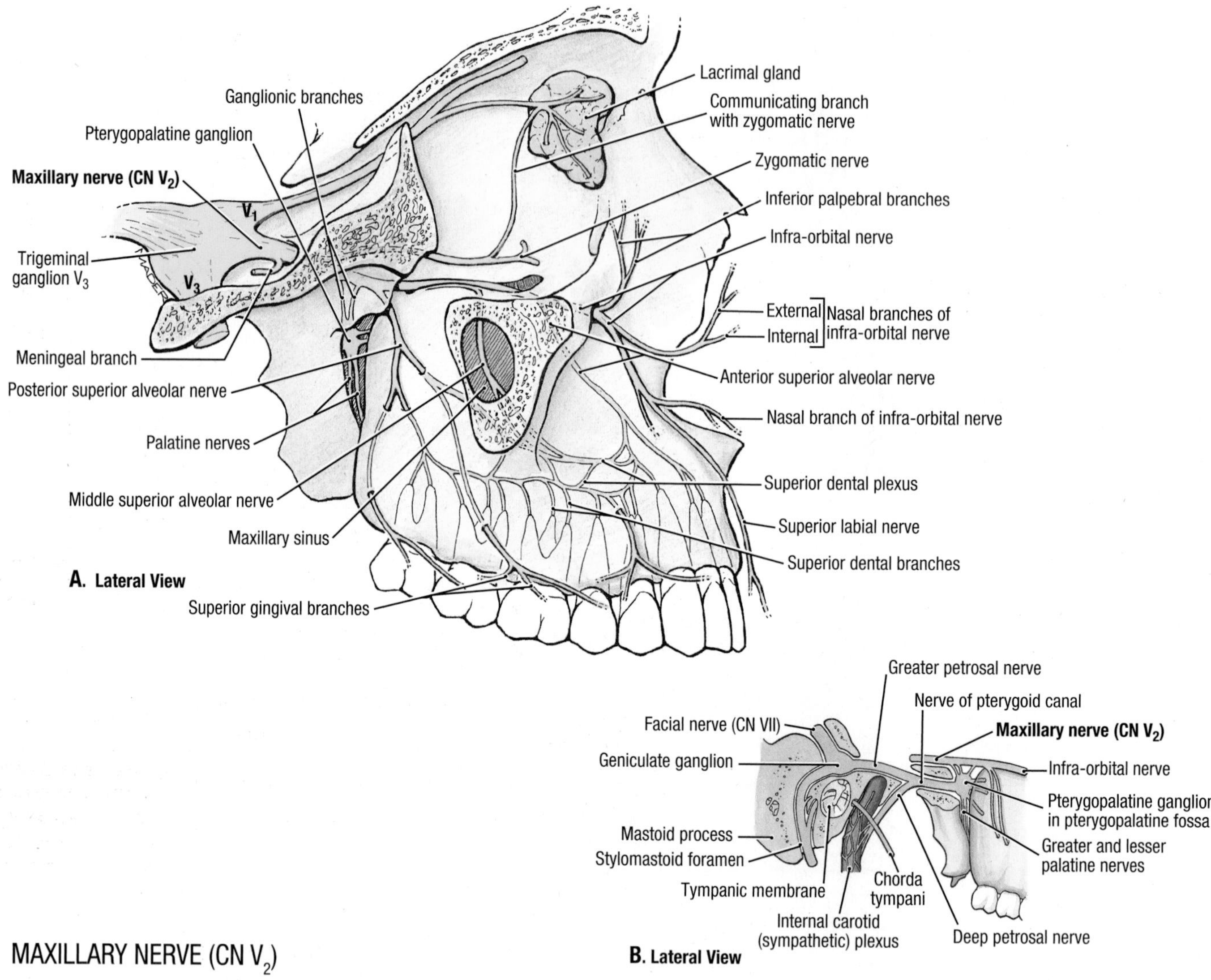
Lacrimal gland
Communicating branch with zygomatic nerve
Ganglionic branches
Pterygopalatine ganglion
Zygomatic nerve
Maxillary nerve (CN V2)
V1
Inferior palpebral branches
Infra-orbital nerve
Trigeminal ganglion V3
V3
External
Internal
Nasal branches of infra-orbital nerve
Meningeal branch
Posterior superior alveolar nerve
Anterior superior alveolar nerve
Nasal branch of infra-orbital nerve
Palatine nerves
Superior dental plexus
Middle superior alveolar nerve
Superior labial nerve
Maxillary sinus
Superior dental branches
A. Lateral View
Superior gingival branches
Greater petrosal nerve
Nerve of pterygoid canal
Facial nerve (CN VII)
Maxillary nerve (CN V2)
Geniculate ganglion
Infra-orbital nerve
Pterygopalatine ganglion in pterygopalatine fossa
Mastoid process
Greater and lesser palatine nerves
Stylomastoid foramen
Chorda tympani
Tympanic membrane
Internal carotid (sympathetic) plexus
Deep petrosal nerve
B. Lateral View

9.13 MAXILLARY NERVE (CN V_2)

TABLE 9.7 BRANCHES OF MAXILLARY NERVE (CN V_2)

Function	Branches
Maxillary nerve (CN V_2) Somatic sensory only (proximally, at origin from trigeminal ganglion) Visceral motor: distally, conveys (1) postsynaptic parasympathetic fibers from pterygopalatine ganglion (presynaptic fibers are from CN VII via greater petrosal nerve and nerve of pterygoid canal); and (2) postsynaptic sympathetic fibers from superior cervical ganglion via internal carotid plexus (presynaptic fibers are from intermediolateral column of gray matter, spinal cord segments T1–T3). Passes through foramen rotundum to enter pterygopalatine fossa Supplies dura mater of anterior aspect of lateral part of middle cranial fossa; conjunctiva of inferior eyelid; mucosa of postero-inferior nasal cavity, maxillary sinus, palate, and anterior part of superior oral vestibule; maxillary teeth; and skin of lateral external nose, inferior eyelid, anterior cheek, and upper lip. Somatic sensory CN V_2	Meningeal branch Zygomatic branch Zygomaticofacial branch Zygomaticotemporal branch Communicating branch to lacrimal nerve Ganglionic branches to (sensory root of) pterygopalatine ganglion Infra-orbital nerve Posterior, middle, and anterior superior alveolar branches Superior dental plexus and branches Superior gingival branches Inferior palpebral branches External and internal nasal branches Superior labial branches Greater palatine nerve Posterior inferior lateral nasal nerves Lesser palatine nerves Posterior superior lateral and medial nasal branches Nasopalatine nerve Pharyngeal nerve

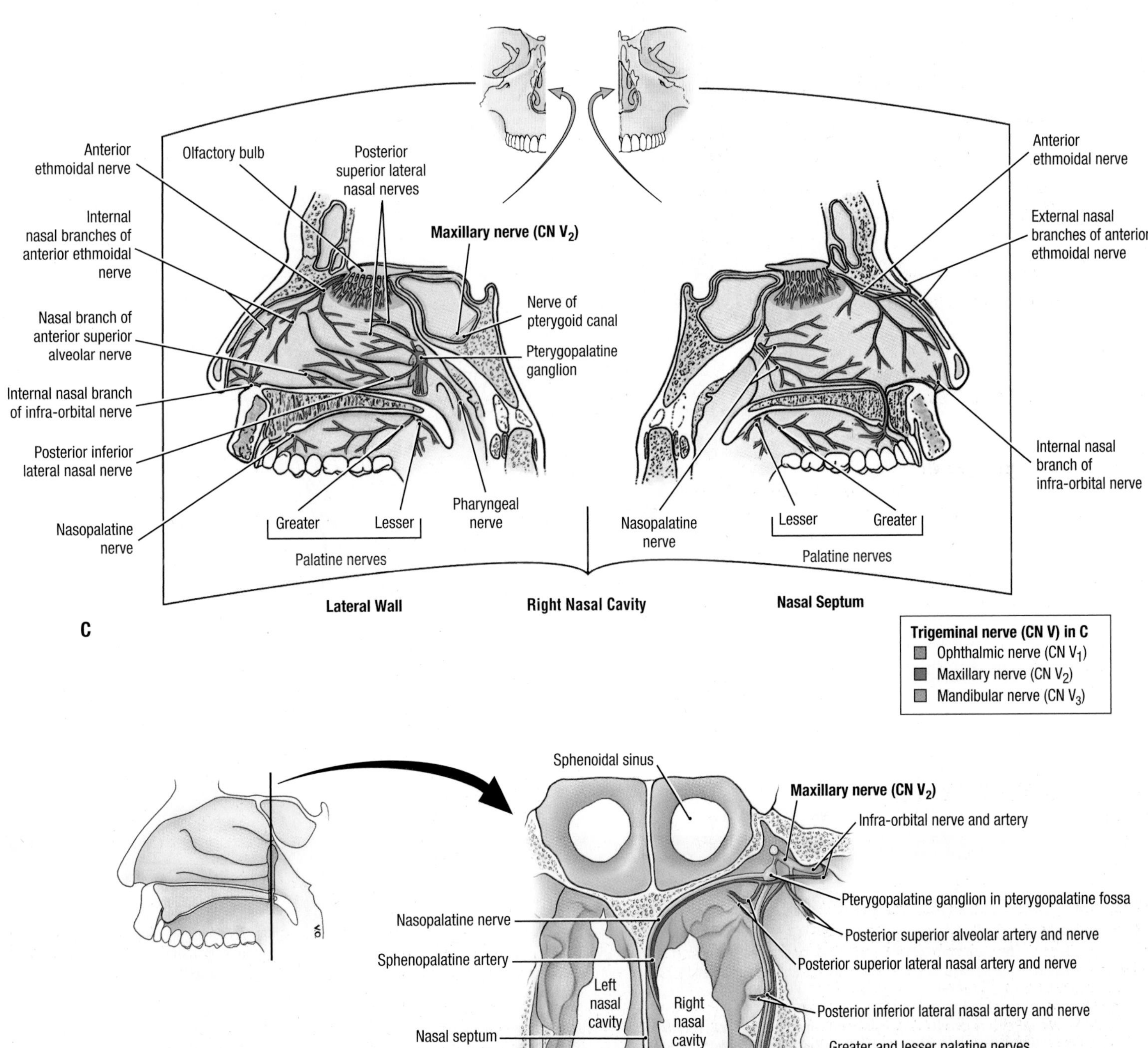
Anterior ethmoidal nerve
Olfactory bulb
Posterior superior lateral nasal nerves
Maxillary nerve (CN V_2)
Internal nasal branches of anterior ethmoidal nerve
Nerve of pterygoid canal
Pterygopalatine ganglion
Nasal branch of anterior superior alveolar nerve
Internal nasal branch of infra-orbital nerve
Posterior inferior lateral nasal nerve
Nasopalatine nerve
Greater
Lesser
Palatine nerves
Pharyngeal nerve
Lateral Wall
Right Nasal Cavity
Nasal Septum
Anterior ethmoidal nerve
External nasal branches of anterior ethmoidal nerve
Internal nasal branch of infra-orbital nerve
Nasopalatine nerve
Lesser
Greater
Palatine nerves
C
Trigeminal nerve (CN V) in C
Ophthalmic nerve (CN V_1)
Maxillary nerve (CN V_2)
Mandibular nerve (CN V_3)
Sphenoidal sinus
Maxillary nerve (CN V_2)
Infra-orbital nerve and artery
Pterygopalatine ganglion in pterygopalatine fossa
Posterior superior alveolar artery and nerve
Posterior superior lateral nasal artery and nerve
Nasopalatine nerve
Sphenopalatine artery
Left nasal cavity
Right nasal cavity
Posterior inferior lateral nasal artery and nerve
Nasal septum
Greater and lesser palatine nerves and artery in palatine canal
Palatine canal
Lesser palatine artery and nerve
Oral cavity
Bony palate
Greater palatine artery and nerve
Posterior view of cranium coronally sectioned through the nasal cavities and pterygopalatine fossa
D

9.13 MAXILLARY NERVE (CN V_2) *(CONTINUED)*

A. Overview. **B.** Nerves of pterygopalatine fossa. **C. and D.** Innervation of lateral wall and septum of nasal cavity and palate.

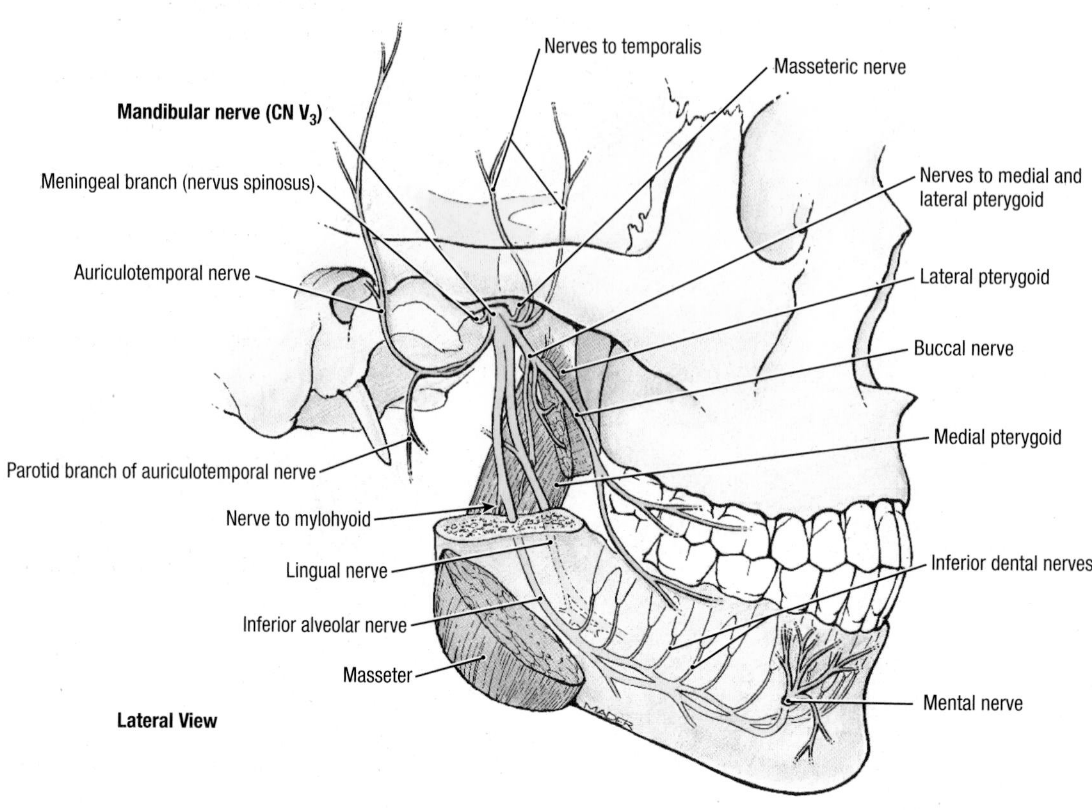
Nerves to temporalis
Masseteric nerve
Mandibular nerve (CN V3)
Meningeal branch (nervus spinosus)
Nerves to medial and lateral pterygoid
Auriculotemporal nerve
Lateral pterygoid
Buccal nerve
Medial pterygoid
Parotid branch of auriculotemporal nerve
Nerve to mylohyoid
Lingual nerve
Inferior dental nerves
Inferior alveolar nerve
Masseter
Mental nerve
Lateral View

9.14 MANDIBULAR NERVE (CN V_3)

TABLE 9.8 BRANCHES OF MANDIBULAR NERVE (CN V_3)

Function	Branches
Maxillary nerve (CN V_3) Somatic sensory and somatic (branchial) motor Special sensory: extracranially, conveys taste fibers (from CN VII via chorda tympani nerve) to anterior 2/3 of tongue Visceral motor: extracranially, conveys (1) presynaptic parasympathetic fibers to submandibular ganglion (presynaptic fibers are from CN VII via chorda tympani nerve); (2) postsynaptic parasympathetic fibers from submandibular ganglion to submandibular and sublingual glands; and (3) postsynaptic parasympathetic fibers from otic ganglion to parotid gland. Passes through foramen ovale to enter infratemporal fossa Supplies general sensory innervation to mucosa of anterior 2/3 of tongue, floor of mouth, and posterior and anterior inferior oral vestibule; mandibular teeth; and skin of lower lip, buccal and temporal regions of face, and external ear (anterior superior auricle, upper external auditory meatus, and tympanic membrane). Supplies motor innervation to all 4 muscles of mastication, mylohyoid, anterior belly of digastric, tensor tympani and tensor veli palatin Somatic sensory CN V_3 Somatic motor CN V_3	*Somatic sensory branches:* Meningeal branch (nervus spinosum) Buccal nerve Auriculotemporal nerve (also conveys *visceral motor fibers*) Superficial temporal branches Parotid branches Lingual nerve (also conveys *visceral motor* and *special sensory fibers*) Inferior alveolar nerve Nerve to mylohyoid Inferior dental plexus Inferior dental branches Inferior gingival branches Mental nerve *Somatic (branchial) motor branches:* Masseteric nerve Medial and lateral pterygoid branches Deep temporal nerves Nerve to mylohyoid Nerve to tensor tympani Nerve to tensor veli palatini

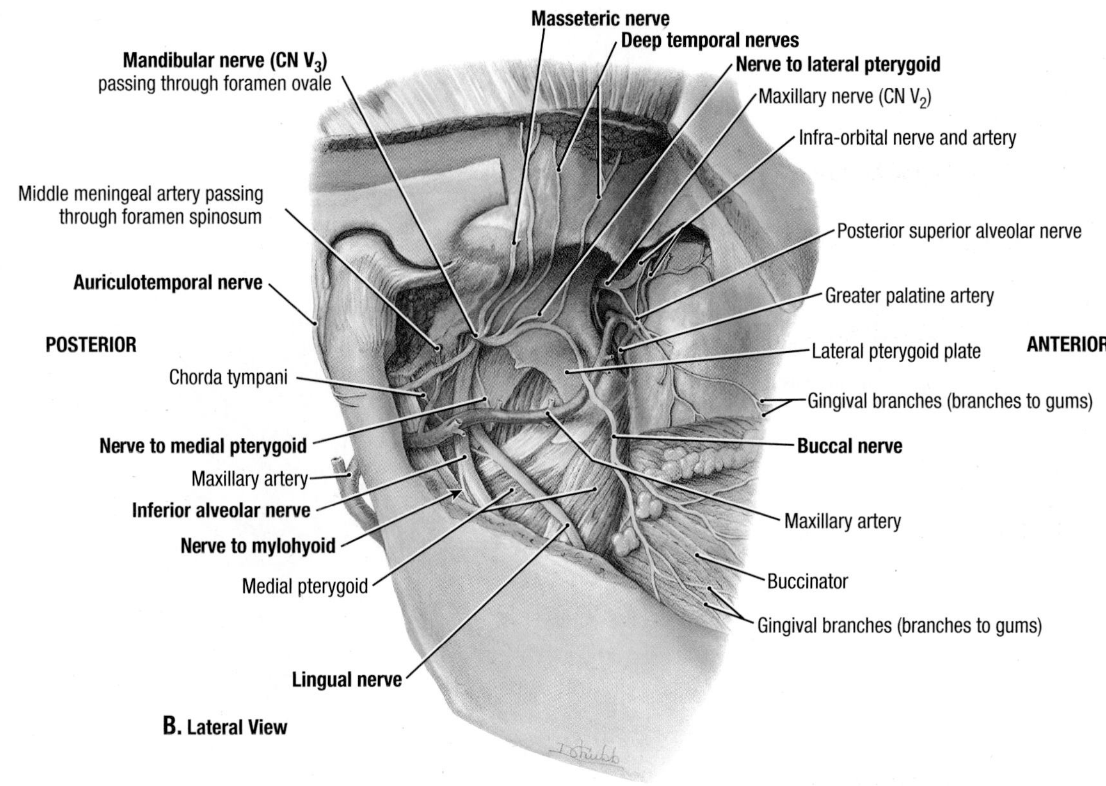
Masseteric nerve
Deep temporal nerves
Nerve to lateral pterygoid
Maxillary nerve (CN V2)
Infra-orbital nerve and artery
Mandibular nerve (CN V3) passing through foramen ovale
Middle meningeal artery passing through foramen spinosum
Posterior superior alveolar nerve
Auriculotemporal nerve
Greater palatine artery
POSTERIOR
Lateral pterygoid plate
ANTERIOR
Chorda tympani
Gingival branches (branches to gums)
Nerve to medial pterygoid
Buccal nerve
Maxillary artery
Inferior alveolar nerve
Maxillary artery
Nerve to mylohyoid
Buccinator
Medial pterygoid
Gingival branches (branches to gums)
Lingual nerve

B. Lateral View

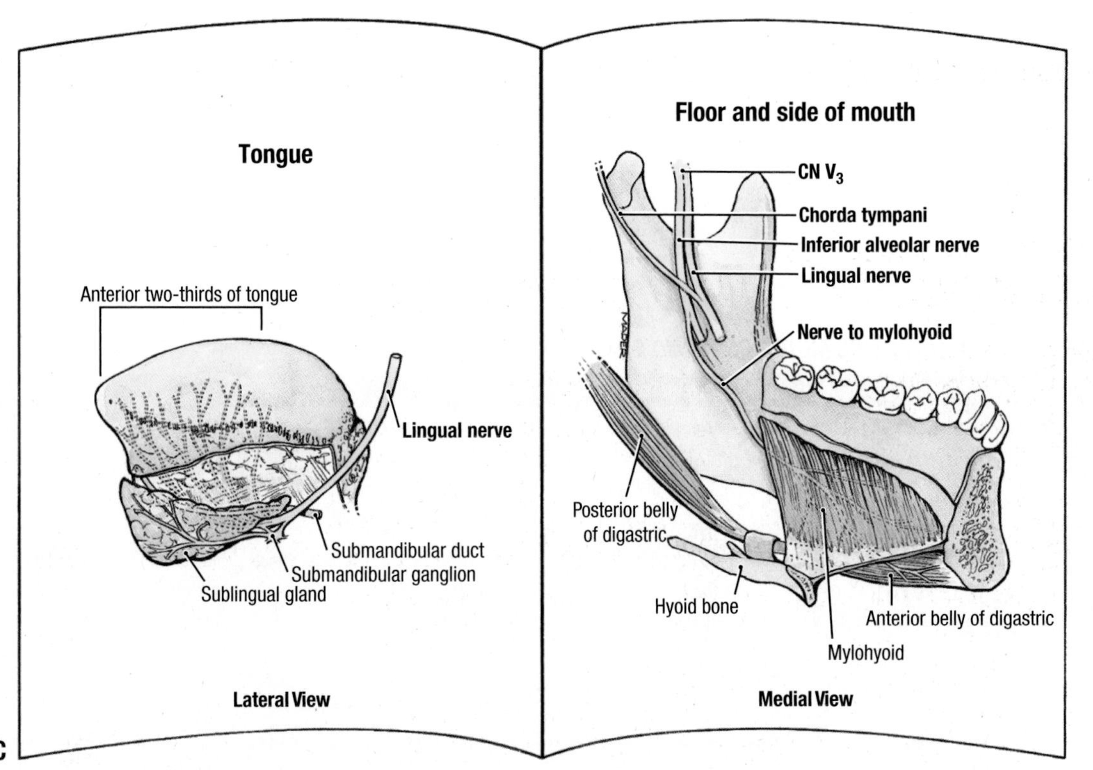
Tongue
Anterior two-thirds of tongue
Lingual nerve
Submandibular duct
Submandibular ganglion
Sublingual gland
Lateral View
Floor and side of mouth
CN V3
Chorda tympani
Inferior alveolar nerve
Lingual nerve
Nerve to mylohyoid
Posterior belly of digastric
Hyoid bone
Anterior belly of digastric
Mylohyoid
Medial View

C

9.14 MANDIBULAR NERVE (CN V_3) *(CONTINUED)*

A. Overview. **B.** Deep dissection of CN V_3 and branches at foramen ovale. **C.** Lateral aspect of tongue and medial aspect of mandible displayed as pages in an open book that is, the tongue has been reflected from the mandible.

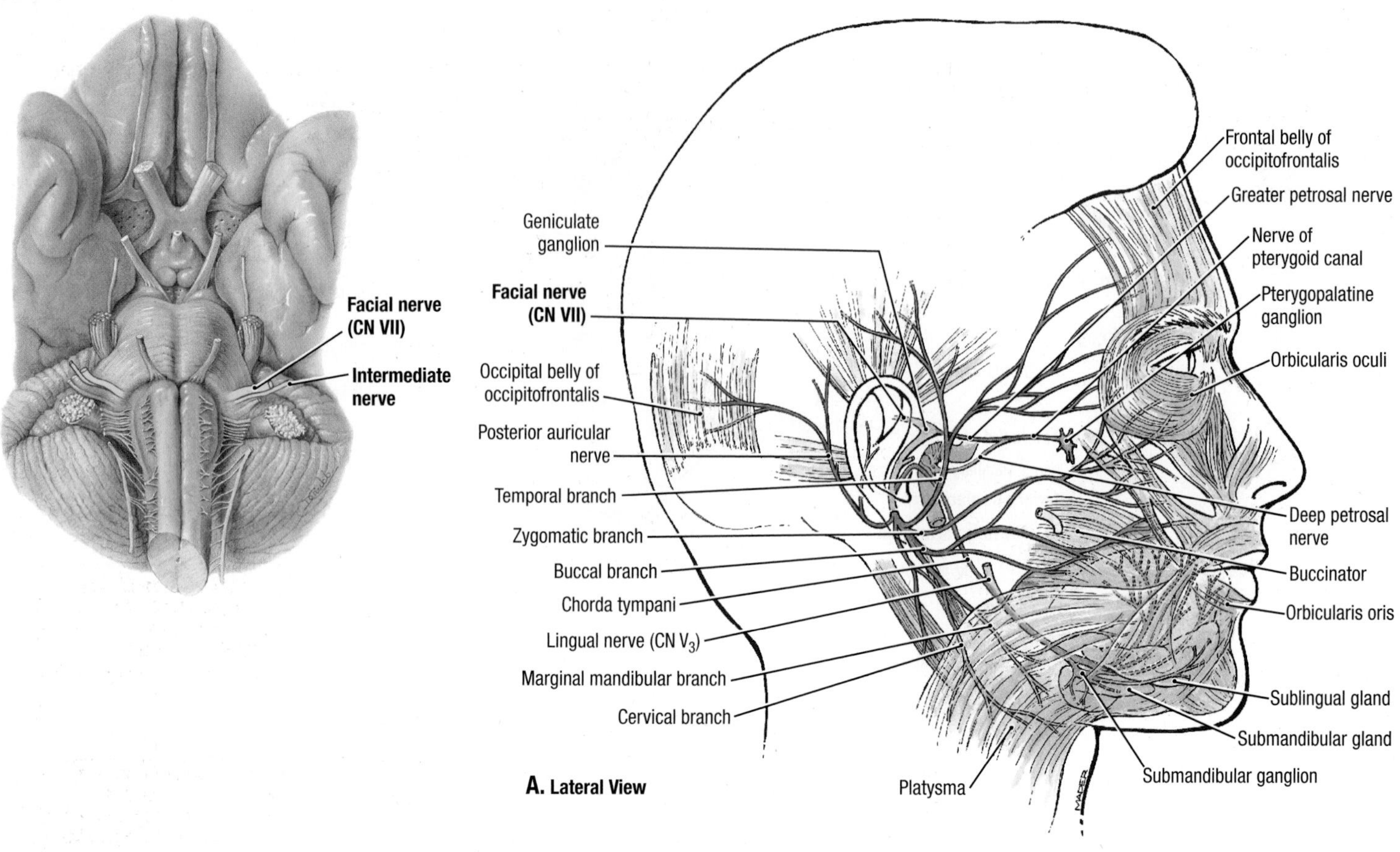

Facial nerve (CN VII)
Intermediate nerve
Geniculate ganglion
Facial nerve (CN VII)
Occipital belly of occipitofrontalis
Posterior auricular nerve
Temporal branch
Zygomatic branch
Buccal branch
Chorda tympani
Lingual nerve (CN V_3)
Marginal mandibular branch
Cervical branch
A. Lateral View
Platysma
Frontal belly of occipitofrontalis
Greater petrosal nerve
Nerve of pterygoid canal
Pterygopalatine ganglion
Orbicularis oculi
Deep petrosal nerve
Buccinator
Orbicularis oris
Sublingual gland
Submandibular gland
Submandibular ganglion

9.15 FACIAL NERVE (CN VII)

A. Overview. **B.** Parasympathetic motor innervation of lacrimal, submandibular, and sublingual glands. **C.** Nerve of pterygoid canal.

TABLE 9.9 FACIAL NERVE (CN VII), INCLUDING MOTOR ROOT AND INTERMEDIATE NERVE[a]

Nerve	Functional Components	Cells of Origin/Termination	Cranial Exit	Distribution and Functions
Temporal, zygomatic, buccal, mandibular, cervical, and posterior auricular nerves, nerve to posterior belly of digastric, nerve to stylohyoid, nerve to stapedius	Somatic (branchial) motor	Motor nucleus of CN VII	Stylomastoid foramen	Motor to muscles of facial expression and scalp;, also supplies stapedius of middle ear, stylohyoid, and posterior belly of digastric
Intermediate nerve through chorda tympani	Special sensory	Geniculate ganglion/solitary nucleus	Internal acoustic meatus/facial canal/ petrotympanic fissure	Taste from anterior two thirds of tongue, through chorda tympani floor of mouth, and palate
Intermediate nerve	Somatic (general) sensory	Geniculate ganglion/spinal trigeminal nucleus	Internal acoustic meatus	Sensation from skin of external acoustic meatus
Intermediate nerve through greater petrosal nerve	Visceral sensory	Nuclei of solitary tract	Internal acoustic meatus/facial canal/ foramen for greater petrosal nerve	Visceral sensation from mucous membranes of nasopharynx and palate
Greater petrosal nerve Chorda tympani	Visceral motor	Presynaptic: superior salivatory nucleus; Postsynaptic: pterygopalatine ganglion (greater petrosal nerve) and submandibular ganglion (chorda tympani)	Internal acoustic meatus/facial canal/ foramen for greater petrosal nerve, (greater petrosal nerve) petrotympanic fissure (chorda tympani)	Parasympathetic innervation to lacrimal gland and glands of the nose and palate (greater petrosal nerve); submandibular and sublingual salivary glands (chorda tympani)

[a]See also Table 9.15.

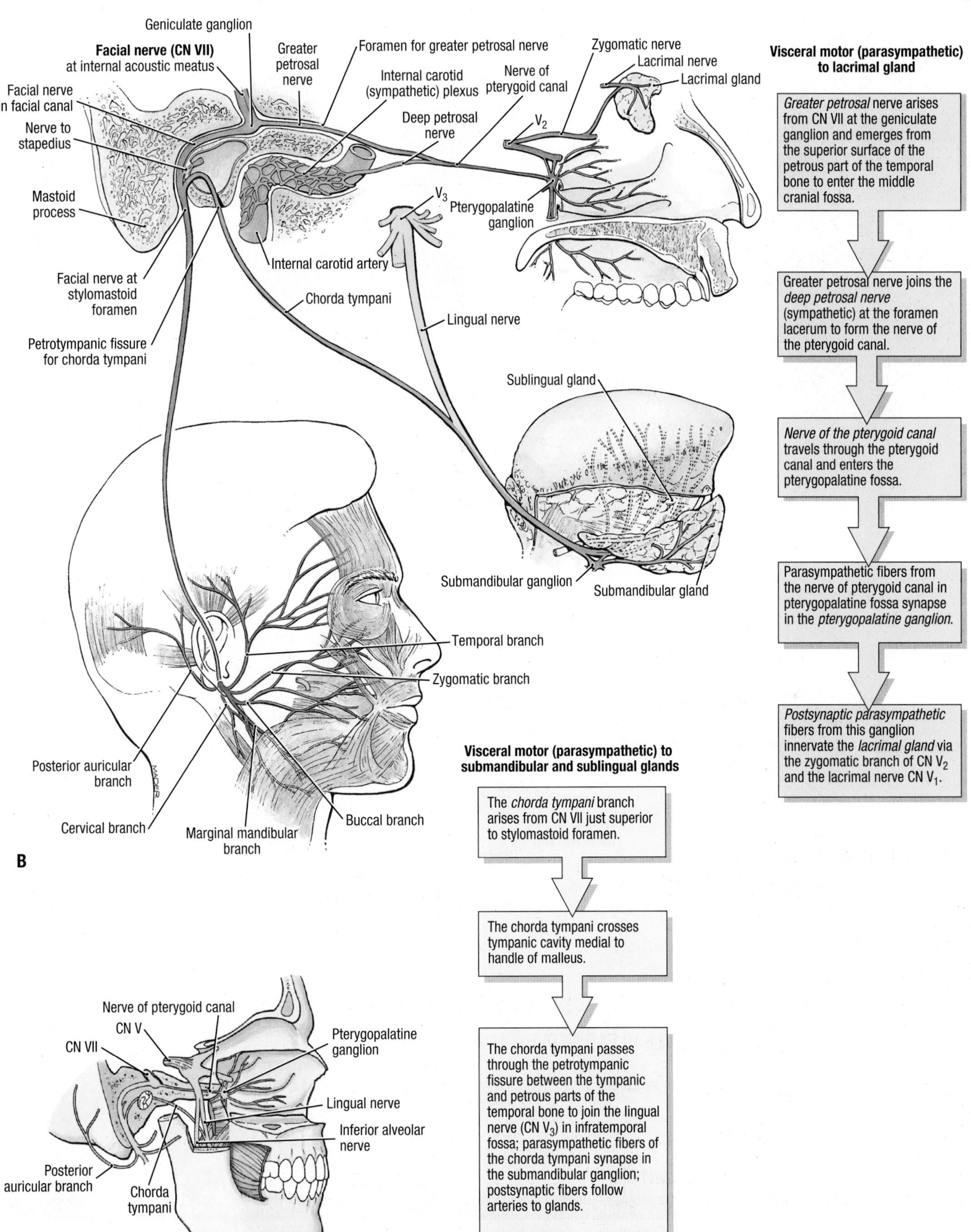
Geniculate ganglion
Facial nerve (CN VII) at internal acoustic meatus
Greater petrosal nerve
Foramen for greater petrosal nerve
Zygomatic nerve
Lacrimal nerve
Lacrimal gland
Facial nerve in facial canal
Internal carotid (sympathetic) plexus
Nerve of pterygoid canal
Nerve to stapedius
Deep petrosal nerve
V_2
Mastoid process
V_3
Pterygopalatine ganglion
Internal carotid artery
Facial nerve at stylomastoid foramen
Chorda tympani
Lingual nerve
Petrotympanic fissure for chorda tympani
Sublingual gland
Submandibular ganglion
Submandibular gland
Temporal branch
Zygomatic branch
Posterior auricular branch
Cervical branch
Marginal mandibular branch
Buccal branch
B
Nerve of pterygoid canal
CN V
CN VII
Pterygopalatine ganglion
Lingual nerve
Inferior alveolar nerve
Posterior auricular branch
Chorda tympani
C

Visceral motor (parasympathetic) to lacrimal gland

Greater petrosal nerve arises from CN VII at the geniculate ganglion and emerges from the superior surface of the petrous part of the temporal bone to enter the middle cranial fossa.

Greater petrosal nerve joins the *deep petrosal nerve* (sympathetic) at the foramen lacerum to form the nerve of the pterygoid canal.

Nerve of the pterygoid canal travels through the pterygoid canal and enters the pterygopalatine fossa.

Parasympathetic fibers from the nerve of pterygoid canal in pterygopalatine fossa synapse in the *pterygopalatine ganglion.*

Postsynaptic parasympathetic fibers from this ganglion innervate the *lacrimal gland* via the zygomatic branch of CN V_2 and the lacrimal nerve CN V_1.

Visceral motor (parasympathetic) to submandibular and sublingual glands

The *chorda tympani* branch arises from CN VII just superior to stylomastoid foramen.

The chorda tympani crosses tympanic cavity medial to handle of malleus.

The chorda tympani passes through the petrotympanic fissure between the tympanic and petrous parts of the temporal bone to join the lingual nerve (CN V_3) in infratemporal fossa; parasympathetic fibers of the chorda tympani synapse in the submandibular ganglion; postsynaptic fibers follow arteries to glands.

9.15 FACIAL NERVE (CN VII) *(CONTINUED)*

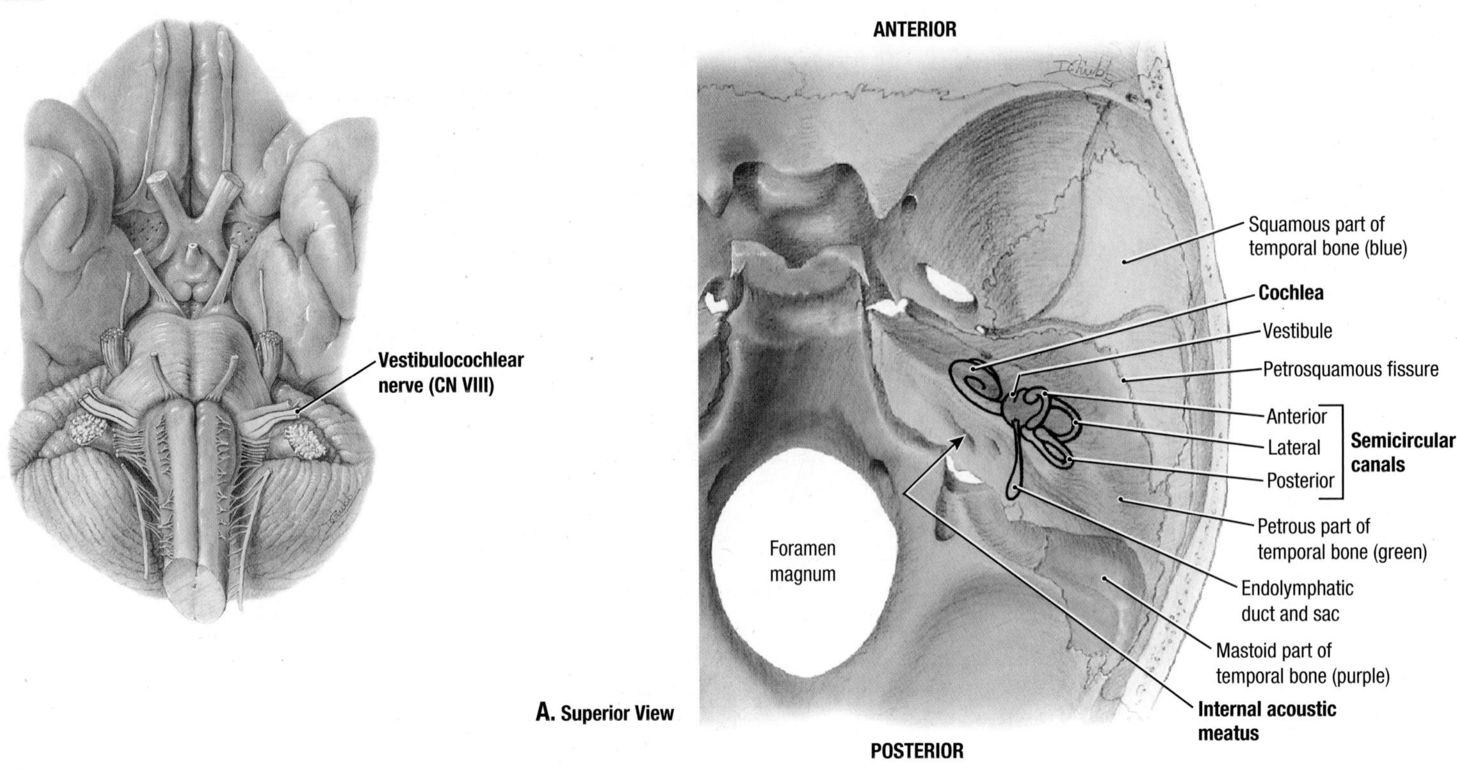
Vestibulocochlear nerve (CN VIII)
ANTERIOR
Squamous part of temporal bone (blue)
Cochlea
Vestibule
Petrosquamous fissure
Anterior
Lateral
Posterior
Semicircular canals
Petrous part of temporal bone (green)
Endolymphatic duct and sac
Mastoid part of temporal bone (purple)
Internal acoustic meatus
Foramen magnum
POSTERIOR
A. Superior View

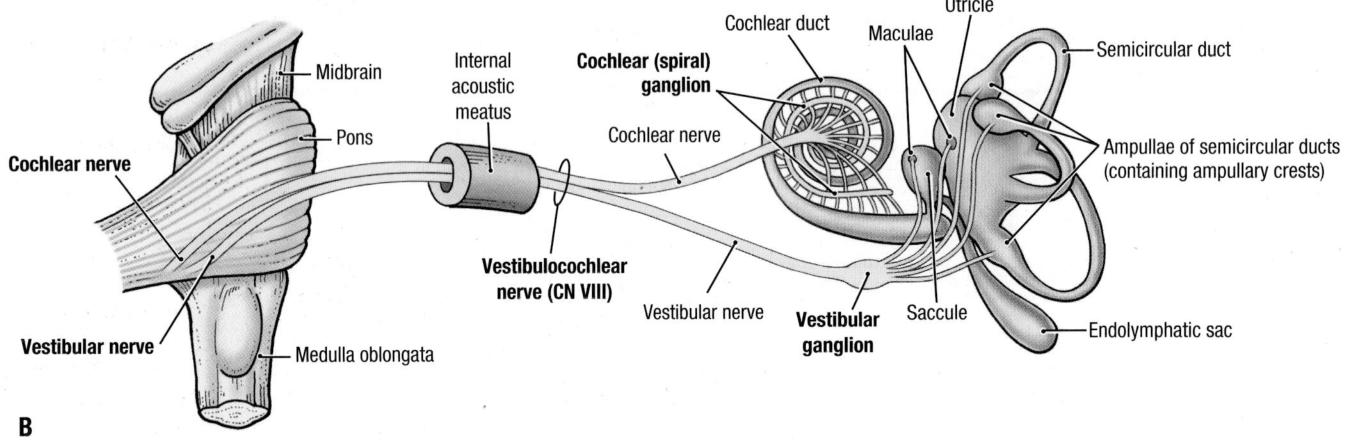
Midbrain
Pons
Cochlear nerve
Vestibular nerve
Medulla oblongata
Internal acoustic meatus
Cochlear (spiral) ganglion
Cochlear nerve
Vestibulocochlear nerve (CN VIII)
Vestibular nerve
Vestibular ganglion
Cochlear duct
Maculae
Utricle
Semicircular duct
Ampullae of semicircular ducts (containing ampullary crests)
Saccule
Endolymphatic sac
B

9.16 VESTIBULOCOCHLEAR NERVE (CN VIII)

A. Cochlea and semicircular canals in situ in the cranium. **B.** Schematic overview of distribution.

TABLE 9.10 VESTIBULOCOCHLEAR NERVE (CN VIII)

Part of Vestibulocochlear Nerve	Functional Components	Cells of Origin/Termination	Cranial Exit	Distribution and Functions
Vestibular nerve	Special sensory	Vestibular ganglion/vestibular nuclei	Internal acoustic meatus	Vestibular sensation from semicircular ducts, utricle, and saccule related to position and movement of head
Cochlear nerve		Spiral ganglion/cochlear nuclei		Hearing from spiral organ

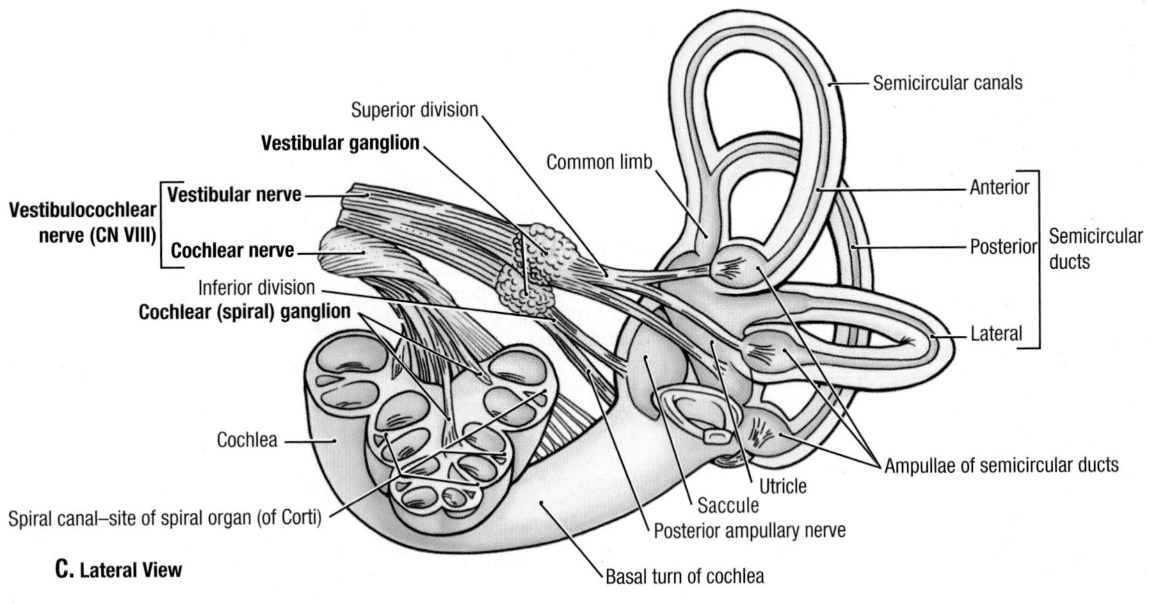
Superior division
Vestibular ganglion
Common limb
Semicircular canals
Vestibulocochlear nerve (CN VIII)
Vestibular nerve
Cochlear nerve
Inferior division
Cochlear (spiral) ganglion
Anterior
Posterior
Lateral
Semicircular ducts
Cochlea
Spiral canal–site of spiral organ (of Corti)
Ampullae of semicircular ducts
Utricle
Saccule
Posterior ampullary nerve
Basal turn of cochlea
C. Lateral View

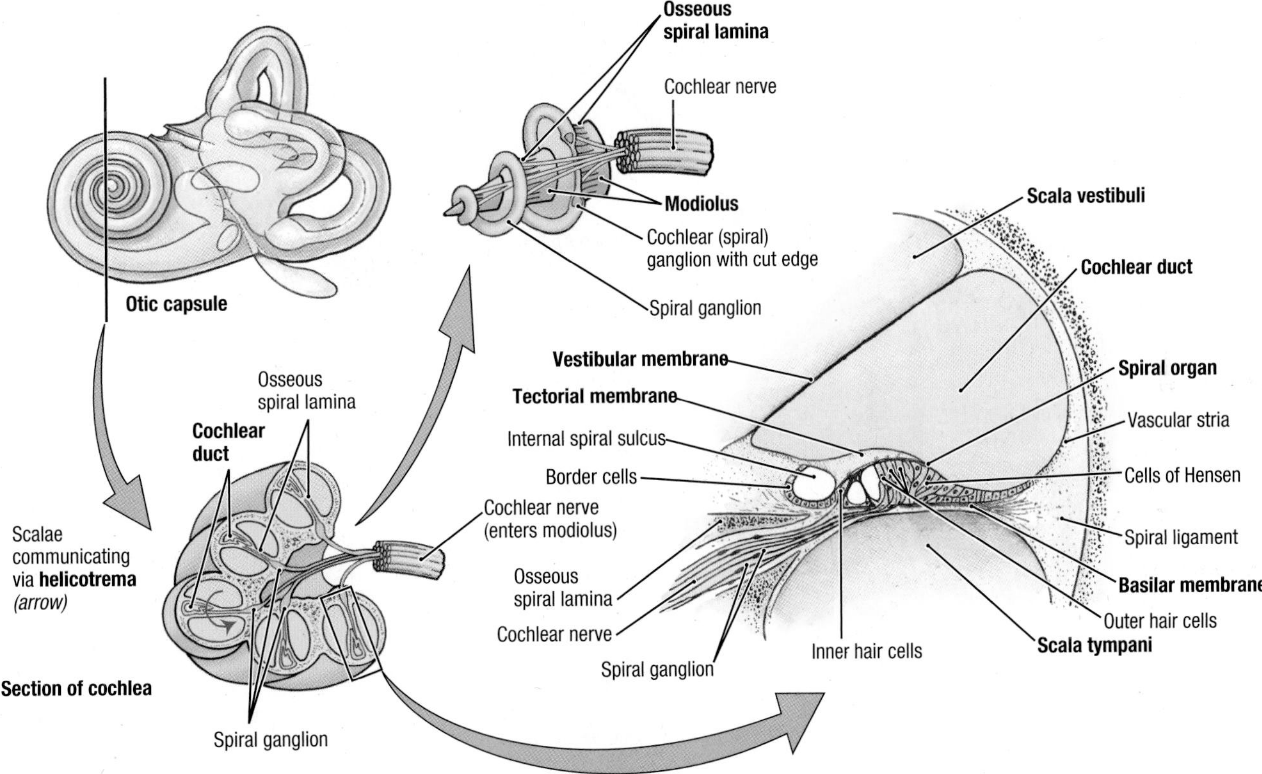
Osseous spiral lamina
Cochlear nerve
Modiolus
Cochlear (spiral) ganglion with cut edge
Spiral ganglion
Otic capsule
Scala vestibuli
Cochlear duct
Vestibular membrane
Tectorial membrane
Spiral organ
Vascular stria
Internal spiral sulcus
Border cells
Cells of Hensen
Spiral ligament
Basilar membrane
Outer hair cells
Scala tympani
Inner hair cells
Spiral ganglion
Cochlear nerve
Osseous spiral lamina
Cochlear nerve (enters modiolus)
Osseous spiral lamina
Cochlear duct
Scalae communicating via helicotrema (arrow)
Section of cochlea
Spiral ganglion
D

9.16 VESTIBULOCOCHLEAR NERVE (CN VIII) *(CONTINUED)*

C. Labyrinthine and cochlear apparatus, nerves and ganglia. **D.** Structure of cochlea. Observe in **D:**

- The cochlear duct is a spiral tube fixed to the internal and external walls of the cochlear canal by the spiral ligament.
- The triangular cochlear duct lies between the osseous spiral lamina and the external wall of the cochlear canal.
- The roof of the cochlear duct is formed by the vestibular membrane and the floor by the basilar membrane and osseous spiral lamina.
- The receptor of auditory stimuli is the spiral organ (of Corti), situated on the basilar membrane; it is overlaid by the gelatinous tectorial membrane.
- The spiral organ contains hair cells that respond to vibrations induced in the endolymph by sound waves.
- The fibers of the cochlear nerve are axons of neurons in the spiral ganglion; the peripheral processes enter the spiral organ (of Corti).

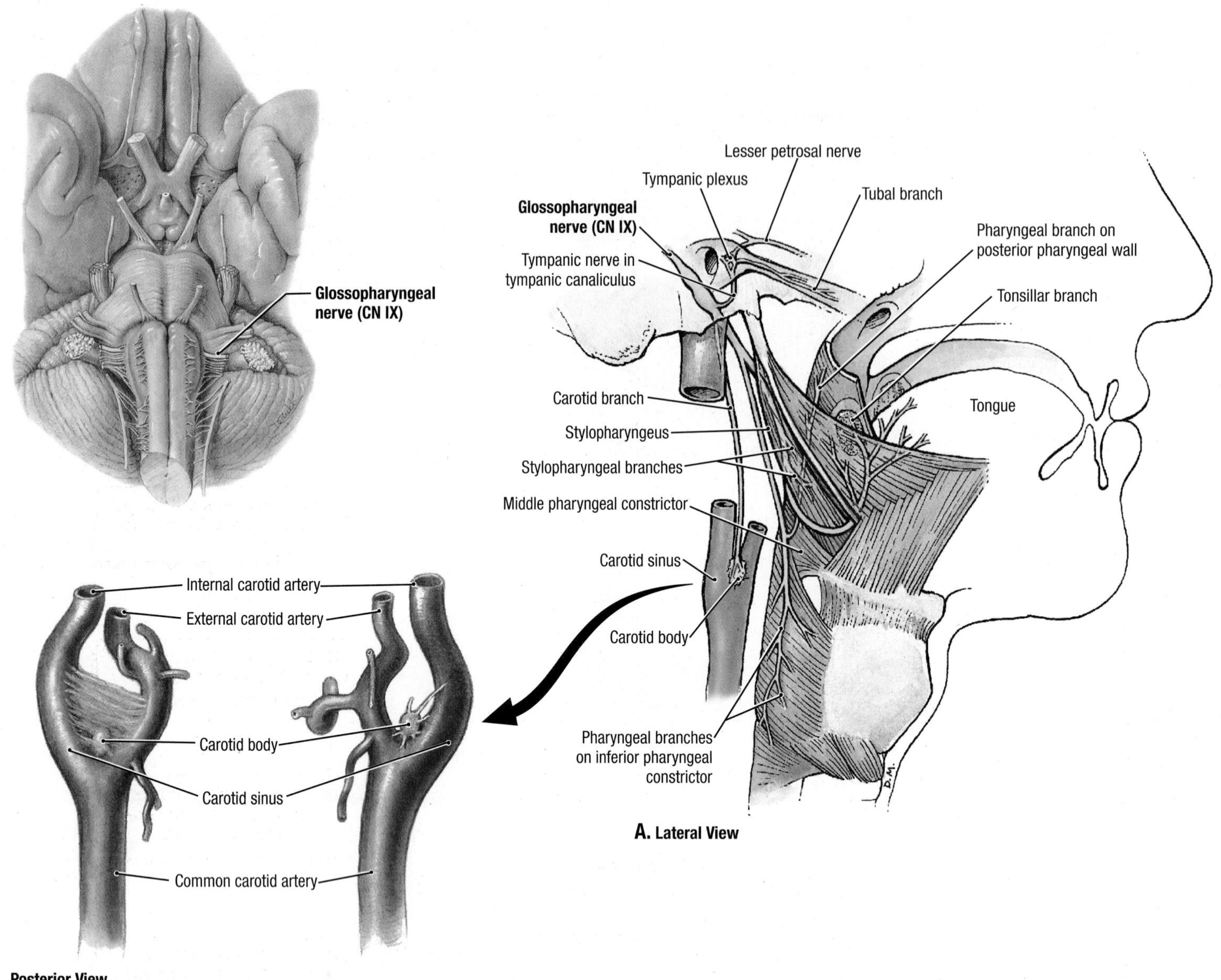
Glossopharyngeal nerve (CN IX)
Lesser petrosal nerve
Tympanic plexus
Tubal branch
Glossopharyngeal nerve (CN IX)
Pharyngeal branch on posterior pharyngeal wall
Tympanic nerve in tympanic canaliculus
Tonsillar branch
Carotid branch
Tongue
Stylopharyngeus
Stylopharyngeal branches
Middle pharyngeal constrictor
Carotid sinus
Carotid body
Pharyngeal branches on inferior pharyngeal constrictor
A. Lateral View
Internal carotid artery
External carotid artery
Carotid body
Carotid sinus
Common carotid artery
Posterior View

9.17 GLOSSOPHARYNGEAL NERVE (CN IX)

A. Overview of distribution. **B. and C.** Parasympathetic innervation.

TABLE 9.11 GLOSSOPHARYNGEAL NERVE (CN IX)[a]

Nerve	Functional Components	Cells of Origin/Termination	Cranial Exit	Distribution and Functions
Glossopharyngeal	Somatic (branchial) motor	Nucleus ambiguus	Jugular foramen	Motor to stylopharyngeus that assists with swallowing
	Visceral motor	Presynaptic: inferior salivatory nucleus; postsynaptic: otic ganglion		Parasympathetic innervation to parotid gland
	Visceral sensory	Nuclei of solitary tract, spinal trigeminal nucleus/ inferior ganglion		Visceral sensation from parotid gland, carotid body, carotid sinus, pharynx, and middle ear
	Special sensory	Nuclei of solitary tract /inferior ganglion		Taste from posterior third of tongue
	General sensory	Spinal trigeminal nucleus/superior ganglion		Cutaneous sensation from external ear

[a]See also Table 9.15.

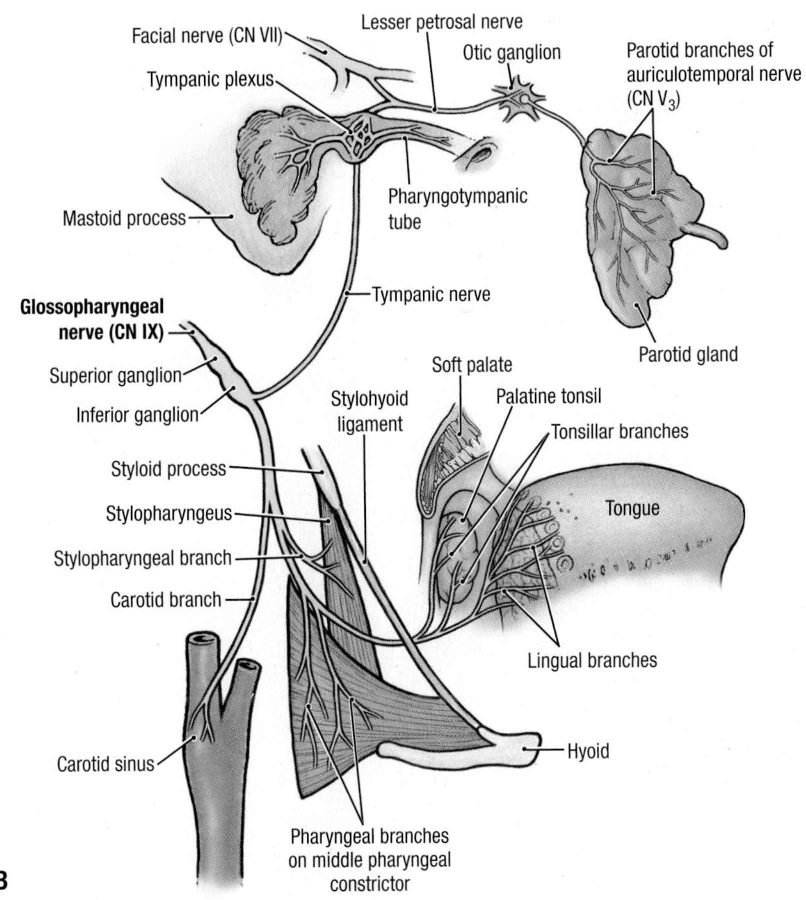
Facial nerve (CN VII)
Lesser petrosal nerve
Otic ganglion
Parotid branches of auriculotemporal nerve ($CN V_3$)
Tympanic plexus
Mastoid process
Pharyngotympanic tube
Tympanic nerve
Glossopharyngeal nerve (CN IX)
Superior ganglion
Inferior ganglion
Parotid gland
Soft palate
Stylohyoid ligament
Palatine tonsil
Tonsillar branches
Styloid process
Stylopharyngeus
Tongue
Stylopharyngeal branch
Carotid branch
Lingual branches
Hyoid
Carotid sinus
Pharyngeal branches on middle pharyngeal constrictor
B

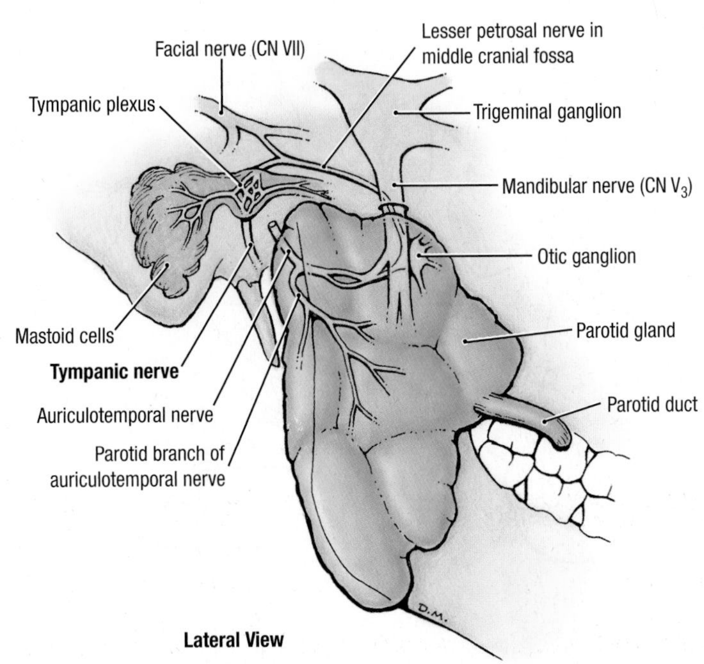
Facial nerve (CN VII)
Lesser petrosal nerve in middle cranial fossa
Tympanic plexus
Trigeminal ganglion
Mandibular nerve ($CN V_3$)
Otic ganglion
Parotid gland
Mastoid cells
Tympanic nerve
Auriculotemporal nerve
Parotid duct
Parotid branch of auriculotemporal nerve
C
Lateral View

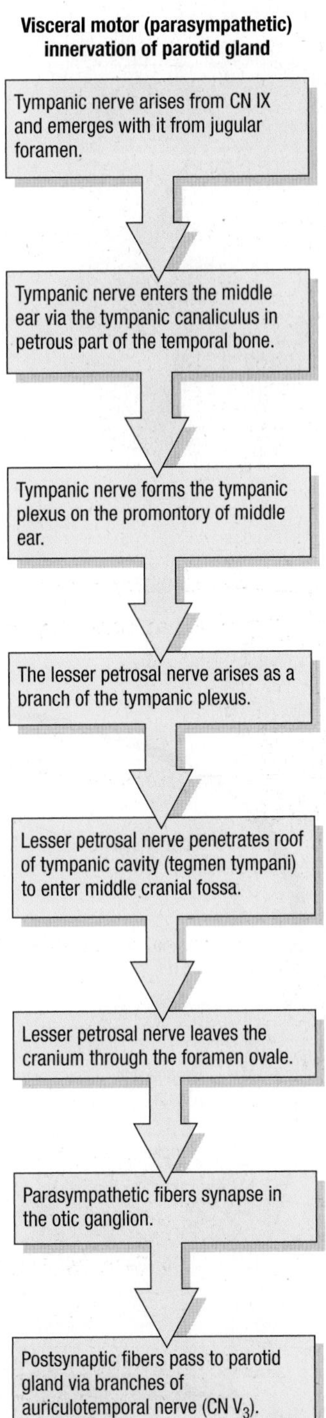
Visceral motor (parasympathetic) innervation of parotid gland
Tympanic nerve arises from CN IX and emerges with it from jugular foramen.
Tympanic nerve enters the middle ear via the tympanic canaliculus in petrous part of the temporal bone.
Tympanic nerve forms the tympanic plexus on the promontory of middle ear.
The lesser petrosal nerve arises as a branch of the tympanic plexus.
Lesser petrosal nerve penetrates roof of tympanic cavity (tegmen tympani) to enter middle cranial fossa.
Lesser petrosal nerve leaves the cranium through the foramen ovale.
Parasympathetic fibers synapse in the otic ganglion.
Postsynaptic fibers pass to parotid gland via branches of auriculotemporal nerve ($CN V_3$).

9.17 GLOSSOPHARYNGEAL NERVE (CN IX) *(CONTINUED)*

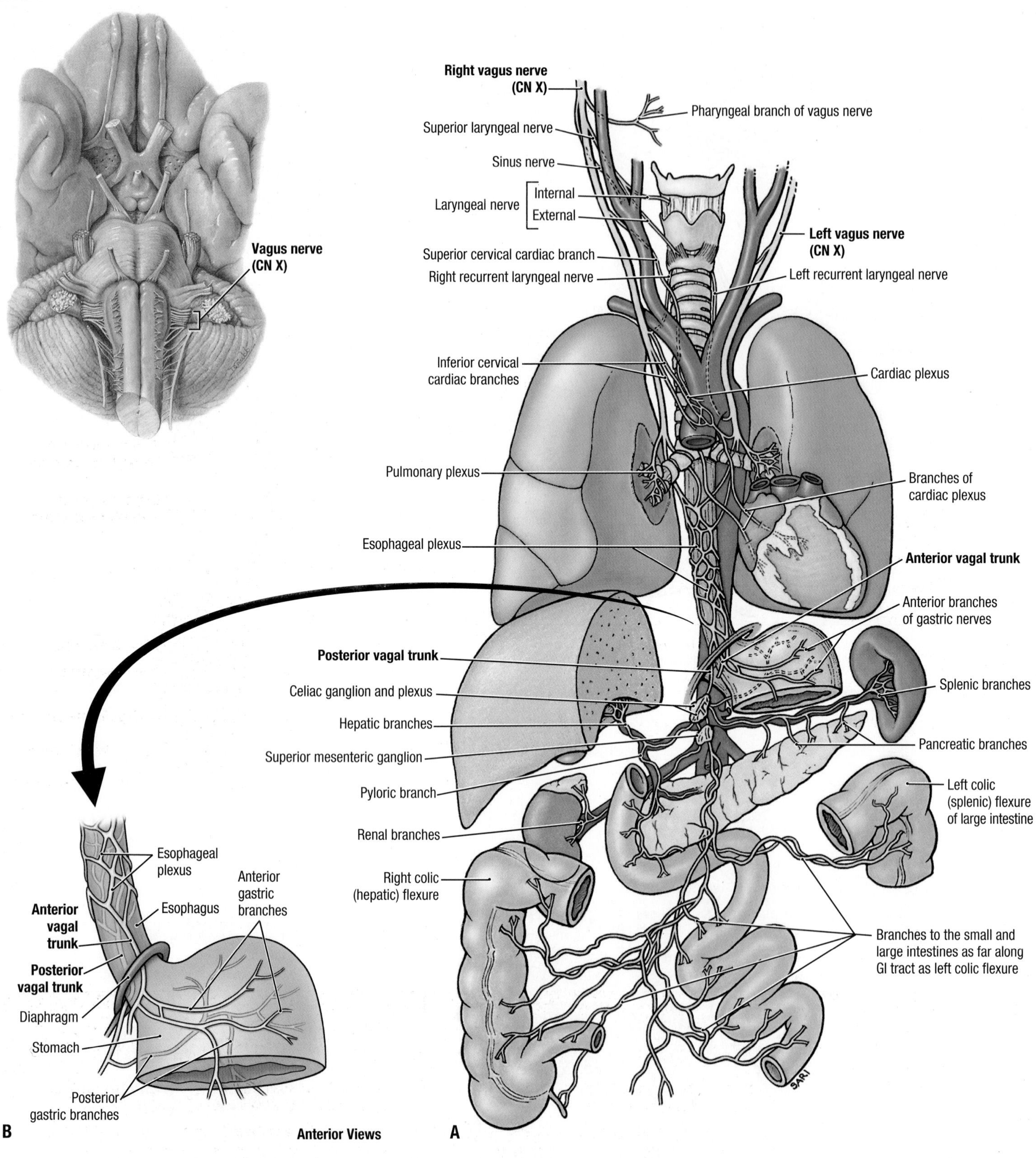
Vagus nerve (CN X)
Right vagus nerve (CN X)
Pharyngeal branch of vagus nerve
Superior laryngeal nerve
Sinus nerve
Laryngeal nerve
Internal
External
Left vagus nerve (CN X)
Superior cervical cardiac branch
Right recurrent laryngeal nerve
Left recurrent laryngeal nerve
Inferior cervical cardiac branches
Cardiac plexus
Pulmonary plexus
Branches of cardiac plexus
Esophageal plexus
Anterior vagal trunk
Anterior branches of gastric nerves
Posterior vagal trunk
Celiac ganglion and plexus
Splenic branches
Hepatic branches
Superior mesenteric ganglion
Pancreatic branches
Pyloric branch
Left colic (splenic) flexure of large intestine
Renal branches
Right colic (hepatic) flexure
Branches to the small and large intestines as far along GI tract as left colic flexure
Esophageal plexus
Esophagus
Anterior gastric branches
Anterior vagal trunk
Posterior vagal trunk
Diaphragm
Stomach
Posterior gastric branches
B
Anterior Views
A

9.18 VAGUS NERVE (CN X)

A. Course in neck, thorax and abdomen. **B.** Anterior and posterior vagal trunks. **C.** Branches in neck. **D.** Superior and inferior ganglia of vagus nerve.

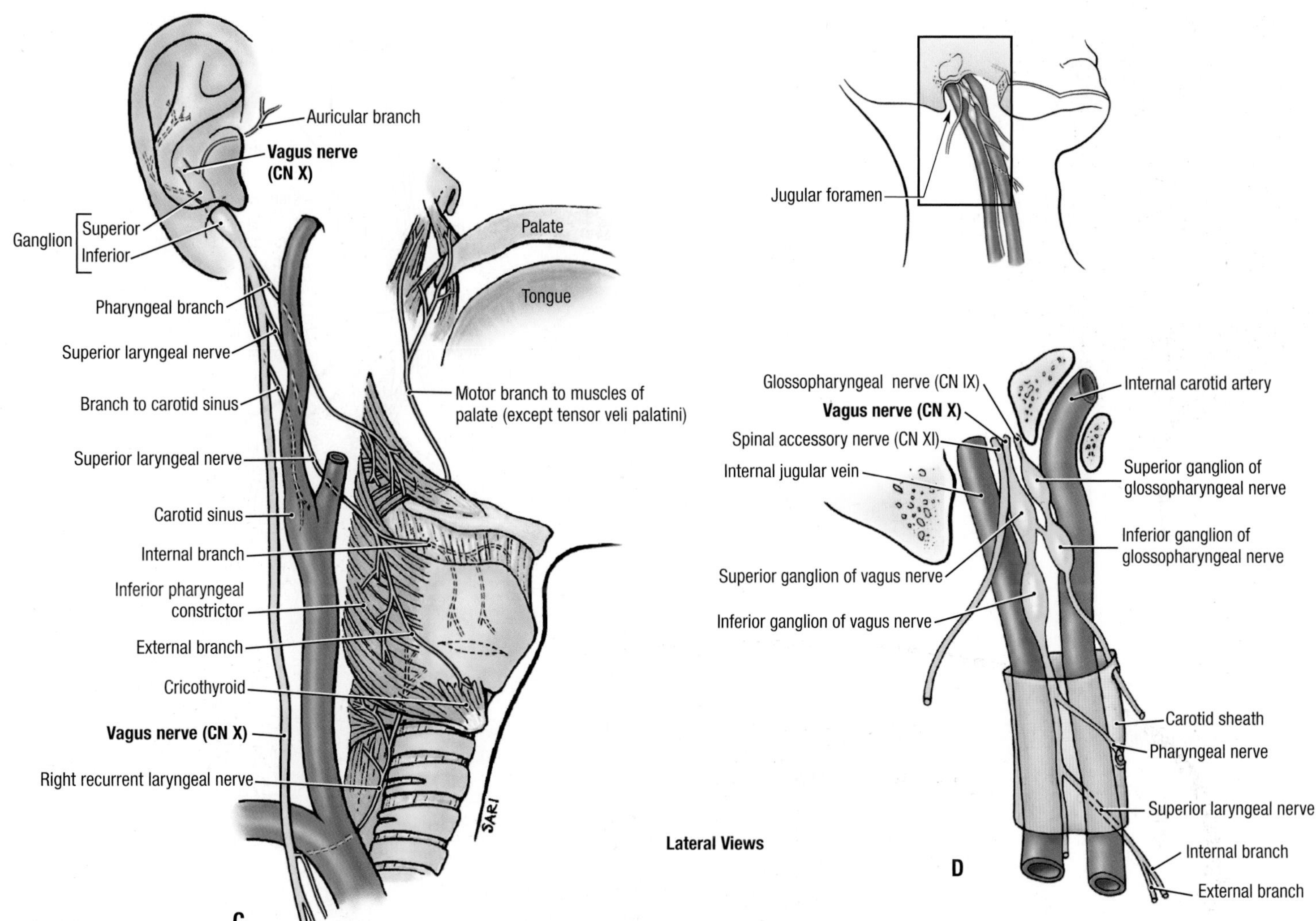
Auricular branch
Vagus nerve (CN X)
Ganglion
Superior
Inferior
Palate
Tongue
Pharyngeal branch
Superior laryngeal nerve
Branch to carotid sinus
Motor branch to muscles of palate (except tensor veli palatini)
Superior laryngeal nerve
Carotid sinus
Internal branch
Inferior pharyngeal constrictor
External branch
Cricothyroid
Vagus nerve (CN X)
Right recurrent laryngeal nerve
SARI
C
Jugular foramen
Glossopharyngeal nerve (CN IX)
Vagus nerve (CN X)
Spinal accessory nerve (CN XI)
Internal jugular vein
Internal carotid artery
Superior ganglion of glossopharyngeal nerve
Inferior ganglion of glossopharyngeal nerve
Superior ganglion of vagus nerve
Inferior ganglion of vagus nerve
Carotid sheath
Pharyngeal nerve
Superior laryngeal nerve
Internal branch
External branch
D

Lateral Views

9.18 VAGUS NERVE (CN X) *(CONTINUED)*

TABLE 9.12 VAGUS NERVE (CN X)

Nerve	Functional Components	Cells of Origin/Termination	Cranial Exit	Distribution and Functions
Vagus	Branchial motor	Nucleus ambiguus	Jugular foramen	Motor to constrictor muscles of pharynx, intrinsic muscles of larynx, muscles of palate (except tensor veli palatini), and striated muscle in superior two thirds of esophagus
	Visceral motor	Presynaptic: posterior (dorsal) nucleus of CN X; Postsynaptic: neurons in, on, or near viscera		Parasympathetic innervation to smooth muscle of trachea, bronchi, and digestive tract, cardiac muscle
	Visceral sensory	Nuclei of solitary tract, spinal trigeminal nucleus/ inferior ganglion		Visceral sensation from base of tongue, pharynx, larynx, trachea, bronchi, heart, esophagus, stomach, and intestine
	Special sensory	Nuclei of solitary tract/inferior ganglion		Taste from epiglottis and palate
	General sensory	Spinal trigeminal nucleus/superior ganglion		Sensation from auricle, external acoustic meatus, and dura mater of posterior cranial fossa

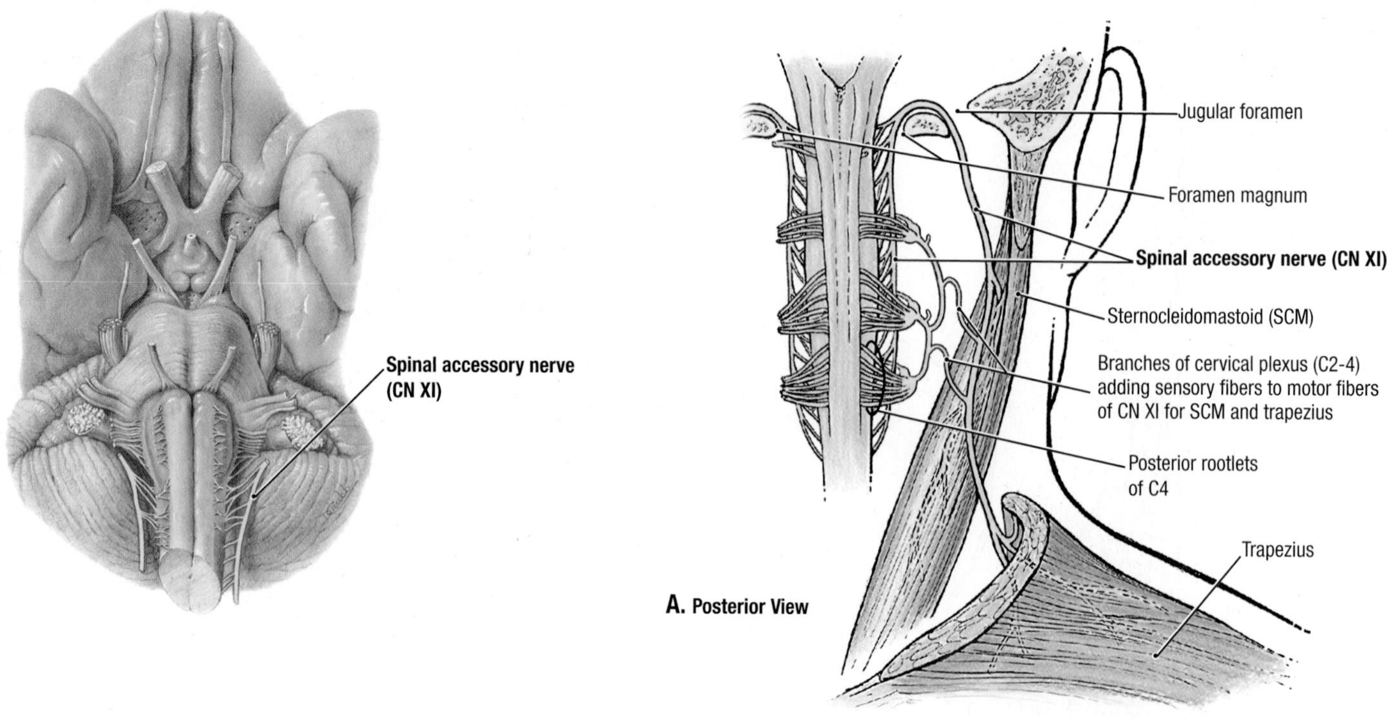

Spinal accessory nerve (CN XI)
Jugular foramen
Foramen magnum
Spinal accessory nerve (CN XI)
Sternocleidomastoid (SCM)
Branches of cervical plexus (C2-4) adding sensory fibers to motor fibers of CN XI for SCM and trapezius
Posterior rootlets of C4
Trapezius

A. Posterior View

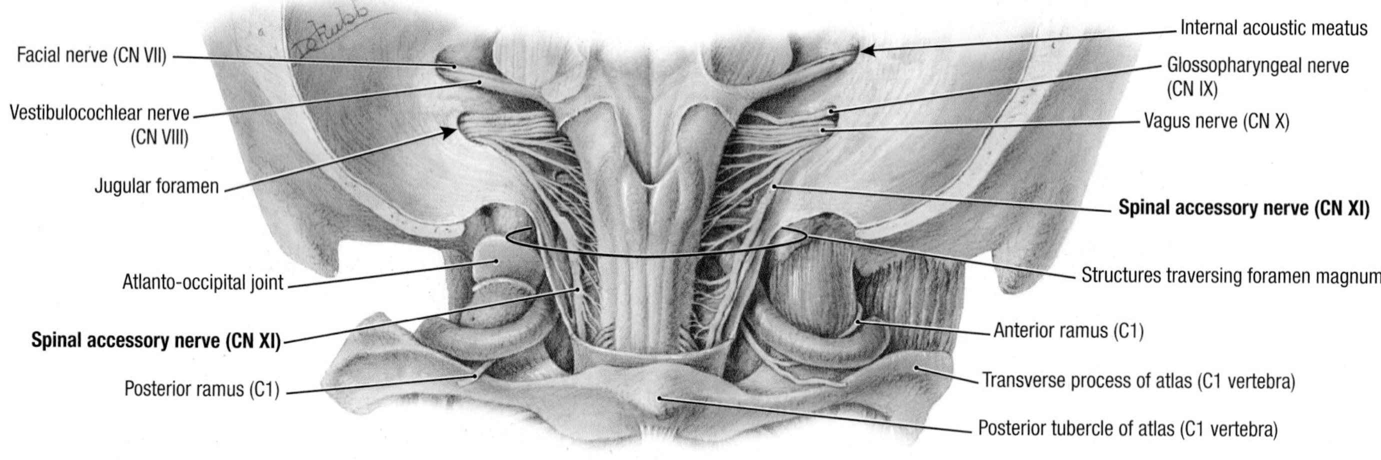

Facial nerve (CN VII)
Vestibulocochlear nerve (CN VIII)
Jugular foramen
Atlanto-occipital joint
Spinal accessory nerve (CN XI)
Posterior ramus (C1)
Internal acoustic meatus
Glossopharyngeal nerve (CN IX)
Vagus nerve (CN X)
Spinal accessory nerve (CN XI)
Structures traversing foramen magnum
Anterior ramus (C1)
Transverse process of atlas (C1 vertebra)
Posterior tubercle of atlas (C1 vertebra)

B. Posterior View

9.19 SPINAL ACCESSORY NERVE (CN XI)

A. Schematic illustration of distribution. **B.** Intracranial course.

TABLE 9.13 SPINAL ACCESSORY NERVE (CN XI)

Nerve	Functional Components	Cells of Origin/Termination	Cranial Exit	Distribution and Functions
Spinal accessory	Somatic motor	Accessory nucleus of spinal cord	Jugular foramen	Motor to sternocleidomastoid and trapezius

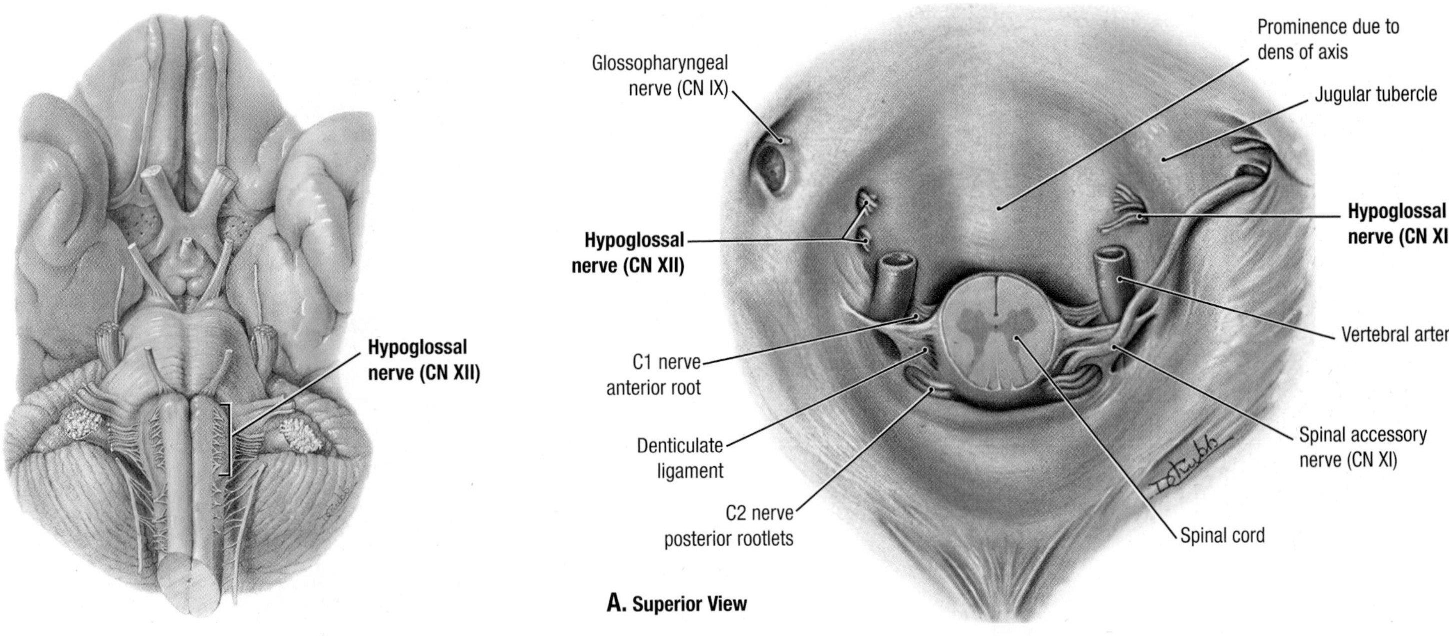
Hypoglossal
nerve (CN XII)
Glossopharyngeal
nerve (CN IX)
Prominence due to
dens of axis
Jugular tubercle
Hypoglossal
nerve (CN XII)
Hypoglossal
nerve (CN XII)
Vertebral artery
C1 nerve
anterior root
Denticulate
ligament
Spinal accessory
nerve (CN XI)
C2 nerve
posterior rootlets
Spinal cord

A. Superior View

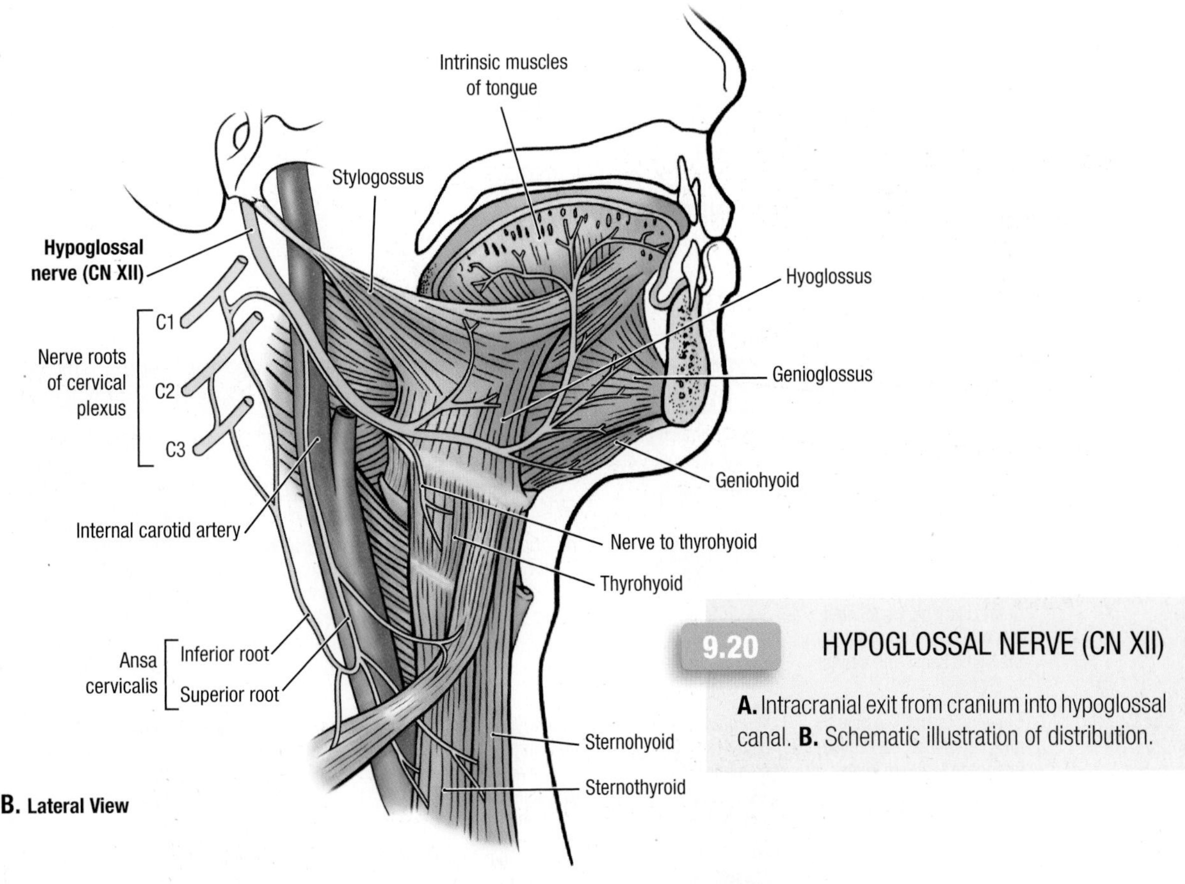
Intrinsic muscles
of tongue
Stylogossus
Hypoglossal
nerve (CN XII)
Hyoglossus
C1
Nerve roots
of cervical
plexus
C2
Genioglossus
C3
Geniohyoid
Internal carotid artery
Nerve to thyrohyoid
Thyrohyoid
Ansa
cervicalis
Inferior root
Superior root
Sternohyoid
Sternothyroid

B. Lateral View

9.20 HYPOGLOSSAL NERVE (CN XII)

A. Intracranial exit from cranium into hypoglossal canal. **B.** Schematic illustration of distribution.

TABLE 9.14 HYPOGLOSSAL NERVE (CN XII)

Nerve	Functional Components	Cells of Origin/Termination	Cranial Exit	Distribution and Functions
Hypoglossal	Somatic motor	Nucleus of CN XII	Hypoglossal canal	Motor to muscles of tongue (except palatoglossus)

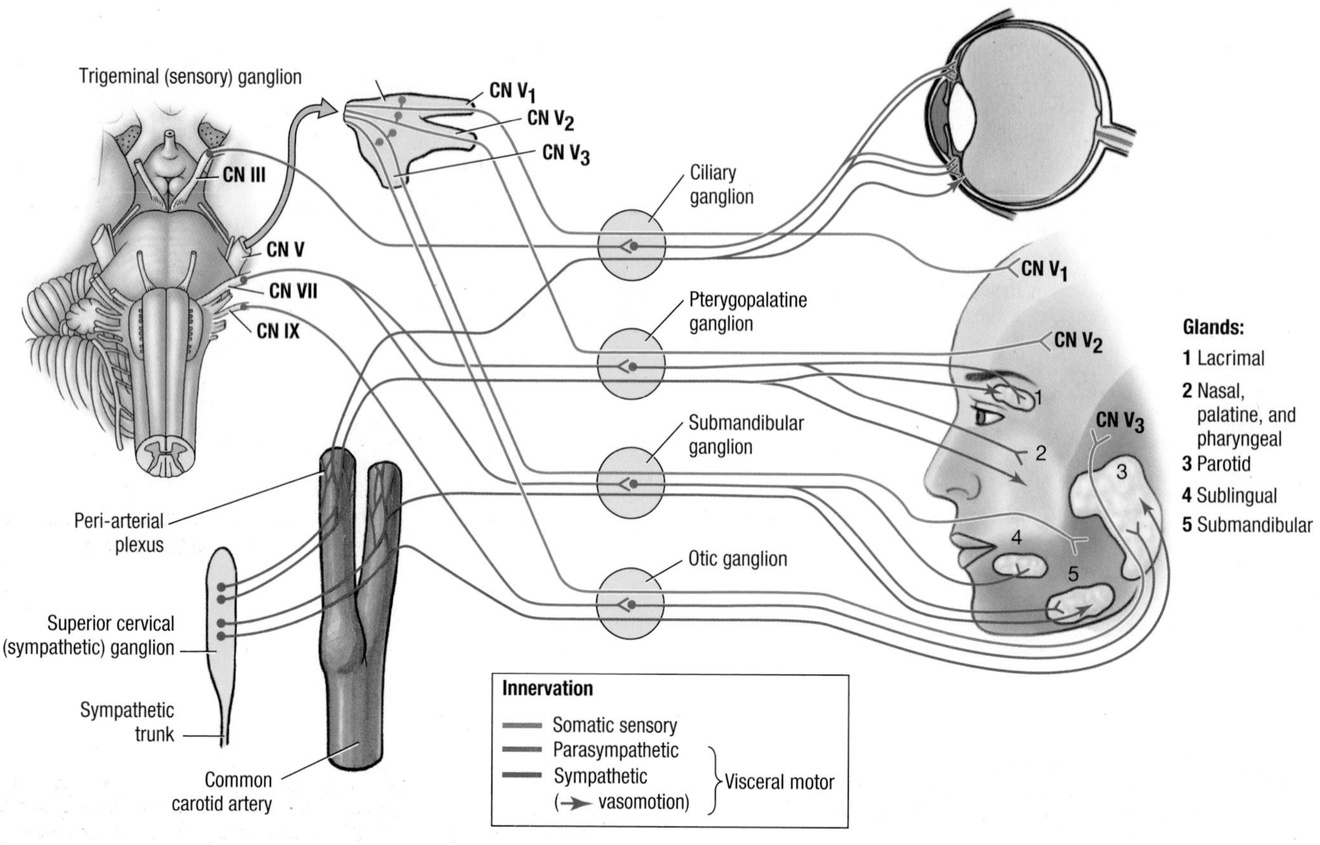
Trigeminal (sensory) ganglion
CN V1
CN V2
CN V3
CN III
CN V
CN VII
CN IX
Ciliary ganglion
Pterygopalatine ganglion
Submandibular ganglion
Otic ganglion
CN V1
CN V2
CN V3
Glands:
1 Lacrimal
2 Nasal, palatine, and pharyngeal
3 Parotid
4 Sublingual
5 Submandibular
Peri-arterial plexus
Superior cervical (sympathetic) ganglion
Sympathetic trunk
Common carotid artery
Innervation
Somatic sensory
Parasympathetic
Sympathetic
(→ vasomotion)
Visceral motor

9.21 SUMMARY OF AUTONOMIC INNERVATION OF HEAD

TABLE 9.15 AUTONOMIC GANGLIA OF HEAD

Ganglion	Location	Parasympathetic Root (Nucleus of Origin)[a]	Sympathetic Root	Main Distribution
Ciliary	Between optic nerve and lateral rectus, close to apex of orbit	Inferior branch of oculomotor nerve (CN III) (Edinger-Westphal nucleus)	Branch from internal carotid plexus in cavernous sinus	Parasympathetic postsynaptic fibers from ciliary ganglion pass to ciliary muscle and sphincter, pupillae of iris; sympathetic postsynaptic fibers from superior cervical ganglion pass to dilator pupillae and blood vessels of eye
Pterygopalatine	In pterygopalatine fossa, where it is attached by pterygopalatine branches of maxillary nerve; located just anterior to opening of pterygoid canal and inferior to CN V_2	Greater petrosal nerve from facial nerve (CN VII) (superior salivatory nucleus)	Deep petrosal nerve, a branch of internal carotid plexus that is continuation of postsynaptic fibers of cervical sympathetic trunk; fibers from superior cervical ganglion pass through pterygopalatine ganglion and enter branches of CN V_2	Parasympathetic postsynaptic fibers from pterygopalatine ganglion innervate lacrimal gland through zygomatic branch of CN V_2; sympathetic postsynaptic fibers from superior cervical ganglion accompany branches of pterygopalatine nerve that are distributed to the nasal cavity, palate, and superior parts of the pharynx
Otic	Between tensor veli palatini and mandibular nerve; lies inferior to foramen ovale	Tympanic nerve from glossopharyngeal nerve (CN IX); tympanic nerve continues from tympanic plexus as lesser petrosal nerve (inferior salivatory nucleus)	Fibers from superior cervical ganglion travel via plexus on middle meningeal artery	Parasympathetic postsynaptic fibers from otic ganglion are distributed to parotid gland through auriculotemporal nerve (branch of CN V_3); sympathetic postsynaptic fibers from superior cervical ganglion pass to parotid gland and supply its blood vessels
Submandibular	Suspended from lingual nerve by two short roots; lies on surface of hyoglossus muscle inferior to submandibular duct	Parasympathetic fibers join facial nerve (CN VII) and leave it in its chorda tympani branch, which unites with lingual nerve (superior salivatory nucleus)	Sympathetic fibers from superior cervical ganglion travel via the plexus on facial artery	Postsynaptic parasympathetic fibers from submandibular ganglion are distributed to the sublingual and submandibular glands; sympathetic fibers supply sublingual and submandibular glands and appear to be secretomotor

[a]For location of nuclei, see Figure 9.3.

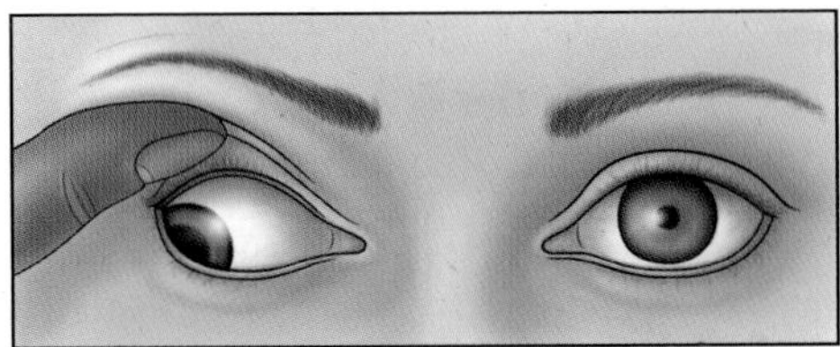
Right eye: Downward and outward gaze, dilated pupil, eyelid manually elevated due to ptosis
Left

A. Right oculomotor (CN III) nerve palsy

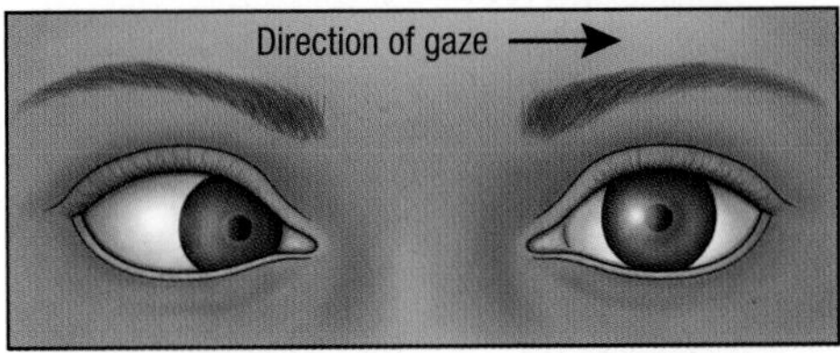
Direction of gaze
Right
Left eye: Does not abduct

B. Left abducent (CN VI) nerve palsy

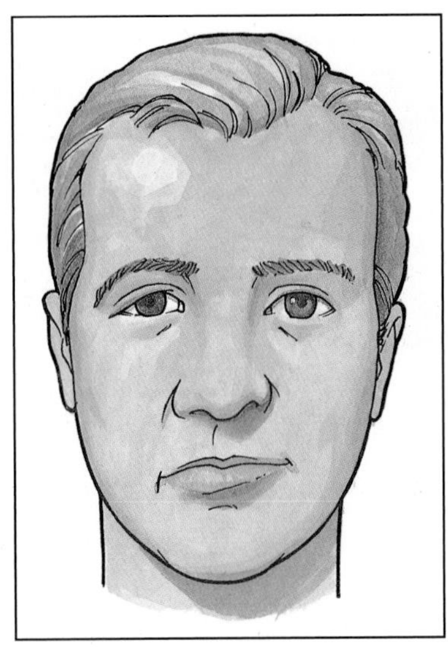

C. Right facial (CN VII) palsy (Bell palsy)

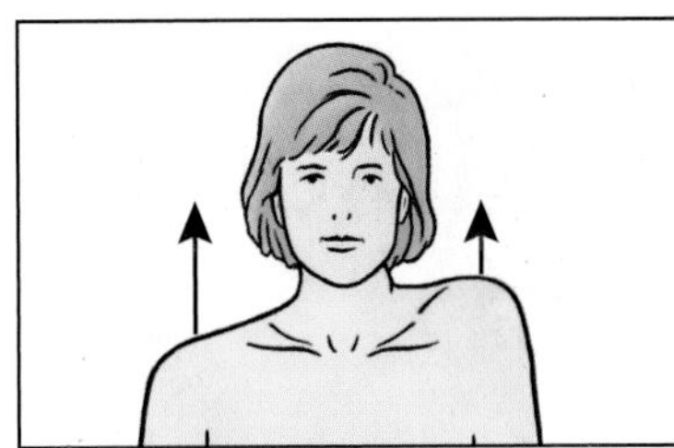

D. Right CN XI lesion

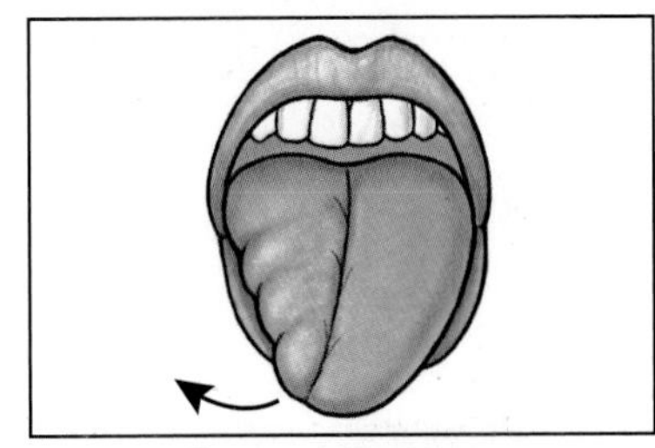

E. Right CN XII lesion

9.22 CRANIAL NERVE LESIONS

TABLE 9.16 SUMMARY OF CRANIAL NERVE LESIONS

Nerve	Lesion Type and/or Site	Abnormal Findings
CN I	Fracture of cribriform plate	Anosmia (loss of smell); cerebrospinal fluid (CSF) rhinorrhea (leakage of CSF through nose)
CN II	Direct trauma to orbit or eyeball; fracture involving optic canal	Loss of pupillary constriction
	Pressure on optic pathway; laceration or intracerebral clot in temporal, parietal, or occipital lobes of brain	Visual field defects
	Increased CSF pressure	Swelling of optic disc (papilledema)
CN III	Pressure from herniating uncus on nerve; fracture involving cavernous sinus; aneurysms	Dilated pupil, ptosis, eye rotates inferiorly and laterally (down and out), pupillary reflex on the side of the lesion will be lost (**A**)
CN IV	Stretching of nerve during its course around brainstem; fracture of orbit	Inability to rotate adducted eye inferiorly
CN V	Injury to terminal branches (particularly CN V_2) in roof of maxillary sinus; pathologic processes (tumors, aneurysms, infections) affecting trigeminal nerve	Loss of pain and touch sensations/paresthesia on face; loss of corneal reflex (blinking when cornea touched); paralysis of muscles of mastication; deviation of mandible to side of lesion when mouth is opened
CN VI	Base of brain or fracture involving cavernous sinus or orbit	Inability to rotate eye laterally; diplopia on lateral gaze (**B**)
CN VII	Laceration or contusion in parotid region	Paralysis of facial muscles; eye remains open; angle of mouth droops; forehead does not wrinkle (**C**)
	Fracture of temporal bone	As above, plus associated involvement of cochlear nerve and chorda tympani; dry cornea and loss of taste on anterior two thirds of tongue
	Intracranial hematoma ("stroke")	Weakness (paralysis) of lower facial muscles contralateral to the lesion, upper facial muscles are not affected because they are bilaterally innervated
CN VIII	Tumor of nerve	Progressive unilateral hearing loss; tinnitus (noises in ear); vertigo (loss of balance)
CN IX[a]	Brainstem lesion or deep laceration of neck	Loss of taste on posterior third of tongue; loss of sensation on affected side of soft palate; loss of gag reflex on affected side
CN X	Brainstem lesion or deep laceration of neck	Sagging of soft palate; deviation of uvula to unaffected side; hoarseness owing to paralysis of vocal fold; difficulty in swallowing and speaking
CN XI	Laceration of neck	Paralysis of sternocleidomastoid and superior fibers of trapezius; drooping of shoulder (**D**)
CN XII	Neck laceration; basal skull fractures	Protruded tongue deviates toward affected side; moderate dysarthria, disturbance of articulation **(E)**

[a]Isolated lesions of CN IX are uncommon; usually, CN IX, X, and XI are involved together as they pass through the jugular foramen.

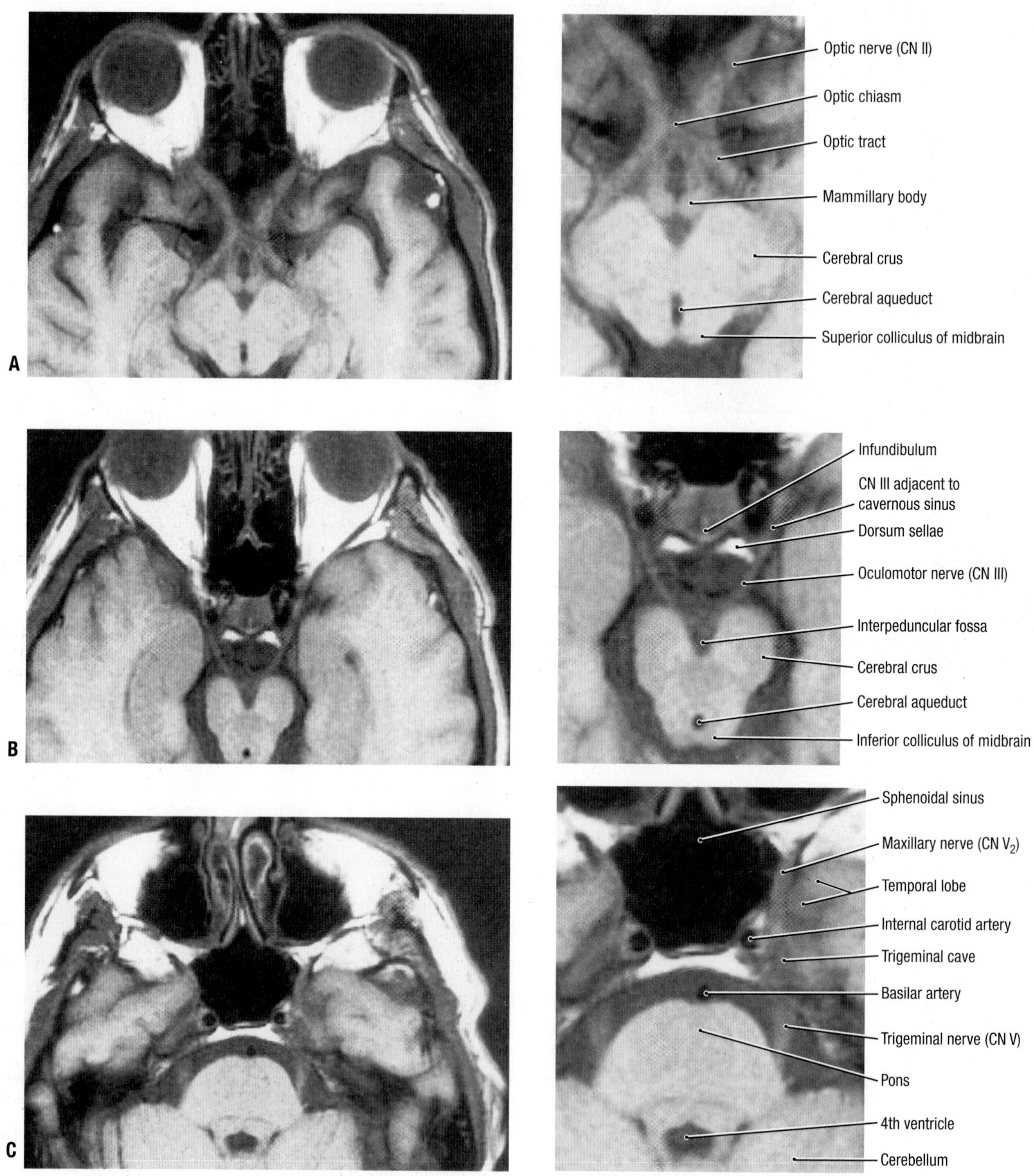
Optic nerve (CN II)
Optic chiasm
Optic tract
Mammillary body
Cerebral crus
Cerebral aqueduct
Superior colliculus of midbrain
A
Infundibulum
CN III adjacent to cavernous sinus
Dorsum sellae
Oculomotor nerve (CN III)
Interpeduncular fossa
Cerebral crus
Cerebral aqueduct
Inferior colliculus of midbrain
B
Sphenoidal sinus
Maxillary nerve (CN V_2)
Temporal lobe
Internal carotid artery
Trigeminal cave
Basilar artery
Trigeminal nerve (CN V)
Pons
4th ventricle
Cerebellum
C

9.23 TRANSVERSE MRIs THROUGH HEAD, SHOWING CRANIAL NERVES

A. Optic nerve (CN II). **B.** Oculomotor nerve (CN III). **C.** Trigeminal nerve (CN V).

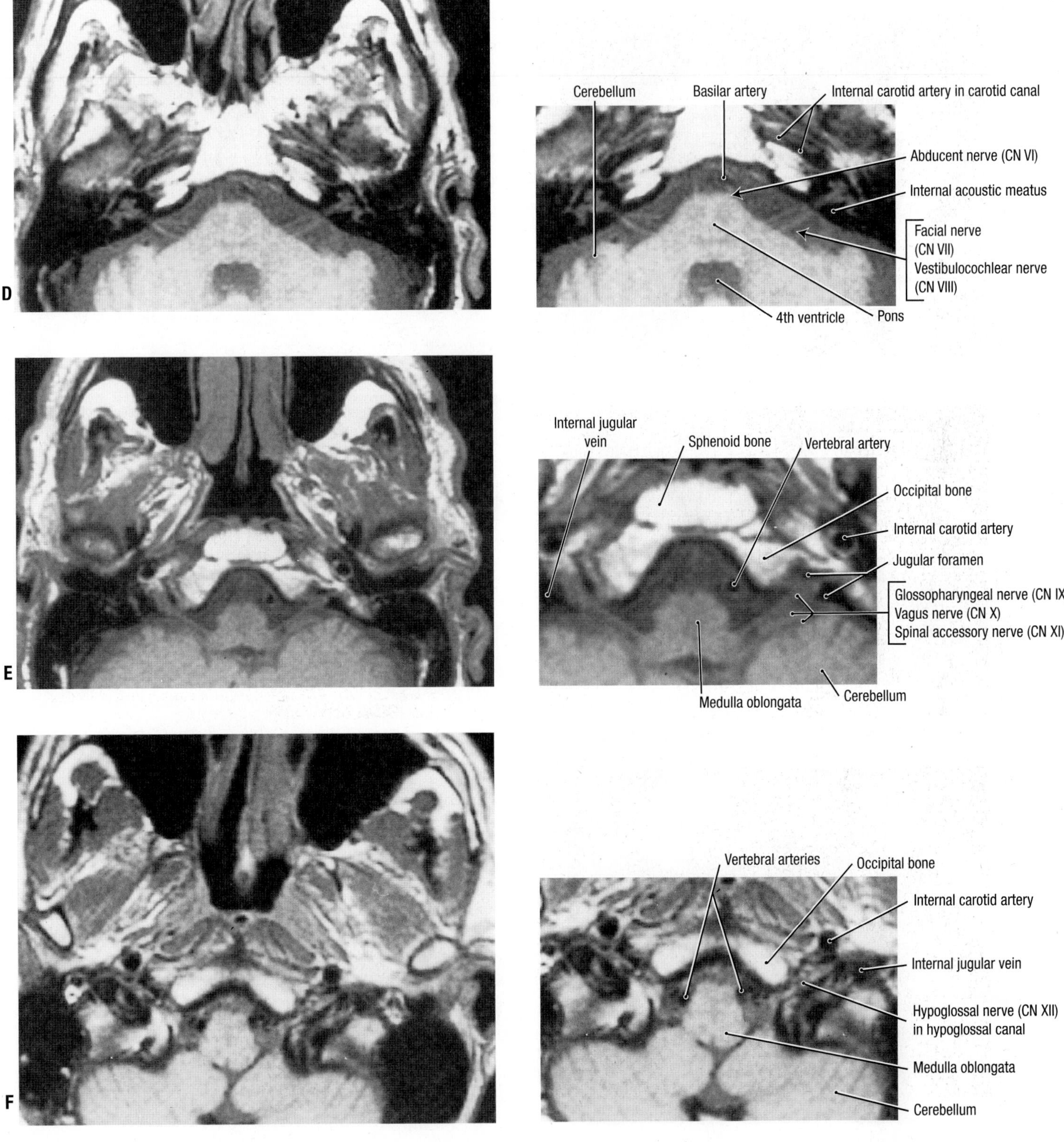
D
Cerebellum
Basilar artery
Internal carotid artery in carotid canal
Abducent nerve (CN VI)
Internal acoustic meatus
Facial nerve (CN VII)
Vestibulocochlear nerve (CN VIII)
4th ventricle
Pons
E
Internal jugular vein
Sphenoid bone
Vertebral artery
Occipital bone
Internal carotid artery
Jugular foramen
Glossopharyngeal nerve (CN IX)
Vagus nerve (CN X)
Spinal accessory nerve (CN XI)
Medulla oblongata
Cerebellum
F
Vertebral arteries
Occipital bone
Internal carotid artery
Internal jugular vein
Hypoglossal nerve (CN XII) in hypoglossal canal
Medulla oblongata
Cerebellum

9.23 TRANSVERSE MRIs THROUGH HEAD, SHOWING CRANIAL NERVES *(CONTINUED)*

D. Abducent (CN VI), facial (CN VII), and vestibulocochlear (CN VIII) nerves. **E.** Glossopharyngeal (CN IX), vagus (CN X), and spinal accessory (CN XI) nerves. **F.** Hypoglossal nerve (CN XII).

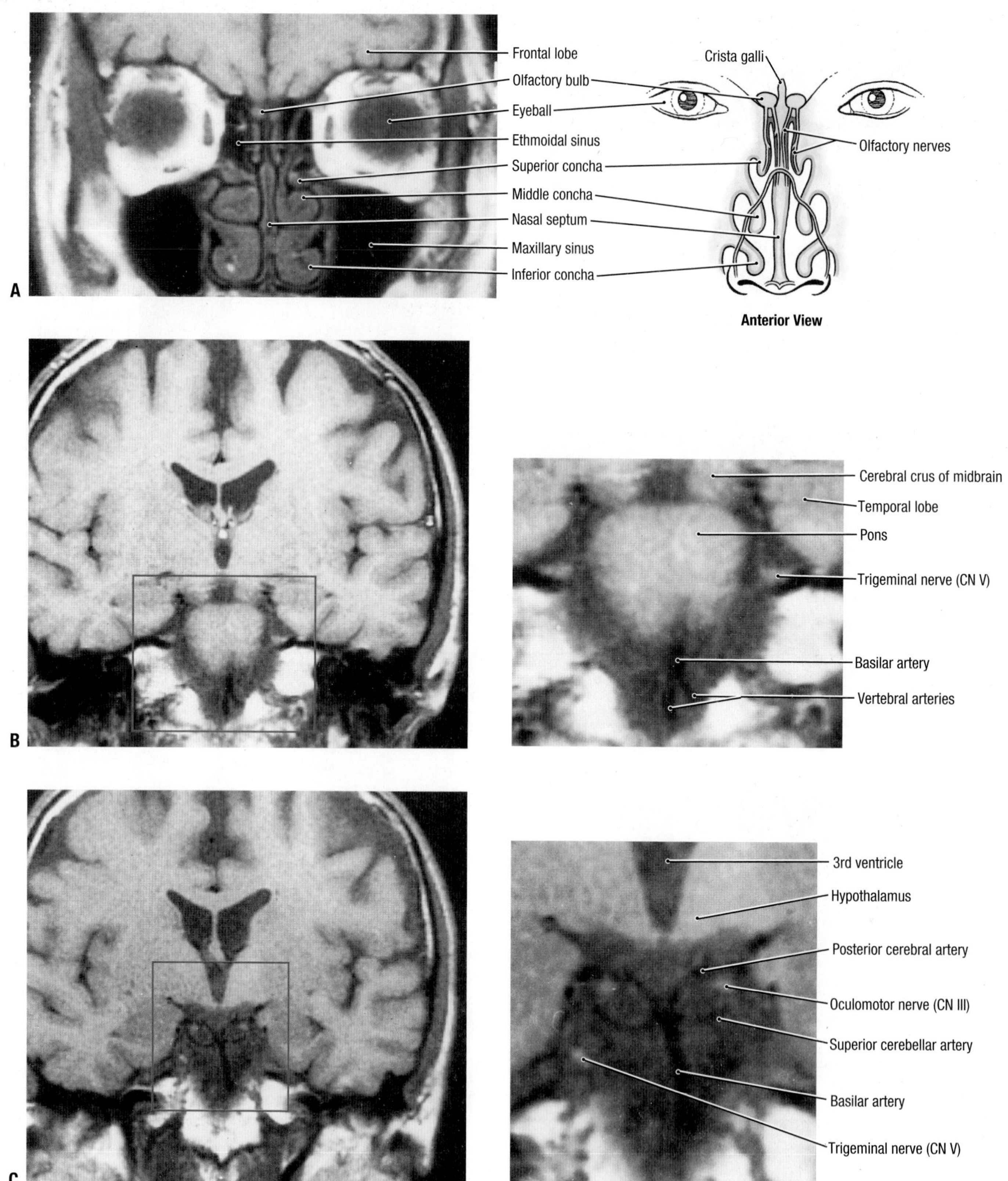
Frontal lobe
Olfactory bulb
Eyeball
Ethmoidal sinus
Superior concha
Middle concha
Nasal septum
Maxillary sinus
Inferior concha
A
Crista galli
Olfactory nerves
Anterior View
Cerebral crus of midbrain
Temporal lobe
Pons
Trigeminal nerve (CN V)
Basilar artery
Vertebral arteries
B
3rd ventricle
Hypothalamus
Posterior cerebral artery
Oculomotor nerve (CN III)
Superior cerebellar artery
Basilar artery
Trigeminal nerve (CN V)
C

9.24 CORONAL MRIs THROUGH HEAD, SHOWING CRANIAL NERVES

A. Olfactory bulb. **B.** Trigeminal (CN V) nerve. **C.** Oculomotor (CN III) and trigeminal (CN V) nerves.

Tribute to Dr. Grant

1. Robinson C. *Canadian Medical Lives: J.C. Boileau Grant: Anatomist Extraordinary.* Markham, Ontario, Canada: Associated Medical Services Inc./Fithzenry & Whiteside, 1993.
2. Grant JCB. *A Method of Anatomy, Descriptive and Deductive.* Baltimore, MD: Williams & Wilkins Co., 1937 (11th ed., Basmajian J, Slonecker C, 1989).
3. Grant JCB. *Grant's Atlas of Anatomy.* Baltimore, MD: Williams & Wilkins Co., 1943 (10th ed., Agur A, Ming L, 1999).
4. Grant JCB, Cates HA. *Grant's Dissector (A Handbook for Dissectors).* Baltimore, MD: Williams & Wilkins Co., 1940 (12th ed., Sauerland EK, 1999).

Chapter 1

Fig. 1.51: Anson BH. The aortic arch and its branches. *Cardiology.* Vol. 1. New York, NY: McGraw-Hill, 1963.

Chapter 2

Fig. 2.49: Couinaud C. Lobes et segments hepatiques: Note sur l'architecture anatomique et chirurgicale du foie. *Presse Med* 1954;62:709.

Fig. 2.49: Healy JE, Schroy PC. Anatomy of the biliary ducts within the human liver: analysis of the prevailing pattern of branchings and the major variations of the biliary ducts. *Arch Surg* 1953;66:599.

Fig. 2.89B: Campbell M. Ureteral reduplication (double ureter). *Urology.* Vol. 1. Philadelphia, PA: WB Saunders, 1954:309.

Chapter 3

Fig. 3.43A: Oelrich TM. The urethral sphincter muscle in the male. *Am J Anat* 1980;158:229.

Fig. 3.43B: Oelrich TM. The striated urogenital sphincter muscle in the female. *Anat Rec* 1983;205:223.

Chapter 4

Fig. 4.48A: Jit I, Charnakia VM. The vertebral level of the termination of the spinal cord. *J Anat Soc India* 1959;8:93.

Note: Page numbers followed by t denote tables.

A

Abdomen
  autonomic innervation. *See* Autonomic innervation
  contents and peritoneum, 123
  magnetic resonance imaging of
    coronal, 192
    sagittal, 193
    transverse or horizontal (axial), 190–191
  ultrasound scans and MR angiogram of, 194–195
  vagus nerves in, 185
  viscera in situ, 98–99
Abdominal aorta, 167, 179, 179t
Abdominal cutaneous branch
  anterior, 103, 104, 106
  lateral, 103
  posterior, 104
Abdominal nerve plexuses and ganglia, 183
Abdominal viscera, 183t
  anterior, 98
  posterior
    and anterior relations, 166
    left kidney and suprarenal gland, exposure of, 168
    vessels of, 167
  presynaptic and postsynaptic fibers, 182
Abdominal wall
  anterior, 106–107
  anterolateral
    arteries, 103
    dermatomes, 102
    lymphatic drainage and subcutaneous (superficial) venous drainage, 105
    muscles of, 108, 108t
    nerves, 103
    posterior aspect of, 122
    regions and quadrants, 101
    structure of, 109
    superficial dissection, 104
    surface anatomy, 100
  posterior, viscera and vessels of, 167
  posterolateral
    diaphragm, lumbar plexus and vertebral attachment of, 176
    kidney, exposure of, 173–175
    lumbar plexus, nerves of, 177
    muscles of, 176t
    renal fascia, exposure of, 174–175
Abdominopelvic nerve plexuses and ganglia, 180
Abducent nerve (CN VI), 646, 650, 651, 660, 818–820, 827–829
  palsy, 847
Abductor digiti minimi, 452, 595
Abductor hallucis, 452
Abductor pollicis brevis, 574
Abductor pollicis longus, 585, 589, 593, 594
Accessory hemi-azygos vein, 80, 81
Accessory pancreatic duct, 137
Acetabular fossa
  blood vessels, 409
Acetabular labrum, 402, 404
Acetabular ligament, 404
Acetabulum, 202, 203
Acoustic meatus, external, 616
Acromion, 33, 448, 486, 487, 506, 519, 521, 524–527, 532, 535, 537, 539–545, 789
Adductor brevis, 383, 388
Adductor hallucis, oblique head, 454
Adductor hallucis, transverse head, 454
Adductor longus, 38, 380, 387
Adductor magnus, 383, 387, 388, 393
Adductor pollicis, 572
Adductor tubercle, 393
Alar ligament, 303
Alveolar nerve, 835
Ampulla
  ductus deferens, 220
  rectum, 236
Anal canal, 265
  innervation, 218
  neurovascular structures, 216
  sphincters, 214–215
Anal column, 215
Anastomosis, 22, 107, 128, 146, 157, 217, 231, 269, 370, 375, 401, 408, 412, 424, 425, 517, 537
Anesthesia
  for childbirth, 274
  local, of intercostal space, 11
  of palatine nerves, 689
  tongue during, 685
Anginal pain, 86
Angiogram
  of abdomen, 194–195
  aortic arch, 72
  coronary circulation, 59
  of thorax, 94–95
  ventricle, 65
Angle
  inferior, 484
  inferolateral, 315
  infrasternal, 12
  left venous, 78
  mandible, 614, 616, 626, 680
  manubriosternal joint, 12, 14, 507
  Q-angle, 326, 415, 416
  of rib, 324
  scapula, 521
  sternal, 304
  subpubic, 200–203
Angular incisure, 133, 135
Angular vein, 639
Ankle
  coronal section, 464
  dislocation, 457
  medial, 446–447
  MRI, 464, 465
  posteromedial aspect, 459
  radiographs, 461
  synovial sheaths and tendons, 438–439
  transverse section, 465
Ankle joint
  anterior view, 358
  articular surfaces, 463
  joint cavity, 456
  ligaments, 457
  medial/deltoid ligament, 460
  posterior aspect, 458
  synovial membrane, 456
Ankle region
  lateral ligaments, 462
  medial ligaments, 460
Ankle sprains, 462
Ansa cervicalis, 769, 772
Antebrachial fascia, 501
Anterior cruciate ligament (ACL), 418, 427, 429
Anterior superior iliac spine (ASIS), 107
Anular ligament of radius, 554–556
Anulus fibrosus, 308–312
Aorta, 76, 340, 370
  abdominal, 167, 179, 179t
  arch of, 27, 48, 49, 51, 69, 71, 76, 83, 494
  ascending aorta, 48
  thoracic aorta, 54, 76, 84
Aortic and pulmonary valve cusps, 66
Aortic aneurysm, 68, 179
Aortic arch, branches of, 72
Aortic hiatus, 178
Aortic valve, 65, 67
Aperture
  anterior nasal, 617
  choana, 796
  of Magendie, 729
  opening of lateral, 728, 729
  posterior nasal, 796
  superior thoracic, 13, 28, 74
  4th ventricle, 818
Apical axillary lymph nodes, 8, 497
Aponeurosis, 109–111, 174, 324, 329
  bicipital, 530, 546, 547
  external oblique, 106
  muscles, 324
  palmar, 501, 569, 571
  plantar, 451
  of transversus abdominis, 113
Appendicular artery, 143
Appendix, 140, 143
  acute inflammation of, 144
  of epididymis, 120
  of testis, 120
Arachnoid mater, 337, 341
Arch
  anterior pancreaticoduodenal, 139
  of aorta, 27, 48, 49, 51, 69, 71, 76, 83, 494
    branches of, 72
  atlas
    anterior, 756
    posterior, 756
  of azygos vein, 82
  carpal, 495
  dorsal carpal, 581
  dorsal venous, 372, 373
  neural, 291
  palatoglossal, 798–800
  palatopharyngeal, 798–800
  palmar, 494, 495, 559, 580
  palmar carpal, 495
  pancreaticoduodenal, 139
  plantar, 370
    deep, 454
    venous, 371
  posterior pancreaticoduodenal, 139
  tendinous, 551
  vertebral, 293
  zygomatic, 616
Arcuate artery, 435
Arcuate ligament, 178
  lateral, 176
  medial, 176
Arcuate line, 107, 122
Areola, 4
Areolar tubercle, 4
Arm
  anterior and posterior compartments of, 529
  dorsal scapular and subdeltoid regions, 536
  muscles, 528
    anterior aspect of arm–I, 530
    anterior aspect of arm–II, 531
    lateral aspect of, 532–533
  posterior view, 483
  and rotator cuff, 524–525
  scapulohumeral muscles, 525

Arm (*Continued*)
suprascapular region, 537
surface anatomy, 534
transverse (axial) MRIs of, 605
triceps brachii and related nerves, 535
Arterial supply
of breast, 10
of kidneys and suprarenal glands, 169
to trachea and esophagus, 77
Artery
abdominal wall, 103
alveolar, inferior, 784
anterior
cerebral, 652
communicating, 652
inferior pancreaticoduodenal, 138
intercostal, 22, 24, 25
interosseous, 559
superior pancreaticoduodenal, 139
of anterolateral abdominal wall, 103
appendicular, 143
arcuate, 435
auricular, posterior, 770
axillary, 494, 511, 517
basilar, 302, 646, 652
brachial, 495, 533, 547, 549, 557, 559
brain, blood supply of, 353t, 653
carotid
common, 769–771, 777, 778
external, 769–771, 788, 811
internal, 769–771, 811
celiac, 134
cervical, deep, 790
circumflex scapular, 518
colic, 144, 146, 147
coronary, 56
cremasteric, 116, 121
cystic, 162
deep circumflex iliac, 103, 113
dorsal
digital, 580
of foot, 370
pancreatic, 139
of penis, 120, 268
dorsalis pedis, 433–435, 448
ductus deferens, 121, 229t, 230
epigastric, inferior, 223, 230
external iliac, 103, 113, 115
and vein, 167
external pudendal, 106
face and scalp, 638, 638t
facial, 632, 784, 788
tonsillar, 786, 802
femoral, 103, 370, 379–381, 388, 390, 401
lateral circumflex, 408, 409
medial circumflex, 408, 409
fibular, 445
gastric, 134
gastroduodenal, 134, 138, 139
gastro-epiploic, 134
gastro-omental, 134, 138
genicular
inferior lateral, 412, 424, 425
inferior medial, 412, 424, 425
middle, 421
superior lateral, 412, 424, 425
superior medial, 412, 424, 425
gluteal
inferior, 216, 230, 396
region, 401, 401t
superior, 216, 230, 397, 401
hand, 581, 581t
hepatic, 131, 134, 136, 157, 162
ileal, 145
ileocolic, 144
iliac
common, 167, 244, 370
external, 219, 222, 244, 370
internal, 216, 219, 229t, 230, 244, 370
iliolumbar, 229t
inferior epigastric, 103, 107, 113, 116
and veins, 112
inferior mesenteric (IMA), 146, 147
inferior pancreatic, 139
internal carotid (ICA), 646, 650, 651
internal thoracic, 24, 25
jejunal, 145
left gastric, 131
left gastro-omental (epiploic), 129
left pulmonary (LP), 70
lingual, 771, 787
deep, 788
lower limb, 370
malleolar, medial, 435
marginal, 145, 146
maxillary, 770
branches of, 676, 677
medullary, anterior segmental, 343
meningeal, 641
mesenteric, inferior, 146
middle colic, 144, 145
middle meningeal, 641
musculophrenic, 103
nasal wall and septum, 699
and nerves, of tongue, 686
obturator, 229t, 230, 409
acetabular branch, 409
posterior branch, 409
occipital, 770
sternocleidomastoid, 768
orbit and eyeball, 665, 665t
palmar digital, 571
pancreaticoduodenal, 139
pelvis
female, 242–247, 247t
male, 228–230, 229t
penis, dorsal and nerve of, 120
perforating, 401
pharyngeal, ascending, 770
phrenic, 169
plantar
deep, 435
lateral, 370, 454
medial, 370, 454
popliteal, 370, 401, 410, 412, 448
posterior
cerebral, 652
circumflex humeral, 535, 536
intercostal, 22, 103
of proximal upper limb, 512, 512t, 513t
pudendal, internal, 217, 229t, 230, 396, 397
pulmonary, 36, 37, 43, 49, 70
radial, 494, 495, 548, 549, 559, 562, 574, 579, 585
radicular, posterior, 343
rectal
inferior, 217
middle, 216, 217, 229t, 230
superior, 216, 217
renal, 169, 178
right pulmonary (RP), 70
of round ligament, 114
sacral, lateral, 229t
scapular, dorsal, 779
sigmoid, 146, 147
spinal
anterior, 343
posterior, 343
splenic, 131, 134, 136, 139, 168
and vein, 129, 168
subclavian, 76, 763, 770, 778
subcostal, 103
sublingual, 788
submental, 784, 788
superficial circumflex iliac, 103
and vein, 106
superficial epigastric, 103
and vein, 106
superficial temporal, 770, 771
superior epigastric, 103, 107
superior mesenteric, 131, 144, 145, 167
and arterial arcades, 144
superior rectal, 146, 147
supraduodenal, 138
suprarenal, 169
suprascapular, 771
testicular, 120, 121, 229t
and vein, 167
thigh, 401, 401t
thoracic, internal, 771
thoraco-acromial, 508
thyroid
ima, 777
inferior, 776, 777
superior, 771, 776, 777
tibial
anterior, 370, 433, 448
posterior, 448, 454
ulnar, 494, 495, 549, 559, 566, 574
umbilical, 122, 223, 229t
upper limb, 494–495
uterine, 244
vertebral, 302, 303, 652, 770, 782, 811
vesical
inferior, 229t, 230
superior, 229t, 230
Articular cartilage, 416
Articular disc, 599
ligamentous border of, 600
Articularis genu, 422
Ascending lumbar vein, 81
Atelectasis, 30
Atlanto-axial joint
ligaments, 303
muscles, 334t
Atlanto-axial membrane
anterior, 302
posterior, 301, 302
Atlanto-occipital joint
ligaments, 303
muscles, 334t
Atlanto-occipital membrane
anterior, 301, 302
posterior, 299, 301, 302, 334, 335, 790
Atlas, 299, 757
anterior arch, 756
anterior tubercle, 781
fracture, 303
posterior arch, 756
transverse process, 756
Atrial septal defects (ASDs), 62
Atrioventricular (AV) node, 60
Atrium, 64, 66
left, 43, 49, 52–54, 57, 62, 64, 66, 67, 81
right, 28, 29, 48, 51, 52, 54, 57, 60, 62, 66, 67, 81, 86, 88, 93, 94
Auricle, 51
Auriculotemporal nerve, 669, 835
Auscultation
heart, areas, 46
triangle of, 520
Autonomic ganglia, of head, 846, 846t
Autonomic innervation
abdominal nerve plexuses and ganglia, 183
abdominal viscera, 182, 183t
abdominopelvic nerve plexuses and ganglia, 180
sympathetic and parasympathetic, 181
of thorax, 86–87
vagus nerves, in abdomen, 185
visceral pain, surface projections of, 184
Axilla, 511
apex of, 510
structures, 511, 516–518

suspensory ligament of, 500
veins, 509
walls and contents of, 510
Axillary artery, 494, 511, 517
Axillary fascia, 500
Axillary fold, 505
anterior, 2
posterior, 2
Axillary fossa, 2, 505
Axillary lymph nodes, 8, 105, 511
Axillary nerve, 489, 490, 514, 518, 535, 536, 544
injury, 536
Axillary process (tail)
of breast, 5
site of, 4
Axillary sheath, 510
Axillary vein, 496, 511
Axis, 299, 756, 757
Azygos vein, 80–82, 84, 85, 340

B

Back
cervical spine
atlanto-axial joint, 301
craniovertebral joints, 302
imaging, 300, 356
ligaments, 299
vertebral artery, 302
coccyx, 314–315
costotransverse ligaments, 327
dermatomes, 348
hip bone, 314
intervertebral disc
ligaments and movements, 310–311
structure, 308–309
lumbar vertebrae, 306–307, 306t, 316–317, 355
muscles
atlanto-axial joint, 334t
atlanto-occipital joint, 334t
base of skull, 334
deep, 330
erector spinae, 325
intermediate, 324, 331t
multifidus, 326, 328
quadratus lumborum, 328
semispinalis, 326
splenius, 325, 331t
superficial, 323
transverse section, 329, 331t
myotomes, 349
nuchal region, 335, 354
pelvis, 313, 316–317
rotatores, 327
sacro-iliac joint
articular surfaces, 318
imaging, 319, 355
sacrum, 314–315
spinal cord
blood supply, 342–343
dural sac, 337–339
nerve roots, 341
prevertebral structures, 340
spinal nerves, 342–343
spondylolisthesis, 321
spondylolysis, 321
strain, 329
suboccipital region-I, 332
suboccipital region-II, 333
surface anatomy, 322
sympathetic nerve fibers, 351
thoracic vertebrae, 304–305, 304t, 356
thoracolumbar fascia, 328–329
vertebral column
anatomy, 290
anomalies, 320
cervical, 298, 298t
curvature, 291
homologous parts, 294
lumbar, 293, 312
movements, 295–297
surface anatomy, 296–297
thoracis, 305
vertebral venous plexuses, 344
visceral afferent and efferent innervation, 352–353
zygapophysial joints, 308–309
Bare areas and peritoneal formations, 124, 124t
Barium enema, of colon, 142
Bartholinitis, 278
Basilar artery, 302, 646, 652
Basilar membrane, 839
Basilic vein, 496, 498, 546
of forearm, 498, 595
Basivertebral vein, 344
Bell palsy, 847
Biceps brachii, 528, 530, 533, 549
short head of, 531
tendon of, 530, 531, 554
Biceps femoris, 389, 392, 395, 410, 411
Bicipital aponeurosis, 530, 546, 547
Bicipital rib, 16
Bifid rib, 16
Bifid ureters, 172
Bile
duct, 138, 156, 160
flow, in liver, 155
and pancreatic ducts, 160
Biliary ducts
biliary passages, radiographs of, 162
of gallbladder and biliary passages, 163
hepatic and cystic arteries, variations in, 162
pancreatic ducts
bile and, 160
development and variability of, 161
variations, of cystic and hepatic ducts and gallbladder, 163
Bipartite patella, 475
Bladder, 169, 209, 212, 213, 226, 236, 254
trigone of, 225
uvula of, 225
Body
hyoid bone, 787
mandible, 784
vertebral, 813
Bones of proximal upper limb, 526
Bony spur/osteophyte, 320
Bony spurs, 320
Bony thorax
anterior view, 12
costovertebral articulations, 17
ligaments of, 18
posterior view, 13
rib and sternum anomalies, 16
ribs, 15
sternum and associated joints, 14
Brachial artery, 495, 533, 547, 549, 557, 559
Brachial fascia, 501
Brachial plexus, 490, 514, 515
anterolateral view, 335
branches of, 515t
lateral cord of, 516
medial cord of, 488, 490, 516
posterior cord of, 517
Brachial veins, 547
Brachialis, 528, 533
Brachiocephalic trunk, 494
Brachiocephalic vein, 68, 69
Brachioradialis, 535, 547, 548, 562, 584
Brain
blood supply of
arteries of, 353t, 653
arteriograms, 654
cerebral arterial circle, 652
head and neck, 655
imaging of, 745–749
Brainstem, 740–741
Branchial motor, 822
Breast
anatomy, 4
anterior view, 4–6
arterial supply and venous drainage of, 10
axillary process (tail), 4, 5
bed of, 11
cancer, 5, 9
imaging of, 7
incisions, 10
lymphatic drainage of, 8–9
mammary gland, 6
posterior, lymph nodes, 8
quadrants of, 5
sagittal section, 6
suspensory ligaments of, 5, 6
Bronchi and bronchopulmonary segments
bronchograms, 41–42
3D volume reconstruction of, 43
pulmonary arteries, relationship of, 43
segmental, 38–39
trachea and bronchi in situ, 40
Bronchomediastinal trunk, 45
Bronchopulmonary (hilar) nodes, 45
Bronchoscopy, 41
Bronchus
intrapulmonary, 71
left inferior lobar, 40, 41, 43, 76
left main, 30, 37, 71, 76
left superior lobar, 40, 41, 43, 76
right inferior lobar, 41, 43
right main, 36
right superior lobar, 76
segmental and bronchopulmonary segments, 38–39
Buccal branches, 668
Buccal nerve (CN VII), 636, 835
Bulb
of penis, 266
vestibule, 276
Bunion, 471
Bursa
gluteofemoral, 396
knee
articularis genu and bursae, 422–423, 423t
lower limb, 422–423, 423t
obturator internus, 403
omentum, 130, 131
inferior recess of, 124
posterior relationships of, 129
posterior wall of, 131
superior recess of, 124, 125, 131
prepatellar, subcutaneous, 416
subacromial, 539, 544
subcutaneous olecranon, 557
suprapatellar, 422, 428
trochanteric, 396

C

Calcaneal bursitis, 444
Calcaneal fracture, 466
Calcaneal tendon, 440–444, 447
Calcaneofibular ligament, 462
Calyx, 170
Canal
anal, 265
innervation, 218
neurovascular structures, 216
sphincters, 214–215
carotid, 620
hypoglossal, 623
inguinal region, boundaries, 112t
lacrimal canaliculi, 657
lower limb, femoral, 381
optic, 623
pterygoid, 621
pyloric, 128, 133
semicircular, 838

Canaliculus
cochlear, 629, 720
tympanic, 629, 716, 717, 840
vestibular, 629
Capitulum, 557
Capsule
external, 732, 737, 739, 747
extreme, 733, 735–737, 739, 747
internal, 737, 739, 747
joint
acromioclavicular, 543
elbow, 556
glenohumeral (shoulder), 536, 538–541
hip, 398, 399, 409
knee, 429
shoulder, 540–541
temporomandibular, 672, 674
zygapophysial, 308, 309
renal, 175
synovial, 570
Carcinoma of tongue, 682
Cardia, 133
Cardiac compression, 50
Cardiac conduction system, 60
Cardiac cycle and cardiac skeleton, 61
Cardiac outflow, surgical isolation of, 52
Cardiac plexuses, 73
and pulmonary arteries, 70
Cardiac referred pain, 86
Cardiac tamponade, 31
Cardial notch, 133
Carotid artery, 76
Carotid canal, 620
Carpal arch, 495
Carpal bones, 482, 483, 487, 601
Carpal tunnel transverse (axial) section, 608–609
Carpi radialis
brevis, extensor, 590
longus, extensor, 590
Carpi ulnaris, extensor, 589
Carpometacarpal (CMC) joints, 601
Cartilages
arytenoid, 804, 805
cricoid, 756, 794, 795, 804, 805
epiglottic, 805
larynx skeleton, 804–805
thyroid, 756, 785, 794, 795, 804, 805
lamina of, 795
Cauda equina, 336, 339
Caudal epidural block, 251
Caval opening, 178
Cavernous sinus, 645
Cavity
ear
right tympanic, 717–719
tympanic, 716
tympanic, tructures of, 714
head, nasopharynx and oral, 724–727
nasal, 30
paranasal sinuses, 703
orbit and eyeball, 656
lateral aspect, 660–661
superior approach, 658, 659
orbital, 612, 615
peritoneum and peritoneal
abdominal contents and, 123
anterolateral abdominal wall, posterior aspect of, 122
formations and bare areas, 124, 124t
omental bursa, 127, 129–131
posterior wall of, 126, 148, 149
stomach and omenta, 128
subdivisions of, 125
transverse sections, 127
pleural cavity, 30, 74
superior mediastinum and great vessels
and roof of pleural cavity, 74
Cecum, 126, 140, 148
vascular fold of, 143
Celiac arteriogram, 136
Celiac artery, 134
Celiac trunk, 131, 134, 136, 178
Central axillary lymph nodes, 8, 497
Central tendon of diaphragm, 75
Cephalic vein, 3, 498, 509, 546
of forearm, 498, 592
Cerebellum, 742–745
Cerebral artery
anterior, 652
middle, 652, 655, 658
posterior, 644, 649, 650, 652, 655
Cerebral compression, 729
Cerebral contusion, 728
Cervical cardiac branches, 44
Cervical fascia
deep, 500
Cervical lordosis, 291
Cervical nerves, 341
Cervical region
anterior, 758, 758t, 766
posterior
muscles, 789
suboccipital, 790
Cervical ribs, 16
Cervical spine
atlanto-axial joint, 301
craniovertebral joints, 302
imaging, 300, 356
ligaments, 299
vertebral artery, 302
Cervical vertebrae, 290, 292, 294
Cervix, 236
Chest radiograph, 29
Choana, 620
Chorda tympani (CN VII), 803, 835
Ciliary vessels, anterior, 667
Circumflex iliac artery
deep, 103, 113
Circumflex scapular artery, 518
Cisterna chyli, 85, 186, 187
Cisternal puncture, 742
Clavicle, 3, 10, 482, 486, 503, 511, 526, 778
Clavipectoral fascia, 508
Clavipectoral (deltopectoral) triangle, 498, 503
Clitoris
body of, 276
crus of, 276
dorsal nerve of, 274
glans of, 276
Clivus, 619
Coccyx, 200, 201, 290–292, 314–315
Cochlea, 838
Cochlear duct, 839
Cochlear (spiral) ganglion, 838
Cochlear nerve, 838
Colic artery, 144, 146, 147
Colic flexure, 140, 148
Collateral ligament, 602
fibula, 417, 418
tibia, 417, 418, 420
Colon, 148
ascending, 98, 99, 123, 126, 132, 137, 140, 142, 144, 148, 149, 164, 187, 189
barium enema, 142
colonoscopy, 142
descending, 126, 140, 141
diverticulosis, 142
sigmoid, 140, 141, 148, 219
sigmoid mesocolon, 126, 141, 148
transverse, 140, 141
transverse mesocolon, 124, 126, 130, 148, 166
Compartments
arm, anterior and posterior, 529
infracolic, 126
lower limb
fascia, 376–377
leg, compartmental infections, 478
musculofascial, 376–377
neck, visceral
alimentary layer, 777
endocrine layer I and II, 774, 775
respiratory layer, 776
perineum
male and female organs/vessels, 258–259, 262–263
supracolic, 126
upper limb, musculofascial, 500, 501
Computed tomography
heart and pericardium, 54
intervertebral discs and zygapophysial joints, 309
lumbar spine, 355
paranasal sinuses and nasal cavity, 703
peritoneum and peritoneal cavity, 127
sacro-iliac joint, 319, 355
temporomandibular joint, 681
Computed tomography angiograms, 94, 95
Concha
inferior, 615, 690, 696, 700
middle, 627
superior, 700
Condyle
epicondyle
humeus, 529, 531, 561, 561t, 565
lateral, 555
medial, 550, 551
femur
lateral, 426
medial, 428
occipital, 620, 621
tibial
lateral, 426
medial, 426, 428
Conjoint tendon, 107, 111, 112
Conus medullaris, 336, 339
Coracobrachialis, 528, 530, 531, 533, 549
Coronal MRI, 608
of abdomen, 192
of cranial nerves, 850
of thorax, 92
Coronal suture, 618
Coronary artery, 56
Coronary ligament, 124, 126, 150
Coronary vessels
arteries, 56
arteriograms, with orientation drawings, 58
cardiac veins, 57
circulation, 59
Corrugator supercilii, 632
Costochondral junction, 28
Costocoracoid membrane, 500
Costotransverse joint, 17
Costotransverse ligament
anterior view, 19
posterior, 327
superior, 18, 19, 327
Costovertebral articulations, bony thorax, 17–18
Cranial nerves, 647, 647t, 820, 821t
abducent nerve (CN VI), 646, 650, 651, 660, 818–820, 828, 828t, 829, 847
auriculotemporal nerve (CN V_3), 669
base, internal aspect of, 819
base of brain, 818
buccal branches, 636, 668
facial nerve (CN VII), 646–648, 668, 669, 818–820, 836, 836t, 837, 847
frontal nerve (CN V_1), 831
gastrocnemius, 389
lateral, 440–443

lateral head, 410, 411, 421
medial, 440–443
medial head, 410, 411
glossopharyngeal nerve (CN IX), 646–648, 669, 818–820, 840, 840t, 841
head, autonomic ganglia of, 846, 846t
hypoglossal nerve (CN XII), 646, 647, 669, 818–820, 845, 845t
infra-orbital nerve (CN V_2), 636
infratrochlear nerve (CN V_1), 636
intermediate nerve (CN VII), 818–820
lacrimal nerve (CN V_1), 636, 831
lesions, 847, 847t
mandibular nerve (CN V_3), 646, 650, 834, 835
maxillary nerve (CN V_2), 646, 650, 677, 707, 832
mental nerve (CN V_3), 636
middle fossa—I, 650
middle fossa—II, 651
MRIs
coronal, 850
lateral view, 823
posterior (dorsal) view, 822
transverse, 848–849
oculomotor nerve (CN III), 646, 647, 649–651, 660, 818–820, 828, 828t, 829, 847
eyeball, innervation of, 829
orbit, muscles and nerves of, 827
olfactory nerves (CN I), 646, 818–820, 824, 824t
ophthalmic nerve (CN V_1), 646, 650
optic nerve (CN II), 646, 647, 818–820, 825–826, 825t
spinal accessory nerve (CN XI), 522, 646–648, 669, 818–820, 844, 844t
supra-orbital nerve (CN V_1), 831
supratrochlear nerve (CN V_1), 636, 831
temporal branches (CN VII), 668
tentorial notch, 649
trigeminal nerve (CN V), 646–650, 818–820, 829, 830, 830t, 832
mandibular nerve, 834t, 835
maxillary nerve, 832t, 833
ophthalmic, 831, 831t
trochlear nerve (CN IV), 646–650, 818–820, 828, 828t, 829
vagus nerve (CN X), 646–648, 669, 818–820, 842, 843, 843t
vestibulocochlear nerve (CN VIII), 646–648, 721, 818–820, 838, 838t, 839
zygomatic branches (CN VII), 660, 668
zygomaticofacial nerve (CN V_2), 636
Cranium
anterior view, 614, 615
base, 781
at birth and in early childhood, 612–613
ethmoid, 626–627
facial (frontal) aspect, 614–615
foramina, 620t–621t
frontal, 626–627
inferior view, 620
interior view, 623–624
lacrimal bones, 626–627
lateral aspect, 616, 617
mandible, 626–627
maxilla, 626–627
nerves and vessels of, 646
nose and infratemporal region, lateral wall of, 628
posterior view, 618, 619
radiographs of, 624–625
sphenoid bone, 630–631
superior view, 622
temporal bone, 629
Cremaster
artery, 116, 121
muscle, 111, 115
within cremasteric fascia, 116, 117
Crest
iliac, 198, 199
urethral, 225
Cribriform plate, 623
Cruciate ligament
anterior, 416–420, 427, 429
posterior, 416–420, 423, 427, 429
Cruciform ligament, 303
Crura, medial and lateral, 106
Crural fascia, 376
Crus, 176
clitoris, 276
diaphragm, 187
penis, 266
CSF rhinorrhea, 622
Cubital lymph nodes, 497
Cubital tunnel, tendinous arch of, 551
Cystic arteries, 162
Cystic duct, 156
variations of, 163

D

3D volume reconstruction, of thorax, 43, 94–95
Deformity of external nose, 697
Deltoid, 503, 508, 509, 521, 525
fascia, 501
Deltopectoral groove, 503
Deltopectoral lymph nodes, 497
Dens of axis, 303, 756
Denticulate ligament, 337
Dermatomes, 102, 348
lower limb, 368, 369
thorax, 11, 75
upper limb, 493, 493t
Descending colon, 126, 140, 141
Descending thoracic aorta, 54, 84
Diaphragm, 26, 99, 176, 178
central tendon of, 75
lumbar plexus and vertebral attachment of, 176
muscular part of, 75
and pericardial sac, 75
right crus of, 187
surface markings of, 47
Diaphragma sellae (sellar diaphragm), 644, 649
Diaphragmatic hernia, 178
Diaphragmatic (anterior and superior) surface, of liver, 150
Diastole, 61
Digestive system, 132
Digiti minimi, extensor, 589
Digitorum
brevis, extensor, 434
longus, extensor, 431, 432, 438, 439, 444
Dilocated epiphysis, femoral head, 360
Disc
articular, 599
intervertebral
ligaments and movements, 310–311
structure, 308–309
Distal humerus, 484
Distal ileum, 140
distal radio-ulnar joint, sacciform recess of, 600
Distal radius, 484
Distal ulna, 484
Diverticulosis, of colon, 142
Dorsal artery and nerve of penis, 120
Dorsal carpal arch, 581
Dorsal digital artery, 580
Dorsal pancreas, 161
Dorsal pancreatic artery, 139
Dorsal scapular vein, 509
Dorsal vein
arch, 372, 373
network, of hand, 496
of penis, deep, 120
Dorsalis pedis artery, 433–435, 448
anomalous, 448
Dorsalis pedis pulse, 434
Dorsum sellae, 619, 649
Duct
accessory pancreatic, 137
bile, 138, 156, 160
cochlear, 839
cystic, 156, 163
ejaculatory, 220, 221, 224, 225
gland
sublingual, 785
vestibular, 276
hepatic, 156, 157, 160
lymphatic, 8, 45, 79
right, 811
nasolacrimal, 657
pancreatic, 137, 160
parotid gland, 633
right lymphatic, 78
submandibular, 786
thoracic, 45, 78, 79, 83–85, 186, 340, 811
vestibular gland, 276
Ductules
prostatic, 224, 225
Ductus deferens, 120, 219–221, 224, 226
ampulla, 220, 224
artery of, 121
Duodenal cap, 135
Duodenal papilla, 137, 160
Duodenojejunal junction, 126, 141, 148
Duodenum, 98, 99, 137, 139, 157
blood supply to, 139
pancreas and, 137–138
parts and relationships of, 137t
radiographs of, 135
Dura mater, 337, 341

E

Ear
auricle, 709
bony and membranous labyrinths, 720
cochlea, 721
external, middle, and internal, 710, 711
middle and inner ear in situ, 715
ossicles of, 713
pharyngotympanic tube, 716–719
right tympanic cavity, 717–719
tympanic cavity, 716
tructures of, 714
tympanic membrane, 712
vestibulocochlear nerve (CN VIII), 721
Ectopic pelvic kidney, 172
Elbow joint
anular ligament, 556, 570
articular surfaces of, 557
bones and imaging of, 552
medial aspect, 554
radio-ulnar joints, 553
synovial capsule of, 556
synovial membrane of, 556
Elbow region
anomalies, 549
anterior view, 546
cubital fossa
deep dissection I, 547
deep dissection II, 548
surface anatomy and superficial dissection, 546
ligaments of, 554, 555
posterior aspect of, 550–551
Eminence
intercondylar, 426
parietal, 613
Endoscopic retrograde cholangiography and pancreatography (ERCP), 160, 163

Epicondyle
humeus, 529, 531, 561, 561t, 565
lateral, 555
medial, 550, 551
Epididymis, 120
Epidural fat, 340
Epidural hematomas, 642
Epigastric artery
inferior, 103, 107, 112, 113, 116
superior, 103, 106, 107
Epigastric vessels
inferior, 122
superior, 103
Epiglottis, 796, 797, 804
Epiphyses, femoral head, 360
Epiphysial plate
tibial fractures, 361
Epistaxis, 699
Erector spinae, 322, 325
Esophageal hiatus, 178
Esophageal vein, 165
Esophagus, 54, 68, 69, 71, 76, 82, 84, 98, 99, 178, 777
arterial supply to, 77
blockage of, 135
radiographs of, 135
Ethmoid bone, 656
Eyeball. *See also* Orbit and eyeball
dissected eyeball, 666
innervation of, 829
ocular fundus and blood supply, 667

F

Fabella, 475
Face and scalp
arteries of, 638, 638t
eyelid, 636
facial expression, 634, 635
muscles, 635t, 636, 640
facial nerve, branches of, 635, 637, 637t, 640
parotid gland and duct, 633
trigeminal nerve, cutaneous branches of, 636
veins of, 639, 639t
Facial artery, 632
Facial nerve (CN VII), 646–648, 668, 669, 818–820, 836, 836t, 837
palsy, 847
Facial vein, 639
Falciform ligament, 123, 150
Fallen arches, 474
Falx cerebelli (cerebellar falx), 644
Falx cerebri (cerebral falx), 644
Fascia
alar, 753
antebrachial, 501, 546, 547, 549, 550, 557, 606
axillary, 500
brachial, 500, 501, 546, 547
buccopharyngeal, 753
Camper, 109, 110, 262, 263
cervical, deep, 753
deep, 376
endopelvic, 252, 255
lata, 376
obturator, 263
omohyoid, 762
parietal abdominal, 223
pelvic, 255
diaphragm, 263
tendinous arch, 223
visceral, 223
perineal, 262, 263
pharyngobasilar, 792, 801
pretracheal, 775
prevertebral, 753, 780
rectal, 263
submandibular gland, 769
superior, 263
thoracolumbar, 323, 328–329
umbilical (prevesical), 255
uterovaginal, 263
vesical, 263
visceral, 775
Fasciotomy, 377
Fat
epidural, 340
paranephric, 175
perinephric, 175
Fat-pad, 114, 115
Fauces isthmus
palatine tonsil, 799
serial dissection
and nasopharynx I lateral wall, 800
and nasopharynx II lateral wall, 801
and nasopharynx III lateral wall, 802
and nasopharynx IV lateral wall, 803
surface anatomy (oropharyngeal), 798
Femoral artery, 103, 370, 379–381, 388
lateral circumflex, 408, 409
medial circumflex, 408, 409
Femoral neck fracture, 408
Femoral nerve, 176, 177
Femoral ring, 380
Femoral sheath, 379, 381
Femur, 359, 390, 391, 412
condyle
lateral, 426
medial, 428
head blood supply, 408
head ligament, 405–407, 409
intermuscular septum
anteromedial, 377
lateral, 377
posteromedial, 377
nerve, 362, 380, 381, 407
transverse sections, 480
vein, 371, 378–381
Fibrous digital sheath, 569, 577
Fibular, 359, 390, 391, 431
collateral ligament, 421, 422, 427
fracture, 441
nerve, 392
peroneal artery, 445
peroneal nerve, 410, 411
common, 362
deep, 362, 432, 433
lesion, 436
superficial, 362, 432, 433, 437
peroneal retinaculum
inferior, 438
superior, 438
peroneal trochlea, 439
peroneus brevis, 431, 434–439
peroneus longus, 436–439
peroneus tertius, 431, 435, 438
vein, 371
Fibularis
brevis 437
longus, 436, 437
Filum terminale externum, 336, 338, 339, 346
Filum terminale
externum, 336, 338, 339, 346
internum, 339
Fissure
horizontal, 34
oblique, 27, 34, 37
superior orbital, 619, 623
Flat feet, 474
Flexor carpi radialis, 562
Flexor carpi ulnaris, 551, 562, 563
Flexor digiti minimi, 454
Flexor digitorum brevis, 452
Flexor digitorum longus, 440, 441, 444, 445, 447, 453
Flexor digitorum superficialis, 563
Flexor hallucis brevis, 454
Flexor hallucis longus, 440, 441, 444–447, 456
tendon, 453
Flexor pollicis brevis, 572, 574
Flexor pollicis longus, 564, 565, 576
Flexor retinaculum, 501
Flexors, deep, 564
Fold
ary-epiglottic, 796, 807, 808, 810
axillary, 2, 505
cecum, vascular of, 143
inferior ileocecal, 143
lateral umbilical, 122
medial umbilical, 122
median umbilical, 122
synovial, infrapatellar, 416
vestibular, 807, 810, 813
vocal, 807, 810
Foot
arches, 474
bones, child, 361
dorsal artery, 370
dorsum, 457
medial, 447
radiographs, 461
region, 358
surface anatomy of, 434, 436, 438, 442, 446, 451
Foramen
jugular, 619, 621, 623, 647t, 716
lacerum, 620, 621t, 623, 628
magnum, 621
omental, 124, 127, 128
ovale, 620
rotundum, 620t, 623, 630, 647, 706
transversarium, 57, 757
Forearm
anterior aspect of, 558, 558t
arteries of, 559
basilic vein of, 546, 595
bones, 560
and muscle attachments on, 582
cephalic vein of, 592
deep structures, extensor aspect of, 585
hand and attachments of forearm muscles, 560
median vein of, 546
muscles, 560, 561t
posterior aspect of, 583, 583t
posterior view, 483
radio ulnar joints, ligaments of, 559
superficial muscles, 562
extensor aspect of, 584
transverse sections and transverse (axial) MRI of, 606–607
Fossa
acetabular, 409
axillary, 2, 505
cranial nerves
middle cranial fossa–I, 650
middle cranial fossa–II, 651
cubital
deep dissection I, 547
deep dissection II, 548
surface anatomy and superficial dissection, 546
ischio-anal, 222, 265
lateral inguinal, 122
mandibular, 620
medial inguinal, 122
muscles, popliteal, 413
nerves
popliteal, 411
pterygopalatine, 705–707
ovalis, 64
pararectal, 219
popliteal, 410–413
pterygopalatine
nerves of, 705–707
sphenoid bone, 708
supraclavicular
lesser, 768

supravesical, 122, 213
temporal, 616
temporal region and infratemporal, 670–679
tonsillar, 800
Fovea, femur head ligament, 402
Fractured mandible, 669
Frontal bone, 612, 613
Frontal nerve (CN V_1), 831
Frontal (metopic) suture, 612
Fundus, 133, 135
of stomach, 135
of uterus, 238

G

Gag reflex, 682
Gallbladder, 156
porta hepatis, 158
variations of, 163
Ganglion
abdominal nerve plexuses and, 183
abdominal viscera, 182
abdominopelvic nerve plexuses and, 180
cervical, superior, 792
cervicothoracic, 782
lymphatic drainage, 187
stellate block, 782
submandibular, 786
Gastric artery, 131, 134
Gastric vein, 131, 165
Gastrocnemius, 389
lateral head, 410, 411, 421, 440–443
medial head, 410, 411, 440–443
strain, 442
Gastrocolic ligament, 123, 128, 131, 148
Gastroduodenal artery, 134, 138, 139
Gastro-epiploic artery, 134
Gastro-omental artery, 129, 134, 138
Gastro-omental vessels, 130
Gastrosplenic ligament, 123
Gemellus
inferior, 396, 397, 399
superior, 393, 396, 397, 399
Genicular artery
inferior lateral, 412, 424, 425
inferior medial, 412, 421, 424, 425
superior lateral, 412, 424, 425
superior medial, 412, 424, 425
Genioglossus paralysis, 685
Geniohyoid, 766
Genitofemoral nerve, 176, 177
femoral branch of, 115
genital branch of, 114
Genu valgum, 415
Genu varum, 415
Gland
bulbourethral, 220
fascia, submandibular, 769
palatine, 800
seminal, 224, 226
sublingual, 785
submandibular, 802
thyroid, 778
inferior pole of, 774
isthmus of, 774
superior pole of, 774
vestibular, 276
Glaucoma, 666
Glossopharyngeal nerve (CN IX), 337, 646–648, 669, 818–820, 840, 840t, 841
Gluteal artery
inferior, 396
superior, 397, 401
Gluteal fascia, 389
Gluteal nerve
inferior, 396, 401
superior, 397
Gluteal region
arteries, 401, 401t
lateral rotators, 398–399
muscles, 392–394, 394t, 396–397
nerves, 400, 400t
Gluteofemoral bursa, 396
Gluteus maximus, 389, 393–394, 396
Gluteus medius, 393, 394, 396, 397
Goiter, 778
Gonads, descent of, 118
Gracilis, 383, 387
Great auricular nerve (C2, C3), 633
Great saphenous vein, 106
Great toe. *See* Hallux
Great vessels, 48–49, 51
Greater curvature, 133, 135
Greater omentum, 124
Greater sac, 124
Greater splanchnic nerve, 84, 85
Greater trochanter, 393
Greater tubercle, 525
Groove
azygos vein, 36
brachiocephalic vein, 36
deltopectoral, 503
iliopsoas, 202
inferior vena cava, 36
lateral meniscus, 417
medial meniscus, 417
obturator, 201
obturator externus, 403
superior vena cava, 36
vertebral artery, 302, 303
Gyrus, 731, 734, 735

H

Hallucis brevis, extensor, 434
Hallucis longus, extensor, 431, 432, 434, 439
Hallux, 471
Hallux valgus, 471
Hamstring strains, 392
Hand
arterial supply of, 580
arteries of, 581, 581t
bones, 596
and muscle attachments on, 582
cutaneous innervation of, 586, 587
dorsal venous network of, 498
dorsum of, 588–590
functional positions of, 604
imaging of bones, 597
lateral aspect, 592–594
medial aspect of, 595
muscles of, 573t
palm, synovial sheaths of, 576
surface anatomy of skeleton of, 568
thumb, movements of, 582
Head
autonomic ganglia of, 846, 846t
autonomic innervation, 723
blood supply, 655
imaging of, 724–727
lymphatic drainage, 722
nasopharynx and oral cavity, 724–727
Heart
conduction system, coronal section, 60
external
and great vessels, 48–49
and pericardium, 50, 52–54
pre-and postnatal circulation, 55
sternocostal (anterior) surface and great vessels in situ, 51
surface markings of, 46–47
innervation of, 86
internal
cardiac cycle and cardiac skeleton, 61
left atrium, 64
left ventricle, 64–65
right atrium, 62
right ventricle, 63
valves of, 66–67
Helicotrema, 839
Hemi-azygos vein, 80, 81, 85
Hemivertebra, 320
Hemopericardium, 53
Hemorrhoids, 231
Hepatic artery, 131, 134, 136, 157, 162
Hepatic branches, 185
Hepatic duct, 156, 157, 160
variations of, 163
Hepatic portal vein, 131, 138, 156, 164, 165
Hepatic segmentation, 154–155, 155t
Hepatic veins, 153
Hepatopancreatic ampulla, 160
Hepatorenal recess, 151
Hernia
hiatal (hiatus), 135
inguinal, direct and indirect, 119, 119t
Hiatal hernia, 135, 178
Hiatus
aortic, 178
esophageal, 178
hiatal hernia, 135
urogenital, 267
High-tone deafness, 721
Hip bone, 198–200, 314, 358, 359, 405
medial view, 318
Hip joint
iliofemoral ligament, 402
ischiofemoral ligament, 403
radiograph and coronal section, 406
transverse section and MRI, 407
Hip prosthesis, 405
Hip replacement, 406
Horseshoe kidney, 172
Housemaid's knee. *See* Prepatellar bursitis
Humeral artery, 544
Humeral (lateral) axillary lymph nodes, 8, 497
Humerus, 482, 483, 486, 526, 527
Hyoid bone, 756, 769, 772, 784, 787, 794
Hypoglossal canal, 623
Hypoglossal nerve (CN XII), 646, 647, 669, 818–820, 845, 845t
Hypothenar fascia, 569
Hysterectomy, 240
Hysterosalpingogram, 288
Hysterosalpingography. *See* Hysterosalpingogram

I

Ileal arteries, 145
Ileal diverticulum, 143
Ileocecal fold
anterior, 244
inferior, 143
Ileocecal orifice, 143
Ileocecal region and appendix, 143
Ileocolic artery, 144
Ileum, 143, 148
Ileus, 145
Iliac artery
common, 370
external, 103, 113, 115, 167, 370
internal, 370
and vein, 167
Iliac crest, 173
Iliac vein
common, 371
external, 115, 167, 371
internal, 371
Iliacus, 381, 383, 385
Iliocostalis, 325
cervicis, 325
lumborum, 325
thoracis, 325
Iliofemoral ligament, 402–404, 407
Iliohypogastric nerve, 103, 111, 112, 174–177

Ilio-inguinal nerve, 103, 106, 111, 112, 176, 177
Iliolumbar ligament, 316, 317
Iliopsoas, 381, 384, 385
Iliopubic tract, 122
Iliotibial tract, 376, 389, 392, 414, 421
Iliotibial tract (band) syndrome (ITBS), 376
Ilium, 200, 405
Incisional nerve injury, of anterolateral abdominal wall, 103
Indicis, extensor, 584, 585, 589
Inferior mesenteric artery (IMA), 146, 147
Inferior vena cava (IVC), 179, 179t
  obstruction of, 81
Inferomedial quadrant, 5
Infracolic compartment, 126
Infra-orbital foramen, 616
Infra-orbital nerve (CN V_2), 636
Infraspinatus, 524
Infratrochlear nerve (CN V_1), 636
Inguinal fossa
  lateral, 122
  medial, 122
Inguinal ligament, 100, 110, 379, 380
Inguinal lymph nodes, 375
  deep, 374
  superficial, 374, 375
Inguinal region
  boundaries, of canal, 112t
  female, 114–115
  gonads, descent of, 118
  hernias, 119, 119t
  male, 110–113
  spermatic cord, and testis, 116–117
Inguinal ring
  deep, 122
  location of, 113
Innermost intercostal, 19–21, 23
Innervation, of lungs, 44
Interchondral joint, 14
Intercondylar eminence, 426
Intercostal artery
  anterior, 22, 24, 25
  posterior, 22, 77, 103, 340, 342
Intercostal nerve, 24, 25
Intercostal spaces
  inferior, anterior ends of, 21
  transverse section, contents of, 22
  vertebral ends
    inferior, external aspect of, 20
    internal aspect of, 19
Intercostal vein, 24, 25
Intercrural fibers, 106, 110
Intermediate muscle, 324, 331t
Intermediate nerve (CN VII), 818–820
Internal carotid artery (ICA), 646, 650, 651
Internal intercostal, 20–22, 24, 25
  interchondral part of, 26
  interosseous part of, 26
  membrane, 19, 20, 22
Internal oblique, 26, 107, 111, 112, 115, 173, 174
Internal spermatic fascia, 116, 117
Internal thoracic artery, 24, 25
Internal thoracic vein, 24, 25
Interosseous artery
  anterior, 559
  posterior, 459, 558
Interosseous ligament, 450
Interosseous membrane, 377, 450, 478, 554, 555
Interpectoral lymph nodes, 8
Interphalangeal joints, 602
Interspinous ligament, 309, 312
Intertransversarii, 328
Intertrochanteric line, 402
Interventricular septum, 65
Intervertebral disc
  ligaments and movements, 310–311
  structure, 308–309
Intestinal lymphatic trunk, 186
Intestines
  anterior view, 140, 141, 148, 149
  barium enema and colonoscopy, 142
  ileocecal region and appendix, 143
  inferior mesenteric arteriogram, 146, 147
  inferior mesenteric artery, 146
  posterior abdominal cavity
    peritoneum of, 148
    with peritoneum removed, 149
  small intestine
    interior of, 140
    sigmoid mesocolon and mesentery of, 141
  superior mesenteric arteriograms, 145
  superior mesenteric artery and arterial arcades, 144
Intra-articular ligament, 18
Intragluteal injection, 396
Intrapulmonary bronchi, 71
Ischemia, 343
Ischial bursitis, 393
Ischial spine, 398
Ischiofemoral ligament, 403
Ischium, 200, 405
Isthmus, 775

J

Jejunal arteries, 145
Jejunum, 135
Joints
  ankle
    articular surfaces, 463
    joint cavity, 456
    ligaments, 457
    medial/deltoid ligament, 460
    posterior aspect, 458
    synovial membrane, 456
  atlanto-axial, 303, 334t
  atlanto-occipital, 303, 334t
  axilla, shoulder, 511
  bony thorax associated, 14
  carpometacarpal (CMC), 601
  craniovertebral, 302
  cubonavicular, 470
  cuneonavicular, 470
  elbow joint, 570
    and anular ligament, 556, 570
    articular surfaces of, 557
    bones and imaging of, 552
    medial aspect of bones, 554
    radio-ulnar, 553
    synovial capsule of, 556
    synovial membrane of, 556
  foot, 467
  forearm, radioulnar, 559
  hip
    iliofemoral ligament, 402
    ischiofemoral ligament, 403
    radiograph and coronal section, 406
    transverse section and MRI, 407
  interphalangeal, 602
  inversion and eversion, 466
  knee
    articular surfaces and ligaments, 417
    cruciate ligaments and menisci, 419
    fibrous layer, 429
    fibrous layer and synovial membrane, 416
    injury, 418
    ligaments, 418
  metacarpophalangeal, 349, 602
  metatarsophalangeal, 471
  midcarpal (transverse carpal), 600
  radiocarpal (wrist), 599, 600
  radioulnar, 559
  sacro-iliac, 318, 319, 355
  scapulothoracic, 482–484, 486, 487, 506, 511, 526, 527
  shoulder region
    acromioclavicular, 539
    imaging of, 544–545
    ligaments and articular capsule of, 540–541
    pectoral girdle, 538
    of rotator cuff, 542–543
    subacromial bursa, 539
  of shoulder region, 538–545
  sternoclavicular, 14, 523, 538, 778
  subtalar, 466
  talocalcaneal, 468
  tarsal, transverse, 469
  tarsometatarsal, 470
  temporomandibular, 616
    coronal section, 680
    mastication, muscles of, 678, 678t
    movements of, 679, 679t
    sectional anatomy of, 681
  tibiofibular, 433, 450
  wrist, radiocarpal, 599, 600
  zygapophysial, 308–310
Jugular foramen, 619, 621
Jugular lymphatic trunk, 78
Jugular vein, 509
  external, 496
  internal, 496
Jumper's knee. *See* Patella
Junction
  costochondral, 28
  duodenojejunal, 126, 141, 148

K

Kidneys, 129, 168, 169, 175, 187
  anomalies of, 172
  exposure of, 168, 173–175
  lymphatic drainage, 186
  segments of, 171
  structure of, 170
  and suprarenal glands, 169
Knee
  anastomoses, 424–425
  anterior aspect, 414–415
  articularis genu and bursae, 422–423, 423t
  clinical imaging, 426
  coronal section and MRI, 427
  lateral aspect, 421
  medial aspect, 420
  posterior view, 410
  radiograph, 428
  sagittal section and MRI, 428–429
Knee joint
  articular surfaces and ligaments, 417
  cruciate ligaments and menisci, 419
  fibrous layer, 429
  fibrous layer and synovial membrane, 416
  injury, 418
  ligaments, 418
Kyphosis
  sacrococcygeal kyphosis, 291
  thoracic kyphosis, 291

L

Lacrimal bone, 615, 656
Lacrimal canaliculi, 657
Lacrimal gland, 657
Lacrimal nerve (CN V_1), 636, 831
Lacrimal sac, 657
Lacunar ligament, 380
Lambda, 618
Lambdoid suture, 618
Laminectomy, 306
Laparoscopy, 237
Larynx, 30
  external and laryngeal nerves, 806
  internal, 807
  laryngoscopic examination and MRI imaging, 810
  muscles, 808t
  skeleton cartilages, 804–805
  sympathetic trunk/peri-arterial plexus, 811

thyroid gland, and trachea lymphatic drainage, 811
Latissimus dorsi, 173, 322, 323, 510, 517, 521, 522, 531
Left pulmonary artery, 70
Left superior intercostal vein, 81
Left suprarenal gland, 185
Leg
anterior aspects
bones and muscle, 431, 431t
muscles, 436
nerves, 432–433, 432t
superficial muscles, 430
compartmental infections, 478
intermuscular septum
anterior, 478
posterior, 478
lateral aspects
muscles, 436–437, 437t
MRI, 479
posterior aspects
arterial supply, 449, 449t
bones, 441
muscles, 440, 440t, 442–445
popliteal arteriogram and arterial anomalies, 448
transverse section, 478
Leg region, 358
Lesser curvature, 133
Lesser omentum, 124, 128, 130
Lesser splanchnic nerve, 84
Levator ani, 208, 222, 254, 265, 276
Levator scapulae, 324, 521, 522
Levatores costarum, 20, 23, 327
Ligaments
acetabular, 404
acromioclavicular, superior, 538
alar, 303
ankle joint, 457
medial/deltoid, 460
ankle region
lateral, 462
medial, 460
anular, radius, 554–556
articular disc, 600
atlanto-axial joint, 303
atlanto-occipital, 303
axilla, suspensoryof, 500
bony thorax, 18
breast, suspensoryof, 6
calcaneofibular, 462
of cervical spine, 299
collateral
fibular, 417, 418, 421, 422, 427
of interphalangeal joints, 602
lateral, of ankle, 458
of metacarpophalangeal joints, 602
radial, of elbow, 551, 555–557
radial, of wrist, 598
tibia, 417, 418, 420, 427
ulnar, of elbow, 554, 557
ulnar, of wrist, 598
conoid, 538, 539, 541
coraco-acromial, 514, 525, 531, 538–541, 543
coracoclavicular, 514, 527, 538, 540
costotransverse, 327
of costovertebral articulations, 18
cruciate
anterior, 417, 418, 427, 429
posterior, 417, 418, 427, 429
cruciform, 303
deltoid, 457, 460
denticulate, 337
elbow joint and anular, 556, 570
elbow region, 554, 555
femur head, 409
forearm, radioulnar joints, 559
glenohumeral, 541, 542
of head of femur, 405–407, 409, 450
iliofemoral, 402–404, 407
iliolumbar, 316, 317
inguinal, 379, 380
interosseous, 450
interspinous, 309, 312
intervertebral disc, 310–311
ischiofemoral, 403
knee joint, 418
lacunar, 380
longitudinal
anterior, 302, 310, 312, 316
posterior, 310–312
lumbar, 316–317
nuchal, 333
palmar carpal, 501
palmar ligament, 600, 602
patellar, 389, 414
pectineal, 380
pelvis, 316–317
pubovesical, 255
radial collateral, 555, 556
radi-oulnar joints, 559
retinacular, 591
sacrococcygeal, 205
anterior, 316
posterior, 317
sacro-iliac, 205, 317
anterior, 316
posterior, 317
sacrospinous, 205, 206, 316, 398
sacrotuberous, 205, 206, 267, 316, 317, 398
shoulder region
ligaments and articular capsule of, 540–541
skin (grayson), 569, 575, 576
sole of foot, 472–473
stylohyoid, 787, 803
supraspinous, 309, 312, 317
suspensory
of axilla, 500
of breast, 5, 6
ovary of, 252
penis of, 268
talofibular, anterior, 462
tibiofibular, anterior, 457
tibionavicular, medial, 460
transverse acetabular, 404, 406, 409
transverse carpal, 501, 600
transverse palmar, 575, 579
trapezoid, 540
ulnar collateral, 554
umbilical, 122, 222, 223
uterosacral, 255
uterus, 212
vestibular, 807
vocal, 807
Ligamentum flavum, 308–310, 312
Ligamentum venosum, 151
Line
pain, pelvic, 230
pectinate, 215
Linea alba, 100
Linea semilunaris, 100
Lingual nerve, 835
Liposuction, 105
Liver, 98
bare area of, 126
biopsy, 151
diaphragmatic (anterior and superior) surface of, 150
flow, of blood and bile in, 155
hepatic veins, 153
porta hepatis
gallbladder and structures of, 158
vessels in, 159
portal triad, exposure of, 156–157
posterior relations, schematic illustration, 152
segmentation, 154–155, 155t
visceral (postero-inferior) surface of, 151
Local anesthesia, intercostal space, 11
Longissimus thoracis, 325
Longitudinal ligament
anterior, 18, 302, 310, 312, 316
posterior, 310–312
Longus capitis, 334
Lower limb
acetabular fossa, 409
acetabular region, 404
ankle
coronal section, 464
dislocation, 457
medial, 446–447
MRI, 464, 465
posteromedial aspect, 459
radiographs, 461
synovial sheaths and tendons, 438–439
transverse section, 465
ankle joint
articular surfaces, 463
joint cavity, 456
ligaments, 457, 460, 462
posterior aspect, 458
arteries, 370
bones
at birth, 360
features, 359
hip, 358
bony anomalies, 475
cutaneous nerves, 364, 365t
deep tendon reflexes, 367
deep veins, 371
dermatomes, 368, 369
dorsum of foot
bones and muscle, 431
muscles, 436
muscles and arteries, 435, 435t
surface anatomy dissection, 434
fascia compartments, 376–377
femoral canal, 381
femoral sheath, 379
femoral triangle, 380
femur
head blood supply, 408
head ligament blood vessels, 409
transverse sections, 480
fibula
transverse sections, 480
foot
arches, 474
dorsum, 457
medial, 447
radiographs, 461
gluteal region
arteries, 401, 401t
lateral rotators, 398–399
muscles, 392–394, 394t, 396–397
nerves, 400, 400t
hip bone, 405
hip joint
iliofemoral ligament, 402
ischiofemoral ligament, 403
radiograph and coronal section, 406
transverse section and MRI, 407
inguinal lymph nodes, 375
knee
anastomoses, 424–425
anterior aspect, 414–415
articularis genu and bursae, 422–423, 423t
clinical imaging, 426
coronal section and MRI, 427
lateral aspect, 421
medial aspect, 420
radiograph, 428
sagittal section and MRI, 428–429
knee joint, 418
articular surfaces and ligaments, 417

Lower limb (*Continued*)
cruciate ligaments and menisci, 419
fibrous layer and synovial membrane, 416
injury, 418
leg
anterior aspects, 430–433, 432t
compartmental infections, 478
lateral aspects, 436–437, 437t
MRI, 479
posterior aspects, 440–444, 448, 449, 449t
transverse section, 478
lymphatic drainage, 374
motor innervation, 362, 363t
musculofascial compartments, 376–377
myotomes, 367
nerve lesions, 366t
nerve root/anterior ramus lesions, 367t
popliteal fossa
anatomy, 410
deep dissection, 412
muscles, 413
nerves, 411
retro-inguinal passage, 380–381
saphenous opening, 378
sole of foot
first layer muscles, 452, 452t
fourth layer muscles, 455, 455t
ligaments, 472–473
second layer muscles, 453, 453t
superficial, 451
third layer muscles, 454, 454t
subtalar joint, 466
superficial inguinal vessels, 378
superficial veins, 372, 373
talocalcaneal joint, 468
thigh
anteromedial aspect, 390
arteries, posterior, 401, 401t
bones, 388–389
lateral aspect, 391
medial aspect, 382–384, 385t, 386–387, 386t
muscles, posterior, 392–393, 395–397, 395t
transverse sections and MRI, 476–477
tibia
transverse sections, 480
tibiofibular joint and syndesmosis, 450
Lumbar cord, 341
Lumbar lordosis, 291
Lumbar lymph nodes, 187
Lumbar lymphatic trunk, 186
Lumbar nerves, 341
Lumbar plexus, 176, 177
Lumbar triangle, 522
Lumbar vertebrae, 290, 292, 294, 306–307, 306t, 316–317, 355
Lumbocostal triangle, 178
Lumborum, quadratus, 175, 328
Lumbosacral trunk, 176, 177
Lumbosacral vertebra, transitional, 320
Lumbricals, 452
and interossei, 573
Lungs
apex of, 28
cancer (carcinoma), 45
inferior lobe of, 27
innervation of, 44
left, 35
lymphatic drainage of, 45
mediastinal (medial) surface and hilum
of left, 37
of right, 36
parietal pleura
extent of, 32–33
surface markings of, 33t
right, 34
surface markings of, 47
topography of, 28
visceral pleura, surface markings of, 33t
Lymph node, 79
apical axillary, 8, 497
axillary, 8, 105, 511
central axillary, 8, 497
cubital, 497
deltopectoral, 497
humeral (lateral) axillary, 8, 497
inguinal, 375
deep, 374
superficial, 374, 375
interpectoral, 8
lower limb, inguinal, 375
lumbar, 187
lymphatic drainage, 187
parasternal, 8, 105
pectoral (anterior) axillary, 8, 497
subscapular (posterior), 8, 497
superficial inguinal, 105
Lymphatic capillaries, 79
Lymphatic drainage, 217, 232–233, 248–249
of anterolateral abdominal wall, 105
of breast, 8–9
breast cancer, 6, 9
gallbladder, 189
of head, 722
large intestine, 189
liver, 189
lumbar and intestinal lymphatic trunks, 188
lumbar lymph nodes, sympathetic trunk, nerves, and ganglia, 187
of lungs, 45
spleen and pancreas, 188
stomach and small intestine, 188
of suprarenal glands, kidneys, and ureters, 186
of testis, 121
of thorax, 88–89
Lymphatic duct, 8, 45, 79
Lymphatic duct, right, 78
Lymphatic plexus
deep, 45
Lymphatic system, posterior thorax, 79
Lymphatic vessels, superficial, 374

M

Macula, 667
Magnetic resonance imaging (MRI)
of abdomen
coronal, 192
sagittal, 193
transverse or horizontal (axial), 190–191
ankle, 464, 465
cervical spine, 356
of cranial nerves
coronal, 850
transverse, 848–849
hip joint, 407
knee, 427–429
leg, 479
thigh, 476–477
of thorax
coronal, 92
sagittal, 93
transverse (axial), 90–91
Malleolar artery, medial, 435
Malleolus
lateral, 358, 372, 373
medial, 358, 370, 372
Mammary gland, 6
Mandible, 612, 615
angle of, 616
body of, 615, 616
coronoid process, 673
head, 670
neck, 670
ramus, 612, 617
Mandibular fossa, 620
Mandibular nerve (CN V_3), 646, 650, 677, 834, 834t, 835
Manubriosternal joint, 14
Manubrium, 14, 50
Marginal artery, 145, 146
Masseteric nerve, 835
Mastication, muscles of, 678, 678t
Mastoid antrum, infections, 717
Mastoid cells, infections, 717
Mastoid process, 616, 620, 621
Mastoiditis, 717
Maxilla, 612
Maxillary artery, branches of, 676, 677
Maxillary nerve (CN V_2), 646, 650, 677, 707, 832, 832t, 833
Maxillary sinusitis, 704
Medial sural cutaneous nerve, 364
Median cubital vein, 546
Median nerve, 514, 547, 557, 600
lateral root of, 516
medial root of, 516
recurrent branch of, 574
Median umbilical fold, 122
Mediastinal silhouette, pathological widening of, 29
Mediastinum, 30, 31, 33
and great vessels, superior
aortic arch, branches of, 72
cardiac and pulmonary plexuses, 73
cardiac plexus and pulmonary arteries, 70
and roof of pleural cavity, 74
superficial dissections, 68–69
and trachea, 70
tracheal bifurcation and bronchi, 71
posterior thorax, 82–85
surface and hilum
of left lung, 37
of right lung, 36
topography of, 28
Mediolateral oblique mammogram, 7
Medulla, 350
Medulla oblongata, 740
Medullary artery, anterior segmental, 343
Membrane
obturator, 205, 206
perineal, 222, 263, 265, 266
quadrangular, 807
thyrohyoid, 776
Meningeal artery, 641
Meninges and meningeal spaces
arachnoid granulations, 643
dura mater, 643, 644
venous sinuses of, 645
middle artery and pterion, 641
scalp, layers of, 642
Meniscus
lateral, 417, 419, 427
medial, 416–420
Mental nerve (CN V_3), 636
Mesenteric arteriogram
inferior, 147
superior, 145
Mesenteric artery
and arterial arcades, 144
inferior, 146
superior, 131, 144, 145, 167
Mesenteric vein
inferior, 131, 164
superior, 131, 138, 164
and artery, 138
Mesoappendix, 143
Mesosalpinx, 240, 241
Mesovarium, 240
Metacarpal bones, 482, 483, 487, 582
Metacarpals, 601

Metacarpophalangeal joints, 349, 602
Metatarsophalangeal, medial, 367
Midarm fracture, 535
Midbrain, 350
Midcarpal (transverse carpal) joint, 600
Middle colic artery, 144, 145
Middle lobe, of lung, 34
Mitral valve, 64, 67
Modiolus, 839
Mons pubis, 273
Motion sickness, 721
MR angiogram, of abdomen, 194–195
Multifidus muscle, 326, 328
  lumborum, 326
  thoracis, 326
Muscles
  of anterolateral abdominal wall, 108, 108t
  aponeurosis, 324
  arm, 528
    anterior aspect of arm–I, 530
    anterior aspect of arm–II, 531
    lateral aspect of, 532–533
    scapulohumeral, 525
  arytenoids, 808t
  back
    atlanto-axial joint, 334t
    atlanto-occipital joint, 334t
    base of skull, 334
    deep, 330
    and deltoid, 521, 521t
    erector spinae, 325
    intermediate, 324, 331t
    multifidus, 326, 328
    and posterior axio-appendicular, 522
    quadratus lumborum, 328
    semispinalis, 326
    splenius, 325, 331t
    superficial, 323
    transverse section, 329, 331t
    transversospinalis, 327, 330, 331t
  of bed of breast, 11
  biceps brachii, 528, 528t, 530, 531, 533, 549, 554, 565
  bulbospongiosus, 259, 260t, 276
  capitis, longus, 780t
  cervical region, posterior, 789
  ciliary, 350, 666, 723
  coccygeus, 206, 208, 209, 211, 258, 267, 287
  colli, longus, 780t
  compressor urethrae (females only), 260t
  costotransverse ligament
    posterior, 327
    superior, 327
  cremaster, 111, 115
    within cremasteric fascia, 117
    and fascia, 116, 117
  crico-arytenoid
    lateral, 808t
    posterior, 808t
  cricopharyngeus, 794t
  cricothyroid, 808t
  deep transverse perineal (male only), 260t
  dilator pupillae, 666, 723, 811
  dorsum of foot, 435, 435t, 436
  erector spinae, 322
  extra-ocular, 633t, 662, 662t, 663
  face and scalp, facial expression, 635t, 636, 640
  forearm, 560, 561t
    bones and attachments on, 582
    hand and attachments of forearm, 560
    posterior aspect of, 583, 583t
    superficial of, 562, 584
  genioglossus, 786
  geniohyoid, 265
  gluteal region, 392–394, 394t, 396–397
  hand, 573t, 582
  hyoglossus, 786
  iliocostalis, 325
  infrahyoid, 767t
  interspinales, 331t, 332
  intertransversarii, 328
  ischiocavernosus, 259, 260t, 275
  larynx, 808t
  latissimus dorsi, 322, 323
  leg
    anterior aspects, 430–431, 436
    lateral aspects, 436–437, 437t
    posterior aspects, 440, 440t, 442–445
  levator costarum longus, 327
  levator scapulae, 324
  longissimus, 789
  longissimus thoracis, 325
  masseter, 668, 672–673, 778
  mastication, 678, 678t
  multifidus, 789
    lumborum, 326
    thoracis, 326
  mylohyoid, 766
  nasal wall, palatine, 702
  oblique
    external, 11, 104, 107, 108t, 173, 174, 504
    inferior, 660, 661, 663, 664, 725, 780t
    internal, 26, 107, 108t, 111, 112, 115, 173, 174
    superior, 658, 662t, 663, 664, 780t
  obliquus
    capitis inferior & superior, 332–334, 790
  obturator
    externus, 386t, 399, 402
    internus, 206, 207, 282, 284, 286, 393, 396, 399
  orbicularis
    oculi, 632, 635t, 661
    oris, 635t, 636, 836
  of orbit, 827
  palatopharyngeus, 794t
  pectoral region
    axio-appendicular, 507, 507t
    scapulohumeral, 507
  pharyngeal constrictor
    inferior, 794t
    middle, 794t
    superior, 794t
  pharynx, 794t
  platysma, 752t
  popliteal fossa, 413
  of posterior abdominal wall, 176t
  posterior median furrow, 322
  posterior superior iliac spine (PSIS), 322
  prevertebral, 780t–781t
  pterygoid
    lateral, 674, 678, 678t
    medial, 674, 675, 678, 678t, 687, 803
  pubococcygeus, 206, 207, 209, 214, 258, 267
  puboprostaticus, 207
  puborectalis, 207, 208, 214
  pubovaginalis, 207, 209, 277
  quadratus lumborum, 328
  quadriceps femoris, 385t, 422, 428
  rectus
    abdominis, 106, 107, 108t
    capitis
      anterior, 334, 335, 780, 781, 791
      lateralis, 335, 648, 780, 781
      posterior, 332–334, 790
    inferior, 659–664
    lateral, 658–664
    medial, 658, 659, 663
    superior, 658, 660, 661, 664
  of respiration, 26, 26t
  rhomboid, 324
  rotatores, 327, 789
  salpingopharyngeus, 794t
  scalene, 762, 780t–781t
    anterior, 781t
    middle, 781t, 783t
    posterior, 781t, 783t
  scapulae, levator, 783t
  semispinalis, 789
  semispinalis capitis, 326
  semispinalis cervicis, 326
  semispinalis thoracis, 326
  serratus posterior superior, 324
  smooth muscle (female only), 260t
  of soft palate, 690, 690t
  sole of foot, 452–455, 452t–454t
  sphincter
    external anal, 214–216, 260t, 265, 266
    external urethral, 220, 258, 260t, 261, 262
    internal anal, 215, 266
    internal urethral, 262, 286
    urethrovaginal, 260t, 261, 263, 277
  spinal (posterior), deltoid, 322
  spinalis, 325
  splenius, 789
    capitis, 783t
  splenius capitis, 325
  splenius cervicis, 325
  stapedius, 714
  sternocleidomastoid, 759
  sternohyoid, 24, 25, 764, 772, 774
  sternothyroid, 24, 25, 764, 772, 774
  stylopharyngeus, 794t
  superficial transverse perineal, 260t
  suprahyoid, 767t
  of temporomandibular joint, 678, 678t
  tensor
    tympani, 687, 690, 690t, 801
    veli palatini, 714, 717
  teres, 322
  thigh
    medial, 386–387, 386t
    posterior, 392–393, 395–397, 395t
  of thoracic wall, 23, 23t
  thoracolumbar fascia, 323, 324
    anterior layer, 329
    middle layer, 328, 329
    posterior layer, 328, 329
  thyro-arytenoid, 808t
  thyropharyngeus, 794t
  of tongue, 683, 683t
  transversospinalis, 330, 331t
  trapezius, 322, 323, 759
    inferior, 322, 323
    middle, 322, 323
    superior, 322, 323
  triceps brachii, 528, 528t, 529, 535
  urethrovaginal sphincter, 260t
  vertical, 780t
  vocalis, 808t
Muscular part of diaphagm, 75
Musculocutaneous nerve, 488, 490, 514, 516, 518, 533
Musculophrenic artery, 103
Mylohyoid nerve, 835
Myotomes, 349, 367

N

Nasal bone, 615, 616, 656
Nasal cavity, 30
  paranasal sinuses, 703
Nasal mucosa, olfactory part, 824
Nasal wall
  palatine muscles, 702
  paranasal sinuses, 702
  rhinits, 701

Nasal wall (*Continued*)
  and septum
    arteries of, 699
    bones of, 697
    innervation of, 698
Nasolacrimal duct, 657
Neck
  anterior region (anterior triangle), 764–767
  blood supply, 655
  bones and cartilages skeleton, 756–757
  cervical region (posterior triangle), lateral, 760–763
  mouth submandibular region and floor
    lingual and facial arteries, 788
    serial dissection, 784–787
  neurovascular structures, carotid triangle
    arteries, 770
    deep dissection, 769, 771
    deep veins, 773
    nerves *vs.* vessels relationships, 772
    superficial dissection, 768
  prevertebral and scalene muscles, 780t–781t
  regions
    cervical, 758t
    sternocleidomastoid and trapezius, 759t
  root region
    brachial plexus and sympathetic trunk, 782
    deep anterior dissection, 779
    right side dissection, 778
  sectional anatomy and imaging
    carotid artery doppler color flow study, 816
    head median and scan, 815
    transverse MRIs, 812
    ultrasound, 816
  subcutaneous structures and cervical fascia
    superficial veins, 753
    surface anatomy and tracheostomy, 755
  suprahyoid and infrahyoid muscles, 764–767
  vertebral muscles, lateral, 783t
  visceral compartment
    alimentary layer, 777
    endocrine layer I and II, 774, 775
    respiratory layer, 776
Nerve
  abducent, 818–820, 829
  alveolar, 835
  anal, inferior, 265, 274
  anococcygeal, 211
  anterior ramus (intercostal), 22
  arm, triceps brachii and related, 535
  auriculotemporal, 835
  axillary, 489, 490, 514, 518, 535, 536, 544
  buccal, 835
  cervical, 341
    transverse, 760
  coccygeal, 210–211, 341
  cochlear, 838
  cranial. *See* Cranial nerves
  cutaneous, 364, 365t, 522
  dorsal
    artery, 120
    of clitoris, 274
    of penis, 120, 268
  eyeball, 664–665
  facial, 818–820, 836, 836t, 837
    branches of, 635, 637, 637t, 640
  femoral, 176, 177, 222, 362, 380, 381, 407
  fibular/peroneal, 410, 411, 436
    common, 362
    deep, 362, 432, 433
    superficial, 362, 432, 433, 437
  frontal, 831
  ganglia
    abdominal plexuses and, 180, 183
  genitofemoral, 176, 177
    femoral branch of, 115
    genital branch of, 114
  glossopharyngeal, 337, 772, 793, 795, 802, 818–820, 840, 840t, 841
  gluteal region, 400, 400t
    inferior, 396, 401
    superior, 397
  great auricular (C2, C3), 633, 760
  greater occipital, 790
  greater splanchnic, 84, 85
  hypogastric, 253
  hypoglossal, 769, 772, 785–787, 818–820, 845, 845t
  iliohypogastric (L1), 103, 111, 112, 174–177
  ilio-inguinal, 103, 106, 111, 112, 176, 177
  incisional injury, 103
  intercostal, 24, 25
  intermediate, 818–820
  interosseous, 565
  lacrimal, 831
  laryngeal
    left recurrent, 776, 777
    right recurrent, 776, 778, 795, 806, 808, 809
    superior, 806
  leg
    anterior aspects, 432–433, 432t
  lesser splanchnic, 84
  to levator ani, 211
  lingual, 785, 786, 803, 835
  lumbar plexus, 177, 341
  mandibular, 677, 834, 834t, 835
  masseteric, 835
  maxillary, 832, 832t, 833
  median, 514, 547, 557, 600
    lateral root of, 516
    medial root of, 516
    recurrent branch of, 574
  musculocutaneous, 488, 490, 514, 516, 518, 533
  mylohyoid, 785, 835
  neck, point of, 760
  obturator, 176, 177, 209, 211, 362
  occipital, 332
    lesser, 760
  oculomotor, 818–820, 827–829
  olfactory, 818–820, 824, 824t
  ophthalmic, 831, 831t
  optic, 818–820, 825–826, 825t
  orbit, 664–665, 827
  palatine nerves, anesthesia of, 689
  palmar digital, 575, 580
  pelvic splanchnic, 253
  penis, dorsal artery, 120
  perineal, 274
    branches of, 274
  peripheral, 347
  peroneal, 362
  phrenic, 82, 761
  piriformis, 211
  plantar
    lateral, 362, 454
    medial, 362, 454
  popliteal fossa, 411
  pterygoid, 835
  pterygopalatine fossa, 705–707
  pudendal, 211, 251, 274, 396, 397
  quadratus femoris, 211
  radial, 489, 490, 514, 517, 518, 535, 536, 548, 557, 563–565, 590
  rectal, inferior, 265, 274
  recurrent laryngeal, 68, 69
  sacral, 210–211, 341
  saphenous, 388, 446
  sciatic, 362, 396–398, 407, 411
  spinal, 342–343, 346, 347
  spinal accessory, 761, 768, 769, 772, 818–820, 844, 844t
  splanchnic, 183t, 187, 352
  stylopharyngeus, 787
  subcostal (T12), 103, 174, 175
  suboccipital, 790
  superior laryngeal, 772
    external branch, 772, 776
    internal branch, 772, 776, 795
  supraclavicular, 502, 760
  supra-orbital, 831
  suprascapular, 489
  supratrochlear, 831
  temporal, deep, 835
  thigh, lateral cutaneous of, 177
  thoracic, 341, 517
  thoraco-abdominal, 103, 104
  to thyrohyoid, 785
  tibial, 392, 410, 411, 442, 443, 445, 446
  trigeminal, 818–820, 829, 830, 830t, 832
    cutaneous branches of, 636
    mandibular, 834t, 835
    maxillary, 832t, 833
    ophthalmic, 831t
  trochlear, 818–820, 827–829
  tympanic, 840, 841
  ulnar, 488, 514, 516, 533, 550, 551, 557, 566, 567, 574, 575, 578, 579, 590, 595
  upper limb, 490, 491t, 603t
    dermatomes of, 493, 493t
    motor innervation of, 488–489
    myotatic reflexes, 492
    myotomes, 492
    nerve root compression, 492t
  vagus, 27, 44, 185, 352, 772, 777, 778, 818–820, 842, 843, 843t
    inferior cardiac branch of, 778
  vestibulocochlear, 818–820, 838, 838t, 839
  zygomaticofacial, 660
Nerve block, pudendal, 251
Nipple, 4
Node
  atrioventricular, 60
  bronchopulmonary, 45
  lymph. *See* Lymph node
  sinoatrial, 60
Notch
  cardial, 133
  clavicular, 14
  interarytenoid, 810
  mandibular, 670
  radial, 556
  sacrococcygeal, 315
  sciatic, 201, 293, 359
  suprasternal, 2, 4, 5
  tentorial, 649
  thyroid, 808
  vertebral, 306
Nuchal ligament, 333
Nuchal line, superior, 618
Nuchal region, 335, 354
Nucleus
  amygdaloid, 733
  cardiorespiratory, 822
  caudate, 733, 736, 737
  cranial nerve, 822–823
  geniculate, 825
  gustatory, 822
  lentiform, 736, 737
  red, 743
Nucleus pulposus, 310, 312

O

Obliquus capitis
  inferior, 332–334
  superior, 332–334

Obturator artery, 399, 409
acetabular branch, 409
posterior branch, 409
Obturator externus, 402
Obturator internus, 393, 399
bursa, 403
tendon, 403
Obturator nerve, 176, 177, 362
Occipital bone, 302, 612, 613, 753
basilar part, 619, 621, 622, 801
jugular process, 648
squamous part, 618, 621, 622
Occipital condyle, 620, 621
Occipital nerve, 332
Oculomotor nerves (CN III), 646, 647, 649–651, 660, 818–820, 827–829
palsy, 847
Olecranon, 486, 487, 527, 529, 534, 535, 550
Olfactory bulb, 818, 824
Olfactory nerves (CN I), 646, 818–820, 824, 824t
Olfactory tract, 824
Omental (epiploic) foramen, 128
Omentum, 123–125, 127–130
bursa, 131
inferior recess of, 124
posterior relationships of, 129
posterior wall of, 131
superior recess of, 124, 125, 131
stomach and, 128
Opening
aortic, 176
caval, 178
coronary sinus, 62
ejaculatory ducts, 225
esophageal, 129, 176
saphenous, 107, 376, 378, 379
Ophthalmic nerve (CN V_1), 646, 650, 831, 831t
Opponens pollicis, 572
Optic canal, 623
Optic chiasm, 825
Optic nerve (CN II), 646, 647, 818–820, 825–826, 825t
Optic tract, 825
Orbit and eyeball, 827, 829
arteries of, 665, 665t
dissected, 666
extra-ocular muscles, 633t, 662, 662t, 663
clinical testing of, 664
eye and lacrimal apparatus, 657
eye surface anatomy, 656
nerves of, 664–665
ocular fundus and blood supply, 667
orbital cavity, 656
lateral aspect, 660–661
superior approach, 658, 659
veins of, 665t
Orbital cavity, 612, 615, 656, 658–661
Orbital fissure
superior, 623
Orbital fractures, 656
Orbitomeatal plane, 616
Orifice
of appendix, 143
coronary artery, 65, 66
ileocecal, 143
urethal
external, 220, 257, 259, 272
internal, 220, 225
vaginal, 259
Os trigonum, 475
Osseous spiral lamina, 839
Osteoarthritis, hip joint, 406
Ovary, 212, 236, 238, 244
suspensory ligament of, 252

P

Palate, 688–690, 690t
Palatine bone, 620, 656, 671, 800
horizontal plate, 688
pyramidal process, 708
Palm
deep dissection of, 578, 579
muscular layers of, 572
superficial dissection of, 574, 575
synovial sheaths of, 576
transverse section, 610
Palmar aponeurosis, 501, 569, 571
Palmar arch, 494, 495, 559, 580
Palmar carpal ligament, 501
Palmar digital artery, 571
Palmar digital nerve, 575, 580
Palmar interossei, 571, 572
Palmar ligament, 600, 602
Palmaris longus, 562
Pampiniform plexus of veins, 120
Pancreas, 98, 99, 129–131, 138, 139, 157, 168
blood supply to, 139
duodenum and, 137–138
uncinate process of, 138
Pancreatic artery, inferior, 139
Pancreatic duct, 137, 160
bile and, 160
development and variability of, 161
Pancreaticoduodenal arch, 139
Pancreaticoduodenal artery, 139
anterior inferior, 138
anterior superior, 139
Papilla
inferior lacrimal, 657
lingual, 682
major duodenal, 137, 160
minor duodenal, 137, 160
renal, 170
Papilledema, 667
Paracentesis, 127
Paracolic gutter, 126
Paranasal sinuses, 703, 704
Paranephric fat, 175
Parasternal lymph node, 8, 105
Parasympathetic innervation, 181
Parasympathetic nerve fibers, 350
Para-umbilical vein, 165
Parietal bone, 613
Parietal eminence, 613
Parietal peritoneum, 122
pain from, 184
Parietal pleura, 44, 98, 99
extent of, 32–33
surface markings of, 33t
Parotid region, 668–669
Parotidectomy, 669
Patella, 359, 383, 390, 414, 426
dislocation of, 417
ligament, 389, 414
retinaculum
lateral, 383, 414
medial, 383, 414
tendinitis, 382
Patellofemoral syndrome, 426
Pectineal ligament, 380
Pectineus, 381
Pectoral fascia, 500, 501
Pectoral region
axilla and clavipectoral fascia, 508
axio-appendicular muscles, 507, 507t
cutaneous branch, anterior, 22
female, 4–5
lymph node, 8, 497
male, 2–3
superficial dissection, 502
surface anatomy, 503
scapulohumeral muscles, 507
serratus anterior, 506
superficial dissection, 3, 5
surface anatomy, 2, 4
trunk
superficial dissection of, 504
surface anatomy of, 505
Pectoralis major, 3, 11, 502, 505, 506, 510, 516
clavicular head of, 2
pectoral fascia covering, 3
sternocostal head of, 2
Pectoralis minor, 508, 510
Peduncle, 740, 743
Pelvis, 313, 316–317
female organs/vessels
arterial supply, 245
arteries and veins, 246–247
autonomic nerves innervation, 252–253
broad ligament and uterus, 240–241
genital, 238
innervation, 250
lymphatic drainage, 248–249
pregnancy and nerve blocks innervation, 251
pregnant uterus, 242–243
in situ, 236–237
ureter *vs.* uterine artery relationship, 244
uterus and adnexa, 239
floor and walls
diaphragm, female, 209
diaphragm, male, 208
diaphragm, muscle, 207
muscles, 207t
obturator internus and piriformis, 206
girdle
anatomical position, 201
bones and divisions, 200
female/surface anatomy, 199
ligaments, 205
male *vs.* female differences, 202–203
male/surface anatomy, 198
radiographs, 204
imaging and sectional anatomy
female, transverse section, 283–285
male, transverse section, 280–282
ultrasound scans, female, 286–287
uterus and uterine tubes radiograph, 288
lesser, 200
male organs/vessels
arteries and veins, 228–229
external genitalia, 220
innervation, 234–235
lymphatic drainage, 232–233
posterior approach, 222–223
prostate and ductus deferens, 221
seminal glands and prostate, 224
in situ and lateral wall, 230
transrectal ultrasound scans, 227
transverse sections, 226
urinary bladder and prostatic urethra, 221, 225
peritoneal reflections
covering organs, female, 212
covering organs, male, 213
portal–systemic (portacaval) anastomoses, 231
posterior neurovascular structures, 216
splanchnic, 211t
subperitoneal region
cervix and upper vagina fascia/supporting mechanism, 255
female pelvis, transverse section, 254
Penis
body, 268
bulb of, 266
corona, 268
corpus cavernosum, 259, 270
corpus spongiosum, 259, 270

Penis (*Continued*)
crus of, 266
deep dorsal vein of, 120
dorsal artery, 120
dorsal nerve, 120, 268
glans, 268, 270
root, 268, 270
suspensory ligament of, 268
Perforating arteries, 401
Pericardial sac, 53
and diaphragm, 75
Pericardium, 31, 50
and heart, 52–54
in relation to sternum, 50
Perinephric fat, 175
Perineum
female organs/vessels
arterial supply, 245
dissection, 273, 275–279
innervation, 274
lymphatic drainage, 248–249
muscles, 260t, 261
pelvis supporting and compressor/ sphincteric muscles, 264
perineal compartments, 258–259, 262–263
surface anatomy, 257
imaging and sectional anatomy
female transverse section, 283–285
male transverse section, 280–282
male organs/vessels
dissection, 265–267
innervation, 234–235
lymphatic drainage, 232–233
muscles, 260t, 261
pelvis supporting and compressor/ sphincteric muscles, 264
perineal compartments, 258–259, 262–263
surface anatomy, 257
urethra, 272
urogenital system, erectile bodies, 270
penis
cross sections, 271
glans, prepuce and neurovascular bundle, 268
layers and nerves, 269
Peripheral nerves, 347
Peritoneum, 213, 220
of posterior abdominal cavity, 148
recto-uterine pouch, 254
Peritoneum and peritoneal cavity
abdominal contents and, 123
anterolateral abdominal wall, posterior aspect of, 122
formations and bare areas, 124, 124t
omental bursa, 127
opened, 130
posterior relationships of, 129, 131
posterior wall of, 126
stomach and omenta, 128
subdivisions of, 125
transverse sections, 127
Peritonitis, 127
Peroneal nerve, 362
Pes anserinus, 387, 420
Pes planus, 474
Petrosal sinus, 645
Phalanx
distal, 361, 435, 580
middle, 452, 474, 576
proximal, 431, 435
Pharyngeal constrictor, 794
inferior, 793, 794, 794t, 795
middle, 792–794, 794t, 795
superior, 793, 794, 794t, 795, 797, 801, 803
Pharynx, 30
external
lateral views, 794–795
posterior views, 792–793
internal, 796–797
muscles, 794t
Phrenic artery, 169
Phrenic nerve, 82
Phrenicocolic ligament, 126, 129
Pia mater, 341
Piriformis, 393, 396, 398
Plane
midclavicular, 101
orbitomeatal, 616, 617
transtubercular, 101
transumbilical, 88, 105
Plantar aponeurosis, 451
Plantar arch, 370
deep, 454
Plantar artery
deep, 435
lateral, 370, 454
medial, 370, 454
Plantar fascia, 451
Plantar fasciitis, 451
Plantar interossei, 455
Plantar nerve
lateral, 362, 454
medial, 362, 454
Plantar venous arch, 371
Plantaris, 440, 441
Plate
cribriform, 623
epiphysial, 361
horizontal, 688
palmar ligament, 577, 579, 602
pterygoid
lateral, 621
medial, 621
tarsal, 636
tibia, 416, 419
Platysma, 3, 502
Pleura
cervical, 68, 70, 71
mediastinal, 75
parietal, 30, 336
cervical, 779
extent of, 32
mediastinal part, 82
sternal reflection of, 75
visceral, 33
Pleural cavity, 30, 74
Pleurisy/pleuritis, 44
Plexus
abdominopelvic nerve and ganglia, 180, 183
brachial, 490, 762, 763, 782
lateral cord of, 516
neck root region, 782
posterior cord of, 517
of upper limb, 514, 515
cardiac, 70, 73
coccygeal, 210–211
lumbar, 176
nerves of, 177
vertebral attachment of, 176
lymphatic
deep, 45
subareolar, 8
pharyngeal, CN IX and CN X forming, 793
pterygoid venous, 773
pulmonary, 44, 73
sacral, 210–211
subareolar lymphatic, 8
subpleural lymphatic, 45
subtrapezial, 522
sympathetic peri-arterial, 811
uterovaginal, 253
venous
pampiniform, 120
rectal, 228
uterus, 246
vertebral, 343, 344
vesical, 228
Pole
caudal, 118
frontal, 734
kidney, 170
temporal, 647
thyroid gland, superior, 774
Pollicis brevis, extensor, 589, 593
Pollicis longus, extensor, 589, 593
Polymastia, 4
Polythelia, 4
Pons, 350
Popliteal aneurysm, 412
Popliteal artery, 370, 401, 410, 412, 448
Popliteal fossa
anatomy, 410
deep dissection, 412
muscles, 413
nerves, 411
Popliteal pulse, 410
Popliteal vein, 371, 410
Popliteus, 422, 440, 441, 449
Popliteus tendon, 421
Porta hepatis, 151
gallbladder and structures of, 158
vessels in, 159
Portacaval system, 165
Portal hypertension, 165
Portal triad, exposure of, 156–157
Portal venous system
anterior view, 164
portacaval system, 165
Posterior clinoid process, 619
Posterior cruciate ligament (PCL), 418, 427, 429
Posterior humeral circumflex artery, 535, 536
Posterior intercostal artery, 103
Posterior median furrow, 322
Posterior superior iliac spine, 322
Posterior vagal trunk, 185
Postsynaptic fibers, abdominal viscera, 182
Pott fracture, 457
Pouch
perineal, 263
recto-uterine, 124, 254
rectovesical, 213
vesico-uterine, 212
Preaortic nodes, 121
Prepatellar bursa, subcutaneous, 416
Prepatellar bursitis, 422
Prepuce, 268
Presynaptic fibers, abdominal viscera, 182
Process
atlas, transverse, 756
axillary
of breast, 5
site of, 4
clinoid, posterior, 619
jugular, 780
mastoid, 616, 620, 621, 756
spinous, 292, 293, 756, 757
styloid, 616, 620, 621, 803
supracondylar, 549
transverse, 292, 756
uncinate, 138
xiphoid, 100
Profunda femoris artery, 370, 388, 401
Profunda femoris vein, 371
Pronator quadratus, 564, 565
Pronator teres, 547, 562, 565
superficial head of, 548
Prostate, 220, 221, 224, 226, 267
Protuberance
external occipital, 299, 330, 332, 333, 618
internal occipital, 623
mental, 614, 616
Proximal ileum and jejunum, 140
Psoas, 222, 381, 383, 385
Pterion, 641
Pterygoid canal, 621
Pterygoid nerves, 835

Pterygopalatine fossa
nerves of, 705–707
sphenoid bone, 708
Pubis, 405
anterior aspect of, 201
branch, 230
hip bone, 200
symphysis, 100, 198, 199, 201
tubercle, 198, 199
Pudendal artery
external, 106
internal, 396, 397
Pudendal nerve, 211, 396, 397
Pudendal nerve block, 251
Pulmonary and aortic valve cusps, 66
Pulmonary artery, 36, 37, 49
and bronchi, relationship of, 43
right, 70
Pulmonary (intrapulmonary) nodes, 45
Pulmonary plexus, 44, 73
Pulmonary trunk (PT), 48, 70
Pulmonary vein, 36, 37, 48, 49
Pulse, carotid (neck pulse), 774
Pyloric antrum, 135
Pyloric canal, 128, 133
Pylorus, 133, 135

Q

Quadrangular space, 518, 535, 536
Quadratus plantae (QP), 447, 453
Quadriceps tendon, 384

R

Radial artery, 494, 495, 548, 549, 559, 562, 579, 585
superficial palmar branch of, 574
Radial collateral ligament, 555, 556
Radial nerve, 489, 490, 514, 517, 518, 535, 536, 548, 557, 563–565
superficial branch of, 590
Radial veins, 496
Radiate ligament, 18, 19
Radicular artery, posterior, 343
Radiocarpal (wrist) joint, 599, 600
Radiograph
ankle, 461
biliary ducts, 162
of biliary passages, 162
caldwell, 624
cervical spine, 296
chest, 29
of chest, 29
cranium, 624–625
duodenum (barium swallow), 135
esophagus, 135
foot, 461
hip joint, 406
knee, 428
pelvic girdle, 204
perineum, 288
stomach, 135
thorax, 29
uterus and uterine tubes, 288
Radio-ulnar joints, ligaments of, 559
Radius, 482, 483, 487, 527
Rami communicantes, 340
Ramus
anterior, 22, 211, 216, 338, 347, 763
abdominal branches of, 107
ischiopubic, 267, 277
posterior, 327, 338, 347
Raphe
palatine, 688
perineal, 256
pharyngeal, 335, 793
pterygomandibular, 671, 794, 803
scrotal, 256
Rebound tenderness, 184
Recess
clinoid process, 704
costodiaphragmatic, 29, 30
epitympanic, 711, 713, 714
hepatorenal, 151, 156
omental bursa
inferior, 124
superior, 124, 125, 131
pharyngeal, 800
sacciform, 600
spheno-ethmoidal, 702
subphrenic, 151
Rectal artery, superior, 146, 147
Recto-uterine pouch, 124
Rectum, 209, 213, 216, 226, 254
ampulla, 219, 236
innervation, 218
neurovascular structures, 216
in situ, 219
vasculature, 217
Rectus
abdominis, 106, 107, 108t
capitis
anterior, 334, 335, 780, 781, 791
lateral, 335, 648, 780, 781
posterior, 332–334, 790
femoris, 383, 384, 414
inferior, 659–664
lateral, 658–664
medial, 658, 659, 663
superior, 658, 660, 661, 664
Rectus sheath
anterior layer of, 106
posterior wall of, 107, 122
Recurrent branch of median nerve, 574
Recurrent laryngeal nerve, 68, 69
Reflected ligament, 111
Renal artery, 169, 178
Renal capsule, 175
Renal fascia, 168, 174–175
Renal transplantation, 169
Renal vein, 179
Respiration, muscles of, 26, 26t
Respiratory system, 30
Retinaculum
lateral patellar, 414
medial patellar, 414
Retrocaval ureter, 172
Retromandibular vein, 639
Retropubic space, 222
Rhinits, 701
Rhomboid, 324, 521, 522
Rib, 3, 12, 13, 15–17, 21, 24, 25, 175
bicipital, 16
bifid, 16
bony thorax, 15
cervical, 16
dislocation/separation, 12
sternum, 15
sternum anomalies, 16
Rima glottidis, 805
Ring
femoral, 380
inguinal
deep, 122
location of, 113
superficial, 106, 114
tracheal, 755, 765
umbilical, 109
Rotatores muscle, 327

S

Sac
dural, 337–339
greater, 124
lacrimal, 657
pericardial, 53, 75
Sacral cord, 341
Sacral nerve, 341
Sacral vertebra, 294, 320
Sacrococcygeal kyphosis, 291
Sacrococcygeal ligament
anterior, 316
posterior, 317
Sacro-iliac joint, 318
anterior, 318
articular surfaces, 318
imaging, 319, 355
Sacro-iliac ligament, 317
anterior, 316
interosseous, 318
posterior, 317
Sacrospinous ligament, 316, 398
Sacrotuberous ligament, 316, 317, 398
Sacrum, 198–201, 290–292, 314–315
lateral view, 318
Sagittal MRIs
of abdomen, 193
of thorax, 93
Sagittal sinus, 645
Sagittal suture, 618, 619
Saphenous nerve, 388, 446
Saphenous opening, 376, 378, 379
Saphenous vein, 372–375, 378, 446
Sartorius, 383, 384, 387
Scala tympani, 839
Scala vestibuli, 839
Scaphoid bone, 593
Scapula, 482–484, 487, 511, 527
coracoid process, 530
spine of, 535, 537
superior angle, 531
winged, 518
Scarpa fascia, 110
Sciatic nerve, 362, 396–398, 407, 411
Sciatic nerve block, 399
Semicircular canals, 838
Semimembranosus, 387, 393, 395, 410, 411, 420
Seminal colliculus, 225
Semispinalis muscle, 326
Semitendinosus, 387, 395, 411
Septal cusp, 67
Septum
intermuscular
anterior, 478
anteromedial, 377
lateral, 377
posterior, 478
posteromedial, 377
transverse, 478
interventricular, 65
nasal wall
arteries of, 699
bones of, 697
innervation of, 698
Serratus
anterior, 2, 11, 104, 504, 506, 510, 517
posterior
inferior, 23
superior, 26, 324
Sesamoid bone, 447, 451, 475
Sheath
axillary, 510
carotid, 753, 775
digital, fibrous, 569, 577
femoral, 379, 381
hypogastric, 222, 255
rectus
anterior, 106
posterior, 107, 122
synovial, 438–439, 576
Shoulder region, joints of
acromioclavicular joint, 539
imaging of, 544–545
ligaments and articular capsule of, 540–541
pectoral girdle, 538
subacromial bursa, 539
Sialography, 686
Sigmoid arteries, 146, 147
Sigmoid colon, 140, 141, 148, 219
Sigmoid mesocolon, 126, 141, 148
Sigmoid sinus, 623, 645
Sinu-atrial nodal branch, 56
Sinu-atrial (SA) node, 60
Sinus
anal, 215
cavernous, 645

Sinus (*Continued*)
maxillary, 704
oblique pericardial, 31, 53, 66
paranasal, 702, 703
petrosal, 645
prostatic, 225
sagittal, 645
sigmoid, 623, 645
sphenoparietal, 645
tonsil, 799
transverse pericardial, 53
venous, 645
Small intestine, 148
interior of, 140
mesentery of, 124, 141
Soleus, 410, 440–444
Somatic sensory nuclei, 823
Space
intercostal, 11
contents of, 21, 22
vertebral ends, 19, 20
meningeal
arachnoid granulations, 643
dura mater, 643–645
middle meningeal artery and pterion, 641
scalp and meninges, layers of, 642
subarachnoid, epidural, 642
perineal, 222–223
quadrangular, 518, 535, 536
retropubic, 222
triangular, 536
Spermatic cord, 106, 112, 113, 116–117, 120
Spermatic fascia, external, 116, 117
Sphenoid bone, 656
Sphenoparietal sinus, 645
Sphincter
external anal, 214–216, 260t, 265
external urethral, 220, 260t
internal anal, 215, 266
urethrovaginal, 260t, 277
Spinal accessory nerve (CN XI), 522, 646–648, 669, 818–820, 844, 844t
Spinal artery
anterior, 343
posterior, 343
Spinal block, 251
Spinal cord
blood supply, 342–343
cervical enlargement, 336
dural sac, 337–339
lumbar enlargement, 336
nerve roots, 341
prevertebral structures, 340
Spinal cord regions, 346
Spinal ganglion, 338
Spinal nerve, 342–343, 346, 347
Spinal (posterior) part, deltoid, 322
Spinal vein, posterior, 343
Spinalis, 325
Spine
iliac, 201
anterior superior, 198, 201
posterior superior, 198
ischial, 274
nasal, 614, 616, 620
Spiral organ, 839
Splanchnic nerve, 183t, 187, 352
Spleen, 98, 99, 129, 136, 168
artery, 129, 131, 134, 136, 139, 168
blood supply to, 139
vein, 129, 131, 164
Splenic branches, 134
Splenius capitis, 325, 334, 761, 783, 789
Splenius cervicis, 325, 789
Splenius muscle, 325, 331t
Splenorenal ligament, 131, 168
Spondylolisthesis, 321
Spondylolysis, 321
Sternal foramen, 16
Sternoclavicular joint, 14
Sternocleidomastoid, 334
Sternocostal joint, 14
Sternum, 2, 12, 14, 25, 50
anomalies and rib, 16
Stomach, 98, 99, 130, 131, 133
celiac artery, 134
greater curvature of, 128
lesser curvature of, 128
radiographs of, 135
Styloid process, 616, 620, 621
Stylomastoid foramen, 620
Subacromial bursa, 544
Subareolar lymphatic plexus, 8
Subclavian artery, 76
Subclavian lymphatic trunk, 78
Subclavian vein, 496
Subcostal artery, 103
Subcostal nerve (T12), 103, 174, 175
Subcostales, 19, 23
Subcutaneous olecranon bursa, 557
Subcutaneous tissue, fatty layer of, 106
Suboccipital region, 332, 333
Subpleural lymphatic plexus, 45
Subscapular lymph nodes, 8, 497
Subscapularis, 510, 517, 524
Subtalar joint, 466
inversion and eversion, 363
Subtrapezial plexus, 522
Sulcus
calcarine, 729
cerebrum, 731, 734–735
coronary, 48
interatrial, 52
intertubercular, 510
parieto-occipital, 729
postcentral, 731
talocalcaneal, 468
terminalis, 51
Superficial back
cutaneous nerves of, 522
and deltoid muscles, 521, 521t
and posterior axioappendicular musclesi, 522
scapula, movements of, 523
surface anatomy of, 520
Superficial circumflex iliac artery, 103
and vein, 106
Superficial epigastric artery, 103
and vein, 106
Superficial epigastric vein, 105
Superficial inguinal lymph nodes, 105, 121
Superficial inguinal ring, 106, 114
Superficial temporal and facial artery pulse, 632
Superficial temporal vein, 639
Superior vena cava (SVC), 48, 49, 82
obstruction of, 81
Supinator, 548
Supraclavicular nerves, 502
Supracolic compartment, 126
Supracondylar process, 549
Supraduodenal artery, 138
Supra-orbital nerve (CN V_1), 831
Supra-orbital vein, 639
Suprapatellar bursa, 422, 428
Suprapatellar bursitis, 422
Suprarenal artery, 169
Suprarenal gland, 167, 187
exposure of, 168
and kidney, 169
lymphatic drainage, 186
right, 185
Suprascapular nerve, 489
Suprascapular veins, 509
Supraspinatus tendon, 525, 539
Supraspinous ligament, 309, 312, 317
Supratrochlear nerve (CN V_1), 636, 831
Supratrochlear vein, 639
Supravesical fossa, 122
Suspensory ligaments of breast, 5
Sustentaculum tali, 456
Suture
coronal, 618
frontal (metopic), 612
lambdoid, 618
sagittal, 619
Sympathetic ganglion, 83, 187
Sympathetic innervation, 181, 351
Sympathetic trunk, 82–84, 340
Synostosis, 320
Synovial capsule, 570
Synovial membrane, 416
Systole, 61

T

Talar neck fracture, 463
Talocalcaneal joint, 468
Talofibular ligament, anterior, 462
Tarsal tunnel syndrome, 459
Tectorial membrane, 302, 303, 839
Teeth
innervation of, 693
permanent teeth-I, 691
permanent teeth-II, 692
primary teeth, 694, 695t
Telencephalon (cerebrum) and diencephalon
caudate and lentiform nuclei, 736, 737
cerebral hemisphere, 731–735, 738, 739
thalamus, 737
ventricular system, 730
Temporal bone, 612, 624, 625, 629
mandibular fossa, 681
mastoid part of, 617
petrous part of, 720
tympanic part, 617, 670
zygomatic process, 617, 670, 680
Temporal branches (CN VII), 668
Temporal fossa, 616
Temporal nerve, deep, 835
Temporal region and infratemporal fossa, 670–679
Temporomandibular joint, 616
coronal section, 680
mastication, muscles of, 678, 678t
movements of, 679, 679t
sectional anatomy of, 681
Tendinous intersection, 106
Tendon
biceps brachii, 530, 531, 554
calcaneal, 440–444, 447
conjoint, 107, 111, 112
deep reflexes, 367
diaphragm, 75
fibularis longus, 437
flexor digitorum longus, 453
flexor hallucis longus, 453
obturator internus, 403
popliteus, 421
quadriceps, 384
supraspinatus, 525, 539
synovial sheaths and, 438–439
triceps, 535
Tensor fasciae latae, 376, 383
Tentorium cerebelli (cerebellar tentorium), 644
Teres major, 322, 510, 517
Teres minor, 524
Testicular artery, 120, 121
Testicular artery and vein, 167
Testis, 116–117, 120, 220
blood supply, 121
lymphatic drainage, 121
spermatic cord and epididymis, 120
Thenar fascia, 569
Thigh
anterior aspects
schematic illustrations, 384, 385t
superficial and deep dissection, 383, 384
surface anatomy, 382

anteromedial aspect, 390
arteries, posterior, 401, 401t
bones, 388–389
lateral aspect, 391
lateral cutaneous nerve of, 177
medial aspect, 382–384, 385t, 386–387, 386t
MRI, 476–477
muscles
medial, 386–387, 386t
posterior, 392–393, 395–397, 395t
transverse section, 476–477
Thoracic aorta, 76
Thoracic cord, 341
Thoracic duct, 45, 78, 79, 83–85, 186, 340
Thoracic kyphosis, 291
Thoracic nerve, long, 517
Thoracic outlet syndromes, 13
Thoracic vertebrae, 290, 292, 294, 304–305, 304t, 356
Thoracic wall
anterior, internal aspect of, 25
external aspect of, 24
inferior intercostal spaces, anterior ends of, 21
intercostal space, transverse section, contents of, 22
muscles of, 23, 23t
muscles, of respiration, 26, 26t
vertebral ends
inferior intercostal spaces, external aspect of, 20
intercostal spaces, internal aspect of, 19
Thoraco-abdominal nerves, 103, 104
Thoraco-acromial artery, 508
Thoracocentesis, 20
Thoraco-epigastric vein, 105
Thoracolumbar fascia, 323, 324, 328–329, 522
anterior layer, 329
middle layer, 328, 329
posterior layer, 328, 329
Thorax
autonomic innervation, 86–87
bony
chest radiograph, 29
lungs and mediastinum, topography of, 28
in situ, 27
3D volume reconstructions and CT angiograms, 94–95
lymphatic drainage, 88–89
MRIs of
coronal, 92
sagittal, 93
transverse (axial), 90–91
posterior
arterial supply, to trachea and esophagus, 77
azygos system, of veins, 80–81
esophagus, trachea, and aorta, 76
lymphatic system, 79
mediastinum, 82–83
structures, of posterior mediastinum, 84, 85
thoracic duct, 78
surgical access to, 24
visceral afferent innervation of, 86
Thumb movement, 582
Thymus, 68, 765
Tibia, 359, 390, 391, 431
anterior, 432, 439
condyles
lateral, 426
medial, 426, 428
fractures, 441
Tibial
artery
anomalous, 448
anterior, 370, 433, 448
posterior, 440, 444, 445, 447–449, 454, 456
collateral ligament, 427
nerve, 392, 410, 411, 442, 443, 445, 446
pulse, posterior tibial, 446
veins, 371
Tibiocalcaneal, 460
Tibiofibular joint, 433
and syndesmosis, 450
Tibiofibular ligament, anterior, 457
Tibiofibular syndesmosis, 433, 450
Tibionavicular, medial ligament, 460
Tissue
extraperitoneal fascia, 222
hepatic, 151
myocardial, 58
subcutaneous, 6, 105
fatty layer, 106, 114
membranous layer, 110
Tongue, 682–687, 683t
Tonsil
palatine, 798, 799
sinus, 799
Tonsillectomy, 799
Trabeculae, 405, 406
Trabeculae carneae, 64
Trachea, 30, 76, 756, 776, 777
arterial supply to, 77
bifurcation and bronchi, 71
and bronchi in situ, 40
and great vessels, 70
Tracheobronchial (carinal) node, 45
Tracheostomy, 755
Tract
iliopubic, 122
iliotibial, 376, 389, 392, 414, 421
olfactory, 824
optic, 825
upper respiratory, 700
Transient ischemic attack, 654
Transumbilical plane, 105
Transversalis fascia, 112, 113, 115, 116, 122
Transverse colon, 140, 141
Transverse fractures, 527
Transverse ligament, of atlas, 303
Transverse mesocolon, 124, 126, 130, 148, 166
Transverse MRI, 608, 609
of abdomen, 190–191
of cranial nerves, 848–849
of thorax, 90–91
Transversus abdominis, 107, 112, 113, 115, 175
and aponeurosis, 113
Transversus thoracis, 23, 25
Trapezius, 322, 323, 334, 522, 523t, 759t
Triangle
carotid, 758
muscular, 758
occipital, 758
omoclavicular, 758
submandibular, 758
submental, 758
Triangular ligament, 126, 150
Triangular space, 536
Triceps brachii, 528, 535
Triceps tendon, 535
Tricuspid valve, 67
Trigeminal ganglion, 650
Trigeminal nerve (CN V), 646–650, 818–820, 829, 830, 830t, 832
mandibular nerve, 834t, 835
maxillary nerve, 832t, 833
ophthalmic nerve, 831t
Trigone
collateral, 733
fibrous, 61
habenular, 736
hypoglossal, 741
urinary bladder, 221, 225
Trochanter, 401, 402
Trochanteric bursa, 396
Trochanteric bursitis, 393
Trochlea, 557
Trochlear nerve (CN IV), 646–650, 818–820, 827–829
Trunk
brachiocephalic, 770
cervicodorsal, 762
costocervical, 771
jugular lymphatic, 811
lumbosacral, 211, 216
sympathetic, 216, 253, 782, 792, 811
thyrocervical, 771
Tubercle
anterior, 756, 757, 781
carotid, 781
corniculate, 810
cuneiform, 810
posterior, 757
Tuberosity
calcaneal, 435, 451
cuboid, 472
deltoid, 487, 521
gluteal, 391
iliac, 314
ischial, 198, 199, 265, 267, 277, 393, 398
metatarsal, 439
radius, 486
sacral, 314
tibial, 414, 429, 430
ulna, 486
Tunica albuginea, 121
Tunica vaginalis, 117, 120
parietal layer, 116
visceral layer, 116
Tympanic membrane, perforation of, 714
Tympanic nerve, 840, 841

U

Ulna, 482, 483, 486, 487, 527, 552
radial notch of, 556
Ulnar artery, 494, 495, 549, 559, 574
Ulnar collateral ligament, 554
Ulnar nerve, 488, 514, 516, 533, 550, 551, 557, 567, 574, 575
and artery, 566
deep branch of, 578, 579
dorsal branch of, 590, 595
Ultrasonography, 815
Ultrasound
abdomen, 194–195
pelvis
female, imaging, 286–287
male organs/vessels, 227
Umbilical artery, 122
Umbilical fold, 122
lateral, 122
Umbilical hernias, 104
Umbilical ligaments, 222, 223
Umbilicus, 100
Upper limb
arteries and arterial anastomoses, 494–495
bones
epiphyses, sites of, 484, 485
features of, 486–487
major joints of, 482, 483
ossification, 484, 485
regions, 482, 483
bones, proximal, 526
imaging and sectional anatomy, 605–610
lesions of nerves, 603t
musculofascial compartments
axillary and clavipectoral fascia, 500
brachial and antebrachial fascia, 501

Upper limb (*Continued*)
nerves
cutaneous, 490, 491t
dermatomes of, 493, 493t
motor innervation of, 488–489
myotatic reflexes, 492
myotomes, 492
nerve root compression, 492t
veins and lymphatics
deep, 496
lymphatic drainage of, 497
superficial venous drainage of, 498–489
Ureter, 167, 169, 187, 219, 230, 244
lymphatic drainage, 186
Urethal orifice, external, 220
Urethra, 169, 226, 236, 254
intermediate, 220
prostatic, 220, 267
spongy, 220
Urinary bladder, 169, 209, 212, 213, 226, 236, 254
trigone of, 225
uvula of, 225
Uterine tube, 212, 236, 238
Uterus, 212, 236, 244
broad ligament of, 212, 238
fundus of, 238
round ligament, 212, 236, 238, 252

V

Vagal trunk, 842
Vagina, 209, 212, 236, 254
Vaginal orifice, 259
Vagus nerve (CN X), 27, 44, 185, 352, 646–648, 669, 818–820, 842, 843, 843t
Valve
anal, 215
aortic, 65–67
mitral, 64, 67
pulmonary, 66
tricuspid, 67
Valvular heart disease, 61
Valvular insufficiency, 61
Varicose veins, 373
Vastus intermedius, 383, 384
Vastus lateralis, 383–385, 414
Vastus medialis, 383–385, 388, 414
Vein
accessory hemi-azygos, 80, 81
angular, 639
anterior intercostal, 24, 25
ascending lumbar, 81
auricular, posterior, 754
axilla, 496, 509, 511
azygos, 80–82, 84, 85, 340
basilic, 496, 498, 546
basivertebral, 344
brachial, 547
brachiocephalic, 68, 69, 773
cardiac, 57
cephalic, 3, 498, 509, 546
cervical, deep, 790
dorsal, of penis, 120, 268
dorsal scapular, 509
epigastric, inferior, 223
esophageal, 165
external iliac artery, 115, 167
face and scalp, 639, 639t
facial, 639, 754
femoral, 371, 378–381
fibular, 371
forearm
basilicof, 546, 595
cephalicof, 592
medianof, 546
gastric, 165
grafts, 372
great saphenous, 106
hemi-azygos, 80, 81, 85
hepatic portal, 131, 138, 156, 164, 165
hepatic, 153
iliac
and artery, 167
common, 371
external, 222, 371
internal, 371
inferior epigastric artery, 112
inferior mesenteric, 131, 164
internal thoracic, 24, 25
jugular, 509
anterior, 754, 773
external, 496, 754, 760, 773
internal, 496, 754, 768, 769, 773, 777, 778
left gastric and artery, 131
left superior intercostal, 81
maxillary, 773
median cubital, 546
occipital, 790
orbit and eyeball, 665t
palatine, external, 802
pampiniform plexus of, 120
para-umbilical, 165
penis, deep dorsalof, 120
popliteal, 371, 410
pudendal, internal, 217
pulmonary, 36, 37, 48, 49
radial, 496
rectal, 217
inferior, 217
middle, 217
superior, 217
renal, 179
retromandibular, 639, 754, 773
saphenous, 372–375, 378, 446
spinal, posterior, 343
splenic artery, 129, 168
splenic, 129, 131, 164
subclavian, 496, 763, 778
left, 779
right, 773
superficial epigastric, 105
superficial temporal, 639
superior mesenteric, 131, 138, 164
supra-orbital, 639
suprascapular, 509
supratrochlear, 639
and testicular artery, 167
thoraco-epigastric, 105
thyroid, 774
tibial, anterior, 371
upper limb, 497
deep veins of, 496
superficial venous, 497
superficial venous drainage of, 498–489
varicose, 373
vertebral, 773
Vena cava
inferior, 48, 80, 82, 179, 371
superior, 27, 29, 48, 69
Venous angle, right, 78
Venous drainage, of breast, 10
Ventral pancreas, 161
Ventricle
fourth, 700, 730, 742
lateral, 730, 733, 735, 736
left, 29, 31, 48, 51, 64–65
right, 31, 48, 51, 66
third, 700, 730, 742
Ventricular septal defects (VSDs), 63
Vermis, 742
Vertebrae
cervical, 290, 292, 294
lumbar, 290, 292, 294, 306–307, 306t, 316–317, 355
synostosis, 320
thoracic, 290, 292, 294, 304–305, 304t, 356
Vertebral arch, 293
Vertebral artery, 302, 303, 652
groove, 302, 303
Vertebral body, 293, 346
Vertebral column
anatomy, 290
anomalies, 320
atlas, 298, 320, 354
axis, 320, 354
cervical vertebra, 298, 298t
curvature, 291
homologous parts, 294
lumbar vertebra, 293, 312
movements, 295–297
surface anatomy, 296–297
thoracic vertebra, 12, 13, 290, 292, 294, 295, 304–305
transverse and spinous process, 292
Vertebral foramen, 293
Vertebral venous plexus, 344
anterior external, 344
anterior internal, 344
posterior external, 344
posterior internal, 343, 344
Vesico-uterine pouch, 212
Vestibular ganglion, 838, 839
Vestibular membrane, 839
Vestibular nerve, 838, 839
Vestibule, bulbs of, 276
Vestibulocochlear nerve (CN VIII), 646–648, 818–820, 838, 838t, 839
Visceral afferent innervation, 352–353
and efferent innervation, 352–353
of thorax, 86
Visceral motor, 837
Visceral motor nuclei, 823
Visceral parasympathetic pathway, 352
Visceral referred pain, 184
Visceral sensory nuclei, 823
Visceral sympathetic pathway, 352
Visual field defects, 826
Visual pathway, 825
Vomer, 615, 621

W

Winged scapula, 518, 519
Wrist
coronal section of, 598
imaging of bones, 597
lateral aspect, 592–594
medial aspect of, 595
radiocarpal joint, 599, 600
structures of anterior aspect, 566, 567
surface anatomy of skeleton of, 568

X

Xiphisternal joint, 14, 50
Xiphoid process, 100

Z

Zygapophysial joint, 308–310
Zygomatic arch, 616
Zygomatic bone, 656, 657
Zygomatic branches (CN VII), 668
Zygomaticofacial nerve (CN V_2), 636, 660